Presented to:

OBSTETRICS AND GYNECOLOGY

EDITOR

DAVID N. DANFORTH

PH.D., M.D., F.A.C.O.G., F.A.C.S.
THOMAS J. WATKINS PROFESSOR EMERITUS OF OBSTETRICS AND GYNECOLOGY
NORTHWESTERN UNIVERSITY MEDICAL SCHOOL
CHICAGO, ILLINOIS

ASSOCIATE EDITORS

WILLIAM J. DIGNAM

M.D., F.A.C.O.G.
PROFESSOR OF OBSTETRICS AND GYNECOLOGY
UNIVERSITY OF CALIFORNIA, LOS ANGELES
SCHOOL OF MEDICINE
LOS ANGELES, CALIFORNIA

CHARLES H. HENDRICKS

M.D., F.A.C.O.G.
ROBERT A. ROSS PROFESSOR OF OBSTETRICS AND GYNECOLOGY
UNIVERSITY OF NORTH CAROLINA SCHOOL OF MEDICINE
CHAPEL HILL, NORTH CAROLINA

JOHN VAN S. MAECK

M.D., F.A.C.O.G., F.A.C.S.
PROFESSOR OF OBSTETRICS AND GYNECOLOGY
UNIVERSITY OF VERMONT COLLEGE OF MEDICINE
BURLINGTON, VERMONT

OBSTETRICS AND GYNECOLOGY

FOURTH EDITION

with 75 authors

1063 ILLUSTRATIONS

Joseph A. Carvelli

HARPER & ROW, PUBLISHERS
PHILADELPHIA

Cambridge
New York
Hagerstown
San Francisco

London
Mexico City
São Paulo
Sydney

1817

The authors and publisher have exerted every effort to ensure that drug selection and dosage set forth in this text are in accord with current recommendations and practice at the time of publication. However, in view of ongoing research, changes in government regulations, and the constant flow of information relating to drug therapy and drug reactions, the reader is urged to check the package insert for each drug for any change in indications and dosage and for added warnings and precautions. This is particularly important when the recommended agent is a new and/or infrequently employed drug.

10   9   8   7   6   5   4   3   2

Obstetrics and Gynecology, Fourth Edition. Copyright © 1982 by Harper & Row, Publishers, Inc. Copyright © 1977, 1971, 1966 by Harper & Row, Publishers, Inc. All rights reserved. No part of this book may be used or reproduced in any manner whatsoever without written permission except in the case of brief quotations embodied in critical articles and reviews. Printed in the United States of America. For information address Harper & Row Publishers, Inc., East Washington Square, Philadelphia, Pennsylvania 19105

Library of Congress Cataloging in Publication Data
Main entry under title:
Obstetrics & gynecology.
   Includes bibliographies and index.
   1. Gynecology.   2. Obstetrics.   I. Danforth, David.   [DNLM: 1.
Genital diseases, Female.   2. Obstetrics. WQ 100 0145]
RG101.023   1982   618   81-6372
ISBN 0-06-140696-1   AACR2

CONTENTS

PART V.   ABNORMAL LABOR AND THE PUERPERIUM   681

AUTHORS

RAJA W. ABDUL-KARIM, M.D.

CHAPTER 27

Professor of Obstetrics and Gynecology, State University of New York Upstate Medical Center; Attending Obstetrician and Gynecologist, Community General Hospital and Crouse–Irving Memorial Hospital, State University of New York Upstate Medical Center, Syracuse, New York

KARLIS ADAMSONS, M.D., Ph.D., F.A.C.O.G.

CHAPTER 42

Professor and Chairman, Department of Obstetrics and Gynecology, The University of Puerto Rico; Obstetrician and Gynecologist-in-Chief, The University Hospital, San Juan, Puerto Rico

GEOFFREY ALTSHULER, M.D.

CHAPTERS 43, 44

Professor of Pathology, University of Oklahoma College of Medicine; Director of Laboratories, Oklahoma Children's Memorial Hospital, Oklahoma City, Oklahoma

A. N. ARNESON, M.D., F.A.C.O.G.

CHAPTER 60

Professor Emeritus of Clinical Obstetrics and Gynecology and Associate Professor Emeritus of Clinical Radiology, Washington University School of Medicine; Associate Obstetrician-Gynecologist, Barnes Hospital, St. Louis, Missouri

RALPH C. BENSON, M.D., F.A.C.O.G., F.A.C.S., F.I.C.S. (Hon.)

CHAPTER 33

Professor and Chairman Emeritus, Department of Obstetrics and Gynecology, University of Oregon Health Sciences Center School of Medicine; Attending Obstetrician and Gynecologist, St. Vincent, Emanual, and Good Samaritan Hospitals, Portland, Oregon

VINCENT J. CAPRARO, M.D., F.A.C.O.G., F.A.C.S., F.I.C.A.

CHAPTER 45

Professor of Obstetrics and Gynecology, State University of New York at Buffalo; Chairman, Department of Obstetrics and Gynecology, Millard Fillmore Hospital; Chief, Division of Pediatric and Adolescent Gynecology, Buffalo Children's Hospital, Buffalo, New York

DENIS CAVANAGH, M.D., F.A.C.O.G., F.A.C.S., F.R.C.O.G.

CHAPTERS 20, 38

Professor of Obstetrics and Gynecology, University of South Florida; Attending Obstetrician and Gynecologist, Tampa General Hospital; Attending Obstetrician and Gynecologist and Director of Medical Education, Women's Hospital, Tampa, Florida

MANUEL R. COMAS, M.D., F.A.C.O.G.

CHAPTERS 20, 38

Associate Professor of Obstetrics and Gynecology, St. Louis University School of Medicine, St. Louis, Missouri

ASHLEY T. COOPLAND, M.D., F.A.C.O.G., F.R.C.S.(C)

CHAPTER 37

Associate Clinical Professor of Obstetrics and Gynecology, Yale University School of Medicine; Director of Obstetrics and Gynecology, Waterbury Hospital Health Center, Waterbury, Connecticut

ROGER C. CRAFTS, Ph.D.

CHAPTER 3

Professor of Anatomy, University of Cincinnati College of Medicine, Cincinnati, Ohio

ROBERT E. CUDDIHEE, M.D.

CHAPTER 38

Assistant Professor of Internal Medicine, St. Louis University School of Medicine; Chief of Nephrology, St. Louis Veterans Administration Hospital, St. Louis, Missouri

DAVID N. DANFORTH, PH.D., M.D., F.A.C.O.G., F.A.C.S.

CHAPTERS 26, 29, 30, 31, 34, 38, 48

Thomas J. Watkins Professor Emeritus of Obstetrics and Gynecology, Northwestern University Medical School, Chicago; Senior Attending Obstetrician and Gynecologist, Evanston Hospital, Evanston, Illinois

JACK DAVIES, M.D.

CHAPTER 4

Professor and Chairman, Department of Anatomy, Vanderbilt School of Medicine, Nashville, Tennessee

EDWARD J. DENNIS, III, M.D., F.A.C.O.G.

CHAPTER 25

Professor and Chairman, Department of Obstetrics and Gynecology, University of South Carolina School of Medicine; Director of Obstetrics and Gynecology, Richland Memorial Hospital, Columbia, South Carolina

RICHARD DEPP, M.D., F.A.C.O.G.

CHAPTER 41

Professor of Obstetrics and Gynecology and Director of Obstetrics, Northwestern University Medical School; Head, Section of Maternal–Fetal Medicine, Prentice Women's Hospital and Maternity Center, Northwestern Memorial Hospital, Chicago, Illinois

GUNTER DEPPE, M.D., F.A.C.O.G., F.A.C.S.

CHAPTERS 54, 55

Assistant Professor of Obstetrics and Gynecology, Mount Sinai School of Medicine; Associate Director of Gynecologic Oncology, Associate Attending Obstetrician and Gynecologist, Mount Sinai Hospital, New York, New York

PHILIP J. DiSAIA, M.D., F.A.C.O.G., F.A.C.S.

CHAPTER 60

Professor and Chairman, Department of Obstetrics and Gynecology, University of California, Irvine, College of Medicine; Chief of Obstetrics and Gynecology, University of California, Irvine, Medical Center, Orange, California

THOMAS E. DOLAN, M.D., F.A.C.O.G.

CHAPTER 57

Associate Professor of Obstetrics and Gynecology and Director of Gynecologic Oncology, Rush Medical College; Attending Obstetrician and Gynecologist, Rush-Presbyterian-St. Luke's Medical Center, Chicago, and Lutheran General Hospital, Park Ridge, Illinois

WILLIAM L. DONEGAN, M.D., F.A.C.S.

CHAPTER 59

Professor of Surgery and American Cancer Society Professor of Clinical Oncology, Medical College of Wisconsin; Attending Surgeon, Milwaukee County Hospital and Columbia Hospital, Milwaukee, Wisconsin

BRUCE D. DOUST, M.B., B.S.

CHAPTERS 28, 58

Associate Professor of Radiology, The Medical College of Wisconsin; Director of Ultrasound and Computed Tomography, Veterans Administration Hospital, Milwaukee, Wisconsin

VIVIENNE L. DOUST, M.B., B.S.

CHAPTERS 28, 58

Assistant Clinical Professor of Radiology, The Medical College of Wisconsin; Staff Radiologist, Veterans Administration Hospital, Milwaukee, Wisconsin

WILLIAM DROEGEMUELLER, M.D., F.A.C.O.G.

CHAPTER 22

Professor and Associate Head, Department of Obstetrics and Gynecology, University of Arizona College of Medicine, Arizona Health Sciences Center, Tucson, Arizona

BRUCE H. DRUKKER, M.D., F.A.C.O.G.

CHAPTER 61

Clinical Professor of Obstetrics and Gynecology, The University of Michigan Medical School, Ann Arbor; Chairman, Department of Gynecology–Obstetrics and Division Head, Gynecologic Oncology, Henry Ford Hospital, Detroit, Michigan

LEO J. DUNN, M.D., F.A.C.O.G.

CHAPTER 39

Professor and Chairman, Department of Obstetrics and Gynecology, Medical College of Virginia, Virginia Commonwealth University; Chairman, Department of Obstetrics and Gynecology, Medical College of Virginia Hospitals, Richmond, Virginia

WILLIAM E. EASTERLING, JR., A.B., M.D., F.A.C.O.G.

CHAPTER 40

Professor of Obstetrics and Gynecology and Vice Dean, The University of North Carolina School of Medicine; Chief of Staff, The North Carolina Memorial Hospital, Chapel Hill, North Carolina

DAVID A. ESCHENBACH, M.D.

CHAPTER 50

Associate Professor of Obstetrics and Gynecology, University of Washington School of Medicine, Seattle, Washington

TOMMY N. EVANS, M.D., F.A.C.O.G., F.A.C.S.

CHAPTER 47

Professor and Chairman, Department of Gynecology and Obstetrics, Wayne State University School of Medicine; Chief of Gynecology and Obstetrics, Harper–Grace Hospital and Hutzel Hospital, Detroit, Michigan

MARTIN FARBER, M.D., F.A.C.O.G.

CHAPTER 49

Associate Professor, Department of Obstetrics and Gynecology, Tufts University School of Medicine; Director, Division of Reproductive Endocrinology, Department of Obstetrics–Gynecology, Tufts New England Medical Center Hospital, Boston, Massachusetts

VINCENT J. FREDA, M.D., F.A.C.O.G.

CHAPTER 23

Associate Clinical Professor of Obstetrics and Gynecology, Columbia University College of Physicians and Surgeons; Associate Attending Obstetrician and Gynecologist, Presbyterian Hospital, New York, New York

JAMES GOLDFARB, M.D.

CHAPTER 46

Assistant Professor of Reproductive Biology, Case Western Reserve University; Associate Director of Gynecology, Mount Sinai Hospital, Cleveland, Ohio

CLIFFORD P. GOPLERUD, M.D., F.A.C.O.G.

CHAPTER 24

Professor of Obstetrics and Gynecology, University of Iowa College of Medicine, Iowa City, Iowa

SAUL B. GUSBERG, M.D., D.Sc. F.A.C.O.G., F.A.C.S., F.R.C.O.G. (Hon.)

CHAPTERS 54, 55

Distinguished Service Professor, Department of Obstetrics and Gynecology, The Mount Sinai School of Medicine of the City University of New York; Consultant, Department of Obstetrics and Gynecology, The Mount Sinai Hospital, New York, New York

E.S.E. HAFEZ, Ph.D.

CHAPTER 4

Professor of Gynecology/Andrology and Reproductive Physiology, Wayne State University School of Medicine, Detroit, Michigan

DOUGLAS M. HAYNES, M.D., F.A.C.O.G., F.A.C.S.

CHAPTER 19

Professor of Obstetrics and Gynecology, University of Louisville School of Medicine; Attending Obstetrician and Gynecologist, University Hospital and Norton–Children's Hospital, Louisville, Kentucky

CHARLES H. HENDRICKS, M.D., F.A.C.O.G.

CHAPTER 35

Robert A. Ross Professor of Obstetrics and Gynecology, University of North Carolina School of Medicine; Attending Obstetrician and Gynecologist, North Carolina Memorial Hospital, Chapel Hill, North Carolina

WILLIAM N. P. HERBERT, M.D., F.A.C.O.G.

CHAPTER 40

Assistant Professor of Obstetrics and Gynecology, University of North Carolina School of Medicine, Chapel Hill, North Carolina

LAWRENCE L. HESTER, JR., M.D., F.A.C.O.G., F.A.C.S.

CHAPTER 25

Professor and Chairman, Department of Obstetrics and Gynecology, Medical University of South Carolina, Charleston, South Carolina

ROBERT D. HILGERS, M.D., F.A.C.O.G., F.A.C.S.

CHAPTER 21

Professor and Chief, Gynecologic Oncology, University of New Mexico School of Medicine; Attending Obstetrician and Gynecologist, University of New Mexico Hospital, Albuquerque, New Mexico

C. PAUL HODGKINSON, M.D., F.A.C.O.G., F.A.C.S.

CHAPTER 61

Clinical Professor of Obstetrics and Gynecology, The University of Michigan Medical School, Ann Arbor; Clinical Professor of Gynecology and Obstetrics, Wayne State University School of Medicine; Emeritus Associate, Department of Gynecology and Obstetrics, Henry Ford Hospital, Detroit, Michigan

ROBERT B. JAFFE, M.D., F.A.C.O.G.

CHAPTER 18

Professor and Chairman, Department of Obstetrics, Gynecology, and Reproductive Sciences and Director, Reproductive Endocrinology Center, University of California, San Francisco, California

L. STANLEY JAMES, M.D., F.A.A.P.

CHAPTER 42

Professor of Pediatrics and Professor of Obstetrics and Gynecology, Columbia University College of Physicians and Surgeons; Attending Pediatrician, Babies Hospital, Columbia–Presbyterian Medical Center, New York

GEORGEANNA SEEGAR JONES, M.D., Sc.D. (Hon.), F.A.C.O.G., F.A.C.S.

CHAPTER 8

Professor of Obstetrics and Gynecology, Eastern Virginia Medical School, Norfolk, Virginia; Professor Emeritus of Obstetrics and Gynecology, Johns Hopkins Medical School, Baltimore, Maryland

IRWIN H. KAISER, M.D., Ph.D., F.A.C.O.G.

CHAPTER 16

Professor of Gynecology and Obstetrics, Albert Einstein College of Medicine of Yeshiva University; Director of Obstetrics and Gynecology, The Hospital of the Albert Einstein College of Medicine, Bronx, New York

ROBERT A. H. KINCH, M.D., F.R.C.O.G., F.R.C.S. (C)

CHAPTER 10

Professor and Chairman, Department of Obstetrics and Gynaecology, McGill University; Obstetrician and Gynaecologist-in-Chief, Royal Victoria Hospital and Montreal General Hospital, Montreal, Quebec, Canada

HOWARD P. KRIEGER, M.D.

CHAPTER 3

Professor of Neurology, The Mount Sinai School of Medicine of the City University of New York; Attending Neurologist, The Mount Sinai Medical Center, New York, New York

WILLIAM J. LEDGER, M.D., F.A.C.O.G., F.A.C.S.

CHAPTER 13

Professor and Chairman, Department of Obstetrics and Gynecology, Cornell University Medical College; Obstetrician and Gynecologist-in-Chief, New York Hospital, New York, New York

JOHN L. LEWIS, JR., M.D., F.A.C.O.G., F.A.C.S.

CHAPTER 21

Professor of Obstetrics and Gynecology, Cornell University Medical College; Chief, Gynecology Service, Memorial Sloan Kettering Cancer Center, New York, New York

A. BRIAN LITTLE, M.D., F.A.C.O.G., F.A.C.S.

CHAPTER 46

Arthur H. Bill Professor and Director, Department of Reproductive Biology, Case Western Reserve University School of Medicine; Director, Department of Obstetrics and Gynecology, University Hospitals of Cleveland, Cleveland, Ohio

HANS LUDWIG, M.D.

CHAPTER 4

Professor and Chairman, Department of Obstetrics and Gynecology, University of Essen School of Medicine, Essen, Germany

JOHN R. MARSHALL, M.D., F.A.C.O.G.

CHAPTER 7

Professor of Obstetrics and Gynecology, University of California, Los Angeles, School of Medicine, Los Angeles; Chairman, Department of Obstetrics and Gynecology, Harbor General Hospital, Torrance, California

KAY F. McFARLAND, M.C., F.A.C.P.

CHAPTER 25

Associate Professor of Obstetrics and Gynecology and Adjunct Associate Professor of Medicine, University of South Carolina School of Medicine, Columbia, South Carolina

JAMES A. MERRILL, M.D., F.A.C.O.G.

CHAPTERS 51, 54, 55, 56, 57

Professor and Head, Department of Gynecology and Obstetrics and Professor of Pathology, University of Oklahoma College of Medicine; Chief of Service, Department of Gynecology and Obstetrics, Oklahoma Memorial Hospital, Oklahoma City, Oklahoma

DANIEL R. MISHELL, JR., M.D., F.A.C.O.G.

CHAPTER 14

Professor and Chairman, Department of Obstetrics and Gynecology, University of Southern California; Chief of Professional Services, Women's Hospital, Los Angeles County—University of Southern California Medical Center, Los Angeles, California

GEORGE W. MITCHELL, JR., M.D., F.A.C.O.G., F.A.C.S.

CHAPTER 49

Professor and Chairman, Department of Obstetrics and Gynecology, Tufts University School of Medicine; Gynecologist-in-Chief, New England Medical Center Hospital, Boston, Massachusetts

KAMRAN S. MOGHISSI, M.D., F.A.C.O.G., F.A.C.S.

CHAPTERS 11, 47

Professor of Gynecology and Obstetrics, Wayne State University; Chief, Division of Reproductive Biology and Endocrinology, Wayne State University School of Medicine and The C. S. Mott Center for Human Growth and Development; Senior Attending Gynecologist and Obstetrician, Harper Hospital and Hutzel Hospital, Detroit, Michigan

HISAYO O. MORISHIMA, M.D.

CHAPTER 32

Associate Professor of Anesthesiology, Division of Perinatal Medicine, Columbia University College of Physicians and Surgeons, New York, New York

JAMES H. NELSON, JR., M.D.

CHAPTER 57

Joe Vincent Meigs Professor of Gynecology, Harvard Medical School; Director, Division of Gynecology, Massachusetts General Hospital, Boston, Massachusetts

ROBERT E. L. NESBITT, JR., M.D., F.A.C.O.G., F.A.C.S.

CHAPTER 27

Professor and Chairman, Department of Obstetrics and Gynecology, State University of New York, Upstate Medical Center; Chief of Obstetrics and Gynecology, State University Hospital; Attending Obstetrician and Gynecologist, Crouse-Irving Memorial Hospital, Syracuse, New York

MICHAEL NEWTON, M.D., F.A.C.O.G., F.A.C.S.

CHAPTER 36

Professor of Obstetrics and Gynecology, Northwestern University Medical School; Attending Obstetrician and Gynecologist and Director, Division of Gynecologic Oncology, Prentice Women's Hospital and Maternity Center, Northwestern Memorial Hospital, Chicago, Illinois

JAMES F. NOLAN, M.D., F.A.C.O.G., F.A.C.S.

CHAPTER 60

Clinical Professor Emeritus, Department of Obstetrics and Gynecology and Department of Radiology, University of Southern California School of Medicine; Medical Director of Southern California Cancer Center, California Hospital Medical Center, Los Angeles, California

JOHN T. QUEENAN, M.D., F.A.C.O.G., F.A.C.S.

CHAPTER 9

Professor and Chairman, Department of Obstetrics and Gynecology, Georgetown University School of Medicine; Obstetrician and Gynecologist-in-Chief, Georgetown University Hospital, Washington, D.C.

EDWARD J. QUILLIGAN, M.D., F.A.C.O.G.

CHAPTER 17

Professor and Head, Division of Maternal–Fetal Medicine, University of California College of Medicine, Orange, California

ELIZABETH M. RAMSEY, M.D., Sc.D., F.A.C.O.G.(A)

CHAPTER 5

Research Associate, Department of Embryology, Carnegie Institution of Washington, Baltimore, Maryland

JIM ROSS, Ph.D., M.D.

CHAPTER 7

Staff Endocrinologist, Department of Obstetrics and Gynecology, Salinas Valley Memorial Hospital, Salinas, California

FELIX RUTLEDGE, M.D., F.A.C.O.G.

CHAPTER 52

Professor of Gynecology, University of Texas System Cancer Center; Head, Department of Gynecology, M.D. Anderson Hospital and Tumor Institute, Houston, Texas

KENNETH J. RYAN, M.D., F.A.C.O.G.

CHAPTER 6

Kate Macy Ladd Professor and Chairman, Department of Obstetrics and Gynecology, Harvard Medical School; Chief of Staff and Director, Laboratory of Human Reproduction and Reproductive Biology, Boston Hospital for Women, Boston, Massachusetts

GLORIA E. SARTO, M.D., Ph.D., F.A.C.O.G.

CHAPTER 2

Professor and Assistant Chairman, Department of Obstetrics and Gynecology, Northwestern University Medical School; Chief of Clinical Services, Prentice Women's Hospital and Maternity Center, Northwestern Memorial Hospital, Chicago, Illinois

JAMES R. SCOTT, M.D., F.A.C.O.G.

CHAPTER 12

Professor and Chairman, Department of Obstetrics and Gynecology, University of Utah Medical Center, Salt Lake City, Utah

HAROLD SPEERT, M.D., F.A.C.O.G., F.A.C.S.

CHAPTER 1

Assistant Clinical Professor of Obstetrics and Gynecology, Columbia University College of Physicians and Surgeons; Assistant Attending Obstetrician and Gynecologist, Presbyterian Hospital, New York, New York

ADOLF STAFL, M.D., Ph.D., F.A.C.O.G.

CHAPTER 54

Associate Professor of Gynecology and Obstetrics, The Medical College of Wisconsin; Senior Attending Obstetrician and Gynecologist, Milwaukee County General Hospital, Milwaukee, Wisconsin

SUZANNE STEINBERG, B.S.C.N., M.N., M.D.C.M., F.A.C.O.G.

CHAPTER 10

Fellow in Obstetrics and Gynaecology and Psychiatry, McGill Faculty of Medicine, Montreal, Quebec, Canada

JOSEPH F. THOMPSON, M.D., M.P.H., F.A.C.O.G.

CHAPTER 15

Professor of Obstetrics and Gynecology, Indiana University School of Medicine, Indianapolis, Indiana

HAROLD M. M. TOVELL, M.D., F.A.C.O.G., F.A.C.S.

CHAPTER 48

Clinical Professor of Obstetrics and Gynecology, Columbia University College of Physicians and Surgeons; Attending Obstetrician and Gynecologist, Women's Hospital, St. Luke's–Roosevelt Hospital Center, New York, New York

DAVID H. VROON, M.D.

CHAPTER 38

Associate Professor of Pathology, Emory University School of Medicine; Director of Clinical Laboratories, Grady Memorial Hospital, Atlanta, Georgia

ANNE COLSTON WENTZ, M.D., F.A.C.O.G.

CHAPTER 8

Professor of Obstetrics and Gynecology, Vanderbilt University School of Medicine and Vanderbilt University Medical Center, Nashville, Tennessee

J. DONALD WOODRUFF, M.D., F.A.C.O.G.

CHAPTER 53

Professor of Obstetrics and Gynecology and Richard W. TeLinde Professor of Gynecologic Pathology, Johns Hopkins Hospital, Baltimore, Maryland

PREFACE

In keeping with the tradition of this book, the purpose of the fourth edition of *Obstetrics and Gynecology* is to provide a comprehensive, authoritative American text that will serve as a central, basic reference to the principles and practice of obstetrics and gynecology. For the editor, each new edition is an exciting challenge: a vast amount of new information must be included, yet the book must be kept to a workable size. To accomplish these objectives, substantial deletions of obsolete material have been made from the third edition to accommodate new material, and particular effort has been made to present the entire text in a style that is crisp, well organized, and readable.

As in previous editions, *Obstetrics and Gynecology* is intended for a wide audience. The emphasis on basic principles and the orderly development of the discussions have caused this book to be adopted by many medical students and recommended as a standard textbook in many medical schools. Residents-in-training find the book to be helpful in the evaluation and management of the day-to-day problems that they encounter, and as a point of departure for subjects they wish to pursue. Practitioners have found this text to be useful as a comprehensive survey of current thought in obstetrics and gynecology.

In any field of medicine a knowledge of basic science relationships is essential to an understanding of normal and abnormal processes. These relationships have been emphasized in each edition, but in the fourth edition new advances have required much change in virtually all of these sections. An important example, which touches much of the book, is ultrasound. Just as radioimmunoassay revolutionized the field of endocrinology, the applications of ultrasound in obstetrics and gynecology have caused an explosive increase in our knowledge of normal and abnormal processes and have altered our approach to many clinical problems. Emphasis was placed on this subject in the third edition, but new advances have required extensive revision of all discussions dealing with topics to which ultrasound has made significant contribution.

The opening section of *Obstetrics and Gynecology* deals with subjects that are applicable to both obstetrics and gynecology. New chapters are included on counseling, nutrition in obstetrics and gynecology, antibacterial therapy in obstetric–gynecologic infections, and immunobiologic considerations in obstetrics and gynecology. The new chapter on gross anatomy of the female reproductive system is intended to be sufficiently precise to serve as a definitive reference source.

The sections dealing with obstetrics have been extensively revised to include the important advances since publication of the third edition and also to recognize the major changes in attitude and technique that have

followed the new emphasis on family-centered obstetric care. Chapters that have been largely rewritten are those that deal with the conduct of pregnancy, complications and disorders due to pregnancy, the physiology of uterine action, preterm labor and the low-birth-weight infant, and the conduct of normal labor. Chapters that have been completely rewritten by new authors include those on ectopic pregnancy, gestational trophoblastic neoplasia, the evaluation of fetal status, obstetric analgesia and anesthesia, coagulation disorders, and abnormalities of the fetus, placenta, membranes, and the newborn.

The chapters on gynecology have been extensively updated and pruned of material that is not essential. A new chapter on endometriosis has been included as well as new chapters, written *de novo* by new authors, on the subjects of gynecologic infections, pediatric gynecology, and diseases of the breast. Several sections from the third edition remain more or less intact in the fourth edition. These include Harold Speert's classic account of the historic aspects of obstetrics and gynecology, and many of the discussions that deal with the basic truths of our discipline.

It is a privilege to introduce many of our modern readers to the work of the incomparable Max Brödel, whose drawings are as fresh and crisp today as when they first appeared more than 75 years ago. The use of these and many other illustrations in the fourth edition follows the editor's conviction that when superior illustrations are available it is much better to use them than to prepare others of lesser quality merely for the sake of originality.

As in previous editions, we have elected to omit reference citations in the text because so many readers find them to be distracting and unnecessary; the categorized reference lists appended to most of the chapters permit easy access to specific subjects and to reviews that contain extensive bibliographies. A particular effort has been made to avoid duplication of material except for a few areas in which this has been let stand deliberately for either emphasis or continuity. The editor is grateful to the authors for their enthusiastic cooperation and for their gracious acceptance of the editing needed to achieve the balance and unity that are vital features of a workable and useful text.

The reception accorded the third edition is gratifying to all who participated in its writing and production. In its periodic recommendation of a "Selected Lists and Journals for the Small Medical Library," *Obstetrics and Gynecology* was listed in the Bulletin of the Medical Library Association among the "items suggested for priority purchase." The book was again among those recommended by the American College of Physicians as most important to the internist for reference use. In the Medical Economics listing of "Books Every Doctor Needs to Own," *Obstetrics and Gynecology* was the only book listed in this field. "The Innominate," a newspaper for medical students, concluded its review with the statement that "I rate this book 10 out of 10." The new and somewhat larger fourth edition follows the tradition of its predecessors, and it is our hope that it, too, will have an important position in the literature of obstetrics and gynecology.

D.N.D.

EXCERPTS FROM THE
PREFACE TO THE FIRST EDITION

A new textbook in a field already noted for the excellence of its literature needs a word of explanation of its background and objectives. In recent years the teaching in our field has been changing, and in all but two American medical schools obstetrics and gynecology are now combined in a single department and taught in a single sequence of courses by the same individuals. It seems a paradox that the student should require two separate books with their differing approaches and their repetition of material to help guide him through his course in the combined subject.

At teaching conferences it has been noted repeatedly that logic, convenience, and efficiency call for a single combined textbook in the interest of the student and the practitioner who require a reference to the basic essentials of the field. The new TEXTBOOK OF OBSTETRICS AND GYNECOLOGY is an attempt to meet this need.

It is designed to cover completely, in logical sequence and with maximum authority, the subject of obstetrics and gynecology in all the areas that are included in today's curriculum and it integrates the thinking of a faculty representing more than 30 medical schools in the U.S.A. and Canada. Each section has been written by an expert with special knowledge and experience in his assigned topic and this authority lends value to the text which could be achieved in no other way.

The scope of this text is wider than in most textbooks of either obstetrics or gynecology. This is deliberate and reflects the growth of knowledge in the field as well as the changing trends in medical education.

Because of the trend toward integrating the basic sciences with clinical problems throughout the medical curriculum, special emphasis is placed on chapters dealing with anatomy, physiology, endocrinology, embryology and genetics. These sections are intended to be sufficiently complete to serve as an authoritative reference source as well as a basis for the material that follows.

Documentation has been confined in most chapters to review articles, monographs, and other key references which will aid the reader in exploring areas of special interest.

Because of its distinguished authorship, and the breadth and detail of its content, it is hoped that the book will be of interest and use to the resident and practitioner as well as to the student. It should provide a central basic reference source around which the graduate can build a library of more specialized works in whatever direction his needs and inclinations may take him.

I am deeply indebted to each of the authors. It is their book and it is their work which has given the text its strength. Any omissions are the responsibility of the editor.

D.N.D.

ACKNOWLEDGMENTS

We are especially indebted to Ranice W. Crosby, Associate Professor and Director of the Department of Art as Applied to Medicine, of the Johns Hopkins School of Medicine, for making available many of the late Max Brödel's original drawings, which are reproduced in several sections of *Obstetrics and Gynecology.* We also wish to express grateful thanks to the many authors and publishers who have granted us permission to reproduce previously published tables and illustrations.

It is again a pleasure to acknowledge the help of Rose Slowinski, Librarian, and Linda Feinberg, of the Evanston Hospital's Webster Medical Library. Their gracious help in obtaining obscure material, verifying references, and all other matters in which skilled library assistance was needed is greatly appreciated.

We wish to express sincere thanks to David N. Danforth, Jr., M.D., whose editorial assistance has been of much help in this and in the previous editions of *Obstetrics and Gynecology.* We are also grateful to Thomas T. Chen, M.D., Lawrence Gratkins, M.D., Scott R. Harriage, M.D., William H. Miller, M.D., David Olive, M.D., and Susan T. Warner, M.D., whose editorial and proofreading assistance was extremely helpful.

We are grateful also to my good friend Richard D. Bryant, M.D., who has read virtually every word of the text and whose acuity has been of great assistance both editorially and in the correction of typographical errors.

The skillful help and expertise of Rebecca D. Rinehart at all phases of the preparation of this fourth edition is most gratefully acknowledged. To her and to the other members of the staff of Harper & Row, as well as to the staff of the J.B. Lippincott Company who contributed so much to the final stages of our work, I wish to express sincere appreciation for their infinite patience and their unusual skill in all matters having to do with the preparation of this volume.

D.N.D.

OBSTETRICS AND GYNECOLOGY

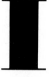

GENERAL
CONSIDERATIONS

HISTORICAL HIGHLIGHTS

Harold Speert

The special field of medicine known as obstetrics and gynecology boasts a background of unsurpassed drama. The discovery of the mammalian egg; the history of the obstetric forceps; the early cesarean sections; the conquest of puerperal fever; the controversy over obstetric anesthesia; the first successful abdominal operation, for ovarian cyst; and the cure of vesicovaginal fistula, one of the most distressing of woman's ills, form threads of a story with few equals in the annals of medicine. At least a superficial knowledge of the specialty's maturation is essential to the physician's general education as well as to an appreciation of his scientific heritage. The already crowded medical curriculum, however, provides scant opportunity for the pursuit of cultural interests beyond the expansive range of twentieth century science. This introduction to the history of obstetrics and gynecology is designed for the busy student with little time, and possibly little taste, for medical history. Contained herein are con-

densed accounts of a few of the major developments that have imparted to obstetrics and gynecology the specialty's distinctive character. The reader stimulated to further inquiry will find ample guidance in the recommended reading list at the end of this chapter.

EARLY MIDWIFERY

The history of obstetrics is the history of civilization itself. In biblical days, before the advent of physicians, labor and delivery were usually supervised by the midwives. These self-styled specialists of the obstetric art, usually without benefit of education or training, exercised a virtual monopoly over their craft until the sixteenth century or later. In 1552 Wertt, a physician in Hamburg, was burned at the stake for having posed as a woman in order to attend a patient in labor. The Old Testament records the role of the midwife in the second labor of Rachel, wife of Jacob (Gen. 35:17) and in Tamar's delivery of twins (Gen. 38:27). During the period of the Hebrews' enslavement in Egypt, when their high birth rate began to pose a threat to Pharaoh's security, he ordered the midwives to destroy all the male children at birth. Not all obeyed, however, and when taken to task for their disobedience, the Egyptian midwives Shiphrah and Puah explained that "the Hebrew women . . . are lively, and are delivered ere the midwives come in unto them" (Exod. 1:15, 19).

The high standards of these Egyptian women did not characterize the practices of all midwives, however (Fig. 1–1); for centuries they were subjected to repeated vilification, and their calling was held in disrepute. At the fall of the Roman Empire, Eusebia, wife of the Emperor Constantius, jealous of her fecund sister-in-law Helen, the wife of Julian the Apostate, induced the midwife to murder Helen's child by allowing it to bleed from the umbilical cord.

As late as the eighteenth century, care of the pregnant woman was generally considered beneath the dignity of the physician, and false notions of modesty barred his participation in the delivery. As a result, the physician was usually summoned only in complicated and neglected cases. Mutilation of both mother and child often followed. The obstetrics of the Middle Ages has been characterized as neglect of normal cases and butchery of abnormal.

The first formal training for midwives was instituted by Hippocrates, in the fifth century B.C., but for several subsequent centuries efforts toward their education were halting and ineffectual. Self-taught or instructed by older midwives, most remained ignorant of the simple principles of obstetrics; many were careless, meddlesome, and dirty. Soranus (A.D. 98–138), the leading Greek authority on obstetrics and gynecology during the reigns of the emperors Trajan and Hadrian, made a noteworthy attempt to elevate the standards of midwifery with his celebrated text, but little improvement

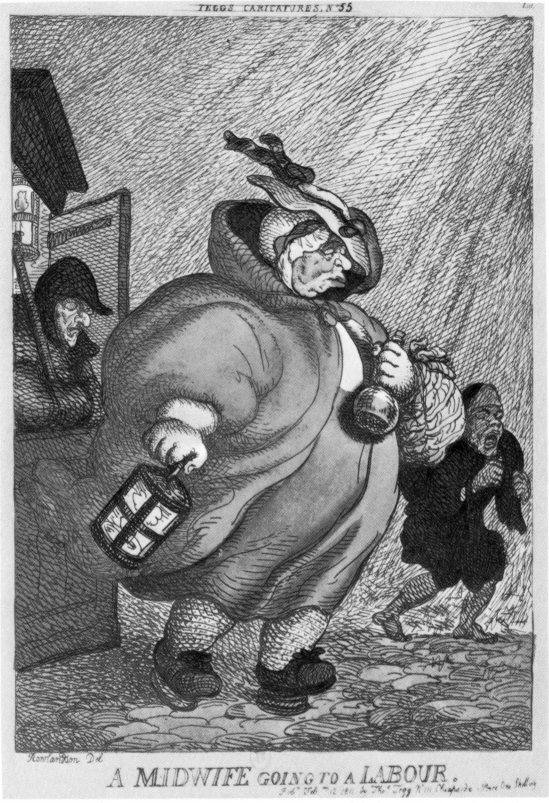

A MIDWIFE GOING TO A LABOUR.

FIG. 1–1. Caricature of "midwife going to a labour"; holding in her right hand a lamp and in her left a flask of alcoholic refreshment, traditional accoutrements of midwives of eighteenth and nineteenth centuries. (Thomas Rowlandson, 1811)

followed for 400 years. A new era in obstetric education was ushered in by the publication of Rösslin's *Der Schwangerenn Frawen und Hebammen Rosengarte* in 1513 (Fig. 1–2). Although it was based in large part on Soranus's *Gynecology* and contained little that was original, Rösslin's book had the great merit of being published in the vernacular German, which the midwives of his land could read and understand. It enjoyed the popularity of numerous editions, and its English translation, *The Byrth of Mankynde*, remained a best seller for 100 years.

Scipione Mercurio, who was born in the very year that *The Byrth of Mankynde* was published, soon introduced into Italy a similar work, *La Commare O'Raccoglitrice* (1595–1596), for the guidance of midwives. Like its German and English counterparts, this book received a warm reception and went into 20 editions. It is still remembered for its description of cesarean section and for the first mentioning of pelvic contraction as an indication for the operation. Obstetrics rapidly acquired the dignity of a clinical science with the publication of more scholarly treatises, outstanding among which were Mauriceau's *Traité des maladies des femmes grosses* (1668), Smellie's *Treatise on the Theory and Practice of Midwifery* (1752–1764), and Denman's *Introduction to the Practice of Midwifery* (1795).

The first obstetric publication in America was reprinted from a London pamphlet of 1663, entitled *A Present To Be Given to Teeming Women by Their Husbands or Friends, Containing Scripture-Directions for Women with Child*. The unhappy recipient was urged to "prayer, repentance, reading of the Scriptures, meditation, resignation, and preparation for death." Sam-

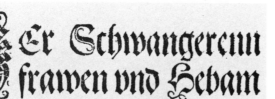

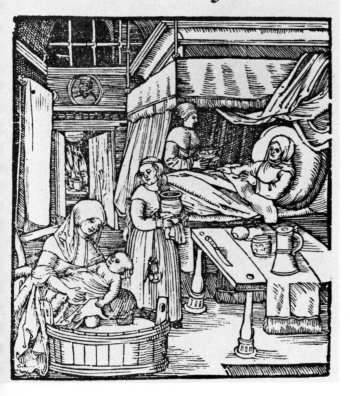

FIG. 1–2. Title page of one of first texts for midwives. (Heinrich Steiner's 1537 edition of Rösslins Rosengarte)

uel Bard's *Compendium of the Theory and Practice of Midwifery*, the first obstetric text by an American author, was published in 1807.

With the practice of obstetrics confined largely to midwives, a few achieved wide renown for their skill, writings, or devotion to their calling. Louise Bourgeois was selected by Henry IV in 1601 to deliver his wife, Marie de Medici, of their son, the future Louis XIII. The candle of this French midwife's fame was rapidly snuffed out, however, in 1627, when another of her fashionable clients, Madame de Montpensier, the Duchess of Orleans, tarnished her attendant's brilliant record by dying of puerperal infection. Perhaps most distinguished of all the French midwives was the scholarly Madame Boivin (1773–1841).

New Orleans was probably the first American community to license midwives, in 1722, but the unlicensed were permitted to practice their craft in the rest of Colonial America unhampered and unsupervised. Scarcely ever was a physician called to attend a woman in childbirth, except in dire emergency. As recently as 1920 no fewer than 4000 midwives were still practicing in North Carolina, where in 1 year they conducted 34,000 deliveries, one-third of all births in that state. In New York City 3000 midwives handled 40% of the deliveries in 1909; in 1956 14 midwives performed a total of only 142 deliveries in the same city. The last of New York's licensed midwives retired in 1963, having attended her final patient in 1961. Superseding this unlamented obstetric guild is a growing corps of well-trained nurse–midwives, some 1900 of whom were practicing in the United States at the end of 1978, about 1700 certified by the American College of Nurse–Midwives.

Early incursions of men into the obstetric domain were bitterly resisted by the women midwives. Their gradual acceptance and ultimate rise to a position of obstetric superiority have been credited to three developments: 1) Ambroïse Paré's popularization of podalic version in the second half of the sixteenth century; 2) the amorous intrigues and resultant obstetric activity in the Court of France during the seventeenth century, which required a high measure of secrecy; and 3) the introduction of the obstetric forceps. In Colonial America the prejudice against male midwives did not begin to melt away until the second half of the eighteenth century. First to penetrate this barrier was John Moultrie, who settled in Charleston, South Carolina, in 1733 and practiced obstetrics successfully there for the next 50 years. In 1765 William Shippen of Philadelphia began a course of lectures on midwifery, the first in America. Before the end of the eighteenth century a lying-in ward had been established in the New York Almshouse, the New York Lying-In Hospital had been organized, and obstetrics had achieved a respected place in American medicine. Yet not until 1813, more than six decades after its inception, did the medical school of the University of Pennsylvania make its course in obstetrics obligatory. At the Harvard Medical School, founded in 1782, no provision was made for instruction in obstetrics until 1815, with the appointment of Walter Channing as lecturer.

ANTENATAL CARE

Only in the present century has medical supervision during pregnancy achieved general acceptance. Earlier, the physician's role was limited to that of accoucheur at the woman's labor and delivery. He was called upon, in addition, when complications arose during pregnancy, but routine antenatal care as it is now understood was unheard of. As early as the seventeenth century, a few obstetricians recognized the importance of preventive midwifery. In Mauriceau's textbook, for example, we find the statement: "The pregnant woman is like a ship upon a stormy sea full of whitecaps, and the good pilot who is in charge must guide her with prudence if he is to avoid a shipwreck." From 1800 to 1840 in France alone no fewer than 55 doctoral dissertations were published on the hygiene of pregnant women, but most contained little that was original or scientifically valuable. A major advance in antenatal care was made in 1843, when the consistent occurrence of proteinuria in patients with eclampsia was noted. Another half-century elapsed before the association of hypertension with this disorder was recorded, but not until almost 20 years later was elevated blood pressure accorded proper significance as a harbinger of eclampsia.

With the dawn of the twentieth century obstetricians finally awoke to an appreciation of their expanding medical responsibility. In 1901 John W. Ballantyne, pleading for hospital facilities for pregnant women, succeeded in having one bed reserved for antenatal patients in the Royal Maternity Hospital in Edinburgh. With eloquence and perseverance he urged the medical supervision of obstetric patients throughout pregnancy rather than only when ill or in labor. Consultations for pregnant and nursing women were initiated in Paris about the same time. A great boon to antenatal care in the United States resulted from the affiliation of the Instructive District Nursing Association of Boston with the Boston Lying-In Hospital in 1901. In 1907 two teacher–nurses were engaged by the Association for Improving the Conditions of the Poor in New York City for the specific purpose of rendering antenatal care and instruction. The death rate among the infants born to the mothers who received this new type of supervision fell from 17.0% to 4.9%. The first maternity center in the United States was established one decade later, by the Women's City Club of New York, with the avowed objective of providing medical and nursing care of every woman in the dis-

trict from the onset of pregnancy until 1 month post-partum. Physicians and clinics soon assumed responsibility for the complete medical care of expectant mothers. Obstetrics had gone beyond the confines of the delivery chamber and acquired the new dignity of preventive medicine.

THE BEGINNINGS OF EMBRYOLOGY

From the time of Aristotle, the development of the mammalian egg was believed to result from the admixture within the uterus of the menstrual blood and the male semen. The female seed was thought to contribute the substance of the embryo, the male the formative impulse to its growth. A somewhat different view was espoused by Galen. The female semen, he taught, originated in the ovarian vessels, and after being separated or strained in the ovaries, which were known in his day as the female testes, passed down the fallopian tubes and into the uterus. Contact with the male semen resulted in a frothy coagulum, from which the embryo evolved. For a thousand years the doctrine of preformation (*emboîtement*) prevailed, which regarded the fetus as the product of the female of the species. Each human being, in compressed form, lay encapsulated within the body of its mother, successive generations resulting from the mere unshelling and subsequent increase in size of the next order of individuals.

The rival theory of *epigenesis,* probably voiced first by Aristotle, was resurrected in the early seventeenth century by William Harvey, best known for his discovery of the circulation of the blood. This doctrine, which denied that the organism exists encased in a preformed state within the mother and which viewed embryogenesis instead as the gradual aggregation and building up of the body's component parts, received almost no attention, however, until revived in 1759 by Caspar Friedrich Wolff's celebrated *Theoria Generationis.* This work antedated Darwin's equally radical *Origin of Species* by exactly 100 years. Peering through his microscope into the chick embryo, Wolff saw no expanding of a prexisting form but instead a host of minute globules that produced the organs of the embryo by growth and multiplication. With the publication of Wolff's treatise the doctrine of *emboîtement* was dealt its final, crushing blow.

Meantime, the unsuccessful quest for the mammalian ovum, which was to engage man's attention for two millennia, continued. Between 1666 and 1672 Jan van Horne and Jan Swammerdam, working together in Leyden, the Danish anatomist Nils Stensen, and the Dutch Reinier de Graaf had developed the idea that the human female testes, like the ovaries of birds, produce eggs. While the others procrastinated and quibbled over priority, de Graaf published his own observations in a brilliant volume entitled *De Mulierum*

Organis Generationi Inservientibus, which resulted in the eponymic association of his name with the ovarian follicles. De Graaf made the great mistake, however, of assuming the entire contents of the mammalian follicle to be the ovum, for when he immersed the ovaries of swine or cows in boiling water, the contents of the follicle coagulated into a white opaque mass, which, when shelled out of the ovary, resembled the boiled albumen of the hen's egg. Another century and a half was to elapse before the actual discovery of the mammalian ovum in 1827.

Karl Ernst von Baer, studying the embryology of the dog, had departed slightly from the usual procedure of examining the embryos in sequential stages of development and was working backward instead, studying the later stages first in order to recognize the next earlier more easily. In this manner he had observed embryos of 24 days, next 12 days, then free blastocysts in the uterus, and finally tubal ova. He recounted:

It remained for me to ascertain the condition of the ova in the ovary, for it seemed clearer than light that the ova were not the very small Graafian vesicles expelled from the ovary, nor did I consider it likely that such solid little bodies had been coagulated in the tubes from the fluid of the vesicles. When I examined the ovaries before incising them, I clearly distinguished in almost all the vesicles, a whitish-yellow point which was in no way attached to the covering of the vesicle, but as pressure exerted with a probe on the vesicle indicated clearly, swam free in its liquid. Led on more by inquisitiveness than by hope of seeing the ovules in the ovaries with the naked eye through all the coverings of the Graafian vesicles, I opened a vesicle, of which, as I said, I had raised the top with the edge of a scalpel—so clearly did I see it distinguished from the surrounding mucus—and placed it under the microscope. I was astounded when I saw an ovule, already recognized from the tubes, so plainly that a blind man could scarcely deny it. It is truly remarkable and astonishing that a thing so persistently and constantly sought and in all compendia of physiology considered as inextricable, could be put before the eyes with such facility.

The origin of the mammalian ovum identified at last, the science of embryology found a new footing and was soon infused with the vigor of fresh discovery. Less than two decades after von Baer's recognition of the ovum, Martin Barry demonstrated a spermatozoan within the egg cell, and in 1875 Hertwig witnessed the actual union of male and female gametes.

THE OBSTETRIC PELVIS

Like the stumps of old trees, notions long sherished are hard to root out. For countless centuries practitioners of the obstetric art remained wedded to the erroneous concept that birth entails the self-propulsion of the fetus through a distensible pelvic girdle, whose bones separate to permit its passenger's easy egress. Difficulty in labor, it followed, resulted from faulty separation at the pelvic joints. This interpretation of the birth

process was first challenged by Vesalius in 1543 and shortly thereafter by his pupil Arantius, but their protestations were ignored for more than a century, until the publication of Deventer's *Novum Lumen* in 1701. Deventer again insisted on the unyielding character of the pelvic inlet, but erred in his belief that the sacrum and coccyx are displaced backward during labor to permit the passage of the infant's head.

Pelvic mensuration was introduced by Levret in 1753, with his elaborate system of pelvic planes and axes, and gained clinical applicability the following year when Smellie proposed the diagonal conjugate as a simple, reliable index of the inlet's capacity. In addition to the impetus it gave clinical pelvimetry, Smellie's *Treatise on the Theory and Practice of Midwifery* is noteworthy for its lucid, accurate, and concise description of the labor mechanism, contained in the first chapter. In the New Sydenham Society's edition of this classic, A. H. McClintock comments that "had Smellie made no other contribution to midwifery than what is contained in this chapter, he would still have placed accoucheurs under a perpetual obligation."

Clinical pelvimetry achieved widespread acceptance and popularization following the publication of Jean–Louis Baudelocque's *L'Art des accouchemens* in 1781, but Baudelocque's best known contribution embodied an error that was to hinder obstetric practice for the next century and a half. The anteroposterior diameter of the pelvic inlet, he taught, could be estimated reliably by subtracting 3 in. from the external conjugate, measured "from the middle of the pubis to the tip of the spine of the last lumbar vertebra." Baudelocque's diameter, as it soon came to be known, could be measured with greater ease for the examiner and less discomfort for the patient than could the internal conjugate, and it rapidly overshadowed the latter in popularity. The obstetric unreliability of external pelvimetry was demonstrated repeatedly in the ensuing years, but so great was the appeal of this simple approach that obstetricians have finally renounced it only within the last generation.

One of the first to stress the unreliability of the external conjugate as a measure of pelvic adequacy was Gustav Adolf Michaelis, in his monumental work, *Das Enge Becken* (1851). This book, based on the study of 1000 patients, provided the basis of modern clinical knowledge of the bony pelvis. It has been recognized as one of the most important contributions to obstetric literature; the late John Whitridge Williams was fond of saying that no obstetrician could pretend to understand contracted pelves until he had read it. *Das Enge Becken* was edited and published 3 years after Michaelis's death by his friend Carl Litzmann, but ironically its value was overlooked for several years. Indeed, only a few copies of the first edition were ever sold, the publisher marking the remainder as unsalable. Not until 1865 had the importance of the book attained sufficient recognition to warrant its reprinting.

Continuing and extending Michaelis's interest, Litzmann contributed another classic to the obstetric literature, *Die Formen des Beckens*, published in 1861. Its very first paragraph contains one of the most lucid and succinct interpretive descriptions of the female pelvis. Wrote Litzmann:

The pelvis fulfills more extensive functions in the female body than in the male. In the female it forms not merely the bony foundation of the trunk . . . to which strong and numerous muscles are attached, but also shelters the largest part of the sexual apparatus in addition to the distal end of the intestinal canal and urinary passages, and thereby assumes great importance in reproduction. In addition to admitting the male organ during coitus, it has to provide space for the whole uterus at the beginning of pregnancy, and later for expansion of the lower uterine segment at least, and at birth a passageway into the outer world for the mature fetus together with its membranes. Nature has understood how to satisfy, in an amazing manner, the diverse and to some degree contradictory demands with which she is thus confronted. She has imparted the necessary firmness to the pelvis with maximal economy in bony substance by giving it an annular shape and supporting its joints with powerful ligaments, but amassing larger concentrations of bone only in the regions exposed directly to pressure. She has placed the canal that opens at the lowermost part of the trunk in such a position that the pelvis can maintain the burden of the abdominal viscera and provide support and purchase for the enclosed organs, by inclining the pelvis anteriorly at a sharp angle to the horizon, bending its axis in a curve convex posteriorly, and covering and finishing its walls with contractile and elastic soft parts; and in this way also achieving adequate capacity and dilatability for the act of birth. However, the space is so proportioned that even a relatively slight deviation from its normal size can interfere with delivery, insofar as a correspondingly more favorable condition in the remaining birth factors does not compensate for the difficulties.

Roentgen pelvimetry, the ultimate in precise mensuration, was introduced in 1897 in Germany by Albert and in France by Budin and Varnier.

THE OBSTETRIC FORCEPS*

The obstetric forceps, the sole surgical device reserved specifically for the obstetrician's use, has been characterized as "this noble instrument, which has done more to abridge human suffering, and to save human life, then any other instrument in the whole range of surgical appliances." Its origins lie buried in antiquity. A prehensile instrument equipped with teeth was probably used by Abrabian physicians in the eleventh and twelfth centuries to extract the head of the dead fetus, for a device of this type is illustrated in an early manuscript of Albucasis, who lived at Cyropolis, a city of Media on the Caspian Sea. Even earlier evidence, from the second or third century, of the use of forceps

---

* The material under the headings The Obstetric Forceps and Puerperal Fever is reprinted from *Clin Obstet Gynecol* 3:761, 788, 1960.

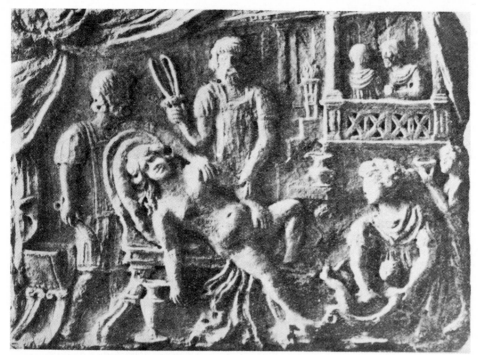

FIG. 1–3. Bas-relief (second or third century A.D.) depicting birth scene. Accoucheur (*center*) holds a pair of obstetric forceps aloft in his right hand.

for delivery of the living child is to be found in a marble bas-relief discovered in the early twentieth century in the vicinity of Rome (Fig. 1–3). Ignored or forgotten, however, the obstetric forceps was not reintroduced into clinical practice until the advent of the colorful Chamberlen family toward the close of the sixteenth century.

In 1569 William Chamberlen fled with his Huguenot family from Paris to Southampton to escape the persecution of Catherine de Medici. Two of his sons, curiously, were given the same name, Peter. These men, both of whom became barber–surgeons, were identified as Peter the Elder and Peter the Younger, and it is the former who invented, and probably constructed with his own hands, the instrument from which the modern obstetric forceps has evolved. Although consisting merely of two curved pieces of iron, shaped like spoons and united at a pivot joint, this invention remained a closely guarded secret, passed from one Chamberlen to another, for three generations and nearly 100 years.

The secret instrument was carried about in a massive wooden chest trimmed with gilt. Two men were required to lift it, and the Chamberlens are said to have used a special carriage for its transport. The eyes of the laboring patient were always blindfolded, lest the secret be discovered.

Peter the Elder achieved renown as a surgeon–midwife and attended both Queen Anne and Henrietta Maria, wife of Charles I. A third Peter Chamberlen, son of Peter the Younger, came to be known as Dr. Peter because of the medical degrees he acquired at Padua, Oxford, and Cambridge. Eccentric in all his activities, Dr. Peter was admitted to fellowship in the Royal College of Physicians on the condition that he "change his mode of dress" and accept "the decent and sober dress of its members." After establishing his reputation as an obstetric surgeon, Dr. Peter, in a manner reminiscent of the twentieth century's labor leaders, attempted to organize the midwives of London. This enterprising Chamberlen, plying the female practitioners of his art with wine and promises of a variety of benefactions, proposed their enrollment in a guild, to be taught and licensed by him. He, in turn, was to be paid a fee for each child they delivered and was to be summoned for consultation in all difficult cases. Only through the intercession of the Archbishop of Canterbury were the midwives able to emancipate themselves from the control of their self-styled benefactor.

The first effort to sell the family secret was made by Hugh Chamberlen, Senior, eldest son of Dr. Peter. While visiting Paris in 1670, he boasted of a device by which, he said, he could deliver any woman in 8 minutes and offered to sell it to the French government for a large sum. A consultation was arranged with Mauri-

ceau, "the oracle of the obstetrics of his century." Mauriceau, coincidentally, had just been called to see a rachitic dwarf whose pelvis was so contracted that after several days of labor vaginal delivery appeared impossible. Chamberlen locked himself in a room with the hapless patient, but after 3 hours of violent struggle, emerged exhausted and unsuccessful. The patient died the following day, undelivered, her uterus ruptured. The Chamberlen invention, needless to say, remained unsold.

Hugh, Senior, enjoyed high political favor. He served as Physician in Ordinary to Charles II and attended Princess Anne of Denmark in childbirth. In Amsterdam he later sold a secret, but probably not the forceps, to Roger van Roonhuyze, a Dutch obstetrician. Roonhuyze seeking to capitalize on his investment, achieved passage of a municipal law in 1747 requiring every practicing physician to purchase this secret under the pledge of silence. One recalcitrant, however, refused to pay this tribute to Roonhuyze and induced the latter's assistant to obtain a sketch of the instrument. The drawing, of a curved lever, was promptly sent to Paris, where a second lever was added by Jean Palfyn, this new instrument being known as the *mains de fer* (iron hands) for grasping the fetal head.

Not until 1813 was the actual instrument of the Chamberlen family revealed. In the house in which Dr. Peter died in 1683 and in which his descendants lived until 1715 when the residence was sold, a Mrs. Kemball, mother-in-law of a later owner of the property, happened upon a previously unknown trapdoor while rummaging one day in the attic. Between the floor and the ceiling she found a box containing a variety of oddments, including letters, fans, trinkets, a Bible dated 1695, and four pairs of obstetric forceps—undoubtedly the Chamberlen secret. These instruments are now in the possession of the Royal Society of Medicine in London.

The design of the obstetric forceps was first made public in 1733 in a book by Edmund Chapman. Since that date it has been modified and redesigned in new form and size probably more times than any other surgical instrument. Hundreds of models have been devised, each identified by the name of its inventor; even now, scarcely a year passes without the addition of at least one new instrument to the obstetrician's forceps arsenal.

PUERPERAL FEVER

Infection of the genital tract has ever been one of the leading causes of death from childbirth. Commonly known as childbed fever, this scourge was believed, from the time of Hippocrates, to result from suppression of the uterine discharge after delivery. Noting the failure of lactation among afflicted women, Hieronymus Mercurialis (1530–1606) concluded that the milk, instead of flowing to the breasts, localized in the uterus and produced the purulent discharge from this organ. "Milk fever" thus arose as an alternate name for the disorder. It assumed epidemic proportions with the establishment of lying-in hospitals, abetted by the frequent internal examinations by unwashed hands; contaminated instruments, dressings, and linens; crowding of patients; and lack of isolation facilities. The first recorded epidemic occurred in the Hôtel Dieu in Paris in 1646. Later statistics from the Allmänna Barnbördhuset in Stockholm reported 1 maternal death for every 5 women delivered. At the Allgemeines Krankenhaus in Vienna an epidemic beginning in 1821 and lasting 20 months took the lives of 829 out of 5139 parturients, a toll of almost 1 in 6. From May 1 to May 10, 1856, 31 deaths occurred among the 32 patients delivered at the Maternité in Paris. The search for an understanding of this disease and the efforts to cope with it have produced some of the warmest debates and most colorful prose in the annals of medicine.

Among the first correctly to call attention to the mode of transmission of childbed fever was Dr. Alexander Gordon of Aberdeen, who wrote in 1795:

This disease seized such women only, as were visited, or delivered, by a practitioner, or taken care of by a nurse, who had previously attended patients affected with the disease. . . . I arrived at that certainty in the matter, that I could venture to foretell what women would be affected with the disease, upon hearing by what midwife they were to be delivered, or by what nurse they were to be attended, during their lying-in: and almost in every instance, my prediction was verified. . . .

In short I had evident proofs of its infectious nature, and that the infection was as readily communicated as that of the small pox or measles, and operated more speedily than any other infection, with which I am acquainted.

. . . I had evident proofs that every person, who had been with a patient in the Puerperal Fever, became charged with an atmosphere of infection, which was communicated to every pregnant woman, who happened to come within its sphere. . . .

It is a disagreeable declaration for me to mention, that I myself was the means of carrying the infection to a great number of women.

Several years later, Gordon's opinions were echoed by James Blundell, in his lectures on midwifery at Guy's Hospital in London:

In my own family, I had rather that those I esteemed the most should be delivered, unaided, in a stable—by the manger side—than that they should receive the best help in the fairest apartment, but exposed to the vapours of this pitiless disease. Gossiping friends, wet nurses, monthly nurses, the practitioner himself, these are the channels by which, as I suspect, the infection is principally conveyed.

Others began to take up the cry. In 1842 Thomas Watson, professor of medicine in King's College, Londin, voiced

the dreadful suspicion, that the hand which is relied upon for succour in the painful and perilous hour of child-birth, and which is intended to secure the safety of both mother and child, but especially of the mother, may literally become the innocent cause of her destruction: innocent no longer, however, if, after warning and knowledge of the risk, suitable means are not used to avert a castastrophe so shocking.

Stimulated by the force of Watson's writing, Oliver Wendell Holmes, then 34 years old, undertook a critical analysis of the recorded experience with childbed fever as published from several European centers. His resulting essay, "The Contagiousness of Puerperal Fever," was read before the Boston Society for Medical Improvement, February 13, 1843, and subsequently published in *The New England Quarterly Journal of Medicine and Surgery*. Although it contained little that was new or original, Holmes's essay has come to be regarded as one of the classics of American medicine, for by its incisive logic and brilliance of statement it roused the profession from its complacent acceptance of epidemics of infection as acts of Providence.

"The recurrence of long series of cases like those I have cited," Holmes wrote,

reported by the most interested to disbelieve in contagion, scattered along through an interval of half a century, might have been thought sufficient to satisfy the minds of all inquirers that here was something more than a singular coincidence. But if on a more extended observation, it should be found that the same ominous groups of cases, clustering about individual practitioners, were observed in a remote country, at different times, and in widely separated regions, it would seem incredible that any should be found too prejudiced or indolent to accept the solemn truth knelled into their ears by the funeral bells from both sides of the ocean—the plain conclusion that the physician and the disease entered hand in hand, into the chamber of the unsuspecting patient.

With an eloquence rarely equaled in medical writing, Holmes emphasized the physician's role as a carrier of infection:

It is as a lesson rather than as a reproach that I call up the memory of these irreparable errors and wrongs. No tongue can tell the heartbreaking calamity they have caused; they have closed the eyes just opened upon a new world of love and happiness; they have bowed the strength of manhood into the dust; they have cast the helplessness of infancy into the stranger's arms, or bequeathed it with less cruelty the death of its dying parent. There is no tone deep enough for regret, and no voice loud enough for warning. The woman about to become a mother, or with her new-born infant upon her bosom, should be the object of trembling care and sympathy wherever she bears her tender burden, or stretches her aching limbs. The very outcast of the streets has pity upon her sister in degradation when the seal of promised maternity is impressed upon her. The remorseless vengeance of the law, brought down upon its victim by a machinery as sure as destiny, is arrested in its fall at a word which reveals her transient claim for mercy. The solemn prayer of the liturgy singles out her sorrows from the multiplied trials of life, to plead for her in the hour of peril. God forbid that any member of the profession to which she trusts her life, doubly precious at that eventful period, should hazard it negligently, unadvisedly, or selfishly!

Holmes's conclusions were published in a journal with a small circulation and one that proved short-lived. Had they not been subjected to bitter attack by Charles D. Meigs and Hugh Lenox Hodge, professors of obstetrics in the Jefferson Medical College and the University of Pennsylvania, respectively, and the leading figures in American obstetrics, probably little attention would have been drawn to the clinical speculations of this young anatomist. Meigs's bombastic denunciation of Holmes's theory, however, brought it into the full daylight of debate. Vigorously denying that the physician might be responsible for the transmission of disease, Hodge lectured:

The mere announcement of such an opinion must strike one with horror, and might induce you, at once to abandon a pursuit fraught with such danger and involving such terrible responsibilities; for what rewards can possibly compensate the obstetrician, who has reason to believe that he has actually poisoned one of those valued and lovely beings who rested confidently and implicitly on him for safety and deliverance?

Many teachers of obstetrics continued to deny that puerperal fever was contagious, and as late as 1854 Meigs advocated copious bloodletting for its cure. In 1855, therefore, after he had been professor of anatomy at the Harvard Medical School for 8 years and its dean for 6, Holmes republished his original essay, together with additional remarks in answer to his adversaries. This pamphlet, entitled *Puerperal Fever as a Private Pestilence,* silenced most of the remaining opposition to his views and led to their final acceptance.

More dissimilar personalities would be hard to picture than the urbane, cultured, and self-possessed Holmes and his European counterpart in the conquest of puerperal fever, the irascible and emotionally unstable Ignaz Philipp Semmelweis, who ultimately became insane. The dedicated role of the latter, emphasized by the tragedy of his personal life, has doubtless gained in drama in the retelling.

In 1846 Semmelweis, a Magyar, was appointed assistant, under Professor Johann Klein, in the first obstetric division of the Vienna Lying-In Hospital, where the medical students received their training. The hospital's second division, identical to the first in all other respects, accepted no medical students, the deliveries being performed by midwives. In the 6-year period 1841–1846, death from puerperal fever had been the lot of 1 woman of every 11 delivered on the first division; the corresponding mortality on the second division was 1 in 29. During 1846 the disparity grew even greater, until the death rate on the first division was ten times that on the second. But Semmelweis made

the interesting observation that the mortality was negligible among the women assigned to his division who delivered before reaching the hospital (and hence without any internal examinations during labor).

Semmelweis struggled with the problem but made no progress toward its solution until the tragic death of his friend and colleague, Professor Kolletschka, who succumbed from a knife scratch accidentally suffered during an autopsy. The pathologic changes in Kolletschka's body, Semmelweis observed, were identical to those in the women dead of peurperal fever. He quickly concluded that the scourge of his clinic was caused by putrid material derived from living organisms and that the poison was transmitted from the dead body to the living patient by the examining finger. The students, who commonly went from the autopsy room directly to the parturient patient, were the obvious connecting link. Almost identical views, it will be noted, had already been voiced by others, but Semmelweis, unschooled in foreign languages and unfamiliar with the English literature, had reached his conclusions independently.

Fired with the elation of discovery, the impulsive Semmelweis promptly posted a notice on the door of his clinic, dated May 15, 1847, ordering every doctor and student to wash his hands thoroughly in a basin of chlorine water before entering the maternity ward. In 6 months, despite the grumbling of the students and the apathy of Professor Klein, the maternal mortality of the first division had dropped to one-fourth its previous level and in 1848 attained a new low of 3%, surpassing the record of the midwives' division.

Like Holmes in America, Semmelweis soon came under the searing attack of reactionary authorities. Refused reappointment in the Vienna Lying-In Hospital, he returned, embittered, to his native Hungary. To Scanzoni, perhaps the outstanding figure in European obstetrics, who had stubbornly opposed the newfangled idea of contagion, the intemperate Semmelweis was goaded to write:

> Your doctrine, Professor, is based upon the corpses of parturient women murdered out of ignorance. If you think my theory wrong, I challenge you to communicate to me your reasons. . . . But should you continue, without having refuted my theory, to teach your pupils the theory of epidemic puerperal fever, I declare you a murderer before God and the world.

Disillusioned and frequently irrational, Semmelweis died August 13, 1865. Like his friend Kolletschka, he had developed septicemia from a cut on his finger.

In the very year of Semmelweis's death, two other principal actors in the drama of puerperal fever were making ready in the wings. Louis Pasteur had already begun his studies in fermentation, which led in 1879 to his demonstration of the villain in the piece, the hemolytic streptococcus. With the introduction of practical methods of asepsis by Joseph Lister, the specter of obstetric as well as surgical infection was laid to rest.

The twentieth century's antibiotics have brought a new air of tranquility to the obstetric scene. Puerperal infection still shows itself, but usually in subdued guise, rarely as a killer.

CESAREAN SECTION

Cesarean section, the most dramatic of all surgical operations, is also one of the oldest (Fig. 1–4). Earliest records trace its origins to the reign of Numa Pompilius (715–672 B.C.), a legendary king of Rome, who decreed that the child be excised from the womb of any woman who died late in pregnancy. Known initially as the *lex regia* (royal law), the requirement for postmortem section continued under the rule of the Caesars, when it acquired the name *lex caesarea*. As late as 1749, a Sicilian physician was condemned to death because of his failure to open the uterus of a recently deceased patient.

As an alternate explanation for the operation's name, some scholars have derived it from the Latin *caedere,* meaning to cut, an abdominal birth being termed *partus caesareus.* No valid basis can be found for the widely held belief that Julius Caesar, who was born about 100 B.C., was delivered by abdominal section and that the operation was named for him; indeed, this myth is controverted by all available evidence. The operation was performed then only on the dead or dying, and for many centuries thereafter was uniformly fatal when attempted on the living woman. Yet Caesar's mother survived his birth by many years, as proved by his letters written to her while he was engaged in his foreign wars. Others of similar or identical name antedated the great emperor; the name Caesar, therefore, could scarcely have been taken from his alleged mode of birth.

According to ancient belief, Buddha was delivered through the flank of his mother (about 563 B.C.), and Brahma is said to have emerged through the umbilicus. Abdominal delivery was also known to the ancient Jews. The Talmud prescribes laws of hygiene for survivors of the operation but provides no clear evidence that cesarean section was actually performed on a living woman.

The celebrated operation on Frau Nufer, in the year 1500, has been interpreted not as a true cesarean section but as a laparotomy for abdominal pregnancy. The patient's husband, a Swiss sowgelder, successfully delivered his wife of a living infant by cutting open her abdomen after 13 midwives and several barbers had failed in their vaginal attempts. Frau Nufer, we are told, lived to bear six more children, including twins.

The first documented, indubitably authentic cesarean operation on a living patient was performed on April 21, 1610, by two surgeons, Trautmann and Gusth. Their patient survived until the 25th postoperative day, longer than the vast majority of the hapless

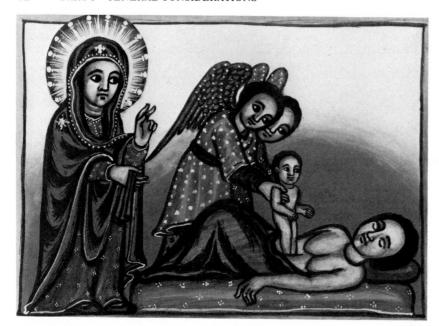

FIG. 1–4. Postmortem cesarean section, from old Ethiopian manuscript. Priest gives his blessing as archangels Michael and Gabriel extract infant from its dead mother's abdomen. Once infant was saved for baptism, purpose of operation was fulfilled. (British Museum, London)

women who were subjected to cesarean section during the next two centuries. Most died either promptly, of hemorrhage, or within a week, of infection; they rarely recovered. From 1750 until the end of the eighteenth century the operation was carried out 24 times in Paris without a single maternal survival, according to Baudelocque. Denman reported a similarly bleak experience in England.

The first half of the nineteenth century saw a little improvement in the operation's record; in 1867 Nuyer reported a mortality of 54% among 1605 cases collected from the literature. In Paris, however, not one mother survived a cesarean section during the 90-year period from 1787 to 1876, and in Great Britain the maternal mortality was recorded at 85%. The American experience was scarcely more encouraging. By 1878 the operation had been carried out only 80 times in the United States, with a maternal mortality of 52.5%. At the Sloane Maternity Hospital (later renamed the Sloane Hospital for Women) not a single cesarean section was performed among the first 1000 confinements. Indeed, the operation was attempted but once from the hospital's founding in 1888 until 1897, and that case ended in disaster. In the entire city of Philadelphia, with a population of 800,000 in 1878, there had likewise been but one cesarean section in the preceding 40 years.

Harris, who reviewed the American cases in 1878, noted that the chances for success seemed greater when the operation was performed remote from the centers of civilization: 5 recoveries occurred among 9 rural patients who had operated upon themselves in desperation or had been gored by a bull, while in New York City during the same period only 1 of 11 survived who were operated upon by physicians. As an example of the former group, Harris cited the case of a woman, who in 1769, "actuated by a frenzied impatience, and violent of temper, to obtain relief in the quickest way, without regard to consequences," performed the operation with the hilt of a broken butcher knife, "cutting at one stroke through the abdominal and uterine walls, and making a two and a half inch incision into the thigh of the foetus." The mother's intestines were replaced and the wound was sutured by a plantation midwife, who failed, however, to remove the placenta. This was done by a surgeon, who reopened the wound and cleaned the blood and dirt from the peritoneal cavity, the original operation having been performed on the ground. The mother recovered and is said to have made preparations for a similar operation upon herself a year or two later, but was forced to submit to a natural delivery.

The first successful cesarean section in the United States, according to one version, was performed in 1794, in a cabin near Staunton, Virginia, by Dr. Jesse Bennett on his own wife. After Mrs. Bennett, a young primigravida, had labored for 3 days without result, consultation was obtained with Dr. Alexander Humphreys, a physician of greater experience, who confirmed Dr. Bennett's suspicion of contracted pelvis and the impossibility of a natural delivery, and proposed a destructive operation on the baby as the only means of saving the mother's life. Having already despaired of her own chances, Mrs. Bennett begged that

a cesarean section be done for the sake of the child. This, however, Dr. Humphreys steadfastly refused, stating that he would not be the cause of his patient's death. Under the importunings of his suffering wife, Dr. Bennett thereupon announced to his older colleague that he himself would perform the operation and, if fate ordained, would assume the full responsibility for her death.

An operating table was improvised with two wooden planks, supported on barrels. Without anesthesia, and while two Negro women held his wife, Dr. Bennett rapidly incised her abdomen and uterus and extracted the living infant. To protect her against a recurrence of this ordeal, should she survive, he then quickly removed his wife's ovaries before closing her abdomen with linen thread. Both mother and child did indeed survive; but despite its successful outcome, Dr. Bennett never reported the case. When questioned years later concerning his reticence, Bennett replied: "No strange doctors would believe that the operation could be done in the Virginia backwoods and the mother live, and I'll be damn'd if I'd give them a chance to call me a liar."

The authenticity of the Bennett case has been questioned by some historians. Better documented as the first cesarean section in America is the operation by John Lambert Richmond of Newtown, Ohio in April, 1827.

To the mid-nineteenth century, and even beyond, surgeons labored under the mistaken notion that the uterine wound at cesarean section required no treatment except cleansing. Sutures were held to be dangerous, leading to peritonitis. From 1769, when the Frenchman Lebas closed a uterine incision with three silk threads, the few attempts at uterine suture during the next century failed to dispel this fear of infection. The nonabsorbable sutures of silk or linen, left long and protruding from the wound to facilitate later removal, almost invariably led to the predicted, feared result. Following prolonged labor, on the other hand, with the uterine musculature lacking adequate retractile power, massive blood loss usually occurred from the edges of the incision if left unsutured. A satisfactory technique of closing the uterine wound therefore constituted one of the major improvements in the cesarean operation.

Silver wire was first used successfully for this purpose in 1852 by Frank E. Polin, a surgeon of Springfield, Kentucky. Although Polin did not bother to report his case, the experiences of less reticent surgeons of pioneer America soon found their way into the literature. Between 1867 and 1880 uterine sutures had been used in at least 16 cesarean sections in the United States. Only in 1882, however, with publication of Max Sänger's widely heralded monograph, was full recognition given to accurate coaptation of the wound edges as an essential part of the cesarean operation. Sänger's technique of longitudinal incision and suture

of the uterine fundus has since been known as the classic cesarean section.

While the fundal incision has been largely superseded by approaches through the lower uterine segment, the cardinal features of Sänger's technique endure—hemostasis by suture and accurate approximation of the muscle edges. The cesarean operation of the mid-twentieth century, aided by the other advances of modern practice, has been shorn of its terror; many obstetric services can now boast of series of 1000 consecutive cases without a single maternal fatality.

The cesarean technique popularized by Sänger sharply reduced the hazard of hemorrhage, but the problem of infection remained. Even before the publication of Sänger's report, Edoardo Porro demonstrated a method of circumventing both dangers of abdominal delivery by the addition of a similarly formidable procedure, hysterectomy. Before 1863 abdominal hysterectomy had proved fatal in seven-eighths of the patients on whom it was attempted; only in three cases had it been performed successfully in the United States. The *London Medico-Chirurgical Review* of 1825 referred to it as "one of the most cruel and unfeasible operations that ever was projected or executed by the head or hand of man."

In Pavia, Italy, the nineteenth century record of cesarean section had been no better than elsewhere. Indeed, no woman had ever survived the operation in that city until the time of Porro. On April 27, 1876, a 25-year-old primigravid dwarf, Julia Cavallini, was referred to Porro's clinic in the university because of the suspicion of a malformed pelvis. She had all the bony stigmas of rickets, and the diagonal conjugate of her pelvis was markedly contracted, measuring only 7 cm. It was obvious to Porro that absolute disproportion existed, and he made elaborate preparations, long in advance, to carry out cesarean section at the time of labor and to amputate the uterus if hemorrhage proved threatening.

Fortunately unknown to Porro, cesarean hysterectomy had been attempted once previously, by Horatio Robinson Storer in 1869, with fatal outcome to both mother and child. Porro's patient went into labor on the morning of May 21, 1876. He had had 4 weeks for rehearsal of his plans. By midafternoon all was ready and cesarean section was carried out, with the delivery of a living female infant weighing 3300 g. Unable to control the bleeding from the cut edges of the uterus, Porro promptly proceeded according to plan. A wire snare was placed around the uterus and drawn tight at the level of the internal os; then the organ was rapidly excised, together with the left ovary. The patient made a complete recovery. During the ensuing years cesarean hysterectomy, which became known as the Porro operation, was adopted in many centers as the preferred method of abdominal delivery. Modern obstetricians continue to employ it, but with sharply modified indications.

ANESTHESIA FOR CHILDBIRTH

In 1591, so it is said, a gentlewoman of Edinburgh, Eufame Macalyane by name, was burned alive on Castle Hill by order of James VI. The lady's crime: she had secretly applied to the midwife for a potion to assuage the pangs of labor. Was this not a clear and flagrant violation of the scriptural injunction: "In sorrow thou shalt bring forth children" (Gen. 3:16)? Not until 1853, when Queen Victoria inhaled the vapors of chloroform during the birth of Prince Leopold, was opposition to pain relief for the parturient effectively silenced. The word "delivery," in the meantime, was used in a more restricted sense than in today's parlance. In the preanesthetic era, it was the mother who was delivered from her travail, at the moment of birth.

The introduction of anesthesia into obstetrics resulted from the efforts of one man, the gifted seventh son of the village baker of Bathgate, Scotland, James Young Simpson (1811–1870). Word had been received from America that sulfuric ether had been employed succeessfully during the excision of a neck tumor at the Massachusetts General Hospital on October 16, 1846. Quick to grasp the significance of this event which, in the minds of many, marks the greatest contribution to mankind in the entire history of medicine, and eager to adapt anesthesia to obstetric use, Simpson successfully employed ether on January 19, 1847, for version and extraction in a patient with a contracted pelvis.

The ensuing controversy over the use of pain-relieving drugs for childbirth has rarely been matched in fervor in the annals of obstetrics. Simpson's principal antagonists were the clergy, but they were ably abetted, on both sides of the Atlantic, by some of the most articulate and influential members of the medical profession. With a biblical knowledge equal to that of the prelates who attacked him, Simpson replied that the Book of Genesis also provided divine sanction for anesthesia. He called their attention to the 21st and 22nd verses of the second chapter, describing the creation of Eve from one of Adam's ribs. Did not the Lord prepare Adam for this ordeal by causing him to fall into a deep slumber?

Charles D. Meigs of Philadelphia, who had also opposed Holmes in the controversy over puerperal fever, referred to the pain of parturition as "physiological pain," insisted upon the serious dangers of anesthetics in labor, compared the unconsciousness resulting from them to the stupor of drunkenness, and asked whether any self-respecting woman could afford to submit to such an influence. Ashwell of London added that to use anesthesia in obstetrics constitutes "unnecessary interference with the providentially arranged process of healthy labour . . . sooner or later, to be followed by injurious and fatal consequences."

Simpson recalled the words of Galen, "pain is useless to the pained," and went on to provide scientific evidence of its mortal potential. Collecting by questionnaire the results of thigh amputations, he showed that ether anesthesia had nearly halved the mortality from this operation. "Bodily pain," he wrote,

with all its concomitant fears and sickening horrors . . . is, with very few, if indeed any exceptions, morally and physically a mighty and unqualified evil. And, surely, any means by which its abolition could possibly be accomplished, with perfect security and safety, deserves to be joyfully and gratefully welcomed by medical science, as one of the most inestimable boons which man could confer upon his suffering fellow-mortals.

In a forceful, impassioned plea to his colleagues, Simpson urged the extension of anesthesia to obstetrics:

Now, if experience betimes goes fully to prove to us the safety with which ether may, under proper precautions and management, be employed in the course of parturition, then . . . instead of determining . . . whether we shall be "justified" in using this agent . . . it will become, on the other hand, necessary to determine whether on any grounds, moral or medical, a professional man could deem himself "justified" in withholding, and *not* using any such safe means (as we at present presuppose this to be), provided he had the power by it of assuaging the agonies of the last stage of natural labour, and thus counteracting what Velpeau describes as "those piercing cries, that agitation so lively, those excessive efforts, those inexpressible agonies, and those pains apparently intolerable," which accompany the termination of natural parturition in the human mother.

As experience had begun to indicate to Simpson some of ether's shortcomings as an obstetric anesthetic, he set out in the autumn of 1847 in quest of a better agent. In collaboration with Drs. Thomas Keith and J. Matthews Duncan, Simpson conducted his experiments at the end of the regular day's work, seated at his dining room table. Countless agents, obtained from the local chemist, were tried. A small quantity of the test liquid was placed in a cup or tumbler, which was then immersed in hot water to increase the volatility. The intrepid trio then proceeded with their hazardous task of inhaling the vapors and recording the effects. In this manner they discovered, for the first time, the anesthetic properties of chloroform.

Exhilarated by the acquisition of this new agent, which appeared superior to ether, Simpson immediately substituted it for the latter in his obstetric practice. On December 1, 1847, with evangelic fervor, he sang the praises of the newly discovered chloroform to his Edinburgh colleagues:

I do not remember a single patient to have taken it who has not afterwards declared her sincere gratitude for its employment, and her indubitable determination to have recourse again to similar means under similar circumstances. All who happen to have formerly entertained any dread respecting the inhalation, or its effects, have afterwards looked back, both amazed at, and amused with, their previous absurd fears and groundless terrors. Most, indeed, have subse-

quently set out, like zealous missionaries, to persuade other friends to avail themselves of the same measures of relief, in their hour of trial and travail. . . . All of us, I most sincerely believe, are called upon to employ it by every principle of true humanity, as well as by every principle of true religion. Medical men may oppose for a time the superinduction of anaesthesia in parturition, but they will oppose it in vain; for certainly our patients themselves will force the use of it upon the profession. The whole question is, even now, one merely of time. It is not—Shall the practice come to be generally adopted? but, When shall it come to be generally adopted?

After slowly gaining acceptance during the next few years, anesthesia became an integral part of obstetric practice. For three-quarters of a century chloroform was employed almost exclusively. It has been supplanted gradually by other agents.

WOMAN'S FERTILITY AND ITS CONTROL

One of the foremost concerns of men and women has ever been their control of reproduction. Both fertility and sterility have been eagerly sought, each at its appointed time and in chosen circumstances. As stated by Norman Himes in his *Medical History of Contraception,* "while women have always wanted babies, they have wanted them when they wanted them. And they have wanted neither too few nor too many."

FERTILITY DEITIES

Until about 6000 or 7000 years ago, man the hunter was probably hungry much of the time, living in daily competition with his fellow men for their dearly won food. With the adoption of an agrarian economy, competition gave way to cooperation. Now help was needed in cultivating the fields and tending the flocks. Fertility of family as well as soil became important. Specific deities were invoked to augment the family. Gifts were offered, amulets worn, and rituals performed. Ceremonies and deities were passed on from generation to generation as tribes migrated, nation conquered nation, and assimilation occurred. The gods and mythology of the early Greeks, for example, were acquired largely from the Egyptians, whose religious heritage had come, in turn, from the Sumerians and Chaldeans.

In the art of the ancients, deities were usually depicted in human form, similar to that of the worshiper; the fertility goddesses were most often shown in frontal view, with exaggerated breasts and pudenda.

With merging and changing of cultures the deities usually acquired new names. To the Semitic peoples of Mesopotamia, for example, the goddess of love, beauty, and fertility was known as Ishtar. To the Phoenicians she was Astarte. Others called her by still other names: Venus by the Romans and Aphrodite by the Greeks. The Egyptian goddess of fertility and love and protectress of women in the vicissitudes of life was Isis, daughter of Qêb and Nut, sister of Osiris, and mother of Horus. Isis was usually shown wearing a crown of two horns embracing a solar disc and often holding a papyrus scepter. After the 25th dynasty (663 B.C.), figures of Isis commonly portrayed her as a nursing mother, with Horus. When Christianity was introduced into Egypt, similarities were soon seen between the new religion and the moral system of the old cult, and many identified the Virgin Mary and her Child with Isis and Horus.

Not until relatively late in Egyptian history were animals worshipped, but they were always accorded a special status close to that of the gods because of their intimate knowledge of nature's laws. Toueris, Egyptian symbol of fecundity and protectress of the pregnant and parturient, was usually shown in the guise of a pregnant hippopotamus standing on her hind legs and holding the hieroglyph meaning protection in one paw, the sign for life in the other. Small figures of Toueris were popular as amulets.

FERTILITY FIGURES, AMULETS, VOTIVES, DOLLS

As man conceived of his deities in human form, so did he likewise endow them with human emotions. Gods and goddesses, like men and women, would surely be flattered by figures in their image and influenced by gifts in their honor. Amulets to curry favor with the gods date back to prehistory; members of some primitive cultures still resort to them to enhance fertility. The Venus of Willendorf, a fertility goddess of the Old Stone Age (40,000–16,000 B.C.), unearthed in Austria in 1908, is believed to be one of the earliest known representations of the human form. Figures of the female torso and breasts, fertility symbols from the seventh millennium B.C., were uncovered in the early 1960s by James Mellaart at Catal Hüyük, a Neolithic city in Anatolia. Three prehistoric statuettes, probably used as amulets, depicting a fertility goddess in advanced pregnancy, were discovered in the caves of Grimaldi, Ventimiglia, in northwest Italy, the home of a negroid race of the late Paleolithic period (before 2500 B.C.). Perhaps most famous of all fertility figures is the marble statue of Artemis (Diana) of Ephesus, showing the goddess with her many breasts symbolizing her reproductive prowess (Fig. 1–5).

Votive tablets and free will offerings, usually in the form of the genital organs, together with torches and wreaths, were carried by the women of ancient Rome and Greece to their temples, beseeching fertility and easy delivery. Outlines of the uterus, as a fertility symbol, were included among the altar decorations of the temple of Babylon in addition to the forms of the deities. The Egyptians later placed the face of Hathor, their mother goddess, within this uterine form, which thus came to be known as Hathor's hairdress.

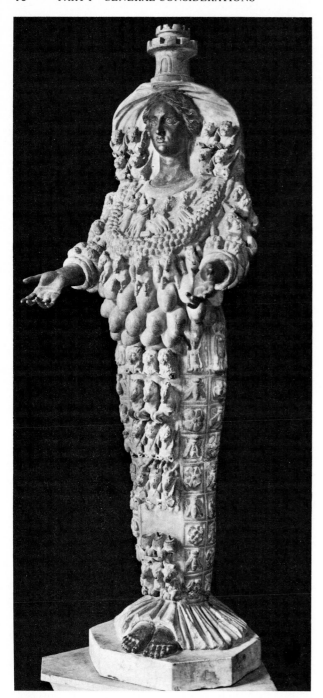

FIG. 1-5. Artemis (Diana) of Ephesus, Greek goddess of fertility. Marble statue with bronze head and hands. (Musei Capitolini, Rome)

Fetishes, usually woodcarvings in human form, considered to be the seat of magic power or the abode of a spirit, are still worshipped in some primitive communities, particularly in Africa. The fetish was almost always endowed with an orifice into which the owner would place his or her own prayerful offerings. Amulets, worn as jewelry, were likewise endowed with magic properties, for example, the power to ward off evil such as infertility. Masks of clay, wood, and animal horns have been worn among the tribes of Africa, New Guinea, and South and Central America for the past 4000 years to dispel the spirits of sickness and death and bring the blessings of fertility. In ancient Mexico fertility figures were sometimes placed in graves as an offering to the dead, to assure fertility to the living.

Among some African tribes, in which a woman's ability to bear children takes precedence over all other wifely functions, a doll was given to her when she was about to marry. Believed endowed with magic powers, the doll was sometimes worn as a necklace or bound to the woman's body to help her become pregnant. Fertility dolls of clay and beads still play an important role in the culture of certain tribes of South Africa. Copies of old beaded fertility dolls are now mass-produced there for sale to tourists.

INFERTILITY

Until the physiologic factors in reproduction began to be recognized, prayer remained the principal resort for relief from infertility. Barrenness was regarded as the supreme curse, as exemplified by Jeremiah's quotation of the Lord, "Write ye this man childless" (Jer. 22:30) and Rachel's entreaty to Jacob, "Give me children, or else I die" (Gen. 30:1). It was God who closed the wombs of Sarah (Gen. 16:2), Hannah (1 Sam. 1:6), Michal (2 Sam. 6:23), and the women in Abimelech's household (Gen. 20:18), while opening up the wombs of Leah (Gen. 24:31) and Rachel (Gen. 30:22). The early Greeks and Romans, in addition to appealing to their gods and goddesses for help in fulfilling their reproductive functions, resorted to theurgic devices including magic formulas, songs and incantations, and the laying-on of hands.

So long as the male partner could perform the conjugal act, infertility in a union was ascribed to the female. Male potency implied virility. Only when coitus could not be consummated because of impotence or anatomic aberration was the husband's role in the reproductive process impugned. The obvious resort was artificial insemination. This was first attempted in 1680, without success, by the Dutch anatomist Jan Swammerdam, with the eggs and sperm of fish. Ludwig Jacobi succeeded in 1742, but not until 1780 was artificial insemination successful in mammals. In that year the Italian anatomist Lazaro Spallanzani impregnated a bitch with the semen of a dog. At about the

same time the illustrious John Hunter impregnated the wife of a man with hypospadias by vaginal injection of her husband's semen.

Attention was later focused on the importance of patency of the woman's reproductive tract. The diagnosis of patency or obstruction of the oviducts, however, depended on the clinical acumen of the examiner and was subject to frequent error. In 1919 the New York gynecologist I. C. Rubin introduced a nonsurgical insufflation test for tubal patency, using oxygen initially but switching later to the more rapidly absorbed and safer carbon dioxide.

CONTRACEPTION

Twentieth century man's unbridled fertility has produced perhaps his most urgent problem. Of the earth's 3 billion inhabitants, more than one-third are sorely malnourished for lack of food. At the current rate of increase the world's population will double in less than 35 years. Demographers, statesmen, theologians, physiologists, chemists, and physicians have joined hands at long last in a hopeful effort to stem this tide, which threatens to engulf mankind.

The Greeks were apparently the first to give serious thought to population control. Most of the early Greek philosophers considered a stable population essential, Plato placing the ideal population of the state at exactly 5040 inhbitants. Reproduction, he suggested, should be legally regulated, with overpopulation being checked by abortion and infanticide; underpopulation, by stimulating fertility and immigration.

In 1798 Thomas Robert Malthus, an English clergyman turned economist, in his *Essay on the Principle of Population,* called attention to the disparity between the geometric rate of population increase and the slower increase of the food supply. War and disease, he pointed out, as had Machiavelli three centuries earlier, were the only alternatives to voluntary limitation of family size in controlling excessive population. Extending the teaching of Malthus, Francis Place, an English sociologist, began to advocate contraception, beginning in the 1820s, as a restraint against population increase. Wrote Place:

Many young men who fear the consequences which a large family produces, turn to debauchery, and destroy their own happiness as well as the happiness of the unfortunate girls with whom they connect themselves.

Other young men, whose moral and religious feelings deter them from this vicious course, marry early and produce large families, which they are utterly unable to maintain. . . . But when it has become the custom . . . to limit the number of children, so that none need have more than they wish to have, no man will fear to take a wife, all will be married while young—debauchery will diminish—while good morals, and religious duties will be promoted. . . .

If, above all, it were once clearly understood, that it was not disreputable for married persons to avail themselves of precautionary means as would without being injurious to health, or destructive to female delicacy, prevent conception, a sufficient check might at once be given to the increase of population beyond the means of subsistence.

Thus was the birth control movement launched, as a social issue.

The earliest known contraceptive formulas are found in the Petrie medical papyrus, an ancient Egyptian manuscript of three large pages from about 1950 B.C. Recommended among other prescriptions were contraceptive pessaries of crocodile dung and honey, and vaginal fumigations with minnis, an ancient drug. Some 2000 years later Soranus of Ephesus advocated, as a barrier to conception, mixtures of honey or cedar wood oil with figs or pomegranate pulp. Lucretius, the Roman poet, suggested violent body movements to shake the semen free after intercourse; while Pliny the Elder recommended wearing as an amulet the worms from the body of a hairy spider, as the most effective means for preventing conception. Blossoms of the palash flower, mentioned as an effective oral contraceptive in the *Kama-Sutra,* a fourth century Hindu love manual, were tested on rats by the Indian Council for Medical Research in the 1960s and found to prevent conception in 80% of the animals.

In the years of the Crusades, when women were viewed as private property, men designed belts and girdles for their wives, mistresses, and unmarried daughters to be worn during their masters' absence, to frustrate the advances of other men. Known as chastity belts, they were made of metal, covered in part with leather, and worn in such a manner as to guard the entrance to the vagina and rectum. The chastity belt consisted of a waistband from which was suspended a metal plate, more often two, fore and aft, connected between the wearer's legs by a joint. In each plate was a serrated opening that provided a portal of egress for the bladder, rectum, and uterus, but prevented the approach of a man. Secured with a lock, the plates could be removed only at the pleasure of the key holder. As recently as 1933 the League of Awakened Magyars advocated that every unmarried girl of age 12 or older be required to wear a chastity belt, the key remaining in the custody of her father or other competent authority.

A linen sheath for coitus, forerunner of the condom, was first described in 1564 by Gabriele Fallopio in his *De morbo gallico.* Penile sheaths were used initially for protection against venereal disease. Not until the eighteenth century did the membranous condom, usually fashioned from an animal's cecum, become popular for contraception. With the vulcanization of rubber in 1884, contraception achieved an explosive popularity because of the sudden cheapness of the new product. At mid-twentieth century the condom was the most widely used of all artificial contraceptives.

By 1880 a variety of chemical agents and mechanical devices, both intravaginal and intrauterine, were in

use. Not enough, however, were the invention and improvement of these contraceptives, for traditional morality posed a formidable barrier to their distribution. Prominent among the opponents of contraception in the United States was Anthony Comstock, anti-sin crusader for whom the federal postal law of 1873 was named; this law prohibited the dissemination of birth control information and contraceptive materials through the mails. Later, as a special agent of the U.S. Post Office, he ordered the destruction of 160 tons of contraceptive literature, which he branded as "lewd, lascivious, and obscene." Not until 1965 did the Supreme Court make possible birth control clinics everywhere in the United States, when it declared unconstitutional Connecticut's law banning the dissemination of contraceptive advice.

Although rigidly opposed by the Catholic Church, the birth control movement received a tremendous boost in 1958 from the Lambeth Conference of Bishops of the Anglican Communion, which resolved:

The responsibility for deciding upon the number and frequency of children has been laid by God upon the consciences of parents everywhere . . . the means of family planning are in large measure matters of clinical and aesthetic choice . . . scientific studies can rightly help, and do, in assessing the effects and usefulness of any particular means; and Christians have every right to use the gifts of science for proper ends.

By the end of 1972 contraceptive advice was being offered by the International Planned Parenthood Federation in more than 100 countries on every continent. In the United States during 1976 an estimated 4.1 million women received contraceptive services from Planned Parenthood affiliates and other organized family planning agencies, more than four times the number served in 1968. At the same time, however, nearly one-half of the medically indigent women in the United States still lacked counsel in the principles and techniques of family planning.

GYNECOLOGY AS A SURGICAL SPECIALTY

Gynecology now seems securely wedded to the practice of obstetrics, but only after a prolonged succession of betrothals to other suitors. For many centuries the diseases of women lay within the province of general medical practice, the meager knowledge and techniques not justifying specialization. During the eighteenth and early nineteenth centuries gynecology, then a nonsurgical discipline, was commonly combined with pediatrics. Many of the textbooks of this era were devoted to "the diseases of women and children," and a large number of professorships were similarly designated. With the introduction of anesthesia and asepsis in the mid-nineteenth century, gynecology abruptly changed in character. The surgeon laid claim to its practice, and in many teaching centers gynecol-ogy became a subdepartment of general surgery. Even though practiced in increasing measure by the obstetrician–gynecologist rather than the general surgeon, the specialty retains today its essentially, but not exclusively, surgical character.

Before the development of a truly rational system of gynecology, fad followed fad in the treatment of woman's ills. Toward the middle of the nineteenth century the Galenic doctrine was revived, attributing to uterine displacements and "uterine sympathies" virtually every sort of female complaint. As a result, the pessary schol of gynecology began to flourish. Fortunes, it is said, were to be made by two groups of gynecologists of that day: those who inserted pessaries and those who removed them. This treatment, if not effective, was at least innocuous. Treatment, fortunately, was largely limited to such nonsurgical measures. From 1848 to 1851, for example, not a single gynecologic operation was performed at the New York Hospital. Shortly thereafter, however, when the surgeon learned how to open the peritoneal cavity with safety, a rash of suspension operations for uterine retroversion broke out, in which the round ligaments were, in the words of Fluhmann, "folded, ligated, plicated, shirred, plaited, planted, transplanted, replanted, drawn over, above, and through the broad ligaments and fastened to the back of the uterus." So popular had uterine suspension become by 1911 that when Mr. Alexander of Liverpool was asked to demonstrate the operation of his invention to a group of visiting surgeons, he was unable to comply. Four assistants, Alexander stated, were sent in quest of a patient, one into the north, one into the east, one into the west, and one into the south of Liverpool; but after diligent search, each returned with the report that in all of that great city he had been unable to find one woman who had not already had the Alexander operation.

Cervical cancer, one of the most important of gynecologic diseases, was attributed by Scanzoni, a leading figure of the mid-nineteenth century, to immoderate coitus and excessive sexual stimulation. For cervical inflammation, leeches were often recommended. Mitchell gave the following instructions for their use:

For the application of leeches, so often necessary in cases of inflammatory congestion of the cervix uteri, the patient should be placed in the same position as for labor, and a conical glass or metal speculum passed up to the uterus; care being taken that no part of the vagina is left around the rim of the instrument, as the bites of the leeches are not painful when the uterus only is wounded, but excessively so if the vagina is. Any adherent mucus is to be carefully wiped off, and the leeches put into the tube in the number required, eight or ten being the usual number. The mouth of the speculum is to be filled with lint, which requires to be pushed towards the extremity applied closely to the uterus, carrying the leeches along with it. In ten minutes the lint may be withdrawn, the speculum being alowed to remain in the vagina until the leeches fill, which will generally occupy from twenty minutes to half an hour. Occasionally, however, it is

necessary to detach an odd one, which may readily be done by dipping a camel-hair pencil in a solution of common salt, and applying it to the head of the leech. . . . I think it is a good plan to apply the speculum so that the mouth of the uterus shall be external to its margin, as in one case I knew of troublesome symptoms arising from a leech crawling into the cervix uteri, and there adhering.

Like all branches of surgery, gynecology burst into flower when anesthesia and asepsis removed the stifling covers of pain and infection. Yet the mores of the times posed a major impediment to the full fruition of this new specialty. Vaginal examination was resorted to only on urgent indication, and even then, under protective drapes that effectively concealed the patient's genitalia from the examiner's eyes (Fig. 1–6). The vaginal speculum was regarded by some as an "instrument of unbridled indecency." Charles D. Meigs, with his characteristic knack for aligning himself on the wrong side of major issues, gave articulate expression to the prevailing puritanical attitudes in his "letters" to his students:

I confess I am proud to say, that, in this country generally, certainly in many parts of it, there are women who prefer to suffer the extremity of danger and pain rather than waive those scruples of delicacy which prevent their maladies from being fully explored. I say it is an evidence of the dominion of a fine morality in our society.

Even after we have been consulted, and where certain concessions are made, there often remains some degree of uncertainty, because we cannot, as we can in persons of our own sex, freely employ every means of research in exploring, and in repeating the explorations of their maladies.

This difficulty is probably greater in this country than it is in Europe. I am rejoiced at it; because, however inconvenient, and however baffling in the particular instances of suffering, it is an evidence of a high and worthy grade of moral feeling. And I hope the day is far distant when the spectacle shall be seen in our hospitals, of troops of women, waiting in succession, for a public examination of their genitals, in presence of large classes of medical practitioners and students of medicine. I regard this public sentiment, as to the sanctity of the female modesty and chastity, as one of the strong safeguards of our spontaneous public polity;—for woman, and man's respect and love for her, are truly at the basis, and are the very corner-stone of civilization and order.

He is but the pander of vice who parades his thousands of uterine cases before the public gaze; and is himself an unchaste man, who ruthlessly insists upon a vaginal taxis in all cases of women's diseases that, however remotely, may seem to have any, the least connexion with the disorders of their reproductive tissues.

Meigs was not alone. In 1850 Dr. James P. White of Buffalo, bitterly attacked for conducting a delivery before a group of students, had to resort to legal action against one of his antagonists. The American Medical Association's Committee on Medical Information, commenting on the matter, stated that the only advantage that might accrue from exposing a patient during delivery was "a somewhat greater facility in protecting the perineum," but held this to be insufficient com-

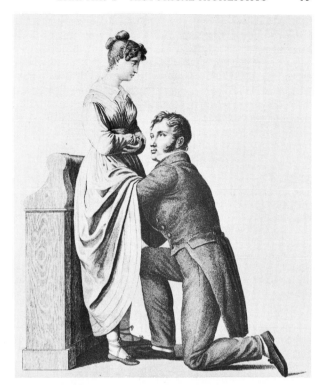

FIG. 1-6. Pelvic examination, early nineteenth century. Modesty precluded inspection. (Maygrier JP: Nouvelles démonstrations d'accouchemens. Paris, Béchet, 1822)

pensation for "the obvious disadvantage." The committee stated further that a physician not prepared to conduct labor by the sense of touch alone was not competent to practice obstetrics.

Similar restrictions, based on a misguided concern for the patient's modesty, prevailed in Europe. Only in the examination of certain socially inferior groups, such as the prostitutes of Paris and the syphilitic women of Berlin, did a laxer attitude prevail toward inspection of the patients' genitals. It was in these groups, therefore, that the bluish coloration of the vagina as a diagnostic sign of pregnancy (subsequently designated Chadwick's sign) was first observed.

The modern era of gynecologic surgery began a few days before Christmas 1809, when Jane Crawford set out on her fateful ride to Danville, Kentucky—a ride that has since been compared with that of Paul Revere, Sheridan's from Winchester, and the charge of the Light Brigade for its historic significance and the courage it took. Dr. Ephraim McDowell's successful operation on Mrs. Crawford, Christmas morning, without anesthesia, marked the beginning of abdominal surgery.

Ovarian cysts had been regarded as incurable. In the few cases where excision had been attempted the result had been uniformly fatal. The only treatment

that could be offered the hapless sufferer was temporary palliation by tapping, to withdraw the rapidly reaccumulating fluid.* In some cases this practice assumed staggering proportions, as in the patient reported by Heidrich, whose ovarian cyst (or peritoneal cavity) was tapped 299 times to remove 9867 lb of fluid. Physicians had been forced to an attitude of fatalism toward this disease.

McDowell's feat is best related by his own account; reported with two additional cases 8 years later:

In December 1809, I was called to see a Mrs. Crawford, who had for several months thought herself pregnant. She was affected with pains similar to labour pains, from which she could find no relief. So strong was the presumption of her being in the last stage of pregnancy, that two physicians, who were consulted on her case, requested my aid in delivering her. The abdomen was considerably enlarged, and had the appearance of pregnancy, though the inclination of the tumor was to one side, admitting of an easy removal to the other. Upon examination, per vaginam, I found nothing in the uterus; which induced the conclusion that it must be an enlarged ovarium. Having never seen so large a substance extracted, nor heard of an attempt, or success attending any operation, such as this required, I gave to the unhappy woman information of her dangerous situation. She appeared willing to undergo an experiment, which I promised to perform if she would come to Danville (the town where I live), a distance of sixty miles from her place of residence. This appeared almost impracticable by any, even the most favourable conveyance, though she performed the journey in a few days on horseback. With the assistance of my nephew and colleague, James McDowell, M.D., I commenced the operation, which was concluded as follows: Having placed her on a table of ordinary height, on her back, and removed all her dressing which might in any way impede the operation, I made an incision about three inches from the musculus rectus abdominis, on the left side, continuing the same nine inches in length, parallel with the fibres of the above named muscle, extending into the cavity of the abdomen, the parietes of which were a good deal contused, which we ascribed to the resting of the tumor on the horn of the saddle during her journey. The tumor then appeared full in view, but was so large that we could not take it away entire. We put a strong ligature around the fallopian tube near to the uterus; we then cut open the tumor, which was the ovarium and fimbrious part of the fallopian tube very much enlarged. We took out fifteen pounds of a dirty, gelatinous looking substance. After which we cut through the fallopian tube and extracted the sack, which weighed seven pounds and one half. As soon as the external opening was made, the intestines rushed out upon the table; and so completely was the abdomen filled by the tumor, that they could not be replaced during the operation, which was terminated in about twenty-five minutes. We then turned her upon her left side, so as to permit the blood to escape; after which we closed the external opening with the interrupted suture, leaving out, at the lower end of the

incision, the ligature which surrounded the fallopian tube. Between every two stitches we put a strip of adhesive plaster, which, by keeping the parts in contact, hastened the healing of the incision. We then applied the usual dressings, put her to bed, and prescribed a strict observance of the antiphlogistic regimen. In five days I visited her, and much to my astonishment found her engaged in making up her bed. I gave her particular caution for the future; and in twenty-five days, she returned home as she came, in good health, which she continues to enjoy.

On the heels of McDowell's triumph similar procedures were soon undertaken by others, especially in England, with encouraging results; and by the middle of the century ovarian excision, the archetype of abdominal surgery, was an established procedure.

Just as Ephraim McDowell was to be named the founder of abdominal surgery, James Marion Sims came to be known as the father of American gynecology because of his success in repairing vesicovaginal fistulas.

In 1835 Dieffenbach wrote this description of the plight of women with urinary fistulas:

A sadder situation can hardly exist than that of a woman afflicted with a vesicovaginal fistula. A source of disgust, even to herself, the woman beloved by her husband becomes, in this condition, the object of bodily revulsion to him; and filled with repugnance, everyone else likewise turns his back, repulsed by the intolerable, foul, uriniferous odor. As a result of the seepage from the opening, whether large or small, the usual retention of the urine in the vaginal folds makes it even sharper and more pungent. The labia, perineum, lower part of the buttocks, and inner aspect of the thighs and calves are continually wet, to the very feet. The skin assumes a fiery red color and is covered in places with a pustular eruption. Intolerable burning and itching torment the patients, who are driven to frequent scratching to the point of bleeding, as a result of which their suffering increases still more. In desperation many tear the hair, which is coated at times with a calcareous urinary precipitate, from the mons pubis. The refreshment of a change of clothing provides no relief, because the clean undergarment, after being quickly saturated, slaps against the patients, flopping against their wet thighs as they walk, sloshing in their wet shoes as though they were wading through a swamp. The bed does not soothe them, because a good resting place, a bed, or a horsehair mattress, is quickly impregnated with urine and gives off the most unbearable stench. Even the richest are usually condemned for life to a straw sack, whose straw must be renewed daily. One's breath is taken away by the bedroom air of these women, and wherever they go they pollute the atmosphere. Washing and anointing do not help; perfumes actually increase the repugnance of the odor, just as foul-tasting things become even worse when coated with sugar. This horrendous evil tears asunder every family bond. The tender mother is rejected from the circle of her children. Confined to her lonely little room, she sits there in the cold, at the open window on her wooden chair with a hole cut in its seat, and may not cover the floor with a carpet even if she could. Indifference overtakes some of these unfortunates; others give themselves over to quiet resignation and pious devotion. Otherwise they would fall victim to despair and would attempt suicide.

* Robert Houstoun successfully evacuated the contents of a large ovarian tumor, probably a mucinous cystadenoma, by laparotomy in August, 1701, but without removal of the ovary. The patient, aged 58, lived in good health until October 1714, when she died of an unknown cause (Philosophical Transactions 7:541, 1734).

Physicians had struggled with vesicovaginal fistulas for centuries, exhausting their ingenuity on countless mechanical devices and surgical procedures, in their vain efforts to reclaim these social outcasts. J. Marion Sims, a young surgeon in Montgomery, Alabama, attacked the problem freshly in 1845, with experiments on the now legendary slaves, Anarcha, Betsy, and Lucy, sufferers from this dreaded affliction. After repeated attempts, about 40 in number, had ended in failure, the persistent Sims ultimately succeeded in developing a surgical technique for fistula repair, with the aid of the rediscovered knee–chest position, a vaginal speculum now named for him, and silver sutures.

Sims reported his success in his historic paper of 1852. The following year he moved to New York, where he founded, in 1855, a small hospital for women, the forerunner of the Woman's Hospital of the State of New York. Here Sims and his colleagues, Thomas Addis Emmet, E. R. Peaslee, and T. Gaillard Thomas, achieved a brilliant record for their fistula repairs and vaginal plastic operations. Gynecology had taken its place as a full-fledged surgical specialty.

REFERENCES AND RECOMMENDED READING

GENERAL

Fasbender HF: Geschichte der Geburtshilfe. Jena, Fischer, 1906

Graham H: Eternal Eve: The History of Gynaecology and Obstetrics. Garden City, NY, Doubleday, 1951

Irving FC: Safe Deliverance. Boston, Houghton Mifflin, 1942

Miller D: Res obstetrica in the Bible. J Obstet Gynaecol Br Emp 60:7, 1953

Ploss HH, Bartels M, Bartels P: EJ Dingwall (ed): Woman: An Historical, Gynaecological and Anthropological Compendium. London, Heinemann, 1935

Preuss J: Biblisch-talmudische Medizin, 3rd ed. (English translation by Fred Rosner, New York, Sanhedrin Press, 1978). Berlin, Karger, 1923

Ricci JV: Development of Gynaecological Surgery and Instruments. Philadelphia, Blakiston, 1949

Ricci JV: Genealogy of Gynaecology: History of the Development of Gynaecology Throughout the Ages. Philadelphia, Blakiston, 1950

Speert H: Obstetric and Gynecologic Milestones: Essays in Eponymy. New York, Macmillan, 1958

Speert H: Obstetrics and Gynecology in America: A History. Chicago, American College of Obstetricians and Gynecologists, 1980

Speert H: Iconographia Gyniatrica: A Pictorial History of Gynecology and Obstetrics. Philadelphia, Davis, 1973

Thoms H: Classical Contributions to Obstetrics and Gynecology. Springfield, Ill, Thomas, 1935

Williams JW: Sketch of the history of obstetrics in the United States up to 1860. Am Gynecol 3:266, 340, 1903

EARLY MIDWIFERY

Bancroft–Livingston G: Louise de la Vallière and the birth of the man–midwife. J Obstet Gynaecol Br Emp 63:261, 1956

Bard S: Compendium of the Theory and Practice of Midwifery, Containing Practical Instructions for the Management of Women during Pregnancy, in Labour, and in Childbed. New York, Collins & Perkins, 1807

Corner BC: William Shippen, Jr., Pioneer in American Medical Education. Philadelphia, American Philosophical Society, 1951

Denman T: Introduction to the Practice of Midwifery. London, Johnson, 1795

Heaton CE: Obstetrics in Colonial America. Am J Surg 45:606, 1939

Mauriceau F: Traité des maladies des femmes grosses et de celles qui sont accouchées. (Chamberlen H [trans], London, Billingsley, 1673). Paris, 1668

Mercurio S: La Commare O' Raccoglitrice. Venice, Ciotti, 1595–1596

Rösslin E: Der Swangerenn Frawen und Hebammen Rosengarte. Strassburg, Flach, 1513

Smellie W: Treatise on the Theory and Practice of Midwifery. London, Wilson & Durham, 1752–1764. (Reprinted with annotations by AH McCintock, London, New Sydenham Society, 1876–1878)

Soranus of Ephesus. Gynecology. Temkin O, Eastman NJ, Guttmacher AF (trans). Baltimore, Johns Hopkins, 1956

ANTENATAL CARE

Ballantyne JW: Plea for a pro-maternity hospital. Br Med J, April 6, 1901, p 813

Ballantyne JW: Visit to the wards of the pro-maternity hospital: A vision of the twentieth century. Am J Obstet 43:593, 1901

Taussig FJ: The story of prenatal care. Am J Obstet Gynecol 34:731, 1937

EMBRYOLOGY

von Baer KE: De Ovi Mammalium et Homini Genesi. O'Malley CD (trans). Leipzig, Voss, 1827

Corner GW: Discovery of the mammalian ovum. Lectures on the History of Medicine: A Series of Lectures at the Mayo Foundation, 1929–1932. Philadelphia, Saunders, 1933

de Graaf R: De Mulierum Organis Generationi Inservientibus. Corner GW (trans). Leyden, Hackiana, 1672

Wolff C: Theoria Generationis. Samassa (trans). Halle, Hendel, 1752

THE OBSTETRIC PELVIS

Baudelocque JL: L'Art des accouchemens. Paris, Méquignon, 1781

van Deventer H: Operationes Chirurgicae Novum Lumen Exhibentes Obstetricantibus, quo fideliter manifestatur ars obstetricandi, et quidquid ad eam requiritur: Instructum pluribus figuris aeri incisis. . . . Leyden, Dyckuisen, 1701

Eastman NJ: Pelvic mensuration: A study in the perpetuation of error. Obstet Gynecol Surv 3:301, 1948

Levret A: L'Art des accouchemens, demontré par des principes de physique et de méchanique. Paris, Le Prieur, 1753

Litzmann CCT: Die Formen des Beckens, insbesondere des Engen Weiblichen Beckens, nach eigenen Beobachtungen und Untersuchungen, nebst einem Anhange über die Osteomalacie. Berlin, Reimer, 1861

Michaelis GA: Das Enge Becken nach eigenen Beobachtungen und Untersuchungen. Litzmann CCT (ed). Leipzig, Wigand, 1851

THE OBSTETRIC FORCEPS

Aveling JH: The Chamberlens and the Midwifery Forceps: Memorials of the Family and an Essay on the Invention of the Instrument. London, Churchill, 1882

Das K: Obstetric Forceps: Its History and Evolution. St. Louis, Mosby, 1929

PUERPERAL FEVER

Blundell J: Lectures on the Principles and Practice of Midwifery, Severn C (ed). London, Masters, 1839

Gordon A: Treatise on the Epidemic Puerperal Fever of Aberdeen. London, Robinson, 1795

Hodge HL: On the Non-contagious Character of Puerperal Fever: An Introductory Lecture. Philadelphia, Collins, 1852

Holmes OW: Contagiousness of puerperal fever. N Eng Q J Med Surg 1:503, 1843 (reprinted in Medical Classics 1:211, 1936)

Holmes OW: Puerperal Fever as a Private Pestilence. Boston, Ticknor & Fields, 1855. Reprint in Medical Classics 1:247, 1936

Semmelweis IP: Semmelweis' Gesammelte Werke. von Györy T (ed). Jena, Fischer, 1905

Watson T: Lectures on the principles and practice of physic, delivered at King's College, London. London Med Gaz (NS) 1:801, 1842

CESAREAN SECTION

Bixby GH: Extirpation of the puerperal uterus by abdominal section. J Gynaecol Soc Boston 1:223, 1869

Eastman NJ: Role of frontier America in the development of cesarean section. Am J Obstet Gynecol 24:919, 1932

Harris RP: Operation of gastro-hysterotomy (true caesarean section), viewed in the light of American experience and success; with the history and results of sewing up the uterine wound; and a full tabular record of the caesarean operations performed in the United States, many of them not hitherto reported. Am J Med Sci 75:313, 1878

King AG: America's first cesarean section. Obstet Gynecol 37:797, 1970

Porro E: Dell' amputazione utero-ovarica come complemento di taglio cesareo. Ann univ Med Chir 237:289, 1876

Sänger M: Der Kaiserschnitt bei Uterusfibromen nebst vergleichender Methodik der Sectio Caesarea und der Porro-Operation. Leipzig, Engelmann, 1882

Young JH: Caesarean Section: The History and Development of the Operation from Earliest Times. London, Lewis, 1944

ANESTHESIA FOR CHILDBIRTH

Simpson JY: Notes on the employment of the inhalation of sulphuric ether in the practice of midwifery. Monthly J Med Sci 7:721, 728, 1847

Simpson JY: Etherization in surgery. Monthly J Med Sci 8:144, 1847

Simpson JY: Account of a new Anaesthetic Agent, as a Substitute for Sulphuric Ether in Surgery and Midwifery. Communicated to the Medico-Chirurgical Society of Edinburgh at Their Meeting on 10th November, 1847. Edinburgh, 1847. Reprint. New York, 1848

Simpson JY: Obstetric Memoirs and Contributions of James Y. Simpson, MD, FRSE, Vol 2. Edited by WO Priestley, HR Storer. Philadelphia, Lippincott, 1865

Watson BP: President's address: Sixty-first annual meeting of the American Gynecological Society. Am J Obstet Gynecol 32:547, 1936

WOMAN'S FERTILITY AND ITS CONTROL

Himes NE: Medical History of Contraception. New York, Gamut Press, 1963

Stopes MC: Contraception (Birth Control): Its Theory and Practice. London, Putnam, 1931

Wood C, Suitters B: The Fight for Acceptance: A History of Contraception. Aylesbury, Medical Technical, 1970

GYNECOLOGY AS A SURGICAL SPECIALTY

Clay C: Results of All the Operations for the Extirpation of Diseased Ovaria, by the Large Incision, from September 12, 1842, to the Present Time. Manchester, Irwin, 1848

Dieffenbach JF: Ueber die Heilung der Blasen-Scheiden-Fisteln und Zerreissungen der Blase und Scheide. Med Zeitung 5:117, 121, 173, 177, 1836

Fluhmann CF: Rise and fall of suspension operations for uterine retrodisplacement. Bull Johns Hopkins Hosp 96:59, 1955

Harris S: Woman's Surgeon: The Life Story of J. Marion Sims. New York, Macmillan, 1950

Heidrich CG: Diss. Sistens Casum Memorabilem Ascitae et Destructionis Ovariorum. Berlin, Brüsch, 1825

McDowell E: Three cases of extirpation of diseased ovaria. Eclectic Repertory Analyt Rev 7:242, 1817

Meigs CD: Females and Their Diseases: A Series of Letters to His Class. Philadelphia, Lea & Blanchard, 1848

Mitchell TR: Practical Remarks on the Use of the Speculum in the Treatment of Disease of Females. Dublin, Fannin, 1849

Peaslee ER: Ovarian Tumors, Their Pathology, Diagnosis, and Treatment. London, Lewis, 1873

Scanzoni FW: A Practical Treatise on the Diseases of the Sexual Organs of Women, 4th American ed. Gardner AK (trans). New York, De Witt, 1861

Sims JM: On the treatment of vesico-vaginal fistula. Am J Med Sci 23:59, 1852

With more successful medical treatment of many acquired serious or fatal diseases, those conditions in which there is a genetic component have gained greatly in relative importance. That genetic and cytogenetic disorders are more important in obstetrics and gynecology than in many other fields of medicine is demonstrated by the fact that after the central nervous and cardiovascular systems, genetic disease most often affects the reproductive system. Clearly, the normal development of this system is determined by a great number of genes distributed on different chromosomes.

The most important role of cytogenetics in clinical medicine lies in genetic counseling. Although chromosome analysis is helpful in diagnosing conditions caused by autosomal abnormalities, such diseases are at present beyond medical help, and chromosome study is valuable chiefly as it enables the physician to counsel the relatives of the affected individual. Chromosome analysis may, however, be very important in diagnosing and treating diseases of the female reproductive system caused by sex chromosome abnormalities.

The recently developed techniques of amniocentesis and amniotic fluid cell culture are powerful adjuncts to genetic counseling. The obstetrician–gynecologist can now use these techniques in collaboration with genetic counseling to provide a high degree of diagnostic accuracy. Instead of the probabilities previously offered, now in many cases it can be determined definitely whether or not an unborn fetus is normal; advice can be founded on facts.

In addition to these practical aspects, information from gynecologic patients with gene and chromosome abnormalities contributes substantially to theoretic genetic research. This is especially true of studies concerning the structure, behavior, and effects of the human X chromosome.

CHAPTER 2

GENETIC CONSIDERATIONS

Gloria E. Sarto

BASIC GENETICS

CYTOGENETICS

HUMAN CHROMOSOMES

Prior to 1940, all knowledge of human chromosomes was based upon the analysis of tissue sections. Squash techniques were used to study chromosomes, but the detail was not good enough for accurate analysis. Since 1952, improvement in media and techniques for tissue culture has made possible the cultivation of cells *in vitro* and has increased the number of tissues that can be studied. The use of colchicine to prevent spindle formation has enabled analysis of cells in the metaphase stage of mitosis. The application of hypotonic solutions to make the cells swell has improved chromosome dispersement. Autoradiographic techniques have facilitated the recognition of individual chromosomes. Only in the last several years, however, has the introduction of banding techniques, such as Giemsa banding or fluorochrome stains and fluorescence microscopy, permitted identification of individual chromosomes.

Karyotype Preparation

Peripheral blood and fibroblasts are the most commonly studied tissues. Blood lymphocytes obtained from 10 ml heparinized blood are induced to divide by adding phytohemagglutinin. Phytohemagglutinin acts as an antigen and stimulates an immunologic response, transforming the lymphocytes into blastlike

cells capable of division in culture. Colchicine is added shortly before harvesting. A hypotonic solution is used to make the cells swell and allow dispersement of the chromosomes for analysis.

Fibroblasts are derived from skin biopsies or from other body tissues, including amniotic fluid. After a monolayer of cells has grown out to cover a glass surface, usually in 2–3 weeks, the cells are subcultured. The peak time for mitosis varies with the tissue, but is usually about 15–24 hours after subculture. The cells are then treated with colchicine and hypotonic solution and fixed, as are the lymphocyte cultures.

Selected cells in metaphase are analyzed and photographed, and a karyotype is prepared. A *karyotype* is composed of chromosomes from one cell arranged according to size, in pairs if possible, and identified by the standard nomenclature.

Chromosome Identification

The size of a specific chromosome is relatively stable within a species; however, chromosome size varies with the stage of mitosis and with some environmental agents. For example, prophase chromosomes are longer and less coiled than metaphase chromosomes; treatment with colchicine and some other agents shortens chromosomes.

The shape of a chromosome is largely determined by the position of the centromere, which is made visible by the so-called primary constriction in the metaphase chromosome. The centromere may be located terminally, subterminally, or in a median position, resulting in acrocentric, submetacentric, or metacentric chromosomes.

Until 1970, only a limited number of chromosomes could be individually identified. They were grouped according to their size and shape. Those identified by morphology alone included Group A (1, 2, 3), Group E (16, 17, 18), and the Y chromosome.

Autoradiographic techniques, introduced in 1957, made it possible to distinguish additional chromosomes. Dividing cells are incubated with a radioactive DNA precursor (usually tritiated thymidine) for a given period (usually 3–7 hours, depending upon the cell type). The cells are treated with colchicine, a hypotonic solution, and a fixative in the usual manner. Slides are coated with a special photographic emulsion, stored at 4 °C in light-tight boxes for varying periods, and then developed. Incorporation of the radioactive precursor is demonstrated by the presence of silver grains over the chromosomes. Plates showing cells in metaphase are photographed and analyzed. Chromosomes synthesize DNA and thus incorporate radioactive thymidine at varying times; this produces characteristic labeling patterns. Autoradiographic techniques allow specific identification of chromosomes in Group B (4 and 5), Group D (13, 14, 15), Group G (21 and 22) and the late-replicating X (Group C).

In 1970, Caspersson *et al.* reported the use of fluorochrome stains and fluorescence microscopy for human chromosome identification. This technique involves staining cells with fluorochromes and exposing them to the ultraviolet light of a fluorescence microscope. With this method basic banding patterns become apparent, each of the 46 chromosomes can be unambiguously identified (Fig. 2–1), and chromosome segments and structural abnormalilties can be detected. A *band* is defined as the part of a chromosome that is distinguishable from its adjacent segments because it appears darker or lighter with one or more banding techniques. The banding patterns are consistent from one individual to another and from one tissue to another; some variations in the intensity of certain fluorescent bands are inherited.

Unfortunately, the fluorescence technique requires expensive equipment, and the fluorescence is not permanent. Another banding technique is by Giemsa stain; the bands are termed G bands and correspond with the Q bands that are demonstrable with quinacrine staining and fluorescence microscopy. Some stains identify only specific bands or structures. These include methods that stain centromeric bands (C bands), telomeric bands (T bands), and nucleolus organizing regions (NORs). Banding techniques have replaced autoradiography as a means of chromosome identification. Although autoradiography is still used to identify the inactive X chromosome (s) in a cell, the inactive X can also be identified by partially quenching the fluorescence of the dye 33258 Hoechst with 5-bromodeoxyuridine (BrdU).

Chromosome Nomenclature

The first conference to standarize chromosome nomenclature was held in 1960 at Denver, Colorado. The Denver system designated each pair of autosomes by number, 1–22, and the sex chromosomes as X or Y. This implied that each chromosome could be identified on a morphologic basis alone, which, as pointed out by Patau, is not the case. Patau suggested that, based on size and location of the centromere, the chromosomes be assigned to one of seven groups, A–G. This nomenclature was accepted at a conference in London in 1963. In 1966, at a conference in Chicago, a uniform system to describe karyotypes was adopted (Table 2–1). The advent of banding techniques made it necessary to agree on additional characteristics. Thus, in 1971 at a conference in Paris, nomenclature for the banding patterns was developed. A committee met in Stockholm in 1977 to review the nomenclature for chromosome and banding patterns. A document entitled *An International System for Human Cytogenetic Nomenclature* (1978), abbreviated ISCN (1978), resulted from that meeting. The ISCN (1978) includes all the major decisions about chromosome nomenclature of the Denver, London, Chicago, and Paris conferences.

FIG. 2-1. 47, XYY karyotype, stained with quinacrine mustard and photographed using ultraviolet light and fluorescence microscope. Each chromosome can be unambiguously identified. (Courtesy K Patau)

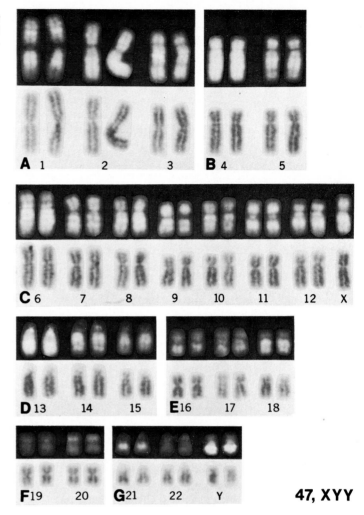

A 1 2 3 B 4 5

C 6 7 8 9 10 11 12 X

D 13 14 15 E 16 17 18

F 19 20 G 21 22 Y

47, XYY

Definitions

Haploid. A set of chromosomes in which each differs from the other, morphologically and genetically. Gametes contain a haploid set (n) of chromosomes. A zygote (fertilized ovum) contains two haploid sets ($2n$), *i.e.*, it is diploid.

Polyploid. A multiple of the basic number of chromosomes higher than diploid, *i.e.*, triploid, tetraploid, etc.

Euploid. A chromosome number that is an exact multiple of the basic haploid number. Cells with n, $2n$, $3n$, $4n$ are euploid.

Aneuploid. A chromosome number deviating from the basic number (n) and from an exact multiple of n, *i.e.*, $2n - 1$; $2n + 1$, etc.

Heteroploid. A chromosome number deviating from the normal chromosome number for the species. This includes aneuploid and euploid.

Mosaic (mixoploid). Two or more cell types derived from same zygote.

Chimera. Two or more genetically different cell types, each derived from different zygotes.

MITOSIS AND MEIOSIS

Normal growth and development are largely determined by genetic makeup. Meiosis brings about the distribution of genes from parent to child. It is through meiosis that the Mendelian processes of segregation and independent assortment occur. Mitosis assures that the exact replication of the genetic material, which takes place prior to cell division, is distributed so that each daughter cell has a genome identical to that of the parent cell. Abnormal chromosome constitutions, which lead to abnormal growth and development, are caused by errors in meiosis and mitosis.

TABLE 2-1. NOMENCLATURE SYSTEM FOR KARYOTYPES

A–G	The chromosome groups
1–22	The autosome numbers (Denver system)
X,Y	The sex chromosomes
+	Indicates extra chromosome
−	Indicates missing chromosome
/	Separates cell lines in describing mosaicism
?	Questionable identification of chromosome or chromosome structure
ace	Acentric
cen	Centromere
dic	Dicentric
end	Endoreduplication
h	Negative-staining region or secondary constriction
i	Isochromosome
inv	Inversion
inv(p+q−) or inv(p−q+)	Pericentric inversion
mar	Marker chromosome
mat	Maternal origin
p	Short arm of chromosome
pat	Paternal origin
q	Long arm of chromosome
r	Ring satellite
t	Translocation
tri	Tricentric

(Chicago Conference, Standardization in Human Cytogenetics. New York, National Foundation March of Dimes, 1966)

Mitosis

Mitosis is only one phase of the cell cycle. The cycle is divided into mitosis, the time between mitosis and the beginning of DNA synthesis, DNA synthesis, and the interval between the end of DNA synthesis and the beginning of mitosis. The total time varies with the type of cell, but is between 12 and 24 hours. The period of DNA synthesis is 7–7.5 hours. Mitosis takes only a relatively short time, 0.5–1.5 hours. Mitosis (Fig. 2–2) itself is divided into several phases—prophase, metaphase, anaphase, and telophase—but, of course, there is no clear-cut separation between successive stages.

Prior to the beginning of mitosis, during interphase, the cell nucleus appears finely granular. The nucleolus is readily visible, as is the heteropyknotic (densely staining) chromatin within the nucleus.

Prophase. The chromosomes coil and become more distinct; they are made up of two chromatids. The nucleolus and nuclear membrane disappear and the centrioles (centrosomes) move to opposite poles.

Metaphase. The spindle is formed between the two centrioles. The centromeres, whose primary function is to attach the chromosomes to the spindle fibers, lie in the metaphase plate, which is equidistant from the two poles (equatorial plane). The centromeres become functionally double; the daughter centromeres immediately repel each other.

Anaphase. The centromeres move to opposite poles with their attached daughter chromosomes. The end of anaphase is marked by the arrival of the daughter chromosomes at the two poles.

Telophase. A nuclear membrane is formed, and the nucleoli are reconstituted. The chromosomes revert to the interphase condition and lose their visible structure. At the end of telophase, the cytoplasm divides into two equal parts (cytokinesis).

Meiosis

Cells that are ready to enter meiosis are known as primary oocytes or primary spermatocytes. The essential characteristics of meiosis (Fig. 2–3), e.g., pairing of homologous chromosomes, crossing over, and reduction of chromosome number (two cell divisions with only one duplication of chromosomes) result in halving the diploid number of chromosomes. Meiosis brings about genotypic diversity by 1) independent assortment of chromosomes and 2) segregation and crossing over or recombination of homologous chromosomes.

Prophase I. Prophase of the first meiotic division (meiosis I) is composed of different stages—leptotene, zygotene, pachytene, diplotene, and diakinesis. Transition from one to the other is gradual and continuous, as in mitosis. Preleptotene and leptotene are characterized by an increase in nuclear volume. The chromosomes appear as fine, single threads coiled and twisted throughout the nucleus. During zygotene, homologous chromosomes pair in a zipper fashion, and they appear somewhat shorter and thicker. At pachytene, pairing is complete, and the number of pairs of homologous chromosomes (bivalents) is half the diploid number of chromosomes. Since each homolog is made up of two chromatids, the paired homologs (bivalents) consist of four chromatids. Diplotene is marked by contraction of the bivalents. The paired chromosomes repulse each other and fall apart, except where they are held together by one or more chiasmata (crossovers). In each crossover only two of the four chromatids are involved. The position and number of chiasmata determine the shape of the bivalents at diplotene. During diakinesis, the chromosomes become shorter and thicker. The nucleolus disappears. The end of prophase I is marked by the disappearance of the nuclear membrane and the division of the centriole.

Metaphase I. The bipolar spindle is formed. The centromeres lie on opposite sides of the equatorial plate.

FIG. 2-2. Schematic diagram of mitosis. (Sharp LW: Fundamentals of Cytology. New York, McGraw–Hill, 1943)

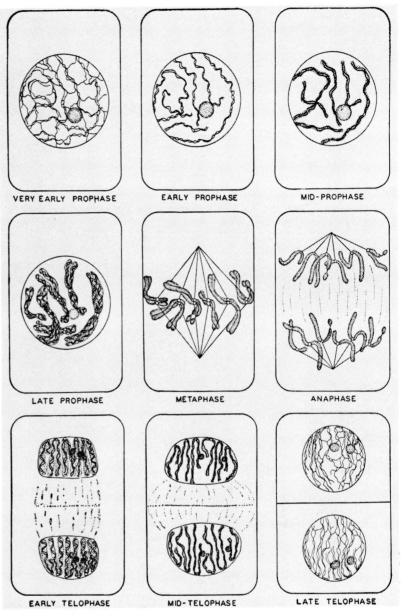

VERY EARLY PROPHASE   EARLY PROPHASE   MID-PROPHASE

LATE PROPHASE   METAPHASE   ANAPHASE

EARLY TELOPHASE   MID-TELOPHASE   LATE TELOPHASE

Anaphase I. As the centromeres separate and move to opposite poles, the chiasmata slip to the ends of the bivalents. When separation is complete, each pole has one-half the diploid number of chromosomes, each consisting of two chromatids. As a result of crossing over, each chromosome has maternal and paternal genetic material.

Telophase I. Cell division takes place, and a nuclear membrane is formed around each nucleus.

Interphase I. The chromosomes do not become extended during interphase I, which is very short. There is no reduplication of chromosomes, and the second meiotic division (meiosis II) begins.

Prophase II. The chromatids are widely separated, but held together by the centromere.

Metaphase II. The nuclear membrane disappears and the spindle develops. The centromeres are lined up on the equatorial plate.

Anaphase II. The centromeres divide and, each with its attached chromatids, move to opposite poles.

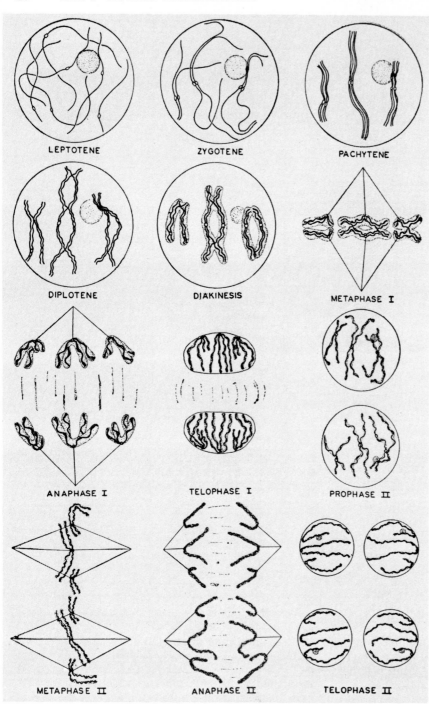

FIG. 2-3. Schematic diagram of meiosis of cell with three chromosome pairs. Telophase II represents gametes. (Sharp LW: Fundmentals of Cytology. New York, McGraw–Hill, 1943)

Telophase II. Cell division takes place and the nuclear membrane is reformed.

NUMERICAL ABNORMALITIES

Aneuploidy

Aneuploidy causes anomalies in man and results from the loss or gain of a chromosome. It may be due to errors in mitosis or meiosis. Monosomy in man is rare, except for X monosomy (which causes Turner's syndrome) and possibly, very rarely, a G monosomy. Several trisomies exist, however, each with a characteristic and relatively well-defined phenotype.

One mechanism known to result in aneuploidy is *nondisjunction,* the failure of sister chromatids to pass to opposite poles of the spindle. Meiotic nondisjunction during gametogenesis can occur during the first or second meiotic division or both. Since oogenesis results in the formation of one functional gamete and three nonfunctional polar bodies and spermatogenesis results in four presumably functional gametes, the consequence of nondisjunction in oogenesis is different from that in spermatogenesis. First division meiotic nondisjunction in spermatogenesis produces either nullisomic or disomic sperm. Second division meiotic nondisjunction produces disomic, nullisomic, and normal sperm (Fig. 2–4). In oogenesis, nondisjunction at either meiotic division produces a disomic or a nullisomic ovum (Fig. 2–5). Therefore, without selection for or against a certain type of gamete, nondisjunction during oogenesis is more likely to result in an abnormal zygote than is nondisjunction during spermatogenesis.

Another cause of aneuploidy is *anaphase lag.* In this instance, a chromosome does not move as readily as others to its pole, and consequently is lost; monosomic and nullisomic gametes result.

Polyploidy

Triploidy can arise from any one of several errors in gametogenesis. For instance, failure of formation of the first or second polar body, with subsequent fertilization, results in fusion of three haploid sets of chromosomes (two maternal, one paternal). Double fertilization of a normally developed oocyte also causes triploidy (two paternal, one maternal). If the second meiotic division in spermatogenesis is aborted, fertilization of a normal oocyte by a sperm with a diploid set of chromosomes produces a triploid cell line. Tetraploidy results from suppression of a division in a diploid zygote or some mitotic mechanism leading to endopolyploidy. Triploidy and tetraploidy are found frequently in plants, but are not compatible with life in mammals; they are found not infrequently in abortuses. Several persons with triploid cells have survived; however, these conditions have been associated with an extensive diploid cell line.

Mosaicism

Mitotic nondisjunction and anaphase lag in the early zygote result in mosaicism (mixoploidy). Diagnosis is based upon the presence of two or more cell types in different tissue and in successive cultures from the same tissues. The abnormalities should be consistent in all the cultures. Sex chromosome mosaicism is much more common than autosome mosaicism.

Chimerism

Chimerism differs from mosaicism in that the cells arise from two independent zygotes. The most common mechanism is thought to be an exchange of cells between dizygotic twins due to placental cross-circulation, which regularly occurs in cattle twins and only rarely in humans.

STRUCTURAL ABNORMALITIES

Intrachromosomal Abnormalities

Deletions and inversions occur as the result of breaks within the same chromosome. *Deletions* can be terminal or interstitial; if interstitial, two breaks occur the intervening segment is lost, and the broken ends rejoin. A *ring chromosome* is caused by a break near the end of each arm of the chromosome and the rejoining of the broken ends. An *inversion* is the result of two breaks, with the segment between the two breaks becoming inverted. If the inverted segment does not involve the centromere, it is a *paracentric inversion;* if it includes the centromere, it is a *pericentric inversion.*

Interchromosomal Rearrangements

Breaks in two chromosomes may result in interchromosomal rearrangements. A *reciprocal translocation* is an exchange of chromosome segments between two chromosomes. If balanced—a mutual exchange with no loss of chromosome segments—there are no ill effects. A specific type of translocation, called *centric fusion,* occurs between two acrocentric chromosomes. An individual carrying a balanced translocation is phenotypically normal (chromosomes are rearranged, but balanced). However, at meiosis the rearranged chromosome is transmitted to the offspring in balanced or unbalanced form (Fig. 2–6). This results in fetal loss, a malformed infant, a phenotypically normal individual with a balanced translocation, or a phenotypically and genotypically normal individual. The chance of each of these occurring depends upon chiasma formation and segregation at meiosis.

Misdivision of the Centromere

Transverse instead of the usual longitudinal division of the centromere results in an *isochromosome.* An isochromosome is metracentric with two identical

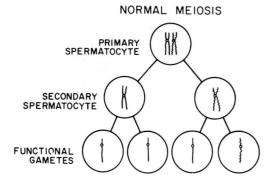

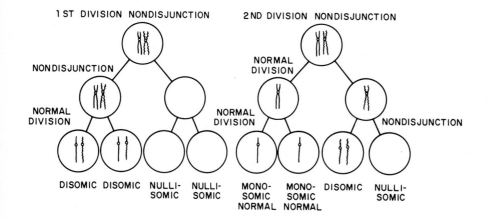

FIG. 2–4. Schematic diagram of spermatogenesis, showing effects of meiotic nondisjunction.

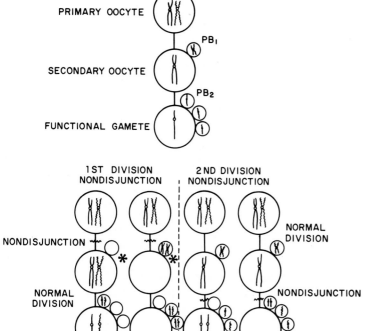

FIG. 2–5. Schematic diagram of oogenesis, showing effects of meiotic nondisjunction. Corresponding types, such as those marked by *asterisks,* may not be equally frequent. This diagram shows division of first polar body (PB_1).

arms formed from the two sister chromatids. In man, the most common isochromosome consists of two long arms of the X.

Chromatid Rearrangements

Breaks in sister chromatids after chromosome doubling may produce chromatid rearrangements. Chromosome breaks and gaps (achromatic regions) without rearrangement occur rarely in normal people. Several inherited disorders (*e.g.,* Bloom's syndrome and Fanconi's anemia) are associated with an increased number of spontaneous chromosome rearrangements. Certain drugs, chemicals, and viruses are known to cause chromosome breaks *in vitro* and *in vivo*. The significance of chromosome and chromatid gaps in peripheral leukocyte cultures is unknown.

MENDELIAN GENETICS

Genes occur in pairs, one inherited from the mother, the other from the father. Those occupying identical positions (*loci*) on a pair of chromosomes are *alleles*. A

mutant gene may be inherited from one or both parents or, very rarely, may arise in the individual. The *genotype* is the genetic makeup of an individual. The *phenotype* is the sum total of all the morphologic or physiologic characteristics of the individual. If one of the two alleles is mutant, then the individual is *heterozygous;* if both alleles are mutant, the individual is *homozygous*. If a disorder is inherited according to Mendelian laws, probabilities of recurrence can be calculated (Table 2–2).

AUTOSOMAL DOMINANT INHERITANCE

The effect of an autosomal dominant disorder is brought about by a single mutant gene situated on an autosome. Characteristics of autosomal dominant inheritance include the following: 1) the trait is transmitted from one generation to the next generation from an affected person to an affected offspring, 2) one-half of the siblings and one-half of the children of an affected person are affected, and 3) the inheritance is usually independent of sex, *i.e.,* both sexes are equally affected. The potential risk for every child of a

FIG. 2-6. Familial Down's syndrome resulting from 15/21 chromosome translocation in more than three generations of a large kindred. (Modified from Macintyre MN, Staples WI, Steinberg AG, Hempil JM: Am J Hum Genet 15:335, 1962)

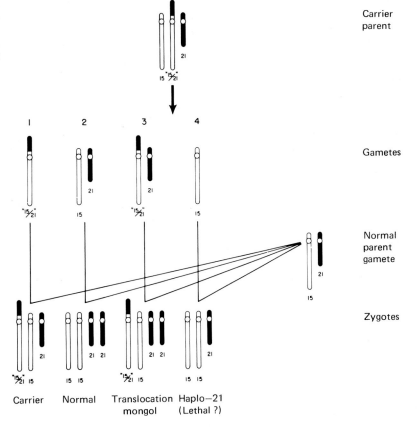

TABLE 2-2. APPROXIMATE RECURRENCE RISKS FOR VARIOUS GENETIC ABNORMALITIES

Abnormality	Risk of Recurrence (%)
MENDELIAN MUTATIONS	
Autosomal recessive	25
Autosomal dominant	50 (unless new mutation or unless penetrance is reduced)
X-linked, for carrier females	25 overall, 50 males
X-linked, for affected males	100 carrier daughters, 100 normal sons
COMMON MULTIFACTORIAL CONDITIONS	2–5 (increases with each affected child)
CHROMOSOME ABNORMALITIES	
Trisomy syndrome (Down's), parents chromosomally normal	1–2
Balanced translocation, carrier parent*	2–100

* See Table 2–5.

person with an autosomal dominant inherited disorder is 50%. This assumes complete penetrance. Family members not suffering from the defect cannot pass it to their offspring.

AUTOSOMAL RECESSIVE INHERITANCE

In autosomal recessive inheritance, the affected individual inherited the mutant gene from each parent and, thus, is homozygous. If the trait is rare, as they usually are, the parents are heterozygous for the mutant gene, *i.e.*, each one carries a mutant gene on one autosome and a normal allele on the other. The effect of the normal gene is dominant to that of the mutant gene; therefore, the heterozygote is phenotypically normal. In autosomal recessive disorders, 1) the carrier parents of the affected child are heterozygous for the mutant gene and are phenotypically normal, 2) one in four individuals is affected in the sibships of affected children, and 3) the children of an affected individual are not affected unless the affected individual has married a carrier (heretozygous for the mutant gene). Since there is small chance of two unrelated parents carrying the same mutant gene, parents of individuals with autosomal recessive inherited disorders often are consaguineous. Many metabolic disorders, *e.g.*, phenylketonuria and cystic fibrosis, are inherited as autosomal recessives.

X-LINKED INHERITANCE

In X-linked inheritance, the mutant gene is on the X chromosome. The characteristics of X-linked inheritance are different for dominant and for recessive genes.

In X-linked recessive inheritance, the chance of manifesting the trait differs in males and females. In the female, an X-linked recessive disorder is usually not expressed because the normal gene on the homologous X chromosome is dominant. In contrast, since there is only one X chromosome in the male, the single (hemizygous) recessive mutant gene on it is expressed. Analyses of many pedigrees with X-linked recessive disorders show that 1) there are more affected males than females, 2) males inherit the disease from carrier mothers, 3) half of the brothers but none of the sisters of an affected male are affected, and 4) carrier females may have affected uncles or affected brothers. In the union of a phenotypically normal, though carrier, female and a normal male, half the sons are affected and half the daughters are carriers. All sons of an affected male are normal, since they inherit only the maternal X chromosome; all daughters of affected males are heterozygous (carriers), since they all inherit the paternal X chromosome also.

In X-linked dominant inheritance, both heterozygous females and hemizygous males manifest the abnormality. All the sons of an affected male are unaffected; all the daughters are heterozygous, and since the mutant gene is dominant, it is expressed, *i.e.*, the daughters are affected. It is sometimes difficult to differentiate between X-linked dominant and autosomal dominant modes of inheritance.

MULTIFACTORIAL INHERITANCE

Many malformations are not inherited in a simple way. Instead, they are determined by the complex interaction of several genes at different loci within the environment. Such traits are considered multifactorial. Anencephaly, spina bifida, cleft palate, and cleft lip are examples. In these conditions, genetic prognosis can be offered only in terms of empiric risks based on the analysis of many pedigrees. After the birth of one affected child, the risk to subsequent siblings is usually about 3%–5%. After two affected children, the risk increases. The exact risk of each disorder must be estimated from the literature.

PENETRANCE, EXPRESSIVITY, SEX LIMITATION, PHENOCOPIES, GENETIC HETEROGENEITY

With some autosomal dominant inherited disorders, an individual may inherit the mutant gene and pass it on, yet be found phenotypically normal. This phenomenon is known as *incomplete penetrance:* The mutant gene is present, but it is not manifested. Penetrance is a statistical concept; for example, if 20 persons have the dominant gene but only 10 express the trait, it is said that the gene shows 50% penetrance. Obviously, it is necessary to study large pedigrees to determine the degree of penetrance.

Some inherited disorders exhibit the phenomenon known as *varying expressivity.* An example is osteogenesis imperfecta. Some family members have blue sclerae, others have brittle bones, and some are deaf; others have two of the three, and some have all three abnormalities characteristic of the disorder. In such an instance, diagnosis can be difficult. A careful physical examination must be done on all possibly affected family members of an affected individual. The basis for this variation in the expression of genes is likely in the interaction of genes and the environment.

If a mutation is expressed in one sex only, it is termed a *sex-limited* disorder. An example is feminizing testis syndrome, a disorder limited to the male sex. It is sometimes difficult to distinguish between autosomal inheritance with male sex limitation and X-linked recessive inheritance.

An environmental agent can cause an abnormality that phenotypically is very similar or identical to an anomaly caused by a gene mutation. Such a disorder is termed a *phenocopy.*

Genetic heterogeneity exists when clinically identical diseases have different modes of inheritance. Data on genetic heterogeneity of a specific disorder must be obtained from the literature.

SEX CHROMATIN

X-CHROMATIN MASS (BARR BODY)

Historical Background and Lyon Hypothesis

The X-chromatin is a sex-specific heterochromatic mass observed in the interphase nuclei of cells of mammalian females. In 1949, Barr and Bertram noticed a dark-staining mass, termed "the nucleolar satellite," in the nuclei of nerve cells from female cats and in human ganglion cells. This body (Barr body) was absent from the nuclei of male cells. Not long thereafter, this sex difference was demonstrated in nuclei of cells from other human tissues.

Though it was first believed that the X-chromatin mass (Barr body) was derived from the heterochromatic regions of the two X chromosomes in females, cytologic and autoradiographic studies proved that it was formed from a single X chromosome. Ohno and collaborators demonstrated that a single heteropyknotic mass was present in diploid cells and that two were present in tetraploid cells. Studies of individuals with an abnormal number of X chromosomes provided additional evidence that the X-chromatin mass was derived from a single X chromosome, since the number of X-chromatin masses was always one less than the number of X chromosomes.

In 1951, the single-active-X-chromosome hypothesis, now called the Lyon hypothesis, was proposed almost simultaneously by Russell and by Lyon. It originated as an explanation of why the homozygous (XX) female shows the same phenotype as a hemizygous (XY) male for X-linked genes.

The Lyon hypothesis may be stated as follows:

1. The normal method of dosage compensation in female mammals depends upon inactivation of the genes on the X chromosome early in embryonic life.
2. Initially, the inactivation of the X chromosome is random, so that in some cells the paternal X is inactivated and in others, the maternal X.
3. Once inactivation has occurred, the descendants of each X chromosome (active or inactive) behave like the parent X. The inactive X forms a sex chromatin and is assumed to be the late-replicating X chromosome found with autoradiography.

The hypothesis that genes on the heteropyknotic X are inactivated is supported by evidence based on genetic and phenotypic studies involving X-linked genes and genes translocated to the X chromosome, on cytologic evidence, and on biochemical studies of X-linked genes in fibroblast cultures. For example, women heterozygous for genes on the X chromosome—two variants of glucose-6-phosphate dehydrogenase (G-6-PD)—give rise to two types of fibroblast clones. Each clone expresses only one of the G-6-PD variants, indicating inactivation of the genes on the other X chromosome. There are exceptions to the inactivation hypothesis, however. For example, the Xg blood group locus does not appear to undergo fixed random inactivation, suggesting that other loci on the X chromosome do not undergo inactivation either. Additional evidence indicating incomplete inactivation of the heteropyknotic X chromosome comes from the study of persons with abnormal numbers of X chromosomes. For example, if all except one X were inactivated, 45,X and 47,XXX karyotypes would not be expected to differ from XX individuals or to have developmental anomalies, as they do. This is also true of the XXXY and XXY states; XXXY is associated with a greater number of somatic anomalies than is XXY.

Structure of the X-Chromatin

The X-chromatin mass is about 1μ in diameter and is generally planoconvex in shape, with the flat portion

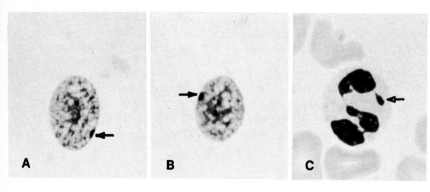

FIG. 2–7. X-chromatin (Barr body) in cell nuclei (*arrows*). *A.* Skin cell of normal female. *B.* Cell of buccal smear from normal female. *C.* Leukocyte from normal female. (Courtesy ML Barr)

against the nuclear membrane and the convex part pointing toward the center of the nucleus (Fig. 2–7). It can be disk-shaped, irregular, spherical, or triangular. It is usually located at the rim of the nucleus of a somatic cell in interphase, but because of the spherical nature of the nucleus, the X-chromatin mass can be seen in the center of a nucleus where, on occasion, it is confused with nonspecific heterochromatic masses. The X-chromatin stains with a number of dyes, including hematoxylin and eosin, methyl green, Feulgen, orcein, and carbolfuchsin.

Correlation of Number and Size of the X-Chromatin Masses with Number and Size of X Chromosomes

There is a correlation between the maximum number of X-chromatin masses and the number of X chromosomes. The number of X-chromatin masses is equal to the maximum number of X chromosomes minus one. Diploid interphase nuclei with two X chromosomes have a single X-chromatin mass, while cells with one X chromosome (XO or XY) have none. More than one X-chromatin mass in a nucleus indicates that there are more than two X chromosomes in the karyotype.

A reasonable correlation exists between larger than normal X chromosomes and larger than normal X-chromatin masses, and between X chromosome deletions and smaller than normal X-chromatin masses. It should be emphasized, however, that the smallness of the X-chromatin masses and the numerous factors affecting its size, density, shape, and disposition against the nuclear membrane and the shape of the nucleus make accurate assessments of its physical dimensions difficult. As an indicator of altered X chromosome structure, the size of the X-chromatin mass in nuclei of cells from a buccal smear is not adequate; for more accurate studies, fibroblast cultures are desirable.

Interpretation of Smears for X-Chromatin

The number of cells that contain the distinctive clump of chromatin in a normal female varies with the tissue being studied. Up to 90% of human amnion cells of female infants contain an X-chromatin mass. This is also true of cultured fibroblasts. In both instances, the high percentage of cells with an X-chromatin mass is probably related to the fact that the cells are in a monolayer with flattened nuclei. The percentage of cells with X-chromatin-positive nuclei in buccal or vaginal smears varies from 20% to 70%. However, in most preparations, the percentage of cells containing X-chromatin is between 20 and 50. Normal males should have no X-chromatin-positive nuclei; indeed, if even 3%–4% of nuclei contain X-chromatin, the individual should have a chromosome analysis to rule out the presence of an XXY cell line. A low percentage of cells with X-chromatin-positive nuclei in a phenotypic female may indicate 45,X/46,XX mosaicism.

The X-chromatin test is valuable for studying individuals with aberrant sexual development. However, it is exceedingly important that the technique be precise so that the results are accurate. Originally, skin biopsies were used, but when it became known that cells scraped from buccal mucosa could be used, this source replaced the skin biopsy.

Although the buccal smear has been a popular method used for nuclear sexing, it is subject to errors in interpretation unless the smears are done with the greatest technical skill. The mucosa must be wiped with a piece of gauze to remove superficial dead cells before it is scraped with a metal spatula to obtain cells for analysis. Once the cells are spread on a clean glass side, they must be placed immediately into a solution of alcohol and ether, or 95% alcohol.

Despite the technical limitations, the buccal smear is useful because of the ease with which it is obtained and prepared. The procedure has enabled surveys of large numbers of individuals, thus providing data on the incidence of sex chromosome abnormalities in different populations.

Mucosal cells from the vagina may be used for X-chromatin analysis; these are best obtained from the lateral vaginal wall with a cotton-tipped applicator. The cotton applicator is rolled across a clean glass slide, which is then placed in the fixative.

DRUMSTICKS
(POLYMORPHONUCLEAR LEUKOCYTES)

Sexual dimorphism also exists in polymorphonuclear leukocytes. The drumstick (Fig. 2–7C), a small lobule on the nucleus of a polymorphonuclear leukocyte, is present if there is more than one X chromosome. As X-chromatin masses vary in size and number, relating to the X-chromosome complement, so do the drumsticks. Assaying for drumsticks is not as popular as the buccal smear assay, primarily because it is not as easy or accurate. A very large number of cells have to be examined, and the interpretations are more difficult.

Y-CHROMATIN (Y BODY)

With fluorescent stains for chromosome identification, Y chromosomes are easily seen; usually the distal part of the long arm in metaphase nuclei stains brightly (Fig. 2–1). The human Y chromosome can be identified also in interphase nuclei as a bright fluorescent body (Fig. 2–8). Thus, with special stains and fluorescence microscopy, the Y chromosome can be identified in some of the same tissues as the X-chromatin mass—buccal mucosa cells, amnion cells, and fibroblast cultures—and in spermatozoa. The number of Y bodies per nucleus equals the number of Y chromosomes.

CLINICAL GENETICS

CHROMOSOME ABNORMALITIES

The incidence of chromosome abnormalities in the newborn population is 6.5/1000. Aneuploidy and unbalanced rearrangements as a cause of congenital malformations occur in approximately 5/1000 newborns (Table 2–3).

SEX CHROMOSOME ABNORMALITIES

A gene (or genes) close to the centromere on the Y chromosome determines maleness in mammals; normally, a 46,XY chromosome constitution is associated with male gonads and genitalia. The development of normal male genitalia requires a fetal testis. Testosterone from the testes stabilizes the wolffian ducts and permits differentiation of the vas deferens, seminal vesicles, and epididymis; müllerian inhibiting factor causes the müllerian ducts to regress. Male differentiation of the external genitalia occurs under the influence of dihydrotestosterone. The male sex determinants on the Y chromosome are so strong that dysgenetic testes are produced even in individuals with an XXXY constitution. On the other hand, the existence of several conditions wherein a nonmosaic 46,-XY chromosome constitution is associated with female or intersex genitalia, with or without female internal genitalia, indicates that gene mutations may influence sex determination and sex differentiation.

While the presence of a fetal testis is essential for male differentiation, the ovary is not essential for female differentiation. Two normal X chromosomes seem to be essential for normal ovarian function. For example, ovarian tissue may differentiate in 45,X individuals and may be present early in development, but the oocytes degenerate before adulthood. A loss of even a portion of one of the X chromosomes results in gonadal dysgenesis of varying degree. Again, the presence of gonadal streaks in some inherited 46,XX disorders indicates that genes, probably both autosomal and those located on the X, affect ovarian differentiation.

The frequency of sex chromosome anomalies in a population varies with ascertainment. The study of abortuses suggests that the incidence of sex chromosome abnormalities in early embryos is about 10%. The 45,X constitution is the most common gonosomal (sex chromosomal) aneuploidy found in aborted material. In newborns, the frequency of sex chromosome abnormalities has been studied by buccal smear analyses, amniotic membrane X-chromatin examination, and chromosome analyses of lymphocyte cultures from cord blood. The overall frequency of sex chromosome abnormalities in the newborn is about 3/1000, excluding mosaicism (Table 2–4). A woman with primary amenorrhea has a one-third probability of possessing an abnormal chromosome constitution or one that disagrees with her phenotype.

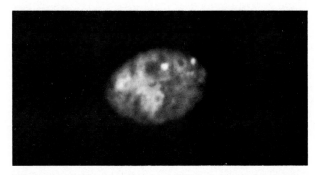

FIG. 2–8. Interphase nucleus from XYY individual, showing two fluorescent Y bodies stained with quinacrine mustard and photographed using fluorescence microscope. (Courtesy K Patau)

TABLE 2-3. OCCURRENCE OF ABNORMAL CHROMOSOME CONSTITUTION IN NEWBORN POPULATION

Type	Incidence per 1000 Newborns	Remarks
ANEUPLOIDY	4.00	See Table 2-4
*Unbalanced rearrangements**		
Centric fusion	0.20	Translocation Down's syndrome and translocation 13 trisomy
5p–	0.15	Deletion causing cri-du-chat syndrome
Other observed	0.22	
Other undetected	0.44	
Total unbalanced	1.01	
TOTAL NEWBORNS WITH CONGENITAL ANOMALIES FROM CHROMOSOME ABERRATIONS	5.01	
BALANCED REARRANGEMENTS*		
Centric fusion	0.75	
Other observed	0.58	
Other undetected	0.16	Conservative estimate
Total balanced	1.49	
TOTAL NEWBORNS WITH SUBSTANTIAL CHROMOSOMAL ABERRATIONS	6.50	

* Considering only substantial rearrangements in the sense that in the unbalanced state they would be expected to cause congenital anomalies.
(Data of K. Patau)

Aneuploidy

45,X. The 45,X sex chromosome constitution is estimated to occur in 1/3000 phenotypic females. The diagnosis may be made at birth, depending upon the presence or absence of associated nongenital anomalies. If the diagnosis is not made at birth, it frequently is made during childhood because of shortness of stature and associated anomalies. In a less affected individual, the disorder may go undiagnosed until adulthood, at which time she consults a physician because of primary amenorrhea.

The anomalies most commonly seen with a 45,X sex chromosome complement are those associated with Turner's syndrome. The patient is significantly short for her age; she often has prominent ears, a narrow highly arched palate, micrognathia, inner epicanthic folds, shortness or webbing of the neck, and a low posterior hairline. A broad chest with widely spaced nipples is also common. Cubitus valgus and hand anomalies, including a short fourth metacarpal and transversely hyperconvexed fingernails, are not uncommon. Frequently, there is an increased number of pigmented nevi. Hypertension, thyroid deficiency, diabetes mellitus, and osteoporosis are common in persons with this disorder. At puberty, secondary sexual development fails to occur. The external genitalia and müllerian ducts are female, though infantile. The gonadal tissue consists of fibrous tissue devoid of germ cells.

Urinary estrogen levels are low and vaginal smears show an atrophic patterrn. Pituitary gonadotropin levels are elevated after puberty. Growth hormone levels are normal; growth hormone administration is of no therapeutic value. Analysis for X chromatin is negative.

47,XXX. The XXX chromosome constitution occurs in 1/1000 phenotypic female newborns. Phenotypically, an XXX female is not distinguishable from a normal female. These individuals have two X-chromatin bodies in a proportion of cells. At birth the only minor anomalies seen with increased frequency are clinodactyly and epicanthic folds. As adults, some have primary and secondary amenorrhea; however, some have had children.

45,X/46,XX; 45,X/47,XXX; 45,X/46,XX/47,XXX. The phenotype associated with X chromosome mosaicism varies from typical Turner's syndrome to normal fertile femaleness. The phenotypic effects depend upon the distribution of the 45,X and 46,XX cells early in development and upon the time of appearance of the 45,X cell line. The physician may be alerted to the possibility of X chromosome mosaicism by a low percentage of X-chromatin-positive nuclei.

47,XXY. The most common chromosome constitution of patients with Klinefelter's syndrome is 47,XXY. It occurs in about 1/800 male newborns. Phenotypically, this syndrome is characterized by male internal and external genitalia, small testes, eunuchoid body proportions, and gynecomastia in adulthood. Microscopic

TABLE 2-4. CONDITIONS CAUSED BY ABNORMAL CHROMOSOME NUMBERS

Type of Chromosomal Aberration*	Incidence per 1000 Newborns	Clinical Name	Remarks and Description
POLYPLOIDY			
Triploidy 69			Aborted (4% of spontaneous abortions) except for extremely rare live-born diploid/triploid mosaics
Tetraploidy 92			Aborted (0.5% of spontaneous abortions)
ANEUPLOIDY			
Gonosomal			
45,X	0.15	Turner's syndrome	Typically short stature, webbed neck, undeveloped breasts, streak gonads (infertile)
45,XXX	0.71		Often normal and fertile; sometimes mentally retarded; children usually have normal chromosomes
47,XXY	0.59	Klinefelter's syndrome	Typically tall, gynecomastia; testes small and histologically abnormal (infertile); sometimes retarded and/or psychotic
47,XYY	0.77		Typically tall, fertile; range from normal to psychotic and/or retarded; children usually have normal chromosomes
Others	Very rare		Generally abnormal and retarded
Autosomal			
47,+21	1.45	21 trisomy, (Down's syndrome, mongolism)	Mentally retarded; numerous anomalies, although individually variable, usually add up to a highly characteristic picture
47,+18	0.20	18 trisomy, (Edwards' syndrome)	Severely retarded, arches on three or more fingers (100%), micrognathia (97%), failure to thrive (97%), flexion deformity of fingers (94%), numerous other anomalies
47,+13	0.13	13 trisomy (Patau's syndrome)	Severely retarded, eye defect (94%), polydactyly (75%), cleft palate (72%), numerous other anomalies
Other trisomies			Practically always lethal
Any monosomy			Practically always lethal
Double aneuploidy	Very rare		For example, 48,XXY,+21
TOTAL ANEUPLOIDY	4.00		

* Mosaicism (mixoploidy) excluded unless stated otherwise.

examination of the testes shows hyalinized seminiferous tubules lined by Sertoli cells. Leydig cells are clumped; spermatogenesis rarely occurs. Pituitary gonadotropin levels are usually elevated. Buccal smear demonstrates X chromatin.

Klinefelter's syndrome with 48,XXXY or a 49,XXXXY chromosome constitution has been described. The developmental abnormalities are more severe with increasing numbers of X chromosomes. Some 6%–10% of oligospermic or azoospermic men may have variants of the XXY chromosome constitution.

45,X/46,XY. The phenotype associated with Y chromosome mosaicism ranges from normal male capable of reproduction through incomplete masculinization manifested as intersexuality to Turner's syndrome.

The 45,X/46,XY sex chromosome constitution is most commonly seen in mixed gonadal dysgenesis (sometimes called asymmetric gonadal dysgenesis). In this disorder, internal genitalia include a uterus, usually with a dysgenetic testis on one side and a streak gonad on the other. Because there is an increased risk of neoplastic degeneration in such gonads, they should be removed.

47,XYY. The 47,XYY chromosome constitution is found in about 1/700 male newborns. First noted with increased frequency among individuals in prisons and in mental hospitals, it was thought to be associated with deviant behavior. Other persons with XYY sex chromosome constitution appear normal, however. There is no XYY syndrome clearly discernible at birth; this condition can be diagnosed only if chromosome studies are performed. As adults, these individuals are generally taller than normal and may have poor coordination and mild facial asymmetry. Most have normal sexual development. A few individuals have been reported with 48,XYYY and 49,XYYYY chromosome constitutions. Like other instances of increasing aneuploidy, these are associated with more severe developmental defects.

Structural Abnormalities of the X Chromosome

In general, the phenotypic expression of X chromosome structural abnormalities depends upon the location and amount of X chromosome lost. Whereas the loss of any part or all of the arms of an X chromosome

is associated with gonadal dysgenesis of varying degree, the Turner phenotype is usually associated with loss of a portion or all of the short arm. Structural abnormalities can occur as a single cell line, but commonly occur with a 45,X cell line; the presence of the 45,X cell line frequently influences the phenotypic expression.

i (Xq) (Long Arm Isochromosome). The most common structural abnormality of the X chromosome is the long arm isochromosome, either as a single cell line or combined with a 45,X cell line. The patient manifests many of the anomalies commonly seen with Turner's syndrome—short stature, skeletal abnormalities, primary amenorrhea. As expected, the X-chromatin mass is larger than normal.

Xp− (Short Arm Deletion). Deletion of the short arm of the X chromosome can occur as a single cell line, but is commonly combined with a 45,X cell line. The individual with a nonmosaic short arm deletion is short of stature and shows anomalies associated with Turner's syndrome. Phenotypically, an individual who lacks the entire short arm of one X chromosome is indistinguishable from a 45,X individual.

Xq− (Long Arm Deletion). Deletion of the long arm of the X chromosome is less likely to be associated with short stature and/or Turner-syndrome-like effects. The phenotype of individuals with Xq− ranges from Turner-like to normal femaleness, except for nondevelopment of secondary sex characteristics. The Turner-like anomalies may be due to an unidentified second 45,X cell line.

r(X) (Ring X Chromosome). The phenotypic effect of a ring X chromosome depends in part upon the size of the missing segments and in part on whether the deletion affects primarily the long arm or the short arm. If a large portion is missing from the short arm, the phenotype is apt to be similar to that of Turner's syndrome.

X Translocations. Translocations between two X chromosomes and between an X and an autosome have been described. Though carriers of balanced translocations between two autosomes are phenotypically normal, individuals with balanced X/autosome translocations have been described with primary amenorrhea and lack of secondary sex characteristics. In some cases, the carrier is fertile, and in general such carriers have few if any extragenital anomalies.

With unbalanced X/autosome translocations, the phenotype varies, depending upon whether X chromosomal or autosomal material is deleted. If autosomal material is deleted, rather severe developmental defects are present; the phenotype associated with X-chromosome deletion depends upon the size of the deleted segment and whether it is from the long or short arm.

AUTOSOMAL ABNORMALITIES

Because a number of autosomal abnormalities occur fairly frequently, it is important that the physician be ble to recognize them (Table 2–4).

21 Trisomy (Down's Syndrome)

Down's syndrome was first described in 1886 by Langdon Down, who noted that it is associated with mental retardation and mongoloid facies. In 1959, Lejeune made the significant discovery that it is associated with a trisomy.

Down's syndrome occurs in approximately 1/800 liveborn infants. The risk of having a child with Down's syndrome increases with maternal but not with paternal age. The risk for women in the 15- to 19-year-old age group is 1/2300, while the risk for women over 45 years of age is 20/1000 (1/46).

Some 95% of individuals with Down's syndrome have 21 trisomy; a translocation between chromosome 21 and another chromosome accounts for some 5%. The latter usually involves a translocation between one of the D-group chromosomes (usually 14) and 21, but may involve the other D-group chromosomes (Table 2–5). If there is maternal transmission of 14/21 translocation, the chance of producing a child with Down's syndrome is approximately 8–10%. If there is paternal transmission, the chance of producing an affected child is less than 5%. Carriers of 21/22 balanced translocations produce both normal and affected offspring. There are insufficient data to give the exact risk for an abnormal child from such a union, but obviously very few affected offspring are produced. A carrier for a translocation between two 21 chromosomes produces gametes that are either disomic or nullisomic for this chromosome. The zygotes are either trisomic or monosomic for 21. All liveborns from such a mating are trisomic and have Down's syndrome; the monosomic zygotes are aborted.

Down's syndrome is characterized by mental retardation, habitually open mouth with a protruding tongue, small teeth, oblique palpebral fissures with inner epicanthic folds, Brushfield spots, small or absent earlobes, flat occiput and flat nasal bridge, short broad hands with short fingers, and clinodactyly. There is a wide space between the first and second toes. Affected children have marked hypotonia, and the newborns lack a Moro reflex. Ventricular septal defects occur, and individuals with Down's syndrome are often troubled by respiratory illness. Dermatoglyphic examination shows simian palmar creases, distal axial triradius, and increased numbers of loops instead of whorls and arches on the fingertips.

TABLE 2-5. GENETIC RISK FOR OFFSPRING OF CARRIERS OF CENTRIC FUSION DISORDERS

| Type of Translocation in Carrier | Liveborn Children of Carrier | | Afflicted with Translocation Trisomy |
| | Phenotypically Normal | | |
	Chromosomally Normal	Carrier	
t (DqDq)*			
13/14 (usual)			<1%
13/15 (rare)	About 2/5	About 3/5	
14/15 (rare)			0
t (Dq21q)†			
Carrier: Mother	Almost 1/2	Almost 1/2	10%–15%
Carrier: Father	Almost 1/2	Almost 1/2	<5%
t (21q22q)‡			
Carrier: Mother	Almost 1/2	Almost 1/2	2/14
Carrier: Father	Almost 1/2	Almost 1/2	1/13

* Incidence: 0.46/1000 births
† Incidence: 0.23/1000 births
‡ Incidence: 0.06/1000 births
(Data of K Patau)

18 Trisomy (Edwards' Syndrome)

In 1960, the 18 trisomy syndrome was described. It is the second most common autosomal trisomy found among liveborn infants, occurring in 1/5000 to 1/8000 live births. The maternal age factor is not as marked as in 21 trisomy, although the mean maternal age is slightly elevated to around 32 years. There is a 3:1 female/male predilection possibly caused by prenatal death of males.

The clinical features of 18 trisomy include failure to thrive, developmental retardation, an elongated skull with lowset and malformed ears, micrognathia, and a shield-shaped chest and a very short sternum. There is a flexion deformity of the fingers. Congenital heart disease is common, primarily ventricular septal defect and patent ductus. Dermatoglyphic examination reveals essentially simple arches on all or nearly all of the fingertips. It is not uncommon for newborns with 18 trisomy to be postmature, although the mean birth weight is less than 2300 g. Mean survival time is about 70 days.

13 Trisomy (Patau's Syndrome)

First described in 1960, 13 trisomy is the third most common trisomy syndrome known, occurring in 1/8000 liveborns (0.13/1000). As is true of most trisomy syndromes, the mean age for mothers of infants with 13 trisomy is somewhat elevated, to about 32 years.

Some 75% of cases are caused by primary nondisjunction. In the remainder, the extra chromosome is translocated to another chromosome, usually another of the D group.

Clinical features include low birth weight, developmental retardation, microcephaly, cleft palate and cleft lip, microphthalmus, colobomas, malformed ears and presumed deafness, capillary hemangiomas, polydactyly, and hyperconvexed nails. Dermatoglyphic examination shows a single palmar crease and distal axial triradius. Congenital heart defect, including atrial septal defect, patent ductus, and ventricular septal defect, occurs in some 80% of the cases. The mean survival time of an infant with the 13 trisomy syndrome is 90 days. Generally, the pregnancy is normal.

5p− Syndrome (Cri-du-Chat)

Described in 1963, 5p− syndrome is caused by deletion of part of the short arm of chromosome 5. Clinical features include low birth weight; failure to thrive; developmental and mental retardation; ocular hypertelorism; epicanthic folds; hypotonia; round, moonlike face; lowset ears; and strabismus. A distinctive, high-pitched cry at birth accounts for the name, "cat-cry syndrome." The characteristic cry disappears later in life, at which time detection of the abnormality is based on physical appearance and mental retardation. Females are affected more often than males, and the infants are born at term. Generally, the mean ages of the parents are normal.

4p− Syndrome

The deletion of part of the short arm of chromosome 4 produces the 4p− syndrome, which was described in 1965. It is far less common than the 5p− syndrome, but the patient is more severely malformed. The syn-

drome is often characterized by microcephaly, ocular hypertelorism, strabismus, ptosis, cleft lip and palate, and micrognathia. There is severe psychomotor and growth retardation. Congenital heart malformations are not uncommon and may cause death early in the first year of life. Birth weight is commonly less than 1 kg, even though delivery occurs at term.

MENDELIAN DISORDERS AFFECTING GENITAL DEVELOPMENT

Abnormalities of sexual differentiation occur as a result of single gene mutations on an autosome, X chromosome, or both. Though many of these patients show intersex external genitalia, some have essentially normal female external genitalia. It is not uncommon for the latter group to go undiagnosed until puberty, at which time aberrant sexual characteristics cause them to seek medical attention.

FEMINIZING TESTIS SYNDROME (TESTICULAR FEMINIZATION)

Feminizing testis syndrome (FTS) is the most common and the best known of the XY female syndromes. Except in those few individuals whose family history suggests the condition or who are seen with an inguinal hernia containing a testis early in life, the disorder often is not diagnosed until puberty. Classically, there are no extragenital malformations. At puberty, body proportions become eunuchoid. Breast development is excellent (see Fig. 46–5); axillary and pubic hair is usually absent or scanty. Primary amenorrhea is present in all patients with FTS. The external genitalia are female, but the vagina ends blindly at varying depths. There is no uterus. Müllerian duct derivatives, if they exist at all, are fibromuscular vestiges. The testes, which may be intraabdominal or in an inguinal position, are accompanied by extremely hypoplastic wolffian duct structures. Though the testes may appear grossly and histologically normal in infants, spermatogonia gradually vanish and tubular adenomas with Leydig cell hyperplasia and degenerative changes of the tubular walls become evident with increasing age.

Persons with FTS are able to synthesize and maintain normal male levels of testosterone. Excretion of 17-ketosteroids is normal or slightly elevated, and urinary estrogen levels are within normal adult range for males.

The testes in individuals with FTS possess a neoplastic potential that increases with age. Investigators agree that the threat of neoplastic change in the gonads is sufficient to warrant orchiectomy. Since the risk of neoplasia is low prior to 20–30 years of age, some physicians think the testes should not be removed until after feminization is complete. Others prefer to perform the orchiectomy early in childhood. The latter approach mandates estrogen replacement therapy as the individual approaches puberty.

Affected individuals have a 46,XY chromosome constitution. "Sisters" and maternal "aunts" may be affected. The disorder is inherited as an X-linked recessive mutation. Future apparent sisters of an affected individual have a one-third chance of being XY.

INCOMPLETE FEMINIZING TESTIS SYNDROME (INCOMPLETE TESTICULAR FEMINIZATION)

Incomplete FTS is a distinct syndrome from FTS. At puberty, individuals with incomplete FTS feminize, *i.e.*, develop breasts, yet the external genitalia show evidence of virilization characterized by clitoral enlargement and partial labioscrotal fusion. Like patients with FTS, these individuals have bilateral testes, no müllerian derivatives, blindly ending vagina, and pubertal breast development. The disorder is inherited in X-linked fashion.

XY PURE GONADAL (TESTICULAR) DYSGENESIS (SWYER SYNDROME)

Characterized by female phenotype and 46,XY chromosome constitution, pure gonadal dysgenesis has been described in both XX and XY individuals. The terms XY pure gonadal (testicular) dysgenesis and Swyer syndrome identify the condition in XY individuals. These individuals have normal female external and internal genitalia, except for the gonads, and have no unusual extragenital anomalies; they have normal intelligence. They are usually of normal height with more or less eunuchoid body proportions. The disorder is characterized by severe early testicular dysgenesis, which results in streak gonads that are devoid of germ cells but sometimes contain undifferentiated hilar mesonephric cells and tissue capable of undergoing neoplasia. Hilar cells may, at times, respond to gonadotropins by androgen production and subsequent clitoral enlargement. Urinary gonadotropin levels are increased after puberty, and 17-ketosteroid levels are low or normal, except in patients with virilization. In the latter, elevated urinary levels of testosterone and 17-ketosteroids have been documented.

Neoplasia can occur in the streak gonads of individuals with XY pure gonadal (testicular) dysgenesis. The risk of gonadal neoplasm begins earlier and appears to be greater than in FTS, and it is recommended that the gonads be removed as soon as possible. Estrogen replacement is indicated to induce female secondary sexual characteristics; it may be given cyclically to induce regular uterine bleeding.

XY pure gonadal (testicular) dysgenesis usually

occurs sporadically, but the syndrome has been reported in sisters and in several sibships of a single family. The disorder appears to be inherited either as an X-linked recessive or as an autosomal dominant gene limited in expression to the male sex, but genetic data presently available to do not exclude the possibility that an autosomal recessive gene produces this disorder.

OTHER XY SYNDROMES

Other, very rare, XY syndromes are associated with primary amenorrhea. An example is pseudovaginal perineoscrotal hypospadias (PPSH). Phenotypically, the syndrome is associated with few, if any, extragenital anomalies, but the patient usually has intersex external genitalia and undergoes masculinization at puberty. The PPSH phenotype may occasionally result from a deficiency of 5α-reductase, the enzyme required for conversion of testosterone to dihydrotestosterone. Another XY syndrome is true agonadism, or XY gonadal agenesis. This condition is characterized by female phenotype; lack of secondary sexual characteristics; female external genitalia; and absence of uterus, vagina, and gonads. It is extremely rare.

XX PURE GONADAL (OVARIAN) DYSGENESIS

Persons with XX pure gonadal (ovarian) dysgenesis are characterized by normal, though somewhat eunuchoid growth, normal intelligence, no extragenital anomalies, lack of secondary sexual characteristics, normal external genitalia, uterus, fallopian tubes, and streak gonads. The streak gonads are usually found at the time of laparoscopy or laparotomy during the investigation for primary amenorrhea and lack of secondary sexual development. Though most reported cases are sporadic, in some instance more than one member of a family has been affected. Available data suggest autosomal recessive inheritance.

TRUE HERMAPHRODITISM

True hermaphroditism implies the presence, in one individual, of both testicular and ovarian tissue. Such an individual may have a testis on one side and an ovary on the other side, an ovotestis bilaterally, or an ovotestis on one side and a testis or an ovary on the other side. Some true hermaphrodites are reared as males; others, as females. The external genitalia tend to be ambiguous. In most cases, there is a uterus and a vagina, which may open into the perineum or into a urogenital sinus. The presence of an ovotestis or pure ovary on a side, determines the extent of differentiation of the fallopian tube. At the time of puberty, depending on the sex of rearing, there may be virilization of a female or feminization of a male.

Therapy is directed toward inducing secondary sexual development to coincide with the sex of rearing. For a male, this includes mastectomy; removal of internal genitalia if there are uterus, fallopian tubes, and ovaries; and efforts toward construction of male external genitalia. If the sex of rearing is female, testicular tissue must be removed and external genitalia constructed to make a sexually functional female.

The most common sex chromosome constitution found in true hermaphroditism is XX; a 46,XY chromosome constitution occurs in some. The finding of three XX true hermaphrodites in one sibship suggests that, at least in some cases, true hermaphroditism is due to a gene mutation. Though XY true hermaphroditism is far less common than the XX type, one instance of familial occurrence has been reported.

ADRENOGENITAL SYNDROME

Adrenogenital syndrome in genetic females is the single most common cause of intersex genitalia in newborns. The mode of inheritance is autosomal recessive. The degree of virilization varies from clitoral hypertrophy to a phalluslike clitoris with a penile urethra. The disorder may be caused by 21-hydroxylase deficiency, 11-β-hydroxylase deficiency, or 3-β-hydroxysteroid dehydrogenase deficiency. Elevated levels of urinary 17-ketosteroids and pregnanetriol are diagnostic. Steroid therapy is simple, may be lifesaving, and will confer normal fertility in affected adults.

GENETICS OF SPONTANEOUS ABORTIONS

The probability that a clinically recognized pregnancy will end in spontaneous abortion is estimated at between 10% and 20%. It has long been thought that the usual cause of fetal death is an abnormality of development. Reports by Hertig and collaborators confirm this. In a study of 1000 spontaneous abortions, an empty embryonic sac was found in 49% of cases, embryos with localized anomalies occurred in 3.2%, and placental abnormalities in 9.6%. Of 34 human embryos less than 17 days of age obtained from uteri removed for medical reasons, 10 showed major abnormalities. Improved technical capability and the burst of interest in cytogenetics resulted in several reports of chromosomally abnormal abortuses. In most instances, the parents of chromosomally abnormal abortuses are chromosomally normal, and the offsprings' abnormalities occur in an unpredictable and sporadic manner. In a small percentage of cases, one member of the couple is a carrier of a balanced translocation. Offspring of these parents may be repeatedly aborted.

CHROMOSOMALLY NORMAL PARENTS

Cytogenetic studies of spontaneously aborted fetuses of chromosomally normal parents show that the incidence of chromosome anomalies varies with the gestational age of the abortus. Depending upon the study, at 4 weeks' gestational age some 75% of abortuses have an abnormal chromosome constitution; at 5–8 weeks, 50%–60%; at 9–12 weeks, 5%–20%. The overall incidence of chromosomally abnormal fetuses is estimated to be about 35%.

Automosomal trisomy occurs in some 40%–50% of chromosomally abnormal specimens and is the most common abnormality found in abortuses. Of the autosomal trisomies, trisomy E (most commonly 16 trisomy), trisomy D, and trisomy G occur in descending frequencies. Some 20% of abortuses have a 45,X chromosome constitution. This is the most common single chromosome abnormality found in aborted specimens. Triploidy is the next most common abnormality found in abortuses. Triploidy is compatible with greater fetal development than tetraploidy, which is also found in aborted material.

CHROMOSOMALLY ABNORMAL PARENTS

Cytogenetic studies have been performed in couples with a history of recurrent abortions or infertility. Though chromosome translocations may not be one of the most common causes of recurrent abortions, in some 3%–6% of couples with such a history, a balanced chromosome translocation exists in one member and is the most probable cause of the repeated early fetal losses.

Chromosome abnormality is not the only genetic aberration that can cause fetal death. X-linked lethal genes in a male or homozygosity for recessively lethal genes in either sex may be the cause.

PRENATAL DIAGNOSIS OF GENETIC DISEASE

HISTORY

Improvements in many cytogenetic and tissue culture techniques, and the widespread acceptance of amniocentesis as a diagnostic aid, have allowed the prenatal detection of many inborn errors of metabolism and of chromosome abnormalities.

As early as 1955, investigators started prenatal sex determination based on the presence of X chromatin in the nuclei of amniotic fluid cells. In 1965, adrenogenital syndrome was diagnosed in an unborn infant by measuring the levels of 17-ketosteroids and pregnanetriol in amniotic fluid obtained in the 39th week of gestation. Not until 1966, however, was the technique

of amniotic fluid cell culture described. Not every laboratory is equipped to do every assay, however. The National Foundation March of Dimes *International Directory of Genetic Services* provides a list of laboratories and their diagnostic capabilities.

The number of disorders that can be diagnosed prenatally is increasing.

TECHNIQUE

Amniocentesis for the purpose of prenatal detection of an inherited disorder is usually performed at 14–16 weeks' gestation, earlier than for Rh alloimmunization. It is done on an outpatient basis. Ultrasonography is used prior to amniocentesis to localize the placenta and fetus. If the placenta is located anteriorly, the risk of fetomaternal bleeding is about 10%. Approximately 10–20 ml fluid are obtained and sent to the laboratory for culture or analysis. The transabdominal route is used instead of the transvaginal route to avoid the risk of infection and the chance of contaminating the specimens. The laboratory time needed to make the diagnosis depends upon the type of analysis to be performed; usually 2–6 weeks are required.

RISKS

Risks of amniocentesis include infection, hemorrhage, fetal damage or abortion, Rh alloimnunization, and possible long-term deleterious effects on the development of the fetus. It appears that there are no statistically significant differences in fetal loss, perinatal problems, birth weights, neonatal complications, or birth defects between pregnant women undergoing second trimester amniocentesis and a group of controls. The overall fetal loss, including abortions and stillbirths was 3.5% for amniocentesis cases and 3.2% in the control pregnancies. When all serious complications are considered, the risks to the pregnancy, fetus, newborn, or infant are approximately 0.5%.

INDICATIONS

Amniocentesis is indicated when the family history suggests that one parent has, or may be a carrier of, a disorder that has a chromosomal or biochemical etiology and for which tests on the amniotic fluid or cultured amniotic fluid cells yield definitive results. For example, severely handicapping autosomal recessive inherited disorders, such as Tay–Sachs disease, Pompe's disease, and Hurler's syndrome, in which the possibility of an abnormal child from normal carrier parents is 25%, are considered to be of high risk, and amniocentesis is indicated. X-linked conditions, such as Lesch–Nyhan's disease and certain of the muscular dystrophies, in which 50% of the male children of

carrier mothers are affected, are also considered high risk. In Lesch–Nyhan's disease and some other X-linked disorders, amniocentesis can provide information, not only about sex, but also whether the male fetus is affected or the female is a carrier. In some X-linked disorders amniocentesis cannot provide a specific diagnosis, only information about the sex of the baby.

Prenatal investigation is also recommended for situations in which the risk of an abnormal child, although low compared with a risk of X-linked or autosomal recessive inherited disorder, is still greater than the risk of fetal abnormalilties in the general population. Such situations include one parent who is a carrier for a balanced translocation, maternal age over 35 years, previous birth of a child with Down's syndrome or any other trisomy syndrome (1%–2% risk), and previous production of a child with a neural tube defect, such as meningomyelocele or anencephaly.

Prenatal genetic diagnosis is performed to forewarn the parents of the presence of the disorder so that they may either choose abortion or make arrangements for the baby's care. In some centers, genetic studies of amniotic fluid are performed only if the patient agrees in advance to abortion if a significant abnormality is found. Many physicians consider this position much too rigid and defer to the wishes of parents who reject abortion but wish to be informed so they can make whatever adjustment and preparation are needed in advance of the baby's arrival.

LIMITATIONS OF THE TECHNIQUE

Prior to performing amniocentesis, it is important to discuss with the couple considering prenatal diagnosis not only the procedure and its hazards, but also its limitations. Rarely, attempts to obtain a viable cell culture are unsuccessful. Minor chromosome abnormalities may not be detected. Diagnosing metabolic disorders on the basis of cultured or uncultured amniotic fluid cells is still somewhat experimental. To ensure accuracy in diagnosis, a nonsuspect amniotic fluid sample of about the same gestation age is cultured and analyzed simultaneously with the specimen suspected of abnormality. Anomalies such as cleft palate or cleft lip cannot be detected by amniocentesis or by chromosome analysis. In multiple gestation, if undetected, the diagnosis may be made on only one fetus.

BENEFITS OF THE TECHNIQUE

Before amniocentesis and prenatal diagnosis became available, couples had to choose whether to proceed with a pregnancy on the basis of risk figures determined from the suspected mode of inheritance of the disease: 50% chance of an affected offspring in autosomal dominant inheritance; 25% chance in autosomal recessive inheritance. In some instances, such as chromosomal translocation, the choice had to be based on empiric risk figures ascertained from families known to have similar abnormalities. Under these conditions, some couples elected not to take the risk and either avoided pregnancy or sought abortion when indeed the fetus may have been normal. Prenatal diagnosis allows the parents to seek abortion only when the infant is known to be affected; the risk of aborting an unaffected infant is reduced to zero.

GENETIC COUNSELING

The aim of genetic counseling is to explain the risk of producing an affected child, to convey the prognosis, and to inform individuals seeking counseling of alternatives for dealing with the risk. Most persons seeking genetic counseling have already had an abnormal child, but as the capability to detect carriers increases, couples will seek counseling prior to any pregnancy.

The prerequisites for genetic counseling include 1) accurate diagnosis, 2) knowledge of the mode of transmission of the disorder, 3) knowledge of the recurrence risk, and 4) insight into the variations of the disease and its prognosis. A correct diagnosis is the single most important prerequisite of genetic counseling. In some instances, the diagnosis is obvious by physical examination; in others, certain biochemical tests are needed; and in some, the diagnosis is not readily made. Persons in the last group are commonly referred to a genetic counselor or counseling center. Often it is only at such a center that a diagnosis can be made, because the counselor has access to diagnostic expertise in pediatrics, neurology, ophthalmology, cardiology, and other disciplines in medicine. Also, individuals expert in syndrome identification and diagnosis are usually located at genetic centers where intensive research into the etiology and epidemiology of birth defects continues.

When an accurate diagnosis has been established, determining the mode of inheritance for a condition due to a single-gene mutation ordinarily presents no problems. Some 2000 disorders due to autosomal dominant, autosomal recessive, and X-linked mutations have been catalogued by McKusick. For those disorders that are rare or unknown to the counselor, the recently published *Birth Defects Atlas and Compendium* is available. This volume describes a large number of malformation syndromes and lists pertinent information about each disorder. Though a detailed family history through three generations should be done in all cases, it is of particular use in those rare disorders where the recurrence risk is unknown. Frequently, a detailed family history elucidates not only the mode of inheritance, but also the risk to the individuals.

Once the diagnosis is known and the mode of trans-

mission determined, recurrence risks can be calculated. For those disorders due to single-gene mutations, the risk for recurrence ranges from 25% for autosomal recessive disorders to 50% for autosomal dominant disorders (Table 2–2). For the common multifactorial conditions such as cleft lip, cleft palate, and anencephaly, empiric risks have been established based on the analysis of a great number of large pedigrees. Risk figures for a specific disorder can be obtained from the literature; most are 2%–5%. This is also true of the multiple congenital anomaly/mental retardation syndromes of the sporadic "idiopathic" type. Recurrence risks for chromosome abnormalities vary from approximately 2% for trisomy Down's syndrome to 100% for a balanced 21/21 translocation in one of the parents. For a balanced translocation which, individually, is so rare that empiric risks are difficult or impossible to determine, the recurrence risk is unknown. Though in such translocation cases a recurrence risk cannot be stated prior to pregnancy, prenatal diagnosis during pregnancy can determine the risk to be either 100% or 0%.

A couple's decision whether to take a risk depends to a great degree upon the burden—physical, emotional, and financial—that an affected child will be to the family. A study of groups of high-risk couples showed that for disorders associated with early death of an affected child, disorders for which treatment is available, and disorders that are relatively mild, parents were not deterred from further reproduction. When the risk of recurrence was high and the disorder severe, approximately two-thirds of parents wished no further children at the time of counseling. Thus, it is important for the adviser to know the prognosis and convey it to the family, for it plays an important role in decision making.

CONCLUSIONS

Advances in biology and medicine that allow control of reproductive capabilities, both quantitatively and now qualitatively, are frequently a cause of concern. Though this seems particularly true in the areas of genetic counseling, screening for genetic diseases, and prenatal diagnosis, it is true of other areas in gynecology and obstetrics as well, *e.g.,* sterilization, artificial insemination, and abortion. In all these areas, there is little need for concern if decision making remains an individual choice; when this choice is lost, all humanity should be concerned.

REFERENCES AND RECOMMENDED READING

Apgar V (ed): Down's syndrome (mongolism). Ann NY Acad Sci 177:303–388, 1970

Barr ML, Bertram EG: A morphological distinction between neurones of the male and female, and the behavior of the nucleolar satellite during accelerated nucleoprotein synthesis. Nature 163:676–677, 1949

Bartsch FK, Lundberg J, Wahlström J: The technique, results and risks of amniocentesis for genetic reasons. J Obstet Gynaecol Br Commonw 81:991, 174

Bergsma D (ed): Birth Defects: Atlas and Compendium. Baltimore, Williams & Wilkins, 1973

Bergsma D, Lynch HT, Thomas RJ et al (eds): Birth Defects: International Directory of Genetic Services, 4th ed. New York, National Foundation March of Dimes, 1974

Carr DH: Genetic basis of abortion. Annu Rev Genet 5:65–80, 1971

Carter CO, Roberts JAF, Evans KA et al: Genetic clinic: A follow up. Lancet 1:281–285, 1971

Caspersson T, Zech L, Johansson C et al: Identification of human chromosomes by DNA-binding fluorescing agents. Chromosomes 30:215–227, 1970

Chicago Conference, Standardization in Human Cytogenetics. Birth Defects. Orig Art Ser II, 2. New York, National Foundation March of Dimes, 1966

DeMars R, Nance WE: Electrophoretic variants of glucose-6-phosphate dehydrogenase and the single-active-X in cultivated human cells. Wistar Inst Symp Monogr 1:35–48, 1964

Denver conference on proposed standard system of nomenclature of human mitotic chromosomes. Lancet 1:1063–1065, 1960

Edwards JH, Harnden D, Cameron A et al: A new trisomic syndrome, Lancet 1:787, 1960

Fairweather DVI, Eshes TKAB (eds): Amniotic Fluid: Research and Clinical Application. Amsterdam, Exerpta Medica, 1973

Ford EHR: Human Chromosomes. New York, Academic Press, 1973

Frøland A: Klinefelter's syndrome: Clinical, endocrinological and cytological studies. Dan Med Bull (Suppl 6) 16:1–108, 1969

Fuchs F, Riis P: Antenatal sex determination. Nature (Lond) 177:330, 1956

Fuhrmann W, Vogel F: Genetic Counselling: A Guide for the Practicing Physician. New York, Springer–Verlag, 1969

Golus M, Laughman W, Epstein CJ et al: Prenatal genetic diagnosis in 3000 amniocenteses. N Engl J Med 300:157–163, 1979

Hammerton JL: Human Cytogenetics, Vol I, General Cytogenetics. New York, Academic Press, 1971

Hamerton JL: Human Cytogenetics, Vol II, Clinical Cytogenetics, New York, Academic Press, 1971

Hertig AT, Rock J, Adams EC et al: Thirty-four fertilized human ova, good, bad and indifferent, received from 210 women of known fertility: A study of biological wastage in early human pregnancy. Pediatrics 23:202–211, 1959

Hertig AT, Sheldon WH: Minimal criteria required to prove prima facie case of traumatic abortion or miscarriage: An analysis of 1000 spontaneous abortions. Ann Surg 117:596–606, 1943

Hirschorn K, Cooper HL, Firschein I: Deletion of short arms of chromosome 4–5 in a child with defects of midline fusion. Hum Genet 1:479–482, 1965

Hook EB, Lindsjö A: Down's syndrome in live births by single year maternal age interval in a Swedish study: Comparison with results from a New York state study. Am J Hum Genet 30:19–27, 1978

International System for Human Cytogenetics Nomenclature. The National Foundation, S. Karger, 1978

Jeffcoate TNA, Fliegner JRH, Russell SH et al: Diagnosis of the adrenogenital syndrome before birth. Lancet 2:553–555, 1965

Kaveggia EG, Durkin MV, Pendleton E, et al: Diagnostic/genetic studies on 1224 patients with severe mental retardation. Proceedings of the Third Int Cong of the International Assn for Scientific Study of Mental Deficiency. The Hague, 1973

Khudi G: Cytogenetics of habitual abortion: A review, Obstet Gynecol Surv 29:299–310, 1974

Langdon Down J: Observations in an ethnic classification of idiots. Lond Hosp Clin Lect Rep 3:259–262, 1866

Lejeune J: Le mongolisme: Premier exemple d'aberration autosimpique humaine. Ann Gen 1:41–49, 1959

Lejeune J, Lafourcade J, Berger R etal: Trois cas de deletion partielle du bras court d'un chromosome 5. C R Acad Sci Paris 257:3098–3102, 1963

London conference on normal human karyotype. Cytogenetics 2:264–268, 1963

Lyon MF: Gene action in the X chromosome of the mouse. Nature 190:372–373, 1961

McKusick V: Mendelian Inheritance in Man. Baltimore, Johns Hopkins Press, 1971

Milunsky A: The Prenatal Diagnosis of Hereditary Disorders. Springfield, Ill, Thomas, 1973

Milunsky A, Atkins L: Prenatal diagnosis of genetic disorders: An analysis of experience with 600 cases, JAMA 230:232–235, 1974

Mittwoch U: Genetics of Sex Differentiation. New York, Academic Press, 1973

Nielson J: Klinefelter's syndrome and the XYY syndrome: Genetical, endocrinological and psychiatric-psychological study of thirty-three severely hypogonadal male patients and two patients with karyotype 47,XYY. Acta Psychiat Scand, Suppl 209, 1971

Ohno S, Kaplan WD, Kinosita R: Formation of the sex chromatin by a single X-chromosome in liver cells of *Rattus nurvegicus*. Exp Cell Res 18:415–418, 1959

Opitz JM, Simpson JL, Sarto G et al: Pseudovaginal perineoscrotal hypospadias. Clin Genet 3:1–26, 1971

Paris Conference, Standardization in Human Cytogenetics. Birth Defects. Orig Art Ser VIII, 7. New York, National Foundation March of Dimes, 1972

Patau K, Smith D, Therman EM et al: Multiple congenital anomaly caused by an extra autosome. Lancet 1:790–793, 1960

Penrose, LS, Smith GF: Down's Anomaly. Boston, Little, Brown, 1966

Race RR: Is the Xg blood group subject to inactivation? Proceedings, Fourth Congress on Human Genetics. Amsterdam, Exerpta Medica, 1973

Robinson A, Puck TT: Studies on chromosomal nondisjunction in man. II. Am J Hum Genet 19:112–119, 1967

Russell LB: Genetics of mammalian sex chromosomes. Science 133:1795–1803, 1961

Sarto GE: Cytogenetics of fifty patients with primary amenorrhea. Am J Obstet Gynecol 119:14–23, 1974

Sarto GE, Opitz JM: The XY gonadal agenesis syndrome. J Med Genet 10:288–293, 1973

Sarto GE, Therman E, Patua K: X inactivation in man: A woman with t(Xq−; 12q+). Am J Hum Genet 25:262–270, 1973

Simpson JL, Christakos AC (eds): Genetics for the obstetrician–gynecologist. Clin Obstet Gynecol 15:107–282, 1972

Steele MW, Breg WR: Chromosome analysis of human amniotic fluid cells. Lancet 1:383–385, 1966

Thompson JS, Thompson MW: Genetics in Medicine. Philadelphia, Saunders, 1973

Van Niekerk WA: True Hermaphroditism: Clinical, Morphologic and Cytogenetic Aspects. Hagerstown, Md, Harper & Row, 1974

Williams DL, Runyan JWJ: Sex chromatin and chromosome analysis in the diagnosis of sex anomalies. Ann Intern Med 64:422–459, 1966

Wolf A, Reinwein H, Porsch R. Schröter T, Baitsch H: Defizienz an den kurzen Armen eines Chromosoms Nr 4. Hum Genet 1:397–413, 1965

Yunis JJ (ed): Human Chromosome Methodology. New York, Academic Press, 1974

CHAPTER

3

GROSS ANATOMY OF THE FEMALE REPRODUCTIVE TRACT, PITUITARY, AND HYPOTHALAMUS

Roger C. Crafts
Howard P. Krieger

THE FEMALE REPRODUCTIVE TRACT*

Roger C. Crafts

The female reproductive tract consists of internal organs, located in the pelvic cavity, and the external genitalia, located in the perineum. The internal organs are the ovaries, uterine tubes, uterus, and vagina. The external genitalia consist of the mons pubis, labia majora, labia minora, the vestibule of the vagina, and related structures.

The new international terminology, introduced in 1955 and modestly revised in 1960 and 1965, has been used in this chapter, with the terms formerly used placed in parentheses.

* Portions of this chapter have been reprinted with permission from *A Textbook of Human Anatomy* by Roger C. Crafts, 2nd edition, published by John Wiley & Sons, Inc., 1979.

PELVIC CAVITY

BONY STRUCTURES

Before the pelvic cavity and perineum can be understood, it is mandatory that one be thoroughly familiar with the bones that form the pelvis. The bony pelvis is made up of the two coxal (innominate) bones which are actually part of the lower limbs, and the sacrum and coccyx, which are parts of the axial skeleton.

Since the shape of a coxal bone is almost indescribable, the following description will be more comprehensible if a model of a bony pelvis is at hand. Care should be taken to hold the pelvis in the position found in the living human body.

Coxal Bones

The coxal bones are made up of three parts: *ilium, ischium,* and *pubis* (Fig. 3–1). The ilium is the wing-shaped superior portion of the coxal bone; the ischium, the short, blunt posteroinferior portion; and the pubis, the anterior inferior portion. These three bones come together at the *acetabulum,* the fossa that articulates with the head of the femur.

On the internal surface of the coxal bone, the *ilium* articulates inferiorly with the pubis and the ischium. This part of the coxal bone flares out into a thin, wing-like portion with a concavity on the medial surface. This concavity is the *iliac fossa.* Following this surface superiorly, one comes to the *iliac crest.* This crest starts anteriorly with the *anterior superior iliac spine* and proceeds posteriorly and laterally until it reaches the *posterior superior iliac spine;* it has an inner and outer lip and an intermediate line. In addition to these two superior spines, the ilium possesses an *anterior inferior iliac spine* and a *posterior inferior iliac spine.* The posterior inferior iliac spine is just posterior to the large surface of the ilium that articulates with the sacrum.

The superior end of the *ischium* is fused with the ilium and pubis. The ischium is the portion of the coxal bone upon which a person sits, and that roughened area located most inferiorly and posteriorly is known as the *ischial tuberosity.* Just superior to the ischial tuberosity is the *lesser ischiadic (sciatic) notch* and, separated from this notch by the *ischiadic spine,* the *greater ischiadic (sciatic) notch.*

The *pubis* articulates with the ilium and the ischium. This part of the coxal bone contains a medial portion—the *body*—and *superior* and *inferior rami.* The inferior ramus is the portion that joins the ischium, while the superior ramus joins the ilium and ischium at the acetabular notch. The superior surface of the body is smooth, while the inferior surface is quite rough because of the attachment of muscles. The articular surface is joined to the pubic bone of the

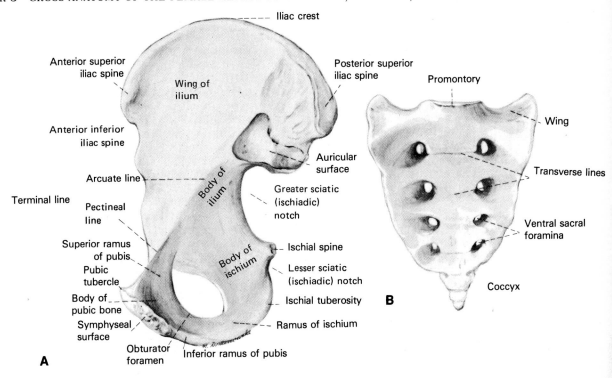

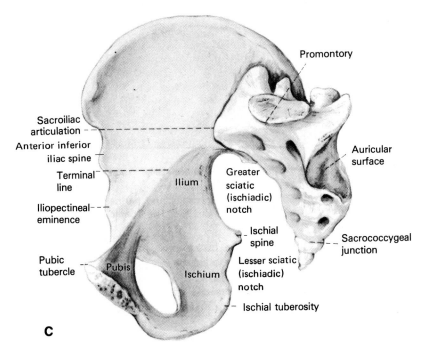

FIG. 3-1. *A.* Coxal bone, medial aspect. *B.* Sacrum, anterior aspect. *C.* Articulated right coxal bone, sacrum, and coccyx, left oblique view.

other side by a fibrocartilage as well as ligaments. The *pubic crest* is that portion of the body of the pubis that is most easily felt and ends laterally in an elevation called the *pubic tubercle*. The superior surface of the superior ramus exhibits a sharp edge called the *pectineal line*. This line runs laterally from the pubic tubercle and joins the *arcuate line* to form the *terminal line*. The two rami of the pubic bone form partial boundaries of a large opening called the *obturator foramen*. The superior edge of this foramen exhibits an *obturator tubercle* and an *obturator sulcus* for passage of vessels and nerves from the pelvis into the lower limb.

Sacrum and Coccyx

The sacral vertebrae are fused into one bone called the *sacrum* (Fig. 3–1*B*), which is broad superiorly and tapers inferiorly; it can be described as having a base superiorly and an apex inferiorly. It is concave anteriorly and convex posteriorly. On the anterior surface, a medial portion is separated from two lateral portions by four *foramina* on each side for passage of ventral rami of the sacral nerves and corresponding vessels. The median portion presents *transverse lines* that indicate the points of fusion of the five vertebrae. The lateral portions possess *articular surfaces* for articulation with the coxal bone. The vertebral canal continues through the sacrum. A *superior facet* serves for articulation with the fifth lumbar vertebra, and an *inferior facet* for articulation with the coccyx.

The *coccygeal vertebrae* (Fig. 3–1*B*) are usually fused into one bone also. The first vertebra is of some size but the remaining three are small rounded bones of various sizes and shapes. Extra bones may be found. The vertebral canal does not continue into these vertebrae.

Pelvis as a Whole

The *pelvis* consists of the two coxal bones anteriorly and laterally and the sacrum and coccyx posteriorly. It is divided into a *true* and *false pelvis*. The *inlet of the true pelvis* is superiorly placed and bounded by the sacral promontory posteriorly, the pubic symphysis anteriorly, and the terminal lines on the sides, the terminal lines being the pectineal lines anteriorly and the arcuate lines posteriorly; the *outlet* is the inferior end and is bounded from anterior to posterior by the pubic arch, inferior ramus of the pubis, ischial tuberosity, lesser ischiadic notch, ischiadic spine, greater ischiadic notch, and the sacrum and coccyx. As can be seen in Figure 3–2, ligaments actually form the boundaries of the outlet rather than the two notches mentioned. The *false pelvis* is that part above the inlet to the true pelvis.

The female pelvis differs from that of the male in several ways, although it is important to realize that there are many degrees of maleness and femaleness. Furthermore, there are racial differences that make measurements in a single sex quite variable.

Lines that have been established to measure the diameters of the pelvic inlet are shown in Figure 3–2. Anthropologists classify pelves into anthropoid, android, gynecoid, and platypelloid types. Figure 3–2 is a drawing of a gynecoid pelvis, typical of that found in most women. Anthropoid has a short transverse (C–D) diameter but a long anteroposterior diameter (E–F), while the platypelloid type is opposite to this, *i.e.,* it has a very long transverse (C–D) diameter and very short anteroposterior (E–F) diameter. Most males are anthropoid or android; most females are android or gynecoid, although mixed types occur with some frequency. The pelvic variations and their obstetric significance are discussed in Chapter 30.

In very general terms, the female pelvis, in comparison with the male pelvis, is lighter, the bones are more slender, and the markings made by the attachments of muscles are less pronounced. The ilium has a greater lateral flair, and the iliac fossa is slightly more shallow. The pubic arch is wider in the female; the ischiadic (ischial) spines do not project toward the center of the pelvis as they do in the male, and the ischial tuberosities are farther apart. The inlet to the true pelvis tends to be oval rather than heartshaped; the ischial spines do not project into the outlet of the pelvis as they do in the male, and the same is true of the sacrum and coccyx. The promontory of the sacrum is less pronounced in the female. This means that all diameters in the true pelvis are longer in the female than in the male.

All of this is of interest to the anatomist or anthropologist, but the obstetrician is interested in comparing the size of the baby's head (fetal cephalometry) with the dimensions of the pelvic outlet (pelvimetry). Therefore, averages are not as important as the dimensions of the pelvic outlet on the particular patient giving birth to a baby. Additional measurements can be made between the pubic symphysis and the tip of the coccyx or the sacrococcygeal joint, transversely between the inside surfaces of the ischial tuberosities, and obliquely between the junction of the pubic and ischial rami anteriorly to the midpoint in the sacrotuberous ligament posteriorly. These are shown in Figure 3–3. All of these measurements can be determined radiologically or by manual palpation via the vagina.

JOINTS AND LIGAMENTS OF THE PELVIS

A knowledge of the ligaments in this area, as well as a clear conception of the bony pelvis, is needed in order to understand the anatomy in this region.

The sacrum articulates with the fifth lumbar vertebra at the lumbosacral joint. The articulation of the

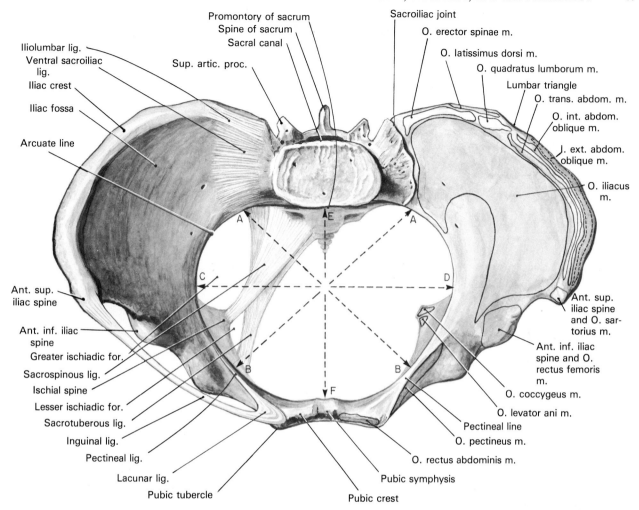

FIG. 3–2. Female bony pelvis, with origins and insertions of muscles indicated *on the left* and the ligaments shown *on the right. A,* Sacroiliac joint. *B,* Iliopubic eminence. *C* and *D,* Middle of pelvic brim. *E,* Sacral promontory. *F,* Pubic symphysis. (Crafts RC: A Textbook of Human Anatomy. Copyright © 1979. Reprinted by permission of John Wiley & Sons, Inc., New York)

coxal bones with each other in the pubic region (the pubic symphysis), and the articulation between the sacrum and these two coxal bones (the sacroiliac joints) remain. Furthermore, there are very important ligaments that connect the sacrum and coccyx to the ischial portion of the coxal bones. In addition, some attention should be given to the articulation of the sacrum and coccyx, and to the obturator membrane.

Pubic Symphysis

A cartilaginous joint, the pubic symphysis, is partially movable (Fig. 3–4*A*). The articular surfaces of each pubic bone are covered with hyaline cartilage, and between these two areas of cartilage is interposed a fibrocartilaginous lamina, the *interpubic disc.* This varies in thickness in different areas and is a very dense and firm structure. In lower animal forms a hormone, re-

laxin, tends to soften this fibrocartilaginous material, allowing the pubic bones to spread apart during parturition. Although this is of a much lesser degree in the human being, it is thought that there is some softening of the fibrocartilage. This interpubic disc is aided by a *superior pubic ligament,* which connects the two pubic bones superiorly, and by the *arcuate pubic ligament,* a thick arch of ligamentous fibers, which connects them inferiorly. The former ligament extends laterally as far as the pubic tubercles. The arcuate ligament forms the superior boundary of the *pubic arch* and continues laterally to be attached to the inferior rami of the pubic bones.

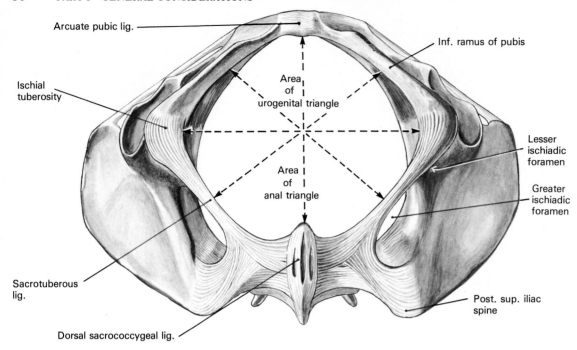

FIG. 3–3. Boundaries of the perineum. Note that a *line* drawn between the two ischial tuberosities divides this area into anterior urogenital and posterior anal triangles. *Dotted lines* represent measurements (pelvimetry) that can be compared with the baby's head (fetal cephalometry). (Crafts RC: A Textbook of Human Anatomy. Copyright © 1979. Reprinted by permission of John Wiley & Sons, Inc., New York)

Sacroiliac Joint

Because they are required to bear great weight, the sacroiliac joints (Fig. 3–4B) are important. These joints are formed by the articulation between the sacrum and the iliac portion of the coxal bones. This joint is *partly cartilaginous* and *partly synovial* in type (Fig. 3–5). Some movement is allowed. Each articular surface is covered with a thin layer of cartilage, and between these cartilages is found a layer of fibrocartilage. The *ligaments* of this joint are the ventral sacroiliac, dorsal sacroiliac, and interosseus ligaments. The *ventral sacroiliac ligament* consists of several thin bands that connect the anterior surface of the sacrum to the anterior surface of the ilium. In contrast, the *dorsal sacroiliac ligament* is quite thick and forms the chief attachment of the sacrum and ilium. It consists of bundles that pass between the bones in several directions. The superior part is the *short posterior sacroiliac ligament,* and the fibers take nearly a horizontal course. They pass between the first and second transverse tubercles on the posterior surface of the sacrum and the tuberosity of the ilium. The inferior part of this ligament—the *long posterior sacroiliac ligament*—

courses obliquely. It courses from the third transverse tubercle on the posterior surface of the sacrum and attaches to the posterior superior spine of the ilium. (This ligament is intermingled with the sacrotuberous ligament.) The *interosseus sacroiliac ligament* is located deep to the posterior sacroiliac ligament just described. The fiber bundles are very short and connect the tuberosities of the sacrum and the ilium.

Several other ligaments serve to attach the coxal bones to the vertebral column. These are the iliolumbar, sacrotuberous, and sacrospinous ligaments. The *iliolumbar ligament* (Fig. 3–4 B and C) is attached superiorly to the transverse process of the fifth lumbar vertebra. It radiates inferiorly and laterally and is attached by two main parts to the coxal bone. The inferior portion courses toward the base of the ilium and blends with the ventral sacroiliac ligament. The superior portion is attached to the crest of the ilium anterior to the sacroiliac articulation. The *sacrotuberous ligament* (Fig. 3–4 B and C) is a large, heavy ligament that attaches over a wide area to the posterior inferior spine of the ilium, to the fourth and fifth transverse tubercles of the sacrum, and to the inferior part of the lateral margin of the sacrum and the coccyx. It passes obliquely inferiorly and laterally, becoming narrower as it proceeds, to attach to the medial side of the ischial tuberosity. The *sacrospinous ligament* (Fig. 3–4 B and C) is much shorter than the sacrotuberous ligament, but it is also triangular in form. Its medial attachment is to the lateral margins of the sacrum and coccyx, and its lateral attachment is to the spine of the ischium. It

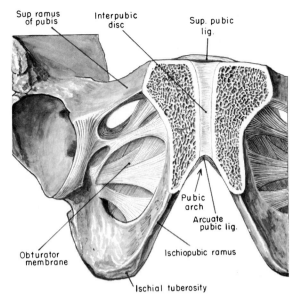

A

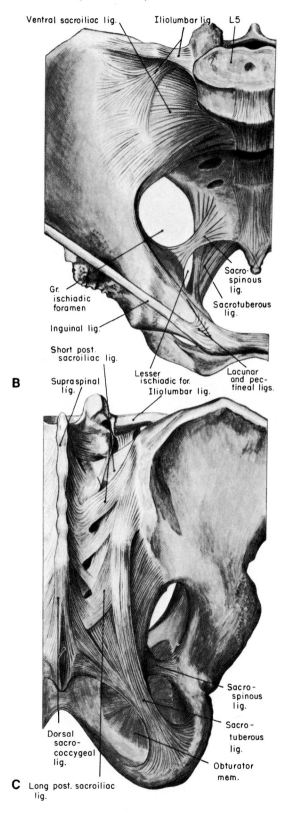

B

C

FIG. 3-4. *A.* Pubic symphysis cut to show interpubic disc. *B.* Anterior view of sacroiliac joints. *C.* Posterior view of sacroiliac joints. (Crafts RC: A Textbook of Human Anatomy. Copyright © 1979. Reprinted by permission of John Wiley & Sons, Inc., New York)

is anterior to the sacrotuberous ligament. These sacrotuberous and sacrospinous ligaments are in such a position that they make foramina out of the greater and lesser ischiadic notches. They also form part of the boundary of the inferior pelvic outlet.

Sacrococcygeal Junction

The cartilaginous joint formed between the inferior articular surface of the sacrum and the base of the coccyx is the sacrococcygeal junction; it is partially movable. In some cases, it is synovial in character, and considerable movement is allowed. Its disc is much thinner than the discs in the rest of the vertebral column. It is supported by ligaments similar to those associated with the rest of the vertebral column. The one that corresponds to the anterior longitudinal ligament is the ventral sacrococcygeal ligament; that which corresponds to the posterior longitudinal and supraspinal ligaments, the deep and superficial portions of the dorsal sacrococcygeal ligament. Lateral sacrococcygeal ligaments connect the transverse processes of the coccyx to the lower lateral angles of the sacrum.

Obturator Membrane

A thin but tough aponeurosis, the obturator membrane (Fig. 3–4*A*) fills in the large bony obturator foramen, except for a small area superiorly for the pas-

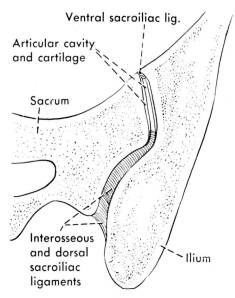

FIG. 3–5. Schematic horizontal section through sacroiliac joint. (Hollinshead WH: Anatomy for Surgeons, Vol 3. New York, Hoeber, 1958)

sage of the obturator vessels and nerve. This structure, consisting of several interlacing bundles, most of which take a transverse direction, really should be considered part of the coxal bone; it serves for the attachment of the obturator internus and externus muscles, which arise from the inside and outside surfaces, respectively, as well as from the surrounding bone.

GENERAL DESCRIPTION

If the pelvis is held in the correct position, it can be seen that it is not a bowl-like area that sits directly superiorly–inferiorly, nor is it one that has its direction anteroposteriorly. As one looks inferiorly through the pelvis, one looks in an inferior–posterior direction. If the pelvic cavity is thought of as a bowl with several holes in the midline, the floor of this bowl resembles the floor of the pelvis (*pelvic diaphragm*), which is made up of muscles. The area superior to this floor of the bowl or the pelvic diaphragm is the pelvic cavity proper; the part inferior and posterior to the bowl is the *perineum.*

The pelvic cavity is never empty. That area that is not filled with the pelvic organs themselves contains the sigmoid colon, cecum, and the ileum, the amount of sigmoid colon and cecum varying considerably.

The *sigmoid colon* continues into the pelvic cavity as the *rectum* and is just anterior to the promontory of the sacrum. The upper two-thirds of the rectum is covered with peritoneum, making it a retroperitoneal organ.

The uterus intervenes between the rectum and the bladder, which divides the pelvic cavity into two pouches, one in which the peritoneum reflects from the rectum to the posterior wall of the vagina and uterus and another in which the peritoneum is reflected from the anteroinferior (vesical) surface of the uterus to the urinary bladder. These pouches are the *rectouterine* and the *uterovesical pouches,* respectively. The *uterine tubes* extend laterally from the fundus of the uterus as far as the lateral pelvic wall. The peritoneum does not simply reflect over the uterus itself, but is also reflected from the floor of the pelvis superiorly and anteriorly over the uterine tubes, and then back to the floor of the pelvis again (the *broad ligaments*). Therefore, the anteflexed uterus and its accompanying uterine tubes and layers of peritoneum cut the pelvic cavity in the female into an anterior and a posterior portion. The uterus bends anteriorly, so the posterior surface is actually a posterosuperior surface and the anterior surface an anteroinferior surface (Fig. 3–6). This is the normal position for the uterus, and it is approximately at right angles to the direction taken by the vagina.

The peritoneum around the rectum is distributed in such a manner as to form *pararectal fossae* (Fig. 3–7). In this same area, two folds of peritoneum (*uterosacral folds*) stretch between the base of the uterus and the sacrum over the *uterosacral ligaments.* In addition, there are *paravesical fossae* on either side of the urinary bladder.

The fimbriated end of each uterine tube is in close approximation to an almond-shaped structure hanging onto the posterior–superior aspect of the broad ligaments (Fig. 3–8). These are the *ovaries,* which are suspended from the broad ligaments by two layers of peritoneum called the *mesovarium* (Fig. 3–9). In addition to this mesentery, the ovaries are attached medially to the uterus by a firm ligamentous structure, the *ligament of the ovary,* and laterally to the lateral pelvic wall by a *suspensory ligament* consisting of a reflection of peritoneum over the vascular system entering and leaving the ovary.

The midline structures, the structures on the lateral pelvic wall, and those on the anterior surface of the sacrum are all embedded in subserous fascia (Fig. 3–8). Indeed, the subserous fascia in the abdominal cavity is directly continuous with similar fascia in the pelvis. It continues into the true pelvis, onto the deep fascia covering the muscles that form the floor of the pelvis, and thence onto the midline organs, where it blends with the capsule of each organ.

The *uterosacral ligaments* are condensations of this subserous fascia. Other condensations of this fascia occur at the point where the blood vessels leave the lateral pelvic wall to course along the floor of the pelvis to reach the uterus (the *cardinal ligaments* of the uterus) and anteriorly from the pubis to the bladder

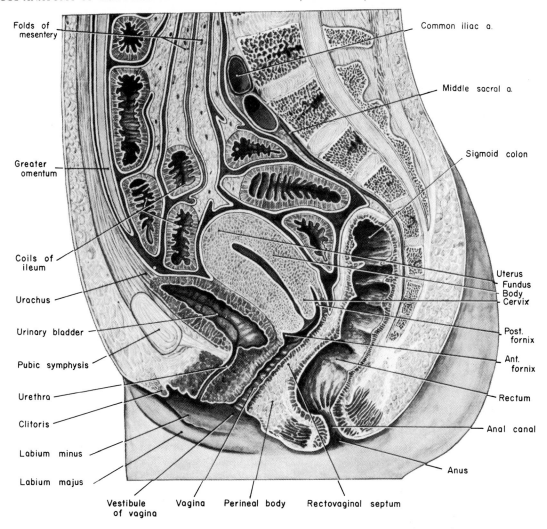

FIG. 3-6. Sagittal section of female pelvic cavity and perineum. (Crafts RC: A Textbook of Human Anatomy. Copyright © 1979. Reprinted by permission of John Wiley & Sons, Inc., New York)

(pubovesical ligaments) and thence to the uterus (uterovesical ligaments). These ligaments are shown diagrammatically in Figure 3–10.

The *ligamentum teres uteri* and *ovarian ligament* are almost continuous structures. The broad ligaments can be divided into an area inferior to the mesovarium and an area superior to this structure (Fig. 3–8). The superior area, between the mesovarium and the tube, is the *mesosalpinx* (mesentery of the tube); the inferior portion is the mesometrium.

The *rectouterine pouch* in reality is an area between the rectum and the superior end of the vagina (Fig. 3–6). This is an important fact to realize, since the very inferior end of the pelvic cavity is often a place where pus can collect as a result of infections of the peritoneum; it can be drained via the vagina. The *ureters* in the female cross the lateral pelvic wall and

course inferior and posterior to the large arteries and veins of the uterus (Fig. 3–11). They also course to the lateral side of the vagina to reach the base of the bladder.

With the exception of the middle sacral artery, which is located on the anterior surface of the sacrum, the *arteries* entering the pelvis follow along the lateral pelvic wall and then the floor of the pelvis to reach the organs to be vascularized (Fig. 3–11). The *veins* take a corresponding pathway in a reverse direction. In fact, the veins form a very profuse network on the floor of the pelvis.

In addition to the vascular system, the *nerves* that

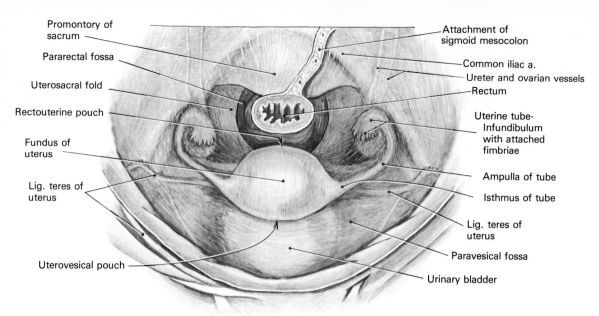

FIG. 3–7. Female pelvic cavity *in situ.* Note structures showing through peritoneum (exaggerated). (Crafts RC: A Textbook of Human Anatomy. Copyright © 1979. Reprinted by permission of John Wiley & Sons, Inc., New York)

FIG. 3–8. Female pelvic cavity. Peritoneum is intact *on left* and has been removed *on right* (Crafts RC: A Textbook of Human Anatomy. Copyright © 1979. Reprinted by permission of John Wiley & Sons, Inc., New York)

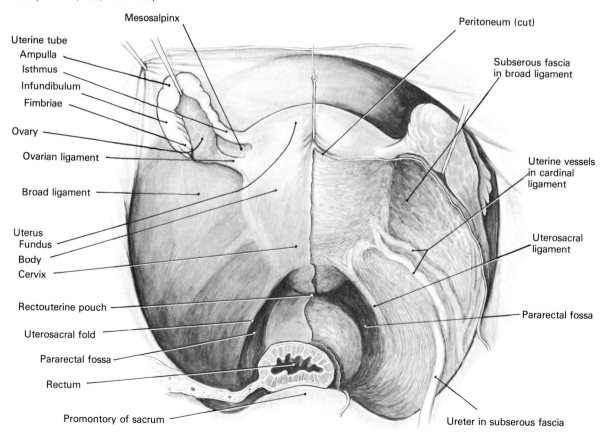

form the visceral afferent and efferent systems are also found in this loose fascia. The hypogastric plexus, on the anterior surface of the sacrum, is made up of contributions from the sympathetic system as well as the parasympathetic. These nerves form a very profuse network of fibers that follow the floor of the pelvis in this loose fascia and reach the organs to be innervated in this manner (see Fig. 3–23). The two sympathetic chains can be seen to be prolonged into the pelvic cavity anterior to the sacrum in this same layer.

The deep fascia is called parietal pelvic fascia as a general term, but it also takes on the name of the particular muscle it covers. If it is on the obturator internus muscle, it is called obturator fascia; if on the levator ani muscle, the supraanal fascia; if on the coccygeus muscle, the coccygeus fascia, *etc.* This fascia is continuous with the transversalis fascia in the abdominal cavity.

The floor and sides of the pelvic cavity are covered by muscles and nerves (Figs. 3–12, 3–13, and 3–14). In the midline posteriorly is the sacrum, and just lateral and anterior to it are the many nerves that make up the *sacral plexus.* Just deep to these nerves is the *piriformis muscle,* arising from the sacrum and extending laterally to leave the pelvis through the greater ischiadic (sciatic) foramen (Fig. 3–14). Anterior to this position, the *coccygeus muscle* (S4 and S5) extends from the ischial spine to the lateral surface of the

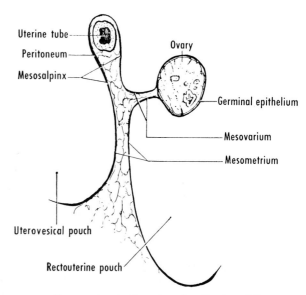

FIG. 3–9. Diagram of sagittal section showing broad ligament and its relations to ovary and uterine tube. Anterior aspect is *on left side* of diagram. (Gardner E, Gray DJ, O'Rahilly R: Anatomy: A Regional Study of Human Structure, 3rd ed. Philadelphia, WB Saunders, 1969)

FIG. 3–10. Diagrammatic presentation of the condensations of the subserous fascia that have been called ligaments. (Crafts RC: A Textbook of Human Anatomy. Copyright © 1979. Reprinted by permission of John Wiley & Sons, Inc., New York)

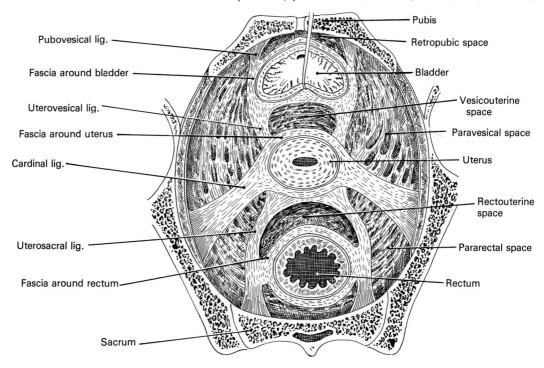

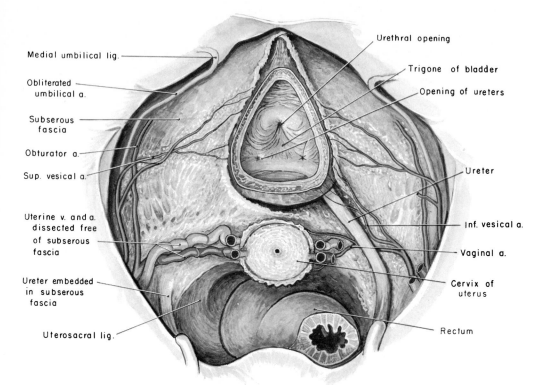

Medial umbilical lig.

Obliterated umbilical a.

Subserous fascia

Obturator a.

Sup. vesical a.

Uterine v. and a. dissected free of subserous fascia

Ureter embedded in subserous fascia

Uterosacral lig.

Urethral opening

Trigone of bladder

Opening of ureters

Ureter

Inf. vesical a.

Vaginal a.

Cervix of uterus

Rectum

FIG. 3-11. Female pelvic cavity. Uterine vessels have been dissected free of subserous fascia in which they course (cardinal ligaments) *on left* and have been removed *on right* to reveal course of ureter. Uterus has been removed to reveal urinary bladder, which has been cut to show its internal structure. (Crafts RC: A Textbook of Human Anatomy. Copyright © 1979. Reprinted by permission of John Wiley & Sons, Inc., New York)

coccyx. Anterior to that, the levator ani muscle (inferior rectal, S2 and S3, plus twigs from S4 and S5) arises from the pubis, lateral pelvic wall, and ischiadic spine, extending inferiorly in a funnel-shaped manner to blend with the organs in the pelvic cavity. This muscle can be divided into *pubovaginal, puborectal, pubococcygeal,* and *iliococcygeal portions* (Fig. 3–12). The pubovaginal portion blends into the vagina. Some fibers of the puborectalis muscle not only blend with the rectum but also meet similar fibers from the opposite side in such a fashion as to form a sling for the rectum just posterior to it. The pubococcygeal and iliococcygeal portions attach to the coccyx. The part of the levator ani muscle arising from the lateral pelvic wall is from the fascia on another muscle that helps to form the walls of the pelvis, the *obturator internus* muscle, and the fascia at this point forms a band called the *arcus tendineus.* The two muscles—the levator ani and the coccygeus muscles on each side—form the floor of the pelvis and are designated as the *pelvic diaphragm.*

In summary, the pelvic floor is formed of these muscles, with the sacrum located posteriorly and the pubic bones anteriorly; these muscles are covered with parietal pelvic fascia that also covers the sacral nerves; the vessels, ureters, and other structures are contained in a layer of subserous fascia; the organs, such as the uterus and vagina in the midline are also covered with a layer of subserous fascia; and then the whole area is covered with peritoneum.

INTERNAL REPRODUCTIVE ORGANS

Ovaries

In the nullipara, the ovaries are smooth, pink in color, and the shape and size of a large almond. In the elderly woman, they are small and quite roughened in appearance. The ovaries are located between the uterus medially and the lateral pelvic wall laterally, and they are suspended from the posterior–superior surface of the broad ligaments by the mesovarium (Fig. 3–15). The ovary is attached to the uterus by a derivative of the gubernaculum; this short ligament is the *ligament of the ovary.* The ovary is also suspended laterally from the pelvic wall by the *suspensory ligament of the ovary,* also referred to as the *infundibulopelvic ligament,* which is made up of peritoneum covering the vascular system entering and leaving this organ. The

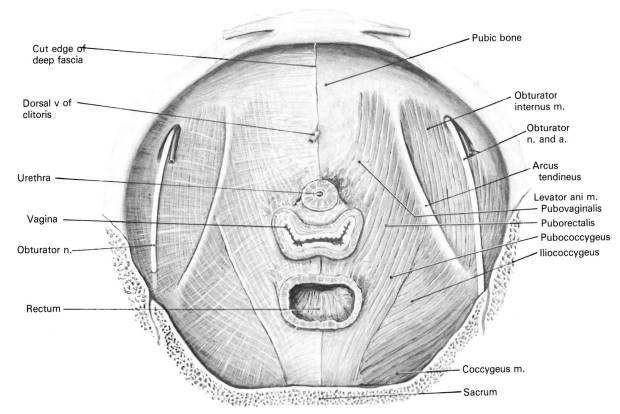

FIG. 3-12. Female pelvic cavity. The midline pelvic organs have been removed. The anterior part of the pelvic floor is seen, with deep fascia present *on the left* and removed *on the right*. Note that removing the subserous fascia has eliminated the blood vessels and the autonomic nerves. (Crafts RC: A Textbook of Human Anatomy. Copyright © 1979. Reprinted by permission of John Wiley & Sons, Inc., New York)

FIG. 3-13. Right half of pelvic diaphragm and sacral plexus, lateral view.

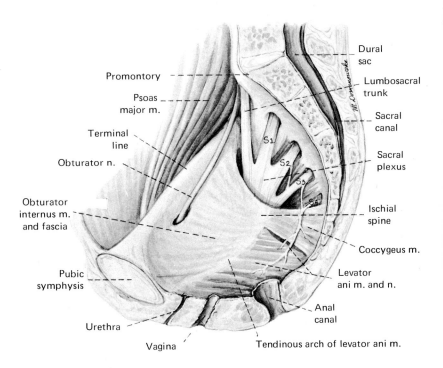

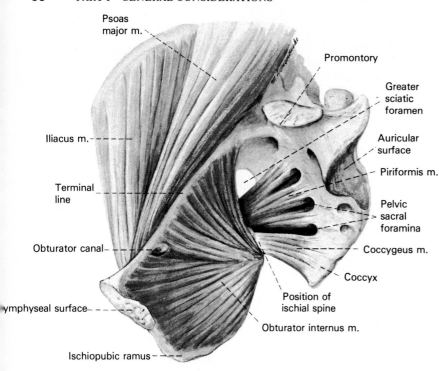

Psoas major m.

Promontory

Greater sciatic foramen

Iliacus m.

Auricular surface

Piriformis m.

Terminal line

Pelvic sacral foramina

Obturator canal

Coccygeus m.

Symphyseal surface

Coccyx

Position of ischial spine

Obturator internus m.

Ischiopubic ramus

FIG. 3-14. Muscles of right half of pelvic wall, anterolateral view.

mesenteries forming the mesovaria are continuous with the germinal epithelial layer on the ovaries themselves.

Since either the ileum or the colon fills in the pelvic cavity, the ovaries are in definite *relation* to either one of these two organs. Each ovary is also close to the lateral pelvic wall and separated only by peritoneum from the umbilical artery, obturator vessels, and nerve on the obturator internus muscle.

The *arteries* to the ovary arise from the aorta just inferior to the origin of the renal arteries. These course retroperitoneally through the abdominal cavity, across the iliac vessels, and approach the ovaries from the lateral side, the peritoneum covering these vessels forming the suspensory ligament of the ovary. The ovarian artery, after supplying the ovary itself, continues just inferior to the tube, between the layers of the broad ligament, supplying branches to the tube itself, and then anastomoses with the uterine artery, which ramifies on the lateral side of the uterus (Fig. 3–16). The ovarian artery sends branches to the ovarian ligament and to the proximal end of the ligamentum teres, as well as to these other structures. The *ovarian veins* form a pampiniform plexus that follows the same course as the arteries, except that the left ovarian vein drains into the left renal vein rather than into the inferior vena cava as does the right.

Since the ovary developed in the vicinity of the kidneys and subsequently migrated, the nerves and blood vessels were carried along. The ovary receives *sympathetic fibers* from the 10th and 11th thoracic segments via the renal plexus and the ovarian plexus on the ovarian artery. The *parasympathetic fibers* are derived from this same ovarian plexus and are vagal in origin. The function of these nerves is problematic; they probably innervate blood vessels only. *Sensory fibers* are more important; they end in the 10th and 11th thoracic segments. Ovarian pain is referred to the skin innervated by these particular segments of the spinal cord.

The lymphatics for the ovary ascend, because of its embryonic development, to lumbar nodes alongside the inferior vena cava and aorta.

Uterine Tubes

Approximately 4 in. long and ¼ in. in diameter, the *uterine tube* (Figs. 3–7, 3–15, and 3–17), is attached to the fundus of the uterus. The tube extends laterally, enters the free edge of the broad ligament, and curls around the ovary to end in approximation with it on the medial surface of that organ. The abdominal end is the funnel-shaped *infundibulum* that ends in many fingerlike processes called *fimbriae,* one of which is attached to the ovary (*fimbria ovarica*). The middle portion of the tube, the *ampulla,* is considerably smaller and is slightly coiled. The medial portion is narrow and straight and is called the *isthmus.* Although the

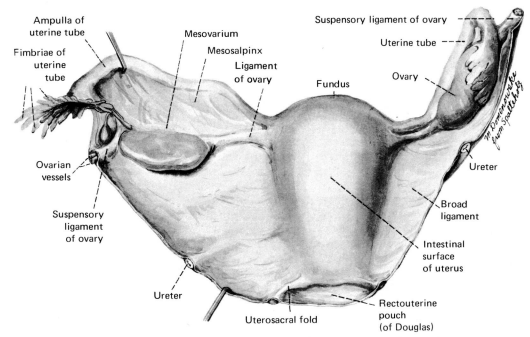

FIG. 3-15. Excised uterus, uterine tubes, and ovaries, posterior aspect.

isthmus attaches to the uterus, the lumen penetrates the uterine wall (*interstitial portion of tube*) to join the uterine cavity. It is obvious that the uterine tube forms a direct connection between the peritoneal cavity at one end and the uterine cavity at the other.

The uterine tube is also related to the ileum and to the cecum. The latter relationship causes confusion between pathology of the appendix and the uterine tube.

The uterine tube contains *smooth muscle* and is lined with a *ciliated columnar epithelium.* At the time of ovulation, the fimbriated end of the tube picks up the ovum; by a combined ciliated action and muscle contraction, the ovum is pushed down the tube toward the waiting uterus.

The *blood supply* to the uterine tube is from the ovarian and uterine vessels (Fig. 3–16).

The *sympathetic nerve* supply to the uterine tube is interesting in that the fimbriated end derives its fibers from the ovarian plexus, while the uterine end receives its sympathetic nerves via the uterine plexus. They arise in spinal cord segments T10–L1. The *parasympathetic nerves* also seem to be dual in nature. The distal end of the tube is innervated by vagal fibers, and the proximal end (near the uterus) by the pelvic nerve. The exact role of these nerves is problematic. *Sensory fibers* end in segments T10–L1, and pain may be referred to areas on the skin innervated by these particular segments.

Lymphatics from the uterine tube terminate in two glands alongside the inferior vena cava and the aorta.

The area of the broad ligament between the mesovarium and the tube contains several *minor tubules* (Fig. 3–17) that correspond to structures in the male. These tubules are remnants of the mesonephric tubules and correspond to the ducts of the testes and to the lobules of the epididymis. They end in a horizontal tubule called the duct of the *epoophoron,* the latter being a remnant of the mesonephric (wolffian) duct and corresponding to the canal of the epididymis. It continues as Gartner's duct. The *paroophoron* consists of a few microscopic tubules, which lie nearer the uterus; these are derived from the mesonephros and correspond to the paradidymis. Abnormal growth can occur in these tubules.

Uterus

Usually described as a pear-shaped organ, the uterus (Figs. 3–6 through 3–8, 3–15, and 3–17) has a comparatively narrow *cervix,* which extends into the vagina, and a wider *body* or *corpus,* which ends superoanteriorly as the *fundus,* to which are attached the uterine tubes. The cervix is divided into vaginal and supravaginal portions, and the point of juncture between it and the body of the uterus is often called the *isthmus.* That part of the vaginal cervix that is anterior to the ostium is the anterior labium; that part posterior, the posterior labium (Fig. 3–17). The normal adult uterus weighs 60–80 g.

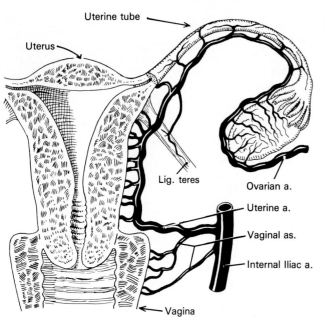

Uterine tube

Uterus

Lig. teres

Ovarian a.

Uterine a.

Vaginal as.

Internal Iliac a.

Vagina

FIG. 3–16. Blood supply to the ovary, uterus, and vagina. (Crafts RC: A Textbook of Human Anatomy. Copyright © 1979. Reprinted by permission of John Wiley & Sons, Inc., New York)

FIG. 3–17. Sectioned female reproductive organs, anterior view.

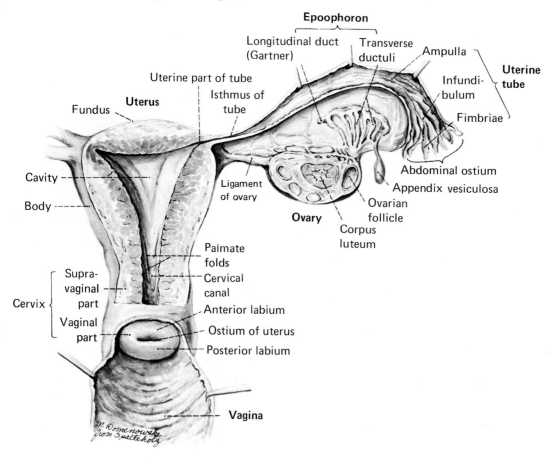

Epoophoron

Longitudinal duct (Gartner)

Transverse ductuli

Ampulla

Infundi-bulum

Uterine tube

Fimbriae

Uterine part of tube

Isthmus of tube

Uterus

Fundus

Cavity

Body

Ligament of ovary

Ovary

Abdominal ostium

Appendix vesiculosa

Ovarian follicle

Corpus luteum

Palmate folds

Cervical canal

Anterior labium

Ostium of uterus

Posterior labium

Supra-vaginal part

Cervix

Vaginal part

Vagina

M. Domenowske from Spalteholz

The uterus is a hollow organ, and the lumina of the uterine tubes are directly continuous with the *lumen* inside the uterus. This, in turn, opens into the vagina through the cervix. The lumen inside the uterus has a different shape in different parts (Fig. 3–16). In the cervix it is a fairly small, narrow opening approximately 2.5 cm in length. Its distal end is called the *ostium* of the uterus. The cavity in the body of the uterus is approximately 4 cm in length and is triangular in shape. The wall of the corpus is rather thick and made up of peritoneum (perimetrium), smooth muscle (myometrium), and a glandular lining on the inside (endometrium). The wall of the cervix, however, is composed almost entirely of dense fibrous connective tissue. The transition from fibrous cervix to muscular corpus is usually abrupt and occurs at about the level of the internal ostium.

The uterus, located between the rectum and the bladder, overhangs the bladder anteriorly (Fig. 3–6). As mentioned earlier, it is normally bent anteriorly and forms approximately a right angle to the vaginal canal. Its vesical surface is in direct relation to the bladder, and the peritoneum on this surface does not cover the entire uterus. The intestinal surface of the uterus is completely covered with peritoneum and is in direct relation to the ileum. It should be noted that the appendix can hang down into the pelvic cavity very close to the uterus.

The *uterus* has five paired ligaments. The *broad ligaments* (Fig. 3–15) are extensions of the peritoneum from the margins of the uterus to the lateral pelvic walls; these two layers stretch over the uterine tubes from the floor of the pelvis. In addition to the uterine tube, these folds of the broad ligament, as just described, enclose embryonic remnants, the ovarian ligament, vessels, lymphatics, and nerves. The *round ligaments* (Fig. 3–7) of the uterus (ligamentum teres uteri) extend laterally from the fundus between the folds of the broad ligament to the lateral pelvic wall, and finally leave the abdominal cavity through the internal ring of the inguinal canal. The two *cardinal ligaments* (Figs. 3–8 and 3–10) extend from the lateral pelvic wall to the cervix of the uterus and are condensations of subserous fascia around the uterine blood vessels. The *uterosacral ligaments* are also condensations of subserous fascia that extend from the sacrum, around the rectum, to the cervix of the uterus. (Similar condensations have been described extending anteriorly from the uterus to the base of the urinary bladder as seen in Figure 3–10; these are *uterovesical ligaments*.) The uterosacral and cardinal ligaments are by far the most important of the ligaments of the uterus. Without these, the uterus tends to pass inferiorly through the vagina, a condition called prolapse of the uterus. The round ligaments are of little value, and the reflections of the peritoneum are equally unimportant. The broad ligaments probably do serve a purpose in holding the uterus in position.

The uterus has a rich blood supply (Figs. 3–8 and 3–16). The uterine arteries are branches of the internal iliac and enter the uterus near its inferior extent at the base of the broad ligaments. This artery then continues superiorly on the lateral side of the uterus, sending branches to the uterus all the way along its course. It anastomoses with the ovarian artery, which courses along the uterine tube. The veins are a plexus of veins that end in the internal iliac.

The *sympathetic* nerves arise from spinal cord segments T12 and L1 and proceed to the uterus through the hypogastric plexus and thence on the uterine arteries. The *parasympathetic* supply is through the pelvic nerve from the second, third, and fourth sacral segments of the cord. The role played by these nerves is problematic, for the uterus can function when denervated. The *sensory nerve supply* is more important. The nerve endings are found associated with the arteries in the myometrium; there are very few in the endometrium. Those from the peritonealized parts of the uterus follow the sympathetic nerves, through the hypogastric plexus, to spinal cord segments T12 and L1; those from the cervix follow the pelvic nerves to the sacral segments. Uterine pain is referred to the sacroiliac and pubic regions.

The *lymphatics* from the uterus end in numerous glands. They are found on the rectum, anterior to the sacrum, around the iliac arteries, and high up in the abdominal cavity close to the inferior vena cava and the aorta. Lymphatics from this organ are known to course along the ligamentum teres to reach the inguinal nodes.

Vagina

The copulatory canal in the female, the *vagina*, starts as an opening in the external genitalia posterior to the urethra and anterior to the rectum (Fig. 3–6). The opening to the vagina in the virgin is usually guarded by a *hymen*, two folds of mucous membrane that extend into the lumen of the vagina from the lateral walls. The hymen may take the form of a complete membrane, which has to be severed at the first menstruation; it may be a sievelike structure; or there may be no hymen at all. After rupture, the fragments of the hymen persist as small nodules designated as *hymenal caruncles*.

The *vagina proper* extends from the hymen to the cervix of the uterus. It traverses a muscular layer in the perineum—the urogenital diaphragm—and then goes through the pelvic diaphragm by passing the inferior edges of the levator ani muscles. These diaphragms are diagrammed in Fig. 3–29 (see p. 78). Since the cervix extends into the anterior aspect of the superior end of the vagina, the anterior wall is shorter than the posterior. The anterior wall is approximately 8 cm long, while the posterior wall is 9–10 cm long (Fig. 3–6). The clefts produced by the cervix projecting into

the vagina are called *fornices;* there are anterior, posterior, and two lateral fornices, the posterior being by far the deepest. The posterosuperior part of the vagina is covered by peritoneum, but the anterior wall makes no contact with it.

The *relations* of the vagina are important, for many structures in the pelvic cavity can be palpated via this canal. These relations are as follows:

Anterior—bladder and urethra
Posterior—the inferior end of the pelvic cavity, small intestine, rectovaginal septum, rectum, and perineal body (a point in the midline between the vaginal and anal openings)
Lateral—broad ligaments, ureters, uterine vessels, pelvic surface of the levator ani muscle, sphincter urethrae muscle, greater vestibular glands, and bulbospongiosus muscles

Thus, any structure in the inferior part of the pelvic cavity can be palpated through the vagina, particularly if bimanual palpation is used (one hand on the anterior abdominal wall). Structures contained in the broad ligaments can be felt, and when the ovary is increased in size from any pathologic condition, it can be felt from the vagina as well. Naturally, the cervix of the uterus is also palpable; it is also visible if the vagina is dilated.

The *walls of the vagina* are in contact with each other except where the cervix intervenes. They are made up of smooth muscle and are lined with stratified squamous epithelium. Ridges (vaginal rugae) are found on the anterior and posterior walls, and several transverse folds around the walls of the vagina connect these ridges. During sexual excitement, the vagina elongates in the area of the posterior fornix, produces a clear fluid by transudation, and the distal third undergoes a vasocongestion, all parasympathetic actions. The vestibule of the vagina has two *greater vestibular* or *bulbourethral glands* that empty just inferior to the hymenal caruncles (see Fig. 3–27); they provide lubrication and are also under control of the parasympathetic system. Several small mucous glands, the *lesser vestibular,* open on the side walls of the vestibule.

The *arteries* to the vagina branch from the uterine arteries, from the internal iliac artery directly, and from the middle rectal; the inferior end derives its blood supply from branches of the internal pudendal artery (see Figs. 3–27 and 3–28).

The vagina obtains its *sympathetic nerve supply* from the hypogastric plexus (L1–L3) and its *parasympathetic* from the sacral region of the cord through the pelvic nerve. The inferior end of the vagina is more sensitive than the superior end, receiving its *sensory branches* from the pudendal nerve.

The *lymphatics* drain to glands on the rectum and along the iliac arteries, but some of the lymphatics from the inferior end of the vagina may drain into the inguinal glands in the groin.

Ureters

In its *course,* the ureter enters the pelvic cavity by crossing the external iliac artery near its branching from the common iliac and follows along the lateral pelvic wall just deep to the peritoneum. It is anterior to the internal iliac artery and vein. Lateral are the psoas major muscle, the obturator internus muscle, and the levator ani. As the ureter approaches the floor of the pelvis, the vessels entering the broad ligament pass superior and medial to the ureter, as does the broad ligament itself. The ureter continues inferiorly and after passing deep to these uterine vessels enters the bladder by passing close to the lateral fornix of the vagina. Although the ovary is not in immediate relation, it is very close to the ureter, being anterior and medial to it. The ureters penetrate the bladder wall in an oblique slanting fashion; this is important in preventing reflux of urine into the ureters when the bladder is distended.

The ureters receive small *arteries* from the renal, ovarian, vesical, and middle rectal arteries.

The ureters receive autonomic innervation from the *sympathetic* nervous system, fibers originating in T12–L2 spinal cord segments. The vagus contributes the *parasympathetic fibers* to the upper part; the pelvic nerve, to the lower part. The ureter can function without a nerve supply; peristalsis will occur. Spasm is induced by stimuli of an unusual nature. *Sensory fibers* return to segments T12–L2.

The *lymphatics* end in glands closest to it in the pelvis and in the abdominal cavity.

Urinary Bladder

Although the urinary bladder is not a reproductive organ, its intimate relation to the reproductive tract warrants its being included in any description of the pelvic cavity. The urethra assumes a similar importance in the perineum.

The *urinary bladder* occupies the anterior portion of the pelvic cavity and is just superior and posterior to the pubic bone (Fig. 3–11). When the bladder is empty, it is said to have an *apex,* a *superior surface,* two *inferolateral surfaces,* a *base* or posterior surface, and a *neck.* The *apex* reaches to a short distance superior to the pubic bone and ends as a fibrous cord, which is a derivative of the urachus (a canal in the fetus that connects the bladder with the allantois). This fibrous cord extends from the apex of the bladder to the umbilicus between the peritoneum and the transversalis fascia; it raises a ridge of peritoneum called the median umbilical ligament. The *superior surface* is the only surface of the bladder covered by peritoneum; it is in relation with the uterus and ileum

in the female. The *base* of the bladder faces posteriorly and is separated from the rectum by the uterus and vagina. The *inferolateral* surfaces on each side of the bladder are in relation with the pubic bone, and with the levator ani and obturator internus muscles, but the bladder is actually separated from the pubic bone by the retropubic space, which contains fat. The *neck* of the bladder is the most inferior part next to the urethra. The bladder is a dilatable structure. When filled with urine, the neck remains in position but the superior part rises into the pelvic cavity.

The loose *subserous fascia* of the pelvic cavity is continuous superiorly over the pelvic organs, and this is true for the bladder as well. Condensations of this fascia form attachments for the bladder, and those running from the levator ani muscle and the pubic bone to the bladder are called the *pubovesical ligaments.*

The *bladder wall* consists of a partial covering of peritoneum, the subserous fascia, a muscular coat made up of intermingling longitudinal and circular fibers of smooth muscle, a submucous layer of connective tissue. and a layer of transitional epithelium.

The interior of the bladder (Fig. 3–6 and 3–11) is wrinkled except at the *trigone,* that area between the openings of the ureters and the opening of the urethra. When the bladder is dilated, all walls become equally smooth in appearance. A ridge is found between the openings of the ureters—the *interureteral ridge.* The trigone of the bladder is an important area in that infections tend to persist at this particular point.

The muscular component of the wall of the bladder—the *detrusor muscle*—consists of three layers of smooth muscle—outer and inner longitudinal layers and a circular layer between them. These layers are not distinct entities, for they tend to form an intermingling meshwork. However, the outer longitudinal layer is continuous with a layer of muscle blended with the vagina. The circular and inner longitudinal layers are continued into the urethra. There seems to be no internal sphincter; in fact, the muscle arrangement at the neck of the bladder is such as to cause an opening of the urethra rather than a constriction. A considerable amount of *elastic tissue* is found at the neck of the bladder, however, and this is arranged in such a manner as to aid in keeping the urethra closed.

The *nerves* to the bladder are part of the nerve plexuses found in the pelvic cavity; they follow the arteries to get to the bladder. The *sympathetic* fibers arise in the last thoracic and the first and second lumbar segments of the spinal cord. They innervate the trigone, the ureteral orifices, and the blood vessels. They also carry pain fibers from the bladder. The *parasympathetic* fibers arise in the second, third, and fourth sacral segments. These fibers innervate the detrusor muscle. Afferent fibers from the bladder wall start as stretch receptors. A full bladder stimulates these receptors, and the impulses follow the pelvic nerve back to the sacral region of the spinal cord.

The *arteries* to the bladder are the superior and inferior vesical branches of the internal iliac artery (Fig. 3–18). There are corresponding *veins* that form a profuse plexus near the base of the bladder; this plexus drains into the internal iliac veins (Fig. 3–19).

ARTERIES

The internal iliac (hypogastric) artery (Fig. 3–18) courses inferiorly into the pelvic cavity in a position posterior to the ureter and anterior to the corresponding internal iliac vein. The internal iliac artery usually divides into anterior and posterior divisions.

Although the branching of this artery is extremely variable, the following branches usually occur:

Branches of posterior division (PD)
1. Iliolumbar
2. Lateral sacral
3. Superior gluteal

Branches of anterior division (AD)
4. Umbilical and superior vesical
5. Uterine and vaginal
6. Middle rectal
7. Obturator
8. Internal pudendal
9. Inferior gluteal

The *posterior division (PD),* lying medial to the sacral plexus, terminates in the large *superior gluteal artery* (3), which exits from the pelvic cavity into the gluteal region through the greater ischiadic (sciatic) foramen in a position superior to the piriformis muscle. The *iliolumbar artery* (1) courses superiorly and laterally between the obturator nerve and the lumbosacral trunk. It is posterior to the common iliac artery. It divides into an iliac branch, which ramifies in the iliac fossa, and a lumbar branch, which ascends superiorly in a position posterior to the psoas muscle. This latter branch sends a spinal branch into the vertebral canal through the lumbosacral intervertebral foramen. Two or more *lateral sacral arteries* (2) course inferiorly and medially, and enter the four anterior sacral foramina supplying structures in the sacral canal; they then emerge through the posterior sacral foramina and supply muscles and skin on the back of the sacrum.

The *anterior division* (AD) of the internal iliac artery continues inferiorly and divides into several branches. The pattern of the branching cannot be relied upon; it is quite variable. The *umbilical artery* and *superior vesical* (4) are usually combined into one stem. It continues along the side wall of the pelvis pos-

FEMALE

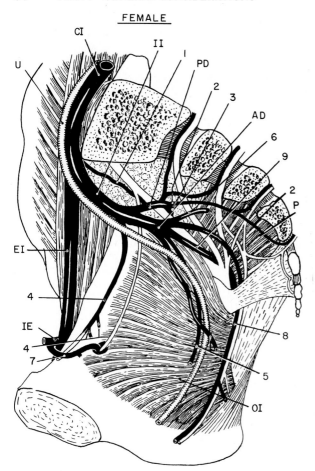

FIG. 3–18. Arteries of the pelvic cavity in the female. The pelvic floor (coccygeus and levator ani muscles) has been removed. Note relation of vessels to piriformis muscle (*P*) as they exit from the pelvic cavity through the greater ischiadic (sciatic) foramen. *AD,* Anterior division. *CI,* Common iliac. *EI,* External iliac. *IE,* Inferior epigastric. *II,* Internal iliac. *OI,* Obturator internus muscle. *PD,* Posterior division. *U,* Ureter. *1,* Iliolumbar. *2,* Lateral sacral. *3,* Superior gluteal. *4,* Umbilical and superior vesical. *5,* Uterine and vaginal. *6,* Middle rectal. *7,* Obturator arising from the inferior epigastric branch of the external iliac—the so-called abnormal obturator artery. *8,* Internal pudendal. *9,* Inferior gluteal. (Crafts RC: A Textbook of Human Anatomy. Copyright © 1979. Reprinted by permission of John Wiley & Sons, Inc., New York. Modified and redrawn after Jamieson.)

medially between the two layers of the broad ligament, superior to the ureter, and on the lateral fornix of the vagina. It supplies branches to the vagina and then continues on the lateral sides of the uterus, between the layers of the broad ligament, to the uterine tube; it gives off branches to these organs and anastomoses with the ovarian artery (Fig. 3–16). The inferior vesical artery in the female usually arises from this uterine artery. The *middle rectal artery* (6) courses medially on the lateral pelvic wall to reach the rectum. The *obturator artery* (7) courses inferiorly and anteriorly along the side wall of the pelvis in company with the obturator nerve. It leaves the pelvis through the obturator foramen. In approximately 40% of bodies, the artery may arise from the inferior epigastric branch of the external iliac (abnormal obturator artery). In this situation, it courses medially in a position posterior to the external iliac vein, and then courses over the brim of the pelvis to enter the obturator foramen. It gives off branches to muscles on the lateral pelvic wall, to the bladder, and a *pubic branch* ramifies on the pelvic surface of the pubis. The *internal pudendal artery* (8) courses inferiorly and slightly posteriorly, and exits from the pelvic cavity into the gluteal region through the greater ischiadic (sciatic) foramen. It is very close to the ischial spine and enters the perineum by coursing through the lesser ischiadic (sciatic) foramen. The *inferior gluteal artery* (9) exits from the pelvic cavity into the gluteal region through the greater ischiadic (sciatic) foramen in a position inferior to the piriformis muscle.

Other arteries contribute to the supply of pelvic structures. The *middle sacral* emerges from the aorta just before it bifurcates, and this branch continues in the midline on the anterior aspect of the sacrum. The *inferior epigastric artery* arises from the distal end of the external iliac and courses superiorly (forming the lateral boundary of the inguinal triangle of Hesselbach) to enter the rectus sheath. The *superior rectal artery,* a branch of the inferior mesenteric, supplies the rectum, coursing just deep to the mucous membrane to anastomose finally with the *inferior rectal arteries* in the anal columns. The *middle rectal arteries* nourish the muscular walls of the rectum and thereby do not play a major role in the anastomosis of arteries on the rectum.*

---

* Uncontrollable bleeding from the arteries supplying the uterus, vagina, superior aspect of the bladder, and midportion of the rectum can usually be stopped by ligating the anterior division of the internal iliac artery just distal to its origin and proximal to the point where its first branch arises. In some cases, anastomosis with the ovarian artery is so rich that the suspensory ligament of the ovary (infundibulopelvic ligament) may also need to be tied. (The collateral circulation is usually sufficient to prevent later disability from the loss of this blood supply.

terior to the obturator nerve and lateral to the ureter and the ligamentum teres. After giving off the superior vesical artery, it becomes the medial umbilical ligament. The *superior vesical arteries* (4) run medially from the umbilical arteries to supply the superior aspect of the bladder. The *uterine artery* (5) is of considerable size and runs anteriorly on the levator ani muscle to the base of the broad ligament. It then courses

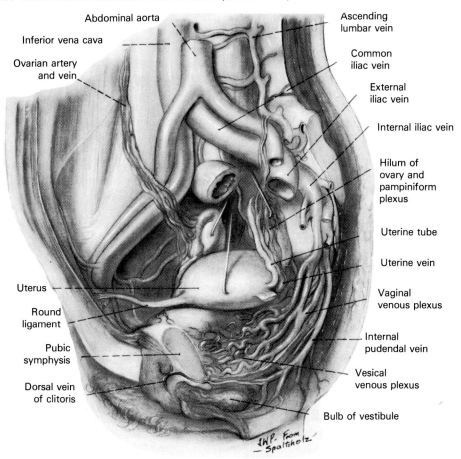

FIG. 3–19. Veins of female pelvic organs.

VEINS

The corresponding veins in the pelvic cavity (Fig. 3–19) form a profuse plexus before ending in the same branches as the arteries. The reproductive organs are surrounded by these plexuses, and parietal and visceral branches anastomose freely. They are located, as expected, in the subserous fascia. The umbilical and iliolumbar arteries have no corresponding veins. It should also be noted that the *deep dorsal vein of the clitoris* drains into the vesical plexus of veins. The *ovarian vein(s)* ascend along with the arteries and drain into the inferior vena cava on the right and the left renal vein on the left.

LYMPHATICS

The major groups of lymph nodes concerned with lymphatic drainage of the female reproductive organs located in the pelvic cavity include the external iliac, internal iliac, common iliac, and lumbar nodes (Fig. 3–20). These are arranged in general along the major

arteries of the pelvic region. Sacral lymph nodes are found on the pelvic aspect of the sacrum, and scattered small nodes lie along parietal arteries (gluteal, pudendal, obturator) and in association with pelvic viscera (vesical, anorectal, parauterine, rectal). The course of lymph through these nodes leads eventually to lumbar nodes and to the thoracic duct.

Lymph vessels from the pelvic organs do not necessarily drain along the lines of the arterial pattern suggested by the arrangement of nodes mentioned above. Lymphatic vessels of the external genitalia, the anus, and the anal canal inferior to the pectinate line (white line of Hilton) drain initially into the superficial inguinal nodes. The lymphatic vessels from the vagina may follow several routes. From the posteroinferior portion of the vagina the drainage may reach the sacral nodes. Other portions of the wall drain to internal, external, or common iliac nodes. The cervix drains to the external or internal iliac nodes and to the sacral nodes. The inferior portion of the body of the uterus drains

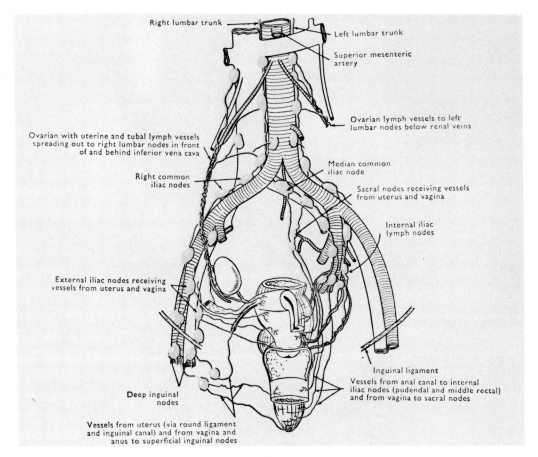

FIG. 3–20. Diagram of lymphatic vessels and lymph nodes of female genital organs. (Romanes GJ [ed]: Cunningham's Textbook of Anatomy, 10th ed. London, Oxford University Press, 1964)

mostly through the external iliac nodes. Lymphatic vessels from the superior body and the fundus pass principally with the ovarian lymphatics to the lumbar nodes. A few vessels, however, go by way of the round ligament to the superficial inguinal nodes. Efferent vessels from the uterine tubes pass toward the ovary and reach the lumbar nodes. Lymphatic vessels from the ovary pass entirely out of the pelvis to the lumbar nodes.

The detailed lymphatic drainage as it is concerned in the spread of gynecologic cancer is considered in the appropriate sections.

NERVES

The nerves that supply the pelvis consist of fibers of several functional types. Striated muscles of the pelvic outlet and the skin of the perineum receive somatic motor and sensory fibers through branches of the lumbosacral plexus. The pelvic viscera are innervated by way of the autonomic plexuses, which convey sympathetic and parasympathetic motor and visceral sensory nerves to the organs. The spinal cord connections of these pathways include the lower thoracic and first lumbar segments, as well as the sacral and coccygeal levels.

Meninges and Spinal Cord

The walls of the vertebral canal (Figs. 3–21 and 3–22), in which the spinal cord is lodged, are formed by the serially arranged vertebral arches of the individual vertebrae. Between adjacent vertebrae, the walls of the canal are completed by the ligamenta flava and interspinous ligaments posteriorly and by the intervertebral discs covered by the posterior longitudinal ligament anteriorly. The canal is continuous from the cranial cavity to the lower end of the sacrum, where it terminates as the hiatus of the sacral canal, an irregular

opening covered by the superficial posterior sacrococcygeal ligament. The portion of the canal within the sacrum is known as the sacral canal.

The *dura mater* (Fig. 3–21) extends inferiorly as a closed tubular sac within the vertebral canal. The sac tapers rather abruptly to end opposite the body of the second sacral vertebra. A fibrous strand, the *filum terminale externum,* continues inferiorly from the sac to fuse to the coccyx. Several additional fibrous strands anchor the dura to the walls of the sacral canal. Sleevelike extensions of the dura also accompany the roots of the spinal nerves as far as the intervertebral foramina. The narrow epidural space (Fig. 3–22) between the dural sac and the walls of the vertebral canal is occupied by fat, small arteries, and the internal vertebral venous plexus.

The thin *arachnoid* membrane (Fig. 3–22) lines the inside of the dural sac and extends a short distance along the nerve roots. Spinal fluid fills the subarachnoid space between the arachnoid membrane and the pia mater covering the spinal cord.

The *pia mater* is the delicate inner layer intimately adherent to the surface of the spinal cord. Lateral fenestrated expansions of the pia mater,the *denticulate ligaments,* attach to the dura mater and help to anchor the spinal cord within the meninges.

The spinal cord (Fig. 3–21) extends inferiorly to the level of the body of the second lumbar vertebra, where it tapers to a cone-shaped termination (the *conus medullaris*), continuous inferiorly with a fibrous strand (the *filum terminale internum*), which extends caudally within the subarachnoid space to fuse with the terminal part of the dural sac.

Sacral and Coccygeal Nerves

The dorsal and ventral roots of the lower lumbar, sacral, and coccygeal nerves descend within the subarachnoid space as elongated filaments known collectively as the *cauda equina.* Each set of roots penetrates the meninges as it approaches its level of exit from the vertebral canal, carrying an extension of the dura and arachnoid as far as the intervertebral foramen. The dorsal root ganglion is located close to the intervertebral foramen. Distal to the ganglion the dorsal and ventral roots join to form the spinal nerve. Each spinal nerve divides promptly into dorsal and ventral rami.

The dorsal rami of the first three sacral nerves emerge through the dorsal sacral foramina to be distributed to the ligaments and periosteum of the sacrum, to the multifidus muscle, and to the skin over the sacral region (middle cluneal nerves). The dorsal rami of the fourth and fifth sacral nerves and the coccygeal nerve are distributed to the skin posterior to the coccyx.

The ventral rami of the lumbar and sacral nerves form the lumbosacral plexus; its branches are distributed to the pelvis and lower limbs. Except for parts of the lumbar plexus (obturator nerve, lumbosacral trunk) and the entire sacral plexus, which pass along the walls of the true pelvis and hence are anatomically related to the pelvic viscera, only certain components of these plexuses are directly involved in pelvic innervation.

The *sacral plexus* (Fig. 3–13) is formed by the confluence of the lumbosacral trunk and the first, second, and third sacral nerves on the anterior aspect of the piriformis muscle. It is covered by the fascia of the piriformis and is, therefore, separated from the pelvic vessels and from the ureter. It is directed inferolaterally into the gluteal region through the greater ischiadic (sciatic) foramen. The superior gluteal nerve emerges from the pelvis superior to the piriformis muscle, whereas the inferior gluteal nerve, the sciatic nerve, the posterior femoral cutaneous nerve, the nerve to the quadratus femoris, the nerve to the obturator internus, and the pudendal nerve course inferior to the piriformis. Small direct branches from the plexus supply the piriformis (S1 and S2), entering its anterior aspect. Branches to the levator ani and coccygeus muscles (S3 and S4) enter the pelvic surface of these muscles. Frequently a perineal branch from S4 passes independently to the sphincter ani externus.

Autonomic Innervation

The nerve plexuses associated with the pelvic organs contain sympathetic and parasympathetic motor pathways as well as numerous visceral sensory fibers (Fig. 3–23). Collections of nerve cells that form irregular ganglionic masses are scattered through these plexuses. Although the exact course of each of the fiber types is difficult to trace with certainty, the following outline indicates the principal pathways and connections of the autonomic nerves to the pelvis.

The ganglionated sympathetic trunks that lie on each side of the vertebral column pass into the true pelvis along the pelvic surface of the sacrum medial to the pelvic sacral foramina. Usually, four sacral ganglia are located along this part of each trunk. The trunks usually unite in front of the coccyx in the small ganglion impar.

Major autonomic plexuses associated with the aorta (celiac, superior mesenteric, aorticorenal, inferior mesenteric, and superior hypogastric) receive connections from the sympathetic trunks through splanchnic nerves. The superior hypogastric plexus lies near the bifurcation of the abdominal aorta in close association with the inferior mesenteric plexus. It continues inferiorly in front of the promontory of the sacrum, where it divides into right and left portions. These strands pass inferiorly on either side of the rectum as the right and left hypogastric nerves. They diverge and swing anteriorly into the uterosacral folds, where an extensive inferior hypogastric plexus is present within

(Text continues on p. 70)

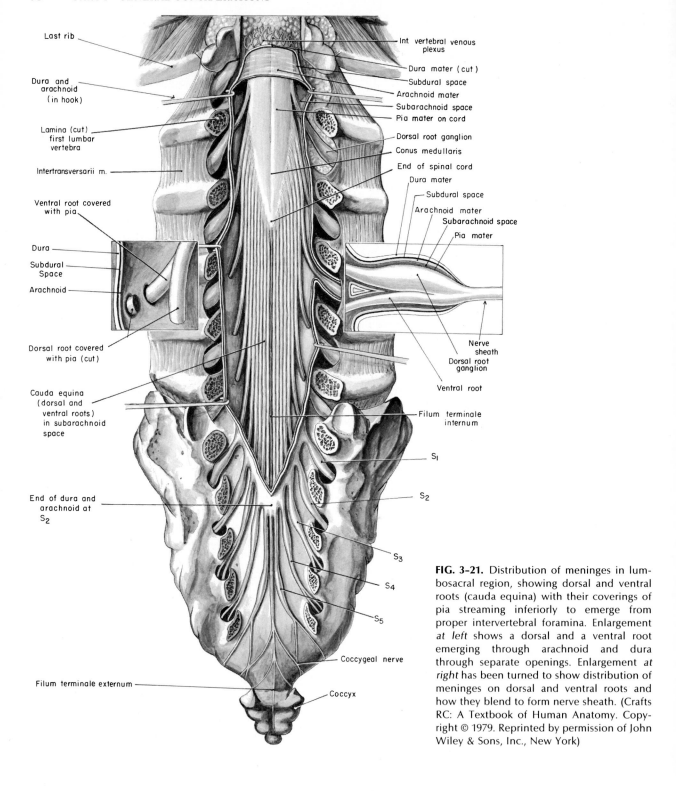

Last rib

Dura and arachnoid (in hook)

Lamina (cut) first lumbar vertebra

Intertransversarii m.

Ventral root covered with pia

Dura

Subdural Space

Arachnoid

Dorsal root covered with pia (cut)

Cauda equina (dorsal and ventral roots) in subarachnoid space

End of dura and arachnoid at S_2

Filum terminale externum

Int. vertebral venous plexus

Dura mater (cut)

Subdural space

Arachnoid mater

Subarachnoid space

Pia mater on cord

Dorsal root ganglion

Conus medullaris

End of spinal cord

Dura mater

Subdural space

Arachnoid mater

Subarachnoid space

Pia mater

Nerve sheath

Dorsal root ganglion

Ventral root

Filum terminale internum

S_1

S_2

S_3

S_4

S_5

Coccygeal nerve

Coccyx

FIG. 3–21. Distribution of meninges in lumbosacral region, showing dorsal and ventral roots (cauda equina) with their coverings of pia streaming inferiorly to emerge from proper intervertebral foramina. Enlargement *at left* shows a dorsal and a ventral root emerging through arachnoid and dura through separate openings. Enlargement *at right* has been turned to show distribution of meninges on dorsal and ventral roots and how they blend to form nerve sheath. (Crafts RC: A Textbook of Human Anatomy. Copyright © 1979. Reprinted by permission of John Wiley & Sons, Inc., New York)

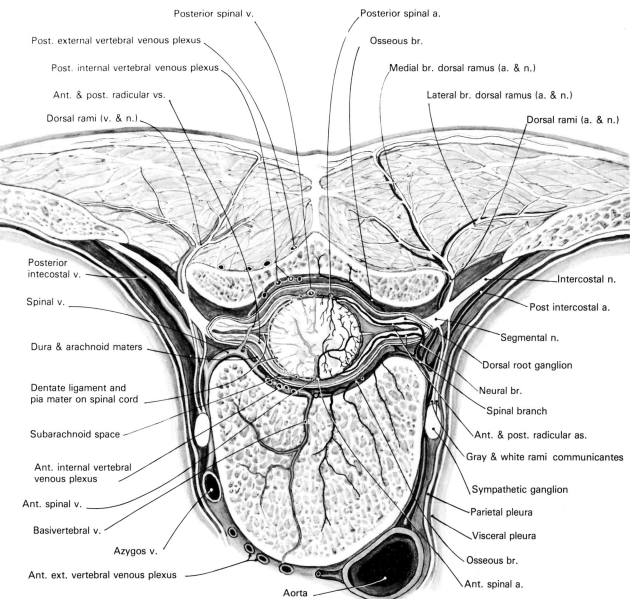

FIG. 3-22. Transverse section of vertebra, spinal cord, and back musculature. Meninges are shown as well as spinal nerves (inferior course naturally taken by nerve roots has been omitted). Spinal arteries and branches are presented *on left side* of body; veins *on right*. (Crafts RC: A Textbook of Human Anatomy. Copyright © 1979. Reprinted by permission of John Wiley & Sons, Inc., New York)

which clusters of ganglion cells (pelvic ganglia) are located. The inferior hypogastric plexus (pelvic plexus) branches into subsidiary plexuses in relation to the sides of the rectum, uterus, vagina, and bladder. These are termed, respectively, the middle and inferior rectal plexus, the uterovaginal plexus, and the vesical plexus. The plexuses ramify along the blood vessels that reach the pelvic organs, including the ureter.

The cell bodies of sympathetic preganglionic fibers concerned with the innervation of the female reproductive tract lie in the intermediolateral cell column (lateral horn) of the spinal cord from the tenth thoracic to the first or second lumbar segments. Fibers from these cells pass through the ventral roots and white rami communicantes to the sympathetic trunks. The distribution of the fibers distally from the sympathetic trunks may follow two general pathways, with synaptic connections to postganglionic neurons possible in the ganglia of the sympathetic trunks or in the ganglia associated with the more peripheral plexuses.

1. Most of the sympathetic preganglionic fibers that supply the internal pelvic organs leave the sympathetic trunks through splanchnic nerves that pass to the aortic plexus. From this plexus delicate postganglionic fibers continue along the ovarian arteries to the ovaries, and a large collection of fibers extends downward as the superior hypogastric plexus described earlier.
2. Other preganglionic sympathetic fibers destined for the pelvic viscera enter the pelvis in the sympathetic trunks, synapse in the chain ganglia, and then pass to the pelvic plexuses directly through small sacral splanchnic nerves to reach the pelvic organs by means of blood vessels. Some fibers may not synapse until small ganglia in the hypogastric plexuses are reached.

The *preganglionic parasympathetic neurons* that supply the ovaries and at least the lateral portions of the uterine tubes arise in the dorsal motor nucleus of the vagus nerve; they accompany these nerves and then the ovarian plexuses to reach ganglia closely associated with these organs. Synapse occurs here, and postganglionic fibers continue to the ovaries and tubes. The preganglionic parasympathetic neurons that supply the remaining pelvic organs lie in the intermediolateral cell columns of the second, third, and fourth sacral segments of the spinal cord and send axons peripherally with the sacral nerves. As the nerves emerge from the pelvic sacral foramina, the parasympathetic fibers pass by way of pelvic nerves* directly into the pelvic plexuses on each side. The pre-postganglionic synapse occurs with cells in the pelvic

---

* Others call these nerves "pelvic splanchnic nerves," but it seems better to restrict the term *splanchnic* to those nerves that leave the sympathetic chain, *i.e.,* greater, lesser, least, lumbar, and sacral splanchnics.

ganglia or in the walls of the organ supplied. It should also be noted that sacral parasympathetic fibers ascend through the hypogastric nerves to reach the inferior mesenteric plexus for distribution to the descending colon and sigmoid colon.

Visceral Sensory Innervation

The cell bodies of visceral sensory fibers, like those of somatic sensory fibers, are located in dorsal root ganglia. In areas reached by spinal nerves, visceral sensory fibers naturally follow the spinal nerves directly to the dorsal root ganglia. The situation is somewhat more complex in the case of sensory fibers from the pelvic organs not directly served by spinal nerves. In this case, the afferent nerves must necessarily follow autonomic plexuses either to reach the sympathetic trunk (ascending to enter spinal nerves T10 to L2 through white rami communicantes) or possibly to enter the sacral nerves through pelvic nerves that also carry parasympathetic fibers.

Relatively little is understood of the anatomic details of the visceral afferent pathways from the reproductive tract. It is known however, that the ovary, uterine tube, fundus, and perhaps the body of the uterus send afferent fibers that carry pain impulses upward through the ovarian plexuses to reach the spinal cord at the level of T10, T11, and T12. Sensory fibers from the cervix ascend through the hypogastric plexuses to enter the spinal cord also at T11 and T12.

PERINEUM

The *perineum* is the most inferior end of the trunk; it is the region between the thighs and between the buttocks. It is *bounded* anteriorly by the pubic arch; laterally by the pubic and ischial rami combined, the ischial tuberosity, and the sacrotuberous ligament; and posteriorly by the sacrum and coccyx (Fig. 3–3). Its *superior limit* is the pelvic diaphragm, consisting of levator ani and coccygeus muscles. If a line is drawn transversely through the point between the anus and the posterior end of the vagina, it will extend laterally to the ischial tuberosities. This line, which bisects the *central perineal tendon (perineal body)*, divides the perineum into a posterior *anal triangle* and an anterior *urogenital triangle*.

ANAL TRIANGLE

The *anal opening* is located in the anal triangle. The sphincter muscles of the anus keep the opening closed, and there are bundles of smooth muscle in the superficial fascia around the anal opening that radiate from the margins of the anus and are attached to the

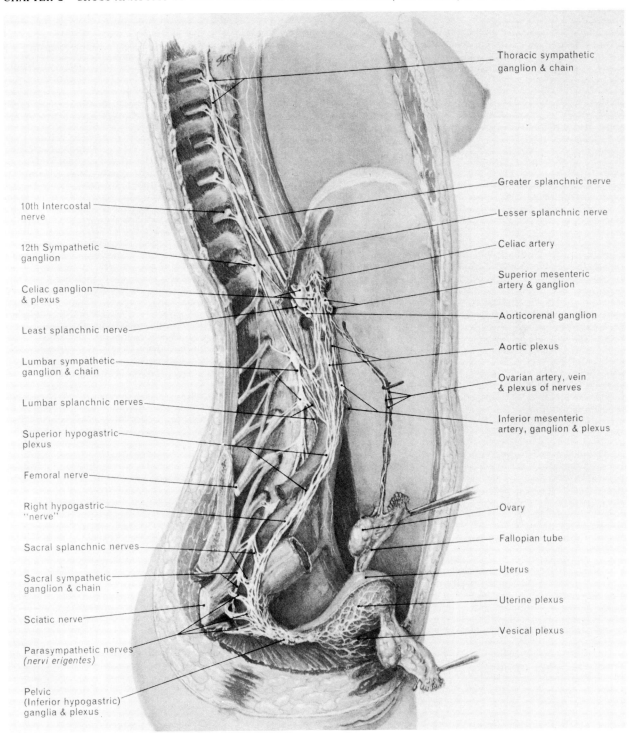

FIG. 3-23. Visceral nerves of female pelvis. (Bonica JJ: Atlas on mechanisms and pathways of pain in labor. What's New, No. 217, 1960)

skin around it. This gives the anus a puckered appearance (Fig. 3–24). The smooth muscles are the *corrugator cutis ani* muscles. A layer of fatty fascia, which is the same as the fatty layer of superficial fascia located in the abdominal wall, lies under the skin of the anal triangle. It is also continuous with a similar fatty layer in the urogenital triangle. This fat fills in a large wedge-shaped area on either side of the anus and rectum—the *ischiorectal fossa* (Figs. 3–25 and 3–26).

The *boundaries* of the ischiorectal fossa are as follows:

Anterior—the transverse muscles of the perineum and the fascia that covers them. (If the finger is pushed anteriorly in the ischiorectal fossa, it can be seen that the finger will be superior to the urogenital diaphragm; this is the anterior recess of the ischiorectal fossa.)

Posterior—the sacrotuberous ligament and the overlying gluteus maximus muscle.

Lateral—the obturator internus muscle with its covering of deep fascia.

Medial—the levator ani and external sphincter muscles covered with deep fascia—the inferior fascia of the pelvic diaphragm.

The *inferior rectal arteries* and *nerves* stream from the lateral superior aspect of the ischiorectal fossa toward the rectum and anus (Fig. 3–25). These nerves and blood vessels supply innervation and vascularity to the inferior end of the anal canal, the circularly arranged external sphincter ani muscle that surrounds the anal opening, and the skin around the anus. These nerves are important, for incontinence results if they are cut. These nerves and arteries are branches of the *pudendal nerve* and *internal pudendal artery,* which course in the layer of fascia on the obturator internus muscle. This canal of fascia is the *pudendal canal* (Fig. 3–26).

In addition to the inferior rectal nerve, a very small

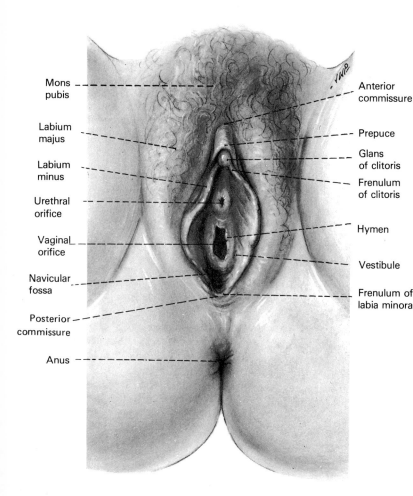

FIG. 3–24. Surface view of female perineum and vulva. Labia have been spread apart.

Mons pubis

Labium majus

Labium minus

Urethral orifice

Vaginal orifice

Navicular fossa

Posterior commissure

Anus

Anterior commissure

Prepuce

Glans of clitoris

Frenulum of clitoris

Hymen

Vestibule

Frenulum of labia minora

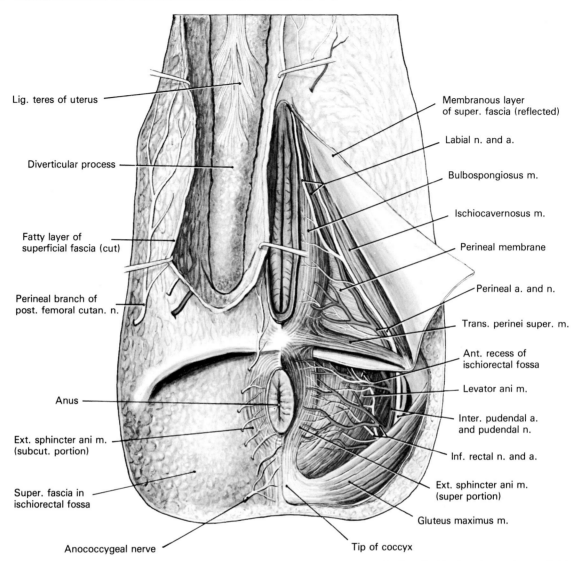

Lig. teres of uterus

Diverticular process

Fatty layer of superficial fascia (cut)

Perineal branch of post. femoral cutan. n.

Anus

Ext. sphincter ani m. (subcut. portion)

Super. fascia in ischiorectal fossa

Anococcygeal nerve

Membranous layer of super. fascia (reflected)

Labial n. and a.

Bulbospongiosus m.

Ischiocavernosus m.

Perineal membrane

Perineal a. and n.

Trans. perinei super. m.

Ant. recess of ischiorectal fossa

Levator ani m.

Inter. pudendal a. and pudendal n.

Inf. rectal n. and a.

Ext. sphincter ani m. (super portion)

Gluteus maximus m.

Tip of coccyx

FIG. 3-25. Perineum in the female. The fatty layer of superficial fascia is intact in the anal triangle *on the right side* of the body, but has been incised in the labium majus to reveal the diverticular process. The fatty layer of superficial fascia has been removed *on the left side* to reveal the contents of the ischiorectal fossa, and the membranous layer of superficial fascia cut and reflected to show contents of the superficial space. (The deep fascia has been removed from the muscles in this space and from the pudendal canal.) (Crafts RC: A Textbook of Human Anatomy. Copyright © 1979. Reprinted by permission of John Wiley & Sons, Inc., New York)

branch, the *coccygeal nerve*, can be found close to the posterior part of the external sphincter muscle of the anus close to where this muscle attaches to the coccyx. This is a sensory nerve to the skin over the coccyx.

The *sphincter ani externus muscle* is divided into subcutaneous, superficial, and deep parts (Fig. 3–26). The *subcutaneous part* completely encircles the anus in a position just deep to the skin. The *superficial portion* has attachments posteriorly to the coccygeal ligament and to the coccyx, and anteriorly to the perineal body, a central fibrous point just anterior to the anus to which several muscles attach. The *deep portion* completely encircles the anal canal (Fig. 3–27); this portion is intimately fused with the puborectal portion of

the levator ani muscle. The latter two parts—superficial and deep—are just lateral to the internal sphincter, which is made up of smooth muscle (Fig. 3–26). The external sphincter is skeletal muscle under voluntary control; *nerve supply*, as mentioned earlier,

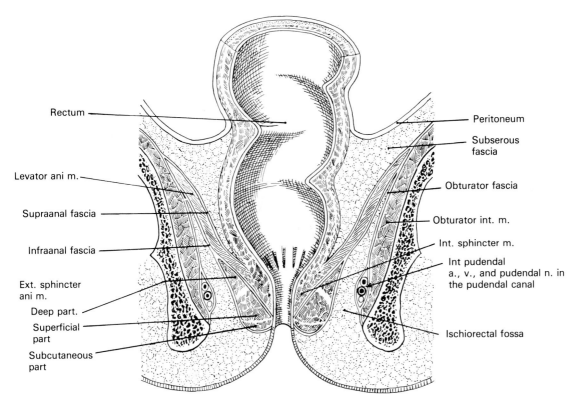

FIG. 3–26. Diagram of a frontal section through the anal triangle of the perineum. (Crafts RC: A Textbook of Human Anatomy. Copyright © 1979. Reprinted by permission of John Wiley & Sons, Inc., New York)

is from inferior rectal branches of the pudendal nerve.

(Abscesses occur in the ischiorectal fossa, and these can spread to the opposite side since the fat pads are continuous both anterior and posterior to the anus. They heal poorly due to the scanty blood supply; they can penetrate the rectum or anal canal between the internal and external sphincter muscles.)

UROGENITAL TRIANGLE

The urogenital triangle in the female contains the *external genitalia* or *vulva* (Fig. 3–24). There is a pad of fat called the *mons pubis* anterior and inferior to the pubic bone. After puberty, this area is covered with hair. This pad of fat can be followed posteriorly to two large lips—the *labia majora*. The point where the lips come together anteriorly is the *anterior labial commissure,* and the region where they come together posteriorly the *posterior labial commissure.* These labia majora are also covered with hair. Medial to the labia majora are two fleshy small lips called the *labia mi-*

nora. These lips are devoid of hair and are usually in contact with one another. The point where the labia minora come together posteriorly is the *frenulum of the labia* while the point where they come together anteriorly is designated as the *frenulum of the clitoris.* The head or glans of the *clitoris* can be seen just at the anterior end of the labia minora, and the fleshy fold just anterior to the glans of the clitoris is the *prepuce of the clitoris.* The space between the labia minora is the *vestibule of the vagina.* This has two openings: 1) the opening of the urethra, which is located about 2.5 cm posterior to the head of the clitoris and appears puckered in the living state, and 2) posterior to that the opening to the *vagina.* If a *hymen* is present, it guards the entrance into the vagina from the vestibule. Just inferior to the hymen on either side are the openings of the *greater vestibular glands.* These glands provide lubrication for the medial sides of the labia minora, being aided in this by small *lesser vestibular glands* opening on the medial sides of the labia minora.

The labia contain an organized process of fat called the *diverticular process* (Fig. 3–25). This is continuous with the fat over the mons pubis and is the structure to which the round ligament of the uterus is attached. The *membranous layer of the superficial fascia* lies deep to the fat and diverticular process; it is exactly

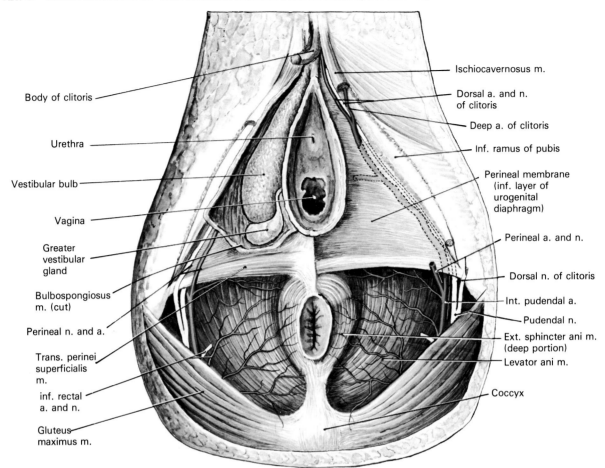

FIG. 3-27. Perineum in the female. The bulbospongiosus muscle has been incised *on the right side* to reveal the vestibular gland and duct, and the bulb. The ischiocavernosus muscle has been removed from the crus of the clitoris. *On the left side* of the body the entire contents of the superficial space has been removed. (Crafts RC: A Textbook of Human Anatomy. Copyright © 1979. Reprinted by permission of John Wiley & Sons, Inc., New York)

the same layer of fascia as found in the abdominal wall. It is attached posteriorly to the posterior edge of the perineal membrane at the line that divides the urogenital triangle from the anal triangle and laterally to the deep fascia on the thigh. Because of these attachments, any matter contained in the area deep to this fascia (the superficial space) is confined to the urogenital triangle, the mons pubis, and the anterior abdominal wall.

In the *superficial space of the perineum,* on either side of the labia minora, are the *bulbospongiosus muscles;* these muscles cover the *vestibular bulb,* which is made up of erectile tissue (Fig. 3–27). Each bulb continues anteriorly and actually joins with that of the opposite side near the head of the clitoris. The *greater vestibular glands* are located just posterior to each bulb. Laterally in the superficial space the *ischiocavernosus muscles* are attached to the ischiopubic rami; these muscles cover the *crura of the clitoris,* which also consist of erectile tissue. Two small muscles run transversely from the perineal body to the inferior pubic rami—the *transversus perinei superficialis*

muscles. The bulbospongiosus muscles form a sort of sphincter around the inferior end of the vagina, the ischiocavernosus muscles may serve to keep the clitoris erect during sexual excitement by compressing the venous return in the crura, and the action of the transversus perinei superficialis muscles is to tense the central point of the perineum, thus aiding in the action of the other muscles.

If the two bulbs and their covering muscles, the two crura with their ischiocavernosus muscles, and the transversus perinei superficialis muscles are removed (Fig. 3–27), the superficial space is seen to be bounded superiorly by a heavy layer of fascia, called the *perineal membrane,* which stretches across the

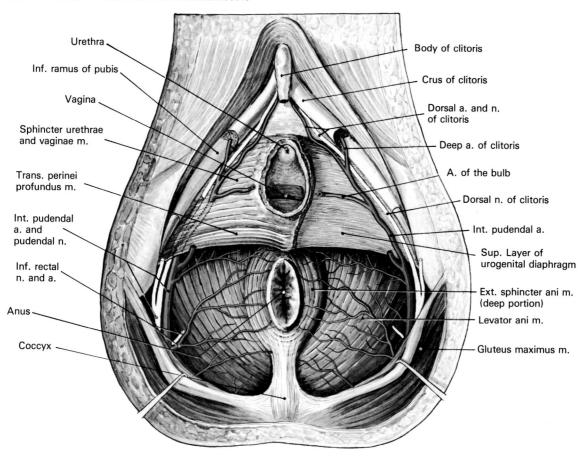

Urethra

Inf. ramus of pubis

Vagina

Sphincter urethrae
and vaginae m.

Trans. perinei
profundus m.

Int. pudendal
a. and
pudendal n.

Inf. rectal
n. and a.

Anus

Coccyx

Body of clitoris

Crus of clitoris

Dorsal a. and n.
of clitoris

Deep a. of clitoris

A. of the bulb

Dorsal n. of clitoris

Int. pudendal a.

Sup. Layer of
urogenital diaphragm

Ext. sphincter ani m.
(deep portion)

Levator ani m.

Gluteus maximus m.

FIG. 3–28. Perineum of the female. The perineal membrane (inferior layer of urogenital diaphragm) has been removed *on the right* to reveal the sphincter urethrae and vaginae muscle and the transversus perinei profundus muscle. *On the left,* these muscles have been removed to reveal the pelvic fascia (superior layer of urogenital diaphragm). (Crafts RC: A Textbook of Human Anatomy. Copyright © 1979. Reprinted by permission of John Wiley & Sons, Inc., New York)

urogenital triangle between the two inferior pubic rami. This is penetrated by both the urethra and vagina.

If the perineal membrane is removed, the contents of the deep space are revealed (Fig. 3–28); it contains a thin sheet of muscle that is divided into two parts: an anterior portion that arises from the inferior rami of the pubis and surrounds the urethra and the vagina (*sphincter urethrae* and *vaginae muscle*), and a posterior component that has been defined as the *transversus perinei profundus muscle.*

If these muscles in the deep space are removed (Fig. 3–28), a layer of *deep fascia* that is continuous with the fascia on the obturator internus muscle (Fig. 3–29) is found. If this deep fascia, in turn, is removed,

the inferior surface of the levator ani muscle is seen.

The layers of the urogenital triangle are, therefore,

1. Skin
2. Fatty layer of superficial fascia
3. Membranous layer of superficial fascia
4. Muscular layer in the superficial space
5. Perineal membrane
6. Muscular layer in the deep space
7. Deep fascia on the superior side of these muscles

These are shown in Figure 3–29. The *superficial space* is the area between layers 3 and 5 in this list, while the *deep space* is between 5 and 7. The perineal membrane, the muscle layer in the deep space, and the deep fascia superior to this muscle (5, 6, and 7) form what is called the *urogenital diaphragm.* Therefore, another name for the perineal membrane is the *inferior layer of the urogenital diaphragm,* and another name for the fascia of layer 7 is the *superior layer of the urogenital diaphragm.* This urogenital diaphragm fills the opening in the pelvic diaphragm between the

two levator ani muscles and supports the pelvic organs.

Clitoris

The *clitoris* (Figs. 3–24 and 3–28) has a structure very similar to that of the penis except that it is much smaller and does not contain the urethra. It is composed of three portions—the *two corpora cavernosa* and the *corpus spongiosum.* The former two arise from the crura of the clitoris in the perineum, and the corpus spongiosum is an anterior continuation of the bulbs in the superficial space of the perineum. The corpus spongiosum, as in the male, ends in a dilated head or *glans.* The organ is erectile in nature. It has a *suspensory ligament,* which suspends the clitoris from the pubic symphysis. The clitoris, which is about 2.5 cm long, takes a sharp bend at the point where the suspensory ligament is attached and heads posteriorly and inferiorly. The loose fold of skin over the clitoris is the *prepuce* of the clitoris.

The nerve and blood supply to the clitoris is discussed below.

Urethra

The urethra in the female is about 4 cm long (Fig. 3–6). It courses inferiorly and slightly anteriorly from the neck of the bladder through the urogenital diaphragm to end in the vestibule of the vagina between the labia minora approximately 2.5 cm posterior to the glans of the clitoris. It is anterior to the opening of the vagina, and its external orifice has firm raised margins. Very small glands open at the sides of the external urethral orifice.

The smooth muscle of the urethra is under control of the *parasympathetic nervous system* (S2, S3, and S4). The external sphincter (sphincter urethrae muscle) is under voluntary control after infancy.

Vessels and Nerves

The *blood and nerve supply* to the urogenital triangle is by branches of the *internal pudendal artery* and *pudendal nerve* (Fig. 3–18), aided by the *perineal branch of the posterior femoral cutaneous nerve* and a branch from the *ilioinguinal nerve.* Although the main role of the *posterior femoral cutaneous nerve* (S2 and S3) is to provide sensory innervation to the posterior surface of the thigh, its *perineal branch* is possibly more important. Because it provides cutaneous innervation to a large part of the perineum (Fig. 3–25), it must be considered in anesthesia of this area. The *ilioinguinal nerve* supplies the mons pubis and the anterior part of the labia majora.

The internal pudental artery and the pudendal nerve arise from the internal iliac artery and the sacral plexus (S2, S3, and S4), respectively, course inferiorly on the inside surface of the piriformis muscle, leave the pelvic cavity through the greater ischiadic (sciatic) foramen in a position inferior to the piriformis muscle to enter the gluteal region, wind around the ischial spine, and enter the lesser ischiadic (sciatic) foramen to become located in the perineum *because they now course beneath the pelvic diaphragm.* The vessel and nerve continue anteriorly and inferiorly on the obturator internus muscle in a fascial canal—the pudendal canal. The first branch of this nerve and artery is the *inferior rectal,* which courses medially through the fat in the ischiorectal fossa to reach the inferior part of the anal canal (Fig. 3–25).

While the internal pudendal artery and pudendal nerve are in the pudendal canal, a *perineal branch* is given off that penetrates the posterior aspect of the membranous layer of the superficial fascia and therefore enters the superficial space (Fig. 3–25). This perineal nerve and artery immediately divide into *muscular branches* to innervate and give blood supply to the muscles already mentioned and into *labial branches,* which carry on to innervate the skin of the posterior surface of the labia and give this area a blood supply. In addition, branches of this perineal nerve enter the deep space to innervate the muscles contained therein, entering the space at its posterior edge.

Returning to the main internal pudendal artery and pudendal nerve, the branching differs after this point. The artery continues anteriorly and enters the deep space, where it occupies a lateral position (Fig. 3–28). In addition to *muscular branches* to the sphincter urethrae and deep transversus perinei muscles contained in this pouch, an *artery to the bulb* emerges, courses medially in the deep space, and then turns inferiorly and penetrates the perineal membrane (inferior layer of urogenital diaphragm) to terminate in the vestibular bulb. The internal pudendal artery continues anteriorly, divides into *deep* and *dorsal* arteries of the clitoris, which then penetrate the perineal membrane to reach this structure. These two vessels course on the dorsum of the clitoris (dorsal branch) and enter the corpora cavernosa of the clitoris (deep branch).

The *pudendal nerve,* in contrast to the artery, terminates before entering the deep space by dividing into the *perineal branch* already mentioned and the *dorsal nerve of the clitoris.* Therefore, the nerve in the deep space is this latter nerve, which then penetrates the perineal membrane to course on the dorsum of the clitoris (Fig. 3–28).

The *external pudendal* arteries also supply perineal structures. These vessels are branches of the femoral artery and supply the mons pubis and the more anterior aspect of the labia majora.

Veins of the perineum accompany arteries usually as double or plexiform vessels. However, the *deep vein of the clitoris,* unpaired, empties directly into the vesi-

FIG. 3-29. Frontal section of the urogenital triangle of the female. *1,* Skin. *2,* Fatty layer of superficial fascia. *3,* Membranous layer of superficial fascia. *4,* Superficial space containing the bulb(s) and bulbospongiosus muscle(s), the crura and ischiocavernosus muscles, transversus perinei superficialis muscles, greater vestibular glands, perineal nerves and vessels. *5,* Perineal membrane or inferior layer of urogenital diaphragm. *6,* Deep space containing the sphincter urethrae and vaginae, and transversus perinei profundus muscles, internal pudendal artery and artery of the bulb, and dorsal nerve of the clitoris. *7,* Pelvic fascia or superior layer of the urogenital diaphram. *8,* Obturator internus muscle covered with pelvic fascia. *9,* Anterior recess of ischiorectal fossa. *10.* Levator ani muscle covered with pelvic fascia (infra- and supraanal fascia). *11,* Subserous fascia. *12,* Peritoneum. Note that the superficial space is between *3* and *5,* the deep space between *5* and *7,* and that *5, 6,* and *7* make up the urogenital diaphragm. (Crafts RC: A Textbook of Human Anatomy. Copyright © 1979. Reprinted by permission of John Wiley & Sons, Inc., New York. Modified after Jamieson.)

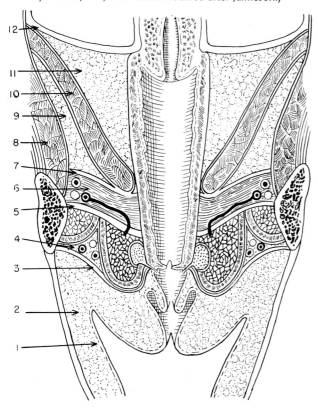

cal plexus by passing superiorly between the urogenital diaphragm and the pubic arcuate ligament. *Superficial dorsal veins* of the clitoris as well as *anterior labial veins* are tributaries of the femoral veins.

The perineal membrane is a relatively thick structure that joins with the pelvic fascia anteriorly and posteriorly to form an enclosed space. The anterior edge of this membrane does not reach the pubic symphysis; this opening is utilized by the dorsal vein of the clitoris to reach the plexus of veins in the pelvic cavity.

The body of the clitoris, the vestibular bulbs, the crura of the clitoris, and the blood vessels in the perineum are innervated by the autonomic nervous system. The sympathetic fibers arise in the upper lumbar segments and ultimately follow the pudendal nerve and internal pudendal arteries to gain their destination. The parasympathetic fibers from S2, S3, and S4 also follow the pudendal arteries and are concerned in erection of these tissues, causing more blood to enter than leave the erectile tissue.

LYMPHATICS

Lymphatics from all structures in the perineum drain into the inguinal nodes.

REFERENCES AND RECOMMENDED READING

Langman J: Medical Embryology. Baltimore, Williams & Wilkins, 1975
Warwick R, Williams PL (eds): Gray's Anatomy, 35th British ed. Philadelphia, WB Saunders, 1973

THE HYPOTHALAMUS AND PITUITARY

Howard P. Krieger

HYPOTHALAMIC–PITUITARY INTERRELATIONS

The pituitary, once considered the master gland, is now known to be functionally dominated by the hypothalamus. The hypothalamus, in turn, is essentially an integrator of influences that arise from the cerebrum (especially the limbic system), from the brain stem (especially the reticular activating system) from the spinal cord, and from the endocrine end organ products carried in the bloodstream.

The functional relations among the nervous structures in the complex system are synaptic. The relation between the hypothalamus and the posterior pituitary is synaptic and secretory (Fig. 3–30). The last synapse in the mechanism is at the supraoptic or paraventricular nuclei, which lie in the anterior part of the hypothalamus. The axons of the neurons in these nuclei collect to form the supraoptic–hypophyseal tract, which traverses the hypothalamus and the pituitary stalk and ends in the posterior pituitary. Here the axon terminals abut upon blood vessels instead of other neurons. The products of these neurons are formed in the nuclei, migrate down the axons, and are secreted into the bloodstream. These neurons are thus a classic example of hypothalamic secretory neurons. The secretory products in this case are antidiuretic hormone and oxytocin (or possibly their precursors).

The anatomic arrangement in the case of the anterior pituitary is basically the same. Neurons from the central nervous system synapse with the axons of neurons of various nuclei of the hypothalamus. The axons end upon blood vessels into which their products are secreted. The hypothalamic–anterior pituitary relation is special because these products are secreted into a portal system (Fig. 3–31), the hypothalamic–pituitary portal system, which arises in the floor of the hypothalamus essentially in the midline just above the pituitary stalk, a region called the median eminence. This portal system descends in and about the pituitary stalk and breaks up into its second capillary system within the anterior pituitary itself. Thus, the products of the hypothalamic secretory neurons (which may be either releasing or inhibiting factors) are delivered from the hypothalamus directly to the pituitary cells. This arrangement allows a very high concentration of these products to enter the anterior pituitary before becoming diluted in the general circulation. Whether the products of small regions of the hypothalamus are selectively delivered to special regions of the anterior pituitary has not been settled, but it seems unlikely. Although there are many nuclei within the hypothalamus and some may have delineated functions, it is still not known whether a given neuron produces only one secretory product (releasing or inhibiting). It also seems that the various functional cell types are not absolutely limited to specific nuclei.

Thus, the basic anatomic plan of the hypothalamus is like that of the rest of the nervous system. The hypothalamic secretory neuron is analogous to a lower motor neuron (*e.g.*, an anterior horn cell of the spinal cord). Both types of neurons are integrators of neuronal information from cerebrum, brain stem, and spinal cord. The result of this neural integration is the production of a secretory factor and its delivery to an effector; in the case of the hypothalamic secretory neuron, the product is delivered either to the anterior pituitary by means of the portal system or to the kidney or the uterus by means of the systemic bloodstream from the posterior pituitary; in the case of the lower motor neuron, the secretory product (acetylcholine) is delivered to a motor end plate across a synaptic cleft.

Although the total pathway is long and complex, the effects can occur with astonishing speed. For example, in the case of cortisol, the original stimulus may arise in the temporal lobe; thereafter, the route is from the temporal lobe through the limbic system to the hypothalamus, over the portal system to the anterior pituitary, and through the bloodstream to the adrenal. In the cat, a stimulus to the temporal lobe is reflected in a rise in blood 17-hydroxycorticosteroids within 1 min. Thus, it appears that the neuroendocrine system is a very rapid organizer of behavioral and physiologic response.

In addition to the central nervous system–pituitary end organ interrelations, the endocrine end organ products act upon the central nervous system. The sites of action are numerous, as can be demonstrated by labeling the cell nuclei that take up hormones made radioactive (Fig. 3–32). The limbic system of the temporal lobe (hippocampus and amygdala), which projects into the hypothalamus, is a major site of cortisol uptake. The hypothalamic preoptic area is a major site of estradiol uptake, but this hormone is also significantly taken up by nuclei of the amygdala and hippocampus. These receptor sites act as sensors of the blood level of the end organ product. The sensors act to excite or dampen hypothalamic and thus pituitary activity. The various endocrine end organ products probably also act directly on the pituitary. In any case, the anatomicophysiologic system is such that endocrine activity can be quickly integrated into the total behavioral response at any time by means of feedback mechanisms and multiple nervous system pathways leading to the hypothalamus.

Clearly, sensory stimuli from essentially the entire

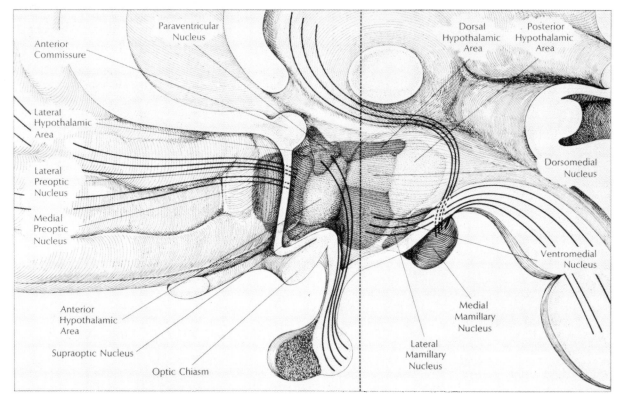

FIG. 3–30. Interconnections of hypothalamus with remainder of central nervous system. (Krieger DT, Hughes JC (eds): Neuroendocrinology. New York, HP Publishing, 1980)

body have potential neuroanatomic access to the hypothalamic–pituitary system. The generally accepted relation of the breast, cervix, and vagina to oxytocin release serves as an example. Although some of the details are not clear, it is suggested that sensory stimuli arising from the nipple, the cervix, or the vagina travel along peripheral nerves to the spinal cord, up to the brain stem, and finally to the hypothalamus to reach the paraventricular nuclei in the anterosuperior aspect of the hypothalamus. There oxytocin or its precursor is formed and transported along the neurons of the supraoptic–hypophyseal tract to the posterior pituitary, where it is released into the blood stream. It is then transported to the breast and uterus. Some of the oxytocin is probably also released into the median eminence and carried over the portal system to the anterior pituitary, where it triggers production of prolactin, which is also carried to the breast. Alterations in the menstrual cycle illustrate the effect of psychic and first cranial nerve stimuli that reach the cerebrum and then are relayed to the hypothalamic–pituitary system. Psychic effects upon the menstrual cycle are well known. Perhaps less well known is that a group of cy-cling females living together, as in a dormitory, may soon have coinciding cycles. In the case of rats, this has been shown to require an intact olfactory nerve and to depend upon pheromones or substances carried through the air from one organism to another.

PITUITARY–JUXTAPITUITARY INTERRELATIONS

A different set of pituitary–hypothalamic–nervous system relations reflects the anatomic juxtaposition of parts of these areas rather than a physiologic relation. Figure 3–33 shows the relations among the hypothalamus, chiasm, pituitary, sella turcica, cavernous sinuses and their contents, sphenoid sinus, and temporal lobes. For the most part, the anatomic juxtaposition of these structures becomes clinically important only in disease. Thus neoplasms in this region (whether they arise in the pituitary, hypothalamus, neighboring meninges, or sphenoid sinus), as well as large aneurysms (such as occur in the carotid artery as it passes lateral to the sella), produce a clinical picture compounded of pituitary–hypothalamic dysfunc-

tion (either hypo- or hyperfunction) and dysfunction (ischemic or destructive) of neighboring neurologic structures. When a mass develops in this region, the most commonly affected nervous system structure is the optic chiasm (producing typically a bitemporal hemianopsia), but any other neighboring structure may be affected. The older literature indicates that during pregnancy the pituitary swells and can produce a visual field defect secondary to chiasmatic compression. We have never seen such a case, and it must be very rare. Temporal lobe seizures are also rare. Various types of third, fourth, and sixth nerve palsies, as well as rupture of the floor of the sella and extension of its contents into the sphenoid sinus, are also uncommon in disease in this area. When masses arise in the hypothalamus, a combination of hypo- and hyperfunction may occur in conjunction with destruction of chiasmatic function.

FIG. 3-31. Main features of unusual circulation that connect hypothalamus and pituitary. *Arrows* indicate direction of blood flow. Blood passing into hypophyseal portal veins from median eminence area is distributed to anterior pituitary through secondary capillary plexuses before draining into general venous circulation; hence, virtually all afferent blood supply of anterior pituitary has first been in contact with hypothalamic median eminence area. Krieger DT, Hughes JC (eds): (Neuroendocrinology. New York, HP Publishing, 1980)

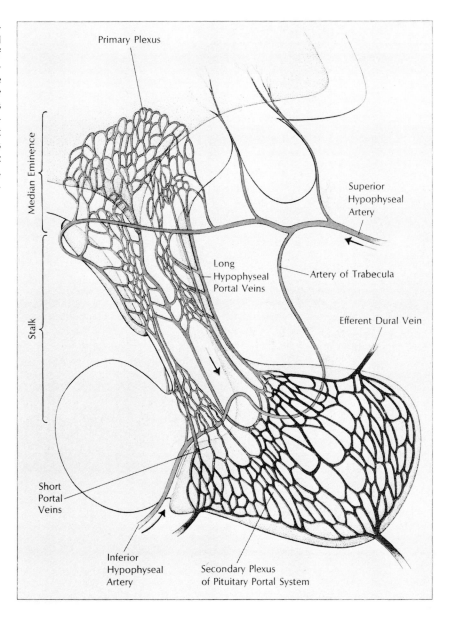

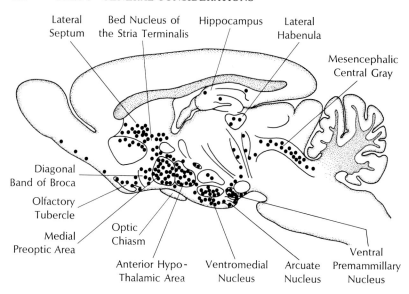

Lateral Septum

Bed Nucleus of the Stria Terminalis

Hippocampus

Lateral Habenula

Mesencephalic Central Gray

Diagonal Band of Broca

Olfactory Tubercle

Medial Preoptic Area

Optic Chiasm

Anterior Hypo-Thalamic Area

Ventromedial Nucleus

Arcuate Nucleus

Ventral Premammillary Nucleus

FIG. 3–32. Estrogen-binding sites in hypothalamic and limbic structures demonstrated by uptake of injected radioactive estradiol in rat. *Black dots* show areas of radioactivity. (McEwen BS: In Krieger DT, Hughes JC (eds): Neuroendocrinology, p 36. New York, HP Publishing, 1980)

FIG. 3–33. Relation of contents of sella turcica to surrounding structures. Disease processes here can compromise optic function, affect nearby cranial nerves, and derange neuroendocrine functions. (Krieger HP: In Krieger DT, Hughes JC (eds): Neuroendocrinology, HP Publishing, 1980)

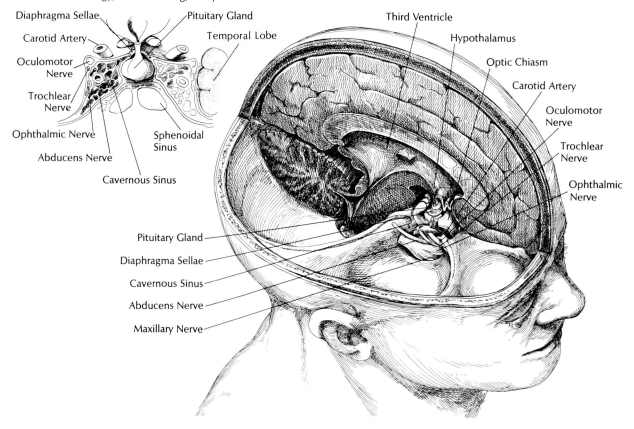

Diaphragma Sellae

Carotid Artery

Oculomotor Nerve

Trochlear Nerve

Ophthalmic Nerve

Abducens Nerve

Cavernous Sinus

Pituitary Gland

Temporal Lobe

Sphenoidal Sinus

Third Ventricle

Hypothalamus

Optic Chiasm

Carotid Artery

Oculomotor Nerve

Trochlear Nerve

Ophthalmic Nerve

Pituitary Gland

Diaphragma Sellae

Cavernous Sinus

Abducens Nerve

Maxillary Nerve

REFERENCES

Krieger DT: The hypothalamus and neuroendocrinology. In Krieger DT, Hughes JC (eds): Neuroendocrinology, p 3. New York, HP Publishing, 1980

Krieger HP: Sellar and juxtasellar disease: A neurologic viewpoint. In Krieger DT, Hughes JC (eds): Neuroendocrinology, p 275. New York, HP Publishing, 1980

Krieger HP, Krieger DT: Chemical stimulation of the brain: Effect on adrenal corticoid release. Am J Physiol 218 (6):1632, 1970

McEwen BS: The brain as a target organ of endocrine hormones. In Krieger DT, Hughes JC (eds): Neuroendocrinology, p 33. New York, HP Publishing, 1980

MICROSCOPIC ANATOMY OF THE FEMALE REPRODUCTIVE TRACT AND PITUITARY

**Jack Davies
E. S. E. Hafez
Hans Ludwig**

HISTOLOGY

Jack Davies

The female reproductive system includes the ovaries, the prime purpose of which is to produce the female germ cells (eggs); the sexual ducts (uterine tubes, uterus, vagina); and the external genitalia. Associated with the latter are certain glandular structures that collectively form the accessory organs of reproduction. The female reproductive system, unlike that of the male, shows cyclic alterations in structure coincident with the phases of the menstrual cycle, which are in turn dependent upon the activities of the estrogenic and progestational hormones of the ovaries. It also shows striking modifications in structure and function during pregnancy.

THE OVARIES

The ovaries are bilateral structures attached to the posterior leaf of the broad ligament in relation to the lateral pelvic wall. Their epithelial covering, or *germinal epithelium* (Fig. 4–1), is a modified area of the celomic lining, which, in the embryo and fetus, gives rise by proliferation to the germinal and supporting elements of the ovary. It is a cuboidal or low columnar epithelium continuous at the hilum with the flat squamous mesothelium of the peritoneal cavity; the transition between the two epithelia is abrupt and marked by Farre's white line. The postnatal origin of the germ cells from the germinal epithelium is disputed, but the weight of evidence is against it. It is probable that the full complement of eggs (estimated as at least 150,000 in the two ovaries) is present at birth and that no further formation of eggs occurs after birth. If this is true, some of the eggs must lie dormant within the ovary for 40 years or more before they complete their maturation in the ovulatory cycle or degenerate. Of this large number of eggs, only about 400 may be successfully ovulated during the sexual life of the woman; the rest degenerate. It is also important to understand that the "eggs" present in the postnatal ovary are primary oocytes, *i.e.,* they have already entered upon the maturation cycle and are arrested in the prophase of the first maturation division (Fig. 4–1). All subsequent divisions of these cells are by reduction division (*meiosis*).

The ovary is customarily described as having a cortex and a medulla. The *medulla,* or central core of the ovary, is continuous with the connective tissue of the broad ligament at the hilum, through which the blood vessels and lymphatics penetrate the organ. Here also are found vestiges of the rete ovarii, homologous with the rete testis of the male, as well as epithelial remnants of the mesonephros (wolffian body) that form the epoophoron.

The ovarian *cortex* in prepubertal and early sexual life contains large numbers of primary oocytes embedded in a highly cellular connective tissue. During sexual life there are also graafian follicles in varying stages of development. The cortical stroma is condensed beneath the germinal epithelium into a tunica albuginea. The germinal epithelium is said not to rest on a basement membrane. This may be true in fetal life, when the germinal epithelium is actively proliferating; however, in the adult ovary a thin basement membrane can always be demonstrated by electron microscopy.

Several stages in the maturation of the primary oocytes and of the graafian follicles may be studied in Figure 4–1, which is from a section of the rabbit ovary; the sequence of events is essentially the same in the human ovary. A group of primary oocytes begins to mature at the beginning of each menstrual cycle under the influence of pituitary gonadotropins, probably chiefly follicle-stimulating hormone (FSH). What

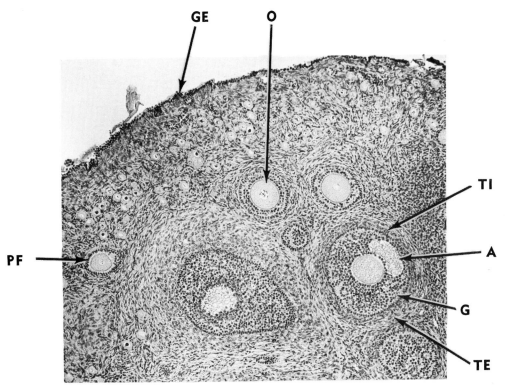

FIG. 4–1. Cortex of ovary of virgin rabbit. Surface germinal epithelium (*GE*) is cuboidal. There is a thin tunica albuginea deep to germinal epithelium. Primary oocytes (*O*) lie embedded in superficial cortex and are surrounded by fibroblastic cells; nuclei of oogonia are in prophaselike state. Primordial follicles (*PF*) lie deeper in cortex. Here also oocyte is larger than in superficial layer and is surrounded by layer of cuboidal granulosa cells. Other follicles are in later stages of development. A follicle with beginning antrum formation (*A*) is shown to right. External to thick layer of granulosa cells (*G*) in larger follicles is theca interna (*TI*), external to which is theca externa (*TE*). A thin zona pellucida is present in oocyte to *right*. (H&E, ×220)

factors are involved in the selection of one group of follicles rather than another are unknown and present an important problem for solution. It is interesting that the number of maturing follicles in any cycle is constant (Lipschutz's law of follicular constancy); and if one ovary is removed, the number of maturing follicles in the remaining ovary is approximately doubled.

DEVELOPMENT OF THE GRAAFIAN FOLLICLE

A *primordial follicle* (Fig. 4–1) consists of a primary oocyte enclosed by a single layer of cuboidal cells derived from the surrounding stroma. The oocyte and the follicular (nurse) cells around it grow *pari passu* until the oocyte is about 80μ and the follicle is about 0.2 mm in diameter. Thereafter, the follicle grows more rapidly than the oocyte. In a fully mature follicle the oocyte is about 120μ in diameter, and the follicle may reach a diameter of 5–10 mm. The cells surrounding the oocyte increase in number by mitosis, and when the follicle is about 0.2 mm in diameter a fluid-filled space (*antrum*) appears. The fluid (*primary liquor folliculi*) is metachromatic at a neutral pH and stains with the periodic acid-Schiff (PAS) method, indicating the possible presence of neutral or weakly acidic mucopolysaccharides. A secondary liquor folliculi of gelatinous consistency is also described in the

antrum of larger follicles. A more watery tertiary liquor folliculi accumulates rapidly within the antrum of a follicle that is destined to rupture at ovulation; it is probably secreted by the lining cells. This preovulatory swelling of the mature follicle is believed to depend upon the action of pituitary luteinizing hormone (LH), which is released into the blood just before ovulation.

In the mature graafian follicle (Figs. 4–1 and 4–2), the cells surrounding the antral cavity are known as the *granulosa cells* or the *membrana granulosa*. The mature oocyte lies within a localized mound of granulosa cells, the *discus proligerus* or *cumulus oophorus* (Fig. 4–2), which is oriented toward the medulla of the ovary. The granulosa cells are avascular and are several layers in thickness; the basal layer of cells rests on a well-marked basement membrane that stains strongly with the PAS method. The stromal elements

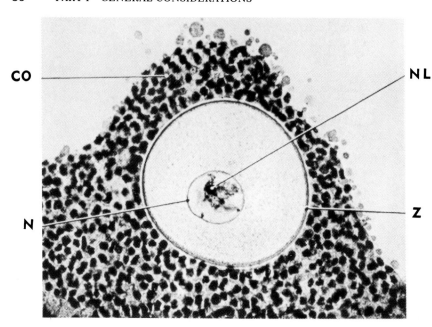

FIG. 4–2. Portion of wall of mature human graafian follicle. Primary oocyte is surrounded by zona pellucida (*Z*). Oocyte is embedded in cumulus oophorus (*CO*). Antral cavity filled with liquor folliculi lies at *top* of picture. N, Nucleus. *NL*, Nucleolus. (Grollman A: Essentials of Endocrinology, 2nd ed. Philadelphia, Lippincott, 1941)

of the ovary are condensed around the follicle in two layers, the theca interna and the theca externa (Fig. 4–1). The *theca externa* is relatively avascular and forms a connective tissue capsule around the follicle. The *theca interna* is vascular, and its cells undergo marked hypertrophy as the follicle matures (Fig. 4–3). The cells become rounded and epithelial in appearance, and sudanophilic droplets appear within their cytoplasm. As ovulation approaches, the hypertrophied thecal cells resemble the luteal cells of the corpus luteum (Fig. 4–4) but are smaller. The luteal hypertrophy of the theca interna probably results from the action of pituitary LH. In some animals, such as the cat, a striking preovulatory luteal hypertrophy of these cells occurs. This may also occur under certain circumstances in the human ovary.

The changes in the primary oocyte during the maturation process are complex. An initial *growth phase,* coincident with the proliferation of the granulosal and thecal elements of the follicle, is followed by a *maturation phase,* in which the growth rate is reduced and in which there is an active synthesis of cytoplasmic proteins and yolk droplets. The nuclei of the oocytes remain in a peculiar prophaselike state both in the dormant phase within the primordial follicle (Fig. 4–1) and during the preliminary phase of maturation. Mitochondria appear in abundance within the cytoplasm, and there is a well-marked Golgi region. When the oocyte has reached a diameter of about 80μ, a highly refractile membrane (*zona pellucida*) appears between the granulosa cells and the oocyte. It may be a secretory product of the granulosa cells, which show increased cytoplasmic complexity in the electron microscope. Microvilli from the surface plasma membrane of the granulosa cells and from that of the oocyte (*vitelline membrane*) are found within the zona pellucida and may make contact with each other, suggesting a possible avenue of transmission of materials between them. The zona pellucida stains strongly with the PAS method and is metachromatic at a low pH, suggesting the presence of strongly acid mucopolysaccharides. Between the zona pellucida and the oocyte is a perivitelline space, which may be exaggerated as an artifact of fixation and dehydration.

A fully mature graafian follicle may reach a size of 5–10 mm in the human ovary. Just before ovulation, the mature oocyte completes the first reduction division, in which the diploid number of chromosomes (46) is halved to the haploid number (23); the smaller daughter cell forms the *first polar body* and lies within the perivitelline space. The egg is now a *secondary oocyte* and is in this stage when ovulation takes place. The second reduction division does not occur until after fertilization of the oocyte in the upper reaches of the uterine tubes. Following sperm penetration, the *second polar body* is formed. This second division of the oocyte nucleus is, however, comparable to a mitotic process with a reduced number of chromosomes, and there is no further alteration in the haploid number.

The secondary oocyte with its polar body enclosed within the zona pellucida is shed at ovulation by rupture of the graafian follicle. The process has been observed by cinephotography in rodents. As ovulation approaches, an area of the follicular wall underlying the germinal epithelium becomes thinned and avascular.

FIG. 4-3. Portion of wall of mature human graafian follicle at about 13th day of cycle, *i.e.,* just before ovulation. Antral cavity at *top* contains coagulated liquor folliculi. Granulosa cells (*G*) form layer five or six cells in thickness; they have small dark nuclei with very little cytoplasm. Basement membrane of granulosa cells is not demonstrated by this stain. External to latter is theca interna (*TI*), made up of epithelium-like cells and containing many blood vessels. Theca externa (*TE*) of condensed connective tissue lies external to theca interna. (H&E, ×100)

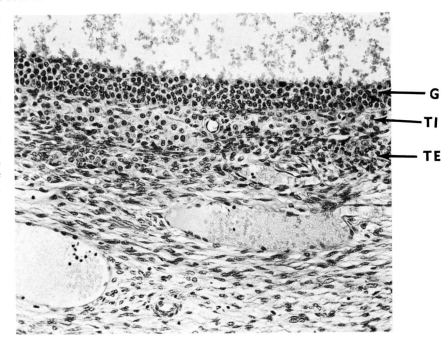

The wall then ruptures at this point, and a mixture of gelatinous and fluid liquor folliculi spurts through the hole. The egg may emerge first or may follow the initial spurt of follicular fluid. The egg carries with it a cluster of cells of the cumulus oophorus (*corona radiata*). It is then carried by fluid currents and ciliary action into the infundibulum of the uterine tube.

FOLLICULAR ATRESIA

A phenomenon of great importance is *follicular atresia*. Of the six or more follicles that begin the growth and maturation process at each cycle, only one as a rule undergoes the preovulatory swelling and ruptures at ovulation. The remaining follicles of the group fail to swell and undergo a degenerative change known as atresia. There is degeneration and nucleus pyknosis of the granulosa cells, beginning in the cells nearest to the antrum. The follicular fluid becomes inspissated, and the entrapped egg degenerates. The zona pellucida may persist for an extended time as a highly refractile, strongly PAS-positive band. The granulosa cells degenerate completely, and the antrum becomes filled with organizing fibrinous material. The basement membrane of the granulosa layer becomes thickened and highly refractile, forming the *glassy membrane;* it also may persist for an extended time as a crumpled refractile homogeneous band. The follicle collapses, and the theca interna and externa are also modified. In some instances, the theca interna may show only fibrotic changes, whereas in others, perhaps

FIG. 4-4. Early stage in luteal transformation of ruptured graafian follicle. Antral cavity at *top* contains organizing fibrinous material. Granulosa cells are hypertrophied and show marked increase in amount of cytoplasm that is acidophilic. Clusters of theca granulosa cells; cells are smaller than granulosa lutein cells. Vessels have grown into modified granulosa layer and are beginning to invest luteal cells with sinusoidal capillary vessels. *TL,* theca lutein cells. (H&E, ×220)

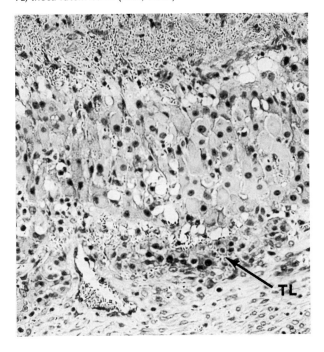

depending on whether an effective luteinizing stimulus is present or not, the theca interna may undergo a luteal hypertrophy. The cells become epithelial and store lipid droplets, and in all respects except size they resemble the luteal cells of the corpus luteum. Such a luteinized follicle is called a *corpus luteum atreticum* and is not to be confused with a true corpus luteum, which is formed only after ovulation. Corpora lutea atretica, as well as atretic follicles in general, are formed in increased numbers in pregnancy in women and in animals with prolonged gestation periods such as the horse. Their appearance in pregnancy may be associated with powerful luteinizing effects emanating from the placenta, which produces human chorionic gonadotropin (hCG) in women and pregnant mare serum gonadotropin (PMSG) in the mare. The rate of follicular atresia is also markedly increased in the postovulatory stage of the menstrual cycle in women and primates and of the estrous cycle in animals, as well as after the administration of progestational compounds. The significance of follicular atresia and the hormonal significance of corpora lutea atretica remain two of the most important unsolved problems of reproductive physiology.

DEVELOPMENT OF THE CORPUS LUTEUM

Following ovulation, the follicle is converted into a true *corpus luteum*. In animals with multiple ovulations, like the rabbit, there are multiple corpora lutea, and their number correlates to a striking degree with the number of viable fetuses at a later stage. Only one, corresponding to the ovulation occurring in that cycle, is present in the human ovary. In rats, which have very short estrous cycles of 4–5 days, there are several generations of corpora lutea, and it may be difficult to identify the ones corresponding to the most recent ovulation.

The manner of formation of the corpus luteum from the follicular elements has been debated for many years. In some animals, such as the rabbit, it is clear that only the granulosa cells are involved in the luteal transformation of the follicle. In the human ovary there are two types of luteal cells, the *granulosa lutein cells* and the *theca lutein cells,* the latter being derived from the theca interna. The cells differ only in size, the theca lutein cells being much smaller in the earlier stages. Later in the development of the corpus luteum it is impossible to identify the two types of cells. Following the rupture of the follicle, the antral cavity collapses and may contain a little extravasated blood. Hemorrhagic cystic follicles without ovulation and associated with theca luteinization are common in animals, such as the rabbit, following coitus or a large dose of a luteinizing preparation. Theca lutein cysts are found in the ovaries of newborn and adult human

beings, but their pathogenesis and hormonal basis are poorly understood.

After collapse of the antral cavity following ovulation, the granulosa cells proliferate by mitosis and undergo a steady hypertrophy and growth. The basement membrane of the granulosa layer is broken in several places, and there is an invasion of capillary sprouts and connective tissue from the theca interna into the granulosa layer (Fig. 4–4). Under the continuing luteal stimulus, both the granulosa cells and the smaller theca cells become slowly transformed into luteal cells, and the two types of cells become closely intermingled. Within 2–3 days the corpus luteum becomes organized into a spherical body in which the luteal cells are arranged in more or less radial cords around the central remnant of the antral cavity. There are coarse septa of connective tissue separating the principal cords of luteal cells that contain the larger vessels, and there are delicate capsules of reticular tissue and capillaries around the individual luteal cells and groups of cells. The structure is highly vascular and bleeds profusely on cutting, so that it may be a source of serious intraabdominal bleeding.

The luteal cells resemble cells of the adrenal cortex in appearance under both light and electron microscopes. These steroid-secreting cells share fine structural characteristics that may tentatively be identified with their function as producers of steroid hormones such as the estrogens and progestational compounds. The mitochondria are rounded and tend to have tubular cristae rather than the usual lamellar type. The cytoplasm is occupied by a honeycomb of small sacs and short tubules of the endoplasmic reticulum. Between these sacs and tubules are numerous ribonucleoprotein granules (ribosomes). There are large lipid inclusions enclosed in membranous sacs, probably representing sites of hormone deposition or synthesis. The droplets of lipid are acetone-soluble, doubly refractile, and autofluorescent; they also give the Schultz reaction for cholesterol and other histochemical reactions considered typical of the ketosteroids, though not specific for them.

Degeneration of the luteal cells is accompanied by changes in the solubility and refractility of the lipid droplets. The droplets also tend to coalesce and form large sudanophilic masses. There are also droplets of the wear-and-tear pigment *lipofuscin;* its presence in the degenerating corpus luteum of the human ovary caused earlier observers to note its yellow color and so to give it its name.

The corpus luteum is formed during the first 3 days after ovulation under the predominant influence of pituitary LH. Thereafter a luteotropic influence is pituitary in origin in the luteal phase of the menstrual cycle. The corpus luteum declines and becomes functionless a few days before the next menstrual cycle,

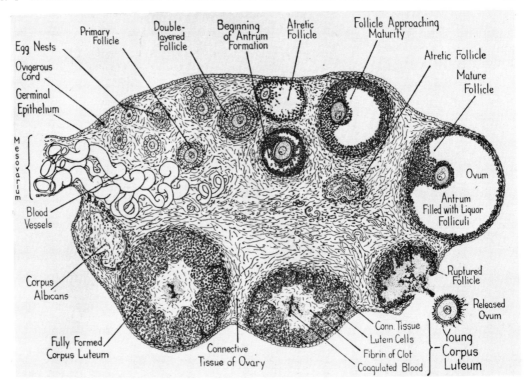

FIG. 4-5. Diagram of ovary, showing sequence of events leading to maturation and rupture of follicles, luteinization, and involution of corpus luteum. Nonruptured follicles undergo atresia. (Patten BM: Human Embryology. New York, Blakiston, 1946)

presumably owing to the withdrawal of the luteotropic stimulus. In the pregnant woman, however, the corpus luteum of menstruation fails to degenerate and increases in size, forming the *corpus luteum of pregnancy.* Its continued life and function depend upon a new luteotropic stimulus, this time emanating from the placenta. This stimulus is probably hCG, which has been identified in the trophoblast soon after implantation and appears in the urine at a slightly later stage. Its effects in animals are predominantly luteinizing; in women large doses have been shown to be luteotropic also. The corpus luteum functions throughout the first third of pregnancy but declines thereafter and has degenerated by the last third. New ovulations with the production of accessory corpora lutea, as in the mare, are not known to occur in women. The final stages in the degeneration of the human corpus luteum of menstruation may last up to a year. They consist of shrinkage and hyalinization of the luteal cells and the intercellular connective tissue and conversion of the corpus luteum into a hyalinized mass (*corpus albicans*). Figure 4-5 diagrams this sequence of events.

INTERSTITIAL CELLS

Interstitial cells of the ovary are abundant in the rabbit, in which they form an interstitial gland and appear to be a source of estrogen and progestational compounds. They are inconspicuous in the human ovary but may be found in considerable numbers in the medulla in the region of the hilum; they are increased in number in the ovary of the patient with the Stein–Leventhal syndrome. Their microscopic appearance is similar to that of the steroid-secreting cells described earlier, and it is reasonable to suppose that they also may be a source of steroid hormones, including estrogenic, progestational, and androgenic compounds.

THE UTERINE TUBES

The oviducts (uterine tubes) are about 10 cm in length. They are bilateral structures and pierce the wall of the uterus at the lateral margins of the fundus on either side. They are divided into three parts: the ampulla, the isthmus, and the intramural part. The uterine tube communicates with the peritoneal cavity close to the ovary through the infundibulum. The margins of the opening are expanded into tentaclelike structures (*fimbriae*) that become turgid at the time

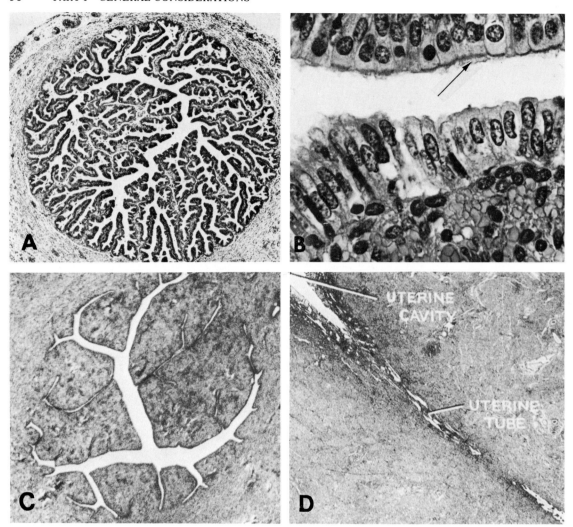

FIG. 4–6. *A.* Transverse section of uterine tube at level of ampulla. *B.* Details of epithelium of ampulla of uterine tube. Ciliated cells are shown at *arrow.* Other cells are secretory in type and there are some narrow peglike cells with dark nuclei. (H&E, approximately ×500) *C.* Isthmus. Note that folding of mucosa is less marked and muscle is thicker. (Leeson TA, Leeson CR (eds): Histology, 2nd ed. Philadelphia, WB Saunders, 1970) *D.* Interstitial or intramural segment of tube. (Greep RO (ed): Histology, 2nd ed. New York, McGraw-Hill, 1966)

of ovulation and closely applied to the rupturing follicle, thereby decreasing the chance of loss of the egg into the peritoneal cavity. The *ampulla* is the relatively dilated lateral half of the tube. Its lumen is wider than the isthmic portion, and the lining mucosal folds are more complex. It is in this portion of the tube that fertilization of the oocyte takes place and in which it completes its second maturation division and later segmentation. The *isthmic portion* of the tube is very narrow, and its lumen is difficult to enter with a probe. The *intramural portion* is about 1 cm in length and penetrates the muscular wall of the uterus.

The epithelium lining all parts of the uterine tube is simple or pseudostratified columnar (Fig. 4–6). Many of the cells are ciliated, while others appear to be secretory or absorptive in type. The ciliated cells occur singly or in islands. The nuclei of the secretory cells show a characteristic tendency to lie close to the lumen of the tube, causing the apical part of the cell to bulge into it. Evidence for the secretory activity of the cells is provided in some animals, such as the rabbit, in which an albuminous coat is added to the zona pellucida during the passage of the fertilized egg through the uterine tube. During estrus in many rodents, large amounts of fluid accumulate within the uterine tubes.

The fundamental importance of the secretions of this part of the reproductive tract in the successful passage and nourishment of the dividing egg and blastocyst in animals and women is only slowly becoming recognized, and much remains to be learned about the nature of these secretions. Of equal importance is the muscular wall of the oviduct, which is responsible for its motility. The tubal transport of the fertilized egg toward the uterus and of the spermatozoa in the opposite direction is poorly understood and appears to depend upon precise patterns of motility of the tube as well as on the presence of fluid currents and ciliary activity. The cilia beat in the direction of the uterus. The bundles of smooth muscle in the wall of the uterine tube consist of mingled outer longitudinal and inner circular and spiral bands.

A thick lamina propria of vascular connective tissue lies between the epithelial and the muscular layer (Fig. 4–6); it is especially dense and tough in the isthmic portion and causes the mucosa to pouch from within the smooth muscle of the wall when the tube is cut transversely. External to the muscular layer is a layer of visceral peritoneum, the epithelium of which is a typical flattened mesothelium and is separated from the muscle by a loose subserous layer of connective tissue rich in blood vessels and lymphatics. Changes in the epithelium have been described in the different phases of the menstrual cycle, but such changes are less evident than in other parts of the reproductive tract.

THE UTERUS

The uterus is a pear-shaped organ lying in the midline enclosed between the two layers of the broad ligament. It consists of a fundus, a body (corpus uteri), and a neck (cervix uteri).

THE CORPUS UTERI

The wall of the uterus consists of three layers: an inner endometrium, a middle myometrium, and an external peritoneal (serous) coat. The endometrium undergoes cyclic changes governed by the interplay of hormones of pituitary and ovarian origin that underlie the menstrual cycle and is profoundly modified in pregnancy. The myometrium also shows cyclic changes, but the most striking changes occur in pregnancy.

Endometrial Changes During the Menstrual Cycle

A menstrual cycle associated with cyclic bleeding from the endometrium is found only in women and primates. The 1st day of the cycle is considered to be the 1st day of external vaginal bleeding. The bleeding phase lasts from several days to a week in normal women and occurs approximately every 28 days. The sequence of events in the cycle is briefly summarized as follows. Under the influence of FSH, several follicles in the ovary begin to grow. The initial maturation of the follicle, up to the early stage of antrum formation, may not be dependent on pituitary gonadotropins, since it occurs in hypophysectomized animals. The later stages of follicular growth and preovulatory swelling are, however, dependent upon the pituitary. As the follicles grow, estrogen is produced from either the thecal or granulosal elements, and this estrogen in turn affects the endometrium. There is a thickening of the endometrial mucosa and an increase in the number and complexity of the glands (Fig. 4–7). This is the *follicular (proliferative) phase* of the cycle. The glands and surface epithelium show intense mitotic activity. The epithelial cells, which are tall columnar, show a marked cytoplasmic basophilia that is abolished by ribonuclease and so is due largely to cytoplasmic ribonucleoprotein (RNP). The stroma becomes vascular and edematous toward the middle of the cycle. Ovulation probably occurs 11–14 days before the next menstrual period, *i.e.,* on about the 17th day of the cycle (Fig. 4–8). The preovulatory swelling of the follicle is associated with the release of LH from the pituitary. There is also good evidence for the production of progestational substances by the follicle before its rupture, probably from the cells of the hypertrophied theca interna.

Ovulation initiates the *luteal (secretory) phase* of the menstrual cycle, which is dependent upon the presence of a functional corpus luteum and the production of progestational hormones. In this phase, the endometrial glands become tortuous and their walls become sinuous, presenting a characteristic sawtooth pattern (Fig. 4–9). The lining cells show evidence of secretory activity, and the glandular lumen becomes distended with secretion that gives a strong PAS reaction and is probably mucopolysaccharide in nature. Glycogen also appears in the glandular epithelium, in the glandular secretion, and in the fibroblastic cells of the endometrial stroma. The latter may show an early decidual reaction in the late secretory (premenstrual) phase of the cycle.

The decline of the corpus luteum of menstruation and the withdrawal of progestational influences from the endometrium are correlated with the involution of the latter and the onset of menstrual bleeding. This phenomenon has been studied in endometrial grafts in the anterior chamber of the eye in monkeys. A day or so before menstrual bleeding, the endometrial transplant shrank markedly (the ischemic phase), presumably because of the withdrawal of water. Throughout the cycle, but most marked before menstruation, there was a rhythmic contraction and relaxation of the endometrial arterioles, which produced an alternate blushing and blanching of the graft. Small petechial hemorrhages then appeared beneath the epithelial surface

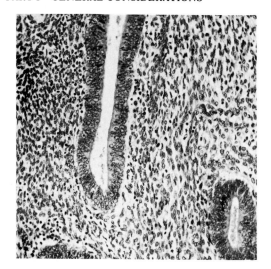

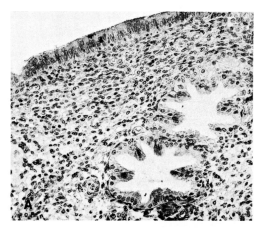

FIG. 4–7. Endometrium in proliferative phase of cycle. Glandular epithelium is tall columnar and shows marked cytoplasmic basophilia. There are numerous mitotic figures in epithelium. Stroma is richly cellular. (H&E, ×220)

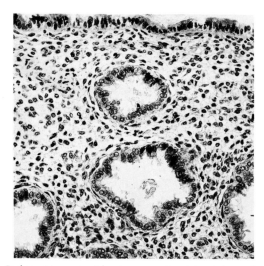

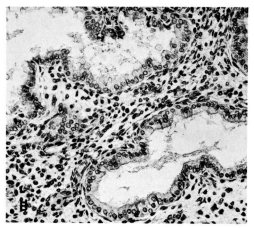

FIG. 4–9. Two sections of endometrium in late luteal or premenstrual phase of cycle. *A.* Surface epithelium is tall columnar (compare Fig. 4–8). Deep to epithelium is zona compacta. *B.* Glands in deeper layers of endometrium (zona spongiosa) are dilated and show characteristic sawtooth pattern. Glandular lumen contains secretion material. Fibroblasts of stroma are hypertrophied but show no decidual change. There is considerable stromal edema (H&E, ×220)

FIG. 4–8. Endometrium at midcycle, approximately at time of ovulation. Surface epithelium is columnar. Glands are dilated and lined by irregular columnar epithelium showing evidence of secretory activity. These cells have lost cytoplasmic basophilia of early proliferative phase. Stroma is edematous, fibroblasts being more widely separated than in early stage (compare Fig. 4–7). (H&E, ×220)

and were shortly followed by bleeding from the graft. The changes in the vascular tone of the endometrial vessels are clearly of great importance and may be associated with an increasing dominance of estrogen over progesterone as the corpus luteum declines.

The human endometrium in the late luteal phase or

in early pregnancy has three layers, beginning at the luminal surface: a *zona compacta* in the region of the mouths of the glands, a deeper *zona spongiosa* in which the glands are tortuous and dilated, and a *zona basalis* adjoining the myometrium. The zona compacta and zona spongiosa are often combined as the *zona functionalis* since they are shed at menstruation. There are two sets of arteries supplying the endometrium (Fig. 4–10). Arteries of one type supply only the zona basalis. This zone accordingly remains intact after menstruation, and the endometrial lining is regenerated from it by the outgrowth of epithelium from the glands. Arteries of the second type are the spiral arterioles, which pursue a tortuous course through the zona functionalis and supply it. These vessels show the

alternate constriction and relaxation described in the terminal (ischemic) phase of the cycle. They also play an important role in the pregnant uterus.

Endometrial Changes in Pregnancy

If the egg is fertilized, it undergoes a series of mitotic divisions, resulting in a ball of cells (*morula*). A cavity then appears within the morula, converting it into the *blastocyst*. The outer wall of the blastocyst (*tropho-blast*) consists of ectodermal cells, which are directly involved in the implantation process and in the later formation of the placenta. Implantation takes place about the 7th day after ovulation.

The presence of the blastocyst within the uterus is directly or indirectly responsible for the transformation of the corpus luteum of menstruation into the corpus luteum of pregnancy, probably because of a luteotropic hormone emanating from the trophoblast. As a result, there is an enhanced output of progestational substances from the corpus luteum, and the endometrium undergoes further transformations. The endometrial stroma shows a *decidual reaction*. Beginning about the 12th day the stromal cells become enlarged and epithelial in appearance, and there is a deposition of cytoplasmic lipid and glycogen. This is illustrated at the 5th month of pregnancy in Figure 4–11. This decidual bed forms an ideal pabulum for the implanted ovum and may also in some way modify or restrain the invasive activities of syncytiotrophoblast. Following the establishment of the mature placenta, there is a complex *junctional zone* between the peripheral trophoblast and the myometrium, consisting of intermingled tro-

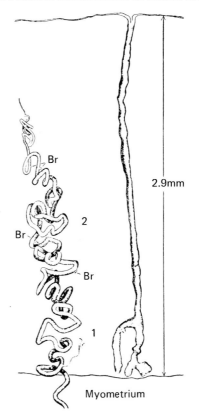

FIG. 4–10. Diagram of spiral arteriole and gland from endometrium at about 4th day. A small branch (type 1) supplies zona basalis close to myometrium. Spiral vessels (type 2) supply zona functionalis. (Daron SH: Am J Anat 58:349, 1936)

FIG. 4–11. Decidual reaction in endometrium at 5th month of pregnancy. Superficial and glandular epithelia appear atrophic. (H&E, ×220)

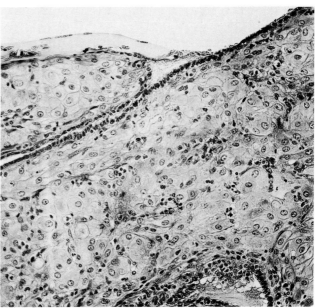

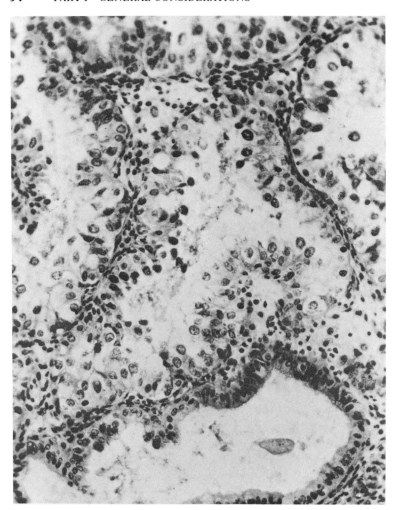

FIG. 4–12. Arias–Stella reaction. Gland at *center* shows proliferative and secretory activity. Some nuclei are about three times as large as those seen in adjacent gland. (Oertel YC: Arch Pathol Lab Med 102:651, 1978)

phoblastic and decidual cells. A *zone of separation* is later formed in this area, and the placenta separates through this zone at parturition. The spiral arterioles of the zona functionalis are the first vessels to be encountered by the invading trophoblast. They are ruptured, and the maternal blood floods into the lacunae within the trophoblastic shell.

Another apparently specific but atypical response of the endometrium to the presence of viable trophoblast is the so-called *Arias–Stella reaction* (Fig. 4–12). In a recent study, the reaction was found in only five of many specimens studied from the Hertig collection at the Carnegie Institution of Washington and was first observed at the 17th day of gestation. It consists of irregular hyperplasia of the superficial epithelial and glandular cells with large, irregular, hyperchromatic nuclei; proliferative appearances in the glands, consisting of villus-like foldings of the cells into the lumen with piling up of cells; and secretory appearance in the glands associated with hyperplasia and cytoplasmic vacuolation. The reaction is usually focal and occurs independently of inflammation.

The Myometrium

The smooth muscle of the wall of the uterus is very thick and is arranged in bundles separated by cellular connective tissue that contains vessels. The inner layers are dispersed in a sphincterlike manner around the intramural portions of the uterine tubes. The intermediate layer is thick and irregularly dispersed with many large venous channels, giving it a spongy texture. The outer layer consists of intermingled longitudinal and circular fibers. There is a serous coat external to the myometrium, except laterally in relation to the attachment of the broad ligament.

The myometrium shows great hypertrophy in pregnancy. Individual smooth muscle fibers may increase in length from 50μ to 500μ, and there may be new formation of muscle fibers.

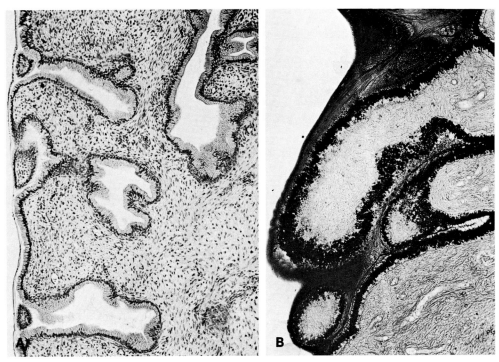

FIG. 4–13. Glands of endocervix at 17th day of cycle. Glands are simple branching in type and are lined by tall clear columnar epithelium (*A*), (×90) which is mucified (*B*), (×220). (*A*, H&E; *B*, PAS.)

THE CERVIX UTERI

The cervix forms a short transition zone between the corpus uteri and the vagina. A portion of it lies above the level of the vaginal vault (*supravaginal cervix*), and a portion lies exposed inferiorly within the vagina and is covered by epithelium of vaginal type (*portio externa*). The cervical lumen is constricted and encroached upon by folds of the mucosal lining that in the virgin form the *plicae palmatae*.

In cross section the cervical lumen presents a complex branching configuration (*arbor vitae*). The *endocervical canal* is about 1 in. long in average women but shows great variation. It is lined by a columnar or pseudostratified columnar epithelium, which is variably mucified (Fig. 4–13). There are deeply penetrating glands of tubular branching type, which are also lined by columnar epithelium. The stroma of the cervix is composed mainly of collagenous connective tissue with a small amount of elastic tissue and occasional smooth muscle fibers. The stroma becomes very vascular during pregnancy.

Mucification of the endocervical epithelium is the salient reaction of this part of the female reproductive tract to cyclic changes in hormone secretion and is maximal just before ovulation, when estrogen is at a high level and progesterone begins to appear. An increase in the amount of mucus at the vaginal introitus is commonly observed by women and appears to coincide more or less closely with ovulation. Ferning of the cervical mucus at about this time is described in Chapter 47, Infertility.

Basally, the endocervical epithelium rests on a continuous basement membrane that is too thin to be resolved by the light microscope. Staining of the basement membrane by such techniques as the PAS method is probably due to polysaccharide materials associated with the basement membrane rather than to the membrane itself. Studies with the electron microscope seem to be essential if statements are to be made with respect to the integrity or lack of integrity of the basement membrane in pathologic processes involving the endocervix or the portio externa. Electron-microscopic studies confirm the virtual absence of smooth muscle from the cervical stroma.

The transition from the columnar epithelium of the endocervix to the stratified squamous epithelium of the portio externa is usually abrupt (Fig. 4–14). The columnar epithelium, however, may extend outside the external os onto the vaginal aspect of the cervix, a common feature of the cervix of the newborn infant and the pregnant woman; it is frequently referred to as physiologic erosion or ectropion. Chronic inflammatory changes are common in the region of the external

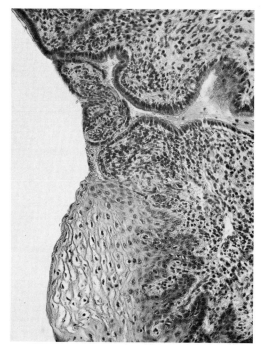

FIG. 4–14. Region of external os of cervix at 17th day of cycle. Transition from columnar epithelium of endocervix to stratified squamous epithelium of vaginal type of portio externa is abrupt. Cervical stroma near external os is infiltrated with leukocytes. (H&E, ×220)

os and are often associated with an actual loss of the epithelium around the external os (*true erosion*) and with an encroachment of stratified squamous epithelium into the endocervical canal. Blocking of the mouths of the cervical glands near the external os may result in the formation of clear cysts (*ovula nabothi*).

The region of the external os is one of the most important junctional regions in the body, comparable to such mucocutaneous junctions as the red margin of the lips and the anus. It shares with these areas a marked predisposition toward cancer. This tendency is enhanced in the case of the cervix by the extreme lability of the junction between the two epithelia involved and by the responsiveness of these to hormonal stimulation.

Other common histologic changes in the region of the cervix are illustrated in Figure 4–15. They are the decidual transformation of parts of the endocervical stroma and the squamous metaplasia of the columnar epithelium. The latter is common in normal cycling women and is almost universal in pregnancy. The nature and significance of this squamous metaplasia have aroused much controversy. Since it often occurs in the depths of the mucosal folds and crypts of the endocervix, far removed from the external os, it cannot

result from an invasion of stratified squamous epithelium from the portio externa. It has been regarded by some as a true metaplasia of the columnar epithelium; by others, as a proliferation of indifferent (reserve) cells lying in the deep layer of the epithelium close to the basement membrane. It is enhanced in the endocervix of the newborn infant, where it appears to be correlated with the intense estrogenic stimulation of the reproductive tract at the time of birth, and in rodents and monkeys receiving large doses of estrogen. It does not appear to be a premalignant change.

THE PORTIO EXTERNA CERVICIS

The portio externa of the cervix is covered by a stratified squamous epithelium identical with that lining the vagina. The reaction of these two identical epithelia to estrogenic stimulation differs fundamentally from that of the endocervical epithelium. The stratified squamous epithelium reacts by thickening and by cornification of the superficial cells; the endocervical epithelium reacts by mucification.

The stratified squamous epithelium of the portio externa (Fig. 4–16) is made up of several layers conventionally described as basal, parabasal, intermediate, and superficial. The *basal layer* consists of a single row of cells and rests on a thin basement membrane. The cells are basophilic, the basophilia being enhanced in pregnancy. The *parabasal* and *intermediate layers* together constitute the prickle cell layer analogous to the same layer in the epidermis. The cells of the parabasal layer show cytoplasmic basophilia that is less in degree than that of the basal layer and decreases toward the intermediate layer. The intermediate layer is vacuolated, largely because of the presence of glycogen which is not stained or dissolved out in the preparation of the sections. The *superficial layer* varies in thickness, depending upon the degree of estrogenic stimulation. It consists of flattened cells that show an increasing degree of cytoplasmic acidophilia in the direction of the surface. The desquamation of surface cells goes on constantly, and the epithelium is replenished by mitotic division of cells in the basal layer and to a lesser extent in the parabasal layer.

The superficial and intermediate layers of the epithelium contain a large amount of glycogen (Fig. 4–17A). This glycogen serves an important function in maintaining the acid pH of the vaginal contents. The glycogen is released by the cytolysis of the desquamated cells and is then acted upon by the glycolytic bacterial flora of the vagina, forming lactic acid. Both the thickness of the epithelium (Fig. 4–16) and the glycogen content of the epithelium are increased following estrogenic stimulation, thus accounting for the therapeutic effect of estrogens in atrophic vaginitis. The staining of glycogen in the normal epithelium of the portio externa is the basis of the Schiller test. Fol-

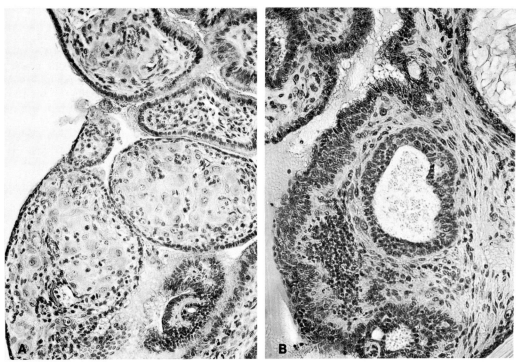

FIG. 4-15. Two patterns of cellular metaplasia in endocervix at 5th month of pregnancy. *A.* Decidual transformation of endocervical stroma. *B.* Squamous metaplasia of columnar epithelium of endocervical glands. (H&E, ×220)

lowing the removal of glycogen by salivary digestion (Fig. 4–16*B*), the intercellular regions stain intensely with the PAS method; the same areas are also sudanophilic. Histochemical studies indicate that the staining material may consist of mucopolysaccharide associated with some kind of lipid. Glycogen is easily identified in the superficial layers.

The superficial cells are desquamated into the vaginal lumen but retain their nuclei, unlike the desquamating cells of a heavily cornified epithelium such as thick skin. There is no stratum granulosum containing electron-dense granules of keratohyalin, as in the epidermis. However, the epithelium of the portio externa and that of the vagina must probably be considered nonkeratinizing epithelia comparable to that of thin skin. The process of cornification is enhanced following estrogenic stimulation, and there seems to be no reason to doubt that cornification of the vaginal epithelium and keratinization of the epidermis are similar processes differing only in degree. Under abnormal circumstances, *e.g.*, prolapse of the uterus in which the vaginal mucosa and vaginal portion of the cervix are exposed to irritation, there is more complete keratinization of the exposed surfaces.

THE VAGINA

The vagina is lined by a stratified squamous, nonkeratinizing epithelium identical in origin, histology, and

fine structure with that covering the portio external of the cervix. It rests on a basement membrane and on a lamina propria of mixed collagenous and elastic connective tissue rich in blood vessels and lymphatic vessels. The lamina propria intrudes into the basal layer of the epithelium in the form of papillae similar to the dermal papillae of the skin. Lymphocytes, singly or in aggregates, are common in the lamina propria and may occasionally be observed migrating through the epithelium. Polymorphonuclear leukocytes are also common in the epithelium and vaginal lumen at certain stages of the cycle. There are no glands in the vaginal mucosa, which is kept moist by the transudation of moisture through the epithelium and by the drainage of mucus from the cervix. As in the portio externa, the epithelium shows changes in thickness in different physiologic states and pathologic conditions. It undergoes thickening under the influence of estrogen and in pregnancy (Fig. 4–16). It is thicker in women who regularly have intercourse than in those who do not. Keratinization of the superficial layers may occur in abnormal circumstances such as excessive exposure to irritation caused by prolapse of the uterus, or in other poorly understood dyskeratotic conditions.

The muscular wall of the vagina consists of bundles of smooth muscle disposed in interlacing circular and

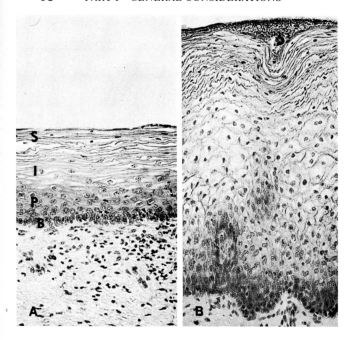

FIG. 4–16. Stratified squamous epithelium of portio externa cervicis following amenorrhea of several months' duration (A) and at 5th month of pregnancy (B). B, Basal layer. I, Intermediate layer. P, parabasal layer. S, Superficial cornified layer. Thickening of all layers in pregnancy striking. (H&E, ×220)

longitudinal layers. These interlace inferiorly with fibers of striated muscle of the levator ani, which forms the principal sphincter of the vagina. External to the muscular layer of the vagina is an adventitial coat of loose connective tissue rich in blood vessels, nerves, and lymphatic vessels. The dead space of the pelvis around the uterus and vagina and other pelvic viscera consists of a richly cellular areolar connective tissue (*parametrium*) which is highly susceptible to infection.

The *hymen* consists of a perforated fold of mucous membrane between the lower end of the vagina and the vestibule. It is covered by stratified squamous epithelium on both its vaginal and vestibular surfaces and encloses a thin lamina of connective tissue in which may be found vestiges of the duct of the mesonephros (*Gartner's duct*).

VAGINAL SMEAR

The changes that occur in the epithelium of the portio externa of the cervix and the vagina under the influence of estrogenic and progestational hormones of the menstrual cycle are reflected in the cells found in the vaginal lumen. Cells derived by exfoliation from the vagina, cervix, endometrium, or even the uterine tube

are obtained from the vaginal fornix by aspiration, or from the external os, endocervix, or endometrial lumen by gently scraping or curetting. They are spread on a glass slide, fixed for about 15 min in alcohol–ether, and then stained with Harris's hematoxylin (for nuclei and cytoplasmic basophilia) and counterstained with a mixture containing either light green or orange G with phosphotungstic acid (for cytoplasmic structures and inclusions).

The interpretation of the cytologic picture requires expert training and judgment, but such a smear can tender valuable information about the hormonal status of the patient, with particular respect to estrogen, and, especially when done sequentially, about the presence of premalignant or malignant changes. Smears are classified in various ways, *e.g.*, that of Papanicolaou: Grade I, no atypical or abnormal cells; Grade II, atypical cells but no evidence of malignancy; Grade III, suggestive but not conclusive of malignancy; Grade IV, strongly suggestive of malignancy; Grade V, conclusive of malignancy. Criteria of malignancy or premalignancy are:

1. Nuclear changes: variation in size (pleomorphism), hyperchromasia, aberrant patterns of chromatin, enlargement of or increase in number of nucleoli, multinucleation, mitosis, thickening of the nuclear membrane, degenerative changes including vacuolation
2. Cytoplasmic changes: pronounced basophilia or acidophilia and vacuolation
3. Changes of the whole cell: enlargement and variation in size, aberrant and bizarre forms, degenerative or necrotic changes, dyskeratotic changes affecting the process of keratinization
4. Interrelations of cells: irregular patterns of clump-

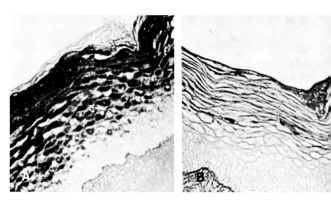

FIG. 4–17. Two sections of portio externa cervicis at 17th day of cycle, stained with PAS method before treatment of section with saliva (A) and after such treatment (B). Note large amount of glycogen revealed in superficial layers of epithelium (A). Following removal of glycogen (B), intercellular areas stain intensely with PAS stain. Basement membrane also stains strongly. (×200)

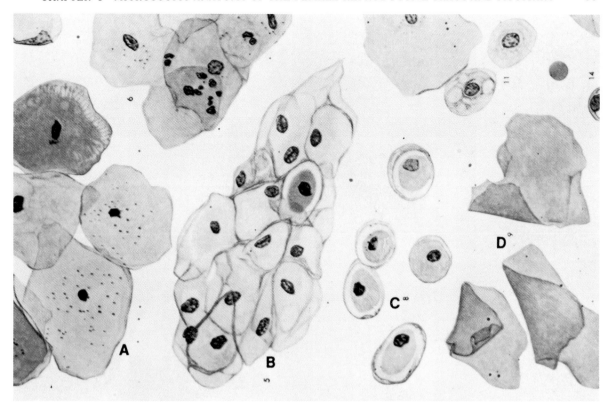

FIG. 4-18. Normal cells in vaginal and cervical aspiration or swab smears. *A.* Superficial squamous cells (late follicular or preovulatory stage of menstrual cycle), stained for glycogen. *B.* Cells of intermediate or navicular type (parabasal), stained for glycogen. *C.* Parabasal cells from ectocervix from patient taking estrogen, stained for glycogen. *D.* Superficial squamous cells showing complete keratinization from 48-year-old woman. (Approximately ×500) (Papanicolaou G: Atlas of Exfoliative Cytology. Cambridge Mass, Harvard University Press, 1954)

ing, variations in size within cell clusters (anisokaryosis and anisocytosis), dense grouping and crowding of cells, engulfment of cells one by another, pronounced stratification

Leukocytic inclusions within cells may be normal, and histiocytes or macrophages with engulfed leukocytes are also not uncommon in normal smears. Intense acidophilia with orange G may be a normal concomitant of keratinization, as in the patient taking high doses of estrogen.

Analysis of the types of cells in vaginal smears or smears of exfoliated cells from the endocervix or uterine body requires an understanding of the normal histology of these areas and their response to sex hormones. These essential details have been illustrated earlier (*e.g.,* Fig 4–16). Cells of strictly vaginal origin, as well as those from the ectocervix, consist of parabasal, intermediate or navicular, and superficial more or less cornified cells (Fig. 4–16). Parabasal cells are rarely shed, being the germinative layer. When they are shed, the parabasal cells are rounded, having lost their intercellular spiny processes when shed. They contain glycogen in proportion to the level of estrogenic stimulation (Fig. 4–18) and have relatively large nuclei. Intermediate cells, including the more superfi-

cial cells that contain keratohyaline granules, are best developed in high estrogenic states. They are moderately flattened, smaller than parabasal cells, and may contain keratohyalin. Their general acidophilia or orangeophilia (with orange G) is a measure of their keratinization; complete keratinization is rare in normal females. The cells from the more superficial zone are flattened with pyknotic nuclei. In high estrogenic states, the keratinized cells appear as squames or scales, intensely acidophilic and lacking nuclei.

Cells derived from the endocervix reflect the normal mucosal pattern of this area, namely, a columnar surface epithelium (simple, mucified, or ciliated) and tubular glands lined by columnar epithelium (Fig. 4–19). Mucification can be identified by appropriate stains. Ciliated cells are rare, but increase in low estrogenic states. Mucified cells are more common in the late luteal phase of the cycle and in pregnancy.

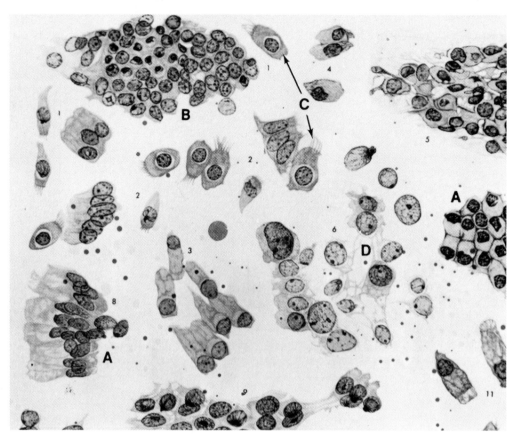

FIG. 4–19. Normal cells in cervical and endocervical smears. *A.* Endocervical mucous columnar cells shown from side and from their basal surfaces. *B.* Cluster of columnar cells from endocervical aspiration (mucous and ciliated). *C.* Ciliated cells. *D.* Endocervical columnar cells showing variation in nuclear size (anisokaryosis) and cytolysis (Approximately ×500) (Papanicolaou G: Atlas Exfoliative Cytology. Cambridge, Mass, Harvard University Press, 1954)

Cells of endometrial origin again reflect the histology of this area (Fig. 4–20). Mucification is rarely seen. Ciliation is very rare, but again is more common in postmenopausal women and in low estrogenic states. The cells are smaller than those of endocervical origin and tend to occur in more compact groups. Rarely, glands or portions of them may be seen. Changes coincident with the menstrual cycle are not of reliable significance in women; in contrast, the vaginal smear in rodents reflects accurately the preovulatory, postovulatory, and resting phases of the estrous cycle. The corpus luteum is short-lived in rodents so that the luteal phase is abbreviated, whereas in women the prolonged luteal phase and the extended action of progesterone causes its own effects on vaginal smear morphology. In particular, the character of the mucus that appears in the smear and emerges from the external os reflects the action of progesterone. It is watery and of low viscosity in the period of high estrogenic activity, *i.e.,* during the follicular phase, and tenacious and sticky during the late luteal stage. During pregnancy there is abundant tenacious mucus and many navicular cells of parabasal type with rather thick cellular walls. Showers of polymorphonuclear cells may appear transiently in the normal smear by the time of ovulation and again in the later luteal phase.

THE EXTERNAL GENITALIA

The *labia minora* are covered by a thin epidermal layer of stratified squamous epithelium continuous with that of the vestibule. The papillae of the submucosal layer are richly developed, and the epithelium may also contain a large amount of pigment. There are scattered glands of sebaceous type, but no hair follicles. The glands secrete a material called *sebum.*

The *labia majora* are covered by thick skin that contains coarse hair follicles and well-developed sweat and sebaceous glands. These glands and the hair follicles

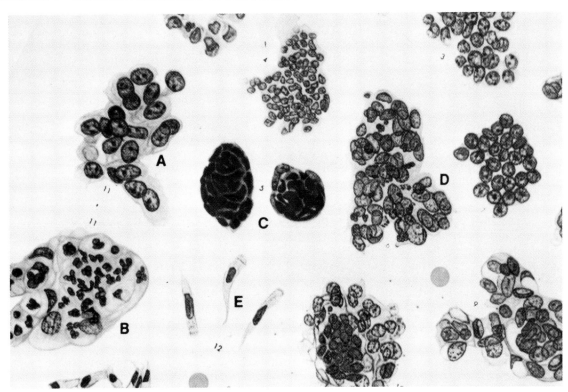

FIG. 4-20. Normal cells in vaginal smear of endometrial origin. *A.* Clusters of endometrial cells, early menstrual cycle. *B.* Cluster of endometrial cells with leukocytic infiltration. *C.* Cluster of endometrial cells showing clumping, shrinkage, and nuclear pyknosis. *D.* Cluster of endometrial cells, late menstrual cycle. *E.* Ciliated and mucous cells, from 55-year-old woman with hyperplasia of endometrium. (Approximately ×500) (Papanicolaou G: Atlas of Exfoliative Cytology. Cambridge, Mass, Harvard University Press, 1954)

are influenced by the sex hormones of the ovary at the time of puberty.

Associated with the vestibule are glandular structures; their principal function is lubrication. The most important of these are the greater vestibular (Bartholin's) gland and the paraurethral (Skene's) glands. The glands are of compound tubuloalveolar type, and the alveoli are lined by mucus-secreting columnar cells. The duct of the greater vestibular gland is lined by stratified squamous epithelium continuous with that of the vestibule.

Surrounding the vestibule are certain modifications of the connective tissue that comprise the erectile tissue of the area: the bulbs of the vestibule, the clitoris, and the pars intermedia. The bulbs of the vestibule are homologous with the corpus spongiosum penis. The crura and glans clitoridis are homologous with the corpora cavernosa and glans penis. The erectile tissue of these organs consists of a spongelike system of vascular spaces lined by endothelium and separated by delicate fibroelastic septa containing blood vessels. The arteries and veins supplying the erectile spaces are so arranged that blood is allowed to enter the spaces while the venous drainage is temporarily obstructed. The erectile tissue is richly supplied with sympathetic and parasymphathetic nerves (nervi erigentes).

PITUITARY-HYPOTHALAMIC SYSTEM

The pituitary gland and its vascular and nervous connections with the hypothalamus are remarkably constant in structure and function throughout the vertebrate phylum, reflecting their fundamental role in the regulation of sexual, metabolic, and osmotic function. The pituitary develops in two parts, both of ectodermal origin: the pars distalis and the pars nervosa. The pars distalis arises as an upgrowth (Rathke's pouch) from the roof of the stomatodeum, or embryonic mouth, which becomes apposed to a downgrowth from the floor of the diencephalon (infundibular process). The pars distalis includes the pars anterior (anterior lobe) and the pars intermedia (intermediate lobe); in some forms, but not in man, there is a remnant of the stomatodeal cleft between the two. The pars anterior extends up toward the base of the brain as the pars tu-

beralis, where it forms a small mass of pituitary tissue that partially encircles the infundibular stalk and median eminence. The pars posterior is essentially a downgrowth of the brain and is connected to the hypothalamus by a leash of nerves, constituting the hypothalamohypophyseal tract.

PARS DISTALIS

The pars distalis stands in intimate relation with the hypothalamus by means of a vascular portal system. The anterior lobe is supplied by superior hypophyseal arteries from the internal carotid, which forms a primary vascular plexus within the hypothalamus. From this plexus a leash of vessels descends into the anterior lobe, forming the hypophyseoportal system. It breaks up within the anterior lobe, where it forms a secondary vascular plexus. This arrangement of vessels, which permits blood to reach an anterior lobe only after it has passed through the hypothalamic plexuses, is remarkably constant throughout the vertebrate phylum. The direction of blood flow has been shown by direct observation. It is now known that regulatory substances (*releasing factors*) are manufactured within the hypothalamic neurons and are transported via the portal vessels to the pars distalis, where they cause the release of hormones. Such releasing factors have been demonstrated for thyroid-stimulating hormone (TSH), adrenocortex-stimulating hormone (ACTH),

lactogenic hormone (prolactin), growth hormone (somatotropin, STH), and the gonadotropins (LH and FSH). In some instances the releasing hormones have been isolated and synthesized. They act in exceedingly minute amounts and will have increasing clinical significance.

The general types of cells within the pars distalis are illustrated in Figure 4–21. Classically, they are described within the anterior lobe as of three types: acidophils (40%), basophils (10%), and chromophobes (50%). The acidophils, which are most numerous posteriorly within the anterior lobe, have granules that stain intensely with acid dyes, *i.e.*, they are themselves basic. They are thought to be the site of growth hormone and prolactin production. Acidophilic adenomas are associated with giantism (acromegaly). The basophils, at least in the rat, are of two types. One group stains with both the PAS and the aldehyde fuchsin methods. These cells are thyrotropes, *i.e.*, secrete TSH. A second type stains with the PAS but not the aldehyde fuchsin method. These are the site of gonadotropic secretion (FSH and LH). In man, the secretion of ACTH appears to be associated with the basophils, and following ACTH or adrenocorticoid administration, these cells undergo a degenerative change (Crooke's hyaline change). The acidophils increase in pregnancy and lactation, probably associated with prolactin production.

The pars intermedia is poorly developed in man. It appears to be a source of melanocyte-stimulating hor-

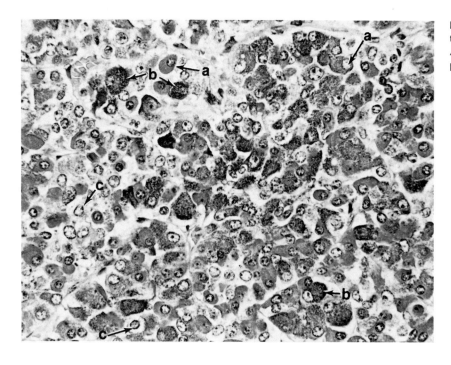

FIG. 4–21. Human pituitary (pars distalis), showing principal cell types. *a*, Acidophils. *b*, Basophils. *c*, Chromophobes. (Halmi, ×300)

mone (MSH), which causes dispersal of melanin in amphibians. Its role in the human is unclear; injection, however, produces hyperpigmentation.

PARS NERVOSA

The pars nervosa or posterior lobe (Fig. 4–22) is made up of clusters or nests of pituicytes, which appear not to have a secretory role in themselves. It now appears certain that the hypothalamohypophyseal tract of nerves is the path by which secretory material of hypothalamic origin reaches the posterior lobe. The "neurosecretory material" that may be observed in the axons of this tract may be shown experimentally to dam up proximal to a point of constriction. It is manufactured within the specialized neurons of the supraoptic and paraventricular nuclei. It is then transferred by axoplasmic flow to the posterior lobe, where the hormones (antidiuretic hormone [ADH] and oxytocin) are released. These materials, which are polypeptides, then enter the perivascular spaces, where they apparently lose their staining properties and are carried into the bloodstream. Vasopressin is identical with ADH and the latter name is preferable. Both the hypothalamic neurons and the posterior lobe cells are influenced to release ADH by changes in the osmolality of the blood. Destruction of the hypothalamohypophyseal tract or lesions in the paraventricular and supraoptic nuclei result in an uncontrolled excretion of large volumes of very dilute urine, a condition known as *diabetes insipidus*. Oxytocin has a contracting effect on the uterus and also causes ejection of milk from the milk ducts.

REFERENCES AND RECOMMENDED READING

Arias–Stella J: Atypical endometrial changes associated with presence of chorionic tissue. Arch Pathol 58:112, 1954

Bamforth J: Cytological Diagnosis in Medical Practice. Boston, Little Brown, 1966

Daron SH: The arterial pattern of the tunica mucosa of the uterus in Macacus rhesus. Am J Anat 58:349, 1936

Fluhman F: The Cervix Uteri and Its Diseases. Philadelphia, Saunders, 1961

Greep RO, Weiss L (eds): Histology, 3rd ed. New York, McGraw–Hill, 1973

Hafez ESE, Blandau RJ (eds): The Mammalian Oviduct. Chicago, University of Chicago Press, 1969

Hafez ESE (ed): Human Reproduction 2nd ed. Hagerstown, Harper & Row, 1980

Ham AW: Histology. Philadelphia, Lippincott, 1974

Harris GW, Donovan BT (eds): The Pituitary Gland. Berkeley, University of California Press, 1966

Markee SH: Menstruation in intraocular endometrial transplants in the rhesus monkey. Contrib Embryol 28:219, 1940

Naeb ZM: Exfoliative Cytology. Boston, Little Brown, 1970

Noyes RW, Hertig AH, Rock J: Dating the endometrial biopsy. Fertil Steril 1:3, 1950

Odell WD, Moyer DL: Physiology of Reproduction. St Louis, Mosby, 1971

FIG. 4-22. Human pituitary (pars nervosa), showing dense feltwork of glial cells (pituicytes) and nerve fibers with abundant blood vessels. (Halmi, ×300)

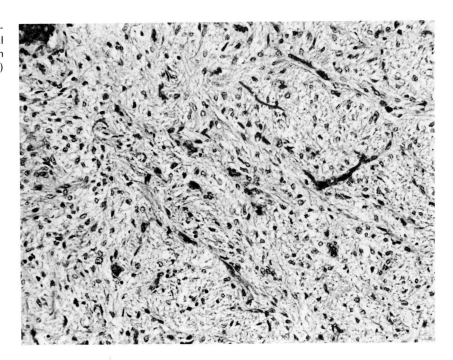

Oertel YC: The Arias–Stella reaction revisited. Arch Pathol Lab Med, 102:651, 1978

Papanicolaou GN: Atlas of Exfoliative Cytology. Cambridge, Mass, Harvard University Press, 1954

Reid DS, Ryan KJ, Bernirschke K: Principles and Management of Human Reproduction. Philadelphia, Saunders, 1972

Reynolds SRM: Physiology of the Uterus, 3rd ed. New York, Hoeber, 1949

Shearman RP (ed): Human Reproductive Physiology. Oxford, Blackwell, 1972

Williams RH (ed): Textbook of Endocrinology. Philadelphia, Saunders, 1974

Woodruff JD, Pauerstein CJ: The Fallopian Tube: Structure, Function, Pathology and Management. Baltimore, Williams & Wilkins, 1969

Wynn RM: Cellular Biology of the Uterus. New York, Appleton, 1967

Zuckerman S (ed): The Ovary. New York, Academic Press, 1962

SCANNING ELECTRON MICROSCOPY OF HUMAN REPRODUCTION

E.S.E. Hafez
Hans Ludwig

Scanning electron microscopy has been used extensively to study the physiomorphology and pathophysiology of human reproduction. Unlike transmission electron microscopy, scanning electron microscopy can be used to investigate the organization of tissues and to observe large intact surface areas with high resolution and depth of field penetration.

FEMALE REPRODUCTIVE TRACT

There are remarkable morphologic differences in tissue organization of the mucosa of different segments of the female reproductive tract. Under the low magnification ($\times 200$) of the scanning electron microscope, the cells of the oviduct and uterus appear uniform in shape and are closely packed, resembling a "cobblestone pattern." In some instances, the borders of the cells are illdefined and covered with short microvilli and residual mucus. Under high magnification ($\times 2,000$–$20,000$) two basic epithelial cell types are observed: ciliated cells and nonciliated secretory cells (Fig. 4–23).[*] Ciliated cells are covered by kinocilia, which overlap the surface of secretory cells that have a dome-shaped surface covered with microvilli. Ciliated cells are found singly or in groups, arranged in rows or

[*] All specimens shown in this section have been fixed in 2.5% glutaraldehyde solution, processed by critical point drying, and gold coated by the sputtering technique.

a mosaic pattern. The percentage of ciliated cells in the tubal epithelium varies in different parts of the tube. The maximal number of ciliated cells is found in the fimbriae, where they are so closely packed it is impossible to distinguish their boundaries. The proportion of ciliated cells decreases gradually from the ampulla to the isthmus, reaching 50% near the ampullary–isthmic junction.

The kinocilia in the female reproductive tract beat rhythmically toward the vagina, creating a directional flow of luminal fluids for the transport of particles and gametes. Two types of ciliary motility are recognized: an effective stroke and a recovery stroke. In the effective stroke, the cilia bend near the basal body, and the degree of bending proceeds as a slow wave toward the tip. In the oviduct, cilia beat some 1200 times/min. Ciliary activity is responsible for the movement of ova into the ostium of the fimbriated tip and through the upper ampulla. Concomitant with this, there is a sharp increase in the intensity of muscular contractions at the time of ovulation and during preliminary migration of the ovum through the tube.

The cilia may facilitate the release of secretory material from the adjacent secretory cells and the distribution of the secretions within the lumen. Infection of the oviduct is associated with the loss of ciliated cells in the oviduct and the accumulation of oviductal fluid and inflammatory exudate, which may contribute to the development of salpingitis. Oviducts taken from patients with endogenous or exogenous estrogenic stimulation possess comparatively more ciliated cells in the ampulla and fimbriae than in the isthmus.

The tubal fluid plays a major role in the transport and maturation of the gametes. The peak of tubal secretory activity coincides with the time of ovulation, indicating that oviductal secretion is mediated by the ovarian hormones of the ovulatory and early postovulatory phase. After menopause, the oviducts become atrophic and the ciliated cells decrease in number.

The surface epithelium of the endometrium undergoes cyclic alterations in cell shape, apical microvilli, ciliation, and secretory activity (Fig. 4–24). These changes are hormone-dependent; lack of estrogens leads to a loss of cilia and cessation of secretory activity, both of which can be restored by exogenous administration of estrogens. Similar cyclic changes appear in the epithelium of the endocervical mucosa and the cervical crypts.

The normal squamous epithelium of the lower vagina is relatively smooth, with very little undulation of the surface. The cells appear flat and polygonal with thin-edged interdigitating borders. The multilayered cells overlap on each other irregularly, similar to the layers of shingles on a roof. The cell edges roll back and lift their borders during the process of exfoliation, Most vaginal cells exhibit delicate interlacing mi-

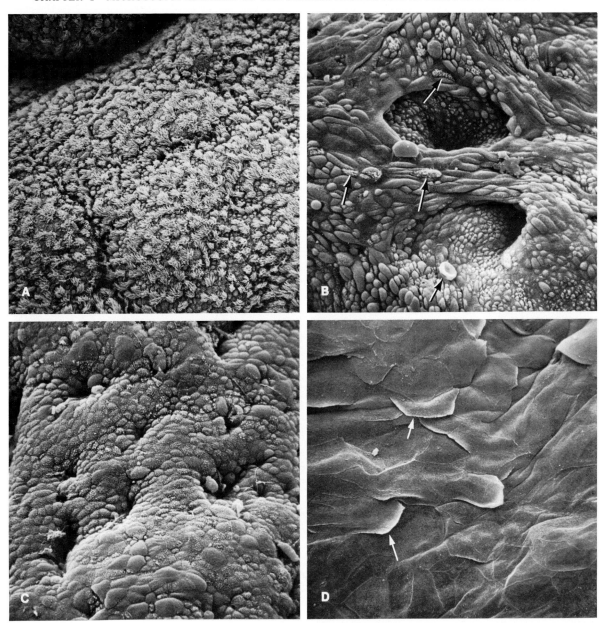

FIG. 4-23. Scanning electron micrographs showing surface ultrastructure of human female reproductive tract during first week of menstrual cycle. Note differences in tissue organization and cell characteristics and differentiations of different organs *at same magnification.* A. Oviduct, ampullar portion. Note ciliated cells surrounding small clusters of secretory cells. (×500) B. Endometrium. Note openings of endometrial glands (50–60 μm), extended ciliated cells with short cilia (*arrows*), and bulging tops of secretory cells. The erythrocyte (*arrow*) gives an idea of size relations. (×500) C. Cervix. Note regular size of cylindric epithelium and small glandular openings. Ciliated cells resemble those in endometrium. (×500) D. Ectocervix. Flat and homogeneous layer of vaginal epithelium, with some cells in process of exfoliation (*arrows*).

croridges with a pattern resembling that of fingerprints. When the exfoliated cells dry, they appear wrinkled and the surface microridges become obscured.

PLACENTA

The primary villi of the human placenta arise from the syncytium of the intervillous space. As soon as mesenchyme develops and invades the primary villi, the fea-

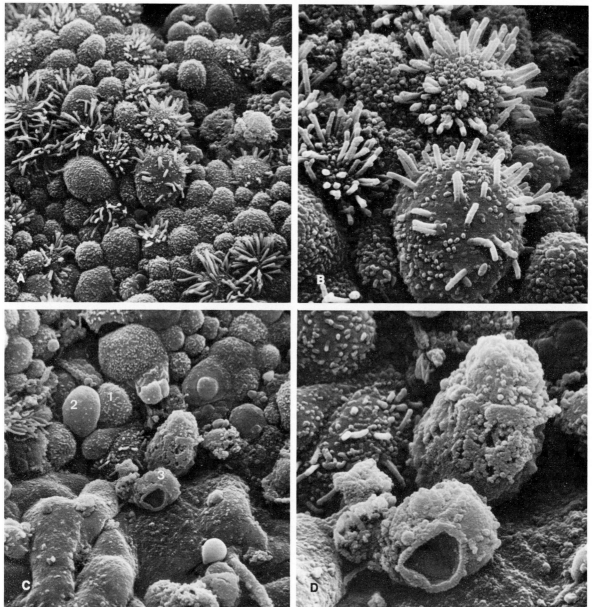

FIG. 4–24. Scanning electron micrographs of human endometrium during midcycle, showing superficial characteristics of individual endometrial cells. *A.* Ciliated and secretory endometrial cells. Note ciliated cells with short cilia of irregular number, unlike those in oviduct. Note microvilli covering secretory cells (×2000) *B.* Detail of *A.* Apical portion of some ciliated cells may be succulent, so that microvillous pattern of surface disappears. (×5000) *C.* Secretory endometrial cells in different stages of activity: (*1*) cell with normal superficial cell membrane, proliferating; (*2*) cell with intact superficial cell membrane but of extreme tension before release of secretory material; (*3*) cell with ruptured superficial cell membrane and clumped secretory material near ruptured surface. (×2000) *D.* Two secretory cells, one with ruptured cell membrane, after release of secretory material. Note difference between normal microvilli (*left* ciliated cell) and secretory material attached to apical cell membrane (*middle*). (×5000)

tures of secondary villi become apparent. The identifying sign of tertiary villi is the presence of fetal vessels in the villous stroma. Quarternary villi are subdivisions of tertiary villi at later stages of pregnancy, when the cytotrophoblastic layer has disappeared. Tertiary and quarternary villi are sometimes referred to as resorptive villi.

As pregnancy advances, there is a decrease in the length and thickness of these microvilli (except for some luxuriant forms that are of extreme length), but their density rises sharply. Clumping of microvilli occurs within marginal zones where basal and chorionic plates are close together. In the term placenta, clumping of microvilli associated with protru-

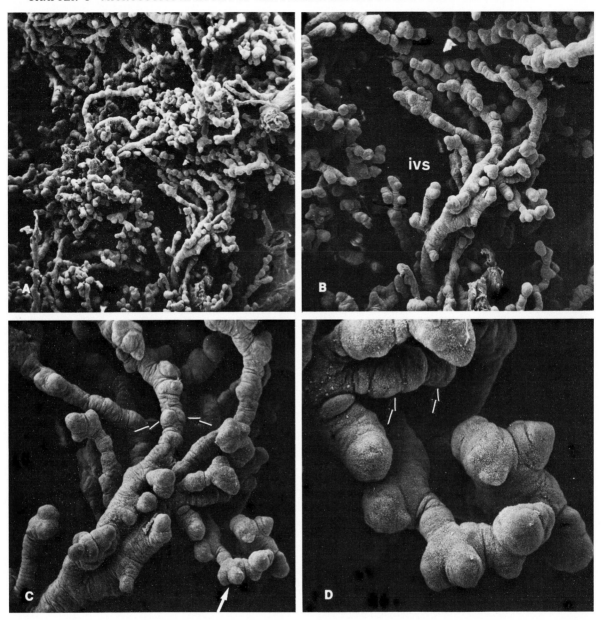

FIG. 4–25. Scanning electron micrographs of normal human term placenta, taken after normal pregnancy and spontaneous delivery. Figures 4–25 and 4–26 show 8 degrees of magnification (×50–20,000). *A.* Placental villi with equal shapes and diameters, but with various depths and widths of intervillous space. (×50) *B.* Ramification of single villous branches. Note terminal subdivisions of villi and various widths of intervillous space (*ivs*). (×100) *C.* Placental villi are continuously covered with velvety layer of syncytiotrophoblast. Note terminal ramification of terminal villi (*large arrow*) and placental knots (*small arrows*). (×200) *D.* Note homogeneity of surface of normal syncytiotrophoblast, which consists of numerous microvillous protrusions. Nuclear areas along flanks create bulging areas (*arrows*) of villous branches (×500)

sions of trophoblastic sprouts indicates maturity (Figs. 4–25 and 4–26).

During the 7th week of gestation, the main villus branches into secondary and tertiary villi that show remarkable variability in size and length. During the 14th week of gestation, the surface of the secondary and tertiary terminal villi are covered with a dense microvillous turf. The microvilli, regular in shape, are more evenly distributed compared with those of the human placenta 4 weeks earlier. At this stage, the mi-

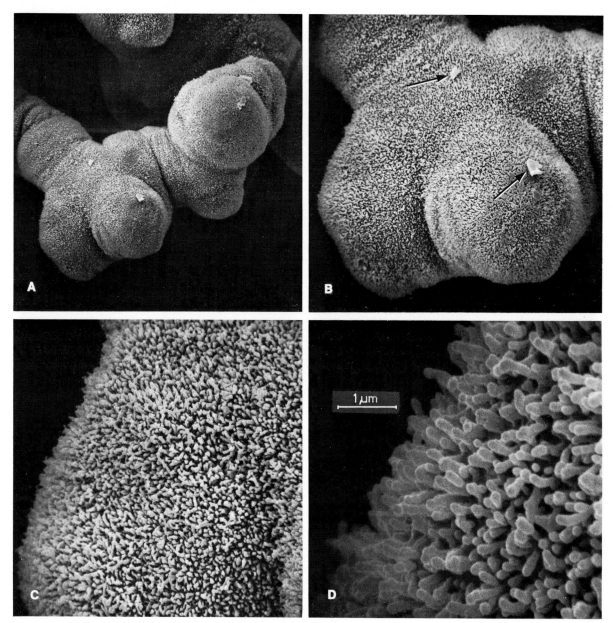

FIG. 4–26. Scanning electron micrographs of surface of placental syncytiotrophoblast from normal human term placenta (continued from Fig. 4–25). *A.* Top of terminal placental villi floating in intervillous space, showing homogeneous layer of syncytiotrophoblast. (×1000) *B.* Syncytiotrophoblast surface consists of a microvillous turf. Note deposits of nonstructured material (*arrows*). (×2000) *C.* Microvilli of syncytiotrophoblast are slender and homogeneous in length and thickness. (×5000) *D.* Single microvilli measure average of 0.65μm in length and 0.15μm in thickness. (×20,000)

crovillous pattern is highly differentiated, and there are protrusions on a syncytiotrophoblast. During the 28th week of gestation, the villous tree is covered by an uninterrupted layer of syncytiotrophoblast differentiated into microvilli.

The cells of the amniotic membrane undergo ultrastructural changes throughout gestation (Fig. 4–27). The changes are adaptive physiologic mechanisms to accommodate the growing fetus and the accumulation of amniotic fluid.

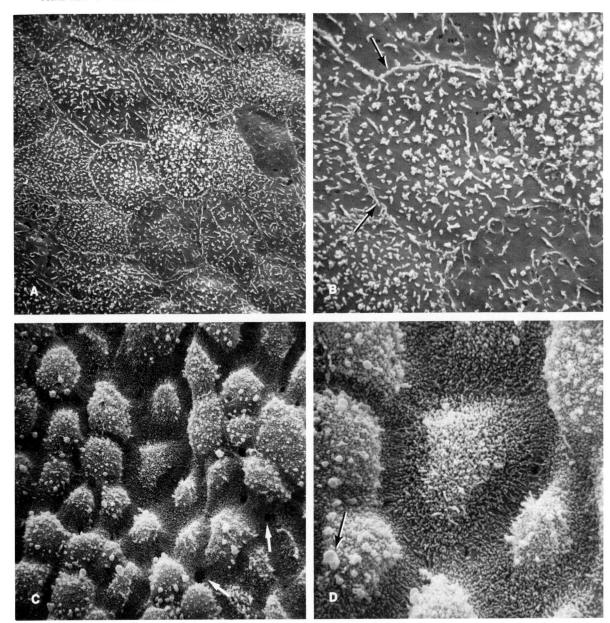

FIG. 4–27. Scanning electron micrographs of human amniotic epithelium, showing development of surface differentiation from first trimester to term pregnancy. *A.* First trimester. Note polygonal, flat epithelial cells and variations in density of microvillous relief. (×2000) *B.* Detail of *A.* Cell borders shown by *arrows.* Note structure of microvilli (×5000) *C.* Term pregnancy. Succulent amniotic epithelial cells with dense microvillous pattern. Cell borders lie in smooth intercellular spaces. Note secretory material (granules) above microvillous relief and openings of intercellular channels (*arrows*). (×2000) *D.* Detail of *C.* Whole cell area, including intercellular space, is covered by microvilli. These are standing densely together in area of cellular nucleus. Secretory granules are shown by *arrow.* (×5000)

SPERMATOZOA

Epididymal spermatozoa undergo cytologic changes that involve dehydration and migration of the cytoplasmic droplet toward the end of the middle piece, narrowing of neck, and reduction of marginal thickening of the acrosomal region (Fig. 4–28). Unlike those of other mammalian species, human spermatozoa show remarkable heterogeneity in the size and shape of sperm heads and mitochondria. There are also signifi-

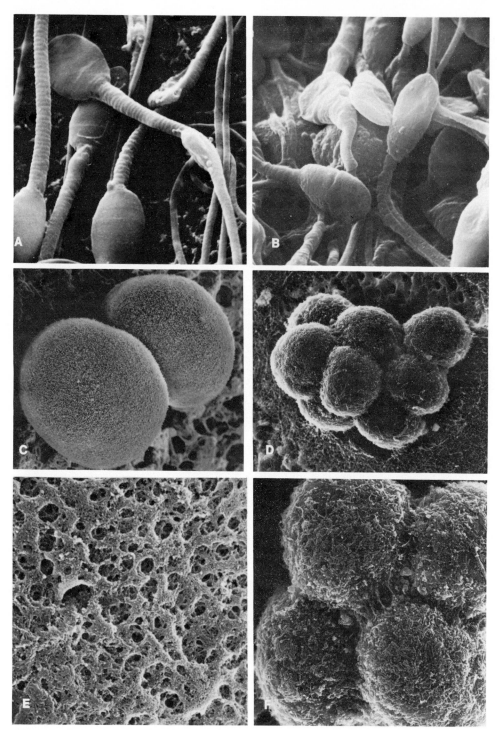

FIG. 4–28. Scanning electron micrographs of mammalian gametes. Species differences in surface ultrastructure are more remarkable in spermatozoa than eggs. *A.* Epididymal spermatozoa from macaque. Note cytoplasmic droplet along midpiece. (×6400) *B.* Human spermatozoa. (×11,000) *C.* Two-cell egg from rat after removal of zona pellucida. Note abundance of microvilli. (×1000) *D.* Morula of baboon after removal of zona pellucida. (×800) *E.* Zona pellucida of rat egg. Note irregular surface. (×8000) *F.* Morula of baboon (same as *D*) after removal of zona pellucida. Note connections between blastomeres. (×2000). (Micrographs courtesy of JE Flechon, ESE Hafez, and D Kraemer)

110

cant regional differences in membrane structure of the spermatozoa. Normal ejaculated spermatozoa are ovoid with slight dorsoventral flattening. The anterior and equatorial segments are not clearly demarcated. A shallow circumferential groove of variable depth is observed between the acrosome and postacrosomal region. The acrosome contains proteolytic enzymes, which probably facilitate sperm penetration in cervical mucus and in luminal fluids in the uterus and the zona pellucida. Closely apposed mitochondria with flattened surface and variable sizes are arranged in a regular or irregular pattern.

Abnormal spermatozoa are observed in all ejaculates of fertile and infertile men. Abnormalities of the head include large deformed spheroid formations or duplicated rudimentary heads. Amorphous spermatozoa have structural defects in the shape or size of the head. Oval, large, small, tapering, and bicephalic forms are also common. Abnormalities of the midpiece include parts of thin and constricted midpieces, enlargement, breakage, and duplication. The morphologic anomalies may result from trauma, illness, or the use of antispermatogenic agents.

CLINICAL CONSIDERATIONS

Scanning electron microscopy, used in combination with other modern techniques (such as immunoelectron microscopy and x-ray dispersive analysis), is a valuable technique for clinical study of human reproduction, diagnosis of female and male infertility, detection of certain types of gynecologic carcinoma and several andrologic and gynecologic disorders, chromsome analysis, and development of new contraceptives. Surface characteristics of amniotic fluid cells (renal epithelium, sebaceous fat cells, pneumonocytes) may be of clinical value comparable to that of biochemical parameters in monitoring fetal maturity.

REFERENCES AND RECOMMENDED READING

Ferenczy A, Richart RM: Scanning Electron Microscopy: Female Reproductive System, Dynamics of Scanning and Transmission Electron Microscopy, p 213. New York, Wiley, 1974

Hafez ESE (ed): Scanning Electron Microscopical Atlas of Mammalian Reproduction. New York, Springer–Verlag, 1975

Hafez ESE (ed): Human Ovulation: Mechanisms, Prediction, Detection and Induction. Amsterdam, Elsevier, 1978

Hafez ESE (ed): Scanning Electron Microscopy of Human Reproduction. Ann Arbor, Ann Arbor Science, 1978

Hafez ESE (ed): Human Reproduction: Conception and contraception, 2nd ed. New York, Harper & Row, 1980

Hafez ESE (ed): Reproduction in Farm Animals, 4th ed. Philadelphia, Lea & Febiger, 1980

Hafez ESE, Barnhart MI, Ludwig H et al : Scanning electron microscopy of human reproductive physiology. Acta Obstet Gynecol Scand [Suppl] 1975

Hafez ESE, Evans TN (eds): Human Vagina. Amsterdam, Elsevier, 1978

Hafez ESE, Kanagawa H: Scanning electron microscopy of human monkey and rabbit spermatozoa. Fertil Steril 24:1776, 1973

Hafez ESE, Ludwig H: Scanning electron microscopy of the endometrium. In Wynn RW (ed): Biology of the Uterus. New York, Plenum Press, 1977

Hafez ESE, Ludwig H, Metzger H: Human endometrial fluid kinetics as observed by scanning electron microscopy. Am J Obstet Gynecol 122:929–938, 1975

Hafez ESE, Thibault C (eds): Biology of Spermatozoa: Maturation, Transport and Fertilizing Ability. Basel, S Karger, 1975

Ludwig H, Metzger H: The human female reproductive tract, A Scanning Electron Microscopic Atlas. New York, Springer–Verlag, 1976

EMBRYOLOGY AND DEVELOPMENTAL DEFECTS OF THE FEMALE REPRODUCTIVE TRACT

Elizabeth M. Ramsey

Familiarity with the embryology of the female reproductive system is as necessary a part of the obstetrician's and gynecologist's armamentarium as are surgical instruments. The notorious "difficulty" of the subject need be no deterrent to attaining this useful familiarity, for confusion can be minimized if four underlying factors are recognized at the outset. Indeed, if these considerations are mastered, the embryology of this tract will be found to be no more difficult than that of any other body system.

1. There is a close relation between the primitive urinary and reproductive systems. Various structures initially formed for excretory functions alone are subsequently used jointly by the two systems or are diverted to reproductive tract use exclusively.
2. Although the sex of the future individual is definitely settled at the time of the union of the nuclei of egg and sperm, reproductive tract structures first appear in a sexually undifferentiated form. During subsequent development, most of the tract is modified to conform to the genetic sex of the individual, but remnants of structures appropriate to the opposite sex persist.
3. Development, particularly of the excretory system, occurs in consecutive but often overlapping waves, each commencing high in the abdominal cavity and progressing toward the pelvis. It thus comes about that structures of quite different stages of developmental maturity may exist simultaneously.
4. The external genitalia owe their origin in part to modification of the primitive cloaca, or joint urinary–intestinal–reproductive receptacle, which is derived at a very early stage from the hindgut.

Figure 5–1 shows, in capsule form, the chronologic relations between developmental events in the four systems involved in genital tract formation. The interrelations and interchanges among elements of the systems are indicated by arrows. The text takes up the systems one by one and carries each from inception to birth. Reference to this chart will make it possible to envisage another dimension, that of relative time, including the sequence or simultaneity of events.

ORIGIN OF PRIMORDIAL GERM CELLS

Conflicting opinions on the origin of primordial germ cells have been voiced for many years. The point at issue is whether all the 300–400 ova a woman sheds in the course of her reproductive years (plus the many thousand others that degenerate in atretic follicles) are formed during her embryonic life, or in any case before puberty, or whether the ovary continues producing ova thereafter. In the embryos of lower vertebrates, birds, and, even more pertinently, mammals (including man), certain distinctive cells appear at a very early somite stage as discrete clumps in the wall of the yolk sac (Fig. 5–2). These cells subsequently migrate through the mesoderm surrounding the hindgut and take up a position within the paired genital ridges from which the gonads are formed (Figs. 5–3 and 5–4). In gonads that become ovaries, these primitive cells are incorporated in the developing stroma and, according to one school of thought, appear eventually as the definitive ova of the ovarian follicles. In gonads that become testes, the primordial germ cells are similarly incorporated in testicular stroma and come to lie in the sex cords. These cords, when subsequently canalized, form the seminiferous tubules, and the germ cells undergo continuous proliferation and maturation into spermatogonia throughout reproductive life.

Certain students of ovarian embryology and physiology, although granting the migration of distinctive primitive cells from the yolk sac to the ovary, have de-

AGE	GLANDS	URINARY TRACT	♂ DUCTS ♀		EXTERNAL GENITALIA
3–4 weeks	PRIMORDIAL GERM CELLS	PRONEPHROS (nonfunctional) Tubules and Ducts	PRONEPHRIC		
4–9 weeks		MESONEPHROS or WOLFFIAN BODY (temporary function) Tubules and Ducts	MESONEPHRIC or WOLFFIAN		CLOACA
5th week	UROGENITAL RIDGE				
6th week	INDIFFERENT GONAD: GERMINAL AND CORE EPITHELIUM	METANEPHROS or KIDNEY (permanent) Tubules and Ducts	PARAMESONEPHRIC or MÜLLERIAN		CLOACA SUBDIVIDES ⎯ ⎯ ⎯ GENITAL TUBERCLE
7th week	MALE TYPE CORDS				ANAL AND URETHRAL MEMBRANES RUPTURE
8th week	TESTIS AND OVARY				URETHRAL AND LABIOSCROTAL FOLDS, PHALLUS AND GLANS
9th week			MÜLLERIAN DUCTS FUSE AT TUBERCLE		
10th week			MÜLLERIAN DUCTS DEGENERATE	WOLFFIAN DUCTS DEGENERATE	
11th week			SEMINAL VESICLES, EPIDIDYMIS, VAS DEFERENS		
12th week	OVARY DESCENT COMPLETE			WALLS FORM	SEX DISTINGUISHABLE
5 months	TESTIS AT INGUINAL RING			SINUS EPITHELIUM GROWS IN VAGINAL CLEFT	
8 months / TERM	TESTIS DESCENT COMPLETE			RAPID UTERINE GROWTH	

FIG. 5–1. Chart showing interrelations and time sequence of events in development of genitourinary system.

nied that these have any kinship with the definitive follicular ova. The latter they regard as products of cyclic proliferation of the coelomic epithelium that originally covers the genital ridges and, in adult life, becomes the germinal epithelium on the surface of the ovary. Studies designed to test this neoformation theory have so far failed to produce evidence of intermediate stages between germinal epithelium and oocytes. Nor have mitoses in oogonia been demonstrated during adult life.

Thus, evidence for neoformation of oogonia is not conclusive, whereas in at least one species (the amphibian *Xenopus laevis*), evidence is strongly in favor of the origin of all oogonia from primordial germ cells and against neoformation. Support for the preformation theory is also found in ablation and transplantation experiments carried out in mammals whose ovaries are closely similar to those of the human being.

For example, if genital ridge tissue of mice is excised and transplanted before the primordial cells have reached it in their migration, no sex cells are formed,

FIG. 5–2. Reconstruction of 25.5-day embryo, showing primordial germ cells (*black dots*) in anterior wall of hindgut and adjacent regions of yolk sac. (Carnegie No. 8005, ×22) (Witschi E: Contrib Embryol 32:67, 1948)

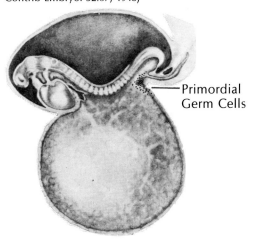

Primordial Germ Cells

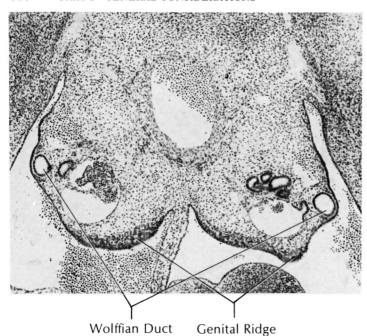

FIG. 5–3. Part of transverse section through 7-week embryo, showing thickening of coelomic epithelium and condensation of underlying mesenchyme that form genital ridge. (Carnegie No. 6524, Sect. 48-3-4, ×250) (Gillman J: Contrib Embryol 32:81, 1948)

Wolffian Duct   Genital Ridge

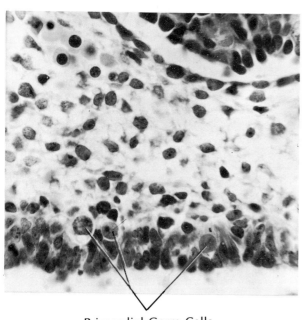

Primordial Germ Cells

FIG. 5–4. Genital ridge of 7-week embryo. (Carnegie No. 8098, Sect. 10-5-4, ×800)

although genital ridge derivatives appear normally. Conversely, if sex cells are present in the ridge tissue when it is transplanted, fully typical gonads form. An additional and more subtle relation is reflected in the following observations: if the primordial sex cells are totally destroyed, the genital ridges themselves do not develop; if, on the other hand, the genital ridges are destroyed before the sex cells reach them, the sex cells undergo degeneration upon arrival at the area. This reciprocal, inductive relation has important implications in certain types of congenital anomalies. In similar fashion, the possibility that ovarian tissue cannot produce new ova in adult life must be borne in mind when ovarian surgery is contemplated.

DEVELOPMENT OF THE OVARY

THE INDIFFERENT GONAD

Gonadal development commences a little later in fetal life than that of the structures giving rise to the reproductive ducts. During the 5th week of embryonic life, when the second of the fetal kidneys has already begun to form, a thickening of the coelomic epithelium occurs on each side of the midline of the dorsal wall. Beneath the epithelium the mesenchyme also proliferates, and the organ thus formed, the indifferent gonad, bulges into the coelomic cavity at the level of the midportion of the mesonephros. A common mesentery suspends the gonad and the mesonephros from the dorsal

body wall. At this time the gonad and the mesonephros bear the joint name *urogenital ridge*. The growth of the gonadal component outstrips that of the mesonephros. Indeed, the latter commences to degenerate fairly soon. In consequence, deep grooves appear in the urogenital ridge, and by the 7th week the gonad has become quite independent, attached to the ridge only by a new mesentery of its own, the *mesorchium* or *mesovarium*, as the case may be, which persists to maturity.

Meanwhile, the thickening of the surface epithelium continues, and fingerlike sprouts begin to penetrate the mesenchymal core of the gonad. The primordial germ cells that had reached the gonadal site just before the epithelial thickening commenced are carried down into the core by the epithelial sprouts and at the same time undergo rapid proliferation of their own (Figs. 5–5 and 5–6).

SEXUAL DIFFERENTIATION

Early in the 7th week in the gonad that will become a testis, the epithelial sprouts assume the form of clearly demarcated epithelial cords with intervening mesenchymal stroma. At the same time, the primordial germ cells disappear from the surface (germinal) epithelium, all of them becoming incorporated in the sex cords. A dense fibrous layer, the *tunica albuginea*, forms beneath the epithelium, separating the sex cords from it (Fig. 5–7).

Distinctive changes in the female gonad do not appear quite as early as those in the male, so that, as Gillman says, "the young ovary is identified chiefly by the fact that it is not a testis." Throughout the 7th week, the epithelial sprouts grow more cordlike (Pflüger's cords), though less dramatically so than in the male (Fig. 5–8). By the end of the 7th week, these break up into discontinuous clumps of cells that become grouped into the *primordial ovarian follicles*, each containing a primordial sex cell (Fig. 5–9). Nothing analogous to the tunica albuginea of the testis separates the germinal epithelium of the ovary from the underlying tissue. Downgrowth and formation of follicles enclosing germ cells may continue to some extent throughout fetal life or even longer.

THE RETE COMPLEX

The differentiation of the sex cords occurs essentially within the future cortex of the gonads, but the epithelial strands continue their growth into the medulla, forming the interlocking networks of the *rete testis* and *rete ovarii*, respectively. The former grows through the mesorchium into the contiguous tissue of the mesonephros and joins the persisting mesonephric tubules. The strands become canalized in the 4th

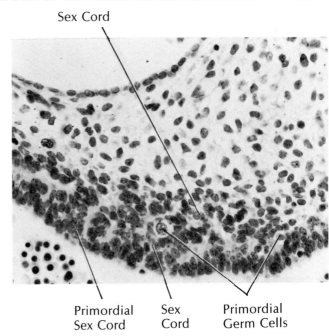

FIG. 5–5. Part of frontal section through 7-week embryo, showing genital ridge at stage slightly more advanced than those shown in Figures 5–3 and 5–4. (Carnegie No. 6516, Sect. 11-1-4, ×500) (Gillman J: Contrib Embryol 32:81, 1948)

FIG. 5–6. Frontal section of gonad in undifferentiated stage (7th week). (Carnegie No. 6507, Sect. 11-1-5, ×100) (Gillman J: Contrib Embryol 32:81, 1948)

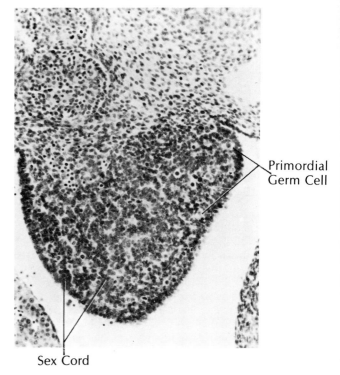

Tunica
Albuginea

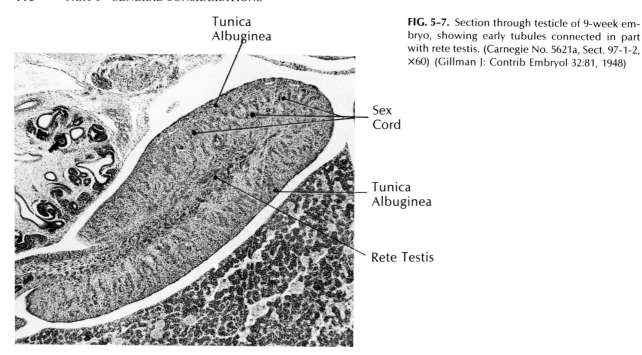

FIG. 5–7. Section through testicle of 9-week embryo, showing early tubules connected in part with rete testis. (Carnegie No. 5621a, Sect. 97-1-2, ×60) (Gillman J: Contrib Embryol 32:81, 1948)

Sex
Cord

Tunica
Albuginea

Rete Testis

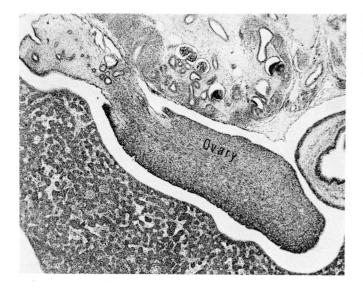

FIG. 5–8. Section through ovary of 9-week embryo. Compare ill-defined rete and very cellular cortex without distinct tubules with condition of testis shown in Figure 5-7. Note that magnifications are same. (Carnegie No. 4304, Sect. 66-3-2, ×60) (Gillman J: Contrib Embryol 32:81, 1948)

month and establish contact through the mesonephric (wolffian) duct with the exterior.

The rete ovarii is less fully formed. Its union with mesonephric tubules is normally sporadic and imperfect, and there is no systematic canalization. The consequent lack of a route to the exterior necessitates the more complicated process of ovarian follicle rupture into the abdominal cavity and transport of ova thence through the lower reproductive tract. The ovarian rete

usually disappears during the course of fetal development, leaving only rudimentary vestiges at the ovarian hilum.

MATURATION OF THE OVARY

Although by the 17th week the ovary and testis can be readily differentiated, numerous developments must

yet take place before the fetal ovary resembles the adult organ. These changes occur in a series of steps, and their sequence is important. First comes encapsulation of the primitive ova by primitive granulosa cells (pregranulosa cells), thus transforming the disorganized cell clumps that were derived from the sex cords into primary ovarian follicles. Coincident with this, the ova swell. Next comes a proliferation of the fetal stroma and its widespread penetration throughout the organ. If these two steps are reversed, the unprotected ova disintegrate upon contact with the stoma.

There is evidence from recent histologic and biochemical studies that this stroma is the precursor of the theca that surrounds the follicles and provides a rich source of estrogens. It follows that the theca is to be regarded as a mesenchymal derivative, whereas the granulosa cells, descendants of the cells composing the sex cords, are of epithelial origin. This concept does much to dispel previous confusion about the origin of the two types of cells, but it must be noted that some authorities continue to contend that granulosa cells as well as the theca are derived directly from the mesenchyme.

About the time these alterations are completed (7th month), proliferation of granulosa occurs in many follicles throughout the ovary, with formation of antra in which fluid collects (*graafian follicles*). The implication seems clear that the ovary has become responsive to maternal gonadotropic hormones. Thus, at birth a small proportion of follicles presents a surprisingly adult appearance (Fig. 5–10), but this normal condition should not be mistaken for a pathologic one. When deprived of maternal hormone stimulation after birth, the follicles regress until puberty.

DESCENT OF THE OVARY

The gonads of both sexes develop high in the abdominal cavity retroperitoneally. They descend into the pelvis, late in fetal life, by different routes; the testes by slipping along the posterior body wall behind the peritoneum, the ovaries by sagging into the peritoneal cavity. In doing so, the ovaries pull the tubes with them, stretch the broad ligaments, and cause an angulation in the round ligaments. These relations are illustrated in Figure 5–11.

The ligaments themselves are formed essentially as a result of the bulging of the ovaries and müllerian ducts into the peritoneal cavity, since they carry a double fold of peritoneum with them. Connective tissue is deposited between the layers, a particularly large amount in the broad ligament, where the mesonephros was originally located. The round ligament is a carryover from the inguinal ligament of the mesonephros, which attached the inferior pole of that organ to the lower margin of the body cavity. The pull of these various ligaments upon the ovaries prevents

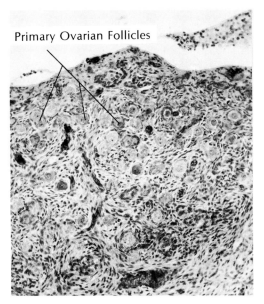

FIG. 5–9. Ovary of 30-week embryo. Fetal stroma has invaded throughout cortex. (Carnegie No. Forbes 12-30, ×200)

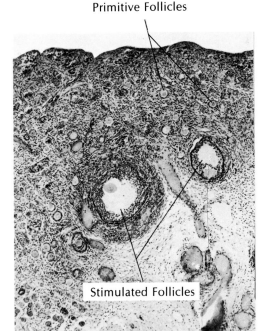

FIG. 5–10. Ovary of full-term fetus. Maternal hormones have stimulated development of two of the follicles shown. (Carnegie No. Forbes 12-14 ×100)

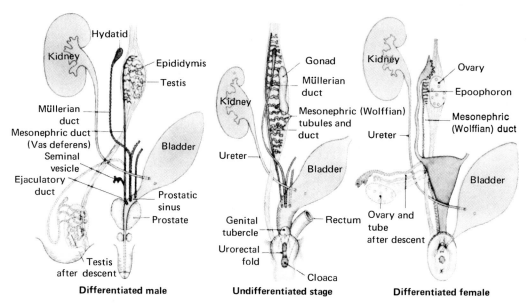

FIG. 5-11. Schematic diagrams showing plan of development of definitive male and female urogenital systems from primitive, undifferentiated state. (Patten BM: Human Embryology, 2nd ed. Philadelphia, Blakiston, 1953)

them from pursuing the same path of descent as the testes.

THE DUCTS

In a brief review of the early development of the urinary tract to make clear its relation with the development of the reproductive system, prime interest focuses upon those urinary tract components that later become functional portions of the reproductive tract, namely, the ducts.

In the development of the mammalian excretory system, three successive kidneys are formed, all of them bilaterally paired. The first, the *pronephros,* probably does not function in the human being. Its first segments appear high in the abdominal cavity during the 3rd week, and development proceeds downward. The organ is composed of tubules whose medial ends meet and fuse to form a common *pronephric duct.* This grows toward the cloaca, into which it eventually opens. As development of the pronephros progresses, the highest tubules commence to degenerate, even before the lowest ones are formed, but the duct does not degenerate.

The second kidney, the *mesonephros,* begins to replace the pronephros in the subdiaphragmatic location in the 4th week. It is composed of tubules similar to those of its predecessor, but instead of elaborating a duct of its own, it appropriates the pronephric duct,

which thereafter is known as the *mesonephric duct* or by the more familiar eponym, the *wolffian duct.* There is evidence that the mesonephros, unlike the pronephros, does have at least rudimentary function for a time, but like the pronephros, it degenerates. The definitive kidney, the *metanephros,* supplants it. The tubules of this final excretory organ form a little lower in the abdominal cavity than those of the previous kidneys and first appear in the 6th or 7th week. Its duct originates as an outpouching of the lower end of the mesonephric duct, the *ureteric bud,* which grows upward, eventually invaginating the metanephros and connecting with the metanephric tubules. The connection of the ureter with the mesonephric duct is interrupted at an early stage by differential growth processes that give the two ducts separate entrances to the urogenital sinus. It is important to emphasize the close association between the definitive urinary tract and those parts of the reproductive tract that are derived from the mesonephric duct. Note in particular the common origin of their lining epithelium.

The foregoing developments are common to both male and female in the early "neuter" stage. With the assumption of all excretory functions by the metanephric complex, the mesonephric duct is used by the male exclusively as the channel through which the sex cells are conducted from the testis to the exterior. Its further course in the male is shown in Figure 5–11. In the female, it gradually degenerates and disappears, except for occasional rests.

The female reproductive duct, the *paramesonephric* or *müllerian duct,* is made afresh for the purpose. It originates during the sexually indifferent period, early in the 6th week, and is therefore present in the future

FIG. 5–12. Reconstructions of müllerian and wolffian ducts in female embryos at 8–14 weeks of development. (After JF Didusch. Koff AK: Contrib Embryol 24:61, 1933)

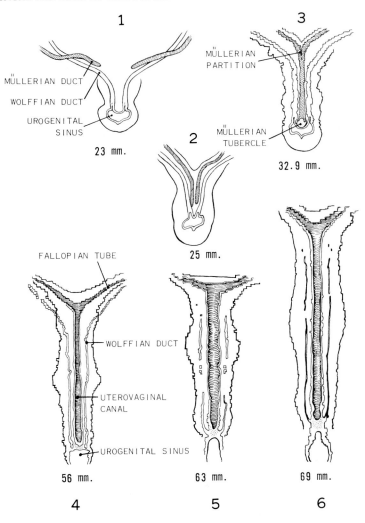

male as well as the future female. In the former, it degenerates about the 10th week, at approximately the time when the mesonephric duct is degenerating in the female. The müllerian duct originates as an invagination of coelomic epithelium lateral to the upper end of the mesonephric duct. The epithelium in the base of the small pit so formed proliferates to form a solid, blind cord that grows downward toward the pelvis. This later becomes canalized. This mechanism, which results in a lining coelomic epithelium, contrasts with the bulging of the gonads into the body cavity, which produces a covering of coelomic epithelium. The müllerian ducts of either side grow toward each other, crossing over the wolffian duct anteriorly to meet and fuse in the midline during the 9th week. The medial walls of the fused ducts gradually disappear, producing a single uterovaginal cavity (Fig. 5–12). The upper portions of the ducts, which do not fuse, remain as the paired uterine (fallopian) tubes, each with a persis-

tent ostium to the peritoneum at its tip (Fig. 5–11). When the lower end of the fused müllerian ducts makes contact with the urogenital sinus, the cell cords are still solid (Fig. 5–12). They merge with the endodermal cells growing back from the sinus to form a temporary barrier between the uterovaginal cavity and the urogenital sinus, the *müllerian tubercle.*

DERIVATIVES OF THE UROGENITAL SINUS

The *cloaca,* the primitive receptacle into which reproductive, excretory, and intestinal tracts open, is the blind end of the hindgut. Hence, the cloaca and its derivatives are lined with endoderm. In the 6th week, the urorectal septum divides the cloaca, separating intestinal and genitourinary compartments. The latter, the *urogenital sinus,* opens exteriorly shortly thereafter as the result of rupture of the urogenital (urethral)

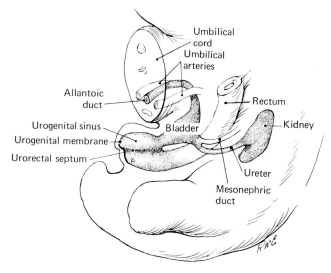

FIG. 5-13. Relations of cloaca and its derivatives.

membrane, and the urogenital duct system thus acquires access to the outside (Fig. 5–13). Previously, certain landmarks appeared in the future perineal region, preeminently a midline protuberance, the *genital tubercle,* precursor of the phallus; the *genital folds;* and the *labioscrotal swellings* lateral to them. The depression between the genital folds is the *primitive urethral groove* (Fig. 5–14). In the female this becomes the outer part of the vestibule, and the rupture of the urethral membrane occurs in its depth. Since this rupture creates a large orifice, the whole urogenital sinus is converted into an open trough that forms the inner portion of the vestibule. The junction between perineal ectoderm and urogenital sinus endoderm occurs on the inner aspect of the genital folds, which become the labia minora.

The opening of the ureter, via its terminal segment, the urethra, occurs in the deep endodermal portion of the vestibule, as does the opening of the uterovaginal cavity. The latter, however, is not entirely simple. Not until the 5th month does sinus epithelium (endodermal in origin) penetrate the wall of the urogenital sinus in the müllerian tubercle where the fused müllerian ducts ended blindly. Subsequent canalization of this barrier opens the vaginal canal into the vestibule. A residue of the barrier still persists in attenuated form as the *hymen.* Thus, the lower portion of the vagina is lined with epithelium tracing its ancestry to gut endoderm, whereas the upper portion, derived from the müllerian duct, originated in coelomic epithelium. The müllerian epithelium becomes columnar and forms a characteristic mucosa. The vaginal epithelium becomes stratified squamous. The junction between the two types, occurring at the site of the future cervix uteri, is not abrupt, and the interaction between the two epithelia is the basis of a number of important pathologic processes that may occur in the adult.

For comparison between male and female development, it may be noted that, although the clitoris is homologous to the penis, the urethral groove at its base is rudimentary only and does not normally deepen or close over in the manner of the penile urethra. Bartholin's glands provide another such comparison between the sexes. They are homologs of the male bulbourethral (Cowper's) glands and, like them, arise by budding from the endodermal epithelium of the portion of the urogenital sinus which forms the urethra.

THE EXTERNAL GENITALIA

The accurate determination of the sex of abortuses is a duty of the obstetrician that may have social, legal, and statistic importance. It is also, in many cases, a source of confusion and error. The difficulty lies, of course, in the fact that the phallus of a female embryo and of an embryo of undifferentiated sex is quite as prominent as that of a true male and in consequence, may be mistaken for a penis. Altogether different landmarks must be used for accurate determinations.

As noted earlier, the genetic sex of the embryo is determined at the time of fertilization, but some weeks of development must pass before what Novak calls "the impress of sex" is made upon various portions of the genital tract. Prior to the 6th week, sex can be determined only by establishing the presence (female) or absence (male) of sex chromatin in the nuclei of resting body cells. From the 7th to the 10th week, differentiation must be based upon the histologic characteristics of the developing gonads (Fig. 5–14). In certain cases, a slightly earlier decision on the basis of external genitalia may appear possible, but this appearance should be distrusted, as relative retardation may occur in males. Since, as indicated previously (Fig. 5–1), the müllerian ducts of the female commence to fuse in the 9th week, gross inspection of the abdominal organs may be of some help in differentiation at about this time. Caution must be observed, however, for entirely male wolffian ducts may lie so closely side by side in the pelvis that they will be mistaken for müllerian ducts about to fuse to form a uterus.

During the 11th week, a series of diagnostic changes in the external genitalia commences, as illustrated in Figure 5–15. In the top row of photographs, showing specimens of the 11th week, male and female can be differentiated. Disregarding the phallus, which is similar in both, it will be noted that in the male the urogenital outlet has become smaller and has apparently migrated toward the tip of the phallus. Actually, the process is a covering over of the lower portion of the primitive urethral groove by fusion of the genital folds. In the female the urogenital opening re-

mains large and continues to be at the base of the phallus. A slight depression separates the posterior ends of the labioscrotal swellings. The closing over of the inferior portion of the outlet in the male brings the scrotolabial folds together in a distinctive band of connective tissue, the scrotal raphe. Since, when diagnosing an individual specimen the obstetrician does not always have an example of the opposite sex at the same stage at hand for comparison, an abolute criterion of sex is more useful than relative ones. The scrotal raphe is perhaps the most reliable such landmark. It is absent in the female at all stages but is detectable early in the male.

By the stage illustrated in the specimens in the middle row of Figure 5–15 (13th week), there is no serious diagnostic difficulty if the foregoing differential points are borne in mind and if, most importantly, the genitalia are examined from the perineal aspect. Diagnosis of the specimens illustrated in the bottom row of photographs, which are of an even later stage (15th week), is equally clearcut, again provided it is made on the basis of perineal examination. Figure 5–16 shows, however, that confusion and error may still result if examination is restricted to the anterior aspect. Here the phallus is the most conspicuous feature and may easily be mistaken for a penis. A characteristically female bending of this organ toward the anus, which is often described, may be obscured by fixation artifact. Even the labial swellings resemble a scrotum if the separation of their posterior ends at the commissure is not observed. The female phallus normally becomes recognizable as a clitoris in the 4th month.

Two small practical points that facilitate diagnosis may be mentioned: 1) it is essential to have a good source of illumination when examining the specimen, if possible a focused beam; and 2) a dissecting microscope or other means of magnification should be employed whenever a case is in doubt.

ANOMALIES

In the transformations and interactions that take place in the course of prenatal growth and development, there are certain points of weakness, certain areas of stress, where departures from the normal course of development may most readily occur (Table 5–1).

ANOMALIES OF MÜLLERIAN DUCTS

At any stage during the course of normal fusion, an impediment may occur. Resultant conditions range from the extreme case of double uterus and double vagina (Fig. 5–17G) to an inconspicuous notching of the fundus of the uterine cavity (Fig. 5–17E) with or without accompanying notching of the uterine wall (Fig. 5–17A). The clinical importance of the various

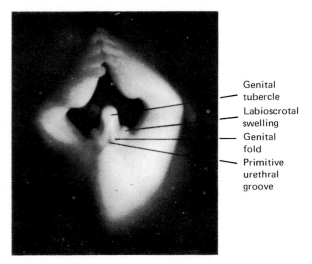

Genital tubercle
Labioscrotal swelling
Genital fold
Primitive urethral groove

FIG. 5–14. Perineal region of $6\frac{3}{7}$-week embryo (24.5 mm), showing undifferentiated precursors of external genitalia. (Carnegie No. 6263)

forms of bicornuate uterus lies in the effect they may have upon the course of pregnancy. The milder degrees of the condition are not uncommon and are often unrecognized clinically unless radiologic study is carried out for some coincidental reason. The more complete partitioning is rare and may present complications. Double pregnancy in two separate cavities with term deliveries at separate times has been reported. Unsuspected cases of this rare circumstance may form the basis of some cases cited as support for the occurrence of superfetation.

Figure 5–17D illustrates a different type of failure of fusion: not, in this instance, failure of two like structures to fuse (e.g., two müllerian ducts) but of two unlike structures to fuse (müllerian ducts and urogenital sinus). The designation *failure to fuse* is perhaps more descriptive of what actually takes place in such cases than the term *atresia*. An anomaly of this sort, of course, precludes pregnancy.

A different sort of müllerian duct anomaly is now thought to underlie the occurrence of adenoma, a condition in which larger or smaller nodules of glandular tissue stud the vagina and cervix. Some of these nodules may undergo malignant transformation.

In 1971, a connection was reported between the occurrence of clear cell adenocarcinoma of the genital tract in young women and the use of diethylstilbestrol (DES) by their mothers during pregnancy. Many, often conflicting, opinions were expressed initially, based in many instances upon limited clinical and statistical data. As more extensive material has become available from the National Cancer Institute and from university-supported studies, greater unanimity of opinion and a more optimistic attitude toward the

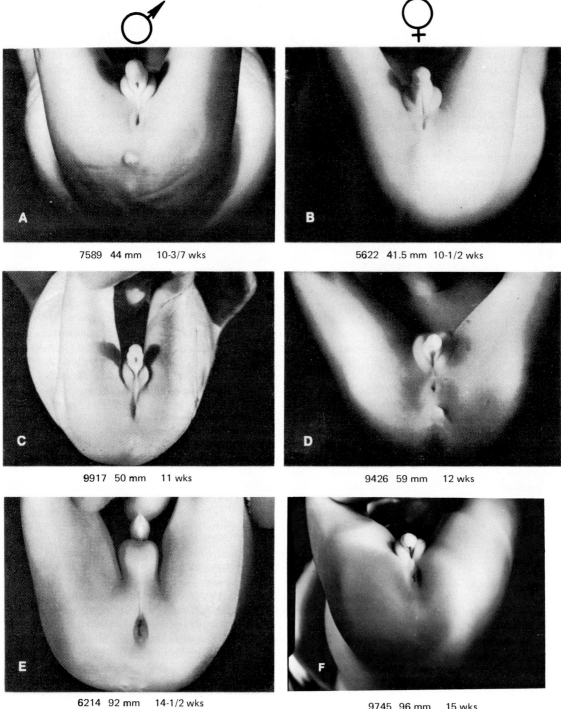

7589   44 mm   10-3/7 wks

5622   41.5 mm 10-1/2 wks

9917   50 mm   11 wks

9426   59 mm   12 wks

6214   92 mm   14-1/2 wks

9745   96 mm   15 wks

FIG. 5-15. External genitalia of male and female embryos. Carnegie numbers and ages as stated.

FIG. 5-16. Two views of external genitalia of female embryo shown in Figure 5-15F, demonstrating masculine appearance of anterior view (A) and emphasizing necessity for examining perineal aspect (B) of all specimens. (Carnegie No. 9745, 96 mm, 15 weeks)

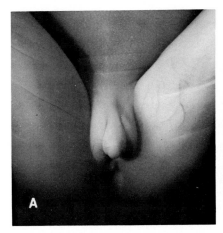
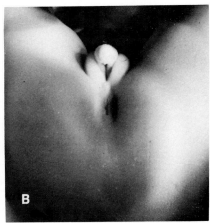

TABLE 5-1. TYPES OF ORIGIN OF ANOMALIES

Type	Example
1. Failure of primordium to appear	Gonadal agenesis
2. Failure of transitory structure to disappear	Persistence of mesonephric tubules or ducts
3. Anomalies of position	Ovary in labium majus
4. Anomalies of fusion	Bicornuate uterus
5. Reduplication of structures	Supernumerary ovaries
6. Overgrowth of structures (usually of hormonal origin)	Hypertrophy of clitoris
7. Chromosomal aberrations	Intersexuality and true hermaphroditism
8. Hormonal disturbances (maternal or fetal)	Hypertrophy of clitoris, true hermaphroditism
9. Breakdown in time schedule	Destruction of ova by proliferating ovarian stroma

problem have become apparent. In brief, the incidence of cancer up to now has been found to be "very low," although dysplasias are relatively common in sons as well as daughters of DES-treated mothers. However, it must be emphasized that the final word has by no means been spoken on this subject. Intensive investigations are still underway, and much more time must elapse before any exposed individual can be completely cleared. Thus, as all are agreed, both mothers and progeny must continue to be examined at regular intervals.

Three types of dysplasia occur in the young women with "adenosis": 1) cervical ectropion, 2) actual adenoma formation, and 3) transverse ridging in the vagina, cervix, or both. All of these varieties of dysplasia are basically a replacement of normal surface epithelial structure by ingrowth of müllerian glandular (columnar) epithelium. In view of the effect of hormonal stimulation upon the normally developing reproductive tract, this aberration resulting from excessive stimulation by administered synthetic hormone is easy to understand. The fact that adenosis results most often when the mother was given the drug early in pregnancy also makes its effect understandable. The clinical evaluation and management of this problem are considered in Chapter 45.

FAILURE OF MESONEPHRIC TUBULES AND DUCTS TO DISAPPEAR

The persistence of vestigial remnants of wolffian ducts and tubules in the female, either with or without symptoms, is more common than anomalies of müllerian duct fusion. The most frequent locations in which these rests occur are the mesovarium and the broad ligament. In the former site, they form the epoophoron (if located high) or the paroophoron (if lower in the ligament). These are often referred to as hydatids of Morgagni, and they occur so regularly that they can hardly be classed as abnormal. Their clinical significance lies in their propensity to cystic dilation and infection, with attendant symptoms. The remnants of the wolffian duct in the broad ligament bear the additional eponym of Gartner's duct. Other, less common residual segments of these ducts occur in the

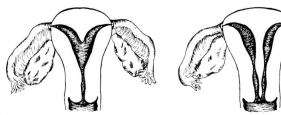

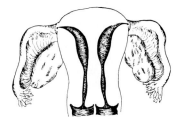

A   Uterus subseptus unicollis

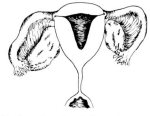

B   Uterus septus duplex

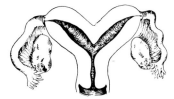

C   Uterus septus duplex with double vagina

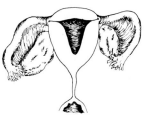

D   Atresia at level of cervix

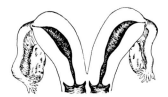

E   Uterus bicornis unicollis

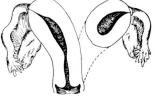

F   Uterus bicornis septus

G   Uterus didelphys with double vagina

H   Uterus bicornis unicollis with one unconnected rudimentary horn

FIG. 5–17. Schematic diagrams of various types of abnormal uteri. (Patten BM: Human Embryology, 3rd ed. Philadelphia, Blakiston, 1968)

walls of the vagina, in the labia minora close to the clitoris, and around the urethra. All are subject to the same clinical symptoms as the cysts of the epoophoron.

Types 1, 3, and 5 in Table 5–1 include anomalies that are more common in other body systems than in the reproductive tract. Anomalies of types 7 and 8 are dealt with elsewhere in this book.

MALFORMATIONS THAT INVOLVE BOTH URINARY AND REPRODUCTIVE TRACTS

The intimate association of the urinary and reproductive tracts gives rise to a number of malformations in which both are involved. These are among the most complex of all anomalies. As classic examples may be cited persistent cloaca, which occurs when the urorectal septum fails to form, and extrophy of the bladder and attendant anomalies of the external genitalia, which results from defective closure of the anterior abdominal wall. Beyond this brief notation, it is recommended that combined genitourinary anomalies be studied, as occasion arises, in specialized texts and reviews.

OVARIAN TUMORS

Related to the congenital malformations of the female genital tract, though not properly described as anomalies, are the special ovarian neoplasms (see Chapter 57, Lesions of the Ovary). These tumors may be composed of one or more of the cell types normally occurring in the gonad at any stage of its development. If

derived from cells of the sexually indifferent stage, the tumor cells may differentiate along the male or the female path, regardless of the fact that the patient's normal gonad became an ovary. A firm grasp of the basic steps of the embryologic development of the gonads renders the complexity of ovarian tumors less baffling. The following points should be noted:

1. Totipotent primordial germ cells migrate from the primitive yolk sac through the gut mesentery to the site of gonad formation. Query: Could a cell, sidetracked during migration, remain viable but dormant until subsequent stimulation to proliferation? Could this account for ovarian type tumors in ectopic locations?
2. The epithelial lining of the müllerian ducts, and therefore of all structures derived from it, originates from the coelomic epithelium. It is unknown at what stage the multipotency of this epithelium ceases or whether subsequent stimulation of any sort can reactivate it. This consideration is allied to the problem of the cause of endometriosis and may be implicated in the histogenesis of certain ovarian tumors, since the germinal epithelium of the ovary has the same origin in coelomic epithelium.
3. Although granulosa cells and theca cells are probably of different origin and not interchangeable, there is evidence that the granulosa cell, at a particular stage of development, induces the differentiation of theca cells from the stroma. Breakdown of the normal time schedule or imbalances in mutual influence might have pathologic consequences.

In conclusion, it may be reiterated that familiarity with the normal development of the reproductive tract and appreciation of the general ways in which developmental processes can go awry are of greater assistance in understanding the complexities of congenital anomalies than the memorizing of individual examples. The multiplicity of eponyms should not be a matter of concern, for once the anatomic definition of a condition is determined, its nature and origin can be comprehended against the background of normal developmental processes. Such analyses are useful because anomalies not infrequently are multiple, and it is important to know for what unsuspected condition any given patient should be examined.

REFERENCES AND RECOMMENDED READING

GENERAL

Arey LB: Developmental Anatomy, 7th ed rev, chaps II, XVII, XVIII. Philadelphia, Saunders, 1974

Corliss CE: Patten's Human Embryology, chaps 2, 19. New York, McGraw–Hill, 1976

Greep RO (ed): Handbook of Physiology, Vol II, Endocrinology, chaps 12–19. Washington, American Physiological Society, 1975

Hamilton WJ, Mossman HW: Human Embryology, 4th ed, chaps II, XII. Baltimore, Williams & Wilkins, 1972

Novak ER, Woodruff JD: Gynecologic and Obstetric Pathology, 7th ed, chaps 17, 25–28. Philadelphia, Saunders, 1974

ORIGIN OF PRIMORDIAL GERM CELLS

Blackler AW: Transfer of primordial germ-cells between two subspecies of *Xenopus laevis.* J Embryol Exp Morphol 10:641, 1962

Mossman HW, Duke KL: Comparitive Morphology of the Mammalian Ovary. Madison, University of Wisconsin Press, 1973

Witschi E: Migration of the germ cells of human embryos from the yolk sac to the primitive gonadal folds. Contrib Embryol 32:67, 1948

DEVELOPMENT OF THE OVARY

Gillman J: Development of the gonads in man, with consideration of the role of fetal endocrines and the histogenesis of ovarian tumors. Contrib Embryol 32:81, 1948

Mossman HW, Duke KL: Comparative Morphology of the Mammalian Ovary. Madison, University of Wisconsin Press, 1973

VanWagenen G, Simpson ME: Embryology of the Ovary and Testis: *Homo sapiens* and *Macaca mulatta.* New Haven, Yale University Press, 1965

DUCTS

Hunter HR: Observations on the development of the female genital tract. Contrib Embryol 22:91, 1930

Koff AK: Development of the vagina in the human fetus. Contrib Embryol 24:59, 1933

Witschi E: Embryology of the uterus: Normal and experimental. Ann NY Acad Sci 75:412, 1959

DERIVATIVES OF UROGENITAL SINUS

Shikinami J: Detailed form of the wolffian body in human embryos of the first eight weeks. Contrib Embryol 18:49, 1926

EXTERNAL GENITALIA

Corliss CE: Patten's Human Embryology, chap 19. New York, McGraw–Hill, 1976

Koff AK: Development of the vagina in the human fetus. Contrib Embryol 24:59, 1933

Spaulding MH: Development of the external genitalia in the human embryo. Contrib Embryol 13:67, 1921 (to be read in conjunction with Gillman, who modifies certain of Spaulding's conclusions)

ANOMALIES

General

Gruenwald P: Relation of the growing müllerian duct to the wolffian duct and its importance for the genesis of malformations. Anat Rec 81:1, 1941

Jones HW, Scott WH: Hermaphroditism, Genital Anomalies and Related Endocrine Disorders. Baltimore, Williams & Wilkins, 1958

McKelvey JL, Baxter JS: Abnormal development of the vagina and genitourinary tract. Am J Obstet Gynecol 29:267, 1935

Marshall FF, Beisel DS: Association of uterine and renal anomalies. Obstet Gynecol 51:559, 1978

Young HH: Genital Abnormalities, Hermaphroditism and Related Adrenal Diseases. Baltimore, Williams & Wilkins, 1937

DES-Associated

Anderson B, Watring, WG et al.: Development of DES-associated clear-cell carcinoma: The importance of regular screening. Obstet Gynecol 53:293, 1979

Bibbo M, Gill WB et al.: Follow-up study of male and female offspring of DES-exposed mothers. Obstet Gynecol 49:1, 1977

Burke L, Antonioli D, Rosen S: Vaginal and cervical squamous cell dysplasia in women exposed to diethylstilbestrol in utero. Am J Obstet Gynecol 152:537, 1978

Johnson LD, Driscoll SG et al.: Vaginal adenosis in stillborns and neonates exposed to diethylstilbestrol and steroidal estrogens and progestins. Obstet Gynecol 53:671, 1979

Prins RP, Morrow P: Vaginal embryogenesis, estrogens, and adenosis. Obstet Gynecol 48:246, 1976

Robboy SJ, Kaufman RH et al.: Pathologic findings in young women enrolled in the National Cooperative Diethylstilbestrol Adenosis (DESAD) project. Obstet Gynecol 53:309, 1979

Scully RE, Robboy SJ: Pathology and pathogenesis of diethylstilbestrol-related disorders of the female genital tract. In Herbst AL (ed): Intrauterine Exposure to Diethylstilbestrol in the Human. Proceedings of "Symposium on DES," 1977. Chicago, Am Col Obstetricians & Gynecologists, 1978

Siegler AM, Wang EF, Friberg J: Fertility of the diethylstilbestrol exposed offspring. Modern Trends 31:601, 1979

Ovarian hormones provide the endocrine base for the development and maturation of the entire female reproductive system, and ovarian germ cells are the essential ingredients of the female contribution to reproduction. The ovary is thus an organ both for germ cell maturation, storage, and release, as well as for cyclic endocrine activity. The two functions are interdependent. Without ova (germ cells), normal ovarian endocrine function cannot develop, since the steroid-producing follicles and corpora lutea are not formed without ova. The ovarian hormones, on the other hand, provide a feedback control of hypothalamic and pituitary function that modulates both germ cell and endocrine activities of the ovary by means of pituitary gonadotropins. An exposition of this complex hypothalamic–pituitary–gonadal interplay is possible in the light of contemporary endocrine knowledge.

NEUROENDOCRINE CONTROL OF OVARIAN FUNCTION

The reciprocal relations of hypothalamus, pituitary, ovary, and endometrium are diagrammed in Figure 6–1. The ovary develops and grows under the influence of the two pituitary gonadotropins, follicle-stimulating hormone (FSH) and luteinizing hormone (LH). Estrogens produced by the ovary also augment ovarian growth as well as ovarian response to gonadotropins—a rare example of a hormone having an effect on its gland of origin.

The major influence of the two gonadotropins is upon the ova-containing follicles. The purposes of the rise in FSH are apparently the induction of LH receptors in the granulosa cells, the increase in steroidogenic capacity of the follicles, especially estrogen production, and the formation of the antral cavity, which leads to the mature graafian follicle. The rise in blood estrogen from the follicle triggers LH release. The mature follicle may then react to the sudden surge of LH (Figs. 6–2 and 6–3) by rupture and expulsion of the egg at the time of ovulation. The ruptured follicle develops into a corpus luteum, which produces progesterone and estrogens and has a limited life span. The cyclic nature of ovarian function is such that many follicles develop each month under the influence of cyclic secretion of pituitary FSH and LH during the so-called follicular phase, which lasts about 14 days. Sudden release of a high level of pituitary LH into the blood stream causes rupture of usually only one follicle, with the formation of a single corpus luteum that has a life span of about 12–13 days. The follicles not ovulated all regress in a process called *atresia*. Why only one follicle ruptures and how that one is selected are at present complete mysteries. The cycle is then repeated each month, with an average total duration of 28 days for the follicular, corpora lutea (luteal), and regression phases. When the corpus luteum regresses

CYCLIC OVARIAN FUNCTION AND ITS NEUROENDOCRINE CONTROL

Kenneth J. Ryan

and its hormones are withdrawn, endometrial shedding (menstruation) occurs (Fig. 6–1).

The pituitary gland does not have an innate capacity either to synthesize or to release these gonadotropins, but is under the influence of the hypothalamus, to which it is attached by the pituitary stalk. The hypothalamus contains hormone-producing neurons that release specific hypophysiotropic hormones into the portal circulation that drains from the hypothalamus to the pituitary. The hypophysiotropic hormones (releasing factors) stimulate production and release of the specific pituitary gonadotropins (Fig. 6–4). If the pituitary is removed from the hypothalamus by transplantation or by cutting the pituitary stalk and circulation, the pituitary gonadotropins are no longer synthesized or released. Capacity to produce gonadotropins can be restored by regrafting the pituitary to the hypothalamus. Pituitary function can also be influenced by experimental lesions, electrical stimula-

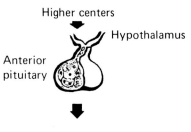

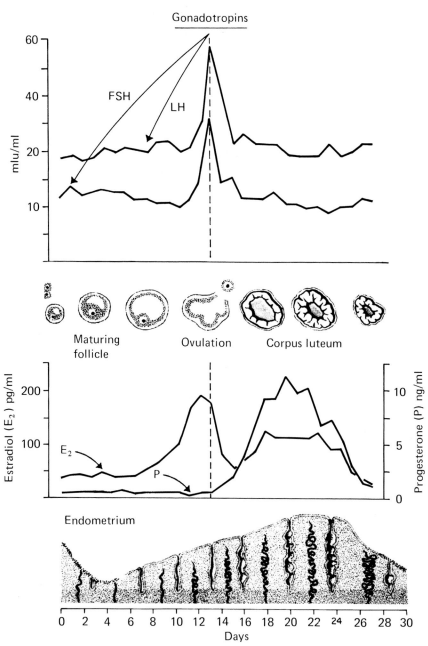

FIG. 6–1. Diagrammatic representation of events of pituitary, ovarian, and menstrual cycle. Note plasma estradiol peak about day 12, plasma FSH and LH peaks about day 13, and ovulation about day 14.

tion, or chemical agents applied locally to the hypothalamus.

The cyclicity or timing of the pituitary gonadotropin secretion, especially the surge of LH that cause ovulation, is determined by programming for this cyclic activity either during fetal life or early in the neonatal period. There is a fundamental difference in cyclicity of pituitary release of gonadotropins between male and female, the female having a preovulatory surge of LH secretion that results in ovulation. The LH surge is clearly a result of the estrogen peak that precedes it by about 24 hours (Fig. 6–3). In experimental animals, females given a single injection of testosterone in the neonatal period have a male pattern at maturity; they cannot respond to positive feedback effects of estrogens by an LH surge. Males deprived of testicular hormone develop a female type of response. If the pituitary of the female rat is transplanted next to a male hypothalamus, it assumes the male programming for pituitary secretion. The converse is also true. This male and female programming of the hypothalamus is less clearly defined in the human.

Mature hypothalamic function is characterized by frequent pulses of releasing hormone into the portal system that drains the hypothalamus. However, the preovulatory release of LH from the pituitary is apparently not due to a surge of releasing hormone into the portal circulation to the pituitary. In rhesus monkeys with destructive hypothalamic lesions, the hourly injection of synthetic gonadotropin-releasing hormone at a level dose for a long period of time is sufficient to reestablish normal ovulatory menstrual cycles. This suggests that the preovulatory surge of gonadotropins is due to the direct effect of estrogens on the pituitary and not a surge in hypothalamic gonadotropin-releasing hormone.

Levels of releasing hormone in the peripheral circulation of women with normal ovulatory menstrual cycles are not related to the levels of gonadotropins in the peripheral circulation. At ovulation, the levels of releasing hormone in the peripheral circulation are, if anything, lower than they are at other times in the cycle.

The role of FSH and LH in developing follicles, increasing estrogen secretion, and finally causing ovulation can be experimentally confirmed by measuring the patterns of these pituitary hormones in the blood during the cycle in relation to the events described (Figs. 6–2 and 6–3). In patients with no hypophyseal function, the ovarian cycle can be mimicked by administration of appropriate amounts of the pituitary hormones.

Furthermore the hypothalamic control of pituitary gonadotropin secretion can be modulated by feedback influences of the steroid hormones on the hypothalamus and on the anterior pituitary. Estrogens have the dual effect of stimulating gonadotropin release by means of positive feedback and inhibiting pituitary se-

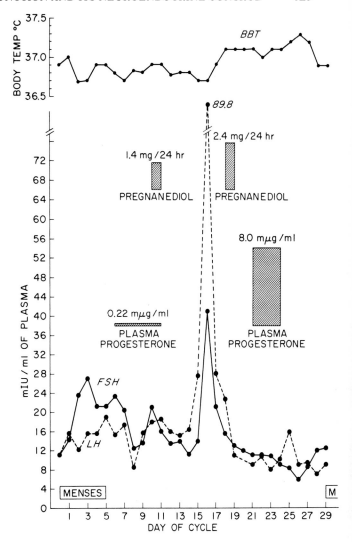

FIG. 6–2. Relation of plasma FSH, LH, and progesterone levels, basal body temperature (*BBT*), and urinary levels of pregnanediol as measured in human subject. Note similarities to and differences from diagrammatic representation in Figure 6–1. (Cargille CM, Ross GT, Yoshimi T: J Clin Endocrinol Metab 29:12, 1969)

cretion by means of negative feedback. Because the latter effect is capable of preventing the LH surge and ovulation, it is the major basis for the contraceptive effect of the birth control pills. The mechanism of this dual effect is not clearly understood, but undoubtedly more is involved than simply control through blood levels of estrogens.

The hypothalamus is also subject to neural influences from higher brain centers, which explains the well-known effects of light, sound, smell, and emotion on the ovarian, and consequently the menstrual, cycle.

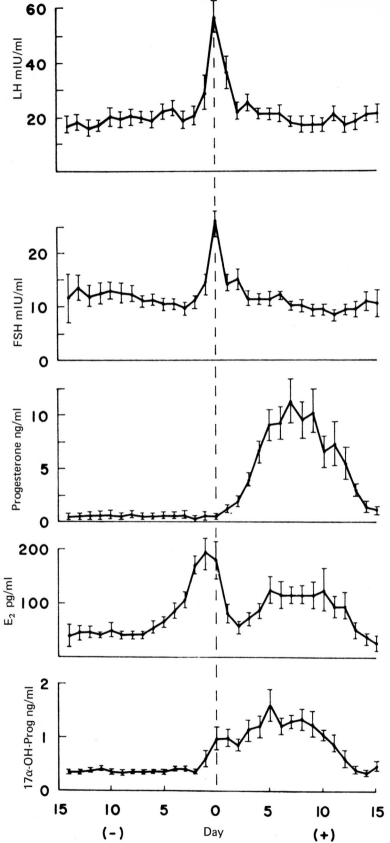

FIG. 6–3. Changes in serum levels of LH, FSH, progesterone, estradiol (E₂), and 17-hydroxyprogesterone (17α-OH-prog) during cycle normalized to day of LH peak as day 0. Note especially peak of estradiol that precedes and causes LH release. (Thorneycroft IH et al.: Am J Obstet Gynecol 111:947, 1971)

FIG. 6-4. Relations between hypothalamus, anterior pituitary, and target glands. Luteotropic hormone (*LTH*) has not been established as a tropic hormone in the human. *TSH*, Thyroid-stimulating hormone. *ACTH*, Adrenocorticotropic hormone. (Modified from Harris GW: Neural Control of the Pituitary Gland. London, Arnold, 1955)

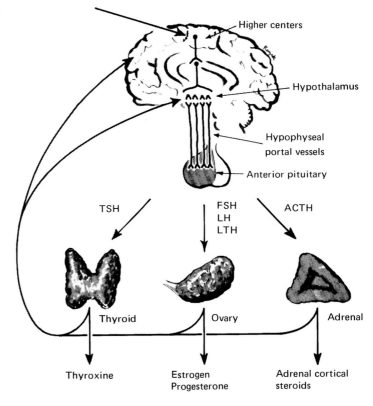

The secretion of gonadotropins has been characterized as having a predominantly negative feedback relation to steroid production. While this is only a crude approximation (since steroids can have a dual effect, as noted), it is a useful concept. After hypothalamic maturation in adolescence, the gonadotropins that are secreted stimulate ovarian steroid production, which in turn modulates the amounts of pituitary hormone released. When ovarian hormones are removed (as after oophorectomy or menopause), gonadotropins rise unchecked and remain elevated. When ovarian hormone levels are high as in pregnancy or following ingestion of birth control pills, the pituitary gonadotropin secretion is depressed. The locus of the steroid effect has been established in both the hypothalamus and pituitary.

HYPOTHALAMIC HORMONES

The hypothalamic factor responsible for control of anterior pituitary gonadotropin synthesis and release has been isolated in animals, identified as a decapeptide, synthesized, and designated luteinizing-hormone–releasing hormone (LHRH). When administered to in-

tact animals or human subjects, it evokes the release of both LH and FSH (Fig. 6–5). Thus far, no discrete FSH-releasing hormone has been identified, and LHRH appears to be involved with both gonadotropins. The effect of LHRH on gonadotropin release from the pituitary is clearly influenced by ovarian steroid hormones acting at both hypothalamic and pituitary sites. It is not known whether there are discrete centers in the hypothalamus that control the negative or positive feedback type of response.

PITUITARY GONADOTROPINS

Both FSH and LH have been isolated and characterized from human material as glycoproteins with a molecular weight of about 30,000. The amino acid composition and carbohydrate content have been described for both gonadotropins, and partial degradation studies have revealed an essential role for the sugar moieties attached to the protein.

For pharmacologic use, FSH and LH can be isolated from human pituitaries, since the gonadotropins do not autolyze prior to autopsy. In addition, high levels of gonadotropins are excreted in the urine of postmeno-

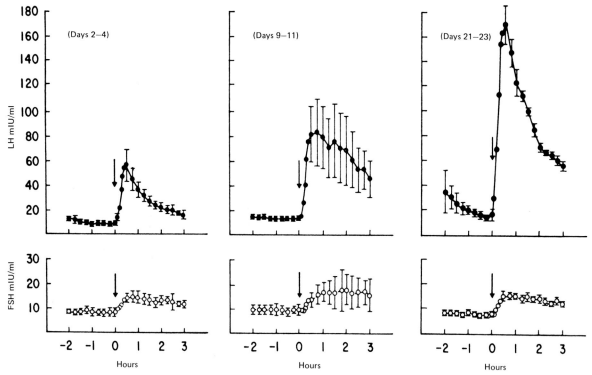

FIG. 6–5. Serum LH and FSH concentrations (mean 1 SE) before and after administration of 150μg LHRH during different phases of cycle studied serially. *Arrow* indicates time of injection of LHRH. It has been suggested that change in gonadotropin release during cycle is due to effects of varying levels of ovarian hormones upon pituitary. (Yen SCC et al.: J Clin Endocrinol Metab 35:931, 1972)

pausal women (owing to lack of the negative feedback mechanism), and these gonadotropins can be extracted and purified for human use.

FSH and LH are available for patients who do not ovulate spontaneously as a result of pituitary or hypothalamic defects. When they are adminstered in a pattern approximating the normal cycle, follicular development occurs and ovulation can be induced by injection of a "surge" level of either LH or human chorionic gonadotropin (hCG), an LH-like hormone produced by the placenta (see Chapter 17). Such treatment occasionally results in multiple ovulation, with as many as six or seven offspring developing. Such multiple pregnancy usually results in early abortion.

Although a specific luteotropic hormone (LTH, prolactin) that maintains the corpus luteum has been described in certain animals, such a role for this hormone has not been described in human or primate reproduction. In the human, LH itself appears to have this luteotropic action. The role of prolactin in control of the human cycle remains to be determined.

OVARIAN HORMONES

The ovary secretes three general classes of steroid hormones: estrogens, androgens, and progestins. All steroid hormones have a common carbon ring structure (Fig. 6–6), and the fundamental differences in the three steroids are in the number of carbon atoms present and the substituents attached. In the numbering sequence illustrated, estrogens have 18 carbons; androgens, 19 carbons (the example given in the left part of Fig. 6–6); and progestins, 21 carbons, consisting essentially of a 19-carbon androgen molecule with a 2-carbon side chain attached to carbon 17 (example in the right part of Fig. 6–6).

ESTROGENS

The estrogens are steroid hormones that produce the characteristic changes in the female reproductive tract and general body metabolism associated with womanhood. The growth and development of the breasts, uterus, fallopian tubes, and vagina are primary estrogen effects. In animals, estrogens can induce sexual receptivity (heat), a property not readily apparent in the human. Typical assays for estrogen biologic activity are based upon changes of the cells lining the vagina (Allen–Doisy test) or growth promotion of the uterus of the immature laboratory animal.

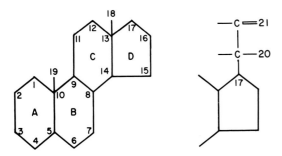

FIG. 6-6. Cyclopentenophenanthrene ring system. Each ring is identified by *letter*, from *A* to *D*. Carbon atoms are numbered in sequence shown.

Estrogens cause proliferation of the endometrial lining of the uterus, and this, like most other estrogen effects, provides a base for subsequent progesterone action on the target tissue. These sequential and synergistic actions of estrogen and progesterone determine the cyclic pattern of endometrial growth, regression, and sloughing (menstruation) (Fig. 6–1).

Estrogens also profoundly affect such general body mechanisms as salt and water balance, insulin and growth hormone secretion, carbohydrate metabolism, calcium dynamics, and cholesterol/phospholipid ratios in blood. These actions account for the side effects occasionally observed when estrogen is used in clinical medicine and for some of the maternal metabolic changes of pregnancy; they also are the basis for estrogen administration following menopause, when the level of estrogens may be deficient. Estrogens may have an augmenting effect on breast or endometrial cancer, and for this reason their use is contraindicated in the presence of these malignancies.

The most potent natural estrogen and the primary ovarian secretory product is 17-β-estradiol. This compound can be converted in the body to estrone or estriol, which are less potent estrogenic substances. The natural estrogens are characterized chemically by an aromatic phenolic A ring and 18 carbon atoms in the steroid skeleton (Fig. 6–7).

Estrogens can be secreted not only by the ovary but also by the adrenal and testis. In some animals, such as the stallion, testicular estrogen production can be considerable. The placenta and the fetal liver can convert blood-borne estrogen precursor steroids into estrogens and are therefore also sources for estrogen production (see Chapter 18). Estrogens can also be formed from androgens in peripheral tissues.

ANDROGENS

The androgens are major determinants of the male habitus and characteristically induce hair growth, lowering of voice, muscularity, development of the male genital system, and a general anabolic or nitrogen-retaining metabolic state. In contrast to the failure of estrogens to induce sexual receptivity in the human female, androgens do increase libido in women and in hypogonadal men.

The major androgen secreted by the ovary is androstenedione (Fig. 6–8), a biologically weak compound but one that can be peripherally converted to testosterone, the potent androgenic substance secreted by the testis. The role of androgens in women has not yet been determined, but the biologic effects of either estrogens or androgens depend on the ratio of the two compounds. Mild hirsutism in women and differences in female development or behavior may be the result of variation in the androgen/estrogen secretion ratio as well as end-organ sensitivity.

The adrenal also secretes androgens in both sexes, the major compounds being androstenedione and dehydroepiandrosterone (Fig. 6–8). In the female, one-third to one-half of the androstenedione is normally secreted by the ovary, the remainder by the adrenal.

The chemical structure of androgens can be altered to a limited degree without altering their biologic activity. If the double bond in the A ring (Figs. 6–6 and 6–8) is reduced either naturally in the body or by chemical means, androgenic potency can be retained. Testosterone is converted in peripheral target tissues to 5α-dihydrotestosterone (DHT), an equally potent androgen. DHT is believed to be the true active hormone in the target tissue rather than testosterone, and conditions such as testicular feminization may reflect a relative inability to convert testosterone to DHT and a failure of the tissue to contain specific receptors for this steroid.

In addition, ovarian and adrenal androstenedione can be converted in amounts of 1%–3% to estrone in peripheral tissues (fat) and can account for most if not all, of the estrogen production in the menopausal state. Occasionally, such a source of estrogen can cause postmenopausal bleeding in women or gynecomastia in adolescent boys. Interestingly, androgens can also be converted to estrogens in the hypothalamus and limbic system of the central nervous system, where they could conceivably exert a local effect.

Androgens may thus act in several ways: as an androgen through the actions of testosterone directly or by conversion to DHT, or as an estrogen through peripheral conversion.

PROGESTINS

Progesterone was first isolated from the corpora lutea of pregnant rabbits. By ovarian extirpation and hormonal replacement studies, this steroid was demonstrated to be important for the maintenance of pregnancy. Progesterone has a characteristic inhibitory action upon the spontaneous contractions of smooth

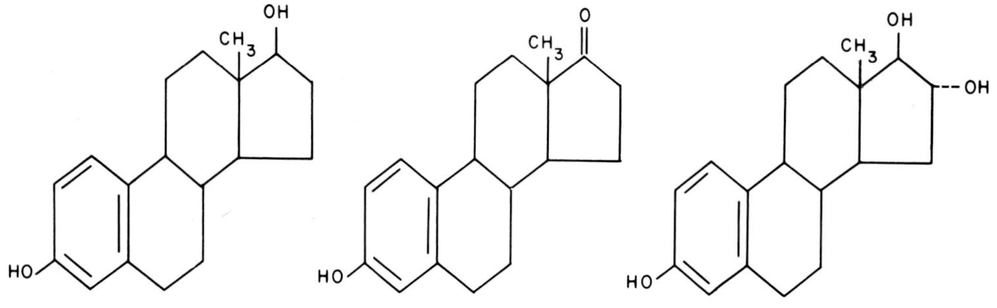

17β - ESTRADIOL ESTRONE ESTRIOL

FIG. 6-7. Structural formulas of three major natural estrogens.

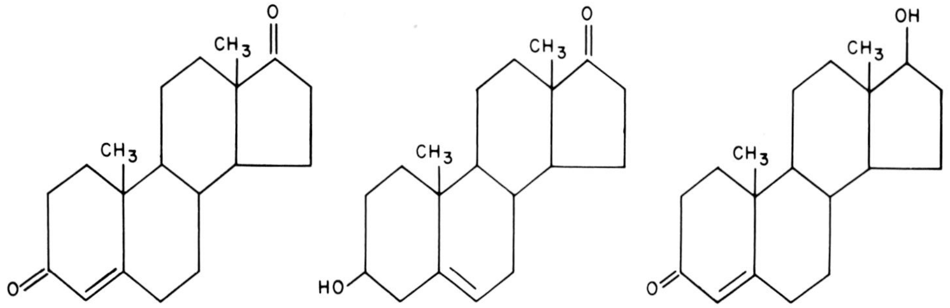

ANDROSTENEDIONE DEHYDROEPIANDROSTERONE (DHEA) TESTOSTERONE

FIG. 6-8. Structural formulas of three natural androgenic compounds.

muscle that is important in the retention of the conceptus within the uterus. Progesterone also has specific effects upon the female genital tract and breasts, causing progestational changes in tissue previously stimulated by estrogen. The so-called secretory endometrium that precedes menstruation is the classic example. The changes in vaginal epithelium and cervical secretions typically evoked by estrogen stimulation are modified when progesterone is added, and the changed appearance of vaginal cells or cervical mucus provides a clinical basis for determining progesterone secretion. Progesterone also has an effect on the central nervous system and hypothalamus that causes an elevation in the basal body temperature of about 0.5° F. When the blood level of progesterone rises after ovulation, owing to its secretion by the newly formed corpus luteum, the accompanying change in basal body temperature can be used as evidence of the event (Fig. 6–2). Daily graphs of the basal temperature are used in infertility work to diagnose ovulation and to suggest optimal timing for coitus.

Progesterone is rapidly and extensively metabolized in the body. One of its metabolites, pregnanediol, is excreted in the urine, where its level can be used as a crude measure of progesterone production.

Progesterone can be synthesized not only by the ovary but by the adrenal and testis as well, although normally in the human these tissues secrete little of the steroid. The placenta in many species, including humans, is a major source of the progesterone produced in pregnancy (see Chapter 18).

The chemical structure of progesterone (Fig. 6–9) is characterized by the basic steroid configuration with a 2-carbon side chain and a double bond in the A ring. Modifications in the molecule may alter and even augment biologic activity.

CYCLE OF OVARIAN STRUCTURE AND FUNCTION

To achieve the fine balance of timing in the development of the entire reproductive tract for mating, conception, and ultimately intrauterine growth of the con-

ceptus, appropriate relative and absolute levels of steroid hormones must be present when needed in relation to the time of ovulation. The ovary is the source of these required steroid hormones, and the secretion of the right hormone or hormones at the right time in relation to ovum discharge is at the heart of ovarian cyclicity. The LH surge in spontaneous ovulation is always preceded by and due to the estrogen rise in blood from ovarian follicle secretion. The ovary achieves its hormone secretion by means of functional subunits and must be considered a heterogeneous tissue with three separate but related steroid-secreting organelles. The three subunits within the normal adult ovary that are responsible for steroid production are the follicle, the corpus luteum, and the stroma.

FOLLICULAR STEROID PRODUCTION

The mature graafian follicle is a fluid-filled cystic structure that contains the ovum, surrounded by a tuft of granulosa cells (cumulus), and is lined by an inner layer of granulosa cells and an outer concentric ring of theca cells (Figs. 4–1 through 4–3). The follicle grows in size in response to FSH and LH; as it does so, rising levels of hormones are released into the follicular fluid and the bloodstream. The major hormone secreted by an ovary containing a mature follicle is 17β-estradiol. The follicular fluid contains this steroid, and the follicle wall contains the enzymes in the granulosa and theca cells that are necessary for estrogen biosynthesis. The follicle also synthesizes small amounts of progesterone, 17-hydroxyprogesterone and androstenedione, and these are also secreted; but estradiol typifies the follicular secretory effort. When the follicles are developing, estrogen is secreted in increasing amounts to reach a peak in both blood and urine just before follicle rupture (Fig. 6–3). During the follicular phase, the effects on the reproductive tract (vaginal cells, endometrium, and cervical mucus) are all estrogen effects. If ovulation does not occur, the anovulatory cycle that ensues is similar to that observed if estrogen alone is given to a castrate animal or person. The endometrial bleeding after estrogen withdrawal is more variable in amount, duration, and interval than that after the estrogen–progesterone withdrawal of an ovulatory cycle.

The capacity of the follicle to produce androstenedione may occasionally be exaggerated, as in polycystic ovarian disease when androstenedione accumulates in the follicular fluid and the ratio of estrogen secretion to androgen secretion is reduced.

CORPUS LUTEUM STEROID PRODUCTION

Following rupture of the follicle and discharge of the ovum, the follicular cells undergo structural and functional changes to form the corpus luteum (Figs. 4–4 and 4–5). The corpus secretes predominantly progesterone, but it also produces estradiol. The ovarian vein blood draining the ovary now contains increased progesterone and estradiol, the progesterone and estrogen levels in peripheral blood rise (Fig. 6–3), and the progesterone metabolite pregnanediol is increased in the urine. The corpus luteum cells contain the enzymes that *in vitro* can cause progesterone and estrogens to be formed from their precursors.

During the luteal phase, all the estrogen effects on the reproductive tract of the preceding follicular period are changed into a progestational type of response. The endometrium becomes secretory, the vaginal cells are altered, and the cervical mucus is affected. The elevated estrogen–progesterone levels now inhibit pituitary secretion, the corpus luteum regresses, the progesterone level declines, the menstrual endometrium is sloughed, and the cycle resumes with another follicular phase. The corpus luteum, effective blood levels of progesterone, and a normal menstrual period are present only in an ovulatory cycle.

STROMAL STEROID PRODUCTION

All the ovarian tissue remaining after the follicles and corpora are removed can be considered the ovarian stroma. The stroma consists of fibroblastic connective tissue cells that have a potential to produce and secrete steroid hormones. Within the stroma there may also occur Leydig-like cells in the hilar region or more highly developed theca cells that also can be responsible for hormone production. The major product of the stroma is androstenedione, but estrogens are also formed by this tissue. The normal role of the stroma is not well defined, but the stroma is, in fact, the only ovarian subunit remaining in the postmenopausal period that could be active in hormone secretion. The stroma may also be active in certain ovarian diseases, but its contribution is difficult to quantitate at this time.

PRODUCTION RATES AND BLOOD LEVELS OF OVARIAN STEROIDS

During the peak of the follicular phase and again in the midluteal phase, estradiol production has been estimated at 200μg–500μg/day, with a peripheral blood level of 100–200 pg/ml.

Progesterone production is 3 mg/day in the follicular phase and 22 mg/day at the peak of the luteal phase. The plasma progesterone concentration is roughly 0.1μg/100 ml in the follicular period and reaches 1μg/100 ml when the corpus luteum is present.

The blood androstenedione level is actually higher in the female than the male, with a concentration of

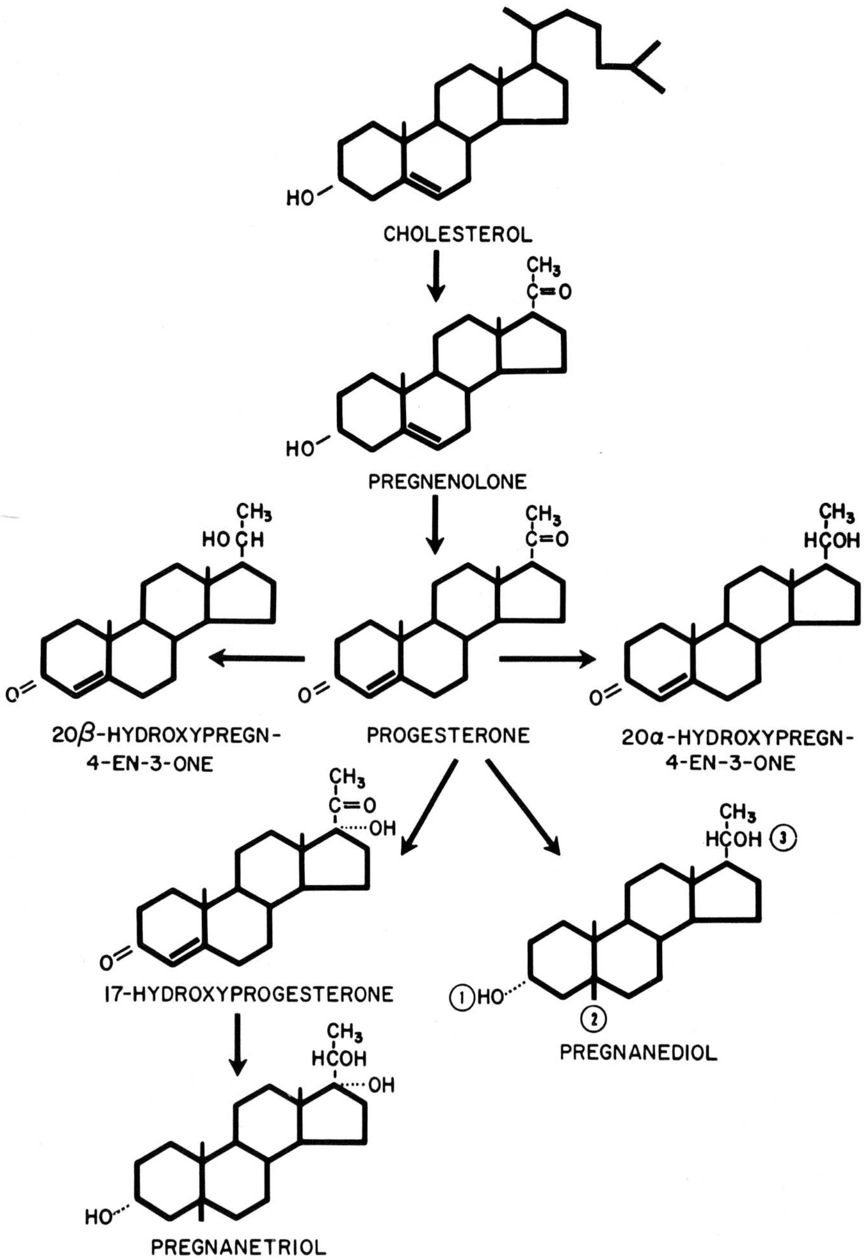

FIG. 6–9. Pathway for progesterone synthesis from cholesterol and its further metabolism. (Ryan KJ: Am J Obstet Gynecol 84:1695, 1962)

$0.1\mu g/100$ ml. The production rate of androstenedione is 3.4 mg/day; that of testosterone, one-tenth the androstenedione level. The adrenal, however, is the major source of these hormones.

BIOSYNTHESIS OF OVARIAN STEROIDS

The ovary's separate functional subunits (follicle, corpus luteum, and stroma) all synthesize hormones in a similar manner. Their differences in endocrine production are more quantitative than qualitative, and steroid biosynthesis can be considered collectively. Any of these three ovarian compartments can synthesize progesterone, androgens, or estrogens in the same way, although the follicle specializes in estrogens, the corpus luteum in progesterone (and estrogen), and the stroma in androgen.

FSH is capable of inducing or activating granulosa cell aromatase activity. There are differences between

the function of the large, dominant follicles in the ovaries and that of the smaller follicles. During follicular development, the granulosa cells produce large amounts of estradiol and small amounts of androstenedione, whereas cells from the large follicles produce progesterone and small amounts of androstenedione. As follicles become atretic, they continue to produce androstenedione but produce much less estradiol. Thecal tissue produces more androstenedione than estradiol when follicles are growing; as they become atretic, however, thecal tissue continues to produce androstenedione but produces much less estradiol. It has been postulated that granulosa cell secretions may accumulate in the follicular fluid, while theca cell secretions may enter the bloodstream so that they may exert their effects at different sites.

The parent compound from which all steroid hormones can be derived is cholesterol, which has a carbon backbone identical to that of the steroid hormones but with a longer side chain. Cleavage of a portion of this side chain in endocrine tissue results in the formation of pregnenolone, the immediate precursor of progesterone (Fig. 6–9).

All steroid hormones, as well as cholesterol, are ultimately derived from the simple 2-carbon compound, acetate. In the stepwise lengthening of intermediate building blocks, 18 2-carbon fragments are joined to form a 30-carbon compound called squalene. In the process of squalene synthesis from smaller molecules, 6 of the carboxyl carbons of acetic acid are lost. Squalene can subsequently be cyclized to form the cyclopentenophenanthrene ring structure of lanosterol, which is then modified to form cholesterol. Subsequent steroid biosynthesis is accomplished by stepwise degradation of the substituents on the steroid ring or insertion of new moieties on the ring structure. The steps for total ovarian steroid biosynthesis are shown in Figure 6–10.

The cholesterol side chain is partially split off to form the C-21 compound pregnenolone, which is readily converted to progesterone by oxidation of the hydroxyl group at position 3 and rearrangement of the double bond (Fig. 6–10). The C-21 compounds, progesterone or pregnenolone, are converted to androgens by complete removal of the side chain to form C-19 series (Fig. 6–11), and finally the C-19 androgens are aromatized to form the estrogens (Fig. 6–12).

Certain cell types of the ovary handle certain steps in the biosynthetic chain more efficiently than others. For example, the granulosa cell of the follicle or the granulosa lutein cell of the corpus luteum is very efficient in the formation of cholesterol from acetate and the conversion of pregnenolone to progesterone. This tends to favor progesterone formation by the corpus luteum.

The follicle is dominated in its synthesis of estrogens by the theca interna cell, which can bypass progesterone in the pathway to androgens and estrogens, but estrogens appear to be most efficiently produced by the combined efforts of both the granulosa and theca cells.

A summary of estrogen biosynthesis using the accompanying figures as a guide includes the following sequential steps: 1) acetate to cholesterol; 2) cholesterol to pregnenolone; 3) pregnenolone to progesterone *or*, bypassing progesterone, to 17-hydroxypregnenolone; 4) 17-hydroxypregnenolone to dehydroepiandrosterone and then to androstenedione and testosterone; 5) progesterone to 17-hydroxyprogesterone and then to androstenedione and testosterone; 6) testosterone to estradiol, androstenedione to estrone (Figs. 6–10 through 6–12).

There is the possibility of synthesizing androgens and estrogens by utilizing steps that bypass progesterone and even 17-hydroxyprogesterone (Fig. 6–11), and this may be a device for regulating the relative amounts of progesterone and estrogens produced by the different subunits of the ovary.

METABOLISM OF OVARIAN STEROIDS

Estradiol is readily converted to estrone by peripheral tissue and thence to estriol in the liver. These are the major metabolites of estradiol (Fig. 6–7). In addition, modifications of the orientation of the substituents at carbons 17 and 16 result in as many as four stereoisomeric forms of estriol. Estriol or its epimers may also be oxidized at position 16 or 17 to form five ketolic steroids. Any of the estrogens may also be hydroxylated at carbon positions 2, 6, 11, or 16 to result in myriad possible metabolites, Suffice it to say that most of these metabolic products do not have biologic activity, and their biologic function, if any, is unknown. At present, they are a measure of estrogen catabolism.

Progesterone is metabolized by reduction of the double bond in ring A and total or partial reduction of the keto groups at positions 3 and 20. These reactions lead to several stereoisomeric forms of pregnanediols and pregnenolones. The compound usually measured in urine as pregnanediol (5β-pregnane-3α, 20α-diol) represents some 20% of the progesterone metabolites, but it suffices as a guide to the extent of progesterone secretion (Fig. 6–9). The 20-keto group of progesterone may be reduced to form a compound (20α-hydroxy-Δ^4-pregnen-3-one) with some progestational activity, but most metabolites are devoid of recognizable hormone function. Progesterone may also be hydroxylated at position 17, and this metabolite ultimately gives rise to pregnanetriols found in the urine during the ovarian cycle and in pregnancy.

Androgen metabolism consists essentially of reduction of the ring A double bond. Although various isomers are possible, the major excretory products are the 17-ketosteroids, androsterone, and etiocholanolone (Fig. 6–13). Since dehydroepiandrosterone and testos-

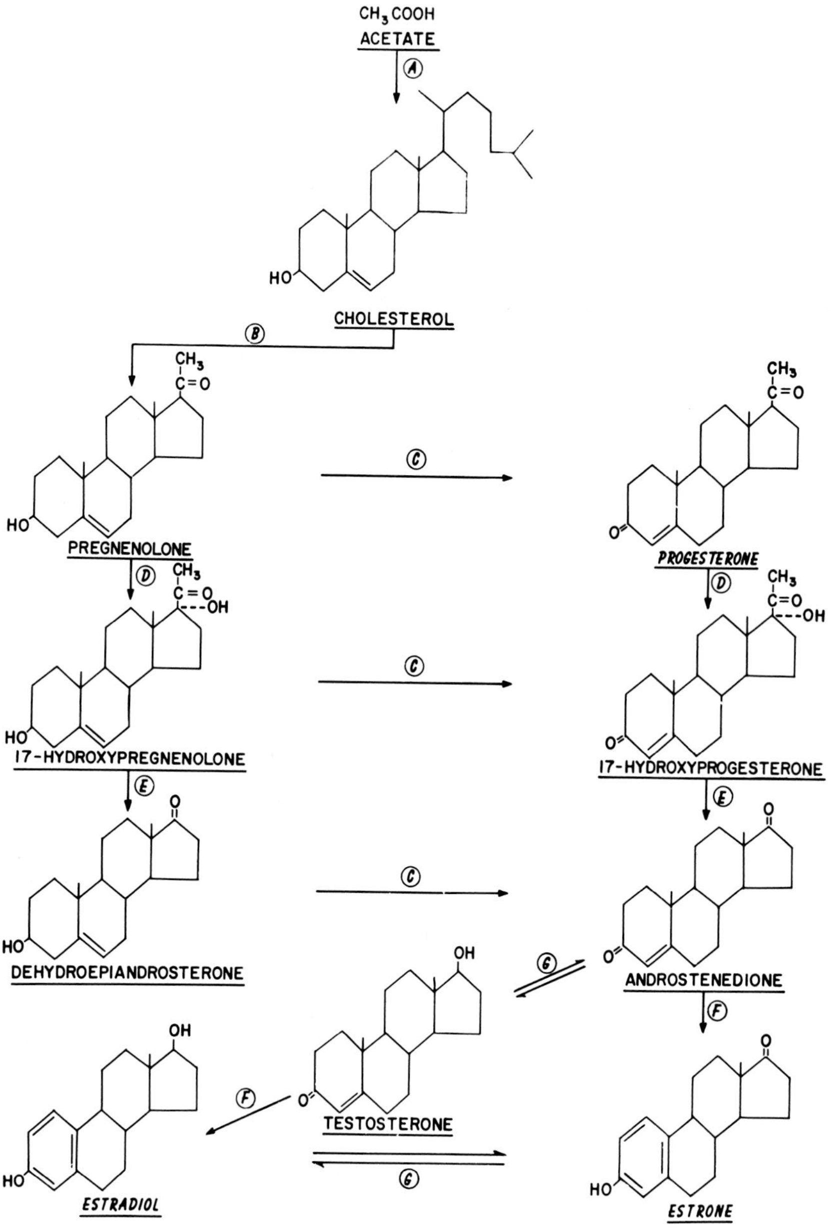

CH₃COOH
ACETATE

Ⓐ

CHOLESTEROL

Ⓑ

CH₃
C=O

PREGNENOLONE

Ⓒ ⟶

CH₃
C=O

PROGESTERONE

Ⓓ

CH₃
C=O---OH

17-HYDROXYPREGNENOLONE

Ⓒ ⟶

CH₃
C=O---OH

17-HYDROXYPROGESTERONE

Ⓔ

DEHYDROEPIANDROSTERONE

Ⓒ ⟶

ANDROSTENEDIONE

Ⓕ

OH

TESTOSTERONE

Ⓖ ⟶ **ANDROSTENEDIONE**

OH

ESTRADIOL

Ⓕ

Ⓖ

ESTRONE

FIG. 6-10. Pathways for biosynthesis of ovarian hormones from acetate and cholesterol. Note alternate routes on *left* and *right sides* of diagram from pregnenolone or progesterone to androgens and estrogens. (Smith OW, Ryan KJ: Am J Obstet Gynecol 84:141, 1962)

terone give rise to androstenedione, the metabolites for all three are similar. The major portion of the 17-keto steroids in urine is derived from adrenal, not ovarian, precursors. As noted earlier, androgens can also be converted to the potent metabolites DHT and estrogens.

Progesterone, estrogen, and androgen metabolites are usually conjugated with either glucuronic or sulfuric acid, rendering them more water-soluble. In addition, the parent hormone or metabolite can be bound in dissociable form to plasma proteins that influence

both blood levels and clearance from the body. The hormonal metabolites may also find their way into the biliary system, from which they are excreted into the intestinal tract for either elimination or reabsorption into the bloodstream. The metabolism of both estrogens and progesterone is extremely rapid, occurring largely in the liver, although other peripheral tissues can participate. The half-life of these hormones after natural secretion or parenteral administration (they do not survive oral administration without extensive destruction) is therefore short. The biologic effects of

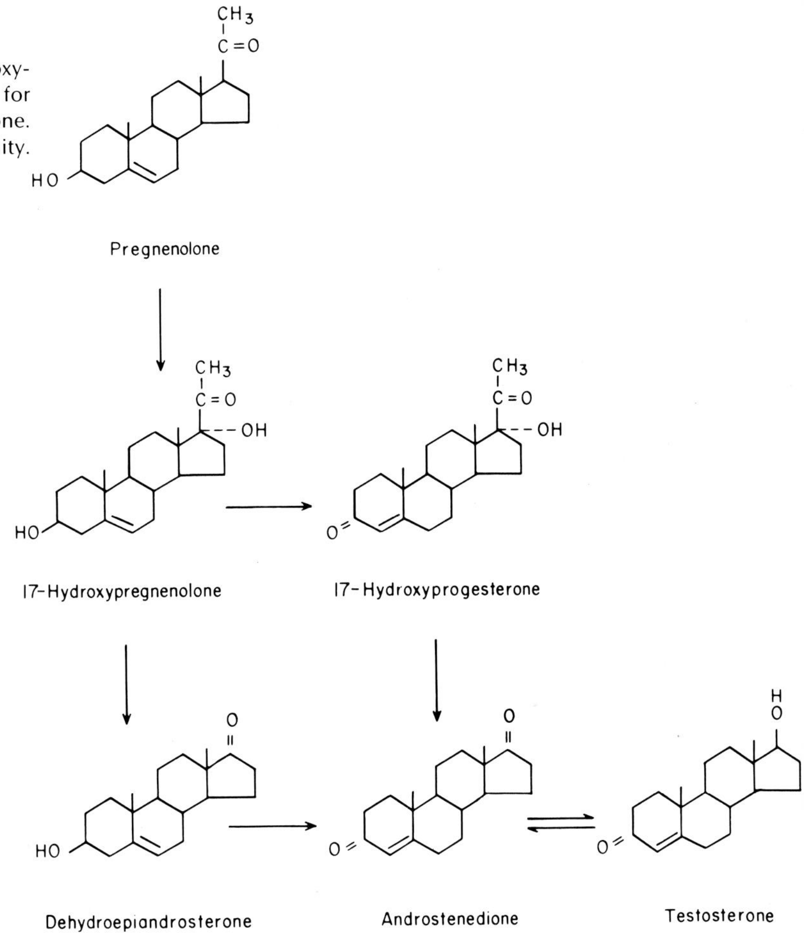

FIG. 6-11. Conversion of pregnenolone to 17-hydroxy-pregnenolone and androgens. Note mechanism for bypassing progesterone or 17-hydroxyprogesterone. (Behrman SJ, Kistner RW [eds]: Progress in Infertility. Boston, Little Brown, 1968)

Pregnenolone

17-Hydroxypregnenolone

17-Hydroxyprogesterone

Dehydroepiandrosterone

Androstenedione

Testosterone

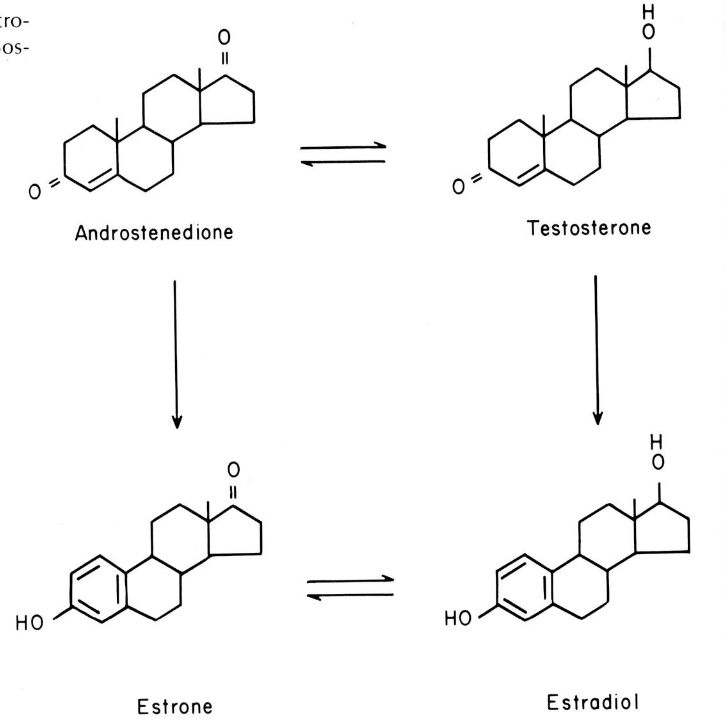

FIG. 6-12. Aromatization: conversion of androgens to estrogens. (Behrman SJ, Kistner RW [eds]: Progress in Infertility. Boston, Little Brown, 1968)

Androstenedione

Testosterone

Estrone

Estradiol

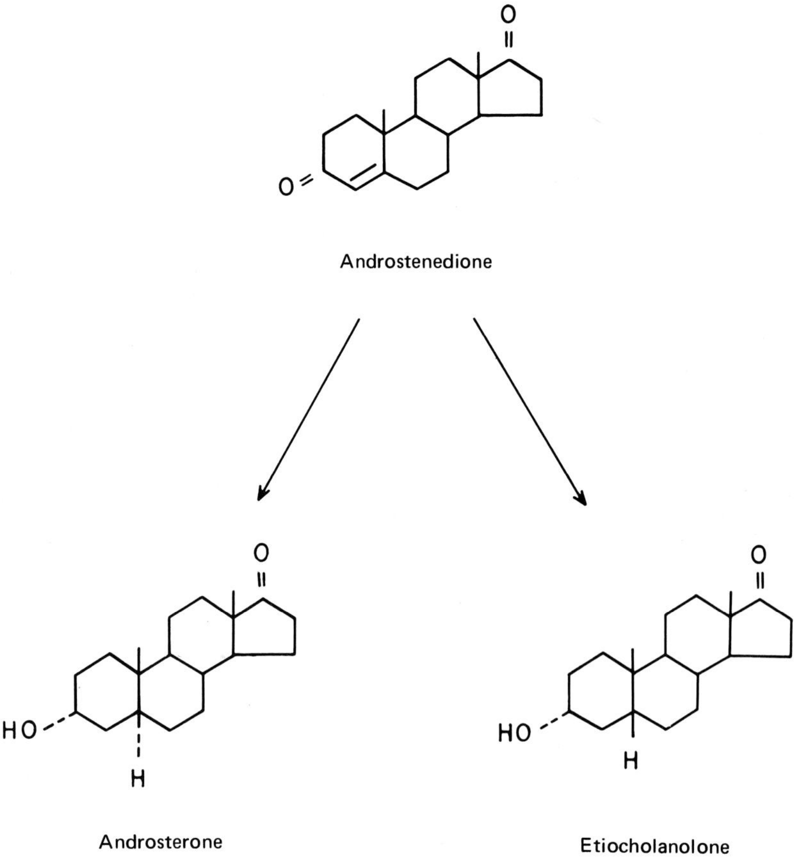

FIG. 6-13. Conversion of androstenedione to 17-ketosteroids. Etiocholanolone is also designated as 3α-hydroxy-5β-androstan-17-one. (Behrman SJ, Kistner RW [eds]: Progress in Infertility. Boston, Little Brown, 1968)

Androstenedione

Androsterone

Etiocholanolone

the natural estrogens and progestins on the genital tissues are also relatively short-lived, since a day or two following withdrawal of hormones, a stimulated endometrium will begin to shed.

SNYTHETIC STEROIDS

Since both natural estrogens and progesterone are largely inactive when given orally and have a short physical and functional half-life in the body, there has been an incentive for the development of orally effective, long-acting substances for clinical use. These are now abundantly available. In the estrogen series, three general types of orally active agents were developed. Diethylstilbestrol, the first of the orally effective agents, has been in use for many years. Subsequently, 17α-ethinylestradiol and its 3-methyl ether, mestranol, were synthesized; they are the most potent oral agents now available. In addition, an extract of pregnant mare's urine, which contains largely potassium estrone sulfate, has been developed as an oral estrogenic preparation. The synthetic estrogenic compounds

have biologic properties quite similar to those of the natural compounds but are less rapidly and extensively degraded.

In the progestin series, a wide array of compounds has been developed. These compounds have varying degrees of similarity or dissimilarity to progesterone's ability to maintain pregnancy, inhabit gonadotropin release and produce a secretory endometrium. The two major types of synthetic progestins are either modifications of the natural progesterone molecule or 19-nor-17α-ethinyl testosterone derivatives (Fig. 6-14).

Since the estrogens and progestins work synergistically, they have been compounded to form the basis of the combination birth control pills (see Chapter 14). Side effects of the use of oral contraceptives are extensions of the general biologic properties of estrogens and progestins. Hence, the tendency to thrombophlebitis, alterations in carbohydrate metabolism, or augmentation of existing breast or genital cancer might be expected and are seen (albeit in a small number of patients) when these agents are used in clinical medicine.

Marder ML, Channing CP, Schwartz NB: Suppression of serum follicle stimulating hormone in intact and acutely ovariectomized rats by porcine follicular fluid. Endocrinology 101:1639, 1977

Martini L: Neuroendocrine control of the pituitary–ovarian axis. In Castelazo–Ayala L et al. (eds): Gynecology and Obstetrics, p 3. Amsterdam, Excerpta Medica, 1977

Naftolin F, Tolis G: Neuroendocrine regulation of the menstrual cycle. Clin Obstet Gynecol 21:17, 1978

Reichlin S: Neuroendocrinology. In Williams RH (ed): Textbook of Endocrinology, p 774. Philadelphia, WB Saunders, 1974

Ross GT, Hillier SG: Experimental aspects of follicular maturation. Eur J Obstet Gynecol Reprod Biol 9:169, 1979

Ross GT, Vande Wiele RL: The ovaries. In Williams RH (ed): Textbook of Endocrinology, p 368. Philadelphia, WB Saunders, 1974

Ryan KJ: Steroid metabolism in the human ovary. In Marcus SL, Marcus CC (eds): Advances in Obstetrics and Gynecology, Vol 1, p 340. Baltimore, Williams & Wilkins, 1967

Ryan KJ: Biosynthesis and metabolism of ovarian steroids. In Behrman SJ, Kistner RW (eds): Progress in Infertility, p 275. Boston, Little Brown, 1968

Ryan KJ, Smith OW: Biogenesis of steroid hormones in the human ovary. Recent Prog Horm Res 21:367, 1965

Savard K, Marsh JM, Rice B: Gonadotropins and ovarian steroidogenesis. Recent Prog Horm Res 21:285, 1965

Sawyer CH: Brain amines and pituitary gonadotrophin secretion. Can J Physiol Pharmacol 57:667, 1979

Thorneycroft IH, Mishell DR, Stone SC et al: The relation of serum 17-hydroxyprogesterone estradiol-17 levels during the human menstrual cycle. Am J Obstet Gynecol 111:947, 1971

Yen SSC: Neuroendocrine regulation of the menstrual cycle. Hosp Pract 15:83, 1979

Yen SSC, Vandenberg G, Rebar R, et al.: Variation of pituitary responsiveness to synthetic LRF during different phases of the menstrual cycle. J Clin Endocrinol Metab 35:931, 1972

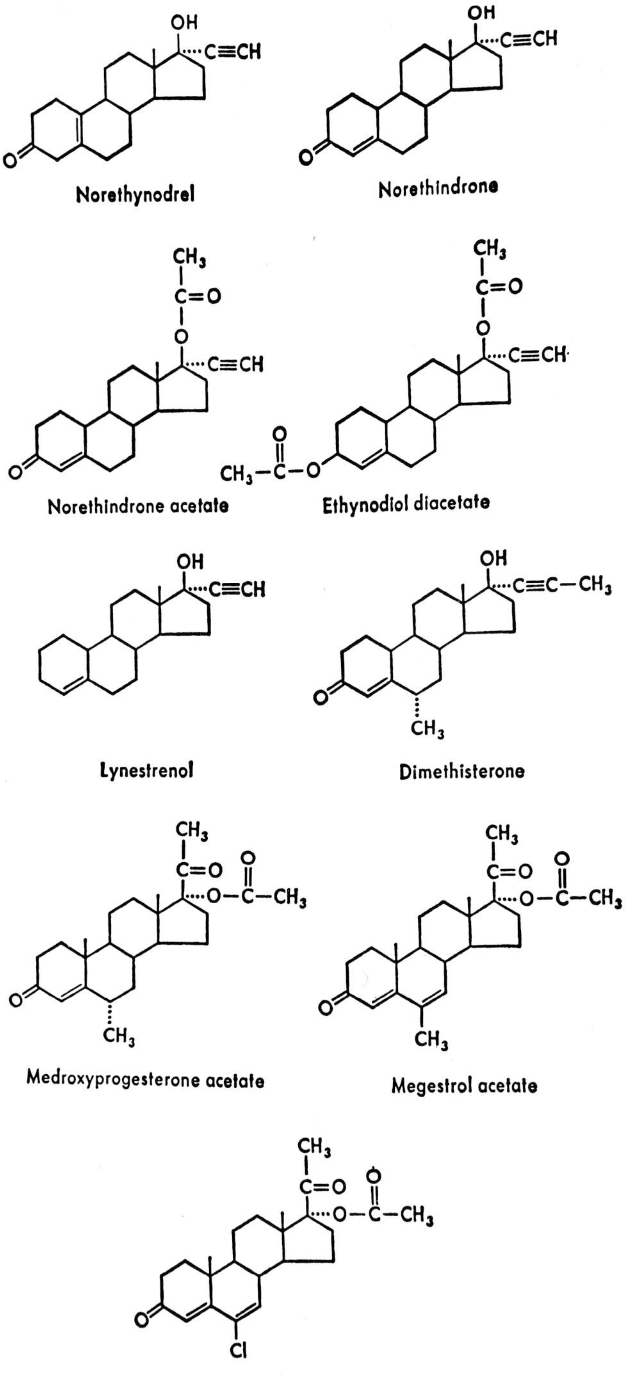

FIG. 6–14. Synthetic progestational agents. *Top six compounds* are structurally related to 19-nortestosterone. *Lower three compounds* are progesterone derivatives. (Oral Contraceptives by Drill VA: Copyright 1966. Used with permission of McGraw–Hill Book Company)

INHIBIN

In addition to steroid hormones, the follicular fluid also contains a protein hormone, inhibin, that is probably produced by the granulosa cells. The effect of inhibin is to suppress FSH production preferentially over LH. It has been presumed that the repression of cohort follicles results from the inhibin produced by the active, dominant follicle. In this way, inhibin may also be concerned in the process of follicular atresia.

REFERENCES AND RECOMMENDED READING

Askel S: Luteinizing hormone-releasing hormone and the human menstrual cycle. Am J Obstet Gynecol 135:96, 1979

Behrman HR: Prostaglandins in hypothalamico-pituitary and ovarian function. Annu Rev Physiol 41:685, 1979

Breitenecker G, Friedrich F, Kemeter P: Further investigations of the maturation and degeneration of human ovarian follicles and their oocytes. Fertil Steril 29:336, 1978

Chari S, Hopkinson CRN, Daume E et al.: Purification of "inhibin" from human ovarian follicular fluid. Acta Endocrinol 90:157, 1979

Dorfman RI, Ungar F: Metabolism of Steroid Hormones. New York, Academic Press, 1965

Fink G: Feedback actions of target hormones on hypothalamus and pituitary with special reference to gonadal steroids. Annu Rev Physiol 41:571, 1979

Gallo RV: Neuroendocrine regulation of pulsatile luteinizing hormone release in the rat. Neuroendocrinology 30:122, 1980

Harris GW, Campbell HJ: The regulation of the secretion of luteinizing hormone and ovulation. In Harris GW. Donovan BT (eds): The Pituitary Gland, Vol 2, p 99. Berkeley, University of California Press, 1966

Henderson KM: Gonadotrophic regulation of ovarian activity. Br Med Bull 35:161, 1979

Heritage AS, Stumpf WE, Sar M, et al.: Brainstem catecholamine neurons are target sites for sex steroid hormones. Science 207:1377, 1980

Hillier JG, van den Boogaard AMJ, Reichert LE Jr, et al.: Intraovarian sex steroid hormone interactions and the regulation of follicular maturation: Aromatization of androgens by human granulosa cells in vitro. J Clin Endocrinol Metab 50:640, 1980

Knobil E, Plant TM, Belchetz PE, et al: Control of the rhesus monkey menstrual cycle: Permissive role of hypothalamic gonadotropin-releasing hormone. Science 207:1371, 1980

Krulich L: Central neurotransmitters and the secretion of prolactin, GH, LH, and TSH. Annu Rev Physiol 41:603, 1979

Lindner HR, Amsterdam A, Salomon Y, et al.: Intraovarian factors in ovulation: Determinants of follicular responses to gonadotrophins. J Reprod Fertil 51:215, 1977

MacDonald PC, Rombaut RP, Siiteri PK: Plasma precursors of estrogen: I. Extent of conversion of plasma androstenedione to estrone in normal males and nonpregnant, normal, castrate and adrenalectomized females. J Clin Endocrinol Metab 27:1103, 1967

McNatty KP, Makris A, DeGrazia C, et al.: The production of progesterone, androgens, and estrogens by granulosa cells, thecal tissue, and stromal tissue from human ovaries in vitro. J Clin Endocrinol Metab 49:687, 1979

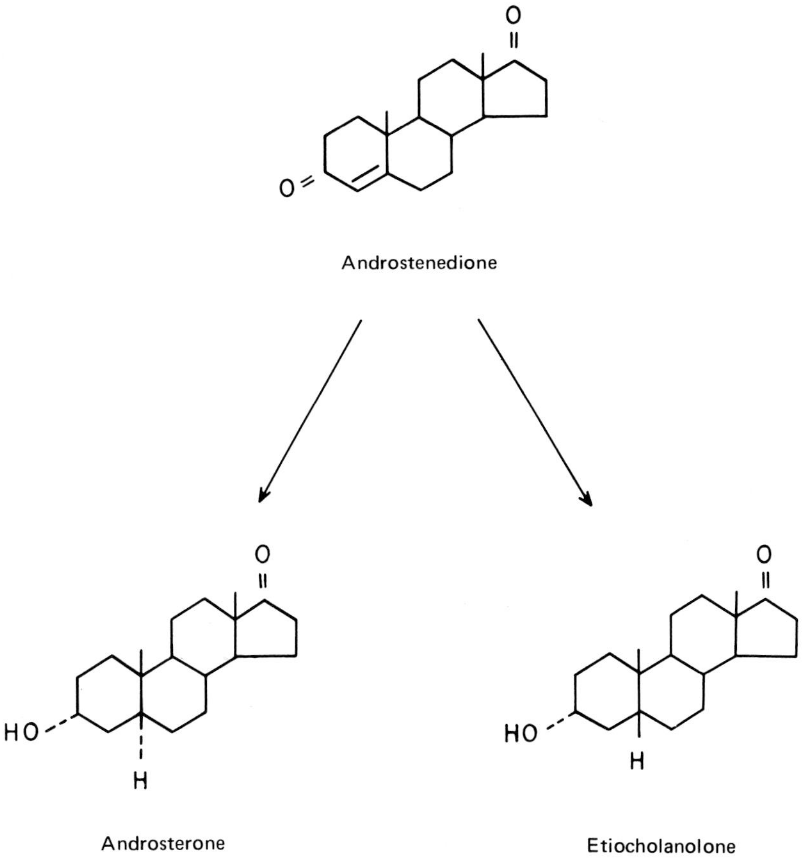

FIG. 6–13. Conversion of androstenedione to 17-ketosteroids. Etiocholanolone is also designated as 3α-hydroxy-5β-androstan-17-one. (Behrman SJ, Kistner RW [eds]: Progress in Infertility. Boston, Little Brown, 1968)

the natural estrogens and progestins on the genital tissues are also relatively short-lived, since a day or two following withdrawal of hormones, a stimulated endometrium will begin to shed.

SNYTHETIC STEROIDS

Since both natural estrogens and progesterone are largely inactive when given orally and have a short physical and functional half-life in the body, there has been an incentive for the development of orally effective, long-acting substances for clinical use. These are now abundantly available. In the estrogen series, three general types of orally active agents were developed. Diethylstilbestrol, the first of the orally effective agents, has been in use for many years. Subsequently, 17α-ethinylestradiol and its 3-methyl ether, mestranol, were synthesized; they are the most potent oral agents now available. In addition, an extract of pregnant mare's urine, which contains largely potassium estrone sulfate, has been developed as an oral estrogenic preparation. The synthetic estrogenic compounds have biologic properties quite similar to those of the natural compounds but are less rapidly and extensively degraded.

In the progestin series, a wide array of compounds has been developed. These compounds have varying degrees of similarity or dissimilarity to progesterone's ability to maintain pregnancy, inhibit gonadotropin release and produce a secretory endometrium. The two major types of synthetic progestins are either modifications of the natural progesterone molecule or 19-nor-17α-ethinyl testosterone derivatives (Fig. 6–14).

Since the estrogens and progestins work synergistically, they have been compounded to form the basis of the combination birth control pills (see Chapter 14). Side effects of the use of oral contraceptives are extensions of the general biologic properties of estrogens and progestins. Hence, the tendency to thrombophlebitis, alterations in carbohydrate metabolism, or augmentation of existing breast or genital cancer might be expected and are seen (albeit in a small number of patients) when these agents are used in clinical medicine.

FIG. 6–11. Conversion of pregnenolone to 17-hydroxy-pregnenolone and androgens. Note mechanism for bypassing progesterone or 17-hydroxyprogesterone. (Behrman SJ, Kistner RW [eds]: Progress in Infertility. Boston, Little Brown, 1968)

Pregnenolone

17-Hydroxypregnenolone

17-Hydroxyprogesterone

Dehydroepiandrosterone

Androstenedione

Testosterone

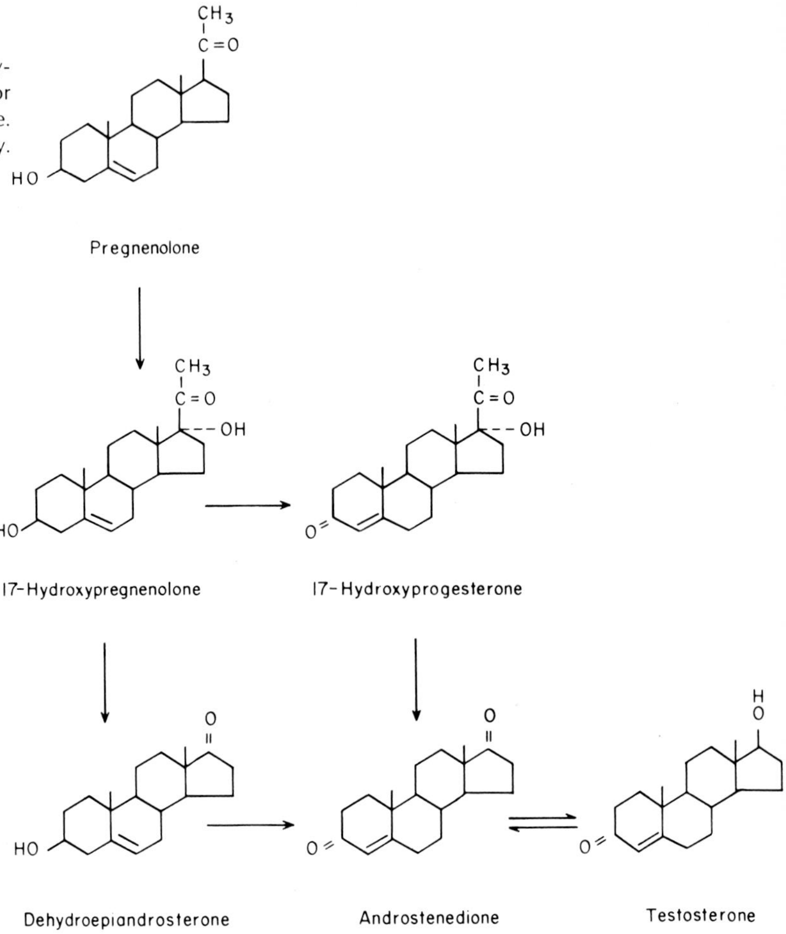

FIG. 6–12. Aromatization: conversion of androgens to estrogens. (Behrman SJ, Kistner RW [eds]: Progress in Infertility. Boston, Little Brown, 1968)

Androstenedione

Testosterone

Estrone

Estradiol

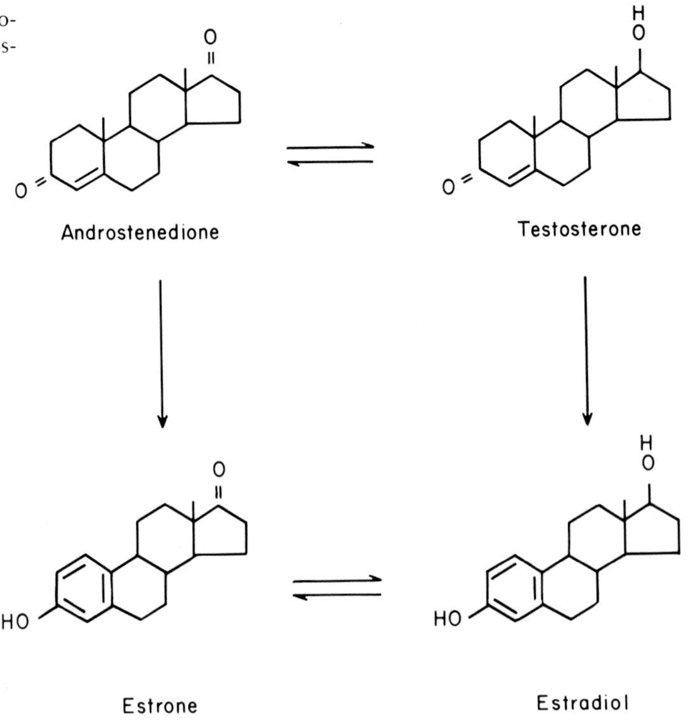

Although usually not considered central in the day-to-day practice of obstetrics and gynecology, an understanding of the adrenal, thyroid, and pineal glands and of the effects of prostaglandins is critical to the diagnosis and treatment of many common gynecologic problems.

THE ADRENAL CORTEX

BIOCHEMISTRY AND PHYSIOLOGY

The adrenal cortex consists of three zones and produces three different functional types of steroids. The three zones can be thought of as three separate glands. The outer zone, the *zona glomerulosa,* produces aldosterone, a mineralocorticoid that affects salt and water metabolism and can be a cause of sodium retention, potassium loss, and hypertension. The middle zone, the *zona fasciculata,* produces hydrocortisone. This glucocorticoid affects carbohydrate, protein, and lipid metabolism. Its overall action is catabolic except in the liver, where it anabolically effects gluconeogenesis. It also suppresses the inflammatory reaction and the body's resistance to infection. The inner zone, the *zona reticularis,* produces sex steroids, predominantly androgens.

An overall view of the biochemistry of adrenocortical hormones is shown in Figure 7–1. Nomenclature and physiologic significance are indicated in Table 7–1. All adrenocortical steroids are synthesized in adrenal cells from either acetate or cholesterol, both of which can be extracted directly from circulating blood. The pathway then proceeds through pregnenolone, the common precursor of all adrenal steroids. Most of the reactions occur in the mitochondria and microsomes. The enzyme systems in the three zones determine the steroid output of the zones and differentiate adrenal steroid production from that of the ovary and testis. The 17-hydroxylating system is present in the zona fasciculata and zona reticularis, as well as in the ovary and testicle, but not in the zona glomerulosa. 11β-Hydroxylase is found almost exclusively in the adrenal and is present in all three zones. 18-Hydroxydehydrogenase is found only in the zona glomerulosa and accounts for the production of aldosterone by that zone. Pathologic lack of any of these enzymes results in overabundance of the precursor steroids and frequently gives rise to elevated serum concentrations that are diagnostic of the specific enzyme deficiency.

Adrenal control mechanisms play an essential role in the normal function of the adrenal cortex. Adrenocorticotropin (ACTH) regulates cortisol output by the zona fasciculata. The control mechanism for aldosterone is also a negative feedback loop but is entirely different and involves renin and angiotensin. Control mechanisms for the androgenic steroids produced by

CHAPTER 7

OTHER ASPECTS OF THE ENDOCRINE PHYSIOLOGY OF REPRODUCTION

John R. Marshall
Jim Ross

the zona reticularis are poorly understood, but they appear to be different from the other two.

In the median eminence of the hypothalamus, corticotropin-releasing factor (CRF) is produced and released into the hypophyseal portal vascular system. CRF is a small polypeptide that acts on the basophilic cells of the anterior pituitary to effect release of ACTH, a 39-amino-acid polypeptide that acts on the adrenal cortex to effect release of cortisol. In the resting state, there is a negative feedback loop that controls cortisol production. When circulating levels of cortisol are low, CRF release increases, resulting in an increase in ACTH release. This brings about increased cortisol production. When high cortisol levels reach the hypothalamic set point, CRF release is normally shut off. This simple servosystem is adequate for routine control but can be overridden by extrahypothalamic neural stimuli. For example, in severe stress CRF secretion is increased even in the presence of high

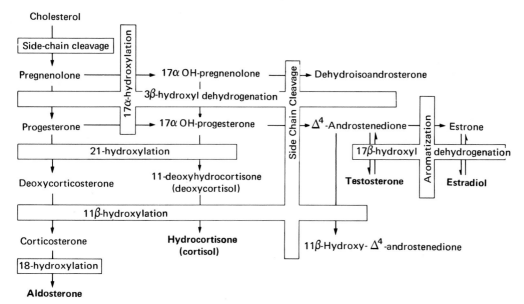

FIG. 7-1. Biochemistry of adrenal corticosteroids. Important biosynthetic steps are shown in *horizontal* and *vertical bars*. (Ezrin C, Godden JO, Volpe R, Wilson R (eds): Systematic Endocrinology, Hagerstown, Harper & Row, 1973)

circulating plasma cortisol levels. This response cannot be blocked by the administration of massive doses of glucocorticoids.

Normally, ACTH and cortisol secretion are episodic. However, overlying these episodic fluctuations is a recognizable diurnal or circadian pattern. Peak values of both ACTH and cortisol occur between 4 and 8 A.M.; lower concentrations are noted in the afternoon and evening. Disturbances in the normal diurnal variation may be important in the genesis of Cushing's syndrome.

The precise mechanism of action of ACTH on the adrenocortical cell is not known; however, it is clear that ACTH is necessary for significant adrenocortical output. ACTH probably acts on the outer cell membrane to activate release of adenylcyclase from the inner cell membrane. Adenylcylase then converts adenosine triphosphate (ATP) to 3'5'-adenosine monophosphate (cyclic AMP), which in turn stimulates protein synthesis by stimulation of enzyme activity. Steroidogenic conversion of acetate to cortisol is the result.

All corticosteroids are relatively insoluble in water and are carried in the blood reversibly bound to an α_2-globulin called transcortin or corticobinding globulin (CBG). Some steroids are also loosely bound to albumin. Approximately 94% of the serum cortisol is bound to CBG, but the free 6% is the active form of the steroid. CBG is always almost entirely saturated so that a rapid release of corticosteroids from the adrenal results in a rapid increase in free cortisol. Pregnancy or estrogen therapy increases the serum concentration of CBG. Therefore, total plasma cortisol is increased in the presence of estrogen, but the concentration of the free or active cortisol is relatively unchanged. Androgens and some disease states decrease serum CBG concentrations.

TESTS OF ADRENAL FUNCTION

Adrenal function is determined most accurately by means of laboratory measurement of corticosteroids. Until recently, this could be accomplished only by measurement of urinary excretory products. The development of the highly sensitive and specific protein-binding test and radioimmunoassay has provided a new dimension for the assessment of endocrine function in general, and one or the other of these two tests is used for each of the specific hormones.

Urine Tests

Measurement of *urinary 17-hydroxycorticosteroids (17-OHCS)* by means of the Porter–Silber chromagen reaction is quite specific for metabolites of cortisol and cortisone. This color reaction depends upon the presence of 17,21-dihydroxy-20-ketone groups.

Measurement of *urinary 17-ketosteroids (17-KS)* is a time-honored method of estimating adrenal androgen production. The test measures predominantly the urinary metabolites of dehydroepiandrosterone, its

TABLE 7-1. NOMENCLATURE AND PHYSIOLOGIC SIGNIFICANCE OF ADRENAL STEROIDS

NORMALLY SECRETED IN AMOUNTS OF PHYSIOLOGIC SIGNIFICANCE
    Hydrocortisone (cortisol, compound F)
    Aldosterone
NORMALLY SECRETED IN AMOUNTS OF LITTLE PHYSIOLOGIC SIGNIFICANCE
    Corticosterone
    Deoxyhydrocortisone (deoxycortisol, compound S)
    Deoxycorticosterone (DOC)
    Progesterone
    Dehydroepiandrosterone (DHEA), free and sulfate
    Δ^4-Androstenedione
    Testosterone
    Estrogens
NORMALLY INACTIVE OR SECRETED IN AMOUNTS OF NO PHYSIOLOGIC SIGNIFICANCE
    Pregnenolone
    17α OH-pregnenolone
    17α OH-progesterone
    18 OH-corticosterone
    11β-OH-Δ^4-androstenedione

(Ezrin C, Godden JO, Volpe R, Wilson R [eds]: Systematic Endocrinology. Hagerstown, Harper & Row, 1973)

sulfate, and androstenedione. Normal values are 8–17 mg/24 hours. The test is of value as a screening procedure, particularly for congenital adrenal hyperplasia and for androgen-producing adrenal tumors, because values are markedly elevated in these conditions. Measurements of 17-ketosteroids cannot always be used to identify tumors that produce predominantly testosterone, however. Testosterone, the most potent androgen, is secreted in only microgram quantities per day. It is not, *per se*, a 17-ketosteroid. Although about 50% of its metabolites are 17-ketosteroids, the microgram quantities of these materials are relatively insignificant when compared to the milligram quantities of the other constituents of the 17-ketosteroid pool. Thus, marked increases in serum testosterone concentrations result in only minimal increases in 17-ketosteroid excretion. Moreover, since both the adrenal gland and the ovary produce steroids that are excreted as 17-ketosteroids, this test alone cannot reliably identify the source of any increased androgen production.

Measurement of *urinary 17-ketogenic steroids* is even less specific and less useful.

Serum Tests

Specific assays are now available for virtually every steroid involved in adrenal steroidogenesis. These tests, which are sensitive and specific, require only small quantities of blood. These tests have largely supplanted tests that use urine for the diagnosis and management of patients with adrenal problems.

Suppression and Stimulation Tests

Adrenal suppression and stimulation tests provide information about the hypothalamic–pituitary–adrenal axis that cannot be obtained by the static measurement of either urinary excretory products or serum concentrations of specific steroids.

The *dexamethasone suppression test* is based on the principles that exogenous glucocorticoid administration suppresses ACTH stimulation and lack of ACTH stimulation results in diminished endogenous adrenal glucocorticoid production. Dexamethasone is used because it is an exogenous corticosteroid that is effective and is not measured by assays used to determine endogenous adrenocortical function. Dexamethasone is administered according to two dose schedules. The low dose, 2 mg/24 hours for 2 days, suppresses the normal but not the hyperplastic adrenal gland (Table 7–2) so that within 2 days the 24-hour 17-OHCS excretion is 3 mg or less. The high dose, 8 mg/24 hours for 2 days, is usually required to suppress the hyperplastic adrenals of Cushing's syndrome. Adrenocortical tumors usually are not suppressed by any dose. Thus, significant suppression of adrenocorticosteroids with dexamethasone practically rules out the presence of an adrenocortical tumor.

Interpretation of the dexamethasone suppression test is greatly facilitated by information about the ovarian and adrenal contributions to the peripheral steroid levels. As shown in Table 7–3, the relative contributions may vary during the menstrual cycle; but, in general, the adrenal contributes 50% of the testosterone, the dihydrotestosterone, and the androstenedione, and 80%–95% of the dehydroepiandrosterone and its sulfate. In addition, the adrenal contributes 100% of the deoxycortisol, whereas the ovary contributes 100% of the estradiol and most of the progesterone and 17-hydroxyprogesterone during the luteal phase.

The *Metopirone (metyrapone) test* assesses pituitary reserve by means of adrenal suppression. Metopirone inhibits adrenal 11β-hydroxylation and thereby decreases the secretion of hydrocortisone. By negative feedback, this, in turn, results in increased pituitary ACTH secretion that, in normal subjects, produces a twofold increase in urinary 17-OHCS and causes elevation of other adrenal steroids (Table 7–2). The usual dose of Metopirone is 500–750 mg every 4 hours for 24 hours. Before it is concluded that a lack of response is secondary to pituitary disease, adrenocortical status should be assessed by the ACTH stimulation test. If the adrenal responds to ACTH but fails to respond to Metopirone, it can be assumed that the Metopirone failure is due to pituitary or hypothalamic malfunction.

The *ACTH stimulation test* measures the adrenal

TABLE 7-2. RESPONSE TO DEXAMETHASONE SUPPRESSION AND METOPIRONE STIMULATION

	Suppression by Dexamethasone		
Type	2 mg	8 mg	Normal or Increased Response to Metopirone
NORMAL ADRENAL	Yes	Yes	Yes
BILATERAL ADRENAL HYPERPLASIA			
Without demonstrable pituitary tumor	No	Yes	Yes
With benign pituitary tumor	No	Variable	No
With malignant pituitary tumor	No	No	No
From ectopic malignant ACTH-producing tumor (e.g., lung cancer)	No	No	No
ADRENAL ADENOMA	No	No	No
ADRENAL CARCINOMA	No	No	No

(Bird CE, Clark AE, Ezrin C, Godden JO, Volpe R, Wilson R [eds]: Systematic Endocrinology. Hagerstown, Harper & Row, 1973)

TABLE 7-3. OVARIAN AND ADRENAL CONTRIBUTIONS TO PERIPHERAL ANDROGENS

	Ovarian Contribution			
Steroid	Early Follicular Phase	Midcycle	Late Luteal Phase	Adrenal Contribution
TESTOSTERONE				
Contribution (ng/ml)	0.1	0.3	0.1	0.2
Percent contribution	33	60	33	40–66
DIHYDROTESTOSTERONE*				
Contribution (ng/ml)		0.1		0.1
Percent contribution		50		50
ANDROSTENEDIONE				
Contribution (ng/ml)	.5	1.5	0.8	0.6
Percent contribution	45	70	60	30–55
DEHYDROEPIANDROSTERONE*				
Contribution (ng/ml)		0.8		3.2
Percent contribution		20		80
DEHYDROEPIANDROSTERONE SULFATE				
Contribution (ng/ml)	80	200	80	2000
Percent contribution	4	10	4	90–96

* Ovarian contribution not influenced by phase of menstrual cycle. (Abraham GE: J Clin Endocrinol Metab 39:340, 1974)

response to administration of exogenous ACTH. Several dose schedules are in use. In a typical schedule, 0.25 mg synthetic ACTH is infused intravenously in 500 ml saline over exactly 8 hours, beginning at 8 A.M. A 24-hour urine sample is collected, beginning 24 hours prior to the onset of the test. This first sample serves as a control. If adrenal function is normal, the 24-hour collection that begins at the onset of the ACTH infusion demonstrates a three- to fivefold increase in 17-OHCS concentrations. Similar increases in serum cortisol occur if it is measured by radioimmunoassay.

DISORDERS OF ADRENAL FUNCTION

Primary disorders that involve aldosterone do not usually affect the reproductive system and are not usually managed by the obstetrician–gynecologist. Disorders that involve glucocorticoids and androgens do affect reproductive function, however.

Hyperfunction

The term *Cushing's syndrome* is generally used to describe any clinical entity associated with excessive and

prolonged action of glucocorticoids. The syndrome, described by Harvey Cushing in 1932, was thought to be due to "pituitary basophilism." It is now recognized that the syndrome of adrenocortical excess can result from any one of a number of conditions that cause an increased secretion of cortisol.

About 75% of patients with Cushing's syndrome have bilateral adrenocortical hyperplasia, probably secondary to an abnormality of the control mechanisms of the hypothalamic–pituitary–adrenal axis. The first change appears to be disruption of the diurnal rhythm, with loss of the usual afternoon decline in serum cortisol concentrations. Eventually, plasma cortisol levels remain elevated throughout the entire day. At this stage of the disease the adrenal is still able to respond to stress with an increased outpouring of cortisol and is still suppressible. With further progression, this responsiveness is lost.

Ectopic ACTH can also be a cause of Cushing's syndrome. Certain nonendocrine tumors that produce polypeptides immunologically and biologically similar to ACTH can cause bilateral adrenal hyperplasia. Oat cell carcinoma of the lungs is the most common nonendocrine cause.

Benign adrenocortical adenomas are responsible for Cushing's syndrome in 10%–15% of patients. Malignant tumors account for 5%–10%. The adenomas are bilateral in approximately 10% of cases and are occasionally associated with adenomatous hyperplasia of the adrenal. Both benign and malignant adrenal tumors secrete cortisol independently of pituitary–hypothalamic control, and accordingly there is no diurnal variability. Moreover, the prolonged hypercorticism results in diminished ACTH secretion by the pituitary and a functional atrophy of the remaining, normal adrenal tissue. Sometimes the adenomas produce excessive androgens, prompting precocious puberty or virilization. Excessive androgen production occurs more frequently with adrenal tumors than with Cushing's syndrome that is secondary to pituitary abnormalities.

The signs and symptoms of Cushing's syndrome result from an excess of glucocorticoids (Table 7–4). The classic features are centripetal obesity, moon facies, purple striae, abnormal glucose tolerance, and hypertension. Oligomenorrhea, amenorrhea, infertility, and hirsutism are also common.

Diagnosis is a two-step process: 1) verification of excess corticosteroid production and 2) determination of the cause. The simplest initial screening test is the measurement of serum cortisol at 8 A.M. and 4 P.M. Normal levels and normal diurnal variation rule out Cushing's syndrome. If results are equivocal, an overnight dexamethasone suppression test is performed: 2 mg dexamethasone is administered at 11 P.M., and a blood specimen for serum cortisol measurement is drawn at 8 A.M. Cortisol levels less than $4\mu g/100$ ml are normal; levels greater than $20\mu g/100$ ml signify Cush-

TABLE 7–4. BIOLOGIC EFFECTS OF EXCESS CORTISOL (CUSHING'S SYNDROME)

PROTEIN METABOLISM
  Reddish striae
  Loss of matrix and demineralization
  Poor wound healing
  Muscle wasting and weakness
  Capillary fragility and bruising
  Thinning of skin
LIPID METABOLISM
  Centripetal fat distribution
  Moon facies
CARBOHYDRATE METABOLISM
  Abnormal glucose tolerance curve
  Overt diabetes mellitus
HEMATOPOIETIC EFFECTS
  Eosinophilia, lymphopenia
  Polymorphonuclear leukocytosis
  Erythrocytosis
ELECTROLYTE BALANCE
  Sodium retention, potassium loss
  Hypertension
  Hypervolemia
GENERAL EFFECTS
  Hypercalcinuria and renal calculi
  Gastric ulceration
  Psychosis
  Impaired immunologic tolerance

(Ezrin C, Godden JO, Volpe R, Wilson R [eds]: Systematic Endocrinology. Hagerstown, Harper & Row, 1973)

ing's syndrome; intermediate values are indeterminant.

Further evaluation and treatment are best carried out in conjunction with an endocrinologist. Bilateral adrenal hyperplasia secondary to pituitary hyperstimulation can be treated by transsphenoidal resection of the pituitary microadenoma, if present, or pituitary irradiation. Bromergocriptine may prove to be useful. Severe disease may require bilateral total adrenalectomy with subsequent lifelong steroid replacement. Adrenal adenomas require surgical removal, which is curative. Adrenal carcinoma is an extremely malignant tumor with a very low 5-year survival rate. Treatment involves excision, if possible, and subsequent treatment with adrenolytic drugs.

Hypofunction

Adrenocortical insufficiency can be either primary or secondary. The primary form (Addison's disease) involves insufficiency of the hormones secreted by all zones of the cortex. Thus, there is a deficiency of adrenal mineralocorticoids, glucocorticoids, and androgens. It is an extremely rare disease and can be due to idiopathic atrophy, bilateral tuberculosis (the major cause in Addison's original description), amyloidosis,

TABLE 7-5. SIGNS AND SYMPTOMS OF PRIMARY ADRENO-CORTICAL INSUFFICIENCY

Sign or Symptom	Occurrence (%)
WEAKNESS	99
PIGMENTATION	98
WEIGHT LOSS	97
HYPOTENSION	90
ANOREXIA	90
VOMITING	84
NAUSEA	81
ABDOMINAL PAIN	34
CONSTIPATION	28
DIARRHEA	21
SYNCOPE	16
VITILIGO	9

(By permission of JE Bethune and Scope® monograph on The Adrenal Cortex, The Upjohn Company, Kalamazoo, Michigan, 1974)

mycotic infections, or possibly an autoimmune phenomenon. Secondary adrenocortical insufficiency occurs as a result of hypothalamic or pituitary malfunction due to disease, trauma, or surgery. Secondary iatrogenic adrenocortical insufficiency can occur following administration of exogenous corticosteroids.

Adrenocortical insufficiency is usually suspected when weakness and tiredness occur in a patient who is hypotensive and has darkly pigmented skin (Table 7-5). The pigmentation is secondary to increased melanocyte-stimulating hormone. Chronic insufficiency results in salt wasting with decreased serum sodium and increased serum potassium values.

An acute, life-threatening episode of adrenal insufficiency (Addisonian crisis) consists of weakness, syncope, hypotension, rapidly progressing pyrexia, vascular collapse, shock, and death. It can occur secondary to the stress of infection or trauma or abrupt cessation of adrenocortical therapy in a patient who has no adrenocortical reserve. Severe preeclampsia sometimes predisposes, resulting in postpartum vasomotor collapse (see Chap. 25). Salt and cortisol are urgently needed. Treatment of an Addisonian crisis requires immediate administration of 100 mg hydrocortisone intravenously, followed by 100 mg intravenously in 1 liter normal saline, which is continued over an 8-hour period. Several liters of saline may be required because of the contracted body fluid compartments.

Less urgent forms of primary adrenocortical insufficiency are diagnosed on the basis of inability of the adrenal to respond to an ACTH stimulation test. The diagnosis of secondary adrenocortical insufficiency is usually suggested by the finding of other, more visible, pituitary tropic hormone deficiencies. Such patients are unable to excrete a water load, but promptly do so following a small dose of cortisol. Additional tests involve insulin stimulation of ACTH production and the

Metopirone stimulation test. Failure to respond to these tests confirms the diagnosis of pituitary insufficiency with secondary adrenal insufficiency.

Treatment of chronic adrenal insufficiency requires the replacement of both glucocorticoids and mineralocorticoids if the adrenal insufficiency is primary, but replacement of cortisol only if it is secondary. Cortisol requirements vary between 15 and 30 mg/day. Because aldosterone is ineffective orally, fluorocortisone, about 0.1 mg/day, is used as mineralocorticoid replacement. Exact dose must be determined on the basis of body weight, blood pressure, and edema.

Congenital Enzyme Block (Congenital Adrenal Hyperplasia)

The essential problem with congenital enzyme block is a congenital deficiency, but not absence, of one or more enzymes required for normal steroidogenesis. Most often, the defect results in deficient cortisol production, which in turn causes increased adrenal stimulation via increased ACTH. In mild cases, enough cortisol is produced to maintain life. However, because of the enzyme block, this increased adrenal stimulation results in excessive levels of the steroids in the metabolic pathways immediately preceding the enzyme defect. In most cases, these steroids are converted to adrenal androgens, which are then peripherally converted to testosterone. Virilization results. In more severe cases, the defects are incompatible with life.

Congenital adrenal hyperplasia is most often seen in infancy or childhood. However, mild forms of the disorder sometimes do not appear until adolescence, when they may be manifest as oligomenorrhea, hirsutism, or both. The sites of severe enzyme deficiencies are shown in Figure 7-1.

Newborns with defective side-chain cleavage (desmolase) produce no steroids and do not survive. At autopsy the adrenals are seen to be large and fat-laden.

Newborns with a 3-hydroxydehydrogenase deficiency do not survive. They are unable to convert pregnenolone to progesterone, or 17-hydroxypregnenolone to 17-hydroxyprogesterone, or dehydroepiandrosterone to androstenedione. Mild virilization may be present. Serum concentrations of pregnenolone, 17-hydroxypregnenolone, and dehydroepiandrosterone are elevated.

Patients with 17-hydroxylase deficiency survive and have primary amenorrhea. The defect, which is present in both the adrenal and the ovary, precludes formation of adequate amounts of both androgens and estrogens. Hydrocortisone production is diminished; deoxycorticosterone and corticosterone production, increased. The weak glucocorticoid effects of these two steroids substitute for the hydrocortisone, but their mineralocorticoid effects result in sodium retention, potassium loss, and hypertension.

The most common defect is the 21-hydroxylase deficiency, an autosomal recessive defect that occurs more often in females; it is found in about 1 of every 5000 liveborn infants. This block inhibits both glucocorticoid and mineralocorticoid production. Serum levels of progesterone, 17-hydroxyprogesterone, and 17-hydroxypregnenolone are elevated, and the first two give rise to increased urinary excretion of pregnanediol and pregnanetriol. Because they are converted to the androgens dehydroepiandrosterone and androstenedione, they result in virilization and increased excretion of urinary 17-KS. The degree of deficiency may vary. Mild deficiency results in androgenic effects manifested at puberty as mild hirsutism, amenorrhea, and poor breast development. An intermediate defect is most common. The infant is born with an enlarged clitoris and, if untreated, precociously develops a male habitus, pubic hair, and deep voice; at puberty she has no menarche. The severe defect, present in about one-third of affected patients, results in severe virilization and mineralocorticoid insufficiency with sodium wasting, hypotension, and dehydration. If untreated, newborns with this severe form of the disorder die.

Patients with an 11β-hydroxylase deficiency are unable to produce hydrocortisone, corticosterone, or aldosterone. Consequently, deoxycorticosterone is produced in excess; virilization, salt retention, hypertension, and hypokalemia ensue.

Diagnosis of all the congenital adrenocortical hyperplasias must be based on the measurement of increased amounts of specific steroids in either serum or urine. The specific steroids measured in serum are dehydroepiandosterone sulfate and 17-hydroxyprogesterone; in urine, 17-ketosteroids and pregnanetriol.

Therapy consists of prompt replacement of the necessary steroids and subsequent maintenance throughout life. Drugs commonly used in treatment of adrenocortical disorders are listed in Table 7–6. With adequate replacement therapy, patients can look forward to normal life and fertility. However, the effects of the increased androgens on the external genitalia may require reparative surgery.

THE THYROID

Since the thyroid influences fertility, pregnancy, and general well-being, an understanding of thyroid function is essential for the obstetrician–gynecologist.

The thyroid gland was the first endocrine gland to evolve in the vertebrate. In lower animals, thyroid hormones have profound effect; in the frog and toad, they cause the metamorphosis from the tadpole to the adult. In humans, they are largely responsible for control of the general level of metabolism. They stimulate calorigenesis, potentiate epinephrine, and are essential for normal central nervous system development. Calcitonin, also secreted by the thyroid, plays a role in

TABLE 7–6. DRUGS COMMONLY USED IN DIAGNOSIS AND TREATMENT OF ADRENOCORTICAL DISORDERS

Drug	Form Supplied
Hydrocortisone	20-mg tablet
Cortisone	30-mg tablet
Hydrocortisone sodium succinate	100 mg/ml
Prednisone	5-mg tablet
Prednisolone	5-mg tablet
Dexamethasone	0.5- or 0.75-mg tablet
Florine (9α-fluorohydrocortisone)	0.1-mg tablet
Deoxycorticosterone	5 mg/ml
ACTH (synthetic B1-24)	0.25 mg
Metopirone	250-mg capsule

(Ezrin C, Godden JO, Volpe R, Wilson R [eds]: Systematic Endocrinology. Hagerstown, Harper & Row, 1973)

calcium and phosphorus metabolism but is not discussed here since it has little bearing on obstetrics and gynecology.

The thyroid develops from an invagination of the pharynx at the base of the tongue and is well differentiated by the 15th week of fetal life.

PHYSIOLOGY AND BIOCHEMISTRY

The thyroid, like the adrenal, ovary, and testis, functions under the feedback control of the hypothalamus and pituitary. In the median eminence, thyrotropin-releasing hormone (TRH), a tripeptide, is synthesized and released into the portal vessels. TRH effects release of thyrotropin or thyroid-stimulating hormone (TSH) from the pituitary, which in turn controls the iodine uptake and the release of the two major thyroid hormones, thyroxine (T_4) and triiodothyronine (T_3) from the thyroid gland. Serum concentrations of T_4 control TRH release by the hypothalamus. Increased serum T_4 levels result in decreased TRH and TSH, whereas decreased serum T_4 levels result in stimulation of the hypothalamus and resultant stimulation of the thyroid. This internal control mechanism tends to maintain a homeostatic level of thyroid function.

TSH is thought to act on the thyroid gland by attaching itself to the cell membrane and stimulating the formation of adenylcyclase, which catalyzes the formation of cyclic AMP, the intracellular "second messenger."

Thyroid biosynthesis can be considered in four steps: 1) iodide transport and trapping, 2) iodination of tyrosine, 3) coupling and storage, and 4) release and secretion of thyroid hormones. Inorganic iodides absorbed from the small intestine are carried in the circulation and trapped by the thyroid gland against a 20:1 gradient. The inorganic iodide is converted in the thyroid to organic iodine, which then combines with tyrosine to form monoiodotyrosine (MIT) and diiodo-

tyrosine (DIT). One molecule of MIT plus one molecule of DIT form T_3, or two molecules of DIT form T_4. T_3 and T_4 combine with thyroglobulin for storage as colloid in the follicles. Release of T_3 and T_4 from the colloid is under the control of TSH. T_3 and T_4 are split from the thyroglobulin, which is recycled within the thyroid cell, and the T_3 and T_4 are released into the thyroid venous circulation.

In the blood, T_3 and T_4 are transported bound to three carrier proteins: thyroxine-binding globulin (TBG), which carries 60% of the bound hormones; a thyroxine-binding prealbumin, which carries 30% of the bound hormones; and an albumin, which carries 10%. More than 99% of the total blood T_3 and T_4 is bound to these three proteins. However, the less than 1% that is unbound or free is the only metabolically active thyroid hormone.

The serum concentrations of these thyroid-binding proteins are increased at least twofold in pregnancy and with estrogen therapy. This profoundly affects the results of thyroid function tests.

T_3 is three to four times more potent than T_4 on a weight basis. Approximately half of the T_4 is converted to T_3. The half-life of T_3 is 1 day or less, whereas the half-life of T_4 is approximately 6–8 days. Approximately 30% of the total body pool of T_4 is in the liver. Both T_3 and T_4 are deactivated by deiodinization and are excreted in the feces.

THYROID FUNCTION TESTS

All tests fall into five main categories: 1) measurement of peripheral effect, 2) measurement of serum-binding protein concentration, 3) measurement of circulating thyroid hormone, 4) measurement of serum thyrotro-

pin, and 5) measurement of thyroidal iodine uptake. Values of the useful thyroid function tests are indicated in Table 7–7. Exact values may vary according to the particular laboratory performing the test.

Tests of peripheral effect include basal metabolic rate, serum cholesterol, and Achilles reflex tests. They are relatively insensitive and inaccurate and have little place in modern clinical medicine.

Serum unsaturated binding protein (TBG) concentration is measured by the resin uptake of T_3 labeled with iodine 131. In this *in vitro* test, T_3 is added to serum that contains radioactive iodine and the unbound radioactive iodine is then picked up by a resin and counted. The test results can be reported as a percentage of normal.

Tests of circulating thyroid hormones can measure either T_3 or T_4 and either total (bound plus free) or free hormones. Tests can be either positively associated with or independent of binding protein concentrations. Because many situations in clinical obstetrics and gynecology are concerned with changes in estrogen concentrations and, consequently, with changes in TBG concentrations, it is necessary to remember the effects of binding protein concentrations on specific tests. The best test of thyroid hormone concentration would be one independent of binding protein concentration.

Tests positively associated with TBG concentrations are the measurement of protein-bound iodine (PBI), the assessment of T_3 by radioimmunoassay, and the assessment of T_4 by the Murphy–Pattee technique or displacement analysis. Increased TBG concentrations result in increased values in each of these tests. The PBI test measures all protein-bound iodine, including organic and inorganic iodine from previously administered radiopaque dyes. Formerly a standby of thyroid-

TABLE 7–7. VALUES OF USEFUL THYROID FUNCTION TESTS

Test	Normal	Hypothyroidism	Hyperthyroidism	Pregnancy
MEASUREMENT OF UNSATURATED SERUM-BINDING PROTEIN CONCENTRATION				
T_3 resin uptake as percent of uptake T_3RU)	25–35	Decreased	Increased	Decreased (<25)
T_3 resin upake as percent of unity (T_3RU%)	0.8–1.2	Decreased	Increased	Decreased
MEASUREMENT OF CIRCULATING THYROID HORMONES				
Positively associated with binding protein concentration				
PBI (mg/100 ml)	4–8	Decreased	Increased	Increased (7–12)
T_4 Murphy–Pattee (T_4) (mg/100 ml)	4–11	Decreased	Increased	Increased
T_3 RIA (T_3) (mg/100 ml)	50–150	Decreased	Increased	Increased
Independent of binding protein concentration				
Free T_4		Decreased	Increased	
Free T_4 index	1.0–3.5	Decreased	Increased	Normal
Effective T_4 (ET_4) (mg/100 ml)	4–11	Decreased	Increased	Normal
MEASUREMENT OF THYROTROPIN				
TSH by radioimmunoassay (μU/ml)	0–10	Increased	Decreased	Normal
MEASUREMENT OF IODINE UPTAKE				
RAI uptake (%)	10–35	Decreased	Increased	Contraindicated

ology, the PBI test has been replaced by more specific tests. The measurement of T_3 by radioimmunoassay uses specific antisera to measure T_3. It is accurate but sometimes difficult to perform and not as readily available as are other tests. The measurement of T_4 by the Murphy–Pattee technique involves the progressive displacement of T_4 from protein-binding sites that measure only T_4. It is not influenced by other iodoproteins; it is relatively easy to perform and readily available.

Tests independent of TBG concentrations measure free T_4, free T_4 index, and effective T_4. Measurement of free T_4 is difficult and is not commonly done. The test measures only the less than 1% of the T_4 that is unbound in the serum. The information it gives is not of sufficient clinical value to compensate for the difficulty of performing the test. The free T_4 index (FTI) is calculated by multiplying the T_4 obtained by the Murphy–Pattee procedure by the T_3 calculated by resin uptake. This test uses the TBG value obtained from resin uptake of T_3 labeled with iodine 131 to compensate for changes in T_4 secondary to changes in TBG. The effective T_4 (ET_4) test utilizes the same Murphy–Pattee measurement of T_4 and the same resin uptake value to compensate for binding. However, the T_3 resin uptake is reported as a percentage of normal, and it is this percent figure that is used in the calculation. Normal values for this test are the same as those found with the usual measurement of T_4 and are not influenced by the effects of estrogen or pregnancy on TBG serum concentrations. This is the best test for following thyroid function during pregnancy or when the patient is undergoing estrogen therapy.

Measurement of TSH utilizes the patient as a bioassay of circulating effective thyroid hormones. TSH is measured by radioimmunoassay, but no radioactive substances are administered to the patient. The test is particularly effective in identifying hypothyroidism because low levels of circulating thyroid hormones result in compensatory elevations of serum TSH. Normal TSH concentrations are $0\mu U$–$10\mu U/ml$. Values greater than $20\mu U/ml$ are usually seen with hypothyroidism. The normal range is unaffected by pregnancy.

Measurement of iodine uptake determines the ability of the thyroid gland to bind administered radioactive iodine. This ability is decreased in hypothyroidism and increased in hyperthyroidism. Results can be recorded as either percentage uptake or as a scan of the thyroid gland that reveals differential uptake. These tests are effective and useful measurements of thyroid function. However, they are all absolutely contraindicated in pregnancy because of placental passage of the radioactive iodine and uptake by the fetal thyroid.

Clinical evaluation of thyroid function for the obstetrician–gynecologist involves a careful history, physical examination, and appropriate laboratory tests. Laboratory evaluation should include measurement of T_4 by the Murphy–Pattee method or of T_3 by radioimmunoassay. If TBG is thought to be elevated, or if increased T_4 or T_3 values suggest the possibility of TBG elevation, a T_3 resin uptake test (indicative of TBG concentrations) should be performed. From the T_4 and the T_3 resin uptake, the FTI or ET_4 can be calculated. If hypothyroidism is a possible diagnosis, a measurement of TSH is indicated. Measurement of radioactive iodine uptake may be helpful in the nonpregnant patient. In a few patients a therapeutic trial of thyroid hormone may be necessary.

DISORDERS OF THYROID FUNCTION

Patients with nontoxic goiter, benign or malignant thyroid neoplasms, or thyroiditis are not usually cared for by the obstetrician–gynecologist. However, patients with hyperthyroidism and hypothyroidism are occasionally seen by the gynecologist because these disorders can result in reproductive abnormalities.

Hyperthyroidism

Hyperthyroidism is found in approximately 0.1% of the general population. It appears to be slightly less common in pregnancy (0.04%–0.075%). The manifestations of hyperthyroidism are always due to excess circulating levels T_3 and T_4.

There are three basic types of hyperthyroidism. Iatrogenic hyperthyroidism is due to excess administration of thyroid hormones, either because of presumed need or for weight reduction.

The more common endogenous form of hyperthyroidism, Graves' disease or diffuse exophthalmic goiter, usually occurs in women under 50 years of age. The hypersecretion of T_3 and T_4 comes from a diffusely hyperplastic gland. The disease is associated with frequent spontaneous remissions and exacerbations and is commonly accompanied by exophthalmos and pretibial myxedema. Excess circulating levels of long-acting thyroid stimulator (LATS) are more commonly noted in patients with exophthalmos and pretibial myxedema.

LATS is a 7S γ-globulin frequently present in the serum of patients with Graves' disease. It appears to arise from lymphocytes as an antibody to one or more components of the thyroid cells. Its exact mode of action is unknown. Although it has been cited as a possible cause of the hyperthyroidism itself as well as of the exophthalmos and neonatal hyperthyroidism frequently associated with Graves' disease, there is a distinct lack of unanimity in these opinions.

The second form of endogenous hyperthyrodism, Plummer's disease or toxic nodular goiter, usually occurs in women over 50 years of age. Thus, it is seldom seen in pregnancy. The hypersecretion of T_3 and T_4 arises from one or more hyperplastic and autonomous areas of the nodular goiter. Signs and symptoms are associated with excess quantities of thyroid hor-

TABLE 7–8. SYMPTOMS OF HYPERTHYROIDISM

INCREASED CATECHOLAMINE EFFECTS
  Nervousness
  Palpitations
  Tachycardia
  Tremor
HYPERMETABOLISM
  Increased perspiration
  Heat intolerance
  Fatigue
  Increased appetite
  Weight loss
INCREASED GASTROINTESTINAL ACTIVITY
  Hyperdefecation/diarrhea
MYOPATHY
  Weakness or paralysis
  Dyspnea
MISCELLANEOUS
  Personality changes or psychosis
  Decreased central nervous system efficiency
  Menstrual irregularities
  Symptoms of congestive heart failure
  Hair loss
  Eyelid retraction, "staring"

(Odell WD, et al.: Calif Med 113:35, 1970)

mones, but exophthalmos is rarely present. This disease is usually of insidious onset and slowly progressive.

The clinical signs and symptoms of hyperthyroidism (Table 7–8) are nonspecific and independent of the cause of the hyperthyroidism. Tachycardia, weight loss, fatigue, or heat intolerance is each seen in more than 80% of patients. Muscle weakness is fairly common but sometimes difficult to demonstrate. It is usually present in the proximal muscles of the trunk and lower limbs. During pregnancy, the weight loss may be obscured by the physiologic weight gain of pregnancy.

An internist or endocrinologist should usually be consulted regarding the treatment of hyperthyroidism. In nonpregnant patients, therapy can consist of administration of radioactive iodine or thyroid-blocking agents, or thyroidectomy. All three have advantages and disadvantages, but radioactive iodine treatment must not be used during pregnancy. During pregnancy, hyperthyroidisim should be treated with propylthiouracil, 100 mg three times a day, to gain control; this is followed by a diminished dose (usually 100 mg propylthiouracil daily) to maintain slight hyperthyroidism. Although thyroidectomy can be considered in the second trimester or postpartum, it is frequently unnecessary because approximately 50% of patients who continue propylthiouracil therapy for 1 year postpartum experience permanent remission.

Both propylthiouracil and methimazole are effective because they block T_4 synthesis; thus, their clinical ef-

fects are not seen until stored hormone is used. Clinical response can be followed by measurement of T_4. Although the most common complication of propylthiouracil and methimazole treatment is a rash, granulocytosis occurs in 0.6% of patients and must be watched for with regular blood counts. Both drugs cross the placenta when given in high doses and can cause fetal goiter. Lower doses do not appear to affect fetal thyroid function. Although some authors recommend concomitant administration of thyroid when these blocking agents are given during pregnancy, there is little evidence to support this practice.

Thyroid storm is a rare, life-threatening, acute worsening of all the symptoms of severe hyperthyroidism. Fever, tachycardia, and severe dehydration are common. Death occurs in about 25% of victims. Storm occurs most often in patients with poorly controlled or undiagnosed disease who are subjected to a stress such as labor, cesarean section, or infection. Treatment consists of 1 g intravenous sodium iodine to block T_4 secretion, large doses of propylthiouracil, 2–4 mg propranolol to control the tachycardia, intravenous cortisol, fluid replacement, and hypothermia.

Hypothyroidism

Hypothyroidism is about one-tenth as common as hyperthyroidism and most frequently occurs in women between 30 and 60 years of age. Most cases occur after the age of childbearing. Medical treatment, thyroidectomy, and administration of radioactive iodine are the most usual causes. End-stage thyroiditis can also result in hypothyroidism.

Clinical signs and symptoms of mild disease consist of paresthesias, cold intolerance, constipation, cool dry skin, coarse hair, irritability, and inability to concentrate. Severe disease is manifest as myxedema, periorbital edema, enlarged tongue, and a hoarse voice. Severe disease is rare during pregnancy. Because so many of the symptoms of mild disease are difficult to distinguish from those of anxiety or depression, the best identifier of hypothyroidism is not any symptom or combination of symptoms but laboratory evaluation of circulating hormone concentrations.

The best test for hypothyroidism is the measurement of serum TSH concentration (Fig. 7–2). Values are unaffected by pregnancy and are usually less than $3\mu U/ml$. Values of greater than $10\mu U/ml$ suggest hypothyroidism. Other thyroid function tests are generally less sensitive indicators of hypothyroidism but can be used both for diagnosis and for monitoring therapy.

Treatment consists of replacement of thyroid hormones. Appropriate therapy returns serum TSH concentrations to normal. Available agents are desiccated thyroid, levothyroxine, liothyronine, and a fixed combination of the last two. Desiccated thyroid USP is the time-honored pharmacologic form of thyroid hormone.

It is inexpensive, but because potency is assayed in terms of protein content rather than T_3 or T_4, effectiveness can vary considerably from lot to lot. Levothyroxine (Synthroid) is synthetic T_4. It is inexpensive and consistent, but administration in doses sufficient to treat hypothyroidism adequately results in serum T_4 levels above the normal range. Thus, measurement of serum T_4 cannot be used to follow patients taking levothyroxine. Liothyronone (Cytomel) is synthetic T_3. It acts quickly but for a short time only and thus is not as useful for long-term therapy as levothyroxine. Patients who are euthyroid on T_3 therapy have subnormal serum T_4 concentrations. Synthetic T_4 and T_3 combined in a 4:1 ratio is marketed as Euthroid. It is expensive and has no advantage over T_4 alone except that administration does not result in distortion of serum T_4 concentrations. Hypothyroid patients who receive thyroid replacement during pregnancy may need increased doses, but requirements may decrease toward term.

THYROID AND REPRODUCTION

The effects of hyperthyroidism on reproductive functions are variable. There is little solid evidence that fertility is affected. Although menstrual irregularities are fairly common and no one type predominates, there is disagreement in the literature about associated fetal wastage and mortality. Mild to moderate hyperthyroidism apparently has no significant effect on pregnancy, but severe disease may be associated with increased fetal wastage.

Hypothyroidism also manifests varied effects on reproduction. The menstrual irregularities, polymenorrhea, oligomenorrhea, or menorrhagia associated with mild disease becomes amenorrhea in 70% of patients with myxedema. Although some reports suggest that women with hypothyroidism have a higher incidence of spontaneous abortion and others attempt to show that hypothyroidism is associated with congenital defects and undifferentiated developmental retardation, several reports detail patients with untreated myxedema who carried apparently normal babies to term.

Pregnancy itself has particular and recognizable effects on thyroid function. Maternal TBG levels rise by 4 weeks of gestation and remain elevated for 1–2 months postpartum. There is a physiologic enlargement of the maternal thyroid associated with pregnancy and an increase in the basal metabolic rate due to the presence of the fetus and not to any metabolic dysfunction. Serum TBG values, total serum T_3 and T_4 values, iodine uptake, and renal clearance of iodide are all increased. Serum concentrations of TSH, free T_3 and free T_4 remain unchanged. Assessments of thyroid function during pregnancy must be based on measured levels of TSH and on calculated FTI or ET_4.

The placenta selectively passes materials important

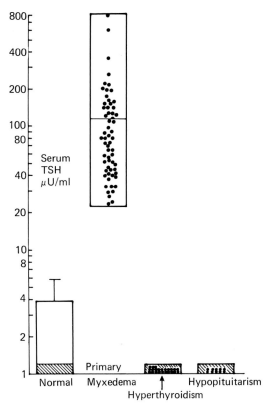

FIG. 7-2. Usefulness of serum thyrotropin (TSH) as diagnostic indicator of hypothyroidism. (Hershman JM, Pittman JA: Ann Intern Med 74:481, 1971)

in thyroid physiology. Iodine and antithyroid blocking agents readily cross the placenta. T_3 and T_4 cross only very slowly; TSH does not cross at all. LATS crosses the placenta and can affect the newborn. Human chorionic gonadotropin (hCG) secreted by the trophoblast has a slight TSH-like effect that can result in clinical hyperthyroidism in some patients with trophoblastic neoplasia and very high serum concentrations of hCG.

Maternal thyroid secretions appear to be required for normal maintenance of early pregnancy. After 12 weeks, the fetal thyroid traps iodine and begins to secrete T_3 and T_4. T_4 appears necessary for the development of the fetal central nervous system but not for fetal growth. The T_4 supplied by the fetal thyroid appears adequate for this purpose.

THE PINEAL

The pineal is a small organ located superior to the entrance of the cerebral aqueduct at the posterior aspect of the third ventricle. It was once thought to be the seat of the soul and to control the flow of conscious

thought. More recently, it has been recognized as an intricate and sensitive biologic clock that converts nervous impulses generated by environmental light into endocrine function.

The pineal originates in the brain of the developing embryo, but it loses its direct nerve connections to the brain soon after birth. Subsequent nerve supply comes from the superior cervical ganglion via the sympathetic nerves that follow the blood vessels through the cranium. Anatomically, this is similar to the arrangement found in the adrenal medulla, where sympathetic fibers end in contact with medullary cells.

The pineal gland is the only organ capable of synthesizing melatonin. The human pineal contains high concentrations of the precursor, serotonin, which is necessary for the production of melatonin, and also the methoxylating enzyme, o-methyltransferase.

In rats and other lower animals, the pineal is important in the control of the secretion of gonadotropic hormones. In these animals, melatonin acts to inhibit hypothalamic release of gonadotropin-releasing factor. Light impulses from the optic nerves stimulate the sympathetic fibers of the superior cervical ganglion. These impulses are then transmitted through the sympathetic chain to the pineal gland, where they inhibit melatonin production. Decreased melatonin frees the hypothalamus from the inhibitory effects of melatonin and results in increased basal secretion of gonadotropin-releasing factor and gonadotropins. This results in subsequent stimulation of the ovaries and increased estrogen production. The net result is the persistent estrus seen in rats under constant illumination. However, when pineal extracts are implanted directly into the median eminence or reticular formation in rats, they inhibit release of luteinizing hormones.

The role of the pineal in humans is even more poorly understood. Boys with tumors that originate from pineal supporting tissues or teratomas near the gland demonstrate precocious puberty. True pineal tumors result in delayed puberty. Girls blind since birth, regardless of the cause, have delayed onset of menses when compared with controls with normal vision. Although these data suggest that the pineal may play some role in the onset of puberty in humans, no abnormalities of adult reproductive function have yet been ascribed to the pineal.

PROSTAGLANDINS

In 1933 Goldblatt and von Euler independently isolated a potent vasopressor and smooth-muscle–stimulating lipid from human seminal plasma and sheep vesicular gland, which von Euler named prostaglandin. In 1959 Bergstrom identified the basic chemical structure as a 20-carbon derivative of prostanoic acid, which contains a five-member ring. The four basic families, prostaglandins A (PGA), B (PGB), E (PGE), and F (PGF), are further subdivided according to chemical structure. The different prostaglandins have strikingly different physiologic and pharmacologic effects. PGE and PGF appear to be most important to obstetrics and gynecology.

Prostaglandins (PGs) can arise from virtually all tissues of the body, but they are present in unusually high concentrations in the male and female reproductive tracts. They appear to be synthesized in the microsomes from arachidonic acid, an unsaturated fatty acid. Release from tissues is enhanced by nervous, humoral, chemical, or physical stimulation. The mere handling of tissue can cause release. The extremely efficient clearance by the lungs, 90% in a single passage, accounts for the short half-life, measured in seconds to minutes, and is the reason that changes in serum or plasma concentrations in antecubital vein blood cannot be measured following release of prostaglandins into the uterine venous circulation.

PGs affect the gastrointestinal and respiratory tracts, the cardiovascular and central nervous systems, the kidneys, and connective tissue. PGs have major effects on the female reproductive system. Particular effects are determined by the tissue, the specific prostaglandin, and the dose. PGs can cause smooth muscle contraction or relaxation, tachycardia, hypotension, nausea, vomiting, diarrhea, bronchodilation, or bronchoconstriction. In the central nervous system, they appear to potentiate polysynaptic transmission. In connective tissue, they are potent inflammatory agents and pyrogens. Aspirin and indomethacin are potent inhibitors of prostaglandin synthesis.

In the female reproductive tract, PGs have multiple effects. Most studies have been done in animals, however, and the role of PGs in human reproduction remains unclear.

PGs may act as central nervous system transmitters, mediating the effects of hypothalamic releasing hormones on the pituitary either by altering vascular permeability or by modifying intracellular concentrations of AMP (CAMP). $PGF_{2\alpha}$ increases pituitary content of luteinizing hormone and both indomethacin and aspirin can block ovulation by blocking the release of luteinizing hormone from the pituitary, presumably by blockage of prostaglandin synthesis.

In the ovary, PGs probably are important in steroidogenesis, particularly of progesterone, and may play a role in luteolysis. PGs incubated with mammalian ovarian tissue slices cause increased production of progesterone. Prostaglandin inhibitors block not only the effects of PGE_1 and PGE_2 but also the effect of luteinizing hormone on cyclic AMP and progesterone production. It has been suggested that luteinizing hormone may act at the cell membrane by stimulating prostaglandin synthesis and subsequent activation of adenylcyclase and CAMP, resulting in steroid produc-

tion. Although PGs are luteolytic in some animals by direct action on the corpus luteum or by changes in ovarian blood flow, no such effects are seen in the human when prostaglandins are administered in the luteal phase. In such circumstances, the induced uterine bleeding appears to be due to a direct effect of the prostaglandins on the endometrium, possibly by means of the endometrial vasculature.

In the fallopian tube, PGE, the prostaglandin present in particulary high concentrations in seminal fluid, causes contraction of the proximal portion and relaxation of the distal portion. These effects may be important in tubal ovum transport and retention, as well as in sperm transport. However, PGF causes contraction of the entire fallopian tube.

PGs have major effects on the uterine musculature and have had their greatest therapeutic usefulness in this area. $PGF_{2\alpha}$, which increases the resting uterine tone and the amplitude of myometrial contractions, reaches its highest concentrations in menstrual endometrium and may be associated with menstrual uterine contractions. It has been suggested that patients with dysmenorrhea produce a higher proportion of PGF compounds, which are responsible for the increased uterine contractility, spasms, and pain.

The role of PGs in the contractions of pregnancy and labor is considered in Chapter 29.

Evidence links PGs to the uterine contractions that follow intraamniotic infusion of hypertonic saline. It is postulated that the saline disrupts the prostaglandin-containing decidual lysosomes. Since $PGF_{2\alpha}$ makes lysosomal membranes unstable, this may be a self-perpetuating process. The delay associated with administration of indomethacin in patients undergoing abortion with hypertonic saline and the increase in

$PGF_{2\alpha}$ concentrations in amniotic fluid associated with the onset of labor support a role for prostaglandins in saline-induced abortion (Fig. 7–3).

It has also been postulated that PGs play a part in eclampsia. The hypothesis proposed by Speroff is indicated in Figure 7–4. According to this hypothesis, PGA is responsible for maintaining a reduced resistance to flow through the uteroplacental vascular bed. Decreased prostaglandin levels would be associated with hypertension. The recent finding of significantly lower PGA levels in patient with essential hypertension and renal artery stenosis supports this hypothesis. If this is indeed true, PGA might be of therapeutic benefit in eclampsia.

PGs are readily absorbed from the vagina after they have been introduced for induction of labor or abortion, or from semen following coitus. Prostaglandin-induced uterine contractions may be the source of the lower abdominal crampy postcoital discomfort noted by some women.

At the present time, the major clinical usefulness of PGs in obstetrics and gynecology is the induction of abortion in midtrimester pregnancy. In approximately 80% of patients, intraamniotic administration of PGF induces uterine contractions that result in cervical dilatation and subsequent delivery of the fetus. Compared with amnioinfusion of hypertonic saline, prostaglandin amnioinfusion is associated with a shorter interval from instillation to delivery, no reported occurrence of maternal disseminated intravascular coagulation, and no other recognized life-threatening maternal side effects. The disadvantages of prostaglandin amnioinfusion are an increased frequency of nausea and vomiting, the occasional delivery of a live fetus, and the rare development of a uterovaginal fistula. PGs

FIG. 7–3. Endocrine basis of mechanism that initiates parturition in sheep. Note that actions of estrogen and progesterone are mediated mainly by $PGE_{2\alpha}$ and that action of oxytocin depends on increase in sensitivity of myometrium. (Liggins GC: Clin Obstet Gynecol 16:152, 1973)

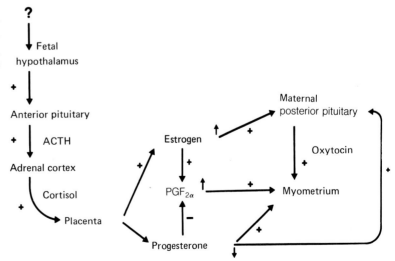

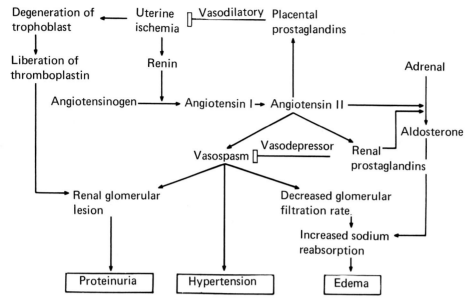

FIG. 7-4. Mechanism of eclampsia may originate in relative ischemia of uteroplacental unit, resulting in degeneration of trophoblastic tissue and release of thromboplastin, followed first by compensatory response and then by aberration of pregnant renin–prostaglandin system. (Speroff L: Am J Cardiol 32:587, 1973)

are also under investigation as a medication to induce uterine contractions at term.

The clinical use of PGs for induced abortion is considered in Chapter 14.

REFERENCES AND RECOMMENDED READING

ADRENAL

Abraham GE: Ovarian and adrenal contributions to peripheral androgens during the menstrual cycle. J Clin Endocrinol Metab 39:340, 1974

Hardling BW: Synthesis of adrenal cortical steroids and mechanism of ACTH effects. In DeGroot LJ et al. (eds): Endocrinology, p 1131. New York, Grune & Stratton, 1979

Krieger DT: Plasma ACTH and steroids, In DeGroot LJ et al. (eds): Endocrinology, p 1139. New York, Grune & Stratton, 1979

Nelson DH: Synopsis of diagnosis and treatment diseases of the adrenal cortex. In DeGroot LJ et al. (eds): Endocrinology, p 1235. New York, Grune & Stratton, 1979

West CD, Meikle AW: Laboratory tests for the diagnosis of Cushing's syndrome and adrenal insufficiency and factors affecting those tests. In DeGroot LJ et al. (eds): Endocrinology, p 1157 New York, Grune & Stratton, 1979

THYROID

DeGroot LJ: Synopsis of diagnosis and treatment of thyroid conditions. In DeGroot LJ et al. (eds): Endocrinology, p 545. New York, Grune & Stratton, 1979

DeGroot LJ: Thyroid physiology. In DeGroot LJ et al. (eds): Endocrinology, p 373. New York, Grune & Stratton, 1979

Prout TE: Thyroid disease in pregnancy. Am J Obstet Gynecol 122:669, 1975

PINEAL

Wartman RJ: The pineal organ. In DeGroot LJ et al. (eds): Endocrinology, p 95. New York, Grune & Stratton, 1979

PROSTAGLANDINS

Arratas WS, Tsai AY: Prostaglandins in reproduction. J Reprod Med 20:84, 1978

Challis JRG, Thorburn GD: Prenatal endocrine function and the initiation of parturition. Br Med Bull 31:57, 1975

Liggins GC: Fetal influences on myometrial contractility. Am J Obstet Gynecol 16:148, 1973

Ramwell PW, Leovey EMK: Prostaglandins and humoral regulation. In DeGroot LJ et al. (eds): Endocrinology, p 1711. New York, Grune & Stratton, 1979

Speroff L: Physiologic and pharmacologic roles for prostaglandins in obstetrics. Clin Obstet Gynecol 16:109, 1973

Speroff L: Toxemia in pregnancy. Am J Cardiol 32:582, 1973

Wiquist N, Widholm O, Nillius SJ, et al: Dysmenorrhea and prostaglandins. Acta Obstet Gynecol Scand [Suppl] 87:1979

Puberty in the human female may be defined as the transiton period between immaturity and attainment of reproductive capacity. This transition period involves complex and dynamic physical, psychologic, and behavioral changes. The most obvious change is the development of secondary sexual characteristics, associated with progressive maturity of the central nervous system and the hypothalamus. Although the menarche is the external manifestation that appears to signal the culmination of pubertal development, puberty is not complete until the normal ovulatory cycle with full luteal development has been attained. An understanding of pubertal development requires a review of the maturational process from conception through the neonatal and childhood stages.

NORMAL ENDOCRINE FINDINGS

THE FETUS

The hypothalamic–pituitary–gonadal axis is functional at birth. Sensitive radioimmunoassays for protein and steroid hormones allow documentation of active hormone production by fetal endocrine glands, which contribute to endocrine regulation even during fetal development.

The hypothalamic hormones for release of luteinizing hormone (LH) and thryoid-stimulating hormone (TSH) have been isolated from fetal brains of 4.5 weeks' gestational age. Cellular differentiation within the gland is completed by 11 weeks and is accompanied by the sequential appearance of pituitary hormones in the fetal circulation. Growth hormone (hGH), prolactin, and TSH have been isolated from fetal pituitary tissue at 9 weeks. Follicle-stimulating hormone (FSH) and LH are detectable at 8 weeks and begin to increase between 12 and 14 weeks' gestational age. Weakly fluorescent cells, suggestive of monoamine content, are found in the pituitary gland as early as 11 weeks, and monoamine-containing structures are demonstrable in the human fetal hypothalamohypophyseal tract at 15 weeks. The 16- to 19-week fetal pituitary responds to hypothalamic releasing hormones, as demonstrated by Tamuar and colleagues with pituitary organ cultures and synthetic hypothalamic LH-releasing hormone (LH–RH). The hypophyseal portal system is fully functional at approximately 20 weeks, and gonadotropin levels rise rapidly thereafter until circulating levels comparable to those in the menopause are seen at 7–8 months' gestationa-

ADOLESCENCE, MENSTRUATION, AND THE CLIMACTERIC

**Georgeanna Seegar Jones
Anne Colston Wentz**

lage. Secretion then begins to decline, but circulating levels remain higher during fetal life than in the neonatal period.

INFANCY AND CHILDHOOD

The high FSH, and to a lesser degree LH, serum values found at birth decline during the first 2 years of life to a nadir at 2 years of age. Higher FSH and LH serum concentrations are seen in female children than in male. Although higher testosterone and androstenedione levels are observed in male neonates, these steroids would tend to suppress LH over FSH. The high serum FSH levels from birth to 2 years in females, in contrast to those in males, may indicate that the follicles in the infant ovary are less efficient in producing "inhibin" than the Sertoli cells of the infant

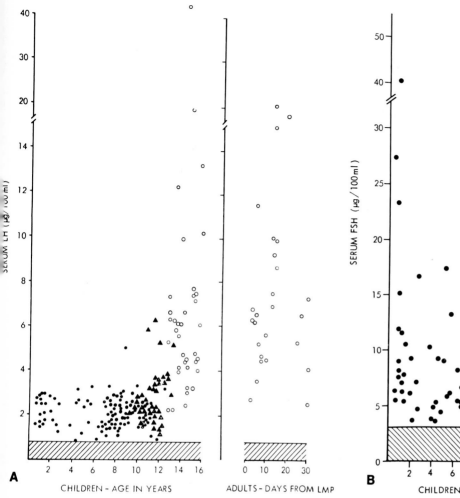

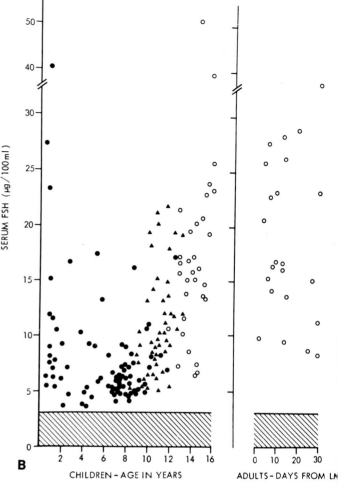

FIG. 8-1. Serum LH (*A*) and FSH (*B*) concentrations in girls at different ages and in adult women. Shaded area shows limit of sensitivity of assay. *Triangles,* Premenarcheal girls. *Circles,* Postmenarcheal girls. *LMP,* Last menstrual period. (Winter JSD, Faiman C: Pediatr Res 7:948, 1973)

testis. Inhibin is the protein hormone that preferentially inhibits pituitary FSH over LH.

Gonadotropin levels are low but measurable between 2 and 8 years, after which FSH and then LH values begin to rise slowly during the prepubertal years (Fig. 8–1). FSH levels in female children are sensitive to estrogen administration. Ethinyl estradiol, 2–5µg daily, lowers urinary FSH excretion in prepubertal children; approximately eight to ten times this dose is required to achieve comparable suppression in adult men. Clomiphene citrate, a weak estrogen that acts as an antiestrogen in the adult by competitive inhibition at the estradiol-binding sites, functions as an estrogen in the child. In the prepubertal female, the administration of clomiphene citrate results in suppression of FSH levels rather than in the stimulation observed in the adult, suggesting no estrogen competition at the estrogen-binding sites.

EARLY PUBERTY

FSH begins to increase again between the ages of 8 and 10 years, while an increase in LH is not demonstrable before the age of 12 years. The LH increase is associated with an increase in circulating estradiol levels, and a study of individual girls suggests that the rise in pituitary hormones precedes the rise in ovarian estrogens. The onset of puberty is marked by periodic secretory episodes of LH output that occur during sleep but are not demonstrable during waking hours. As puberty advances, the pattern shifts to episodic re-

FIG. 8-2. Serum FSH and LH values at 2- to 3-day intervals in perimenarcheal girls. *Hatched bars* denote menses. (Winter JSD, Faiman C: Clin Endocrinol Metab 37:714, 1973)

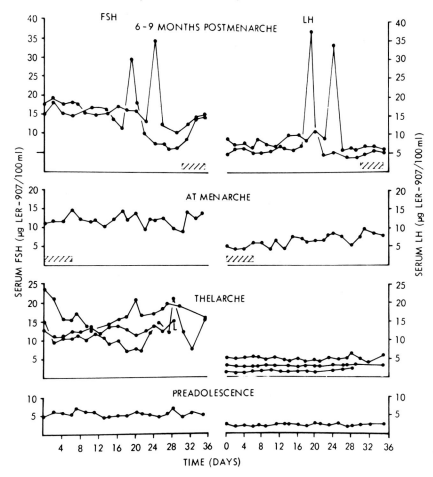

lease of LH irrespective of sleep stages. The midcycle LH surge is the characteristic feature of puberty; however, the occurrence of vaginal bleeding associated with low levels of gonadotropins without a surge is not unusual shortly after the menarche and, indeed, such anovulatory bleeds may be the rule rather than the exception (Fig. 8–2).

Evidence has accumulated suggesting that hypothalamic catecholamines play a role in the neuroendocrine mechanisms that control the release and, perhaps, synthesis of hypothalamic hormones and subsequent pituitary gonadotropin secretion. Partanen and Hervonen localized catecholamines in both the fetal pituitary and later in the fetal hypothalamus and median eminence. Ruf has suggested that a gradual growth and development of the adrenergic nervous system after birth are responsible for the continuously evolving developmental processes that occur from birth to puberty. These catecholamines, synthesized in the cortex and such sensory nerve endings as the ret-

ina, are then funneled down the axons, probably by way of large nerve tracts such as the stria terminalis and the hypothalamohypophyseal tract, into the hypothalamus. Muller has demonstrated a steady increase in brain catecholamine content until puberty. As these biogenic amine neurotransmitters reach adequate levels, sufficient hypothalamic hormone (LH–RH) is released into the pituitary portal system to cause FSH and LH pituitary discharge responsible for follicle growth and development. The subsequent increased ovarian steroidogenesis then produces the "positive" estrogen feedback that induces the LH surge and triggers ovulation.

The interesting patterns of gonadotropic secretion associated with the prepubertal age in both males and females may well be a signal of this increasing catecholamine hypothalamic content. Recent studies of human sleep indicate that sleep is not merely the absence of wakefulness, but rather a qualitatively unique state of activation of the central nervous system in-

fluenced by particular biogenic amine nerve transmitters. Not only is there a sleep-related increase in LH secretion in all early pubertal subjects, but there is also an increase in hGH in prepuberty and adolescence. Both these findings indicate the important role of the central nervous system in initiating the development of secondary sexual characteristics and growth in the prepubertal state. Prolactin and adrenal corticotropin (ACTH) release is also sleep-related, being highest just before waking.

Although the mechanisms that determine the onset of this sleep-related pituitary or hypothalamic secretory function at puberty are unknown, various correlations have been made. Like older pubertal boys, young patients with untreated congenital adrenal hyperplasia and advanced bone age show augmented LH secretion synchronous with sleep. Thus, the prolonged exposure to increased concentrations of adrenal androgen may result in 1) premature central nervous system maturation, 2) stimulation of hGH, or 3) events initiated by hGH stimulation that may activate the pubertal LH response. In support of the latter theory, chronically ill children undergoing adrenal suppression with cortiosteroids have a suppressed hGH output. This may explain the growth retardation and delayed maturation of these children.

THYROID PHYSIOLOGY DURING PUBERTY: PROLACTIN

Thyroid pathology is more frequent among females, and abnormalities of thyroid function have long been recognized as related to the changing hormonal patterns in female reproduction. Thus, both hypo- and hyperthyroidism occur most commonly at the menarche, during pregnancy, and in the perimenopause.

Winter and coworkers have demonstrated the presence of both LH–RH and thyrotropin-releasing hormone (TRH) in the human fetal brain as early as 4.5

weeks' gestation. At birth, there is a marked rise in TSH and thyroid function. This acute functional change may be important for thermal regulation in the newborn.

One wonders if TRH is also increased and responsible for the greatly increased prolactin values (between 123 and 222 ng/ml) in the newborn. This elevated prolactin level may in fact be the initial cause of "witchs' milk." The elevated serum values found at term, perhaps related to the stress of labor, fall rapidly; by 6 weeks after delivery a level of 17 ng/ml is reached. From the ages of 2–12 years, values remain at about 5 ng/ml. In the adult male, prolactin remains at 5 ng/ml; in the adult female, however, it is slightly higher (8 ng/ml). This difference is apparently due to the increased estrogen milieu of the female, as lower values, *e.g.*, 6 ng/ml, are seen in the menopausal woman.

The percentage uptake of triiodothyronine (T_3) is maximum at 2–3 days of life, begins to decrease thereafter, and then increases progressively from low levels at 120 days of age to adulthood (Table 8–1). In premenarcheal and menarcheal girls, Lamberg *et al.* have shown a decreasing level of TSH from a high value of 7.4 μU/ml in the youngest skeletal age group of 9 years until the menarche, when there was an abrupt increase. Following this, values again decreased to the adult levels. Mean values in pre- and postmenarcheal girls did not differ but were significantly higher than the adult value of 3.4 μU/ml (Fig. 8–3). The prepubertal, pubertal, and postpubertal values in boys showed no variation and were substantially lower than those of girls, the mean being 3.9 μU/ml. The authors concluded that girls, but not boys, show a significant change in thyroid physiology during puberty. At the menarche a second dramatic change is seen. It could be expected that these fluctuations must be estrogen-related. However, if this is so, it is apparently independent of the estrogen effect on binding proteins, according to Lamberg *et al.*

TABLE 8–1. AGE VARIATION IN THYROID TESTS IN FEMALES

	Serum T_4 Values (μg/100ml)			T_3 Uptake Values (%)			Free Thyroxin Index (FTI)		
	No.	Mean	SD	No.	Mean	SD	No.	Mean	SD
1 day	12	6.4	±1.47	12	40.8	±6.90	12	5.2	±0.78
2–3 days	5	11.2	±2.83	5	53.0	±4.69	5	12.3	±2.47
4–10 days	10	10.1	±2.29	10	44.7	±5.89	10	9.3	±2.40
11–45 days	13	7.2	±1.35	13	44.5	±4.48	13	6.7	±1.28
46–90 days	15	7.5	±2.19	15	39.5	±6.90	15	5.9	±0.68
121 days–1 yr	9	5.5	±1.74	9	39.7	±4.90	9	4.7	±1.84
1–13 yr	17	6.3	±1.77	17	44.6	±6.81	17	5.7	±1.30
13–20 yr	10	5.6	±1.08	10	46.0	±3.80	10	5.4	±1.02
Over 20 yr	16	6.0	±1.47	16	48.7	±7.48	16	6.1	±1.66

(Adapted from Hays GC, Mullard JE: J Clin Endocrinol Metab 39:958, 1974)

FIG. 8-3. Serum TSH values (*A*) and free thyroxin index (*B*) before and after menarche. Mean 1 SEM. Numbers above points represent numer of samples at each age. Skeletal age is the same as bone age. Gynecologic age is time elapsed since menarche. (Lamberg BA, Kantero RL, Saarinen P, Widholm O: Acta Endocrinol (Copenh) 74:685, 1973)

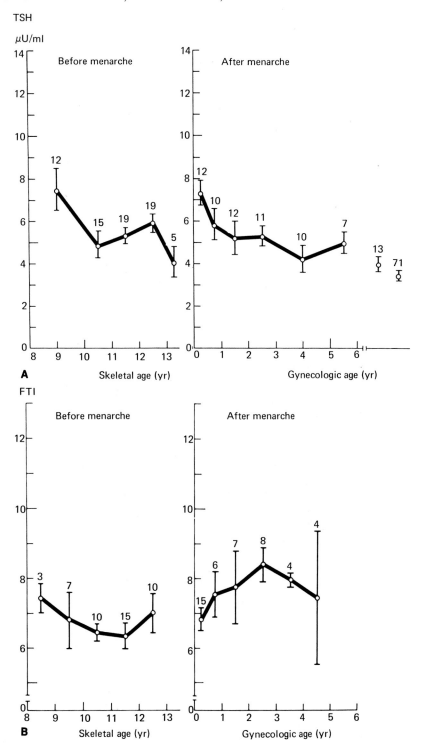

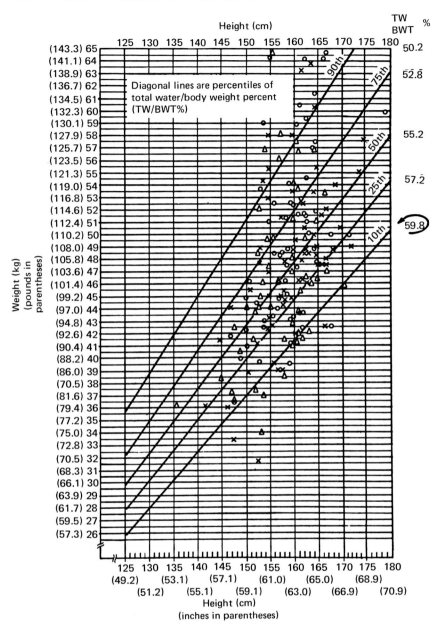

FIG. 8-4. Minimal weight necessary for particular height for onset of menstrual cycles indicated on weight scale by tenth percentile diagonal line of total water/body weight percent as it crosses vertical height lines. A 15-year-old girl whose completed height is 63 in should weigh at least 91 lb before menstrual cycles can be expected to start. (Frisch RE, McArthur JW: Science 185:949, copyright 1974 by the American Association for the Advancement of Science)

MENARCHE

The menarche, the appearance of periodic vaginal bleeding, is the clinical indicator of sexual maturity in females. The onset of the first menstrual period usually implies ovulation and the ability to conceive. These first cycles may be anovulatory, or at least aluteal, with a short and inadequate luteal phase, however. That patients with these cycles are infertile is not well documented; if fertilization does occur, the chorionic gonadotropin (hCG) may in fact "rescue" the corpus luteum.

The menarcheal age is reported to vary from a mean of 12.3 years in England and America to an average of 18.8 years in the New Guinea islands. This may perhaps be related to the small size of these indigenous peoples. The menarcheal age has been steadily and consistently decreasing during the past 100 years. Although the reason is unknown, it is recognized that heritable factors may be one important influence. Frisch, in a series of studies undertaken over many years, has shown that the age of menarche is highly sensitive to protein-calorie malnutrition and correlates well with body mass or weight; undernutrition delays

menarche and the adolescent growth spurt. Frisch and McArthur report that amenorrhea accompanies the self-inflicted starvation of anorexia nervosa and that an increase in food intake associated with a gain of body weight restores normal menstrual function after a predictable interval of time. These authors propose that a minimal level of stored, easily mobilized energy is necessary for ovulation and menstrual cycles (Fig. 8–4), although they accept that other factors, particularly emotional stress, can affect the maintenance or onset of menstruation.

CLINICAL CHANGES IN PUBERTY

SECONDARY SEXUAL DEVELOPMENT

The onset of puberty is associated with striking physical and behavioral changes that accompany or parallel the alterations of circulating gonadotropic and gonadal hormone levels. Marshall and Lund, as well as Tanner, in longitudinal studies, have described the temporal relations among thelarche (development of the breasts), pubarche (development of the pubic hair), the adolescent growth spurt, and menarche. The stages in breast development (Fig. 8–5) are

1. Preadolescent; elevation of papilla only
2. Breast bud stage; elevation of breast and papilla in a small mound, enlargement of areola diameter
3. Further enlargement of breast and areola, with no separation of their contours
4. Projection of areola and papilla to form a secondary mound above the level of the breast
5. Mature stage; projection of papilla only, due to recession of the areola to the general contour of the breast

The stages of development of pubic hair are

1. Preadolescent; no pubic hair
2. Sparse growth of long, slightly pigmented, downy hair, appearing chiefly along the labia
3. Considerably darker, coarser, and more curled hair spreading sparsely over the junction of the pubes
4. Adult-type hair, but area covered is less, with no spread to medial surface of the thighs
5. Adult in quantity and type, distributed to medial surface of the thighs, but not up to the linea alba

There is wide variation among normal girls in the correlation of these parameters. Although the first sign of puberty is usually breast development, which may reach stage 4 before pubic hair appears, pubic hair may occasionally reach stage 3 or even 4 in normal girls before there is any development of the breasts. The menarche usually occurs during breast develop-

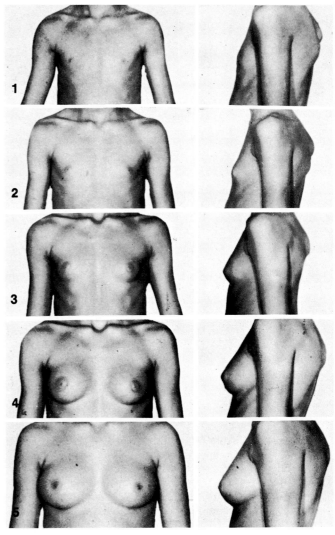

FIG. 8–5. Standards for evaluating breast development. (Tanner JM: Growth at Adolescence, 2nd ed. Oxford, Blackwell, 1962)

ment stages 3 or 4, but some girls do not menstruate until the breasts are fully mature. Although the average interval from the first sign of puberty to menarche is approximately 2 years, the extremes in Tanner's study were between 1.5 and over 6 years (Fig. 8–6).

The physical manifestations of puberty reflect the increased secretory activity of the adrenals and the ovaries. Ovarian estrogens stimulate the growth and maturation of the reproductive organs, influence fat deposition, and accelerate epiphyseal closure, thus ending linear growth. The major ovarian estradiol production, which occurs late in pubertal development, stimulates a follicle to the preovulatory stage. The pubarche, frequently the first sign of beginning maturity,

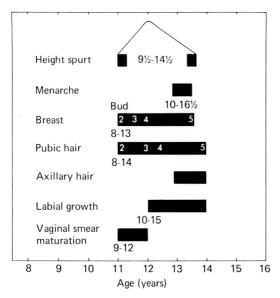

FIG. 8–6. Sequence of events that occur in girls at puberty. *Numbers* under each event are normal range of ages within which event may occur. (Tanner JM: Growth at Adolescence, 2nd ed. Oxford, Blackwell, 1962)

is characterized by the growth of pubic and axillary hair. The steroids responsible for this development are derived from the adrenal androgen precursors dehydroepiandrosterone (DHEA) and its sulfate, DHEAS. A measurable increase in these steroids can be demonstrated in the prepubertal stage. The mechanism by which this adrenal pathway is activated remains unknown, however, as there is no associated change in the rate of cortisol or adrenocorticotropic hormone (ACTH) production. It has been suggested that prolactin may be the trigger mechanism; although there are some provocative *in vitro* and clinical findings to support this theory, it has not been possible to detect a prepubertal rise in prolactin production. Also, the sleep-induced prolactin stimulation is present by at least the age of 1 year. An adrenal androgen corticotropin (AACSH) has been postulated.

BEHAVIORAL DEVELOPMENT

Adolescence is characterized not only by the magnitude and rapidity of somatic changes of sexual maturation but also by an important process of psychic maturation. There are qualitative and quantitative changes in the sexual drive that affect the behavior of the adolescent. A change in role from dependent child to independent, autonomous adult slowly occurs. Social interactions change, with a shift in personal relations and a search for identity. Intellectual performance increases, reaching its maximum in the early twenties.

Abstract thinking develops, which explains the adolescent's interest in philosophical, ethical, and moral issues.

Kastenberg and Blos described the menarche as a necessary organizer that for the young girl, crystallizes and defines body boundaries. There is a reorganization of the ego around a clearer, better defined body image. Concurrently, confusion increases concerning the definition of femininity and the female role. These conflicts are partially determined by maternal attitudes and education toward femininity and by the changing role of the female in society. Although the menarche is a landmark in female physical development, the adolescent psychology is characterized by contradictions in actions and words. The adolescent needs information presented in such a fashion that solutions to problems are self-evident and inescapable. Solutions must not be offered, nor advice given about specific behavior. The facts must be sufficiently convincing to allow the adolescent to make the correct judgment. Value judgments placed upon adolescent behavior by the physician are inappropriate and should be carefully avoided. Key features of the successful interview with the adolescent patient are

1. The patient should be seen alone initially, without parents present.
2. The basis of confidentiality should be stated early and adhered to strictly.
3. A relaxed, open, flexible, and unhurried approach is essential.
4. The adolescent should be spoken with on her own level, not as a younger child, which is disrespectful, or as an adult, which is confusing.
5. At the end of the interview, if her parents are in the waiting room, it is well to ask the patient if she would like to have certain facts explained to them in her presence. Observing the parent–adolescent relationship under these conditions is often very revealing and sometimes provides the basis for improvement in attitudes on both sides.
6. Questions should be answered honestly, simply, and completely.
7. Information, knowledge, and factual advice should be provided.
8. The adolescent's point of view should be respected; if the physician disagrees this should also be stated and explanation provided.
9. The patient should be trusted.

For the physical examination of the adolescent, the following are important:

1. Discuss what is to be done and how it is to be done—models or diagrams are helpful.
2. Carefully respect the modesty of the patient.
3. Focus on the area of the chief complaint, but pay special attention to blemishes, deformities, and areas of concern to the patient.

PATHOLOGY OF PUBERTY

PREDICTION OF ADULT HEIGHT: THE TOO TALL GIRL

The psychologic disadvantage of height to the adolescent taller than her peers may bring the child or her parents to the gynecologist for consultation concerning estrogen therapy. According to the Bayley and Pinneau tables, adult height can be predicted from the correlation between skeletal age, as read from hand x-rays, and the proportion of adult stature achieved by the child at the time the x-ray was taken (Table 8–2). Estrogen therapy induces epiphyseal closure and may thus influence predicted height by decreasing linear growth potential. The work of Frasier and Smith, and of Whitelaw, has indicated that treatment must be begun early, usually prior to 12 years bone age for successful reduction of final height. Often, neither family nor patient focuses on this problem until too late. If therapy is begun early enough, at about the age of 9–10 years, however, the child herself is not at all interested and frequently resents the necessary medical details, such as pelvic or rectal examination. The premature onset of menstruation may also be undesirable.

DELAYED PUBERTY

Puberty is considered delayed in girls, according to the standards of Marshall and Lund and of Tanner, if breast budding has not occurred by the age of 13 or if more than 5 years have elapsed between beginning breast growth and menarche. Delayed puberty may result from intrinsic gonadal disease or from relative or absolute deficiency of gonadotropin stimulation, as outlined in the following:

I. Lesions of central origin
  A. Functional and organic brain disease
    1. Traumatic, toxic, and infectious lesions, including tumors
    2. Congenital anomalies
      a. Isolated releasing hormone deficiencies
      b. Kallman's syndrome
    3. Constitutional delay
  B. Psychogenic factors
    1. Major and minor psychoses, emotional shock
    2. Malnutrition, including anorexia nervosa
  C. Pituitary disturbances
    1. Tumors
    2. Congenital defects
      a. Isolated gonadotropin deficiency
II. Lesions of intermediate origin
  A. Chronic illness
  B. Metabolic diseases
    1. Thyroid disease
    2. Diabetes mellitus
    3. Adrenal disease
  C. Nutritional disturbances
    1. Malnutrition
    2. Exogenous obesity
III. Lesions of peripheral origin
  A. Ovarian disorders
    1. Congenital developmental defects
      a. Ovarian dysgenesis
      b. Hermaphroditism, true or male
    2. Tumors
    3. Insensitive ovary syndrome (Savage syndrome)
    4. Trauma, including portion of ovary
  B. Vaginal and uterine defects
    1. Congenital defects
      a. Absence of vagina or uterus
      b. Malformation of uterus
    2. Traumatic and infectious lesions
      a. Stenosis of vagina or cervix
      b. Asherman's disease or endometrial sclerosis and tuberculosis

In girls, gonadal dysgenesis, the most common form of primary hypogonadism, may be associated with 45 XO or other abnormal sex chromosome karyotypes and may be detected even before the age of puberty. The diagnosis may be made at a relatively early age by the measurement of serum FSH and LH levels, which are well above expected levels.

More difficult to diagnose are the clinical syndromes associated with hypogonadotropism, which may be secondary to failure of either hypothalamic or pituitary function. Gonadotropin deficiency may accompany a lack of other pituitary tropic hormones and may be secondary to panhypopituitarism, tumor, trauma, or infectious disease of the gland. Isolated hypogonadotropism, which may be familial, may be related to a developmental abnormality of the nervous system or hypothalamus as in Kallman's syndrome. This condition, transmitted as an autosomal dominant trait with variable expressivity, manifests gonadotropin deficiency in association with anosmia and color blindness.

Finally, physiologic delayed puberty is relatively common and is difficult to differentiate from true, anatomic gonadotropin deficiency. A constitutional delay in growth and development occurs, but these children eventually undergo normal sexual maturation. Genetic factors may be responsible, as evidenced by a family history of late menarche. More commonly, however, severe malnutrition, chronic disease, hypothyroidism, hypoadrenocorticism, or poorly controlled diabetes mellitus is the cause.

Difficulties in the differential diagnosis of the syndromes of delayed puberty complicate decisions about therapy. In general, adolescence is a difficult time of adjustment, and delay in evaluation much beyond the

TABLE 8-2. PREDICTION OF ADULT HEIGHT FROM CORRELATION OF SKELETAL AGE AND PROPORTION OF ADULT STATURE ACHIEVED*

SKELETAL AGE (yr)	6-0	6-3	6-6	6-10	7-0	7-3	7-6	7-10	8-0	8-3	8-6	8-10	9-0	9-3	9-6
PERCENT OF MATURE HEIGHT	72.0	72.9	73.8	75.1	75.7	76.5	77.2	78.2	79.0	80.1	81.0	82.1	82.7	83.6	84.4
PRESENT HEIGHT (in.)															
37	51.4														
38	52.8	52.1	51.5												
39	54.2	53.5	52.8	52.0	51.5	51.0									
40	55.6	54.9	54.2	53.3	52.8	52.3	51.8	51.2							
41	56.9	56.2	55.6	54.6	54.2	53.6	53.1	52.4	51.9	51.2					
42	58.3	57.6	56.9	55.9	55.5	54.9	54.4	53.7	53.2	52.4	51.9	51.2			
43	59.7	59.0	58.3	57.3	56.8	56.2	55.7	55.0	54.4	53.7	53.1	52.4	52.0	51.4	
44	61.1	60.4	59.6	58.6	58.1	57.5	57.0	56.3	55.7	54.9	54.3	53.6	53.2	52.6	52.1
45	62.5	61.7	61.0	59.9	59.4	58.8	58.3	57.5	57.0	56.2	55.6	54.8	54.4	53.8	53.3
46	63.9	63.1	62.3	61.3	60.8	60.1	59.6	58.8	58.2	57.4	56.8	56.0	55.6	55.0	54.5
47	65.3	64.5	63.7	62.6	62.1	61.4	60.9	60.1	59.5	58.7	58.0	57.2	56.8	56.2	55.7
48	66.7	65.8	65.0	63.9	63.4	62.7	62.2	61.4	60.8	59.9	59.3	58.5	58.0	57.4	56.9
49	68.1	67.2	66.4	65.2	64.7	64.1	63.5	62.7	62.0	61.2	60.5	59.7	59.3	58.6	58.1
50	69.4	68.6	67.8	66.6	66.1	65.4	64.8	63.9	63.3	62.4	61.7	60.9	60.5	59.8	59.2
51	70.8	70.0	69.1	67.9	67.4	66.7	66.1	65.2	64.6	63.7	63.0	62.1	61.7	61.0	60.4
52	72.2	71.3	70.5	69.2	68.7	68.0	67.4	66.5	65.8	64.9	64.2	63.3	62.9	62.2	61.6
53	73.6	72.7	71.8	70.6	70.0	69.3	68.7	67.8	67.1	66.2	65.4	64.6	64.1	63.4	62.8
54		74.1	73.2	71.9	71.3	70.6	69.9	69.1	68.4	67.4	66.7	65.8	65.3	64.6	64.0
55			74.5	73.2	72.7	71.9	71.2	70.3	69.6	68.7	67.9	67.0	66.5	65.8	65.2
56				74.6	74.0	73.2	72.5	71.6	70.9	69.9	69.1	68.2	67.7	67.0	66.4
57						74.5	73.8	72.9	72.2	71.2	70.4	69.4	68.9	68.2	67.5
58								74.2	73.4	72.4	71.6	70.6	70.1	69.4	68.7
59									74.7	73.7	72.8	71.9	71.3	70.6	69.9
60										74.9	74.1	73.1	72.6	71.8	71.1
61												74.3	73.8	73.0	72.3
62														74.2	73.5
63															74.6
64															
65															
66															
67															
68															
69															
70															
71															
72															
73															
74															

* Predicted adult height in inches is read off directly at point of intersection of skeletal age and present height. Table shown is for average girls with skeletal age within 1 year of chronologic age. Other tables, presented in original article, are to be used if skeletal age is either accelerated or retarded 1 or more years. (Bayley N. Pinneau SR: J Pediatr 40:432, 1952)

age of 16 may be associated with psychologic or behavioral problems related to anxieties about development that lags behind that of peers. Any young girl who has failed to develop must undergo a physical and pelvic examination to rule out chronic illness and to document normality of the external genitalia and the presence of a uterus. Gonadotropin assay, estimation of estrogen milieu by vaginal smear, and radiologic evaluation of bone age constitute baseline studies. In some patients, documentation of thyroid or adrenal function, radiologic examination of the sella turcica, or karyotyping might be indicated by associated clinical signs or symptoms. A prolactin assay must always be considered.

Management of the patient with delayed puberty depends upon the presumed cause. Patients with gonadal dysgenesis will never develop without administration of exogenous estrogen, preferably in associa-

9-9	10-0	10-3	10-6	10-9	11-0	11-3	11-6	11-9	12-0	12-3	12-6	12-9	13-0	13-3	13-6	13-9	14-0
85.3	86.2	87.4	88.4	89.6	90.6	91.0	91.4	91.8	92.2	93.2	94.1	95.0	95.8	96.7	97.4	97.8	98.0
51.6	51.0																
52.8	52.2	51.5															
53.9	53.4	52.6	52.0	51.3													
55.1	54.5	53.8	53.2	52.5	51.9	51.6	51.4	51.2	51.0								
56.3	55.7	54.9	54.3	53.6	53.0	52.7	52.5	52.3	52.1	51.5	51.0						
57.4	56.8	56.1	55.4	54.7	54.1	53.8	53.6	53.4	53.1	52.6	52.1	51.6	51.1				
58.6	58.0	57.2	56.6	55.8	55.2	54.9	54.7	54.5	54.2	53.6	53.1	52.6	52.2	51.7	51.3	51.1	51.0
59.8	59.2	58.4	57.7	56.9	56.3	56.0	55.8	55.6	55.3	54.7	54.2	53.7	53.2	52.7	52.4	52.1	52.0
61.0	60.3	59.5	58.8	58.0	57.4	57.1	56.9	56.6	56.4	55.8	55.3	54.7	54.3	53.8	53.4	53.2	53.1
62.1	61.5	60.6	60.0	59.2	58.5	58.2	58.0	57.7	57.5	56.9	56.3	55.8	55.3	54.8	54.4	54.2	54.1
63.3	62.6	61.8	61.1	60.3	59.6	59.3	59.1	58.8	58.6	57.9	57.4	56.8	56.4	55.8	55.4	55.2	55.1
64.5	63.8	62.9	62.2	61.4	60.7	60.4	60.2	59.9	59.7	59.0	58.4	57.9	57.4	56.9	56.5	56.2	56.1
65.7	65.0	64.1	63.3	62.5	61.8	61.5	61.3	61.0	60.7	60.1	59.5	58.9	58.5	57.9	57.5	57.3	57.1
66.8	66.1	65.2	64.5	63.6	62.9	62.6	62.4	62.1	61.8	61.2	60.6	60.0	59.5	58.9	58.5	58.3	58.2
68.0	67.3	66.4	65.6	64.7	64.0	63.7	63.5	63.2	62.9	62.2	61.6	61.1	60.5	60.0	59.5	59.3	59.2
69.2	68.4	67.5	66.7	65.8	65.1	64.8	64.6	64.3	64.0	63.3	62.7	62.1	61.6	61.0	60.5	60.3	60.2
70.3	69.6	68.7	67.9	67.0	66.2	65.9	65.6	65.4	65.1	64.4	63.8	63.2	62.6	62.0	61.6	61.3	61.2
71.5	70.8	69.8	69.0	68.1	67.3	67.0	66.7	66.4	66.2	65.5	64.8	64.2	63.7	63.1	62.6	62.4	62.2
72.7	71.9	70.9	70.1	69.2	68.4	68.1	67.8	76.5	67.2	66.5	65.9	65.3	64.7	64.1	63.7	63.4	63.3
73.9	73.1	72.1	71.3	70.3	69.5	69.2	68.9	68.6	68.3	67.6	67.0	66.3	65.8	65.1	64.7	64.4	64.3
	74.2	73.2	72.4	71.4	70.6	70.3	70.0	69.7	69.4	68.7	68.0	67.4	66.8	66.2	65.7	65.4	65.3
		74.4	73.5	72.5	71.7	71.4	71.1	70.8	70.5	69.7	69.1	68.4	67.8	67.2	66.7	66.5	66.3
			74.7	73.7	72.9	72.5	72.2	71.9	71.6	70.8	70.1	69.5	68.9	68.3	67.8	67.5	67.3
				74.8	74.0	73.6	73.3	73.0	72.7	71.9	71.2	70.5	69.9	69.3	68.8	68.5	68.4
						74.7	74.4	74.1	73.8	73.0	72.3	71.6	71.0	70.3	69.8	69.5	69.4
									74.8	74.0	73.3	72.6	72.0	71.4	70.8	70.6	70.4
											74.4	73.7	73.1	72.4	71.9	71.6	71.4
												74.7	74.1	73.4	72.9	72.6	72.4
														74.5	73.9	73.6	73.5
															74.9	74.6	74.5

tion with a progestational agent. Constitutional delay in growth and development is best treated with reassurance and correction of attendant problems such as malnutrition or obesity. Girls with documented abnormalities of the hypothalamic–pituitary axis require estrogen therapy for development. Induction of ovulation is not indicated except in the rare case when it may be attempted either as a diagnostic tool or as a psychologic tool for reassurance of the patient.

PRECOCIOUS PUBERTY

In the female, true precocious puberty, the most common form of sexual precocity, is defined as a premature initiation of the normal physiologic and endocrinologic processes of puberty before the age of 8 years. Premature activation of the hypothalamic–pituitary–gonadal mechanism occurs with no demonstrable organic lesion of the central nervous system, no gonad-

otropin-secreting tumor, and no adrenal or gonadal disorder. True precocious puberty culminates in the capability of reproduction, which in the female implies ovulation. Historically, this has resulted in parenthood at a very early age, as classically illustrated by Lena Medina, delivered at age 5 years by cesarean section of a 3000-g male infant.

Isosexual pseudoprecocious puberty is development appropriate to the sex in the presence of any or all of the lesions mentioned. Gametogenesis does not occur, and development of sexual characteristics may be isolated. For instance, premature thelarche may occur in the absence of pubarche or *vice versa*.

The differential diagnosis of precocious puberty, includes the true or complete form, implying activation of the hypothalamic–pituitary–gonadal axis, and so-called pseudoprecocious or incomplete puberty, independent of stimulation by the central nervous system:

I. Complete, true precocious puberty
   A. Idiopathic or constitutional
   B. Neurogenic, cerebral lesions
      1. Tumors of hypothalamus, pineal, or cortex
      2. Infections, including toxoplasmosis, encephalitis, and meningitis
      3. Inherited disease such as neurofibromatosis
      4. Developmental defects, including microcephaly, aqueduct stenosis, craniostenosis
      5. Trauma
      6. Miscellaneous (Sturge–Weber syndrome, diffuse encephalopathy, idiopathic epilepsy)
   C. McCune–Albright syndrome
   D. Juvenile hypothyroidism
   E. Silver's syndrome (craniofacial disproportion, small stature, retarded bone age, increased gonadotropin levels)
II. Incomplete or pseudoprecocious puberty
   A. Premature pubarche
   B. Premature thelarche
   C. Adrenal lesions, including congenital adrenal hyperplasia, Cushing's syndrome, and tumors
   D. Ovarian tumors (steroid producing)
   E. Iatrogenic (androgen or estrogen administration, geriatic vitamins, oral contraceptives)
III. Extrapituitary gonadotropin production
   A. Gonadotropin-secreting tumors
   B. Exogenous gonadotropin administration

The diagnosis of true isosexual precocious puberty is one of exclusion. The evaluation of this condition must include the following:

1. History: sequence of sexual development, onset and characteristics of vaginal bleeding, and possibility of exogenous hormone administration
2. Physical examination: weight, height and span, skeletal abnormalities, café-au-lait spots, stage of secondary sexual development, possible abdominal or pelvic masses, and local vaginal lesions or foreign bodies that could result in external bleeding
3. Measurement of serum gonadotropins FSH and LH
4. Skull series including sella turcica; tomography if necessary
5. Bone survey to determine bone age
6. Thyroid studies, including free T_4, thyroid index, total T_4, and TSH
7. Vaginal maturation index; possibly daily urinary cytography
8. Urinary 17-ketosteroid and 17-hydroxysteroid values, or serum androgen index and AM and PM serum cortisol
9. Basal body temperature

Idiopathic precocious puberty is graphic demonstration that the anterior pituitary and gonads are capable of responding and maturing in a normal manner long before puberty generally occurs. The changes of precocious puberty follow the same sequence and occupy a similar time period as those of normal puberty, although the pattern can vary considerably. There is a definite female predisposition; however, idiopathic precocious puberty in boys may occur as a familial disorder, inherited as a mendelian trait.

The influence of the pineal gland on sexual maturation, both normal and abnormal, remains a matter of controversy. Pineal tumors in children are rare, but approximately 30% of these patients, almost exclusively boys, have shown precocious sexual development. Hamartomas or ganglioneuromas in the posterior region of the tuber cinereum or near the mammillary bodies have been associated with precocious pubertal development. The mechanism by which these tumors cause precocious puberty is often unknown.

The treatment of true precocious puberty is aimed at inhibiting sexual development and retarding steroid-induced bone maturation. Although the first objective can be satisfactorily accomplished, the second is as yet not attainable.

Treatment with medroxyprogesterone acetate (Depo-Provera), a synthetic progestin, induces a fall in gonadotropin excretion. Signs of precocity diminish, as judged in females by cessation of menses, decreased breast size, and regression of estrogenic effects on the vaginal mucosa; but the rate of linear growth and skeletal maturation is not significantly decreased. Richman *et al.* have reported that some patients develop signs suggestive of Cushing's disease and corticoid excess. Danazol and cyproterone acetate, both steroids with apparent antigonadotropin activities, also induce a decrease in circulating gonadotropins but no decrease in bone maturation. Thus, with all current forms of therapy, the adult height is approximately 5 ft. The use of synthetic long-acting LH–RH analogs is another possible therapeutic approach.

Juvenile hypothyroidism as the cause of precocious puberty is a favorable finding, since treatment with thyroid hormone normalizes serum concentrations of gonadotropins and allows catch-up linear growth. Some of these girls lactate, presumably because elevated thyroid-hormone–releasing hormone results in increased prolactin as well as TSH. With replacement thyroid hormone, galactorrhea ceases, menstruation stops, and enlarged polycystic ovaries return to normal size.

MENSTRUATION

The classic definition of normal menstruation is a bloody vaginal discharge that is spontaneous, periodic, and represents endometrial shedding following ovulation. The precise diagnosis can be made only from histologic evaluation of endometrial tissue. Thus, *menstruating endometrium* is diagnosed when the secretory pattern implies that ovulation has occurred. *Bleeding endometrium*, by contrast, is diagnosed when a proliferative pattern is present, implying unopposed estrogen activity without ovulation.

The normalcy of a cycle is judged by the duration, amount, and periodicity of flow. Associated symptoms of menstruation and the menstrual cycle, including pain with menses and recurrent cyclic manifestations, are to be regarded as within or outside normal limits according to the woman's ability to function.

CHARACTERISTICS OF NORMAL MENSTRUATION

INTERVAL AND DURATION OF BLEEDING

The most common interval between menstrual periods is 28 days, cycle day 1 being defined as the 1st day of bleeding. However, Ross and associates found the average cycle length to be 29.1 ± 0.6 days, and an extensive study of some 20,655 cycles in 2316 women indicated a variation between 24 and 32 days, with less than one-sixth of the cycles being the lunar 28 days. Although variations of this degree among normal women are not unusual, variations in the same woman are remarkably slight.

The duration of normal ovulatory menses is usually 3–7 days. This is confirmed by Rybo's report that 19.2% of Scandinavian women had periods lasting 2–3 days, 57.5% had periods lasting 4–5 days, 21.8% had periods lasting 6–7 days, while only 1.5% had periods lasting longer than 1 week.

Menstrual cycles are less regular in interval and du-

ration at both extremes of menstrual life. Dewhurst and colleagues documented irregular and increased cycle length most commonly in postmenarcheal girls and next in perimenopausal women. Concern about menstrual irregularities during the first 2 years of menstrual life and in the perimenopausal era is, therefore, unnecessary, provided the periods are not unduly frequent, prolonged, or excessive.

AMOUNT OF BLOOD LOSS

Various methods have been used to quantitate menstrual blood loss, *e.g.*, estimating the hemoglobin on pads, on tampons, or in cups and whole body counting after administration of alkaline hematin, radioactive iron, or of red cells tagged with ^{59}Fe or [51]Cr. All studies, regardless of technique, have arrived at approximately the same estimations. The amount of blood lost in a normal menstrual period averages approximately 33 ml, with the top normal values between 60 and 80 ml. Rybo found a mean value of 43.4 ml for menstrual blood loss in 476 randomly selected Swedish women. Excluding those women with abnormalities, the average menstrual blood loss was found to be 33.2 ± 1.6 ml in 183 women. The 95th percentile was calculated to be 76.4 ml, and blood loss greater than 80 ml was considered abnormal. Of the total menstrual blood loss, 78% was lost during the first 2 days and 91% during the first 3 days of menses.

Circulating hemoglobin concentration varies with measured menstrual blood loss. A decrease in hemoglobin is usually evident when blood loss exceeds 80 ml, but such a decrease may be seen when blood loss reaches 60 ml or above. Beaton and associates calculated that the average iron intake is 12.4 mg/day and the menstrual iron loss averages 0.44 mg/day. Menstrual loss may not be compensated for, and iron depletion will result, if iron intake is below 11 mg/day.

COMPOSITION OF MENSTRUAL BLOOD

Menstrual blood does not coagulate and contains no fibrinogen. Characteristically dark red, it contains red blood cells, endometrial tissue, cervical mucus, cervical and vaginal cells, bacteria, and enzymes. Among those identified are alkaline and acid phosphatases, high levels of β-glucuronidase, acid cathepsin D, plasminogen, and fibrinolysins.

The fluidity of the menstrual blood and the lack of gross clot formation within the uterus may be explained by the rapid activation of intrauterine fibrinolytic systems as evidenced by the lack of fibrinogen and the large amounts of fibrinolysis breakdown products in the menstruum. Beller suggests that intrauterine clotting is a limited process in which fibrin forma-

tion does not go beyond the monomer stage and that a variety of mechanisms inhibit the coagulation scheme.

Although the lack of fibrinogen in the menstrual discharge is well documented, clot formation in the vagina is not infrequent. Beller demonstrated that the vaginal clots are not composed of fibrin. They are red cell aggregations to mucoid substances, mucoproteins, or glycogen, rather than the end product of the coagulation scheme. Clots associated with dysfunctional bleeding and heavy blood loss are also free from fibrin and are indistinguishable from normal menstrual clots on both histologic and histopathologic examination. Fibrin clots, however, do occur following curettage.

MECHANISMS INVOLVED IN MENSTRUATION

Coupled with the electron-microscope studies of Henzl *et al.*, the known characteristics of normal menstruation make it possible to describe the dynamics of menstrual bleeding. Under the influence of estrogen, the Golgi apparatus in the epithelial cells becomes progressively more complex. The numbers of lysosomes and other vesicles that contain acid hydrolytic enzymes increase. These changes are accentuated in the postovulatory phase and become most marked in the late secretory phase. As estrogen and progesterone decrease during corpus luteum involution, a series of reactions is initiated that eventually leads to endometrial desquamation. Protracted contractions of the spiral arteries associated with hormone deprivation cause a decreased endometrial blood supply. The resulting hypoxia increases the fragility of the lysosomal membranes, allowing a gradual release of their destructive hydrolytic enzymes. These enzymes further digest cellular membranes, causing endothelial breakdown of the small arterioles. Red cells are released from breaks in the capillaries and from defects in the arterioles and venules. Plasminogen activators from the lysosomes convert plasminogen into plasmin, which digests fibrin and perhaps fibrinogen, prior to fibrin polymerization. The fibrinolytic system, activated by cellular necrosis, together with the lysosomal acid hydrolytic enzymes, causes a consumption of plasma clotting factors, leading to a decreased concentration of factors II, VIII, and X in menstrual blood, absence of fibrin, and increased fibrinogen degradation products.

The endometrial prostaglandin (PG) is synthesized by the action of prostaglandin synthetase enzyme (released from lysosomes) on the arachidonic acid released by breakdown of cell membranes (lipids). The highest concentrations of $PGF_{2\alpha}$, PGE_1, and PGE_2 are found in the menstrual flow. These concentrations apparently result in vasoconstriction, causing slowing of the blood flow in the venous lacunae of the endometrium and permitting increased aggregation of platelets at the points of vascular rupture. This prevents too

rapid blood loss and ensures orderly desquamation of the endometrium in the process of tissue digestion. Thus, the platelet plug is reinforced by small amounts of monomer fibrin formed probably by both tissue and blood thromboplastin. Plasmin digests the fibrin clot, thrombin is lysed, blood again flows from the endometrial vessels, the platelet plug is again formed, and the process is repeated. The resulting fibrinolytic activity contributes to the complete breakdown of fibrinogen and fibrin before blood leaves the uterine cavity. The clotting and fibrinolysis, which continue side by side, allow the endometrium to be gradually desquamated down to the basalis. If the fibrinolytic activity, which is apparently dependent upon the plasminogen activators and acid hydrolytic enzymes from the lysosomes, is inadequate and incompletely redigested fibrin is deposited in the stroma, abnormal bleeding associated with incomplete endometrial shedding may occur, as described by Picoff and Luginbuhl.

MENSTRUATION IN HEMATOLOGIC DISORDERS

Abnormalities of menstrual flow may occur in patients with hemorrhage diseases. Normal mechanisms involved in hemostasis are usually evoked only in response to injury. These mechanisms can be classified under four major headings: (1) *tissue resistance,* which limits the extravasation of blood; 2) *capillary permeability,* rather poorly understood and known to be dependent upon adequate amounts of vitamin C and normal plasma proteins; 3) *blood platelets,* which maintain normal capillary resistance; and 4) *blood coagulation,* the result of a complex enzymatic conversion of fibrinogen to fibrin that requires the presence of multiple clotting factors.

Disturbances of those factors related to fibrin clot formation are usually unassociated with menstrual bleeding problems, while those related to vessel fragility or platelet insufficiency are associated with abnormal uterine bleeding. For instance, patients being treated with sodium warfarin (Coumadin) or heparin may have serious problems with hematuria, epistaxis, and bleeding into muscles, but usually have normal menses. Patients with congenital afibrinogenemia (factor I deficiency), hypoprothrombinemia (factor II deficiency), or deficiencies of factors III, IV, VI, VIII, IX, and possibly XII have no problems with menstruation. On the other hand, patients with deficiencies of factors V, VII (proconvertin), and X—factors concerned with hemostasis rather than coagulation—may have menorrhagia.

Patients with von Willebrand's disease, an autosomal dominant heritable bleeding disorder in which a prolonged bleeding time is the only demonstrable abnormality, have severe menorrhagia. Although von Willebrand's disease was originally thought to be a

factor VIII deficiency, the two conditions have now been distinguished clinically by Henson *et al.* Baugh *et al.* have separated factor VIII coagulant activity from von Willebrand's antigen by ion exchange chromatography. Excessive blood loss at menstruation is also seen with disturbances that cause platelet deficiency. Acute leukemia, lupus erythematosus, and infrequently pernicious anemia may be present with menorrhagia because of associated thrombocytopenic purpura.

SYMPTOMS RELATED TO MENSTRUATION

DYSMENORRHEA

Some discomfort normally accompanies ovulatory menstruation. This varies with the woman and may be manifested as lower abdominal cramping, backache, and aching of the thighs. Nausea, vomiting, diarrhea, headache, and anorexia are not uncommon. When symptoms become so troublesome that they cause loss of time from work or school, especially if 2 days or more in duration, menstrual discomfort may be termed dysmenorrhea. Primary dysmenorrhea is defined as painful menstruation unrelated to an obvious physical cause such as endometriosis, uterine polyps, pelvic inflammatory disease, or uterine myomas. Secondary dysmenorrhea is diagnosed when pelvic disease is demonstrable.

The discomfort of menstruation is now thought to be related to PG release. Under the influence of progesterone during the luteal phase, the potential endometrial content of $PGF_{2\alpha}$ is increased. The secretion is maximum at the onset of menstruation. $PGF_{2\alpha}$ administered intravenously to normal women reproduces many of the symptoms of dysmenorrhea, including nausea, vomiting, diarrhea, cramping due to increased uterine contractility, irritability, and poor concentration. Because of the coincidence in the temporal relation and the similarity of the symptoms, a cause and effect relationship may be assumed between the release of PG from the endometrium at the time of tissue desquamation, and the local and systemic symptoms of menstruation.

With a better understanding of the etiology of dysmenorrhea, it is now possible to direct treatment toward the cause rather than to resort to nonspecific analgesics, potent endocrine drugs, and surgical therapy. PG synthetase inhibitors, *e.g.,* ibuprofen (Motrin), 400 mg every 5–6 hours when menstrual pain occurs, usually control the most severe symptoms. Mild cases may still be successfully treated by the local use of heat and drugs with analgesic, sedative, or antispasmodic properties *e.g.,* meprobamate and ethoheptazine citrate (Equagesic) or ethoheptazine citrate (Zactirin Compound-100), or propoxyphene hydrochloride (Darvon). Habit-producing drugs, such as morphine or alcohol, should be vigorously discouraged; the possibility of addiction is extremely worrisome. Phenobarbital or sodium amobarbital may be indicated occasionally.

Endocrine treatment for dysmenorrhea should be reserved for the case in which PG synthetase inhibitors are ineffective and pain is incompatible with lifestyle or career necessities. Since ovulation is a primary requisite for dysmenorrhea, the continuation of symptoms while the patient is taking ovulation-suppressing agents should suggest either a fixed psychoneurosis or a secondary physical or mechanical cause. Progestational agents alone have been utilized with moderate success, as inhibition of ovulation is accomplished by relatively small doses with few side effects or complications. Dydrogesterone (Duphaston) is not an ovulation inhibitor, but it apparently interferes with ovarian steroidogenesis to prevent dysmenorrhea. Daily use of 10–20 mg from cycle day 5 to 25 is usually effective but may be complicated by bleeding.

If contraception is indicated, combined oral contraception is a convenient therapy for dysmenorrhea. Since the indication for an oral contraceptive is prevention of unwanted pregnancy and since it has been documented that these drugs change metabolic parameters, their use as a primary prevention of dysmenorrhea is unwarranted. Short-term use of oral contraception to provide relief may be indicated, however, if only to show the patient and physician that cyclic bleeding can occur without severe symptoms. Once this psychic alteration has occurred, the patient may find she is able to control her symptoms with milder therapy.

Presacral neurectomy or sympathectomy surgically interrupts the innervation of the uterus, resulting in almost complete pain relief in 70% of women with intractable dysmenorrhea. It should be considered as the last therapeutic resort.

PREMENSTRUAL TENSION SYNDROME

The premenstrual phase of the cycle, that time during which progesterone and estrogen are falling from peak luteal values, is associated with bursts of energy, activity, and creativity. Occasionally, these changes are interpreted as increased nervousness and moodiness or even irritability. Women may both laugh and cry more readily, and judgment is sometimes thought to be less acute. Mild insomnia or a decreased need for sleep may interfere with a woman's ability to function to her own satisfaction or to that of her associates. Mood swings may be noticed for the first time in postmenarcheal girls. These cyclic recurrent manifestations just prior to menstruation are classified as premenstrual tension. In contrast to dysmenorrhea, which is an acute, easily recognized entity associated with menstrual bleeding, premenstrual tension is much more

diffuse in its symptoms, onset, and duration in relation to menstruation. Thus, although occasionally confused or used synonymously, the two entities are etiologically distinct and not necessarily or even usually associated.

The most frequent complaints of the premenstrual tension syndrome can be divided into three major categories: 1) those related to edema, *e.g.,* abdominal bloating, swelling of the extremities, breast tenderness, and weight gain; 2) those related to emotional instability (*e.g.,* irritability, depression, insomnia, inability to reason, feelings of unreality and panic); and 3) headache. Coppen and Kessel, using psychologic testing, concluded that those women with dysmenorrhea and those with premenstrual tension had different personality types. The syndrome of premenstrual tension seems to depend upon a specific, apparently heritable, type of sympathetic nervous system that hyperresponds when subjected to factors that must be considered normal stimuli. As with dysmenorrhea, no abnormality of ovarian hormone production or metabolism has been demonstrated, and a normal hormonal balance is suggested by the occurrence of ovulation. However, secondary aldosteronism under the influence of estrogen and progesterone during the luteal phase may explain the syndrome. Increased aldosterone secretion has indeed been demonstrated in normally menstruating women during the premenstrual phase, resulting in edema formation due to fluid and sodium retention. Certainly, fluid retention and edema are almost constant features of the syndrome, although not always the primary complaint. The fluctuation of aldosterone in a normal cycle is compatible with the theory. Although increased aldosterone levels have not been demonstrated during a premenstrual tension episode, these hormonal values are so dependent upon external factors that it would be difficult to design a satisfactory experiment to demonstrate an abnormality. The investigative situation frequently sequesters the individual from the environment. Although the sympathetic nervous system probably initiates, and normal menstrual physiology triggers, the premenstrual tension syndrome, it is the conjunction with environmental factors that evokes the seriousness of the reactions.

Symptomatic treatment should be directed toward the major complaint. For premenstrual swelling and edema, salt restriction and diuretics are most useful. When recurrent depression or irritability is the major manifestation, lithium carbonate, 300 mg three times daily, is sometimes extremely effective. If headache is the chief symptom and not over 5 days are involved, methyltestosterone in high doses, 25 mg/day for fewer than 5 days a month, is effective. No treatment should be given until the woman's entire life situation has been carefully analyzed by the gynecologist, in conjunction with an internist or psychiatrist. The patient must be aware that the basis of the symptoms is a "reactive" nervous system. She must, therefore, understand the role of symptomatic therapy and realize the necessity of readjusting her habit patterns to avoid the everyday stresses and strains with which she is apparently unable to cope when the physiologic factor is added during the premenstruum.

Prolactin has been implicated as an etiologic factor in premenstrual tension. There is some indication that patients with hyperprolactinemia show a mood swing with depressive tendencies; however, although the initial studies indicated that hyperprolactinemia occurred in patients with the premenstrual tension syndrome, subsequent investigators have failed to confirm this. Nevertheless, this possibility must be considered, as it is extremely difficult to study the syndrome without causing the highly subjective symptomatology to disappear. Bromocriptine therapy would be specific if such an etiology could be proved.

THE MENOPAUSE AND CLIMACTERIC

The menopause, defined as the physiologic cessation of menses associated with failing ovarian function, may be diagnosed in retrospect when a year has passed with no menses. The climacteric is defined as the transitional period in the life of a woman during which the reproductive function gradually diminishes and is lost. It is unique to the human, apparently because of longevity, and begins with a critical loss of oocytes associated primarily with follicular atresia. It is eventually manifested by the lack of cyclic estrogen secretion. The decrease in circulating estrogen results in specific symptoms, but certain psychic or related symptoms that may also occur during this period cannot be attributed strictly to lowered estrogen levels. Although the initial specific symptoms may sharply diminish with time, the metabolic changes inexorably progress.

Cessation of ovarian function may be produced prematurely by surgery, radiation, immunologic disease, and bacteriologic or viral agents. Rarely, it is associated with genetic defects, and most commonly the cause is unknown. The term *premature menopause* has been attached to these nonphysiologic events.

According to the 1970 census, there were 104 million women in the United States. Of these, 27.2 million, or approximately 26.2%, were 50 years of age or older. Thus, the average woman can expect to live some 25 years beyond her menopause, and one-eighth of the population of the United States is made up of menopausal women.

PSYCHOLOGY OF THE MENOPAUSE

The cessation of menses brings a woman face to face with the reality of aging. This realization may precipitate the depressions, anxiety, and tension associated with the menopause, which often have their basis in loss of reproductive status, which may produce a feeling of diminution of her biologic role; loss of dependent children, which may deprive her of ego support; loss of attainable goals, especially in the woman who has toyed with an occupational drive but never come to grips with its problems and solutions; loss of a husband's attainable goals, often a source of satisfaction and excitement during his years of occupational attainment; loss of protection by the husband, who is becoming more and more dependent upon her; and finally a loss of sexual vigor, not necessarily because of a loss of sexual desire, but more often because this desire is thwarted by the constantly diminishing sexual activities of the husband or the discomfort of atrophic vaginitis.

A variety of fears are associated with the menopause—fear of death; fear of dependence upon children; fear of loneliness, helplessness, and failure of physical and financial resources. All these factors should be understood and dealt with appropriately by the physician who is treating the menopausal woman.

PHYSICAL CHARACTERISTICS OF THE MENOPAUSE

SYMPTOMS

A multiplicity of symptoms has been attributed to the menopause, but when these are recorded on the basis of frequency (Table 8–3), only flushing is ubiquitous. Thus, the hot flush may be considered the characteristic symptom of estrogen deprivation, while the rest of the symptoms are referable to the autonomic nervous system, to physiologic and hormonal changes (including those of aging), and to psychologic or emotional factors.

The flushing occurs first in the perimenopausal time bracket and may last for only a few months or for many years. In those patients with persistent symptoms, the severity and frequency seem to decrease with time. The flush is best described as a sensation of warmth that begins in the upper part of the chest, characteristically spreads to neck, face, and upper extremities, and is followed by profuse perspiration and sometimes chilliness. The actual cause of the flush is unknown. It appear to be due to an instability of the autonomic nervous system, probably because of a lowering of the total estrogen level. The elevated gonadotropin level is apparently not responsible for this symptom, as hot flushes do not occur in untreated

TABLE 8-3. FREQUENCY OF SYMPTOMS DURING THE CLIMACTERIC

Symptom	Incidence (%)
FLUSHING	67.0
DEPRESSION	38.5
SWEATING	31.0
INSOMNIA	26.0
ATROPHIC VAGINITIS	20.0
FATIGUE	18.5
HEADACHE	11.0
ALL OTHER	<10.0

(Kaufman SA: Obstet Gynecol 30:399, 1967)

women with Turner's syndrome, who classically have the most elevated gonadotropin values, nor are hot flushes induced by administration of exogenous gonadotropins. The hot flush occurs only when estrogen has been withdrawn in a previously estrogen-sensitized woman. For instance, this situation can be seen in patients with Turner's syndrome who have been treated with estrogen for a number of years and then had therapy discontinued. Flushes may also be induced in women following treatment with clomiphene citrate, an antiestrogen that blocks estrogen at the level of its receptor protein.

Physical changes in menopausal women are frequently as much a part of a physiologic aging process as of estrogen deficiency. Dyspareunia, leukorrhea, and pruritus, symptoms referable to atrophic vaginal changes and directly related to estrogen deprivation, rarely occur prior to 10 years after cessation of menses. Atrophic vaginitis is characterized by thinning of the mucosa and disappearance of rugae. The occasional narrowing and shortening of the vagina are probably related to disuse, although there is evidence that the muscular layer in the submucosa is sometimes replaced by fibrous tissue, which results in loss of elasticity. Because of these changes, the vaginal canal is easily traumatized and susceptible to infection and adhesion formation. Atrophy of the urethral mucosa may also occur and is frequently associated with urethritis.

ENDOCRINE CHANGES

The two cardinal endocrinologic findings in menopausal women are the presence of a low tonic estrogen output in conjunction with an elevation of the serum gonadotropins, FSH and LH. The first indication of failing ovarian function is an elevation of FSH, while LH values remain within normal limits. This is a result of the failure of inhibin to inhibit FSH preferentially over LH. These abnormally high levels may return to normal, as homeostatic mechanisms reestablish the

normal ovarian–pituitary relations. When the ovary can no longer be stimulated to follicle maturation, the FSH again rises; an LH rise follows; and both remain permanently elevated during the rest of the woman's life.

Although the estrogen levels in the menopause are low, circulating estrogen *is* present and peripheral estrogenic effects continue to be manifested. McLennan and McLennan report that 40% of menopausal women maintain moderate levels of estrogen activity during their remaining years of life. Urinary estrogen excretion is maintained in the range of 5 μg–15μg/24 hours. A number of studies have attempted to determine the source of circulating estrogens in menopausal women. Poliak and coworkers have demonstrated that hCG administration to postmenopausal women results in excretion of appreciable amounts of estrogens in the urine, accompanied by changes in the vaginal smear cornification. Histologic and histochemical examinations of the ovaries in these women suggest a secretory activity. In a follow-up study 6 months postcastration, hCG was administered and followed a week later by ACTH. Administration of hCG produced no effect, while ACTH administration caused an increase in the urinary estrogens. Poliak concluded that the postmenopausal ovary is capable of being stimulated to produce either an estrogen or, more compatible with current knowledge, a preestrogen, androstenedione.

Mattingly and Huang studied the hormonal activity of ovarian stroma *in vitro* and concluded that menopausal and postmenopausal ovarian stroma produces androgenic steroids, primarily androstenedione and testosterone. Although they felt that the ovarian contribution of androgens to the circulating pool would be sufficient to allow for extraglandular conversion to estrogens, no aromatization of androgens to estrogens occurred in the ovarian stroma. Baird and Guevara found that the serum concentration of estrone was greater than the concentration of estradiol in postmenopausal women and that the estrone/estradiol ratio was approximately doubled. Grodin *et al.* showed that the principal estrogen formed in menopausal women is estrone and that it is derived by aromatization of plasma androstenedione in the periphery. This conversion occurs more frequently with age and obesity. Neither adrenal nor ovarian secretion of estrone or estradiol contributed significantly to the total postmenopausal estrogen production.

OSTEOPOROSIS

Characterized by a reduction in the quantity of structural bony material, osteoporosis is a disorder that causes bone fragility and thus is a predisposing factor to fracture. Although symptomatic osteoporosis is relatively uncommon and may be familial or associated with hypoparathyroidism, asymptomatic osteoporosis, diagnosed by x-ray evidence, is clearly age-related, is almost universal, and encompasses all bones except the skull. The importance of this condition is emphasized by the finding that 80% of all patients with hip fracture have preexisting osteoporosis and that one-sixth of such patients die within 3 months of injury. About 25% of all white women over age 60 have spinal compression fractures due to osteoporosis. A loss of bone mass as a result of an excess of bone resorption over bone formation is an essential characteritic of osteoporosis. Although this process can be influenced by estrogen, other hormones, such as parathyroid hormone and thyrocalcitonin, nutritional and metabolic factors, and exercise may have as great or greater effects. Excessive smoking has also been shown to be a major predisposing factor to osteoporosis.

The elegant studies of Rasmussen and Bordier indicate that bone formation by the osteocyte and bone resorption by the osteoclast are not independent functions, as thought by Albright and coworkers, but rather are coupled and interdependent. In the postmenopausal female, there is a delay between the resorption phase and the formation phase, but the total active resorption area is not increased. Thus, with increasing age, the problem is a decrease in the rate of bone formation, which leads to a net skeletal loss.

Parathyroid hormone causes calcium depletion and bone resorption, apparently related to its ability to cause citrate accumulation, both by inhibiting citrate oxidation and increasing citric acid accumulation through the glycolysis cycle. Calcitonin decreases calcium resorption but does not increase bone formation. Estrogen also decreases bone decalcification and resorption, apparently by decreasing glycolysis and thereby interfering with the action of parathyroid hormone to increase citric acid accumulation. Thus, if administered prior to the onset of active osteoporosis, estrogen may delay the acute phase of bone loss, cause a positive calcium balance, and reduce bone resorption. However, bone formation is not increased. After 3–9 months of estrogen therapy, the result is a stabilized bone turnover at a new level without a significant net increase in bone mass in the osteoporotic patient. Thus, there is no evidence yet that estrogen administration can totally prevent osteoporosis.

Two major methods of investigation have been employed to clarify the role of estrogen in osteoporosis: 1) study of the onset of osteoporosis in relation to decrease or failure of ovarian function and 2) investigation of the arrest of osteoporosis by estrogen replacement therapy. Most studies, although not all, indicate that increased osteoporosis parallels the duration of estrogen deprivation, and the high incidence of osteoporosis in relatively young women with Turner's syndrome is one of the most convincing statistics. However, it might be argued that there is perhaps some metabolic bone defect in these patients, as evidenced

by their short stature. Saville compared a group of patients who had a natural menopause with a group who had a surgical menopause and found that the mean age at onset of osteoporotic symptoms in both groups was between 62.7 and 65.4 years, respectively, but it was not recorded whether oophorectomy had been performed in these patients. In another study, however, 72 women with symptomatic osteoporosis were found to have experienced menopause at the same average age as 97 control women without osteoporosis. Aitkin et al. performed bone density measurements in 258 oophorectomized women and found that, if oophorectomy has been performed before the age of 45 years, there was a significantly increased prevalence of osteoporosis within 3–6 years of the operation. Note that this is *asymptomatic* osteoporosis. Bone density measurements in women oophorectomized after the age of 45 years were indistinguishable through the 6 years after surgery from those found in healthy women with intact ovaries. Riggs et al. concluded that the menopause was one of the factors responsible for postmenopausal osteoporosis. The menopause appeared to accelerate bone loss, and the accelerated loss could be slowed by estrogen replacement therapy. However, serum concentrations of estrogen, testosterone, and gonadotropins were similar in the osteoporotic and nonosteoporotic menopausal women. Some factor, in addition to the menopause or estrogen deficiency, must therefore have been present in the osteoporotic patients to accelerate their bone loss.

A study by E. Smith on the effects of physical activity in the aged led him to conclude that physical activity slowed the process of bone loss and demineraliation and caused active bone accretion with remineralization. Although this study was carried out only over a 9-month period, it nevertheless emphasizes the importance of exercise and increased stress on muscle mass in decreasing postmenopausal osteoporosis. If it can be corroborated that exercise does indeed *increase* bone formation, this would be the therapeutic method of choice. As stated by Jowsey, bone is not only a supportive tissue but also is the major calcium reservoir of the body. Calcium is stored in the lacunae and released on demand. As calcium is an extremely important electrolyte for many physiologic functions, including mental activity, a sufficient calcium uptake must be maintained to ensure an adequate calcium reserve that can be readily mobilized. This adequate reserve depends on the dietary calcium intake and a normal calcium absorption from the gut, which, in turn, depends on a normal absorption of vitamin D. The conversion of the vitamin D precursor is dependent on the kidney enzyme, 1-α-hydroxycholesterolase. As prolactin activates this enzyme, the lowered prolactin level that occurs at the menopause, probably due to the lowered estrogen level, might be associated with a decreased vitamin D absorption from the gut. Calcium malabsorption because of an intestinal lactase deficiency and

inability to digest milk may also cause a dietary calcium deficiency. Any or all of these factors may contribute to the decreased intestinal absorption of calcium in older people.

In summary, estrogen can be shown to decrease bone resorption, and thus arrest or slow the process of osteoporosis. If estrogen is given, however, it would seem that there should also be an adequate dietary calcium intake and adequate vitamin D to ensure absorption from the gut. Only with these precautions can the physician be sure that there is a sufficient calcium reserve for other metabolic functions. Some systematic exercise program should be undertaken, and excessive smoking should be precluded.

CORONARY HEART DISEASE

Coronary heart disease is said to increase markedly following the menopause, suggesting that estrogen administration may prove prophylactic against this disease. However, the cause of coronary heart disease is far from clear. Certain risk factors are thought to contribute to its development, including hyperlipidemia, diabetes mellitus, obesity, hypertension, smoking, physical inactivity, and psychic stress. These multiple variables make it difficult to study the influence of the menopause on heart disease.

Study of the mortality rates from coronary disease shows that the risk for females steadily rises, but there is no abrupt upward trend at the time of the menopause. The graph for males is somewhat different. There is a break in the steep slope at the fourth to fifth decade, indicating that some males who are at high risk die in the third and fourth decades and that the risk for the remaining population increases slowly paralleling the rate for menopausal women. The sex difference in coronary disease mortality rates is negligible in populations that lack the affluence and "high standard of living" of the United States, where the male/female ratio is 5:1. This is not an absolute correlation, however, as in Italy the ratio is 2:1 and in Japan 1:1.

It has been postulated that oophorectomy predisposes women to mortality or morbidity from coronary heart disease. The reports are conflicting and suffer from bias, however. Ritterband et al. in 1962 studied 267 women who were oophorectomized and a similar group of women who underwent hysterectomy without castration. Arteriosclerotic cardiovascular disease and myocardial infarction prevalence rates were similar in the two groups, excluding evidence of an estrogen or gonadal effect. Coronary heart disease incidence increased with age, and mortality was similar.

Studies designed to demonstrate the value of estrogen in secondary prophylaxis of coronary artery disease and stroke have yielded clear-cut answers. Although estrogen doses have been relatively high, the

results are worth noting. Stampler *et al.,* in a 5-year study of 275 men treated with Premarin in doses of 1.25–10 mg/day, showed that the treated group suffered a large number of fatal and nonfatal cardiovascular and renal complications. The Coronary Drug Project involved 53 centers that collaborated in evaluating certain pharmacologic agents in the secondary prophylaxis of myocardial infarction in men. Males treated with estrogens had a higher incidence of nonfatal myocardial infarction, pulmonary embolism, and thromboembolism. McDowell administered Premarin, 1.25 mg/day, to 176 men and women under the age of 75 who had had nonembolic cerebral infarction, mild or moderate strokes, and who were expected to survive at least 6 months. The incidence of death from recurrent stroke and myocardial infarction was significantly *increased* in the estrogen-treated group. Oliver and Boyd treated 100 men with previous myocardial infarction with either ethinyl estradiol or placebo. No difference between the two groups was observed with respect to fatal myocardial infarction, sudden death, or nonfatal myocardial infarction, but cerebral vascular accidents, arteriothrombosis, and other thrombotic complications increased markedly.

Estrogen administration is known to increase certain blood clotting factors, notably factors VII and X, and to accelerate platelet aggregation. Estrogen administration accelerates vascular occlusion, apparently as a result of locally formed thrombi and embolization associated with these changes in clotting mechanisms and with damage to the endothelial wall caused by the arteriosclerotic process.

The initial arteriosclerotic changes are thought to be associated with hypercholesterolemia or hyperlipidemia. As cholesterol is carried on the lipoproteins, these fractions have been closely examined. Premenopausal women have less plasma lipid in the form of low-density lipoproteins, (LDL), accounting for lower serum triglyceride concentrations. Men and postmenopausal women have higher concentrations of high-density (HDL), low-density and very low density lipoprotein (VLDL) fractions, which ultimately results in increased serum cholesterol, phospholipid, and triglyceride. The functions of these various lipid fractions, high-density lipoprotein and very low density lipoprotein, are just beginning to emerge. It seems that there is a clear interrelationship among them. Most observers believe a high level of low-density lipoprotein and a low level of high-density lipoprotein are associated with arteriosclerotic vascular disease. However, it would seem that various enzyme defects in lipid metabolism, such as a lecithin/cholesterol acyltransferase deficiency, may also contribute to the changes in these ratios. Although it can be shown that estrogen increases high-density lipoprotein and decreases low-density lipoprotein, causing a decreased cholesterol/phospholipid ratio, the significance of such changes in the course of arteriosclerotic cardiovascular disease is undetermined and perhaps depends on the etiology of the abnormal lipid metabolism.

Estrogen administration delays the exit from the bloodstream of triglyceride-rich very low density lipoproteins responsible for the higher concentrations of serum triglycerides. High-density lipoprotein increases the α-lipoproteins and serum triglyceride levels, causing a fall in the cholesterol/phospholipid ratio. As estrogen seems to have little effect on cholesterol in the woman with *normal* cholesterol levels, it does not establish a premenopausal lipid/lipoprotein profile. A lowered cholesterol level in women with abnormally *elevated* lipoprotein values may result.

Because of its effect on the renin–angiotensin system, estrogen may precipitate hypertension in some women prone to this disease. A family history of essential hypertension is a contraindication for estrogen therapy. Blood glucose, but not serum insulin, increases with age in both sexes. Therefore, glucose tolerance tends to decrease with age, and the incidence of diabetes mellitus increases. There is no evidence that the menopause or estrogen deficiency *per se* is related to these changes. Weight gain, hypertension, and physical inactivity are all age-dependent. It would, therefore, seem that factors predisposing to arteriosclerotic vascular disease are related to aging rather than to estrogen withdrawal.

There is little substantive evidence to warrant the use of estrogens as prophylactic therapy for cardiovascular disease. Although estrogen lowers the level of low-density lipoprotein and raises the level of high-density lipoprotein, until the basic function of these lipoproteins in the metabolism of lipids is better understood and perhaps until specific populations at risk can be identified, it will not be possible to say if such reversals are helpful. Once arteriosclerotic changes have been established, estrogen seems to be contraindicated because of the possibility of thromboembolic disease.

CARCINOGENESIS AND ESTROGEN

ENDOMETRIAL CARCINOMA

Anecdotal evidence linking exogenous estrogen to endometrial carcinoma has accumulated throughout the years. As long ago as 1918, Loeb suggested the possibility that estrogen might act as a carcinogenic agent in estrogen growth-dependent target tissues. In 1932, Taylor reported the association of endometrial carcinoma and adenomatous hyperplasia, a pathologic entity considered to be estrogen-dependent. The belief that unopposed estrogen is an etiologic factor in endometrial carcinoma was consistently held by Emil Novak, and Edmund Novak continued to insist upon the correlation. Gusberg's systematic perusal of the problem throughout the years has tended to substan-

tiate the belief. The report of endometrial carcinoma in patients with Turner's syndrome who had received estrogen replacement therapy was perhaps one of the first important anecdotal documentations of this possible relationship.

In a Johns Hopkins study of the endometrial findings in patients with Turner's syndrome who had received estrogen therapy for long periods of time, it was found that the response of the endometrium was directly related to the total estrogen dosage calculated in both amount and duration of therapy. The patient who had received the highest dosage, over the longest period of time had an endometrial cancer. Patients who had received the lowest dosage, 0.3 mg/day of conjugated estrogen or its equivalent, showed no evidence of increased endometrial growth.

A number of reports in the literature indicate that the risk of endometrial cancer for women who have received estrogen is between 2.2 and 15 times that of women who have never received estrogen therapy (Table 8–4). Many objections have been raised to the type of control used in most of these reports, however. Horwitz and Feinstein, using an alternate sampling method devised to eliminate detection bias, found a risk of 2.3. The odds ratio calculated by conventional methods in this study was 11.98. Thus, the type of case control selection does influence the risk ratio; but even in the series with most rigorous control, risk is still present. Duration of exposure has been related to the risk, a 5.6 risk ratio being found in women who used estrogens between 1 and 5 years and a 13.9 risk ratio in women who used them for 7 years or longer, but the findings do not indicate the incidence of carcinoma in estrogen users. In spite of numerous objections to these studies, the most serious being the suggestion that the diagnosis is pathologically unsubstantiated, the evidence nevertheless seems too overwhelming and too consistent with the physiologic facts to permit any trivial explanation for the findings. Estrogen may

not be a cause of endometrial cancer, but rather an association. However, until the facts underlying such an association are sufficiently understood to identify an at risk population, caution must be used in the amount and duration of estrogen prescribed for a specific indication.

The question of the value of progestational drugs as endometrial growth inhibitors is still unresolved. The Johns Hopkins study in patients with Turner's syndrome indicated that the conventional dose of a C-21 progestational drug for 5 days is insufficient to influence the endometrial pattern, nor does it protect against endometrial cancer. However, in the Duke study, no patient who had received supplemental cyclic progestational agents developed carcinoma of the endometrium. The development of carcinoma in patients using sequential oral contraceptives indicates that total protection is not obtained by some progestational therapy. If one remembers that, in the normal cycle, high levels of estrogen may be unopposed only during a 6-day period immediately prior to ovulation, a more physiologic comprehension of estrogen replacement therapy might be obtained.

As estrogen is a growth stimulant and the carcinogenic potential is still equivocal, it seems wise to examine the risks versus the benefits and to use the lowest possible dose compatible with relief of symptoms. It should be remembered that the amount of estrogen necessary for skeletal and supportive tissue maintenance or repair is far below that necessary for the support of the reproductive function.

CARCINOMA OF THE BREAST

The breast is also a target organ for estrogen. At the present time, however, there has been only one report that shows a possible relationship between estrogen administration and breast cancer. Such an effect, if it

TABLE 8-4. ESTROGEN AND RELATIVE RISK OF ENDOMETRIAL CANCER

	Exposure Time	Cancer Patients (No.)	Estrogen Exposed (%)	Relative Risk
Smith et al., 1975	6 + mo	317	48	4.5
Ziel and Finkle 1975	Ever	94	57	7.6
Mack et al., 1976	Ever	63	89	8.0
McDonald et al., 1977	Ever	145	27	0.9
Gray et al., 1977	3 + mo	205	16	3.1
Hoogerland et al., 1978	Ever	587	18	2.2
Horowitz and Feinstein, 1978	6 + mo	119	32	11.98*
	6 + mo	149	33	2.3†
Autunes et al., 1979	< 1 yr	274	4	2.2
	5+	274	14.6	15.0

* Conventional statistics
† Alternative statistics
(Novak E, Jones G, Jones H: Novak's Gynecology, 10th ed. Baltimore, Williams & Wilkins, 1980)

exists, is apparently extremely difficult to document. If there is an association, the latent period is 20 years or more after the initiation of therapy. A report by Symmers of bilateral carcinoma of the breast in two transsexual patients receiving estrogens is strong anectodal evidence that estrogen can augment abnormal breast growth patterns, including carcinoma. Care must therefore be taken to avoid excessive estrogen stimulation, even in patients without a uterus. This is especially so in patients who have a family history of breast cancer.

TREATMENT OF THE MENOPAUSE

As previously stated, of the multiple symptoms attributed to the menopause, only two—the hot flush and senile atrophic vaginitis—can be attributed to estrogen deprivation. Therefore, only these two symptoms can be statistically shown to respond to estrogen therapy. Nevertheless, estrogen therapy has a cascade effect that cannot be disregarded. The relief of flushes, which may be severe enough to impair sleep, improves sleep, which improves energy, which improves the level of activity, which improves interpersonal relationships, which improves mood.

The acutely symptomatic patient, who requires estrogen therapy, must be investigated for factors contraindicating such treatment. Any such factors found then must be evaluated in relation to the severity of symptoms. Absolute contraindications to postmenopausal estrogen replacement therapy are 1) a history of or existence of breast or genital cancer, except some cases of cervical cancer; 2) a history of recent or old thromboembolism; 3) fluid retention due to congestive heart failure or to renal or liver disease; and 4) abnormal liver function. Relative contraindications to estrogen therapy are 1) uterine fibroids or endometriosis, 2) hypertension (as estrogen has been shown to increase aldosterone excretion), and 3) insulin-requiring diabetes mellitus.

When bleeding is not a problem, estrogens should be administered at a dose that will rapidly control symptoms. This dose should then be substantially reduced over the next 6 months, but symptoms should not be allowed to recur. Usually 1.25 mg/day conjugated estrogen or its equivalent from the 1st through the 24th day of each month, reduced over the 6-month period to 0.3 mg constitutes an effective regimen. After 6 months, medication can be taken according to symptoms. Pills should be counted every 3 months by the physician in order to obtain some estimate of the patient's progress. Many women will not need additional therapy. If symptoms recur or persist, 0.3 mg conjugated estrogen or its equivalent daily, or even less frequently, 3 weeks of each month keeps most patients symptom-free and maintains the vaginal mucosa

with a maturation index of between 0/100/0 and 0/90/10. When estrogen therapy is to be continued over protracted periods of time, *e.g.,* longer than 1 year, a progestational drug (5 mg norethindrone or its equivalent) should be added the last 10 or 14 days of therapy as an antimitotic agent. An endometrial biopsy or wash should be obtained once a year.

Regular withdrawal "bleeding" following progestational drug administration does not equate to complete endometrial shedding. Adenocarcinoma may be associated with either no bleeding, regular "withdrawal" bleeding, or, as a late sign, excessive irregular bleeding. Monitoring by endometrial biopsy is essential before estrogen therapy is initiated as well as when it is discontinued. In prolonged therapy, as stated earlier, routine endometrial biopsy should be taken at regular intervals.

In symptomatic women who are still having some menstrual function, bleeding can be a serious problem and treatment should be deferred whenever possible. If symptoms are severe enough to warrant hormone therapy, it is wise to give an estrogen–progesterone regimen, and smaller amounts of conjugated estrogen can usually be given under these circumstances. A conjugated estrogen or its equivalent (0.625 mg/day) for 21 days, with a nonestrogenic progestational agent such as norethindrone (5 mg/day) added during the last 10 days, is usually satisfactory. This therapy should be interrupted periodically to determine if the patient will menstruate and if she is still symptomatic.

When atrophic vaginitis or urethritis is the only symptom, estrogenic vaginal creams or suppositories provide effective and rapid relief. A urethral suppository is available for atrophic urethritis. Administration can be daily for approximately a week and, thereafter, once or twice a week, depending on the patient's response.

Androgens, particularly methyltestosterone, may produce a sense of well-being in menopausal women, but the increased hirutism, which may already be a problem, can be distressing. Increased libido at this age is also occasionally undesirable.

POSTMENOPAUSAL BLEEDING

If abnormal bleeding occurs during estrogen therapy, treatment should be discontinued immediately and diagnostic curettage performed. It must not be taken for granted that the bleeding is iatrogenic in nature. One of the potential dangers of estrogen therapy in the postmenopause is that the statistical frequency of bleeding secondary to estrogen therapy may mask serious disease. The rule of thumb is that bleeding after menopause is secondary to cancer until proved otherwise. Of 574 patients with postmenopausal bleeding studied, 222 had no demonstrable disease, 148 had be-

nign disease of the corpus, 55 of the cervix, and 45 of the vagina. However, 53 had malignant disease of the corpus, 34 of the cervix, 6 ovary, and 1 of the vulva, which indicates the seriousness of the symptom of bleeding.

CONCLUSION

There is no firm evidence that the development of osteoporosis, arteriosclerotic heart disease, or hyperlipidemia can be prevented by systemic therapy. The amelioration of symptomatic osteoporosis does seem to be clinically substantiated, and there is laboratory evidence to support the efficacy of estrogen therapy pharmacologically in this disease. For the relief of acute symptoms, a wise dictum is to prescribe the lowest adequate dose over the shortest possible time. In patients who require prolonged therapy, periodic endometrial biopsy is mandatory.

The administration of a pill is no substitute for the physician's time and attention. The menopausal patient should be allowed to voice her fears and concerns, whether they be real or imagined. Sympathetic concern and common sense advice often relieves anxieties far better than sedatives and tranquilizers. A new intellectual interest or increased exercise may be more effective and less complicated long-range therapy than estrogen. Finally, cigarette smoking is the common denominator for patients at risk both for postmenopausal arteriosclerosis and osteoporosis. Cigarette smoking should therefore be discouraged in the postmenopausal woman.

REFERENCES AND RECOMMENDED READING

ADOLESCENCE

Aubert ML, Grumbach MM, Kaplan SL: Heterologous radioimmunoassay for plasma human prolactin (hPRL): Values in normal subjects, puberty, pregnancy and in pituitary disorders. Acta Endocrinol (Copenh) 77:460, 1974

Bayley N, Pinneau SR: Tables predicting adult height from skeletal age: Revised for use with the Greulich–Pyle hand standards. J Pediatr 40:432, 1952

Blos P: On Adolescents. New York, Macmillan, 1962

Boyar RM, Finkelstein JW, Rolfwarg H et al: Synchronization of augmented luteinizing hormone secretion with sleep during puberty. N Engl J Med 287:582, 1972

Curtis EM: Normal ovarian histology in infancy and childhood. Obstet Gynecol 19:444, 1962

Duncan JW: An essay on adolescent girls. Med Clin North Am 58:847, 1974

Frasier FD, Smith FG, Jr: Effect of estrogens on mature height in tall girls: A control study. J Clin Endocrinol Metab 28:416, 1968

Frisch RE, McArthur JW: Menstrual cycles: Fatness as a determinant of minimum weight for height necessary for their maintenance or onset. Science 185:949, 1974

Frische RE, Revelle R: Height and weight at menarche and a hypothesis of menarche. Arch Dis Child 46:695, 1971

Frisch RE, Wyshak G, Vincent L: Delayed menarche and amenorrhea in ballet dancers. N Engl J Med 303:17, 1980

Greulich WW, Pyle SI: Radiographic Atlas of Skeletal Development of the Hand and Wrist, 2nd ed. Stanford, Stanford University Press, 1959

Hays GC, Mullard JE: Normal free thyroxin index values in infancy and childhood. J Clin Endocrinol Metab 39:958, 1974

Judd HL, Parker DC, Silver TC et al: The nocturnalization of plasma testosterone in pubertal boys. J Clin Endocrinol Metab 38:710, 1974

Kato J, Atsumi Y, Inaba M: Estradiol receptors in female rat hypothalamus in the developmental stages and during pubescence. Endocrinology 94:309, 1974

Lamberg BA, Kantero RL, Saarinen P et al: Endocrine changes before and after the menarche. III. Total thyroxin and "free thyroxin index" and the binding capacity of thyroxin binding proteins in female adolescents. Acta Endocrinol 74:685, 1973

Lamberg BA, Kantero RL, Saarinen P et al: Endocrine changes before and after the menarche. IV. Serum thyrotropin in female adolescents. Acta Endocrinol 74:695, 1973

Libertun C, Timiras PS, Kragt CL: Sexual differences in the hypothalamic cholinergic system before and after puberty: Inductory effect of testosterone. Neuroendocrinology 12:73, 1973

Marshall WA, Lund JM: Variations in pattern of puberty changes in girls, Arch Dis Child 44:291, 1969

Reyes, FI, Boroditsky RS, Winter JSD et al: Studies on human sexual development. II. Fetal and maternal serum gonadotropin and sex steroid concentrations. J Clin Endocrinol Metab 38:612, 1974

Richman RA, Underwood LE, French SS et al: Adverse effects of large doses of medroxyprogesterone (MPA) in idiopathic isosexual precocity. J Pediatr 79:963, 1971

Root AW: Endocrinology of puberty. I. Normal sexual maturation. J Pediatr 83:1, 1973

Root AW: Endocrinology of puberty. II. Aberrations of sexual maturation. J Pediatr 83:187, 1973

Ruf KB: How does the brain control the process of puberty? Z Neurol 204:95, 1973

Sadeghi-Nejad A, Kaplan SL, Grumbach MM: The effect of medroxyprogesterone acetate on adrenocortical function in children with precocious puberty. J Pediatr 78:616, 1971

Santen RJ, Paulsen CA: Hypogonadotropic eunuchoidism. I. Clinical study of the mode of inheritance. J Clin Endocrinol Metab 36:47, 1973

Tanner JM: Growth at Adolescence, 2nd ed. Oxford, Blackwell, 1962

Van Wyk JJ, Brumbach MM: Syndrome of precocious menstruation and galactorrhea in juvenile hypothyroidism: An example of hormonal overlap in pituitary feedback. J Pediatr 57:416, 1960

Whitelaw MJ: Experiences in treating excessive height in girls with cyclic estradiol valerate. Acta Endocrinol 54:472, 1967

Winter JSD, Faiman C: The development of cyclic pituitary–gonadal function in adolescent females. J Clin Endocrinol Metab 37:714, 1973

Winter JSD, Faiman C: Pituitary–gonadal relations in female children and adolescents. Pediatr Res 7:948, 1973

Zachmann M, Sobradillo B, Frank M et al: Bayley–Pinneau, Roche–Wainer–Thissen, and Tanner height predictions in normal children and in patients with various pathologic conditions. J Pediatr 93:749, 1978

MENSTRUATION

Andersen AM, Larsen JF, Steenstrup OR et al: Effect of bromocriptine on the premenstrual syndrome. A double-blind clinical trial. Br J Obstet Gynaecol 84:370, 1977

Beaton GH, Thein M, Milne H et al: Iron requirements of menstruating women. Am J Clin Nutr 23:275, 1970

Beller FK: Observations on the clotting of menstrual blood and clot formation. Am J Obstet Gynecol 111:535, 1971

Chan WY, Dawood MY, Fuchs F: Relief of dysmenorrhea with prostaglandin synthetase inhibitor ibuprofen: Effect on prostaglandin levels in menstrual fluid. Am J Obstet Gynecol 135:102, 1979

Chiazze L, Jr, Brayer FT, Macisco JJ, Jr et al: The length and variability of the human menstrual cycle. JAMA 203:377, 1968

Coppen A, Kessel N: Menstruation and personality. Br J Psychiatry 109:711, 1963

Dewhurst CJ, Cowell CA, Barrie LC: The regularity of early menstrual cycles. J Obstet Gynaecol Br Commonw 78:1093, 1971

Halbreich V, Assael M, Ben–David M et al: Serum prolactin in women with premenstrual syndrome. Lancet 2:654, 1976

Hanson FW, Izu A, Henzl MR: Naproxen sodium in dysmenorrhea. Its influence in allowing continuation of work/school activities. Obstet Gynecol 52:583, 1978

Henzl MR, Buttram V, Segre EJ et al: Treatment of dysmenorrhea with naproxen sodium: Report on two independent double-blind trials. Am J Obstet Gynecol 127:818, 1977

Henzl MR, Oretga–Herrera E, Rodriquez C et al: Anaprox in dysmenorrhea: Reduction of pain and intrauterine pressure. Am J Obstet Gynecol 135:455, 1979

Henzl MR, Smith RE, Boost, G et al: Lysosomal concept of menstrual bleeding in humans. J Clin Endocrinol Metab 34:860, 1972

Larkin RM, VanOrden DE, Poulson AM et al: Dysmenorrhea: Treatment with an antiprostaglandin. Obstet Gynecol 54:456, 1979

McLennan MT, McLennan CE: Estrogenic status of menstruating and menopausal women assessed by cervical vascular smears. Obstet Gynecol 37:325, 1971

Picoff RC, Luginbuhl WH: Fibrin in the endometrial stroma: Its relation to uterine bleeding. Am J Obstet Gynecol 88:642, 1964

Quick AJ: Menstruation in hereditary bleeding disorders. Obstet Gynecol 28:37, 1966

Ross GT, Cargille CM, Lipset MB et al: Pituitary and gonadal hormones in women during spontaneous and induced ovulatory cycles. Recent Prog Horm Res 26:1, 1970

Rybo G: Clinical and experimental studies on menstrual blood loss. Acta Obstet Gynaecol Scand 45, Suppl 7, 1966

Sommer B: The effect of menstruation on cognitive and perceptual–motor behavior: A review. Psychosm Med 35:515, 1973

CLIMACTERIC

Aitken JM, Hart DM, Andersen JB et al: Osteoporosis after oophorectomy for non-malignant disease in premenopausal women. Br Med J 2:325, 1973

Albright F, Smith PH, Richardson AM: Postmenopausal osteoporosis: Its clinical features. JAMA 116:24, 1941

Alvia JF et al.: Prevention of involutional bone by exercise. Am Int Med 89:356, 1978

Antunes CMF, Stolley PD, Rosenshein NB et al: Endometrial cancer and estrogen use. Report of a large case control study. N Engl J Med 300:9, 1979

Baird BT, Guevara A: Concentration of unconcentrated estrone and estradiol in peripheral plasma in non-pregnant women throughout the menstrual cycle, castrate and post-menopausal women and in men. J Clin Endocrinol Metab 29:149, 1969

Crilly R, Cawood M, Marshall DH et al.: Hormonal status in normal osteoporotic corticosteroid treated post-menopausal women. J R Soc Med 71:733, 1978

Daniell HW: Osteoporosis and the slender smoker. Arch Intern Med 136:298, 1976

Grodin JM, Siiteri TK, MacDonald TC: Source of estrogen production in postmenopausal women. J Clin Endocrinol Metab 36:207, 1973

Gusberg SB: Hormone dependence of endometrial carcinoma. Obstet Gynecol 30:287, 1967

Hammond CB, Jelovsek FR, Lee KL et al: Effects of long-term estrogen replacement therapy. II. Neoplasia. Am J Obstet Gynecol 113:537, 1979

Hoover R, Gray LA, Cole P et al.: Menopausal estrogens and breast cancer. N Engl J Med 295:401, 1976

Horwitz RI, Feinstein AR: Alternative analytic methods for case-control studies of estrogens and endometrial cancer. N Engl J Med 299:1089, 1978

Hulka BS: Effect of exogenous estrogen on postmenopausal women: the epidemiologic evidence. Obstet Gynecol Surv 35:389, 1980

Jowsey J: Why is minimal nutrition important in osteoporosis? Geriatrics 33:39, 1978

Mattingly RF, Huang WY: Steroidogenesis of the menopausal and postmenopausal ovary. Am J Obstet Gynecol 103:679, 1969

Newcomer ED et al: Lactase deficiency: Prevalence in osteoporosis. Ann Intern Med 89:218, 1978

Poliak A, Jones GS, Goldberg B et al: Effect of human chorionic gonadotropin on postmenopausal women. Am J Obstet Gynecol 101:731, 1968

Poliak A, Smith JJ, Friedlander D et al: Estrogen synthesis in castrated women: The action of human chorionic gonadotropin and corticotropin. Am J Obstet Gynecol 110:376, 1971

Rasmussen H, Bordier P: The Physiological and Cellular Basis of Metabolic Bone Disease. Baltimore, Williams & Wilkins, 1974

Rosenwaks Z, Wentz AC, Jones GS et al: Endometrial pathology and estrogens. Obstet Gynecol 53:403, 1979

Schiff I, Ryan KJ: Benefits of estrogen replacement. Obstet Gynecol Surv 35:400, 1980

Smith DC, Rose P, Thompson DJ et al: Association of exogenous estrogen and endometrial carcinoma. N Engl J Med 293:1164, 1975

Smith EL: The Effects of Physical Activity on Bone in the Aged. International Conference on Bone Mineral Measurement, Chicago, October 12–13, 1973. DHEW Publication No. (NIH) 75-683. Bethesda, Public Health Service, 1974

Ziel HK, Finkle WD: Increased risk of endometrial carcinoma among users of conjugated estrogens. N Engl J Med 293:1167, 1975

MISCELLANEOUS REFERENCES

Baugh R, Brown J, Sargeant R et al: Separation of human factor VIII activity from the von Willenbrand's antigen and ristocetin platelet aggregating activity. Biochim Biophys Acta 371:360, 1974

Chari S, Hopkinson CRN, Duane E et al: Purification of "in-

hibin" from human follicular fluid. Acta Endocrinol (Copenh) 90:157, 1979

Coronary drug project: Initial findings leading to modification of its research protocol. JAMA 214(7):1303, 1970

Cutler BS, Forbes AP, Ingersol FM et al: Endometrial carcinoma after stilbestrol therapy in gonadal dysgenesis. N Engl J Med 287:628, 1972

Guyda HJ, Friesen HG: Serum prolactin levels in humans from birth to adult life. Pediatr Res 7:534, 1973

Henson A, Mattern MJ, Laliger EA: Hemophilia A with apparently autosomal dominant inheritance: Evidence for a second autosomal locus involved in factor VIII production. Thromb Diath Haemorrh 14:341, 1965

Levina SE: Times of appearance of LH and FSH activities in human fetal circulation. Gen Comp Endocrinol 19:242, 1972

Partanen S, Hervonen A: Monoamine-containing structures in the hypothalamohypophyseal system in the human fetus. Z Anat Entwicklungs Gesch 140:52, 1973

Payne AH, Jaffe RV: Androgen formation from pregnenolone sulfate by the human fetal ovary. J Clin Endocrinol Metab 39:300, 1974

Rubin RT, Poland RE, Rubin LE et al: The neuroendocrinology of human sleep. Life Sci 14:1041, 1974

Sassin JF, Fratz AG, Weitzman ED et al: Human prolactin 24 hour pattern with increased release during sleep. Science 177:1205, 1972

Seigel S, Corfman P: Epidemiological problems associated with studies of the safety of oral contraceptives. JAMA 203:148, 1965

Siler–Khodr PM, Morgenstern LL, Greenwood FC: Hormone synthesis and release from human fetal adenohypophysis in vitro. J Clin Endocrinol Metab 39:891, 1974

Spanos E, Pike JW, Hausslen MR et al: Circulating 1,25-dihydroxy-vitamin D in the chicken: Enhancement by injection of prolactin during the egg laying. Life Sci 19:1751, 1976

Steinberger A, Steinberger E: Secretion of an FSH inhibiting factor by cultured Sertoli cells. Endocrinol 99:918, 1976

Symmers W St C: Carcinoma of breast in transsexual individuals after surgical and hormonal interference with the primary and secondary sex characteristics. Br Med J 2:83, 1968

Tamura T, Minaguchi H, Sakamoto S: Responsiveneess of human fetal pituitary to hypothalamic hormones in vitro. Endocrinol Jpn 20:545, 1973

Veterans Administration Cooperative Study: An evaluation of estrogenic substances in the treatment of cerebral vascular disease. Circulation 33:(5) S II:2, 1966

Wilkinson EJ, Friedrich R, Jr, Mattingly RF et al: Turner's syndrome with endometrial adenocarcinoma and stilbestrol therapy. Obstet Gynecol 42:193, 1973

Winters AJ, Eskay RL, Porter JC: Concentration and distribution of TRH and LRH in the human fetal brain. J Clin Endocrinol Metab 39:960, 1974

THE PATIENT

John T. Queenan

THE PHYSICIAN-PATIENT RELATIONSHIP

More than is true of most physician–patient dialogues, a woman's initial visit to the gynecologist's office can be fraught with anxiety, concern, and even humiliation. Whatever her age, social background, or previous experience—and all these influence her reaction—she usually expects the encounter with the gynecologist and the examination to be uncomfortble both emotionally and physically. Unfortunately, misapprehensions about the experience are all too common; rumor and hyperbole often heighten a young patient's fears. Even more unfortunately, previous experiences may have given this anxiety a very real foundation. It is the physician's responsibility to allay undue apprehension, dispel false impressions, and make the visit as comfortable and informative as possible so that the patient leaves the office calm and in an improved frame of mind. This is best achieved by an understanding atti-

tude and a matter-of-fact approach. Condescension and domination have no place in the physician–patient relationship.

Even under the best of circumstances, the patient is likely to find the visit disagreeable. Soon after entering the office or clinic, she is asked to discuss her most personal problems, which she has mentioned to few, if any, others. Then, after verbally exposing herself, she must undress, put on the most unappealing of garments, and be examined by a complete stranger. No wonder the visit to the gynecologist for an annual checkup or for help with a pressing problem is rarely anticipated with enthusiasm. Indeed, subsequent visits are usually as trying as the first.

The patient is sensitive to subtle nuances in the physician's words or facial expression, a fact rarely appreciated by the busy practitioner. The physician's demeanor is extremely important in allaying the patient's anxiety and in establishing rapport; the physician who appears abrupt, preoccupied, hurried, hesitant, embarrassed, or flippant can destroy the possibility of a satisfactory physician–patient relationship. Frivolity and lightheartedness rarely have a place in the initial evaluation. The seriousness of the moment for the patient should be foremost in the physician's mind. Propriety of address and composure are qualities all patients appreciate and respect. The physician should express sincere concern in a friendly, direct atmosphere.

There are other rules for the relationship of an obstetrician–gynecologist with the patient. Many women have expressed resentment toward physicians who address their patients by first names, or as "dear" or whatever, considering this an undue familiarity. Use of surnames also has a practical value, for a midnight call from "Janet" may be recognized less quickly than a call from "Janet Henderson" or "Mrs. Henderson." While conducting the examination the physician should not "think out loud," articulating possible diagnoses, for needless and disturbing explanations may be required later. Finally, the physician should evaluate the patient's mien and attitude, and make every effort to adjust to it. Patients will not alter or adjust their personalities to conform to the wishes of the physician; any adjusting that is needed must be done by the physician.

Today, women are more curious and more knowledgeable about anatomy and physiology than ever before. Voluminous data, both accurate and inaccurate, are readily available to them. Lay periodicals abound in articles on contraception, sexual function, abortion, obstetric practices, and gynecologic operative procedures. The physician must often correct misinformation and educate. A forthright dialogue with full explanation of the diagnosis and rationale for therapy is essential to effective physician–patient communication. An explanation of what medications are being prescribed and why, and a straightforward discussion

of anticipated surgical procedures, duration of hospital stay, potential complications, and possible sequelae constitute the minimum information a gynecologist owes the patient.

The physician must be honest and forthright in answering the probing questions asked by today's woman. If the physician is not familiar with certain matters, it is acceptable to admit the lack of knowledge and to express a willingness to obtain the appropriate information. A vague answer or avoidance of the question altogether is unacceptable.

Every patient is a combination of anatomic, physiologic, endocrinologic, and psychologic components. In evaluating her condition, the physician must not let the parts obscure the whole patient. She can well appreciate that one component is diseased, but it is the whole person who wishes to know what is happening, what is to be done, and what will be the results. This is the minimum information she deserves.

THE HISTORY

When large numbers of patients are involved, as in a clinic setting or a very busy office, certain basic information (*e.g.,* age, ethnic background, marital status, obstetric history, and whatever the patient may wish to divulge about the problem for which she consults the physician) is often obtained by interview with an office nurse or by a questionnaire the patient is asked to fill out. Although these devices are sometimes considered essential, it is astonishing how little time they really save; and by obtaining these data personally, the physician provides a logical opening for the interview and establishes a preliminary rapport with the patient. In addition, the manner in which she answers these mundane questions may alert the physician to areas that should be probed more deeply.

The setting for the history taking is important. A quiet area where distractions (telephone calls, interruptions) can be kept to a minimum and where privacy is ensured promotes a comfortable dialogue between physician and patient. The foundation for rapport in a continuing relation can be established during these 15–30 minutes of the initial history taking. This is perhaps the most critical time the physician spends with most patients.

HISTORY OF THE OBSTETRIC PATIENT

The patient's initial obstetric visit does not usually pose a diagnostic problem. She may have been referred by another physician who has already confirmed her pregnancy, or she may have made the diagnosis herself on the basis of a home pregnancy test kit. The obstetrician, however, should review recent events and confirm the probability of pregnancy, the current sta-

tus of the pregnancy, the patient's general well-being, and her feelings about the pregnancy. The obstetrician should never accept another's diagnosis. While the occasion would certainly be uncommon, the patient's presumption of pregnancy can be in error—based merely on an overdue period coupled with the fear of or desire for a pregnancy.

The obstetric history should include the following information:

History of current pregnancy
    Date of last menstrual period
    Bleeding, spotting, or staining since last normal period
    Pelvic cramps noted since last period
    Documentation of positive result on pregnancy test
    Findings of previous pelvic examinations during this pregnancy and relative uterine size
    Whether this pregnancy was planned
    Patient's attitude to the pregnancy
History of menstrual function
    Age of menarche
    Regularity of menstrual cycle
    Frequency of menstrual flow
    Use of contraceptives, in particular birth control pills, and how long since these were discontinued
    Whether pregnancy immediately followed discontinuance of oral contraception or progesterone withdrawal
    History of dysmenorrhea
Past obstetric history
    Number of pregnancies
    Number of living children
    Number of abortions, spontaneous or induced
    History of preceding pregnancies (duration of pregnancy, antepartum complications, duration of labor, type of delivery, anesthesia employed, intrapartum complications, postpartum complications, hospital, physician, time when deliveries occurred)
    Perinatal status of fetuses (birth weights, comments pediatrician may have made, and perhaps comments about early growth and development of children, including feeding habits, growth, and overall well-being)
Previous gynecologic history
    Date on pelvic examinations, uterine size
    Vaginal infections
    Previous pelvic surgery
    Abnormal results of cytologic examinations
    Treatment of cervical disease (cauterization, cryosurgery)
    Use of hormone agents, including birth control pills and fertility pills, and when discontinued
    Treatment for venereal disease
Current medical history
    Medications currently taken (sedatives, hypnotics, psychotropic agents)

Allergy to medications and specific reactions to them

Potential teratogenic events during this pregnancy (viral infections, roentgenographic examinations, medications)

Past medical history

Conditions for which physician treatment or hospitalization has been required

Surgical history (type of operation, anesthesia employed, problems related to anesthesia, postoperative complications)

Bleeding disorders or tendency

Requirement for blood transfusions (blood type and Rh status, if known)

Review of systems

Neurologic disorders

Pulmonary disorders

Cardiac disorders

Gastrointestinal disorders (nausea, vomiting, constipation, diarrhea, melena)

Genitourinary disorders (frequency, nocturia, dysuria, incontinence)

Cardiovascular symptoms (edema, leg cramps, history of phlebitis, fainting, other signs of vascular instability)

Social history

Drug use

Smoking habits

Alcohol use

Family history

Preeclampsia, diabetes, hypertension, hematologic disorders

Occurrence of twins, impression of weights of babies in family

Dietary history

Maternal food ingestion, fads, cravings

Vitamin ingestion

History taking should be a dialogue conducted with a minimum of stress. The physician should use terms the patient can understand. He or she should not assume that the patient understands the relevance of the questions and should follow questions with explanations, when needed, of why they are asked. Professional people, nurses and physicians should be treated the same way. The obstetrician must not assume that they know what to mention. If it appears that the questions are not clearly understood, they must be rephrased. The more questions asked during the course of the interview, the more answers and data are accumulated.

HISTORY OF THE GYNECOLOGIC PATIENT

There can be no set pattern for the gynecologic history taking. Certain obvious medical data should be obtained in a straightforward manner. However, appreciation of subtle aspects of the patient's history, social circumstances, and functioning requires time and subsequent visits.

The patient's own description of her primary symptoms is the first matter for discussion. It is wise for the physician to say as little as possible and allow the patient to elaborate. General questions can be asked to help her expand on a subject, but judgmental comments should not be made. The physician should not exhibit amazement no matter how bizarre the information unearthed by the history. Neither should practices that do not conform to the physician's own moral code be criticized, unless they are detrimental to the patient's health, in which case their unsuitability should be explained in these terms.

Duration, severity of the disorder, frequency of occurrence, and what aspect is most bothersome to the patient constitute the basic information that can be elaborated on by guided questioning. After the patient has had her say, the physician should pursue pertinent questions, not only to complete the clinical picture but also to demonstrate concern for the patient. The comfort and confidence that can be established in the history taking can make the examination easier and more productive.

The gynecologic history should include the following information:

Chief complaint

The primary problem

Its duration

Its severity

Occurrence in relation to other functions (menstrual cycle, coital activity, gastrointestinal activity, voiding, or other pertinent functions)

Any previous similar symptom and its diagnosis and management

Change in normal lifestyle resulting from the complaint

Menstrual history

Date of onset of last menstrual period

Frequency of menstrual periods

Duration of flow

Degree of discomfort

Menarche

Regularity of menstrual flow

Quantity of menstrual flow (number of pads used per day)

Obstetric history

Number of pregnancies

Miscarriages

Obstetric problems

Response to pregnancies

Gynecologic history

Galactorrhea

Findings of previous gynecologic examinations

Previous gynecologic surgery, including details

Vaginal infections, abnormal results of cytologic examinations
Venereal disease
Medical history
Medical symptoms for which care was required
Surgical history
Any operative procedures
Review of systems
Pulmonary disorders
Cardiac disorders
Gastrointestinal disorders
Genitourinary disorders
Vascular disease, especially circulatory defects affecting extremities
Leg cramps
Phlebitis
Social history
Drug use
Alcohol use
Smoking habits
Marital status
Number of years married
Coital activity (libido, dyspareunia, orgasm)
Family history
Significant medical and surgical disorders in family members
Nutrition
Assessment of dietary habits, affection for fad diets
Use of vitamins
Medications taken
Hormone pills, birth control pills, fertility pills
Medications employed on a long- or short-term basis, especially sedatives, hypnotics, psychotropic agents

The history provides information about the total patient and is perhaps the most important part of the gynecologic evaluation. It enables the patient to become acquainted with the physician in a nonthreatening situation. In most cases, it gives the physician data to establish a tentative diagnosis before the physical examination. In many respects, the gynecologist who takes a history is like the detective who keeps the various clues that are pertinent and discards those that are deliberately or inadvertently misleading. If the gynecologic history is sufficiently penetrating, it should in almost all cases permit the physician to narrow the likely possibilities to one, or at most two, probable diagnoses. This preliminary opinion may not always be correct, but the history-taking session should not be ended until a tentative diagnosis has been made.

Like a hospital chart, the office history is a legal, as well as a medical, record. As such, it is subject to subpoena, and whatever is recorded in it may at some future date need to be defended in court. It should not contain extraneous or casually written material, and the notes should be sufficiently complete that the case can be readily reconstructed.

TYPES OF PATIENTS

The *neonate* is occasionally brought to the gynecologist's office because of vaginal discharge or bleeding. The true patient is not the infant, who is responding physiologically to the withdrawal of maternal estrogen, but an anxious and justifiably apprehensive mother who needs reassurance.

The *young child* is frequently brought to the office because of a mother's concern about a genital problem, such as pruritus or discharge, that she cannot explain. In dealing with a young child, the gynecologist's primary responsibility is to avoid creating fear or apprehension. Gentleness is mandatory, but the examination should never be compromised because of the child's possible sensitivity. On rare occasions significant pathology, such as sarcoma botryoides, may be present. Overnight hospitalization and pelvic evaluation under anesthesia may be required, but in the long run this will be far less traumatic than examining a frightened child in the office.

Today, an increasing number of mothers are bringing an *adolescent* daughter to the gynecologist for her first examination. Simple problems of breast development, vaginal discharge, irregularity of menses, and painful menstruation should be discussed openly and treated appropriately. Reassurance is important, regardless of the findings. Minutes spent in such education and preparation of the maturing adolescent can do much to establish a healthy attitude toward reproductive functions and should set the stage for good gynecologic care in the future.

Occasionally, a teenager is brought to the gynecologist in the hope that responsibility for sex education can be shifted from parents to physician. While this is certainly not the ideal approach, the responsibility for sex education cannot be ignored. In such a case it is appropriate for the physician, in the quiet atmosphere of a discussion (preferably without a parent present), to explain such matters as menstrual function, the physiology of maturation, pregnancy, and contraception. There may also be opportunity to discuss venereal disease and, in some cases, the psychologic maladjustments that can result from the new freedom of sexual expression. Adolescence is not the time to correct educational and cultural maladjustments that have been established over the years, but it is of great value for the teenage girl to have access to a person who is knowledgeable and concerned about her well-being.

The *mature woman* does not have the identical complaints of her adolescent counterpart, although some of the symptoms may be similar. She does require, however, the same care and consideration. It is a mistake to presume that, because a woman is sexually active, has borne children, seems familiar with contraceptive agents, and has undergone multiple gynecologic evaluations, she will be at ease with the present examination. When the physician undertakes

the pelvic examination as a routine and perfunctory procedure, the patient immediately senses it and her response is quite negative.

Some of the problems of the *postmenopausal woman,* notably hot flashes and atrophic vaginitis, are the direct result of estrogen deficiency. But it is a serious error to presume that all emotional and physical problems that arise in this age group are "due to the change." Of special importance are depression, irritability, and anxiety. Sometimes they result from the woman's conviction that the menopause marks the onset of senility and that her years of attractiveness and femininity are past. Reassurance and an explanation of the positive and rewarding aspects of the menopausal years can be of much help. Emotional problems are often the direct result of the stresses that commonly beset women of this age group: responsibility for aging parents, sons and daughters whose attitudes seem unacceptable, and marital problems that may be compounded by the demands of the patient's or her husband's employment. In a few cases, the stage is already set for mental illness, and the menopause is a nonspecific precipitating factor. It is, of course, idle to presume that problems such as these can be solved by prescribing estrogens, and it is axiomatic that physical and emotional disorders arising in the menopausal or postmenopausal years should be investigated on their own merits. Problems of patients in this age group deserve the same consideration accorded problems of younger patients.

Perhaps no single condition is responsible for more obstetric and operative morbidity than obesity. Our culture accepts overweight as a fact of life. In no other nation is obesity more of a problem. It is truly remarkable that, even though so many medical disorders are related to obesity, an intensive effort has not yet been made to combat overweight. For the gynecologic as well as the obstetric patient, obesity predisposes not only to simple problems of hygiene and a greater frequency of vaginitis, but also to more significant intra- and postoperative complications. The physician should suggest diet control and a program of physical activity for such a patient. Here, as in few other circumstances in medicine, a potentially hazardous clinical problem must be approached aggressively.

OFFICE OPERATIONS

Today, many procedures heretofore considered hospital practices are performed in the physician's office. Cervical biopsy, endometrial aspiration, and cryosurgery for chronic cervicitis are now routinely done in the gynecologist's office. It is not uncommon for amniocentesis to be performed in the office, and the colposcopically directed biopsy is also an office operation. These procedures involve equipment unfamiliar to most patients. The purpose of the procedure and the functioning of the equipment should be explained to the patient.

SEXUALITY

Major cultural changes in recent years have allowed women to express their individuality more freely. The Women's Movement, a rebellion against traditional male domination, is one aspect of this change. Many women today resent and distrust men who are in positions of authority. The male gynecologist is in just such a position, and he must learn not only to respect his patient's individuality but also to deal with his own discomfort in the face of her hostility.

Cultural change has also sanctioned greater sexual freedom for women and a code of sexual morality that conflicts with traditional values. Though the patient may not specifically refer to sexual attitudes, it is safe to assume that many young women experience serious anxiety in this area. The physician's role is never to judge. It is to counsel and educate—forthrightly if the patient asks, tactfully if she only hints at questions.

The enormous amount of popular writing about sex and sexuality may be the source of the patient's questions. The gynecologist should be prepared to discuss masturbation, orgasm, coital positions, and sexual techniques—topics once rarely mentioned but now commonplace.

In addition, the gynecologist is often the first physician whose advice is sought regarding marital and sexual problems. For the busy practitioner this is time-consuming and frustrating. The physician's degree of involvement, of course, is related to interest and time available, but a request for help must not be passed off with the suggestion that the problem will take care of itself in time. The gynecologist should be versed in basic counseling and questioning techniques and should be able to offer some elementary recommendations. He or she must be prepared to evaluate the severity of such problems and to direct the troubled patient or couple to another physician or an appropriate agency for help.

THE PHYSICAL EXAMINATION

It is important for the obstetrician–gynecologist to know the physical condition of the patient. In the case of the obstetric patient, a complete physical examination and appropriate laboratory tests should be performed at the first visit. A complete physical examination may or may not be a part of the first or subsequent office visit of the gynecologic patient. For the woman in good health who has consulted an internist recently or is under the care of an internist for some on-going disorder, such as hypertension or diabetes, a complete physical examination is not needed. For the woman

with an endocrine disorder, a complete physical examination clearly should be a part of the gynecologist's evaluation. The designation of the obstetrician–gynecologist as a "primary physician for women" is variously interpreted by the practitioners of this discipline. An important part of this responsibility is referral to other physicians for such special examinations as may be needed, including referral to a family practitioner or an internist for periodic physical appraisal. Except for the breasts, which should be examined at every gynecologic visit, the detail of the physical evaluation of gynecologic patients varies according to the circumstances.

Upon entering the examining room, the physician should make some brief comment to put the patient at ease, but to expect the patient to "relax" is probably out of the question. During the physical examination another woman participant, usually a nurse or aide, must be present. Not only can this woman assist the physician, but she lends an element of psychologic support to the patient. Her presence is also of legal importance to the physician as a guard against accusations that may be initiated by an unscrupulous or disturbed patient. The dialogue between physician and patient should continue during the examination. Distracting conversation with the nurse or aide tends to influence the patient adversely and detracts from the physician–patient rapport.

EVALUATION OF GENERAL APPEARANCE

A general impression should be recorded of the color, texture, and coarseness of the patient's skin, of birth marks, of the condition of her fingernails, and of her state of nutrition.

EXAMINATION OF THE HEAD AND NECK

The patient's hair should be examined for cleanliness, texture, and scalp health. Eye examination should include funduscopy to detect retinal aberrations. The patient's nose, throat, and teeth should be checked. Otoscopy should be performed, and the anterior cervical, posterior cervical, and supraclavicular nodes should be palpated. The thyroid gland should be palpated both in the direct anteroposterior position and with the patient's head turned.

CHEST EXAMINATION

From the back, the vertebral column can be assessed and degree of curvature noted. The chest should be percussed and auscultated, and the breasts examined (see Ch. 59). The heart should then be percussed and auscultated.

EXAMINATION OF THE ABDOMEN

The patient should be positioned supine, with her arms against her body, in order to relax the abdominal musculature. The knees should be elevated and flexed, also to decrease abdominal wall tone. In methodical and consistent fashion, all quadrants of the abdomen should be examined, percussed, and palpated. Relaxation of the abdomen to elevate a suspected mass can be assisted by having the patient breathe deeply and then exhale. After all quadrants have been examined, the inguinal nodes should be palpated. Abdominal scars should be discussed; even though the surgery has been noted during history taking, new information may be learned at this time.

EXAMINATION OF THE LOWER EXTREMITIES

Examination of the lower extremities supplies important information regarding the cardiovascular system. The presence of significant varicosities, for example, would be a disturbing finding in a multigravida. Peripheral pulses should be checked.

PELVIC EXAMINATION

The pelvic examination consists of inspection and palpation. To allow adequate exposure, the patient should be placed in the lithotomy position. She should be reasonably comfortable and properly draped.

Except in special circumstances, a deftly performed bimanual pelvic examination should not be painful. Special circmstances might involve the patient who is virginal and has not used tampons for menstrual protection and the woman with an inflammatory or other painful condition. Such a patient should understand in advance the nature of the information needed and the probability that the examination will be uncomfortable. In some cases sufficient information can be obtained by using the index finger only for the bimanual examination instead of inflicting the discomfort of the more customary index and middle fingers.

The vulva should be examined for general state of hygiene, growth of hair, regions of ulceration, rash, discoloration, labial abnormalities, excessive vaginal discharge, evidence of perineal trauma from previous deliveries, and evidence of rectal disease such as hemorrhoids. Bartholin's and Skene's glands can be inspected and palpated. The labia should be spread apart for inspection of the labia minora as well as the urethra. Severe vesicovaginal or rectal prolapse can be appreciated at this point. Having the patient strain down may allow better assessment of anatomic distortion.

The physician should prepare the patient for any pelvic manipulation by warning her in advance of examining fingers and speculum. This is important not

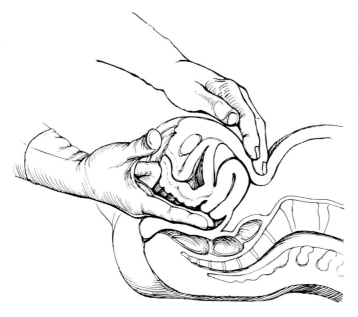

FIG. 9–1. Bimanual examination, *first step.* Vaginal fingers first feel consistency and symmetry of cervix and its axis in relation to axis of vagina. They then elevate uterus toward abdominal wall so total length of uterus can be determined. (Modified from Duncan AS. In Bourne A: British Gynaecological Practice, 1st ed. Philadelphia, Davis, 1955. Figure drawn by G McHugh)

only because the patient cannot see what is going on but also because the area to be examined is extremely sensitive, both psychologically and physically.

A Graves bivalve speculum is employed for visualization of the vagina and cervix. Several points of technique should be remembered. If material is to be obtained for cytologic examination, the speculum should be rinsed in warm water; if not, the instrument should be lubricated. By spreading the labia and placing some tension on the posterior fourchette, the speculum can be gently inserted downward at an angle of about 45° to avoid the urethra. This angled insertion is necessary because, with the patient in a supine position, the vagina is not horizontal. The speculum should be completely inserted and rotated to the horizontal plane. In most patients, it should now lie inferior to the cervix. With the gentle opening of the speculum, the valves separate and the cervix can be visualized.

The cervix should be inspected for color, erosion, degree of dicharge, evidence of trauma, presence of lesions. Two smears are usually taken: 1) a scraping from the region of the squamocolumnar junction of the cervix and 2) a collection of cells from the posterior fornix. Each is smeared on a glass slide and fix-dried by an aerosol spray. When the vaginal sidewalls have been examined, the speculum may be gently rotated to get a more complete view of the superior and inferior surfaces of the vaginal vault.

In the patient with severe vaginitis, when immediate microscopic assessment is desirable, the secretions that have pooled in the inferior valve of the speculum can be used as the sample for microscopic study; otherwise, a vaginal aspirate may be obtained. The speculum should then be withdrawn over the cervix and

slowly removed; during withdrawal the walls of the vagina can be visualized and the supporting structures assessed for cystocele and rectocele. Incontinence may be demonstrated by asking the patient to cough after the speculum has been removed, provided the bladder contains sufficient urine. Usually, however, the patient has voided before the examination and this assessment is not possible.

Various authors describe different techniques for the bimanual examination. One method is illustrated in Figures 9–1 through 9–5. Generally, the physician should acquire proficiency with the index and middle fingers of one hand and then always use that hand for the vaginal examination. After the speculum has been withdrawn, the physician should gently insert the index and middle fingers along the posterior wall of the vagina. It is helpful to place a stool at the base of the examining table and support the examining arm and elbow during the examination. This support of the elbow allows greater sensitivity in the examining fingers. At the same time, a second dimension is added by pressing on the patient's abdomen with the other hand. The first palpable structure is the cervix. Next is the anteriorly placed uterine fundus. The bimanual technique can outline its position, size, shape, consistency, and degree of mobility. Uterine or cervical mobility can be further assessed by placing the fingers on one side of the structure and moving it to the contralateral side. This can be done on both right and left sides to detect chronic or acute inflammatory changes and fixation. The abdominal hand is then placed on one lower quadrant and slowly worked inferiorly and medially to meet the examining fingers of the vaginal hand. In this way, adnexal structures on that side can

FIG. 9-2. Bimanual examination, *second step.* Vaginal fingers are moved into anterior fornix to permit palpation of uterine corpus. If abdominal wall is thin and well relaxed, it is possible by this maneuver to define even minor irregularities in contour or consistency of uterus. *Third step.* With vaginal fingers still in anterior fornix and with aid of abdominal hand, uterus is moved gently toward retroverted position and then from side to side to determine its mobility and presence or absence of pain on movement of uterus. (Figure drawn by G McHugh)

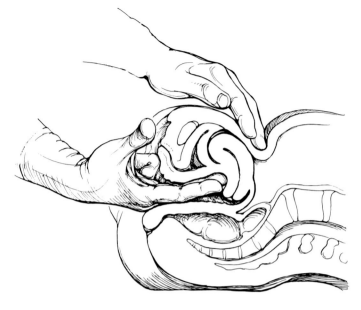

FIG. 9-3. If fingertips of abdominal and vaginal hands come together in carrying out step 2, it can be concluded that uterus is retroverted; vaginal fingers are then moved to posterior fornix to outline symmetry, consistency, and mobility of retroverted corpus. (Figure drawn by G McHugh)

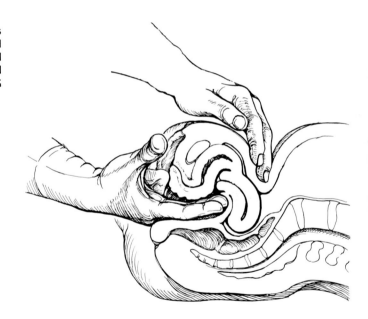

be appreciated. The degree of adherence of an adnexal structure to the uterus can be ascertained. Enlargement, consistency, and position of ovaries and tubes can be noted. Expressions of pain and discomfort should be heeded. The ovary is a sensitive structure, and patients differ in tolerance to palpation. The contralateral side should be similarly examined.

A third dimension in the bimanual examination is the rectovaginal examination. A fresh glove is donned, and the lubricated middle finger is inserted in the pa-tient's rectum and the index finger in the vagina. Hemorrhoids, sphincter tone, and perineal integrity are evaluated. The pouch of Douglas is checked for masses. Uterosacral ligaments can be palpated for tone and nodularity. This examination permits palpation a little higher than is possible in vaginal bimanual examination and should be employed in almost all patients, repeating the steps noted earlier.

When the patient is apprehensive and difficult to examine, the procedure is sometimes facilitated by

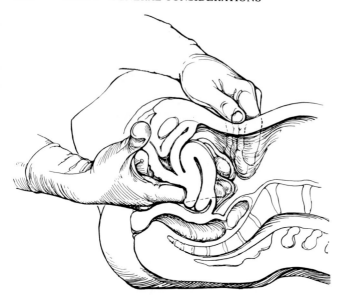

FIG. 9-4. Bimanual examination, *fourth step.* To outline adnexa, vaginal fingers are moved to right fornix, and examiner attempts to bring abdominal and vaginal fingers together at a point presumed to be superior to tube and ovary. (Figure drawn by G McHugh)

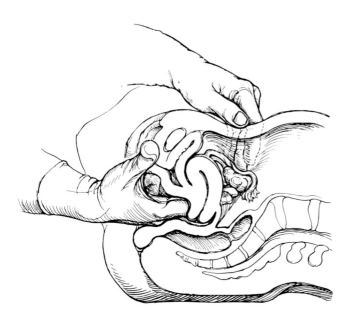

FIG. 9-5. Bimanual examination, *fifth step.* When fingers of abdominal and vaginal hands are quite close together (it is desirable, but not always possible, to approximate these fingers), they are then moved gently toward examiner so adnexa slip between fingers and can so be outlined. (Figure drawn by G McHugh)

having the patient place her hands on her abdomen, inhale deeply, and then exhale completely. Hyperventilation must be avoided, however.

After the examination is completed, the physician should assist the patient to a sitting position and leave the examining room.

The information gained from the pelvic examination can be recorded in the following outline form:

Perineum
    Old lacerations

External genitalia
    Stage of development
    Color
    Evidence of lesions
    Bartholin's glands
Vestibule
    Skene's glands
    Urethral orifice
    Hymenal ring
Vagina
    Presence of leukorrhea

Color
Lesions
Tone
Rugae
Cervix
    Shape
    Consistency
    Mobility
    State of parity
    Lesions
Uterus
    Position
    Mobility
    Size
    Shape
    Consistency
Adnexa
    Position and mobility of ovaries and tubes
    Presence of masses or tenderness
Results of rectovaginal examination
    Degree of confirmation of previous findings
    Statement about additional pathology

When the patient rejoins the physician in the consultation room, diagnosis and findings should be explained in terms she can understand. The implications of the findings should be carefully detailed. It is occasionally helpful to have the patient paraphrase what the physician has said to make certain she understands. This is especially relevant when surgery is contemplated, for the nuances of an operation and its results may be unclear to the patient. At this time, the use of medications and the duration of their use must be explained. The physician should also carefully explain the symptoms that may be expected after any treatment given during the office visit (*e.g.,* heavy leukorrhea following cryosurgery or bleeding following cervical biopsy). Advice against coitus should be given when appropriate, and the duration of abstinence should be made clear. The importance of a follow-up examination should be stressed. Prescriptions for hormones should be adequately detailed and restrictions on refills explicitly stated.

RAPE*

Many gynecologists are reluctant to become involved in cases of alleged rape because the time required for courtroom procedures infringes on their other professional duties. Nevertheless, as physicians, their primary responsibility is the care of their patients, and when this care extends outside the hospital and into a court of law, the responsibility remains.

Rape is a legal rather than a medical diagnosis. The physician can testify about the findings at the time of

---

* See also ACOG Technical Bulletin #52 (November, 1978).

examination, but the court must decide whether rape occurred. The record of the examination of a rape victim, whether emergency room record or physician's office chart, should be complete in every respect. It is the responsibility of the physician to document fully the state of the patient, from her emotional composure to her physical appearance. Data should be recorded as fact; allegations should be recorded as allegations, since the legal status of the situation is undefined at the time of the examination.

HISTORY

A thorough history of the episode should include locale, time, description of the assailant, and description of the alleged assault with particular reference to penetration and ejaculation. While this interrogation will probably have been done earlier by police authorities, the physician's interview supplies corroborating evidence in a court of law.

PHYSICAL EXAMINATION

The record should note the patient's overall appearance and the state of her clothing, composure, and attitude. Physical examination should include a search for evidence of trauma and recent injury. Pertinent negative points should be noted. All data, from vital signs to the findings of a thorough physical examination, should be documented. The record of the pelvic examination should include all findings that support the allegation of rape, such as evidence of trauma and lacerations.

LABORATORY DATA

In some cities, local crime laboratories have attained great expertise in the processing of evidence in cases of rape and have prepared detailed instructions for obtaining the materials for analysis. When appropriate, they wish to have and are equipped to take photographs that can later be used as evidence. If specimens are sent to the crime laboratory, duplicates should also be submitted to the hospital laboratory.

Laboratory evaluations should include a complete blood count, a serologic test for syphilis, blood typing, Rh determination, and blood tests for alcohol and drugs. Vaginal aspirate should be studied for mobile sperm, acid phosphatase, and ABO antigens. Cervical and vaginal material should be cultured for gonorrheal organisms. Slides should be obtained for permanent fixation to show the presence of sperm. Other specimens that should be obtained include clippings and washings from pubic hair, debris from beneath fingernails, and washings of blood or foreign material obtained from clothes.

TREATMENT

Treatment consists of medication to prevent pregnancy. Common prescriptions are diethylstilbestrol, 25 mg twice daily for 5 days; conjugated estrogen, 10 mg/day for 5 days; or conjugated equine estrogen, 50 mg injected intravenously (see page 269). The oral medication should be prescribed with an antiemetic. Prophylactic penicillin or other antibiotic must be employed according to the apparent need, depending on the circumstances of the incident and the physician's judgment. Since many persons are allergic to this agent, its routine use is not recommended.

The physician should be aware that many, perhaps most, women involved in assault episodes require comfort, understanding, and emotional support. These should be supplied initially by the physician, but many victims also need the help of a crisis counselor, an appropriately trained social worker, or a psychiatrist.

FOLLOW-UP

A repeat examination of the patient should be performed approximately 6 weeks after the episode to ensure resumption of menstrual function. At this visit, the serologic test for syphilis and culture of cervical material for *Neisseria gonorrhoeae* should be repeated.

Obstetrics and gynecology is one of the most demanding specialties in medicine. In order to cope with the volume of requests for attention, the physician must set priorities, and for the most part, counseling never ranks at all. Counseling is perceived as a separate entity, one that requires time unavailable to the physican and skills of questionable validity. On a rare occasion, when convinced that surgery or drugs will not provide a cure, the obstetrician-gynecologist refers the patient to a psychiatrist. A change in perspective is needed, since counseling is an inherent part of a woman's medical care, regardless of her age and her predicament.

Counseling is not to be done in a vacuum, but simultaneously with other forms of care. The pregnant patient makes numerous antenatal visits. The patient with premenstrual tension wishes relief from her misery. The patient with sexual problems arrives with vague complaints that are difficult and frustrating to unravel without a counselor's approach. The patient who has had a hysterectomy is depressed and wishes help. The patient is accidentally pregnant, but ambivalent about abortion. The patient has tried almost all forms of contraception and is not satisfied with them. What alternatives are still available? The patient has cancer but does not want to die; what are her chances? The obstetrician–gynecologist who wishes to provide care of high quality must recognize the social and psychologic needs of the patient and must realize that these needs are the context for her care. They represent the person behind the specific obstetric or gynecologic problem.

CHAPTER 10

COUNSELING IN OBSTETRICS AND GYNECOLOGY

Robert A. H. Kinch
Suzanne Steinberg

SEXUAL COUNSELING

THE THEORY OF SEXUALITY

Masters and Johnson have evolved a four-stage division of the sexual cycle: 1) excitement, 2) plateau, 3) orgasm, and 4) resolution. The first three phases coincide with two distinct and relatively independent components of the sexual response: 1) a genital and vasocongestive reaction that produces penile erection in the male and vaginal lubrication and swelling in the female and 2) the reflex clonic muscular contractions that constitute orgasm in both sexes. The resolution occurs quickly in the male, while the female returns to the nonsexual stage more slowly and can continue to experience orgasms at this time. It is now believed that female orgasms are physiologically identical to those of the male. Orgasm in the female is produced primarily by stimulation of the clitoris. The vagina is sensitive to touch only near its entrance, and such stimulation produces pleasure different from that produced by clitoral stimulation and is not essential for orgasm.

The biphasic concept has very important clinical applications. In the male, impotence is associated with failure of the first phase and is usually psychogenic.

Disorganization of the second phase produces premature and retarded ejaculation. The treatment is different in each phase. In the female, there are two syndromes produced by a disturbance in phase 1 of the sexual response. In one syndrome, the woman responds to an erotic stimulus with lubrication and vasocongestion and yet is not orgasmic. The other is quite different, the woman is not stimulated at all when her partner makes love to her, a more profound disturbance. The major disorder of the second phase is vaginismus. Based on these theoretical concepts, Kaplan defines six sexual malfunctions:

1. Premature ejaculation: inability to control orgasm
2. Male impotency: inability to produce or maintain an erection
3. Retarded ejaculation: inability to trigger orgasm
4. General female sexual dysfunction: lack of erotic response to sexual stimulation, commonly called frigidity

5. Female orgasmic dysfunction: difficulty in reaching orgasm
6. Vaginismus: a spasm of the muscles at the entrance of the vagina, preventing penetration

There are numerous causes for these sexual malfunctions. First, they can be caused by medical problems and drug effects. Psychodynamic etiology should not be considered until pathology and iatrogenic effects are ruled out. Antihypertensives in the male and oral contraceptives in the female can be the culprits. Diabetes, pelvic surgery, and atherosclerosis are often implicated. Second, there may have been negative conditioning in childhood. Most women who report sexual dysfunction have suffered from a nonpermissive parental approach toward their sexual behavior, as well as from a complete lack of education on the topic. This often is accompanied by a permissive attitude toward the young man in the family—the familiar double standard.

Traumatic early experiences may lead to sexual dysfunction. Sexual experimentation by young adolescents often leads to disillusionment. A young girl may agree to intercourse in order to keep a relationship intact. A young boy may be so anxious to succeed that he develops premature ejaculation persisting into adult life. If adequate help were available to young people at these critical points, many serious sexual problems might be prevented.

Another cause of sexual problems is the ignorant lover syndrome. In many cases, both partners are ignorant of sexual techniques. The man may feel that the woman's sexual response is exactly the same as his; acting on this assumption, he satisfies himself before he has even brought his partner to the phase of excitement, or worse still, leaves her on the plateau. She may be unable to ask for the right kind of stimulation, never having masturbated or been brought to orgasm before. He may not even know that the clitoris exists. He may feel that, because he needs a fair amount of rough stimulation in order to ejaculate, she may need exactly the same treatment. Neither understands that they are ineffective lovers, so, in silence, they continue their unsatisfactory sexual habits. Nonverbal communication is very romantic but completely useless in sexual relationships.

Sexual dysfunction may also be caused by the fear of pregnancy. This is very real in early marriage and in later marriage, when the family is considered complete. Exploration of this area—improved contraception—may solve the problem.

Excessive goal orientation may cause problems. The couple who is generally ambitious may be achievement-oriented sexually as well. They may define the *best* orgasm as one that occurs at the same time as the partner's. Anything different, regardless of how pleasurable, is classified as failure. He is an inadequate lover. She is physiologically imperfect. Most couples experiencing performance anxiety fill their time with compulsive activities that leave little time for lovemaking, so the clue to their difficulties may be in their everyday lifestyles. Most couples understand the significance of prime time for the best television programs; rarely do they understand the importance of prime time for love-making. It may be difficult to make them understand.

The greatest immediate cause of orgasmic dysfunction in the female and impotence in the male is the fear of failure, that is, of being unable to perform the sexual act. This anticipatory anxiety starts a vicious cycle of fear of impotence, consequent impotence, fear of impotence and so forth. If stressed, it turns one failure into a chronic and serious case of impotence. In an attempt to improve the situation, the partners try to observe their performances objectively. All spontaneity is lost with this "spectatoring," and more impotence results.

Of course, the absolute basis of all sexual difficulties is the failure to communicate. This takes many forms, one being the pretended orgasm, which is extremely common and reasonably easy to treat. In most cases, the woman has concealed her anorgasmic state to save her partner's pride and to relieve herself of the need to try to reach a climax. She comes to the physician when she wishes sexual satisfaction yet finds it difficult to untangle herself from her perpetuated lie.

SEXUAL HISTORY

The essential factor in sexual counseling is the allocation of adequate time. By interviewing each partner alone on one or two occasions before beginning conjoint therapy, the physician becomes informed about each partner's impression of the relationship and possibly about some issues that have been concealed. Consequently, the physician has a better overview of the marriage than does either participant and is in an improved position to counsel.

The following outline for sexual history taking presupposes that the gynecologist is working with a woman patient, alone. Having realized the importance of inquiring into this patient's sexual history, the physician will have examined personal biases, has accepted them, and is determined not to let them affect advice on sexual matters. The physician will therefore be comfortable with the patient; will put forward warm, accepting vibrations; and will be capable of listening to her story without embarrassment. Aware of the therapeutic value of "letting go and weeping," the physician will be happy helping unhappy women. Having reached this stage, each physician will obviously have an individual approach to learning about the sexuality of patients, but certain guidelines can be helpful.

It is most important that the physician limit note

taking to the minimum. The use of a tape recorder is permissible, providing the patient agrees. It is important to schedule a 10-minute break between patients so that the physician can synthesize the information obtained from the session.

A sexual history is not taken in a prescribed sequence with a prescribed set of questions. The history should be allowed to evolve, following the patient's lead and yet still covering the ground. The physician should encourage the patient to describe her problem in detail in her own words. Since the current difficulties may have roots in her past, the physician may inquire into her relations with her parents and siblings as a child. Points of particular importance include parental attitudes toward toilet training and masturbation; her memories of her parents' sexual relationship; their attitude toward sexuality, particularly her activity in this area; and their part in her sexual education.

A natural sequel to this discussion is the exploration of her first sexual encounter and then other such experiences, either homosexual or heterosexual. The physician should encourage the patient to reveal in detail her satisfaction with her partner's love-making techniques, with the strength of her libido, with her ability to respond with orgasms, with the degree of her assertiveness in love-making. She may describe her most important sexual fantasies. When the topic of sex appears temporarily exhausted, the physician may ask about other aspects of the relationship. This leads into the areas of discord with her partner, and the discussion moves to the emotional problems. The physician thus has the opportunity to assess the quality of the relationship and may be able to determine to what extent the sexual difficulties are a part of a more complex problem.

Throughout the entire conversation the physician is collecting information almost more important than the facts themselves. The completeness of the patient's sexual education can be ascertained. The emotional overtones that accompany the various topics under discussion as well as those feelings directed at and aroused in the physician, can be noted. These are clues to areas of sensitivity for her and her partner for the latter is also a recipient of her messages. Finally, the physician is searching for patterns in the patient's behavior that are the bases of her difficulties.

There are three situations in which the taking of a sexual history is important. The first is when the patient has come with a specific sexual problem, and the physician feels sufficiently knowledgeable in this field to become a sexual counselor. The patient's motivation for assistance may come from within or from some significant other. The partner involved may be equally or more in need of counseling than the woman herself. The question of incentive should be clarified at the onset of the interview. For this type of history taking, both the physician and the patient should be assured of undisturbed privacy, and a time should be set not only for the onset of the session but also for its termination.

The second type of patient whose sexual history should be explored is the one in whom the physician has detected beneath her presenting complaint an emotional disturbance, which in gynecologic practice is often in the sexual field. This patient may come to the office repeatedly with the same complaint, although there is no observable physical explanation. These complaints are often those which the physician seems incapable of curing, *e.g.*, recurrent *Monilia* vaginitis, recurrent urgency and frequency of urination, recurrent backache, pruritis vulvae, and recurrent right lower quadrant pain. Under these circumstances, the complaints may be considered psychosomatic; before assuming that the problem is sexual; however, the physician should explore other aspects of the patient's emotional, vocational, and social life. Alternatively, an introductory question such as "Are you happy with your life?" may be enough to release the flood gates. Should a sexual problem be disclosed at this time, arrangements should be made for deeper exploration, as previously outlined.

The third group of patients from whom a sexual history may be required are those who come for their regular annual checkup. Again, the physician must follow the patient's lead. If the woman states that all is well, she is closing a conversation. If the woman says that she has numerous problems and she is under psychotherapy, the gynecologist's job is also done. The physician who does not probe sufficiently to identify the status quo however, is shirking responsibility. The annual checkup is an ideal time to inquire openly, but tactfully, into marital experience, and this easily leads to its sexual side.

In the case of widows, a much neglected group, inquiry might be made into their social life. So often they spend their time primarily with other women, and a door can be opened to allow them to talk about their actual or fantasized relationships with men. There appears to be no reason why the single woman cannot be asked straightforward questions about sexual relationships. This gives the patient the option to discuss any problems. Denial of problems does not always mean that there are none; it may mean that the patient is not at ease with the particular physician, is not ready to discuss the problem, or feels that the physician does not have time. There is no point in insisting, but the mere attempt at evincing such information may make her feel more comfortable so that she will be able to discuss problems at the next visit.

As far as the adolescent is concerned, neither the topics of sexuality nor heterosexual relationships should be considered taboo. The most important things to find out are how much she knows, how much she has experienced, and how much she has enjoyed it. The physician can give her the opportunity to share her experiences with an accepting adult, as well as to

have some questions answered. There may be occasions when the physician and the patient elect to invite the involved partner to join the conversations.

SEXUAL COUNSELING

One of the major functions of the gynecologist is to sanction certain taboos. It should be explained to the patient that

1. Women can be self-assertive without destroying masculinity.
2. Masturbation in order to produce orgasm is permissible. The physician may even recommend the use of a vibrator.
3. The patient should please herself, for her pleasure will enhance her partner's enjoyment. This is in contradistinction to the traditional emphasis on satisfaction of the mate.
4. Noncoital and orogenital orgasms can be sanctioned.
5. Striving for a simultaneous orgasm with the penis in the vagina is not the be-all and end-all of lovemaking; orgasms are essentially egocentric and selfish, and it is very difficult to share them. Moreover, the feeling of togetherness and gratitude is exactly the same, whether orgasm occurs sequentially or simultaneously.
6. It is important that the patient cease feigning orgasm.
7. Romance in love-making will not be lost if each partner makes the other aware of his or her most erotic zones.
8. Libido is innate, but skillful love-making is a learned art. There is the art of touching, teasing, sensing, massaging, and caressing.

The gynecologist who has developed an interest and skill in this area may wish to follow Kaplan's approach to the following sexual malfunctions.

Disorders in the Male

Premature Ejaculation. Kaplan states that premature ejaculation is one of the most common and easily treated of male complaints. Many men with this problem have a homemade cure; they may employ distraction, such as nonerotic thoughts, or infliction of pain, such as digging their fingernails into their palms. Kaplan recommends that a man with this problem learn to recognize his own erotic preorgasmic sensations. With the help of his partner, he is stimulated almost to the verge of orgasm. Following this, stimulation stops and the erection subsides. He is then restimulated. As he recognizes the point "of almost no return," he signals his partner to stop. Eventually, by this noncoital approach, the man learns to control his orgasm. With confidence comes the ability to carry out

coital exercises, starting with the woman in the superior position, increasing in stimulation until the partners are on their sides, and finally with the man on top.

Masters and Johnson described a "squeeze" technique in which, just prior to orgasm, the man signals his partner to squeeze the penis just below the corona. Apparently, this immediately inhibits erection and produces the same effect as the approach outlined by Semans. Kaplan, however, considers it more important that the man concentrate on his erotic feelings rather than invoke any anxiety that he might signal too late or that his partner might not be an expert in the squeeze technique.

Impotence. The major nonphysical factor that produces impotence is fear of failure. Fear may be dispelled by reassurance from a supportive partner that it is not really important whether the man achieves erection or not. To be convincing, the partner must be free of the often present resentment of her partner's impotence, which demands a totally unselfish attitude. Unless the man can depend upon complete cooperation from his mate in his rehabilitation, it is very difficult to cure the symptom of impotence. The man is also reassured if he can have an erection with masturbation or even experience morning erection.

The couple is then advised as to noncoital pleasuring activities. This provides some consolation for the absence of an erection and often produces one in the process. To give the man confidence that he can lose his erection and regain it satisfactorily, the partner stimulates him to an erection, allows it to subside, and then promptly stimulates him again to show that the disappearance of the erection is no great problem. He should not worry about trying to please his partner. Again, this cure really depends on total support from a possibly already dissatisfied partner. In most cases, psychotherapy is necessary along with the treatment.

Retarded Ejaculation. Less common than the two problems previously discussed, retarded ejaculation is often associated with a strict religious upbringing. This disorder develops when a man has been severely restricted in his sexuality. The treatment is a combination of psychotherapy and desensitizing behavioral therapy to enhance existing ejaculation capacity. These patients are probably best left to the experts—unless therapeutic response is rapid.

Disorders in the Female

In the female there are also three disorders.

General Sexual Dysfunction. Probably the most severe of all female inhibitions is general sexual dysfunction. Women with this problem do not seem to experience

any erotic pleasure from sexual stimulation of any type. They often respond to premarital love-making short of intercourse, but as soon as the main interest is intercourse they lose their response.

The first approach is to have the partners communicate openly about their sexual technique, making sure to exploit maximally anything that turns the woman on. It may be difficult to find anything that arouses her; however, they should openly tell each other what pleases them most. Following this, they are led through nongenital caressing. If this arouses her, it is followed by light genital caressing and, finally, by coitus with the woman in control. This condition is the analog of male impotence, and the male partner also must be supportive and not resentful. This kind of approach may produce resistance, and if so psychotherapy can be extremely beneficial.

Female Orgasmic Dysfunction. This patient falls in love, enjoys sex play, lubricates copiously, and loves the sensation of penetration by the penis, but she does not experience coital orgasm. If orgasm can be obtained any other way, these women can be reassured and the importance of coital orgasm played down. If not, the first goal is to eliminate her inhibitions and encourage her to learn about orgasm by masturbation, first manually and, if this is unsuccessful, then with a vibrator. When she can stimulate herself easily without anxiety or guilt, her partner is brought into the program. She will then be able to teach him to bring her to orgasm in the most pleasurable way. Many couples are quite satisfied at this point, and the therapist should also be satisfied. If there is a demand for coital orgasm, further behavioral exercises can be employed.

Vaginismus. The easiest form of sexual dysfunction to treat, vaginismus, usually occurs early in a sexual relationship. It results from a woman's fear or anticipation of pain at penetration. The most important thing for the gynecologist to do is to carry out gentle vaginal examination. In many cases, the physician can reassure the patient of the normal caliber of the vagina; in almost all cases, the patient with this problem is gynecologically normal. The gynecologist must not either anesthetize her "to stretch the hymen" or operate on her to enlarge the introitus.

After reassurance, the patient is instructed to dilate her vagina with a well-lubricated finger and move it gently around in the passage. Many women have never felt inside the vagina. From there, she graduates to having her partner gently stretch her vagina with one finger, followed by two, followed by gentle stretching and rotating movements. Should this produce spasm at any point the treatment is discontinued. If confidence for penetration is not obtained by these simple measures, vaginal dilators can be recommended. In most cases, with constant reassurance by the therapist and gentle help from the partner, the patient is cured

by these measures. If not, she needs desensitizing behavioral therapy.

Referral

It is imperative for those gynecologists without further time or inclination for counseling to know when to refer. Four groups of patients need referral:

1. Patients who have never had an orgasm, either by themselves or with the help of a partner
2. Patients who have not responded to the efforts outlined
3. Patients who need sophisticated behavioral modification therapy
4. Patients whose problems are beyond the personal competence of the counselor, *i.e.,* those with deep psychodynamic problems

CONTRACEPTION

The first issue to consider in contraceptive counseling is whether the patient wants birth control. There are at least three groups of women who do not. Some women reject the concept on moral or religious grounds. Others have tried everything once, have had a poor experience in each case, and refuse to expose themselves to further problems. Still others are content to utilize therapeutic abortion as their method of contraception.

If the woman does want birth control the physician's role initially is to assess what she knows about the methods on the market and to ascertain if she already has a preference. The patient who is uninformed needs facts. The more acquainted she is with the options, the more appropriate her choice will be. She needs to know the efficacy of the method to guard against pregnancy versus the risks involved in its use. A too complete list of side effects would discourage all women from all methods at all times.

The following factors influence the patient's choice: 1) her attitude toward contraception, 2) the physician's choice, 3) her motivation and, consequently, her reliability in the use of contraception, 4) her previous experience with contraception, and 5) her partner's attitude. It is understandable that physicians have definite opinions about each method. How far should they go toward determining the choice rather than influencing it? It is important to recognize the weight of the physician's word in the decision-making process and bring it to bear only when necessary. It is equally important to recognize the variable influence of the partner; at times he dictates the choice, and at times he is not consulted at all.

In some instances, women make decisions repeatedly over the years. A pattern emerges. The young woman adamantly opposed to pregnancy begins with the safest reversible method, the contraceptive pill.

For various reasons, the first pill is not satisfactory, and another one is described. She stops the pill to become pregnant, conceives, delivers, and reconsiders her position on birth control methods. She decides on the intrauterine device. After a time, this produces problems. She has it removed and resorts to barrier techniques. Eventually, the patient tires of the barrier technique and opts for sterilization. The physician should be aware of this progression, for with every change, there is a hiatus; with every hiatus, there is a definite possibility of pregnancy.

The role of the physician is not finished once the choice is made. Counseling may be needed on follow-up visits. For example, the birth control pill may suppress the libidinal urges, and such a complaint would warrant a trial period without the pill to rule it out as the cause. The role of the gynecologist involves more than simply writing a prescription or inserting a device. It is one of a counselor on family planning throughout the childbearing years.

ABORTION

A decade ago, abortion was an unacceptable procedure except under the most extenuating circumstances. Although it has become more accepted and more widely performed, views on the matter range from one extreme to the other among both physicians and consumers.

Some physicians may be so strongly in favor of abortion that they accept without discussion a woman's request for the procedure. For those women who are comfortable with their decision to have an abortion, such a physician is ideal. Other physicians may accept abortion but feel a responsibility to distinguish the patient with firm convictions from the one who is ambivalent. They are not interested in persuading women not to have an abortion but in assisting women to live easily with their decisions. Recognizing the patient whose mind is set, such a physician leaves well enough alone. Still other physicians approve abortions only for concrete medical reasons, *e.g.*, rubella exposure, ingestion of teratogenic drugs, Down's syndrome, hemophilia, and congenital defects that tend to be repetitive. These physicians recommend pregnancy termination, even insist on it, for these indications and reject it completely on sociopsychologic grounds. Some physicians oppose abortion as a form of murder. Recognizing the multitude of opinions, however, they refer patients to colleagues for this form of care. Finally, there are physicians who reject the idea so completely that they try to make the patient see sense, *their sense*. Each obstetrician must make a personal decision on the matter and then advise his or her patients accordingly.

The attitudes of patients are as variable as those of physicians. There is the woman who feels guilt and embarrassment, who whispers when the subject is broached, who keeps it secret from her close relatives, and who never loses the feeling that she has committed a crime. Another woman, totally depressed by a pregnancy, feels a sense of enormous relief when assured of an abortion. Still another patient thinks that abortion is her right and demands it; such women receive a great deal of publicity but are relatively few in number. Finally, there is the casual patient who returns regularly for pregnancy termination. For her, this is the perfect form of contraception.

There are no unbiased guidelines available to help the physician differentiate between the patient who needs an abortion and the one who does not, except in the rare case of clear-cut medical indications. The decision to abort is essentially the decision of the patient. It is the physician's responsibility to provide information and warn of the possible hazards, and possible obstetric sequelae, such as cervical incompetence and preterm labor. Finally, the physician should support the patient once her choice is made in the hope that postabortion guilt or depression can be avoided.

PREGNANCY

Pregnancy is one of the crucial periods in a woman's life; it is a time when disorders in relationships are most apt to occur. Caplan's main technique in correcting these disturbances is anticipatory guidance. He recommends that the physician have a joint interview with the husband and wife early in pregnancy. He points out that women may be more sensitive than usual during pregnancy and that emotional lability should not be confused with preliminary signs of psychiatric illness. At this initial conference, the physician should mention the possible changes in the pregnant woman's sexual desire and performance. The woman who loses her sexual desire and her capacity for orgasm may imagine either that she is permanently frigid or that she has lost her love for her husband. The husband may feel rejected and search elsewhere for gratification. The couple may think that sexual activity is taboo during pregnancy. Such thinking can be altered. The physician can also help both parties become aware of the stresses imposed by pregnancy and, consequently, of the added support each needs from the other. Factors of this kind balance the general societal view of motherhood and pregnancy as a form of utopia.

On the initial antenatal visits, the physician should counsel the patient regarding alcohol ingestion, smoking, and drug use. Counseling on these issues is uncomplicated. Alcohol has been found to be detrimental to the offspring and is not recommended during pregnancy. It has been demonstrated that cigarette smoking produces infants small for their gestational age. Many drugs have known teratogenic effects, and many

have not been proved free of such effects. It is strongly recommended that the patient consult with her physician prior to using any drugs while pregnant.

The second joint interview is best held in the middle trimester. Caplan finds women become more passive and demanding of affection, often a dramatic change from their former manner. Studies have shown that satisfaction of these needs not only makes the woman more comfortable but also prepares her for adequate motherhood after delivery. The physician's role is to help her get what she needs from the significant others about her. The husband may be irritated by his wife's petulant behavior, sexually frustrated, frightened by her increasing demands and apparent personality change, and unsure of his role as an expectant father. The physician must reassure the husband of the self-limited nature of this change and enlist his aid in building his wife's resources in preparation for the baby's arrival. The physician should convey respect for the father's role; in this way, problems of jealousy that interfere with the development of a father–child relationship may be avoided. At this stage, the woman recognizes the changes in her body; in some cases, with dismay. Some men find a pregnant woman attractive; others do not. She must deal with her own feelings regarding her loss of shape, as well as those of her husband. She may be surprised by some ambivalence toward this budding offspring. She may question how the baby will alter her relationship with her husband and her lifestyle; how will she manage as a parent?

A final interview held in the third trimester elicits still other responses. The woman is often impatient for delivery. Behind her impatience is fear—fear of never delivering, fear of having a deformed offspring, fear of pain in labor, fear of not recognizing the onset of labor. It is not unusual for the mother to feel she can communicate with her fetus once she can feel movement. The father, too, can be involved in these communications and may feel a desire to caress the mother and child. This is also the time for organizing for the birth, often a redundant activity—usually, all is prepared months earlier. When preparations are incomplete, this may be one manifestation that the mother is denying or rejecting the infant's arrival. The husband is just as anxious to see the end of the process and to have the memory of having been adequately supportive, of having reached the hospital in good time, of his wife having tolerated the labor and delivery well, and of having handled the infant without catastrophe.

Specific counseling regarding women's behavior during labor and delivery may alleviate some postpartum concern. At present, there is an increased emphasis on breathing exercises for coping with pain and on deliveries free of instrumentation. So thorough is some antenatal teaching that some women who opt for analgesia or lose control without it feel a sense of failure and humiliation. It is difficult to understand why a pain-free labor is any less "natural" than one that is painful. Nor is it easily understood why some prenatal instructors take a condemning attitude to forceps or episiotomy when these are at times indicated for fetal well-being. Such teaching only adds to the burdens of expectant parents.

The physician may briefly discuss the initial parent–child relationship, another subject that is often poorly handled by the formal classes. The parents' initial reaction to the newborn is disbelief and insecurity. Bonding is not an instantaneous process that occurs at first sight but a gradual one that begins at delivery and develops with each interaction. Women who believe that maternal instinct instantaneously produces love and efficiency in infant care and relationships should be corrected. Instead, the idea of learning from experience, which is more realistic and definitely less defeating, should be offered.

The postpartum emotional disorders, not well defined, are described in Chapter 40. At one end of this spectrum is "the postpartum blues," suffered by some 60% of patients. It involves a transient depressed mood and crying spells, and it is considered "normal." Postpartum depression and postpartum psychoses are more severe. The depressive forms are more common. The onset of postpartum emotional disorders may be sudden or slow and insidious. Of women who have suffered from postpartum depression, 20%–30% will have a recurrence in subsequent pregnancies. The obstetrician–gynecologist is responsible for identifying the patients at risk. Braverman and Roux, in a small sample of women, found that marital difficulty and a lack of enthusiasm for the offspring are significantly correlated with postpartum emotional disorders. They suggest that women with such indicators and those with a history of postpartum emotional disorders fared better in later pregnancies when they were treated by a psychotherapist. Therefore, the second responsibility of the obstetrician–gynecologist is to recognize if counseling is needed and, if so, to refer the patient to a therapist.

TUBAL LIGATION

The question of sterilization is not dissimilar from the issue of abortion. The woman requests a tubal ligation. If she already has six offspring and is without the resources to support a seventh, the physician may encourage sterilization. If she is 28, single, and without children but has a history of four previous abortions, one self-inflicted, the physician may feel justified in consenting to surgery; she has proved her lack of interest in parenthood. If she is 35, single, and nulligravid, she is old enough to know her own mind and is close enough to menopause to dissipate any reluctance on the part of the physician. *But,* if she is 24, single, and

convinced that she never, never wants children, her physician becomes cautious. She has obviously thought this over for some time, and she has probably been refused by other physicians. While the physician would be reassured by the partner's support of the sterilization, his involvement in the issue is entirely the patient's prerogative. The physician's role is merely to provide this woman with all the information available so that she can make a well-informed decision. The procedure should be described, the success rate defined, and the lack of effect on menstrual and ovarian function underlined.

The difficulty of reversing this procedure should be emphasized, although tuboplasty by microsurgery is improving the success rate. The woman who appears overly concerned about reanastomosis should take time to reconsider the surgery. Women who will regret their decision are not easily identified. Most often, they are unexpectedly remarried after a divorce and wish to have a child with their new partner.

PELVIC SURGERY

Hysterectomy has been performed so frequently that questions have been raised regarding whether all these operations were really necessary. Studies have demonstrated that in 12.5%–30.8% of cases, there are no abnormal pathologic findings. For many, perhaps most, of the indications in these cases, *i.e.*, dysfunctional uterine bleeding or as a part of plastic repair, surgery is the treatment of choice, but the truly unnecessary hysterectomy must be avoided. What are the most common circumstances under which unnecessary surgery is recommended? First is the patient with the premorbid hysterical personality who develops vague symptoms. She has a dramatic, persuasive manner, and she demands action. Action is taken in the form of hysterectomy four times as often in this type of person as in normal subjects. Second is the patient with current psychiatric illness and gynecologic symptoms. Many of these depressed women have undergone gynecologic surgery in the year preceding admission to a psychiatric hospital. Third, there is always the gynecologist who rationalizes that the woman wishes sterilization, she is inconvenienced by menstruation, and she would be protected from cancer; why not take it out?

COUNSELING FOR SURGERY

Once the indications for surgery have been established, counseling is necessary. The physician presents the findings, and the recommendation may come as a shock. Some women comply immediately. Others want time to adjust, to make their own decisions, and possibly to consult another physician. It is the physi-

cian's role to perceive this need and accept it, thus enhancing the patient's cooperation and trust. The operation is then scheduled.

Often a total hysterectomy is misconstrued as the removal of the uterus, tubes, and ovaries, while removal of the uterus only is considered a partial hysterectomy. Such false beliefs are best dispersed by explanation, unless the patient shows a lack of interest. The extent of detail presented must depend upon the wish of the woman. Other information, such as the length of the surgery, the hospitalization, and the convalescent period, should be offered to dispel the unknown and to permit the patient some control and the chance to make appropriate plans.

The patient is now educated, but how does she feel? She may experience fear. She may be frightened by the surgery itself, the loss of control under anesthesia, the possibility of death, the possibility of malignancy, the severity of postoperative pain and a loss of dignity if she is unable to deal with it, or the idea of addiction to analgesia. Her concerns may revolve around the notions that she will lose her capacity to function, that she will be obese, that she will no longer attract a lover, that she will experience diminished libido, and that she will not have the energy to work. The physician should listen to her and reassure her but should not offer false expectations, such as describing this surgery as a preventive measure against cancer. The timing of this discussion is important. The need may appear shortly after the news of impending surgery; it may be delayed until admission to the hospital, recovery from surgery, or the follow-up visit; or it may never arise at all. The precise moment is determined by the patient. The physician's responsibility is to provide the opportunity. Furthermore, the information may require repetition. She may have been too anxious to absorb it the first time. She may have been overwhelmed with all that was presented to her and forgotten details that are of later significance. The physician must be patient and review on request.

All these considerations apply with even more force when mutilating operations, such as vulvectomy, and extensive operations, such as radical hysterectomy or exenterative surgery, are involved.

POSTHYSTERECTOMY SYNDROME

A thorough assessment is important not only to prevent unnecessary surgery, but also to identify the patient at risk for the posthysterectomy syndrome. With this syndrome, the patient suffers with an endogenous depression characterized by agitation, somatic symptoms, depressive mood, and insomnia. Relapses are similar in nature. The depression is severe and is more refractory to treatment than other depressions. Patients who undergo hysterectomy are at greater risk than those who require other surgery, *e.g.*, cholecys-

tectomy. A woman is most vulnerable to this syndrome in the first 6 months following surgery, although studies have documented its appearance as late as 1.5 years after the procedure. The women at risk are those who have a history of depression or unstable personality; those who are in the throes of marital disruption; those who are in the 35–45 age group, definitely premenopausal; those who have been found to have no organic pathology; and those who have experienced illegitimate births.

Why does this syndrome occur? There is no conclusive evidence, only theories. Perhaps the patient feels that the loss of the uterus symbolizes the loss of her femininity or is an indication of advancing age; perhaps the loss produces a sense of incompleteness that calls for a readjustment of body image. Studies have shown that the incidence of depression following tubal ligation is significantly less than that following hysterectomy. Can this be explained by the fact that the first group have opted for sterilization, whereas the latter group have been compelled by apparent disease to sacrifice their ability to reproduce? Does the explanation rest in the discovery that women with ligated tubes retain a fantasy of future pregnancy, while those without a womb do not?

PREMENSTRUAL TENSION

The greatest problems in counseling for premenstrual tension are the facility many physicians have in denying its existence, and the difficulty many women have in recognizing its presence. Both are faced with the dilemma of not knowing the components of the syndrome. A week to 10 days prior to menstruation, the woman suffers symptoms that spontaneously resolve with the onset of a period. She may feel depressed, anxious, irritable, tired, irrational, and either sexually aroused or indifferent. She may experience peripheral edema, weight gain, breast tenderness, acne, back pain, constipation, abdominal bloating, headache, dizziness, and palpitation. It is the physician's responsibility to distinguish premenstrual tension from psychiatric disorder. For the physician to make this distinction, it may be necessary for the patient to keep a daily diary of her moods and behavior for several months. Once this task is accomplished, the patient who has no psychiatric problems can be reassured. She is not losing her sanity, nor is she the least bit strange. In fact, 40% of women share her feelings. She will feel a great sense of relief just "confessing" and finding someone who believes and understands it all. After diagnosing premenstrual tension, the physician can then provide the patient with the information available on the syndrome. Facts can help her to accommodate changes in herself. Premenstrual tension is variable in intensity and frequency. It appears to be more pronounced in the mid-30s and is aggravated by environmental stress. It produces no intellectual impairment, despite its reputation.

Premenstrual tension is more easily appreciated by intimates at times than by the women herself. The best time to work out the turmoil premenstrual tension creates between partners is usually at a time when it has subsided. The couple may begin by developing a system of acknowledging the onset of premenstrual tension to avoid possible misunderstanding. The husband can be informed of its self-limited nature, of how she feels, and what her special needs are at the time. Then, if she needs solitude, he will not perceive it as rejection; if she needs tender loving care, he will not be discouraged by her irritability. If she becomes angry, he will realize the folly of blaming it all on premenstrual tension. Sometimes a woman is better able to communicate a concern when her defenses are lowered by premenstrual tension than at other times of the month. If this is the case, such revelations can be useful in the growth of the relationship. Finally, the physician can offer some symptomatic relief for anxiety with tranquilizers, and for fluid retention and breast tenderness with diuretics. Symptomatology may be generally diminished with oral contraception.

THE MENOPAUSE

The menopause is a time of change, both physical and psychologic. The postmenopause years occupy one-third of a woman's life and therefore demand a considerable investment in management by the physician. The way women cope with this phase of their existence is largely determined by their basic personality pattern, by their past and present environmental stresses, and by their expectations of the menopause.

One of the earliest symptoms, although sometimes unnoticed, is the distinct loss of libido. If the menopause alone accounts for the diminution in sexual drive, then there is a resurgence of interest after menopause. Kaplan reports that erotic fantasies of men or masturbation are not unusual in women during this period. Physiologic changes have been documented as well. Vaginal lubrication tends to occur more slowly and clonic contractions of the pelvic platform during orgasm are less vigorous and less frequent. There is a general lessening of muscular response to sexual excitement, and erotic sensations are reported to be less intense. Nevertheless, elderly women remain capable of enjoying orgasm. Apart from the sexual aspects of menopause, it may be accompanied by fatigue, suboccipital headaches, hot flushes, and irritability. The fatigue may be inherent to the estrogen deficiency or secondary to insomnia associated with nocturnal hot flushes. The suboccipital headaches are possibly related to irritability.

To these changes of the menopause add a lifetime difficulty with "frigidity" and the resulting feelings of

insecurity and inadequacy. Or add to this a lifetime belief in Victorian morality—sexual release for the male, sexual disinterest in the female, sex for procreation only; with menopause, these women may regret never having ventured to their full potential. Or add to this the youth mania, the husband who has grown more dignified with age, the parents who have died or are now dependent on her, and the children who have departed. She is left to face her own aging, loss of attractiveness, loss of usefulness. Add to this a lost mate, either through death, divorce, impotence, or satisfaction of his sexual desires away from home. She is left with unfulfilled sexual desire, mourning for a loss, and busy activities to fill time.

This description emphasizes the extreme importance of counseling in the general management of the menopausal woman. It is the physician's responsibility to encourage the patient to ventilate and then to clarify her problem. Once defined, it is simpler to plan an approach to the dissolution of the difficulty. Depression may require psychotherapy. Sexual dysfunction may require behavior or couple therapy. Ignorance may require information and reassurance. The essential difference in counseling this age group is that the opportunity for prevention is past; there is only the chance for amelioration of sequelae, sequelae of a lifetime's experience and a set personality.

REFERENCES AND RECOMMENDED READING

Adams D, Gold AR, Burk Ad: Rise in female initiated sexual activity at ovulation and its suppression by oral contraceptives. N Engl J Med 299:1145, 1978

Ananth J: Hysterectomy and depression. Obstet Gynecol 51:724, 1978

Braverman J, Roux JF: Screening the patient at risk for post-partum depression. Obstet Gynecol 52:731, 1978

Caplan G: An Approach to Community Mental Health. Tavistock, 1961

Easley E: Sex problems after the menopause. Clin Obstet Gynecol 21:269, 1978

Frank E, Anderson C, Rubenstein D: Frequency of sexual dysfunction in "normal" couples. N Engl J Med 299:111, 1978

Green R (ed): Human Sexuality. A Health Practitioner's Text. Baltimore, Williams & Wilkins, 1975

Kaplan, HS: The New Sex Therapy. New York, Brunner Mazel, 1974

Kolodny RC, Masters WH, Johnson VE: Textbook of Sexual Medicine. Boston, Little, Brown, 1979

Sarrel PM, Sarrel L: Orgasmic difficulties. The role of the gynaecologist. Clin Obstet Gynecol 21:191, 1978

Semans H: Premature ejaculation: a new appraoch. South Med J 49:353, 1956

Sloan D: Emotional and psychological aspects of hysterectomy. Am J Obstet Gynecol 131:598, 1978

Vincent CE: Sexual and Marital Health: The Physician as a Consultant. New York, McGraw-Hill, 1973

Inadequate or inappropriate nutrition may be responsible for many disorders of the reproductive process, as well as for other health problems at all ages. Special nutritional demands are imposed on women throughout their life span. An adequate supply of food is needed not only to maintain all bodily functions and daily activities at maximum efficiency but also to meet increased dietary needs imposed by pregnancy or lactation.

ADOLESCENCE

Adolescence, the period of life between childhood and adulthood, is characterized by a rapid increase in the rate of physical growth, initiation of the reproductive process, and profound endocrine changes. The details of these dramatic changes are considered in Chapter 8. Nutrition in this age group is influenced by family tradition, by cultural factors, by peer group preferences, and by fadisms. Adequate intake of nutrients is necessary for the rapid linear growth that is the hallmark of this period of life.

Normal biologic growth follows an orderly series of events that relates physical growth and development with endocrinologic and sexual maturation. In the female, the onset of puberty and the menarche are the important markers. For the average adolescent girl, the growth spurt begins at age 10; rapidly increases to the time of peak growth, which is usually 12–13 years of age; and then gradually declines, terminating at the age of about 17. After the menarche, further increase in height is limited to about 4 or 5 cm. All the organs of the body except the thymus and the lymphatic glands participate in the growth spurt, which contributes about 15% to adult height and about 40%–50% to adult weight. The large increase in body mass that occurs during these years requires considerable amounts of nutrients.

In the United States, as well as in some Western European countries, the age of menarche has progressively declined, an effect that is generally attributed to improved nutrition. Malnutrition or undernutrition may delay the menarche and the onset of regular ovulation. It may also interfere with postmenarcheal and postovulatory physiologic maturation and optimum readiness for reproduction. Furthermore, undernutrition can modify the pattern and timing of skeletal growth.

Until recently, it was considered that variations in the age of menarche were determined principally by genetic factors. Nutrition is now recognized as a major contributing factor, however, and the existence of a threshold of percent body fat and weight for hypothalamic–pituitary maturity and initiation of menstrual cycles and ovulation is strongly supported by experimental and clinical data. Establishment of a postmen-

NUTRITION IN OBSTETRICS AND GYNECOLOGY

Kamran S. Moghissi

archeal normal ovulatory pattern is also believed to be related to the age of menarche.

Increasing concern about the nutritional status of adolescent females and about the rising pregnancy rate in this age group has led to special emphasis on the importance of correct nutrition and the avoidance of pregnancy until physical and reproductive maturation are complete. Most large-scale nutrition programs are now directed largely to pregnant women, but adolescent and preadolescent females should also be regarded as prime targets. Moreover, the time during which adolescent girls are exposed to such programs can be used to discourage pregnancy.

NUTRITIONAL REQUIREMENTS

Data regarding the minimal nutritional requirements for teenagers are scant. Most recommended daily di-

etary allowances for adolescents are based on extrapolation from infant or adult studies. To estimate caloric need, variables such as climate and physical activity must be considered.

Calories and Basic Nutrients

Healthy young females have a peak daily caloric need at menarche (12–13 years) of 2400 kcal. This need slowly declines to 2100 by age 16. Protein requirement is in direct proportion to needs for other nutrients and should provide approximately 12%–15% of the total caloric intake. Carbohydrates should supply 40%–50%; fats, 30–45% of caloric needs (Table 11–1).

Micronutrients

The diet of most American teenagers and those in developed countries contains almost all the vitamins and minerals needed for maintenance and growth. One possible exception is iron. Because of the frequency of anovulatory cycles and excessive menstrual bleeding in this age group, or even because of normal menstrual blood loss, some female adolescents are unable to replenish their iron loss from dietary sources alone. Most female adolescents thus benefit from iron supplements. Also, because vitamin B_{12} occurs almost exclu-

TABLE 11-1. RECOMMENDED DAILY DIETARY ALLOWANCES FOR FEMALES AGED 11-18

	11–14	15–18
WEIGHT (lb.)	97	119
HEIGHT (in.)	62	65
ENERGY (kcal)	2400	2100
PROTEIN (g)	44	48
FAT-SOLUBLE VITAMINS		
Vitamin A (IU)	4000	4000
Vitamin D (IU)	400	400
Vitamin E activity (IU)	12	12
WATER-SOLUBLE VITAMINS		
Ascorbic acid (mg)	45	45
Folacin (g)	400	400
Niacin (mg)	16	14
Riboflavin (mg)	1.3	1.4
Thiamin (mg)	1.2	1.1
Vitamin B_6 (mg)	1.6	2.0
Vitamin B_{12} (μg)	3.0	3.0
MINERALS		
Calcium (mg)	1200	1200
Phosphorus (mg)	1200	1200
Iodine (μg)	115	115
Iron (mg)	18	18
Magnesium (mg)	300	300
Zinc (mg)	15	15

(Based on recommendations of the Food and Nutrition Board, National Academy of Sciences, National Research Council, Revision 1974).

sively in foods of animal origin, vegetarian teenagers may be deficient in this vitamin and need supplementation. Supplementation of other micronutrients also may be necessary when dietary sources are deficient.

SPECIAL PROBLEMS

Although malnutrition is uncommon among teenagers in the United States and other developed nations, there are special circumstances when undernutrition may become a problem. This occurs most often in the 13- to 16-year-old girl who perceives her enlarging body with alarm at a time when she is particularly sensitive about her appearance. She may attempt to change her body image by restricting her food intake. A potentially more serious problem is posed by the increasing number of adolescents who, for emotional or ideologic reasons, decide to follow a very restricted or pure vegetarian diet. If such diets are adhered to over a long period, they can lead to various vitamin deficiencies, anemia, hypocalcemia, hypoproteinemia, emaciation, or other forms of starvation. Finally, mention should be made of *anorexia nervosa*, the relentless pursuit of weight loss through self-starvation, which may result in severe malnutrition, disturbances of metabolic and endocrine functions, and even death.

Another nutritional problem encountered among teenagers is food fadism characterized by avoidance of certain types of nutrients, exclusive use of processed foods, or overzealous consumption of other foods, particularly vitamins and minerals. Other adolescents may indulge in excessive consumption of "junk food" or calories, with resultant obesity.

Well-balanced meals and proper nutrition during adolescence should result in normal biologic growth and reproductive function. However, nutritional problems are intimately related to the familial, cultural, environmental, socioeconomic, educational, and iatrogenic influences to which females are exposed from childhood through the teens. A concerned and knowledgeable physician can play a major role in improving the nutritional health of the adolescent by providing needed counsel.

ADULTHOOD

The healthy woman should consume a well-balanced diet that contains all the basic food groups and required micronutrients. The United States Food and Nutrition Board of the National Academy of Sciences recommends that an average, healthy woman weighing 128 lb (58 kg), measuring 65 in. (162 cm) tall, and aged 23–50 years follow a diet containing 2100 kcal, 46 g protein, 18 mg iron, and the recommended daily allowances (RDA) of other minerals and vitamins. Since the iron needs of women are usually not

met by dietary sources, periodic iron supplementation may be required, particularly for those women who have prolonged or excessive menstrual blood loss.

NUTRITIONAL NEEDS IN USERS OF HORMONAL CONTRACEPTIVES

Steroidal contraceptives cause metabolic changes that may influence a woman's requirements for certain nutrients, vitamins, and minerals. A decrease in glucose tolerance has been observed in approximately 10% of oral contraceptive users who have taken these preparations for 1 year. Abnormal glucose tolerance is seen most often in users of combined estrogen–progestogen agents, but it appears to depend on the specific progestogen as well. It has also been noted in women who have received long-acting injectable progestogens. For this reason, prediabetic and diabetic patients should use other contraceptive methods. If they are given steroidal contraceptives, glucose metabolism should be carefully monitored.

Some studies suggest that the impairment of glucose metabolism in some women may be associated with the alteration of tryptophan metabolism that accompanies oral contraception, and with a relative or absolute vitamin B_6 deficiency.

Hormonal contraceptives may increase the serum levels of triglycerides, cholesterol, phospholipids, and lecithin. Elevated serum lipids have been associated with an increased risk of vascular occlusive diseases, such as myocardial infarction. The significance of the rise in triglycerides and other lipids in normal women has not been determined, however, nor has it been established whether such changes occur in women on low-fat diets.

The effect of hormonal contraceptives on protein metabolism is similar to that of pregnancy. Serum levels of some amino acids and albumin are generally decreased, while those of many of the other proteins formed in the liver are increased.

Oral contraceptives have no effect on hemoglobin, hematocrit, or erythrocyte count, but serum iron levels and total iron-binding capacity may become elevated with the use of certain preparations. Plasma copper levels usually increase and plasma zinc levels decrease, but no effect has been observed on plasma levels of calcium and magnesium. Generally, plasma vitamin A increases and carotene levels decrease when oral contraceptives are used, but plasma levels of vitamin C remain the same. A significant reduction of plasma pyridoxal phosphate, as well as in red cell and serum folate levels, in pill users suggests a relative deficiency in vitamin B_6 and folic acid. Oral contraceptive use has no significant effect on vitamin B_{12} serum levels.

At present, nutritional supplements to the diet of steroidal contraceptive users are not recommended on a routine basis. However, such supplements are advised for high-risk groups in whom chronic nutritional inadequacies, repeated pregnancies, or various disorders could increase the risk of a deficiency.

NUTRITIONAL NEEDS IN PREGNANCY

Adequate fetal growth and development depend on a steady supply of nutrients from the mother to the fetus. Deficient dietary intake; inadequate absorption of nutrients from the gut; abnormal metabolism of proteins, lipids, carbohydrates, and micronutrients in the mother; insufficiency of placental circulation; and abnormal use of nutrients by the fetus may impair fetal development. For a long time, it was believed that the fetus, as a parasite, was able to draw all of its dietary needs from the mother, regardless of her nutritional status. Studies performed during the last two decades have demonstrated, however, that inadequate or deficient maternal nutrition during pregnancy may lead to intrauterine stunting and impairment of fetal brain development.

For all mammalian species, fetal life begins as one cell; this cell multiplies several billion times before birth. The rate at which this multiplication proceeds determines the substantial variation in birth weight and mean daily increment in fetal body weight among different species. Between conception and birth the nutritional needs of the fetus are met by three different mechanisms. During the preimplantation phase, the blastocyst presumably absorbs nutrients from the reproductive tract fluids through its outer layer of cells, the trophoblast. From implantation until establishment of the placental circulation, the embryo receives nutrients directly from the maternal blood through a sinusoidal space between the fetal and maternal tissues. When the placenta is developed, the fetus receives its nutrients by means of the placental circulation. Thus, the placenta has a central function in pregnancy, being involved in the transfer of nutrients to the fetus and inducing many of the metabolic changes in the mother that are essential for fetal survival and well-being.

ENERGY REQUIREMENTS DURING PREGNANCY

During the course of pregnancy, the mother undergoes considerable physiologic adjustment in order to supply the fetus with necessary dietary ingredients while maintaining her own homeostasis. Additional energy is required for the growth of the fetus, placenta, and maternal tissues, as well as for support of increased maternal metabolic processes (see Figure 17–7). The *total extra energy cost attributable to pregnancy needs* was formerly thought to be approximately 27,000 kcal. The Committee on Maternal Nutrition of

the National Research Council has expanded this figure and estimates the extra metabolic requirements of pregnancy to be approximately 40,000 kcal for a woman performing average housework and gaining 11.4 kg (25 lb) during pregnancy. This amounts to 200 kcal/day during pregnancy to meet additional energy needs.

Caloric expenditure is minimal during early pregnancy, increases sharply during the second trimester, and remains fairly constant to term. During the second trimester, the extra caloric requirements are due principally to maternal needs, such as the expansion of blood volume, uterine and breast hypertrophy, and accumulation of adipose tissue. In the third trimester, fetal and placental growth account for most of the additional energy needs.

The basic nutritional needs of the fetus at different gestational ages are unknown. In the past, glucose was thought to supply all of the substrate required for fetal oxidative metabolism, but amino acid catabolism may supply a considerable amount of substrate for aerobic metabolism. Thus, the adequate supply and transfer of glucose and amino acids to the fetus is essential for normal fetal growth.

EFFECT OF DIETARY DEFICIENCY ON FETAL GROWTH AND DEVELOPMENT

Animal models have been a major source of information relative to the role of nutrition in human pregnancy. Numerous animal experiments suggest that dietary deprivation in general and protein restriction in particular during pregnancy impair fetal growth and development. Protein and other nutritional deficiencies in rodents lead to growth retardation, increased mortality, lower intelligence, and physical and behavioral abnormalities. Animals born of protein-restricted mothers have permanent impairment in their ability to use nitrogen and a deficit in the total number of brain cells that can still be observed at weaning, even if they have been nursed by normal foster mothers receiving adequate nutrition. Related studies have clearly demonstrated that the physical growth of the brain can be seriously restricted by comparatively mild undernutrition during the periods of its fastest growth and that such restrictions have certain permanent sequelae. The greatest increase in mass in the human fetus, particularly in that of its brain, occurs during the last few weeks of gestation and the first 4 months after birth.

Unlike investigations in animals, studies in women are inexact since the experimental conditions cannot be precisely regulated. Human malnutrition is commonly associated with such factors as poverty, lack of education, social deprivation, and an increased incidence of infection and chronic disease. It is difficult to dissociate the mutual influence of these factors on one another. Despite these handicaps, indirect data indicate that the physical and mental well-being of infants subjected to malnutrition during fetal life may be impaired, just as in other mammalian species. The following conditions are known to make greater demands on maternal nutritional reserve, and, hence, predispose to fetal growth retardation and in many cases, subsequent impairment of mental development:

Multiple pregnancy
Maternal acetonuria during pregnancy with or without diabetes (third trimester)
Rapid succession of pregnancies
History of low birth weight in previous pregnancies
Low prepregnancy weight
Inadequate pregnancy weight gain
Malabsorption
Smoking

Nutrients are distributed from the maternal bloodstream into the various tissues according to metabolic needs; thus, tissues that are more active metabolically receive a greater proportion of materials. During pregnancy, the conceptus participates in this partition and, based on its higher metabolic rate, receives more nutrients per unit of weight than the mother. If nutrients become less available, the fetus competes advantageously with the mother. As the limitations become more severe, the fetus receives a proportionately larger share of nutrients. Fetal growth is affected only when the restriction of calories or proteins during pregnancy is extreme. Under conditions of severe protein or dietary restriction during pregnancy, the mother does not use a significant amount of her own tissues to support fetal growth, and the deprivation is proportionately greater for the conceptus than for the mother.

PROTEINS AND AMINO ACID CHANGES DURING PREGNANCY

The nitrogen balance is positive during pregnancy because of the requirements of the fetus and the growth of the reproductive tract. Nitrogen may also be retained for other maternal organs, such as the alimentary tract and liver. The amount of retained nitrogen has been estimated to be 1.17–1.3 g/day, which exceeds fetal needs by a considerable margin if protein intake is adequate.

Pregnancy brings about considerable change in serum protein levels. There is a progressive decline in total protein and albumin concentrations and a steady decrease in the albumin/globulin ratio. Late in the puerperium, total protein and albumin levels return to prepregnancy levels, and the albumin/globulin ratio assumes the prepregnancy relationship. Serum concentrations of many globulins are also altered in the

course of gestation. A pregnancy zone protein that migrates electrophoretically in the α_2-globulin region has been observed in the serum of the majority of pregnant women. Large-molecular-weight proteins are selectively transported across the placental barrier in varying amounts.

It is generally accepted that the free α-amino acid concentration is reduced in the maternal plasma during pregnancy. The level of free amino acid nitrogen is about 25% lower than that in the plasma of nonpregnant women. The reduction in concentration is not the same for all amino acids, however. Amino acids pass freely and rapidly across the placenta by active transport and usually have a higher concentration in fetal than in maternal plasma. The ratio of essential amino acid concentrations in the umbilical vein to those in the maternal antecubital vein is lower in pregnancies complicated by intrauterine growth retardation than it is in normal pregnancies. Increased amino aciduria during pregnancy is well documented.

AMNIOTIC FLUID PROTEINS

A progressive decrease in the amount of proteins in amniotic fluid is observed in the course of gestation. During the first 6 months of pregnancy, the levels vary between 0.6–1.8 mg/100 ml. A plateau is reached prior to 32 weeks, after which there is a progressive decrease. Higher levels of proteins have been found when the fetus has been critically affected by erythroblastosis. An inverse relationship between amniotic fluid protein levels and infant birth weight has been demonstrated.

Several studies suggest that amniotic fluid proteins originate from both mother and fetus. The bulk of the amniotic fluid proteins comes directly or indirectly from the mother, but fetal urinary proteins also contribute to the pool. However, the α_1-fetoprotein present in the amniotic fluid is almost exclusively of fetal origin; it is passed into the amniotic fluid by means of fetal urine and possibly by other routes as well.

The major process involved in clearance of amniotic fluid protein is fetal swallowing. The absorption of intact proteins from amniotic fluid by fetal lung, cord, or skin appears to be negligible. All of the proteins leaving amniotic fluid are not cleared by fetal swallowing; approximately 10%–15% are probably cleared by diffusion through fetal membranes. The amniotic fluid protein swallowed by the fetus is subsequently hydrolyzed to amino acids, absorbed, and used by the fetus for the synthesis of body proteins. Only a fraction of the ingested and absorbed proteins is subsequently excreted into the amniotic fluid. Thus, amniotic fluid proteins swallowed by the fetus are not merely recycled but are, for the most part, a contribution by the mother to fetal nutrition and metabolism.

WEIGHT GAIN

For many years pregnant women were advised to limit their weight gain during pregnancy to less than 20 lb and to restrict their dietary intake to achieve this goal. This practice was based on the assumption that excessive weight gain in pregnancy might in some way be associated with or lead to the development of preeclampsia. Many studies in the last decade have shown that arbitrary weight restriction does not influence the incidence of preeclampsia and that it is potentially harmful to both mother and fetus.

It is generally agreed that for a woman of standard weight before pregnancy, a gain of 24–27 lb (11–13 kg) is associated with the most favorable maternal and fetal outcome. The rate of weight gain must also be taken into account. The usual pattern consists of minimal weight accumulation (1–2 kg) during the first trimester and a progressive increase thereafter to term, although the greatest accumulation rate of weight gain is linear from approximately 10 weeks until term (see Fig. 17–8).

Prepregnancy weight and pregnancy weight gain have been shown to be significantly related to infant birth weight. Prepregnancy weight indicates maternal nutritional status before pregnancy, and pregnancy weight gain is indicative of caloric intake during gestation. Other studies have demonstrated that infant birth weight is positively correlated with IQ. Maternal height shows no significant correlation with infant development.

DIETARY REQUIREMENTS IN PREGNANCY

Proteins

Considerable evidence suggests that protein deprivation during pregnancy has deleterious effects on the course of pregnancy and fetal development. Also, the levels of certain maternal blood amino acids and proteins correlate significantly with infant birth weight, length, cranial volume, and motor and mental development. Additional proteins are needed during pregnancy for both mother and fetus. Amino acids derived from dietary proteins are used for expanded maternal blood volume and other tissues, as well as for fetal synthesis of its own proteins.

The optimal protein requirement during pregnancy has not been precisely determined and probably varies depending on the woman's age and nutritional status prior to pregnancy. The current RDA is 1.3–1.7 g/kg/day or, for most women, in excess of 75 g/day (Table 11–2).

Carbohydrates

Sufficient carbohydrate in the diet is required to prevent ketosis and excessive breakdown of proteins. The

TABLE 11-2. REQUIRED NUTRIENTS DURING PREGNANCY AND LACTATION

Nutrients	RDA Nonpregnant	RDA Pregnant	RDA Lactation
TOTAL CALORIES (kcal)	2100	2400	2600
PROTEINS (g)	46	76	66
IRON (mg)	18	36	18
CALCIUM (mg)	800	1200	1200
IODINE (μg)	100	125	150
MAGNESIUM (mg)	300	450	450
PHOSPHORUS (mg)	800	1200	1200
ZINC (mg)	15	20	25

mother may store calories ingested in any form early in pregnancy, and these calories may be used for subsequent fetal growth. A supply of sufficient calories in the form of carbohydrate usually makes it unnecessary to use more important nutrients such as proteins for growth. A minimum of 50–200 g/day of digestible carbohydrates should be provided during pregnancy.

Fats and Essential Fatty Acids

Linoleic acid and arachidonic acid are the only fatty acids known to be essential for the human fetus. The diet of pregnant women must contain 1%–2% essential fatty acids to prevent deficiency. Vegetable oils (*e.g.,* corn, cotton seed, peanut) are the best source of linoleic acid. Arachidonic acid is usually found in animal fats. A sample meal pattern for pregnant women is shown in Table 11–3.

Effect of Dietary Supplementation on Fetal Growth and Development

Controlled studies in several large population groups in developing countries have shown that food supplementation of undernourished women during pregnancy improves fetal outcome. For example, in studies performed with a chronically malnourished population in rural Guatemala, it was observed that women whose diet was supplemented consistently delivered infants with higher birth weight who scored better on mental and motor tests. Furthermore, infant mortality was significantly decreased as the level of maternal supplementation during pregnancy and lactation increased. In developed countries, specific inquiry should be made as to dietary habits. Supplementation should be used if RDAs are not met.

Effect on Newborn of Maternal Alcohol Ingestion During Pregnancy

The effects of alcohol in pregnancy and the "fetal alcohol syndrome" are considered in Chapter 19. Total abstinence appears to be the best policy in pregnancy.

Trace Elements and Vitamins

Minerals and vitamins play a major role in regulating metabolic processes of living organisms. In pregnancy, more of these nutrients are required to satisfy the needs of the growing fetus and to maintain the optimal nutritional status of the mother. Vitamins and minerals cannot be synthesized *de novo* in the human organism. Thus, an increased demand can only be met by available reserves or additional supply. Fortunately, these substances are found in abundance in the average diet.

Minerals. Trace elements serve a variety of functions but act primarily as catalysts in enzyme systems in the cells. In the metalloenzymes, the metal moiety is firmly associated with a protein from which it cannot be easily dissociated.

Under normal circumstances, a deficiency of a trace element is uncommon, even though the supply may be insufficient during pregnancy. However, a deficiency may develop when an inadequate body reserve (before pregnancy) of a trace element is followed by a deficient supply during pregnancy.

Iron. An essential component of hemoglobin, iron is a large-molecular-weight substance responsible for oxygen transport to all organs, tissues, and cells. When there is an iron deficiency, sufficient hemoglobin cannot be synthesized and anemia results.

During pregnancy, two factors contribute to greater demands for iron: 1) a quantity of iron amounting to 300–400 mg is diverted to the fetus for its development, and 2) approximately 500 mg iron are required for expansion of the maternal hemoglobin mass if hemoglobin and hematocrit values are to remain within normal limits in the face of increased plasma volume. Further, variable amounts of blood loss sustained during delivery and in the postpartum period (200–250 mg iron) make additional iron supplies necessary. Thus, at least 500–600 mg iron are lost during each pregnancy. Few women have these quantities in reserve, and iron deficiency anemia is the consequence. Rapid succession of pregnancies imposes repeated demands on maternal iron reserves, which cannot be replaced by dietary iron alone. Because of dietary factors and losses sustained during menstruation and pregnancy, all women are prone to iron deficiency.

Prevention of iron deficiency involves administration of an iron supplement to every pregnant woman. It is recommended that 30–60 mg ferrous salt be supplied daily. In addition, the pregnant woman should consume a well-balanced diet containing adequate amounts of proteins, fruit, and vegetables (Table 11–2).

All iron preparations are potentially and equally toxic. In adult, iron poisoning is very rare. Iron supplementation in physiologic and pharmacologic doses

TABLE 11-3. SAMPLE MEAL PATTERN

Meal	Nonpregnant Woman	Pregnant Woman
BREAKFAST	1 serving of vitamin C rich fruits & vegetables 1 serving of grain products 1 serving of milk & milk products	1 serving of vitamin C rich fruits & vegetables 1 serving of grain products 1 serving of milk & milk products
MORNING SNACK	Optional	Optional
LUNCH	2 servings of grain products 1 serving of protein foods 1 serving of other fruits & vegetables 1 serving of milk & milk products	2 servings of grain products 1 serving of protein foods 1 serving of other fruits & vegetables 1 serving of milk & milk products
AFTERNOON SNACK	1 serving of protein foods ½ serving of milk & milk products	1 serving of protein foods ½ serving of milk & milk products
DINNER	1 serving of protein foods 2 servings of leafy green vegetables	2 servings of protein foods 2 servings of leafy green vegetables 1 serving of milk & milk products
EVENING SNACK	½ serving of milk & milk products	½ serving of milk & milk products

(Adapted from Nutrition During Pregnancy and Lactation, California State Department of Public Health, 1975)

during pregnancy has not been found to be associated with any untoward effects in the mother or fetus. A suggestion that iron ingestion during pregnancy may be teratogenic has been refuted by several studies.

Copper. Hemoglobin formation, autooxidation (conversion of atmospheric oxygen to water), reproduction, and several other functions require copper. Blood copper concentration is influenced by the level of dietary copper and by its ratio to other components of the diet, notably molybdenum, inorganic sulfate, zinc, and iron. Serum copper rises dramatically during pregnancy and returns to normal slowly in the 1st weeks postpartum. These changes may be due to increased endogenous estrogens, since administration of oral contraceptives and estrogen preparations causes similar effects.

A drop in the copper level during pregnancy has been proposed as an index of placental insufficiency and as an indicator of impending fetal death. A rise in serum copper levels above the normal pregnancy level is found in preeclampsia. *Chloasma*, a darkening of the skin commonly observed in pregnancy and in estrogen users, appears to result from oxidation of tyrosine to melanine by tyrosinase, a copper-containing enzyme. Copper and zinc are antagonists, and an excess of one can cause a relative deficiency of the other. Thus, copper excess may contribute to human zinc deficiency with well-known consequences.

Zinc. Zinc is a normal constituent of many metalloenzymes, including carbonic anhydrase, alkaline phosphatase, alcohol dehydrogenase, and pancreatic peptidase. It is essential for growth of all tissues, since it is required for normal mobilization of vitamin A from the liver and for synthesis of nucleic acid. It also participates in protein synthesis and carbohydrate metabolism. Zinc is absorbed in the small intestine, predominantly in the duodenum. Its absorption is adversely affected by high calcium intake and by high levels of copper, cadmium, and phytate, which bind the zinc in a form from which it is not readily released and absorbed. Absorption of zinc increases when there is a deficiency and declines when zinc intake is higher. The plasma zinc level declines gradually during pregnancy, reaching its lowest concentration in the third trimester. Zinc is rapidly transported through the placental barrier to the fetus.

Nutritional deficiency of zinc is known to occur in humans. Clinical manifestations in patients from the Middle East included short stature, marked hypogonadism, rough skin, hepatosplenomegaly, and iron deficiency anemia. Fetal growth, as determined by adjusted birth weight, seems to be related to maternal plasma zinc levels. Reduced serum zinc concentration during early pregnancy has been linked to preterm birth, abnormal labor, or atonic bleeding. The current RDA for zinc in pregnancy is 20 mg daily, an increase of 5 mg daily over the allowance for nonpregnant

women (Table 11–2). Common foods vary greatly in zinc content. Animal proteins are the principal dietary source of zinc. Most mixed diets in human adults supply from 12–15 mg/day of zinc. Thus, supplementation may be necessary in pregnant women with substandard or protein-deficient diet.

Fluorine. Fluorine is known to affect the activity of several enzymes, and has a role in absorption or utilization of other dietary nutrients. Daily supplemental administration of fluorine (NaF 2.2 mg) during pregnancy has been suggested to improve dental hygiene and to prevent dental caries in offspring. The need for additional intake of fluorine in pregnancy remains to be confirmed.

Iodine. The importance of iodine in the synthesis and metabolism of thyroid hormone is well known. Deficiency of iodine inevitably leads to enlargement of the thyroid and goiter. In areas of endemic goiter, each person should receive supplements of not less than 100 μg iodine daily. In the United States, Canada, and most countries of Latin America, salt is iodinized at a level of 1 part in 10,000, providing a supplement of about 200 μg/day (Table 11–2).

Analysis of data collected by the Collaborative Perinatal Project suggested an association between iodine-containing drugs and fetal malformations. However, the data were clearly insufficient to justify anything more than a suspicion of possible teratogenicity, which requires confirmation.

Magnesium. One of the most plentiful elements on earth is magnesium, which is associated with many biologic processes. In humans, magnesium deficiency may be manifested by muscular twitching and tremor, muscle spasms similar to those of tetanus, cardiac arrhythmia, ventricular fibrillation, and even death. Intoxication and hypermagnesemia occur mainly in patients with serious renal insufficiency, preeclampsia, or eclampsia when large doses of magnesium salts are administered. Serious complications of magnesium toxicity include respiratory paralysis and cardiac arrest.

Calcium. Pregnancy is accompanied by extensive adjustment in calcium metabolism. The rate of bone turnover is enhanced progressively throughout pregnancy, apparently as a result of human chorionic somatomammotropin. Estrogen inhibits bone resorption, inducing a compensatory increase in the output of parathyroid hormone—which maintains the serum calcium level—as well as enhancing intestinal absorption and decreasing urinary excretion of calcium. There is probably also some increase in calcitonin, which preserves the maternal skeleton in the face of elevated parathyroid hormone. The net effect of these alterations is to promote progressive calcium retention during pregnancy. The changes begin well in advance of the time of fetal skeletal mineralization and appear to represent anticipatory adjustments. The maternal total serum calcium level declines during pregnancy, but the fall is apparently related to the physiologic hypoalbuminemia that involves only the protein-bound portion. Ionic calcium levels remain constant due, in part, to increasing maternal parathyroid hormone output. The placenta transports calcium ions from mother to fetus against a concentration gradient, making the fetus hypercalcemic with respect to its mother. The amount of additional calcium stored in the products of conception is approximately 30 g.

The current RDA for calcium during pregnancy is 1200 mg daily, an increase of 400 mg over the allowance for the nonpregnant adult (Table 11–2). Dairy products are the principal food source of calcium. Cow's milk contains an average of 120 mg calcium/100 ml. A quart of milk (approximately 1 liter) provides the exact RDA for calcium in pregnancy. Thus, in women who have an adequate intake of dairy products, calcium supplementation may be unnecessary. Pregnant women who are unwilling or unable to ingest a diet rich in milk or milk products may need supplemental calcium.

Severe calcium deficiency in pregnancy occurs only with sustained dietary inadequacy and may lead to osteomalacia.

Vitamins. Adequate supplies of vitamins during pregnancy are necessary to ensure normal development and viability of the offspring (Table 11–4). Some surveys have found that mothers who had not taken any iron or vitamin supplement during pregnancy delivered more preterm infants. Also, an association between low folic acid levels and pregnancy wastage has been suggested by a few studies. Most of the evidence suggests that despite a higher demand for vitamins in pregnancy, under normal circumstances and with an adequate, well-balanced diet, most women do not require supplemental vitamins in pregnancy.

Fat-Soluble Vitamins. The fat-soluble vitamins (A, D, E, and K) are stored principally in the liver and are readily available for increased demands. Therefore, deficiencies are not known. However, since urinary excretion is limited, toxicity from overdosage is a potential danger.

Vitamin A (Retinol). Several physiologic functions require vitamin A, *e.g.,* vision, growth, and development of epithelial tissue and bone, spermatogenesis, and fetal development. Maternal serum concentrations of vitamin A decrease during early pregnancy, rise in late pregnancy, fall during labor, and increase again postpartum. Alterations in this pattern have been observed in pathologic conditions and in poor nutritional circumstances. The levels may also be affected by factors such as socioeconomic status, fetal sex, and vitamin

TABLE 11-4. VITAMINS IN PREGNANCY AND LACTATION

Vitamin	Changes in Pregnancy (Blood Level)	RDA in Women/Day		
		Nonpregnant	Pregnant	Lactating
FAT-SOLUBLE				
Vitamin A (IU) (retinol)	Decrease in early pregnancy; increase in late pregnancy	4000	5000	6000
Vitamin D (IU)	Unchanged	400	400	400
Vitamin E (IU) (tocopherol)	Increase of 40%–50%	12	15	15
WATER-SOLUBLE				
Vitamin B_1 (mg) (thiamine)	Usually decreased	1.1	1.4	1.4
Vitamin B_2 (mg) (riboflavin)	Decreased	1.4	1.7	1.9
Vitamin B_3 (pantothenic acid)	Decreased			
Vitamin B_5 (mg) (niacin)	Increased urinary excretion	14	16	18
Vitamin B_6 (mg) (pyridoxine)	Progressive decline during pregnancy	2	2.5	2.5
Vitamin B_7 (biotin)				
Vitamin B_{12} (μg) (cobalamin)	Marked decrease	3	8	6
Folic acid (μg)	Decreased	400	800	600
Vitamin C (mg) (ascorbic acid)	Decreased	45	60	60
Vitamin K				

supplementation. Both vitamin A and its precursor, carotene, cross the placental barrier. Serum concentration of vitamin A in the newborn is slightly lower, and that of carotene is considerably lower, than concentrations of these substances in maternal serum. The RDA for vitamin A during pregnancy is 5000 IU daily, an increase of 25% over the allowance for nonpregnant adult females. Dietary sources can readily provide the necessary amount of vitamin A, and there is usually no need for supplementation. Animal studies have shown that vitamin A deficiency is teratogenic, but there is no confirmatory evidence in humans.

Hypervitaminosis A is associated with teratogenicity in experimental animals. Renal and central nervous system anomalies in human neonates have been reported after large doses of vitamin A were administered to the pregnant mother. Some food faddists advocate massive amounts of vitamin A; patients should be cautioned against this practice, particularly during pregnancy.

Vitamin D. A deficiency in vitamin D is uncommon in the adult unless exposure to sunlight is restricted. The principal circulating metabolite of vitamin D in human plasma is 25-hydroxycholecalciferol (25-OHC). The importance of vitamin D in calcium metabolism has long been recognized; it promotes calcium absorption and regulates bone mineralization. Studies have demonstrated its role in promoting positive calcium balance in pregnant women. Vitamin D requirements are not usually increased in pregnancy. In fact, there is evidence that markedly excessive intake may cause maternal hypercalcemia, predisposing the fetus to severe forms of infantile hypercalcemia. The RDA for vitamin D is 400 IU/day for both pregnant and nonpregnant women (Table 11–4).

Water-Soluble Vitamins. The B complex vitamins, B_6, ascorbic acid, and folic acid are water-soluble. These vitamins, in contrast to fat-soluble ones, are readily excreted in urine, and are not stored in the body in significant amounts. Because of the lack of reserves, they must be supplied frequently; also, deprivation is more likely to lead to deficiency, and toxicity and overdosage are less likely.

Vitamin B_1 (Thiamine). In carbohydrate metabolism, thiamine pyrophosphate functions as a coenzyme in decarboxylation of α-ketoacids. Pyruvic acid tends to accumulate in tissues that are thiamine-deficient. Most investigations have shown that an increased amount of thiamine is required throughout pregnancy. By the last month of pregnancy, 30%–80% of pregnant women are probably biochemically thiamine-deficient. The current RDA for thiamine in the nonpregnant female is 1 mg daily, to which the addition of 0.3 mg daily is recommended during pregnancy. This amount can readily be provided by the diet, at least in developed countries. Severe thiamine deficiencies can occur in neglected hyperemesis gravidarum, and in extreme cases, gestational polyneuritis (see Chapter 26) can result.

Vitamin B_2 (Riboflavin). As a coenzyme or flavoprotein, riboflavin functions in tissue oxidation and respiration; it is involved in both protein and energy metabolism. Riboflavin deficiency in humans is characterized by lesions of the lips, fissures at the angles of the mouth, localized seborrheic dermatitis of the face, and glossitis. Riboflavin deficiency, however, is seldom seen without other nutritional deficiencies.

In pregnant women, hypovitaminosis B_2 is not rare; in contrast to the findings in animal experiments, however, a relationship between riboflavin deficiency and fetal malformation has not so far been recognized in

humans. Since riboflavin depletion may occur in pregnancy, some investigators have recommended supplementation for pregnant women. RDA for nonpregnant women is 1.4 mg between ages 15 and 22 and 1.2 mg daily thereafter, to which 0.3 mg daily is added during pregnancy.

Vitamin B₅ or Nicotinic Acid (Niacin). Niacin functions in the body as a component of two important coenzymes in glycolysis and tissue respiration. A progressive increase in urinary excretion of niacin metabolites has been observed during pregnancy. Large doses of niacin, up to 2 g/kg body weight, have not been found to have any toxic effect in human subjects.

Vitamin B₆ (Pyridoxine). There are no definitive clinical manifestations of vitamins B₆ deficiency. Oral lesions similar to those induced by riboflavin deficiency have been demonstrated during experimentally induced vitamin B₆ deficiency. A progressive decline in plasma pyridoxal phosphate levels during pregnancy has also been observed. (Several studies have shown that women taking oral contraceptives require substantially larger amounts of vitamin B₆ to maintain serum levels and biochemical normalcy than do nonpregnant controls.) Estimates of requirements during pregnancy range from 2.5–20 mg/day. For reasons that are not apparent, levels of vitamin B₆ in cord blood are double the levels found in maternal blood.

Vitamin B₁₂ (Cobalamin). The antipernicious anemia vitamin, B₁₂, is the extrinsic factor required for hematopoiesis. Vitamin B₁₂ deficiency in humans is usually due to poor absorption rather than to inadequate dietary intake. Malabsorption of cobalamin leads to megaloblastic anemia and its associated neurologic complications. Other conditions described in association with vitamin B₁₂ deficiency include infertility in females, and semen and sperm anomalies in males. The RDA for vitamin B₁₂ has been established at 3 µg. During pregnancy, 8 µg/day is recommended. Dietary intake alone supplies sufficient vitamin B₁₂.

Folic Acid. A member of the vitamin B complex, folic acid acts as a cofactor in deoxyribonucleic acid (DNA) synthesis. In folic acid deficiency, DNA is replicated at a reduced rate, and mitotic activity of individual cells is delayed. Specific morphologic changes occur in virtually all cells in the body when DNA formation is slowed; cell maturation is dysplastic, megaloblasts appear in the bone marrow, and anemia develops. Megaloblastic anemia as a result of folic acid deficiency occurs in a substantial proportion of pregnant women in developing countries; it is less common, although it does occur, in developed nations. It is much more common in multiple pregnancy and in conditions associated with abnormally high rates of erythropoiesis, *e.g.,* hemolytic anemia. The incidence of megaloblastic marrow in pregnant women follows a pattern parallel to the fetal growth curve. Folic acid deficiency may occur as a result of inadequate diet, defects in absorption and use, or a combination of these factors.

Considerable evidence indicates that folic acid requirements are substantially increased in pregnancy; among the factors potentially responsible are impaired absorption, defective utilization, and increased demand. Defects in utilization or metabolism of folic acid may be related to increased estrogen levels in pregnancy, since similar alterations are observed in oral contraceptive users. It appears, however, that increased metabolic demand is the most important factor.

The current RDA for folic acid in pregnancy is 800 µg/day. Several studies have correlated folic acid deficiency in nonanemic patients with certain complications of pregnancy, such as abruptio placentae, spontaneous abortion, fetal malformation, and preeclampsia. Other investigators have been unable to confirm reproductive wastage or complications as a result of this deficiency. The preponderance of current opinion is that, because of the increased folic acid needs during pregnancy and the marginal amounts of this substance contained in the average American diet, there should be routine folic acid supplementation of all pregnant women.

Vitamin C (Ascorbic Acid). The major function of ascorbic acid is formation of tissue collagen. In addition, vitamin C with ferrous iron has been shown to catalyze the hydroxylation of proline and possibly lysine in collagen formation. There is also evidence that ascorbic acid is involved in the metabolism of folic acid and in the absorption and utilization of iron, and that it regulates cholesterol metabolism.

A deficiency in vitamin C is characterized by the appearance of scurvy. Ascorbic acid levels in maternal plasma decline progressively during pregnancy. Values at term are approximately half those of midpregnancy. Fetal serum levels are 50% higher than maternal values. Ascorbic acid deficiency during pregnancy is almost nonexistent in developed countries. A possible relationship between low plasma levels of this vitamin and premature rupture of the membranes, as well as between low levels and preeclampsia, has been suggested. The RDA for nonpregnant and pregnant women is 45 mg/day and 60 mg/day, respectively (Table 11–4).

MATERNAL NUTRITION DURING LACTATION

Maternal milk is usually considered the best source of nutrition for the newborn infant. Breast-feeding fortunately appears to be on the rise in the United States. In developing countries, breast-feeding is an important and inexpensive source of proteins and other nutrients for the infant. Additionally, a prolonged lactation period may be a safe and reasonably effective means of birth control for populations of women who would otherwise be likely to become pregnant again after a very short time. Lactation, however, imposes consider-

able nutritional demands on the mother. It is believed that the needs of an infant will be satisfied by a milk output of 850 ml/day. This would amount to a total dietary supplement of 21,775 kcal for the lactating mother who nurses her infant for a period of 1 year. In an assessment of the nursing mother's dietary needs, allowances should be made for individual patterns of absorption, depletion of tissues because of repeated childbearing, existing degrees of malnutrition, and the amount of energy expended.

CALORIES

Caloric supplies during lactation should be sufficient to provide for milk production and to meet the increased calorific demands on the mother to produce the calories in the milk. The present RDA, consisting of an additional 500 kcal (Table 11–2), takes into account the presence of a pregnancy "fat bank" of 3.5 kg, which is deposited in well-nourished women and is believed to subsidize lactation at the rate of 300 kcal/day for 3–4 months. It is important therefore to pay adequate attention to individual circumstances. If the amount of fat laid down during pregnancy is insufficient, more dietary energy is needed during lactation.

PROTEINS

Human milk contains approximately 1.1%–1.2% protein. The additional protein needed by a lactating mother for a year is estimated to be 3.3 kg. This would translate to a supplement of 20 g protein/day for nursing women (Table 11–2).

MICRONUTRIENTS

The need for additional minerals, trace elements, and vitamins in lactation depends on any existing deficiencies. The concentrations of vitamins in milk is influenced by maternal dietary intake. Deficiencies of water-soluble vitamins, mainly riboflavin, thiamine, and ascorbic acid, have been noted. In most cases, the RDAs of vitamins are similar to those in pregnancy (Table 11–4). The concentration of calcium in the breast milk varies. In studies of malnourished women, normal to low concentrations have been reported. The amount of calcium secreted in the milk daily represents a net loss of 250–300 mg to the lactating woman. For this reason, an extra 400 mg calcium/day is added to the RDA of nursing mothers.

The amount of iron required by nursing women is similar to that required by nonlactating women. Considerably enhanced allowances are, however, recommended for zinc, phosphorus, magnesium, and iodine (Table 11–2).

NUTRITION IN POSTMENOPAUSAL WOMEN

Menopause is characterized by the cessation of menstrual cycles and the cessation or considerable decrease of ovarian function. The extent of physiologic and metabolic changes that occur after the menopause varies among different women. Some of these changes, such as atrophy of the reproductive organs, are related to the lack of estrogen stimulation; others seem to be a part of the general process of aging. Endocrine and metabolic alterations observed during menopause have been the subject of numerous studies in recent years and are discussed in Chapter 8.

Increased morbidity and mortality in postmenopausal women owing to cardiovascular disease have been repeatedly documented. Atherosclerosis is recognized as a major underlying cause of cardiovascular disease, and there is strong evidence that nutrition and metabolism are centrally involved. Beneficial results in control of atherogenesis have been reported from diets of limited fat and cholesterol intake.

Osteoporosis, a condition characterized by reduced bone tissue relative to the volume of anatomic base and increased radiolucency of the skeleton, commonly appears among women after menopause. Osteoporotic women show an increased bone resorption, although their serum calcium, phosphorus, and alkaline phosphatase remain within normal limits. Osteoporosis is a major health hazard in postmenopausal women. The condition is responsible for a variety of atraumatic fractures, and such fractures occur in approximately 25% of postmenopausal women. Low calcium content of the diet may play a role. Other factors considered important include decreased activity or immobilization, loss of muscle tone, and lack of estrogen and nutrients such as vitamin D and phosphate.

NUTRITIONAL REQUIREMENTS

As mentioned earlier, some menopausal changes are associated with the aging process, and others are distinct from the aging process. Nutrient requirements of menopausal and older women are influenced by several factors: 1) nutritional status at the time of menopause, 2) body weight and body composition, 3) degree of physical activity, and 4) metabolic and endocrine changes. RDAs for older women do not differ from those for premenopausal women. In general, the quantitative requirements for essential amino acids, proteins, and calories decline with age. Because of the reduction in caloric consumption with increasing age, greater care must be taken in selection so that the nutrient intakes are not decreased. The most neglected food groups in the diet of older women are proteins, dairy products, and the green leafy and yellow vegetables.

The vitamin requirements of women over 50 are believed to be the same as those for younger women (Table 11–4). Older women who spend little or no time in the sunshine may be low in vitamin D. There is also some evidence that they use thiamine less efficiently and that vitamin B_6 requirements increase with age and with high-protein diets. Drugs commonly prescribed in old age may interfere with folic acid metabolism. Finally, those women who do not have a daily intake of fruits and vegetables may develop a deficiency of ascorbic acid.

The mineral elements that are most commonly lacking in the diet of older people are calcium and iron. The appearance of thin osteoporotic bones and the increased incidence of fractures among older women may be related to the meager supply of calcium in their diet as well as to diminished physical activity and estrogen deficiency.

SPECIAL NUTRITIONAL PROBLEMS

Overnutrition and undernutrition can occur in older women. Obesity is common in this age group, but undernutrition is a more frequent problem. Undernutrition can range from mild subclinical deficiencies to overt malnutrition. Malnutrition in the elderly is frequently related to socioeconomic, psychologic, or biomedical problems. It is important that the physician involved in the care of the elderly be prepared to evaluate nutritional deficiencies and to provide dietary advice and supplemental nutrients as needed.

NUTRITIONAL SUPPORT IN GYNECOLOGIC SURGERY

Six to eight hours before surgery the patient begins a period of partial starvation that lasts for an indefinite period until nutriment is either administered or is taken by mouth. The magnitude of the resulting changes depends upon the degree of the insult imposed by the surgery as well as the patient's nutritional status prior to surgery.

Three postoperative phases are recognized: an acute, or catabolic phase; an adaptive, or early anabolic phase; and a convalescent, or late anabolic phase. The *catabolic phase* is characterized principally by a sharp and immediate increase in metabolic demands. Catecholamines are immediately released into the circulation, stimulating ACTH release and consequently liberating adrenal corticosteroids. Retention of water and sodium results from the action of the mineralocorticoids and the renal hormones renin and angiotensin, accounting for the low urine output of the first several postoperative hours. Muscle protein is mobilized as a result of glucocorticoid-induced catabolism, and a negative nitrogen balance and also a negative potassium balance follow promptly. The *early anabolic phase* is characterized by withdrawal of the corticoid influence, synthesis or new protein, and reversal of the previously negative nitrogen and potassium balances and the previously positive sodium balance. Appetite, muscle strength, weight, and activity are increased, and it is at this point that patients are usually discharged from the hospital. The *convalescent phase* is characterized by a gain in body fat, a slow weight increase, and a gradual return to normal activity.

Most gynecologic surgical procedures are performed in 1 to 2 hours and, for the most part, the nutritional status of the patients is good. Most of the operations are elective, the catabolic phase is brief, and blood loss is rarely sufficient to require replacement. Among such patients the maintenance of nutritional balance is not a major problem, but due attention should be given to the several imbalances that do occur. Although most healthy, well-nourished women can withstand the protein catabolism and nitrogen loss for 5 to 7 days without notable effect, nevertheless the maintenance of normal nutritional balance can minimize the loss of muscle protein, improve wound healing, and hasten recovery. The protein-sparing effect of glucose is such that the administration of 100 g can reduce protein catabolism by about 50% in the presence of starvation; the effect is somewhat less in surgical patients, but it is still significant. In the uncomplicated gynecologic laparotomy, a sufficient source of energy and also compensation for the loss of fluid and sodium in the first 24 hours after surgery is supplied by an infusion of 1000 ml of 5% dextrose in 0.45N saline, repeated twice at 8-hour intervals. After 24 hours, sips of water, broth, tea, and carbonated liquids are taken by mouth, supplemented by 1500 ml of the above infusion. As a rule, progressive oral feedings suffice after 48 hours, and the infusion should be discontinued. (Thrombophlebitis at the infusion site is a significant threat after 48 hours; if an infusion is still needed, a new site should be selected.)

If there should be complications such that the gastrointestinal tract cannot be used for nutritional purposes and it is presumed that the patient will be eating again within 1 week, specific nutriments (amino acids, electrolytes) can be added to the infusion fluid for this short period. Blood and plasma must, of course, be administered when they are specifically indicated, but their use as nutritional supplements is neither indicated nor necessary. When caloric or protein needs are especially urgent, the use of *total parenteral nutrition (TPN; hyperalimentation)* should be considered. TPN, administered by a central venous catheter, is a major therapeutic regimen and it has been suggested that the results are vastly improved if it is carried out by a "nutrition support team" comprised of an attending physician, a pharmacist, a nurse, a clinical dietician, and an infection control coordinator. TPN is finding increased usefulness in selected postoperative

gynecologic patients, for example, ileal or mechanical intestinal obstruction, to avoid colostomy after extensive rectovaginal fistula repair, and exenterative or other extended oncologic procedures. (TPN has also been recommended for selected obstetric problems, including severe hyperemesis gravidarum, inflammatory bowel disease, and in certain cases in which the fetus is considered to be at risk because of estriol levels below the tenth percentile.)

REFERENCES AND RECOMMENDED READING

Benny PS, Legge M, Aickin DR: The biochemical effects of maternal hyperalimentation during pregnancy. New Zealand Med J 88:283, 1978

Ferguson DJ: Total parenteral nutrition and the team. JAMA 243:1931, 1980

Glenn F: The rationale for the administration of a NaF tablet supplement during pregnancy and postnatally in a private practice setting. J Dent Child 48: 118, 1981

Halpren SL: Quick Reference to Clinical Nutrition. Philadelphia, JB Lippincott 1979

Hew LR, Deitel M: Total parenteral nutrition in gynecology and obstetrics. Obstet Gynecol 55:464, 1980

Laboratory Indices of Nutritional Status in Pregnancy. Washington, DC, National Academy of Sciences, 1978

Maternal Nutrition and the Course of Pregnancy. Washington, DC, National Academy of Sciences, 1971

Moghissi KS: Maternal nutrition in pregnancy. Clin Obstet Gynecol 21:297, 1978

Moghissi KS, Churchill JA, Kurrie D: Relationship of maternal amino acids and proteins to fetal growth and development. Am J Obstet Gynecol 123:398, 1975

Moghissi KS, Evans TN (eds): Nutritional Impact on Women. Hagerstown, Harper & Row, 1977

Moore FD: Metabolic Care of the Surgical Patient. Philadelphia, WB Saunders, 1959

Mosley WH (ed): Nutrition and Human Reproduction. New York, Plenum Press, 1978

Naeye RL: Weight gain and the outcome of pregnancy. Am J Obstet Gynecol 135:3, 1979

Nehme AE: Nutritional support of the hospitalized patient. JAMA 243:1906, 1980

Pitkin RM: Vitamins and minerals in pregnancy. Clin Perinatol 2:221, 1975

Pitkin RM: Nutritional support in obstetrics and gynecology. Clin Obstet Gynecol 19:489, 1976

Shires T, Canizaro PC: Fluid, Electrolyte, and Nutritional Management of the Surgical Patient. In Schwartz SI (ed), Principles of Surgery, 3rd ed. New York, McGraw–Hill, 1979

Steffee WP: Malnutrition in hospitalized patients. JAMA 244:2630, 1980

IMMUNOBIOLOGIC ASPECTS OF OBSTETRICS AND GYNECOLOGY

James R. Scott

The obstetrician is in a unique position to observe the only natural grafting of tissue from one person to another—pregnancy. Since tissue grafts exchanged between mother and infant following delivery are doomed to failure, the immunobiologic mechanism that allow the maternal–fetal parabiotic relationship to prosper for 9 months are all the more intriguing. Nevertheless, interest in immunology developed relatively slowly in obstetrics and gynecology until the field was legitimized by the understanding, treatment, and finally the remarkably effective prophylaxis against Rh immunization (see Ch. 23). This disorder demonstrated to physicians for the first time that maternal–fetal immunology was of more than academic interest and suggested that other problems in obstetrics and gynecology should be studied from the immunologic standpoint. Although still in its infancy, reproductive immunology has now become a rapidly changing and expanding area of investigation and clinical application.

FUNDAMENTAL IMMUNOBIOLOGY

The principal function of the host immune system is to maintain the body's integrity by repelling and destroying invaders or antigens of extrinsic origin. However, abnormal cells, foreign tissues, and organs vary in their ability to withstand rejection by a host with an intact immune system, depending on such properties as inherent antigenicity, or, in the case of grafted tissue, the ability of the tissue to endure ischemia and the type of vascular and lymphatic anastomosis developed at the graft site. Even more important is the genetic relationship between donor and recipient; a major role of the immune system is to distinguish, in a biologic sense, "self" from "nonself." If the ability to distinguish self from nonself antigens is disturbed, autoimmune disease can result.

Autografts, where the recipient receives a graft of his or her own tissue, and syngeneic grafts exchanged between monozygotic twins or members of inbred strains of animals survive indefinitely. Conversely, allografts, which are those exchanged between genetically dissimilar members of the same species, are ultimately rejected after a transient period of viability. The antigens of the human leukocyte antigen system (HLA antigens) are products of a gene complex located on the short arm of chromosome 6 and constitute the major histocompatibility system of man. These antigens, associated with certain diseases that appear to have immunologic overtones, are cell membrane–associated glycoproteins of 45,000 molecular weight expressed by all nucleated human cells.

The characteristic cells of the immune system are derived from undifferentiated stem cells that originate in the fetal yolk sac, whence they migrate to the fetal thymus (T cells) or to bursa-equivalent structures (B cells). (The term *bursa-equivalent* takes its origin from the bursa of Fabricius, a primary lymphoid organ in the avian hind gut that mediates humoral immunity in birds. In the human, this term refers to such tissues as bone marrow, liver, spleen, Peyer's patches, and the pharyngeal tonsils.) After partial maturation in thymus or bursa-equivalent areas, the cells migrate to the secondary lymphatic structures where they undergo further maturation and differentiation when they are confronted by an antigen.

NORMAL IMMUNE REACTIONS

Primary allograft rejection and elimination of foreign cells of any origin require three essential processes that occur in sequence and involve chiefly the lym-

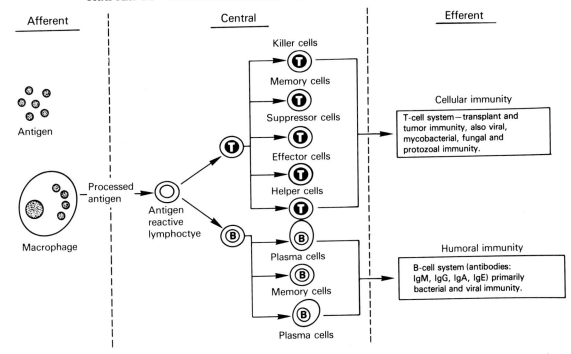

FIG. 12-1. Schematic view of cellular (T cells) and humoral (B cells) components of the immune system.

phatic system (Fig. 12–1): 1) the action of the afferent limb, 2) central processing, and 3) the action of the efferent limb. In the *afferent limb,* the foreign antigens are identified by tissue macrophages, and some of the alien antigenic material is carried to the draining lymph nodes.

The antigen provokes a reactive response in the lymphoid organs, and clones of small lymphocytes divide and differentiate for certain specialized functions. Differentiation proceeds along two general lines, producing either "sensitized" lymphocytes (T cells) or plasma cells (B cells). This is central processing.

T cells are involved principally in *cellular response.* They represent roughly 60%–80% of the lymphocytes in the peripheral blood and characteristically bind sheep red blood cells to form rosettes that can be seen by light microscopy and readily counted. At least five categories of T cells, differing from one another both in function and in cell surface features, have been identified:

1. *Effector cells* are an immunologically specific population of lymphocytes activated and generated predominantly in regional lymph nodes. It is thought that effector cells may be the precursors of the other categories of T cells.
2. *Killer cells,* which destroy foreign cells by elaboration of a cytotoxin, are largely responsible for allograft rejection.
3. *Memory cells* provide the cellular basis for anamnestic ("remembered") responses, by which an anti-

gen that was introduced in the past is quickly recognized if it is reintroduced.
4. *Suppressor cells* are regulatory cells that modify or suppress the formation of humoral antibody by B cells, thus modulating the humoral antibody response. This is one of the ways in which there is interdependence between B cells and T cells.
5. *Helper cells* promote the formation of antibody by enabling the B cells to respond to antigens that they would otherwise not recognize.

B cells are plasma cells that produce large amounts of surface immunoglobulins (Ig). These immunoglobulins circulate in the blood and other body fluids, and they can be detected with fluorescent antiimmunoglobulin serum (Fig. 12–2). It is these cells that give rise to the *humoral antibody response.* Also, some B cells are specialized, having been modified by the action of helper T cells so that they can recognize a reintroduced antigen.

In the *efferent limb,* the specially committed small lymphocytes leave the node through the efferent lymphatics, where they migrate to and infiltrate the parenchyma of the foreign tissue or confront invading organisms; they initiate the mechanism of destruction by direct binding with target cells, production of lymphotoxin, and secretion of soluble factors that activate macrophages and cause them to accumulate. The plasma cells, on the other hand, produce specific anti-

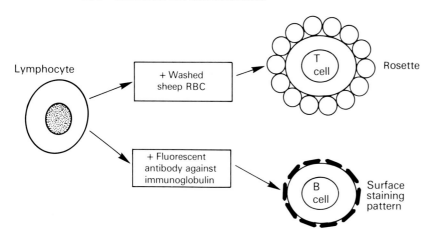

FIG. 12-2. Methods of identification of T cells and B cells. *RBC,* Red blood cells.

body that circulates through the bloodstream and destroys target cells, usually in concert with complement.

The primary humoral antibody response to an antigen in the adult is in the IgM fraction, which is soon superseded by a predominantly IgG response. Because the lymphoid system is capable of remembering its first contact with the antigen, a second exposure results in an accelerated and intensified anamnestic response. Antibodies themselves are heterogenous proteins composed of several different classes of immunoglobulins (Table 12–1). Four different subclasses of human IgG, each with slightly different properties, can be distinguished on the basis of differences in the heavy polypeptide chain of the Ig unit. In addition, human immunoglobulins carry highly specific labels, termed allotypic markers, that can be used to analyze the genetic control of immunoglobulin structure. Although complement, a collective term for a group of at least 11 distinct serum protein fractions, is the principal humoral mediator of the antigen–antibody reaction, the functional role of complement and antibodies in allograft rejection is still not clear.

IMMUNOLOGIC UNRESPONSIVENESS

It is obvious that the human being has a very elaborate and efficient immune system. Nevertheless, tumors grow, allografts are accepted, patients die of infections, and immunologic attack on the fetus is apparently infrequent. These dichotomies indicate that the immune apparatus is capable of responses ranging from sensitization to complete tolerance; the specific response depends on such variables as the strength, dose, physical form, route of administration, and age of the host at the time of antigen exposure. At times, the humoral mechanism may obstruct cell-mediated destruction of allogeneic cells through the production of blocking antibodies or formation of antigen–antibody com-

plexes. This mechanism of immunologic enhancement may involve 1) the afferent limb, if the antibody binds with the antigen and inhibits its antigenicity; 2) the central processing, if antibodies react with and inhibit the immunologically competent cells; or 3) the efferent limb, if antibodies coat target antigens and prevent interaction with the lymphoid cells. Host suppressor T cells and their factors can also undermine effective immune responses. These thymus-derived cells can inhibit antibody synthesis by B lymphocytes, exert a suppressive or restraining influence on mixed lymphocyte reactions, promote tumor cell proliferation, and establish unresponsiveness to certain antigens when adoptively transferred.

REPRODUCTIVE IMMUNOLOGY

MORPHOLOGY OF LYMPHOID TISSUE IN THE FEMALE GENITAL TRACT

There is a marked contrast between the highly organized lymphoid tissue in the gut and lung mucosa and the sparse lymphoid content in the much less studied female reproductive tract. The lymphatic drainage and main regional lymph nodes potentially involved in local and systemic immune responses in the human female genital tract are shown in Figure 12–3.

Although IgA and IgG immunoglobulins have been detected in vaginal secretions, it has been difficult to ascertain their origin. In view of the paucity of immunocompetent tissue in the vaginal epithelium and the constant contamination of the vagina by cervical secretions, it is likely that vaginal immunoglobulins are products of the cervix and endometrium. In cervical mucus, the ratios of IgA to IgG appear to be much higher than those observed in the serum, and variations in immunoglobulin levels have been demonstrated during the menstrual cycle. The concept of local synthesis of antibodies is supported by reports

TABLE 12-1. COMPARISON OF PROPERTIES OF VARIOUS IMMUNOGLOBULINS

Immunoglobulin Class	Cross Placenta?	Molecular Weight	Primary Location	Serum Concentration (mg/dl)	Antibody Activity
IgG	Yes	140,000	Intravascular	1000–1500	Most antibodies to bacterial and viral infections; major part of secondary response; Rh isoagglutinins; lupus erythematosus factor
IgM	No	900,000	Intravascular	50–110	First antibody formed; ABO isoagglutinins; rheumatoid factor
IgA	No	350,000	Seromucous	170–300	Major antibodies of external secretions—milk, colostrum, saliva, and secretions of GI, reproductive, respiratory tracts
IgD	No	180,000	Interstitial membrane-bound	0.3–40	Antibody activity rarely demonstrated; found on lymphocyte surfaces
IgE	No	200,000	Skin and epithelium	0.01–0.07	Reaginic antibodies

showing the presence of IgA and IgA-containing cells in cervical tissues. IgA and IgG have also been found in the human endometrium during the proliferative, secretory, and decidual phases. The immunoglobulins are distributed in the stroma between the glands and along the basement membrane of glandular epithelium. Although various tissues from the human genital tract are capable of *in vitro* synthesis of secretory immunoglobulins, IgG predominates in all endometrial specimens. Immunoglobulins in tubal fluid are also thought to be derived from serum.

FETOPLACENTAL ANTIGENICITY

The processes of fertilization and implantation constitute the two essential and specific acts of immunologic recognition between genetically dissimilar cells. The fertilized ovum undergoes fundamental changes in organization that render it potentially vulnerable to a maternal immune reaction, since minor and subsequently major transplantation antigens appear sequentially on the plasma membranes of embryonic cells from at least the two-cell stage onward. There is evidence, however, that early embryonic tissue is functionally hypoantigenic: ectopic pregnancies in many different sites are normally successful for considerable periods, even in presensitized hosts, and small grafts of pure trophoblastic tissue obtained from ectoplacental cones are invulnerable to transplantation immune reactions.

Further evidence that trophoblast becomes an immunologically privileged tissue comes from studies on plasma membranes prepared from human placentas that express very low levels of inherited HLA antigens. Trophoblastic cells contain an extracellular layer of

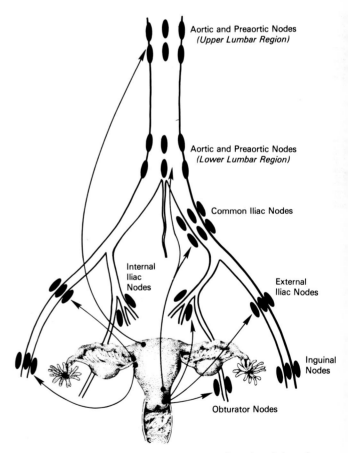

FIG. 12-3. Lymphatic drainage system and regional lymph nodes of female genital tract.

sialomucin, and, although all mammalian cells possess a net negative surface charge, lymphocytes and trophoblast excel in this biologic property. This strong electrostatic force at the cell surface may prevent antigen-reactive lymphocytes from reacting with trophoblastic cells. Moreover, cell surface determinants appear to be internalized into the villus and out of the trophoblastic epithelium as pregnancy progresses. The intrinsic loss or dilution of antigenic determinants from the trophoblastic plasma membrane, resulting in low antigen density, may create a situation in which the determinants are too widely spaced for linkage with lymphocytes, antibody, or complement.

It is essential to mention that, although antigenic peculiarities are associated with trophoblastic tissue, gestating mothers normally respond immunologically to the presence of allogeneic fetuses in their uteri, as evidenced by hypertrophy of the lymph nodes draining the uterus and the production of circulating cytotoxic antibodies. Definite Rh antigens have been found on human embryonic red cells by the 38th day of life, the embryo possesses a number of iso- and autoantigens by at least 6 weeks, and fetal tissues implanted outside the uterus are rejected.

FETAL IMMUNOCOMPETENCE

During the 2nd and 3rd weeks of gestation in the human fetus, pluripotential yolk sac stem cells form the precursors of all the blood cell series. The thymus develops at about 6 weeks' gestation and lymphocyte differentiation proceeds in the complete absence of foreign antigens. Small lymphocytes appear in the peripheral blood at about 7 weeks and in connective tissue around lymphocyte plexuses by 8 weeks. Primary lymph node development and lymphopoeisis do not occur until at least 12 weeks; but, as early as 13 weeks' gestation, T cells capable of responding to mitogens and recognizing histoincompatible cells begin to appear. In the spleen, lymphocyte aggregates form at 14 weeks, and by 20 weeks' gestation the human fetus can respond to congenital infections with the production of plasma cells and antibody.

The fetus generally enjoys a high degree of protection from infectious organisms in its isolated intrauterine environment and is not often called upon to demonstrate its immunologic capabilities, but immunologic maturation proceeds in preparation for exposure to a highly contaminated world. The transition of the fetus from immunologically incompetent to immunologically competent has a profound influence on disease processes. Immunologic immaturity and susceptibility of organizing fetal tissues are factors that make first trimester congenital rubella infection such a severe teratogenic process as compared with the relatively benign adult disease. Conversely, an active fetal immune response can actually contribute to the patho-

logic process in certain situations. For example, the changes caused by *Treponema pallidum* after it has crossed the placenta and gained access to the fetus are probably not due to adverse effects of the organism on fetal cells but rather to widespread inflammatory responses. Thus, the infection may occur at a much earlier stage but follow a benign course until the fetal host develops the capacity to respond to the organism during the 5th month of gestation.

In contrast to the response in an adult, the dominant humoral antibody response in the fetus is the IgM immunoglobulin fraction. Indeed, it is the presence of circulating IgM of fetal origin in umbilical cord blood that assists in the clinical diagnosis of such congenital infections as rubella, toxoplasmosis, syphilis, and cytomegalovirus. Since the large IgM molecule does not cross the placenta and immunoglobulins are not synthesized prior to antigenic stimulation, IgM is usually not detected in the fetal circulation or amniotic fluid of normal pregnancies. Conversely, the smaller IgG molecule, by virtue of its Fc fragment, is specifically selected for placental transfer. Fetal IgG, usually about 10% of adult levels by the middle of the first trimester, gradually increases throughout pregnancy, and a significant number of newborns have IgG levels higher than those of the mother.

Thus, adequate humoral immunity in the newborn period depends on the circulating maternal antibodies that have crossed the placenta. However, fetal blood levels of IgG tend to reflect maternal levels, and specific antibody protection in turn depends on the mother's own total antigenic experience. Moreover, maternal IgG antibodies, in addition to their primary role of protecting the neonate from infections, can result in disease syndromes such as neonatal thrombocytopenia, hyperthyroidism, and erythroblastosis fetalis.

MATERNAL IMMUNOLOGIC REACTIVITY

It is at once apparent that the placenta implanted on the maternal endometrium is in many respects analogous to a skin graft (Fig. 12–4), but it is also clear that the fetoplacental unit does not behave like most other conventional allografts. Of the many theories that have been put forward over the years to account for survival of the conceptus, none appears to explain it completely. The fetus and its placenta with self-protecting properties is not a vascularized intercommunicating graft and may not sensitize the host in the usual way, but the uterus is endowed with a vascular supply and lymphatic drainage system capable of eliciting classic transplantation immunity. Thus, most recent studies have focused on the possibility that maternal serum contains nonspecific or immunologically specific factors that protect the fetus from rejection.

During pregnancy there is an increased production

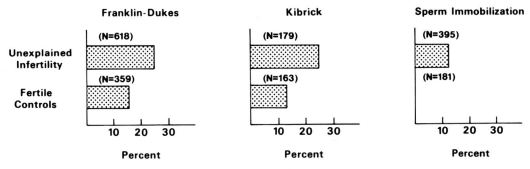

FIG. 12-8. Percentages of fertile and infertile women in whom sperm antibodies were found in three tests. (Scott JR: Semin Perinatol 1:149–160, 1977)

FIG. 12-9. Pregnancy rates in "immunologic" infertility with various modalities of therapy. Patients treated with condom therapy and corticosteroids have positive sperm antibody tests and patients treated with intrauterine insemination had poor postcoital tests.

Pregnancy rate in "immunologic" infertility
with various modalities of therapy.

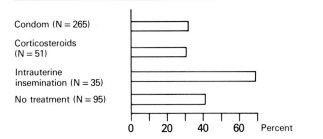

The most benign and commonly used treatment is condom therapy, the rationale being that it protects the woman from contact with seminal antigens until her level of immunity against these antigens is diminished. Over a period of 6–12 months, antisperm activity is monitored periodically; when the titer is significantly reduced or drops to zero, unprotected coitus is resumed at midcycle. Timing the first intercourse at the time of ovulation theoretically maximizes the chance of conception before the patient can develop an anamnestic response to the seminal antigens. Since corticosteroids have antiinflammatory and immunosuppressive properties and are successfully used clinically to treat a variety of immunologic disorders, it is possible that they could be utilized to suppress humoral or cellular responses to sperm antigens in either the man or woman. The two regimens used to date have been prednisolone, 5 mg three times per day for 2 weeks prior to ovulation, and methylprednisolone, 96 mg/day for 7 days. In order to bypass the "hostile" cervical mucus, artificial methods of intrauterine in-

semination have also been tried. However, very small amounts of semen must be used to avoid adverse side effects, such as uterine pain and anaphylactic reactions. There is considerable controversy over whether the pregnancy rates with these treatments result from placebo therapy, since none of the studies have been randomized or controlled and women with idiopathic infertility who are not treated in any way eventually have pregnancy rates in the range of 28%–42%.

Immunologic causes of infertility remain speculative at the present time, and no consistently reliable diagnostic tests have yet emerged from numerous investigations. It is intriguing that the fertilization process is so successful in the vast majority of cases and that there is no evidence that fertility decreases with multiparity. Treatment modalities currently in use are nonspecific and of uncertain clinical value, and this will remain the case until evidence is collected that definitely implicates immune mechanisms as a cause of infertility.

ABORTION

Since the immunologic mechanisms that allow a mother to tolerate her fetus are incompletely understood and alloantigens are only weakly expressed on preimplantation embryos, it is difficult to assess to what extent the failure of one of these factors might be responsible for spontaneous abortion. Despite the general resistance of fetuses to rejection, there are some indications from experimental animal studies that implantation and fetal survival can be influenced by the maternal immune response. In exaggerated maternal–fetal incompatibility models, illustrated by the transfer of fertilized sheep ova into the goat uterus, implantation occurs but the gestation usually fails by the 60th day of pregnancy. The death of the embryo and associated infiltration of adjacent maternal tissues by lymphocytes could be interpreted as evidence for a local immunologic response by the mother that is initiated by organ-specific or species-specific antigens of the trophoblast. Further evidence for this concept has come from studies in which abortion has been artifi-

typing of husband and wife is still being performed in some infertility evaluations, this practice is of doubtful value. Since HLA differences between husband and wife are the rule rather than the exception, it can safely be predicted that histoincompatibility must be an extremely rare cause of infertility.

There have been many attempts to measure serum antibody to sperm antigens, but the results have been inconclusive. Data from recent investigations in which patients with unexplained infertility were compared with fertile controls are shown in Figure 12–8. The controls were usually pregnant patients because of their proved fertility, but the immunologic alterations that occur during gestation may make them less than optimum control subjects in this case. There are marked differences in the results, and only the sperm immobilization test seems to have no false-positives. Proponents of sperm antibody testing maintain that these discrepancies can be explained by flaws in technique, study design, or interpretation. However, it has been reported that the Franklin–Dukes method measures a lipoprotein–steroid conjugate rather than true antibody, which casts some doubt on the significance of follow-up pregnancy rates in couples studied only by this method. The other tests measure an IgG or IgM antibody, but which of the multiple antigens present in semen provokes the antibody response is not well understood. It is even possible that current sperm antibody tests may have no relationship to infertility, but simply assay "nonspecific immunologic noise" from repeated exposure to sperm, somewhat analogous to the development of clinically insignificant HLA antibodies in many multiparous females. It has also been suggested recently that sperm antibodies as presently measured are simply cross-reacting antibodies to various bacteria commonly found in the vaginal flora and that they merely reflect exposure to these organisms. Possibly women who do develop isoimmunity to spermatozoa may represent a genetically determined subgroup of individuals prone to develop immunity to specific antigens.

Since the tissues and secretions of the female reproductive tract contain antibodies, antibody-forming cells, macrophages, and T lymphocytes, the possibility of local immunity at the site where spermatozoa are deposited and processed is potentially more relevant than systemic immunity. This is supported by the poor correlation between serum sperm antibody levels and antibody activity in cervical mucus or postcoital tests. It should be noted, however, that the status of the postcoital test and its role in infertility investigations is in question, since sperm can be recovered from the peritoneal cavity in most patients with a negative or poor postcoital test. Unfortunately, studies to date on sperm antibodies in cervicovaginal secretions are no more revealing than those done on serum from infertile women. Moreover, the complement cascade components necessary for antibody-mediated sperm cyto-

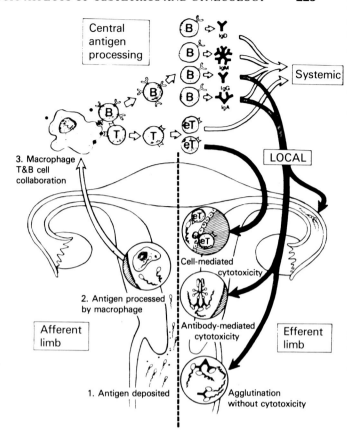

FIG. 12–7. Elicitation and expression of systemic and local immune responses following local challenge of the reproductive tract of the female with a foreign antigen. (Beer AE, Neaves WB: Fertil Steril 39:3, 1978)

toxicity are normally absent from cervical mucus, and semen itself has properties that are markedly inhibitory to the elicitation and expression of local immune responses.

Investigation of cell-mediated immunity (CMI) has been relatively neglected in infertility problems, particularly in view of the fact that spermatozoa are cellular transplants analogous to those of a kidney graft or tumor cells. Although CMI of peripheral blood lymphocytes to sperm antigens correlates poorly with the presence of sperm antibodies, too few studies have been done to determine whether CMI has any association with infertility.

It is apparent from the foregoing discussion that interpretation of results of immunologic tests and even the question of whether there is a true immunologic cause of infertility present a dilemma for the clinician. Nevertheless, because sperm antibody titers and abnormal postcoital tests in some infertile women suggest a correctable condition, various treatments have been advocated (Fig. 12–9).

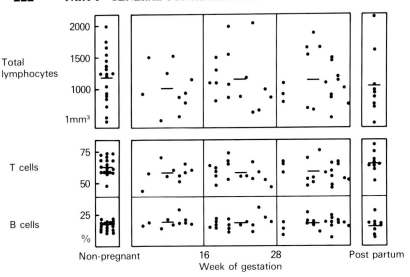

FIG. 12-5. Total lymphocytes and percent of T and B lymphocytes throughout gestation. (Scott JR, Feldbush TL: JAMA 239:2770, 1978. Copyright © 1978, American Medical Association)

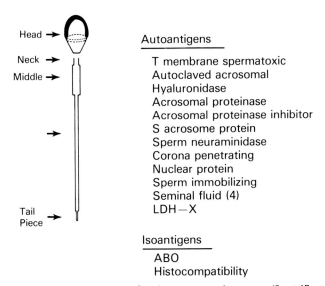

FIG. 12-6. Various types of antigens present in semen. (Scott JR: Semin Perinatol 1:149, 1977)

any stage in the human reproductive process, but there is little evidence that a host response to the ovum or maternal hormones, tissues, or secretions plays a significant role in infertility. If women commonly developed an immune response to gonadotropins or ovarian steroids, it is assumed that the ensuing menstrual abnormalities and anovulation would have more resistance to standard treatment regimens than usually occurs (see Ovarian Failure, page 915).

Through sexual activity, the female reproductive tract is repeatedly inoculated with millions of immunogenetically alien spermatozoa. Whole semen chemically and physiologically is a very complex material

that contains a variety of antigens variously distributed in the sperm head, acrosome, tail, and seminal fluid (Fig. 12-6). Introduction of spermatozoa directly into the uterine cavity of rodents elicits regional node hypertrophy, transplantation immune reaction, and a local hypersensitivity reaction. Consequently, it is curious that allergic reactions occur so infrequently in women. After degradation, spermatozoa are presumably processed in a manner that involves the afferent, central, and efferent pathways, providing the basis for a local or systemic immune response on the part of the female host (Fig. 12-7).

Many, but not all, workers have described varying degrees of reduced fertility in female animals following immunization with seminal or testicular material. Nevertheless, the relevance of many of these studies to the human situation can be questioned because adjuvants are virtually always necessary to produce this effect, and parenteral routes are used for injection. Without the use of adjuvants, infertility is rarely produced in female animals by sensitizing them to male antigens; when spermatozoa are introduced directly into the uterus, the number of implantations is actually enhanced. The establishment of an association between immune phenomena and infertility in humans has been hampered by the lack of definition of the antigen–antibody or cell-mediated immune systems involved and by the lack of standardization or refinement of techniques utilized for assessing the alleged immune reactions in infertile subjects.

By chance alone, about 20% of couples could be expected to be ABO incompatible; if erythrocyte antibodies were important in the etiology of this problem, these couples would be infertile. However, most studies on infertile married couples have failed to reveal any excess ABO incompatible matings. Although blood

of adrenocortical steroid, ovarian, and placental hormones, as well as a temporary involution of some of the maternal lymphoid tissues. It is now generally agreed that placental protein hormones, fetal embryonic antigens, and sex steroids in the maternal blood can at best provide only a weak ancillary protective mechanism for prevention of maternal alloimmunization. A more attractive hypothesis is that some of the hormones produced in high concentrations by the trophoblast may have a local immunosuppressive effect, preventing immunologically significant interactions between maternal lymphocytes and trophoblast. Although there is a wide variation in placental architecture and intimacy of encounter of the trophoblast with the uterus among different mammalian species, a common theme shared by all is progesterone production by the trophoblast during some portion of gestation. Recent studies support the concept that local suppression of the maternal cellular immune responses by high tissue concentrations of progesterone may contribute to acceptance of the conceptus. However, it has been difficult to document the effect of these nonspecific factors on the maternal immune system, since parameters such as the percentage of circulating T and B cells do not change significantly during pregnancy (Fig. 12–5).

It has been shown *in vitro* that the maternal host can develop sensitized T cells capable of destroying embryonic cells, but the lymphocytes are prevented from interacting with the fetal cells by blocking antibody, excess antigen, or antigen–antibody complexes suggestive of immunologic enhancement. In humans, IgG eluted from placentas has complement–dependent cytotoxic effects on lymphocytes that are capable of inhibiting mixed lymphocyte culture reactions and prolonging the survival of skin allografts. These antibodies may protect the conceptus by binding to receptors on the trophoblast cells, but a relationship between the recently described suppressor T-cell system and the success of the fetus as an allograft must also be considered.

Even the stimulus for maternal unresponsiveness to fetoplacental antigens is not known. It is possible that the unique method by which "transplantation" antigens are presented to the host in pregnancy might determine the type of reaction they evoke. Spermatozoa phagocytosed in the reproductive tract could cause the initial stimulus. Moreover, in a fertilized ovum there is only a minute quantity of antigenic material foreign to the host, and exposure to those antigens is not only gradual as fetal tissue grows, but it is extended over a long period of time. Trophoblasts are demonstrable in maternal circulation as early as 10–14 days after implantation; since the intravenous route is the most efficient way to induce either sensitization or tolerance, this could also be important in the production of maternal blocking factors or suppressor T cells.

In summary, the mechanisms that prevent rejection of the fetus are, extremely complex, but the most im-

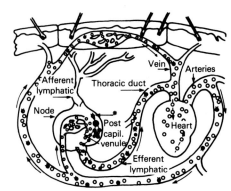

Skin allograft

*Effector cells
°Small lymphocytes

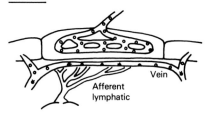

Placenta

FIG. 12–4. Anatomic differences between a skin allograft and the placental allograft.

portant of them at present seem to be 1) decreased antigenicity of trophoblast at the maternal–fetal junction, 2) separate maternal and fetal circulations and lymphatic drainage systems, and 3) the maternal production of blocking factors or suppressor T cells.

POTENTIAL IMMUNOBIOLOGIC DISORDERS

INFERTILITY

Approximately 15% of married couples in the United States have an infertility problem, and the standard infertility workup identifies the cause (*e.g.*, male, tubal, or hormonal abnormalities) in the vast majority of cases. It has often been stated that about 15% of infertile couples are found to have no definite cause for their problem; the incidence is now probably less than 5%, however, because of the development of laparoscopy and more sophisticated methods of evaluation. Largely by the clinical process of exclusion, immunologic mechanisms have been suspected or implicated in these patients.

Theoretically, immunologic factors could operate at

sialomucin, and, although all mammalian cells possess a net negative surface charge, lymphocytes and trophoblast excel in this biologic property. This strong electrostatic force at the cell surface may prevent antigen-reactive lymphocytes from reacting with trophoblastic cells. Moreover, cell surface determinants appear to be internalized into the villus and out of the trophoblastic epithelium as pregnancy progresses. The intrinsic loss or dilution of antigenic determinants from the trophoblastic plasma membrane, resulting in low antigen density, may create a situation in which the determinants are too widely spaced for linkage with lymphocytes, antibody, or complement.

It is essential to mention that, although antigenic peculiarities are associated with trophoblastic tissue, gestating mothers normally respond immunologically to the presence of allogeneic fetuses in their uteri, as evidenced by hypertrophy of the lymph nodes draining the uterus and the production of circulating cytotoxic antibodies. Definite Rh antigens have been found on human embryonic red cells by the 38th day of life, the embryo possesses a number of iso- and autoantigens by at least 6 weeks, and fetal tissues implanted outside the uterus are rejected.

FETAL IMMUNOCOMPETENCE

During the 2nd and 3rd weeks of gestation in the human fetus, pluripotential yolk sac stem cells form the precursors of all the blood cell series. The thymus develops at about 6 weeks' gestation and lymphocyte differentiation proceeds in the complete absence of foreign antigens. Small lymphocytes appear in the peripheral blood at about 7 weeks and in connective tissue around lymphocyte plexuses by 8 weeks. Primary lymph node development and lymphopoeisis do not occur until at least 12 weeks; but, as early as 13 weeks' gestation, T cells capable of responding to mitogens and recognizing histoincompatible cells begin to appear. In the spleen, lymphocyte aggregates form at 14 weeks, and by 20 weeks' gestation the human fetus can respond to congenital infections with the production of plasma cells and antibody.

The fetus generally enjoys a high degree of protection from infectious organisms in its isolated intrauterine environment and is not often called upon to demonstrate its immunologic capabilities, but immunologic maturation proceeds in preparation for exposure to a highly contaminated world. The transition of the fetus from immunologically incompetent to immunologically competent has a profound influence on disease processes. Immunologic immaturity and susceptibility of organizing fetal tissues are factors that make first trimester congenital rubella infection such a severe teratogenic process as compared with the relatively benign adult disease. Conversely, an active fetal immune response can actually contribute to the patho-

logic process in certain situations. For example, the changes caused by *Treponema pallidum* after it has crossed the placenta and gained access to the fetus are probably not due to adverse effects of the organism on fetal cells but rather to widespread inflammatory responses. Thus, the infection may occur at a much earlier stage but follow a benign course until the fetal host develops the capacity to respond to the organism during the 5th month of gestation.

In contrast to the response in an adult, the dominant humoral antibody response in the fetus is the IgM immunoglobulin fraction. Indeed, it is the presence of circulating IgM of fetal origin in umbilical cord blood that assists in the clinical diagnosis of such congenital infections as rubella, toxoplasmosis, syphilis, and cytomegalovirus. Since the large IgM molecule does not cross the placenta and immunoglobulins are not synthesized prior to antigenic stimulation, IgM is usually not detected in the fetal circulation or amniotic fluid of normal pregnancies. Conversely, the smaller IgG molecule, by virtue of its Fc fragment, is specifically selected for placental transfer. Fetal IgG, usually about 10% of adult levels by the middle of the first trimester, gradually increases throughout pregnancy, and a significant number of newborns have IgG levels higher than those of the mother.

Thus, adequate humoral immunity in the newborn period depends on the circulating maternal antibodies that have crossed the placenta. However, fetal blood levels of IgG tend to reflect maternal levels, and specific antibody protection in turn depends on the mother's own total antigenic experience. Moreover, maternal IgG antibodies, in addition to their primary role of protecting the neonate from infections, can result in disease syndromes such as neonatal thrombocytopenia, hyperthyroidism, and erythroblastosis fetalis.

MATERNAL IMMUNOLOGIC REACTIVITY

It is at once apparent that the placenta implanted on the maternal endometrium is in many respects analogous to a skin graft (Fig. 12–4), but it is also clear that the fetoplacental unit does not behave like most other conventional allografts. Of the many theories that have been put forward over the years to account for survival of the conceptus, none appears to explain it completely. The fetus and its placenta with self-protecting properties is not a vascularized intercommunicating graft and may not sensitize the host in the usual way, but the uterus is endowed with a vascular supply and lymphatic drainage system capable of eliciting classic transplantation immunity. Thus, most recent studies have focused on the possibility that maternal serum contains nonspecific or immunologically specific factors that protect the fetus from rejection.

During pregnancy there is an increased production

TABLE 12-1. COMPARISON OF PROPERTIES OF VARIOUS IMMUNOGLOBULINS

Immunoglobulin Class	Cross Placenta?	Molecular Weight	Primary Location	Serum Concentration (mg/dl)	Antibody Activity
IgG	Yes	140,000	Intravascular	1000–1500	Most antibodies to bacterial and viral infections; major part of secondary response; Rh isoagglutinins; lupus erythematosus factor
IgM	No	900,000	Intravascular	50–110	First antibody formed; ABO isoagglutinins; rheumatoid factor
IgA	No	350,000	Seromucous	170–300	Major antibodies of external secretions—milk, colostrum, saliva, and secretions of GI, reproductive, respiratory tracts
IgD	No	180,000	Interstitial membrane-bound	0.3–40	Antibody activity rarely demonstrated; found on lymphocyte surfaces
IgE	No	200,000	Skin and epithelium	0.01–0.07	Reaginic antibodies

showing the presence of IgA and IgA-containing cells in cervical tissues. IgA and IgG have also been found in the human endometrium during the proliferative, secretory, and decidual phases. The immunoglobulins are distributed in the stroma between the glands and along the basement membrane of glandular epithelium. Although various tissues from the human genital tract are capable of *in vitro* synthesis of secretory immunoglobulins, IgG predominates in all endometrial specimens. Immunoglobulins in tubal fluid are also thought to be derived from serum.

FETOPLACENTAL ANTIGENICITY

The processes of fertilization and implantation constitute the two essential and specific acts of immunologic recognition between genetically dissimilar cells. The fertilized ovum undergoes fundamental changes in organization that render it potentially vulnerable to a maternal immune reaction, since minor and subsequently major transplantation antigens appear sequentially on the plasma membranes of embryonic cells from at least the two-cell stage onward. There is evidence, however, that early embryonic tissue is functionally hypoantigenic: ectopic pregnancies in many different sites are normally successful for considerable periods, even in presensitized hosts, and small grafts of pure trophoblastic tissue obtained from ectoplacental cones are invulnerable to transplantation immune reactions.

Further evidence that trophoblast becomes an immunologically privileged tissue comes from studies on plasma membranes prepared from human placentas that express very low levels of inherited HLA antigens. Trophoblastic cells contain an extracellular layer of

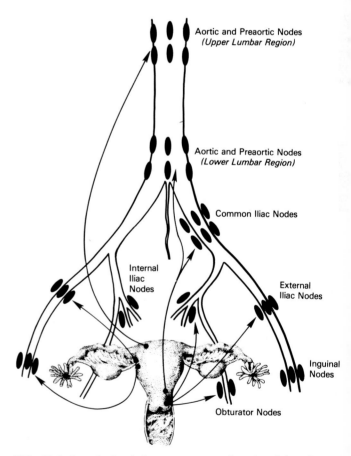

FIG. 12-3. Lymphatic drainage system and regional lymph nodes of female genital tract.

cially produced in rodents and primates by active or passive immunization against a variety of placental antigens.

Although it seems clear that maternal–fetal ABO and histoincompatibility have no influence on fertilization, some epidemiologic data have suggested that they may be predisposing factors in human spontaneous abortion. Furthermore, women with antisperm antibodies and otherwise unexplained infertility who subsequently conceive have a high incidence of spontaneous abortion, again suggesting immunologic incompatibility that involves paternal antigens.

Recently, it has been reported that women with recurrent abortions lack an immunologic "blocking factor" that is present in the serum of women who have had successful pregnancies. The blocking factor was shown to be an immunoglobulin, almost certainly IgG, and could be specific for antigens coded at the HLA-D locus, a gene exerting some control over immune response. Primigravidas were not tested, and it is possible that the presence of the blocking factor is the result rather than the cause of a successful pregnancy. Nevertheless, if blocking antibody is found to be important in the prevention of abortion, this would provide new therapeutic possibilities, such as the administration of serum from women with successful gestations to women with recurrent pregnancy wastage.

It is important to point out that an immunologic cause of intraspecies abortion is not shown in all studies. T- and B-cell levels, lymphocyte blast transformation, and response to mutogens are not altered in these patients. Several authors have disputed the evidence that either ABO or HLA incompatibility is relevant to the abortion problem. The most recent information indicates that antigen incompatibility between the parents within the ABO, HLA, Rhesus, MN, S, Lewis, Kell, P, and Duffy systems is not of significance. Indeed, one investigator has found that a higher percentage of couples with repeated abortion have common HLA antigens, suggesting an increased incidence of homozygotic fetuses in these cases. Animal studies also point toward a more successful pregnancy outcome in hybrid matings as compared with more compatible inbred matings, and successful pregnancies also follow the transfer of eggs of maximal immunogenetic disparity to foster mothers. These pregnancies proceed normally even when the foster mother has been presensitized with skin grafts from both the father and mother of the transferred ovum. It is therefore difficult to attribute abortions exclusively to immunologic factors, since many studies have shown that the majority of such conceptuses are chromosomally abnormal. In addition, histologic examination of the products of conception rarely reveals any lymphocyte infiltrate to suggest a rejection reaction. Yet even this conclusion may be premature, since autoimmune disease may interfere with gamete development and

result in aneuploidy; also, there is *in vitro* evidence that chromosomal abnormalities can at times by immunologically induced.

PREECLAMPSIA

Although the frequency and risks of preeclampsia have been reduced through modern obstetric care, the etiology of this disease, which occurs only in the human and only during gestation, is still poorly understood, thereby precluding specific treatment or effective prevention. An immunologic cause has long been suspected; but, because of the broad clinical spectrum of hypertensive diseases of pregnancy, it is more likely that both immunogenetic and nonimmunologic factors are involved.

There is growing evidence that immunocompetence is genetically controlled and that diseases caused by immune responses to certain antigens are hereditary. There is a familial predisposition for both essential hypertension and preeclampsia, but environmental rather than inherited factors could be the common theme in these families. Indeed, most investigations of genetically inherited antigens have not shown any unusual distribution of erythrocyte or histocompatibility antigens in preeclamptic or eclamptic women. However, women with essential hypertension are more likely than normal controls to have rheumatoid factors, thyroid and other autoantibodies, and raised concentrations of IgG and IgA in their serum. Nonspecific effector mechanisms that may have hypertensive effects include increased viscosity, increased peripheral resistance, release of vasoactive substances, or ischemia of pressure-sensitive organs, such as the kidney; specific effector mechanisms could involve the production of autoantibodies with direct vasopressor activity.

The protective effect of prolonged exposure to sperm antigens and the fact that the incidence of preeclampsia in women pregnant for the second time in the same marriage is markedly reduced as compared to that in primigravidas suggests that exposure to paternal antigens or a previous pregnancy in some way alters a woman's response or introduces other variables that modulate the development of the disease process.

Speculation regarding the etiology of preeclampsia has often centered on properties of the placenta, since the signs and symptoms regress when the uterus is emptied. In addition, "hyperplacentosis" obstetric conditions, such as diabetes mellitus, multiple gestations, hydatidiform mole, and neglected hydrops fetalis, are more frequently associated with preeclampsia. In normal pregnancy, trophoblast cells are shed continuously into the maternal circulation, beginning soon after implantation; in preeclamptic patients, the magnitude of this process is significantly increased. The progressively increased incidence of preeclampsia

from singleton to twin to triplet pregnancies suggests that a possible increased antigenic challenge to the maternal host plays some role in the underlying pathogenesis. This mechanism could also explain why preeclampsia does not usually occur until the third trimester, *i.e.*, when the placenta reaches a certain critical size.

Many of the clinical features of preeclampsia also involve the kidney, and the elucidation of the nature and distribution of antigens apparently shared in common by placenta and kidney has been the subject of numerous studies. An analogy could be drawn between the response to placental antigens and the immune response to a number of other cross-reacting antigens known to be nephrotoxic, such as nuclear deoxyribonucleic acid (DNA), streptococci, and exogenous serum or haptene conjugates that have been implicated in human immunologically mediated glomerulonephritis. The diagnosis of immunologic causes of renal disease is usually dependent on fluorescent antibody study of tissue obtained by renal biopsy. Unfortunately, immunofluorescent studies designed to demonstrate immunoglobulin, complement, and fibrinogen deposition in the glomeruli, as well as reports on circulating immune complexes in preeclamptic women, have been conflicting.

Histologic changes in the vasculature in placental vessels similar to those in rejected renal allografts have been taken as evidence that an active immunologic process is present in preeclampsia. It has been suggested that preeclampsia could occur when a young, often submaximally nourished primigravida is confronted with a large placental mass, its size and extent of trophoblastic invasion determined by histocompatibility or organ-specific antigenic differences between graft and host. Since not all primigravidas are affected, this premise would require the presence of placentas with certain unique or predisposing antigens, or it would imply that unaffected women are "nonresponders" analogous to Rh-negative women who are unresponsive to Rh antigens. If this were the situation, the normal maternal–fetal immunologic homeostasis could be overwhelmed in "responding" primigravidas so that effector lymphocytes or specific antibodies of maternal origin were then free to attack, damaging the trophoblast and basement membrane of the renal glomerulus and producing placental insufficiency, maternal proteinuria, and hypertension. Sufficient blocking factors may be evoked during or after the first pregnancy to prevent the initiation of this same process in a second pregnancy.

More recently, it has been proposed that the protective response generated by the maternal immune recognition of fetal–placental antigens in normal pregnancy is imperfectly developed in preeclampsia because of maternal hyporesponsiveness. Evidence for this hypothesis includes findings of maternal HLA and A and B homozygosity that reduce the number of antigen disparities between preeclamptic women and their husbands. Lymphocytes from preeclamptic women are also hyporesponsive when cultured with their spouse's lymphocytes, and few lymphocytotoxic antibodies are detectable at the end of preeclamptic pregnancies.

It should be emphasized that by no means does all evidence favor an immunologic contribution to the pathogenesis of preeclampsia/eclampsia. However, one important reason for the persistent exploration of any potential immunologic cause is the possibility that therapeutic regimens to alleviate or prevent the disease might be developed. For example, whether preeclampsia involves hypo- or hyperresponsiveness to fetal–placental antigens, it might be possible to help a woman establish a more satisfactory immunologic homeostasis with her conceptus by immunizing her prior to or early in the first pregnancy with antigenic material from either her husband or trophoblastic tissue. Alternatively, the disease might be amenable to abrogation by the passive administration of specific immune serum.

SPECIFIC CLINICAL IMMUNOLOGIC PROBLEMS

TRANSPLANT PATIENTS

More physicians are now being confronted with disorders encountered in allograft recipients. For example, over 25,000 kidney transplants have been performed and the number is rapidly increasing.

Disorders of the reproductive tract in nonpregnant transplant patients, although more frequent, have not attracted the same publicity nor received the same emphasis in the literature as have the pregnancies in these women. Female renal allograft recipients may have any gynecologic disease that afflicts the general population, but a number of problems are specifically related to the immunosuppressive drugs they receive (Table 12–2). The physician caring for these patients is therefore wise to review the side effects of the drugs to determine whether they can account for the symptoms the patient is experiencing or whether they will affect the management plan.

Menstrual abnormalities are common in women with chronic renal disease, and amenorrhea usually occurs when the serum creatinine rises to 5–10 mg/dl. Amenorrhea often persists during hemodialysis treatment, and the most common serum gonadotropin pattern is a normal concentration of follicle-stimulating hormone (FSH) and a moderately elevated level of luteinizing hormone (LH) similar to the tonic profile found in the male and in females with polcystic ovarian disease. More of a problem to the physician are women who develop dysfunctional uterine bleeding, specifically hypermenorrhea, while they undergo dialysis treatment and are markedly anemic. Although no hor-

TABLE 12-2. PROPERTIES OF IMMUNOSUPPRESSIVE AGENTS COMMONLY USED IN RENAL TRANSPLANTATION

	Prednisone	Azathioprine (Imuran)	Cyclophosphamide (Cytoxan)	Antilymphocyte Globulin
CLASS	Corticosteroid	Purine antimetabolite	Alkylating agent	Immune serum
PRINCIPAL ACTION	Antiinflammatory	↓Primary immune response	↓On-going immune responses	↓Lymphocytes
MAINTENANCE DOSE/DAY	5–25 mg	75–150 mg	50–150 mg	2.5 mg/kg
HAZARDS				
Immunosuppression	Infection Neoplasia (?)	Infection Neoplasia	Infection Neoplasia	Infection Neoplasia
Other activities	Fluid and electrolyte disturbances, myopathy, osteoporosis, peptic ulcer, impaired wound healing, carbohydrate intolerance, cataracts, glaucoma, negative nitrogen balance	Bone marrow depression, mutagenesis, anorexia	Bone marrow depression, mutagenesis, teratogenesis, hemorrhagic cystitis, gonadal suppression, alopecia, anorexia	Reversed anaphylaxis, thrombocytopenia
Idiosyncracy hypersensitivity	Pancreatitis	Drug fever, rash, myopathy, arthralgia pancreatitis, hepatic cholestasis or fibrosis	Inappropriate antidiuretic hormone secretion	Serum sickness, fever, anaphylaxis

monal regimens are competely successful, the oral contraceptives or intramuscular medroxyprogesterone can be used to decrease the frequency and quantity of menstrual bleeding, produce therapeutic amenorrhea, and prevent hemorrhagic dysfunctional ovarian cysts, a troublesome syndrome in women taking anticoagulants and undergoing intermittent dialysis. Following renal transplantation, resumption of ovulatory cycles and regular menses correlates relatively closely with the level of renal function. With less successful transplants, many women continue to have amenorrhea or irregular menses. Nevertheless, effective contraception is necessary in all women who have received a renal transplant.

The incidence of cancer in renal transplant patients taking immunosuppressive drugs is approximately 100 times greater than that observed in the general population in the same age range. The most common gynecologic neoplasms in these patients have involved the cervix, and it has been estimated that the risk of intraepithelial cervical carcinoma is increased nearly 14-fold over that of the general population. Therefore, all women receiving immunosuppressive drugs should have regular pelvic examinations and Pap smears at 6-month intervals.

Several hundred women with renal allografts from living or cadaver donors (and one liver allograft recipient) have now become pregnant. Although the general tone in the literature is one of optimism, this is a high-risk situation that requires expert obstetric and pediatric care in addition to superior perinatal facilities. The 50%–60% long-term graft survival rate makes the prognosis for these women somewhat guarded. It is likely that some transplant recipients may not live long enough to raise their children to adulthood and may leave the surviving spouse the problem of raising the child. There is unanimous agreement that a good graft is essential before pregnancy should be considered. In order to assess renal function adequately, the patient must be followed for at least 1–2 years after transplant. Pregnancy should probably not be attempted in any patient with serum creatinine above 1.5 mg/dl. Other medical problems such as diabetes mellitus, recurrent infections, or serious side effects from the immunosuppressive drugs also make pregnancy inadvisable.

Early diagnosis of pregnancy is important so that meticulous antepartum care can be given and an accurate date of delivery can be calculated, because intervention may be necessary should complications arise. The following prenatal care regimen is suggested for renal transplant patients:

I. First antepartum visit
  A. Routine prenatal history
  B. Physical and pelvic examination: establish estimated date of confinement and compatibility of uterine size with date of last menstrual period
  C. Record of weight
  D. Baseline laboratory values
    1. Urinanalysis
    2. Urine culture
    3. Total protein (24-hour urine specimen)
    4. Creatinine clearance

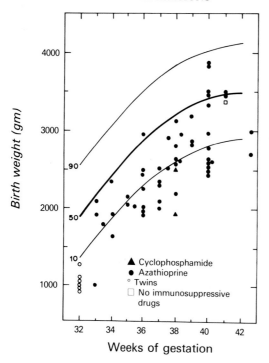

FIG. 12–10. Birth weight and week of gestation of infants born to mothers taking azathioprine or cyclophosphamide throughout pregnancy. All azathioprine-treated women were renal transplant patients, and the two mothers treated with cyclophosphamide had multiple myeloma and Hodgkin's disease, respectively.

5. Complete blood count
6. Blood type and Rh
7. Test for venereal disease
8. Serum Na, K, Cl, CO_2, BUN, creatinine, glucose, SGOT, alkaline phosphatase, bilirubin
9. Cervical cytology

II. Subsequent visits at least every 3 weeks until 28 weeks, gestation, then weekly
   A. General health and evaluation of any infections
   B. Weight, blood pressure, urinary protein and glucose
   C. Fundal height and fetal heart tones
   D. Periodic creatinine clearance and urine culture
   E. Ultrasound for placental localization and biparietal diameter of fetal head in midtrimester; repeat for biparietal diameter at 32 and 36 weeks
   F. Cervical cultures for viruses at 28 weeks
   G. Repeat CBC, cervical cytology at 32 weeks
   H. Fetal maturity studies and hospitalization as necessary

Immediate hospitalization should be considered if any complications arise.

Normal pregnancy is associated with elevated glomerular filtration rate (GFR), which is observed at about 8–10 weeks and persists until term. In transplant patients, very few have shown even a moderate increase of the GFR; in most, it has decreased during the third trimester, although this deficit has been reversible after delivery except in a few cases. Preeclampsia, preterm delivery, small-for-gestational-age infants, and premature ruptured membranes have been the most common obstetric complications in these women. Figure 12–10 illustrates the week of delivery and the birth weight of the infants of mothers with renal allografts. Of 57 pregnancies that progressed to the third trimester, the percentage of preterm births (before the 37th week) was 35%. Excluding the three sets of twins, 48 (89%) of the infants were below the 50th percentile for weight, and 26 (48%) below the 10th percentile were definitely small for their gestational age. Although animal experiments suggest that immunosuppressive drugs decrease both placental and fetal weight, it is not clear in the human whether the drugs or the underlying maternal disease is responsible for this phenomenon.

The position of the kidney in the pelvis is not usually a major obstacle to normal vaginal delivery, nor is the kidney damaged. If the fetal head is not engaged when labor begins, the possibility of soft tissue dystocia can be assessed by obtaining simultaneous x-ray pelvimetry and intravenous pyelography. Indications for cesarean section must be studied on a case-by-case basis and the decision made primarily on obstetric factors.

Despite studies in animals showing anomalies in the offspring secondary to corticosteroids and azathioprine, no statistical increase in congenital anomalies in the human has been attributed to these agents. However, single cases of pulmonary artery stenosis, diaphragmatic hernia, and pyloric stenosis have occurred in infants delivered from mothers who took these drugs during pregnancy. Chromosomal changes, adrenocortical suppression, and infection with cytomegalovirus have also been observed. Since the incidence of infections and neoplasms is increased in association with primary immunologic deficiencies and administration of immunosuppressive drugs, it is imperative that any child exposed to these agents *in utero* have a careful evaluation of the immune system and longterm followup.

AUTOIMMUNE DISEASES IN PREGNANCY

Autoimmunity is the process by which a humoral or cellular response is directed against a specific component of the host. Cells that are capable of recognizing self-antigens and producing an immune response seem to be present in all normal people, but they are actively regulated by a process involving antigen–antibody complexes or suppressor T cells. *Autoimmune*

diseases apparently result from a breakdown in this regulatory mechanism, leading to the inability to discriminate between self and nonself, and the formation of endogenous antibodies, antigen–antibody complexes, or sensitized lymphocytes that react with the host's own cells or tissues. Since these disorders have a predilection for women in their reproductive years, associations with gestation are not uncommon. Pregnancy may affect the disease process; in turn, some of the disorders adversely influence the course of pregnancy or are detrimental to the fetus (Table 12–3).

Systemic Lupus Erythematosus

A chronic multisystem inflammatory disease, systemic lupus erythematosus (SLE) is one of the most frequent serious disorders in women of childbearing age. Despite the general impression that the disease is rare, more than 250,000 people are known to have SLE, and an estimated 50,000 new cases are diagnosed each year. The pathogenesis involves the development of antibody to autologous DNA, perhaps under the influence of some triggering mechanism such as a virus, leading to the deposition of antigen–antibody complexes and resultant inflammatory responses in target tissues. The frequency of SLE among identical twins and familial aggregations, as well as abnormal distributions of HLA antigens in these patients also strongly implicates genetic factors.

The disease is easily overlooked because it may begin with mild symptoms, such as fatigue, but it eventually affects a variety of organs. It is characterized by a series of exacerbations and remissions. In order to standardize the diagnosis of SLE, a subcommittee of the American Rheumatism Association has proposed the following criteria:

I. Systemic lupus erythematosus (the presence of four or more criteria is strongly suggestive of SLE)
   A. Facial erythema
   B. Discoid lupus
   C. Raynaud's phenomenon
   D. Alopecia
   E. Photosensitivity
   F. Oral or nasopharyngeal ulceration
   G. Arthritis without deformity
   H. Lupus erythematosus cells
   I. Chronic false-positive serologic test for syphilis
   J. Profuse proteinuria
   K. Cellular casts
   L. Pleuritis or pericarditis
   M. Psychosis or convulsions
   N. Hemolytic anemia, leukopenia, or thrombocytopenia
II. Rheumatoid arthritis (classic RA-7 criteria, RA-5 criteria, probable RA-3 criteria)
   A. Morning stiffness
   B. Pain, tenderness in at least one joint
   C. Swelling, one joint, lasting at least 6 weeks
   D. Swelling, another joint
   E. Symmetrical joint swelling
   F. Subcutaneous nodules
   G. Periarticular osteoporosis, bony erosions
   H. Poor mucin precipitate or synovial fluid
   I. Positive test for rheumatoid factor
   J. Typical histologic appearance of synovium
   K. Typical histologic appearance of nodule

The diagnosis is further supported by the presence of antinuclear antibodies in high titer, antibodies against DNA and ribonucleic acid (RNA), lowered serum complement evels, reduced creatinine clearance, and biopsy evidence of renal involvement. With an increased awareness of the disease, more sophisticated diagnostic methods, and improved drug therapy, the outlook for these patients has greatly improved. The survival rate in SLE is now more than 90% for 5 years; more than 80% of patients are living 10 years after diagnosis.

Most patients should be counseled to postpone conception until at least 2 years after the diagnosis. At that time, if the disease has been in good control on low

TABLE 12-3. AUTOANTIBODIES IN PREGNANCY AND THEIR EFFECT ON THE FETUS

Autoimmune Disorder	Cross Placenta	Fetal Effect	
		Clinical Manifestations	Frequency
SYSTEMIC LUPUS ERYTHEMATOSUS	++++	Discoid lupus, anemia, neutropenia, thrombocytopenia, congenital heart block	+
RHEUMATOID ARTHRITIS	0	None	—
HYPERTHYROIDISM	+	Thyrotoxicosis	+
MYASTHENIA GRAVIS	++	Weak cry, suckling, facial muscles, respiratory problems	++
IMMUNOLOGIC THROMBOCYTO-PENIC PURPURA	+++	Thrombocytopenia; petechiae; GI, GU, intracranial bleeding	+++

doses of corticosteroids, pregnancy may be reasonably considered. Diaphragm, condom, intrauterine devices, and sterilization are the preferred methods of fertility regulation for these patients. Oral contraceptives have occasionally caused exacerbations, can themselves lead to positive LE tests, and may induce antinuclear antibodies.

Although the effect of pregnancy on SLE seems inconsistent, most maternal deaths have occurred during the puerperium. A substantial proportion of patients are in remission during pregnancy but the disease may flare postpartum or after therapeutic abortion. The high rate of spontaneous abortion in these patients has recently been related to the presence of a trophoblast-reactive lymphocytotoxic antibody. Maternal complications correlate most closely with cardiac or renal involvement. Diffuse proliferative lupus glomerulonephritis carries a very poor prognosis; these patients have a high incidence of renal failure, hypertension, and death. When the kidneys are affected, superimposed preeclampsia, stillbirths, preterm delivery, and small-for-gestational age infants are frequent. Nevertheless, in most stable SLE patients there is only a slight risk that the disease will become worse with pregnancy.

The obstetric management of SLE patients includes surveillance of the renal status, serial ultrasonic estimations of fetal growth, and fetal heart rate monitoring before and during labor. Since a fall in complement levels and elevated antinuclear antibody titers may herald the onset of an exacerbation, these assays are useful indicators of disease activity during pregnancy and after delivery. The mainstay of therapy in active SLE is corticosteroids. An initial regimen of prednisone in the range of 60–100 mg daily induces remission in most patients. With a satisfactory response, the dosage can usually be gradually tapered over several weeks to 10–15 mg daily. Increased doses, such as hydrocortisone, 100 mg intravenously every 8 hours, during labor and delivery and continuation of adequate corticosteroid treatment during the first 2 months postpartum is recommended to limit the chance of exacerbation.

Antinuclear antibodies and LE cells can be found in the blood of infants born to women with SLE. The maternal autoantibodies disappear after several weeks, and these babies are generally asymptomatic. However, a number of cases of congenital atrioventricular heart block have now been diagnosed before and after delivery, and a few of these infants have died of extensive subendocardial fibroelastosis.

Rheumatoid Arthritis

Rheumatoid arthritis is a chronic inflammatory process that can affect several organ systems but primarily involves synovial-lined joints, which become swollen and painful. Fortunately, most cases are mild and require little or no medical treatment; in others, however, the disease is characterized by an intermittent course with ultimate progression over many years to typical joint deformities and the findings listed previously. Since the disease affects 1% of adults and exhibits a threefold female preponderance, rheumatoid arthritis is a common complication of pregnancy.

The signs and symptoms gradually improve in the majority of pregnant patients, which may be related to increased blood levels of free cortisol or to enhanced phagocytosis of immune complexes. The rheumatoid factors (IgM antibodies against autologous IgG) do not cross the placenta, and there is no fetal or neonatal involvement.

Proper management of rheumatoid arthritis during pregnancy includes an appropriate balance of rest and exercise, heat and physical therapy, and salicylates 3–6g/day as tolerated. Despite some concerns, such as mild hemostatic changes in the infant and an increase in the average length of gestation attributed to maternal ingestion of large doses, aspirin probably remains the safest and most useful antiinflammatory drug in these patients. Systemic corticosteroids can reduce the inflammatory response; but, because of the complications with chronic use, their place in rheumatoid arthritis is limited to acute situations in which other methods are ineffective.

Hyperthyroidism

Although disorders of thyroid function are covered more completely in Chapters 7 and 27, it should be mentioned here that hyperthyroidism is unique among autoimmune diseases because immunoglobulins that have biologic effects similar to those of thyrotropin are frequently present. There is now considerable evidence implicating both cellular and humoral immunity in hyperthyroidism and Hashimoto's thyroiditis. Both have familial associations, and many patients have demonstrable antibodies to thyroid antigens. This suggests that the two diseases are primarily due to genetic defects in immunologic surveillance, resulting in an inability to destroy or control a specific clone of lymphocytes that arises by random mutation.

Long-acting thyroid stimulator (LATS) is an IgG immunoglobulin frequently present in the serum of patients with hyperthyroidism, and the transplacental passage of such immunoglobulins has a significant impact on the fetus. It is now recognized that mothers who have thyrotoxicosis during pregnancy may give birth to infants who have manifestations of the disease. Likelihood of hyperthyroidism in the neonate can be predicted by antepartum observations of the fetal heart rate for tachycardia and by tests for circulating maternal thyroid-stimulating immunoglobulins. A reasonable approach is to obtain LATS levels in pregnant women with hyperthyroidism, obtain a serum thyroxine level from cord blood immediately after delivery,

and follow the infant carefully during the first 2 weeks of life for signs of thyrotoxicosis. The neonate with this condition is a jittery, underweight baby with tachycardia, tachypnea, goiter, and diarrhea. The duration of the neonatal disease is almost always less than 3 months, and most affected infants recover without incident.

Myasthenia Gravis

Myasthenia gravis is a relatively rare chronic disease characterized by fatigue and weakness, typically of the extraocular, facial, pharyngeal, and respiratory muscles. It is worsened by exertion and relieved by rest. The presence of a circulating IgG immunoglobulin capable of blocking acetylcholine effects at the neuromuscular junction forms the basis for the presumed immunologic etiology. In addition, the disorder is associated with HLA-Cw3 haplotype and is often accompanied by a thymoma, thymic hyperplasia, or hyperthyroidism.

The functional abnormalities associated with the disease are similar to those induced by curare. The course during pregnancy is variable, although there is a tendency for relapse during the puerperium. The cholinesterase inhibiters most commonly utilized to alleviate symptoms are neostigmine, 60 mg/day, and pyridostigmine bromide, 240 mg/day, in four divided doses. Treatment with high-dose corticosteroids has also been used successfully in some patients. Regular rest periods with limited physical activity should be prescribed for the pregnant myasthenia gravis patient, and aggressive treatment of any infections in indicated, since they appear to predispose to exacerbation. Some antibiotics, such as the aminoglycosides, may produce a myasthenic crisis and should be avoided.

In the management of the pregnant myasthenia gravis patient, three types of crises may occur:

1. Myasthenic—an acute intensification of symptoms and a need for increased doses of anticholinesterase medication and supportive care.
2. Cholinergic—decreased requirement for anticholinesterase medication manifested by such symptoms as abdominal pain, diarrhea, nausea, vomiting, and increased skeletal muscle weakness. This is treated by administering atropine and by withholding anticholinesterase medication.
3. Refractory—periods when the myasthenic symptoms become relatively or totally unresponsive to anticholinesterase medication.

Careful plans should be made for drug therapy during pregnancy, labor, delivery, and the postpartum period. Labor typically progresses normally or even more rapidly than usual, since smooth muscle is unaffected. Vaginal delivery is the rule; cesarean section is reserved for obstetric reasons. Assisted ventilation

should be available in the event of respiratory difficulty. During labor, the patient's oral dose of anticholinesterase should be discontinued and replaced with an intramuscular equivalent. Myasthenic patients are often very sensitive to sedatives, analgesics, tranquilizers, and especially narcotics. Muscle relaxants should be avoided, if possible; local or regional anesthesia is preferable. It should also be noted that magnesium sulfate is contraindicated, since the drug diminishes the acetylcholine effect and has been known to induce a myasthenic crisis.

Approximately 12%–20% of infants born to myasthenic women exhibit neonatal myasthenia, which lasts from a few hours to several days. The manifestations are due to the transplacental transfer of acetylcholine-blocking factor. Interestingly, neonatal myasthenia may not occur in all infants of the same myasthenic patient. The classic features of neonatal myasthenia gravis differ from those seen in the adult form. Usually, the symptoms do not develop until the 1st or 2nd day of life, probably because of some protection to the baby from the maternal blood levels of anticholinesterase agents. It is clinically important to recognize this phenomenon, since a baby who appears healthy at birth may later develop respiratory failure with asphyxia. In the involved infant, there is a generalized muscular weakness, the limbs are hypotonic, and the baby is limp and motionless. The Moro reflex is often weak or absent, and there may be a feeble cry, inability to suck, and associated difficulty in swallowing and breathing.

Immunologic Thrombocytopenia Purpura

The most common autoimmune hemolytic disorder encountered during pregnancy is immunologic thrombocytopenia purpura (ITP). Platelets form complexes with endogenous antiplatelet antibodies and are sequestered and destroyed in the reticuloendothelial system at a rate that exceeds the compensatory ability of the bone marrow. This results in the hemorrhagic consequences of abnormally low platelet levels in peripheral blood. The diagnosis is based on 1) a platelet count repeatedly less than $100,000/mm^3$ with or without megathrombocytes on the peripheral smear, 2) a bone marrow aspirate with normal or increased numbers of megakaryocytes that are otherwise normal, and 3) exclusion of other diseases or drugs associated with thrombocytopenia. Corticosteroids are the mainstay of drug therapy, but splenectomy is utilized for those patients who fail to respond to steroid therapy or for those who develop serious complications from this.

The overall course of ITP does not differ in pregnant and nonpregnant women. Gestation appears to exert little influence on the disease. The principal maternal risk is that of bleeding from lacerations of the birth canal, episiotomy, or cesarean section.

The most serious clinical problem regarding the ob-

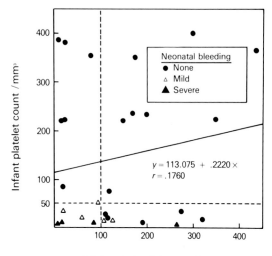

FIG. 12-11. Relationship of maternal and infant platelet counts in pregnant patients with immunologic thrombocytopenic purpura from a series of patients managed at the University of Utah Medical Center and the University of Iowa Hospitals.

stetric management of these patients involves the transplacental passage of the maternal antiplatelet antibody, which results in a platelet count of less than $100,000/mm^3$ in approximately 50% of infants born to these women. Unfortunately, it is impossible to predict which baby will be thrombocytopenic, but those with low platelet counts often have clinical bleeding manifestations such as purpura, hematuria, melena, or intracranial bleeding (which is also the most common cause of perinatal death). Largely because of the unpredictable nature of fetal thrombocytopenia and the suspected but not proved relationship between neonatal intracranial hemorrhage and the trauma of vaginal delivery, the optimum method of delivery for these women has become controversial. If, as some authors have proposed, universal cesarean section is used to avoid trauma to the fetal head during vaginal delivery, the operation will be performed unnecessarily in the 50% of cases where the infant platelet count is normal. If, as others have suggested, the decision for cesarean section is based on a maternal platelet count less than $100,000/mm^3$, a significant number of infants delivered abdominally will have normal platelet counts. There is some correlation between the maternal platelet count at delivery and the infant platelet count (Fig. 12–11), but this is not a reliable predictor in individual cases. Moreover, unless there is a definite benefit to the infant in each case, cesarean section cannot be advised lightly in any patient with a coagulopathy because of the risk of maternal bleeding at the time of surgery. Because of these difficulties, studies

are currently underway to determine whether fetal scalp blood sampling for platelet determinations early in labor or at the time of elective induction might be a safe and practical method to determine whether cesarean section is necessary. Regardless of the method of delivery, whole blood, platelets, and fresh-frozen plasma should be available for the mother, and a pediatrician or neonatologist should be present to provide prompt treatment for any hemorrhagic complications in the neonate.

TUMOR IMMUNOLOGY

Oncologists have long hoped for a screening test for cancer, a means to assess the patient's condition more precisely after definitive treatment, and an effective immunologic method for eradicating malignant tissue. Most investigations of the immunologic reaction against cancer cells have been based on the belief that some unique factor distinguishes a cancer cell from a normal cell and that this difference can be recognized by the body's immune system. Tumors induced in animals by chemical carcinogens generally have cell surface antigens (Fig. 12–12) that are specific for a given tumor, while viruses produce common antigens even when different organs or tissues are involved. In humans, the occurrence of tumor-specific transplantation antigens is more difficult to establish, because of histocompatibility differences between patients, but evidence that suggests their existence comes from a number of studies. The concept of immunologic surveillance attributes the evolution of adaptive immunity, and the host's ability to recognize nonself antigens, to the need to detect cells with a malignant potential, which may arise as a result of somatic mutation. Such cells may then be eliminated by immunologic mechanisms. Escape mechanisms not yet understood and failure of the immune response on the part of the host undoubtedly play a role in the development of some human neoplasms. For example, in patients with immunodeficiency disorders and in transplant patients receiving immunosuppressive drugs, the incidence of cancer is markedly increased.

Immunodiagnosis

Because of the difficulty in early diagnosis and effective therapy of ovarian carcinoma once signs and symptoms occur, most investigations into the antigenicity of tumors and immunocompetence of the host have been in patients with this disease. The detection of tumor-specific or tumor-associated antigens must fullfill several criteria to be clinically useful: 1) the antigens must pass from the tumor into body fluids, 2) they should be cancer-specific and ideally site- or tumor-specific, 3) they should decline in amount with successful therapy and rise again with recurrence, and

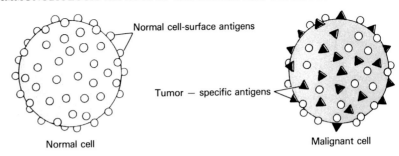

FIG. 12-12. Tumor-specific antigens that appear on the surface of most and perhaps all cancer cells as a consequence of the malignant transformation. Like the transplantation antigens on both normal and cancer cells, the tumor-specific antigens are thought to be complexes of protein and carbohydrate that have been synthesized within the cell and inserted into the cell membrane. (Old LJ: Sci Am 236:64, 1977)

4) they must be readily measurable by routine methods.

None of the substances for which assays are currently available completely fulfill these criteria. Although the development of radioimmunoassay procedures for *carcinoembryonic antigen* and *α-fetoprotein* provide a routine laboratory technique for their assessment, neither is sufficiently specific for gynecologic neoplasms to be ideal as a routine screening procedure. A review of work to date, in which both heterologous antibody and human antibody have been used, suggests that the common epithelial ovarian tumors produce at least one surface-specific antigen. However, purification and characterization of the antigen are necessary before it can be used in radioimmunologic studies.

If the theoretic model of immunosurveillance in which cellular mechanisms destroy tumors is valid, then the clinical recognition of a malignant tumor of the reproductive tract implies abrogation of the cell mediated immunity of the host. Studies of response to multiple skin test antigens have shown that lack of immunity is associated with a poor prognosis. An unsolved dilemma is the demonstration of apparently normal cell-mediated immunity to specific tumor antigens in some patients with progressive tumors. Answers may come from more detailed examination of the components in the cellular immune response, particularly as new information becomes available about effector cells, suppressor cells, and the mechanisms involved with tumor kill and cell migration.

Immunotherapy

Although immunotherapy in gynecologic oncology is still in the experimental stage, enthusiasm for such a concept is based on the presumption that the immunologic attack could be directed specifically against the malignant cells without the attendant damage to normal tissues that is inherent to all other forms of cancer therapy. The possible forms of immunotherapy are

1. *Specific*
   a. *Active*—inoculation with tumor cells, extracts, or chemically modified tumor antigens
   b. *Passive*—administration of antitumor sera of allogeneic or xenogeneic origin
   c. *Adoptive*—the use of allogeneic or xenogeneic sensitized lymphocytes, immune RNA, transfer factor.
2. *Nonspecific*
   a. *Active*—nonspecific stimulation of immune responsiveness with bacille Calmette Guérin, (BCG), *Corynebacterium parvum,* or other immunity-stimulating agents.
   b. *Passive*—employment of nonspecific serum factors such as properdin or interferon
   c. *Adoptive*—transfer of normal lymphoid cells from allogeneic or xenogeneic donors

Assessment of the value of immunotherapy is difficult, since in most instances it has been employed only in cases of advanced malignancy. It should be noted that a theoretic danger with immunotherapy is that it could produce immunologic enhancement, which could actually enhance tumor growth. A recent development is the concept of *immunochemotherapy,* whereby cytotoxic drugs are coupled with specific antitumor antibodies in order to direct the chemotherapeutic agent more precisely to tumor cells. At present, it seems doubtful that immunotherapy is capable of producing a cure when there is a large volume of tumor in the host, but it may be able to stimulate the host's immune response to eliminate small numbers of malignant cells once the tumor mass has been reduced by conventional measures, such as surgery, radiation, or chemotherapy.

Choriocarcinoma

The unique importance of choriocarcinoma from an immunologic standpoint is that it links two apparent anomalies. The first is that many neoplasms have been demonstrated to have tumor-specific antigens and are

therefore antigenically different from the rest of the host's tissues, but an effective immune response to them does not appear to occur in the host. The second is that malignant trophoblastic tissue of fetal origin derives half of its genetic material from the father and is therefore foreign to the mother, but it also escapes immune rejection. However, it seems somewhat pointless to argue that choriocarcinoma should be immunologically rejected when it is not known exactly why normal trophoblastic tissue is not rejected in the usual pregnancy. Patients with choriocarcinoma have not been reported to have impaired responses to other antigens, and the development of this tumor can be attributed to a maternal immunologic failure only with caution. Nevertheless, complete cure with chemotherapy and the association of choriocarcinoma with occasional spontaneous regression has suggested that the host's immune mechanism might be involved.

Since choriocarcinoma is abnormal placental tissue, at least partially paternal in origin, it must possess tissue antigens similar to those of other allografts. Direct evidence of HLA antigens on choriocarcinoma cells is at present restricted to one reported case, but HLA antibodies against the antigens present on the paternal lymphocytes have been found in women with persistent trophoblastic disease following a first pregnancy with a hydatidiform mole. Choriocarcinoma also appears to contain a tumor-associated antigen that is missing from normal placental tissue, as demonstrated by immunoelectrophoresis, immunodiffusion, and a cytotoxic effect of the antiserum on choriocarcinoma cells cultured *in vitro*.

Since this trophoblast malignancy does not occur naturally in other species, it has not been possible to study its immunologic activity in a meaningful manner. However, when human choriocarcinoma is transplanted to the hamster cheek pouch, an immunologically privileged site, its growth follows a characteristic pattern; there is a short latent period, after which it grows to 50–150 times its original volume. After approximately 10 days of rapid growth, it is infiltrated with host mononuclear cells, becomes necrotic, and is sloughed, probably because at that stage it outgrows the privileged site, having grown into the underlying adipose tissue, and is immunologically rejected. The animals given antilymphocyte serum have a much poorer response to methotrexate than do those not treated with the serum, again suggesting that the host's own immunologic response is important in the control and treatment of this tumor.

The hypothesis that progressive tumor growth is dependent on tumor–host histocompatibility has been substantiated by some studies, but not confirmed by others. Recent large series of patients have shown no association of HLA or ABO compatibility in the occurrence of gestational trophoblastic neoplasia. About 2% sharing of paternal haplotypes is estimated for a random mating of Caucasians. This represents a 1:50 incidence of compatibility, yet the incidence of trophoblastic neoplasia is 1:12 to 1:40,000. Recent investigations, however, have correlated the morbidity of trophoblastic disease with maternal antibody to particular HLA phenotypes.

To date, reports of immunotherapy in patients with advanced trophoblastic disease that is resistant to multiple drug therapy reveal only transient successes in small numbers of patients. Paternal lymphocytes, paternal skin grafts, and the use of nonspecific stimulants of cell mediated immunity such as *C. parvum* and BCG have produced variable results. Nevertheless, it seems possible that a potent heterologous antiserum directed against tissue-specific antigens and trophoblast- or tumor-specific antigens in malignant trophoblastic tissue could be the ultimate treatment in this disorder.

Maternal Neoplasms and the Fetus

Immunologic competence is greatest during young adulthood when neoplasms are uncommon; as immunologic competence decreases with aging, the incidence of cancer increases. Nevertheless, the incidence of malignancy in the 25–35 age group is approximately 0.06%, and this is not altered by pregnancy. Gestation does not change the 5-year survival rates of women with leukemia, Hodgkin's disease, and various solid tumors, even when the malignancy is one that is frequently affected by the endocrine milieu, such as carcinoma of the breast.

Relatively little attention has been focused on the possibility of fetal–placental metastasis in women with common types of malignancies during pregnancy because it has never become a clinical problem. For example, carcinoma of the cervix occurs once in every 2000–6000 pregnancies, but there has never been a verified report of placental or fetal invasion by this tumor. Although leukemia and Hodgkin's disease are not uncommon in women of reproductive age and as many as 1 in every 35 patients with carcinoma of the breast is pregnant, transmission of these malignancies to the fetus is also exceedingly rare. This is particularly surprising in the case of hematologic malignancies in which there are relatively large numbers of malignant stem cells in the maternal bloodstream. There is a possibility that diseases such as leukemia are oncogenic viral diseases and that the virus is occasionally transmitted early in fetal life.

Although the spread of cancer to the placenta is unusual, it can occur, as illustrated by the cases listed on Table 12–4 in which the placenta and fetus were studied in detail. It is apparent that the representation of melanoma is out of proportion to its incidence, but the reason for this phenomenon is unknown. Careful histologic observations in these patients have shown that tumor cells may be present in the intervillous spaces, but only rarely is there actual invasion of the villi.

TABLE 12-4. REPORTED CASES OF METASTASIS OF NEOPLASTIC DISEASE TO PLACENTA OR FETUS

Malignancy	Total Number	Placental Metastasis	Fetal Metastasis
MALIGNANT MELANOMA	15	9	6
HEPATIC CARCINOMA	2	1	1
SARCOMA	2	1	1
LEUKEMIA	7	5	2
HODGKIN'S DISEASE	1	0	1
BRONCHIAL CARCINOMA	3	3	0
BREAST CARCINOMA	6	6	0
GASTRIC CARCINOMA	2	2	0
PANCREATIC CARCINOMA	1	1	0
ETHMOID CARCINOMA	1	1	0
ADRENAL CARCINOMA	1	1	0
OVARIAN CARCINOMA	1	1	0
Totals	40	31	11

Moreover, in the extremely unusual instances of congenital neoplasia such as neuroblastoma, melanoma, or leukemia, the tumor does not spread from the fetus to the mother. The placental villus thus appears to be an effective barrier to the spread of tumor cells from the maternal-to-fetal circulation, as well as in the opposite direction. Once malignant tumor cells enter the fetal bloodstream, however, they can be disseminated throughout the entire fetus and are usually sequestered in the liver.

Since fetal and maternal tissues are genetically dissimilar, maternal–fetal metastasis can logically be considered an allograft or the transplantation of foreign cells. The rare cases of fetal dissemination of maternal malignant disease may be isolated examples of acquired tolerance in which fetuses were exposed to maternal antigen prior to immunologic competency and as a result did not recognize the maternal tumor cells as foreign. Conversely, those cases in which maternal malignant melanoma has widely metastasized to the fetus and then regressed spontaneously after birth are probably examples of true allograft rejection. This phenomenon could also explain what may be underdiagnosed cases of placental transmission of other maternal malignant diseases, particularly during the latter half of pregnancy—after the establishment of fetal immunocompetence.

REFERENCES AND RECOMMENDED READING

FUNDAMENTAL IMMUNOBIOLOGY

Feldbush TL, Lubaroff DM: Fundamental immunobiology. Semin Perinatol 1:113, 1977

Gell PGH, Coomes RRA, Lachmann PJ (eds): Clinical Aspects of Immunology, 3rd ed. Oxford, Blackwell, 1975

Sells S (ed): Immunology, Immunopathology and Immunity, 2nd ed. Hagerstown, Harper & Row, 1975

REPRODUCTIVE IMMUNOLOGY

Beer AE, Billingham RE (eds): The Immunobiology of Mammalian Reproduction. Englewood Cliffs, NJ, Prentice-Hall, 1976

Gall SA: Maternal immune system during human gestation. Semin Perinatol 1:119, 1977

Scott JR: Reproductive immunology. In Wynn RM (ed): Obstetrics and Gynecology Annual, p 101. New York, Appleton-Century-Crofts, 1974

Infertility

Beer AE, Neaves WB: Antigenic status of semen from the viewpoints of female and male. Fertil Steril 29:3, 1978

Jones WR: Immunological aspects of infertility. In Scott JS, Jones WR (eds): Immunology of Human Reproduction, p 375. London, Academic Press, 1976

Lande IJ, Scott JR: Immunology and the infertile female. Current Prob Obstet Gynecol 1 (4):3, 1977

Abortion

Rocklin RE, Kitzmiller JL, Carpenter CB et al: Maternal–fetal relation: Absence of an immuno-logic blocking factor from the serum of women with chronic abortions. N Engl J Med 295:1209, 1976

Scott JR: Potential immunopathological pregnancy problems. Semin Perinatol 1:149, 1977

Preeclampsia

Scott JS, Jenkins DM, Need JA: Immunology of pre-eclampsia. Lancet 1:704, 1978

Beer AE: Possible immunologic bases of preeclampsia/eclampsia. Semin Perinatol 2:39, 1978

TRANSPLANT PATIENTS

Sciarra JJ, Toledo-Pereyra LH, Bendel RP et al: Pregnancy following renal transplantation. Am J Obstet Gynecol 123:411, 1975

Scott JR: Gynecologic and obstetric problems in renal allograft recipients. In Buchsbaum HG, Schmidt J (eds): Gynecologic and Obstetric Urology, p 423. Philadelphia, WB Saunders, 1978

AUTOIMMUNE DISORDERS

Carloss HW, McMillan R, Crosby WH: Management of pregnancy in women with immune thrombocytopenic purpura. JAMA 244:2754, 1980

Pitkin RM: Autoimmune diseases in pregnancy. Semin Perinatol 1:161, 1977

Plauché WC: Myasthenia gravis in pregnancy: An update. Am J Obstet Gynecol 135:691, 1979

Scott JS: Immunological diseases in pregnancy. Prog Allergy 23:321, 1977

Kitzmiller JL: Autoimmune disorders: Maternal, fetal, and neonatal risks. Clin Obstet Gynecol 21:385, 1978

OBSTETRIC AND GYNECOLOGIC INFECTIONS: GENERAL CONSIDERATIONS AND ANTIBACTERIAL THERAPY

William J. Ledger

There has been an explosion of new information in the past decade on the nature of bacterial infections in women. Practitioners must struggle with the significance of such new and unfamiliar microinvaders as anaerobic bacteria, chlamydia, and mycoplasma in pelvic infections. As in any period of rapid change, a new and broader data base must be assimilated, and new therapeutic strategies that reflect the new realities must be formulated. Much has been learned, but much is still unclear about the pathophysiology of pelvic infections.

MICROBIOLOGY OF PELVIC INFECTION

There has been a complete change in our understanding of the microbiology of pelvic infection. The emphasis in the early years of bacteriology was on single bacterial pathogens. Since the development of any new medical science, whether it be cell biology or microbi-

ology, can be justified only by its significance in the understanding of disease, there is little wonder that early workers like Koch and Pasteur focused upon individual bacterial species to demonstrate the importance of microbiology. These investigators isolated bacterial species from the site of recognized clinical infections, cultured these isolates in artificial media, and showed that the bacteria could reproduce pathologic states when reinoculated into animals or human volunteers. The concept that single bacterial species, pathogens, caused diseases became the dominant theme of microbiology.

This model fit closely many clinical entities. Infections, including pneumococcal pneumonia or an *Escherichia coli* pyelonephritis, became the model for the therapeutic approach to all bacterial infections. One pathogenic species caused a disease, and the selection of an appropriate antibiotic effective against this one species would result in a cure for that disease. It was a simple, straightforward model of infection; however, both laboratory and clinical studies in the last few years have shown the limitations of this concept when applied to such soft tissue pelvic infections as the infected abortion, salpingo-oophoritis, postpartum endomyometritis, and postoperative pelvic infection. These infections have a diffuse microbiologic etiology with multiple bacterial isolates, and anaerobic bacteria are present in most of the patients.

Many aspects of these mixed bacterial soft tissue infections are not completely understood. Many feared anaerobic bacteria do not fulfill Koch's postulate. When injected alone, *Bacteroides fragilis* without a capsule do not produce disease in animals. Is it a nonsignificant contaminant? That is unlikely, for these same organisms combined with an enterococcus or a gram-negative aerobe result in an overwhelming infection. The confusion about the pathophysiology of these infections is not limited to research in animal models. Clinical cures can be seen in patients who are treated with antibiotics that are not effective against all of the bacterial isolates obtained from the site of infection. In contrast, therapeutic failures can be seen in women with a pelvic abscess who fail to respond to antibiotics, despite the presence of bacteria within the abscess that are susceptible to the antibiotics employed. There is no adequate scientific explanation for these findings at present, although many theories have been advanced.

A major drawback in the clinical evaluation of infectious disease in obstetrics and gynecology has been the paucity of accurate microbiologic data. The standard investigations of the impact of antibiotics on bacterial infection have used microbiologic data to help in the assessment of clinical results. The antibiotic susceptibility of the bacteria isolated from the site of infection and the bloodstream is measured, and a test of the apparent clinical cure is the elimination of the bacterial pathogen from the infection site. Such microbiologic

data can seldom be obtained for the evaluation of pelvic infections in the human. These infections are internal, and attempts at bacterial sampling have to traverse the abundant surface bacterial contamination of the lower genital tract. Attempts to distinguish the bacteria on the surface of the endometrial cavity of non-infected postpartum women from the bacteria similarly recovered from women with a diagnosis of postpartum endomyometritis have not been successful. The same kinds of bacteria have been isolated in both infected and noninfected women.

The only reliable microbiologic data on pelvic infection are obtained from women who fail to respond to systemic antibiotic therapy and require operative intervention for the drainage or removal of an abscess. Although these cases provide excellent bacteriologic information, since large amounts of purulent material can be obtained directly, this patient population is small and unique. These women represent the infrequent treatment failures and are not representative of the majority of women with pelvic infections, who respond to antibiotic therapy. When there have been difficulties with the collection of human data, one commonly employed approach to gain insight has been the use of an animal model of infection.

A popular model of intraabdominal infection in the rat has been developed by Gorbach and Bartlett. Pooled rat feces and barium sulfate were encased in a gelatin capsule and used as the bacterial innoculum. These capsules were inserted into the peritoneal cavity of rats. As the gelatin dissolved, there was a uniform response to the presence of the feces, with huge bacterial counts of both aerobes and anaerobes in the peritoneal cavity. All of the animals developed peritonitis; when their bloodstreams were sampled, gram-negative aerobic organisms were recovered. This peritonitis and the associated bacteremia were lethal to approximately 40% of the rats, and none of those that died had abscesses. The survivors appeared better for 1–2 days and then developed symptoms of an intraabdominal infection. Sacrificed, they were found to have intraabdominal abscesses in which anaerobes were the predominant organisms. These investigators postulated a biphasic response to this mixed bacterial insult, *i.e.*, early onset sepsis in which gram-negative aerobes predominated and late onset abscess formation in which anaerobes predominated. The major appeal of the model was the reproducibility of the results.

The next step in experimental design was to determine if this response could be modified by the use of systemic antibiotics. When an aminoglycoside such as gentamicin, which has antibacterial activity against gram-negative aerobes, was given systemically at the time of the bacterial insult, the early onset phase was largely eliminated; but the survivors went on to develop intraabdominal abscesses. If an antibiotic with antibacterial activity against anaerobes, *i.e.*, clindamycin, was given at the time of the bacterial insult, there

was no impact on the early onset phase, but the late onset development of intraabdominal abscesses was largely eliminated. These observations influenced many infectious disease experts to recommend a combination of clindamycin and gentamicin for the treatment of soft tissue pelvic infections in humans.

There are distinct variations between the animal model and human experience that must be accounted for in any prospective judgment about appropriate antibiotics. The animal model involves a massive bacterial insult that is seldom reached in human infection. Deaths from sepsis were seldom seen on an obstetric–gynecologic service in the 1970s, and patients with an intraabdominal abscess are a tiny proportion of the total population of women with a pelvic infection. These differences do not negate the lessons of the animal model, but suggest that individual risk factors must be considered in each of the human infections that require treatment.

COMMUNITY-ACQUIRED INFECTIONS

INFECTED ABORTION

Patients with infected abortion are a much less common problem for the obstetrician–gynecologist in the 1980s than they were in the 1960s. Not only is the number of patients with infected abortion lower, but also death from sepsis occurs far less frequently than in previous decades. Center for Disease Control statistics indicate a dramatic drop in the number of maternal mortalities from sepsis after a termination of pregnancy.

There are several obvious influences on these encouraging statistics. One was the development of better contraceptive methods in the late 1960s and early 1970s. These new and better methods of contraception were rapidly introduced into clinical practice. In addition, considerable effort was put into the delivery of contraceptive care to populations at high risk for an unwanted pregnancy; family planning for the urban poor became a reality. These developments gave a greater proportion of sexually active women more control over their reproductive destinies. There was also a breakthrough in the availability of definitive care for the woman with an unwanted pregnancy. Pregnancy termination by licensed physicians became legal. Although no termination technique is free of complications, the incidence of difficulties is, of coure, lower when abortion procedures are performed by qualified medical personnel. Because of the availability of legal abortion, patients sought confirmation of pregnancy at an early date; unwanted pregnancies were terminated early, when complications are much less frequent. The net result has been a dramatic fall in both the number of women with pelvic infection following abortion and the number of women with life-threatening infection.

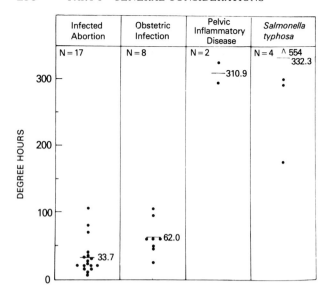

FIG. 13–1. Fever indices in degree hours of patients with bacteremia from a community infection. *Salmonella typhosa* refers to patients with an enterocolitis. The mean fever index is indicated for each group. (Ledger WJ, Kriewall TJ, Gee C. Obstet Gynecol 45:603, 1975)

Despite all this, some women with infected abortion will be seen by the obstetrician–gynecologist.

Evaluations of infected abortions in the 1970s indicate this is a low-risk infection. Generally, these women respond rapidly to medical and surgical therapy and recover without serious complications. Figure 13–1 shows the fever index of patients hospitalized with a community-acquired infection and an associated bacteremia. In general, bacteremia has been a marker for the patients most seriously ill with infection on an obstetric–gynecologic service, so this analysis includes only a small group of the total number of women with infection. The fever index is a quantitative measure of patient response to infection, and the clinical response of patients with infected abortion is usually the least serious of the responses to all the major categories of community-acquired infections (Fig. 13–1).

Treatment

Patient responses to infected abortion are different from responses to most other pelvic infections. The patient usually responds rapidly to medical and operative therapy. One study by Chow *et al* indicated that curettage was a more important component in the cure than systemic antibiotics. This is probably related to the efficient bacterial-clearing mechanism of the pregnant uterus. Successful responses to therapy, based on microbiologic data, are seen in situations in which an inappropriate antibiotic was used. Many women with a

B. fragilis bacteremia become afebrile and are cured despite the use of systemic antibiotics that do not cover this microorganism. This is an important observation, for Rotheram and Schick have shown that *B. fragilis* is the second most common bloodstream isolate in patients with infected abortion. If cures could not be achieved without specific antibiotic coverage, there would be more widespread use of such agents as clindamycin and chloramphenicol in these patients. These potentially toxic agents are seldom needed; in one woman with infected abortion and an associated *B. fragilis* bacteremia, however, chloramphenicol was necessary to achieve a cure (Fig. 13–2). Usually, these women can be treated with a single agent, such as a cephalosporin, or a combination of penicillin and an aminoglycoside. If they fail to respond to this or are critically ill on admission, clindamycin or chloramphenicol should be prescribed as initial therapy.

Factors That Impose Special Risk in Infected Abortion

Some situations increase the risk of serious infection for patients with infected abortion. Identification of these possibly serious problems is an indication for more aggressive antibiotic and operative therapy. Any evidence of *infection beyond the limits of the uterus* puts the patient in a high-risk category. This is usually secondary to damage to the uterus, particularly perforation at the time of induced abortion, and it provides a setting in which the patient is more likely to develop a pelvic abscess. In these women, antibiotics that are effective against both gram-negative aerobes and anaerobic organisms should be ordered to prevent abscess formation.

Another subgroup of women at high risk includes those with a clinical picture of *endotoxic shock*. In these clinical situations, therapy should be directed primarily toward gram-negative aerobic organisms, for these are most frequently the culprits. On occasion, however, the only isolate from the bloodstream is an anaerobe. Therefore, antibiotic coverage effective against anaerobes should be employed at the initiation of therapy. Even in these high-risk patients, the clinical prognosis is still more favorable than it is in other serious infections seen on an obstetric–gynecologic service. Figure 13–3 documents the fever index response of seriously ill patients treated with a combination of antibiotics and either clindamycin or chloramphenicol as coverage for *B. fragilis*. Again, uncomplicated posttreatment courses were seen in the patients with infected abortion, and none of these women developed a pelvic abscess that required operative drainage.

A final group of high-risk patients includes *women who are critically ill, with evidence of myometrial gas formation,* and an "onion skin" appearance on roentgen examination, which is pathognomonic of a *Clostri-*

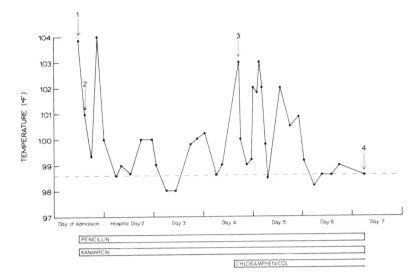

FIG. 13-2. Infected abortion, *B. fragilis* bacteremia. Chloramphenicol was required for cure. (Ledger WJ: Am J Obstet Gynecol 123:111, 1975)

dium perfringens infection. These infections can be lethal as a result of the toxins produced by these organisms, and they require an aggressive operative approach when they are extensive. The recovery of *C. perfringens per se* from a site of infection or the identification of gram-positive rods in the purulent exudate is not an indication for hysterectomy. There should be clinical evidence of extensive infection with intravascular hemolysis and renal failure or roentgen evidence of extensive pelvic infection before hysterectomy is performed. In these critically ill patients, antibiotic coverage should be directed against gram-positive and gram-negative aerobes as well as all anaerobes. Curettage is important, with hysterectomy reserved for the patients whose condition continues to deteriorate after the curettage. However, this aggressive approach is not universally accepted for critically ill patients with renal failure following pregnancy termination. In one series of cases from England 17 of 19 women with this problem survived with treatment limited to antibiotics and supportive measures while awaiting return of renal function, results that are far superior to the usually quoted mortality rate of nearly 100% when these patients are treated without surgery. Further studies are needed in other medical centers before this medically oriented therapy will be accepted in the United States.

SALPINGO-OOPHORITIS

There are many current controversies about the etiology and treatment of salpingo-oophoritis. The microbiologic basis for the syndrome of salpingo-oophoritis has not been firmly established. In the past decade, the nongonococcal nature of many cases of salpingo-oo-

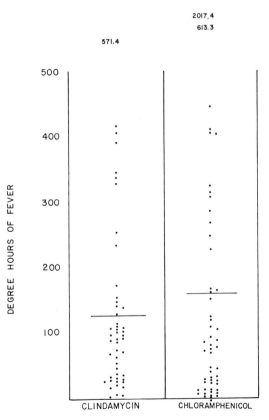

FIG. 13-3. Fever index response to clindamycin and chloramphenicol in patients seriously ill with *B. fragilis* infection. (Ledger WJ, Moore DE, Lowensohn RI et al: Obstet Gynecol 50:523, 1977)

phoritis has become increasingly clear but all the potentially causative organisms have not been identified. For example, one Swedish study established a major role for *Chlamydia* nongonococcal salpingitis, but this was not confirmed in investigations by Sweet and coworkers. Some of the clinical bases for the diagnosis of salpingitis have been challenged. Afebrile salpingitis is reported to be common, particularly in the woman with an intrauterine device in place. It may be impossible to differentiate afebrile salpingitis from other noninfectious causes of pelvic pain, particularly if a diagnostic culdocentesis cannot be performed. All reported treatment regimens represent best guesses; they are not based on firm scientific data. Should patients with salpingitis be treated as outpatients? This controversy can be resolved only by a careful prospective treatment study to determine the effectiveness of an inpatient versus an outpatient treatment regimen.

There are no data available on the most important aspect of medical care, the future fertility of the woman. Westrom has shown the impact of repeated episodes of salpingitis upon future fertility (Table 13–1). These data make the dangers of salpingitis obvious. None of the many alternative therapeutic regimens currently employed has been evaluated for this important end point. Until this is done, any treatment recommendations remain empirical. This is an important fact to acknowledge, for a rapid clinical response does not necessarily indicate better tubal function in the future. For example, patients treated with steroids plus antibiotics had a better initial clinical response than did patients treated with antibiotics alone in Falk's study; they became afebrile more rapidly, and pelvic tumors regressed in size more rapidly. However, on follow-up laparoscopic examination, the incidence of adhesion formation and blocked tubes was no different in the two treatment groups. Future studies of drug therapy will require evaluation of future tubal function as a definitive measure of therapy effectiveness.

Classification

Any acceptable method of classification of salpingo-oophoritis should be based upon methods that are both reproducible and available to all clinicians. Monif has championed the concept of endometritis–salpingitis–peritonitis (ESP), but a classification based upon (1) the presence or absence of a pelvic mass and (2) the recovery or nonrecovery of *Neisseria gonorrhoeae* from the endocervical culture seems preferable. In addition, such a classification can be used as a guide to therapy. Prior to the initiation of therapy, a pelvic examination should be performed to determine whether the patient has a pelvic mass. This information is important, for women with a pelvic mass are in a higher risk category and may require an operation for the drainage of a pelvic abscess. There is not total agree-

TABLE 13-1. FERTILITY FOLLOWING SALPINGITIS

TYPE OF INFECTION	Incidence of Involuntary Sterility with Tubal Occlusion
Gonococcal	6%
Nongonococcal	17%
NUMBER OF EPISODES OF SALPINGITIS	
One	13%
Two	35%
Three	75%

(Modified from Westrom L: Am J Obstet Gynecol 121:707, 1975)

ment on the significance of a pelvic mass, for an ultrasound study by Spaulding *et al* did not show any poorer outcomes in women with a fluid-filled pelvic mass. However, since such a mass may be a pelvic abscess with anaerobes, particularly *B. fragilis,* as the predominant organisms, therapy should be initiated with either clindamycin or chloramphenicol to cover these organisms, as well as an antibiotic effective against gram-negative aerobes. Even so, many patients fail to respond to medical therapy and for cure require operative intervention in the form of drainage or extirpation of the abscess.

For those women who do not have a pelvic mass prior to the initiation of therapy, another factor is important—whether or not *N. gonorrhoeae* can be recovered from the endocervical culture. Women who have an infection that involves this microorganism become afebrile more rapidly with antibiotic therapy, rarely develop abscesses, and have a more favorable prognosis for future fertility. The male partner should be treated before the patient resumes sexual activity.

It is difficult for the clinician to differentiate between gonococcal and nongonococcal salpingitis on the first examination of the patient. Some have suggested that this diagnosis can be made on the basis of a Gram stain of an endocervical smear, *i.e.,* that a positive smear correlates with a positive culture. The difficulty lies with the patient with a negative smear, for a positive culture can be obtained in some women with a negative smear. In addition, others found poor correlations between both positive and negative smears and cultures. It is hoped that some fluorescent staining technique will be developed to identify women with gonococcal salpingitis. In any event, women with no pelvic masses have a favorable response to therapy, for few go on to develop a pelvic abscess that requires operative drainage.

Treatment

The widely divergent treatment regimens employed in patients without a pelvic mass is a good indication that

a controlled study to demonstrate immediate and long-term effectiveness of specific regimens has not yet been done. Outpatient studies in which the effectiveness of ampicillin was compared with that of a standard tetracycline showed equivalent results with both gonococcal and nongonococcal salpingitis. An inpatient study that evaluated ampicillin and doxycycline in gonococcal and nongonococcal salpingitis showed a better response as indicated by the fever index, in the women treated with doxycycline. Monif *et al.* prefer a combination of penicillin and doxycycline in hospitalized patients, while Sweet has preferred a combination of penicillin and an aminoglycoside.

A major problem in the evaluation of the antibiotic treatment of salpingo-oophoritis is the lack of microbiologic information about this disease. The internal anatomic location of the fallopian tubes and ovaries makes it difficult to obtain culture material. A commonly employed diagnostic technique is *culdocentesis*. Since peritoneal fluid is sterile in the asymptomatic woman, any bacteria recovered from the peritoneal fluid aspirate are assumed to be the same as those causing the inflammation in the endosalpinx. Unless the cul de sac is not free, this procedure should be done in afebrile women with pelvic pain who are suspected of having salpingitis. Some physicians are reluctant to diagnose salpingitis unless there is evidence of infection, *i.e.*, bacteria and white blood cells in the peritoneal fluid smear, although Monif in his ESP classification would classify the disease of the patient with negative peritoneal fluid as simply endometritis–salpingitis (ES). Unfortunately, there seem to be major limitations in the microbiologic evaluations of fluid obtained by culdocentesis. Using direct aspiration of peritoneal fluid at the time of laparoscopy, Sweet *el al* have found poor correlation with the bacteria recovered from the peritoneal fluid and that recovered from the endosalpinx fluid obtained from the fimbria.

One confusing issue in the microbiologic etiology of salpingo-oophoritis is the role of *Chlamydia*. Clinically, *Chlamydia* appear to be important because of the favorable response of patients with salpingitis to doxycycline, which is effective against *Chlamydia*. Mardh *et al.*, using fimbrial biopsy via laparoscopy, recovered *Chlamydia* from 30% of women with nongonococcal salpingitis. However, Sweet *et al.* have not yet recovered *Chlamydia* from the endosalpinx cultures of patients with salpingitis.

The *intrauterine contraceptive device* affects both the frequency and the type of pelvic infections seen in nonpregnant women. A number of studies done in the past few years indicate that women who use the intrauterine device (IUD) for contraception have a higher frequency of pelvic infection, particularly if they are young and unmarried. In addition, there is evidence that the host response to infection is altered when an IUD is present. Pelvic infections due to *Actinomyces*

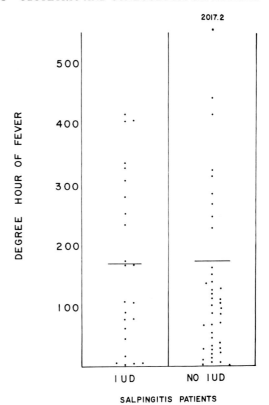

FIG. 13-4. Response to triple antibiotic therapy for salpingo-oophoritis in patients with and without an IUD. (Ledger WJ, Moore, DE, Lowensohn RI et al: Obstet Gynecol 50:523, 1977)

bovis are much more frequently seen in IUD users. The unilateral tuboovarian abscess occurs more frequently in IUD users, and the pathophysiology of this unilateral problem resembles that of the ovarian abscess more than it resembles the ascending types of infection seen with salpingitis. IUDs do not always cause a more severe infection. An evaluation of the response to triple antibiotic therapy for salpingo-oophoritis showed no difference between patients who were using an IUD and patients who were not (Fig. 13-4).

Operative treatment of patients with salpingo-oophoritis remains an important component of therapy. Women who have clinical evidence of a ruptured tuboovarian abscess, such as diffuse peritonitis and a tachycardia out of proportion to their temperature, are critically ill. Failure to operate could mean their demise, and the operation should include hysterectomy and bilateral salpingo-oophorectomy for cure. The problem is not as simple in women who fail to respond to antibiotic therapy and show no signs of a tuboovarian abscess rupture. For years, physicians have been reluctant to perform surgery in the acute phase of infection because of the increased incidence of com-

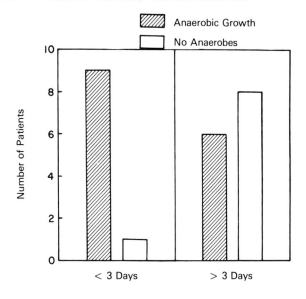

FIG. 13–5. Isolation of anaerobes from abscesses, depending upon the length of preoperative exposure to clindamycin or chloramphenicol. Increase in the recovery of anaerobes is significant when preoperative duration of therapy is 3 days or less. $P < 0.01$ by the Fisher exact test. (Ledger WJ, Gee C, Pollin P et al: Am J Obstet Gynecol 125:677, 1976)

plications and mortality associated with surgery at this time. In recent years, however, it has been shown that operations can be performed in the acute phase of infection without serious complications. This is undoubtedly related to the availability of antibiotics that are effective against the organisms involved in these acute infections. Although the operations can be performed, they are seldom necessary and should be reserved for patients who fail to respond within 72 hours to antibiotic therapy that includes clindamycin or chloramphenicol. Figure 13–5 shows the recovery of anaerobes in such situations, and the reason that 72 hours of medical therapy are recommended to eliminate anaerobes from the site of infection.

HOSPITAL-ACQUIRED INFECTIONS

HOSPITAL PERSONNEL

Despite continued emphasis on the importance of asepsis, some of the standard hospital rules are repeatedly disregarded. Shoe covers, caps, and masks should be discarded immediately when the wearer leaves the operating or delivery room. Scrub suits should not be worn outside the operating rooms and delivery rooms except in special circumstances, and the wearer must change to a fresh scrub suit before reentering an aseptic or controlled area. Abundant facial hair can be a collector, and a shedder, of bacteria, especially the gram-positive, coagulase-positive type; men with beards or mustaches should use a antistaphylococcus shampoo regularly and should exercise special care in the use of operating room cap and mask. Medical attendants who develop skin infections, even if they are hidden from view, should not be directly involved in patient care. One hospital outbreak of group A β-hemolytic streptococcal infections was traced to an anesthesiologist who was an aymptomatic anal carrier of this organism. One series of coagulase-positive staphylococcal wound infections was related to a surgical resident's contaminated beard; another, to a pustule on the hand of an anesthesiologist.

INFECTION AFTER PREGNANCY TERMINATION

With the liberalization of the abortion laws in the 1960s, infectious morbidity following pregnancy termination became an entity to be coped with by the practicing obstetrician–gynecologist. A number of observations about these infections seem universal. The later in pregnancy the termination occurs, the more frequently the infections, but serious infections following therapeutic abortion are rare. Because of the infrequency of infection following pregnancy termination before 12 weeks, there has been little enthusiasm for the use of prophylactic antibiotics; however, one study showed that tetracycline was effective when used in this manner. A more logical approach would be to screen patients for *N. gonorrhoeae* before curettage; those whose test results are positive should be treated with antibiotics, for this population has increased postoperative morbidity. The most serious infections, which have resulted in disseminated intravascular coagulation and death, have occurred after hysterotomy in women over 38 years of age. Therefore, hysterotomy has been largely abandoned as a termination procedure. Recently, evacuation of the uterus by suction curettage has been used in women beyond 12 week's gestation. Although this technique compares favorably with prostaglandin and saline abortion techniques, serious soft tissue injury and subsequent serious pelvic infection is possible.

In all women with a postabortion infection, the basic therapeutic approach is the same: antibiotic coverage followed by operative intervention to remove any retained products of conception. If there is evidence of infection beyond the confines of the uterus, antibiotics that are effective against *B. fragilis* should be used and laparotomy utilized for the patient who fails to respond to therapy or shows any evidence of clinical deterioration.

PUERPERAL ENDOMYOMETRITIS

The greatest problem of hospital-acquired infections on the obstetric–gynecologic service in the 1980s is puerperal endomyometritis. These infections occur frequently and may become the most serious infections seen on the inpatient service. Because of their importance, the clinician should have a clear view of the risk factors, modes of prevention, and the treatment of these problems. The clinical features of this important disease are considered in Chapter 40.

The established *risk factors* for patients with puerperal endomyometritis are few in number. There is good evidence that both the rate of infection and severity are greater following cesarean section than following vaginal delivery (Fig. 13–6). Other factors that influence puerperal infections are not as obvious. There is evidence that the incidence of puerperal endomyometritis following cesarean section increases as the time interval between membrane rupture and delivery lengthens, but these longer time intervals are not associated with more severe infections (Fig. 13–7). The relationship of the invasive intrauterine monitoring catheter and postpartum infection is also unclear. Several studies have suggested that there is no correlation between intrauterine monitoring and the rate of infection, but two studies in private patients demonstrated a greater frequency of infection when this technique is used. It is possible that the multiple factors associated with infection in a lower socioeconomic population prevent discrimination of individual factors.

The high risk of *infection following cesarean section*, particularly when the procedure is performed on women in labor, has generated a great deal of interest in *prophylactic antibiotics*. Clinical experience with prophylactic antibiotics in vaginal hysterectomy has been favorable. Almost without exception, therapeutic results with prophylactic antibiotics have been better than those with a placebo. Despite this, there are still concerns about the uniform use of prophylactic antibiotics in order to prevent infections. A most important concern is the timing of the antibiotic administration. In prior clinical evaluations of prophylactic antibiotics, the medication has been given just before the operative procedure. In cesarean section, this produces therapeutic levels of antibiotics in the fetus. Since mothers at high risk for infection also deliver babies with a greater than usual chance for infection, the presence of measurable levels of antibiotic in the fetus complicates evaluation of the blood culture in the infant with suspected sepsis. The administration of antibiotics after cord clamping may produce results equivalent to those obtained by the more standard preoperative administration. This avoids any dosage to the fetus, but intravenous administration of antibiotic to an anesthetized patient may not be the most acceptable approach to the problem; two deaths have been

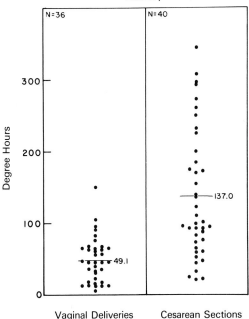

Bacteremia by Route of Delivery

FIG. 13–6. Fever indices in degree hours of patients with puerperal bacteremia, comparing patients with a vaginal delivery to those delivered by cesarean section. The mean is indicated. (Ledger WJ, Gee C, Pollin P et al: Am J Obstet Gynecol 125:677, 1976)

reported with this technique. Because prophylactic antibiotics in cesarean section seem to have little impact on the number of serious infections in patients who have received this type of therapy, alternative approaches to prevention or therapy appear to be preferable.

A different approach to this problem has been the extraperitoneal cesarean section. This does not avoid postoperative infection, but it transforms an intraperitoneal infection to an extraperitoneal infection, which is better tolerated by the human host. Although a whole generation of obstetrician–gynecologists lacks experience with the technique, it remains a viable alternative.

Another approach has been to employ different therapeutic strategies in the treatment of patients with puerperal endomyometritis following cesarean section. DiZerega *et al* found that a clindamycin–gentamicin combination produced more favorable results than did a penicillin–gentamicin combination (Table 13–2). Although not statistically significant in this study, the prevention of serious infection would seem to be the most significant aspect of the study. The 4% rate is exactly the same as that reported by Gibbs *et al* in pa-

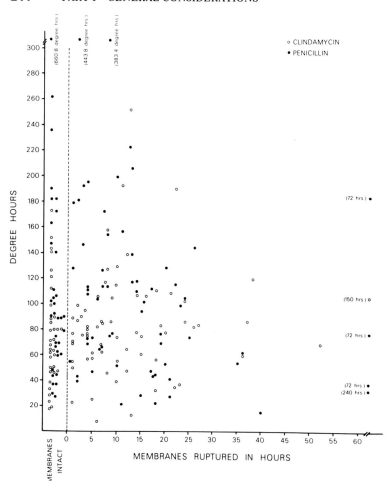

FIG. 13–7. Scattergram of patient's febrile response to endomyometritis after cesarean section compared to the length of time of membrane rupture. (DiZerega G, Yonekura L, Roy S et al: Am J Obstet Gynecol 134(3):238, 1979)

tients treated with penicillin–kanamycin. Similarly, the same results were seen when clindamycin–gentamicin was compared to cephalothin–gentamicin in a study from Newark. In making the final judgment on the use of this regimen, the physician must weigh the potential toxicity of clindamycin against the possibility of preventing serious infection in a small percentage of patients.

Although they occur infrequently, serious infections following cesarean section can be devastating to the patient. The unfortunate women who develop septic pelvic thrombophlebitis face exposure to multiple antibiotics with toxic potential for long periods of time, as well as a prolonged hospital stay of 10–14 days for a full treatment course of heparin. Even more distressing is a pelvic abscess that develops after cesarean section. Not only must these patients endure the protracted hospital stay and treatment that may have unpleasant side effects, but also they are subjected to the risks of a second operation. If they are fortunate, they need only vaginal drainage of a pelvic abscess. If there is an extensive uterine infection or tuboovarian abscesses, ex-

tirpation of the pelvic organs is required. This invariably results in a cure, but the therapeutic success leaves the patient with no hope for future childbearing.

The therapy of the patient with puerperal endomyometritis following vaginal delivery is much simpler than that for a patient with the same condition following cesarean section. There is no need for frequent use of the first line agents used so successfully in post–cesarean section patients. Those who develop infection after vaginal delivery usually respond favorably to single antibiotic treatment such as ampicillin, cephalothin, or metronidazole. Rarely are additional antibiotics necessary for cure.

POSTOPERATIVE INFECTIONS

The surgical technique has much to do not only with the postoperative course in general, but with infection in particular: the longer the operative procedure, the greater the incidence of postoperative infection. As

TABLE 13-2. COMPARISON OF CLINDAMYCIN–GENTAMICIN REGIMEN WITH PENICILLIN–GENTAMICIN REGIMEN

	Clindamycin–Gentamicin	Penicillin–Gentamicin	Significance
NO. OF PATIENTS	100	100	N.S
THERAPY COMPLETED, NO PROBLEMS	86	64	p < 0.001
POOR CLINICAL RESULTS			
No response—third antibiotic	5	29	p < 0.001
Abdominal wound infection	8	16	N.S.
Operative drainage only	6	4	N.S.
Prolonged febrile course after drainage	2	12	p < 0.02 (Fisher's exact test)
SERIOUS PROBLEMS	0	4	p < 0.06
Pelvic abscess, total abdominal hysterectomy, bilateral salpingo-oophorectomy	0	1	
Wound evisceration	0	1	
Heparin	0	2	
REACTION DURING ANTIBIOTICS	4	3	N.S.
Rash	2*	2	
Hematuria	0	1†	
Diarrhea	2	0	
INDIRECT MEASURES OF MORBIDITY			
Hospital days	7.4	8.7	p < 0.01 (Mann–Whitney U test)
Fever index in degree hours			
Median	77.3	91.3	p < 0.02
Mean	81.2	110.7	
±SD	±40.6	±89.6	
±SE	± 4.06	± 9.0	

N.S., Not significant.
* Drug continued, rash disappeared, one patient.
† Drug continued, hematuria stopped.
(DiZerega G, Yonekura L, Roy S et al: Am J Obstet Gynecol 134:238, 1979)

Victor Bonney noted many years ago, "an operation rapidly yet correctly performed has many advantages over one technically as correct, yet laboriously and tediously accomplished." Until the time of his retirement, the surgeon should strive continuously to improve the precision of his technique, and to reduce his operating time, not by increased speed of action, but by avoiding unnecessary movements that do not advance the procedure and can significantly prolong it.

Hospital-acquired infections are frequent problems following gynecologic operations. The abundant bacterial flora of the lower genital tract may multiply and invade the crushed and necrotic tissue left behind after a pelvic operation. Many of the operative procedures in gynecology involve sites close to the urinary tract, often necessitating the use of a catheter to maintain bladder drainage. This markedly increases the risk of a urinary tract infection. All of these factors make a knowledge of infection control and treatment important for the obstetrician–gynecologist.

URINARY TRACT INFECTION

A frequent source of postoperative morbidity is the urinary tract infection. In order to deal properly with this problem, the physician must have a knowledge of techniques for both the prevention and treatment of infection. The *prevention of urinary tract infection* in the postoperative gynecologic patient must be focused on the care of the catheter. A catheter should be inserted only when necessary and then with meticulous care. A closed drainage system not only decreases the total number of urinary infections, but also delays the entry of bacteria into the urinary tract. This is an important consideration for the gynecologist who frequently uses short-term bladder drainage in postoperative patients. Despite these precautions, urinary tract infections will still occur, particularly when the catheter must remain in place for longer than 48 hours. In postoperative patients who are likely to have the catheter removed by the 4th or 5th postoperative day, there is evidence that the *systemic use of nitrofurantoins as prophylaxis* dramatically reduces the subsequent incidence of urinary tract infection.

Women who develop a postoperative urinary tract infection should be approached by the physician in a logical, structured way to acquire the necessary diagnostic information before therapy is begun. Urine should be obtained for culture and susceptibility testing before a systemic antimicrobial agent is prescribed. Since there is a good correlation between the presence

of bacteria on microscopic high-power magnification of centrifuged urine and subsequent bacterial colony counts of greater than 10^5/ml, this evaluation should be done immediately. If any postoperative patient complains of costovertebral angle pain, an intravenous pyelogram should be taken to search for the possibility of operative ureteral damage with obstruction rather than to assign a diagnosis of pyelonephritis. When the evaluation is complete, these patients should be treated with drugs such as the sulfas or the nitrofurantoins. These drugs are as effective as oral penicillin or cephalosporin, and their antibacterial activity is limited to the urinary tract. Broad spectrum agents may mask symptoms of infection and make it impossible for the physician to delineate the infection site clinically. The most important evaluation of treatment is the urine culture obtained after 36–48 hours of therapy. If this is free of bacteria, the patient should not have prolonged difficulties with recurrent infection. If bacteria are present, susceptibility testing should be carried out to determine if alternative agents should be employed.

RESPIRATORY TRACT INFECTIONS

Postoperative respiratory tract infections are relatively infrequent problems for the gynecologist. Most elective operative procedures are done on women in good health, and the incidence of postoperative respiratory difficulties is understandably lower after pelvic operations than after operations that require an upper abdominal incision, *e.g.*, cholecystectomy. The major concern in postoperative patients is aspiration, which is usually recognized immediately or within 24 hours of the operation. Such patients may require supportive respiratory measures if a large amount of material was aspirated. Other patients may develop a postoperative pneumonia because of difficulty in establishing a normal breathing pattern postoperatively. Since there is an increase in the gram-negative aerobic respiratory flora of hospitalized patients, antibiotic therapy should include agents effectively against these aerobes.

PELVIC INFECTIONS

Postoperative pelvic infections occur with some frequency, and therapy usually prolongs the patient's stay in the hospital. These pelvic infections may take many forms with different prognoses. An infected collection of material in the vaginal cuff after hysterectomy can often be treated by simple operative drainage alone. A diffuse pelvic cellulitis always requires systemic antibiotics; heparin is required if the infection progresses to septic pelvic thrombophlebitis. Postoperative pelvic abscesses can be lethal if they rupture into the peritoneal cavity. If this occurs, immediate laparot-

omy must be performed to remove the infected pelvic organs. Patients with unruptured abscesses usually do not respond to medical therapy and require operative intervention, with all of the risks of a second anesthetic and major operation, for drainage or removal of the abscess.

Widely diverse techniques have been employed to prevent postoperative pelvic infections. The most popular technique has been systemic antibiotic prophylaxis, particularly in the premenopausal woman undergoing vaginal hysterectomy. A wide variety of antibiotics has been used successfully in this situation, including penicillin, cephalosporin, tetracyclines, and metronidazole. There is evidence that a short course of prophylaxis limited to the day of the operation is just as effective as therapy for 3–5 days postoperatively. In fact, one study of vaginal hysterectomy in which patients were given only 1 g cefazolin intramuscularly just prior to the operation showed outstanding results. All of these prophylactic regimens have been associated with a reduction in the number of postoperative pelvic infections. There are alternative methods of prevention of post-operative pelvic infection, however. Using closed suction T-tube drainage of the space between the peritoneum and vaginal cuff in abdominal and vaginal hysterectomy, Swartz and Tanaree have shown a marked reduction in postoperative pelvic infections. The addition of systemic antibiotic prophylaxis to the closed suction drainage system did not result in further lowering of the postoperative infection rate. A very different approach to the prevention of infection was championed by Osborne *et al.* By performing hot conization of the cervix just before hysterectomy to remove the potential bacterial contamination from the endocervix, they demonstrated a sharp reduction in the number of postoperative pelvic infections.

The patient with a postoperative pelvic infection requires careful evaluation before therapy is instituted. A pelvic examination should be performed to determine the location of the infection. If purulent material can be aspirated directly from the vaginal cuff, it should be cultured for aerobic and anaerobic bacteria. If there is a suggestion of a pelvic mass, ultrasonography may be a helpful diagnostic tool to determine if there is a fluid-filled mass in the pelvis. Several antimicrobials have been successfully employed in patients with pelvic cellulitis. These include ampicillin alone, penicillin and an aminoglycoside, a cephalosporin alone or with an aminoglycoside, or tetracyclines. If there is evidence of a widespread infection on the initial examination or if the patient shows no response after 48–72 hours of the initial therapy, then either chloramphenicol or clindamycin should be added to the regimen for coverage of *B. fragilis*. Whether better results would be achieved in these women by the initial use of either clindamycin or chloramphenicol has not been evaluated by prospective study.

If patients continue a febrile course after antibiotics effective against *B. fragilis* have been given, then the possibility of either septic pelvic thrombophlebitis or a pelvic abscess should be considered. There are no specific diagnostic techniques to confirm the presence of septic pelvic thrombophlebitis, but a tentative diagnosis can be made if the patient has a persistent fever and no evidence of a pelvic mass. Such a patient should be treated with intravenous heparin by continuous pump infusion; dosage should be determined by pretreatment and intratreatment coagulation studies. The continuous infusion method should be employed instead of intermittent bolus therapy because it decreases the risk of serious bleeding in these postoperative patients. In the patient who remains febrile after 36–48 hours of heparin therapy or who has a pelvic mass, the diagnosis to be considered is a pelvic abscess. Operative drainage or removal is indicated.

ABDOMINAL WOUND INFECTIONS

The drainage of an infected abdominal wound is not only a distressing psychologic event for a patient, but also it prolongs her stay in the hospital. A serious infection with synergistic bacteria may result in necrotizing fasciitis and death, while badly infected abdominal wounds may progress to dehiscence and evisceration. This serious problem of abdominal wound infection requires knowledge of techniques of prevention as well as a reasoned clinical approach.

Methods of prevention have been detailed by Cruse and Ford, whose studies have implicated a series of pre- and intraoperative rituals with an increase in the abdominal wound infection rate. They showed that a prolonged preoperative stay in the hospital; shaving the incision site the day before the operation instead of the day of the operation; using an electrocautery knife, plastic wound drapes instead of towels, and a wound drain through the abdominal wound all resulted in a higher number of postoperative wound infections. Elimination of these factors, as well as other preventive techniques, may decrease the number of abdominal wall infections. In the very obese patient or the patient with massive intraoperative bacterial contamination, a delayed primary closure of the wound with reapproximation of the subcutaneous tissue and skin 3 days after the operation has been associated with a low abdominal wound infection rate. Another variation in preventive care of the massively obese woman who requires laparotomy has been the use of closed suction drainage of the wound site, with the drainage tube exit away from the operative incision.

Despite all of these attempts to prevent operative site infections, some abdominal wound problems are seen. The first task of the physician attending a woman with an infected abdominal wound is to establish drainage and determine that the fascial incision is intact. Careful assessment is necessary to be certain that the drainage is not secondary to an evisceration, rather than the supposed infection. Antibiotics are rarely needed for the treatment of an abdominal wound infection, but they should be prescribed whenever inflammation of the skin appears to be spreading. Since a coagulase-positive *Staphylococcus* may be involved in this event, the use of a cephalosporin is preferable to the use of a penicillin in these women. Women with evidence of skin inflammation should be carefully monitored, for rapid spread may denote a necrotizing fasciitis that necessitates operative debridement for cure.

SUPERFICIAL THROMBOPHLEBITIS OF THE UPPER EXTREMITY

The long-term use of intravenous infusion lines is responsible for a relatively new syndrome, superficial thrombophlebitis of the upper extremity, which may give rise to fever on the 3rd postoperative day. A simple preventive measure is to prohibit the use of intravenous infusion lines for longer than 48 hours after surgery.

ANTIBIOTICS

The basic judgment every physician must make when prescribing a drug is whether the benefits of the agent outweigh its dangers. To make an intelligent choice of antibiotics, a physician must know the antibacterial spectrum of activity, the organisms most frequently involved in the infection to be treated, the appropriate route of administration, and the toxicity of the drugs.

THE PENICILLINS

The penicillins are still the most valuable single group of antibiotics. Because of the vast difference between therapeutic levels and toxic levels, these antibiotics have a wide range of safety. In addition, they have not been specifically prohibited from use in obstetric patients. Also, they are the drugs of choice for the treatment of infections due to *N. gonorrhoeae* and *Treponema pallidum*. One of the great developments in applied research has been the discovery of new congeners of penicillin that have broadened its spectrum of activity. Penicillin G is primarily effective against gram-positive aerobes, although it has some gram-negative aerobic rod coverage when very high doses are given intravenously. Problems with penicillin-resistant coagulase-positive staphylococci have been largely eliminated by the introduction of the new semisynthetic penicillin. The introduction of ampicillin in the early 1960s provided better coverage of gram-negative

aerobes, and the later development of carbenicillin improved the coverage of *Pseudomonas aeruginosa*. All of the penicillins are effective against anaerobes, with the exception of gram-negative anaerobic rods like *B. fragilis*. There is good laboratory evidence, however, that an increasing number of strains of *B. fragilis* is responsive to the high levels of carbenicillin that can be achieved by megadose therapy. This broad spectrum of activity make the various penicillins attractive as therapy for the obstetric–gynecologic patient with a bacterial infection.

The penicillins are versatile drugs because of the varied routes of administration that can be used. The intravenous route should be used for the hospitalized patient with an infection, although intramuscular therapy can be used for either an inpatient or an outpatient. The oral forms of penicillin are especially helpful for the patient who requires prolonged outpatient therapy. They have not been shown to be more effective than either the sulfa drugs or nitrofurantoins in the treatment of lower urinary tract infections, however, and the nitrofurantoins remain the drugs of choice for this condition because they have a more limited effect on bowel flora than does ampicillin.

There are a number of *toxic reactions* to penicillin. Such reactions may be allergic, or they may be directly related to toxic effects of the drugs. The allergic reactions are most easily categorized as either immediate or late. Immediate reactions, *i.e.*, anaphylaxis, are the most feared, for they can result in the death of the patient. Late reactions, such as a maculopapular eruption, are not life-threatening, but they prolong the patient's discomfort and distress. Ampicillin is the penicillin that is most likely to produce these late appearing skin eruptions, although most such reactions are related to some substance in the ampicillin other than the penicillin molecule itself. The toxic reactions to the penicillin vary with the form employed. Very high doses of intravenous penicillin, in excess of 40 million units per day, may produce very high serum levels in elderly patients with reduced renal function and may result in convulsions because of the increased excitability of the central nervous system in these patients. Intravenous methicillin may result in nephropathy. Ampicillin has caused fatal pseudomembranous enterocolitis in one patient following abdominal hysterectomy. The high dosages of intravenous carbenicillin therapy can be associated with many serious side effects. The huge sodium load with these megadoses may be poorly tolerated by a cardiac patient. Hypokalemia can occur in up to 20% of women who have received a high dosage of intravenous carbenicillin therapy. In addition, carbenicillin affects platelets, and administration of the drug may be accompanied by unexpected bleeding. The physician must be aware of these side effects and be on the alert for their appearance.

THE CEPHALOSPORINS

Although introduced primarily as alternative bactericidal antibiotics for the penicillin-allergic patient, the cephalosporins have been widely used by obstetrician–gynecologists as primary therapeutic agents. There are a number of reasons for this popularity. The cephalosporins have a broad spectrum of antibacterial activity, similar in many respects to that of the penicillins. They are effective against the coagulase-positive *Staphylococcus* and all gram-positive aerobes except the enterococci. They are also effective against gram-negative aerobes, especially *Klebsiella*, which is so often resistant to ampicillin, but they have not been effective against *P. aeruginosa*. Against the anaerobes, their action is very similar to that of penicillin, but they are much less effective against *B. fragilis* than is carbenicillin. These are versatile drugs, for they can be given intravenously, intramuscularly, and orally. The oral form has no advantages over sulfa or nitrofurantoin in the treatment of urinary tract infection. Despite these favorable activities, potential toxicity causes the cephalosporins not to be the drug of choice for single infections in obstetrics–gynecology if other drugs are appropriate. One of the most common reasons for the prescription of cephalosporins is prophylaxis for elective pelvic operations.

A second generation of cephalosporins has recently been approved by the Food and Drug Administration (FDA). Cefamandole provides broader coverage of gram-negative aerobic organisms, as shown in clinical tests with obstetric–gynecologic infections. Cefoxitin, a cephamycin, has the distinct advantage of good activity against *B. fragilis* and is similarly effective in the treatment of soft tissue infections. This antibiotic, a cephamycin, is unique among the cephalosporins currently available because of its activity against *Bacteroides fragilis*. Clinical studies of patients with soft tissue pelvic infections have demonstrated a high degree of effectiveness. Since there are many strains of *Bacteroides fragilis* that are less susceptible to cefoxitin than to clindamycin, chloramphenicol, and mentronidazole, it is not the drug of choice in seriously ill patients. In addition, clinical experience has confirmed less than optimal results when this antibiotic has been prescribed in patients with well-established infections. Fortunately, most patients with soft tissue pelvic infections are not seriously ill and do not have well-established infections. For these women, cefoxitin is an excellent antibiotic to employ.

Notwithstanding the widespread interest of clinicians in the cephalosporins, there can be *toxic side-effects*. Immediate reactions can occur, and death has been reported as a result of cardiovascular collapse after the intravenous administration of a cephalosporin. Anaphylaxis is a possibility, and there is danger of cross reactivity in the woman with a history of peni-

cillin anaphylaxis. Late reactions range from a mild allergic skin reaction to death from pseudodmembranous enterocolitis, probably from alterations in the bacterial flora of the gut. Renal toxicity has been reported, particularly with cephaloridine, but all of the cephalosporins have this potential, especially when used in combination with aminoglycosides.

THE AMINOGLYCOSIDES

A valuable family of antibiotics for the obstetrician–gynecologist, aminoglycosides are highly effective against gram-negative aerobes, particularly the more resistant ones found in hospitalized patients. This is really the sole reason for their use. However, their use presents many problems. They are the least versatile of the classes of antibiotics discussed thus far, for they can be given only intravenously and intramuscularly. More importantly, the range between therapeutic levels and toxicity both to the eighth cranial nerve and to the kidney is quite narrow. In addition, predictions of serum levels based upon the patient's weight have not always been accurate. To avoid serum levels so high that toxicity results or so low that therapy is ineffective, peak and trough levels should be obtained in patients undergoing a therapeutic course. These complicated safeguards make it necessary to limit the use of these antibiotics to seriously ill, hospitalized patients.

TREATMENT OF SOFT TISSUE INFECTIONS

An awareness of the importance of anaerobes, particularly B. fragilis, in pelvic infections has led to the use of many agents, some unfamiliar, in the *treatment of soft tissue infections.*

The *tetracyclines* are a unique group of antibiotics. They are the drugs of choice for only a few exotic infections, but they are second line drugs for many common obstetric–gynecologic infections. Because of their toxicity to the pregnant woman when given intravenously for pyelonephritis, with maternal death from fatty liver, they are contraindicated in pregnancy. In the laboratory, the newer tetracyclines are more active against all anaerobic strains than standard tetracycline. In addition, all these agents are highly effective against *Chlamydia.* Because of these factors, the most frequent infection to be treated with tetracycline is nongonococcal salpingitis. Generally, the therapeutic results have been favorable in this population.

Clindamycin is one of the most popular drugs for the treatment of anaerobic infections, particularly those due to B. fragilis. It is highly effective and can be administered intravenously or orally. There are problems related to the use of this drug, however, particularly in the gastrointestinal tract where pseudomembranous enterocolitis can develop. The cause of this reaction has now been determined. The enterocolitis is caused by a specific strain of *Clostridium difficile,* which is resistant to clindamycin and produces an enterotoxin. This strain of clostridia is susceptible to vancomycin, and it is hoped that treatment with vancomycin will diminish the severity of the gastrointestinal effects of clindamycin. It is important for the physician prescribing clindamycin to be alert to any changes in the patient's gastrointestinal function. Consequently, every patient taking the drug should make a daily record of her bowel movements. If she has more than five, the drug should be stopped, and in this way, progression of the gastrointestinal difficulties may be halted. If diarrhea persists, then sigmoidoscopy should be performed.

Chloramphenicol is a valuable drug for the treatment of anaerobic infections. It is highly effective against anaerobes involved in pelvic infections, particularly B. fragilis. Since there is no evidence that chloramphenicol is superior to clindamycin in serious pelvic infections, the decision regarding which drug to use must be based upon the physician's concern about the toxicity of the two agents. An occasional patient, somewhere between 1/20,000–100,000 of those receiving chloramphenicol, will develop an aplastic anemia that may be fatal. This complication is not dose-dependent and cannot be prevented by pretreatment laboratory screening. This rare event is devastating when it occurs. Although it does not absolutely prevent the problem, intravenous chloramphenicol for the total length of therapy is preferable because it appears to be associated with a lower incidence of aplastic anemia than the oral route. This complication is rare, but its severity has led many physicians to use clindamycin in all patients except those with preexisting gastrointestinal difficulties.

Metronidazole may be the anaerobic antibiotic of the future. It is the most bactericidal of any agent in the laboratory to B. fragilis and has been successfully employed clinically in soft tissue pelvic infections. The drug shows great promise, and the intravenous form, now approved by the FDA for such problems, has been well tolerated in clinical studies. Metronidazole also presents problems, however. It should be used with other antibiotics, since an increasing number of gram-positive anaerobes show resistance to it; its lack of activity against gram-negative aerobes means that a second and third antibiotic will be necessary for the treatment of seriously ill patients. In addition, although not demonstrated to date in humans, the drug is carcinogenic in animals and mutagenic for bacteria. These are disturbing findings that mandate continued observation of women who have received the drug in the past.

As noted earlier, *cefoxitin* is highly active against B. fragilis and may have increasing usefulness in management of soft tissue infections.

REFERENCES AND RECOMMENDED READING

Bartlett JG, Chang TW, Taylor NS et al: Colitis induced by *Clostridium difficile.* Rev Infect Dis 1:370, 1979

Burkman RT, Tonascia JA, Atienza MG et al: Untreated endocervical gonorrhea and endometritis following elective abortion. Am J Obstet Gynecol 126:648, 1976

Chow AW, Marshall JR, Guze LB: A double blind comparison of clindamycin with penicillin plus chloramphenicol in treatment of septic abortion. J Infect Dis 135:535, 1977

Collins CG, Nix FG, Cerha HT: Ruptured tubo-ovarian abscess. Am J Obstet Gynecol 72:820, 1956

Cruse PJF, Ford R: A five year prospective study of 23,649 surgical wounds. Arch Surg 107:206, 1973

Cunninham FG, Hauth JG, Strong JD et al: Tetracycline or penicillin–ampicillin for pelvic inflammatory disease. N Engl J Med 296:1380, 1977

Dawood MY, Birnbaum SJ: Unilateral tubo-ovarian abscess and an intrauterine contraceptive device. Obstet Gynecol 46:429, 1975

Dineen P, Druzin L: Epidemics of postoperative wound infections associate with hair carriers. Lancet 2:1157, 1973

DiZerega G, Yonekura L, Roy S et al: A comparison of clindamycin–gentamicin and penicillin–gentamicin in the treatment of post cesarean section endometritis. Am J Obstet Gynecol 134:238, 1979

Eschenbach DA, Harnisch JP, Holmes KK: Pathogenesis of acute pelvic inflammatory disease: Role of contraception and other risk factors. Am J Obstet Gynecol 128:838, 1977

Falk V: Treatment of acute non-tuberculous salpingitis with antibiotics alone and in combination with glucocorticoids. Acta Obstet Gynecol Scand 44:Suppl 6, 1965

Gibbs RS, Jones PM, Wilder CJ: Antibiotic therapy of endometritis following cesarean section. Obstet Gynecol 52:31, 1978

Gibbs RS, Listria HM, Read JA: The effect of internal fetal monitoring on maternal infection following cesarean section. Obstet Gynecol 48:653, 1976

Gibbs RS, Weinstein AJ: Bacteriologic effects of prophylactic antibiotics in cesarean section. Am J Obstet Gynecol 126:226, 1976

Golde SH, Israel F, Ledger WJ: Unilateral tubo-ovarian abscess: A distinct entity. Am J Obstet Gynecol 127:807, 1977

Goldman P: Drug Therapy: Metronidazole. N Engl J Med 303:1212, 1980

Gorbach SL, Thadepalli H: Clindamycin in the treatment of pure and mixed anaerobic infections. Arch Intern Med 134:87, 1974

Gordon HR, Phelps D, Blanchard K: Prophylactic cesarean section antibiotics: Maternal and neonatal morbidity before and after cord clamping. Obstet Gynecol 53:151, 1979

Hagen D: Maternal febrile morbidity associated with fetal monitoring and cesarean section. Obstet Gynecol 46:269, 1973

Hawkins DF, Levitt LH, Fairbrother PF et al: Management of septic chemical abortion with renal failure: Use of a conservative regimen. N Engl J Med 282:722, 1975

Kaplan AL, Jacobs WM, Ehresman JB: Aggressive management of pelvic abscess. Am J Obstet Gynecol 98:482, 1967

Kunin CM, McCormack RC: Prevention of catheter induced urinary tract infection by closed sterile drainage. N Engl J Med 274:1155, 1966

Ledger WJ: Anaerobic infection. Am J Obstet Gynecol 123:111, 1975

Ledger WJ, Gee C, Lewis WP: Guidelines for antibiotic prophylaxis in gynecology. Am J Obstet Gynecol 121:1038, 1970

Ledger WJ, Gee CL, Lewis WP: Bacteremia on an obstetric–gynecological service. Am J Obstet Gynecol 121:205, 1975

Ledger WJ, Gee CL, Lewis WP et al: Comparison of clindamycin and chloramphenicol in treatment of serious infections of the female genital tract. J Infect Dis 135:530, 1977

Ledger WJ, Gee CL, Pollin P et al: The use of pre-reduced media and a portable jar for the collection of anaerobic organisms from clinical sites of infection. Am J Obstet Gynecol 125:677, 1976

Ledger WJ, Kriewall TJ, Gee C: The fever index: A technique for evaluating the clinical response to bacteremia. Obstet Gynecol 43:603, 1976

Ledger WJ, Lewis W, Golde S et al: The use of metronidazole in obstetric and gynecologic infections. Proceedings of the International Metronidazole Conference, Montreal, Canada, p 356. Excerpta Medica, 1976

Ledger WJ, Moore DE, Lowensohn RI et al: A fever index evaluation of chloramphenicol or clindamycin in patients with serious pelvic infections. Obstet Gynecol 50:532, 1977

Ledger WJ, Sweet RL, Headington JT: The prophylatic use of cephaloridine in the prevention of pelvic infection in premenopausal women undergoing vaginal hysterectomy. Am J Obstet Gynecol 115:776, 1973

Mardh PA, Ripa T, Svensson L et al: Role of *Chlamydia trachomatis* infection in acute salpingitis. N Engl J Med 296:1377, 1977

Monif GRG, Welkos SL, Baer H et al: Cul de sac isolates from patients with endometritis–salpingitis–peritonitis and gonococcal endocervicitis. Am J Obstet Gynecol 126:158, 1976

Morrow PJ, Hernandez WL, Townsend DE et al: Pelvic celiotomy in the obese patient. Am J Obstet Gynecol 127:335, 1977

Onderdonk AB, Kasper DL, Cisneras RL et al: The capsular polysaccharide of *Bacteroides fragilis* as a virulence factor: Comparison of the pathogenic potential of encapsulated and unencapsulated strains. J Infect Dis 136:82, 1977

O'Neill RT, Schwarz RH: Clostridial organisms in septic abortions. Obstet Gynecol 35:458, 1970

Osborne NG, Wright RC, Dubay M: Pre-operative hot conization of the cervix. Am J Obstet Gynecol 133:374, 1979

Rotheram EB, Schick SF: Non clostridial anaerobic bacteria in septic abortion. Am J Med 46:80, 1969

Schultz JC, Adamson JS, Workman WW et al: Fatal liver disease after intravenous administration of tetracycline in high dose. N Engl J Med 269:499, 1963

Sen P, Apuzzio J, Reyelt C et al: Prospective evaluation of combination of antimicrobial agents in cesarean section endometritis. SGO (in press)

Simpson FF: The choice of time for operation for pelvic inflammation of tubal origin. Surg Gynecol Obstet 9:45, 1909

Spaulding LB, Gelman SR, Wood, SO et al: The role of ultrasonography in the management of endometritis/salpingitis/peritonitis. Obstet Gynecol 53:442, 1979

Spruill FG, Minelte LJ, Stumer WC: Two surgical deaths associated with cephalothin. JAMA 229:440, 1974

Subbagha RE, Hyashi TT: Disseminated intravascular coagulation complicating hysterectomy in elderly gravidas. Obstet Gynecol 38:844, 1971

Swartz WH, Tanatee P: Suction drainage as an alternative to prophylactic antibiotics for hysterectomy. Obstet Gynecol 45:305, 1975

Sweet RL, Ledger WJ: Cephoxitin: Single agent treatment of mixed aerobic–anaerobic pelvic infections. Obstet Gynecol 54:193 1979

Sweet RL, Mills J, Hadley MK et al: Use of laparoscopy to determine the microbiologic etiology of acute salpingitis. Am J Obstet Gynecol 134:69, 1979

Weinstein WM, Onderdonk AB, Bartlett JG: Antimicrobial therapy of experimental sepsis. J Infect Dis 132:282, 1975

Weinstein WM, Onderdonk AB, Bartlett JG et al: Experimental intra-abdominal abscesses in rats: Development of an experimental model. Infect Immun 10:1250, 1974

Westrom L: Effects of acute pelvic inflammatory disease on fertility. Am J Obstet Gynecol 121:707, 1975

Westrom L, Bengtsson LP, Mardh PA: The risk of pelvic inflammatory disease in women using intra-uterine contraception devices as compared to non-users. Lancet 2:221, 1976

Wong R, Gee CL, Ledger WJ: Prophylactic use of cefazolin in monitored obstetric patients undergoing cesarean section. Obstet Gynecol 51:407, 1978

CONTROL OF HUMAN REPRODUCTION: CONTRACEPTION, STERILIZATION, AND INDUCED ABORTION

Daniel R. Mishell, Jr.

The term *family planning* implies that the birth of each child is planned and desired by the parents. To prevent unplanned or unwanted children, a couple can use *contraception* (the temporary avoidance of pregnancy), *sterilization* (the permanent prevention of pregnancy), or *induced abortion* (voluntary evacuation of the fetus from the uterus before it has attained viability).

CONTRACEPTION

An ideal method of contraception has not yet been developed. All existing contraceptive techniques have advantages and disadvantages. Therefore, the physi-

cian's advice about contraception should include an explanation of the advantages and disadvantages of each method so that the patient is fully informed and can rationally choose the method most suitable for her. If there are medical reasons for not using certain methods, the physician should inform the patient and offer her alternatives.

Except for the condom, no acceptable method has been developed for use by the male. A great deal of research effort is currently being expended to develop one or more methods of contraception for the male, but there are several problems that will be difficult to overcome. These include 1) difficulty in separating suppression of the major testicular functions, spermatogenesis and androgen production; 2) the long lag period from initiation of treatment until the elimination of sperm from the ejaculate, usually about 3 months; 3) the problems of reversibility, including a variable delay in the time required for restoration of fertility as well as the possibility that abnormal sperm may be produced initially; and 4) the lack of motivation of most men to use a contraceptive, as the male is not the member of the couple who becomes pregnant. For these reasons, even if a male contraceptive such as a combination progestin–androgen agent is developed, its use will be limited.

In order of popularity the methods of contraception most widely used by married couples in the United States are as follows: oral steroids (∿30%), condom (∿10%), intrauterine device (IUD) (∿8%), diaphragm (∿4%), foam (∿4%), and rhythm (∿3%; Table 14–1). Between 1975 and 1979 retail pharmacy purchases of oral contraceptives in the U.S. have declined about 40%. This decline in use of oral contraceptives is partially due to both an increase in voluntary sterilization, mainly by couples of older reproductive age, and also concern by women about the serious, but infrequent, side effects of oral contraceptives.

The use of sterilization has increased about fourfold during the past decade, with men and women being sterilized in approximately equal numbers. In 1975, the percentage of couples sterilized to prevent pregnancy was similar to the percentage of those using oral contraceptives. The percentage of couples using each method varied according to the duration of marriage and whether or not the couple intended to have more children. Use of oral contraceptives was greatest in the first 5 years of marriage and declined steadily thereafter, while use of IUDs was greatest in the second 5 years of marriage. Both male and female sterilization steadily increased with increasing duration of marriage. Either the husband or wife had been sterilized in about half the couples who had completed their families. About 15%–20% of couples use barrier methods (condom, diaphragm, and foam) irrespective of the duration of marriage.

TABLE 14-1. METHODS USED TO PREVENT CONCEPTION BY WHITE MARRIED WOMEN IN THE UNITED STATES (PERCENTAGE OF WOMEN USING CONTRACEPTION)

Method	1965	1970	1975
ORAL STEROIDS	28.4	35.4	34.3
CONDOM	22.0	14.8	10.9
IUD	1.1	7.5	8.7
DIAPHRAGM	10.5	5.7	3.9
FOAM	3.1	6.6	3.6
RHYTHM	11.5	7.1	2.8
WITHDRAWAL	4.0	2.3	2.0
OTHER	10.5	6.6	2.6
WIFE STERILIZED	4.7	6.8	16.3
HUSBAND STERILIZED	4.1	7.2	15.0

(Adapted from Westoff CF, Jones EF: Fam Plann Perspect 9:153–157, 1977)

CONTRACEPTIVE EFFECTIVENESS

It is difficult to determine the actual effectiveness of various methods of contraception because of a large number of factors that affect contraceptive failure. The terms *method effectiveness* and *use effectiveness* (or *method failure* and *patient failure*) have been used to differentiate between conception occurring with correct use of the method and that occurring with incorrect use. In general, methods used at the time of coitus, such as the diaphragm, condom, foam, rhythm, and withdrawal, have a much greater method effectiveness than use effectiveness; *i.e.*, many more pregnancies occur because the couple failed to use the method than would have occurred if the method had been used correctly. With methods in which coitus-related activities are not needed, such as oral contraceptives and IUDs, there is less difference between method and use effectiveness. With less motivation required, their overall effectiveness is greater than that of coitus-related methods.

The overall value of a contraceptive method as used by a couple (correctly or incorrectly) is determined by calculation of actual effectiveness as well as the continuation rate. To determine these rates, actuarial (life table) methods instead of the Pearl Index should be used. Even with the use of these excellent statistical techniques, it is difficult to determine what the effectiveness of the various methods is in actual practice. Most studies undertaken to determine effectiveness of a contraceptive method are performed in carefully controlled clinical trials, during which frequent contact and support by clinic personnel results in lower failure rates and higher continuation rates than occur in actual uncontrolled clinical use.

Several other factors influence failure rates. One of the most important is motivation. The failure rate is higher when a method is used by couples seeking to delay a wanted birth than it is when the same method is used by those seeking to prevent any more births. Age of the woman also has a strong negative correlation with contraceptive failure. The level of education has consistently been found to have a negative correlation with the rate of contraceptive failure for several methods. Thus, many variables must be considered before the effectiveness of any method of contraception can be determined for an individual patient.

VAGINAL FOAMS, CREAMS, AND SUPPOSITORIES

All vaginal foams, creams, and suppositories contain a spermicidal ingredient, usually nonoxynol-9, which immobilizes or kills sperm on contact. They also provide a mechanical barrier to sperm. They must be placed in the vagina 10–15 min prior to each coital act. There are no data comparing the efficiency of the various types of vaginal spermicides, but their effectiveness increases greatly with increasing age of the woman and approaches that of the IUD in the woman over 30. This is probably due to increased motivation. Also, acts of coitus are usually more planned and less frequent in older women than in younger women.

DIAPHRAGM

The diaphragm must be carefully fitted, and the largest size that causes no discomfort or undue pressure on the vaginal mucosa should be used. After the fitting, the patient should remove the diaphragm and reinsert it herself. The physician should then examine the patient to make sure the diaphragm is covering the cervix. When the woman is wearing the diaphragm, she should not be aware of its presence or have any discomfort. The diaphragm should be used with contraceptive cream and should remain in place for at least 8 hours after the last coital act.

In 1974, Vessey and Wiggins reported the experience of 4052 women who had used the diaphragm in a British Family Planning Association study for a total of 5909 woman-years of exposure. All women were over 25 and had used the diaphragm for at least 5 months prior to entering the study. They all had been carefully instructed in its use and were strongly advised to use a spermicide. Life table analysis of the data revealed a use–effectiveness pregnancy rate of only 2.4/100 woman-years. This low rate was partially attributed to the age of these women and their previous experience with the diaphragm. The risk of accidental pregnancy with the diaphragm is greatest in the first few months of use. The failure rate in women who used the diaphragm after entering the study declined with age and

with duration of use. The results of this study indicate that the diaphragm is an effective method of contraception, especially after the first few months of use.

CONDOM

Patients who have multiple sexual partners should be encouraged to use the condom, as it is the method of contraception that is most effective in preventing transmission of venereal disease. The condom should not be applied tightly. The tip should extend beyond the end of the penis by about 1 cm to collect the ejaculate. Care must be taken not to spill the ejaculate upon withdrawal. In the British Family Planning Association study referred to earlier, 2057 couples used the condom, all at some time after entering the study. All had previously used another method, mainly oral contraception. During 1543 woman-years of exposure, 62 unplanned pregnancies occurred, a use–pregnancy rate of 4/100 woman-years. This study is one of the largest to be published, and the results are consistent with those of several older studies that show a similar high level of effectiveness for the condom in couples with enough motivation for the wife to attend a family-planning clinic.

RHYTHM

The Roman Catholic church officially proscribes all methods of contraception except rhythm, or periodic abstinence. The rationale for the rhythm method is based upon three assumptions: 1) the human ovum is capable of being fertilized for only about 24 hours after ovulation; 2) spermatozoa retain their fertilizing ability for only about 48 hours after coitus; and 3) ovulation usually occurs 12–16 days (14±2) days before the onset of the subsequent menses. According to these assumptions, after a woman records the length of her cycles for several months, she can establish her fertile period by subtracting 18 days from the length of her previous shortest cycle and 11 days from the length of her previous longest cycle. In each subsequent cycle, the couple abstains from coitus during this calculated fertile period.

The effectiveness of this calendar method of periodic abstinence is poor. Failure rates are reported to vary between 21/100 woman-years and 47/100 woman-years. The failure rate in one large U.S. study was reported to be 30/100 woman-years. In another study, 21% of American women who used rhythm to prevent an unwanted pregnancy were reported to be unsuccessful. The reasons for this lack of success, as summarized by Mastroianni, are numerous, despite advances in knowedge of human reproductive physiology. First, there is no good evidence that the three assumptions upon which the rhythm method is based have scientific validity. Second, since menstrual cycle length is highly irregular, a woman with previously regular cycles may occasionally have marked variations in cycle length. Cycle irregularity is very common in perimenarchal and perimenopausal women, two times of life when most pregnancies are unwanted. In addition, because a woman is menstruating during several of the nonfertile days and most couples do not have coitus during this time, the period of abstinence is frequently greater than the period in which the couple may have sexual relations.

To increase the effectiveness of the rhythm method, instead of relying solely on the calendar calculations, it is also advisable for the woman to measure her basal body temperature every day. Since progesterone causes an increase in basal temperature, if the couple abstains from intercourse from the start of menses until at least 48 hours after the rise in basal body temperature (2 days after ovulation), sexual relations will take place only after the ovum is no longer capable of being fertilized. Data from several sources indicate that the use of daily basal temperature for determining the days of periodic abstinence increases the effectiveness of the rhythm method. One British study reported a failure rate of only 6.6/100 woman-years among women practicing the temperature method to determine the time of periodic abstinence.

Recent reports suggest that a woman can detect changes in her own cervical mucus. By learning to analyze the quality and quantity of the cervical mucus, the woman can predict the time when ovulation is going to occur. Although reports of extraordinary success have come from some enthusiasts, careful analysis of their results suggests that the actual effectiveness of this modification is substantially less than claimed.

Thus, periodic abstinence (the rhythm method) requires a high degree of motivation, communication, and sophistication. Even for a couple with these qualities, the rhythm method of family planning is associated with a very high failure rate, and this should be understood by all couples who choose it.

ORAL STEROIDS

The steroid contraceptive pill is the most widely used method of pregnancy prevention in the United States. There are two major categories of oral steroid contraceptives: combination and gestagen-only (progestin, progestogen). With the combination contraceptive, the most widely used and the most effective type, tablets that contain both an estrogen and a gestagen are taken daily for 3 weeks. No medication is given for the next 7 days to allow withdrawal bleeding. With the other method, a small dose of gestagen without estro-

FIG. 14-1. Formulas of the five progestins used in combination oral contraceptives in the United States. (Diczfalusy E, Borell U (eds): Nobel Symposium 15: Control of Human Fertility. New York, Wiley, 1971)

NORETHINDRONE   NORETHYNODREL   NORETHINDRONE ACETATE

ETHYNODIOL DIACETATE   NORGESTREL

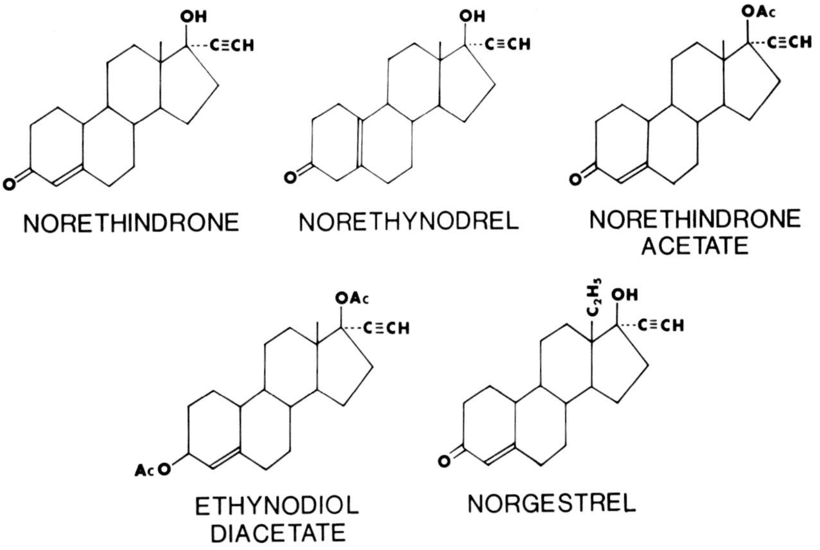

gen is ingested every day, preferably at the same time of day. This method is used by only about 0.2% of oral contraceptive users.

PHARMACOLOGY

Presently used oral contraceptives do not contain natural estrogens or gestagens, but are formulated of synthetic steroids. The two major types of synthetic gestagens are derivatives of 19-nortestosterone and derivatives of 17α-acetoxy progesterone. The latter group of C-21 gestagens, consisting of steroids such as medroxyprogesterone acetate and megestrol acetate, is no longer utilized in present contraceptive formulations because, when these agents were given to female beagle dogs, the animals developed an increased incidence of mammary cancer. The 19-nortestosterone derivatives did not produce this effect. Thus, all of the oral contraceptive formulations marketed in the United States consist of varying doses of one of the following five 19-nortestosterone gestagens: 1) norethindrone, 2) norethynodrel, 3) norethindrone acetate, 4) ethynodiol diacetate, or 5) norgestrel (Fig. 14–1). Except in two daily gestagen-only formulations, the gestagens are combined with varying doses of two estrogens, either ethinyl estradiol or ethinyl estradiol-3-methyl ether (mestranol; Fig. 14–2). Each of these seven compounds has an ethinyl group at the 17 position.

The presence of the ethinyl group enhances the activity of the synthetic agents when taken orally, since the essential functional groups of the agents are less rapidly hydroxylated and then conjugated as they pass through the portal system than are those of the natu-

FIG. 14-2. Formulas of the two estrogens used in combination oral contraceptives in the United States. (Diczfalusy E, Borell U (eds): Nobel Symposium 15: Control of Human Fertility. New York, Wiley, 1971)

Mestranol   Ethinyl Estradiol

rally occurring steroids. When ingested, the synthetic steroids thus have greater potency per unit weight than natural steroids.

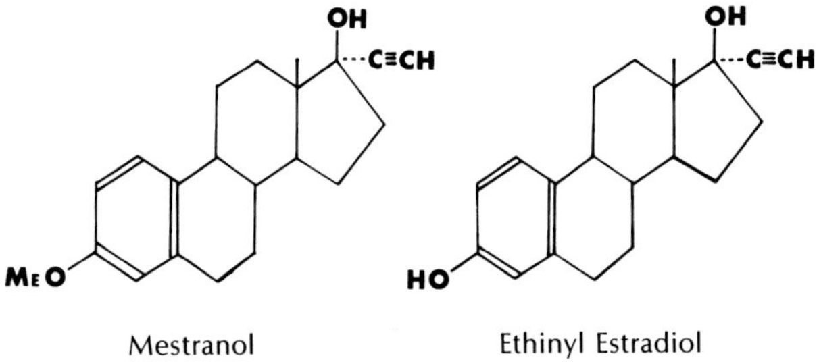

The various modifications in chemical structure of the synthetic gestagens and estrogens alter their biologic activity. For these reasons, the pharmacologic activity of the gestagen or estrogen in a particular contraceptive steroid cannot be predicted solely on the basis of the amount present in the formulation. The biologic activity of the various steroids must also be considered. With the endometrial response as a reference point, it has been shown that norethindrone and norethynodrel are approximately equal in activity, while norethindrone acetate is twice as active. Ethynodiol diacetate is about 15 times as potent and norgestrel is about 30 times as potent as an equivalent weight of norethindrone.

The two estrogens present in oral contraceptives,

ethinyl estradiol and mestranol, also have different biologic activity in the human. To become biologically effective, mestranol must be demethylated to ethinyl estradiol, as mestranol does not bind with cytosol estrogen receptors. The degree of conversion of mestranol to ethinyl estradiol varies among patients; some are able to convert all of it, while others can convert only half of it. Thus, in some patients a given amount of mestranol is as potent as the same amount of ethinyl estradiol, while in others it is only about half as potent. On the basis of the human endometrial response and the effect on liver corticosteroid-binding globulin (CBG) production, it has been estimated that ethinyl estradiol is about 1.7 times as potent as an equivalent amount of mestranol. When deciding which contraceptive steroid to prescribe initially, the physician must evaluate both the quantity and biologic activity of each steroid component in the formulation.

MECHANISM OF ACTION

The combination preparations are the most effective oral contraceptives because they consistently inhibit the midcycle gonadotropin surge and thus prevent ovulation. In addition, they act on other steps in the reproductive process. They alter the cervical mucus, making it consistently thick, viscid, and scanty, and thus retard sperm penetration. They alter the endometrium so that glandular production of glycogen is diminished and less energy is available for the blastocyst to survive in the uterine cavity. Finally, they alter ovarian responsiveness to gonadotropin stimulation. Nev-

ertheless, neither gonadotropin production nor ovarian steroidogenesis is completely abolished, and levels of those endogenous hormones in the peripheral blood during ingestion of combination oral contraceptives are similar to those found in the early follicular phase of the normal cycle (Fig. 14–3).

Contraceptive steroids prevent ovulation mainly by interfering with the release of gonadotropin-releasing hormone (GnRH) from the hypothalamus. Studies in rats, as well as a few studies in humans, show that the inhibitory action of the contraceptive steroids can be overcome by the administration of GnRH. However, in other studies, it has been found that the release of luteinizing hormone (LH) and follicle-stimulating hormone (FSH) is suppressed following GnRH infusion in most women who have been ingesting combination contraceptive steroids, indicating that the steroids have a direct inhibitory effect on the pituitary as well as on the hypothalamus. It is possible that, when the hypothalamus has been inhibited for a prolonged time, the mechanism for synthesis and release of gonadotropins becomes refractory to the normal amount of GnRH stimulation. In a few oral contraceptive users studied after serial daily administration of GnRH, there was still a refractory response to GnRH infusion. It is thus probable that the combination contraceptive steroids do have a direct inhibitory effect on the gonadotropin-producing cells of the pituitary, in addition to their effect on the hypothalamus. This direct pituitary effect occurs in about 80% of women ingesting combination steroids. This is not related to the age of the patient or the duration of steroid use, but depends on the potency of the preparations; it is more frequent with

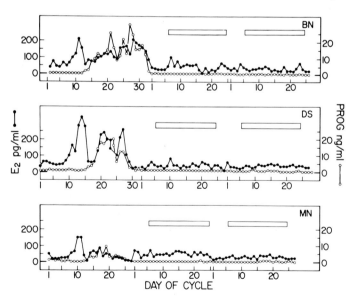

FIG. 14–3. Daily serum estradiol and progesterone levels in the three subjects. (Mishell DR Jr, et al.: Am J Obstet Gynecol 114:923, 1974)

formulations that contain 50μg estrogen or more, as well as the more potent gestagens. It is not known whether or not the degree of pituitary suppression is related to the syndrome of postpill amenorrhea.

The daily use of gestagen preparations does not consistently inhibit ovulation; these agents exert their contraceptive action via other mechanisms. Because of the inconsistent ovulation inhibition, the effectiveness of these formulations is significantly less than that of the combined type.

The combined type of oral contraceptive is the most effective type of contraception currently available. Although there has been no significant difference in clinical effectiveness demonstrated among the various combination formulations marketed in the United States (Table 14–2) the formulations containing only 20μg ethinyl estradiol may be slightly less effective. Provided no tablets are omitted, the pregnancy rate is less than 0.2/100 women at the end of 1 year, no matter which formulation is used.

EFFECTS OTHER THAN CONTRACEPTION

In addition to their effects on the female genital tract, both the estrogen and progestin components of the oral contraceptive pills have a wide range of activities that affect nearly every organ system of the body. More than 52 metabolic alterations have been reported in users of oral contraceptives. As a result of these metabolic changes, patients frequently experience undesirable symptoms when taking these medications.

Although unwanted symptoms associated with oral contraceptive agents are fairly common, serious complications associated with their use are relatively rare. Because of the rarity of these effects, it is difficult to establish a definite causal relationship to steroid ingestion. In most instances, a relationship has been inferred on the basis of a series of case reports followed by a retrospective case comparison or case control study. These studies compare drug (oral contraceptive) use in patients having a certain disease (cases) with a group of controls carefully matched for other variables, such as age, parity, and socioeconomic class. The results show the relative risk of developing the disease between drug users and nonusers. They do not provide information on incidence. Although the validity of the case comparison studies has been questioned by some epidemiologists, nearly all their results have been confirmed by three large ongoing prospective cohort studies. The largest of these, the Royal College of General practitioners study, as well as the Oxford Family Planning Association study, were initiated in the United Kingdom in 1968. The Kaiser–Permanente Contraceptive Drug study, also called the Walnut Creek study, was initiated in the United States in 1969. From published reports of these studies, as well as from other studies in the literature, the metabolic alterations and clinical changes associated with oral contraceptive use have been evaluated. For convenience these effects are classified into three categories: 1) effects on the primary target organs of the female reproductive system, 2) general metabolic effects, and 3) effects on other organ systems.

Effects on Organs of the Female Reproductive System

There are several studies which indicate that the incidence of functional ovarian cysts is reduced in oral contraceptive users. Their use is unrelated to the risk of developing benign ovarian neoplasms, but two recent studies indicate that the use of oral contraceptives may prevent the development of ovarian cancer.

There have been several recent studies clearly demonstrating that oral contraceptives prevent the development of salpingitis. A recent, well-performed study from Sweden has shown that oral contraceptive users infected with gonorrhea are only one-half as likely to develop laparoscopically confirmed salpingitis as women using no method of contraception. A large prospective study from Britain has shown that oral contraceptives protect individuals from developing salpingitis to about the same extent as does the diaphragm.

Myometrium. Leiomyomas may enlarge with oral contraceptive use, but rarely to the extent that they become symptomatic. Nevertheless, their presence is one of the relative contraindications to the use of contraceptive steroids. If women with leiomyomas do use oral contraceptives, they should be examined at frequent intervals, usually every 3 months. Since the gestagenic component of the oral contraceptive formulation diminishes the synthesis of the myometrial cytosol estrogen receptor protein, the estrogen mitogenic effect on the cells of the leiomyoma is usually slight. However, the newer formulations, which contain lower doses of estrogen, should cause less growth than formulations with more estrogen, and patients with leiomyomas should be treated with formulations that have a low estrogen/gestagen ratio.

Endometrium. Endometrial changes caused by oral contraceptives may result in hypomenorrhea, amenorrhea, or lack of withdrawal bleeding, as well as intermenstrual bleeding. Usually, these symptoms are caused by insufficient estrogen or excessive gestagen and can be ameliorated by increasing the amount of estrogen in relation to the amount of gestagen. The steroids in the pill produce these effects through direct action on the endometrium and not through the hypothalamic–pituitary axis. Thus, lack of withdrawal bleeding during oral contraceptive therapy is not related to postpill amenorrhea.

Amenorrhea in a patient who is taking the pill is only of concern because it must be differentiated from

TABLE 14-2. RELATIVE POTENCY OF ORAL CONTRACEPTIVE STEROIDS CURRENTLY MARKETED IN THE UNITED STATES

Brand Name	Company	Estrogens (µg)		Gestagens (mg)					Potency Ratio† (E/G × 10⁻³)
		Mestranol 1.0	Ethinyl Estradiol 1.7–2.0	Norethindrone 1	Norethynodrel 1.09	Norethindrone Acetate 2	Ethynodiol Diacetate 15	Norgestrel 30	
COMBINATION **STANDARD OR HIGH DOSE**									
Demulen	Searle		50				1.0		6.7
Enovid-E	Searle	100			2.5				36.7
Enovid-5	Searle	75			5.0				13.8
Norinyl 1/50	Syntex	50		1.0					50.0
Norinyl 1/80	Syntex	80		1.0					80.0
Norinyl 2	Syntex	100		2.0					50.0
Norlestrin 1	Parke–Davis		50			1.0			50.0
Norlestrin 2.5	Parke–Davis		50			2.5			20.0
Ovcon 50	Mead/Johnson		50	1.0					50.0
Ovral	Wyeth		50					0.5	6.7
Ovulen	Searle	100					1.0		6.7
Ortho-Novum 1/50	Ortho	50		1.0					50.0
Ortho-Novum 1/80	Ortho	80		1.0					80.0
Ortho-Novum 2	Ortho	100		2.0					50.0
Ortho Novum 10	Ortho	60		10.0					6.0
LOW DOSE									
Brevicon	Syntex		35	0.5					140.0
Loestrin 1/20	Parke–Davis		20			1.0			20.0
Loestrin 1.5/30	Parke–Davis		30			1.5			20.0
Lo-Ovral	Wyeth		30					0.3	6.7
Modicon	Ortho		35	0.5					140.0
Norinyl 1/35	Syntex		35	1.0					70.0
Ortho Novum 1/35	Ortho		35	1.0					70.0
Ovcon 35	Mead/Johnson		35	0.4					175.0
GESTAGEN ONLY									
Micronor	Ortho			0.35					
Nor-Q-D	Syntex			0.35					
Ovrette	Wyeth							0.075	

* Estrogens, based on uterine volume analysis by histometric technique in human females (Delforge JP, Ferin J: Contraception 1:57, 1970); gestagens, based on a delay in menses test in human females. (Greenblatt RB: Med Sci 18:37, 1967).

† A dimensionless number calculated by converting the estrogens to mg and using the relative potency of 2.0 for ethinyl estradiol. This number should be used with caution, since some gestagens are inherently estrogenic (e.g., norethynodrel), while others have antiestrogenic effects (weak: e.g., norethindrone; strong: e.g., norgestrel and norethindrone acetate).

pregnancy. Oral steroids should not be ingested during pregnancy because of a reported increased incidence of fetal malformations. Therefore, if pregnancy has been ruled out, it is best to induce withdrawal bleeding cycles by increasing the estrogenic component or using a less potent gestagen. If a woman experiences gradual decreases in withdrawal bleeding followed by amenorrhea, the endometrium can be built up by adding 20μg estradiol to the previously used formulation for about 3 months. Withdrawal bleeding will usually be reinstated. If a woman who has had regular withdrawal bleeding suddenly has none, the oral contraceptive should be stopped, a barrier method used, and a sensitive pregnancy test performed.

Although the sequential type of oral contraceptive was associated with an increased risk of cancer of the endometrium when compared to the combination type, there is recent evidence that use of the latter is associated with decreased risk of endometrial cancer in comparison with controls.

Oral Contraceptives as a Cause of Cancer of the Uterus. There is no evidence of an increased incidence of carcinoma of the endometrium in oral contraceptive users. As a matter of fact, two recently published epidemiologic studies indicate that women who are using oral contraceptives are one-half as likely to develop cancer of the endometrium as are a control group of women who do not use oral contraceptives. The mistaken belief that oral contraceptives increase the incidence of cancer of the uterus arose because of recent findings indicating that postmenopausal women who were taking estrogen had an increased incidence of cancer of the endometrium when compared to controls. Oral contraceptives contain estrogen but they also contain a progestogen, and the progestogen counteracts the stimulatory effect of the estrogen on the endometrium. In order for estrogen to cause growth of the endometrium it has to react with a receptor protein in the endometrial cell. Progestogens inhibit the development of these estrogen receptors and, thus, when given with an estrogen, prevent the growth-promoting action of the estrogen.

Cervix. Polypoid adenomatous hyperplasia of the endocervical glands has been reported in association with contraceptive steroids. Although somewhat similar in appearance to adenocarcinoma of the endocervix, this change is neither malignant nor premalignant and usually regresses after treatment is stopped. There is no evidence that oral contraceptives cause an increased incidence of epidermoid carcinoma of the cervix or carcinoma in situ. Generally, patients who choose oral contraceptives have a higher incidence of abnormal cervical cytology than women who chose other types of contraception, but the abnormal cytology has not been shown to be causally related to oral contraceptive use. In one report, however, it was suggested that, if dysplasia exists when oral contraception

begins, it may progress more rapidly to carcinoma *in situ* than would occur among nonusers.

Vagina. There are numerous reports of changes in the vaginal flora with an increased incidence of vaginitis, especially moniliasis, in women taking contraceptive steroids. However, one prospective study has shown that contraceptive steroids do not increase the incidence of monilial vaginitis. If recurrent monilial vaginitis develops in oral contraceptive users, a glucose tolerance test should be performed, since the incidence of abnormalities in glucose tolerance tests is increased in oral contraceptive users and recurrent moniliasis occurs more commonly in diabetics.

Breasts. The increased incidence of breast tenderness in women who use oral contraceptives is mainly related to the estrogenic component of the pill. Among puerperal lactating women, the amount of milk produced is diminished by oral contraceptives, and the concentration of both proteins and fats is reduced. Also, the steroids are found in measurable amounts in the milk of lactating women, and their long-term effects on the developing infant are not known. Oral contraceptives are therefore not advised for patients who wish to breast-feed their infants.

Development of inappropriate lactation is an uncommon side effect associated with hormonal contraceptives. Although serum prolactin levels are slightly elevated in oral contraceptive users, the increased amounts of exogenous estrogen suppress the action of prolactin on the target tissue (breast), as occurs during pregnancy. If galactorrhea appears during oral contraceptive therapy, the contraceptive should be stopped and the serum prolactin measured. If galactorrhea persists and the prolactin level continues to be elevated after the steroids are stopped, a diagnostic evaluation should be initiated (see Chap. 46).

In none of the prospective and retrospective studies thus far reported has there been any clear evidence of either an increase or decrease of malignant breast disease in users of oral contraceptives. However, there is evidence from both retrospective studies and the British prospective studies that the incidence of benign breast disease, mainly fibrocystic disease, is reduced in oral contraceptive users and that this reduction is directly related to the amount of gestagen in the formulation.

Hypothalamus. The incidence of amenorrhea lasting more than 6 months after oral contraceptives are discontinued ranges from 0.2%–0.8% in different populations. The incidence is higher in patients who have oligomenorrhea or amenorrhea prior to oral contraceptive therapy than in those with a history of regular menses. About 35%–45% of women who develop amenorrhea after taking oral contraceptives have a prior history of menstrual irregularity. It is not known

whether postpill amenorrhea is caused by continued suppression of the hypothalamic–pituitary axis, whether the periodic withdrawal bleeding produced by oral contraceptives masks amenorrhea that would have occurred if the steroids were not ingested, or whether both mechanisms are operative. Regardless of its cause, the relationship is clear, and the use of any oral contraceptive steroid is contraindicated for women who have a history of oligomenorrhea or amenorrhea. If such women desire regular menses, treatment with a gestagen alone for 5 days each month is usually sufficient to induce menses without suppressing hypothalamic function or masking the development of amenorrhea associated with low estrogen production. If they also desire contraception, it is best to use a method other than hormonal steroids, preferably a barrier method, since among these women ovulation occurs infrequently, if at all, and the chance of conception is small.

General Metabolic Effects

Serum Proteins. As in pregnancy, blood amino acid levels are lowered when oral contraceptives are used; blood protein concentration is also changed, but the changes are of less magnitude. Thus, there are increases in β-globulins and α_2-globulins, blood coagulation factors, and the carrier proteins (cortisol-binding globulin, thyroid-binding globulin, transferrin, and ceruloplasmin). The pre-β-lipoprotein and haptoglobin levels are also increased, while albumin levels are decreased. These changes are due mainly to the fact that the estrogen component of the oral contraceptive has a direct effect on the endoplasmic reticulum of the liver, which alters protein production. For the most part, these changes do not involve a medical hazard, but they do alter the results of some clinical laboratory tests. For example, serum levels of copper and iron are increased, while the results of tests of thyroid function are similar to those found in pregnancy. There is no evidence, however, that the oral steroids alter thyroid function itself. Although there may be a slight increase in the free as well as the bound plasma cortisol levels, the increase in free cortisol is not as great as that which occurs in pregnancy and is within the normal range for nonpregnant women. Thus, it is of little practical significance. In addition to these effects, these protein changes have been shown to be concerned in two significant clinical problems: thromboembolism and hypertension.

Carbohydrate Metabolism. A body of evidence documents alterations in glucose metabolism associated with oral contraceptive use—both impairment of glucose tolerance and increased plasma insulin levels. Whether these changes are related to the estrogen or the gestagen component of the formulation, or to both,

has not been established. There is some indication that different gestagens may have different adverse effects upon glucose tolerance, and that lower dosage formulations do not affect glucose tolerance as much as higher dosage formulations. However, it is probably best not to prescribe oral contraceptives for patients who previously have shown abnormal glucose tolerance, *e.g.,* a woman with prior gestational diabetes; the oral contraceptives are likely to induce the same alterations in glucose metabolism that developed during pregnancy, and if used, glucose tolerance should be monitored. An annual glucose tolerance test is recommended for all women who use this type of contraceptive and are at risk to develop diabetes, *e.g.,* those with a family history of diabetes, high-birth-weight babies, unexplained fetal deaths, and obesity. Other users should have an annual fasting blood glucose determination.

If oral contraception is to be used in insulin-dependent diabetics, it may be necessary to change the dose in subsequent months. It has been suggested that use of oral contraceptives may increase the incidence of myocardial infarction in women with insulin-dependent diabetes and may hasten the progression of other vascular changes. For these reasons it is better for women with diabetes mellitus to use another form of contraception.

Lipid Metabolism. Certain serum lipid levels, mainly triglycerides, are elevated to some extent in most users of oral contraceptives. Some women also have an increase in serum cholesterol concentration, although it is not as great as the increase in triglycerides. The increase in triglycerides appears to be due mainly to the effect of estrogen on the liver, which causes an increased production of low-density lipoproteins. The estrogenic component causes an increase in the beneficial high-density lipoproteins, while most gestagens cause a decrease. Thus, different formulations, depending on their steroid ratio, have varying effects on lipoprotein levels.

Water and Electrolyte Metabolism. The effect of oral contraceptives on salt metabolism is poorly understood, but their use does result in a decrease of sodium excretion accompanied by water retention. Some users develop edema and an associated weight gain of 3–5 lb.

Body Weight. Because the gestagens in current formulations are chemically related to testosterone, they are anabolic. Some women have an increase in body weight beyond 3–5 lb. Metabolic balance studies have shown an increase in nitrogen retention in patients who use oral contraceptives. Thus, if a woman gains more than 10 lb in a year, oral contraceptives should be discontinued or a formulation that contains a less potent gestagen should be utilized.

Tryptophan Metabolism. Tryptophan is normally metabolized by two pathways: a major nicotinic acid–ribonucleotide metabolic pathway in the liver and a minor serotonin metabolic pathway in the brain. The estrogen component of oral contraceptives diverts tryptophan from the minor to the major pathway by increasing liver tryptophan oxygenase activity and lowers serotonin levels in the brain. Certain of these metabolic changes in tryptophan metabolism are also noted in pyridoxine deficiency, and most oral contraceptive users have low levels of pyridoxine. It has been postulated that the pyridoxine deficiency may be responsible for the disturbance of tryptophan metabolism in the serotonin pathway. The resulting lower serotonin levels in the brain are associated with depression and sleep disturbances, and it is thought that this mechanism may explain some of the neuropsychiatric symptoms noted in oral contraceptive users. The British prospective studies confirmed the causal relationship between oral contraceptives and neurotic depression. Symptoms of depression in oral contraceptive users can be alleviated by treatment with high doses of pyridoxine (vitamin B_6), but it is best to discontinue the steroid medications if the patient develops symptoms of depression. High doses of vitamin B_6 result in high transaminase activity, which, by amino acid metabolism, could further reduce the already lowered levels of plasma amino acids found in oral contraceptive users.

Vitamins and Minerals. In addition to pyridoxine, decreases occur in plasma levels of other B vitamins, including B_2, folic acid, and B_{12}, as well as ascorbic acid. Levels of vitamin A are increased in oral contraceptive users. The clinical significance, if any, of these changes is unknown at present, and routine vitamin supplements for oral contraceptive users have not been shown to be beneficial if the diet is adequate. Serum iron and copper levels are increased due to increases in their binding protein, while levels of manganese, calcium, and zinc are decreased.

Effects on Other Organ Systems

Cardiovascular Systems. *Thromboembolism.* Several retrospective studies indicate that the incidence of thromboembolic disease in oral contraceptive users is about four times as high as that in nonusers. The risk of suffering clinically significant venous thromboembolism attributable to the use of oral contraceptives is about 1/10,000 users annually. Mortality from thromboembolic disease associated with the use of hormonal contraceptives is estimated to be about 3/100,000 women/year. Results from these retrospective studies were confirmed by the British prospective studies, but not by the Walnut Creek study. The Royal College study indicated that the development of thromboem-

bolism was related to age, but not to parity, smoking, or duration of oral contraceptive use. The etiology has been attributed to an increase in blood-clotting factors, in the number of platelets, and in platelet adhesiveness, as well as to a decrease in antithrombin-III. However, the actual cause of increased thromboembolism in oral contraceptive users has not been established.

All these changes are produced by the estrogenic component of the formulation, and there is evidence that the increased incidence of thromboembolism is related to the amount of estrogen and that formulations containing more than 50μg estrogen are associated with a higher incidence of thromboembolic phenomena. Therefore, it is best not to prescribe pills with more than 50μg estrogen unless it is absolutely necessary for short intervals to prevent breakthrough bleeding. Recent data suggest that any of the products with less than 50μg of estrogen have a lower incidence of vascular disease including both thromboembolism and myocardial infarction than products with 50μg of the same estrogen. If this is confirmed, it would appear best to use formulations with less than 50 μg of estrogen.

Patients who develop pulmonary emboli while taking oral contraceptives do not necessarily have clinical evidence of deep vein thrombophlebitis of the lower extremities prior to the development of the emboli. Also, there is no evidence that the incidence of thromboembolism is increased in women with varicosities of the lower extremities. Patients who develop chest pain while taking contraceptive steroids should discontinue therapy at once, and diagnostic studies, including a lung scan, should be made. Finally, several reports link use of oral contraceptives prior to surgical procedures to an approximate twofold increase in incidence of postoperative venous thromboembolism. For this reason, oral contraceptives should be discontinued at least 1 month prior to elective surgical procedures.

Hypertension. One of the α_2-globulins, the serum level of which is increased in women taking oral contraceptives, is angiotensinogen, a plasma renin substrate. In women without a normally functioning feedback mechanism, plasma renin and angiotensin levels are also increased; these women therefore develop a significant but reversible hypertension after contraceptive steroid therapy is initiated. Rarely, a marked rise in blood pressure occurs soon after therapy is begun. More commonly, the degree of hypertension is slight and occurs after prolonged use of the oral contraceptive.

The incidence of hypertension during treatment of previously normotensive women with oral contraceptives is relatively low. In the Royal College prospective study, it was estimated that the incidence of hypertension in the 1st year of oral contraceptive use is less than 1%, but a relationship between the duration of

oral contraceptive use and the development of hypertension was demonstrated. Data from this study indicated that about 5% of oral contraceptive users develop hypertension after 5 years of usage, an incidence about 2.6 times greater than that in controls. Since these women cannot be identified in advance, the blood pressure of all patients treated with oral steroids should be monitored regularly. Because a larger proportion of women with preexisting hypertension may have a further increase in blood pressure with oral contraceptive therapy, preexisting hypertension is a contraindication to this kind of contraception. The Walnut Creek study revealed that the hypertension associated with oral contraceptive use disappears after the drugs are stopped. The incidence of hypertension in oral contraceptive users was 4%, compared to an incidence of 1.5% in both nonusers and former users.

Myocardial Infarction. Several studies have suggested that women over 35–40 years of age who use oral contraceptives have an increased incidence of myocardial infarction if certain risk factors are also present. The major factor is heavy cigarette smoking; the others include hypertension, hypercholesterolemia, and possibly diabetes. Women over 35 who have these associated risk factors and use oral contraceptives are about three times as likely to die of a myocardial infarction as women who do not use oral contraceptives. Several epidemiologists who have analyzed the data conclude that women with these risk factors should not use oral contraceptives at any age, especially after age 35. Although the data do not reach statistical significance, there is some evidence that older women without risk factors who use oral contraceptives may also have a slightly greater chance of having a myocardial infarction as nonusers. On the basis of these studies, the Food and Drug Administration (FDA) has advised that the use of oral contraceptives is hazardous in women over age 40 and that other forms of contraception should be recommended.

Mortality Risks. Recent data obtained from both British prospective oral contraceptive studies indicate that the risk of death due to circulatory diseases is also increased in users of oral contraceptives. In the Royal College study, the mortality rate for women with circulatory diseases who had ever used oral contraceptives was 4.2 times that of women in the control group. For nonrheumatic heart disease and hypertension, the death rate was 5.6 times that of the control group; for cerebrovascular diseases, mainly subarachnoid hemorrhage, it was 2.9 times that of the control group. These differences were significant (Table 14–3). Researchers in the Family Planning Association study observed a nonsignificant increase in the incidence of death from cardiovascular diseases among oral contraceptive users. Of the 81 total deaths in this study group, 10 deaths due to cardiovascular disease occurred among the oral contraceptive users and none among the IUD or diaphragm users.

Recent data from the Walnut Creek study, however, did not confirm these findings. There was no significant increase in circulatory disease among oral contraceptive users in this 10-year prospective study. However, there was a trend toward increased risk among older women (>40) who smoked. The Royal College study also showed that the high mortality rate due to cardiovascular causes in women who had used oral contraceptives increased with the patient's age and that most of the deaths occured in women over 35 who smoked. There was not a significantly increased incidence of death from circulatory disease in nonsmoking oral contraceptive users. The risk of death increased markedly in women over 35, and in this older age group only. Furthermore, the increased risk of death from subarachnoid hemorrhage occurred both in current users of oral contraceptives and those who had previously used oral contraceptives but no longer took them; this finding suggests a persistent adverse effect on the cardiovascular system. Since the metabolic changes that occur during oral contraceptive use generally regress within 3 months after the medication is discontinued, the findings of this study indicate that certain circulatory alterations may be present for longer periods or may be irreversible. Except for subarachnoid hemorrhage, there was no increased incidence of death from circulatory disease in women who had stopped using oral contraceptives; hence the

TABLE 14–3. RCGP OC STUDY 1969–1979: MORTALITY RATES/100,000 + (NO. DEATHS)

	Ever-Users	Controls	Ratio
CANCER	30.0 (53)	31.5 (46)	1.0
CIRCULATORY	29.9 (55)	7.2 (10)	4.2*
PREGNANCY	1.0 (2)	0.8 (1)	1.2
ACCIDENTS	18.2 (34)	12.6 (17)	1.5
OTHER	7.8 (12)	11.2 (11)	0.7
TOTAL	87.7 (156)	64.4 (93)	1.4

(Lancet 1:541, 1981)
* p < 0.05

cause is probably thrombolic and not atherosclerotic. Smoking acts synergistically with the oral contraceptives to cause these thrombi.

The extent to which death due to circulatory disease is associated with the use of oral contraceptives in women without predisposing causes (under 35 years of age and nonsmokers) has not been answered by these studies, as there were so few deaths in younger, nonsmoking women. If there is an increased risk, it is probably very small. Furthermore, mortality data from the United States and Great Britain have shown a falling death rate from circulatory disease in the past decade, despite a marked increase in oral contraceptive usage. The decrease in death rate from cardiovascular disease in the United States is equal among men and women, indicating the oral contraceptives probably do not cause a large number of deaths. Thus, the incidence of death due to cardiovascular disease associated with oral contraceptive use is small and is limited for the most part to specific subgroups of women: those who are over 35, those who smoke, and those with predisposing causes. *In light of this information, it is now recommended that women over 35 who smoke should discontinue oral contraceptives in favor of another method and that women under 35 with hypertension, diabetes, and hyperlipidemia not use oral contraceptives.*

Liver. There is an increased incidence of abnormalities in the results of some liver function tests in oral contraceptive users, mainly tests measuring bile excretion. The steroids adversely affect the function of enzymes that aid in the excretion of bile, similar to the changes that occur in pregnancy. Both a collaborative retrospective study in the United States and the prospective British studies indicate that oral contraceptive users have twice the risk of developing cholelithiasis as do controls. However, the actual number of patients who develop this condition is small, estimated as 49–68/100,000 users/year in the two studies.

It has recently been shown that oral contraceptives cause marked alterations in the composition of gallbladder bile, mainly an increase in the concentration of cholesterol. Women who develop idiopathic recurrent jaundice of pregnancy frequently develop jaundice when treated with oral contraceptive steroids, and the use of these steroids is thus contraindicated in such patients. Active liver disease is also a contraindication to hormonal contraceptive therapy, but its use is not restricted in women who have a history of hepatitis but currently have normal liver function. Nevertheless, these patients in particular should have periodic tests of liver function at regular intervals while receiving oral steroids.

A rare complication that has been linked to long-term use of oral contraceptives is the benign liver cell adenoma. The incidence of these tumors, which can cause pain and can result in rupture with intraperi-

toneal bleeding and, rarely, death, is not presently known; but it is probably no more than 1/100,000 users under age 30, annually. The risk is higher in women over 30, and the magnitude of the risk increases both with increased dose of steroids and increased duration of use. These tumors cannot be detected by changes in tests of liver function, but because they can become large, routine annual palpation of the liver should be performed in all women ingesting oral contrceptives. If an adenoma is suspected, its presence can be confirmed by a liver scan. After the steroids are discontinued, most of these tumors regress spontaneously.

Central Nervous System. The tryptophan relationships, with resulting depression and sleep disturbances, were previously mentioned.

There is an increased incidence of nausea and vomiting, migraine headaches, and cerebrovascular accidents in women receiving oral contraceptives. Nausea, which is thought to be due to the estrogen component, is greater in the first few cycles of use. There is an increased incidence of migraine headaches in oral contraceptive users, but there is apparently no relationship between oral contraceptive use and other types of headaches. Women who have migraine headaches before oral contraceptive therapy is initiated may note a change in time of occurrence, *e.g.*, from the premenstrual portion of prior untreated cycles to the medication-free intervals following therapy.

In the Duke University retrospective collaborative study on stroke in young women, it was estimated that the incidence of cerebral thrombosis in women who use oral contraceptives is about nine times greater than that in nonusers, while the risk of developing a cerebral hemorrhage is doubled. The prospective British studies confirmed the increased occurrence of cerebrovascular disease in oral contraceptive users, but a significantly increased risk of thrombotic stroke was not found in the Walnut Creek study. If there is an increased risk of cerebral thrombosis in oral contraceptive users, the incidence is very low, about 1/30,000 users.

Data from the Duke Collaborative Study revealed a strong positive correlation between increased blood pressure and relative risk for developing thrombotic or hemorrhagic stroke in both oral contraceptive users and nonusers. The increased risk in oral contraceptive users, be they normotensive or hypertensive, is relatively constant in comparison with normotensive or hypertensive controls. The authors of this study stated that oral contraceptives should not be used by women with any degree of hypertension. They also found that heavy cigarette smoking in oral contraceptive users and preexisting migraine headaches may also increase the likelihood of stroke. Therefore, oral contraception should be discontinued in women who develop an increased incidence of severe or migraine headaches, or

any peripheral neurologic changes, while taking oral steroids, since these symptoms may be prodromes of cerebrovascular accidents.

Oral contraceptives do not increase the incidence of epileptic seizures in women with preexisting epilepsy. Therefore, the presence of epilepsy is not a contraindication to the use of oral contraceptives.

Skin. Melasma, similar to that which develops in pregnancy, occurs in some patients who use oral contraceptives. This change is accentuated by exposure to sunlight and takes a long time to disappear after the patient stops taking the medication. There is no specific treatment for this cosmetic problem. The gestagen component of the contraceptive increases sebum production and exacerbates acne, while the estrogen component exerts an ameliorative effect. Therefore, patients with acne or those who develop acne with contraceptive steroid therapy should be given a formulation with a greater estrogen/gestagen ratio.

Genitourinary Tract. The Royal College prospective studies have shown a definite association between oral contraceptive usage and urinary tract infection. The incidence of both pyelitis and cystitis was significantly increased in users as compared to controls. The reason for this is not established, but it may be due partly to increased sexual activity among pill users.

Gastrointestinal Tract. Several case reports indicate possible changes in the gastrointestinal tract related to oral contraceptives, particularly an increased incidence of mesenteric thrombosis and, possibly, ulcerative colitis. A causal relationship between these entities and oral contraceptive use is doubtful, according to the findings of the British studies. Nevertheless, patients who develop these disorders while they are receiving oral contraceptive therapy should discontinue the medication.

Eye. Several adverse ophthalmic effects, including retinal artery thromboembolism, have been reported to occur in oral contraceptive users. Again, no causal relationship can be established, and in two well-controlled studies no significant differences in eye abnormalities were found between groups of women using oral steroids and those not taking the drugs.

Immune Mechanism. The British Royal College study showed a significant increase in the frequency of gastric influenza, hay fever, and recurrent chickenpox in oral contraceptive users. This increased frequency was also found for other viral diseases and may be related to alterations in the immune mechanism brought about by oral steroid use.

Effect on Subsequent Fertility

After oral contraceptive use is discontinued, resumption of fertility is delayed for 2 or 3 months in about 20% of users. In the British study, about 20% of nulliparous women and 10% of parous women who stopped taking the pill in order to become pregnant had not conceived at the end of 1 year. However, 2 years after discontinuing the medication, 85% of nulliparous women and 93% of parous women had conceived. In the Oxford Family Planning study, conception rates were compared between women who stopped taking oral contraceptives and those who stopped using the IUD or diaphragm in order to conceive. There was a delay in resumption of fertility in the oral contraceptive users; 32 and 42 months later in nulliparas and primiparas, respectively, the conception rates were similar, however, indicating that oral contraceptives do not cause permanent infertility.

There is no evidence that oral contraceptive use adversely affects the outcome of subsequent pregnancies. In the British study, the total abortion rate in women who discontinued oral contraceptives in order to conceive was 13%, similar to the normal incidence of spontaneous abortion. No significant difference in congenital abnormalities was found in babies born to women who had been oral contraceptive users when they were compared with a control group. There is some evidence, however, that the ingestion of oral contraceptives during pregnancy may cause masculinization of the external genitalia of female fetuses. Therefore, women should not take oral contraceptives if they are pregnant of if they fail to have withdrawal bleeding and there is a possibility of pregnancy.

Earlier reports suggested that the incidence of chromosomal abnormalities is increased in spontaneous abortions that occur in women who conceived shortly after discontinuing oral contraceptives, but more recent studies have failed to confirm this finding.

Since the return of ovulation is delayed for variable periods of time after oral contraceptives are discontinued, it is difficult to estimate the expected date of delivery if conception takes place before spontaneous menses resume. For this reason, if a woman stops taking oral contraceptives in order to conceive, it is probably best that she use barrier methods for the first month.

CHOICE OF FORMULATION AND INITIATION OF PROGRAM

In some discussions regarding which of the currently available combination preparations to prescribe initially, it has been suggested that preparations with greater amounts of gestagens be given to "estrogen-dominant" women and *vice versa*. There are no factual data to demonstrate that the incidence of side effects is significantly reduced by such a treatment plan. Many

of the common annoying side effects, such as nausea and breast tenderness, as well as the uncommon serious side effects, such as thromboembolism, are related to the dose of estrogen in the formulation. Government regulatory agencies of several countries have reported that preparations containing 50μg estrogen or less are associated with a significantly reduced incidence of thromboembolism. For these reasons, the FDA in 1970 recommended that, in choosing among the oral contraceptives, the physician should consider prescribing a product that contains a lower dose of estrogen if it is otherwise effective and acceptable to the patient. The higher dose products should be reserved for use only when necessary.

Although most of the serious adverse metabolic and clinical alterations are related more to the estrogen than to the gestagen component of the formulation, some, such as alterations in carbohydrate metabolism, may be caused by the gestagen component. The British study demonstrated an apparent correlation between gestagen dose and the incidence of hypertension, although it is believed that a minimum concentration of estrogen must be ingested with the gestagen if hypertension is to occur. This study also showed the incidence of gallbladder disease to be related to gestagen dosage.

For these reasons, when deciding which contraceptive preparation to prescribe initially, the physician should use the formulation with the least potency (considering the potency per unit weight) of both estrogen and gestagen that does not cause breakthrough bleeding or amenorrhea. The potencies shown in Table 14–2, although not precise because of the difficulty of determining metabolic activity of these steroids in the human, do provide a guideline for the clinician.

The formulations that contain gestagens without estrogen obviously have a lower incidence of adverse metabolic effects. Since the factors that predispose to thromboembolism are caused by the estrogen component, the incidence of thromboembolism in women ingesting these compounds is probably not increased. Furthermore, blood pressure is not affected, serum lipids are unchanged, nausea and breast tenderness do not occur, and milk quantity and quality are unchanged. These agents also have serious disadvantages, however. There is a very high frequency of intermenstrual and other abnormal bleeding patterns, including amenorrhea, and the rate of effectiveness is lower, both of which markedly limit their use. The failure rate of these preparations is reported to vary between 2%–8%/year, and many of these pregnancies are ectopic.

One possible candidate for a gestagen-only preparation is the nursing mother who wishes to use an oral contraceptive. Since nursing mothers have reduced fertility and are amenorrheic, the major disadvantages of these preparations are minimized. Furthermore,

since gestagens, unlike the combination pills, do not affect milk quantity or quality, the formulations with gestagens alone may be offered to these women while they are nursing. However, small amounts of these synthetic steroids have been detected in breast milk, and the long-term effects, if any, on the infant are not known. Thus, caution must be used in prescribing any synthetic steroids to nursing mothers. Barrier methods are an acceptable alternative while the woman is nursing.

In deciding which combination drug to prescribe initially, the clinician should choose the one with the lowest effective dose and an acceptable level of side-effects. It is probably best to prescribe initially a formulation with 30 or 35 μg of ethinylestradiol. A recent study from great Britian has indicated that the incidence of total deaths, as well as death due to venous causes alone, was significantly decreased in patients using formulations with 30 μg of ethinylestradiol compared to those with 50 μg of ethinylestradiol and the same amount of progestin. Furthermore, the incidence of ischemic heart disease and stroke was also significantly decreased in women using the lower-dose estrogen formulations. Although mestranol, a component of many 50 μg formulations, is about 1.7 times less potent than ethinylestradiol, there is no evidence that formulations with 50 μg of mestranol are less harmful than those with a lower dose of ethinylestradiol. Very few randomized studies have been performed comparing the different formulations currently marketed in the United States. Unless acne is present, there is no evidence that some patients do better with more estrogenic formulations while other patients do better with formulations that are more gestogenic. Until large-scale comparative studies are performed, the clinician must decide which formulation to use, based upon which ones appear to have the least adverse effects among patients in his individual practice.

Oral contraceptives do produce certain adverse effects, although their incidence has been exaggerated, and in most instances the more common adverse effects are relatively mild. About half are produced by the estrogenic component of the formulation and half by the gestogenic component either alone or in combination with estrogen. The most frequent symptoms produced by the estrogenic component are nausea, breast tenderness, and fluid retention, which usually does not exceed 3–4 lb of body weight. Another is the temporary hypertension produced by the estrogen-induced increase in the production of antiotensinogen, which causes about 5% of oral contraceptive users to develop some degree of hypertension after 5 years of use. When the estrogen is stopped, both angiotensinogen levels and blood pressure return to normal. Still another adverse effect of estrogen is mood changes and depression caused by a diversion of tryptophan metabolism from its minor pathway in the brain to its

major pathway in the liver; the end product of tryptophan metabolism, serotonin, is thus decreased in the central nervous system. The resultant lowering of serotonin can produce depression in some women and sleepiness and mood changes in others. This is an uncommon reversible symptom that disappears when oral contraceptives are stopped. If women develop one or more of these estrogenic symptoms, oral contraceptives should be either discontinued and another method of contraception used, or a different formulation with a lower estrogen/gestogen ratio prescribed. Alternatively, the physician can prescribe a formuation of a gestogen alone to be taken daily; unfortunately the incidence of abnormal bleeding and accidental pregnancy is increased with use of these formulations, since ovulation is frequently not inhibited.

Because the gestogens are structurally related to testosterone, they produce certain adverse anabolic effects, including weight gain, acne, and a symptom perceived by some women as nervousness. If these systoms occur, changing to a more estrogenic formulation may rectify the problem. Some women gain a considerable amount of weight when they take oral contraceptives, a result of the anabolic effects of the gestogenic component. If the woman has substantial weight gain, the physician should consider stopping oral contraception. Although estrogens decrease sebum production, gestogens increase it and can cause acne to develop or worsen. Thus, patients who have acne should be given a formulation with a high estrogen/gestogen ratio.

The final symptom produced by the gestogenic component is failure of withdrawal bleeding. Although this symptom is not medically important since bleeding serves as a signal that the patient is not pregnant, it is desirable to have some amount of periodic withdrawal bleeding during the days when she is not taking the steriods. Adding 30 μg of ethinylestradiol to the present formulation or changing the formulation to one with a higher estrogen/gestogen ratio will build up the endometrium and produce withdrawal bleeding. Finally, the estrogen/gestogen formulation can act together to produce irregular bleeding or chloasma. Breakthrough bleeding, usually produced by not enough estrogen, too much gestogen, or a combination of both, can be alleviated by increasing the amount of estrogen in the formulation or switching to a more estrogenic formulation. The symptom of chloasma (pigmentation of the malar eminences) is accentuated by sunlight and usually takes a long time to disappear after oral contraceptives are stopped. Therefore, when chloasma becomes apparent, it is best to stop oral contraceptives.

Drug Interactions

Although synthetic sex steroids can retard the biotransformation of certain drugs such as phenazone and meperidine by substrate competition, such interference is not clinically important. Oral contraceptives have not been shown to inhibit the action of other drugs. However, certain drugs can interfere clinically with the action of oral contraceptives by causing the liver enzymes to convert the steroids to more polar and less biologically active metabolites. Barbiturates, sulfonamides, cyclophosphamide, and rifampicin have been shown to accelerate the biotransformation of steroids in humans. Several investigators have reported a relatively high incidence of oral contraceptive failure in women ingesting rifampicin, and these two agents should not be given concurrently. The data are less clear concerning oral contraceptive failure in users of other antibiotics, such as penicillin, ampicillin, sulfonamides, and analgesics such as phenytoin and phenobarbitone. A few anecdotal studies have appeared in the literature, but good evidence for a clinical inhibitory effect, such as occurs with rifampicin, is not available for these drugs. Until controlled studies are performed, it seems prudent when both agents are given simultaneously to suggest use of a barrier method in addition to the oral contraceptives because of possible interference in action of the oral contraceptive.

During Adolescence

In deciding whether the pubertal, sexually active girl should utilize oral steroids for contraception, the clinician should be more concerned about compliance than possible physiologic harm. Provided the postmenarcheal girl has demonstrated maturity of the hypothalamic–pituitary–ovarian axis by having at least three regular, presumably ovulatory cycles, it is safe to prescribe oral contraceptives; they cause no harm to her reproductive process. As mentioned earlier, oral contraceptives should not be prescribed to women of any age with oligomenorrhea because of the increased risk of postpill amenorrhea, and oligomenorrhea is more frequent in adolescence than in later life. There is no need for concern about accelerating epiphyseal closure in the postmenarcheal female; endogenous estrogens have already initiated the process a few years prior to menarche, and the contraceptive steroids will not hasten epiphyseal closure.

Following Pregnancy

The relationship between the return of ovulation and bleeding in the woman who has had an abortion is different from that in the woman who has had a term delivery. The first episode of menstrual bleeding in the postabortal woman is usually preceded by ovulation. Following a term delivery, the first episode of bleeding is usually, but not always, anovulatory. Ovulation occurs sooner after an abortion, usually between 2 and 4 weeks, than after a term delivery, when ovulation is usually delayed beyond 6 weeks but may occur 4–5 weeks after delivery.

If abortion occurs at less than 12 weeks' gestation,

oral contraceptives should be started immediately after the abortion to prevent conception following the first ovulation. In patients who have a delivery after 28 weeks' gestation and are not nursing, the combination pills should be initiated 2 weeks after delivery. If the termination of pregnancy occurs between 12 and 28 weeks, contraceptive steroids should be started 3 weeks after delivery. The reason for delay in the latter instances is that the normally increased risk of thromboembolism postpartum may be further enhanced with steroid ingestion. As the first ovulation is delayed for a period of at least 4 weeks, there is no need to expose the patient to this increased risk.

SAFETY, CONTRAINDICATIONS, PATIENT MONITORING

The safety of oral contraceptives must be considered in relation to the potential harmful effects of unwanted pregnancy. The risk of morbidity and death associated with induced abortion or pregnancy in the woman under 40 is greater than that associated with hormonal contraceptive use. When prescribing oral contraceptives, the physician must weigh the benefits against the risks for the individual patient. It is the opinion of the FDA that oral contraceptives are safe inasmuch as their benefits outweight their risks. Nevertheless, there are certain absolute and relative contraindications to their use.

The FDA lists seven *absolute contraindications* to the use of oral contraceptives:

1. Known or suspected estrogen-dependent neoplasia
2. Known or suspected cancer of the breast
3. Thrombophlebitis or thromboembolic disaese
4. A history of thrombophlebitis, thromboembolism, or thrombotic disease
5. Cerebrovascular and coronary artery disease
6. Abnormal uterine bleeding from an unknown cause.
7. Known or suspected pregnancy

Additional contraindications that should be added to this list include congenital hyperlipidemia, hypertension, diabetes mellitus, liver disease, cholestatic jaundice of pregnancy, and (except for patients with polycystic ovarian disease) amenorrhea. *Relative contraindications* include depression, migraine headache, leiomyomata of the uterus, heavy cigarette smoking, and oligomenorrhea. Patients with these conditions who do ingest oral contraceptives should be seen at least every 3 months.

All patients who use these potent pharmaceutic agents should be seen by a physician and examined regularly, at least 3 months after therapy is begun and annually thereafter. Before therapy is initiated, as well as during these checkups, a pelvic examination should be performed and the patient's blood pressure and weight should be recorded. A breast examination and palpation of the right upper quadrant of the abdomen should also be performed. In women less than 35 years of age, 2-hour postprandial blood glucose should be obtained if there is a family history of diabetes mellitus or prior unexplained stillbirth. Liver function tests should be performed in women with a past history of liver disease. If either of the patient's parents suffered a myocardial infarction before the age of 65, a lipid profile should be obtained. In all women over 35 who use oral contraception, 2-hour postprandial blood glucose and lipid profile should be measured annually. If any of these tests is abnormal, another method of contraception should be used. If these examinations are performed in all women who use contraceptive steroids, some of the serious uncommon side effects can be avoided.

There are no documented benefits to be derived from intermittently stopping therapy, and there is a risk of unwanted pregnancy. In the Royal College study, women who discontinued steroids while requiring contraception had a pregnancy rate of 20/100 woman-years.

The analysis of earlier data by Tietze and associates indicated that, while the risk of mortality with use of oral contraceptives increases with age, the risk of death with IUDs declines and the risk of death with tubal sterilization remains low. Because of the increasing risk of death in older women who use oral contraceptives, as well as the increased incidence of systemic disease among older women, oral contraceptives should be used mainly by young, healthy women for the purpose of family spacing. When childbearing is completed, alternative forms of contraception, mainly the IUD or a barrier method, may be adjusted, or sterilization performed for either member of the couple. Use–failure rates of both the IUD and barrier methods are only slightly higher than that of oral contraceptives in the older age groups. Sterilization is now the most frequently used method of preventing pregnancy in women who do not intend to have more children. If they have no associated risk factors, women who wish to continue using oral contraceptives after their family is complete may continue to do so with careful monitoring, but their use after the age of 35 should be discouraged in smokers, and after 40 in all women.

INJECTABLE STEROIDS

Four injectable steroid contraceptive formulations have undergone extensive clinical trials. Depomedroxyprogesterone acetate (DMPA), a microcrystalline suspension of the gestagen, administered in a dosage of 150 mg every 3 months, is marketed in many countries but has not been released for use as a contraceptive in the United States. Studies have also been undertaken with 300 mg DMPA administered every 6

months: norethindrone enanthate (NET-EN), 200 mg every 12 weeks; combinations of dihydroxyprogesterone acetofenide and estradiol enanthate; and medroxyprogesterone acetate (MPA) and estradiol cypionate, administered monthly. NET-EN is formulated in an oily suspension, and its duration of action is shorter than that of DMPA. It is marketed as a contraceptive in some European countries.

EFFECTIVENESS

DMPA is given by deep gluteal intramuscular injection without manual massage in a dosage of 150 mg every 3 months. This drug has been evaluated in more than 14,000 women for more than 150,000 woman-months of experience, and it has been shown to provide a very effective method of contraception. Pregnancy rates from individual clinics with substantial numbers of patients vary from 0.0–0.5/100 woman-years. As the contraceptive action of 150 mg DMPA usually lasts longer than 3 months, patients who delay receiving their next scheduled injection for a few weeks are still protected against accidental pregnancy. This enhances the effectiveness of the preparation.

NET-EN in a dosage of 200 mg every 12 weeks is slightly less effective than DMPA. In a randomized trial of the two agents conducted by the World Health Organization (WHO), the pregnancy rate with DMPA was 0.7/100 woman-years, significantly less than that of NET-EN, which was 3.6/100 woman-years (Table 14–4). Because most pregnancies occurred in the last 4 weeks of the first injection interval, NET-EN is now being administered every 2 months for the first 6 months and every 3 months thereafter.

MECHANISM OF ACTION

The large dose of gestagen alone is very effective because of the multiple mechanisms of action, similar to those of the combination oral steroids. They inhibit secretion of gonadotropins, including the midcycle release of LH, and thus prevent ovulation. DMPA and the combination oral steroids are the only steroid contraceptive formulations developed to date that consistently inhibit ovulation, a quality that appears to be essential for complete effectiveness of steroid contraceptives. Estradiol levels measured daily during treatment with DMPA show only slight fluctuation and usually approximate those found in the early follicular phase of the normal menstrual cycle, which are significantly higher than the levels in postmenopausal women. Uterine size was smaller in patients who had received the drug for long periods of time, but there were no other signs or symptoms of deestrogenization. There was no subjective decrease in breast size, and the vagina remained moist and well rugated.

The delay in resumption of ovulation after DMPA administration is due to the slow release from the injection site and prolonged presence of effective MPA levels in the serum. In clinical studies, resumption of ovulation and fertility occurs in the majority of women within 1 year after treatment is discontinued. Because of the unpredictable length of this delay in resumption of ovulation in the individual patient, this method of contraception is usually restricted to women whose childbearing is completed.

METABOLIC EFFECTS

In contrast to the metabolic effects noted with the combination estrogen–gestagen oral contraceptives, no changes in liver function, lipid metabolism, or blood pressure have been noted during DMPA treatment. There is some evidence, however, that DMPA at a dosage of 150 mg every 3 months, but not NET-EN, may cause some deterioration of glucose tolerance and an increase in plasma insulin levels. Also, there is some evidence that DMPA has a glucocorticoid effect at this dose. Nearly all clinical studies with DMPA indicate that an increase in body weight occurs during therapy, according to the duration of use. In the WHO comparative study, the average weight gain after 1 year of DMPA was 2 kg; with NET-EN, it was 1.5 kg.

Beagle dogs treated with high doses of DMPA have an increased incidence of mammary cancer. Similar tumors in dogs have also been noted following administration of high doses of other related C-21 gestagens, but not with the 19-nortestosterone gestagens such as NET-EN. Studies with DMPA in the monkey, as well as in humans, have to date shown no increased incidence of mammary carcinoma, although adequate long-term epidemiologic studies in the human have not been undertaken. The relevance of the carcinogenic effect of DMPA in the beagle to the development of breast cancer in humans is not known. Because of these findings, the FDA has not approved the use of DMPA as a contraceptive, despite its availability in the United States for treatment of other disorders. NET-EN is not available for any use in the United States.

BLEEDING PATTERN

Patients who receive DMPA and those who receive NET-EN have complete disruption of the normal menstrual cycle and a totally irregular bleeding pattern. During the 3 months after the first injection of DMPA, most patients bleed from 8–30 days of each 30-day time period. Thereafter, the incidence of amenorrhea gradually increases in direct proportion to the amount of time the patient has received the drug, while the incidence of increased bleeding steadily diminishes (Fig. 14–4). In the WHO comparative study, bleeding with

TABLE 14-4. WORLD HEALTH ORGANIZATION RANDOMIZED STUDY OF USE OF DMPA AND NET-EN IN 10 CENTERS (12 MONTHS TERMINATION RATES PER 100 WOMEN)

	DMPA (150 mg Every 12 Weeks) Number of Patients = 846	NET-EN (200 mg Every 12 Weeks) Number of Patients = 832
PREGNANCY RATE	0.7	3.6
DISCONTINUATION (MEDICAL)	23.4	16.9
Bleeding	9.3	10.3
Amenorrhea	11.5	1.8
DISCONTINUATION (NONMEDICAL)	7.7	9.5

World Health Organization Expanded Programme of Research Development and Research Training in Human Reproduction: Task Force on Long-Acting Systemic Agents for the Regulation of Fertility: Contraception 15:513, 1977)

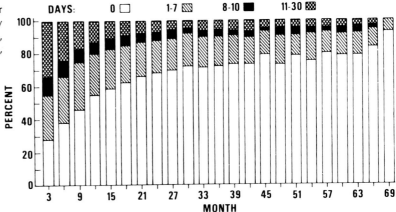

FIG. 14-4. Percent of patients with bleeding or spotting on 0, 1–7, 8–10, 11–30 days per 30-day cycle while receiving injectable DMPA, 150 mg, every 3 months. (Schwallie PC: Fertil Steril 24:335, 1973)

DMPA tended to be somewhat more irregular than that with NET-EN. DMPA was associated with more frequent days of spotting and fewer normal cycles. Nevertheless, the discontinuation rate due to bleeding problems for both drugs was similar, 9.3/100 women for DMPA and 10.3/100 women for NET-EN at 1 year. When bleeding does occur, it is usually not excessive and is frequently characterized as spotting. Periodic bleeding can be regulated by the cyclic administration of oral estrogen, and some have advocated that it be used in conjunction with DMPA for this purpose.

After discontinuing DMPA treatment, about half of the patients resume a regular cyclic menstrual pattern within 6 months; about three-quarters have regular menses within 1 year. When bleeding does resume after the effect of the last injection is dissipated, it is initially regular in about half the patients. In one study, some of the women with irregular bleeding after discontinuation of therapy had to be treated with hormonal steroids for a short duration. Resumption of regular menses may be delayed for more than a year in 20%–25% of women.

INTERCEPTION (POSTCOITAL CONTRACEPTION)

Morris and van Waganen suggested that estrogen in high dose given in the early postovulatory period will prevent implantation. Morris suggests that the term *interception* be used for what is commonly called the "morning-after pill." The estrogen compounds used by various investigators for interception include diethylstilbestrol, 25–50 mg/day; diethylstilbestrol diphosphate, 50 µg/day; ethinyl estradiol, 1–5 mg/day; and conjugated estrogens, 20–25 mg/day. Treatment is continued for 5 days. If treatment is begun within 72 hours after an isolated midcycle act of coitus, its effectiveness is very good. If more than one episode of coitus has occurred or if treatment is initiated later than 72 hours after coitus, the method is much less effective.

In 1973, Morris and van Waganen summarized the literature and found that, in 9000 midcycle exposures treated with estrogen, there was a total of 29 pregnan-

cies, *i.e.*, a pregnancy rate of approximately 0.3%. Only three of the pregnancies appeared to be due to method failure, a Pearl Index of 0.4/100 woman-years. Of the 29 pregnancies, 3 were ectopic, an incidence of approximately 10%.

Side-effects associated with this therapy are, as expected, nausea and vomiting, breast soreness, and menstrual irregularities. Because of the high dose of estrogen and the unpleasant side effects, interception should be used only as an emergency treatment; other methods should be used if the patient has a continuing need for contraception. Some women fail to complete the 5-day course because of the side effects of high-dose estrogen; therefore, a regimen of two tablets ethinyl estradiol 0.05 mg and dl-norgestrel 0.5 mg (Ovral) given twice with an interval of 12 hours has been tested in Canada. Effectivenes is comparable to the high-dose estrogen regimen with a short duration of adverse symptoms. Because of the teratogenic potential of these agents, the woman should agree to termination of pregnancy if interception should fail.

INTRAUTERINE DEVICE

In 1975, the IUD was used by an estimated 6.4% of married women under the age of 45 in the United States, a total of about 1.74 million women. Although the IUD was not as popular as oral contraceptives, from 1965 to 1970 the rate of increase in use of the IUD was more rapid than that of any other contraceptive method. During this time period there was a six-fold increase in use of the IUD, from 1.1% to 7.5% of married women. In 1975, the IUD was used by 8.7% of married women practicing contraception, a slight decrease from the peak of 9.5% in 1973.

The main benefits of IUDs are the paucity of associated systemic metabolic effects and their excellent effectiveness. These two characteristics account for a very high continuation rate. Women using the nonmedicated IUDs must make only a single visit to a health care facility; with medicated devices, visits related to the IUD are necessary only at intervals of several years. Of course, it is desirable for all women to make at least annual visits to a health care facility, but in some areas of the world this is not possible. With an IUD, there is no need for continued motivation to ingest a pill daily or to follow a coitus-related procedure consistently. Thus, for IUDs, the method–effectiveness rates and use–effectiveness rates are similar. Although 1st year failure rates generally range 2%–3%, the annual incidence of accidental pregnancy decreases steadily after the 1st year; after 6 years of use of the loop-type of IUD, the cumulative annual failure rate is less than 1%. With increasing age, the incidence of abnormal bleeding or pain steadily decreases (Table 14-5). Thus, the IUD is especially suited for older parous women who wish to delay or prevent further pregnancies.

MECHANISM OF ACTION

It is generally accepted that the contraceptive action of the IUD is due to a local sterile inflammatory reaction caused by the presence of the foreign body in the uterus. Nearly a 1000% increase in the number of leukocytes present in uterine washings of the human endometrial cavity has been found 18 weeks after insertion of an IUD, compared to washings prior to insertion. Tissue breakdown products of these leukocytes are toxic to all cells, including sperm and the blastocyst. Small IUDs do not produce as great an inflammatory reaction as larger devices and, therefore, have higher pregnancy rates than larger devices of the same design. The addition of copper increases the inflammatory reaction. Whether or not fertilization is usually prevented in women wearing an IUD has not been determined, although the short phase of sperm transport from the cervix to the oviduct is not present in women wearing an IUD. In rabbits, the sterile inflammatory reaction changes the receptivity of the endometrium for nidation of the blastocyst, preventing implantation. The same effect is believed to occur in humans if fertilization does occur. Both copper ions and locally released progesterone probably also act to prevent the normal process of implantation.

Upon removal of the IUD, the inflammatory reaction rapidly disappears. Resumption of fertility following IUD removal is not delayed and occurs at the same rate as resumption of fertility following discontinuation of mechanical methods of contraception, such as the condom or diaphragm. Tietze and Lewit reported that, of a group of 378 women who had had IUDs removed in order to conceive, 59.4% had done so at the end of 3 months and 88.2% at the end of 1 year, rates similar to those found with women who discontinued barrier methods.

TABLE 14-5. TWO-YEAR NET CUMULATIVE EVENT RATES WITH THE LOOP D PER 100 WOMEN

	Age at Insertion			
	15–24	25–29	30–34	35–49
PREGNANCIES	5.8	4.7	2.8	1.5
EXPULSIONS	17.4	9.8	7.1	5.4
REMOVALS FOR BLEEDING/PAIN	18.0	17.7	16.8	16.2
CONTINUATION RATE	58.0	66.7	72.0	75.4
FIRST INSERTIONS	2,753	2,082	1,397	1,187
WOMAN-MONTHS OF USE	41,758	34,574	23,874	19,912

FIG. 14-5. IUDs currently approved for use in the United States. *Top row,* double coil and copper T. *Bottom row,* loop, copper 7, and progesterone-releasing IUD.

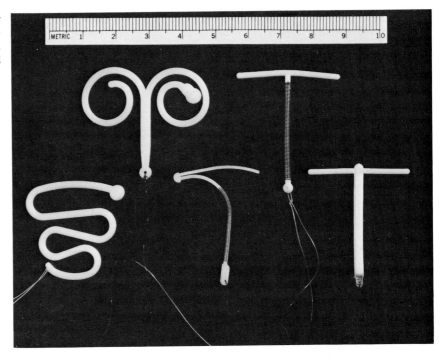

TYPES OF IUDs

In the last 15 years, many models of IUDs have been designed and used clinically; however, at present only five types are available for unrestricted use in the United States (Fig. 14–5). These forms of IUD are the nonmedicated loop and double coil, the medicated copper 7 and copper T 200, and the progesterone-releasing T. Production and distribution of the shield with a multifilament tail has been permanently discontinued. All IUDs now approved for distribution have a monofilament tail.

The T- and 7-shaped plastic devices are smaller than the other types of IUD. When T-shaped devices without copper underwent clinical trials, they were found to have a much higher pregnancy rate than the larger loops and coils. With the addition of copper wire, their effectiveness was increased and is now comparable to that of other IUDs.

Because the copper component dissolves (to the extent of a daily amount less than that ingested in the normal diet) the copper IUDs must be replaced at periodic intervals. The necessary interval was originally estimated to be 2–3 years, but it is now believed to be 4–5 years. The annual pregnancy rates with the copper 7 IUD are reported to remain nearly constant for 4 years after insertion. When the copper is gone, the effectiveness of these small IUDs diminishes greatly.

Adding a reservoir of progesterone to the vertical arm of the T also increases its effectiveness. The presently marketed progesterone IUD releases 65μg pro-

gesterone daily. This amount is sufficient to prevent pregnancy by local action in the endometrial cavity but is not enough to cause a measurable increase in peripheral serum progesterone levels. The currently approved model of the progesterone-releasing IUD needs to be replaced annually, as the reservoir of progesterone is depleted after about 18 months of use.

Because of the small size of these T and 7 devices, there is much less pain during and following their insertion than with the larger devices. Therefore, they are suitable for nulliparous women and provide these women with an effective alternative to the oral contraceptive steroids.

A plastic IUD need not be changed unless the patient develops increased bleeding after the IUD has been in place for more than a year. Calcium salts are deposited on the plastic in time, and the roughness can cause ulceration and bleeding of the endometrium. If increased bleeding develops after a loop or double coil has been in the uterus for a year or more, the old IUD should be removed and a new one inserted.

ADVERSE EFFECTS

In general, in the 1st year of use, IUDs have about a 2% pregnancy rate, a 10% expulsion rate, and a 15% rate of removal for medical reasons—mainly bleeding and pain. The incidence of each of these events, especially expulsion, diminishes steadily in subsequent years.

TABLE 14–6. NET ANNUAL AND CUMULATIVE RATES OF EVENTS AND CLOSURES PER 100 WOMEN USING THE LOOP-D IN 6 YEARS OF USE

| Year | Pregnancy | Expulsions | | Removals | | | | Total Closures | Active |
		Initial	Later	Bleeding and Pain	Medical	Planned Pregnancy	Personal		
FIRST	2.4	2.9	1.9	10.4	2.5	0.6	1.9	22.6	77.4
SECOND	1.5	0.9	0.7	6.3	2.2	1.5	2.1	15.3	65.6
THIRD	1.0	0.5	0.6	6.4	1.3	1.9	1.9	13.6	56.6
FOURTH	1.1	0.3	0.2	5.0	1.2	1.9	2.2	11.9	49.9
FIFTH	0.4	0.1	0.0	2.2	2.1	2.2	1.6	8.6	45.4
SIXTH	0.6	0.0	0.0	2.2	0.3	1.1	2.1	6.3	42.6

(Adapted from Tietze C, Lewit S: Stud Fam Plann 1:55, 1970)

Since the most extensively studied type of IUD is the loop D, more information is available concerning event rates with this device than any other. A large enough population of women have had this device inserted that reliable data for 6 years of use is available (Table 14–6). As reported by Tietze and Lewit, at the end of the 1st year, 22.6% of the women had discontinued use of this device, and the rate of discontinuation declined steadily thereafter. At the end of 6 years, 42.6% of women were still wearing the device. A total of 5.4% of the terminations during 6 years were due to pregnancy, a little less than 1% per year. Thus, although the pregnancy rate in the 1st year is greater with the IUD than with oral contraceptives, within the framework of longer time periods the use–pregnancy rate with the IUD is similar to that of the combination oral contraceptives. Although the incidence of expulsion is about 10% during the 1st year, most of these women have the IUD reinserted. Therefore, at the end of 6 years, only about 7% of women discontinued use of the loop D because they had expelled it one or more times. About one-half of all women who had discontinued use of the loop D after 6 years did so because of bleeding, pain, other medical reasons, or a combination of these factors.

Long-term studies on the use of other IUDs are not available. It appears, however, that there are no significant differences in the rates of adverse events associated with their use (mainly pregnancy and removal for bleeding or pain), with the possible exception of expulsion. This assumption was made after careful evaluation of reports of IUD performance in multiclinic studies, as well as in single clinic studies; this evaluation showed that variations in event rates are as great or greater among different clinics using the same type of IUD as among different types of IUDs used in the same clinic.

The reasons for these marked variations among clinics include differences in 1) patient populations, since both age and parity have been shown to affect IUD performance; 2) physician skill, since the device must be inserted into its correct high fundal position in order to avoid downward displacement, expulsion, and pregnancy: 3) tolerance of side effects by patients, nurses, and physicians; and 4) use of additional methods of contraception, mainly vaginal foam. For these reasons, the only valid way to compare different IUDs is by randomized insertion of the devices in the same clinic by personnel during the same time period and analysis of the effectiveness of the various devices by life table analysis. Published reports claiming superior performance for any IUD cannot be considered valid unless randomized studies are conducted with another type of IUD that has previously undergone extensive clinical testing for comparison. Statistical analysis is necessary to determine the significance of differences in event rates.

RISKS OF IUD USE

Risks associated with IUDs include excessive bleeding, displacement of the device, uterine and cervical perforation, pregnancy-related complications and pelvic infection.

Uterine Bleeding

The amount of blood lost in each menstrual cycle is significantly increased in women wearing an IUD compared with that lost by controls. In a normal cycle, about 35 ml blood is lost. In women wearing a coil or a loop, about 70–80 ml blood is lost; in those wearing a copper T, 50–60 ml is lost per cycle. Liedholm and associates reported at the Third International Conference on Intrauterine Contraception that the mean increase of menstrual blood loss after insertion of a copper T was 26 ml, corresponding to an 84% increase over control cycles. The amount of the increase remained stable 1 month, 6 months, and 1 year after insertion. In these Swedish women, there was no signifi-

cant change in mean hemoglobin concentration, serum iron, and total iron-binding capacity determined 6 and 12 months after IUD insertion as compared to mean values measured prior to insertion. In a study from England, reported at the same conference, Morehead and colleagues found that use of the IUD caused a mean hemoglobin decrease of about 0.5 g/dl in the first 6 months but that the reduction was not sufficient to produce anemia in these healthy, well-nourished women. The IUD rarely causes anemia to develop when there are adequate amounts of iron in the diet. If menorrhagia develops while a patient is using an IUD, her hemoglobin level should be measured; if it is low, the IUD should be removed and iron supplementation given.

Patients may develop more frequent or excessive vaginal bleeding with an IUD, and efforts to control this with ancillary therapeutic formulations have in general been unsatisfactory. Antifibrinolytic agents, particularly tranexamic acid, have ameliorated the bleeding problems, but these potent agents may be associated with adverse systemic effects. Excessive bleeding in the first few months after IUD insertion should be treated expectantly with reassurance and supplemental oral iron, since the bleeding usually diminishes as the uterus adjusts to the presence of the foreign body. Excessive bleeding that continues or develops several months or more after IUD insertion is best treated by removal of the device; if the patient still wishes to use an IUD for contraception, another device may be inserted 1 month later. If the patient originally had a plastic device, the reinsertion should be done with a copper or progesterone-releasing IUD; these types are associated with less blood loss than the larger plastic devices.

Displaced Device (The Missing IUD String)

If the string of a previously inserted IUD cannot be seen within or protruding through the external os of the cervix, the possibilities to be considered are that the device was expelled spontaneously; that the string has receded into the uterine cavity, *e.g.,* because the device has turned; that the woman may be pregnant and the enlarging uterus has caused the string to recede; or that the device has penetrated the uterine wall and lies free in the peritoneal cavity.

If the device is in the uterine cavity, it can usually be felt with a uterine sound. Even if it is not, ultrasound will not only clarify the position of the device but also determine the presence of early pregnancy. The IUD can usually be removed, if necessary, by use of a retrieval hook or grasping instrument. If this fails, hysteroscopy is probably preferable to an attempt to remove the device after dilatation of the cervix under anesthesia, since the latter effort is often unsuccessful, especially if the device is embedded in the uterine wall.

Perforation

Although uncommon, one of the potentially serious complications associated with the IUD is perforation of the uterus. Perforation occurs at insertion and can best be prevented if the physician first determines whether the uterus is anteflexed, in midposition, or retroverted; uses traction with a tenaculum to straighten the axis of the uterine cavity; and then probes the cavity with a uterine sound before IUD insertion. Sometimes only the distal portion of the IUD penetrates the uterine muscle at insertion, and the uterine contractions over the next few months force the device into the peritoneal cavity. IUDs correctly inserted entirely within the endometrial cavity do not wander through the myometrium into the peritoneal cavity.

The incidence of perforation is generally related to the shape of the device and the amount of force used during its insertion. The perforation rate with the loop is about 1/1000 insertions. The perforation rates for the copper 7 and the copper T in large multiclinic studies are in the same range as those for the loop.

Perforation should be suspected if a patient states she cannot feel the appendage but did not notice the device was expelled. The physician should not assume that an unnoticed expulsion has occurred. Frequently, the device has rotated 180° and the appendage is withdrawn into the cavity. In this situation, after a pelvic examination has been performed and the possibility of pregnancy has been excluded, the uterine cavity should be probed. If the device cannot be felt with a uterine sound or biopsy instrument, an x-ray or sonograph should be obtained. With x-rays, it is best to take both anteroposterior and lateral views with contrast media or a uterine sound inside the uterine cavity; the IUD may be located in the cul-de-sac, and the diagnosis may be missed with only an anteroposterior film.

If the IUD is found to be outside the uterus, it should be removed because adhesions and bowel obstruction can result. The copper IUDs have been found to produce especially severe peritoneal reactions; therefore, it is best to remove these devices as soon as possible after the perforation is diagnosed. Unless severe adhesions have developed, most intraabdominal IUDs can be removed by laparoscopy, avoiding the need for laparotomy.

Perforation of the cervix by devices that have a straight vertical arm, such as the T or 7, has also been reported. The incidence of downward perforation of these devices into the cervix has been reported to range from about 1/600 to 1/1000 insertions. When follow-up examinations are performed on patients with these devices, the cervix should be carefully inspected and palpated, as the perforation does not always extend completely through the ectocervical epithelium. Cervical perforation is not a major problem, but devices that have perforated downward should be re-

moved with a uterine packing forceps because their downward displacement reduces contraceptive effectiveness. Posterior cervical perforation can also occur when an IUD is removed. This possibility can be minimized by tenaculum traction to the cervix to straighten its axis before the device is removed.

Pregnancy-Related Complications

Congenital Anomalies. When pregnancy occurs with an IUD in place, implantation occurs away from the device, which therefore remains extraamniotic. Although there is a paucity of published data, to date there is no evidence of an increased incidence of congenital anomalies in infants who developed with IUD *in utero*.

Tatum and associates reported that, of 166 fetuses conceived while an intrauterine copper T IUD was in place who grew to a size that permitted adequate examination of anomalies, only one had a congenital anomaly, a fibroma of the vocal cords. Although these numbers are small, there is no evidence to indicate that the presence of copper in the uterus has a deleterious effect on fetal development.

Spontaneous Abortion. In all series of pregnancies with any type of IUD in situ, the incidence of fetal death was not significantly increased; however, a significant increase in the incidence of spontaneous abortion has been consistently observed. If a patient conceives with an IUD in place and the IUD is not removed, the incidence of spontaneous abortion is about 55%, approximately three times greater than that of patients who conceive without an IUD. If the IUD is spontaneously expelled after conception or if the appendage of the device is visible and the IUD is removed by traction, the incidence of spontaneous abortion is significantly reduced.

Septic Abortion. The risk of septic abortion may be increased if the IUD remains in place. Most of the evidence indicating an increased risk of sepsis is based on data from women who conceived with the now obsolete shield type of IUD in the uterus. This device, which has a filament tail, was widely used throughout the world from 1971–1974. A retrospective study from the Center for Disease Control indicated that the risk of death from spontaneous abortion was 14.8/100,000 women/year with an IUD in place compared with a mortality rate of 0.28/100,000 pregnant women without an IUD, a 52.8-fold increased risk of death with the IUD. Nearly all of these additional deaths were associated with the shield device (Table 14–7).

Although there is evidence that there is an increased risk of septic abortion if a patient conceives with a shield IUD in place, there is no conclusive evidence that a patient who conceives with a device other than the shield in the uterus has an increased risk of

TABLE 14-7. MORTALITY FROM SPONTANEOUS ABORTION STUDY OF THE CENTER FOR DISEASE CONTROL (1972–1974); NUMBER OF PATIENTS

	Number of Patients	Estimated Deaths per 100,000	Relative Risk
NO IUD	33	0.28	
IUD (shields)	13 ⎫	14.80	5.2
IUD (other)	4 ⎭		1.0

(Adapted from Cates W, Jr, et al.: N Engl J Med 295:1155, 1976)

septic abortion. In one series of cases, there was no significant difference in the incidence of septic abortion in women who conceived with an IUD in place compared with the incidence in women who conceived while using other contraceptive methods. When Tatum *et al.* studied 918 women who conceived with a copper T in situ, they found only two cases of septic abortion, both occurring in the first trimester. This evidence does not suggest that there is an increase in sepsis in pregnancy because of the presence of the copper T.

Thus, if a patient conceives with a shield *in utero* and the device cannot be removed without entering the uterine cavity, she should be fully informed about the increased risk of sepsis, the device should be removed, and the pregnancy should be terminated. Although, as noted earlier, there is no conclusive evidence that the incidence of sepsis is increased with other types of IUDs, the patient should be informed of the possibility. If she wishes to continue the pregnancy, she should report symptoms of infection promptly. If intrauterine infection does occur with an IUD in the pregnant uterus, the endometrial cavity should be evacuated after a short interval of appropriate antibiotic treatment, similar to treatment of uterine sepsis without an IUD in place.

Ectopic Pregnancy. The IUD prevents intrauterine pregnancy more effectively than it prevents ectopic pregnancy. It has been estimated that, if the rate of fertilization in the 300,000 women enrolled in the Population Council IUD study had not been changed by use of the IUD, about 180,000 fertilized ova and 900 ectopic pregnancies would be expected during the 45,000 woman-years of use (Table 14–8). Of the ectopic pregnancies, 845 would be tubal and approximately 5 would be ovarian. Actually, during this time there were 1046 pregnancies with the device in situ, 50 of which were ectopic (45 tubal and 5 ovarian). It was concluded that use of the IUD reduces uterine implantation by 99.5%, tubal implantation by about 95%, and ovarian pregnancy not at all. Thus, a pregnancy that occurs with an IUD in place is more likely to be ectopic than a pregnancy that occurs without an

TABLE 14-8. EFFECT OF IUD ON FERTILIZATION RATE AND OCCURRENCE OF ECTOPIC PREGNANCY (NUMBER OF PATIENTS = 300,000; 45,000 WOMAN-YEARS)

	Expected	Observed	Reduction
TOTAL PREGNANCIES	180,000	1,046	99.5
TUBAL PREGNANCIES	900	45	95.0
OVARIAN PREGNANCIES	5	5	0.0

(Adapted from Lehfeldt H, Tietze C, Gorstein F: Am J Obstet Gynecol 108:1005, 1970)

IUD in place. Additional studies have confirmed these findings. If a patient conceives with an IUD in place, her chances of having an ectopic pregnancy range from 3%–9%, an incidence about ten times greater than the reported ectopic pregnancy frequency of 0.3%–0.7% of total births in similar populations. Thus, the possibility of ectopic pregnancy should be considered if a patient conceives with an IUD in place.

Preterm Delivery. In the study of conceptions with a copper T IUD in the uterus, performed by Tatum and associates, the rate of preterm delivery among live births was four times greater when the copper T was left in place than when it was removed. Therefore, if it is not possible to remove the IUD and the patient wishes to continue her pregnancy, she should be warned of the possible increased risk of preterm delivery in addition to the increased risk of spontaneous abortion. She should also be informed about an increased risk of ectopic pregnancy and possible septic abortion; she should be instructed to report the first signs of pelvic pain or fever.

Infection

Despite great concern among gynecologists in the 1960s that use of the IUD would markedly increase the incidence of salpingitis, there was little evidence of such an increase. In 1966, we performed aerobic and anaerobic cultures of endometrial homogenates obtained transfundally after hysterectomy at varying intervals after insertion of a loop. In the first 24 hours following insertion, the normally sterile endometrial cavity was consistently infected with bacteria. Nevertheless, the natural defenses destroyed these bacteria within 24 hours in 80% of cases. In our study, the endometrial cavity, the IUD, and the portion of the thread within the cavity were found to be consistently sterile when transfundal cultures were obtained more than 30 days after insertion.

These findings agree with the incidence of the clinical diagnosis of pelvic inflammatory disease (PID) found in a group of 23,977 mainly parous women analyzed by Tietze and Lewit in 1970. In this group, there were 239 cases of PID in which the device was removed and 437 in which the device remained in situ during and following treatment. When PID rates were computed according to duration of time the IUD was in place, the rates were higher in the first 2 weeks after insertion and then steadily diminished. Rates after the 1st month were on the order of 1–2.5/100 woman-years. The results of both these studies provide evidence that an IUD should not be inserted in a patient who may have been recently infected with a gonococcus, as insertion of the device could transport these pathogens into the upper genital tract. If there is clinical suspicion of a gonococcal endocervicitis, cultures should be obtained, and the insertion of the IUD should be delayed until negative results are obtained.

Following the introduction and widespread use of the shield, particularly among nulliparous women, several studies suggested that use of the IUD increased the relative risk of developing salpingitis or PID. Tatum *et al.* carefully examined the sheaths of the appendage of both new shields in their sterile packages and those removed from patients. He found that 34% of the former and 9% of the latter had breaks in the sheath around the knot attaching it to the device. These breaks would allow bacteria continuous access from the vagina into the endometrial cavity and thus increase the risk of upper genital tract infection. *For this reason, all of the shield-type IUDs currently in place should be removed.*

Faulkner and Ory performed a prospective case controlled study of patients attending an emergency room in Atlanta. They demonstrated a relative risk of 5.1 for IUD-related febrile PID versus non-IUD–related febrile PID. In the prospective British Family Planning cohort study based on inpatient illness, the incidence of salpingitis was about three times greater in IUD users than in diaphragm or oral contraceptive users. In a prospective case controlled study from Sweden, performed by Weström and associates, the diagnosis of salpingitis was made by laparoscopy while the controls were chosen by questionnaire. Analysis of the data by Ory showed that the relative risk for development of salpingitis in IUD users versus non-IUD users was 2.9 for all women, 6.8 for nulliparous women, but only 1.7 for parous women (Table 14–9). A retrospective case controlled study conducted in Seattle by Eschenbach and coworkers, showed the relative risk for PID among IUD users versus non-IUD users to be 4.4 for all women, 2.8 for those having gonococcal PID, and 6.5 for nongonococcal PID. This study also showed an increased risk of PID in nulliparous versus parous IUD users. The increased incidence of salpingitis in nulliparous IUD users is possibly related to the greater number of sexual partners in this group of women.

There are several problems with these studies. One problem is that the guidelines for the diagnosis of salpingitis or PID were not uniform. Salpingitis may be diagnosed in patients with lower abdominal pain who

TABLE 14-9. RELATIVE RISKS OF PID FOR IUD USERS COMPARED TO NON-USERS BY AGE AND PARITY

	Age			Age
Parity	<20	20–25	26+	Standardized*
NULLIPAROUS	7.7	7.5	3.0	6.8 (4.1–11.4)
MULTIPAROUS	1.1	1.8	1.9	1.7 (1.2–2.6)
PARITY STANDARDIZED*	4.0	3.1	2.0	2.9 (2.1–4.0)
	(2.2–7.2)	(2.0–5.0)	(1.1–3.5)	

* Standardized relative risks calculated by the method of Mantel and Haenzsel. Ninety-five percent confidence intervals are shown in parentheses. They were calculated by the method of Miettinen.

(Adapted by Ory HW: J Reprod Med 20:200, 1978, after Weström L et al.: Lancet 2:221, 1976)

have only minimal or no temperature elevation more often if an IUD is in the uterus. A second problem is the likelihood that the use of oral contraceptives or the diaphragm provide some protection against salpingitis. In the British Family Planning study, the incidence of hospitalized cases of PID with these two methods of contraception was similar. The data from the study by Faulkner and Ory indicated that the incidence of both febrile and nonfebrile PID in women using oral contraceptives and barrier methods was about half the incidence in women using no method of contraception. Yet, women using mainly oral contraceptives or barrier methods were compared with IUD users in studying the incidence of PID. Finally, in all of the studies except the one from Sweden, the shield was the method employed by a high percentage of IUD patients, and this device is more likely to have a causal relationship with salpingitis than other devices.

Nevertheless, the results of studies performed by several different investigators in three different countries provide some evidence that there is a cause-and-effect relationship between the use of an IUD and the development of PID in women infected with pathogenic organisms (see Chap. 50), and that the magnitude of increased risk is about threefold. Actual risk must be considered in terms of the incidence rate of PID in a particular population, however. Ory has shown that, if only 1 of every 1000 women develops PID annually, in a particular population, a threefold increased risk in IUD users will result in an overall incidence rate of only 3/1000, which is relatively small (Table 14–10). However, if the underlying rate of PID is 15/1000 women, IUD users would develop PID at the rate of 45/1000 or 4.5% per year. Thus, although the relative risk is the same, the incidence in the latter group is greater because of the greater underlying incidence of the disease.

The populations at high risk for developing PID include those who have had a prior history of PID, nulliparous women under 25 years of age, and women with multiple sexual partners. Until more definitive data are available, it seems prudent to avoid the use of

an IUD in a nulliparous woman. The risk of salpingitis or ectopic pregnancy, which may impair future fertility, must also be taken into account when an IUD is considered for a nulliparous woman.

Symptomatic salpingitis can usually be successfully treated with antibiotics without removing the IUD until the patient becomes asymptomatic. In those patients who have clinical evidence of a tuboovarian abscess or who have a shield in place, the IUD should be removed only after a therapeutic serum level or appropriate parenteral antibiotics has been reached and preferably after a clinical response has been observed. An alternative method of contraception should be used by patients who develop salpingitis with an IUD in place or by those with a past history of salpingitis.

SAFETY

Several long-term studies have indicated that the IUD is not associated with an increased incidence of carcinoma of the cervix or endometrium. Jain estimated that IUD users have a mortality rate of three to five deaths per million women annually, mainly due to infection. However, he demonstrated that, as far as mortality is concerned, the IUD is as safe or safer than other methods of contraception, including sterilization, and safer than no contraception at all at any age. Kahn and Tyler estimated that the IUD causes more morbidity resulting in hospitalization, with a rate of about 5/1000 woman-years of use, than do oral contraceptives, with a rate of about 1/1000 woman-years of use.

The main causes for hospitalization in IUD users, in decreasing order of magnitude, were pelvic infection, complications of pregnancy, uterine perforation, and hemorrhage. Despite the increased morbidity with IUDs, the actual incidence of these problems is low and is probably decreasing now that the shield is no longer distributed and physicians are aware of the potential complications associated with IUDs in pregnancy. The IUD is a particularly useful method of con-

TABLE 14–10. INTERRELATIONSHIP BETWEEN PID INCIDENCE, RELATIVE RISK, AND INCIDENCE OF PID ATTRIBUTABLE TO IUD USE

(1) PID Incidence Rate in Nonusers	(2) Relative Risk of PID in IUD Users	(3) PID Incidence Rate in Users*	(4) PID Incidence Rate Attributable to IUD Use†
1/1000	3	3/1,000	2/1,000
15/1000	3	45/1,000	30/1,000

* Column 1 × column 2.
† Column 3 − column 1.
(Ory HW: J Reprod Med 20:204, 1978)

traception for women who have completed their families and do not wish to undergo sterilization, as well as for older women in whom the risk of taking steroid contraceptives is increased.

STERILIZATION

In 1975, one partner had been sterilized in nearly one-third of all married couples in the United States who were using a method of contraception. Sterilization was the most popular method of preventing pregnancy a) if the wife was over 30, b) if the couple had been married more than 10 years, and c) if the couple desired no further children. In contrast to the other methods of contraception, which are reversible or temporary, sterilization should be considered permanent. Although reanastomosis following vasectomy or tubal ligation is possible, the reconstructive operation is much more difficult than the original sterilizing procedure and the results are uncertain. Pregnancy rates following reanastomosis of either vas or oviduct average only about 50% and depend on the amount of tissue damage associated with the original procedure.

Voluntary sterilization is legal in all 50 states, and the decision to be sterilized should be made solely by the patient in consultation with the physician. Since all sterilization procedures require surgical techniques, patients who request sterilization should be counseled regarding both the risks and the irreversibility of the procedures. It is advisable to inform the patient fully, and the spouse if possible, of the benefits and risks of these voluntary surgical procedures. In addition, it has been useful to have more than one physician decide whether sterilization should be performed if the woman is less than 25 years of age and has fewer than three living children. At least two physicians should concur in the propriety of sterilization before it is performed.

REVERSIBILITY CONSIDERATIONS

The rationale for such careful scrutiny of younger candidates for sterilization is that they tend to change their minds more often, their attitudes may be less fixed, and they face a longer period of reproductive life during which divorce, remarriage, or death among their children can occur. About 1% of sterilized women subsequently request reversal. Based on a 1975 survey, this means that approximately 7000 women request reversal each year.

The most effective, least destructive method of tubal occlusion is the most desirable in younger patients, since ovarian dysfunction and adhesion formation are diminished, while the incidence of successful reversal procedures is increased. The effective clip and band techniques or the modified Pomeroy technique (see Figure 61–30) should be used in patients who are less than 25 years of age. Reversal after this method of sterilization is followed by pregnancy in about 50% of cases, a rate that is higher than that reported following laparoscopic fulguration. Many patients in the latter group are not candidates for any reversal since so little viable tube remains.

MALE STERILIZATION

Sterilization in the male is performed by vasectomy, an outpatient procedure that takes about 20 min and requires only local anesthesia. The vas deferens is isolated and cut. The ends of the vas are closed, either by ligation or by fulguration, and are then replaced in the scrotal sac and the incision closed. Complications of vasectomy include hematoma (in up to 5% of subjects), sperm granulomas (inflammatory responses to sperm leakage), and spontaneous reanastomosis (if this is to occur, it usually does so within a short time after the procedure). Hematoma is best prevented by ligating all small vessels in the scrotal wall. The occurrence of sperm granuloma is minimized by cauterizing or fulgurating the ends of the vas instead of ligating them. After the procedure, the man is not

considered sterile until two sperm-free ejaculates have been produced. Semen analysis should be performed 1 and 2 months after the procedure. It usually requires about 15–20 ejaculations after the operation before the man is sterile. Although in the United States requests for reversal range from 6%–7%, vas reanastomosis is a difficult procedure that requires meticulous surgical technique and has a success rate of only about 30%.

FEMALE STERILIZATION

Sterilization of the female is more complicated, requiring a transperitoneal incision and general anesthesia. Postpartum sterilization is usually performed by making a small infraumbilical incision and performing either a Pomeroy or an Irving type of tubal ligation. These simple and rapid procedures can be performed either in the delivery room immediately after delivery or in the operating room the following day without prolonging the patient's hospital stay. The same operative techniques can be used for female sterilization at times other than the puerperium, but additional techniques are also used for what has been termed "interval sterilization." Ligation of the oviducts in these cases can usually be easily and rapidly performed through a colpotomy incision or through an abdominal incision.

The development of fiberoptic light sources has made laparoscopy a popular gynecologic operative technique. By utilizing various accessories, in addition to the laparoscope, the operator can fulgurate and cut the oviducts without making an intraperitoneal incision other than one or two small punctures. Most gynecologists find the two-puncture technique for laparoscopy sterilization easier to learn and associated with fewer complications than the single-puncture technique. General anesthesia is advised for laparoscopic sterilization, but overnight hospitalization is usually unnecessary. The failure rate following this technique is about 1/1000 procedures. Since the pregnancy rate following fulguration and transection is lower than that following fulguration alone, it is recommended that the oviducts be cut following fulguration. The incidence of complications following laparoscopic fulguration ranges from 1%–6%; major complications (hemorrhage, puncture or cautery of bowel) occur in about 0.6% of cases.

In an attempt to eliminate the problem of bowel injury, bipolar forceps were developed to replace the unipolar apparatus, which has a grounding plate attached to the patient through which the current passes; in the bipolar system, the current passes into one prong of the forceps, through the tissue, and out the other prong, thus producing a limited coagulation with destruction of a small segment of the oviduct. After coagulation, if division is to be performed, scissors are introduced to cut the oviduct. If division is not to be performed, some operators perform a two-burn coagulation on each oviduct to ensure adequate obliteration of the lumen. When the unipolar apparatus is used, a single burn on each oviduct suffices. Local tissue damage following these procedures is extensive. Attempts at reanastomosis have a very low rate of success, and both techniques should be considered irreversible.

Because of the problems of electrocoagulation, efforts have been made to develop safer methods that destroy less tissue. One of these is low thermal coagulation. Nonelectrical tubal occlusion techniques that may be performed through the laparoscope are the tantalum, plastic, and spring-loaded clips, and the Silastic band, or Falope ring. All of these techniques require a modification of the conventional laparoscope, as well as specialized training in their use. The failure rate for the clip and band techniques averages about 2/1000 procedures, with a range of 1–6/1000.

Elective vaginal hysterectomy for sterilization is an accepted procedure in many communities. Although the morbidity, blood loss, and hospital stay are greater after hysterectomy than after tubal ligation, there are long-term benefits, such as the elimination of menstrual disorders, which in some women make hysterectomy the procedure of choice for sterilization.

INDUCED ABORTION

When contraception or sterilization is not used or fails, abortion may now be legally performed in the United States and many other countries. After the first trimester of pregnancy, each state, in promoting its interest in the health of the mother, may regulate the abortion procedure in ways that are reasonably related to maternal health.

Since 1973 the number of legal abortions performed in the United States has steadily increased. In 1977, there were an estimated 1.3 million legal abortions; in the same year, 28% of all pregnancies were terminated by induced abortion, a rate of 26/1000 women between the ages of 15 and 44, and 385 abortions were performed for every 1000 live births. About one-third of the abortions were in women under age 20, another third in women aged 20–24. One-fourth of these abortions were obtained by married women. About 90% of abortions were performed at 12 weeks' gestation or earlier, and nearly half were performed at 8 weeks' gestation or less. About 85% of abortions were performed by suction curettage, 10% by surgical curettage, and 5% by saline infusion. Less than 2% were terminated by prostaglandins.

METHODS OF ABORTION

There are three major methods for termination of pregnancy: 1) instrumental evacuation by the vaginal route, 2) stimulation of uterine contractions, and 3) major surgical procedures.

VAGINAL EVACUATION

Vaginal evacuation by either dilatation and curettage or vacuum aspiration (suction) is mainly limited to abortion in the first trimester. In the first few weeks of gestation, endometrial aspiration, sometimes misnamed "menstrual extraction," can be done with a small flexible plastic cannula without dilatation or anesthesia. Abortions 8 or more weeks after the onset of the last menses require dilatation of the cervix and general or local paracervical anesthesia. Mechanical dilatation of the cervix can be facilitated or avoided entirely by insertion of laminaria tents for several hours before evacuation of the uterus. Use of these tents is particularly helpful in the nulliprous woman, and their routine use allows the majority of first trimester abortions to be performed without anesthesia. Beyond 7 to 9 weeks, it is advisable to evacuate the uterus in the operating suite, but overnight hospitalization is usually not necessary.

Formerly, suction curettage was largely restricted to cases in which gestation was less than 13 weeks. Recent studies have shown that dilatation and evacuation can be performed in the second trimester by means of either graduated dilators or preinsertion of several laminaria, a larger suction cannula, and crushing forceps. At 12–16 weeks' gestation, it is safer, more rapid, and less expensive than the infusion technique or major surgical techniques. Between 16 and 20 weeks, the minor risks are probably similar to those of saline or prostaglandin infusion, but the major risks are probably greater. Disadvantages include the greater technical expertise that is required, the emotional trauma to participating physicians and paramedical personnel, and the possible long-term effects of cervical trauma.

STIMULATION OF UTERINE CONTRACTIONS

Second trimester abortion is usually initiated by the stimulation of uterine contractions. The most commonly used method is the replacement of 100–200 ml amniotic fluid with up to 200 ml 20% saline solution. Labor usually starts within 12–24 hours after the instillation, and evacuation of the uterine contents usually follows 12–24 hours later. The delay can usually be shortened by the concomitant use of oxytocin; however, the addition of oxytocin increases the incidence of complications, especially consumption coagulopathy and cervical rupture that results in cervicovaginal fistula.

Intraamniotic administration of 40 mg prostaglandin $F_{2\alpha}$ is also used to stimulate uterine contractions in the second trimester. This technique has a slightly higher success rate (90%–95%) than saline instillation (85%–90%), and the infusion–abortion time interval is somewhat shorter.

Other solutions that have been injected into the amniotic fluid to induce abortion include urea and hypertonic glucose. The former is frequently used in Great Britain, but the latter is associated with a high incidence of infection and is not recommended.

Transvaginal extraamniotic administration of Rivanol or prostaglandin $F_{2\alpha}$ and placement of a metreurynter into the lower uterine segment are also used to initiate uterine contractions in the second trimester. These procedures are usually recommended for use early in the second trimester, at 12–16 weeks' gestation, as it is easier to avoid the amniotic sac prior to the 16th week (see Figure 29–0). Recently developed analogs of prostaglandins, especially (15S)-15-methyl prostaglandin, are particularly successful when used in this time period. When administered as a single extraamniotic injection in pregnancies of 13–16 weeks, these analogs are nearly 100% successful, and multiple administration intramuscularly in patients from 12–20 weeks' gestation is also nearly completely effective, with a mean injection–abortion time of 12 hours.

Two additional prostaglandins have been approved for abortion. These are vaginal suppositories of prostaglandin E_2 (20 mg), and intramuscular 15 methyl prostaglandin $F_{2\alpha}$. Both are noninvasive techniques with a decreased morbidity, primarily infection, and ease of administration. They should not be used in patients with asthma or those with prior uterine surgery, but otherwise they have a success rate greater than 95% with a rapid abortion time of 8–12 hours. Repeated insertion or injection is necessary for both. Also, both have a high incidence of gastrointestinal side effects, primarily nausea, vomiting, and diarrhea, which can usually be controlled by appropriate premedication. The E_2 suppositories also cause a chilly sensation and temperature elevation.

These new approved methods are particularly suitable for late first and second trimester pregnancy termination. After 18 weeks, it is probably best to use saline, as it is more effective than the prostaglandins; between 12 and 18 weeks, however, intramuscular prostaglandin is probably the method of choice.

Hysterectomy or hysterotomy can be performed in both the first and second trimester. Hysterotomy has a high incidence of morbidity and should be avoided if possible. Despite the increased morbidity of the procedure, however, hysterectomy has the advantage of sterilizing the patient without problems of subsequent menstrual disorders. Abortion hysterectomy has been

performed both abdominally and vaginally in both the first and early second trimester in relatively large numbers of patients with a low incidence of morbidity.

COMPLICATIONS

The possible immediate complications of evacuation of the uterus include perforation of the uterus, hemorrhage, and cervical laceration. Hypertonic saline may cause consumption coagulopathy with severe hemorrhage, as well as adverse central nervous system effects. Complications of prostaglandins include hypertension, tachycardia, bronchoconstriction, nausea, vomiting, and diarrhea, as well as development of slow-healing cervicovaginal fistulas. The possible delayed complications of all therapeutic abortions include retention of a portion of the placenta, which causes bleeding problems; infection; thrombophlebitis; a possible increased incidence of preterm labor in subsequent pregnancies; sensitization of RH-negative women; and a possible increased incidence of sterility, especially in those patients who develop infection and perhaps in others who develop intrauterine synechiae.

Complication rates are three to four times higher for second trimester abortions than for first trimester abortions. By technique, complication rates are lowest for vacuum aspiration, followed in order by dilatation and curettage, hypertonic saline, hysterotomy, and hysterectomy. The complication rate for abortion by saline is two to three times higher than the usual high rates for second trimester abortion by other methods.

In young women, the incidence of both serious complications and death is higher for abortion than for any method of contraception. For this reason, contraception or sterilization should be employed to prevent unwanted pregnancy, and therapeutic abortion should be reserved for failure of these safer techniques.

REFERENCES

Eschenbach D, Harnish J, Holmes K: Pathogenesis of acute pelvic inflammatory disease: Role of contraception and other risk factors. Am J Obstet Gynecol 128:883, 1977

Faulkner W, Ory H: Intrauterine device and acute pelvic inflammatory disease. JAMA 235:1851, 1976

Flesh G, Weiner JM, Corlett RC Jr: The intrauterine contraceptive device and acute salpingitis. A multifactor analysis. Am J Obstet Gynecol 135:402, 1979

Forrest JD, Tietze C, Sullivan E: Abortion in the United States, 1976–1977. Fam Plann Perspect 10:271, 1978

Hefnawi F, Segal SD (eds): Analysis of intrauterine contraception. Proceedings of the Third International Conference on Intrauterine Contraception, Cairo, December 12–14, 1974. New York, American Elsevier, 1975

Jain AK: Safety and effectiveness of intrauterine devices. Contraception 11:243, 1975

Jick H, Dinan B, Rothman KJ: Oral contraceptives and nonfatal myocardial infarction. JAMA 239:1403, 1978

Kahn HS, Tyler CW: IUD-related hospitalizations. JAMA 234:53, 1975

Layde PM, Beral V, Kar CR: Further analyses of mortality in oral contraceptive users. Royal College of General Practitioners' Oral Contraceptive Study. Lancet 1:541, 1981

Mann JI, Inman WHW, Thorogood M: Oral contraceptive use in older women and fatal myocardial infarction. Br Med J 2:445, 1976

Mastroianni L, Jr: Rhythm: Systematized chance-taking. Fam Plann Perspect 6:209, 1974

Meade TW, Greenburg G, Thompson SG: Progesterogens and cardiovascular reactions associated with oral contraceptives and a comparison of the safety of 50- and 30-µg preparations. Br Med J 280:1157, 1980

Millen A, Austin F, Bernstein GS: Analysis of 100 cases of missing IUD strings. Contraception 18:485, 1978

Mishell DR, Jr: Assessing the intrauterine device. Fam Plann Perspect 7:103, 1975

Mishell DR, Jr: The effects of contraceptive steroids on hypothalamic–pituitary function. Am J Obstet Gynecol 128:60, 1977

Mishell DR, Jr, et al.: The intrauterine device: A bacteriologic study of the endometrial cavity. Am J Obstet Gynecol 96:119, 1966

Morris JM, vanWaganen G: Interception: The use of postovulatory estrogens to prevent implantation. Am J Obstet Gynecol 115:101, 1973

Nash HA: Depo-provera: A review. Contraception 12:377, 1975

Nissen ED, Kent DR, Nissen SE: Association of liver tumors with oral contraceptives. Obstet Gynecol 48:49, 1976

Oral Contraceptives and Health: An Interim Report from the Oral Contraceptive Study of the Royal College of General Practitioners. New York, Pitman, 1974

Ory HW: A review of the association between intrauterine devices and acute pelvic inflammatory disease. J Reprod Med 20:200, 1978

Ory HW, Rosenfield A, Landman LC: The pill at 20: An assessment. Fam Plann Perspect 12:278, 1980

Ramcharan S, Pellegrin FA, Ray RM et al: The Walnut Creek contraceptive drug study. J Reprod Med 25 (suppl) 6, 1980

Schwallie PC, Assenzo JR: The effect of depomedroxyprogesterone acetate on pituitary and ovarian function, and the return of fertility following its discontinuation: A review. Contraception 10:181, 1974

Steroid Contraception and the Risk of Neoplasia. Report of a WHO Scientific Group. World Health Organization Technical Report Series, No. 619, 1978

Tatum HJ, Schmidt FH, Phillips D, et al.: The Dalkon shield controversy. JAMA 231:711, 1975

Tatum HJ, Schmidt FH, Jain AK: Management and outcome of pregnancies associated with the copper T intrauterine contraceptive device. Am J Obstet Gynecol 7:869, 1976

Tietze C, Bongaarts J, Schearer B: Mortality associated with the control of fertility. Fam Plann Perspect 8:6, 1976

Vessey MP, Mann JI: Female sex hormones and thrombosis. Br Med Bull 34:157, 1978

Vessey MP, McPherson K, Johnson B: Mortality among women participating in the Oxford Family Planning Association Contraceptive Study. Lancet 2:731, 1977

Vessey M, et al.: A long-term follow-up study of women using different methods of contraception—An interim report. J Biosoc Sci 8:373, 1976

Vessey MP, Wiggins P: Use-effectiveness of the diaphragm in a selected family planning clinic population in the United Kingdom. Contraception 9:15, 1974

Vessey MP, Wright NH, McPherson K et al: Fertility after stopping different methods of contraception. Br Med J 1:265, 1978

Westoff CF, Jones EF: Contraception and sterilization in the United States, 1965–1975. Fam Plann Perspect 9:153, 1977

Traditionally, the obstetrician–gynecologist's concern is with the patient as an individual and with her particular medical problem. Public health agencies, through their function of analyzing routinely collected vital data, have fostered awareness of gynecologic and obstetric problems of population groups identified by certain common racial, ethnic, socioeconomic, geographic, or reproductive characteristics. The health facts of an individual patient are described in terms of single events: a birth, a death, a diagnosis, an abortion, a cure, a 5-year survival. Health facts describing populations are presented as rates, ratios, and percentages. This is necessary because populations differ in numbers. To compare data from one year with those from the next, or from one group with those from another, the number of events in question per unit of population must be determined. For rates, ratios, and percentages to be meaningful, the original data, gathered from year to year or in two areas simultaneously, must be obtained with comparable methods, similar diligence, and identical definitions.

The gathering of health data about the obstetric and gynecologic problems of groups has created an awareness of similar and dissimilar trends of disease, morbidity, and mortality rates among groups studied. This knowledge has had several important, highly practical effects on the community and public health aspects of medicine. It has demonstrated that certain patients, because they are members of characteristic groups, have a greater or lesser probability of a particular obstetric or gynecologic insult. It has also shown that certain diseases are more important than others as causes of morbidity or mortality, and it has provided a basis for accurate prediction of and effective preparation for expected events in future years. Moreover, it has demonstrated that there are adverse environmental factors affecting medical events that cannot be completely neutralized by intensifying medical care.

This knowledge has led to more effective methods of prevention and treatment, to research directed at the more disabling problems, and to more intensified care in areas or groups showing the most need or the poorest results.

The purpose of this chapter is to indicate the kinds of information that can be obtained from the local, state, and federal health agencies and the trends of recent years.

VITAL DATA AND THEIR COLLECTION

Vital records consist of certificates of birth, death, stillbirth, marriage, and divorce. In the United States, legal responsibility for the collection of such data rests with the states. In all states it is the responsibility of the one who attends the birth or death to report this event to the legal authority. Certain additional data are required. Information about age, residence, cause of

THE VITAL STATISTICS OF REPRODUCTION

Joseph F. Thompson

death, and length of gestation are in this category. The reporting of information such as the legitimacy of the pregnancy, the number of living children, and the date of the last delivery is not required in all states. There are other variations. For example, not all states use the same measure for gestation period for registration purposes. In some states gestation is measured in weeks; in some, by weight. In most, however, gestations exceeding 20 weeks' duration or 500 g in weight are reported.

Fortunately most states use the same basic definitions of stillbirth and live birth. These definitions, recommended by the World Health Organization in 1950, are:

Live birth is the complete expulsion or extraction from its mother of a product of conception, irrespective of the duration of pregnancy, which after such separation, breathes or shows any other evidence of life such as beating of the heart, pulsation of the umbilical cord, or definitive movement of vol-

untary muscles, whether or not the umbilical cord has been cut or the placenta is attached; each product of such a birth is considered liveborn.

Fetal death [*stillbirth*] is death prior to the complete expulsion or extraction from its mother of a product of conception, irrespective of the duration of pregnancy; the death is indicated by the fact that after such separation, the fetus does not breathe or show any other evidence of life such as beating of the heart, pulsation of the umbilical cord, or definite movement of voluntary muscles.

After the certificate of registration is completed and signed by the attendant, it is sent to the local health department, either city or county, where certain data are recorded and a copy of the certificate may be retained. The original is then forwarded to the state health department, which in most states has the legal responsibility and authority for collecting and storing the data. In 1902, Congress authorized the Bureau of the Census to begin collection of individual birth and death data from the states. The states had to fulfill certain accuracy and reliability requirements before the federal government would accept their data. All states had met these requirements by 1933. The National Center for Health Statistics of the Public Health Service now has the responsibility for gathering state data on individual births and deaths. It is also a source of a great deal of other health data, which it gathers directly.

REPRODUCTIVE RATES

The *birth rate* is the number of births per 1000 total population for a particular unit of time, usually 1 year. For rates to be comparable, the definitions of "births" (*i.e.,* whether live births only or live births plus stillbirths) must be the same, and there must also be agreement on the minimum period of gestation necessary for the designation of birth in contradistinction to abortion. Accurate birth data covering almost all the states have been available only since 1930, when 46 states were included in the birth registration area. The birth rate during this period has varied from a low of 14.8 in 1976 to a high of 26.6 in 1947 (Fig. 15–1).

The *fertility rate* is the number of births per 1000 women aged 15–44 per year. This is a more accurate index than the birth rate for comparing the reproductive results of two different groups. For example, if the two populations to be compared contained markedly different percentages of women aged 15–44, they might well exhibit marked differences both in birth rate and in actual number of births, but have a similar fertility rate. The fertility rate also makes it possible to compare data on a single population group that over a period of years has experienced a change in the percentage of women of childbearing age. Since 1930, the fertility rate has varied from a low of 65.8 in 1976 to a high of 122.9 in 1957 (Fig. 15–2).

Other rates are frequently used to describe reproductive characteristics of populations. One of these, the *gross reproduction rate,* is essentially a fertility rate for female births only.

The accurate forecast of the approximate number of births in any geographic area 2 or 3 or even 15 or 20 years in advance used to be quite simple when fertility rates were reasonably predictable and basic census trends were stable. The increasing availability and absolute certainty of contraception and abortion and the increasing prevalence of sterilization have caused modern demographers to be cautious indeed in predicting the numbers of births that will occur in the future. Using Marion County, Indiana, as an example, Figure 15–3 illustrates the problems of forecast. On the basis of the 1970 fertility rate (90), 26,000 births would be predicted for the year 1990. However, the fertility rate dropped to 75 in 1973, causing the prediction to be revised downward by more than 3000 deliveries; had the 1973 fertility rate increased to 100, about 30,000 births would have been predicted for 1990. Actually in 1976, there were 11,191 births in a population of 179,860 women aged 15–44. Thus, the fertility rate was 62.2, making further revisions necessary in predicting the future number of births.

OBSTETRIC AND GYNECOLOGIC MORBIDITY RATES

HOSPITAL MORBIDITY RATE

The classic definition of hospital morbidity is the elevation of the body temperature, after the first 24 hours, above 100.4° F on two occasions 24 hours apart in the postoperative or postpartum period. This rate is usually computed as a percentage of the total patients in each of these groups and is used to compare the occurrence of operative or puerperal infection in different institutions or in the same institution over a period of time. With the introduction of antibiotics, the importance and usefulness of this rate has declined. However, the hospital morbidity rate is a figure in which local health departments maintain continuing interest.

PRETERM DELIVERY

Attempts are now being made to introduce for routine use comparable and more accurate methods of identifying physiologic immaturity. The most generally acceptable, easily definable, error-free measure of physiologic immaturity is the weight of the infant at birth. Infants weighing less than 2500 g (5 lb 8 oz) are identified as preterm. The use of such a simple method exclude some physiologically immature infants and includes some physiologically mature infants, but the definition is useful for evaluation of large numbers of babies.

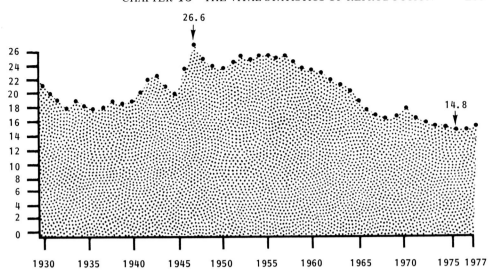

FIG. 15-1. Birth rates (births per 1000 population), United States, 1930–1977. (Vital Statistics of the United States, 1930–1977, Vol 1. US Department of Health, Education, and Welfare)

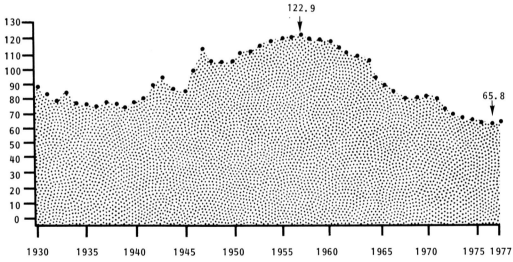

FIG. 15-2. Fertility rates (births per 1000 women ages 15–44 years), United States, 1930–1977. (Vital Statistics of the United States, 1930–1977, Vol 1. US Department of Health, Education, and Welfare)

A refinement was developed by Yerushalmey *et al.* These authors divided all newborns into five groups according to length of gestation and weight (Table 15-1). This classification identifies those infants with differing intrauterine growth rates but comparable periods of gestation. When this is done, differences in prognosis, as shown by relative mortality, become evident. The effect of weight alone (intrauterine growth) on all gestations of similar length can be seen by comparing the relative mortality of Group III with that of Group V and the relative mortality of Group II with that of Group IV. The effect of length of gestation alone can be seen when Group II is compared with Group III and Group IV with Group V. This classification also tends to collect infants with major congenital anomalies in Group III, because they characteristically exhibit intrauterine growth retardation, and to collect infants born to diabetics and isoimmunized infants in Group IV, because they are pathologically excessive in size and weight for the length of their gestation.

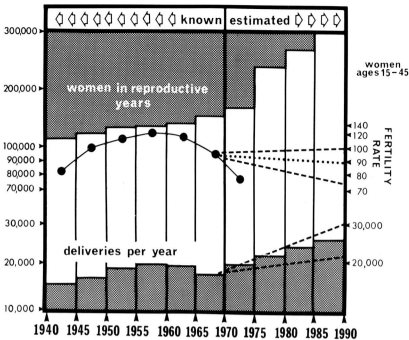

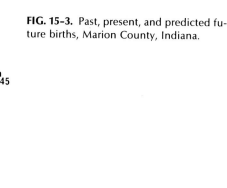

FIG. 15-3. Past, present, and predicted future births, Marion County, Indiana.

TABLE 15-1. RELATION OF BIRTH WEIGHT, LENGTH OF GESTATION, AND MORTALITY

Classification	Birth Weight (g)	Gestation (wk)	Relative Mortality
GROUP I	Less than 1588	All gestations	139.6
GROUP II	1617–2500	Less than 37	19.9
GROUP III	1617–2500	More than 37	6.4
GROUP IV	More than 2524	Less than 37	2.9
GROUP V	More than 2524	More than 37	1.0

(Data from Yerushalmey J. van den Berg BJ, Erhardt CL, Jacobziner H; Am J Dis Child 109:43. Copyright 1965, The American Medical Association)

CONGENITAL ANOMALY RATE

The rate of congenital anomaly is usually computed as a percentage of total births. All states have a reporting system for congenital anomalies, usually in the form of an additional certificate filed in a manner similar to that used for the birth certificate. It is, however, a medical record and not a vital record. These data, while available, are not routinely published. Major inaccuracies in comparability arise because of variations in definitions, methods of classification, diligence in examining the infant, and time period over which examinations are made. Similarly, there is no good means for reliable collection of data on the rates of cerebral palsy, central nervous system damage, or birth trauma.

SOCIAL MORBIDITY RATES

The concept of measuring social morbidity on the basis of vital data is relatively new to obstetricians and gynecologists. Information about the legitimacy of a pregnancy, a social fact, is required on birth certificates by 34 states and the District of Columbia. Other data from the certificate that may be used to indicate social morbidity associated with the birth are maternal age, previous pregnancy loss, date of previous delivery, address, number of prenatal visits, month of first prenatal visit, and educational attainment of the mother. The variable accuracy and completeness of the reporting affect greatly the comparability of specific items. However, such information is important as an index of social morbidity associated with birth and death.

FIG. 15-4. Illegitimacy: possible errors affecting comparability of reporting.

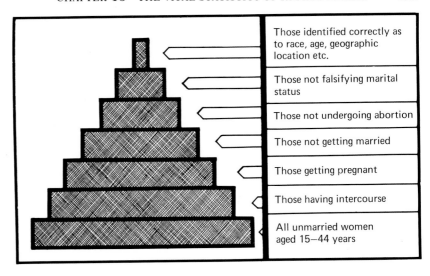

Those identified correctly as to race, age, geographic location etc.

Those not falsifying marital status

Those not undergoing abortion

Those not getting married

Those getting pregnant

Those having intercourse

All unmarried women aged 15–44 years

TABLE 15-2. ILLEGITIMATE BIRTHS, MARION COUNTY, INDIANA, 1961–1977

Year	Total Live Births	Illegitimate Births	Illegitimate Births/1000 Live Births	Percent Unmarried Gravida 1	Percent Unmarried Under 20 yr
1961	17,783	1359	76.4	50.3	50.5
1962	17,359	1366	78.7	50.3	50.1
1963	17,030	1525	89.5	49.1	51.9
1964	16,566	1653	99.8	51.7	55.1
1965	15,249	1618	106.1	53.0	55.8
1966	14,930	1718	118.4	55.1	59.1
1967	14,779	1829	123.7	57.8	60.0
1968	14,184	1909	134.5	61.3	61.9
1969	14,414	2010	139.4	61.5	61.5
1970	15,740	2392	152.0	62.1	64.5
1971	14,555	2429	166.9	60.0	64.0
1972	13,295	2505	188.4	59.3	65.5
1973	12,240	2411	197.9	58.5	63.3
1974	11,937	2428	211.8	58.0	65.5
1975	11,774	2663	226.1	56.8	63.8
1976	11,191	2571	229.7	54.8	62.8
1977	12,050	2960	245.6	53.8	61.3

(Annual Reports, Health and Hospital Corporation of Marion County, Indiana)

Illegitimacy may be measured as a rate (number of births per 1000 unmarried women aged 15–44) or as a ratio (number of illegitimate births per 1000 total live births). It is difficult to draw conclusions from such data because of inaccuracy in collection and reporting. Figure 15–4 illustrates some of the possible errors in reporting that may occur between identification of the population at risk (at the base of the pyramid), the occurrence of what is initially a conception out of wedlock, and the correctly recorded illegitimate birth. Illegitimacy rates, as they are presently gathered, probably more accurately indicate the variable environmental pressures upon geographically, socioeconomically, and racially identified groups than the occurrence of conception among unmarried women.

Table 15–2, showing total births and recorded illegitimate births according to maternal age and parity, gives some idea of the immensity of this problem in urban areas, in this case, Marion County, Indiana. These data also show that a recent trend in Marion County is for women under the age of 20 and pregnant for the first time to account for a decreasing percentage of total illegitimate births. This is a reverse of the previous trend.

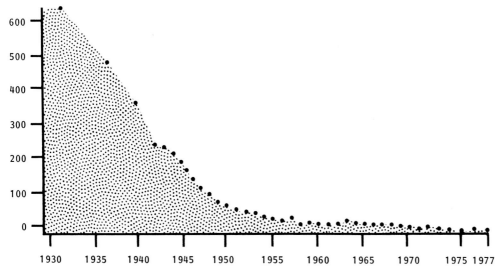

FIG. 15-5. Maternal mortality rates (per 100,000 live births), United States, 1930–1977. (Vital Statistics of the United States, 1930–1977, Vol 2. US Department of Health, Education, and Welfare)

MORTALITY RATES

MATERNAL MORTALITY

Maternal death is usually defined as death during pregnancy or as a result of pregnancy or its complications. Sometimes a distinction is made between *maternal death* and *obstetric death*. The former includes death from any cause during pregnancy; the latter, only death directly related to the pregnancy or its complications. In this context, the death of a pregnant woman from injuries resulting from an automobile accident would be a maternal death; death from hemorrhage following vaginal delivery would be an obstetric death.

The *maternal mortality rate* used to be the number of maternal deaths per 10,000 births. Because the rate nationally is in the range of 1–6, the National Center for Health Statistics now uses a base of 100,000 births to give the number more realistic variation. The rate may be computed with either live births or total births as the denominator and either obstetric deaths or maternal deaths as the numerator. Presently most states have a committee that reviews the facts surrounding maternal deaths. Deficiencies, responsibilities, and preventability in relation to each death are studied. These state committees were first established in the 1930s and have been instrumental in bringing to the attention of the medical community preventable factors associated with maternal death. The maternal mortality rate has gradually decreased over the years

(Fig. 15–5), and in 1977 in the United States there were 9.4 maternal deaths for each 100,000 births.

This decrease has resulted in large measure from the emergence of obstetrics and gynecology as a recognized specialty, the greater use of hospitals for delivery, the recognition and special care of pregnant women at high risk, the availability of antibiotics to combat infection and of blood for transfusions, the use of postpartum recovery units, improvement in the quality of anesthesia, and the intensive study of the preventable causes of maternal death. Recent data from the larger urban areas, when excessive numbers of maternal deaths used to result from infected extralegal abortions, show a considerable decrease in maternal deaths. This decline has been attributed to the availability of safe legal abortions. In 1963, 201 maternal deaths resulted from abortion with sepsis; in 1971, only 99 maternal deaths were associated with abortion in the United States; and in 1977; only 27.

Hemorrhage and preeclampsia–eclampsia are still the most common causes of death among pregnant women. The leading causes of maternal death in the United States in 1974 are listed in Table 15–3.

ABORTION

The termination of pregnancy prior to the 20th week of gestation is in most states termed abortion. *Spontaneous abortion* identifies those pregnancies that terminate as a result of abnormal fetal development or other frequently unidentifiable or unknown uterine, fetal, or maternal conditions. A fetus may or may not be involved or identified; in some cases the pregnancy may have been so abnormal that a fetus did not exist. There are no routinely collected vital data concerning sponta-

TABLE 15-3. CAUSES OF MATERNAL DEATH IN WOMEN OF ALL AGES, UNITED STATES, 1974

Cause	No. of Deaths	Rate
ECTOPIC PREGNANCY	51	1.6
PREECLAMPSIA–ECLAMPSIA	91	2.9
HEMORRHAGE	74	2.3
ABORTION	27	0.9
SEPSIS	30	0.9
MISCELLANEOUS COMPLICATIONS	188	5.9
UNKNOWN	1	0.0
TOTAL	462	14.6

(Vital Statistics of the United States, 1974, Vol 2. US Department of Health, Education, and Welfare)

neous abortions. On the basis of hospital records from the Illinois Department of Health, it appears that about 10% of known pregnancies terminate in hospitals as incomplete or complete abortions. Shapiro *et al.*, in a study of members of a prepayment medical insurance group, found that 11.5% of known pregnancies terminated by the end of the 20th week of gestation. In the United States data are almost nonexistent concerning trends, socioeconomic variation, and geographic differences in abortion ratios.

Pregnancies that terminate prior to the 20th week of gestation when the fetus weighs about 500 g almost never produce a surviving infant. While some infants weighing less than 500 g at birth have survived, this medical curiosity is disregarded for the purposes of routine data collection.

Legal abortion identifies those pregnancies that are terminated legally by physicians or other health professionals using mechanical or pharmacologic means. Some authors have further subdivided legal abortions into therapeutic and elective, the former denoting pregnancies terminated because of complicating medical factors that compromise the life or health of the mother and the latter denoting those terminated upon request of the patient for socioeconomic or other environmental reasons.

The actual *abortion rate* is the number of abortions computed as a percentage of total pregnancies. Since the total number of pregnancies in a geographic area is almost impossible to determine accurately, the *abortion ratio* is used. This is the number of abortions per 1000 live births. The spontaneous abortion ratio is usually given as a percentage of live births, while legal abortions are reported as a ratio of the number of legal terminations per 1000 live births. Most, but not all, states require the reporting of legal abortions. The completeness of the reporting is unknown and may be variable. In some states, all legal abortions must take place in a licensed health facility, while in others this is not a requirement. Unless there is a pathologic examination, the presence of a conceptus at the time of

"menstrual extraction" would in some instances be unknown. Calculated from available data, the legal abortion ratio for the United States in 1976 was 313 per 1000 live births.

STILLBIRTH

An infant born after the 20th week of gestation who shows no sign of life at birth is termed stillborn. The *stillbirth rate* is the number of stillborn infants per 1000 live births. Although there are notable exceptions, the almost universal acceptance of the World Health Organization definition of stillbirth has done much to permit international comparison of rates. In the United States the stillbirth rate has shown a decreasing trend (Fig. 15–6), reaching an all-time low of 10.3 in 1976. A further decline can be expected as greater use is made of intrapartum fetal monitoring and other devices of this kind. The major causes of stillbirth in Indiana in 1977 are listed in Table 15–4.

NEWBORN MORTALITY

The *infant mortality rate* is the number of liveborn infants that die within the 1st year of life per 1000 births. The *neonatal mortality rate* is the number of liveborn infants that die within the first 28 days of life. The *hebdomadal death rate* is the number of liveborn infants that die within the first 7 days of life per 1000 live births.

Newborn mortality rates are computed from death certificates. In many cases, additional information is obtained by studying the birth certificate along with the death certificate. Formal committees for the study of the facts surrounding a stillbirth or the death of a newborn infant came into existence shortly after the formation of committees to investigate maternal mortality. Because of the openness of the deliberations and the practicality of each hospital having such a committee, these groups, frequently termed perinatal mortality committes, became valuable sources of continuing education for all who participated. Such committees also were instrumental in raising the standards of care of the pregnant woman and the newborn child. Data for 1977 reveal an infant mortality rate of 14.0 and a neonatal mortality rate of 9.8 (Fig. 15–7).

The major causes of infant death are 1) postnatal asphyxia and atelectasis, 2) immaturity (unqualified), 3) congenital malformations, 4) influenza and pneumonia (including pneumonia of the newborn), and 5) maternal complications. Infants do not die at a uniform rate during the 1st year of life; also, the leading causes of death in one period may vary from those in another. For purposes of study, the 1st year may be divided into the first 24 hours, the remainder of the 1st

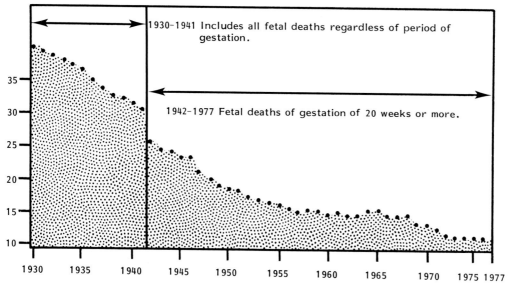

FIG. 15–6. Stillbirth rates (per 1000 live births), United States 1930–1976. (Vital Statistics of the United States, 1930–1976, Vol 2. US Department of Health, Education, and Welfare)

TABLE 15–4. CAUSES OF STILLBIRTH AND STILLBIRTH RATE, INDIANA, 1977

Cause	Number	Stillbirth Rate/1000 Live Births
PLACENTAL AND UMBILICAL CORD ABNORMALITIES	347	4.1
UNKNOWN OR ILL-DEFINED CAUSES	212	2.5
FETAL DISEASE	14	0.2
MATERNAL OBSTETRIC COMPLICATIONS	68	0.8
CONGENITAL MALFORMA-TIONS OF FETUS	44	0.5
MATERNAL MEDICAL DIS-EASES	92	1.1
PREGNANCY TERMINATION	8	0.1
TOTAL	785	9.2

(Indiana Vital Statistics, 1977. Indiana State Board of Health)

week, the remainder of the 1st month, and the remainder of the 1st year. About 40% of infant deaths occur within the first 24 hours of life. At this time, the leading cause of death is unqualified immaturity. About 25% of infant deaths occur during the remainder of the 1st week, when the leading causes are postnatal asphyxia and atelectasis. During the remainder of the 1st month, another 8% die; during the subsequent 11 months, the final 27% die. The leading causes of death for each period are given in Table 15–5. These data are compiled on a nationwide basis from death certificates.

The causes of death are not exclusive of other associated or underlying causes. Variability in accuracy, interest, and diagnostic criteria may affect these data.

After the 1st year of life and up to about the 40th year of life, accidents are the leading cause of death.

PERINATAL MORTALITY

The number of stillbirths plus the number of neonatal deaths per 1000 live births is the *perinatal mortality rate.* The logic of such a rate becomes apparent when it is considered that an obstetric complication in its severest form may kill both the mother and her unborn child, and in lesser degrees of severity may result in a stillborn infant, a preterm liveborn infant who dies, a preterm infant who lives with disabling central nervous system damage, or a term infant with minimal central nervous system impairment. To Yankhauer must be given credit for pointing out the amount of life lost during the period extending "from the 20th week of gestation to the seventh day of life." He states that there are more lives lost during this period than in the next 40 years.

PREGNANCY WASTAGE

It seems logical to combine the stillbirth rate with the neonatal mortality rate to arrive at a figure that represents pregnancy loss between the 20th week of gestation and the 28th day of life. It appears just as logical to start routine data collection in pregnancies that terminate prior to the 20th week and to add these pregnancy losses (abortions) to the perinatal rate. From a combi-

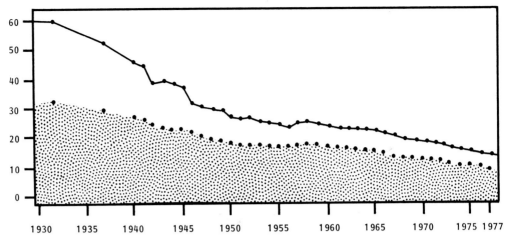

FIG. 15-7. Infant and neonatal mortality rates (per 1000 live births), United States, 1930–1977. (Vital Statistics of the United States, 1930–1977, Vol 2. US Department of Health, Education, and Welfare)

nation of such data, *total pregnancy wastage* could be ascertained. This concept is shown in Figure 15–8. Figure 15–9 indicates the number involved in total pregnancy wastage, from known conception to completion of the 1st year of life. This figure is a hypothetical cohort of 1000 known conceptions, their spontaneous and legal termination, and the resultant infant survival at the end of the 1st year of life. It assumes a 10% spontaneous abortion ratio, a legal abortion ratio of 313, a stillbirth rate of 10, a neonatal mortality rate of 10, and a postneonatal mortality rate of 4. Pregnancy wastage from conception to the first missed menses has not been considered.

EPIDEMIOLOGY OF PREGNANCY MORBIDITY AND MORTALITY

The identifying characteristics used in classic descriptive epidemiology are time, place, and person.

TIME

As noted, the secular trends of morbidity and mortality rates show a progressive decrease over time. This probably results from improved medical care and an increase in the general resistance of the population to obstetric health hazards. This increase in the general resistance has been facilitated by an improvement in the health environment and nutritional status of the population that has also lowered many other morbidity and mortality rates.

PLACE

Making comparisons of reproductive rates of geographically identifiable populations, along with as-

TABLE 15-5. CAUSES OF DEATH DURING 1ST YEAR OF LIFE, IN ORDER OF FREQUENCY FOR EACH PERIOD

Under 1 Day	1–6 Days	7–27 Days	28 Days–11 Months
Immaturity (unqualified)	Postnatal asphyxia and atelectasis	Congenital malformation	Influenza and pneumonia*
Postnatal asphyxia and atelectasis	Immaturity (unqualified)	Influenza and pneumonia*	Congenital malformation
Birth injuries	Maternal complications	Maternal complications	Accidents
Maternal complications	Congenital malformation	Immaturity (unqualified)	Residual of accidents
Congenital malformation	Birth injuries	Postnatal asphyxia and atelectasis	Gastrointestinal infections

* Including pneumonia of the newborn.
(Infant and Perinatal Mortality in the United States. National Center for Health Statistics, Series 3, No 9, 1965, p 17. US Department of Health, Education, and Welfare)

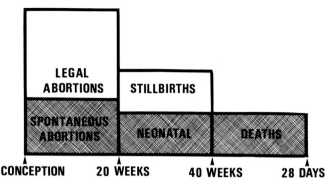

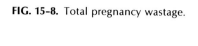

FIG. 15-8. Total pregnancy wastage.

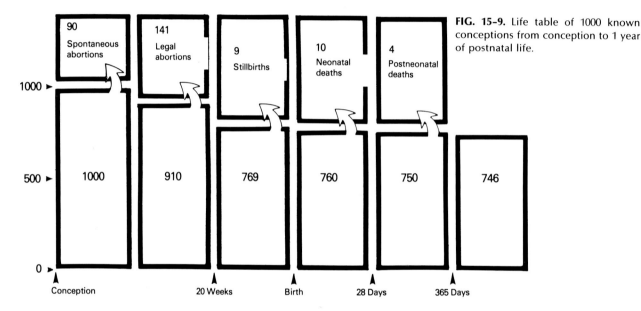

FIG. 15-9. Life table of 1000 known conceptions from conception to 1 year of postnatal life.

sumptions and explanations for the differences noted, has become a common pastime. It is important to remember, however, that for data to be meaningful they must be obtained using comparable methods, similar diligence, and identical definitions.

International Differences

The neonatal and infant mortality rates of the United States and some other countries are presented in Table 15–6. These rates are based on live births. Although the differences are probably real, there are several reasons why they cannot be taken absolutely at face value. In a special study in Sweden in 1956, 17% of "stillborn" infants breathed and therefore should have been classified as liveborn infants who died, thus raising Sweden's infant and neonatal mortality rates. In many Western European countries, it is the responsibility of the parents to report the birth. In the Netherlands, birth weight is not reported; the extent of un-

derreporting is unknown, and registration of fetal death is required only for gestations of 28 weeks or more. In Norway, birth registration is an ecclesiastical function.

These are examples of some differences in methods, diligence, and definitions. However, those who have studied these discrepancies conclude that more is concerned than differences in the collection of data. These matters are discussed at length in *International Comparison of Perinatal and Infant Mortality,* published by the U.S. Department of Health, Education, and Welfare.

Urban-Rural Differences

Arranging identifiable geographic areas according to population density and then studying the associated pregnancy wastage rates can also provide insight into the relation between environment and reproductive loss. A strong positive association has been shown be-

TABLE 15-6. NEONATAL AND INFANT MORTALITY RATES IN VARIOUS COUNTRIES, 1971

Country	Infant Mortality	Country	Neonatal Mortality
Sweden	11.1	Japan	8.2
Finland	11.8	Sweden	8.8
Netherlands	12.1	Netherlands	9.1
Japan	12.4	Norway	9.4
Norway	12.5	Switzerland	9.9
Denmark	13.5	England and Wales	11.6
Switzerland	14.4	Ireland	12.0
France	17.3	Hong Kong	12.1
Canada	17.5	Singapore	14.0
England and Wales	17.5	United States	14.3
Hong Kong	17.7		
Ireland	18.0		
Spain	18.4		
United States	19.2		

(World Health Statistics Report, Vol 26, No 12, 1973, pp 787–788. World Health Organization)

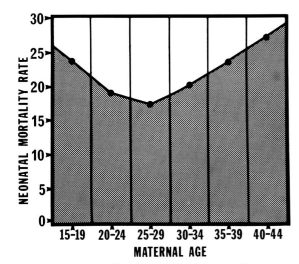

FIG. 15–10. Maternal age and neonatal mortality rate. (Infant and Perinatal Mortality in the United States, Series 3, No 4, 1965, p 77. US Department of Health, Education, and Welfare)

tween preterm delivery and population density and between perinatal mortality and population density.

PERSON

For purposes of epidemiologic investigation, the patient may be identified by certain personal characteristics such as age, race, socioeconomic status, previous pregnancy loss, and interval since last delivery, and the pregnancy may be identified by such factors as breech presentation, premature rupture of membranes, repeat cesarean section, or labor in excess of 18 hours. Figure 15–10 shows the relation of neonatal mortality to one of these parameters, maternal age. These data indicate that reproductive wastage is lowest among gravidas who are in the third decade of life.

REFERENCES AND RECOMMENDED READING

Abortion Surveillance: 1976. US Department of Health, Education, and Welfare, Center for Disease Control, 1978

Annual Summary of Selected Activities in Hospital Maternity Service. Department of State, State of Illinois

The Facts of Life and Death. US Department of Health, Education, and Welfare, 1965, p 6

Fielding JE: Adolescent pregnancy revisited: Trends in births to adolescents. N Engl J Med 299:893, 1978

International Comparison of Perinatal and Infant Mortality, Series 3, No 6. US Department of Health, Education, and Welfare, 1967

Shapiro S, Jones E, Densen P: A life table of pregnancy terminations and correlates of fetal loss. Milbank Mem Fund Q 40:1, 1962

State Definitions of Livebirths, Fetal Deaths, and Gestation Periods at Which Fetal Deaths Are Registered. US Department of Health, Education, and Welfare, 1966, p xii

Statistical Abstract of the United States. US Bureau of the Census, 1978

Thompson J: Some observations on the geographic distribution of premature births and perinatal deaths in Indiana. Am J Obstet Gynecol 101:43, 1968

Yankhauer A: The public health aspect of perinatal mortality. NY State J Med 57:2499, 1957

Yerushalmey J, van den Berg BJ, Erhardt CL et al: Birth weight and gestation as indices of "immaturity." Am J Dis Child 109:43, 1965

PART **II**

NORMAL PREGNANCY

16

FERTILIZATION AND THE PHYSIOLOGY AND DEVELOPMENT OF FETUS AND PLACENTA

Irwin H. Kaiser

EVENTS SURROUNDING FERTILIZATION

The anatomy and physiology of ovulation are discussed in Chapters 4 and 6. The events of ovulation, fertilization, and implantation are diagramed in Figure 16–1.

The ovum, with the mass of surrounding granulosa cells that formed the cumulus oophorus, is shed into the fimbriated end of the tube. It is moved by muscular and ciliary activity into the ampulla. There it encounters the spermatozoa that have ascended through the uterus. The mobility of ovaries and tubes apparently makes it possible for an ovum from one ovary to enter the opposite tube. It is not known whether sperm can migrate from one tube to the other.

Spermatogenesis (Fig. 16–2) occurs in the tubules of the testis under the influence of follicle-stimulating hormone and of the testosterone formed by the adjacent Leydig cells, which are under the influence of luteinizing hormone. Secretion of these hormones is es-

sentially continuous after the pubarche. The maturation from spermatogonium to spermatozoan goes through several distinct stages—spermatocyte and spermatid—during which reduction division is accomplished, so that the spermatozoan has a haploid number of chromosomes. The nuclear mass becomes the head of the sperm. X-bearing sperm are minutely heavier than Y-bearing sperm. The cytoplasm of the spermatid makes up the spiral midpiece and the elongated tail of the mature sperm.

A spermatozoan has an outer plasma membrane and an outer coat that may contain antigenic material. The acrosome, a minute structure, is situated at the very tip of the head of the sperm and contains the hyaluronidase that initiates the dispersion of cells that surround the ovum. It may also contain an enzyme that causes the zona pellucida to become readily permeable to the head of the sperm and its chromosomal material.

Behind the head of the sperm is the coiled helix of the midpiece, which consists of mitochondria. These generate most of the energy responsible for tail motion. The tail proper consists of two long longitudinal fibers surrounded by nine pairs of shorter fibers. These are the contractile units that generate both forward motion and rotation. This motion is essential to fertilization.

A spermatozoan is able to maintain motility for as much as a week in the fallopian tube, but is probably actually fertile for less than half that time. It cannot repair damage, having lost its ribonucleic acid (RNA), and its energy systems are needed only to maintain motility. Once the stored adenosine triphosphate is exhausted, cell death ensues. There is some intracellular lipid, but extracellular substances, principally fructose, are essential to support glycolysis. When the sperm is immobile, its energy consumption is virtually nil, and it can therefore survive for several weeks in the male reproductive tract after release from the seminiferous tubule.

The suspending material for the sperm, the seminal plasma, is derived from epididymis, vas deferens, seminal vesicle, prostate, and urethral glands. It has a characteristic odor due to unique amines, and it contains considerable fructose. It also contains prostaglandins, whose physiologic function is still unclear, and considerable amounts of amino acids.

In coitus, 2–4 ml semen is deposited in the vagina at the cervix. It contains more than 50 million sperm. In healthy fertile specimens, more than 75% of these spermatozoa are of normal morphology and more than half of these are motile. Of the motile sperm, more than half exhibit forward motion and rotation.

If the cervical mucus is favorable, as it is at midcycle, some of these sperm penetrate and ascend the female tract at a rate of about 5–6 mm/min. It is thought that uterine contractions assist in sperm progress, but nonmotile sperm do not reach the fallopian tubes.

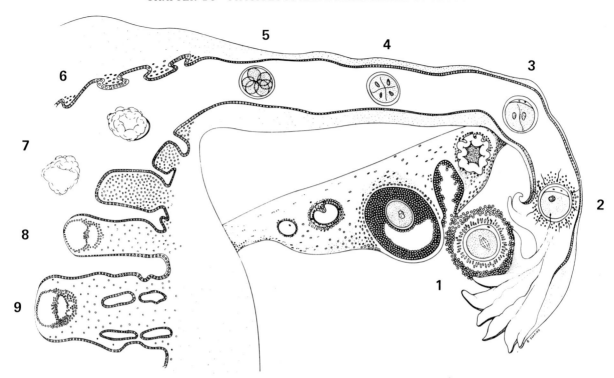

FIG. 16–1. Schematic representation of events of ovulation, fertilization, and implantation. *1.* Extrusion of ovum, with first polar body and cumulus oophorus, which then forms corona radiata. *2.* Cells of corona have become loosened, a sperm has penetrated zona pellucida and entered ovum, and second polar body has formed. *3.* Cleavage of fertilized ovum has begun, and ovum has moved well into fallopian tube. *4.* Further cleavage proceeds. About 24 hours have elapsed since fertilization. *5.* By 48 hours, many cells are present and zona begins to fragment. *6.* At 72–84 hours, zona has fallen away and ovum has entered uterine cavity. Central cavity begins to form in ovum. *7.* By 120 hours, there is a distinct cell mass on one side of ovum, which is still free in uterine fluid. *8.* At 7 days, implantation has taken place. Ovum is promptly covered over by surface epithelium. Trophoblast burrows into endometrial stroma and starts to form syncytiotrophoblast. Primitive amniotic and chorionic cavities have begun to form, and a germ disk is recognizable. *9.* By 9 days, lacunae have begun to appear in syncytiotrophoblast. They will form intervillous space. Germ disk is well formed, as is amnion. (Modified from Dickinson RL: Human Sex Anatomy, 2nd ed. Baltimore, Williams & Wilkins, 1949)

There is an effect of the fluid in the uterus or tubes that makes the sperm capable of fertilization. This process is called *capacitation* and requires some hours. One of the major problems in achieving *in vitro* fertilization has been the production of artificial capacitation.

When the spermatozoan and ovum meet in the tube, syngamy takes place. It is known that a number of sperm can make contact with the cumulus and corona radiata and penetrate to the zona pellucida (Fig. 16–3). In some species, the zona consists of two layers, and sperm must penetrate both to enter the cytoplasm of the ovum. Once one sperm has entered, a reaction occurs in the zona that renders it impervious to other sperm. A diploid chromosome number is reestablished, and mitotic cell division of a new individual can begin.

TIMING OF PREGNANCY

In the precise timing of pregnancy, the initial event is considered to be ovulation, and physicians may refer to *ovulation age.* When the time of fertile coitus is known, especially with laboratory animals, this time may be used as well, stated in hours, days, or weeks.

Clinically, however, pregnancy is dated from the 1st day of the last menstrual period, when this is known. From this, an expected date of labor or confinement (EDL or EDC) is calculated by assuming a duration of 280 days. Nägele's rule, by which 3 is subtracted from the original number of the month and 7 is added to the date, is based on this estimate. Clearly, since in an idealized cycle ovulation occurs on the 14th day, the actual duration of pregnancy is 266 days. Where cycles

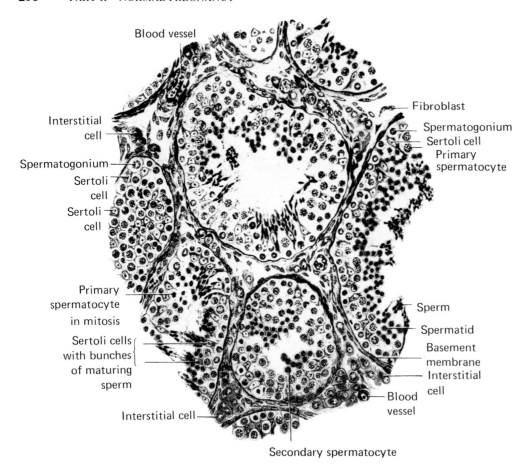

Blood vessel

Interstitial cell

Spermatogonium

Sertoli cell

Sertoli cell

Primary spermatocyte in mitosis

Sertoli cells with bunches of maturing sperm

Interstitial cell

Secondary spermatocyte

Fibroblast

Spermatogonium

Sertoli cell

Primary spermatocyte

Sperm

Spermatid

Basement membrane

Interstitial cell

Blood vessel

FIG. 16–2. Section of human testis. Transected tubules show various stages of spermatogenesis. (×170) (Bloom W, Fawcett DW: A Textbook of Histology, 9th ed. Philadelphia, Saunders, 1968)

are very irregular or artificially induced, timing must be based on a presumed date of ovulation or fertilization and 266 days added.

Although actually the duration of pregnancy may vary by several weeks, these estimates of expected duration are accurate enough for clinical use. The embryologist and reproductive endocrinologist prefer the more precise statement, however.

THE FERTILIZED OVUM

THE HERTIG–ROCK SERIES

Information about human pregnancy is obviously difficult to obtain, and most of our present knowledge is based upon what is referred to as the Hertig–Rock series of ova. A large number of women who were awaiting hysterectomy for gynecologic disease, but who were normally fertile and within the reproductive epoch, were asked to report their menstrual and coital dates to these researchers. At the time of hysterectomy, the most meticulous study of the uteri and fallopian tubes was made for evidence of early ova. A remarkably large number were recovered and were described in great detail in a series of publications in the *Contributions to Embryology* of the Carnegie Institution of Washington. Because the women studied were all essentially normal from a reproductive standpoint, great reliance can be placed on the normality of this material, in contrast to material obtained at the time of spontaneous abortion or uterine curettage for bleeding.

EARLY FETAL LOSS

The remarkably high fetal loss originally observed in the pig (*i.e.,* a greater number of corpora lutea in the pig's ovary than viable fetuses in the uterus) has, on the basis of the Hertig–Rock series, been found to apply to the human being as well. Too few ova have

been examined prior to implantation to allow generalization, and indeed it is difficult to adduce entirely satisfactory criteria of normality in such a group. However, if consideration is restricted to implanted ova recovered up to the 14th day following ovulation (obtained, therefore, from patients who had no way of knowing they were pregnant), major disturbances of differentiation of the germ disk or of implantation or proliferation of the trophoblast are observed in more than 40%. Those ova with marked hemorrhage at the implantation site or marked deficiency in formation of trophoblast and villi are probably lost at the time of the next menstrual period, and the mother has no way of knowing she was ever pregnant. The remainder probably account for the greater portion of the abortions resulting from defective germ plasma, which constitute most of the spontaneous abortions.

EARLY DEVELOPMENT AND TRANSPORT OF OVUM

After fertilization, mitotic division begins, slowly at first but gradually increasing in speed. During its life in the fallopian tube, the ovum undergoes considerable growth, more in terms of the number of cells than in actual size, although the latter also increases (Figs. 16–4 and 16–5). During most of the period of its existence in the tube, the fertilized ovum is a solid mass of cells. Blastocyst formation begins at about the 5th day. On the 5th or 6th day, the blastocyst (Fig. 16–6) arrives in the uterine lumen, where it continues a free-floating existence for at least 24 hours. The outermost layer of the blastocyst is one or two cells thick, with a central cell mass located somewhere on the inner surface. This central mass consists of cells that are not themselves much more differentiated than those elsewhere in the blastocyst. Some investigators believe that the fertilized ovum spends 3–4 days within the uterine cavity; however, the fact that Hertig and Rock failed to find a substantial number of unattached ova in that location makes this appear unlikely.

IMPLANTATION OF OVUM

The formation of the corpus luteum in the ovary and the consequent secretion of progesterone in large quantities begin to alter the endometrium in preparation for implantation. Since the uterine cavity is only potential at this time and for practical purposes consists only of an anterior and a posterior wall, the initial implantation of the ovum tends to take place on one of these two surfaces of endometrium. Implantation most often occurs at about the middle of the roughly triangularly shaped uterine wall but the reason for this is not completely understood. There are deviations from the pattern, but implantation does not appear to be entirely random.

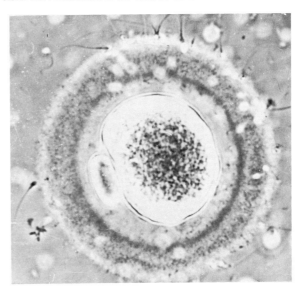

FIG. 16–3. Human ovum. Polar body is on *left*. Many spermatozoa are visible in and around zona pellucida. (Shettles LB: Ovum Humanum. New York, Hafner, 1960)

FIG. 16–4. Two-cell human conceptus, washed from fallopian tube within 36 hours of conception. Polar body can be seen *below*, still within zona pellucida. (Carnegie No. 8698, ×500) (Hertig AT, Rock J, Adams EC, Mulligan WJ: Contrib Embryol 35:199, 1954)

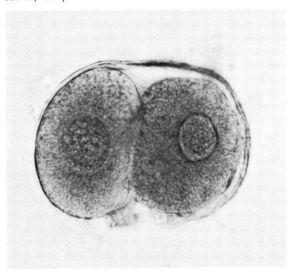

Implantation ordinarily takes place on the surface epithelium at a point midway among a series of openings of endometrial glands, *i.e.*, directly over endometrial stroma (Fig. 16–7). At this time in the development of the endometrium, the coiled arteries approach closer and closer to the surface, and capillary sprouts,

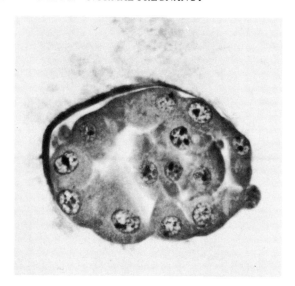

FIG. 16-5. Section of fixed, stained 58-cell human conceptus, found in uterine cavity within 4 days of conception. Zona pellucida is intact and cells appear to be differentiating into outer and inner group. (Carnegie No. 8794, ×600) (Hertig AT, Rock J, Adams EC, Mulligan WJ: Contrib Embryol 35:199, 1954)

FIG. 16-6. Section of 107-cell human blastocyst approximately 1 day older than embryo in Figure 16-5. This embryo was also found in uterine cavity. Zona pellucida is now gone, and differentiation into inner cell mass, which will form embryo, and outer layer, which forms trophoblast, has taken place. (Carnegie No. 8663, ×600) (Hertig AT, Rock J, Adams EC, Mulligan WJ: Contrib Embryol 35:199, 1954)

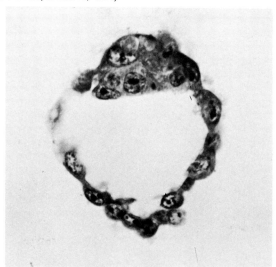

which come off the distal ends of the arteries, reach up almost to the lining epithelium. Thus, the area in which implantation takes place is likely to have, on a microscopic scale, an immediately available blood supply. The ovum up to this point has been leading a relatively anaerobic existence and probably does not experience any sudden increase in requirements for gas exchange. On the other hand, it has probably begun to approach the limits of its ability to continue to exist and grow as a free-floating organism, so it can be assumed that implantation improves the metabolic circumstances of the ovum. If the trophoblast invades the blood vessels prematurely, however, the effect is deleterious rather than favorable; hematomas are likely to form under the implantation site and, consequently, implantation is defective. It is also of some interest that decidual alteration of endometrial stroma, which is greatest in the vicinity of the coiled arteries, appears after, rather than before or simultaneous with, implantation.

Within 24 hours the blastocyst is apparently able to burrow down into the endometrium, and the surface epithelium of the endometrium has begun to proliferate over the top of the blastocyst. By 7.5 days after ovulation, this implantation, which is referred to as interstitial since the blastocyst burrows into the endometrium, is complete. Shortly thereafter, the surface epithelium is healed over the blastocyst. As can be seen from the illustrations, the blastocyst tends to bulge above the normal surface of the epithelium, and the implanted ovum can be seen under the dissecting microscope and, in favorable conditions, with the naked eye.

DEVELOPMENT OF PRIMITIVE PLACENTA

The advancing trophoblast, which consists almost entirely of syncytiotrophoblast at this stage, being provided with ready gas exchange and, in the glycogenrich endometrium, a ready source of energy, begins to develop rather rapidly into the primitive placenta (Figs. 16–8 and 16–9). This consists of large masses of syncytiotrophoblast among which spaces begin to form. These are the primitive lacunae, which are destined to form the intervillous space. Columns of trophoblast, the primary villi, then form, and some attach themselves to the decidua as anchoring villi. In these villi, central cores of connective tissue develop to give rise to the secondary villi.

On about the 11th day, the advancing cytotrophoblast penetrates a maternal capillary and initiates a flow of blood into the lacunae of the primitive placenta (Fig. 16–10). The circulation in this early placenta is necessarily sluggish and the pressure of blood extremely low. This is almost certainly desirable, since penetration of an arteriolar structure by the early trophoblast would presumably release blood into this

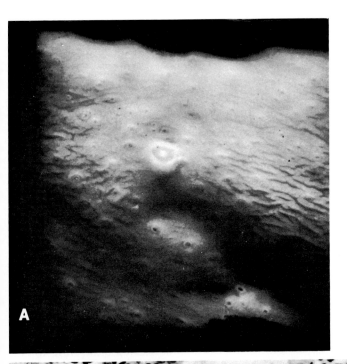

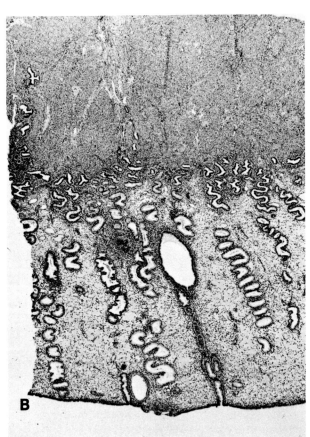

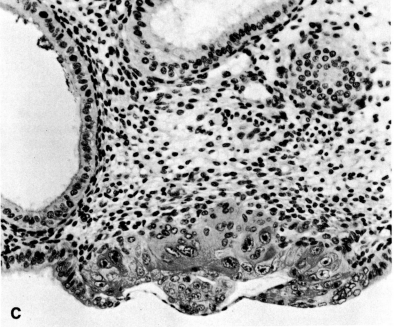

FIG. 16–7. Human conceptus 6.5–7 days old. *A.* Surface view of collapsed blastocyst attached to endometrium. Note position away from gland mouths and clearly seen inner cell mass. *B.* Low-power view of perpendicular fixed and stained section directly through conceptus. Condition of endometrium and superficial location of implantation are clear. *C.* Higher power view of same section as in *B.* Bilaminar nature of germ disk is evident, as is variegated nuclear morphology of advancing syncytiotrophoblast. Surface epithelium is not complete over embryo. Endometrial stroma directly under trophoblast is more compact than deeper. (Carnegie No. 8020. *A,* ×22; *B,* ×30; *C,* ×250) (Hertig AT, Rock J: Contrib Embryol 31:65, 1945)

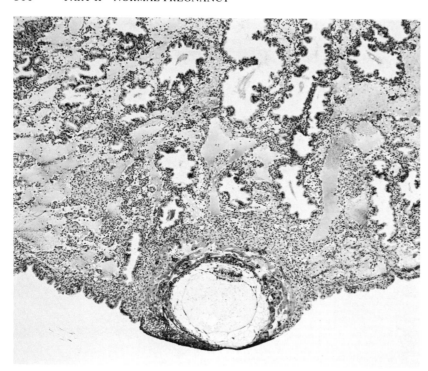

FIG. 16–8. Human conceptus, estimated 12 days of age. Trophoblast has now formed lacunae that contain maternal blood from sinusoid on *right*. Endometrium is much more advanced. Trophoblast has differentiated into cytotrophoblast and syncytiotrophoblast. Germ disk is formed, and several extraembryonic structures such as extracelomic membrane and amnion have differentiated. Compare with Figures 16–7 and 16–9. (Hertig AT, Rock J: Contrib Embryol 29:127, 1941)

primitive placenta at a pressure that might dislocate the ovum. The perforation of maternal blood vessels by the syncytiotrophoblast also makes possible the direct injection into the maternal circulation of human chorionic gonadotropin, which within the next few days is able to convert the corpus luteum in the ovary into a corpus luteum of pregnancy, thereby preventing the withdrawal of hormonal support from the endometrium and allowing the continuation of the pregnancy. This, of course, results in failure to menstruate, one of the obvious signs of early pregnancy.

The proliferation of syncytiotrophoblast can go on throughout the entire surface of the sphere of the blastocyst. However, there is very little growth on the surfaces most remote from maternal circulation; the greatest growth is toward the endometrium. This growth differential, which is apparently determined mostly by the availability of nutrients, sets the stage for the development of the definitive placenta at the site of implantation. Because implantation is interstitial in the human being, ordinarily there is only one placenta at the site of implantation. The healing of surface epithelium over the ovum effectively keeps the trophoblast from contact with the opposite uterine wall in the course of its further growth and development, and hence the placenta forms on only one side.

By about the 18th day, as a result of local angiogenesis, capillaries have developed within what are now the tertiary villi. The primitive heart of the embryo is simultaneously forming, along with islands of hemato-poiesis, and together these establish the fetal side of the placental circulation.

As pregnancy advances, the endometrium is virtually entirely changed into decidua. Although the term *decidua* means that which is shed, areas of decidua are retained within the uterus, both at the placental site and elsewhere, and are later the source of relining of the uterine cavity by endometrium at the conclusion of pregnancy. The gradual expansion of the membranes flattens the decidua into a layer to which the chorion is rather loosely attached. Scattered throughout this area there may be ghosts of the villi that at one time covered the entire surface of the chorion as the chorion frondosum (Fig. 16–11).

THE DEFINITIVE PLACENTA

LOCATION

The definitive placenta apparently tends to form and to delimit itself in the area where blood supply is most satisfactory. In the corpus, this is under the developing embryo at the site of the original interstitial implantation. When implantation takes place in the lowermost portion of the uterus, which almost certainly is the anatomic antecedent of placenta previa, the blood supply is not as efficient as in the corpus, and the placenta ordinarily is much larger in area and less in thickness. Since, however, the entire surface of the chorion is in

FIG. 16-9. Artist's reconstruction of Carnegie No. 7700. (×160) (Hertig AT, Rock J: Contrib Embryol 27:127, 1941)

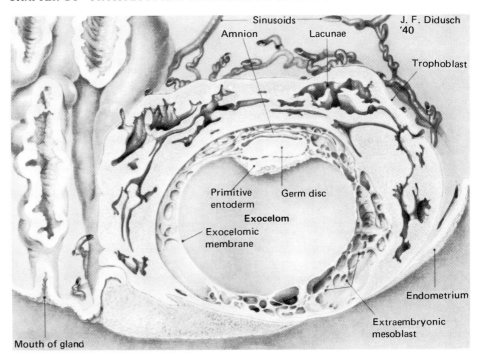

FIG. 16-10. Human conceptus about 16.5 days old. Note formation of primitive villi around much of periphery of trophoblast. Further development in germ disk has produced much larger amnion and early yolk sac. (Carnegie No. 7802, ×30) (Heuser CH, Rock J, Hertig AT: Contrib Embryol 31:185, 1945)

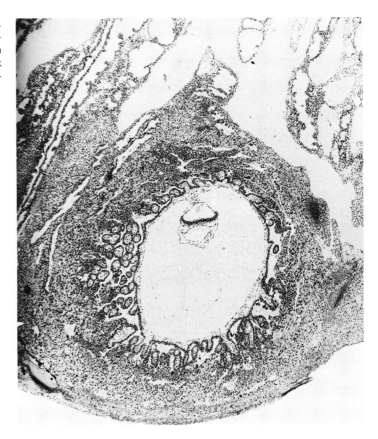

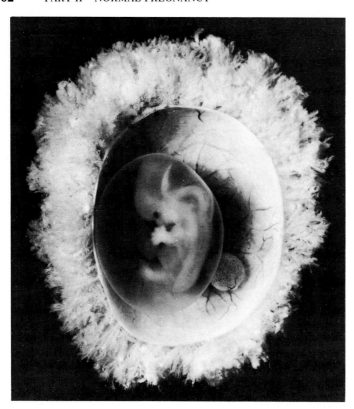

FIG. 16–11. Well-differentiated human embryo, approximately 40 days old, with portion of chorion frondosum dissected away to show amnion and yolk sac. Formation of villi over entire surface is evident. (Carnegie No. 8537A, ×1.5)

its primitive stages covered with placental villi that participate in the fetal circulation and then are lost secondarily, it is possible for the placenta to occur almost anywhere (Fig. 16–11). It is undoubtedly in this fashion that separate small islands of placenta, known as *placenta succenturiata,* are formed. In rare instances, placental tissue persists over almost the entire surface of the chorion; this is known as *placenta membranacea.*

INSERTION OF CORD

The factors that determine the site of insertion of the umbilical cord on the placenta are not entirely known. The primitive germ disk differentiates with what is destined to be the dorsal surface of the fetus closest to the uterus so that the ventral surface, which eventually differentiates the umbilical cord, is directed toward the uterine cavity. Rotation of the germ disk or the embryo takes place as the amnion differentiates. If the orientation of the embryo within its membranes influences the direction of the umbilical cord, failure of the embryo to achieve 180° rotation might direct the umbilical cord to a point other than what is destined to be the center of the definitive placenta. It seems equally possible that such an event is result rather

than cause and that the site of insertion of the umbilical cord on the amnion in relation to the placenta is an entirely random event, since some length of umbilical cord is necessary for the growth and development of the fetus and insertion of the umbilical cord must, in fact, occur. In the case of twins, one of the cords ordinarily inserts near the margin of one of the placentas or the main placenta, and in the placenta associated with placenta previa there is also a higher than ordinary incidence of marginal insertion. In rare circumstances, the cord may insert away from the placenta, a velamentous insertion, so that the vessels run along the membranes from the site of cord insertion to the surface of the placenta. When the insertion of the cord is over the cervix, a condition known as *vasa previa,* rupture of the membranes prior to delivery may disrupt the blood vessels and cause fetal hemorrhage. This is a rare event that is almost impossible to diagnose and treat.

SIZE

Early in the second trimester, the placenta approximately equals the size of the infant; as pregnancy advances, it becomes relatively smaller, although it continues to grow until term (Fig. 16–12). The placenta

FIG. 16-12. Placental growth by weeks of gestation, based on over 11,000 births at University Hospitals of Cleveland, 1956–1962. *Solid line,* mean; *dashed line,* ±1 standard deviation; *dotted line,* 12 standard deviations. (Hendricks CH: Obstet Gynecol 24:360, 1964)

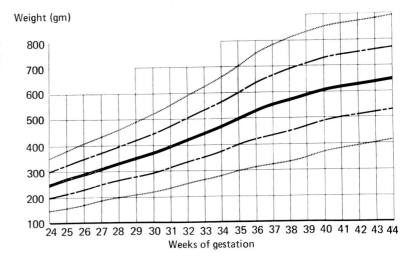

eventually attains a size approximately 15 cm in diameter and 2 cm in thickness. At term the ratio of its weight to that of the fetus is about 1:6 but may vary from 1:2 to 1:10 (Fig. 16–13). The weight of the membranes and cord is trivial. At term the placenta may weigh 300–1200 g. The smaller placentas are associated with smaller infants. Extensive placental infarction is not responsible for any striking decrease in weight of the placenta. Placental edema, however, sometimes causes an increase in weight, as well as alteration in color.

The observation that the placenta continues to grow in size leaves unsettled one curious but clinically important point. It is clear that the fetus depends for its welfare on the growth of the placenta and that the growth of the placenta must keep pace with that of the fetus. Should the placenta fail, the fetus must either be born or experience intrauterine starvation or asphyxiation. There seems little question that in unusual instances the placenta does fail to grow sufficiently to meet the needs of the infant, and the result is either a wizened, malnourished-looking newborn devoid of subcutaneous fat and obviously mature beyond its size or a stillborn fetus. There is, however, little evidence that placental growth is limited under normal conditions or that such limitation restricts fetal growth.

MORPHOLOGY

Normally, the placenta consists of blood vessels and vascular spaces, with a small amount of supporting connective tissue and a relatively transparent endothelium on the surface of the villi. The maternal surface of the placenta normally has the dark red color of venous blood. The fetal surface is shiny and consists

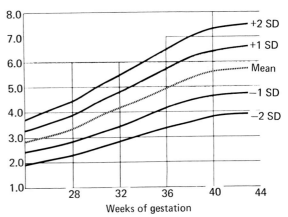

FIG. 16-13. Ratio of fetal-to-placental weight, based on over 11,000 births at University Hospitals of Cleveland, 1956–1962. **SD,** standard deviation. (Hendricks CH: Obstet Gynecol 24:361, 1964)

of large opaque-walled blood vessels coursing on the dense opalescent surface of the thickened chorion. The pale color of the edematous placenta is ordinarily enhanced on the fetal surface because many conditions that produce placental edema are also associated with fetal anemia.

The placenta, on the maternal surface, is ordinarily broken up into 12–20 subdivisions, referred to as *cotyledons.* There is no consistent pattern of anchoring villi or connective tissue septa that establishes the cotyledon arrangement. A further, functional subdivision has been demonstrated by angiography and dissection. (Fig. 16–14). The arborizing fetal vessels eventually are distributed to small units of the placenta, each of which is irrigated by a coiled artery on the maternal side. The jet of maternal blood enters the middle of the

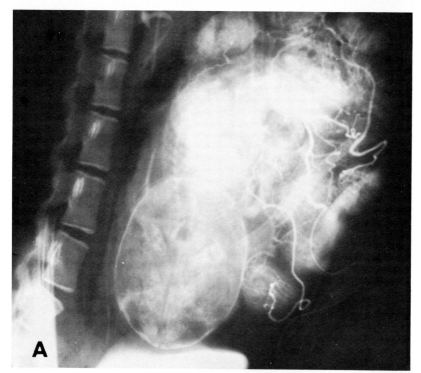

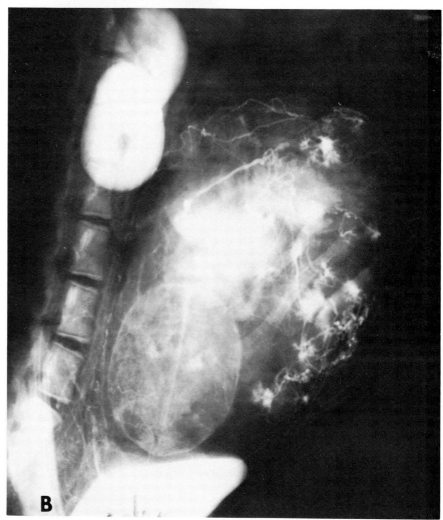

FIG. 16–14. Lateral radiographs of 152-day pregnancy in a macaque. Fetal head and spine can be readily seen. *A* was taken 3 sec after injection of radiopaque material into an interplacental (umbilical) artery to display fetal side of placental circulation. Note several well-filled fetal cotyledons. *B* was taken 2 sec after injection of radiopaque material into maternal uterine arteries. It can be seen that there are functional cotyledons without functional maternal arterial entry tracts, and *vice versa*. (Ramsey EM, Martin CB, Jr, Donner MW: Am J Obstet Gynecol 98:419, 1967)

unit and spreads out from there. There are about 50 such lobules in the human placenta.

HISTOLOGY

Changes in the microscopic appearance of the placenta occur with time. The primitive villi are replaced by villi that contain blood vessels and a relatively large amount of connective tissue. Their surface is covered by a double layer of epithelium, the innermost being the cytotrophoblast (Langhans' layer) and the outer the syncytiotrophoblast. There is now overwhelming evidence that the syncytiotrophoblast is all derived from cytotrophoblast; presumably, this may still be true even late in pregnancy when the cytotrophoblast can no longer be readily identified in microscopic sections. Some of the villi extend down to the decidua basalis, and their connective tissue cores become the anchoring areas of the placenta. Others form main stems through which large fetal blood vessels travel and from which secondary and tertiary branching occurs. As pregnancy proceeds, the villi contain relatively less and less connective tissue; toward term, the outermost villous twigs consist of very little more than fetal capillaries surrounded by the syncytiotrophoblast, which is equivalent to the endothelial lining of the intervillous space.

Two cells that may be found in the connective tissue are worthy of special mention. One of these is the plasma cell, which ordinarily is quite rare but which has been identified beyond question in an instance of maternal agammaglobulinemia. The other is the Hofbauer cell, which has a varied appearance, depending upon the type of preparation in which it is seen. Ordinarily, it has a small amount of eosinophilic cytoplasm and a dense basophilic nucleus. It stands in contrast to the ordinary connective tissue cells of the villus, which contain very little cytoplasm and have smaller, more pyknotic nuclei. The Hofbauer cell is a phagocyte and has been shown to have IgG surface receptors.

As pregnancy advances, the trophoblast is spread ever thinner over the surface of the villi, and its nuclei tend to accumulate in localized areas (Fig. 16–15). This gives rise to what is referred to as a *syncytial knot*. In the face of injury, the trophoblast tends to revert to a more primitive type, and with fetal disease, cytotrophoblast may occasionally be readily seen. A more common event, however, is the deposition of maternal fibrin on the surfaces of villi. Apparently, it is possible for this to build up, perhaps by interference with flow in the intervillous space, so that eventually large areas of a cotyledon may be deprived of normal maternal circulation. This, in turn, appears to be followed by a shutdown of activity on the fetal side, and eventually a large inactive area of placenta that is slowly undergoing involution can be seen.

AREA AVAILABLE FOR EXCHANGE

In the presence of all these changes, apparently the area available for diffusion increases slowly but steadily, at least until the last few weeks of pregnancy. Regardless of the gross size or weight of the placenta, what is really important in terms of fetal welfare is the area available for diffusion. Such processes as intervillous fibrin deposition and the calcification that occurs within the intervillous space under these circumstances reduce the area for diffusion, but whether the net effective area of normal placenta is reduced is not known.

The concept of *aging of the placenta* has in part been based upon anatomic evidence. In addition, studies of placental exchange have shown some decreases in exchange near term. There is some question whether enough data have been obtained from these studies to permit the generalization that there is a diminution in function, comparable to senescence, which is a simple consequence of the age of the placenta. Nevertheless, this concept, which suggests an increasing precariousness of intrauterine life as term approaches, has great appeal, and the concept of placental senescence as a basis for clinical management still dominates a good deal of thinking. It may be correct, but most of the evidence for it is still intuitive.

CIRCULATION

The circulation through the placenta on the fetal side is simple. The umbilical arteries divide as the umbilical cord reaches its attachment to the membranes and subdivide continuously to supply arterial blood to all portions of the placenta. The arteries proceed down intervillous stems into precapillary arterioles and then into the capillaries traversing the villi themselves. These capillaries then empty into venules, which join to form veins and eventually give rise to the umbilical vein. There are also arteriovenous anastomoses that permit bypass of villous capillaries.

On the maternal side, the original circulation comes from the capillary extensions of the endometrial arterioles. As the placenta grows and as the placental circulation becomes more complex, the rather sluggish capillary circulation through the trophoblastic lacunae is succeeded by a circulation arising from the endometrial arterioles themselves. This is, of course, under greater pressure, since it empties into venules without the intervention of a capillary bed. As demonstrated in Figure 16–16, blood enters the intervillous space under the pressure of maternal arterial systole. Blood almost certainly enters the intervillous space continuously, but under much greater force and at a greater speed during systole. The blood thus injected through the open tips of the arterioles mixes in the intervillous space and leaves the placenta through veins at the

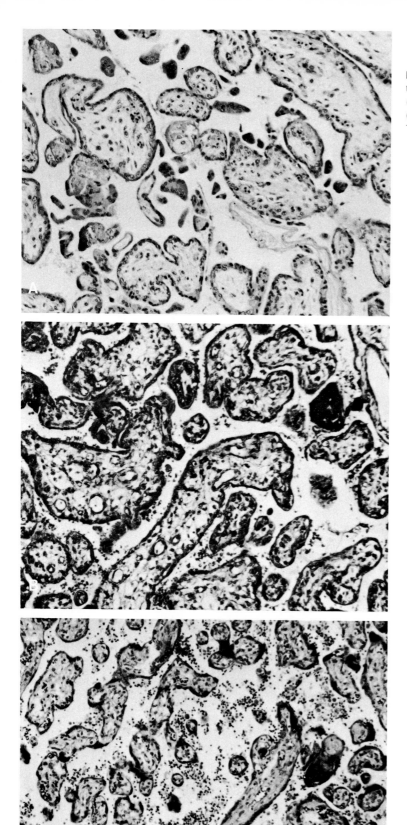

FIG. 16–15. Photomicrographs, at same magnification, of villous substance of placenta at 6 weeks (*A*), at 6 months (*B*), and at term (*C*), (×200). (Wilkin P: Pathologie du Placenta. Paris, Masson, 1965)

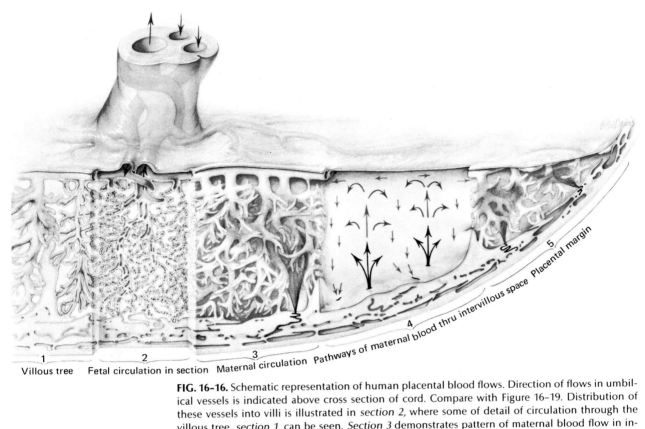

FIG. 16–16. Schematic representation of human placental blood flows. Direction of flows in umbilical vessels is indicated above cross section of cord. Compare with Figure 16–19. Distribution of these vessels into villi is illustrated in *section 2*, where some of detail of circulation through the villous tree, *section 1*, can be seen. *Section 3* demonstrates pattern of maternal blood flow in intervillous space; for clarity, finer villi are omitted so that the intervillous space appears more empty than it is in fact. *Section 4* shows maternal intervillous space flow schematically, making clear that outflow proceeds through subchorionic lake and through basal veins. *Section 5* depicts these same arrangements at margin of placenta. Marginal sinus is inconstant feature of widely varying size. (Ramsey EM, Davis RB: Carnegie Institution of Washington Year Book 61. Washington, DC, Carnegie Institution, 1962)

base of the cotyledons. Some of the blood in the intervillous space mixes just under the fetal surface of the chorion in the subchorionic lake and, indeed, may flow transversely across the placenta to enter the marginal vein at its edge.

There is some evidence that not all endometrial arterial jets are functional at all times and that the rate of flow from each endometrial artery is under some form of local control, either by the muscles in the wall of the artery itself or by localized contraction of the myometrium through which the artery must pass before reaching the intervillous space. It is, therefore, likely that under normal conditions the entire placenta is not in a state of maximum function at any single time. Furthermore, since intrauterine pressure during uterine contractions may approach or even exceed maternal systolic pressure, there are periods when there is no inflow to the placenta. Very little is known about the venous outflow from the placenta; there is evidence that this outflow is also influenced by uterine contractions (Figs. 16–17 and 16–18).

The biochemical characteristics of the blood in the portions of the intervillous space quite near the inflow tracts are necessarily different from those of the blood in the outflow tracts. Thus, the composition of intervillous space blood is not uniform, but varies from place to place within the intervillous space and from time to time, related to changes in local vascular control and in uterine contractility. There is, of course, an average value, but from a practical standpoint there is no possiblity of obtaining blood samples that will assuredly represent it.

Since villi in immense numbers are present in the intervillous space, where they serve as baffles, it is by no means unusual for fragments of trophoblast, or even whole villi, to break off and enter the maternal circulation. Some of these are trapped in blood vessels within the uterine wall; indeed, this is where they are

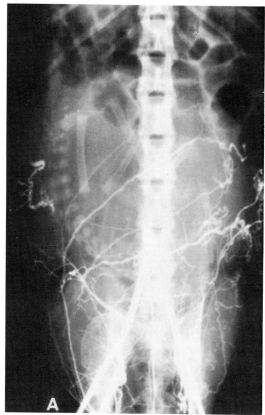

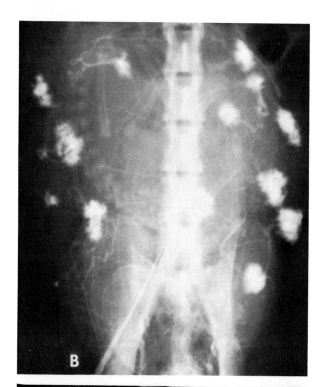

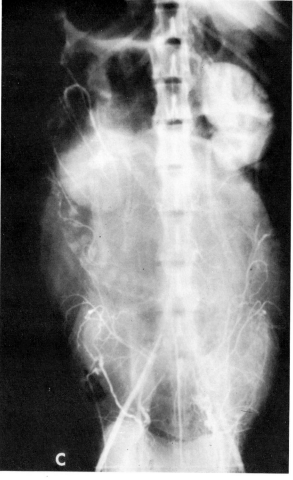

FIG. 16–17. Radiographs taken following injection of radiopaque material into aorta of macaque on 130th day of pregnancy. Fetal spine and extremities are clearly seen. *A* and *B* were taken 2 and 6 sec, respectively, after injection during uterine relaxation. In *A*, femoral and uterine arteries are well opacified, and many small uterine arterial branches to both placentas can be seen. In *B*, spurts of material into intervillous space are clearly shown. In *C*, taken 4 sec after injection during a strong uterine contraction, spurts previously seen are no longer visible. (Courtesy EM Ramsey and Carnegie Institution of Washington)

most commonly found when suitable material is available for examination. However, a trophoblast fragment can reach the maternal lungs, where it may be found at autopsy performed on an otherwise normal pregnant woman who has died suddenly. When the placenta is normal, this trophoblast apparently does not have the capacity to implant in or invade the structures of the lung.

MATERNAL-FETAL BLOOD EXCHANGE

It is possible, with gross breaks in the placenta, for maternal blood to enter the fetal circulation or fetal blood to enter the maternal circulation. In view of the pressure relations involved, the latter event is more

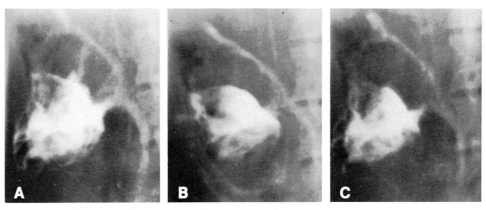

FIG. 16-18. Radiographs taken after slow injection of radiopaque material into intervillous space of macaque placenta on 99th day of pregnancy. In *A*, several drainage channels can be seen. In *B*, taken during uterine contraction, size of intravillous space pool has changed little, but drainage tracts are emptied. In *C*, taken as uterus relaxed, drainage tracts are restored. (Ramsey EM, Martin CB, Jr, McGaughey HS, Kaiser IH, Donner MW: Am J Obstet Gynecol 95:948, 1966)

likely, but it is also more difficult to prove. The fetus must lose a relatively large amount of blood into its mother's circulation before it is demonstrable by analysis of the concentration of fetal hemoglobin in maternal blood or by differential blood typing.

It is likely that the incidence of fetomaternal exchange has been exaggerated on the basis of the frequently observed increased concentration of hemoglobin F in the circulation of the pregnant woman. In supposing that this event proves the presence of fetal blood in the maternal circulation, many authors have overlooked the fact that increased maternal production of hemoglobin F is a response to a high chorionic gonadotropin concentration, combined with the stress on the bone marrow caused by the need to keep up with drainage of iron by the fetus. It is noteworthy that the highest concentrations of hemoglobin F observed in the pregnant woman have occurred in the presence of hydatidiform mole, in which case there is no fetal erythropoiesis and the hemoglobin F must arise from the woman's own bone marrow.

For the perfusion of any sizable amount of blood from fetus to mother, the break in the fetal circulation must occur in the fetal arteriole. This does take place; there are now a large number of unquestionably demonstrated instances of fetomaternal transfusion, provable because, among other things, a severely anemic infant was born. This may account for a certain number of otherwise unexplained stillbirths as well.

There is also a substantial body of evidence for transmission of maternal erythrocytes, leukocytes, and platelets to the fetus, so there can be no doubt about the transfer of solutes such as antibodies from mother to fetus.

Transfer of formed fetal blood elements to the mother in immunologically significant amounts is most likely to occur at the time of placental separation. For this reason, the administration of anti-D (anti-Rh) globulin to prevent D sensitization in an unsensitized D-negative mother who has borne a D-positive child is undertaken in the early puerperium.

EXCHANGE ACROSS THE PLACENTA

Ever since it was established that the maternal and fetal circulations are separate, the phenomenon of exchange across this intact membrane has fascinated investigators. There are many analogies between exchange across the lung and exchange across the placenta, particularly in regard to the transfer of gases. The difference lies primarily in the fact that in the placenta the exchange occurs in a water-to-water system, whereas in the lung the exchange occurs in an air-to-water system. It is also highly probable that the functions of lung and placenta are different. Since it has been proved that exchange across the lung takes place by passive diffusion in proportion to gradients, it is tempting to extend this without argument to the placenta; in fact, this mechanism does apply for a number of substances. The placenta, however, is a more complex structure than the lung, and the exchange process is not the same for all substances. Page has suggested that placental exchange be discussed in terms of four groups of substances:

Group I: Substances Concerned with Maintenance of Biochemical Homeostasis or Protection Against Sudden Fetal Death. For these substances the rate of transfer is measured in milligrams per second, and the predominant mechanism is rapid diffusion. In this category are the electrolytes, water,

and the respiratory gases. In regard to oxygen, the gradient on the two sides of the placenta is considerable, corresponding to a very rapid rate of exchange. On the other hand, although the gross exchange of water is immense, the gradient is quite small because the net exchange is relatively small. The best estimate is that the gross transfer of water in one direction across the placenta is in excess of 500 ml/sec. Carbon dioxide, which is more soluble in water than oxygen, has a very small gradient but a very large gross transfer. An electrolyte such as sodium travels at its peak rate at about 1 mg/sec, so the range of transfer in this class of substances is rather large. Finally, because some substances that are probably exchanged at these rates are metabolized in the placenta, the net transfer appears to be negligible. Examples are 5-hydroxytryptamine and possibly epinephrine, which can be affected by the very high concentration of monoamine oxidase in the placenta.

Group II: Substances Concerned Primarily with Fetal Nutrition. Exchange of these substances is measured in milligrams per minute. They are primarily moved by carrier systems, although the process of diffusion is also involved. Examples are the amino acids, sugars, and most of the water-soluble vitamins. For some substances there may be carrier systems operating equally in both directions; this appears to be the case, in some species, in regard to glucose, because the transfer of this substance is far in excess of what can be accounted for by diffusion alone. Some materials, such as the amino acids, are found in greater concentration in fetal than in maternal plasma; these substances are likely moved by carrier systems that operate against a concentration gradient. A third type of material is exemplified by riboflavin. The total content of riboflavin in fetal blood is 20% higher than that in maternal blood, whereas the free riboflavin content is 300% greater. There appears to be, therefore, an unequal distribution of these substances, with some sort of alteration of the riboflavin molecule or its precursor during active transport across the placenta.

Group III: Substances Concerned Primarily with Modifications of Fetal Growth and Maintenance of Pregnancy. Transfer of these substances is measured in milligrams per hour. The predominant mechanism of transport is probably slow diffusion of relatively large molecules. Most of the hormones are in this group. The most satisfactory information currently available relates to labeled thyroxine and estrogen and progesterone.

Group IV: Substances of Immunologic Importance Only. Transfer of these substances is measured in milligrams per day and may occur by leakage through large pores in the placenta or by droplet transfer by pinocytosis. There is evidence that particles as large as red cells can traverse the placenta through breaks in its membrane. There is also, however, some evidence that this is not normal, and using Group IV substances to illustrate exchange under physiologic conditions might be questioned. Also included in this group are plasma proteins, which may be exchanged by means of the droplets in the vesicles that have been observed in the placental epithelium under the electron microscope.

PLACENTAL HORMONE PRODUCTION

The role of the placenta as an important endocrine gland is considered in Chapter 18.

PLACENTAL METABOLISM

The placenta is endowed with an incredible variety of enzyme systems. These have been studied mostly *in vitro*. It is a safe generalization that, given appropriate conditions in a Warburg apparatus and given a substrate and suitable cofactors, living placenta will manifest almost any enzymatic reaction that has been observed in other tissues. The conclusions to be drawn from this and related observations are limited.

The intrinsic metabolic activity of the placenta is rather low. There is good evidence that most of the activity of the placenta in the genesis of hormones and the exchange of materials resides in the trophoblast and that the connective tissue stroma and the walls of the fetal blood vessels are inactive. Under these circumstances, the energy consumption of the placenta is not great, although, like the lung, it has an immense blood flow. So far there is little evidence to suggest a correlation between any known abnormality of pregnancy and change in placental metabolism. Since intervillous fibrin and infarcts are undoubtedly metabolically inert, when they make up a sizable fraction of placental weight, activity per gram is low. It is, therefore, difficult to determine the metabolic activity of the living fraction of placenta.

One placental enzyme, diamine oxidase, which is actually a histaminase, is found in steadily increasing amounts in the maternal plasma as pregnancy proceeds. Its concentration has been used, along with other findings, as an indicator of fetoplacental well-being.

PREGNANCY-SPECIFIC β-1 Glycoprotein

Pregnancy-specific β-1-glycoprotein (PSβG) is produced by the trophoblast and is secreted primarily into the intervillous space, quickly reaching both the ma-

TABLE 16-1. PS/βG CONCENTRATIONS (μG/LITER) IN VARIOUS BODY FLUIDS DURING PREGNANCY

Body Fluid	Concentration
MATERNAL BLOOD	
21–24 days postovulation	50–100
10–11 weeks	10400 ± 3100
20 weeks	33500 ± 970
20–21 weeks	53000 ± 16900
38 weeks	250000 (50th centile)
38 weeks	159000 ± 48000
38 weeks	199300 ± 48600
38 weeks	139300 ± 42500
AMNIOTIC FLUID	
15–22 weeks	616 ± 180*
27–40 weeks	300–3800
TERM	1400
TERM	1260 ± 120
TERM	938 ± 534*
CORD BLOOD	
17–22 weeks	116 ± 65
25 weeks	66
27–40 weeks	100 − 600
TERM	295
TERM	327 ± 150
BREAST MILK	
Colostrum 25 weeks	135
TERM	160
URINE	
3–8 weeks postovulation	0–400*
early pregnancy	0–4000
late pregnancy	0–30000
TERM	0–8000

* Figures given here were calculated from data shown graphically (adopted from Horne CHW, Towler CM: Obstet Gynecol Surv 33:761, 1978)

ternal bloodstream and the amniotic fluid. The substance can be detected in maternal serum as early as 7 days after ovulation, and thereafter it increases very rapidly in the various body fluids (Table 16–1). Its function is not known; but, since PSβG is of placental origin, it has been suggested that the body fluid levels may provide an index of placental function. The serum level has been correlated with fetal weight, indicating a possible application in the diagnosis of intrauterine growth retardation. Since it is unique to pregnancy and appears very early, it has been suggested as a simple, rapid, specific test for pregnancy.

THE UMBILICAL CORD

LOCATION

The umbilical cord runs from the infant's umbilicus to the point of its insertion in the membranes or placenta. The origin of the umbilical cord from the umbilicus is subject to few variations; the most common is *omphalocele*. In this condition, the ring of connective tissue of the anterior abdominal wall at the point of the umbilicus fails to close, and a certain portion of the intestinal contents are not in the abdomen proper but in the sac, which is lined by peritoneum and covered by a thin layer that resembles amnion. This sac joins the skin of the infant at the level of the anterior abdominal wall. The cord ordinarily inserts on the apex of this mass, and the vessels than run along the mass between the two thin covering layers. This does not seem to interfere with the function of the umbilical cord during intrauterine life.

ANATOMY AND HISTOLOGY

The cord itself consists of the umbilical vessels, ordinarily two arteries and one vein. A small amount of connective tissue, within which is distributed a gelatinous material known as *Wharton's jelly*, supports these structures. All this is covered by a thin layer of amnion.

The microscopic appearance of the umbilical cord varies according to whether it has been fixed in the

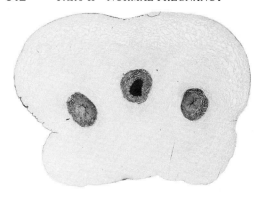

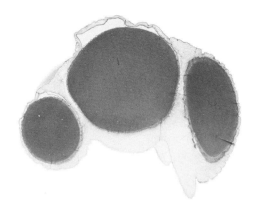

FIG. 16–19. Cross sections of umbilical cord fixed after collapse (*above*) and in distended state (*below*). Vein is between two arteries here. Cord is distended during function *in utero*. (Reynolds SRM: Anat Rec 113:368, 1952)

distended or collapsed state (Fig. 16–19). If the cord is clamped while in a state of distention and then fixed, it is clear that the vessels are huge relative to the connective tissue, Wharton's jelly, and amnion. On the other hand, in cross sections of the collapsed umbilical cord, which are the kind ordinarily studied in the pathology laboratoy, the vessels look rather trivial.

The arteries have characteristic arterial walls. The vein has more than the expected amount of connective tissue and muscle in its wall. The stroma contains very few cells, and these have scanty cytoplasm. Occasionally, on the surface of the cord the cells of the amnion are slightly piled up, which creates the appearance of small squamous plaques. In contrast to the fetal villi, there are ordinarily no wandering cells in the stroma of the umbilical cord.

LENGTH

Umbilical cords have been observed to vary from 20–150 cm in length. The normal length is in the range of 50–70 cm. As the umbilical cord reaches a greater length, the incidence of complications, such as cord obstruction due to wrapping of the cord around the baby's neck or over the extremities and prolapse of the cord, increases. Such complications are still relatively infrequent, however. The umbilical cord, being an erectile structure maintained in a state of turgor during normal intrauterine life, does not tend to fall loosely from one place to another as it does after delivery. If its blood flow is obstructed, the cord may become flaccid and more liable to accident; it may be that cord abnormalities are the consequence of primary interference with cord circulation. However, the presence of cord wrapped around the neck one, two, three, or more times is not presumptive evidence of fetal difficulty and may in fact cause no trouble at all.

An unusually short cord may be responsible for dystocia, since it may literally restrict the descent of the fetus, much as a dog is restricted by the length of the chain attached to its collar.

DISTRIBUTION OF BLOOD VESSELS

Within the umbilical cord, the distribution of blood vessels is subject to a number of variations. For one thing, the vessels tend to coil around one another. Although it is generally supposed that the vein is interposed between the two arteries, this is ordinarily not the case. The vein is subject to more twists and turns than the arteries and may produce rather complex structures in which it is coiled upon itself, producing what is called a *false knot*. The thickness of the arterial walls and the greater force of blood flowing through them apparently endow the umbilical arteries with greater resistance to this kind of reduplication. Although from time to time it has been proposed that the pulsatile flow through the umbilical arteries may have some influence in maintaining flow through the umbilical vein in the opposite direction, the complexities of the umbilical vein provide so many exceptions to the anatomic relationships between it and the umbilical arteries that the general proposition is probably incorrect. False knots are, of course, of no clinical consequence. On the other hand, if the cord is long, it is possible, particularly in the middle trimester of pregnancy, for the infant to pass through a loop of the cord and thereby create a *true knot*. In fact, this may occur more than once, and several true knots may be encountered in the cord. Since the cord is an erectile structure, it is unusual for a true knot to be pulled tight enough to produce irreversible cord obstruction.

BLOOD FLOW

Total blood flow through the umbilical cord has been estimated approximately 125 ml/kg/min, or approxi-

mately 500 ml/min in the average human fetus at term. Within the fetus the umbilical arteries are the main branches of the dorsal aorta, arising from the external iliacs just beyond the bifurcation of the common iliac arteries and constituting their major branches. The systolic pressure in the umbilical arteries is about 60 mm Hg and the diastolic about 30 mm Hg. There is a pressure drop across the placental capillary bed such that the pressure in the umbilical vein is about 20 mm Hg and is not pulsatile. As the blood enters the abdominal wall of the fetus in the umbilical vein, it enters the liver, where it can flow either into the substance of the liver or directly into the inferior vena cava. Between the umbilical vein and the inferior vena cava is interposed the ductus venosus, in which is located a sphincteric mechanism that is at least partly under nervous control. Under certain circumstances contraction of the ductus venosus diverts blood into the substance of the liver, whence it returns to the systemic circulation through the hepatic vein. Under other circumstances the ductus relaxes and allows blood to flow directly into the right atrium. This structure, therefore, is located in such a position as to have a regulatory influence on the pressure in the umbilical vein. As mentioned earlier, the umbilical vein must have an elevated blood pressure, since the blood vessels in the villi have to be maintained in a state of patency while within the intervillous space, which is itself under pressure greater than the venous pressure of the mother.

Under steady-state conditions, there is evidence that the placental blood flow is near maximal. There is no known mechanism by which the fetus can alter blood flow under stress and only inferential evidence of major vascular bed shunts within the fetus.

THE FETAL MEMBRANES

ANATOMY AND HISTOLOGY

In the ordinary course of events, the fetal membranes line the uterine cavity and completely surround the fetus. The chorion, the outer membrane, forms a good deal of the connective tissue thickness of the placenta on its fetal side and is the structure in and through which the major branching umbilical vessels travel on the surface of the placenta. The remnants of the yolk sac are found resting on top of the chorion, ordinarily near the insertion of the umbilical cord. Occasionally, small fluid-containing cysts are formed by duplications of the chorion on the placental surface. When felt grossly, this membrane is quite thin but obviously more than a single layer of cells in thickness.

The outer side, which is ordinarily applied to the decidua reflexa (the area of the altered endometrium that is not the site of the implantation of the placenta), is a little roughened and may be adherent in areas

where more than the ordinary degree of villous penetration by the chorion frondosum took place. The chorion does not ordinarily have a fetal blood supply except in cases of velamentous insertion; even then, the fetal blood vessels do not have branches to the chorion, and it is reasonable to suppose that the vascular support of the chorion is provided primarily by blood vessels arising from the decidua. On its inner (fetal) side, the chorion is juxtaposed to the outer layer of amnion (Figs. 16–20 and 16–21).

These two membranes slide upon each other readily; indeed, there is only trivial connective tissue attachment between the two. This looseness of attachment between amnion and chorion may not only provide some safety features for the fetus in the course of its growth but also may permit differential sliding in the event the chorion ruptures while the amnion remains intact in the course of labor and delivery. The inner surface of the amnion has a smooth, slippery lining and is shiny in appearance under normal circumstances. The strength of the membranes is imparted by the layer of dense connective tissue to which the amnion epithelial cells are attached.

MEMBRANES IN MULTIPLE PREGNANCY

In multiple pregnancy, the membranes may be duplicated; the ultimate number of amnion and chorion layers depends on the number of eggs from which the multiple pregnancy was derived. In the case of monozygotic (derived from a single egg) twins, it depends on the stage of gestation at which splitting took place. Since secondary resorption of some of the layers can also occur, dizygotic twins (derived from two separate eggs) are occasionally found lying within a single chorion but, of course, separate amnions. Examination of the membranes can be considered conclusive proof of monozygotic twinning only when both infants are found within a single amniotic sac. If infants are found within a single chorion, it is likely that they are monozygotic twins. When chorion and amnion are both unquestionably duplicated, it is likely that the twins are dizygotic, but this again is not conclusive (see Chap. 43).

FUNCTION

The principal functions of the membranes appear to be to retain and to assist in forming the amniotic fluid. This provides for growth and development of the fetus in a stable, mechanically buffered environment and in a state of relative weightlessness, since the specific gravity of the infant is, for practical purposes, the same as the specific gravity of the amniotic fluid. Growth and development of extremities are therefore unimpeded, and resistance to fetal muscular activity is di-

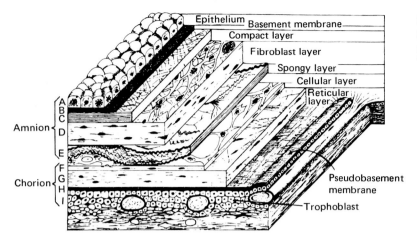

FIG. 16-20. Composite diagram showing relationships of layers of amnion and chorion. (Bourne GS: Am J Obstet Gynecol 79:1070, 1960)

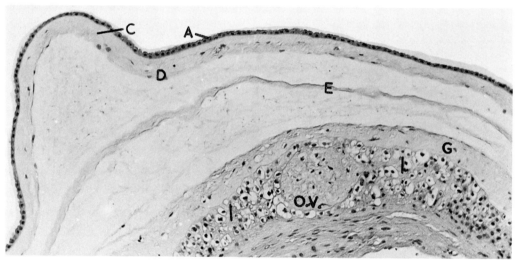

FIG. 16-21. Human amnion and chorion. *A,* Epithelium. *C,* Compact layer composed of dense connective tissue. *D,* Fibroblast layer. *E,* Spongy layer. *G,* Reticular area. *I,* Trophoblast. *OV,* Obliterated villus. (×90, reduced) (Reproduced by kind permission from The Human Amnion and Chorion, 1962, by Gordon Bourne. London, Lloyd–Luke Medical Books)

minished compared with what would be present in the uterus without an interposing buffer of fluid. The amniotic sac is also a repository for a number of secretions and excretions from the fetal urinary, respiratory, and alimentary tracts. Exchange of materials between the fetus and amniotic fluid is essentially rather sluggish, but there is rapid transfer of water between the amniotic fluid and the mother, presumably across the amnion and chorion in the large surface area applied to the decidua.

During most of gestation, amniotic fluid is similar to plasma in total osmolarity and electrolyte content, al-

though it has a relatively low protein content. Near term it becomes hypotonic relative to plasma, and the sodium concentration drops, the decrease in cations accounting for virtually all the drop in osmolarity. The cause of the drop in osmolarity is not known. Fetal urine undoubtedly contributes to, but hardly accounts for, the observed hourly water turnover of 350–600 ml. The exchange of water may occur by simple diffusion, but there is a characteristic differential in the transfer rate of certain tagged substances. In the rat, there are differences in protein fractions between amniotic fluid and maternal serum, which suggests that the exchange process is neither by transudation nor by the ultrafiltration of plasma. The demonstration of special amnion cells that overlie the placenta and are believed to have secretory properties (Fig. 16–22) suggests that the membranes themselves play an important role in amniotic fluid formation.

FIG. 16–22. Isolated cells from placental surface of amnion. Brush type border is evident in cells, canalicular apparatus in focus in one cell. (Original mag. ×323) (Danforth DN, Hull RW: Am J Obstet Gynecol 75:541, 1958)

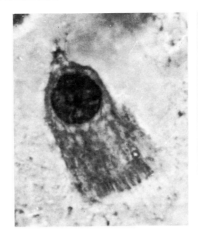
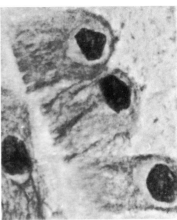

THE AMNIOTIC FLUID

Amniotic fluid is derived from maternal and fetal sources. The major portions are a maternal plasma filtrate and a fetal urinary contribution. Exchange of water takes place from the cavity across the amnion and chorion into the maternal decidua and into the placenta itself. Some exchange occurs across the umbilical cord. There is a flow of fluid into and out of the respiratory passages, and the fetus swallows a considerable fraction. Thereafter, exchange takes place across fetal mucous membranes. All the components of amniotic fluid are simultaneously being exchanged in the intervillous space between fetus and mother. This has been idealized and studied as a three-compartment system, as illustrated in the classic figure of Hutchinson *et al.* (Fig. 16–23).

At term, the gross exchange of water between fetus and mother is about 3500 ml/hour in each direction. Between fetus and amniotic fluid, it is about 225 ml/hour in each direction. The normal fetus is believed to swallow about 20 ml fluid an hour, but exchange in the respiratory tree of the fetus is still unmeasured. The gross exchange between amniotic fluid and maternal decidua, presumably directly across the membranes, is also about 225 ml in each direction. In normal pregnancy at term, the net turnover of fluid is probably no more than 10 ml/hour. The total volume at term is variable but generally less than 1 liter.

In the first half of pregnancy, the fluid is similar to maternal plasma, but the osmolarity declines steadily to term. This is attributed to dilution with increasing amounts of fetal urine, since the concentrations of urea and creatinine rise and those of sodium, potassium, and chloride fall. The exchange rates appear to be specific for each solute.

Various clinical observations, some confirmed by experimental study, have shed some light on this most complex relation. Fetuses lacking kidneys have virtually no amniotic fluid. When a fetus has no hypothalamus, excessive fluid is present. Hydramnios is common in diabetic pregnancy. In severe hemolytic disease, hydramnios may accompany hydrops fetalis and placental edema. This is usually due to fetal hypoproteinemia and cardiac failure. The hydramnios and hydrops may occur without fetal hemolysis and are then of unknown cause.

Amniotic fluid has an odor and a distinct faint yellow or greenish yellow color; the nature and source of the responsible substances are not known. Near term, the fluid becomes opalescent, probably because of the presence of vernix caseosa.

The pH of the fluid is 7.22 early in pregnancy and falls to 7.11 at term. Carbon dioxide pressure correspondingly rises from 41–51 mm Hg, while the bicarbonate concentration falls slightly. Oxygen pressure is always quite low, usually below 10 mm Hg. Bilirubin is present at midpregnancy but gradually decreases to almost nil at 36 weeks. Protein follows a similar course.

The formed elements are all of fetal origin. Viable cells can be cultured and stained for genetic studies. As the fetus becomes older, however, laboratory culture is less successful. As term approaches, there are increasing amounts of fat derived from the fetus's vernix caseosa, a fatty material coating the skin, principally over the vertex, back, and extremities. Occasionally several millimeters thick, it is vigorously antibacterial.

There is no known physiologic or pharmacologic means of affecting amniotic fluid volume. Early in pregnancy, the ratio of fluid to fetus is large. At about 20 weeks, it is approximately 3:2. Thereafter, the rate of fetal growth exceeds that of fluid accumulation, and at term there is ordinarily no more than a few hundred milliliters. The volume of amniotic fluid at the different stages of pregnancy is shown in Figure 16–24.

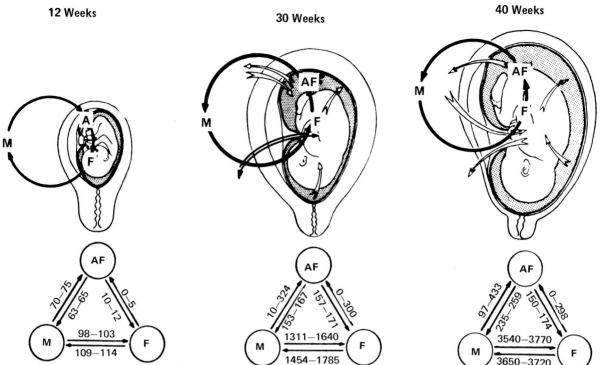

FIG. 16–23. Schematic representation of water exchange among mother (M), fetus (F), and amniotic fluid (AF) in pregnancy. *Arrows* in the lower diagrams indicate directions; *numbers,* hourly gross transfer in milliliters. *Heavy circles* on *left* of upper diagrams indicate direction of net transfer. (Hutchinson DL et al.: J Clin Invest 38:979, 1959)

THE FETUS

The somatic growth and development of what eventually will be the newborn infant can be divided into three major stages. The first is the period of differentiation, which begins at the time of fertilization and ends when the last structure destined to be present at birth has formed. Streeter devoted the latter years of his distinguished career as an embryologist to the delineation of events during this period and was satisfied that the final structure to make its appearance in the human fetus is the nutrient artery of the humerus, which appears toward the end of the 11th week after ovulation.

In the second period, a time of rapid growth that extends from the 11th to approximately the 27th week after ovulation, the fetus reaches a weight of approximately 850 g but has still not developed to the point where it is likely to survive if born. Few fetuses in this age range survive birth.

From the 27th week after ovulation until term, al-

though the rate of growth necessarily slowly decreases, the absolute growth increases rapidly to eventual term size of approximately 3300 g, with increasing physiologic maturity, survival becomes increasingly possible (Figs. 16–25 and 16–26). Among the factors concerned in fetal growth, insulin appears to have an important role. This is supported by the finding of very high concentrations of high-affinity receptors for insulin on fetal cells.

DIFFERENTIATION

Streeter's greatest contribution was the delineation of what he referred to as the *horizons of embryonic development.* Not only does each organ system have a definite time sequence for its appearance and differentiation and, as in the case of the urinary apparatus, for the disappearance of primitive early structures and their replacement by later definitive ones, but also the sequence of events in one system is related to the sequence of events in other systems. If deviations occur from these normal sequences and relationships, fetal abnormality results.

The sequential and predetermined nature of fetal development has two practical corollaries: 1) a noxious event cannot influence the development of a structure

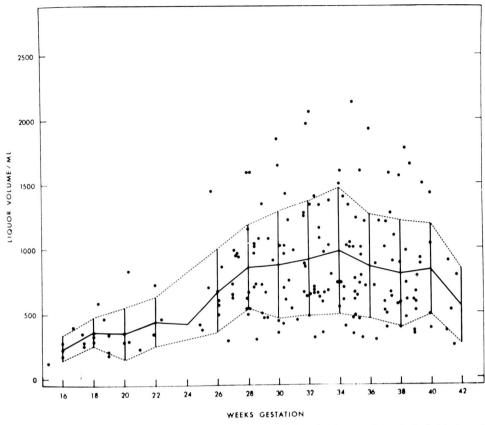

FIG. 16-24. Range of normal volumes of amniotic fluid plotted against weeks of gestation. (Queenan JT, Thompson W, Whitfield CR et al.: Am J Obstet Gynecol 114:34, 1972)

if the event takes place prior to the appearance of the structure in the embryo, and 2) if the noxious event occurs well after the structure has been differentiated and it is undergoing growth only, deletion of the structure is exceedingly unlikely. Thus, rubella causes congenital cataracts only if the fetus is infected at the precise time when the lens is developing; infection earlier or later does not produce the defect. Table 16–2 indicates the period of gestation during which certain common malformations may occur.

DEVELOPMENT SUBSEQUENT TO DIFFERENTIATION

When differentiation is completed (11th week), the eventual infant should no longer be referred to as an embryo; it should be called a fetus. Its growth continues in terms of increasing development of organ systems to a degree of maturity that will permit extrauterine survival.

Intrauterine circulation, respiratory gas exchange, and thermoregulation are discussed in Chapter 42 in

FIG. 16-25. Fetal growth by weeks of gestation, based on over 11,000 births at University Hospitals of Cleveland, 1956–1962. *Heavy solid line* indicates mean; *dashed line,* 11 standard deviation; *light solid line,* 12 standard deviations. Compare with Figure 16–13. (Hendricks CH: Obstet Gynecol 24:358, 1964)

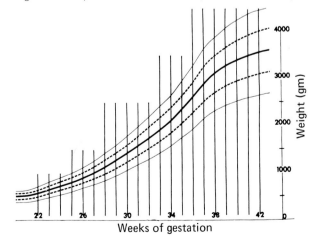

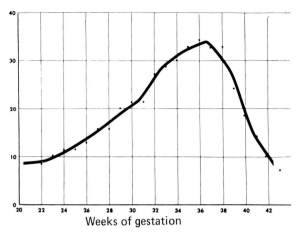

FIG. 16-26. Mean daily fetal growth in grams during previous week of gestation, based on same data as Figure 16-25. (Hendricks CH: Obstet Gynecol 24:358, 1964)

TABLE 16-2. PERIOD OF GESTATION DURING WHICH CERTAIN FETAL MALFORMATIONS OCCUR

Week Since Ovulation	Potential Malformation
3	Ectopia cordis
	Omphalocele
	Ectromelia
	Sympodia
4	Omphalocele
	Ectromelia
	Tracheoesophageal fistula
	Hemivertebra
5	Tracheoesophageal fistula
	Hemivertebra
	Nuclear cataract
	Microphthalmia
	Facial clefts
	Carpal or pedal ablation
6	Microphthalmia
	Carpal or pedal ablation
	Harelip, agnathia
	Lenticular cataract
	Congenital heart disease
	Gross septal and aortic anomalies
7	Congenital heart disease
	Interventricular septal defects
	Pulmonary stenosis
	Digital ablation
	Cleft palate, micrognathia
	Epicanthus, brachycephaly
8	Congenital heart disease
	Epicanthus, brachycephaly
	Persistent ostium primum
	Nasal bone ablation
	Digital stunting

connection with the changes in these mechanisms associated with birth. Intrauterine development of the other organs and systems is discussed in the following.

Heart

The function of the myocardium is the same in the fetus as in the infant or adult. Of all the characteristics that can be observed before birth, the fetal heart rate is the most susceptible to quantitation.

The heartbeat can be detected by ultrasound devices, which use the Doppler principle, as early as the 9th menstrual week of pregnancy. Then and for the remainder of pregnancy, the heart rate is between 120 and 160 beats/min. There is no trend in rate with time for an individual fetus or for fetuses as a group, and a fetus may exhibit much fluctuation in rate from week to week. Contrary to persistent superstition, the rate is not related to the sex of the fetus.

The fetal electrocardiogram is essentially indistinguishable from that of the newborn, except that multiple leads cannot be studied. An occasional instance of complete fetal heart block is observed, manifest by a steady heart rate of 60 or below when there has been no obstetric accident and persisting for days and weeks. This continues during labor and into the newborn period and may be associated with anatomic defects. Even rarer instances of *in utero* atrial tachycardia with rates up to 220 beats/min have been seen. This can result in intrauterine cardiac failure. The rate may revert to normal after birth, with complete recovery. Rarer still are irregularities of rate, sometimes due to a wandering pacemaker. These also ordinarily vanish shortly after birth.

Abnormalities of fetal heart rate associated with the acute changes of labor or cord obstruction are described in Chapter 41.

Fetal Blood Analysis

It is possible, once labor has begun, to obtain small samples of fetal blood directly from the fetal scalp or buttock. The use of an analysis of this blood as an early warning of fetal distress, especially in correlation with changes in fetal heart rate, has been intensely investigated. It is important in these studies to determine that the mother's acid–base balance is normal, since maternal acidosis is rapidly reflected in the fetus.

In normal early labor, the pH of fetal capillary blood

is about 7.30; the lower limit is about 7.20. The carbon dioxide pressure is about 40 mm Hg, and the base deficit 6.5 mEq. The oxygen pressure is 22 mm Hg. As labor progresses, the fetal pH tends to decrease.

Lungs

Although they are present quite early in fetal life, the lungs are lined at first by columnar epithelium in the upper reaches of the respiratory tree and by transitional cuboidal epithelium in its lower portions. Gradually, the alveolar ducts differentiate from the terminal bronchioles, and the epithelium thins out. At the same time, capillaries proliferate toward the surfaces of the air sacs. Eventually, rudimentary alveolar sacs make their appearance, but these are not present in large numbers prior to the 32nd week (Fig. 16–27).

Anatomic maturity is, of course, essential for extrauterine survival, but the lungs must also be functionally prepared. Functional maturity depends largely on the formation of *surfactant*, a surface-active material that lines the pulmonary alveoli and reduces surface tension at the tissue–air interface. The alveolar epithelium consists of squamous lining cells (type I) and septal cells (type II). The main characteristic of the type II cells is the presence of osmiophilic lamellar inclusion bodies (Fig. 16–28), which are responsible for the synthesis of surfactant. The type I and type II cells differentiate between 20 and 24 weeks' gestation, and the lamellar bodies make their appearance shortly thereafter. The number of type II cells rapidly increases, and increasing numbers of inclusion bodies are discharged into the alveoli and thence to the amniotic fluid, correlating with the increasing alveolar surfactant and the increased amounts of surface-active lecithin in the amniotic fluid.

Gluck and Kulovich noted a rapid late gestational surge of total amniotic fluid phospholipids and observed that the ratio of amniotic fluid lecithin to sphingomyelin (L/S ratio) correlated directly with pulmonary maturity and, hence, with the likelihood that the preterm newborn would develop respiratory distress syndrome (RDS). In this syndrome, surfactant deficiency leads to incomplete postnatal lung expansion, expiratory atelectasis, and impaired gas exchange. The following L/S ratios are found in normal, uncomplicated pregnancy: At 12 weeks, 0.5:1; at 31 weeks, 1:1; at 31–33 weeks, 1:1; at 35 weeks, 2:1; and at term 4:1. RDS does not occur in the newborn if the L/S ratio is 2:1 or higher. The L/S ratio and cortisol levels in amniotic fluid show high correlation, and the evidence suggests that fetal cortisol is probably the important physiologic regulator of surfactant production. Hence, preterm infants suffer a serious anatomic disadvantage in effecting gas exchange across the lung.

It is likely that vigorous respiratory activity conditioned by effective central nervous system stimulation

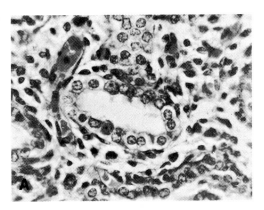

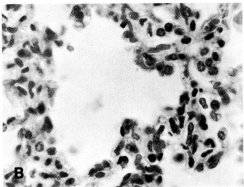

FIG. 16-27. *A.* Section of lung of 18-week stillborn infant. Air space is lined with cuboidal epithelium. *B.* Section of lung of 38-week stillborn infant. Lumen of air space is much greater, but lining cells are so dispersed that they are not visible. (Both ×541, reduced) (Valdes–Dapena MA: Atlas of Fetal and Neonatal Histology. Philadelphia, Lippincott, 1957)

and an adequate circulation may facilitate the expansion of alveoli and the progressive thinning of the epithelial lining. Thus, there is a fine interdependence among the general condition of the baby at birth, the anatomic and functional maturity of the lungs, and the infant's chances for survival. The maturity of the epithelial lining of the lung probably establishes the lower limit for viability of the human newborn, since this structure's prompt function for gaseous exchange is absolutely essential to the maintenance of homeostasis once the placental circulation has been interrupted. Recent studies of fetal breathing suggest that the respiratory movements of the human fetus can be a valuable aid in determining fetal well-being (see Chapter 41).

Kidneys

Although the preterm kidney is not efficient, it suffices for the limited needs of a normal fetus, provided acid–base regulation can be achieved by gas exchange

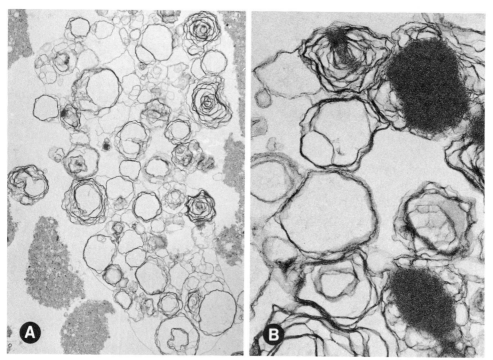

FIG. 16–28. *A.* Large cluster of lamellar bodies from a term infant. Peripheral lamellae of adjacent lamellar bodies are closely associated with each other in this complex. Amorphous flocculent debris is also present. (×5250) *B.* Laminar strands formed by "unwinding" of peripheral portions of lamellar bodies. Two lamellar bodies exhibit conspicuous electron-opaque cores that are also continuous with laminar strands. Same specimen shown in *A.* (×20800) (Lee W, Bell M, Novy MJ: Am J Obstet Gynecol 136:60, 1980)

in the lung. The kidney excretory system is fully differentiated quite early in fetal life, but the renal cortex is by no means fully formed even at the time of birth. Grossly, there persist irregularities in the surface that are referred to as *fetal lobulations* (Fig. 16–29). At the time of birth and for several weeks thereafter, glomeruli continue to differentiate from the area immediately under the renal cortex. This provides a microscopic appearance that is characteristic of the newborn kidney and distinguishes it from that of the adult. Remarkably enough, these anatomic changes are not accompanied by striking alterations of function. Obviously, there are sufficient numbers of glomeruli to produce a large glomerular filtrate, and the tubules are sufficiently differentiated to perform efficiently in the reabsorption of essential materials. There may be minor limitation in the ability of the fetal and newborn kidney to retain electrolytes, but it is certainly able to dilute and concentrate urine immediately after birth even in the preterm infant; failure to survive is never attributable to renal immaturity.

Adrenals

The adrenals of the human fetus in the third trimester and at delivery are remarkable structures; they are very nearly the same size as the kidneys. Almost all this bulk is made up of the fetal, or X, zone, which is part of the adrenal cortex. The adrenal medulla is unremarkable, and all the normal infant and adult layers of the adrenal cortex are present. In addition to this, there is a wide zone of cells that do not differ in microscopic appearance from those of the zona glomerulosa. Involution of this zone begins shortly after birth and is completed within the first few weeks of life, reducing the adrenals to their normal size proportionate to the kidneys.

This zone is absent only from the grossly abnormal adrenals associated with major defects of the central nervous system, such as anencephaly. At the present time, however, nothing is known with assurance about the function of this fetal adrenal zone. It is not observed in most other mammalian fetuses. There are no unique adrenal steroids excreted by the human fetus or newborn that could conceivably be produced in this zone, nor does there seem to be any unique function associated with intrauterine life that is suddenly lost at the time of birth when this zone begins to undergo regression. The normal human newborn, furthermore, does not exhibit signs of adrenal insufficiency, so the necrosis of the adrenal cortex in the newborn is apparently a selective process. The nature of the stimu-

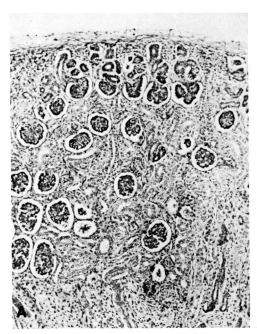

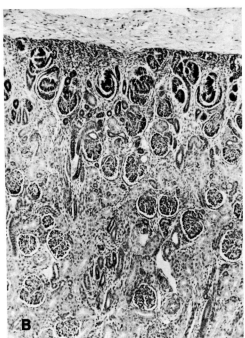

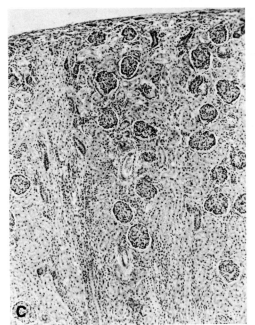

FIG. 16–29. *A.* Section of kidney of 16-week still-born infant. Many glomeruli are incompletely differentiated and tubules are not developed. *B.* Section of kidney of 24-week infant who lived 4 hours. Glomeruli are still forming from cortex and are much more developed than at 16 weeks (*A*). Tubules occupy more space in parenchyma. *C.* Section of 40-week infant who lived 2.5 days. Glomerular formation from cortex is still in progress, but cortex has achieved almost adult appearance. (All ×68, reduced) (Valdes–Dapena MA: Atlas of Fetal and Neonatal Histology. Philadelphia, Lippincott, 1957)

lus for this regression is unknown; it has never been observed prior to birth and does not fail to occur after birth.

As outlined in Chapter 18, the fetal adrenals, in conjunction with the fetal liver and the placenta, play a key role in the production of estrogens in pregnancy. As pregnancy advances, they are also a potent and increasing source of cortisol, much of which finds its way into the amniotic fluid. The increasing cortisol concentration in amniotic fluid correlates well with the L/S ratios, and it has been suggested that the demonstrated increase in cortisol production by the fetal adrenals may be responsible for inducing fetal lung maturation. Specifically, the evidence supports the hypothesis that one function of the fetal adrenal cortex is to control the differentiation of the alveolar epithelium

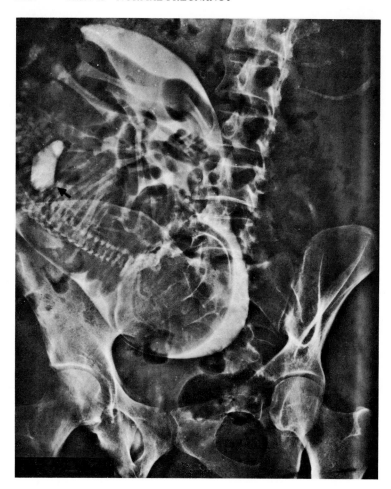

FIG. 16–30. Roentgenographic demonstration of radiopaque medium in amniotic fluid and stomach of fetus at 35–36 weeks' gestation. Hypaque was injected into amniotic fluid by transabdominal amniocentesis 1 hour earlier. Head can be seen in contrast; *arrow* indicates stomach. (McLain CR: Am J Obstet Gynecol 86:1079, 1963)

and, hence, the synthesis of phospholipid surfactant.

The possible role of the fetal adrenal in precipitating the onset of labor is considered in Chapter 29.

Central Nervous System

The central nervous system of the fetus is functional well before birth. The strongest evidence of this is that electroencephalograms have been obtained from the fetus *in utero*. The low amplitude and random nature of the waves suggest that there is little sensory input to the central nervous system. However, the diencephalon is not essential for fetal growth and development; infants who are born with cerebral agenesis may appear almost entirely normal in the neonatal state and may exhibit no external anomalies. It is unlikely that function of the midbrain is necessary for normal fetal development, although this is difficult to decide inasmuch as anomalies of the development of the midbrain are often associated with other congenital defects.

Gastrointestinal Tract

The gastrointestinal tract, which is almost completely developed rather early in fetal life, is also functional well before term. This has been demonstrated by the injection of radiopaque material into the amniotic fluid (Fig. 16–30). The opaque medium can be observed to enter the fetal stomach and pass down the fetal gastrointestinal tract.

The solid material in amniotic fluid that is available for fetal swallowing consists primarily of the desquamated surface epithelium of the fetus, fetal hairs, and particles of vernix caseosa. The remaining material in amniotic fluid is in solution or suspension but, in either event, is available for absorption through the small intestine. Since under ordinary circumstances defecation does not take place *in utero,* the large intestine becomes packed with the partially digested or undigested remnants of the solid material of the amniotic fluid mixed with bile pigment and unaltered by bacte-

rial decomposition. This viscid greenish black material is known as *meconium.* A certain portion of the material reabsorbed from the gastrointestinal tract is excreted by the fetal kidney into the excretory apparatus and thence into the amniotic fluid, from which it is reabsorbed. The same material, of course, also enters the fetal circulation and is available for exchange back into the mother directly through the intervillous space. The material in the amniotic fluid is available for direct transfer to the maternal circulation across the membranes.

To the gastrointestinal system for the turnover of water and electrolytes may be added absorption of these materials in the respiratory tree and the contributions of the secretory areas of the upper respiratory passages to the material found in amniotic fluid. The importance of these mechanisms in the normal turnover of amniotic fluid can be appreciated from the impact of anomalies on that system. Atresia high in the gastrointestinal tract, *e.g.,* in the esophagus, stomach, or duodenum, which interferes with the swallowing of amniotic fluid and its passage into the small intestine, is frequently associated with marked hydramnios. Obstruction lower down in the gastrointestinal tract, the most striking example of which is imperforate anus, has no such result. On the other hand, agenesis of the kidneys or marked obstruction in the excretory system from the kidney is ordinarily associated with severe oligohydramnios. That the unusual quantities of amniotic fluid are a direct result of the organ defect and not associated anomalies has been demonstrated by the artificial production of oligohydramnios in the primate fetus by *in utero* bilateral nephrectomy.

Musculoskeletal System

Normal differentiation of the musculoskeletal system is essential for the fundamental framework for fetal growth. The skull forms mostly from membranous bone, whereas the spinal column and the extremities form primarily from cartilaginous bone. For this reason, the ossification centers of the spinal column can be identified roentgenographically far earlier than the skull itself. This evidence of the existence of the fetus can sometimes be seen as early as the 14th week of pregnancy and almost always by the 18th week.

Capacity for Antibody Formation

The fetus synthesizes its own proteins, and there is little evidence of placental transfer of intact proteins from the mother. The concentration of albumin and globulins other than the γ-immunoglobulins of the fetus is about equal to the mother's throughout the last trimester, while that of the γ-globulins is much lower.

Transfer of maternal immunoglobulins, specifically

IgG, is accomplished by a splitting of the parent molecule into an Fab fragment, which contains the antigen-binding activity, and an Fc fragment, which contains the biologic activity in an inactive form. The Fc then crosses the placenta and presumably unites with Fab of fetal origin to reconstitute IgG. Such proteins as albumin and human growth hormone, which are smaller than IgG, do not cross the placenta.

The molecular weight of IgG is 144,000, and its half-life is 23–30 days. There is a rising curve of transfer (as Fc) as term approaches, and the IgG level in newborns is 700–1300 mg/100 ml. The IgG level is about 90 mg/100 ml in colostrum. The IgG falls after birth, depending principally on breast-feeding and minimally on infant production. By 6 months of age, levels vary from 200–1200 mg/100 ml. IgG has marked activity against bacterial toxins.

IgM has a molecular weight of 880,000 and does not cross the placenta in any form. It has a half-life of 5 days. The response of IgM production is very rapid, and mole for mole it is much more potent than IgG. The latter gradually replaces IgM in the antibody response to a given antigen.

IgM manifests marked activity against gram-negative bacilli and minimal antitoxin potency. In the newborn, IgM levels range from 0–30/100 ml in contrast to 10–90 mg/100 ml at 6 months of age. Curiously, perhaps as a reflection of the short half-life, IgM levels may not be elevated with proved but mild infections, so a low level does not rule out infection. The IgM level in colostrum is 40–50 mg/100 ml.

The normal fetus and newborn can synthesize IgG, but the rate by body weight is less than 1% of that of an adult. The extent of newborn protection, with a half-life of IgG of 30 days, is directly proportional to maternal plasma concentrations. Furthermore, to achieve proper active immunization of infants, it is necessary to wait after birth until the IgG level has fallen below threshold.

The maternal antibody responsible for isoimmunization and erythroblastosis fetalis is an IgG and consequently transfers readily to the fetus.

Alpha-Fetoprotein

α-Fetoprotein (AFP) is formed by the yolk sac and fetal liver, beginning as early as the 4th week of pregnancy. It increases rapidly in the fetal serum and makes its appearance in the amniotic fluid shortly thereafter. AFP can be detected in the serum of nonpregnant women at levels up to 10 ng/ml, but the higher levels in pregnancy are due specifically to production of this protein by the fetus. The first elevation of the AFP level in maternal serum is detected after 10 weeks; at 12 weeks, the level is approximately 25 ng/ml. Serum levels may vary from one laboratory to another, but serial tests show that they rise rapidly in

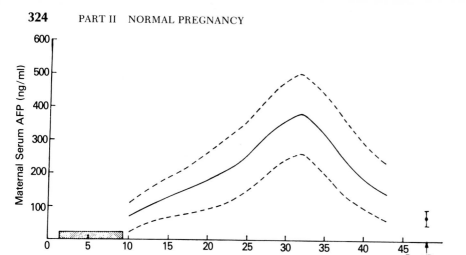

FIG. 16–31. Normal range for maternal serum α-fetoprotein according to gestation. (Hay DM, Forrester PI, Hancock RL et al.: J Obstet Gynaecol 83:534, 1976)

the second trimester and more slowly thereafter, reach a maximum at about 32 weeks, and then decline toward term (Fig. 16–31). The serum levels of AFP are elevated in certain circumstances (*e.g.*, recent transplacental amniocentesis, endothelial changes in the placental vessels as in Rh disease or preeclampsia, fetal death, neural tube defects, twins) and may have diagnostic usefulness (see Figure 44–00). Serum levels of AFP are also elevated in the presence of ovarian tumors that contain a significant vitelline component, *e.g.*, an endodermal sinus tumor.

Enzyme Systems

There is considerable evidence that not all enzyme systems are functioning at maximum efficiency at the time of birth. Perhaps the most important of these is the glucuronyl transferase system in the liver. In many newborn infants, this functions quite efficiently; but the less mature the infant, the less effective is the glucuronyl transferase system. As a consequence, substances in the blood that pass through the glomeruli and become available for renal excretion only when they are conjugated as glucuronides are not efficiently conjugated and tend to accumulate in the circulation. They may then be able to pass through capillary membranes and into the tissues in high concentration. The classic example of such a substance is bilirubin, which, under ordinary circumstances, is conjugated to a diglucuronide and readily excreted in the urine. If the glucuronyl transferase system is inefficient, either because it is not mature or because other substances are competing with bilirubin for its activity, the bilirubin may accumulate in the blood. The adaptive importance of this can be appreciated in light of the fact that conjugated bilirubin is highly polar and hence, when excreted into the intestines, is not readily reabsorbed. The unconjugated form, being lipid-soluble, crosses the placenta easily and the mother disposes of fetal unconjugated bilirubin efficiently. This system is limited not by enzymatic immaturity, but by the availability of transport protein in the fetus.

Relation of Fetal Maturity to Survival

The physiologic maturity of the fetus is directly related to its ability to survive in an extrauterine environment. However, the curve describing the relation of fetal age to survival is asymptotic. There is a striking increase in survival from the 33rd to the 37th week, but beyond that time changes are trivial.

REFERENCES AND RECOMMENDED READING

Adamson YR, Bowden DH: Reaction of cultured adult and fetal lung to prednisolone and thyroxine. Arch Pathol 99:80, 1975

Adamsons K (ed): Diagnosis and Treatment of Fetal Disorders. New York, Springer–Verlag, 1968

Assali NS (ed): Biology of Gestation, Vols 1, II. New York, Academic Press, 1968

An assessment of the hazards of amniocentesis. Report to the Medical Research Council by their working party on amniocentesis. Br J Obstet Gynaecol 85, Suppl 2, 1978

Benirschke K, Driscoll SG: Handbuch der speziellen pathologischen Anatomie und Histologie, Vol 7, Part 5, pp 98–616. Berlin, Springer, 1967

Boddy K: Fetal breathing: Its physiologic and clinical implications. Hosp Prac 89, 1979

Bourne G: Human Amnion and Chorion. London, Lloyd–Luke, 1962

Cowchock FS: Use of maternal blood protein levels in identification and management of high risk obstetric patients. Clin Obstet Gynecol 21:341, 1978

Danforth DN, Hull RW: Microscopic anatomy of the fetal membranes with particular reference to the detailed structure of the amnion. Am J Obstet Gynecol 75:536, 1958

Fencl M deM, Tulchinsky D: Total cortisol in amniotic fluid and fetal lung maturation. N Engl J Med 292:113, 1975

Fox H: Pathology of the Placenta. Philadelphia, WB Saunders, 1978

Freese UE, Maciolek JJ: Plastoid injection studies of the uteroplacental vascular relationship in the human. Obstet Gynecol 33:160, 1969

Gluck L, Kulovich M: Lecithin sphingomyelin ratios in amniotic fluid in normal and abnormal pregnancy. Am J Obstet Gynecol 115:539, 1973

Golbus MS, Louchman WD, Epstein CS et al.: Prenatal genetic diagnosis in 3000 amniocenteses. N Engl J Med 300:157, 1979

Grudzinskas JG, Evans DG, Gordon YB et al.: Pregnancy specific beta$_1$ glycoprotein in fetal and maternal compartments. Obstet Gynecol 52:43, 1978

Hay DM, Forrester PI, Hancock RL et al.: Maternal serum alpha-fetoprotein in normal pregnancy. Br J Obstet Gynaecol 8:534, 1976

Hendricks CH: Patterns of fetal and placental growth: The second half of pregnancy. Obstet Gynecol 24:357, 1964

Horne CHW, Towler CM: Pregnancy-specific beta$_1$ glycoprotein: A review. Obstet Gynecol Surv 33:761, 1978

Hutchinson DL, Gray MJ, Plentl AA et al.: The role of the fetus in the water exchange of the amniotic fluid of normal and hydramniotic patients. J Clin Invest 38:971, 1959

Hytten FE, Leitch I: Physiology of Human Pregnancy, 2nd ed. Oxford, Blackwell, 1971

Lee W, Bell M, Novy MJ: Pulmonary lamellar bodies in human amniotic fluid: Their relationship to fetal age and the lecithin/sphingomyelin ratio. Am J Obstet Gynecol 136:60, 1980

McLain CR: Amniography studies of the gastrointestinal mobility of the human fetus. Am J Obstet Gynecol 86:1079, 1963

Moghissi KS, Hafez ESE: Biology of Mammalian Fertilization and Implantation. Springfield, IL, Thomas, 1972

Moskalewski S, Pitak W, Czarnik Z: Demonstration of cells with IgG receptor in human placenta. Biol Neonate 26:268, 1975

Page EW: Transfer of materials across the human placenta. Am J Obstet Gynecol 74:705, 1957

Queenan JT, Thompson W, Whitfield CR et al.: Amniotic fluid volumes in normal pregnancies. Am J Obstet Gynecol 114:35, 1972

Ramsey, EM, Houston ML, Harris JWS: Interactions of the trophoblast and maternal tissues in three closely related primate species. Am J Obstet Gynecol 124:647, 1976

Ramsey EM, Martin CB, Jr, Donner MW: Fetal and maternal placental circulations. Am J Obstet Gynecol 98:419, 1967

Report of UK Collaborative Study on alpha-fetoprotein in relation to neural-tube defects. Lancet 1:1323, 1977

Reynolds SRM: The care and feeding of embryos. Int J Gynaecol Obstet 7:43, 109, 1969

Reynolds SRM: Mechanisms of placentofetal blood flow. Obstet Gynecol 51:245, 1978

Shields JR, Resnick R: Fetal lung maturation and the antenatal use of glucocorticoids to prevent the respiratory distress syndrome. Obstet Gynecol Surv 34:343, 1979

Streeter GL: Developmental horizons in human embryos: Age Groups XI to XXIII. Contrib Embryol, Vol II. Washington, DC, Carnegie Institution, 1951

Thorrson AV, Hintz RL: Insulin receptors in the newborn. N Engl J Med 297:908, 1977

Valdes–Dapena MA: Atlas of Fetal and Neonatal Histology. Philadelphia, Lippincott, 1957

Van Herendael BJ, Oberti C, Brosens I: Microanatomy of the human amniotic membranes. Am J Obstet Gynecol 131:872, 1978

Warkany J, Monroe BB, Sutherland BS: Intrauterine growth retardation. Am J Dis Child 102:294, 1961

Wilkin P: Pathologie du placenta. Paris, Masson, 1965

CHAPTER 17

MATERNAL PHYSIOLOGY

Edward J. Quilligan

The pregnant patient presents many symptoms and physical findings that are quite different from those of the nonpregnant patient. It is only with thorough knowledge of the changing physiology during pregnancy that the physician can understand and evaluate these symptoms and findings satisfactorily. Further, the physician must know physiology to recognize pathology, for pathology is, after all, only sluggish or overexuberant physiology. In general, the normal physiologic processes in the pregnant woman function at an increased level of activity; however, there are notable exceptions to this rule, particularly in the systems dominated by smooth muscle (*e.g.,* gastrointestinal and urinary tracts).

In the past, the reasons for the physiologic alterations of pregnancy were explained rather simply by the observation that all maternal systems are now working for two—mother and fetus. In this equation, the fetus is considered the extra and is therefore responsible for the changes. Recent knowledge has not really altered, but has only refined, this concept. It now appears that many pregnancy changes are the direct result of steroid or protein hormones from the fetoplacental unit acting on maternal systems. Taken a step further, this statement raises the interesting speculation that the fetus is in a sense at the controls during pregnancy. This leads to the question: Can the fetus control to some extent its own environment by altering maternal physiology?

In the consideration of each organ system, it should be remembered that in the final analysis all the pregnancy changes must be integrated to produce the functioning whole.

CENTRAL NERVOUS SYSTEM CHANGES

Many of the changes that occur in the central nervous system are manifest as emotional in character. During the first trimester, the patient experiences easy fatigability and has a desire to spend a larger proportion of her time sleeping. The cause of this is unknown, but it is postulated that the increased levels of progesterone in pregnancy play a role. Progesterone in high doses can cause somnolence, and the hormone has even been used in some instances as an anesthetic agent. Another common symptom in the first trimester is nausea with occasional vomiting. This probably is also central in its origin and is related to the increased level of estrogen in early pregnancy.

During the second trimester, the patient frequently experiences a period of euphoria and extreme well-being. The cause of this emotional state is unknown.

During the third trimester, there are again some elements of depression and chronic fatigue. Here the cause is perhaps simply that the patient is approaching the end of a 9-month period of stress and is carrying an increased amount of weight. It should be pointed out that the somnolence of the first trimester, the euphoria of the second, and the slight depression of the third are not universal; a woman may go through pregnancy with few or none of these apparently emotional reactions.

The severe emotional and psychiatric disturbances that may occur in pregnancy were once thought to be due to pregnancy *per se;* however, recent investigation has demonstrated that in all women so affected there is a background of emotional disturbance and that pregnancy simply acts as a trigger.

Physical coordination may be impaired in pregnancy, even before the uterine bulk is sufficient to constitute a mechanical impediment. Accordingly, pregnant women are advised to avoid any physical activity in which their safety may depend upon fine coordination or timing. Neuromuscular and reflex response are obviously involved, but the mechanism is obscure.

Measurements of blood flow to the central nervous system, using the nitrous oxide technique, have demonstrated no difference in this parameter between men and pregnant women.

RESPIRATORY SYSTEM CHANGES

The most obvious change that might be expected as pregnancy progresses is a gradual elevation of the diaphragm, and this indeed does occur. It is accompanied by compensatory flaring of the ribs, so there is no significant deficit in intrathoracic volume.

The respiratory rate remains unchanged throughout pregnancy. The *tidal volume* (that volume of air moved with each normal inspiration and expiration) gradually increases throughout pregnancy so that at term it is 30%–40% above the baseline levels. Milne *et al.* measured specific airway conductance in a group of women each month during pregnancy and for 3–5 months after delivery, and found no significant changes.

As pregnancy progresses, there is a gradually decreasing *expiratory reserve volume* (the maximum amount of air that can be expired after normal expiration), which reaches a maximum 20% decrease at term. There is a comparable decrease in the *residual volume* (volume of gas remaining in the lungs, not including anatomic dead space, at the end of maximum expiration). Since the functional residual capacity is the sum of the expiratory reserve plus the residual volume, there is a decrease in functional residual capacity as the pregnancy approaches term, this decrease being approximately 20% at term. The inspiratory capacity increases by about 10% in pregnancy, reaching a maximum at 22–24 weeks' gestation.

The timed vital capacity, as well as the *maximum breathing capacity* (the maximum amount of ventilation achieved by forced voluntary breathing in 15 sec) remain unchanged throughout pregnancy (Fig. 17–1).

The increase in respiratory tidal volume associated with the normal respiratory rate necessarily results in an increase in respiratory minute volume, the magnitude of this increase being approximately 26%. This increase in the respiratory minute volume is the *hyperventilation of pregnancy*, which is responsible for a decreased concentration of carbon dioxide in alveoli. The decreased concentration of carbon dioxide in the alveoli causes a lowered carbon dioxide tension in the blood of the pregnant woman. The oxygen tension in the alveoli remains within normal limits. The hyperventilation of pregnancy is apparently due to the increased levels of progesterone, as it has been mimicked in males given progesterone.

Dyspnea is common in pregnancy, but its cause is largely unknown. It is not due to encroachment of the enlarging uterus on the diaphragm, because almost

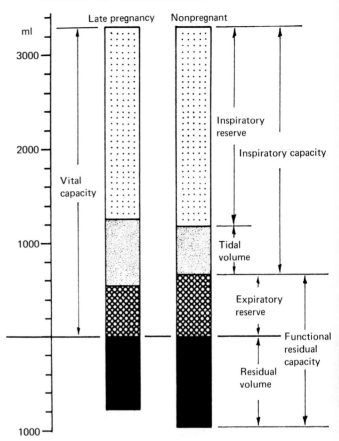

FIG. 17-1. Components of lung volume in late pregnancy and in nonpregnant state (Hytten FE, Leitch I: the Physiology of Human Pregnancy. Blackwell, Oxford, 1964)

half of Milne's subjects experienced dyspnea before 20 weeks' gestation, and 76% reported this symptom before 30 weeks. The time course of dyspnea fits fairly well with alveolar PCO_2 measurements, which reach their lowest levels before the third trimester. Among those who complain of dyspnea in pregnancy, measurements of respiratory function are usually normal for the stage of gestation. Campbell and Howell proposed that the sensation of dyspnea occurs when the ventilatory response is inappropriate to the demand, a theory that helps to explain many, but not all situations in which dyspnea occurs.

CARDIOVASCULAR CHANGES

HEART CHANGES

The changes in the configuration of the heart seen on x-ray film are fundamentally those caused by elevation of the diaphragm, *i.e.,* the heart appears larger since it

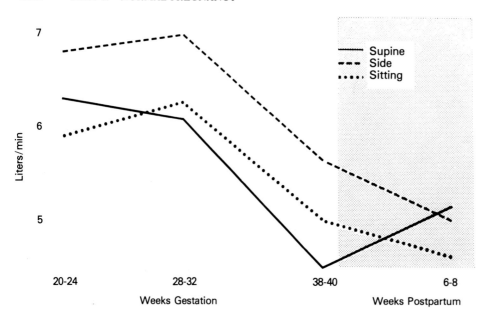

FIG. 17–2. Cardiac output at different stages of pregnancy and puerperium according to patient's position. (Ueland K, Novy MJ, Peterson EN, et al: Am J Obstet Gynecol 104:856, 1969)

is pushed upward and to the left, and the apex beat moves laterally. A number of investigators have actually found an increase in heart volume of the order of 10%–12%. The increase in volume may be due both to an increase in filling volume and to hypertrophy of cardiac muscle.

Systolic murmurs are common in pregnancy, probably because of changes in both the circulatory dynamics and the position of the heart as pregnancy advances. A pulmonic murmur can be heard at one time or another in almost all pregnant women; an apical systolic murmur, in about 60%. It is important that they be distinguished from organic murmurs, which tend to be present both when the woman is in the upright position and when she is supine, to be heard on both inspiration and expiration, and to become louder as the rate increases.

The heart rate increases during pregnancy by 10%–15%, reaching a maximum between 13 and 23 weeks' gestation. When the heart rate is measured only when the woman is in the lateral position, the increase throughout pregnancy appears to be gradual and progressive, reaching its maximum at term.

Premature ventricular contractions are sometimes troublesome in pregnancy; the woman may report that she has the sensation of her heart "doing a flip-flop" from time to time. These contractions are of no concern if they are infrequent and if there is no associated cardiac disease. It is not known why they are more common in pregnancy.

The changes in blood pressure during pregnancy are small in normotensive women, but there is general agreement that a slight decrease normally occurs, to the extent of 2–3 mm Hg in the systolic and 5–10 mm

Hg in the diastolic pressures. Both values tend to rise toward prepregnancy levels as term is approached. Women with essential hypertension may show a significant decrease in both systolic and diastolic pressures during the first two trimesters, with a return to the hypertensive state during the third trimester. This finding may make the differential diagnosis between preeclampsia and essential hypertension difficult.

The stroke volume increases to a maximum of about 30% between 13 and 23 weeks' gestation. From 19 weeks' gestation until term, some authors report that the stroke volume remains relatively unchanged; others report that it progressively decreases, reaching normal (prepregnancy) levels at term. The discrepancy between the various stroke volume findings can be explained by the position of the patient when the measurements of stroke volume or cardiac output were made (Fig. 17–2). Those who have reported a decrease in stroke volume as term approaches invariably made the measurements in the supine pregnant woman, while those reporting the stroke volume to be unchanged until term made their determinations with the patient in the lateral position. In any tests of cardiovascular dynamics in pregnancy, the position of the patient can markedly alter the results (Table 17–1).

The cardiac output has been measured during pregnancy in a variety of ways. More recently, a noninvasive technique, echocardiography, has permitted repeated measurements on the same woman throughout pregnancy, with minimal likelihood that their accuracy will be influenced by stress. In general, all techniques demonstrate that the cardiac output begins to increase early in the first trimester and rises fairly rapidly during this first 13 weeks (30%–50% above nor-

TABLE 17-1. HEMODYNAMIC PARAMETERS THROUGHOUT PREGNANCY

	Patient Position	1st Trimester	2nd Trimester	3rd Trimester	Postpartum
HEART RATE (beats/min)	L	77 ± 2	85 ± 2	88 ± 2	69 ± 2
	S	76 ± 2	84 ± 2	92 ± 2	70 ± 2
STROKE VOLUME (ml/min)	L	75 ± 3	86 ± 4	97 ± 5	79 ± 3
	S	82 ± 5	85 ± 4	87 ± 5	79 ± 3
CARDIAC OUTPUT $1/min/m^2$	L	3.53 ± 0.21	4.32 ± 0.22	4.85 ± 0.27	3.30 ± 0.17
	S	3.76 ± 0.24	4.19 ± 0.21	4.54 ± 0.28	3.33 ± 0.21
LEFT VENTRICULAR EJECTION TIME (msec)	L	302 ± 2	290 ± 5	281 ± 4	310 ± 5
	S	301 ± 3	286 ± 4	260 ± 4	307 ± 5
SYSTOLIC BLOOD PRESSURE (mm Hg)	L	98 ± 2	91 ± 2	95 ± 2	97 ± 2
	S	106 ± 2	102 ± 2	106 ± 2	110 ± 2
DIASTOLIC BLOOD PRESSURE (mm Hg)	L	53 ± 2	49 ± 2	50 ± 2	57 ± 2
	S	57 ± 2	60 ± 1	65 ± 2	65 ± 1

L, Lateral. **S,** Supine.
(Adapted from Katz R, Karliner JS, Resnick R: Circulation 58:434–441, 1978)

mal). During the third trimester some authors report a slight to moderate decline in cardiac output (5%–10%); others, an increase. Those reporting a decrease find values that are still above those of the nonpregnant woman; however, the actual values depend on the position of the patient when the measurements are made (Table 17–1 and Fig. 17–2). The change associated with position is undoubtedly at least partially due to compression of the vena cava by the pregnant uterus, which traps blood in the lower extremities and reduces venous return. Since the majority of pregnant patients, particularly at term, do not often lie supine, it is proper to consider that the cardiac output remains elevated at approximately 30% above baseline levels from about 30 weeks until term.

The cause of the increased cardiac output is incompletely understood. Two principal theories have been proposed. The first and oldest considers the placenta to be an arteriovenous shunt. Since there is in the strictest sense no capillary bed in the hemochorial placenta of the human, it has been held that the intervillous space is a functional arteriovenous shunt. However, both injection models and models of blood flow studied using cineangiography techniques have shown that flow through the intervillous space is not sufficiently rapid to produce this kind of change in cardiac output. The second theory proposes that the increase in cardiac output is a response of the heart to the increased levels of circulating estrogen during pregnancy. Supporting this thesis is the finding of Ueland and coworkers that in experimental animals a significant rise in cardiac output follows the injection of estrogens. Its mechanism is obscure.

TABLE 17-2. CHANGE IN CARDIAC OUTPUT WITH UTERINE CONTRACTIONS

	Percent Change in		
Position of Patient	Cardiac Output	Stroke Volume	Pulse
SUPINE	+24.8	+33.1	−15.0
LATERAL	+ 7.6	+ 7.7	− 0.7

(Ueland K, Hansen JM: Am J Obstet Gynecol 103:1, 1969)

Remarkable changes in cardiac output occur during labor. If the patient lies on her back, the cardiac output increases by 30% with each uterine contraction. If the patient lies on her side, cardiac output is also elevated, but only by 8%. The increase in cardiac output with each uterine contraction is fundamentally due to an increase in stroke volume, since with each uterine contraction during labor there is a slight or moderate decrease in the pulse rate, as well as an increase in blood pressure (Table 17–2). It has also been estimated that each labor contraction at term squeezes 400 ml blood into the general circulation.

In late pregnancy and labor there may be an accentuation of the vena cava compression syndrome referred to earlier, resulting in a significant drop in blood pressure. This *supine hypotensive syndrome* occurs in about 10% of pregnant women at or near term. The patient's blood pressure drops precipitously when she is lying supine, because blood is trapped in the lower extremities, venous return is diminished, and cardiac output is decreased (Figs. 17–3 and 17–4). This is

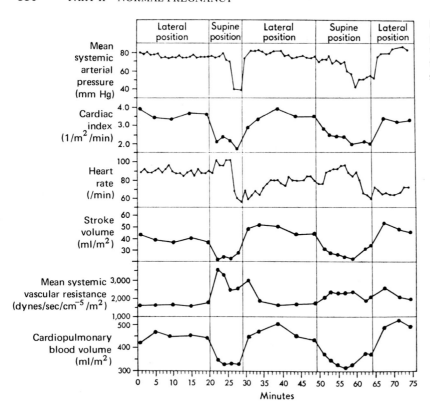

FIG. 17-3. Serial hemodynamic studies in patient with supine hypotension. After patient has been lying supine for 6 min, a profound fall in arterial blood pressure can be seen. (MG Kerr)

perhaps the easiest shock of all to treat; one simply turns the patient to the lateral position.

UTERINE BLOOD FLOW CHANGES

There is a dramatic increase in blood flow to the uterus during pregnancy. In the nonpregnant woman uterine blood flow is probably less than 50 ml/min. At 10 weeks' gestation, Assali *et al* found the flow to be about 50 ml/min, increasing gradually thereafter to 500 ml/min at term. The nitrous oxide equilibration method used in these studies provides only indirect measurement, and is less accurate than the measurements made in the sheep by use of a flow meter applied directly to the uterine artery. In the human, the pregnancy changes in uterine blood flow are probably similar to those found in the sheep: in the nonpregnant, 35 ml/min; at term, 1000 ml/min, of which 35% is directed to the placenta. In the sheep it has also been shown that the uterine vascular bed is widely dilated at term, and responds to α-adrenergic but not to β-adrenergic stimulators. In women, the uterine blood flow can be significantly increased by estradiol, a change that also occurs in pregnancy but to a lesser extent.

During labor in the sheep and monkey, blood flow diminishes as the uterus contracts, the reduction in flow being proportionate to the intensity of the contraction. In the human, using x-ray and dye-injection, Barell has shown that blood flow through the intervillous space either slows or stops completely during the contractions of labor.

VASCULAR SYSTEM CHANGES

The incidence of dissecting aneurysm of the aorta and rupture of aortic and splenic artery aneurysms is higher in pregnant women than in nonpregnant women of equivalent age. This difference appears to be due to pregnancy-associated change in the walls of the blood vessels. During pregnancy, the vessels have a looser overall texture and seem to be thinner; there is an increase in the smooth muscle in the vessel walls; the reticular fibers of the vessels are much more lacy and finely fragmented; acid mucopolysaccharides are decreased markedly in the larger vessels and to a lesser extent in the smaller vessels.

There is generalized peripheral vessel dilatation during pregnancy that results in a sixfold increase in peripheral blood flow. This rise is most marked during the last trimester and is due to decreased resistance in the precapillary arteries and arterioles; since there ap-

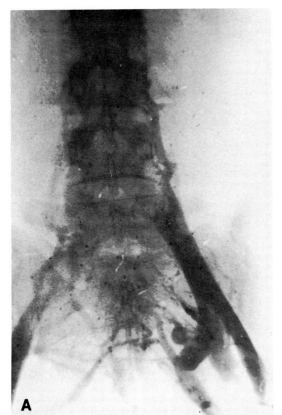
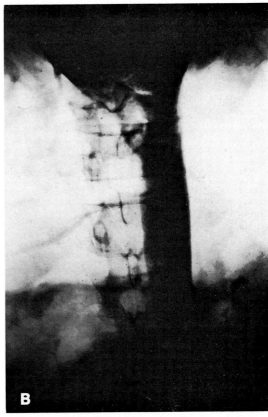

FIG. 17-4. *A.* Caval angiogram taken with patient in supine position before delivery by cesarean section. Note occlusion of inferior vena cava and prominent collateral venous circulation. *B.* Caval angiogram taken after delivery of same patient. Note normally patent inferior vena cava. (Kerr MG: Br Med Bull 24:19, 1968)

pears to be no increase in capillary filtration during pregnancy, it must be assumed that precapillary shunting is increased.

Venous distensibility increases progressively throughout pregnancy, reaching its maximum at term. This is due in large measure to the vascular changes and is responsible for the high incidence of varicosities in the lower extremities and anus during pregnancy. There is an increase in venous blood flow in the arm during pregnancy. There appears to be no increase in blood flow in the calf; however, in the study reporting this, there is no indication whether the patient's position was supine or lateral when the calf measurements were made. Position of the patient (lateral or supine) must influence determinations of blood flow in that area. The same study reported an increase in linear velocity of blood flow of the calf during pregnancy; however, this is not found in the forearm and again may be subject to change according to the patient's position.

BLOOD CHANGES

There is a marked increase in blood volume during pregnancy. A slight rise occurs during the first trimes-

ter, a more marked rise in the second trimester, a major increase up to 48% by the end of the second trimester, and a slight further rise in the third trimester. In the first half of pregnancy the increase in blood volume is greater than that in the red cell mass; later in pregnancy the reverse is true, *i.e.,* the red cell mass increases more rapidly. Overall, however, the increase in plasma volume slightly exceeds the increase in red cell mass so that the hematocrit value falls during pregnancy. If iron stores are adequate, the drop in hematocrit is minimal. In Pritchard's study, the decrease in hematocrit value was from an average of 41.7% in the nonpregnant state to approximately 37% late in pregnancy (Table 17-3). The iron demands of pregnancy and the changes that often lead to iron deficiency anemia are discussed on page 483.

The cause of the hypervolemia is at present unknown; however, there are several theories. It is known, for example, that in primary aldosteronism there is a marked increase in blood volume. Pregnancy

TABLE 17-3. BLOOD CHANGES IN PREGNANCY

Parameter	Late Pregnancy	Nonpregnant State	Percent Increase
BLOOD VOLUME (ml)	4820	3250	48
RBC VOLUME (cells/cu mm)	1790	1355	32
HEMATOCRIT (%)	37.0	41.7	

RBC, Red blood cell.
(Data from Pritchard JA: Anesthesiology 26:393, 1965)

is accompanied by an increase in aldosterone production, and it may be this hormone that is responsible for the hypervolemia. It is also known that blood volume can be increased by administration of large doses of estrogens, and indeed pregnancy is a hyperestrogenic state. Finally, large arteriovenous shunts are invariably accompanied by hypervolemia; and, as mentioned previously, the intervillous space may constitute an arteriovenous shunt.

During pregnancy, the leukocyte count increases from a prepregnancy mean of 4500 cells/cu mm to about 7500 cells/cu mm and may be as high as 15,000 cells, making a diagnosis of infection somewhat difficult during pregnancy. Polymorphonuclear leukocytes primarily are increased; there is little or no change in the lymphocyte series. Since the distribution of polymorphonuclear leukocytes in the differential count does not normally exceed the level for the nonpregnant state, any shifts in this parameter should be considered significant, not the result of pregnancy.

It has long been recognized that the pregnant woman is more susceptible to venous thrombosis. Fibrinogen increases from the normal value of 350 mg/100 ml to approximately 500 mg/100 ml, and both factor VII (proconvertin) and fibrinolytic activity decline. These factors, together with the expected venostasis in the lower extremities, would seem to provide ample reason for the noted increase in thrombophlebitis. Platelets have also been reported to increase by approximately one-third. The presence of large depots of tissue thromboplastin in the placenta, plus the hypercoagulable state of the pregnant woman's blood account for the intravascular coagulation that may be associated with abruptio placentae, the dead fetus syndrome, and amniotic fluid embolism.

Acid–base changes that occur during pregnancy are primarily the result of the respiratory changes mentioned previously. The increased ventilation and consequent blowing off of excessive amounts of carbon dioxide result in a compensated respiratory alkalosis. The carbon dioxide tension in the blood decreases from a normal prepregnancy value of about 38.5 mm Hg to approximately 31.3 mm Hg at term. There is a slight drop in standard plasma bicarbonate level from 23.4 mEq/liter in the nonpregnant state to 21.2

mEq/liter at term, and there is a concomitant fall in base excess from -0.7 mEq/liter in the nonpregnant state to about -3.5 mEq/liter at term (Table 17–4). All this leads to partially compensated respiratory alkalosis and elevation of blood pH from 7.35, the average nonpregnancy value, to 7.42 as term approaches. Most of this change has occurred by the 20th week of gestation. Hyperventilation, which is responsible, results from an increased sensitivity of the central nervous system to carbon dioxide tension in the blood, which in turn is thought to be due to elevated blood progesterone. This type of hyperventilation, although to a lesser degree, is also seen in the luteal phase of a normal menstrual cycle.

There are no characteristic changes in the *electrolyte* composition of the blood during pregnancy. Sodium, potassium, chlorides, and magnesium all remain within normal limits. There are changes, however, in *plasma and serum proteins.* The magnitude of the reduction of total proteins in plasma and serum has been the subject of some controversy, various authors reporting values between 0.15 and 1 g/100 ml. If the total proteins are considered according to their various fractions (albumin and α_1-α_2-, β_2-, and γ-globulins), there are differences in both magnitude and direction of change. Serum albumin decreases about 1 g/100 ml. The α_1- and α_2-globulins remain relatively unchanged during pregnancy, but they make up a higher proportion of total protein because of the drop in albumin. β-globulin rises conspiciously during pregnancy both as a proportion of the total protein and in absolute concentration. γ-Globulin remains relatively stable throughout pregnancy.

The blood level of *total lipids* rises during pregnancy from a mean prepregnancy value of 650 mg/100 ml to about 1000 mg/100 ml at the end of pregnancy. The total lipids are composed of several fractions, of which a major one is cholesterol. Serum cholesterol rises from a mean prepregnancy value of 180 mg/100 ml to 260 mg/100 ml at term. The major increment occurs after the 12th week of pregnancy; there may even be a decrease in cholesterol during the first 12 weeks of pregnancy. The phospholipids also rise from about 250 mg/100 ml at term. The lipids are carried in blood attached to proteins. These are α-lipoproteins

TABLE 17-4. ACID-BASE CHANGES IN PREGNANCY

Time	pH	pCO_2 (mm Hg)	Plasma Base Excess (mEq/liter)	Plasma Standard Bicarbonate (mEq/liter)
7–20 WK PREGNANCY	7.411	34.1	−2.5	22.0
21–30 WK PREGNANCY	7.402	33.6	−3.0	21.5
31–40 WK PREGNANCY	7.416	31.3	−3.5	21.2
2–5 MO POSTPARTUM	7.348	38.5	−0.7	23.4

(Modified from MacRae JJ, Palavradji D: J Obstet Gynaecol Br Commonw 74:11, 1967)

and β-lipoproteins. There is a larger rise in the β-lipoprotein so that the ratio of β- to α-lipoproteins increases during pregnancy. The mechanism for these changes in blood lipids may result from the increased estrogen levels in pregnancy. Similar changes have been observed in women taking oral contraceptives.

GASTROINTESTINAL CHANGES

There is frequently a marked increase in appetite during pregnancy. This may be an emotional reaction or may result from stimulation of the appetite center in the central nervous system. Occasionally, this increase in appetite assumes bizarre forms (*pica*) in which the patient has an overwhelming desire to eat foods not normally eaten. An example of pica is the desire to eat laundry starch, which may result in severe anemia in the pregnant patient. The cause of pica is at present unknown.

In the oral cavity during pregnancy there is a tendency to hypertrophy of the gums, sometimes sufficiently marked to produce bleeding. The cause is unknown but may be the high estrogen levels, as similar changes occur in women taking oral contraceptives. There are no fundamental changes in the teeth in pregnancy. Calcium in the teeth is stable and is not in constant circulation as is the calcium of the bones. Any tendency to caries in pregnancy results not from changes in the teeth, but from alterations in the composition of the saliva.

The remainder of the gastrointestinal tract is characterized by a decline in activity. Esophageal function in pregnancy has been studied by means of catheters to record the speed and amplitude of peristalsis and the pressure of the lower esophageal sphincter. Both peristaltic speed and amplitude are unchanged in early pregnancy, but they are reduced in late pregnancy. Although lower esophageal sphincter pressure is reduced, it is still higher than the slightly increased intragastric pressure. If a reversal of these pressures should occur, as in Ulmsten and Sundström's patients, severe heartburn may result.

It might be assumed that there is increased secretion of gastric acid during pregnancy, since heartburn is such a common symptom; however, this is not the case. Indeed, there is a decrease in the amount of acid secreted.

The general decrease in motility of the alimentary tract gives rise to constipation, another common symptom in pregnancy. The slower passage of food through the large bowel may permit an increased absorption of water with the result that the feces are dry, hard, and difficult to expel.

The gallbladder also suffers the smooth muscle lethargy of pregnancy, and x-ray studies demonstrate impaired emptying of the gallbladder at this time. Because of incomplete emptying, the large residual volume of bile may cause cholesterol crystals to be retained, increasing the risk of cholesterol gallstones.

The transport of food substances across the intestinal mucosa has not been extensively studied; however, some animal and some *in vitro* studies suggest that carbohydrate transport is not increased during pregnancy. There does appear to be an increase in iron absorption during pregnancy, but this is probably on the basis of increased demand for iron. Such a demand influences the absorption of iron in the nonpregnant as well as the pregnant state.

URINARY TRACT CHANGES

Marked changes in renal function occur in pregnancy. The renal plasma flow increases by 25%–50%. The sharpest increment occurs in the first trimester. There is little change from this high level in the second trimester and a decrease toward normal as term approaches. There is also an increase of about 50% in the glomerular filtration rate (Table 17–5). This too occurs early in pregnancy and remains at elevated levels until term. Values for the renal function tests, such as urea clearance and uric acid clearance, that depend primarily on filtration rate increase in pregnancy.

Hydroureter is a normal finding in pregnancy (Fig.

TABLE 17-5. CHANGES IN KIDNEY FUNCTION IN PREGNANCY

Time	Renal Plasma Flow (ml/min)	Glomerular Filtration Rate (ml/min)
13.0 WK PREGNANCY	804.67	161.33
20.8 WK PREGNANCY	749.13	157.11
38.0 WK PREGNANCY	589.00	146.00
20 WK POSTPARTUM	491.00	100.00
80 WK POSTPARTUM	549.00	97.00

(Modified from Sims EAH, Krantz KE: J Clin Invest 37:1764, 1958)

17–5), and it is almost invariably more marked on the right side. The cause is thought to be primarily mechanical obstruction of the ureter by the uterus as the ureter crosses the pelvic brim; however, it develops before the uterus is large enough to impinge upon the pelvic brim, and it progresses during pregnancy in the monkey despite reduction of uterine volume by removal of the fetus. Another possible cause of this physiologic hydroureter is the elevated progesterone level; however, studies have shown that large doses of progesterone in the nonpregnant woman do not cause hydroureter. Uterine dextrorotation may explain the customary exaggeration of the process on the right side. Ureteral motility remains normal in most of the ureter. There is, however, some reflux of urine from the bladder into the lower portion of the ureter during pregnancy.

All the foregoing may contribute to relative stasis of urine in the ureters, kidney pelvis, and at times, in the bladder; which, in turn, predisposes to urinary tract infection. Indeed, there is in pregnancy an increased incidence in both asymptomatic bacteriuria (6%) and acute pyelonephritis (1.5%). In the latter case, the predominant physical finding (costovertebral angle tenderness) is almost always more marked on the right side.

The patient frequently complains of increased micturition during pregnancy; frequency of urination is common and may be confused with one of the early symptoms of cystitis. This increase in micturition probably results from the increased vascularity of the trigone of the bladder, as well as the decrease in bladder capacity produced by the developing fetus.

CHANGES IN THE INTEGUMENT

The changes in the skin during pregnancy are more evident in some patients than in others and are sometimes quite bothersome. An increase in pigment deposition occurs on the face in a masklike distribution around the eyes and over the cheekbones. This is the characteristic mask (*chloasma*) of pregnancy, which occurs to some extent in most women, but is marked in some (Fig. 17–6). The mask usually disappears at the termination of pregnancy. There is also increased deposition of pigment in the areola of the breasts and in the line alba of the lower abdomen (which then becomes the linea nigra). The areolar and linea nigra changes may not regress completely after pregnancy is terminated.

In some patients, there appears to be a breakdown in subcutaneous tissue over the abdomen as the uterus enlarges. This produces the striae of pregnancy (Fig. 17–7), sometimes referred to as stretch marks. Actual stretching of the skin may be involved, but this is surely not the fundmental change. Striae are rarely found in the presence of abdominal distention by ascites or large ovarian tumors, and they are often found on the inner thighs and over the iliac crests where there is no stretching in pregnancy. Striae occur commonly after excessive weight loss and in conditions associated with high levels of adrenal steroids, such as Cushing's disease. Elevated levels of adrenal steroids in pregnancy may be responsible for striae gravidarum; an alteration in collagen–ground substance relation may also be concerned. During pregnancy, the striae frequently assume a purple color due to increased venous distention beneath the skin. After pregnancy terminates, the striae gradually become whitish in color; however, they do not disappear.

GENERAL CHANGES

The weight gain during pregnancy should be at least 15 lb or more above the prepregnancy weight. The fetus accounts for approximately 7 lb of the increase, amniotic fluid for about 2 lb, placenta for about 1.5–2 lb, uterine enlargement for about 2 lb, and breast enlargement for about 1 lb (Fig. 17–8). The remainder of the weight gain results from an increase in total body water, divided as shown in Table 17–6.

NITROGEN

The pregnant woman is anabolic in that she stores protein. This has been measured in various balance studies as the *total nitrogen* accumulated during pregnancy. In one large series of pregnant women, the total nitrogen accumulation from the 4th to the 10th month of gestation was found to be 515 g. Approximately 145 g of this could be accounted for by increases in growth of tissues, such as the uterus and breasts; however, 370 g nitrogen accumulation was totally unaccounted for. This large unaccountable accumulation of nitrogen has been confirmed in other studies.

FIG. 17–5. Intravenous pyelogram show-ing normal urinary tract changes at 7.5 months of pregnancy. Note excessive dilatation of renal pelvis (*upper arrow*) and ureter (*lower arrow*) on right. Note also ureteral kink (asymptomatic) owing to ureteral lengthening and dis-tortion of bladder by fetal head.

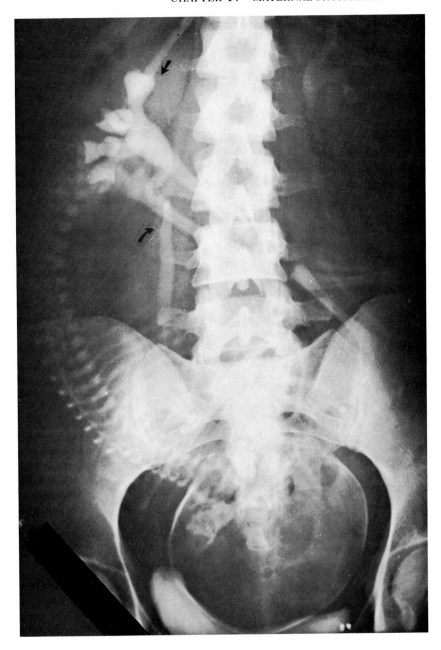

FAT

Fat storage is also a common finding. While most re-ports are not of serial studies on the same patient (and thus are open to some criticism), they do demonstrate an increase in total body fat. This increase obviously varies with the total weight gain of the patient. The obese patient who loses a great deal of weight during pregnancy may have an actual reduction of total body fat. In a study in which serial measurements of skin thickness were used as a manifestion of body fat, in-creases of 20%–40% were found, depending on the area of skin measured.

INSULIN–CARBOHYDRATE

Pregnancy is often considered diabetogenic. While there is considerable controversy about this, there seems no doubt that latent diabetes is frequently un-

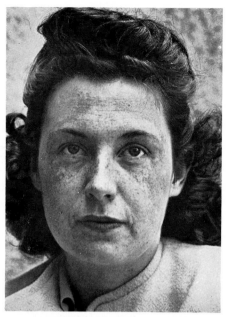

FIG. 17-6. Chloasma, mask of pregnancy. Pigmentation is often most prominent on bridge of nose and forehead. (Bookmiller MM, Bowen GL: Textbook of Obstetrics and Obstetric Nursing. Philadelphia, WB Saunders, 1963)

FIG. 17-7. Abdomen of patient at term, showing striae gravidarum and prominent linea nigra. (Bookmiller MM, Bowen GL: Textbook of Obstetrics and Obstetric Nursing. Philadelphia, WB Saunders, 1963)

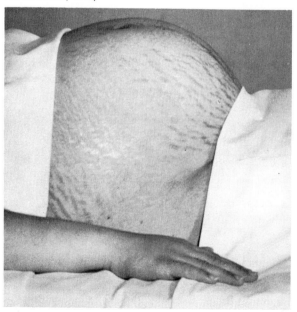

masked during pregnancy. *Plasma insulin* is elevated during pregnancy, and the insulinogenic response to an injected load of glucose appears to increase during pregnancy. There is a diminished reduction in blood glucose to a given insulin load. These two factors surely impose a stress upon the islet cells and may indeed be the factors responsible for unmasking a latent deficiency in islet cell secretion. In pregnancy, response to the glucose tolerance test performed with oral loading of glucose is similar to the response in the nonpregnant state; however, with intravenous loading, glucose disappears from the bloodstream faster in the pregnant than in the nonpregnant state. This is particularly true in the first trimester of pregnancy, and the glucose disappearance rate diminishes as term approaches. Even by 40 weeks' gestation, however, it is still elevated above prepregnancy levels.

MINERALS

Increased amounts of the *minerals* sodium, potassium, and calcium are stored in various compartments during pregnancy. While the greatest portion of these minerals is stored in the developing fetus (33% of the sodium, 48% of the potassium, and 90% of the calcium), there are also large amounts of sodium in the placenta, the amniotic fluid, and the edema fluid that collects in pregnancy. Increased amounts of potassium accumulate in the placenta, uterus, and breasts. Total serum calcium declines progressively during pregnancy, but both serum ionized calcium and parathyroid hormone increase progressively until delivery. In the serum of the newborn, total and ionized calcium, magnesium, and phosphorus are all significantly elevated, compared with the mother's serum at the time of delivery.

Iron, not stored during pregnancy, must obviously be supplied in increasing amounts to meet the needs of the expanding red cell mass, as well as those of the placenta and fetus. The increment of iron necessary for pregnancy has been calculated to be about 1000 mg, of which half is in the fetus and placenta and the remainder in the expanded red cell mass. Of the latter, about 150+ mg is lost at delivery, and the remaining 450 mg enters the mother's iron stores. (See also page 483).

OXYGEN CONSUMPTION

The pregnant woman's oxygen consumption increases by about 14%. The components of the increase in oxygen consumption are detailed in Figure 17–9. It is apparent that about half the increase in oxygen consumption is due to the products of conception, the remaining increase being due to the added uterine muscle and breast tissue, the increased work of respiration, and the increased cardiac work.

FIG. 17-8. Components of weight gain in normal pregnancy. (Hytten FE, Leitch I: The Physiology of Human Pregnancy. Oxford, Blackwell, 1964)

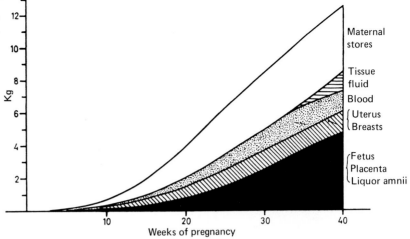

TABLE 17-6. ESTIMATE OF EXTRACELLULAR AND INTRACELLULAR WATER ADDED DURING PREGNANCY

	Total Water (ml)	Extracellular (ml)	Intracellular (ml)
FETUS	2343	1360	983
PLACENTA	540	260	280
LIQUOR AMNII	792	792	0
UTERUS	743	490	253
MAMMARY GLAND	304	148	156
PLASMA	920	920	0
RED CELLS	163	0	163
EXTRACELLULAR EXTRAVASCULAR WATER	1195	1195	0
TOTAL	7000	5165	1835

(Hytten FE, Leitch I: The Physiology of Human Pregnancy. Oxford, Blackwell, 1964)

FIG. 17-9. Components of increased oxygen consumption in pregnancy. (Hytten FE, Leitch I: The Physiology of Human Pregnancy. Oxford, Blackwell, 1964)

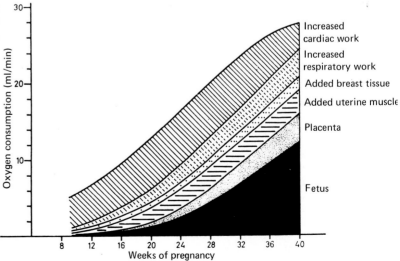

Weeks

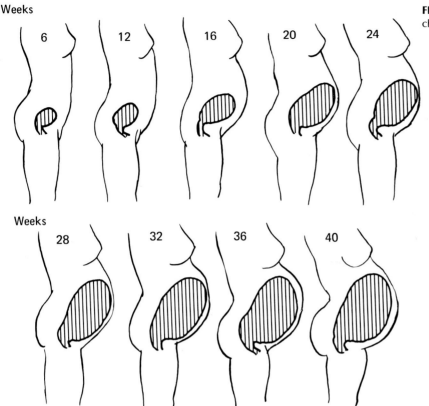

FIG. 17-10. Development of postural changes during pregnancy.

Weeks

BREASTS

The breasts undergo marked enlargement during pregnancy. This enlargement, associated with some tingling and occasionally pain, may be one of the very early signs of pregnancy. The enlargement of the breasts is due to an increase in the amount of ductal tissue, as well as to an increased deposition of fat. A clear substance, *colostrum,* can frequently be expressed from the breasts early in pregnancy. The breast tissue does not usually produce milk until about the 2nd or 3rd day after delivery. The pigmentation changes discussed earlier occur in the areola. Also in this area there are multiple small papules, called the *glands of Montgomery.* These are hypertrophied sebaceous glands.

POSTURE

The significant changes in *posture* during pregnancy are associated with one of the most common complaints—low back pain. The fundamental change is lumbar lordosis. This increase in curvature of the lumbar spine occurs because the patient's enlarging

uterus tends to change her center of gravity; therefore, she must lean backward to keep her balance (Fig. 17–10).

Some of the measurable pregnancy changes discussed in the foregoing sections are summarized in Table 17–7.

CHANGES IN THE REPRODUCTIVE TRACT

VULVAR CHANGES

Edema and increased vascularity are the major vulvar reactions to pregnancy. In multiparous women especially, the edema may be such that the patient feels, whenever she sits down, as though she were "sitting on something." Except in the grand multipara, vulvar varices are rarely seen in the nonpregnant state. They are common in pregnancy, however; and, although they are often large enough to be troublesome, phlebitis, rupture, or other secondary reactions are extremely unusual. Regardless of size, the varices usually regress completely when the pregnancy is over and, in fact, may vanish before the patient leaves the delivery table.

TABLE 17-7. SUMMARY OF MEASURABLE PREGNANCY CHANGES

Parameter	Percent Increase	Percent Decrease	Unchanged
RESPIRATORY SYSTEM			
Tidal volume	30–40		
Respiratory rate			x
Resistance of tracheobronchial tree		36	
Expiratory reserve		40	
Residual volume		40	
Functional residual capacity		25	
Vital capacity			x
Respiratory minute volume	40		
CARDIOVASCULAR SYSTEM			
Heart			
Rate	0–20		
Stroke volume	x		
Cardiac output	20–30		
Blood pressure			x
Peripheral blood flow	600		
Blood volume	48		
Blood constituents			
Leukocytes	70–100		
Fibrinogen	50		
Platelets	33		
Carbon dioxide		25	
Standard bicarbonate		10	
Proteins		15	
Lipids	33		
Phospholipids	30–40		
Cholesterol	100		
Clotting factors I, VII, VIII, IX, X, XIII	x	x	
GASTROINTESTINAL SYSTEM			
Cardiac sphincter tone		x	
Acid secretion		x	
Motility		x	
Gallbladder emptying		x	
URINARY TRACT			
Renal plasma flow	25–50		
Glomerular filtration rate	50		
Ureter tone		x	
Ureteral motility			x
METABOLISM			
Nitrogen stores	x		
General stores of			
Sodium	x		
Potassium	x		
Calcium	x		
OXYGEN CONSUMPTION	14		

VAGINAL AND UTERINE CHANGES

The vagina becomes edematous and more pliable. The squamous epithelium lining the vagina is increased in thickness and cornification, and vascularity beneath the mucous membranes is greatly augmented. The color, ordinarily pink, becomes dusky in early pregnancy and by term is almost purple. This congestion may result in vaginitis, which can rarely be cured until the pregnancy is over; in the formation of varices, which may rupture and cause vaginal hemorrhage; or in the formation of large clusters of veins, which simulate hemangiomas. The supporting structures of the vagina, along with the other connective tissues, acquire great distensibility; at term, the vagina can readily accommodate the fetal head without rupturing.

Gestational changes in the uterus are described in Chapter 29. Endometrial changes and the Arias–Stella phenomenon are described in Chapter 4.

CHANGES IN THE UTERINE TUBES

Except for edema, hyperemia, and the change in location occasioned by the growth of the uterus, the fallopian tubes undergo virtually no gross changes in pregnancy. Microscopic examination may show occasional patches of decidual tissue on the surface and some flattening of the lining epithelium, but there is no alteration in the distribution of epithelium within the tubes or in the number or complexity of the epithelial folds protruding into the lumina.

OVARIAN CHANGES

Consideration of ovarian changes associated with pregnancy properly begins with the alterations in the graafian follicle to form a corpus luteum (see page 88). As soon as the syncytiotrophoblast penetrates maternal blood vessels, the secretion of chorionic gonadotropin into the maternal bloodstream becomes possible. This hormone immediately replaces the pituitary gonadotropins and acts to maintain the corpus luteum, which is then referred to as the *corpus luteum of pregnancy* or *corpus luteum vera*.

Regressive changes begin as usual in the corpus luteum on about the 8th day of its existence, since at that time not enough trophoblast is in contact with maternal tissue to produce sufficient chorionic gonadotropin to alter events. However, by the 12th day, secretion by the trophoblast into the maternal bloodstream is sufficient to halt regression of the corpus luteum. By the 6th or 7th week following the last menstrual period, the production of steroids by the placenta is sufficient to ensure the continuation of a normal pregnancy. This has been repeatedly demonstrated in human beings by the survival of the infant after accidental or deliberate extirpation of the gonads at this stage of pregnancy. However, there is also strong evidence that in the ordinary course of events the corpus luteum continues to contribute to steroid production until about the 12th week. After that time, the total production of estrogen and progesterone becomes far greater than the largest amount ever measured from a corpus luteum. Chorionic gonadotropin

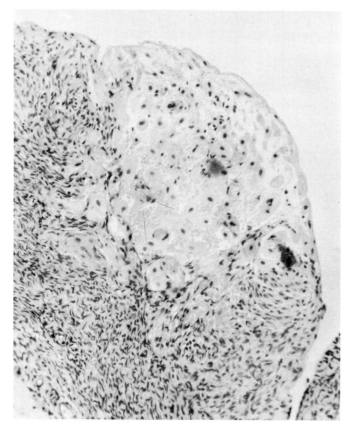

FIG. 17-11. Decidual reaction on surface of ovary. (Huffman JW: Gynecology and Obstetrics. Philadelphia, WB Saunders, 1962

excretion then begins to decline. As a consequence, the corpus luteum undergoes regression, becoming smaller in size and losing a good deal of its lipoid content. At term, the corpus luteum is less than half its maximal size and is pale pink and convoluted on its cut surface. It does not protrude above the surface of the ovary and may be overlooked on casual inspection. Following delivery, regression is completed, and the corpus luteum of pregnancy is gradually converted into an ordinary corpus albicans.

On the surface of the ovary, and indeed on almost any other peritoneal surface in the pelvis (but particularly on the posterior surface of the broad ligament), sheets of cells that are indistinguishable from the decidua of the uterine cavity may appear (Fig 17–11). In some patients, these cells represent pregnancy alterations in areas of endometriosis. Microscopic examination of these areas shows a mixture of partially altered endometrium and tissue that is completely changed to decidua. However, small patches of decidual alteration are also observed in patients in whom there is no likelihood, on the basis of previous history or physical examination, that endometriosis existed. It must be supposed, therefore, that such decidual changes arise by metaplasia of the peritoneum or the germinal epithelium of the ovary under the heavy hormone stimulus of pregnancy. This endocrine stimulation may also cause changes resembling luteinization of atretic and partially developed graafian follicles in the ovary.

REFERENCES AND RECOMMENDED READING

Alaily AB, Carrol KB: Pulmonary ventilation in pregnancy. Br J Obstet Gynaecol 85:518, 1978

Assali NS, Douglass RA, Baird WW, et al.: Measurement of uterine blood flow and uterine metabolism: IV. Results in normal pregnancy. Am J Obstet Gynecol 66:248, 1953

Braverman DZ, Johnson ML, Kern F, Jr: Effects of pregnancy and contraceptive steroids on gallbladder function. N Engl J Med 302:362, 1980

Campbell EJM, Howell JBL: The sensation of breathlessness. Brit Med Bull 19:36, 1963

Carey HM: Modern Trends in Reproductive Physiology. London, Butterworth, 1963

Danforth DN, Buckingham JC: Connective tissue mechanisms and their relation to pregnancy. Obstet Gynecol Surv, 19:715, 1964

Danforth DN, Manalo-Estrella P, Buckingham JC: The effect of pregnancy and of Enovid on the rabbit vasculature. Am J Obstet Gynecol 88:952, 1964

Dunlop W: Renal physiology in pregnancy. Postgrad Md J 55:329, 1979

Fried AM: Hydronephrosis of pregnancy: Ultrasonographic study and classification of asymptomatic women. Am J Obstet Gynecol 135:1066, 1979

Hytten FE, Leitch I: The Physiology of Human Pregnancy, 2nd ed. Oxford, Blackwell, 1971

Katz R, Karliner JS, Resnick R: Effects of natural volume overload state (pregnancy) on left ventricular performance in human subjects. Circulation 58:434, 1978

Kjeldsen J: Hemodynamic investigations during labour and delivery. Acta Obstet Gynecol Scand 58:3, 1979

Lindheimer M, Katz AI: Renal function in pregnancy. In Wynn R (ed): Obstetrical and Gynecological Annual 1:139, 1972

Macgillivray I, Rose GA, Rowe B: Blood pressure survey in pregnancy. Clin Sci 37:395, 1969

Metcalf J, Ueland K: Maternal cardiovascular adjustments to pregnancy. Prog Cardiovasc Dis 363, 1974

Milne JA, Howie AD, Pack AI: Dyspnoea during normal pregnancy. Br J Obstet Gynaecol 85:260, 1978

Milne JA, Mills RJ, Howie AD et al.: Large airways' function during normal pregnancy. Br J obstet Gynaecol 84:448, 1977

Pritchard JA: Change in the blood volume during pregnancy and delivery. Anesthesiology 26:393, 1965

Prowse CM Gaensler EA: Respiratory and acid–base changes during pregnancy. Anesthesiology 26:381, 1965

Reitz RE, Daane TA, Woods JR et al.: Calcium, magnesium, phosphorus, and parathyroid hormone interrelationships in pregnancy and newborn infants. Obstet Gynecol 50:701, 1977

Sims EA, Krantz KE: Serial studies of renal function during pregnancy and the puerperium in normal women. J Clin Invest 37:1764, 1958

Taylor GO, Modie JA, Agbedana EO et al.: Serum free fatty acids and blood glucose in pregnancy. Br J Obstet Gynaecol 85:592, 1978

Ulmsten U, Sundström G: Esophageal manometry in pregnant and nonpregnant women. Am J Obstet Gynecol 132:260, 1978

18

ENDOCRINE PHYSIOLOGY OF PREGNANCY

Robert B. Jaffe

The hypothalamic–pituitary–ovarian relations in the nonpregnant woman and the consequences of cyclic ovarian activity are outlined in Chapter 6. During pregnancy a new group of protein hormones, of placental origin, makes its appearance. In addition, there is a marked increase in the concentration of circulating sex steroids that are derived from the maternal–fetal–placental complex. Much remains to be learned of the physiologic role of these hormones, even though a great deal is already known of their origin, concentrations, and actions. Among their actions it is clear that they play a major role in the maintenance of pregnancy and in the initiation of labor, as outlined in Chapter 29.

PROTEIN HORMONES

HUMAN CHORIONIC GONADOTROPIN
Origin and Chemistry

In 1927, Aschheim and Zondek described a hormone, human chorionic gonadotropin (hCG), in the urine of pregnant women. Initially, they believed the hormone to be produced by the anterior pituitary gland of the mother. Subsequently, the findings that hCG is produced by trophoblastic cells in tissue culture and that urinary excretion of hCG is maintained at normal levels following hypophysectomy at the 26th week of human gestation have established the placenta as the source of this hormone. Ultrastructural and immunofluorescent studies point to the syncytiotrophoblast as the source of the hormone.

A glycoprotein of 36,000–40,000 molecular weight, hCG consists of two glycoprotein chains dissociable in 8M urea solution: an alpha subunit that is structurally similar to that found in all three pituitary glycoprotein hormones and a beta subunit (β-hCG) that is structurally similar to the β-subunit of pituitary luteinizing hormone (LH) and confers the specific biologic character of the hormone.

Measurement

Detection and measurement of hCG is of practical importance, since this determination forms the basis for most commonly employed pregnancy tests, as noted on page 359, and for the evaluation and treatment of certain trophoblastic diseases. Initially, various biologic procedures were used; today, immunologic determinations and radioreceptor assays are employed in many centers.

The commonly employed tests for pregnancy do not separate hCG from LH, but usually this does not affect the tests because of the very low concentration of LH, compared with that of hCG, in the body fluids of pregnant women. The biologic test described by Aschheim and Zondek (AZ test) used 21- to 28-day-old mice that were given subcutaneous injections of urine in six divided doses for 2 days. The ovaries of the animals were examined 96 hours after the initial injection, and the presence of corpora lutea or bleeding points was interpreted as a positive reaction (*i.e.*, pregnancy). Current biologic tests employ the weight of the immature rat uterus, the weight of the immature rat prostate and seminal vesicles, or the presence of ovarian hyperemia in the rat, as described by Riley *et al.* These tests have a high degree of reliability and also may be employed quantitatively. Qualitative tests based upon an ovulatory response to hCG by the South African toad or the initiation of ejaculation by the male American frog also are utilized.

FIG. 18-1. Serum gonadotropin concentrations (log scale) during normal menstrual cycle and early period of ensuing pregnancy, as determined by radioimmunoassay. 2nd IRP-HMG is standard preparation, referring to Second International Reference Preparation of human menopausal gonadotropin. Each vial has been assigned a potency of 40 IU of LH activity and 40 IU of FSH activity. *mIU,* milli International Units. (Jaffe RB, Lee PA, Midgley AR, Jr: J Clin Endocrinol 29:1281, 1969)

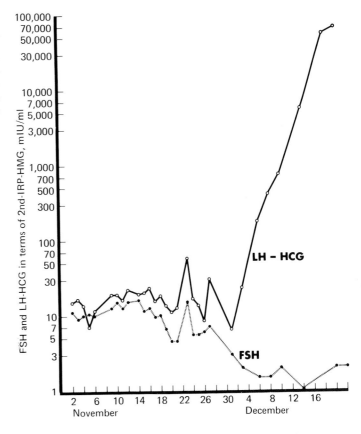

Immunologic methods for detection and measurement of hCG in blood and urine by radioimmunoassay, radioreceptor assay, hemagglutination inhibition, and complement fixation techniques obviate the necessity of using animals and have been modified to provide relatively rapid and reliable tests for pregnancy. The hemagglutination inhibition and complement fixation tests have approximately 90% accuracy 10–14 days after a missed menstrual period. On the other hand, the radioimmunoassays for β-hCG and the radioreceptor assays, performed on blood samples, have great sensitivity, permitting the diagnosis of pregnancy even before a menstrual period is missed. Their accuracy following a missed menstrual period approaches 99%.

Radioimmunoassay techniques have demonstrated detectable serum concentrations of hCG 9 days after the surge of pituitary gonadotropins at midcycle, corresponding to 8 days after ovulation and only 1 day after implantation (Fig. 18–1). By conventional, less sensitive techniques, the excretion of hCG in the urine is first detectable at approximately the 26th day after conception. The concentration gradually rises, reaching a peak value between the 60th and 70th days of gestation. Thereafter, the concentration falls slowly,

reaching a low level between the 100th and 130th days of pregnancy. This low level persists during the remainder of pregnancy, and hCG vanishes about 2 weeks after delivery (Fig. 18–2).

By means of radioimmunoassay, it has been found that the rate at which hCG disappears from the serum following delivery decreases with time, resulting in an apparent progressive increase in the half-life of hCG during the first 3 days. The composite disappearance curve appears to be the result of two linear components, the first corresponding to a half-life of 8.9 hours and the second to a half-life of 37.2 hours. These are much longer half-life values than those of most other hormones.

Yen and co-workers demonstrated the utility of the radioimmunoassay procedure for determining hCG concentrations in patients treated for trophoblastic disease. They suggested that the method is an accurate, sensitive, and quantitative means of determination useful for diagnosis, assessment of efficacy of therapy, and patient follow-up. Concentrations of hCG above normal may be found in trophoblastic disease, pregnancy with multiple fetuses, and Rh-isoimmunization.

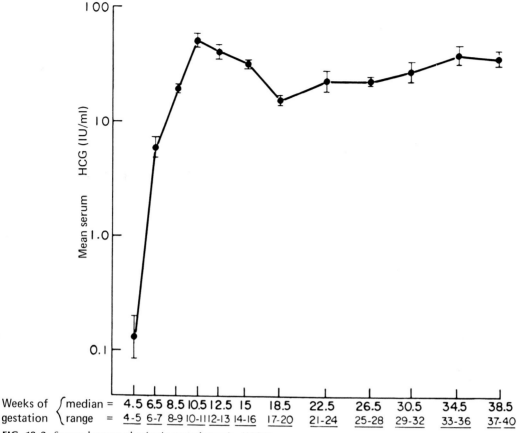

FIG. 18-2. Serum human chorionic gonadotropin (*HCG*) concentrations during pregnancy, as determined by radioimmunoassay. (Goldstein DP, Aono T, Taymor ML, Jochelson K, Todd R, Hines E: Am J Obstet Gynecol 102:110, 1968)

Physiologic Role

The major known action of hCG appears to be its ability to maintain the corpus luteum, although it does not appear to influence the maturation of the follicle and seems unable to restore a regressing corpus luteum. Thus, it appears to be luteotropic in function, responsible for the early development and maintenance of the corpus luteum of pregnancy. Recent studies by Huhtaniemi and colleagues have demonstrated that hCG binds specifically to the human fetal testis and stimulates testosterone production by the fetal testis. In addition, Serón–Ferré *et al.* demonstrated that hCG could stimulate androgen production by the fetal zone of the fetal adrenal gland. Thus, hCG also plays a role in stimulating fetal steroidogenesis.

Recent studies suggest that, since hCG has been found to inhibit chemically induced mitosis *in vitro*, its secretion might be responsible for the well-known protection against rejection of the allogenic fetal graft

during pregnancy. The fact that large concentrations of commercial (*i.e.*, impure) hCG are required to reduce mitosis to a great degree, as well as the lack of relation between lymphocyte mitosis and secretion of antibody, suggests that further studies should be carried out with hCG and related proteins before conclusions are drawn concerning its immunosuppressive role.

HUMAN CHORIONIC SOMATOMAMMOTROPIN

In the early 1960s, several investigators, including Higashi, Josimovich and MacLaren, and Grumbach and coworkers, showed that the human placenta produces a protein hormone that has lactogenic properties and is similar to pituitary growth hormone immunologically and in some aspects of its metabolism. Josimovich and MacLaren found this protein in peripheral maternal and retroplacental serum, as well as in the placenta. It was found to be lactogenic in the pigeon crop sac assay and to promote milk production by the mammary gland of the pseudopregnant rabbit. For this reason, although its lactogenic properties in the human remain

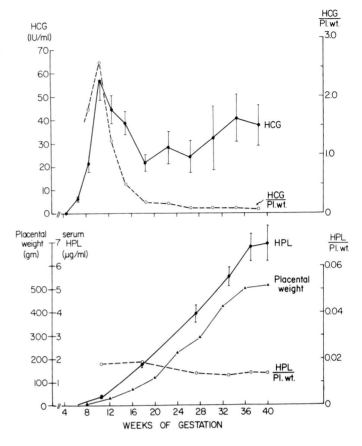

FIG. 18-3. Levels of human chorionic gonadotropin (*HCG*) and human chorionic somatomammotropin (here called *HPL*) during normal pregnancy. (Selenkow HA, Saxena BM, Dana CL, Emerson K, Jr: In Pecile A, Fenzi C (eds): The Foeto-Placental Unit. Amsterdam, Excerpta Medica, 1969)

to be established, the hormone was designated *human placental lactogen* (hPL) by Josimovich and his colleagues. They also demonstrated that the hormone has luteotropic properties in the pseudopregnant hypophysectomized rat. Grumbach *et al.* have suggested that this placental hormone, because of its immunochemical similarity to growth hormone and its possible metabolic effects on the mother, may have an important anabolic function in pregnancy and therefore have proposed the designation *human chorionic growth hormone–prolactin* (CGP). More recently, the term *human chorionic somatomammotropin* (hCS) has been used; although complex, this term more adequately defines the hormone's origin and function. Accordingly, the designation hCS is used in the following discussion.

Origin

HCS is synthesized by the syncytiotrophoblast of the placenta. It is present in the serum and urine during normal pregnancy and molar pregnancy. It disappears rapidly from the serum and urine after delivery of the placenta or evacuation of the uterus. Following normal delivery, it is no longer detectable in the serum after the first postpartum day. *In vitro* biosynthesis of this hormone has been accomplished.

Measurement

To date, the most satisfactory method for the measurement of hCS in biologic fluids is a radioimmunoassay procedure that is extremely sensitive and permits accurate measurement of microgram quantities in a milliliter of maternal or fetal plasma or urine. A hemagglutination inhibition test also has been developed for the assay of hCS in pregnancy urine.

During the first trimester, hCS is present in microgram quantities per milliliter of plasma. Its concentration increases as pregnancy progresses, and peak levels occur at term (Fig. 18–3). From the first to the third trimesters there may be a tenfold or greater increase in measurable blood levels. The urinary excretion parallels the serum concentrations, with several micrograms of hormone measurable per day during the first trimester and a progressive increase until term. There is some disagreement about whether there is a significant relationship between placental weight and blood levels of hCS.

The concentration of hCS in maternal peripheral

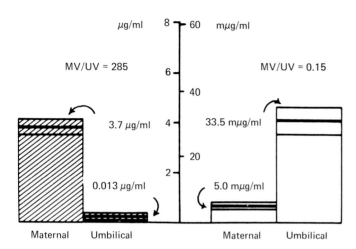

Ratio of CGP/HGH	
Maternal venous serum	Umbilical venous serum
740	0.39

FIG. 18–4. Concentrations of human chorionic somato-mammotropin (here called *chorionic growth hormone–prolactin, CGP*) and human growth hormone (*HGH*) in maternal and fetal circulation. (Grumbach MM, Kaplan S: Ann NY Acad Sci 148:501, 1968)

blood is about 300 times that in umbilical vein blood (Fig. 18–4). Also, blood leaving the gravid uterus has a considerably higher concentration of hormone than peripheral blood.

The half-life survival of this compound in the maternal circulation has been estimated as 13–23 min. For maintenance of circulating hormone levels, this suggests that the placenta produces hCS at a rate of 1–4 g/day at term. If this is true, production of this hormone must be one of the major metabolic and synthetic activities of the syncytiotrophoblast.

Several studies of hCS have been performed in abnormal pregnancies. It has been found in extracts prepared from a hydatidiform mole, in the serum of patients with molar pregnancies, and in the urine of patients harboring trophoblastic tumors. It also has been found in male patients with choriocarcinoma of the testis. Thus, like hCG, this protein hormone appears to be elaborated by all varieties of trophoblastic tissue.

Control of Secretion

A variety of factors known to alter pituitary growth hormone secretion has been found ineffective in altering hCS levels. There are exceptions, however. Prolonged fasting at midgestation and hypoglycemia produced by large doses of insulin raise hCS levels, while intraamniotic injection of prostaglandin $F_{2\alpha}$ causes a marked reduction in hCS concentrations.

Physiologic Role

Because of the immunologic and chemical similarities between hCS and human growth hormone, there has been considerable interest in the general metabolic role of hCS in normal pregnancy. It has been suggested that hCS may be a "metabolic hormone of pregnancy" with an essential role in the anabolic state of the pregnant woman. According to this concept, the hormone may ensure adequate maternal storage of nitrogen and minerals, as well as adequate mobilization of fat, to meet the requirements for fetal growth and development. This kind of regulatory role for hCS seems likely in light of its complete independence of the neural regulatory mechanism of the maternal pituitary.

Also of obvious interest is the possible role of hCS in certain of the diabetogenic features of normal pregnancy. *Normal* pregnancy is associated with a pronounced resistance to exogenous and endogenous insulin and is characterized by increased levels of circulating insulin or insulinlike activity and a rise in circulating free fatty acids. In many ways these modifications in carbohydrate and lipid metabolism in pregnancy are similar to the metabolic modifications in-

duced in nonpregnant subjects by the administration of human growth hormone; hCS may be associated with these changes in normal pregnancy. The fact that administration of this hormone produces a rise in plasma fatty acid levels in both animals and humans strengthens the hypothesis that it is related to the diabetogenic features of normal pregnancy. Other relations may be relevant to the increased resistance to insulin-induced hypoglycemia that characterizes the last trimester of normal human pregnancy.

The possible mammotropic effects of hCS also have been investigated. It has been shown that hCS synergizes with hydrocortisone and insulin to cause development of mammary gland alveoli that is histologically indistinguishable from that produced by prolactin. The evidence suggests that hCS is a potent prolactinlike hormone that is not species-specific and may be important in mammary gland development during normal human pregnancy. The possible physiologic role of hCS in the initiation of lactation in the postpartum period awaits further exploration.

It remains to be seen whether hCS plays a role in steroidogenesis in the fetoplacental unit. The marked luteotropic effect of hCS in rodents has been noted. In mice and rats, ovarian conversion of 20α-dihydroprogesterone is apparently inhibited by lactogenic hormones, allowing greater support of gestational changes in the reproductive tract. Thus, the luteotropic effects of hCS in these species suggest a possible inhibitory role for this hormone in human gestation in which placental or fetal conversion of progesterone to the less biologically active steroid might be effected.

HUMAN CHORIONIC THYROTROPIN

A third protein hormone that is immunologically similar to pituitary thyrotropin (TSH) has been shown to be synthesized and secreted by the placenta. This compound, human chorionic thyrotropin (hCT), is thought by some to have hormonal activity and physicochemical properties similar to those of pituitary TSH. The data suggest that the active principle is a glycoprotein; with some exceptions, the chromatographic and electrophoretic properties also resemble those of human pituitary TSH. Surprisingly, hCT seems immunologically more closely related to bovine and porcine TSH than to human pituitary TSH.

Biologically, hCT has been demonstrated to increase the secretion of thyroid hormone, to stimulate incorporation of inorganic phosphate into the thyroid, and to be neutralized by highly specific antipituitary TSH. Thus, the thyroid-stimulating activity of hCT appears to be due to a factor structurally related to TSH. Hennen and associates noted that the thyroid-stimulating activity in the serum of pregnant women is particularly high during early pregnancy and decreases in subsequent months to reach a minimum at term. They sug-

gested that hCT may play a role in the well-known variations in parameters of thyroid function and the incidence of thyroid enlargement during pregnancy, although they emphasized that the levels of hCT during pregnancy are not sufficient to induce clinical hyperthyroidism. More recent studies strongly suggest that much of the thyrotropic activity of the placenta is actually a function of hCG, which may explain the increased incidence of hyperthyroidism seen in patients with trophoblastic diseases.

HUMAN CHORIONIC CORTICOTROPIN

Liotta and colleagues have obtained data suggesting that the placenta also may be the source of yet another pituitary-like hormone, chorionic corticotropin. They demonstrated both immunoassayable and bioassayable adrenocorticotropic hormone (ACTH) activity in extracts of extensively washed human placental tissue and dispersed viable trophoblasts. When the trophoblasts were incubated in tissue culture medium, the ACTH content of both the cells and medium was significantly greater than the preincubation level, suggesting its synthesis by trophoblastic cells. The physiologic role, if any, of chorionic corticotropin and its regulation remain to be elucidated.

OTHER PLACENTAL PROTEIN AND POLYPEPTIDE HORMONES

Recent studies have suggested that the placenta has the capacity to synthesize hypothalamic-like gonadotropin-releasing hormone (GnRH). It may be that the placenta has the capacity to produce a wide array of pituitary- and hypothalamic-like protein and polypeptide hormones.

STEROID HORMONES

Previously, the placenta was thought to be one of the four steroid-producing glands, each complete in itself and all having similar metabolic pathways of hormone synthesis. However, evidence suggests that the manner in which the placenta produces estrogen and progesterone may be significantly different from the manner in which the ovaries produce these hormones. The concept has evolved that *the placenta is an incomplete endocrine organ*, relying for much of its hormone synthesis on precursors that reach it from the maternal and fetal compartments. It is now evident that the constant interaction of fetus, placenta, and mother, rather than the autonomous action of the placenta, is responsible for the marked increase in steroid hormone production characteristic of pregnancy. Therefore, the *fetal–placental–maternal unit*, not the pla-

centa alone, is the major source of steroid hormones during pregnancy.

ESTROGENS

More than 25 different estrogens have been isolated from the urine of pregnant women. Most are maternal and fetal metabolites of hormones secreted by the placenta. The three classic estrogens (estrone, 17β-estradiol, and estriol) have been shown to be secreted by the placenta, and most studies have involved these three hormones.

Source

There is good evidence that the placenta produces estrogen and that the syncytiotrophoblast is the site of production. This placental source is suggested by 1) the significantly higher levels of the three classic estrogens in the umbilical vein than in the umbilical arteries and 2) the rapid decrease in estrogen concentration in both fetal and maternal urine immediately after delivery.

Recent work has clarified the pathways for estrogen production by the placenta. Although ovarian tissue *in vitro* has the capacity to utilize progesterone in the formation of estrogens, similar incubations with placental tissue do not result in the transformation of progesterone into estrogens. Various *in vivo* approaches, including placental perfusion with progesterone, intraamniotic progesterone infusion, and simultaneous introduction of progesterone into the maternal and fetal circulations, produced no evidence of any significant conversion to estrogen. It is now apparent that progesterone in the umbilical circulation and in the maternal blood does not serve as a significant precursor of placental estrogens in human pregnancy.

In contrast, there is good evidence that the placenta can make estrogens by conversion of circulating androgens. Thus, the production of estrogens by the placenta appears to depend upon the availability of androgen precursors from the fetus and the mother. Moreover, the blood level of natural androgens and the production of estrogens by the placenta are quantitatively interrelated.

In both circulations that perfuse the placenta, *i.e.*, fetal and maternal, there is a high level of sulfoconjugated androgens, particularly dehydroepiandrosterone sulfate (DHAS) and 16α-hydroxydehydroepiandrosterone sulfate (16-OH-DHAS). DHAS is present in higher concentration in cord than in maternal plasma, and there is an arteriovenous difference in the umbilical circulation that suggests both fetal production and placental use of this compound.

Urinary and plasma 17-ketosteroids usually are lowered during pregnancy. The primary constituent of

the 17-ketosteroids in women is the DHAS produced in the adrenal gland, and it is probable that the use of DHAS by the placenta in forming estrogen is largely responsible for the decreased urinary 17-ketosteroids. As pregnancy progresses, increasing amounts of maternal DHAS are converted to estrogen, particularly 17β-estradiol. This is reflected in decreasing blood concentrations of DHAS and increasing production rates of estradiol with advancing gestation. Fetal DHAS also contributes to the placental production of estradiol. The rate of conversion of fetal DHAS to total estrogens approximates 80%, which is much higher than the corresponding 30% conversion rate for maternal DHAS. In pregnancy, over 90% of the total estrogen excretion in the maternal urine is estriol, and most of the 80% conversion of fetal DHAS to estrogen is concerned in estriol production.

In the production of estriol, just as in the production of estradiol, the placenta is dependent upon androgenic precursors that originate in the fetal and maternal compartments. In nonpregnant women, estriol is primarily a metabolic product of estrone and estradiol. In pregnancy, however, estriol released into the circulation by the placenta is not derived in appreciable amounts from estradiol or estrone, but primarily from 16-OH-DHAS. In the fetus, the 16-hydroxylated compound can be formed in the liver and adrenal from DHAS that has been synthesized in the fetal adrenal gland. The fetal source of estriol precursors appears to be higher than the maternal, at least in the latter stages of pregnancy (Fig. 18–5). It has been suggested that estriol may function to increase uteroplacental blood flow.

The conversion of 16-OH-DHAS to estriol by the placenta (Fig. 18–5) depends first on removal of the sulfate moiety by an enzyme, steroid sulfatase. A deficiency of this substance can block the synthesis of estriol. The cases of *sulfatase deficiency* reported have been associated with healthy male infants; during pregnancy, there was no evidence of jeopardy except extremely low estriol excretion. Spontaneous labor was frequently delayed or did not occur at all.

Clinical Application of Estriol Determinations

Both an intact fetus and an intact placenta appear necessary for the synthesis of normal amounts of estriol. Thus, compromise of either or both should be reflected in decreased estriol values. Estriol is secreted by the placenta into the maternal circulation, and is transferred into the amniotic fluid. It is excreted in the maternal urine primarily in a conjugated form.

Measurement of estriol to assess fetoplacental function has been performed on urine, plasma, and amniotic fluid. To date, the most extensive measurements of estriol have been carried out on maternal urine. Estriol is measured in milligram rather than microgram quantities, its concentration in the pregnant woman

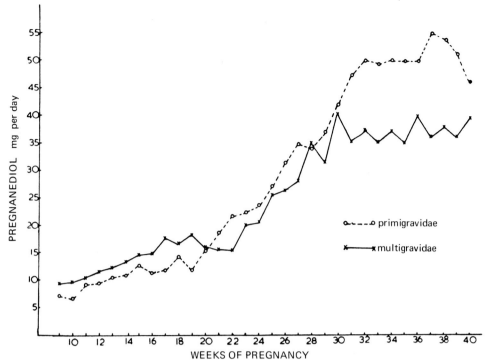

FIG. 18–8. Urinary pregnanediol excretion during pregnancy in primigravid and multigravid patients. (Shearman RP: J Obstet Gynaecol Br Emp 66:1, 1959)

Recent studies suggest that low-density lipoprotein cholesterol is the primary precursor of placental progesterone.

The work of Siiteri and colleagues suggests that progesterone produced by the placenta, ovaries, or both is the essential hormone of mammalian pregnancy because of its ability to inhibit T lymphocyte cell-mediated responses involved in tissue rejection. They have suggested that a high local (intrauterine) concentration of progesterone can effectively block cellular immune responses to foreign antigens. Siiteri points out that progesterone has been aptly called the hormone of pregnancy in all mammals examined and its presence has been detected in species representing all classes of vertebrates and lower forms.

CHANGES IN OTHER ENDOCRINE GLAND FUNCTIONS

As discussed in Chapters 7 and 14, thyroid and adrenal function in nonpregnant women may be altered by the use of steroidal contraceptives or estrogen therapy. Similarly, during pregnancy, when elevated levels of estrogen apparently induce increased serum levels of thyroxine-binding and corticosteroid-binding globulins, increased levels of total serum thyroxine and cortisol are seen. Of the more active fractions, the non–protein-bound thyroid hormone is not increased, while the free corticosteroids are apparently elevated.

It is apparent that both hCS and progesterone may be responsible for enhanced insulin release in response to a glucose load in normal pregnant women. This process counteracts the estrogen–hCS-enhanced insulinase mechanisms that cause resistance to insulin in late pregnancy. Enhanced release, balanced by insulin resistance, results in an essentially normal glucose tolerance test during pregnancy.

Lastly, maternal pituitary release of gonadotropins and growth hormone (Fig. 18–4) is apparently suppressed during gestation.

REFERENCES AND RECOMMENDED READING

Adcock EW, III, Teasdale F, August CS et al: Human chorionic gonadotropin: Its possible role in maternal lymphocyte suppression. Science 181:845, 1973.

Aschheim S, Zondek B: Anterior pituitary hormone and ovarian hormone in the urine of pregnant women. Klin Wochenschr 6:1322, 1927

Bahl OP: Human chorionic gonadotropin: I. Purification and physicochemical properties. J Biol Chem 244:567, 1969

Bahl OP: Human chorionic gonadotropin: II. Nature of the carbohydrate units. J Biol Chem 244:575, 1969

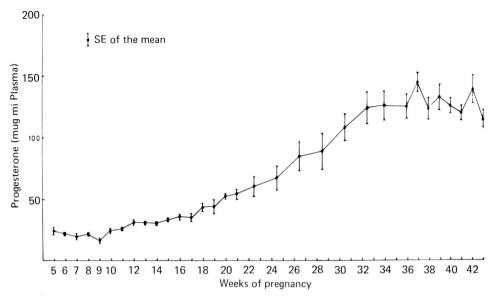

FIG. 18-7. Plasma progesterone concentrations during pregnancy. (Johansson EDB: Acta Endocrinol 61:607, 1969)

surement. Also, because of the very low concentration of estriol in blood, radioactive estriol conjugates may have to be added to the plasma samples to evaluate recovery. Finally, when estriol concentration is assessed at only one point in time, rather than over an entire day, changes occurring at other times of the day and diurnal variation may not be appreciated.

Amniotic fluid estriol determinations, primarily by gas–liquid chromatography, also have been reported. It has been suggested that these determinations may be of value in following the progress of Rh-isoimmunized pregnancies because they may provide a more accurate index of the status of the erythroblastotic fetus *in utero* than do urinary values.

Thus, estriol determinations may be helpful in the management of certain complications of pregnancy. At present, it is suggested that their measurement be used as an adjunct to, not as a replacement for, clinical management. It is conceivable that another compound, which may or may not be hormonal in nature, will eventually be found that will more adequately reflect fetal status. Also, as more is learned of the clinical implications of the fetal heart reactions to nonstress, contraction stress, and oxytocin challenge tests, it is entirely possible that these tests will replace serial estriol determinations for evaluating the fetus at risk.

PROGESTERONE

Serum progesterone levels have been measured at various stages of gestation. Average concentrations range from approximately 25 mμg/ml at 37 weeks (compared with an average nonpregnancy luteal phase

value of 5 mμg/ml; Fig. 18–7). The total 24-hour production of progesterone near term is approximately 250 mg.

Pregnanediol, a major metabolite of progesterone in maternal urine, also has been measured throughout pregnancy (Fig. 18–8). Daily pregnanediol excretion fluctuates quite markedly during pregnancy. It has been demonstrated that pregnanediol is not solely a metabolite of progesterone, but also may be formed from other steroids.

In the production of certain estrogens, the placenta uses precursors that reach it from both the maternal and the fetal circulations. It is less certain that circulating precursors, at least from the fetus, are needed for the placental production of progesterone. Interruption of the umbilical circulation by clamping the cord and allowing the placenta to remain *in situ* is not followed by a marked diminution in pregnanediol excretion. Neither is there a significant change in pregnanediol excretion in abdominal pregnancy following the removal of the fetus without disturbing the placenta or after intrauterine fetal death while the placenta is still functioning. Thus, it appears that the progesterone production is not markedly affected by the absence of the fetus. However, studies involving placental perfusion with cholesterol and the classic work of Bloch, who gave radioactive cholesterol to pregnant women, suggest that the placenta can use circulating cholesterol in the synthesis of progesterone. Work by Hellig and colleagues provides strong evidence that cholesterol in the maternal circulation accounts for most of the progesterone produced by the placenta.

TABLE 18-1. AVERAGE ESTRIOL EXCRETION IN NORMAL PREGNANCY

Gestation (weeks)	Mean Estriol Excretion (mg/24 hr)	Standard Deviation (mg)	No. of Subjects
6	0.05		3
7	0.06		3
8	0.09		4
9	0.15	0.079	7
10	0.16	0.085	7
11	0.23	0.255	7
12	0.28	0.153	8
13	0.58	0.249	9
14	0.70	0.354	10
15	1.15	0.425	7
16	1.95	0.760	8
17	2.40	0.775	10
18	3.65	0.899	15
19	4.36	1.339	29
20	5.59	1.932	31
21	6.70	2.256	11
22	7.59	1.904	9
23	9.36	2.221	12
24	10.04	2.144	11
25	10.57	3.228	11
26	12.98	1.612	11
27	13.75	2.100	10
28	12.96	3.465	19
29	14.67	3.266	42
30	15.21	3.490	41
31	15.24	3.604	18
32	17.51	4.265	11
33	18.12	4.197	15
34	18.82	3.571	16
35	22.55	3.040	15
36	23.39	3.928	19
37	28.61	7.652	24
38	31.33	6.565	42
39	33.34	9.373	46
40	34.49	9.352	25
41	33.22	7.935	16

(Klopper A, Billewicz W: J Obstet Gynaecol Br Commonw 70:1024, 1963)

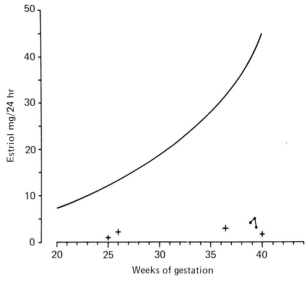

FIG. 18-6. Curve of average maternal urinary estriol excretion during normal pregnancy and after intrauterine fetal death (+). *Connected points* from 38.5 to 39.5 weeks' gestation represent estriol excretion in a patient with sarcoidosis and clinical adrenocortical insufficiency who had a viable fetus. Curve based upon estriol concentrations in Table 18–1; values corrected to 100%.

decreased. Again, serial determinations are of greater value than an isolated measurement.

When placental function is compromised or when the placenta undergoes excessive senescence, as in the postmaturity syndrome, estriol excretion may decline significantly. A finding of low estriol excretion after the expected date of confinement or when the uterus ceases to enlarge is an indication for termination of the pregnancy.

Estriol excretion is decreased in the presence of an anencephalic fetus, probably because of the marked hypoplasia of the fetal adrenal frequently found in this condition. Estriol excretion is also decreased in patients receiving large doses of adrenal corticosteroids, presumably because this medication suppresses adrenal androgenic precursors of placental estriol. Estriol excretion has been reported low in anemic patients, in those with nutritional deficiencies, and in those living at high altitudes. Urinary estriol excretion may be elevated in pregnancy with multiple fetuses. Varying levels of urinary estriol excretion are found in pregnancies complicated by erythroblastosis fetalis. In these clinical situations, measurement of urinary estriol excretion has been of only limited help in assessing the status of the fetoplacental unit.

Several reports have dealt with the use of plasma estriol determinations to monitor the progress of certain complicated pregnancies. These measurements have generally been used in the same clinical situations in which urinary estriol determinations have been employed. The stated advantages of plasma over urinary estriol measurements include elimination of the need for 24-hour urine collection, the ability to obtain two or more plasma samples for analysis in a single day, and the fact that, in view of the short half-life of estriol in plasma, a decreasing rate of estriol synthesis is reflected more rapidly in a single plasma sample than in a pooled urine collection. Among the disadvantages of plasma estriol determinations are the considerable diurnal variation in plasma estriol levels and the greater technical skill required to perform this mea-

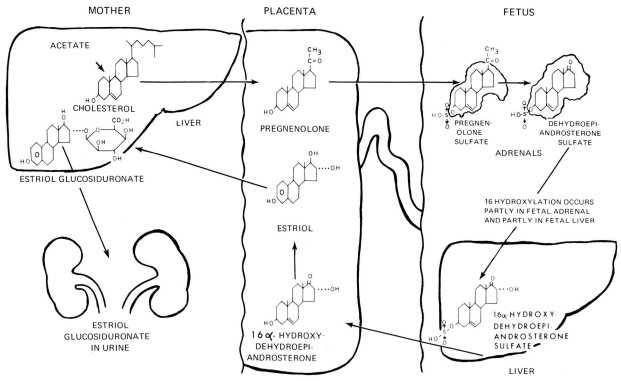

FIG. 18–5. Pathway of estriol biosynthesis in late pregnancy. (Modified from Taylor ES: Obstet Gynecol Surv 24:320, 1969. Baltimore, © The Williams & Wilkins Co)

being some 1000-fold greater than that in the non-pregnant woman. Because of these relatively large concentrations, it has proved feasible to perform serial urinary estriol determinations as a routine clinical procedure. A variety of techniques, including spectrophotometry and gas–liquid chromatography, has been used for its measurement. A radioimmunoassay technique also has been described. One drawback to estriol determinations, sometimes unrecognized and uncorrected, is the variability of recovery. Use of radioactive internal standards obviates this problem.

As can be seen in Table 18–1 and Figure 18–6, under normal circumstances urinary estriol excretion increases with advancing gestation. Day-to-day variation during the course of a normal pregnancy is seen, but the general trend is upward. There appears to be a correlation between estriol excretion and fetal weight. Serial determinations are of far greater value than a single estimation. Normal estriol excretion values and fiducial limits have been established; a 30–40% decrease from these values in a patient whose previous estriol determinations were within the normal range suggests possible compromise of fetoplacental status.

There are four disorders associated with pregnancy in which serial measurement of urinary estriol excretion may be of aid in assessing pregnancy status: 1) diabetes mellitus, 2) hypertension and preeclampsia–eclampsia, 3) "placental insufficiency" (including

intrauterine growth retardation and postmaturity syndrome), and 4) suspected intrauterine fetal death.

Several investigators have reported the use of serial urinary estriol determinations in the management of pregnancy complicated by maternal diabetes. Although there is no evidence of greatly increased fetal salvage when estriol is monitored, these measurements are a useful adjunct in assessing the intrauterine status of the fetus. Additionally, estriol measurement may be helpful in selecting the optimal time for termination of pregnancy. It has been suggested that the pregnancy of a diabetic woman should be terminated promptly in the face of a falling estriol concentration. Ideally, these determinations should be performed at least every other day.

It also has been suggested that maternal urinary estriol measurement is of value in the management of pregnancy complicated by hypertensive vascular disease and the preeclampsia–eclampsia syndrome. Here, too, estriol measurement is an aid in assessment of fetoplacental status and in determination of the optimal time for pregnancy termination. One investigator has suggested that in a patient with hypertension and preeclampsia–eclampsia, pregnancy should be terminated within 4–5 days after estriol values have significantly

centa alone, is the major source of steroid hormones during pregnancy.

ESTROGENS

More than 25 different estrogens have been isolated from the urine of pregnant women. Most are maternal and fetal metabolites of hormones secreted by the placenta. The three classic estrogens (estrone, 17β-estradiol, and estriol) have been shown to be secreted by the placenta, and most studies have involved these three hormones.

Source

There is good evidence that the placenta produces estrogen and that the syncytiotrophoblast is the site of production. This placental source is suggested by 1) the significantly higher levels of the three classic estrogens in the umbilical vein than in the umbilical arteries and 2) the rapid decrease in estrogen concentration in both fetal and maternal urine immediately after delivery.

Recent work has clarified the pathways for estrogen production by the placenta. Although ovarian tissue *in vitro* has the capacity to utilize progesterone in the formation of estrogens, similar incubations with placental tissue do not result in the transformation of progesterone into estrogens. Various *in vivo* approaches, including placental perfusion with progesterone, intraamniotic progesterone infusion, and simultaneous introduction of progesterone into the maternal and fetal circulations, produced no evidence of any significant conversion to estrogen. It is now apparent that progesterone in the umbilical circulation and in the maternal blood does not serve as a significant precursor of placental estrogens in human pregnancy.

In contrast, there is good evidence that the placenta can make estrogens by conversion of circulating androgens. Thus, the production of estrogens by the placenta appears to depend upon the availability of androgen precursors from the fetus and the mother. Moreover, the blood level of natural androgens and the production of estrogens by the placenta are quantitatively interrelated.

In both circulations that perfuse the placenta, *i.e.*, fetal and maternal, there is a high level of sulfoconjugated androgens, particularly dehydroepiandrosterone sulfate (DHAS) and 16α-hydroxydehydroepiandrosterone sulfate (16-OH-DHAS). DHAS is present in higher concentration in cord than in maternal plasma, and there is an arteriovenous difference in the umbilical circulation that suggests both fetal production and placental use of this compound.

Urinary and plasma 17-ketosteroids usually are lowered during pregnancy. The primary constituent of the 17-ketosteroids in women is the DHAS produced in the adrenal gland, and it is probable that the use of DHAS by the placenta in forming estrogen is largely responsible for the decreased urinary 17-ketosteroids. As pregnancy progresses, increasing amounts of maternal DHAS are converted to estrogen, particularly 17β-estradiol. This is reflected in decreasing blood concentrations of DHAS and increasing production rates of estradiol with advancing gestation. Fetal DHAS also contributes to the placental production of estradiol. The rate of conversion of fetal DHAS to total estrogens approximates 80%, which is much higher than the corresponding 30% conversion rate for maternal DHAS. In pregnancy, over 90% of the total estrogen excretion in the maternal urine is estriol, and most of the 80% conversion of fetal DHAS to estrogen is concerned in estriol production.

In the production of estriol, just as in the production of estradiol, the placenta is dependent upon androgenic precursors that originate in the fetal and maternal compartments. In nonpregnant women, estriol is primarily a metabolic product of estrone and estradiol. In pregnancy, however, estriol released into the circulation by the placenta is not derived in appreciable amounts from estradiol or estrone, but primarily from 16-OH-DHAS. In the fetus, the 16-hydroxylated compound can be formed in the liver and adrenal from DHAS that has been synthesized in the fetal adrenal gland. The fetal source of estriol precursors appears to be higher than the maternal, at least in the latter stages of pregnancy (Fig. 18–5). It has been suggested that estriol may function to increase uteroplacental blood flow.

The conversion of 16-OH-DHAS to estriol by the placenta (Fig. 18–5) depends first on removal of the sulfate moiety by an enzyme, steroid sulfatase. A deficiency of this substance can block the synthesis of estriol. The cases of *sulfatase deficiency* reported have been associated with healthy male infants; during pregnancy, there was no evidence of jeopardy except extremely low estriol excretion. Spontaneous labor was frequently delayed or did not occur at all.

Clinical Application of Estriol Determinations

Both an intact fetus and an intact placenta appear necessary for the synthesis of normal amounts of estriol. Thus, compromise of either or both should be reflected in decreased estriol values. Estriol is secreted by the placenta into the maternal circulation, and is transferred into the amniotic fluid. It is excreted in the maternal urine primarily in a conjugated form.

Measurement of estriol to assess fetoplacental function has been performed on urine, plasma, and amniotic fluid. To date, the most extensive measurements of estriol have been carried out on maternal urine. Estriol is measured in milligram rather than microgram quantities, its concentration in the pregnant woman

duced in nonpregnant subjects by the administration of human growth hormone; hCS may be associated with these changes in normal pregnancy. The fact that administration of this hormone produces a rise in plasma fatty acid levels in both animals and humans strengthens the hypothesis that it is related to the diabetogenic features of normal pregnancy. Other relations may be relevant to the increased resistance to insulin-induced hypoglycemia that characterizes the last trimester of normal human pregnancy.

The possible mammotropic effects of hCS also have been investigated. It has been shown that hCS synergizes with hydrocortisone and insulin to cause development of mammary gland alveoli that is histologically indistinguishable from that produced by prolactin. The evidence suggests that hCS is a potent prolactinlike hormone that is not species-specific and may be important in mammary gland development during normal human pregnancy. The possible physiologic role of hCS in the initiation of lactation in the postpartum period awaits further exploration.

It remains to be seen whether hCS plays a role in steroidogenesis in the fetoplacental unit. The marked luteotropic effect of hCS in rodents has been noted. In mice and rats, ovarian conversion of 20α-dihydroprogesterone is apparently inhibited by lactogenic hormones, allowing greater support of gestational changes in the reproductive tract. Thus, the luteotropic effects of hCS in these species suggest a possible inhibitory role for this hormone in human gestation in which placental or fetal conversion of progesterone to the less biologically active steroid might be effected.

HUMAN CHORIONIC THYROTROPIN

A third protein hormone that is immunologically similar to pituitary thyrotropin (TSH) has been shown to be synthesized and secreted by the placenta. This compound, human chorionic thyrotropin (hCT), is thought by some to have hormonal activity and physicochemical properties similar to those of pituitary TSH. The data suggest that the active principle is a glycoprotein; with some exceptions, the chromatographic and electrophoretic properties also resemble those of human pituitary TSH. Surprisingly, hCT seems immunologically more closely related to bovine and porcine TSH than to human pituitary TSH.

Biologically, hCT has been demonstrated to increase the secretion of thyroid hormone, to stimulate incorporation of inorganic phosphate into the thyroid, and to be neutralized by highly specific antipituitary TSH. Thus, the thyroid-stimulating activity of hCT appears to be due to a factor structurally related to TSH. Hennen and associates noted that the thyroid-stimulating activity in the serum of pregnant women is particularly high during early pregnancy and decreases in subsequent months to reach a minimum at term. They sug-

gested that hCT may play a role in the well-known variations in parameters of thyroid function and the incidence of thyroid enlargement during pregnancy, although they emphasized that the levels of hCT during pregnancy are not sufficient to induce clinical hyperthyroidism. More recent studies strongly suggest that much of the thyrotropic activity of the placenta is actually a function of hCG, which may explain the increased incidence of hyperthyroidism seen in patients with trophoblastic diseases.

HUMAN CHORIONIC CORTICOTROPIN

Liotta and colleagues have obtained data suggesting that the placenta also may be the source of yet another pituitary-like hormone, chorionic corticotropin. They demonstrated both immunoassayable and bioassayable adrenocorticotropic hormone (ACTH) activity in extracts of extensively washed human placental tissue and dispersed viable trophoblasts. When the trophoblasts were incubated in tissue culture medium, the ACTH content of both the cells and medium was significantly greater than the preincubation level, suggesting its synthesis by trophoblastic cells. The physiologic role, if any, of chorionic corticotropin and its regulation remain to be elucidated.

OTHER PLACENTAL PROTEIN AND POLYPEPTIDE HORMONES

Recent studies have suggested that the placenta has the capacity to synthesize hypothalamic-like gonadotropin-releasing hormone (GnRH). It may be that the placenta has the capacity to produce a wide array of pituitary- and hypothalamic-like protein and polypeptide hormones.

STEROID HORMONES

Previously, the placenta was thought to be one of the four steroid-producing glands, each complete in itself and all having similar metabolic pathways of hormone synthesis. However, evidence suggests that the manner in which the placenta produces estrogen and progesterone may be significantly different from the manner in which the ovaries produce these hormones. The concept has evolved that *the placenta is an incomplete endocrine organ,* relying for much of its hormone synthesis on precursors that reach it from the maternal and fetal compartments. It is now evident that the constant interaction of fetus, placenta, and mother, rather than the autonomous action of the placenta, is responsible for the marked increase in steroid hormone production characteristic of pregnancy. Therefore, the *fetal–placental–maternal unit,* not the pla-

Beck P, Parker ML, Daughaday WH: Radioimmunologic measurement of human placental lactogen in plasma by a double antibody method during normal and diabetic pregnancies. J Clin Endocrinol 25:1457, 1965

Bloch K: Biological conversion of cholesterol to pregnanediol. J Biol Chem 157:661, 1945

Bolté E, Mancuso S, Eriksson G et al: Aromatisation of C-19 steroids by placentas perfused in situ. Acta Endocrinol 45:535, 1964

Bolté E, Mancuso S, Eriksson G et al: Over-all aromatisation of dehydroepiandrosterone sulphate circulating in the foetal and maternal compartments. Acta Endocrinol 45:576, 1964

Cassmer O: Hormone production of the isolated human placenta: Studies on the role of the foetus in the endocrine functions of the placenta. Acta Endocrinol (Supp) 45:15, 1959

Doe RP, Zinneman HH, Flink EB et al: Significance of the concentration of non–protein-bound plasma cortisol in normals, Cushing's syndrome, pregnancy and during estrogen therapy. J Clin Endocrinol 20:1484, 1960

Dowling JT, Freinkel N, Ingbar SH: Thyroxine-binding by sera of pregnant women, newborn infants and women with spontaneous abortion. J. Clin Invest 35:1263, 1956

Fuchs F, Klopper A (eds): Endocrinology of Pregnancy. New York, Harper & Row, 1971

Gaspard U, Sandront H, Luyckx A: Glucose–insulin interaction in the modulation of human placental lactogen (HPL) secretion during pregnancy. J Obstet Gynaecol Br Commonw 81:201, 1974

Genazzani AR, Cocola F, Neri P et al: Human chorionic somatomammotropin (HCS) plasma levels in normal and pathological pregnancies and their correlation with the placental function. Acta Endocrinol 71 (Suppl 167):1, 1972

Got R, Bourrillon R: New physical data concerning human chorionic gonadotropin. Biochim Biophys Acta 39:241, 1960

Grumbach MM, Kaplan SL, Sciarra JJ et al: Chorionic growth hormone–prolactin (CGP): Secretion, disposition, biologic activity in man, and postulated function as the "growth hormone" of the second half of pregnancy. Ann NY Acad Sci 148:501, 1968

Hanson F, Powell J, Stevens V: Effects of HCG and human pituitary LH on steroid secretion and functional life of the human corpus luteum. J Clin Endocrinol 32:211, 1971

Hellig A, Lefevbre Y, Gattereau D et al: Placental progesterone synthesis in the human. In Pecile A, Fenzi C (eds): The Foeto-Placental Unit, p 152. Amsterdam, Excerpta Medica, 1969

Hennen G, Pierce JG, Freychet P: Human chorionic thyrotropin: Further characterization and study of its secretion during pregnancy. J Clin Endocrinol 29:581, 1969

Higashi K; Studies on the prolactin-like substance in human placenta. Endocrinol Jpn 8:288, 1961

Huhtaniemi IT, Korenbrot CC, Jaffe RB: hCG binding and stimulation of testosterone biosynthesis in the human fetal testis. J Clin Endocrinol Metab 44:963, 1977

Jaffe RB, Lee PA, Midgley AR, Jr: Serum gonadotropins before, at the inception of, and following human pregnancy. J Clin Endocrinol 28:1281, 1969

Jaffe RB, Peterson EP: In vivo steroid biogenesis and metabolism in the human term placenta. 2. In situ placental perfusion with cholesterol-7α-³H. Steroids 8:695, 1966

Jaffe R, Pion R, Eriksson G et al: Studies on the aromatisation of neutral steroids in pregnant women: Lack of oestrogen formation from progesterone. Acta Endocrinol 48:413, 1965

Josimovich JB: Placental protein hormones in pregnancy. Clin Obstet Gynecol 16:46, 1973

Josimovich JB, MacLaren JA: Presence in the human placenta and term serum of a highly lactogenic substance immunologically related to pituitary growth hormone. Endocrinology 71:209, 1962

Kim YJ, Felig P: Plasma chorionic somatomammotropin level during starvation in mid-pregnancy. J Clin Endocrinol 32:864, 1971

Kosasa TS, Levesque LA, Taymor ML et al: Measurement of early chorionic activity with a radioimmunoassay specific for human chorionic gonadotropin following spontaneous and induced ovulation. Fertil Steril 25:211, 1974

Landesman R, Saxena BB: Radioreceptor assay of human chorionic gonadotropin as an aid in miniabortion. Fertil Steril 25:1022, 1974

Liggins GC, Fairclough RJ, Grieves SA et al: Parturition in the sheep. In The Fetus and Birth, p 5. Ciba Foundation Symposium 47. Amsterdam, Elsevier, Excerpta Medica, 1977

Liotta A, Osathanondh R, Ryan KJ et al: Presence of corticotropin in human placenta: Demonstration of in vitro synthesis. Endocrinology 101:1552, 1977

Little B, Smith OW, Jessiman AG et al: Hypophysectomy during pregnancy in a patient with cancer of the breast. J Clin Endocrinol 18:425, 1958

Midgley AR, Jr, Fong IF, Jaffe RB: Gel filtration radioimmunoassay to distinguish human chorionic gonadotropin from luteinizing hormone. Nature 213:733, 1967

Midgley AR, Jr, Jaffe RB: Regulation of human gonadotropins: II. Disappearance of human chorionic gonadotropin following delivery. J Clin Endocrinol 28:1712, 1968

Midgley AR, Jr, Pierce GP, Jr: Immunohistochemical localization of human chorionic gonadotropin. J Exp Med 115:289, 1962

Nachtigal L, Bassett M, Hogsander V et al: A rapid method for the assay of plasma estriol in pregnancy. J Clin Endocrinol 26:941, 1966

Pearlman WH: 16-³H-progesterone metabolism in advanced pregnancy and in oophorectomized–hysterectomized women. Biochem J 67:1, 1957

Pérez-Palacios G, Pérez AE, Jaffe R: Conversion of pregnenolone-7α-³H-sulfate to other Δ⁵-3β-hydroxysteroid sulfates by the human fetal adrenal in vitro. J Clin Endocrinol 28:19, 1968

Riley GM, Smith MH, Brown P: The rapid rat test for pregnancy: the ovarian hyperemia response as a routine diagnostic procedure. J Clin Endocrinol 8:233, 1948

Ryan KJ: Biological aromatization of steroids. J Biol Chem 234:268, 1959

Selenkow HA, Saxena BM, Dana CL et al: Measurements and pathophysiologic significance of human placental lactogen. In Pecile A, Fenzi C (eds): The Foeto-Placental Unit. Amsterdam, Excerpta Medica, 1969

Serón-Ferré M, Lawrence CC, Jaffe RB: Role of hCG in the regulation of the fetal zone of the human fetal adrenal gland. J Clin Endocrinol Metab 46:834, 1978

Siiteri PK, Febres F, Clemens LE, et al.: Progesterone and maintenance of pregnancy: Is progesterone nature's immunosuppressant? Ann NY Acad Sci 286:384, 1977

Siiteri PK, MacDonald PC: Utilization of circulating dehydroisoandrosterone sulfate for estrogen synthesis during human pregnancy. Steroids 2:713, 1963

Siiteri PK, MacDonald PC: Placental estrogen biosynthesis during human pregnancy. J Clin Endocrinol 26:751, 1966

Simmer HH, Easterling WE, Jr, Pion RJ et al: Neutral C-19 steroids and steroid sulfates in human pregnancy. Steroids 4:125, 1964

Suwa S, Friesen H: Biosynthesis of human placental proteins and human placental lactogen (HPL) in vitro: I. Identification of ³H-labelled HPL. Endocrinology 85:1028, 1969

Teoh ES, Spellacy WN, Buhi WC: Human chorionic somatomammotropin (HCS): A new index of placental function. J Obstet Gynaecol Br Commonw 78:673, 1971

Turkington RW, Topper YJ: Stimulation of casein synthesis and histological development of mammary gland by human placental lactogen in vitro. Endocrinology 79:175, 1966

Tyson JE, Austin KL, Fairholt JW: Prolonged nutritional deprivation in pregnancy: Changes in human chorionic somatomammotropin and growth hormone secretion. Am J Obstet Gynecol 109:1080, 1971

Vaitukaitis JL, Braunstein GD, Ross GT: A radioimmunoassay which specifically measures human chorionic gonadotropin in the presence of human luteinizing hormone. Am J Obstet Gynecol 113:751, 1972

Wislocki GB, Dempsey EW: The chemical histology of human placenta and decidua with reference to mucoproteins, glycogen, lipids and acid phosphatase. Am J Anat 83:1, 1948

Yen SSC, Pearson OH, Rankin JS: Radioimmunoassay of serum chorionic gonadotropin and placental lactogen in trophoblastic disease. Obstet Gynecol 32:86, 1968

Ylikorkala O, Pennanen S: Human placental lactogen (HPL) levels in maternal serum during abortion induced by intra- and extra-amniotic injection of prostaglandin $F_{2\alpha}$. J Obstet Gynaecol Br Commonw 80:827, 1973

DIAGNOSIS OF PREGNANCY

Pregnancy is diagnosed from the history of certain subjective symptoms noted by the patient together with objective signs observed by the physician while performing the physical examination. Laboratory tests are of special importance early in the course of pregnancy.

SUBJECTIVE SYMPTOMS

Cessation of Menses

Pregnancy is suspected whenever a woman who has had regular menstrual cycles notices abrupt cessation of her periods. This symptom is difficult to evaluate in a patient with a previously irregular bleeding pattern. Other causes of amenorrhea must be ruled out. Some women have unexplained cyclic bleeding throughout an apparently normal pregnancy and thus do not have this symptom.

Morning Sickness

Many women tend to develop morning sickness, *i.e.,* symptoms of nausea, often with vomiting, between the 2nd and 12th weeks of pregnancy. Usually, the nausea is most marked on awakening in the morning and tends to remit as the day progresses. About half of all pregnant women complain of this symptom.

Bladder Irritability

In early pregnancy the enlarging uterus presses on the bladder. The resulting bladder irritability and reduced capacity are noticed by the patient as urinary frequency and nocturia during the first trimester. The symptoms disappear during the second trimester but commonly reappear in the third trimester at the time of lightening.

Breast Changes

Shortly after the first missed period, the pregnant woman notices a heavy sensation in the breasts, accompanied by tingling and soreness. These symptoms are related to hormonal stimulation of the ducts and alveoli of the breast parenchyma and may occur in identical form just before a menstrual period.

Enlargement of the Abdomen

Even before external evidence of abdominal enlargement can be seen, the patient may experience a sensation of tightness or heaviness in the pelvis that alerts her to the fact that she has a mass in the abdomen.

CHAPTER **19**

COURSE AND CONDUCT OF NORMAL PREGNANCY

Douglas M. Haynes

Quickening

At about the 18th week of pregnancy, the patient becomes aware of a peculiar sensation in the abdomen, often described as suggestive of the fluttering of a bird in the hand. The feeling is produced by the mother's perception of the movements of the fetus. Multiparas tend to notice quickening somewhat earlier than primigravidas, presumably because the symptom is remembered from a previous pregnancy.

Lightening

About 2 weeks from term, many patients, especially in the first pregnancy, note a sudden sensation of heaviness in the pelvis produced by dropping of the baby's head into the pelvis.

OBJECTIVE SIGNS

Changes in Uterine Consistency

Softening of the cervix (*Goodell's sign*) can be detected by the beginning of the 2nd month. The fibrous cervix of the nonpregnant woman normally feels like the tip of the nose. The effects of pregnancy on the cervix alter its consistency to approximate that of the lips.

FIG. 19-1. Early uterine signs of pregnancy. *A.* Piskaček's sign. *B.* Braun v. Fernwald's sign.

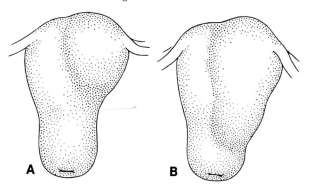

Hegar's sign is a palpable softening of the lowermost portion of the corpus, which appears at about the 6th week of gestation. To elicit this sign, the examiner places two fingers of one hand behind the cervix in the posterior vaginal fornix, then compresses the lower part of the corpus anteriorly by retropubic pressure with the other hand. In this way, a distinct area of uterine softening is noted between two firmer structures, the fundus above and the cervix below. An experienced examiner can place great reliance on Hegar's sign, since very few conditions apart from pregnancy simulate it. A somewhat subtler manifestation of early softening of the uterus is *Ladin's sign*, a soft spot in the anterior midline of the uterus between the corpus and the cervix. This finding may be present shortly before the appearance of Hegar's sign, but it is easily overlooked and hence of less clinical value.

Piskaček's sign can be elicited when the implantation of the ovum has taken place near one of the uterine cornua (Fig. 19–1A): the uterus is felt as an asymmetric organ with a well-defined soft prominence of the cornu on the side of implantation. A little later, one lateral half of the uterus is softer than the other throughout its entire length, and there may be a separatory groove between the soft and firm halves (*Braun v. Fernwald's sign;* Fig. 19–1B). This finding may be present even earlier than Hegar's sign and is evidence of probable pregnancy unless there has been an antecedent irregularity of the uterus such as may be produced by myomas. *McDonald's sign*, positive when the uterine body and cervix can be easily flexed against one another, depends on the localized softening responsible for Hegar's sign.

Changes in Mucosal Appearance

Between the 6th and 8th weeks, the mucous membranes of vulva, vagina, and cervix become congested and take on a bluish violet hue. This is *Jacquemier's* or *Chadwick's sign.* It is especially well defined in the tissues about the vaginal opening and in the anterior vaginal wall, but it is also present to some extent throughout the vagina and on the cervix.

Changes in Uterine Size

A few weeks after implantation, distinct enlargement of the uterus can be felt on vaginoabdominal palpation. The organ remains in the pelvis until the 3rd month, when the fundus becomes palpable above the pubic symphysis. Progressive enlargement noted on several occasions several weeks apart is especially helpful as a diagnostic sign. The early asymmetry disappears promptly, usually by the 3rd month, and from this time on the enlarging organ is symmetric. Some diagnostic confusion is occasionally encountered in differentiating between pregnancy enlargement and other causes of uterine enlargement such as myomas or other

FIG. 19-2. Pregnancy hypertrophy of axillary breast tissue.

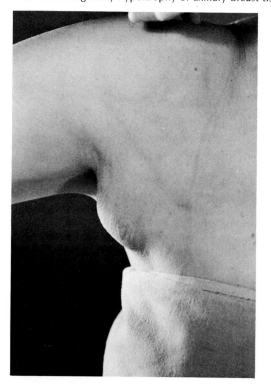

FIG. 19-3. Internal ballottement of fetus in early pregnancy.

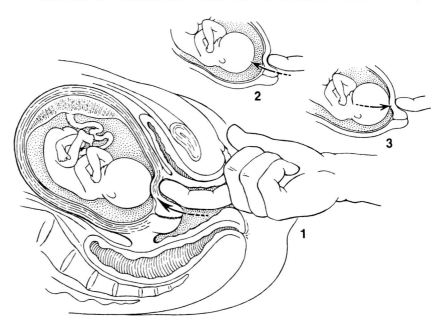

tumors; ovarian neoplasms not easily distinguishable from the uterus may complicate the picture.

Changes in Uterine Shape

The uterus changes in pregnancy from its pear-shaped configuration to a globular contour, passing through a transient asymmetric phase. In later months, the uterus is elongated as the fundus grows upward toward the xiphisternum.

Contractions of the Uterus

Soon after implantation, intermittent, irregular, painless uterine contractions are palpable from time to time, beginning near the end of the first trimester. These constitute *Braxton Hicks' sign*. Such contractions occur periodically throughout pregnancy. Since they occur also in the nonpregnant state, they are not a sure sign of pregnancy.

Breast Changes

From the 2nd month or even earlier, progressive enlargement of the breasts can be observed. In patients with well-developed axillary breast tissue, its hypertrophy may give rise to symptomatic lumps in the armpits (Fig. 19–2). The modified sebaceous glands in the area of the areola known as Montgomery's glands become prominent. The nipples are pink and flushed at first, especially in primigravidas; later, the areola becomes darker, and an area of increased pigmentation of the adjacent skin (*secondary areola*) becomes apparent.

No fluid can ordinarily be expressed from the nipples during the early part of pregnancy except in multigravidas with persistent breast secretion following previous pregnancies. The characteristic breast secretion of late pregnancy, *colostrum,* a thin, yellowish fluid containing epithelial cells, leukocytes, and "colostrum corpuscles," makes its appearance too late to be of much diagnostic value. The venous patterns of the skin of the breasts become prominent as the result of dilation early in the first trimester.

Changes Noted on Abdominal Examination

On palpation of the abdomen, the examiner notes progressive uterine enlargement reflected in bulging of the anterior abdominal wall. Externally visible protrusion begins at about the 3rd month and increases in prominence as the uterine fundus enlarges upward. By about the 20th week, fetal movement can often be felt by the physician. Passive fetal movements may be elicited by internal ballottement (Fig. 19–3), in which the anterior vaginal wall and the lower pole of the uterus are tapped sharply upward by two fingers in the vagina. This maneuver pushes the fetal body up; it will fall back promptly and will be felt to bump against the examiner's fingertips in the vagina. The details of the clinical methods used to determine intrauterine fetal relations are given later in this chapter under Prenatal Care.

The presence of a fetus can be confirmed by auscultation about the 20th week of gestation. At this time, the fetal heart sound can be heard through a specially designed stethoscope, the fetoscope (Fig. 19–4). The normal fetal heartbeat is a rapid tick-tock sound with a

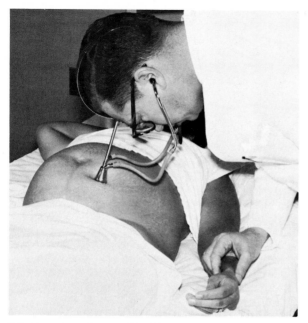

FIG. 19-4. Auscultation of fetal heartbeat with DeLee–Hillis fetoscope. Maternal pulse is checked simultaneously.

FIG. 19-5. Points of maximum intensity of fetal heartbeat in various presentations, positions, and attitudes of fetus. *RSA,* Right sacrum anterior. *LSA,* Left sacrum anterior. *ROP,* Right occiput posterior. *LOP,* Left occiput posterior. *RMA,* Right mentum anterior. *ROA,* Right occiput anterior. *LMA,* Left mentum anterior. *LOA,* Left occiput anterior.

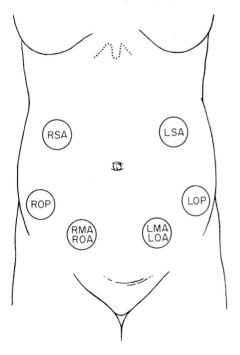

rate varying between 120 and 160 beats/min. When it is first audible at 20 weeks, the fetal heartbeat is best heard in the midline just above the symphysis. Later, it is loudest over the most convex part of the fetal body and hence will vary with the presentation, position, and attitude of the fetus. Many circumstances may obscure the fetal heart sounds, but heart sounds definitely heard constitute positive proof of a live fetus. The points of maximum intensity of the fetal heartbeat in the various presentations, positions, and attitudes of the fetus are illustrated in Figure 19–5.

Although the fetoscope is the time-honored instrument for detecting the fetal heartbeat, its reliability is weakened by such variables as the patient's size and degree of obesity, hydramnios, changes in fetal position, and various extraneous factors such as environmental noise. The latter also interferes with the effectiveness of phonocardiography, the results of which are inconsistent and unsatisfactory for early detection of the fetal heart sounds. Fetal electrocardiography, in its most recent modification, is an excellent research tool in later pregnancy and reliably demonstrates fetal complexes from 18–20 weeks from cessation of menses; but the high cost of the instrument, together with the necessity for special skill in both use and interpretation, restrict its practical usefulness.

Callagan and associates, in 1964, suggested the possibility of ultrasonic methods for the early detection of fetal life, and several practical instruments have since been developed for this purpose. All use the Doppler phenomenon, which depends on the physical principle that sound (or radio) waves reflected from a moving object return to a transmitting source at a slightly altered frequency, while waves reflected from a stationary object return at exactly the same frequency. The Doptone fetal pulse detector is one of the instruments designed for this purpose. It transmits a sound wave at a constant frequency of 2.25 megacycles with an intensity of 2.6 mw/sq cm and receives only deviations from this pattern. When the ultrasound is transmitted into the body, its reflection from immobile structures returns at the same frequency and is not converted to an audible signal, while its reflection from moving structures is slightly shifted in frequency; this difference in frequency is converted into audible sound by the Doptone. This method can detect the fetal pulse occasionally at 10 weeks' gestation and consistently at 12 weeks'. The instrument is also of great value if fetal heart sounds cannot be heard and intrauterine death is suspected, *e.g.,* in certain cases of premature separation of the placenta; if the fetal pulse cannot be detected by this method, intrauterine death is a virtual certainty.

Another uterine sound is the *funic souffle,* a hissing sound synchronous with the fetal pulse. This sign is of minor diagnostic importance, since it is heard in only 15% of patients; when heard, it has the same positive diagnostic significance as the fetal heartbeat. The

TABLE 19-1. PREGNANCY TESTS

Trade Name	Manufacturer	Principle	Method Sensitivity (mIU/ml)	Reaction Time
PREGNOSIS (SLIDE)	Roche	AI	1500–2500	2 min
SENSI-TEX (TUBE)	Roche	AI	250	1½ h
GEST STATE (SLIDE)	Fisher	AI	2000–4000	2 min
HCG TEST	Hyland	AI	2000–8000	2 min
PREGNOSTICON (TUBE)	Organon	AI	750	2 h
PREGNOSTICON (ACCUS-PHERES)	Organon	AI	750–1000	2 h
PREGNOSTICON (SLIDE)	Organon	AI	1000–2000	2 min
PREGNOSTICON DRI-DOT	Organon	AI	1000–2000	2 min
GRAVINDEX	Ortho	AI	3500	2 min
DAP URINE	Wampole	DA	2000	2 min
DAP SERUM	Wampole	DA	2000	2 min
UCG (TUBE)	Wampole	AI	1500	2 h
UCG (SLIDE)	Wampole	AI	2000	2 min
BIOCEPT-G	Wampole	RRA	200	1 h
HCG (β-SUBUNIT, QUALITATIVE)	RSL, Inc.*	RIA	40	2 h
PREG/STAT β-HCG (QUALITATIVE)	Serono	RIA	15	1 h
β-HCG (quantitative)	Serono	RIA	3.12	3 h
β-HCG (quantitative)	Serono	RIA	1.56	18 h

* Radioassay Systems Laboratories, Inc. *AI,* Agglutination inhibition. *DA,* Direct agglutination. *RRA,* Radioreceptorassay. *RIA* Radioimmunoassay.
(Data from published reports or manufacturers' information.)

sound is produced by the rush of blood through the umbilical arteries.

A soft murmur synchronous with the maternal pulse, the *uterine bruit,* results from the passage of blood through the dilated uterine vessels. It is loudest on either side of the midline just above the symphysis.

In midpregnancy, sudden movement of the fetus during auscultation may give rise to a characteristic fetal shock sound. The quality of this sound can be simulated by placing the palm of one hand over an ear and tapping the dorsum of that hand with one finger of the other. The sign is a late one; but, when heard, it is a reliable indication that the fetus is alive.

TESTS FOR PREGNANCY

Tests for pregnancy are based on analyses for human chorionic gonadotropin (hCG), which is elaborated by the trophoblast in minimal but detectable amounts as early as 1 day after implantation, increases rapidly to peak serum levels of about 50,000 mIU/ml about 65 days after implantation, and slowly declines to low levels between the 100th and 130th days of pregnancy. It disappears from the bloodstream and urine 10–14 days after delivery.

As noted in Chapter 18, precise and rapid tests are now available for the diagnosis of pregnancy. Tests in current use are listed in Table 19–1. The biologic tests (*e.g.,* Aschheim–Zondek test; Friedman test) are no longer used. The immunologic tests have the advantages of speed; reasonable accuracy, provided hCG levels are not lower than the tests' limit of sensitivity (about 1500 mIU/ml); and simplicity, since they can be readily performed in the physician's office. Both radioreceptorassay (RRA) and radioimmunoassay (RIA) have the advantage of great sensitivity, but they require expensive equipment and skilled technicians. Because the RRA test cross-reacts with luteinizing hormone (LH), the limit of sensitivity for this test is set at 200 mIU/ml serum, which is sufficiently higher than the LH midcycle peak of about 175 mIU/ml to avoid confusion with ordinary serum levels of LH. The RRA test can be performed in 1 hour. Newer RIA tests for the beta subunit of hCG (β-hCG) can also be performed in about 1 hour and have sensitivity of 15 mIU/ml. Optional quantitative tests have extreme sensitivity: a 3-hour test is sensitive to 3.12 mIU/ml, an 18-hour test to 1.56 mIU/ml, levels that might be found on the 1st day after implantation. The β-hCG RIA test also cross-reacts with LH, but in amounts so minimal that for practical purposes the test can be considered specific.

Physicians employing hCG tests should know the general range of hCG levels that they wish to detect and the sensitivity of the test that is used. In general,

tests for home or office use are suitable for diagnosis of pregnancy at 6+ weeks gestation. RRA tests are suitable if greater precision is required and hCG levels are known or expected to be higher than the standard for the test, usually about 200 mU/ml serum; examples include most cases of ectopic pregnancy, the diagnosis of pregnancy from 4–6 weeks gestation, and trophoblastic disease in which hCG levels are higher than 200 mU/ml. RIA tests are used for cases in which hCG levels are known or expected to be lower than the standard for RRA tests; examples include pregnancy before 3–4 weeks gestation, known or suspected trophoblastic disease in which the RRA test is negative, and suspected ectopic pregnancy in which the RRA test is negative.

Recent studies suggest that determination of serum *pregnancy-specific β_1 glycoprotein* may serve as a sensitive pregnancy test. This substance has been detected by RIA as early as 7 days after ovulation, but the scarcity of purified antigens has hampered its widespread use. It is presumed that simple latex agglutination tests will ultimately be available.

ULTRASOUND DIAGNOSIS OF PREGNANCY

Ultrasound has simplified many aspects of obstetric diagnosis and has rendered unnecessary many tests previously used (see Chapter 28). Use of the Doppler effect for detection of the fetal pulse at 12 weeks' gestation was mentioned earlier. Scanning methods can detect a gestational sac as early as 6 weeks after the last menstrual period; this provides evidence of pregnancy, but gives no indication whether the fetus is living. Real-time methods can detect the fetal cardiac pulsations at 8 weeks in about half the cases and almost uniformly by 10 weeks. Fetal movements are readily detected by this method, beginning at about 12 weeks' gestation.

X-RAY DIAGNOSIS OF PREGNANCY

It is potentially hazardous to expose patients to x-rays during pregnancy, and such exposure should be avoided except when clearly indicated. It may be justified, for example, when ultrasonography is unavailable and visualization of the fetal skeleton after the 16th week is necessary to differentiate pregnancy from a large abdominal tumor.

DIFFERENTIAL DIAGNOSIS OF PREGNANCY

Although the progressive changes that occur during pregnancy are characteristic, difficulty may be encountered in differentiating pregnancy from other conditions at the early examination.

Uterine Leiomyomas

Uterine enlargement because of leiomyomas can simulate the enlargement of pregnancy. With myomas, however, amenorrhea is only coincidental. The breast does not change as it does in pregnancy, and the myomas are firmer than the pregnant uterus and often irregular in outline. The tests for pregnancy are negative unless the patient is also pregnant. The asymmetric cornual enlargement of Piskaček's sign may closely resemble a myoma in that location; here the differential diagnosis depends on recognition of the peculiar elastic consistency of the pregnant uterus.

Ovarian Cysts

The soft consistency of an ovarian cyst can closely resemble that of the pregnant uterus. There is usually no amenorrhea, however, and neither softening of the cervix nor bluish discoloration of the vagina is present. With large tumors, failure to hear the fetal heart sounds and inability to outline the fetal body or to feel active movements help to rule out pregnancy. Tests for pregnancy are negative, and the fetal skeleton cannot be visualized on an x-ray film.

Ascites

When the abdomen is distended by ascitic fluid, a fluid wave can be detected by palpation. Amenorrhea, vaginal changes, and breast enlargement and tingling do not occur and pregnancy tests are negative. The abdominal wall is tense and fails to show the loosening and relaxation characteristic of pregnancy.

Hematometra

An imperforate hymen or vaginal or cervical stenosis may result in an enlarged, intermittently contractile uterus associated with amenorrhea. Breast, cervical, and vaginal changes of pregnancy do not appear, and pregnancy tests are negative. The underlying lesion responsible for blocking the uterine outflow can be diagnosed by history, examination, or both.

Pseudocyesis

Although most often found in women nearing the menopause, pseudocyesis (imaginary pregnancy) occurs also in young women who have a strong, unfulfilled desire for pregnancy. It is associated with all the subjective symptoms of true pregnancy. The abdomen may appear enlarged. The patient interprets gas in the intestines or other abdominal sensations as fetal movements. On examination, the uterus is not enlarged, and there are no pelvic signs of pregnancy. There is no objective evidence of a fetus, and the pregnancy tests are negative. The physician may encounter difficulty

in convincing the patient with pseudocyesis that she is not pregnant; when this is the case, a psychiatrist should be consulted.

The signs and symptoms of pregnancy are classed as presumptive, probable, and positive in order of reliability. They are summarized in Table 19–2.

DIAGNOSIS OF PREVIOUS PREGNANCY

If the patient is unwilling to admit to a previous delivery, the physician must rely on objective signs involving many body structures. Systematic examination permits an accurate diagnosis.

Abdomen

The multiparous patient usually has a lax, flabby abdomen as the result of stretching of the anterior abdominal wall; often, her abdomen is pendulous. The primigravida has a firm, unrelaxed contour. Fresh pinkish blue striae may be seen in the abdominal skin of the primigravida; in the multipara, old silvery white striae are also present.

Breasts

In the multipara, the breasts are often less firm than those of a primigravida and have scars of striae from previous pregnancies, as well as fresh striae from the present one.

External Genitalia

The torn hymen of the primigravida is replaced in the multipara by the characteristic carunculae myrtiformes. The labia majora are loose and pigmented after pregnancy and may show varicosities. The perineum is intact in the primigravida, while that of the multipara may show an old tear or the scar of a repaired episiotomy.

Cervix

In the primigravida, the external os has a circular pinpoint appearance, and the cervical canal is tightly closed. After childbirth, the os is apt to be patulous and shows a transverse laceration at 3 and 9 o'clock. The multiparous os usually admits a fingertip, and when the transverse laceration is a deep one, there may be distinct formation of anterior and posterior lips separated by a groove.

Vagina

The vagina in the primigravida is narrow, with prominent crested folds; in the multipara, however, the folds are smooth and flattened, and the entire vaginal canal is widened.

TABLE 19-2. SUMMARY OF SYMPTOMS AND SIGNS OF PREGNANCY

Symptoms and Signs	Approximate Time of Appearance (weeks)
PRESUMPTIVE	
Amenorrhea	2
Morning sickness	3–5
Bladder symptoms	4–6
Early breast symptoms	3–4
Soft spot on uterus	6
Braxton Hicks contractions	6
Bluish discoloration of vagina	6
Quickening	16
Abdominal enlargement	16
PROBABLE	
HCG (RIA, RRA)	3–5
Routine immunologic tests	6
Increased compressibility of isthmus	8
Asymmetric uterine enlargement	6–8
Internal ballottement	16–20
Uterine bruit	16
Palpation of active fetal parts	16
POSITIVE	
X-ray demonstration of fetal parts	16
Fetal heart sounds	20
Palpation of active fetal movements	20–24
Ultrasound scan	10

DIAGNOSIS OF LIFE OR DEATH OF THE FETUS

SIGNS OF FETAL LIFE

Proof of a living fetus is provided by hearing the fetal heartbeat, palpating active movements, and observing progressive increase in size of the fetus on successive examinations several weeks apart.

After 20 weeks' gestation, the fetal heartbeat can be detected with the stethoscope; even before this time, the pulse can be detected by Doptone or an equivalent instrument. As mentioned previously, real-time ultrasound provides positive evidence of both movements and beating of the fetal heart usually after 10 weeks' gestation, but invariably after 12 weeks' gestation.

SIGNS OF FETAL DEATH

The earliest indication of fetal death is cessation of growth of the uterus, followed by regression in uterine size, as detected by repeated examinations over several weeks. At the same time, retrogressive changes can be observed in the breasts, notably diminution in overall size. Later in pregnancy, the mother may report that she feels no fetal movements; this is suggestive of fetal death when the physician can find no fetal heartbeat and can corroborate the cessation of fetal movements

already noted by the mother. Death of the fetus is confirmed most readily by a real-time scan that fails to demonstrate either fetal movements or contractions of the fetal heart. If this instrument should not be available, failure to detect the fetal pulse with a Doptone or equivalent instrument strongly suggests the baby has died. Serial estriol determinations decline rapidly; later, abdominal x-ray shows overlapping of the cranial bones (*Spalding's sign*) and gas, thought to be nitrogen, in the fetal circulation. Pregnancy tests may remain positive for extended periods after fetal death because of the persistence of viable chorionic tissue.

ESTIMATION OF DURATION OF PREGNANCY

Pregnancy begins with fertilization of the ovum. Since this event cannot be timed accurately, the exact duration of pregnancy is unknown. Several methods can be used to estimate the duration of pregnancy with reasonable accuracy.

NÄGELE'S RULE

The average length of pregnancy is approximately 266 days after the date of the fruitful coitus, with lower and upper limits of authenticated cases at 230 and 349 days, respectively. A rough but practical estimation of

FIG. 19-6. Height of fundus at comparable gestational dates varies greatly from patient to patient. Those shown are most common. Convenient rule of thumb is that at 5 months' gestation, fundus is usually at or slightly above umbilicus.

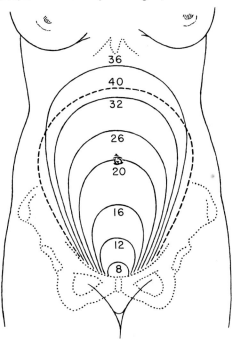

the duration of pregnancy in a given patient can be made by applying Nägele's rule: To the 1st day of the last normal menstruation, add 7 days, subtract 3 months, and add 1 year to obtain the expected date of delivery. This method is a formula for counting forward 280 days from the beginning of the last period. About 60% of patients can be expected to deliver within 1 week of the estimated date of delivery calculated by Nägele's rule, but less than 5% will deliver on the actual date itself after spontaneous labor.

TIMING FROM QUICKENING

Maternal perception of fetal movements (quickening) sometimes furnishes a rough estimate of the duration of pregnancy. Although it may occur any time between 3.5 and 5 months, quickening usually occurs at about the 18th week in the multigravida and a week or two later in the primigravida. This method should be used *only* as a rough check of other calculations and with full knowledge of its variability.

HEIGHT OF FUNDUS

Progressive palpable enlargement of the uterus can be followed during pregnancy by feeling the height of the fundus on the abdomen (Fig. 19-6). The fundus can be felt just above the pubic symphysis at about the 10th week of gestation. At 16 weeks, it rises to approximately halfway between the symphysis and the umbilicus, and it is at the umbilicus at 20 weeks. At 28 weeks, it is 3 fingerbreadths above this point and rises a further 3 fingerbreadths during the ensuing 4 weeks. At the 36th week, the fundus is just below the ensiform cartilage, where it may remain until the onset of labor in the multipara; in the primigravida, the fundal height drops at the time of lightening to about 2 fingerbreadths below its maximum height.

SPIEGELBERG'S MEASUREMENTS

Spiegelberg compiled a table relating the distance from the symphysis to the fundus to the duration of gestation (Table 19-3). A modified form of this method is incorporated in *McDonald's rule* (Fig. 19-7), which states that the fundus-to-symphysis distance in centimeters divided by 3.5 gives an approximation of the lunar month of pregnancy after the 6th month.

ULTRASONOGRAPHIC MEASUREMENTS

Ultrasound techniques (see Chapter 28) should be used to assist in establishing an estimated date of labor

TABLE 19-3. SPIEGELBERG'S TABLE OF RELATIONS BETWEEN LINEAR DISTANCE FROM SYMPHYSIS TO FUNDUS AND LENGTH OF GESTATION

Linear Distance, Symphysis to Fundus (cm)	Estimated Fetal Age (weeks)
26.7	28
30.0	32
32.0	36
37.7	40

1) if the woman is unsure of the date of her last menstrual period, 2) if an oral contraceptive was used immediately before conception and the timing of the pregnancy is uncertain, 3) if the dates are suspect because the first visit is after 20 weeks' gestation, or 4) if the size of the uterus appears not to conform to the menstrual dates. A single scan (real-time or B scan) is helpful, but accuracy is higher if a first scan is made when the uterus conforms to 20–24 weeks' size, and a second scan at about 30–33 weeks'. The two scans provide a growth-adjusted gestational age (GASA), as discussed in Chapter 41.

PRENATAL CARE

One of the most important contributions of modern obstetrics to mothers and babies has been the systematization of prenatal care. The beginnings of this doctrine are outlined in Chapter 1. As a result of careful examination of the pregnant patient at frequent intervals throughout the period of gestation, abnormalities can be detected and dealt with before difficulties arise, and catastrophic occurrences can be almost eliminated. Conscientious prenatal care not only protects the health and well-being of the mother, but also significantly reduces perinatal morbidity and mortality. The beneficial effects of properly conducted prenatal care programs are documented by the great reduction in avoidable complications in populations that use such programs, as contrasted with the problems reported from areas of the world in which prenatal care is either unavailable or not widely sought.

INITIAL HISTORY

The first step in the workup of an obstetric patient consists of the taking and recording of a careful general history of her medical background before the present pregnancy, as well as of events that have occurred during the current gestation. The details of this history are outlined in Chapter 9. A standard printed form may be used to record the data. It is important for the physician to develop the habit of methodically recording clinical data.

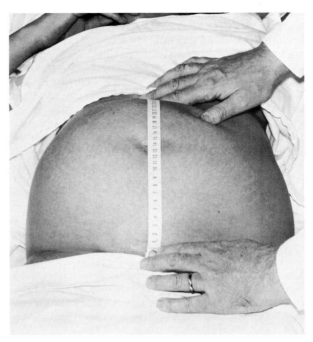

FIG. 19-7. Measuring fundus-to-symphysis distance by McDonald's method.

The expected date of delivery is calculated by Nägele's rule from the 1st day of the last normal menstrual period. The date of quickening is recorded if the patient has noted fetal movements. Systems are reviewed for recent symptoms, and specific questions are asked about cardiorespiratory symptoms (dyspnea, edema, orthopnea); gastrointestinal upsets (nausea, vomiting, constipation); genitourinary complaints (vaginal discharge, bleeding, pruritus); neuromuscular disturbances (headache, dizziness, syncope, visual defects); and discomfort of bones and joints (backache).

INITIAL PHYSICAL EXAMINATION

Vital Signs

Blood pressure, pulse rate, temperature, and respiration per minute constitute an important series of baseline measurements, even when they are entirely normal at the first visit.

Weight

Observation of weight gain during pregnancy is an important part of prenatal care, and the weight of the obstetric patient is checked and recorded from the outset.

General Physical Survey

A thorough general physical examination is performed at the initial visit of each obstetric patient. Notes are made in the record of the patient's general appearance and state of nutrition, and the condition of her skin and hair. The ears, eyes, nose, and throat are inspected by standard techniques and any abnormalities recorded. The condition of the teeth is noted, especially fillings, caries, and soft tissue abnormalities about the mouth. The size of the thyroid gland is estimated by palpation, and the neck is checked for lymphadenopathy. The heart and lungs are evaluated by careful percussion and auscultation. The legs are inspected for evidence for varicosities, skeletal deformities, or edema.

Examination of the Abdomen

The abdomen is described with special attention to the height of the uterine fundus, the number and distribution of striae, and the firm or soft consistency of the rectus abdominis muscles. Diastasis recti is noted if present. If the initial visit has been delayed until after the 20th week of gestation, the fetal heartbeat is auscultated. From the 32nd week to term, systematic examination of the abdomen is carried out using Leopold's maneuvers. The details of this examination are outlined under Subsequent Examinations.

Breast Examination

The breasts are examined systematically for masses, skin lesions, and axillary extension. Erectility and eversion of the nipples are noted, together with any local lesions.

Pelvic Examination

With the patient in the lithotomy position and with the aid of a good light for the initial inspection, pelvic examination is performed. The configuration of the outlet is noted; it may be relaxed or tightly supported. Bartholin's and Skene's glands are inspected and palpated, and any enlargement or induration is described. Varicosities of the vulva or vagina are noted and their size and distribution described. A speculum is then inserted into the vagina and the vaginal walls examined for evidence of discharge, local lesions, or prolapse. The cervix is visualized, and a Pap smear is taken. Any lesions or bleeding are described. The location and extent of previous cervical lacerations are of particular importance. After removal of the speculum, the uterus is examined by bimanual palpation. The height of the fundus is related to the symphysis or umbilicus (in late pregnancy, to the ensiform cartilage) and its consistency and general contour noted. Attempts to palpate the adnexa often fail during pregnancy, especially after the first few weeks, but an attempt should be made in order to disclose tumor masses separate from the uterus. If the patient is approaching term at the first visit, the degree of cervical effacement and the patulousness of the external os are pertinent observations. The final step in the pelvic examination is the palpation of the parametria by combined rectovaginal touch to rule out neoplastic or inflammatory infiltrations of the broad ligament bases. Manual mensuration of certain obstetrically significant diameters is carried out at this point. The procedure involved is described in the discussion of clinical examination of the pelvis (see Chapter 30).

INITIAL LABORATORY STUDIES

Several basic laboratory tests form a part of the initial workup of each obstetric patient. Those summarized in the following should be performed as early in pregnancy as possible.

Serologic Test for Syphilis

Not only is a serologic test for syphilis a legal requirement in all states in the United States, it is an essential feature of good prenatal care. The most commonly used test is the precipitin (VDRL) test, but a complement fixation test such as the Kahn or Kolmer test is equally acceptable.

Blood Count

The basic tests for detection of maternal anemia are hematocrit and packed cell volume (PC) determinations. Hemoglobin determination is less accurate, although it offers a rough guide to the patient's hematologic status and is widely used. ABO and Rh typing of both the patient and her husband are routinely done at this time. White cell and Schilling differential cell counts are necessary only if infection or blood dyscrasia is suspected.

Urinalysis

A clean voided specimen of urine is evaluated for protein, glucose, specific gravity, and blood, pus, or casts in the microscopic sediment. If proteinuria is present in early pregnancy, further tests are indicated to rule out renal disease. As term is approached, proteinuria can be a sign of preeclampsia. If glucose is present in the first specimen studied, the patient is instructed to return next day with a 2-hour postprandial specimen for further analysis. If this contains glucose, arrangements are made to perform a glucose tolerance test to evaluate the possibility of diabetes mellitus.

X-Ray Studies

It is generally agreed that chest x-ray, formerly considered an essential part of pregnancy evaluation, is not routinely needed. Pulmonary tuberculosis has become a rare disease in the United States; when it is suspected, skin testing, preferably with the Mantoux test, should be used for screening.

The fetal and gonadal doses of diagnostic x-ray examinations are listed in Table 60–1. These and the tests discussed in Chapter 28 must not be used promiscuously in pregnancy (or at any other time), but the physician should not hesitate to use them if they are essential to the proper diagnosis and management of obstetric complications.

SUBSEQUENT EXAMINATIONS

The routine examination of the obstetric patient on subsequent visits is less detailed and time-consuming than the initial workup, but its basic steps are essential for proper supervision of the patient.

Weight

Limitation of weight gain is of less importance than was formerly thought. It is the physician's responsibility, however, to provide instruction in optimum dietary intake to avoid both nutritional deficiencies and excessive caloric intake. Sharp increases in weight exceeding 0.5–1 lb/week are usually due to water retention, and in the last month this may herald the onset of preeclampsia. Bedrest is an excellent diuretic if it should be needed and is feasible.

Blood Pressure

Elevation of the blood pressure in pregnancy carries with it the possibility of serious complications. Patients with basic hypertensive disease have an increased tendency to develop preeclampsia, and this itself is signaled by hypertension. Blood pressure elevation in pregnancy requires careful evaluation of its cause and may require special treatment.

Urinalysis

Small amounts of protein can appear in the urine as a result of contamination by a vaginal discharge; significant amounts accompanied by hypertension are ominous, suggesting severe preeclampsia. A large protein spill without hypertension suggests a nephrotic syndrome. Glycosuria is an indication for fasting and 2-hour postprandial blood sugar measurements.

Systematic Examination of the Abdomen

By midpregnancy, the fetus can usually be palpated through the anterior abdominal and uterine walls. After the fetal body becomes palpable, its position within the uterus is determined and recorded at each prenatal visit. The fetal position is mapped out by means of a systematic sequence of maneuvers, the *maneuvers of Leopold*. The first three maneuvers are carried out with the physician facing the patient's head and standing to one side of her as she lies supine on the examining table; the fourth maneuver is done with the examiner facing the patient's feet. Each maneuver is designed to answer by palpation a specific question regarding the relation of the fetal body to that of the mother.

First Maneuver (Fig. 19–8). The first maneuver answers the question: What fetal part occupies the fundus? The examiner palpates the fundal area and distinguishes between the irregular, nodular breech and the hard, round, mobile, and ballottable head.

Second Maneuver (Fig. 19–9). The second maneuver answers the question: On which side is the fetal back? The palms of the hands are placed on either side of the abdomen. On one side, a linear, bony ridge is felt, the back, while on the other side are numerous nodular masses corresponding to the small parts. This maneuver also determines the position by disclosing anterior, transverse, or posterior orientation of the back.

Third Maneuver (Fig. 19–10). The third maneuver answers the question: What fetal part lies over the inlet? A single examining hand is placed just above the symphysis so as to grasp between thumb and third finger the fetal part that overrides the symphysis. If the head is unengaged, it will be readily recognized as a round, ballottable object that can be easily displaced upward. After engagement, a shoulder is felt as a relatively fixed, knoblike part. In breech presentations, the irregular, nodular breech is felt in direct continuity with the vertebral column in the dorsoanterior position. In frank and complete breech presentations, a knee or a foot may be felt in the dorsoposterior position.

Fourth Maneuver. The fourth maneuver answers the question: On which side is the cephalic prominence? The examiner faces the patient's feet and places both hands on either side of the lower pole of the uterus just above the inlet. If the presenting part is floating, the maneuver cannot be performed; it applies only when the head is engaged. When pressure is exerted in the direction of the inlet, one hand can descend further than the other. The other part of the fetus that prevents deep descent of one hand is called the *cephalic*

prominence. In flexion attitudes, it is on the same side as the small parts (Fig. 19–11), while in extension attitudes, it is on the same side as the back (Fig. 19–12).

If the foregoing maneuvers disclose a significant abnormality (*e.g.,* transverse or oblique lie, breech presentation), its disposition depends upon the imminence of labor as judged by both the duration of pregnancy and the condition of the cervix. If labor is considered *not* imminent, the abnormality should be noted in the patient's record; but nothing more need be made of it, since the problem may correct itself before the onset of labor. If the cervix is soft and partly dilated and there is reason to presume labor is imminent, then specific evaluation and management should be followed as though the patient were indeed in early labor (see Chapter 34).

It is a moot question whether the patient should be informed of abnormal findings such as these. In the writer's opinion, she should definitely be advised if cesarean section is seriously contemplated; she *may* be advised if the findings suggest clearly that the baby is in jeopardy, although in some circumstances it is preferable to discuss this with the husband; she should usually *not* be advised, nor is there reason to inform the husband, if the case is to be managed expectantly because the problem may correct itself or because there is at the time neither reason for intervention nor likelihood that labor is imminent.

External Cephalic Version. When abdominal examination after 34 weeks' gestation reveals a breech presentation, the question arises whether an attempt should be made to convert this to the vertex presentation, a technique referred to as external cephalic version. Over the years, the maneuver has enjoyed sporadic and spotty enthusiasm. Eastman, the leading obstetrician of his time, interpreted the available data to show that, if it is done gently enough to be innocuous, many of the attempts fail; of those that are successful, most in later weeks revert to breech presentation or would have spontaneously turned later to a vertex presentation. In addition, he believed that the mother's awareness of something clearly wrong may produce much psychologic stress. If a serious effort at version is made, the hazards of separation of the placenta, cord entanglement, premature rupture of the membranes, and rupture of the uterus may be encountered. The pendulum seems again to be moving, however, and many physicians now believe that everything possible should be done to avoid breech presentation and that it can be done with little risk. The question remains unsettled; some obstetricians attempt external version routinely, while others prefer to deal with a breech presentation at term by vaginal delivery if the conditions are perfect or otherwise by cesarean section.

If external version is contemplated, it should be preceded by an ultrasound scan to confirm the presentation, to rule out multiple pregnancy, and to localize the placenta (of which about 40% are on the anterior uterine wall). The procedure should not be done if the placenta is on the anterior wall or in the lower pole of the uterus; if the membranes have ruptured; if there is a multiple pregnancy; if the patient has hypertensive vascular disease or preeclampsia; if the uterus is too irritable to permit the procedure to be done easily; if there is a history of antepartum bleeding, cesarean section, or myomectomy; or if the possibility of delivery by cesarean section is already being considered (*e.g.,* elderly primigravida, prior infertility problem, prior vaginal plastic operation).

In performing the procedure, two factors are of special importance. First, the uterus must be sufficiently relaxed to permit the manipulations without inciting a uterine contraction, a condition that is increasingly unlikely as term is approached. Second, the breech must be mobilized from the pelvis, which is facilitated if the version is done after the woman has been in a modified Trendelenburg posture for 10–30 min. The breech is displaced from the pelvis. The version is done toward the side of the baby's face, since this increases flexion of the head and improves the chance of success. Having displaced the breech from the pelvis, the physician moves it laterally toward the side of the back with one hand, while *at the same time* the opposite hand moves the head in the direction the face "looks," as in a forward somersault. The operation is done gently and smoothly, with frequent monitoring of the fetal heart, until the head comes to lie over the inlet and the breech to occupy the fundus. The fetal heart should be monitored before and during the version, and the attempt should be discontinued if there is any abnormality that persists for more than a minute. The fetal heart rate may slow after the version is completed; if this persists longer than 5 min, the possibility of cord entanglement should be considered, and the baby should be gently turned back to the breech presentation.

Detection of Fetal Movements. Abdominal palpation may be used to detect active intrauterine fetal movements after the 4th month of gestation. Such movements are positive indications of fetal life.

Estimation of Fetal Size

Unfortunately, no clinical method for estimating the size of the fetus is accurate, and errors are common. If needed, the information provided by ultrasound scans is accurate within limits. However, the physician should usually be content if the uterus continues to enlarge at a normal rate.

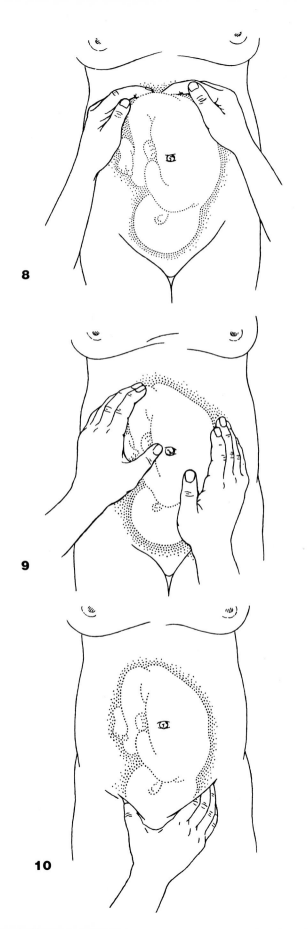

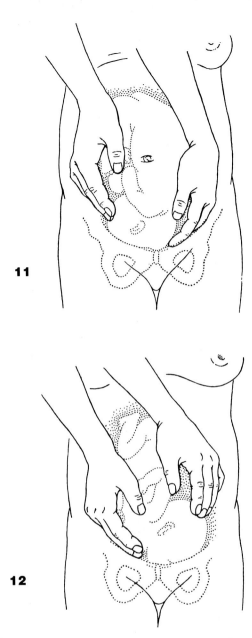

FIG. 19-8. Leopold's first maneuver. Answers question: What fetal part occupies fundus?

FIG. 19-9. Leopold's second maneuver. Answers question: On which side is fetal back?

FIG. 19-10. Leopold's third maneuver. Answers question: What fetal part lies over pelvic inlet?

FIG. 19-11. Leopold's fourth maneuver. Answers question: On which side is cephalic prominence? In flexion attitude, cephalic prominence is on same side as small parts.

FIG. 19-12. Leopold's fourth maneuver. Answers question: On which side is cephalic prominence? In extension attitude, cephalic prominence is on same side as back.

Auscultation

At each prenatal visit, the fetal heartbeat is auscultated and counted, as is the funic souffle.

Vaginal Examination

Vaginal examination may be performed at any time during pregnancy to determine the presenting part, to estimate its degree of descent into the pelvis (station), and to evaluate the degree of effacement of the cervix. These observations become more important as term is reached, and they are essential if induction of labor is contemplated.

Other Tests in Pregnancy

Aside from the routine laboratory baseline studies that are performed at the time of the initial prenatal visit, various other tests may subsequently be indicated during pregnancy. Some of these are summarized in Table 19–4. Of particular usefulness is ultrasonography, to confirm the early diagnosis of pregnancy in equivocal cases, to follow the progress of fetal growth, and to establish the diagnosis of multiple pregnancy.

The advisability of routine screening for α-fetoprotein by immunoassay to detect fetal neural tube defects, particularly spina bifida and anencephaly, is currently controversial. Arguments against the routine use of this test are that it would be too costly for the yield of affected cases to be anticipated and might in addition be psychologically harmful to some women. The problem is compounded by the fact that α-fetoprotein elevations in maternal serum are also encountered in multiple pregnancy, threatened abortion, fetal death, Rh disease, some congenital malformations other than those involving the neural tube system (*e.g.,* exomphalos), and some maternal diseases (*e.g.,* viral hepatitis). Although it is unlikely that maternal α-fetoprotein screening will be instituted on a national basis in the immediate future, it may well become part of routine obstetric practice after reagents have been licensed by the Food and Drug Administration (FDA).

Frequency of Visits with Advancing Pregnancy

Before the 32nd week, monthly prenatal visits are adequate to safeguard the patient from asymptomatic pregnancy complications. She should be instructed to come in if untoward symptoms develop. From the 32nd to the 36th week, it is best to see the patient at 2-week intervals. Weekly visits are appropriate for the final month.

REASSURANCE

An important function of the physician during all prenatal visits is to listen to the patient's symptoms or complaints and to answer her questions regarding the progress of her pregnancy. Neglect of this aspect of prenatal care can lead to numerous problems, ranging from an unfortunate physician–patient relationship to complications of labor and delivery caused in part by the patient's apprehension and lack of psychologic preparation.

GENERAL INFORMATION NEEDED BY THE OBSTETRIC PATIENT

At the initial prenatal visit, the obstetrician should supply the new obstetric patient with a set of written instructions for her guidance in understanding the course of a normal pregnancy. These instructions outline in simple language all the points enumerated here. The patient should be told that the booklet is simply a reminder of matters that might otherwise be forgotten and does not mean that the physician is unwilling to answer her questions.

WEIGHT GAIN

In the past, obstetricians commonly advised their patients to make every effort to restrict weight gain during pregnancy, often to the extent of 15–18 lb above the normal prepregnant weight. Only in recent years has it become apparent that insufficient weight gain during pregnancy may be a significant cause of small, preterm, and high-risk infants. Thus, current thought indicates that the optimal weight gain during pregnancy, calculated on the basis of the lowest rate of complications and low birth-weight babies, is 24.0–27.5 lb.

In general, it seems true that marked deviation from the ideal weight in either direction is associated with an increased risk of various complications. Of particular importance in this regard is the evidence that high prepregnancy weight correlates significantly with an increased risk of preeclampsia. Sudden weight gain in the third trimester is usually caused by fluid retention and may constitute a warning sign of impending preeclampsia. Apart from this transient cause of weight gain, many women tend to add to their body fat stores during pregnancy, and weight gained in this way may not be entirely lost after delivery. This permanent weight gain may be lessened in mothers who nurse their babies, since the secretion of milk requires a sizable amount of energy. Breast-feeding also acts as a preventive measure against obesity in the baby; bottle-feeding has been shown to be an important cause of overfeeding in infants, laying the foundation at an early age for a lifetime obesity problem.

TABLE 19–4. TESTS THAT ARE OR MAY BE APPLICABLE IN APPARENTLY NORMAL PREGNANCY*

Test	Timing	Indication
WEIGHT	Each office visit	Routine
BLOOD PRESSURE	Each office visit	Routine
URINE FOR GLUCOSE AND PROTEIN	Each office visit	Routine
PHENYLKETONURIA (PHENOSTIX RX)	1st visit	Routine
HEMOGLOBIN OR HEMATOCRIT	1st visit and at 32 weeks	Routine
RUBELLA TITER	1st visit	Routine; required in some states
ROLL-OVER TEST	28–32 weeks	Routine (?)
FASTING AND 2-HOUR POSTPRANDIAL BLOOD SUGAR		Glycosuria at any time
REAL-TIME OR B SCAN†		
Diagnose intrauterine pregnancy	6+ weeks	Question of normal intrauterine pregnancy
Rule out missed abortion	8–12 weeks	Apparent failure of uterus to grow and recession of pregnancy symptoms
Diagnose twins or hydatidiform mole	12 weeks on	Uterus apparently too large for dates
Localize placenta	15 weeks to term	Preliminary to amniocentesis
Assess fetal growth	20–24 weeks *and* 30–33 weeks	History of low birth weight, uterus small for dates, or appropriate risk factors
ALPHA FETOPROTEIN	15–19 weeks	Serum: risk of fetus with neural tube defect
		Amniotic fluid: probably advisable as routine if amniocentesis for karyotype or other reason
AMNIOCENTESIS FOR LECITHIN/SPHINGOMYELIN RATIO	Before delivery	Contemplated induction or repeat cesarean section before labor
ESTRIOL (URINARY 24-HOUR)	2–3 times weekly after 32 weeks	Postterm pregnancy or risk factors (No longer used in many centers, superseded by NST, CST, OCT‡)
NST, CST, OCT‡	Usually after 36 weeks	Risk factors, postterm pregnancy, apparent intrauterine growth retardation
TAY SACHS (BLOOD FOR HEXOSAMINE A) TO DETERMINE CARRIER STATE	Preferably before pregnancy or at first visit	Woman of Ashkenazi Jewish heritage
AMNIOCENTESIS FOR HERITABLE DISORDERS	15–18 weeks	Risk of heritable disorders

* These tests apply to pregnancies that appear to be and probably are entirely normal, or in which there may be some question that needs evaluating. The tests to be used in clearly abnormal, complicated, or high-risk pregnancies are listed in the appropriate chapters.

† Real-time and B scan can sometimes be used interchangeably, but one may be better suited than the other for a particular problem.

‡ *NST* = nonstress test; *CST* = contraction stress test; *OCT* = oxytocin challenge test.

DIET

The nutritional requirements for pregnant women and sample diets are given in Chapter 11. Providing nutritional advice is an essential part of the obstetrician's responsibility, and it must never be assumed, merely because a woman appears to be well nourished and not economically deprived, that her nutritional reserves and intake are appropriate for pregnancy. Specific inquiry must be made, and the recommendations outlined in Chapter 11 must be followed. In addition to the customary supplementation with vitamins, minerals, and folic acid, Glenn has reported that a daily supplement of 2.2 mg sodium fluoride is effective in the prevention of caries in the offspring, regardless of whether fluorinated water is used during pregnancy. Confirmation of this work is needed, as well as assurance that the supplement has no deleterious effects. If these are forthcoming, the work may have extremely important public health significance.

BOWEL FUNCTION

Pregnancy-induced increases in steroid metabolism promote bowel sluggishness by suppressing smooth muscle motility. The resulting constipation may be aggravated by displacement of the intestines by the enlarging uterus. Constipation also aggravates hemorrhoids. Control can be attained in most cases by liberal water intake and generous amounts of fruits, vegetables, and salads in the diet. Mild laxatives may be used in sufficient doses to secure one daily evacuation of the bowel, preferably in the morning after breakfast. Enemas or strong cathartics are to be avoided.

HEARTBURN AND NAUSEA

Heartburn (*pyrosis*), a burning sensation in the stomach often accompanied by a feeling of epigastric fullness, is a frequent minor complaint during pregnancy. It can be relieved by a glass of milk or appropriate antacid preparations as needed for control. The patient should be warned not to rely on baking soda or proprietary preparations recommended for heartburn or flatulence, since many of them contain large amounts of sodium.

The frequently encountered nausea of early pregnancy (morning sickness) responds well to repeated small feedings of dry foods such as crackers and cookies along with ample fluids (water or carbonated beverage). Bendectin (two tablets at bedtime) may be extremely helpful, but the FDA has recently narrowed its indications; it should be used only if simple measures do not suffice, or if the problem interferes with normal eating habits or is sufficiently distressing to require drug therapy.

URINARY SYMPTOMS

Pressure of the presenting part against the bladder may produce a variety of urinary symptoms, including frequency, urgency, and stress incontinence, often to a troublesome extent. Severe discomfort or pain demands investigation to rule out urinary tract disease, as does hematuria. If nothing is found, reassurance that the symptoms are temporary and will regress after delivery is helpful in allaying the patient's anxiety about her urinary symptoms.

CARE OF BREASTS AND NIPPLES

Engorgement of the breasts associated with tingling sensations is especially likely to occur in early and late pregnancy. A supporting brassiere worn throughout pregnancy will minimize discomfort. Fluid discharge from the nipples is normal, and the patient should be told not to be concerned about it. The nipples should be kept clean and dry but require no other special care.

EXERCISE AND REST

A moderate amount of exercise is beneficial during pregnancy; the extent to which it should be prescribed depends on the patient's habits before pregnancy. The patient should walk as much as she wishes, as long as she does not become tired. Stairs can be climbed whenever necessary. Strenuous exercise such as tennis, horseback riding, and skiing are best avoided for at least two reasons: the pelvic ligaments loosen in pregnancy and are easily strained, and both timing and coordination may be altered. Driving an automobile is harmless. Light housework is beneficial, but heavy forms of work about the house should be given up during pregnancy. The patient should get an adequate amount of rest and avoid becoming overtired.

Recent interest in jogging has raised a question of its safety during pregnancy. No detrimental effects have been documented to date, and many women have jogged throughout pregnancy without reported mishap. However, the pregnant woman should be advised to stop if she is unable to carry on an ordinary conversation while jogging. Also, in view of the increase in cardiac output at rest with advancing pregnancy and the concomitant decrease in functional residual capacity of the lungs, it is perhaps wise to suggest to women accustomed to regular jogging to substitute less strenuous exercise, such as walking, after the 6th month of pregnancy.

At the present time, no data are available on the safety of scuba diving in pregnancy. The sharp pressure changes, with their attendant effects on acid-base and nitrogen balance, would appear to contraindicate this form of activity.

SMOKING IN PREGNANCY

Accumulated data summarized in the Surgeon General's 1973 report, *The Health Consequences of Smoking,* support the observation that babies born to women who smoke during pregnancy are on the average 200 g lighter than babies born to nonsmoking mothers. This reduction in birth weight appears to be independent of other identifiable factors that influence this parameter. Further, the more a woman smokes during pregnancy, the greater is the birth weight reduction; cessation of smoking during pregnancy has been shown to reduce the chance of delivering a low-birth-weight baby to the same as that of a nonsmoker. In addition, a landmark study by the Ontario Department of Health has indicated that maternal smoking level is correlated with a number of other pregnancy complications, notably preterm delivery, placental abnormalities, pregnancy bleeding, and premature rupture of the membranes (Table 19–5).

The mechanisms whereby maternal smoking leads to perinatal loss are complex and poorly understood, but from a practical point of view it is reasonable to include cigarette smoke in the list of drugs that adversely affect the outcome of pregnancy. Pregnant women should be especially cautioned against smoking if they have a history of previous prenatal loss, bleeding, or placental complications, or if they are in the older age group. Heavy smokers should be referred to local smoking cessation clinics whenever possible.

CARE OF THE TEETH

At least one dental visit should be advised during the course of pregnancy. Minor dental difficulties may arise, notably hypertrophy and irritation of the gums. Tooth decay may progress more quickly during pregnancy than at other times if cavities are already present at the beginning of the gestation. Dental repair and extraction, preferably under local anesthesia, may be carried out without harm during pregnancy.

ALCOHOL CONSUMPTION

Like many other agents and practices long thought to be harmless in pregnancy, alcohol has now surfaced as deleterious. The *fetal alcohol syndrome* was first noted among offspring of women who consumed 6 drinks per day (equivalent to 3 oz absolute alcohol) or more. The characteristics of this syndrome include 1) persisting growth deficiency for length, weight, and brain, of prenatal onset; 2) facial abnormalities, including short palpebral fissures, epicanthal folds, maxillary hypoplasia, micrognathia, and thin upper lip; 3) cardiac, primarily septal, defects; 4) minor joint and limb abnormalities; and 5) delayed development and mental deficiency varying from borderline to severe. Because of these findings, the FDA recommends that pregnant women limit alcohol consumption to 2 drinks per day. Later work suggested that even lesser amounts, of the order of 1 or 2 drinks per day, may produce the fetal alcohol syndrome. Moreover, the days surrounding implantation appear to be critical, since the syndrome is reported to occur with some frequency according to the drinking habits of women in the weeks before pregnancy is suspected. These reports indicate that alcohol intake should be at least sharply reduced, preferably eliminated, during pregnancy and, if possible, for 1 month before conception.

CAFFEINE

Preliminary animal studies (rats, mice, hamsters, rabbits) have suggested that caffeine administered during pregnancy may produce birth defects and delayed

TABLE 19–5. RATES OF PERINATAL MORTALITY, PRETERM BIRTH, AND CERTAIN PREGNANCY COMPLICATIONS PER 1000 BIRTHS BY MATERNAL SMOKING LEVEL

Outcome	Smoking level (packs/day)			Chi Square*
	0	<1	1+	
	28,358 Births	15,328 Births	6,581 Births	
PERINATAL MORTALITY	23.3	28.0	33.4	24.7
GESTATION LESS THAN 38 WEEKS	76.6	93.2	119.9	141.8
PLACENTA PREVIA	6.4	8.2	13.1	28.5
ABRUPTIO PLACENTAE	16.1	20.6	28.9	47.4
BLEEDING DURING PREGNANCY	116.5	141.6	180.1	201.3
RUPTURE OF MEMBRANES OVER 48 HOURS	15.8	23.3	35.8	110.2

* $p<0.00001$, Cochran's chi square for trends

(Ontario Perinatal Mortality Study Committee: Supplement to the Second Report of the Perinatal Mortality Study in Ten University Teaching Hospitals. Toronto, Ontario, Department of Health, 1967)

skeletal development in the offspring. An unpublished study under the auspices of the Food and Drug Administration was sufficiently suggestive that the Commissioner of Food and Drugs felt constrained to issue a press release "advising pregnant women to avoid caffeine-containing foods and drugs, or to use them sparingly."* There are no data regarding the effects, if any, of caffeine in human pregnancy.

CLOTHING

The patient's regular clothes can be worn in early pregnancy, but they should be replaced by specially designed maternity clothes as soon as they become at all tight, usually by the 4th month. As pregnancy advances, the most appropriate clothing is of a design that is supported from the shoulders. The shoes should be as comfortable as possible. A maternity garter belt will minimize troublesome varicosities that would be aggravated by constricting garters. Corsets and girdles are rarely essential during a first pregnancy, but may be helpful in later pregnancies. A maternity corset sometimes helps to reduce a feeling of lack of support or persistent backache. The purpose of a corset or girdle during pregnancy is support rather than concealment, and this principle should be made clear to the patient.

CIRCULATORY DISTURBANCES

Varicosities due to congenital or acquired weakness of the vein walls, to increased venous stasis, or to inactivity or obesity may trouble the pregnant patient, especially as term is approached. These involve principally the lower extremities, but may also be encountered on the vulva and as hemorrhoids about the anus. Troublesome varicosities of the legs can be managed by the use of elastic stockings and by instructing the patient to lie down as often as possible and to prop the legs up at a level higher than the rest of the body. Painful hemorrhoids are rendered more tolerable by keeping the bowels regular and the feces soft. Discomfort that arises from large vulvar varices can be relieved by a vulvar pad held in place by a T binder.

MARITAL RELATIONS AND VAGINAL HYGIENE

In recent years, it has been generally accepted that sexual intercourse in pregnancy is not harmful, except possibly to susceptible patients in whom the prostaglandin content of semen could contribute to the pre-

* Goyan JE, Commissioner of Food and Drugs, Food and Drug Administration: Press release of September 4, 1980 regarding possible teratogenic effects of caffeine.

cipitation of labor. This concept is now challenged by Naeye in his analysis of data from the Collaborative Perinatal Project that covered the years 1959–1966. The implication of the study is that frequent intercourse (at least four times per month or once per week) during the month before delivery may cause amnionitis or even neonatal death. Since the preterm infant would be most vulnerable, it could be inferred that intercourse should be forbidden after the 20th week of pregnancy. Some have questioned whether the results are valid and, if they are, whether they should be applied to the modern era in view of the extremely low perinatal death rates and new knowledge of the management of infection. Moreover, the summary prohibition of intercourse is not to be taken lightly; its effects may vary from mild annoyance to the disruption of a family. In the meantime, the practitioner is left with allegations that, if true, are extremely serious. It is to be hoped that the matter will be settled by a modern and carefully controlled study.

If the patient has had several early abortions, intercourse should be avoided until after the third missed period. Tub baths may be taken at will throughout pregnancy, as bath water does not enter the vagina under usual circumstances. Douches are best avoided entirely during pregnancy unless prescribed for some particular purpose.

TRAVEL

Travel by any customary means does not jeopardize the pregnancy directly and cannot be implicated as a cause of abortion or preterm labor. The disadvantages of long journeys during pregnancy are all indirect ones. If an obstetric emergency should arise, the patient may be in a place where competent care is not immediately available. Long, tiring trips may interfere with the maintenance of a well-supervised diet and with regular periods of exercise. Tension and fatigue are more likely to become extreme under travel conditions.

Long automobile trips are likely to be fatiguing and are best avoided. Air travel is far less tiring and in no way harmful even in the last month of pregnancy, but many airlines will not permit women to fly at that time because of the possibility that labor may begin during a flight. Short rides or drives are harmless. If it is necessary for the patient to make a long journey for an urgent reason, she should ask her physician to recommend a competent obstetrician in the community she plans to visit.

EMPLOYMENT

Categorical statements about the safety of continued employment during pregnancy cannot be made. Some

kinds of work are dull, stressful, and arduous, while some are easy, pleasant, and intellectually stimulating. The physician should make recommendations only after inquiry into the details of each case. *Guidelines on Pregnancy and Work,* published by the American College of Obstetricians and Gynecologists, provides an overview of this question and may help to determine the propriety of a particular kind of employment.

BACKACHE AND PELVIC PAIN

The weight of the pregnant uterus can cause discomfort or pain in the pelvis, especially on the right side. As term is approached, the Braxton Hicks contractions may become painful, and the patient should be warned that such contractions may mean that labor is imminent. Pain in the low back is a troublesome complaint during pregnancy. It results from poor posture, fatigue, lack of abdominal support, and relaxation of the pelvic joints. It can usually be relieved effectively by an abdominal or sacroiliac support, by increasing the daily rest period, or by changing the shoe style. Gentle massage may relieve backache and leg cramps when they occur.

DANGER SIGNALS

At the initial visit, the physician must instruct the patient to report certain symptoms *immediately*. The following symptoms are potential danger signals and require prompt investigation:

Vaginal bleeding of any amount.
Spontaneous rupture of the membranes. This is signaled by a sudden, uncontrollable gush of a large amount of clear fluid.
Oliguria. The patient must report to the physician any marked reduction in the amount of urine passed, as oliguria may be the first sign of fulminant preeclampsia the patient can observe.
Headaches. Any headache that does not respond promptly to simple household remedies warrants a visit to the obstetrician's office. This symptom can represent the aura of the first eclamptic convulsion even without any other warning.
Cerebral and visual disturbances. Dizziness, mental confusion, or spots before the eyes are signs of severe preeclampsia and should be reported.
Edema. Swelling of the feet and ankles or of the hands and face sufficiently marked to be noted by the patient should be reported to the physician.
Cramping. Recurrent pelvic or abdominal cramping should be reported immediately, regardless of the duration of pregnancy, as such symptoms may represent the onset of abortion in early pregnancy or of labor in the later months.

SIGNS OF BEGINNING LABOR

The patient should be carefully instructed regarding the signs of the onset of labor. The principal sign is the onset of cramping pains in the back, the lower abdomen, or both these areas at intervals of 8–20 min. When the contractions recur at 8–12 min in a primigravida, the patient should be instructed to go to the hospital after first notifying the obstetrician by telephone. Since labor may be very rapid in a multigravida, such a patient should call the physician when she notices any unusual pain or distress in the lower abdomen or back near the expected date of delivery. The patient should eat sparingly as soon as she has reason to think labor is starting.

PREPARED CHILDBIRTH

Over the years, several programs of preparation for childbirth have been developed. Their objectives are to reduce or eliminate the pain of labor and the need for analgesia, as well as to reduce or eliminate the need for intervention by the obstetrician. *Lamaze's method* of *psychoprophylaxis* (apparently a restatement of the Russian doctrine outlined much earlier by Velvovsky and by Nikolayev) is most widely used. Virtually all health organizations and obstetric centers urge pregnant women and their husbands (or "supporting others") to participate in preparatory educational courses of which psychoprophylactic instruction is usually a part. The courses are designed to impart information about pregnancy, labor and the role of the attendants, thus removing fear of the unknown. The instruction provided to minimize the pain that does occur in labor is based on Pavlov's principle of the conditioned reflex. Most women believe that labor is painful and therefore experience pain. Psychoprophylaxis is intended to decondition them so that this belief is no longer held and to recondition them to the principle that uterine contractions in labor need not be painful.

A typical course consists of six sessions.* The first session includes basic definitions of the stages of labor and a general description of the maternal body changes of normal pregnancy. In the second session, relaxation exercises, drill for coach reinforcement, and basic exercises designed to prepare the body for childbirth are described. In the third session, the couples are instructed in the technique of breathing to be followed during the early stages of labor, and the coach learns to time the contractions. In the fourth session, different methods of breathing to be used in the late phase of the first stage are taught, along with rapid breathing for use during the transition phase of cervi-

---

* The general program and the specific exercises are outlined in a booklet, *Preparation for Childbirth,* which can be obtained from the Maternity Center Association, 48 East 92nd St., New York, NY 10028.

cal dilatation. In the fifth session, exercises are described to promote relaxation of the rectal and vaginal muscles during the bearing-down phase, as well as use of the diaphragm and abdominal musculature for expulsion of the fetus in correlation with the uterine contractions. In the final session, the couple learns the signs and symptoms of true labor, the use of medication, and practical matters such as the necessary preparations for coming to the hospital.

For the most part, couples who conscientiously participate in these courses appear to derive significant benefits; less analgesia and anesthesia may be needed, and spontaneous delivery may occur more frequently. Unfortunately, as Beck and Hall have emphasized, these and the other allegedly salutary effects of the method do not lend themselves to experimental or statistical verification, despite many attempts to provide objective evidence of their efficacy. Perhaps the couples who elect and adhere to these programs are most highly motivated and at lowest obstetric risk.

REFERENCES AND RECOMMENDED READING

GENERAL AND MISCELLANEOUS

ACOG Technical Bulletin No. 58: Pregnancy, Work, and Disability. American College of Obstetricians and Gynecologists, May, 1980

Bonebrake CR, Noller KL, Loehnen CP et al: Routine chest roentgenography in pregnancy. JAMA 240:2747, 1978

Chamberlain G: A re-examination of antenatal care. J Soc Med 71:662, 1978

Christakis G (ed): Maternal nutritional assessment. Am J Public Health (Suppl) 63:57, 1973

Department of Health and Human Services (FDA): Caffeine; Deletion of GRAS (Generally Recognized as Safe) status, proposed declaration that no prior sanction exists, and use on an interim basis pending additional study. Fed Register 45:69817, 1980

Food and Drug Administration: Caffeine and pregnancy. FDA Drug Bulletin, 10:19, 1980

Glenn FB: Immunity conveyed by sodium-fluoride supplement during pregnancy. Part II. ASDC J Dent Child, Jan–Feb, 1979

Golbus MS: Teratology for the obstetrician. Obstet Gynecol 55:269, 1980

Hadlock FP, Seung KP, Wallace RJ: Routine radiographic screening of the chest in pregnancy: Is it indicated? Obstet Gynecol 54:433, 1979

Jacobson HN: Current concepts in nutrition. N Engl J Med 297:1051, 1977

Lindheimer MD, Katz AI: Sodium and diuretics in pregnancy. N Engl J Med 288:891, 1973

Milunsky A, Alpert E: Maternal serum AFP screening. N Engl J Med 298:738, 1978

Nadler HL, Simpson JL: Maternal serum alpha-fetoprotein screening: Promise not yet fulfilled. Am J Obstet Gynecol 135:1, 1979

Naeye RL: Maternal weight gain and outcome of pregnancy. Am J Obstet Gynecol 135:3, 1979

Naeye RL: Coitus and associated amniotic-fluid infections. N Engl J Med 301:1198, 1979. See also letters to the Editor. N Engl J Med 302:632, 633, 1980

National Research Council Committee on Maternal Nutrition: Maternal nutrition and the course of pregnancy, summary report. Washington, DC, National Academy of Sciences, 1970

Ontario Perinatal Mortality Study Committee: Supplement to the second report of the perinatal mortality study in ten university teaching hospitals. Toronto, Ontario Department of Health, 1967

Pitkin RM, Wamintsy RA, Newton M et al: Maternal nutrition: A selective review of clinical topics. Obstet Gynecol 40:773, 1972

Ryan GM, Jr, Sweeney PJ, Solola AS: Prenatal care and pregnancy outcome. Am J Obstet Gynecol 137:876, 1980

Taylor ES: Editorial Comment on Nutrition in Pregnancy. Obstet Gynecol Surv 33:384, 1978

PREGNANCY TESTS

Berry CM, Thompson JD, Hatcher R: The radioreceptor assay for hCG in ectopic pregnancy. Obstet Gynecol 54:43, 1979

Boyko WL, Barrett B: Detection and quantitation of the β-subunit of human chorionic gonadotropin in serum by radioimmunoassay. Fertil Steril 33:141, 1980

Boyko WL, Russell HT: Application of the radioreceptor assay for human chorionic gonadotropin in pregnancy testing and management of trophoblastic disease.

Boyko WL, Russell HT: Evaluation and clinical application of the quantitative radioreceptorassay for serum hCG. Obstet Gynecol 54:737, 1979

Boyko WL, Russell HT: Letters to the Editor. Obstet Gynecol 53:699, 1979

Landesman R, Saxena B: Results of first 1000 radioreceptorassays for determination of human chorionic gonadotropin: New, reliable and sensitive pregnancy test. Fertil Steril 27:357, 1976

Lorenz RP, Work BA, Menon KMJ: A radioreceptor assay for human chorionic gonadotropin in normal and abnormal pregnancies: A clinical evaluation. Am J Obstet Gynecol 134:471, 1979

Roy S, Klein A, Scott JZ et al: Diagnosis of pregnancy with a radioreceptorassay for hCG. Obstet Gynecol 50:401, 1977

Saxena BB, Landesman R: Diagnosis and management of pregnancy by radioreceptorassay of human chorionic gonadotropin. Am J Obstet Gynecol 131:97, 1978

Sullivan WF, Bart WF, Jr, Stiles GE: Evaluation of a new rapid slide test for pregnancy. Am J Obstet Gynecol 133:411, 1979

ALCOHOL EFFECTS

Hanson JN, Streissguth AP, Smith DW: The effects of moderate alcohol consumption during pregnancy on fetal growth and morphogenesis. J Pediatr 92:457, 1978

Jones K, Smith DW, Ulleland CN et al: Pattern of malformations in offspring of chronic alcoholic mothers. Lancet 1:1267, 1973

Kline J, Shrout P, Stein Z, et al: Drinking during pregnancy and spontaneous abortion. Lancet 2:176, 1980

Little RE: Moderate alcohol use during pregnancy and decreased infant birth weight. Am J Public Health 67:1154, 1977

Mulvihill JJ, Klimas JT, Stokes DC et al: Fetal alcohol syndrome: Seven new cases. Am J Obstet Gynecol 125:937, 1976

Streissguth AP, Herman CS, Smith DW: Intelligence, behavior and dysmorphogenesis in the fetal alcohol syndrome: A report on 20 patients. J Pediatr 92:363, 1978

CIGARETTE SMOKING IN PREGNANCY

Fielding JE: Smoking and pregnancy. N Engl J Med 298:337, 1978

Krishna K: Tobacco chewing in pregnancy. Br J Obstet Gynaecol 85:726, 1978

Lehtovirta P, Forss M: The acute effect of smoking in intervillous blood flow through the placenta. Br J Obstet Gynaecol 85:729, 1978

Meyer MB, Tonascia JA: Maternal smoking, pregnancy complications and perinatal mortality. Am J Obstet Gynecol 128:492, 1977

Naeye RL: Effects of maternal cigarette smoking on fetus and placenta. Br J Obstet Gynaecol 85:732, 1978

United States Public Health Service: Smoking and pregnancy. In The Health Consequences of Smoking, A Report of the Surgeon General. US Department of Health, Education and Welfare Publication No. (HSM) 73-8704, 1973

EXTERNAL VERSION

Eastman NJ: Editor's note on external version. Obstet Gynecol Surv 76:196, 1952

Fall O, Nilsson BA: External cephalic version in breech presentation under tocolysis. Obstet Gynecol 53:712, 1979

Ranney B: The gentle art of external cephalic version. Am J Obstet Gynecol 116:239, 1973

Ylikorkala O, Hartikainen–Sorri A–L: Value of external version in fetal malpresentation in combination with use of ultrasound. Acta Obstet Gynecol Scand 56:63, 1977

PREPARED CHILDBIRTH

Beck NC, Hall D: Natural childbirth, a review and analysis. Obstet Gynecol 52:371, 1978

Hughey MJ, McElin TW, Young T: Maternal and fetal outcome of Lamaze-prepared patients. Obstet Gynecol 51:643, 1977

Velvovsky IZ: Psychoprophylaxis in obstetrics: A Soviet method. In Howells JG (ed): Modern Perspectives in Psycho-obstetrics. Edinburgh, Oliver & Boyd, 1972

PART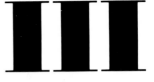

ABNORMAL
PREGNANCY

20

SPONTANEOUS ABORTION

Denis Cavanagh
Manuel R. Comas

Spontaneous abortion is defined as the natural termination of pregnancy prior to the 20th week of gestation. The products of conception may or may not be expelled.

CLASSIFICATION

Abortions may be classified according to gestational age, fetal weight, etiology, or clinical picture.

GESTATIONAL AGE

Although helpful, gestational age may not be entirely accurate, as a woman frequently does not remember the exact date of her last menstruation. The World Health Organization divides abortion into *early* and *late,* depending on whether it occurs before 12 weeks or between 12 and 20 weeks of gestation. The designation "early" or "late" must be applied to each abortion, for it may have important implications with regard to both etiology and management.

FETAL WEIGHT

Another factor frequently used to classify abortions is fetal weight. Infants weighing less than 500 g are abortuses, those weighing 500–1000 g are immature infants, and those weighing 1000–2500 g are preterm infants. Infants weighing more than 2500 g are classified as mature, although some may indeed be less than mature. This classification is attractive because an exact determination of fetal weight can be made, thereby ruling out possible error in the patient's recall of her last menstruation. It has also close correlation with fetal survival: with optimal care the outlook for a baby weighing less than 1000 g is better than it was a few years ago, but it is almost unheard of for one weighing less than 400 g to be salvaged. Nonetheless, exceptions do occur, and at least one baby weighing 397 g on the 2nd day of life has not only survived but developed normally. For this very durable infant the term *abortus* is scarcely appropriate.

ETIOLOGY

On the basis of cause, abortions are divided into two general categories: *spontaneous,* in which no active interference has precipitated the abortion, and *induced,* in which a deliberate attempt has been made to terminate the pregnancy. Induced abortions are further divided into therapeutic, criminal, and elective. *Therapeutic abortion* is the legal deliberate termination of pregnancy for such reasons as a serious maternal illness. *Criminal abortion* is the illegal termination of pregnancy. The term *elective abortion* describes the legal termination of pregnancy when there is no medical indication for so doing.

CLINICAL PICTURE

According to the clinical picture, abortions are divided into the categories *threatened, inevitable, incomplete, complete,* and *missed.* The term *septic* is added to these designations whenever signs of infection complicate the clinical picture. *Habitual abortion* is a condition in which spontaneous abortion has occurred in at least three consecutive pregnancies.

It should be stressed here that the term *abortion* may have connotations of criminality for nonmedical persons. In conversations with patients and other lay people, the term *miscarriage* is preferable. A patient may deny indignantly that she has ever had an "abor-

tion," but the same woman will admit readily to prior "miscarriages."

INCIDENCE

It is impossible to establish the exact incidence of abortion. A woman may abort without knowing she has been pregnant; she may not suffer severe symptoms and may interpret the abortion as a delayed, heavy period. Of more importance, a criminal abortion is unlikely to be reported to a physician by the patient or her agent unless life-threatening complications arise.

Traditionally, the incidence of abortion is reported as the ratio of the number of abortions to the number of live births in a given hospital. This *abortion rate* is usually 10%–20%. In a series from the Jackson Memorial Hospital, Miami, covering a 28-month period, 1549 women were admitted with vaginal bleeding occurring before the 20th week of pregnancy; of these, 1459 were admitted with a diagnosis of abortion. During the same period there were 12,963 live births at this hospital, so the spontaneous abortion rate was approximately 11.3%. Table 20–1 summarizes the final diagnosis in these patients.

ETIOLOGY

As a rule, an abortion cannot be ascribed to any single cause. Usually, there is a failure of many closely related factors, and the study of the causes of abortion is handicapped by difficulty in evaluating the impact of the individual factors. This difficulty stems from two reasons: 1) abortion occurs in a developing organism, and the evaluation of pathologic changes in embryonic structures is always less accurate than that in completely differentiated organs; and 2) abortion is usually

preceded by fetal death, so by the time the conceptus is delivered assessment of individual influences is frequently impossible.

FETAL FACTORS

In 1943, Hertig and Sheldon published their classic study of specimens obtained from 1000 women consecutively admitted to the Boston Lying-In Hospital with a diagnosis of abortion. They found developmental anomalies incompatible with human life in 61.7% of cases. These defects were distributed in three general categories: 1) pathologic ova, either without embryos or with defective embryos (48.9%); 2) embryos with localized anomalies (3.2%); and 3) placental abnormalities (9.6%). Hydatidiform (hydropic) degeneration of villi occurred in 63% of the cases. In contrast, these degenerative changes occur in only 4% of normal products from therapeutic abortions. The two most likely mechanisms for these changes appear to be 1) the contribution of a defective germ cell by either parent and 2) injury of a normal embryo by accidents in the internal or external environment at a critical time in development.

Spontaneously aborted embryos and fetuses often show chromosomal abnormalities. Lauritsen, in a study of 288 abortuses and their parents, found an incidence of chromosome anomalies of 61% in first trimester abortions and 55% in the entire series of spontaneous abortions. The frequency of chromosome aberrations in the parents was only 0.76%. The role of genetic influences as a cause of spontaneous abortion is considered in Chapter 2.

Abnormalities of the umbilical cord have been shown to be another important cause of the pathologic fetus. Javert and Barton reviewed 297 abortuses who had umbilical cords sufficiently complete for analysis. Of this number, 35% were abnormal, in contrast to 4.8% in a control group of therapeutic abortions. Most of the cord complications compromised the fetal circulation and produced death *in utero*. Approximately 64% of the fetal cord disorders were congenital, and 36% were acquired.

MATERNAL FACTORS

More is known about maternal factors that produce abortion than about fetal or environmental factors.

Systemic Diseases

Although systemic diseases have been shown to interfere with the entire course of pregnancy, they usually have their greatest effect in the last trimester. Occasionally, however, they may be the cause of spontaneous abortion. Maternal infection probably carries the

TABLE 20–1. CAUSES OF VAGINAL BLEEDING BEFORE 20TH WEEK OF PREGNANCY

Final Diagnosis	No. of Patients	Percent of Patients
THREATENED ABORTION*	211	13.6
INEVITABLE AND INCOMPLETE ABORTIONS	951	61.4
COMPLETE ABORTION	203	13.1
SEPTIC ABORTION	67	4.3
MISSED ABORTION	27	1.7
BENIGN HYDATIDIFORM MOLE	12	0.8
TUBAL PREGNANCY	78	5.1
Total	1549	

* Includes all patients in whom bleeding stopped and pregnancy continued and in whom no other cause for bleeding was found. (Cavanagh D, Fleisher A, Ferguson JH: Am J Obstet Gynecol 90:216, 1964)

greatest risk to the developing conceptus. Acute febrile infections like pneumonia, typhoid, pyelonephritis, and influenza occasionally lead to abortion. It is unknown whether the conceptus becomes infected itself or whether toxins liberated by the agent cause fetal death.

Many viruses are known to be capable of causing congenital malformations or abortion through infection of the fetus. The most important are rubella virus, cytomegalovirus, and herpes simplex virus. Other viruses that can infect the fetus and cause abortion or congenital disease are mumps, coxsackie virus, varicella zoster, vaccinia, variola, measles, hepatitis, polio, western equine encephalomyelitis, echovirus, and perhaps influenza. There is no treatment for these diseases of the fetus once the infection has been established. Fortunately, most of these are relatively uncommon during pregnancy, although the rise in the number of pregnancies among teenagers will probably increase the magnitude of the problem.

Rubella (German measles) is the viral disease that has received the most attention. Most investigators agree that if a woman is infected with rubella during the first 12 weeks of pregnancy there is at least a 20% chance of fetal abnormality. This risk is greatest during the first 4 weeks (about 60%), falling progressively to about 7% at 13–16 weeks. Similar data are not readily available for abortion following maternal infection with rubella, although Siegal and coworkers report an overall incidence of 20.4% in the first 12 weeks of pregnancy.

The most important aspect in the control of this problem is prevention. A patient who is susceptible to the disease can be identified because she lacks rubella antibodies. Every woman of childbearing age should be screened at her first visit to a gynecology clinic with the hemagglutination inhibition test for rubella. She should be vaccinated against rubella between pregnancies if the test result shows no immunity.

Benirschke has suggested that infection with *Listeria monocytogenes* is probably a more common cause of abortion than previously suspected. *Toxoplasma gondii* was initially implicated in Thalhammer's series. Kimball and coworkers reported a prospective study of congenital toxoplasmosis in 4048 obstetric patients. No evidence was obtained to contradict the generally accepted views that a mother must acquire toxoplasmosis during pregnancy in order to transmit it to the fetus and that the disease is not transmitted in a subsequent pregnancy. Only six patients showed definite serologic evidence of having acquired toxoplasmosis during the observation period (23 weeks), and only three infants were shown to be infected.

Until recently, the best known method of acquiring *T. gondii* was the ingestion of insufficiently cooked meat. A second source has now been established. The cat discharges oocysts in its fecal stream. These oocysts, after a few days of maturation outside the body, remain infectious for several months and may contaminate the environment. It is agreed that a pregnant woman who has a cat should not feed it uncooked meat and should not herself clean the litter area. Other measures for the prevention of toxoplasmosis are outlined in Table 27–6 (page 499).

Syphilis is no longer believed to be a cause of abortion; if untreated, however, it may cause congenital anomalies, preterm labor, or late fetal death.

Diabetes mellitus is associated with an increased incidence of abortion. This is related particularly to the severity and degree of control of the disease. The exact mechanism in the fetus is unknown, but it may be assumed that hypoglycemia or acidosis wreaks havoc on fetal metabolism at this critical period of intrauterine life.

Hypothyroidism and hyperthyroidism are both implicated as causes of abortion. The exact nature of this mechanism is unknown, but medical restoration of the euthyroid state sometimes restores normal childbearing capacity.

Hypertensive vascular disease, particularly in association with glomerulonephritis, may result in late abortion. This is probably mediated through vascular changes that result in placental insufficiency or through a premature separation of the placenta.

Any severe long-standing illness may be responsible for an abortion.

Endocrine Disorders

Progesterone, at first produced by the corpus luteum and later by the placenta, is necessary for the maintenance of pregnancy. Inadequate production of progesterone is estimated to be the cause of about 4% of early spontaneous abortions.

Nutritional Defects

There is no proved relation between any single nutritional factor and successful pregnancy in the human. At one time or another a variety of conditions, such as hypoproteinemia and hypovitaminosis (A, C, E, and folic acid), has been considered associated with abortion. Owing to difficulties of actual proof, these associations are merely suggested and cannot be translated into definite recommendations for therapy.

Immunologic Factors

Parental ABO system incompatibility appears to be associated with a higher incidence of spontaneous abortion than parental ABO system compatibility. Circulating hemolysins have been demonstrated in a high percentage of women with abortions associated with ABO incompatibility and are presumed to be the cause. Because of this early finding, other types of blood group incompatibility have been evaluated in relation

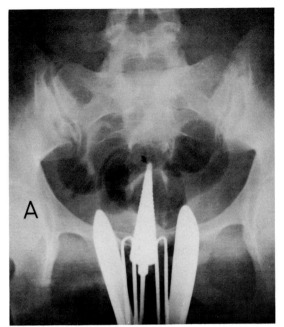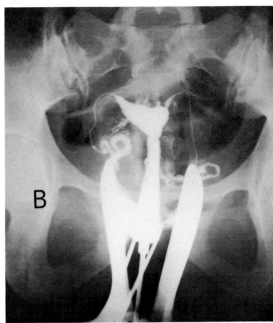

FIG. 20-1. *A.* Hysterosalpingogram of patient with Asherman's syndrome. *B.* Hysterosalpingogram in same patient after cervical dilatation and lysis of intrauterine synechiae, showing improvement in uterine filling.

to abortion. Recent results seem to indicate that antigen incompatibility between parents in the HLA, Rh, M, N, S, Lewis, Kell, P, and Duffy systems may not be significant in the etiology of early spontaneous abortion. In some series, Lutheran system incompatibility seems to be implicated.

Whether parts of the fetal mass can be rejected as foreign protein is debatable. Each successful pregnancy might be considered a failure of the maternal immunologic mechanisms. In certain cases of infertility, the spermatozoa are rejected by local antibodies in the cervix. Improved methods for typing tissue factors, among other recent advances, make the relationship of immunologic factors to unsuccessful pregnancy and infertility an important field for future investigation. This subject is discussed at greater length in chapter 12.

Trauma

The number of *bona fide* traumatically caused abortions is much rarer than is supposed by the average lay person. Hertig and Sheldon, in their previously mentioned analysis of 1000 abortions, found only one case (an apparently normal twin pregnancy) in which abortion could be reasonably ascribed to a combination of external and psychic trauma. These authors recommend the following criteria to prove abortion due to trauma: 1) the ovum must be shown by expert pathologists to have been developing normally up to the time

the abortion occurred, and 2) the onset of signs or symptoms leading to abortion must follow the causative trauma within minutes to hours.

Travel (by air, rail, or car) has *not* been shown to be associated with an increased incidence of abortion.

Uterine Disorders

Many uterine defects affect the growth and development of the fetus by their action on its immediate environment. Leiomyomas that distort or intrude upon the endometrial cavity may interfere not only with nidation of the fertilized ovum, but also with the early growth of the fetus. Malformations of the uterine cavity have long been recognized to be associated with an elevated rate of abortion and preterm labor. Occasionally, an incarcerated fixed retroverted uterus may cause abortion; but, with this exception, uterine malpositions are unrelated to abortion. Intrauterine synechiae (*Asherman's syndrome*) have been reported associated with abortion, probably merely on a spatial basis. Their presence can be confirmed by hysterosalpingography (Fig. 20-1).

Cervical incompetence may be a major cause of late abortion. A congenitally weak cervix, or one weakened by surgical or obstetric trauma, may fail to retain the increasing bulk of the growing conceptus.

Surgery

The corpus luteum is necessary for support of the endometrium in early pregnancy, but how early it can be dispensed with appears to vary from patient to patient. Removal of an ovary containing the corpus luteum verum before the 8th week after the last menstruation usually, but not always, leads to abortion. By the 12th week after the last menstruation, the contribution of the corpus luteum to the maintenance of pregnancy is negligible. If it must be removed before the 12th week, the pregnancy should be supported by parenteral administration of progesterone.

Intraabdominal surgical procedures and operations performed on the uterus during pregnancy may be followed by abortion, probably as the result of stimulation of uterine contractions by direct handling or incision of the uterus or by visceral peritonitis. However, most acute surgical problems can now be resolved without interfering with pregnancy.

Psychosomatic Factors

That a woman approaches pregnancy with mixed feelings is not surprising. Her happiness at starting or enlarging her family may fade as the fact of pregnancy intrudes. Rejection of pregnancy at some time is not at all unusual. Although the feeling is common, it does not significantly affect most pregnancies. Emotional stress and psychogenic dysfunction can probably influence the duration of pregnancy in some women. The mechanism of action is unclear and, indeed, debatable. Since the pituitary gland is activated by the hypothalamus, the hormonal changes that deleteriously influence pregnancy may be mediated by unbridled emotions. However, so many women subjected to major emotional stress in the first trimester do not abort that the influence of this factor must be seriously questioned.

EXTERNAL FACTORS

Ionizing radiation, drugs, and other chemicals have been implicated in abortion. The problem of wholesale radiation to the fetus in the course of diagnostic roentgenography has been somewhat ameliorated by the installation of better shielding in the machines, the use of lead abdominal aprons to protect the conceptus, and an increased awareness on the part of physicians and technicians of the hazards to the fetus when roentgenography is done during pregnancy. In women of reproductive age, nonurgent abdominal diagnostic x-ray films should be taken only during the week after menstruation in order to avoid radiation of an unsuspected embryo. A dose of 1–10 rad to the conceptus in the first 9 weeks of pregnancy may damage the fetus, and larger doses may produce miscarriage. The weight of evidence at the present time suggests that diagnostic ultrasound, as now employed, is much safer than diagnostic roentgenography, and over the next decade its use will become more widespread.

The list of drugs implicated as abortifacients, if not teratogens, is increasing (see chapter 27). Except for the treatment of serious maternal disease, no drug should be used before the 16th week of pregnancy until it has been specifically shown to be harmless to the conceptus.

Cohen and coworkers have evaluated the possible relation between spontaneous abortion and exposure to the operating room. Abortions occurred more frequently and earlier in a group of operating room nurses and anesthetists in comparison with control groups. These results implicate the inhalation of anesthetic gases in abortion, although the studies do not incriminate any specific anesthetic agent and a cause–effect relation has not been definitely established.

PATHOLOGY

Most spontaneous abortions occur soon after the death of the fetus or of the rudimentary analog. This is followed by hemorrhage into the decidua basalis, then by necrotic changes at the implantation area, infiltration by acute inflammatory cells, and ultimately external (vaginal) bleeding. The conceptus becomes detached totally or in part, uterine contractions begin, and soon afterward expulsion occurs. It is emphasized that, in spontaneous early abortion, death of the embryo usually *precedes* the appearance of vaginal bleeding by as much as 2 weeks. Hence, active treatment to retain the conceptus is not appropriate if heavy bleeding has already started and abortion is inevitable.

Hydropic degeneration of the villi is a common finding in abortion. Seen under the microscope, the villi are much enlarged because of overdistention with fluid. This degeneration follows the death of the fetus and is caused by retention of tissue fluid. Figure 20–2 shows the histologic changes.

The gross specimens of abortions present four distinct patterns:

1. Amniotic rupture occurs with tearing of the umbilical cord and expulsion of the fetus but retention of the remainder of the amnion and chorion (Fig. 20–3).
2. The amniotic sac and its contents are extruded, leaving the chorion and decidua (Fig. 20–4).
3. The conceptus is stripped off and passed, leaving the decidual remnant behind (Fig. 20–5).
4. The entire conceptus and the attached decidua are extruded intact (Fig. 20–6).

By far the greatest number of abortions are of the first three types, and curettage is therefore necessary

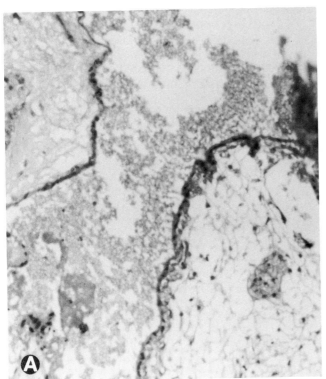

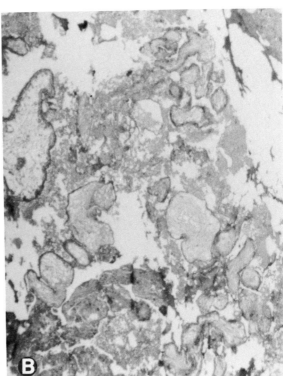

FIG. 20-2. Curettings from incomplete abortion, showing cellular debris, blood, and chorionic villi in varying stages of degeneration. *A.* Hyaline (*left*) and hydropic (*right*) degeneration. (× 250) *B.* Villi, showing hyaline degeneration and necrosis. (× 90)

to empty the uterus and prevent further bleeding or infection.

Most abortuses show gross embryonic malformations. The abnormalities are grouped in what is known as the Carnegie classification, originally proposed by Mall and Meyer and modified by Hertig as follows:

Group I: Chorionic villi only
Group II: Empty chorionic vesicle
Group III: Chorion containing empty amnion
Group IV: Chorion and amnion containing nodular embryo
Group V: Chorion and amnion containing cylindrical embryo
Group VI: Chorion and amnion containing stunted embryo

Most of the abnormal conceptuses are in Groups II, III, and IV. Although few clinicians and pathologists concern themselves with these details, classifying the expelled products in this manner may ultimately be helpful in determining which etiologic factors apply in any particular case. Perhaps a common denominator can be found.

When expulsion of the conceptus does not occur for a prolonged period after embryonic death (missed abortion), hemorrhage around the ovum may result in the formation of a firm, nodular, fleshy mass. This is the *carneous* or *blood mole* (Breus' mole). Rarely, the loss of placental circulation may result in the drying up of the fetus, giving it the appearance of parchment. This is the *fetus papyraceous.*

CLINICAL ASPECTS AND TREATMENT

To diagnose a complication of pregnancy, the physician must first diagnose pregnancy. A history of a missed period or an abnormal period is suggestive evidence. Symptoms of bladder irritability, breast tenderness or engorgement, a feeling of lassitude, and some nausea or vomiting support the probability of pregnancy. Chadwick's and Hegar's signs are usually positive; and, unless tissue has been lost, the uterus is symmetrically enlarged to a size that corresponds to the gestational age. Later in pregnancy, fetal parts may be balloted, and at 20 weeks the fetal heart can usually be heard with the stethoscope.

The cardinal sign of abortion is vaginal bleeding. Initially, this may be a dark spotting; it may increase to frank, bright red hemorrhage. The hemorrhage may be enough to cause shock, and this may be life-threat-

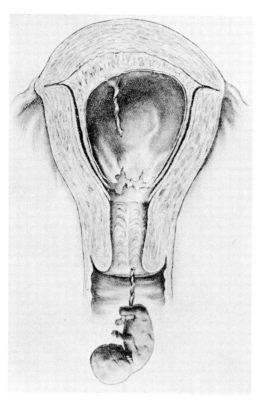

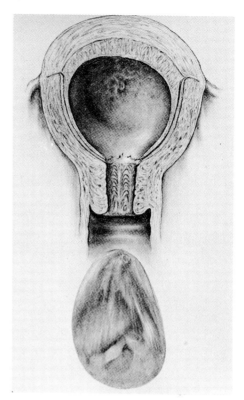

FIG. 20-3. Incomplete abortion in which fetus only has been expelled.

FIG. 20-4. Incomplete abortion in which fetus covered by amnion has been expelled. Placenta remains within uterine cavity.

FIG. 20-5. Early incomplete abortion in which entire chorionic vesicle has been expelled, leaving decidua in place.

FIG. 20-6. Complete abortion following retention of conceptus some weeks after death of embryo.

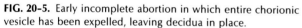

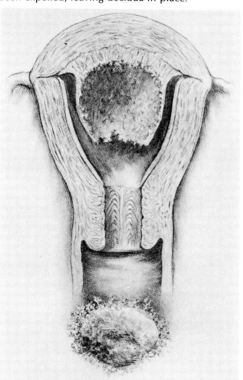

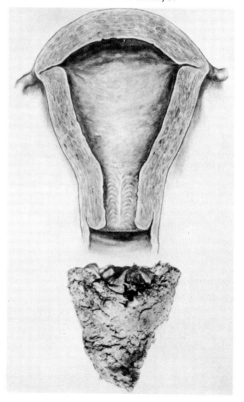

ening without immediate surgical intervention. Clots and tissue may be passed. Pain, which is common, is usually of a cramping nature, suprapubic in location, and sometimes referred to the lower back. The patient may compare it to severe menstrual cramps or a "little" labor pain. The added presence of fever and constant hypogastric or generalized abdominal pain, accompanied by guarding and rebound, should suggest peritonitis, probably due to criminal interference. When there are no complications, abortion is characterized by a paucity of severe abdominal signs and symptoms.

The cervix should be closely inspected for tenaculum marks or other signs of previous instrumentation. The patency of the cervix should be carefully evaluated with the tip of the index finger, as this is the single most important means of distinguishing a threatened abortion from one that is inevitable or incomplete.

Laboratory examinations are of little help in evaluating the problem. The hemoglobin level is low if there has been significant blood loss. The leukocyte count is normally increased during pregnancy and is especially high after a hemorrhage, but a white cell count over 16,000/mm^3, accompanied by fever, should be regarded as evidence of sepsis. Results of pregnancy tests are not often helpful in the differential diagnosis of the various types of abortion, and even in the event of fetal death they may remain positive for as long as 2 weeks.

THREATENED ABORTION

When vaginal bleeding occurs in the first 20 weeks of pregnancy, threatened abortion is diagnosed. Lower abdominal cramps or backache may be present. The bleeding associated with threatened abortion is usually scanty and may occur repeatedly in the course of many days. It may vary from bright red spotting to a dark vaginal discharge. The cervix is closed and no tissue has been lost.

Other causes of vaginal bleeding in early pregnancy, such as other stages of abortion, cervical erosions or polyps, vaginal ulceration, trophoblastic disease, ectopic pregnancy, and carcinoma of the cervix, must be ruled out. Pelvic examination (including a Papanicolaou smear), cervical biopsy, and culdocentesis when indicated, will usually clarify the cause.

Some bleeding, in greater or lesser amount, occurs in early pregnancy in 20% of all patients. Approximately half of these ultimately abort and half do not. There is no good evidence that drugs or other therapy affect the course of threatened abortion or improve the salvage rate. When slight bleeding is reported, the patient should be advised to remain at home, to do no heavy work, to avoid intercourse, and to report again in 24 hours—or sooner if the bleeding increases or if she

becomes febrile. She should be advised that, if the bleeding reaches the proportions of a normal menstrual period, hospitalization will be desirable.

In a given case of threatened abortion, prediction of outcome is sometimes, but not always, possible. Tests that suggest the pregnancy is doomed are lack of movement after 8 weeks' gestation as noted by real-time ultrasound, low serum levels of beta subunit of hCG on three successive tests taken 3 days apart, and abnormally low levels of serum estradiol. Other tests reported to give evidence of the status of the conceptus early in pregnancy include serum human placental lactogen (human chorionic somatomammotropin), plasma progesterone, and urinary estrone, but there is not full agreement as to their reliability.

In the past, progestational agents were used extensively in an effort to salvage the pregnancy in cases of threatened abortion. The grounds for this were dubious, since not more than 4 of every 100 miscarriages are believed to result from progesterone deficiency. Of more importance, the conceptus is usually dead by the time the bleeding starts. Finally, a report that alleges a teratogenic effect (phocomelia) from administered progestational agents in early pregnancy has caused the Food and Drug Administration (FDA) to recommend that these preparations not be used in this way.

South and Naldrett collected information on the effect of vaginal bleeding in early pregnancy on infants born after the 28th week of gestation. They surveyed 1226 mothers who had had some bleeding in early pregnancy. Their findings confirm that bleeding during pregnancy is associated with an increased incidence of preterm labor, small babies, congenital abnormalities, and perinatal deaths. Whereas there was no increase in congenital anomalies when the bleeding occurred before 16 weeks, there was a high rate when bleeding occurred between the 16th and 28th weeks of pregnancy. In addition, the perinatal death rate was three times that of the general population when the bleeding occurred during the latter period. In view of these statistics, strenuous efforts to maintain a pregnancy are not wise when bleeding occurs between the 16th and 28th weeks of pregnancy. Moreover, most efforts are unavailing.

INEVITABLE AND INCOMPLETE ABORTIONS

Although different clinically, inevitable and incomplete abortions present the same problem and are treated in the same way. An abortion is considered inevitable when the internal cervical os is dilated to the point that a finger can be introduced, and the patient has painful uterine contractions and vaginal bleeding. This is a contrast to cervical incompetence, in which the internal os may dilate without either uterine contractions or vaginal bleeding. An abortion is considered incomplete when fragments of the products of concep-

TABLE 20-2. POSTOPERATIVE COMPLICATIONS AFTER AGGRESSIVE MANAGEMENT OF INEVITABLE AND INCOMPLETE ABORTIONS IN 951 PATIENTS

Complication	No. of Private Patients	No. of Staff Patients	Total No. of Patients
AFEBRILE			
Pulmonary distress	2	3	5
Cystitis	1	2	3
Secondary anemia	2	12	14
Other conditions	1	7	8
Total	6 (1.5%)	24 (4.5%)	30 (3.2%)
FEBRILE			
Pulmonary distress	0	2	2
Septicemia	0	2	2
Peritonitis	0	2	2
Pelvic abscess	0	1	1
Other conditions	0	1	1
Unknown origin	2	10	12
Total	2 (0.5%)	18 (3.4%)	20 (2.1%)

(Cavanagh D, Fleisher A, Ferguson JH: Am J Obstet Gynecol 90:216, 1964)

tion protrude from the external os, are found in the vagina, or have been passed. A gentle vaginal examination under aseptic conditions is usually enough to establish the diagnosis. There is no fetal survival in inevitable or incomplete abortions, so attempts at preservation of the pregnancy are contraindicated. The aim of therapy is prompt evacuation of the uterus to prevent complications from further hemorrhage or infection. As can be seen from Table 20-2, complications are relatively uncommon following vigorous treatment.

Because hemorrhage may be brisk and even life-threatening, hospitalization is required. Blood should be administered to attain a hemoglobin level above 10 g/100 ml, and 1 liter blood should be cross-matched and kept readily available. An intravenous infusion of 10 units oxytocin in 1000 ml 5% dextrose in normal saline is helpful in reducing the rate of bleeding and in contracting the uterus so that the curettage is relatively safe. Placental tissue retained in the lower uterine segment and cervical canal may prevent complete uterine emptying and encourage hemorrhage. Thus, it should be removed with ovum or sponge forceps.

Prompt curettage affords the best opportunity for completely emptying the uterus and avoiding complications. If blood replacement has not been adequate or if the uterus is larger than 12 weeks' gestational size, sharp curettage is postponed. Suction curettage is sometimes applicable if there is urgency and the uterus is larger than 12 weeks' size.

Neither inevitable nor incomplete abortion should ever be taken lightly, but with adequate management the danger is soon over and the patient can usually be discharged from the hospital 4–6 hours after treatment if no complications are encountered. Before discharge, a hemoglobin or hematocrit determination should be obtained. Iron deficiency anemia should be treated with a suitable iron preparation. It is usually wise to prescribe methylergonovine maleate tablets, 0.2 mg, orally every 4 hours for six doses, as this will keep most postoperative bleeding to a minimum.

Most authorities agree that anti-D γ-globulin should be administered prophylactically to Rh-negative women with spontaneous abortions. Recent small series, however, suggest that this may be unnecessary in women who have early spontaneous abortions of less than 12 weeks by dates or 8–10 weeks by uterine size.

If hospital space is not available, the patient can be treated on an outpatient basis if the uterus is small and the patient is not anemic or infected. Curettage is carried out under paracervical block anesthesia in the emergency room, and the patient is discharged from the hospital after a period of observation of at least 4 hours, if no complications are encountered. However, this is second best; hospitalization is desirable.

SEPTIC ABORTION

Any abortion associated with fever and signs of pelvic or generalized peritonitis is considered an infected abortion. Most septic abortions result from criminal (and inept) interference, but sepsis may follow elective or spontaneous abortion. The patient must be admitted to the hospital and aggressive treatment begun immediately.

Diagnosis of Septic Abortion

The clinical manifestations of septic abortion are varied. The amount of bleeding may be slight or severe. If the uterus has been perforated in a criminal abortion attempt, there may be a hidden internal hemorrhage, and the extent of cardiovascular collapse may not be entirely commensurate with the amount of external blood loss. Shock in such a patient may also be due to endotoxins liberated by gram-negative microorganisms, in which case blood transfusion will have little or no effect on the patient's general condition. On admission, the patient's temperature usually ranges 100°–105° F. Hypothermia should be considered a bad prognostic sign, as it may indicate endotoxin shock. The patient may complain of constant lower abdominal pain, in addition to the usual uterine cramps. On examination, the abdomen is often distended. Suprapubic and lower abdominal rebound tenderness are present. Pelvic examination may be consistent with threatened, inevitable, or incomplete abortion, but there is characteristically severe parametrial and uterine tenderness in septic abortion. Movement of the cervix usually produces severe pain in these patients, while in a woman with spontaneous abortion the same

procedure produces little distress. A foul discharge is frequently seen with septic abortion, but it is not pathognomonic of the condition. Gas bubbles are rarely seen on speculum examination, but their presence suggests clostridial infection. Much more commonly, tenaculum marks may be noted on the anterior lip of the cervix, or lacerations of the vagina may be observed.

In advanced septicemia due to *Clostridium welchii* infection, hemolytic anemia is common and skin icterus may be present. Oliguria in association with septic abortion may be due to hypovolemia secondary to blood loss, but it may also indicate acute renal failure with hemorrhagic shock, clostridial infection, or endotoxin shock. Diminished urinary output should be considered a bad prognostic sign if it is not promptly responsive to blood transfusion and hydration with intravenous fluids.

Useful laboratory procedures are

1. *Complete blood count.* It is not uncommon to find a hemoglobin level of less than 8 g/dl or a hematocrit value of less than 24%, although occasionally these values may be falsely high owing to hemoconcentration. A red cell count should be done as a baseline, as fall of this parameter accompanied by spherocytosis may be the earliest indication of hemolysis due to *C. welchii* (*clostridium perfringens*).
2. *Urinalysis.* Urobilinogen is commonly found, but not bile. Microscopy is important in a febrile patient, since urinary tract infection may account for fever in association with a spontaneous abortion. A gram-stained smear should be made from a clean-caught or catheter-obtained specimen of urine, and a portion of the specimen should be sent for culture and antibiotic sensitivity determination.
3. A specimen of the uterine discharge should be obtained for *Gram stain,* aerobic and anaerobic *culture,* and *sensitivity* determinations. The gram-stained smear is useful as a guide in selecting the antibiotic for the immediate treatment of the patient. It becomes crucially important when gram-positive, encapsulated, spore-forming bacilli are seen, as this should alert the physician to the possible presence of *C. welchii* infection.
4. Samples for *blood culture* should be obtained before starting antibiotic therapy and at the time of chills or peaks of fever. The types of organisms found in the blood of patients with septic abortion in one study are listed in Table 20–3. Note that in almost half these patients results of blood culture were negative. The use of anaerobic methods of culture increases the yield of organisms from the bloodstream.
5. If possible, an *upright film of the chest* should be obtained. Not only can this serve as a baseline study, but it facilitates the diagnosis of pneumonia associated with spontaneous abortion or multiple

TABLE 20-3. RESULTS OF BLOOD CULTURES IN PATIENTS WITH SEPTIC ABORTION WITH ENDOTOXIN SHOCK*

Organisms	Incidence (%)
ESCHERICHIA COLI	27
AEROBACTER-KLEBSIELLA GROUP	19
PROTEUS	17
PSEUDOMONAS	13
OTHERS	14

* The blood culture was positive in 21 of 39 patients (56%). (Cavanagh D, Singh KS, Ostapowicz F, Woods R, DeCenzo J: Aust NZ J Obstet Gynaecol 10:160, 1970)

pulmonary embolization from septic pelvic thrombophlebitis. Air seen under the diaphragm should be considered evidence of perforation of the uterus or vaginal vault in an attempt at abortion. If the patient is too sick to stand for an upright film, a lateral decubitus film of the abdomen may show free air under the flanks. In any case, the abdomen should always be radiographed in cases of septic abortion. The presence of a foreign body, such as a catheter in the peritoneal cavity, calls for abdominal exploration and possible hysterectomy (Fig. 20–7). Physometra may occasionally be seen.

6. *Serum electrolyte, blood urea nitrogen,* and *creatinine levels* should be determined as baseline studies.
7. Determination of *platelet count, clotting time,* and *clot lysis time,* and examination for *fibrin split products,* serve as an initial screening battery for the detection of disseminated intravascular coagulation (see Chapter 38).

Management of Septic Abortion

Successful management of the patient with a septic abortion depends upon prompt treatment once the diagnosis is established. The treatment should be individualized. The aim of the initial medical management is to control the infection by the use of appropriate antibiotics and, in inevitable and incomplete abortions, to correct the blood volume, prevent further bleeding, and begin emptying the uterus medically in preparation for curettage.

Since many patients with septic abortion lose a considerable amount of blood, compatible blood should be available for replacement. Whole blood should usually be given when the patient is judged to have lost 500 ml blood or more. Transfusion should usually be carried out before the patient is taken to the operating room and anesthesia begun. Some patients may need transfusions before, during, and after surgery. Blood may have to be given by intravenous cutdown, and a needle smaller than 18 gauge should not be used when a blood transfusion may be required.

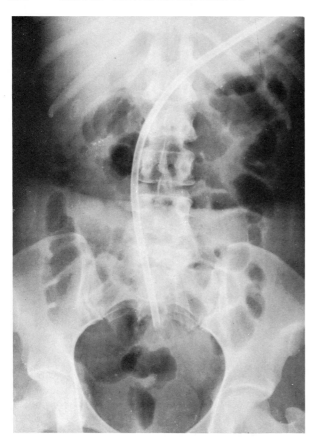

FIG. 20-7. Catheter lying free in abdominal cavity following perforation of uterus as result of criminal abortion. (Cavanagh D, Woods RE, O'Connor TCF: Obstetric emergencies. 2nd ed Hagerstown, Harper & Row, 1978)

Initially, and while blood is being given, 5% dextrose in saline with 10–20 units oxytocin should be started, beginning at 20 mIU/min intravenously, and increasing as needed to maintain firm uterine contraction. In calculating the patient's fluid intake, the central venous pressure (CVP), the urinary output, and the blood volume estimation should be taken into account. An attempt should be made to correct the fluid and electrolyte imbalance, but the patient should not be overhydrated. The CVP is an adequate measure of the circulating blood volume. It should be monitored constantly, and pulmonary edema is usually prevented if the CVP is maintained in the range of 5–15 cm H_2O. Pulmonary artery pressure and pulmonary wedge pressure, as measured with a Swan–Ganz catheter, are more exact in the detection of cardiopulmonary embarrassment than is CVP. Oxytocin administration should be continued for about 8 hours following curettage.

Before the culture and antibiotic sensitivity reports are available, antibiotic treatment based upon the gram-stained smear of the uterine discharge should be begun. Usually, broad spectrum antibiotic combinations are necessary. A combination of bactericidal antibiotics, such as penicillin (or ampicillin) and tobramycin, is preferred. Provided there is no history of sensitivity, 15 million units crystalline penicillin should be given every 6 hours. The sodium rather than the potassium salt should be used, as renal shutdown and hyperkalemia may develop in these patients. Alternatively, 2 g ampicillin can be given intravenously every 6 hours. If gram-negative organisms are present in the smear, a second drug, such as tobramycin (80 mg every 8 hours) should be given intravenously. If anaerobic infection is suspected, bacteroides is frequently involved, so clindamycin (600 mg every 8 hours) or chloramphenicol (1 gm every 8 hours) should be given intravenously. The clinical response and antibiotic sensitivity tests provide the basis for changing the initial antibiotic regimen. Penicillin and ampicillin (or, in the event of sensitivity, erythromycin) are the drugs of choice when *C. welchii* (*perfringens*) is the offending organism, although antibiotic therapy should only be used as an adjuvant to surgery in these cases.

In cases of this kind, it is essential to be alert for the appearance of septic shock, a condition that is discussed on page 756.

Tetanus antitoxin, 30,000 units, should be given intramuscularly after careful skin testing if the patient is not actively immunized. Gas gangrene antitoxin is of dubious value and may produce anaphylactoid reactions; hence, it is not recommended.

When a patient is severely ill with septic abortion, it can be assumed that placental and fetal infection have advanced to the stage where abortion is inevitable, and the uterus should be expeditiously emptied of all infected tissue (Table 20–4). The patient should be treated as any other woman with an inevitable or incomplete abortion; following an oxytocin infusion, careful curettage should be carried out within 6 hours of admission, provided the uterus has diminished in size to at least a 14 weeks' gestation and the patient is

TABLE 20-4. RESULTS OF SURGICAL TREATMENT OF SEPTIC ABORTION WITH ENDOTOXIN SHOCK*

Type of Surgery	No. Survived	No. Died	Total No.
DILATATION AND CURETTAGE	29	2	31
DILATATION AND CURETTAGE WITH HYSTERECTOMY	6	1	7
NONE	0	1	1
TOTAL	35	4	39

* Overall mortality, 11.4% (Cavanagh D, Singh K, Ostapowicz et al.: Aust NZ J Obstet Gynaecol 10:160, 1970)

fit for anesthesia. If tissue is protruding through the cervical canal, removal of as much as possible should be attempted with ring forceps without anesthesia, so as to aid the contraction of the uterus and the expulsion of any residual products of conception. Hysterectomy is indicated in septic abortion complicated by 1) *C. welchii* infection, 2) traumatic uterine perforation, 3) formation of pelvic abscess, 4) development of septic shock unresponsive to medical management, or 5) development of oliguria in an apparently normovolemic patient.

Inferior vena cava ligation and high ligation of the ovarian veins should be carried out at the time of hysterectomy if there is clinical or surgical evidence of septic pelvic thrombophlebitis. Anticoagulants should be given in therapeutic dosage for septic pelvic thrombophlebitis, and the preferred operation is vena caval ligation and not plication. Also, unless the ovarian veins have been previously ligated, the surgical approach should be transperitoneal, not extraperitoneal.

COMPLETE ABORTION

Until recently, an abortion was considered complete if upon gross examination it appeared that the fetus, cord, placenta, and membranes had been delivered intact. It was believed that hospitalization and curettage were not necessary in these cases. Even though the conceptus appears to have been passed intact, however, necrosis of the decidua remaining in the uterus (Fig. 20–5) is a common cause of postabortion bleeding and infection, and it is only rarely that the decidua is passed as a cast along with the rest of the conceptus (Fig. 20–6). For these reasons, *abortion is now considered incomplete until curettage is performed.* This principle of "curettage for all" carries small risk and shortens the recovery time.

MISSED ABORTION

Retention of the conceptus in the uterine cavity for 4 weeks or longer after the death of the embryo is classified as missed abortion. Typically, the patient with a missed abortion reports that abdominal swelling has ceased and that breast changes have regressed. No fetal movements are felt, and often a brownish vaginal discharge appears. Results of a pregnancy test are negative when chorionic function has ceased.

The diagnosis can usually be made from the history, the breast and pelvic examination, and the negative result of the pregnancy test. In the latter part of the second trimester, a plain film of the abdomen may show overlapping of the fetal skull bones. Examination with an ultrasound pulse detector reveals no fetal pulse. Bidimensional real-time ultrasonic scanning usually confirms the diagnosis.

Most women with a missed abortion abort spontaneously within 6 weeks of intrauterine death, so no attempt should be made at induction unless a definite indication is present. The patient may remain at home for this period.

Profuse hemorrhage may occur in missed abortion as a result of a coagulation defect. This is due to the absorption of thromboplastins released in the process of fetal autolysis. It is most likely to occur in the second trimester and is rarely seen within 6 weeks of intrauterine death.

If there is laboratory evidence of significant disseminated intravascular coagulation, if there is clinical evidence of a coagulation defect, or if the patient becomes anxious at the prospect of carrying a dead fetus or facing coagulation difficulties, evacuation of the uterus is indicated. High doses of oxytocin may be used to empty the uterus, and this is followed by curettage. Concomitant use of estrogen in large dosage may improve the uterine response to oxytocin. The use of prostaglandins E_2 and $F_{2\alpha}$ may be advantageous in missed abortion. Since the basic defect is usually consumption coagulopathy, the use of heparin to stabilize the clotting factors prior to induction is indicated, unless the uterus can be evacuated promptly.

CRIMINAL ABORTION

The deliberate termination of pregnancy under circumstances not legally acceptable in the state in which the abortion is done is a criminal abortion. The implication is that it is done in improper and clandestine circumstances and probably by someone not technically qualified to do an operation of this kind. The incidence of infection, and indeed of all complications, is high. Although most women escape without serious or permanent damage, the most grotesque mutilations have been described as the result of criminal abortions.

Because of the danger of septic shock, any patient who is febrile and displays the signs and symptoms of incomplete abortion must be suspected of having a septic abortion. Unless some unrelated cause can be found for the fever, the patient should be managed as if she had a septic abortion.

CERVICAL INCOMPETENCE

Cervical incompetence may be the cause of repeated late abortions. In this situation, a weakened cervix fails to retain the increasing bulk of the growing conceptus, and a relatively painless and bloodless slipping out of the conceptus occurs. This usually happens in the second trimester when the conceptus is of sufficient volume to put the weakened cervix to the test (Fig. 20–8).

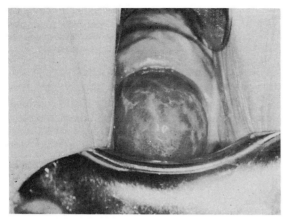

FIG. 20–8. Cervical incompetence with bulging membranes at 20 weeks' gestation. (Barter R, Dusbabek JA, Riva HL, Parks J: Am J Obstet Gynecol 75:511, 1958)

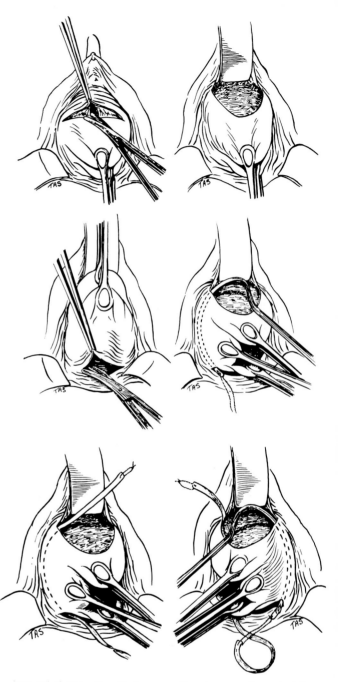

FIG. 20–9. Shirodkar–Barter operation to correct cervical incompetence. Incision in anterior and posterior mucosa. Aneurysm needle loaded with Mersaline tape is passed through anterior incision, under vaginal mucosa, and out through posterior incision. (Barter R, Dusbabek JA, Riva HL, Parks J: Am J Obstet Gynecol 75:511, 1958)

The cervix may be weakened for a variety of reasons. Danforth and Buckingham discussed the need for an anatomic fibrous cervical ring and maintained that this necessary sphincter can be destroyed or eliminated by mechanical injury, congenital defect, or the chronologically premature triggering of those factors that normally result in softening, effacement, and progressive dilatation of the cervix. Obstetric trauma in the form of cervical lacerations associated with the birth of an extremely large infant and surgical trauma from cone biopsy or excessive dilatation for curettage may result in cervical incompetence. Patients exposed to diethylstilbestrol in utero may develop a hypoplasia with resulting cervical incompetence.

The diagnosis of cervical incompetence can be inferred from a history of repeated, relatively painless, relatively bloodless second trimester abortions, sometimes associated with bulging membranes. A woman with such a history should be examined repeatedly during the second trimester. Speculum examination may reveal the bulging membranes typical of this condition. Progressive effacement and dilatation of the cervix noted during serial examinations confirms the diagnosis.

If the patient is not pregnant, admission of a No. 8 Hegar dilator effortlessly through the internal os is presumptive evidence of cervical incompetence, but more important than this finding is the typical history of repeated second trimester abortions or preterm deliveries.

Management is usually surgical and is designed to reinforce the weakened cervix by adding suture material and fibrous tissue at the level of the internal os. The Shirodkar–Barter operation commonly used to reinforce the internal os is illustrated in Figures 20–9 and 20–10. The Wurm procedure (through-and-

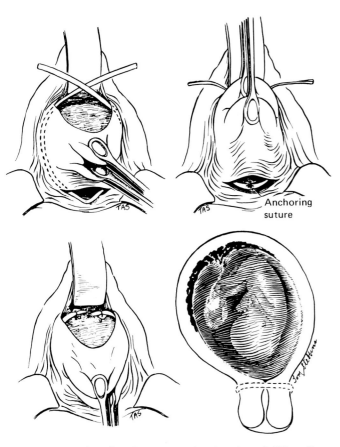

FIG. 20-10. Shirodkar–Barter operation (*continued*). When ligature has been pulled through incisions on patient's *right,* same procedure is carried out on *left* side. Ligature is anchored to anterior and posterior cervix by a silk ligature to prevent it from slipping over cervix. (Barter RH, Dusbabek JA, Riva HL, Parks J: Am J Obstet Gynecol 75:511, 1958)

through sutures anteroposteriorly and transversely) is also employed for this purpose. The McDonald–Hofmeister procedure is preferred by many. The basic technique consists of the placement of two purse-string sutures of No. 1 braided silk around the cervix. The first suture, at the level of the internal os, is inserted by taking superficial bites through the mucosa at 12, 9, 6, and 3 o'clock; the suture is tied tight enough that the cervix will be slightly constricted, but loose enough that the operator's fingertip can be interposed between the cervix and the suture. The suture ends are left 1.5 cm long. A second suture, similarly fixed, at the same tension, and with ends left 1.5 cm long, is placed 1 cm inferior to the first. The sutures are cut at 38 weeks' gestation or at the onset of labor and are removed upon termination of pregnancy. If the repair is successful and the patient is to be delivered vaginally, the reinforcing suture is cut and removed at term. Labor soon ensues and an easy vaginal delivery

follows unless there are other complications. If other pregnancies are desired, cesarean section is the better method of delivery. The reinforcement suture *should not* be employed if the diagnosis is in doubt, if membranes are ruptured, if vaginal bleeding and cramping are part of the clinical picture, or if the cervix is dilated beyond 3 cm and effaced beyond 50%.

When patients are carefully selected, this type of management may be up to 90% successful in preventing abortion from this uncommon complication of pregnancy. The importance of cervical incompetence lies not in its frequency, but in its often iatrogenic origin and its amenability to correction by appropriate surgical procedures.

HABITUAL ABORTION

The occurrence of three or more *consecutive* spontaneous abortions is called habitual abortion. The term is usually restricted to early abortion, during the first trimester; as noted earlier, most repeated abortions that occur in the second trimester are due to cervical incompetence, whereas those in the first 3 months are not so easily explained. The incidence of this condition is estimated at 0.41% of all pregnancies. Assuming that about 10% of abortions are due to recurrent factors, Malpas calculated that the hypothetical chance of a normal pregnancy occurring after three consecutive abortions is about 27%. Fortunately, the actual outlook is not so bleak; regardless of what treatment is used, about 75% of women with a history of habitual abortion eventually have a normal pregnancy. This is not to suggest that nothing need be done in the fourth pregnancy; to the contrary, a careful and thorough inquiry should be made into each case.

The treatment of habitual abortion should begin between pregnancies with a careful history and physical examination. The physician not only should delve into possible local and systemic causes, but also should encourage a frank discussion of any personal problems affecting the couple. This should not be minimized. A considerable number of women treated only with psychologic support conceive and carry a pregnancy to full term. The husband should also participate in these discussions, as his support and understanding of the patient often prove invaluable. At the time of the initial interview, attention should be paid to the patient's nutritional habits, and proper nutrition (especially with proteins, iron, and vitamin supplementation as needed) and normal weight should be advised. Rest patterns should be explored and the patient counseled about methods of relaxation.

Thyroid function should be evaluated. Frequently, treatment to establish the euthyroid state is all that is necessary to ensure a normal, fruitful pregnancy. Diabetes mellitus must be ruled out.

The adequacy of the progestational or ovulatory half

of the cycle should be investigated at this time. Basal temperature charts, vaginal cytology, endometrial biopsies, and pregnanediol excretion estimations should be obtained as baseline studies and repeated early in pregnancy. For a patient who may have inadequate corpus luteum function, the administration of progesterone for the first 20 weeks of pregnancy may be indicated; however, the need for this therapy must be weighed against the FDA admonition against its use.

Local anomalies of the uterus such as fibroids, a uterine septum, or a bicornuate uterus may be evident on pelvic examination, hysterography, or at the time of curettage. Repair should be attempted upon diagnosis in a patient with a history of habitual abortion who wants to have a baby.

Possible local causes in the cervix should be treated. Chronic cervicitis and extensive cervical lacerations are frequently associated with habitual abortion.

Rocklin and coworkers have published work that has important therapeutic implications for the chronic aborter. One explanation for the failure of the mother to reject the fetus, in spite of fetal antigens that are foreign to her, may be the presence of a serum blocking factor that prevents either the recognition or the effector arm of the immune response. Rocklin *et al.* found that women with recurrent abortion lacked a "blocking factor" that is present in the serum of multiparous women. If a blocking factor is confirmed to be important in the prevention of abortion, this would suggest new therapeutic possibilities, such as the administration of serum from women with successful pregnancies to women with recurrent pregnancy wastage.

Lastly, the physician should keep in mind the possibility of genetic incompatibility between the prospective parents. The G-banded chromosome technique has shown translocations in a sufficient number of couples with recurrent pregnancy wastage that it has been suggested as a part of the initial evaluation. Although knowledge of this matter is incomplete, karyotypic analysis of the husband and wife should be performed when there is a history of repeated abortion, particularly if the abortuses show a consistent abnormal development.

REFERENCES AND RECOMMENDED READING

Abaci F, Aterman K: Changes of the placenta and embryo in early spontaneous abortion. Am J Obstet Gynecol 102:252, 1968

Barnes AC: Prevention of congenital anomalies from the point of view of the obstetrician. Presented at the Second International Conference on Congenital Malformation, July 1963

Benirschke K: A review of the pathologic anatomy of the human placenta. Am J Obstet Gynecol 84:1595, 1962

Carr DH, Bateman AJ, Murray AB: Analysis of data from abortuses which failed to grow in culture. Obstet Gynecol 28:611, 1966

Cavanagh D, Fleisher A, Ferguson JH: Inevitable and incomplete abortion. Am J Obstet Gynecol 90:216, 1964

Cavanagh D, Talisman MR: Prematurity and the Obstetrician. New York, Appleton, 1969

Cavanagh D, Woods RE, O'Connor TCF: Obstetric Emergencies, 2nd ed. Hagerstown, Harper & Row, 1978

Cohen EN, Bellville JW, Brown BE: Anesthesia, pregnancy and miscarriage: A study of operating room nurses and anesthetists. Anesthesiology 35:343, 1971

Danforth DN, Buckingham JC: Cervical competence: A reevaluation. Postgrad Med 32:345, 1962

DeCenzo JA, Cavanagh D: Management of incomplete abortion on an outpatient basis. Am J Obstet Gynecol 97:17, 1967

Goldstein DP: Incompetent cervix in offspring exposed to diethylstilbestrol in utero. Obstet Gynecol 52:735, 1978

Hertig AT, Sheldon WH: Minimal criteria to prove prima facie case of traumatic abortion or miscarriage. Ann Surg 117:596, 1943

Karjalainen O, Stenman U, Wickmann K et al: Evaluation of outcome of pregnancy in threatened abortion by biochemical methods. Ann Chir Gynaecol Fenn 63:457, 1974

Kimball AC, Kean BH, Fuchs F: Congenital toxoplasmosis: A prospective study of 4048 obstetrical patients. Am J Obstet Gynecol 111:211, 1971

Lauritsen JG: Etiology of spontaneous abortion: Cytogenetic and epidemiologic study of 288 abortuses and their parents. Acta Obstet Gynecol Scand (Suppl) 52: 1976

Lauritsen JG, Jorgensen J, Kissmeyer-Nielsen F: Significance of HL-A and blood group incompatibility in spontaneous abortion. Clin Genet 9:575, 1976

McLennan MT, McLennan CE: Failure of vaginal wall cytologic smears to predict abortion. Am J Obstet Gynecol 103:228, 1969

Matsunaga E, Itoh S: Blood groups and fertility in a Japanese population with special reference to intrauterine selection due to maternal–fetal incompatibility. Ann Hum Genet 22:111, 1968

Mennuti MT, Jingeleski S, Schwarz RH et al: An evaluation of cytogenetic analysis as a primary tool in the assessment of recurrent pregnancy wastage. Obstet Gynecol 52:308, 1978

Monro JS: Premature infant weighing less than one pound at birth who survived and developed normally. Can Med Assoc J 40: 69, 1939

Rendle-Short J: Maternal rubella. The practical management of a case. Lancet 2:373, 1964

Rocklin RE, Kitzmiller JL, Carpenter CB et al: Maternal–fetal relation: Absence of an immunologic blocking factor from the serum of women with chronic abortions. N Engl J Med 295:1209, 1976

Schweditsch MO, Dubin NH, Jones GS et al: Hormonal considerations in early normal pregnancy and blighted ovum syndrome. Fertil Steril 31:252, 1979

South J, Naldrett J: Effect of vaginal bleeding in early pregnancy on infant born after 28th week of pregnancy. J Obstet Gynaecol Br Commonw 80:236, 1973

Tho PT, Byrd JR, McDonough PG: Etiologies and subsequent reproductive performance of 100 couples with recurrent abortion. Fertil Steril 32:389, 1979

Trophoblastic neoplasms are by tradition divided into three groups: 1) hydatidiform mole, 2) invasive mole (chorioadenoma destruens), and 3) choriocarcinoma. Before the advent of chemotherapy, approximately 90% of women with metastatic trophoblastic neoplasms died of their disease. The discovery by Li, Hertz, and Spencer in 1956 that methotrexate may cure patients with metastases not only provided the first dramatic evidence of the efficacy of chemotherapy in malignant disease, but it is also the basis for the present understanding of trophoblastic neoplasia. In 1961, Hertz and his coworkers reported the first 5-year study of the effect of methotrexate in metastatic choriocarcinoma and presented evidence of the interrelationship of the three pathologic entities. They concluded that strict segregation of the three entities obscured the important fact that these tumors comprise a continuing spectrum, each merging imperceptibly with the other. This dynamic process became known as "gestational trophoblastic disease," and the concept of "gestational trophoblastic neoplasia" was introduced to emphasize a developmental relationship between the benign and the malignant processes. The qualifying term *gestational* is needed because trophoblastic disease is not always associated with pregnancy; it may occur in the testicle or the ovary. Because these tumors produce human chorionic gonadotropin (hCG) and respond predictably to therapy, it has been possible to develop a new classification that includes the entire pathologic spectrum and also permits categorization according to both prognosis and selection of treatment. At present, complete remission can be achieved in 75% to 90% of the cases of metastatic gestational trophoblastic disease, depending upon the distribution of patients in the high-risk category.

GESTATIONAL TROPHOBLASTIC DISEASE

Robert D. Hilgers
John L. Lewis, Jr.

PATHOLOGY

The histopathologic features of gestational trophoblastic disease are quite straightforward, but they do not necessarily bear any relationship to the biologic behavior of the lesions. Although the three traditional categories of gestational trophoblastic disease are not useful for decisions regarding management or surveillance, they are useful for purposes of description.

HYDATIDIFORM MOLE

Also called hydatid mole or vesicular mole, hydatidiform mole is a pathologic pregnancy characterized by innumerable avascular hydropic vesicles derived from chorionic villi (Fig. 21–1). A coexistent fetus, usually malformed, can occur, but this is extremely rare. The characteristic smooth, translucent, pale gray vesicles, which are held together by tenuous stems of connective tissue, vary in size from microscopic to more than 2 cm in diameter. The larger vesicles resemble white grapes; if such tissue is passed vaginally, the diagnosis is hydatidiform mole. The conglomerate mass of vesicles grows rapidly in the 1st weeks of pregnancy, filling and distending the uterine cavity and usually, but not always, causing the uterus to be larger than would be expected from the menstrual dates. Since there is no definitive placenta, the intervillous space is in disarray, and all of the maternal blood arriving from the spiral arterioles is not directed back through veins of the placental site. Rather, some of it is retained within the molar tissue and eventually finds its way into the vagina. Bleeding may be dark brown or bright red, scanty or profuse.

In addition to distention and edema of the chorionic villi, and the defective vasculature, there is a third characteristic—trophoblastic proliferation. Extremely

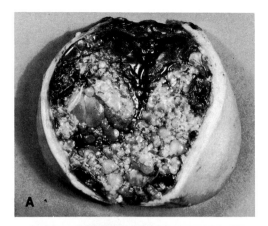

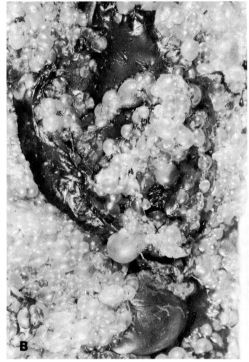

FIG. 21-1. *A.* Uterine cavity filled with hydatidiform mole. *Dark areas* denote hemorrhage. *B.* Vesicular appearance of hydropic villi.

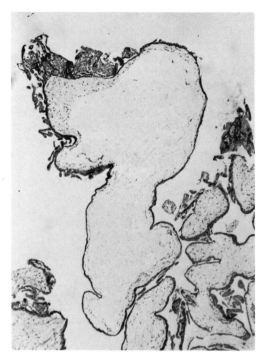

FIG. 21-2. Hydatidiform mole. Chorionic villus demonstrates marked interstitial fluid accumulation, and there are no fetal vessels. Area of trophoblastic proliferation is seen at one margin of villus. (H&E, ×40)

variable in amount (Fig. 21–2), it is analogous to the trophoblastic proliferation noted in the previllous stages of implantation (see Figure 16–7C), and in isolated high-power fields, the distinction may be impossible. One or both layers of trophoblast may be involved in the proliferation. Proliferating syncytium appears as sheets of vacuolated pink-staining cytoplasmic masses spotted with numerous hyperchromatic nuclei without mitoses; the Langhans' cells appear as closely packed cuboidal or polyhedral cells with large deeply staining nuclei. Although such changes are much more common and more marked in trophoblastic neoplasia, they are also found in normal pregnancy.

The degree of trophoblastic proliferation associated with a hydatidiform mole has been identified as a possible risk factor in the development of persistent malignant disease. While there is a general correlation between morphologic and clinical malignancy, histologic grading of trophoblastic proliferation cannot be used to predict malignant potential.

In about 90% of hydatidiform moles, 46XX diploid and chromatin-positive cellular patterns are found. As the histopathologic picture progresses toward malignancy, the percentage of aneuploid cells increases. To account for the dominance of female sex patterns, it has been theorized that hydatidiform moles arise as a result of endoreduplication of the haploid cells of the second polar body.

INVASIVE MOLE (Chorioadenoma destruens)

An invasive mole is a hydatidiform mole that has invaded the myometrium. The reason for penetration

may lie in an immunologic alteration of host resistance to the developing trophoblast (see Chapter 12) or in a malignant potential that cannot be histologically defined. Regardless of the cause, plaques and columns of molar tissue penetrate the myometrium and invade the blood vessels, resulting in local hemorrhage and, in some cases, metastatic transport of fragments to other parts of the body. The advancing mole may penetrate the entire thickness of the myometrium, causing uterine rupture with intraabdominal hemorrhage and secondary involvement of adjacent pelvic structures.

The histologic characteristics of an invasive mole are identical to those of a hydatidiform mole that is confined to the uterine cavity. The villous pattern is well preserved. Abnormal mitotic figures do not accompany either hydatidiform mole or invasive mole. Curettings are helpful in making the diagnosis only if they include a sample of myometrium that is large enough to demonstrate actual invasion (Fig. 21–3).

CHORIOCARCINOMA

Choriocarcinoma is a highly malignant, pure epithelial tumor derived from uncontrolled proliferation of trophoblastic cells. The chorionic villi almost invariably have no connective tissue core; there are only sheets of anaplastic trophoblastic tissue intermixed with areas of necrosis, hemorrhage, and vacuolation that form the plexiform cellular pattern which characterizes this tumor (Fig. 21–4). Abnormal mitoses, multinucleated cells, hyperchromatism, and anisonucleosis are characteristic. Grossly, the cut surfaces of the lesions have a red granular appearance (Fig. 21–5). The malignant tissue invades the myometrium and blood vessels, and metastases quickly follow. The most common sites are the lungs and vagina, although the brain, kidney, liver, and vulva are other possible sites of metastatic lesions. The malignant transformation of the chorionic tissue may occur either in the uterus (or fallopian tube) or, when benign trophoblast reaches the maternal circulation, in the bloodstream or in target tissues.

Although the microscopic findings of choriocarcinoma are characteristic, it may be difficult to diagnose from curettings unless the entire specimen is carefully processed. The lack of chorionic villi is a striking and diagnostic feature; but curettage may have dislodged the foci of trophoblastic cells from underlying villi that would have been evident if the entire uterine specimen had been available for study. When curettage is done for postpregnancy bleeding, it is important to process the entire material histologically, since small isolated areas of choriocarcinoma may be found. The similarity of the trophoblastic cells of an implanting blastocyst to the proliferation of trophoblastic disease was mentioned earlier, but this should not cause confusion in diagnosis.

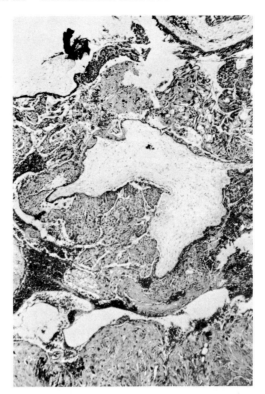

FIG. 21-3. Invasive mole (chorioadenoma destruens) invading myometrium. Villous architecture is preserved. (H&E, ×30)

Unlike invasive mole, choriocarcinoma can follow any kind of pregnancy: hydatidiform mole, tubal pregnancy, blighted ovum, spontaneous or induced abortion or term pregnancy. Latent choriocarcinoma has been observed several years after the last known pregnancy. Spontaneous regression has also been known to occur, and some metastases have disappeared after removal of the primary tumor, which accounts for the occasional cures that were achieved before the advent of chemotherapy.

INCIDENCE

Hydatidiform moles occur in approximately 1/1500 pregnancies in the United States; a coexistent fetus occurs in approximately 1/20,000 pregnancies. The risk of developing a second mole is four to five times higher than the risk of the first. The possibility of three independent moles in the same patient is 1500^3 (1/3,375,000,000). There is marked geographic variation in the incidence of hydatidiform mole in relation to the known number of pregnancies. The incidence is 5–15 times higher in the Far East and Southeast Asia than it is in the Western world; as a consequence, the inci-

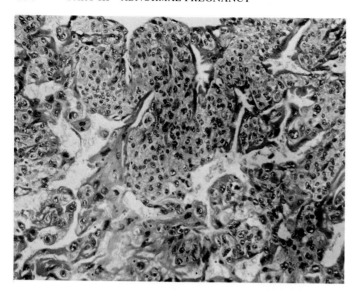

FIG. 21–4. Choriocarcinoma. Cords of cytotrophoblasts are surrounded by syncytiotrophoblasts, with intervening vascular spaces (H&E, ×120)

dence of all types of malignant trophoblastic neoplasia is similarly increased. Approximately 80% of hydatidiform moles regress spontaneously; 15% continue as nonmetastatic gestational trophoblastic disease, and 5% become metastatic gestational trophoblastic disease. Of patients with metastatic trophoblastic disease, 50% develop the tumors as sequelae of a molar pregnancy.

Invasive mole occurs in approximately 1/15,000 pregnancies, or one-tenth as frequently as noninvasive mole.

It has been estimated that in the United States 1 in 40 moles, 1 in 5000 ectopic pregnancies, 1 in 15,000 abortions, and 1 in 150,000 normal pregnancies result in *choriocarcinoma*. Choriocarcinoma is preceded by hydatidiform mole in 50%, by abortion in 25%, by normal pregnancy in 22.5%, and by ectopic pregnancy in 2.5%.

Approximately 3000 new cases of hydatidiform mole and 500–750 new cases of malignant gestational trophoblastic neoplasia are expected to occur in the United States each year.

According to incidence figures for all pregnancies, 67 cases of gestational trophoblastic neoplasia should be encountered among every 100,000 induced abortions. This number is small, but it indicates the need for gross and microscopic examination of every induced abortion specimen.

PATHOPHYSIOLOGY

Since the three major trophoblastic neoplasms are part of a continuing spectrum of trophoblastic proliferation, it follows that the systemic responses to the three neoplasms are similar.

HUMAN CHORIONIC GONADOTROPIN

There is no documented exception to the observation that human trophoblastic cells produce (hCG) when they grow. The formation, function, and detection of hCG in normal pregnancy are discussed in Chapter 18. The amount of hCG produced correlates directly with the amount of viable trophoblastic tissue present (Table 21–1). In trophoblastic neoplasia, the hCG production greatly exceeds that of normal pregnancy, providing the single most important measure for evaluating the response to therapy.

In normal pregnancy, hCG is produced in minimal but detectable amounts as early as 1 day after implantation, increases rapidly to peak levels of about 50,000 mIU/ml serum about 65 days after implantation, and declines for the remainder of pregnancy to levels that vary from 15,000–30,000 mIU/ml. It disappears from the maternal bloodstream and urine 10–14 days after delivery or after the successful treatment of trophoblastic neoplasia.

Early in the course of trophoblastic disease, hCG levels are not helpful in diagnosis unless they exceed 100,000 mIU/ml serum, since such levels are sometimes found in normal pregnancy. However, if a hydatidiform mole has been evacuated, if choriocarcinoma is suspected after a normal pregnancy, or if there is a possibility of metastasis from an invasive mole, hCG levels assume preeminent importance. The available tests and their range of sensitivity are discussed on page 359 and listed in Table 19–1. Since in the aforementioned cases the amounts of hCG may vary widely at either high or low levels, it is apparent that a sensitive and specific test is needed and that ordinary tests for the diagnosis of pregnancy are not appropriate. When hCG levels are extremely high, as in the early

FIG. 21–5. Surgical specimen. After evacuation of hydatidiform mole, hCG titers dropped progressively for 4 weeks, then increased. Hysterectomy specimen showed no trophoblastic tissue in uterine cavity; intramural nodule (*arrow*) proved microscopically to be choriocarcinoma. Titers are shown in Figure 21–7.

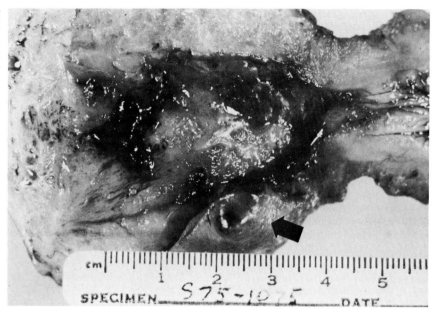

TABLE 21-1. TUMOR hCG PRODUCTION*

Volume	No. of Cells	hCG (IU)
1 MG	10^6	10^2
1 G	10^9	10^5
1 KG	10^{12}	10^8

* Based on exponential growth of tumor cells.

stages of trophoblastic neoplasia, rapid radioreceptorassay tests (RRA) or immunologic agglutination assays can be used. However, when hCG levels below 1000 mIU/ml are encountered, it is preferable to employ radioimmunoassay (RIA) for the beta subunit of hCG in order to avoid confusion with hLH. For practical purposes, the RIA β–hCG test is specific, and it can detect hCG concentrations of less than 2 mIU/ml serum. Immediate availability of these tests is an essential part of the armamentarium for management and follow-up of trophoblastic neoplasia.

Preliminary studies suggest that as the assays for pregnancy-specific β_1-glyco-protein become more specific, tests for this protein may serve as a useful adjunct to hCG for the evaluation and monitoring of trophoblastic disease.

THECA LUTEIN OVARIAN CYSTS

Because of the intense stimulation of the theca interna by very high levels of hCG, theca lutein cysts are a common finding in gestational trophoblastic neoplasia. They occur in at least 30% of cases. The cysts are multilocular, bilateral, red gray to purple gray in color, and of sizes up to 10–12 cm in diameter. The locules are lined by plump theca interna or granulosa cells, and the cyst contents often test positively for gonadotropins. Such cysts sometimes become refractory to hCG and may subside during the course of the disease. They invariably regress spontaneously after removal of all trophoblastic tissue and are to be left in place even if encountered in the course of laparotomy for evacuation of a hydatidiform mole (a procedure that is used less often now than in the past) (see Fig. 57–7).

THYROID-STIMULATING ACTIVITY

Thyroid-stimulating activity has been observed in patients with extensive trophoblastic neoplasia and approximately 5% of patients with metastatic disease suffer from thyrotoxicosis. Recent evidence suggests that the thyroid-stimulating hormone (TSH) of trophoblastic disease is chemically different from the similarly acting hormones secreted by the placenta (see page 347) and the pituitary, and that it is hCG *per se* that has this quality. Compared to pituitary TSH, its activity is estimated to be approximately 1:4000. The condition clears dramatically after eradication of all trophoblastic tissue.

ESTROGENS

The estrogens (notably estriol) that require fetal participation in synthesis are decreased in patients with hydatidiform mole. Total estrogen level is low normal

for early pregnancy, and estradiol is somewhat increased, especially in the presence of theca lutein cysts. This leads to a reversal of the pregnancy ratio of estriol:estradiol + estrone.

SERUM PROGESTERONE

Significant increases in serum progesterone levels occur with both hydatidiform mole and choriocarcinoma. Both molar trophoblast and theca lutein cysts contribute to the elevated progesterone levels. In choriocarcinoma, the ovaries are the major source of progesterone. Since progesterone levels are invariably elevated in trophoblastic disease, they have been used to monitor the course of the disease; however, they are far less reliable than hCG determinations.

PREECLAMPSIA

Preeclampsia occurs in about 15% of women with hydatidiform mole, the only circumstance in which this complication occurs before 20 weeks' gestation. Its cause is unknown. Factors that may be concerned are uterine distention, excessive levels of hCG, and immunobiologic phenomena.

CLASSIFICATION

As noted earlier, the course of gestational trophoblastic disease is so variable and so unpredictable that the pathologist's classification in three major categories (hydatidiform mole, invasive mole, and choriocarcinoma) is not adequate either for evaluating an individual case or for outlining or monitoring therapy. Clinical findings are of major importance in categorizing patients for treatment, and a classification must take them into account to be clinically useful.

The major headings that immediately suggest themselves are 1) disease that is confined to the uterus and 2) disease that has metastasized. The recommended classification is shown in Table 21–2. In addition to encompassing the ordinary manifestations of the disease, this classification permits categorization of bizarre circumstances, *e.g.*, coexisting benign molar tissue in the uterus and choriocarcinoma in the lungs, or pulmonary choriocarcinoma months after a normal pregnancy or evacuation of a hydatidiform mole. It also takes into account the fact that metastatic lesions, regardless of whether histologic choriocarcinoma or invasive mole, respond to therapy in the same way. Among the latter, low-, intermediate-, and high-risk categories can now be defined. The importance of this classification is in the categorization of individual patients and selection of therapy.

TABLE 21-2. CLINICAL CLASSIFICATION

I. Nonmetastatic trophoblastic disease
   A. Hydatidiform mole
      1. Undelivered
      2. Delivered (<8 weeks)
   B. Persistent mole (>8 weeks)
   C. Invasive mole or choriocarcinoma confined to the uterus
II. Metastatic trophoblastic disease
   A. Low-risk metastatic
      1. Short duration (<4 months)
      2. Low hCG titer (<100,000 IU/24 hrs)
      3. Lung or vaginal metastasis
   B. Intermediate-risk metastatic
      1. Long duration (>4 months)
      2. High hCG titer (>100,000 IU/24 hrs)
      3. Metastasis other than central nervous system or liver
   C. High-risk metastatic
      1. Central nervous system metastasis
      2. Liver metastasis

(Modified from Lewis JL, Jr: *Ann Clin Lab Sci* 9:387–392, 1979)

NONMETASTATIC GESTATIONAL TROPHOBLASTIC DISEASE

Non-metastatic trophoblastic disease refers to the gestational trophoblastic lesions that are confined to the uterus. They include hydatidiform mole (either pre- or postevacuation), invasive mole confined to the uterus, and choriocarcinoma confined to the uterus.

HYDATIDIFORM MOLE

Symptoms and Signs

In the early stages, hydatidiform mole is indistinguishable from a normal pregnancy. Ultimately, *vaginal bleeding* occurs in virtually all cases. It may be dark brown ("prune juice") or bright red and may continue for only a few days or intermittently for weeks. Scant bleeding occurs in 10% of all early pregnancies, but prolonged bleeding should raise the question of hydatidiform mole. Many moles are aborted spontaneously.

At the first examination, only half the patients have a uterus significantly larger than would be expected from the menstrual dates. The percentage of patients with an excessively enlarged uterus increases as the length of time from the last menstrual period increases.

Anemia from blood loss, nausea and vomiting, and *abdominal cramps* due to uterine distention are relatively common. *Preeclampsia* occurs in about 15% of cases, usually between 9 and 12 weeks. *Hyperthyroidism* and *pulmonary embolization* of trophoblastic fragments are less common but serious manifesta-

tions. *Ovarian enlargement* due to theca lutein cysts is detected in about 10% of women at the time of uterine evacuation. In 20% of cases, ovarian enlargement can be detected 1–4 weeks after a mole is evacuated.

Diagnosis

The *finding of one or more grapelike hydatid vesicles* in the vagina or passed vaginally is diagnostic of hydatidiform mole.

Ultrasonography (see page 565) is not pathognomonic, since similar pictures can be produced by uterine fibroids, intrauterine death, and, rarely, a normal intrauterine pregnancy. However, the problem is usually clarified by an accurate clinical history and, if needed, by a repeat examination by both real-time and B scan 2 weeks later. *Amniography* (see Fig. 28–9) is reported to have an error rate of 3%, but for practical purposes the test is almost invariably diagnostic. The technique is rarely needed if ultrasonography is available.

Serum hCG determinations are rarely needed for diagnosis since the necessary information is usually provided by the ultrasound scan and the clinical picture. If both the scan and the clinical picture are equivocal, hCG concentrations that are significantly higher than those of normal early pregnancy can be very suggestive. The customary hCG level in hydatidiform mole of 6–8 week's duration is from 200,000–300,000 mIU/ml serum, but in occasional cases much higher values may be found, especially if the mole is very large.

Treatment

In the past, dilatation and curettage (D and C) was recommended if the uterus was the size of a 12 weeks' pregnancy or less, and abdominal hysterotomy if it was larger. More recently, *suction curettage* has been found to be safe and effective for most hydatidiform moles, regardless of size. For those larger than 12 weeks' size, however, a laparotomy setup should be immediately available; the larger the uterus, the greater the possibility of perforation and uncontrollable hemorrhage. An oxytocin infusion (30 U/liter 5% DW, 40–60 drops/min) should be started when the mole is about 50% evacuated or if disturbing bleeding should occur. After the mole is evacuated by suction curettage, *sharp curettage* is performed gently. The curettings are submitted for separate study, since this tissue could provide the evidence of an invasive mole if one is present. The hCG level should drop sharply after evacuation of a benign mole, and should return to nonpregnant levels within 8 weeks.

Although suction curettage is usually appropriate, *hysterectomy* should be considered for patients who are of high parity, for those who are 40 years of age or over, and for those who have completed their desired childbearing. In women of high parity, regardless of age, the malignancy rate approximates 15%. In women over 40, it reaches 35%. Women over 40 are not only more likely to develop malignant sequelae after a molar pregnancy, but also have more problems with chemotherapy, which may be avoided by surgery. Surgical removal of the uterus does not dismiss the need for careful follow-up, however.

Chemotherapy is not recommended for either prophylaxis or therapy of uncomplicated hydatidiform mole. In 80% of cases, retained molar tissue regresses spontaneously; of those who do develop malignant sequelae, all can be cured by presently available techniques.

Subsequent Clinical Course

Eighty percent of patients with a hydatidiform mole undergo spontaneous regression following uterine evacuation with prompt decline in serum hCG (Fig. 21–6), and resumption of cyclic menses and no subsequent development of malignant disease. The rate and constancy of hCG production by any remaining viable tumor cells predict the outcome. If the hCG level re-

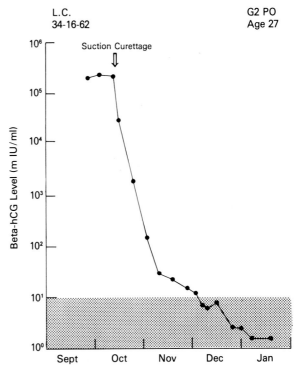

FIG. 21-6. *β*-hCG levels in 27-year-old G2 PO after evacuation of hydatidiform mole by suction curettage. Values returned to within normal range (below 10 mIU/ml serum) in about 7 weeks.

mains elevated 8 weeks after evacuation of a hydatidiform mole and there is no evidence of extrauterine disease, then a persistent mole, invasive mole, or a nonmetastatic gestational choriocarcinoma is assumed to be present. The clinical features of patients at greatest risk for the development of malignant sequelae are a large uterus and bilateral ovarian enlargement. In two recent reviews of hydatidiform mole, 57% and 62% of patients with these characteristics required chemotherapy for persistent trophoblastic disease. Approximately 30% of patients with nonmetastatic and 25% of patients with metastatic disease have an enlarged uterus and theca lutein cysts.

Follow-up

The principal objective of follow-up is to detect persistent uterine or metastatic disease at the earliest possible time. Approximately 20% of patients with hydatidiform mole have an elevated hCG titer 8 weeks after evacuation. Of these, 50% develop clinical or histologic malignancy, i.e., invasive mole or choriocarcinoma. The initial pathologic diagnosis is of little value in predicting whether an individual patient will develop subsequent trophoblastic malignancy. Clinical findings such as prompt uterine involution, regression of enlarged ovarian cyst(s), and cessation of bleeding are all optimistic clinical signs, but definitive follow-up after molar pregnancy requires serial gonadotropin assays. Figure 21–6 illustrates a normal β-hCG regression curve in a patient with a hydatidiform mole treated by suction curettage.

The following protocol should be rigidly adhered to in the follow-up of all patients with hydatidiform mole:

1. *Weekly hCG assay until complete remission* (bleeding stopped, uterus involuted, adnexa normal, hCG level normal for 3 consecutive weeks). RRA is suitable if hCG levels exceed 1000 mIU/ml serum; RIA for β-hCG should be used for levels below 1000 mIU/ml. *After complete remission, RIA (β-hCG) should be done every month for 6 months and then every 2 months for the next 6 months. In patients who require chemotherapy or who develop malignant disease, RIA for hCG should be made every 6 months for 5 years after remission.
2. *Physical and pelvic examination every 2 weeks until complete remission.*
3. *Chest x-ray at time of evacuation of mole.* Further chest x-ray is not needed if hCG level continues to fall spontaneously and complete remission follows. When chemotherapy is required, chest x-ray is necessary for staging purposes and thereafter as indicated.
4. *Avoidance of pregnancy* for 1 year after evacuation of a hydatidiform mole. Oral contraception is not

necessarily contraindicated, but recent evidence suggests that trophoblastic tissue may regress more slowly if oral contraception is started before elevated hCG levels return to normal.
5. Prompt institution of *chemotherapy* if hCG levels plateau or rise, or if metastases appear.

A *cure* is defined as complete absence of all clinical and humoral evidence of disease for 5 years.

PERSISTENT HYDATIDIFORM MOLE

Retention of molar tissue and continued elevation of hCG level 8 weeks after evacuation of a hydatidiform mole is referred to as a persistent hydatidiform mole. Clinically, uterine bleeding is unabated, and the uterus remains soft and enlarged. Theca lutein cysts may be palpable. Under these circumstances, it is essential to rule out extrauterine disease by physical examination, chest x-ray, intravenous pyelogram, liver and brain scans, liver and kidney function tests, and ultrasound and selected computerized axial tomography (CAT) scan of the abdomen and pelvis. If the results of these tests are negative, it can be presumed that the disease is limited to the uterus. Persistent hydatidiform mole is one of the three conditions that can produce this picture. The other two possibilities are invasive mole and choriocarcinoma limited to the uterus. Regardless of the diagnosis, the clinical approach is the same.

Treatment

Chemotherapy. It is emphasized that chemotherapy, like surgery and radiation therapy, is a major therapeutic modality and should be used only by those who are properly schooled in its effects and side effects, who are knowledgeable in the nuances of trophoblastic disease, and who have at hand the supporting services required. Brewer *et al* have shown a significant difference in remission rate between those originally treated at the Northwestern Trophoblastic Disease Center and those who were referred after treatment failure. Of those who died, 34% were in the latter group and 21% in the former.

Single agent chemotherapy is used as a first treatment modality for persistent hydatidiform mole, as well as for invasive mole and choriocarcinoma confined to the uterus, and should be started at once. The two agents that are used for this purpose are methotrexate and dactinomycin (actinomycin D). Either methotrexate or Dactinomycin can be used initially if renal and hepatic function are normal. If renal and hepatic function are abnormal or impaired, the use of methotrexate is to be avoided. The two drugs have similar response rates, and there is no crossover in drug resistance.

Toxicity is a major problem in the use of all chemotherapeutic agents that are appropriate for treatment of trophoblastic neoplasia. Appropriate precautions against toxicity must be taken before each course of therapy; if precautions are not taken, it can be fatal. Predictable and usually not limiting side effects include loss of hair, dermatitis of various sorts, and, occasionally, vulvovaginitis and conjunctivitis. The drugs should be discontinued if the patient develops more serious side effects, *e.g.*, ulcerative stomatitis, severe gastroenteritis, or bone marrow suppression. All of these are serious, but bone marrow suppression is the most common factor that limits the use of these drugs.

The following tests should be made before the first dose of chemotherapy is administered and should be repeated before each new course is started: hemoglobin; white blood cell count (WBC); granulocyte count; platelet count; serum glutamic–oxaloacetic transaminase (SGOT); serum urea; serum creatinine. The drug should be withheld until the results are as follows: hemoglobin above 10 g/dl; WBC above 3500/µl; granulocyte count above 1500/µl; platelet count above 100,000/µl; SGOT below 50 units; serum urea and serum creatinine stable and not rising.

The regimen for single-agent methotrexate and dactinomycin therapy is as follows: *Methotrexate* should be prescribed in a dosage of 0.4 mg/kg/day/ by deep intramuscular injection (not to exceed 30 mg/day) for 5 days. Maximum toxicity occurs 5–10 days after the conclusion of a course of therapy; the tests mentioned earlier, plus serum hCG, are made on the 7th day. If the patient's hCG level is within normal range for each of three consecutive weeks, it is our practice not to use further chemotherapy, but to perform routine follow-up for hydatidiform mole. The criteria for changing the chemotherapeutic agent or regimen, in this case to dactinomycin, are 1) excessive drug toxicity, 2) weekly hCG levels that are on a plateau or rising, or 3) clinical advancement of the disease. Dactinomycin should be prescribed in a dosage of 12 µg/kg/day through intracatheter tubing (placed deeply in the vein) for 5 days. If the drug extravasates, a slough will occur.

Dilatation and curettage. D. and C. should be performed on the 3rd day of chemotherapy. The purposes of the D. and C. are 1) to be certain all ordinary molar tissue has been removed from the uterus and 2) to determine whether invasive mole or choriocarcinoma may be present. Although myometrial fragments showing actual invasion by chorionic villi are needed for the diagnosis of invasive mole, it is not prudent to deliberately make deep swipes with the curette in order to obtain a sample. If an invasive mole is present the evidence is likely to be obtained in the course of an ordinary curettage. If choriocarcinoma is present it should be disclosed when the curettings are examined microscopically.

Hysterectomy. Instead of D. and C., hysterectomy is appropriate with presumptive diagnosis of persistent hydatidiform mole if the patient is 40 years of age or older, is of high parity, or desires no further pregnancies. This operation provides an intact uterus for exact pathologic diagnosis of the extent of the disease and, assuming that extrauterine extension has already been ruled out, terminates the problem. Hysterectomy does not, however, eliminate the need for rigid follow-up, according to the protocol outlined for hydatidiform mole. If hysterectomy is indicated, it is performed on the 3rd day of chemotherapy or, if done because the initial course of treatment failed, on the 3rd day of the second course.

INVASIVE MOLE

When an invasive mole is confined to the uterus, there are no symptoms to distinguish it from hydatidiform mole except that bleeding may be very heavy because the myometrial vasculature is involved. Large intramural nodules may cause the uterus to be irregular, suggesting the presence of leiomyomas. An arteriogram can provide a definitive diagnosis if it should be needed, but this information is usually academic. If the diagnosis is made on the basis of curettings from evacuation of a hydatidiform mole (which, as noted earlier, is often not the case), *hysterectomy* should be performed if the patient is 40 years of age or more, if she is of high parity, or if she desires no further pregnancies. In some of the cases, hysterectomy is urgently needed to control hemorrhage. If bleeding is not a factor and the patient desires to have more children, *single agent chemotherapy* is usually effective in eradicating the intramural lesions of invasive mole. This is administered according to the protocol outlined earlier. Regardless of whether the lesion is treated by hysterectomy or by chemotherapy, the same follow-up is needed as for uncomplicated hydatidiform mole.

NONMETASTATIC CHORIOCARCINOMA

The woman with a choriocarcinoma limited to the uterus presents a somewhat more difficult problem. In 2%–5% of patients with persistent hydatidiform mole, the tumor undergoes transition to gestational choriocarcinoma. Of more concern diagnostically is the problem of choriocarcinoma that develops after a term delivery or a spontaneous abortion. When the tumor is confined to the uterus, uterine subinvolution and bleeding may be present. The diagnosis is based on an

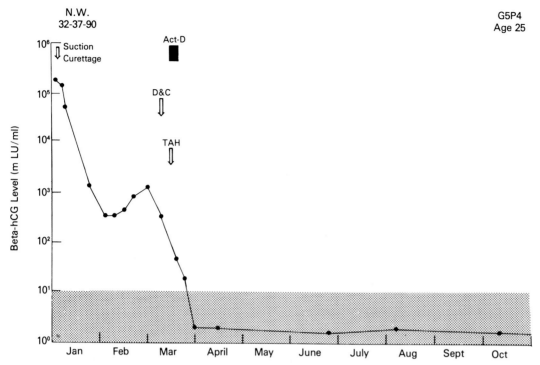

FIG. 21-7. β-hCG regression curve. Following suction curettage of molar pregnancy, serial β-hCG values declined as expected, but 4 weeks later began to rise. Studies revealed no evidence of extrauterine disease. No trophoblastic tissue on uterine curettage. Hysterectomy specimen (Fig. 21–5) showed intramural choriocarcinoma.

elevated hCG titer, histologic diagnosis of choriocarcinoma, and the lack of extrauterine metastases. Seldom is tissue passed spontaneously as in a hydatidiform mole, and establishing the diagnosis of choriocarcinoma by curettage may be difficult.

Treatment of nonmetastatic gestational choriocarcinoma depends on the desire of the patient to retain her ability to have children. If she desires more children, it is reasonable to start treatment with chemotherapy alone; however, it may not be safe to wait until after the patient's disease has been shown to be noncurable by chemotherapy before turning to hysterectomy, as metastasis during chemotherapy has been reported. If no further children are desired, the wise policy is to perform a hysterectomy on the 3rd day of the first course of chemotherapy. Figure 21–7 illustrates a β-hCG regression curve, showing a rise in titer. Because the patient desired no further children, a hysterectomy was performed on the 3rd day of chemotherapy. The surgical specimen (Fig. 21–5) showed a solitary intramural nodule of choriocarcinoma. When further childbearing is important, chemotherapy is recommended until the disease clears or until it becomes evident that the patient is not responding to that particular drug, in which case hysterectomy should be performed during the first course of the subsequent drug selected.

METASTATIC GESTATIONAL TROPHOBLASTIC DISEASE

Metastatic gestational trophoblastic disease is defined as trophoblastic disease which exists beyond the limits of the uterus. The diagnosis of metastatic disease is easier, and usually earlier, if there is a prior history of hydatidiform mole; these patients are observed more closely because of the known risk of malignant sequelae. Metastatic disease may be the first evidence of choriocarcinoma following a full-term delivery or abortion. The tumor commonly metastasizes to the lungs, and less frequently to the vagina, brain, or liver. Metastases may occur in multiple sites and have been observed in unusual areas such as the breast, bone, lymph nodes, or a branch of the coronary artery. Their growth pattern often leads to unexpected manifestations of disease if the first symptoms are due to metastases in organs distant from the reproductive tract.

While symptoms of trophoblastic neoplasms usually develop soon after delivery, long asymptomatic intervals may occur; in the interim, normal menstruation may resume and pregnancy tests may remain negative. It is in cases of this kind that diagnostic errors are

especially common. Unfortunately, the diagnosis is often not made in these cases until after the patient has undergone a craniotomy, thoracotomy, resection of a segment of the small bowel, or a nephrectomy. One-third of patients with metastatic gestational trophoblastic disease seek medical care because of symptoms due to metastases, making it especially critical to recognize the nongynecologic manifestations of this disease. (Table 21–3). *Any woman with bleeding or a tumor in any organ who has a recent or even remote history of molar pregnancy, abortion, or term delivery should have at least one hCG assay to be sure that metastatic gestational trophoblastic disease is not the cause of her problem.*

The following should be used to determine the existence of metastatic disease: history and physical examination, chest x-ray, intravenous pyelogram, liver scan, liver and kidney function tests, and ultrasound and selected CAT examination of the pelvis and abdomen. There are usually no brain metastases if the chest x-ray is normal; if pulmonary metastases are found, however, a brain scan, CAT scan of the brain, and determination of cerebrospinal fluid hCG may be needed to rule out cerebral metastases. The prognosis depends upon the duration of disease following the antecedent pregnancy, the height of the hCG titer, the site of metastases, and the patient's response to any previous chemotherapy.

Patients with metastatic gestational trophoblastic disease are divided into low-, intermediate-, and high-risk groups according to the probability of cure in response to chemotherapy. (Table 21–4). In low-risk and intermediate-risk cases, the rate of cure approaches 100%. In the high-risk group, the outlook is much less favorable.

LOW-RISK METASTATIC DISEASE

Patients with metastatic gestational trophoblastic disease who are considered at low risk of failing to respond to single agent chemotherapy (Table 21–4) are treated initially with single agent chemotherapy, either methotrexate or actinomycin D. Some patients fail to respond to one drug and require treatment with the other. Serum hCG and the size of the metastatic lesion(s) are measured serially to determine response. In this group, single agent chemotherapy produces a complete remission rate of 100% when treatment is given in the appropriate manner.

From the standpoint of response to chemotherapy, a *ruptured uterus due to invasive mole* must be placed in the low-risk category, and it must be classified as metastatic because of the extrauterine spill of chorionic material. These cases are characterized by peritonitis and major intraabdominal hemorrhage. Hysterectomy is not only mandatory, but also it is usually extremely urgent. After this immediate problem is dealt with, the management is according to the protocol for low-risk metastatic disease.

INTERMEDIATE-RISK METASTATIC DISEASE

The patients with intermediate-risk gestational trophoblastic disease (Table 21–4) usually require combination chemotherapy. Chemotherapy is more effective when used early, and single agent chemotherapy is associated with poor response rates when treatment is delayed. Accordingly *combination chemotherapy* is used if initial treatment is delayed more than 4 months, if hCG levels are above 100,000 mIU/ml serum, or if there are metastases to lung, vagina, or pelvis. This therapy should yield a prognosis equivalent to that of the low-risk group. For the intermediate-risk group, combination therapy usually takes the form of methotrexate 15 mg/day intramuscularly for 5 days, and dactinomycin 0.5 mg intravenously daily for 5 days, and chlorambucil 10 mg orally for 5 days.

TABLE 21-3. EXTRAUTERINE MANIFESTATIONS OF METASTATIC TROPHOBLASTIC DISEASE

I. Pulmonary: coin lesion, progressive dyspnea or hemoptysis, x-ray appearance of pneumonia, unexplained pulmonary hypertension

II. Central nervous system: signs of an expanding lesion, hemorrhage (intracerebral, subarachnoid, or subdural)

III. Gastrointestinal: hemorrhage (lesions of small or large bowel)

IV. Genitourinary: hemorrhage (renal or bladder), ureteral obstruction

TABLE 21-4. RISK FACTORS IN METASTATIC GESTATIONAL TROPHOBLASTIC DISEASE

Low Risk	Intermediate Risk	High Risk
Chemotherapy started within 4 months of antecedent pregnancy	Chemotherapy started more than 4 months after antecedent pregnancy	Brain or liver metastases
Serum hCG less than 100,000 mIU/ml	Serum hCG more than 100,000 mIU/ml	Previous inadequate therapy
Metastases limited to lungs, vagina, pelvis	Metastases limited to lungs, vagina, pelvis	

The next course of chemotherapy is begun when the toxic response to the first course has subsided. Other doses and combinations of other agents have been employed for the treatment of intermediate-risk gestational neoplasia, but they are rarely needed at this level of risk.

HIGH-RISK METASTATIC DISEASE

The presence of metastatic choriocarcinoma in the brain and liver significantly increases the severity of the disease but does not preclude cure. Metastatic choriocarcinoma in the brain should be considered in any woman of reproductive age with a brain tumor, increased intracranial pressure, or intracranial bleeding. Brain metastases are diagnosed in approximately 10%–20% of patients with metastatic gestational trophoblastic disease. A significant number of patients who die of trophoblastic disease develop brain metastases, apparently after metastatic lesions in other sites have become drug-resistant. Hemorrhage into a metastatic brain lesion is a common fatal event.

Liver metastases are insidious in onset. Hepatic involvement is often extensive before symptoms appear. A palpable abdominal mass or evidence of intraabdominal hemorrhage may be the first sign of liver metastasis. Abnormal liver function values are seldom observed in early disease, and transient abnormalities may follow chemotherapy; if they persist, the possibility of extensive liver metastasis should be considered. When asymptomatic metastases are suspected, the physician must rely on the liver scan. Pain and intraabdominal bleeding following acute distention and rupture of Glisson's capsule often indicates extensive hepatic metastases. Ordinarily, such bleeding can be controlled with primary suture of the lesion or hepatic artery ligation and packing. Radiation therapy and chemotherapy must also be used.

Patients with brain or liver metastases are started at once on whole organ *radiation therapy* (2000–3000 rads over 10–14 days) *and combination chemotherapy.* Dexamethasone is given to prevent the side effects of radiation therapy to the brain. Craniotomy is not recommended for a space-occupying lesion of the brain if the hCG titer is elevated or if pulmonary metastases are present. Chemotherapy consists of dactinomycin, methotrexate, and chlorambucil given simultaneously in 5-day courses. When hepatic enzymes are elevated, double agent therapy with dactinomycin and 6-mercaptopurine is employed.

The complete remission rate for intermediate- and high-risk metastatic gestational trophoblastic disease varies between 70% and 80% with first line chemotherapy. If single agent chemotherapy fails to cure the patient, the remission rate drops to 15%–20%. One of the worst prognostic factors is inappropriate chemotherapy given unsuccessfully prior to referral.

REFERENCES AND RECOMMENDED READING

Baggish MS, Woodruff JD, Tow SH et al: Sex chromatin pattern in hydatidiform mole. Am J Obstet Gynecol 102:362, 1968

Bagshawe KD: Trophoblastic tumors: Chemotherapy and developments. Br Med J 2:1303, 1963

Bagshawe KD: Choriocarcinoma. In The Clinical Biology of the Trophoblast and Its Tumors. Baltimore, Williams & Wilkins, 1969

Bagshawe KD: Risk and prognostic factors in trophoblastic neoplasia. Cancer 38:1373, 1976

Bagshawe KD, Harland S: Immunodiagnosis and monitoring of gonadotropin-producing metastases in the central nervous system. Cancer 38:112, 1976

Bardawil WA, Toy BL: The natural history of choriocarcinoma: Problems of immunity and spontaneous regression. Ann NY Acad Sci 80:197, 1959

Beischer N: Hydatidiform mole with co-existent fetus. Aust NZ J Obstet Gynaecol 6:127, 1966

Beling C: Estrogens. In Fuchs F, Klopper A (eds): Endocrinology of Pregnancy, 2nd ed, pp 76–98. Hagerstown, MD, Harper & Row, 1977

Beling CG, Weksler MD: Suppression of mixed lymphocyte reactivity by human chorionic gonadotropin. Clin Exp Immunol 18:537, 1974

Braunstein GD, Grodin JM, Vaitukaitis J et al: Secretory rates of human chorionic gonadotropin by normal trophoblast. Am J Obstet Gynecol 115:447, 1973

Brewer JI, Rinehart JJ, Dunbar R: Choriocarcinoma. Am J Obstet Gynecol 81:574, 1961

Brewer JI, Smith RT, Pratt GB: Choriocarcinoma: Absolute five year survival rates of 122 patients treated by hysterectomy. Am J Obstet Gynecol 85:841, 1963

Brewer JI, Torak EE, Webster A: Hydatidiform mole: A follow-up regimen of identification of invasive mole and choriocarcinoma and for selection of patients for treatment. Am J Obstet Gynecol 101:557, 1968

Closset J, Hennen G, Lequin RM: Human luteinizing hormone: The amino acid sequence of the beta subunit. FEBS Lett 29:97, 1973

Cohen BA, Burkman RT, Rosenshein NB et al: Gestational trophoblastic disease within an elective abortion population. Am J Obstet Gynecol 135:452, 1979

Cotton DB, Bernstein SG, Read JA et al: Hemodynamic observations in evacuation of molar pregnancy. Am J Obstet Gynecol 138:6, 1980

Curry SL, Hammond CB, Tyrey L et al: Hydatidiform mole: Diagnosis, management, and long term follow-up of 347 patients. Obstet Gynecol 45:1, 1975

Dawood MY: Evaluation of serum progesterone during treatment of malignant trophoblastic disease. Am J Obstet Gynecol 123:291, 1975

Dawood MY: Serum progesterone and serum human chorionic gonadotropin in gestational and non-gestational choriocarcinoma. Am J Obstet Gynecol 123:762, 1975

Dawood MY, Ratnam SS, Teoh ES: Serum estradiol-17β and serum human chorionic gonadotropin in patients with hydatidiform moles. Am J Obstet Gynecol 119:904, 1974

Decherney AL, Silverman BB, Mastroianni L: Abortions and unrecognized trophoblastic disease. N Engl J Med 285:407, 1971

Delfs E: Quantitative chorionic gonadotropin: Prognostic value in hydatidiform mole and chorionepithelioma. Obstet Gynecol 9:1, 1957

Douglas GW: The diagnosis and management of hydatidiform mole. Surg Clin North Am 37:379, 1957

Duke PC, Fink LM: Latent choriocarcinoma. Cancer 20:150, 1967

Elston CW, Bagshawe KD: Cellular reaction in trophoblastic tumours. Br J Cancer 28:245, 1973

Everson TC, Cole WH: Spontaneous Regression of Cancer, p 221. Philadelphia, WB Saunders, 1966

Goldstein DP: Neutrophile alkaline phosphatase activity in patients with choriocarcinoma and related trophoblastic tumors, undelivered hydatidiform mole, and in normal pregnancy. Am J Obstet Gynecol 92:1014, 1965

Goldstein DP, Goldstein PR, Bottomley P et al: Methotrexate with citrovorum factor rescue for non-metastatic gestational trophoblastic neoplasms. Obstet Gynecol 48:321, 1976

Green RR: Chorioadenoma destruens. Ann NY Acad Sci 80:143–151, 1959

Hammond CB, Borchert LG, Tyrey L et al: Treatment of metastatic trophoblastic disease: Good and poor prognosis. Am J Obstet Gynecol 115:451, 1973

Hammond CB, Lewis JL, Jr: Gestational trophoblastic neoplasms. In Carter AB (ed): Davis's Gynecology and Obstetrics, Vol I, pp 1–30. Hagerstown, MD, Harper & Row, 1972

Hammond CB, Parker RT: Diagnosis and treatment of trophoblastic disease: A report from the Southeastern Regional Center. Obstet Gynecol 35:132, 1973

Hertig AT, Mansell H: Tumors of the female sex organs: I. Hydatidiform mole and choriocarcinoma. In Atlas of Tumor Pathology. Washington, DC, Armed Forces Institute of Pathology, 1956

Hertig AT, Sheldon WH: Hydatidiform mole: A pathologicoclinical correlation of 200 cases. Am J Obstet Gynecol 53:1, 1947

Hertz R: Biological aspects of gestational neoplasms derived from the trophoblast. Ann NY Acad Sci 172:279, 1971

Hertz R: Choriocarcinoma and Related Gestational Trophoblastic Tumors in Women. New York, Raven Press, 1978

Hertz R, Lewis JL, Jr, Lipsett MB: Five years' experience with the chemotherapy of metastatic choriocarcinoma and related trophoblastic tumors in women. Am J Obstet Gynecol 82:631, 1961

Hertz R, Ross GR, Lipsett MB: Primary chemotherapy of nonmetastatic trophoblastic disease in women. Am J Obstet Gynecol 86:808, 1963

Javey H, Borazjani G, Behmard et al: Discrepancies in the histological diagnosis of hydatidiform mole. Brit J Obstet Gynaecol 86:480, 1979

Jones, WB: Treatment of chorionic tumors. Clin Obstet Gynecol 18:247, 1975

Jones WB: Gestational trophoblastic neoplasms: The role of chemotherapy and surgery. Surg Clin North Am 58:167, 1978

Jones WB, Lewis JL, Jr, Lehr M: Monitor of chemotherapy in gestational trophoblastic neoplasm by radioimmunoassay of the beta subunit of human chorionic gonadotropin. Am J Obstet Gynecol 121:669, 1975

Kenimer JG, Herschmen JM, Higgins HP: The thyrotropin in hydatidiform moles in human chorionic gonadotropin. J Clin Endocrinol Metab 40:482, 1975

Klinefelter HF, Jr, Albright F, Griswold GC: Experience with quantitative test for normal or decreased amounts of follicle-stimulating hormone in urine in endocrinological diagnosis. J Clin Endocrinol 3:529, 1943

Kohler PO, Bridson WE: Isolation of hormone-producing clonal lines of human choriocarcinoma. Comments 22:683, 1971

Lewis JL, Jr: Serum leucine aminopeptidase values in patients with trophoblastic tumors and in normal pregnancy. Am J Obstet Gynecol 84:1407, 1962

Lewis JL, Jr: Lymphocyte transformation studies in pregnant women and women with gestational trophoblastic neoplasms. In Lund CJ, Choalte JW (eds): Transcript of the Fourth Rochester Trophoblast Conference. Rochester, University of Rochester, 1967

Lewis, JL, Jr: Choriocarcinoma task force. Transactions of the annual meeting of the Society of the Alumni of the Sloane Hospital for Women. Bull Sloane Hosp Women 15:75, 1969

Lewis JL, Jr: Human leukocyte antigens and ABO blood groups in gestational trophoblastic neoplasms. In Seventh National Cancer Conference Proceedings, pp 205–211. New York, American Cancer Society, 1973

Lewis JL, Jr: Current status of treatment of gestational trophoblastic disease. Cancer 38:620, 1976

Lewis JL, Jr: Treatment of gestational trophoblastic neoplasms: A brief review of development in the years 1968 to 1978. Am J Obstet Gynecol 136:163, 1980

Lewis JL, Jr, Davis RC, Ross GT: Hormonal, immunologic and chemotherapeutic studies of transplantable human choriocarcinoma. Am J Obstet Gynecol 104:472, 1969

Lewis JL, Jr, Gore H, Hertig AT et al: Treatment of trophoblastic disease with rationale for use of adjunctive chemotherapy at the time of indicated operation. Am J Obstet Gynecol 96:710, 1966

Lewis JL, Jr, Terasaki, PI: HL-A leukocyte antigen studies in women with gestational trophoblastic neoplasms. Am J Obstet Gynecol 111:547, 1971

Li MC, Hertz R, Spencer DB: Effect of methotrexate therapy upon choriocarcinoma and chorioadenoma. Proc Soc Exp Biol Med 93:361, 1956

Louvet J, Harman SM, Nisula BC et al: Follicle stimulating activity of human chorionic gonadotropin: Effect of dissociation and recombination of subunits. Endocrinology 99:1126, 1976

Magrath IT, Golding PR, Bagshawe KD: Medical presentations of choriocarcinoma. Br Med J 2:633, 1971

Makino S, Sasaki MS, Fukuschima T: Preliminary notes on the chromosomes of human chorionic tissues. Proc Jpn Acad 39:54, 1963

Maroulis GB, Hammond CB, Johnsrude IS et al: Arteriography and infusional chemotherapy in localized trophoblastic disease. Obstet Gynecol 45:397, 1975

Marshall JR, Hammond CB, Ross GT et al: Plasma and urinary chorionic gonadotropin during human pregnancy. Obstet Gynecol 32:760, 1968

Midgley AR, Pierce GB: Immunohistochemical localization of human chorionic gonadotropin. J Exp Med 115:289, 1962

Miller JM, Surwit EA, Hammond CB: Choriocarcinoma following term pregnancy. Obstet Gynecol 53:207, 1979

Miyakawa I, Yagi K, Nakayama M et al: Plasma levels of human chorionic somatomammotropin, progesterone, unconjugated estradiol and estriol and alpha fetoprotein in patients with hydatidiform moles. J Endocrinol 72:371, 1977

Morrow CP, Kletzky OK, DiSaia PJ et al: Clinical and laboratory correlates of molar pregnancy and trophoblastic disease. Am J Obstet Gynecol 128:424, 1977

Nathanson L, Fishman WH: New observations on the Regan isoenzyme of alkaline phosphatase in cancer patients. Cancer 27:1388, 1971

Nelson JH, Jr, Lu T, Hall JE et al: The effect of trophoblast on immune state of women. Am J Obstet Gynecol 117:689, 1973

Nisula BC, Morgan FJ, Canfield RE: Evidence that chorionic gonadotropin has intrinsic thyrotropic activity. Biochem Biophys Res Commun 59:86, 1974

Nisula BC, Taliadouros GS: Thyroid function in gestational trophoblastic neoplasia: Evidence that the thyrotropic activity of chorionic gonadotropin mediates the thyrotoxicosis of choriocarcinoma. Am J Obstet Gynecol 138:77, 1980

Novak E, Seah CS: Choriocarcinoma of the uterus. Am J Obstet Gynecol 67:933, 1954

O'Brien TJ, Engvall E, Schlaerth JB et al: Trophoblastic disease monitoring: pregnancy-specific β_1-glycoprotein. Am J Obstet Gynecol 138:313, 1980

Osathanondh R, Goldstein DP, Pastorfide GB: Actinomycin D as the primary agent for gestational trophoblastic disease. Cancer 36:863, 1975

Park WW: Choriocarcinoma: A general review, with analysis of 516 cases. Arch Pathol 49:73, 1951

Pastorfide GB, Goldstein DP: Pregnancy after hydatidiform mole. Obstet Gynecol 42:67, 1973

Patillo RA, Gey GO, Delfs E et al: Human hormone production in vitro. Science 159:1467, 1968

Patillo RA, Gey GO, Delfs E et al: The hormone-synthesizing trophoblastic cell in vitro: A model for cancer research and placental hormone synthesis. Ann NY Acad Sci 172:288, 1971

Robinson E, Ben–Hur N, Zuckerman H et al: Further immunologic studies in patients with choriocarcinoma and hydatidiform mole. Cancer Res 27:1202, 1967

Ross GT: Congenital anomalies among children born of mothers receiving chemotherapy for gestational trophoblastic neoplasms. Cancer 37:1043, 1976

Ross GT: Clinical relevance of research in the structure of human chorionic gonadotropin. Am J Obstet Gynecol 129:795, 1977

Ross GT, Goldstein DP, Hertz R et al: Sequential use of methotrexate and actinomycin D in the treatment of metastatic choriocarcinoma and related trophoblastic diseases in women. Am J Obstet Gynecol 93:223, 1965

Ross GT, Hammond CB, Hertz R et al: Chemotherapy of metastatic and non-metastatic gestational trophoblastic neoplasms. Tex Rep Biol Med 24:326, 1966

Sasaki M, Fukuschima T, Makino S: Some aspects of the chromosome constitution of hydatidiform moles and normal chorionic villi. Gann 53:101, 1962

Saxena BN, Goldstein DP, Emerson K, Jr et al: Serum placental lactogen levels in patients with molar pregnancy and trophoblastic tumors. Am J Obstet Gynecol 102:115, 1968

Seppala M, Bagshawe KD, Ruoslahti E: Radioimmunoassay of alpha-fetoprotein: A contribution to the diagnosis of choriocarcinoma and hydatidiform mole. Int J Cancer 10:478, 1972

Siris ES, Nisula BC, Birken S et al: New evidence for intrinsic FSH-like activity in HCG and LH. Abstracts of the 58th Meeting of the Endocrine Society, 1977

Smith JP: Chemotherapy in gynecologic cancer. Clin Obstet Gynecol 18:109, 1975

Soules MR, Tyrey L, Hammond CB: The utility of a rapid assay for human chorionic gonadotropin in the management of trophoblastic disease. Am J Obstet Gynecol 135:384, 1979

Stone M, Dent J, Kardana A et al: Relationship of oral contraception to development of trophoblastic tumor after evacuation of a hydatidiform mole. Br J Obstet Gynaecol. 83:913, 1976

Surwit EA, Hammond CB: Treatment of metastatic trophoblastic disease with poor prognosis. Obstet Gynecol 55:565, 1980

Szulman AE, Surti U: Syndromes of hydatidiform mole: I. Cytogenetic and morphologic correlations. Am J Obstet Gynecol 131:665, 1978

Tow W: The influence of the primary treatment of hydatidiform mole on its subsequent course. J Obstet Gynaecol Br Commonw 73:544, 1966

Twiggs LB, Morrow CP, Schlaerth JB: Acute pulmonary complications of molar pregnancy. Am J Obstet Gynecol 135:189, 1979

Vaitukaitis JL: Human chorionic gonadotropin. In Fuchs F, Klopper A (eds): Endocrinology of Pregnancy, 2nd ed, pp 63–75. Hagerstown, MD, Harper & Row, 1977

Van Thiel DH, Grodin JM, Ross GT et al: Partial placenta accreta in pregnancies following chemotherapy for gestational trophoblastic neoplasms. Am J Obstet Gynecol 112:54, 1972

Vaughn TC, Surwit EA, Hammond CB: Late recurrences of gestational trophoblastic neoplasia. Am J Obstet Gynecol 138:73, 1980

Walden PAM, Bagshawe KD: Reproductive performance of women successfully treated for trophoblastic tumors. Am J Obstet Gynecol 125:1108, 1976

Weed JC, Jr, Hammond CB: Cerebral metastatic choriocarcinoma: Intensive therapy and prognosis. Obstet Gynecol 55:89, 1980

Ectopic pregnancy is a pregnancy that is implanted outside the uterine cavity, *i.e.*, at a site that is not designed either to receive the conceptus or to permit it to develop. The most common site for ectopic pregnancy is the fallopian tube (Fig. 22–1). Most of the cases culminate in disaster of one kind or another; the conceptus is almost invariably lost, and the condition may also be fatal for the mother. With modern care, the death rate from ectopic pregnancy is about 3/1000 cases. From 4%–10% of all maternal deaths and about 16% of deaths from hemorrhage during pregnancy are due to ectopic pregnancy. There has been a slight decrease in mortality from this cause, but even so, in a recent series of cases, 75% of the deaths were considered to have been preventable. The major sources of morbidity and mortality are patient delay in reporting early symptoms and physician delay in making the diagnosis and instituting appropriate treatment.

The true incidence of ectopic pregnancy is difficult to determine. It varies from one population to another, and some of the cases, notably tubal abortion, may resolve spontaneously without diagnosis. In recent years, the incidence of diagnosed cases has been increasing. Although there are many causes, the increasing incidence is believed to be related especially to the greater frequency of pelvic inflammatory disease and the increasing use of certain modern contraceptives, particularly the intrauterine device and the progestin-only oral contraceptive.

From 25,000–30,000 ectopic pregnancies occur in the United States each year. The reported incidence ranges from 1/80 to 1/200 live births. Ectopic pregnancy is more common among the poor than the affluent. Jamaica has one of the highest incidences of ectopic pregnancies in the world—1/28 live births.

Almost 100 years have passed since the publication of Tait's classic paper on the *Modern Management of Ectopic Pregnancy.* He discussed the difficulty of making the diagnosis but emphasized the importance of early surgery. "If an operation is to be done, it must be done without delay." Tait was the first to establish the importance of exploratory laparotomy if ruptured tubal pregnancy is a reasonably possible diagnosis. Prior to his paper, most women died of either hemorrhage or infection.

Ectopic pregnancy, "the great masquerader," can mimic many other abdominal and pelvic problems. If patients report symptoms early, if the physician has a high index of suspicion, and if modern methods of diagnosis are used, the diagnosis is missed in only a few cases. Early diagnosis depends on the clinical caveat: "think ectopic." In all women between menarche and the menopause who complain of lower abdominal pain, the possibility of ectopic pregnancy should be considered, and discarded only if it is untenable.

22

ECTOPIC PREGNANCY

William Droegemueller

TUBAL PREGNANCY

ETIOLOGY

The common denominator in most theories of etiology is delay in ovum transport, but several other factors have been associated or implicated in women who develop ectopic pregnancy. There is no suitable animal model, as ectopic pregnancy is unknown in lower animals and is a rarity in subhuman primates. Only 3 tubal pregnancies have been reported in 3000 pregnancies observed in monkeys in captivity.

Tubal Abnormalities

Chronic pelvic inflammatory disease is a common cause of tubal pregnancy. The adherent mucosal folds may either trap the fertilized ovum or alter its trans-

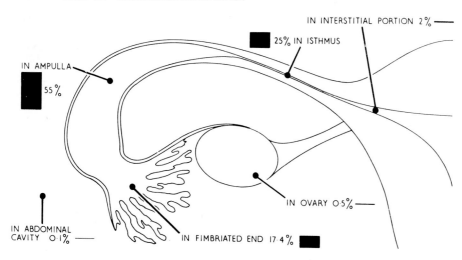

FIG. 22-1. Sites of ectopic gestation implantation with relative frequency of occurrence. (Llewellyn-Jones D: Fundamentals of Obstetrics and Gynaecology, Vol 1, Obstetrics. London, Faber and Faber, 1969)

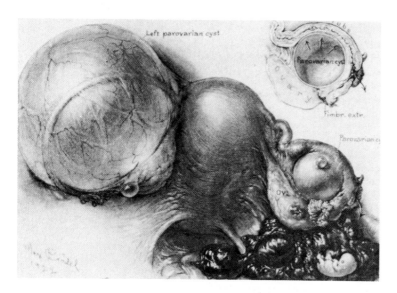

FIG. 22-2. Ruptured tubal pregnancy (*right*), possibly caused by a parovarian cyst. The pelvic organs are viewed from behind. The pregnancy was situated in the ampulla of the right tube, which has ruptured at a point 2 cm from the fimbriated end (*arrow*). The blood, fetus, and products of conception are collected behind the right broad ligament. The right tube is drawn over the parovarian cyst and compressed proximal to the point of nidation (*insert*). The corpus luteum of pregnancy is located in the right ovary near the fimbria. On the *left* side, is a larger parovarian cyst, with the fallopian tube drawn out over its surface, and the ovary underneath it. This case illustrates the relation of tubal constriction to tubal pregnancy. (Brady L: Bull Johns Hopkins Hosp 33:442, 1933. Drawing by Max Brödel)

port. Cases of acute pelvic inflammatory disease are reaching epidemic numbers in the United States, and many epidemiologists relate this disease directly to the increase in the incidence of ectopic pregnancy. A history of prior salpingitis is obtained from 30%–50% of women operated upon for ectopic pregnancy. In tubes excised for ectopic pregnancy, histologic evidence of chronic salpingitis is found in approximately half the cases. Prior to the advent of antibiotic therapy, gonorrheal infections usually resulted in total occlusion of the tube. On the women now treated with antibiotics for acute pelvic inflammatory disease, complete tubal occlusion occurs in only about 15%. In the remainder, some escape with no tubal lesion, but others may be left with lesions that interfere with function of the epithelium and agglutination of adjacent mucosal folds,

with the formation of blind pockets. Pregnancies following tuberculous salpingitis are at an even higher risk of ectopic location, perhaps one pregnancy of every three being located in the tube.

Peritubal adhesions can distort tubal anatomy and function. The initial insult may have been from either postpartum or postabortion pelvic inflammatory disease, previous ruptured appendix, or sterile inflammation produced by endometriosis.

Other anatomic abnormalities that may lead to ectopic pregnancy include accessory tubal ostia, convolutions, and diverticula. Tubal diverticula can be congenital, or acquired as a result of infection. Extrinsic masses, such as uterine or tubal myomas, and adnexal masses (see Fig. 22–2) may cause kinking or displacement of the tube.

Other often mentioned but less popular theories on the etiology of ectopic pregnancy include the *mechanical effect of retrograde menstrual bleeding* and *endometriosis.* There is speculation as to the exact pathophysiology that relates endometriosis to ectopic pregnancy. Possibly the chemotaxis of the aberrant endometrium attracts the conceptus to the ectopic location.

Abnormalities of the Zygote

Various developmental abnormalities of the zygote, including an abnormal zona pellucida, have been implicated in tubal pregnancy. Chromosomal analysis of material from such a pregnancy reveals an abnormal karyotype in approximately one-third of the cases. Detailed morphologic studies of the embryos have revealed in many cases grossly disorganized growth and a high incidence of neural tube defects. Whether or not the defects result from the poor vascular supply of the ectopic implantation is not known.

A male factor has been implicated in some cases. The incidence of ectopic pregnancy is reported to be highest if the male has an abnormal sperm count and especially if he has a high percentage of abnormal spermatozoa.

Endocrine Disorders

Some investigators have related ectopic pregnancy to inadequacy of the corpus luteum or to delayed ovulation, which, because of altered estrogen–progesterone relationships, may affect tubal and cilial motility and ovum transport. An increased incidence has been reported to follow ovulation induction with human pituitary and chorionic gonadotropin. Prostaglandins, catecholamines, and other substances can also affect tubal motility and function so that the fertilized ovum is trapped in the tube. It has been estimated that hormonal factors may be responsible for about 50% of cases in which no recognizable mechanical or structural abnormality can be found.

Prior Tubal Pregnancy

Regardless of the cause, the history of a prior ectopic pregnancy is an important etiologic factor. A woman who has had one ectopic pregnancy has a 10%–20% chance that her subsequent pregnancies will be ectopic.

Contraceptive Failure

Intrauterine Device. Of pregnancies that occur in women using intrauterine devices 4%–9% are ectopic; one of eight is a primary ovarian pregnancy. The risk of ectopic pregnancy among women using intrauterine devices is estimated to be 12 times that of those using barrier methods. Approximately two ectopic pregnancies occur per 1000 intrauterine device users per year. Although the incidence of pregnancy diminishes with long-term use of the intrauterine device, among those who do become pregnant the likelihood of ectopic pregnancy increases. The cause of the high incidence of ectopic pregnancy among users of intrauterine devices is unsettled. Some have suggested that the effect of the intrauterine foreign body on tubal motility delays ovum transport or that tubal infection may be the cause.

There is little difference in the incidence of ectopic pregnancy according to the type of intrauterine device, except for the progesterone-bearing Progestasert; in one series, 16% of the pregnancies that occurred were extrauterine.

Progestin-Only Oral Contraception. The minipill or progestin-only oral contraceptive has been associated with an incidence of ectopic pregnancy about five times as high as the customary incidence. In women taking the minipill, 4%–6% of pregnancies are ectopic. There is no increased incidence of ectopic pregnancy with combination oral contraceptives.

Tubal Ligation. Sterilization by tubal ligation may fail because of fistula formation and recanalization. Approximately 15% of pregnancies following tubal ligation or application of spring-loaded clips are ectopic. When silastic rings fail, more than 50% of the resulting pregnancies are ectopic.

Tubal Surgery. With the recent advances in microsurgery and changes in our society, many more women are requesting reversal of a previous sterilization operation. Approximately 5% of women who conceive following a tuboplasty operation have an ectopic implantation.

"Morning-After Pill." Pregnancy is rare after the postcoital administration of large doses of estrogen. However, when this contraceptive method fails, there is a ten-fold increase in the incidence of ectopic pregnancy.

Elective Abortion

Studies differ as to whether elective abortion increases or does not significantly change the incidence of ectopic pregnancy. One study suggested an increased relative risk of ectopic pregnancy after elective abortion. However, this report comes from Greece, a country in which elective abortion is illegal, and therefore its conclusion may be related to an increase in postabortal infection. In countries where early abortion is legal and is usually performed by suction curettage, no increase in later ectopic pregnancy has been reported.

PATHOLOGY

As the trophoblast penetrates the wall of the tube, hemorrhage is inevitable as a consequence either of erosion of capillaries or blood vessels, or rupture of the viscus containing the conceptus. The stroma adjacent to the conceptus may show a feeble decidual response that is insufficient to nurture or to limit advancement of the conceptus, leading to its early death and also to the erosion of its blood supply. There is some evidence to suggest that even after the death of the embryo, the trophoblast may remain viable for a time and continue its erosive activity.

At first, the tube enlarges locally at the point of implantation, but there is little discoloration; later, the whole tube is usually distended, has a dark red to purple gray color, and contains both clotted and fresh blood. A gestational sac is sometimes seen, but no embryo may be evident. If the tube is ruptured or if a great deal of blood has escaped from the ostium, the tube may be surrounded by clot. If chorionic villi cannot be found in the tubal lumen, the surrounding debris must be searched for evidence of the pregnancy. The presence of an embryo is, of course, proof of pregnancy. If none can be found, the mere presence of he-

matosalpinx is not sufficient for diagnosis, since at least one chorionic villus, either within the tube or among the extruded clots, is needed for diagnosis.

The course and outcome of tubal pregnancy, and consequently the clinical picture, vary according to the site of implantation.

Ampullar Implantation

Ampullar pregnancy is by far the commonest of ectopic pregnancies, but its true incidence is unknown because the manifestations in many cases are so trivial that they are not observed by the patient. As noted in Figure 22–3, a very early conceptus may die and be absorbed without producing any notable symptoms; another conceptus, also quite early, may be extruded into the abdominal cavity and be absorbed without incident (*complete tubal abortion*). If there is extensive erosion of capillaries or if a major tubal vessel is opened, free blood may collect at the fimbriated end of the tube. Some of this leaks into the cul-de-sac, and some of it organizes around the conceptus, which may be partially extruded through the ostium (*incomplete tubal abortion*). In some cases, repeated choriodecidual hemorrhages occur around the dead conceptus,

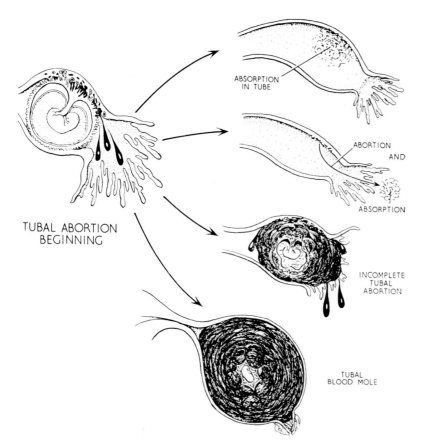

FIG. 22-3. Sequelae of tubal abortion. (Llewellyn-Jones D: Fundamentals of Obstetrics and Gynaecology, Vol 1, Obstetrics. London, Faber and Faber, 1969)

TUBAL ABORTION
BEGINNING

ABSORPTION IN TUBE

ABORTION AND ABSORPTION

INCOMPLETE TUBAL ABORTION

TUBAL BLOOD MOLE

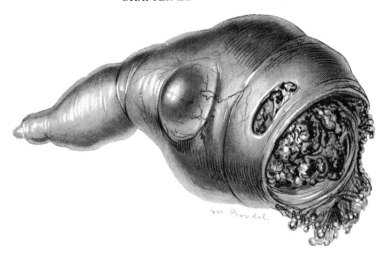

FIG. 22-4. Tubal blood mole. The bleeding is checked by a large coagulum distending and thinning out the tube; the fimbriated opening is greatly distended, but the greater diameter of the clot in the ampulla prevents its escape. Wall of tube averaging 1 mm in thickness. Operation. Recovery, July 7, 1896. Natural size. (Kelly HA: Operative Gynecology. New York, D Appleton, 1898. Drawing by Max Brödel)

giving rise to a *tubal blood mole* or carneous mole (Fig. 22–4). The amount of blood reaching the cul-de-sac varies in amount, being least in cases of complete tubal abortion and greater (*pelvic hematocoele*) in incomplete tubal abortion.

Isthmic Implantation

The lumen of the isthmic portion of the tube is quite narrow and is much less distensible than the ampullary portion. Implantation in this area predisposes to early and dramatic tubal rupture (Fig. 22–5) as a result of either erosion of the trophoblast through the tubal wall or distention by the conceptus and by rapidly collecting blood. (According to Munro Kerr's clinical grouping, it is usually in isthmic pregnancy that "the woman is struck down suddenly with abdominal pain and becomes collapsed.") The site of the rupture is ordinarily toward the peritoneal cavity (Figs. 22–6 and 22–7), but in some cases rupture occurs between the leaves of the broad ligaments. In either case, bleeding is usually heavy and may be fatal if it is not dealt with promptly. Intraligamentous bleeding may diminish as the pressure builds in the broad ligament, but the anterior or posterior leaf may ultimately give way in response to recurrent hemorrhage.

Interstitial Implantation

In interstitial pregnancy, the implantation site is partially surrounded by myometrium, which can hypertrophy to an extent to accommodate the enlarging conceptus. Rupture therefore occurs later than when implantation occurs in the isthmus, being delayed usually until 12–14 weeks. When the disaster occurs, it is no less dramatic, however; indeed, rupture of the rich blood supply of the cornual area leads quickly to intraabdominal hemorrhage that can be massive, and must be dealt with at once if the patient is to survive.

CHANGES IN THE UTERUS

The response of the myometrium to the hormones of early tubal pregnancy is identical to its response to the hormones of intrauterine pregnancy. The uterus first becomes softened and then enlarges as a result of both hypertrophy and hyperplasia of the myometrial cells. If the tubal pregnancy declares itself at a very early stage, the uterine enlargement may not be clinically detectable (Table 22–1), just as it may be difficult to discern uterine enlargement before 6 weeks, in a normal intrauterine pregnancy; if a tubal pregnancy extends beyond 6 weeks, the uterus is usually found to be slightly enlarged. (In an interstitial pregnancy of 6–8 weeks' duration, an irregularity may be found at one side of the fundus. This gradually enlarges and becomes tender, making it difficult to determine whether there is a combination of degenerating fibroid and intrauterine pregnancy, or an interstitial pregnancy.)

The endometrium also responds to a tubal pregnancy as it does to an intrauterine pregnancy: the stroma is transformed to decidua, and the endometrial glands assume the feathery pattern commonly found in early pregnancy. The atypical glandular patterns that characterize the Arias–Stella reaction (see page 94) may also be found. However, in tubal pregnancy, the gestational changes usually last for only a short time, because the early death of the embryo and trophoblast results in the withdrawal of the hormones responsible for the endometrial changes. In one series of cases in which curettage was performed before lap-

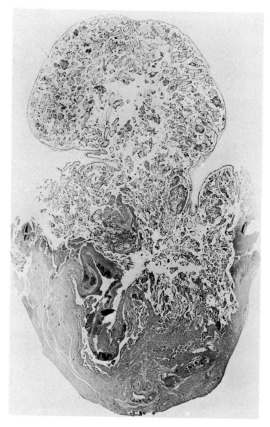

FIG. 22-5. Ruptured tubal pregnancy, 7 weeks' gestation. Note contraction of tubal musculature opposite rupture. (×3) (DN Danforth)

arotomy for tubal pregnancy, no decidua was found in more than 80% of the cases. Usually, the decidua breaks down gradually over the course of days or weeks, giving rise to the *intermittent,* occasionally heavy *vaginal bleeding* that occurs commonly in ectopic pregnancy. In some cases, the decidua may be cast off abruptly in the form of a flat, triangular, reddish brown, shaggy *decidual cast* of the uterine cavity. It is comprised of two layers of tissue each made up of decidual cells, sparse endometrial glands in varying stages of collapse, thin-walled blood vessels that are either thrombosed or filled with red cells, and scattered areas of lymphocytes, plasma cells, and neutrophils. Passage of a decidual cast should alert the physician to the possibility of ectopic pregnancy, but it should not be considered diagnostic since endometrial casts may also be passed at the time of normal menstruation.

SYMPTOMS AND SIGNS

Like appendicitis, the myriad clinical pictures presented by tubal pregnancy can be divided into two major groups: 1) those that follow the classic "textbook" picture or a recognizable variation thereof, and 2) those that are entirely bizarre and cannot be solved by logic alone. Wharton recalled that the preeminent Howard A. Kelly once remarked in the course of one of his clinics that a physician who is confronted with a pelvic problem that follows no rules and conforms to no standards should think first of ectopic pregnancy and second of pelvic tuberculosis. Classically, the first symptoms of tubal pregnancy are the first symptoms of any early pregnancy (nausea, breast tenderness, over-

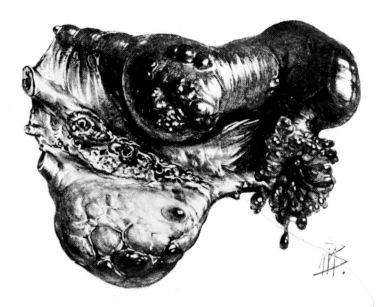

FIG. 22-6. Ruptured left extrauterine pregnancy with large, free intraperitoneal hemorrhage. The rupture is at the junction of the ampulla and the isthmus; the rest of the ampulla is dilated and infiltrated down to a narrow neck just behind the fimbriated end. Enucleation; saline infusion. Recovery. Feb. 25, 1895. Natural size. (Kelly HA: Operative Gynecology. New York, D Appleton, 1898. Drawing by Max Brödel)

eral adnexal pain, and both adnexa are extremely tender. There is usually no history of amenorrhea or fainting, the breasts are soft and not tender, and the results of the hCG test are negative. The traditional gonorrheal salpingitis is accompanied by fever, leukocytosis, and dysuria. Other organisms that cause salpingitis and some gonorrheal strains may produce a lesser systemic reaction; in one series, 50% of proved cases had no fever or leukocytosis. Although the manifestations of salpingitis and tubal pregnancy may seem to be so different that there should be no difficulty in distinguishing them, this is not true. In emergency rooms, this can be one of the most puzzling of diagnostic problems.

Acute Appendicitis. In some cases, appendicitis may be confused with tubal pregnancy, since appendicitis may produce bizarre clinical pictures. Typical cases of appendicitis differ from cases of tubal pregnancy in that vomiting is more likely, fainting and amenorrhea do not occur, low-grade fever and leukocytosis are much more common, the breasts are soft and nontender, and right lower quadrant rigidity and rebound tenderness are usually more pronounced.

Degenerating Fibroid. Fibroids tend to become painful and to enlarge in pregnancy. If such a tumor is small in early pregnancy and is located in the cornual area of the uterus, it may be impossible to distinguish it from an interstitial pregnancy. Ultrasound should be helpful in determining the nature of the enlarging mass. If the matter is not solved by 10 weeks' gestation, the diagnosis should be made by laparotomy (not laparoscopy).

Normal Intrauterine Pregnancy and an Associated Abdominal or Pelvic Problem. As Osler emphasized, the physician should be loath to assign two simultaneous causes for a single group of symptoms. However, in considering the differential diagnosis of tubal pregnancy, it is important to consider such possibilities as a normal intrauterine pregnancy with torsion of the tube and ovary, torsion of an ovarian cyst, or a pedunculated fibroid. Finally, a normal intrauterine pregnancy *and* a tubal pregnancy may coexist, a rare combination but by no means a medical curiosity.

Intrauterine Device. Spotting, pelvic pain, and unilateral pelvic infections are complications that can result from the use of an intrauterine device (IUD). Tubal pregnancy is also more common in women using an IUD. The distinction between IUD complications and tubal pregnancy is extremely important and may be difficult. When the patient does not have amenorrhea or any other signs of early pregnancy, and the results

of a test for hCG are negative, she is unlikely to have a tubal pregnancy.

TREATMENT

Routine Procedure

Laparotomy is urgently indicated as soon as the diagnosis of tubal pregnancy is made. In the past, the presence of massive intraabdominal bleeding and shock led to debate over whether the first step should be to stop the bleeding, or whether surgery should be deferred until the circulation is restored. Before blood and blood substitutes were readily available, a prompt clinical diagnosis and rapid, skillful surgery were usually rewarded by a healthy patient. In one series of 174 ectopic pregnancies reported in 1947, most of the operations were done in 20 min or less, and 17 patients were transfused. Four women died. Of these, it is reasonable to presume that two, and possibly three, would have survived had modern methods of circulatory support and monitoring been available. At present it is usually possible for medical and surgical therapy to be started simultaneously.

If the woman's condition is at all precarious, the simplest procedure that will control the bleeding should be selected. A midline incision can usually be made more rapidly than a transverse one. Sufficient blood is cleared away so that *both* adnexa can be readily visualized. The operation of choice is a total salpingectomy. The tube is removed from the mesosalpinx by clamping with successive Kelly clamps and placing transfixation sutures of 2-0 chromic catgut (Fig. 22–8).

It is preferable to resect the uterine cornu. This should be superficial in order to avoid a myometrial defect that could rupture in a subsequent pregnancy. Following the cornual resection, it is important to peritonealize this area; the adjacent round ligament can be used for this purpose. (Fig. 22–8C). All old blood and clots are removed from the peritoneal cavity, and the pelvis is irrigated with warm saline. This step is important for future fertility, as it reduces the possibility of damage as a result of pelvic adhesions. The ipsilateral ovary is not removed unless there is an extensive hematoma of the infundibulopelvic or broad ligaments. The contralateral tube and ovary should be inspected. Hematosalpinx of the contralateral tube is a frequent finding in acute tubal pregnancy, but it requires no treatment. Several years ago, some physicians recommended that the ovary on the side of the ectopic pregnancy be routinely removed so that all future ovulations would occur from the ovary with the remaining tube, thus preventing loss of ova from the opposite side and improving fertility. This theoretic concept is interesting, but there is no proof of its efficacy.

tured tubal pregnancy is suspected or is even considered as part of the differential diagnosis of some other pelvic problem. Before the advent of laparoscopy, most of the suspected cases were managed by observation and repeated pelvic examination; at present, such problems can be quickly solved by laparoscopy, permitting early laparotomy and, in some of the cases, preservation of the affected tube.

Pregnancy Tests

A positive result to the test for human chorionic gonadotropin (hCG) confirms pregnancy, but gives no indication whether the pregnancy is intra- or extrauterine. In tubal pregnancy, the need for diagnosis usually arises at 6 or 7 weeks' gestation when hCG levels are relatively low either because it is so early in the pregnancy or because the trophoblast has undergone abruption or degeneration. Such low levels of hCG are readily detectable by radioimmunoassay (RIA) and also by radioreceptorassay (RRA; see page 359 and Table 19–1). If a urine slide or tube agglutination test yields positive results, they can be relied on; but negative results do not rule out the presence of hCG in amounts below the sensitivity of the test. Consequently, it is important to select a test with sensitivity of 200 mIU hCG/ml serum or less. Even at sensitivity of 200 mIU/ml, the test is negative in 5% of ectopic pregnancies.

It has been suggested that analyses for pregnancy-specific β-glycoprotein (see page 310) may be a useful adjunct to hCG testing in ectopic pregnancy, but sufficient data are not yet available to evaluate this.

Dilatation and Curettage

In cases in which the leading symptom is abnormal bleeding, dilatation and curettage (D. and C.) may be performed with a presumptive diagnosis of dysfunctional uterine bleeding or incomplete abortion. In the presence of an unsuspected tubal pregnancy, the returns are usually scant, consisting only of decidua in which the Arias–Stella reaction (see page 94) may be noted. If no chorionic villi are found in such a case, it may be prudent to request that the pathologist make deeper cuts in the paraffin block, for the finding of even one chorionic villus in the curettings establishes the diagnosis of intrauterine pregnancy. If none are found in the presence of decidua with or without the Arias–Stella reaction, the possibility of ectopic pregnancy must be considered and steps taken to establish or rule out the diagnosis.

Posterior Colpotomy

Prior to laparoscopy, posterior colpotomy was an excellent method of directly visualizing the pelvic organs.

Occasionally, definitive surgery for tubal pregnancy was accomplished through the posterior cul-de-sac. Obviously, it should be used with caution if there is frank hemorrhage.

Ultrasound

The place of ultrasound in the diagnosis of tubal pregnancy is discussed on page 567. Occasionally, the procedure can be definitive, but more frequently, its value is in demonstrating the presence of an intrauterine pregnancy, which would cause the possibility of a simultaneous tubal pregnancy to be extremely unlikely.

Differential Diagnosis

A careful and painstaking history is of more value than physical findings in raising the question of tubal pregnancy and ruling out other conditions that may be confused with it. The following conditions are among those most frequently confused with tubal pregnancy.

Corpus Luteum Cyst. Amenorrhea, spotting, and unilateral pelvic pain are common. The patient does not have the symptoms and signs of early pregnancy, the pain is less severe than that in tubal pregnancy, there is no history of faintness, and RIA or RRA tests for hCG are negative. The uterus is firm and not enlarged, and the adnexal mass of a corpus luteum cyst is usually well defined, smooth, cystic in consistency, and very freely movable. A ruptured corpus luteum cyst with intraabdominal hemorrhage is usually a surgical emergency; unless bleeding stops spontaneously, as it does occasionally, laparotomy is usually performed with a presumptive diagnosis of ruptured tubal pregnancy. The corpus luteum of pregnancy may attain a size of 3+ cm and is usually an incidental finding at a first pelvic examination in early pregnancy. There is no pain, and the structure is round, usually nontender, freely movable, with a cystic consistency. Ultrasound usually discloses the nature of the contents and also permits diagnosis of an early intrauterine pregnancy.

Threatened or Incomplete Abortion. The period of amenorrhea in threatened or incomplete abortion is usually longer than that in tubal pregnancy. The pain, if any, is midline and crampy, and it is less severe; bleeding is usually heavier and is not accompanied by fainting. There is no vaginal or adnexal tenderness, and no adnexal mass unless a corpus luteum of pregnancy should be palpated. The uterus is usually larger and softer than in tubal pregnancy.

Pelvic Inflammatory Disease. Salpingitis is usually bilateral, movement of the cervix produces equal bilat-

TABLE 22-1. ADMITTING SIGNS AND SYMPTOMS IN 300 CONSECUTIVE CASES OF ECTOPIC PREGNANCY

Sign or Symptom	Cases (%)
ABDOMINAL PAIN	99.3
Generalized abdominal	44.3
Unilateral abdominal	32.7
Radiating to shoulder	22.3
ABNORMAL UTERINE BLEEDING	74.3
AMENORRHEA $\angle$ 2 WEEKS	68.3
SYNCOPAL SYMPTOMS	37.0
ADNEXAL TENDERNESS	96.3
UNILATERAL ADNEXAL MASS	53.7
UTERUS	
Normal size	70.7
6–8 weeks' size	25.7
9–12 weeks' size	3.3
UTERINE CAST PASSED VAGINALLY	6.7
ADMISSION TEMPERATURE > 37°C	2.3

(Modified from Brenner PF, Roy S, Mishell DR, Jr: JAMA 243:673, 1980)

cus), if it appears, is striking evidence of extensive intraabdominal hemorrhage; but it is found so rarely, even when the hemorrhage is massive, that its absence by no means rules out extensive bleeding.

On *pelvic examination,* the findings vary from the presence of a large mass to completely negative findings. As noted in Table 22–1, tenderness is present in most of the cases, and a mass in about half. In many cases, the mass is vague and ill defined; it may consist not only of the tubal pregnancy, but also of adherent omentum, blood clots, and small bowel. A tender, boggy mass in the cul-de-sac, when present, is due to the collection of blood in this area, a pelvic hematocoele.

When an adnexal mass is suspected, it is not uncommon for the physician to repeat the examination under anesthesia with the intent to avoid laparotomy if nothing is found. This practice is extremely dangerous if there is a reasonable possibility of tubal pregnancy. A tube about to rupture may indeed rupture if the slightest pressure is exerted on it; no mass is felt, and, since the patient cannot react or protest, the incident is unnoticed until shock ensues. Ian Donald records two fatal cases of this kind, and Jeffcoate refers to three cases in which the patient died within 30 min of being moved from the operating room. In suspected tubal pregnancy, pelvic examination should be done under anesthesia only if laparotomy is to be done immediately, regardless of the findings.

Culdocentesis

The value of culdocentesis is emphasized in Table 22–2, since blood appeared in the fluid obtained by this method in 95% of 300 proved cases. The procedure is simple and rapid, and it can be diagnostic of intraperitoneal bleeding. When blood escapes into the abdominal cavity, it undergoes the clotting process and subsequent fibrinolysis, after which it fails to clot. With the patient's legs in stirrups and her hips slightly lower than her thorax so that any blood will pool in the cul-de-sac, a tenaculum is placed on the cervix and, with slight traction, an 18-gauge needle is introduced through the posterior vaginal vault without anesthesia. If the aspirated blood clots, its probable source is a vessel that was punctured en route to the cul-de-sac. Failure to obtain any fluid may suggest that the cul-de-sac was not entered. Culdocentesis is a valuable diagnostic aid, especially when unclotted blood with an hematocrit value of 15% or higher is obtained. The purpose of the procedure is to determine whether there is any free blood in the abdomen. Of course, there will be none if a tubal pregnancy is unruptured or has not leaked from the ostium. If it is negative, further diagnostic tests should be made; if it is positive, laparotomy should be performed at once.

Laparoscopy

Laparoscopy is not needed if culdocentesis reveals free blood in the abdominal cavity or if the clinical picture of tubal rupture is classic. It is invaluable if unrup-

TABLE 22-2. ADMITTING LABORATORY AND OTHER DATA IN 300 CONSECUTIVE CASES OF ECTOPIC PREGNANCY

Laboratory or Other Data	Cases (%)
PREGNANCY TEST (HI, urine, sensitive to 700 mIU hCG/ml)	
Positive	82.5
Negative	17.5
Not done (surgical emergency)	16.3
HEMATOCRIT	
> 30%	72.3
Between 21% and 30%	23.0
< 21%	4.7
WHITE BLOOD CELL COUNT	
< 10,000/mm³	49.0
Between 10,000 and 15,000/mm³	35.7
Between 15,000 and 20,000/mm³	10.7
> 20,000/mm³	4.7
CULDOCENTESIS	
Nonclotting blood obtained	95.0
Hematocrit value on blood > 15%	97.5
Hematocrit value on blood < 15%	2.5
No blood or fluid obtained	5.0

HI, Hemagglutination inhibition test
hCG, Human chorionic gonadotropin
(Modified from Brenner PF, Roy S, Mishell DR, Jr: JAMA 243:673, 1980)

FIG. 22-7. Sequelae of tubal rupture in cases of ectopic gestation. *A.* Intraperitoneal hemorrhage and pelvic hematocoele: *B.* Broad ligament hematoma. (Llewellyn–Jones D; Fundamentals of Obstetrics and Gynaecology, Vol 1, Obstetrics. London, Faber and Faber, 1969)

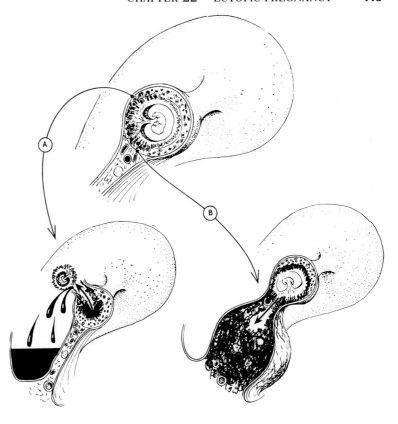

due menstruation). They are followed, in order, by lower quadrant discomfort, spotting, faintness, and, finally, sharp exacerbation of pain as rupture occurs or is imminent, and syncope with shoulder pain as the abdomen fills with blood that finds its way between the liver and diaphragm. In such cases, the diagnosis can be made over the telephone; but usually, the picture is less tidy. The variations are due principally to the unpredictable character of vaginal bleeding and abdominal pain, the differences in the anatomic location of the tubal implantation, the abruptness of tubal rupture or distention, and the magnitude and speed of hemorrhage.

The admission symptoms and signs in 300 consecutive surgically treated cases of ectopic pregnancy are listed in Table 22–1. It should be noted that abdominal pain was more commonly diffuse than localized; that abnormal uterine bleeding and amenorrhea of at least 2 weeks' duration occurred in most of the cases; that adnexal tenderness occurred in almost all cases, but an adnexal mass could be felt in only half; that in two-thirds of the cases the uterus was thought to be of normal size; that leukocytosis appeared in only half the cases; and that fever was extremely unusual.

DIAGNOSIS

Although the diagnosis is obvious, in occasional cases, more often it is not. A sufficiently penetrating history usually leads to at least a suspicion of tubal pregnancy that makes it mandatory to proceed at once to more definitive diagnostic measures.

Physical Examination

Depending on the rate and amount of bleeding, the patient's general status may vary from only slight pallor to hemorrhagic shock. Since bleeding tends to be recurrent as successive clots are dislodged, serial determinations of pulse and blood pressure should be made while the patient is being prepared for surgery. Progressive loss of fluid from the circulatory compartment may become evident by first noting the pulse and blood pressure in the reclining posture, then in the sitting posture.

The *abdominal signs* vary. Deep lower quadrant tenderness is usually present; occasionally, guarding and rebound tenderness are also seen. *Cullen's sign* (bluish discoloration of the skin around the umbili-

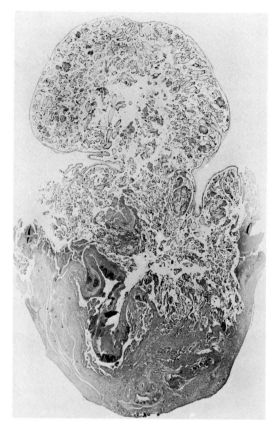

FIG. 22–5. Ruptured tubal pregnancy, 7 weeks' gestation. Note contraction of tubal musculature opposite rupture. (×3) (DN Danforth)

arotomy for tubal pregnancy, no decidua was found in more than 80% of the cases. Usually, the decidua breaks down gradually over the course of days or weeks, giving rise to the *intermittent,* occasionally heavy *vaginal bleeding* that occurs commonly in ectopic pregnancy. In some cases, the decidua may be cast off abruptly in the form of a flat, triangular, reddish brown, shaggy *decidual cast* of the uterine cavity. It is comprised of two layers of tissue each made up of decidual cells, sparse endometrial glands in varying stages of collapse, thin-walled blood vessels that are either thrombosed or filled with red cells, and scattered areas of lymphocytes, plasma cells, and neutrophils. Passage of a decidual cast should alert the physician to the possibility of ectopic pregnancy, but it should not be considered diagnostic since endometrial casts may also be passed at the time of normal menstruation.

SYMPTOMS AND SIGNS

Like appendicitis, the myriad clinical pictures presented by tubal pregnancy can be divided into two major groups: 1) those that follow the classic "textbook" picture or a recognizable variation thereof, and 2) those that are entirely bizarre and cannot be solved by logic alone. Wharton recalled that the preeminent Howard A. Kelly once remarked in the course of one of his clinics that a physician who is confronted with a pelvic problem that follows no rules and conforms to no standards should think first of ectopic pregnancy and second of pelvic tuberculosis. Classically, the first symptoms of tubal pregnancy are the first symptoms of any early pregnancy (nausea, breast tenderness, over-

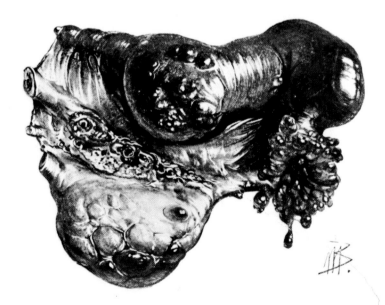

FIG. 22–6. Ruptured left extrauterine pregnancy with large, free intraperitoneal hemorrhage. The rupture is at the junction of the ampulla and the isthmus; the rest of the ampulla is dilated and infiltrated down to a narrow neck just behind the fimbriated end. Enucleation; saline infusion. Recovery. Feb. 25, 1895. Natural size. (Kelly HA: Operative Gynecology. New York, D Appleton, 1898. Drawing by Max Brödel)

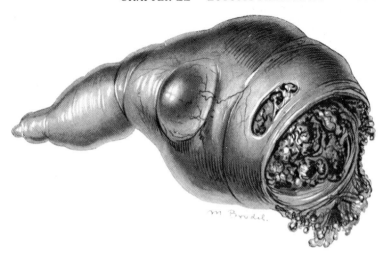

FIG. 22-4. Tubal blood mole. The bleeding is checked by a large coagulum distending and thinning out the tube; the fimbriated opening is greatly distended, but the greater diameter of the clot in the ampulla prevents its escape. Wall of tube averaging 1 mm in thickness. Operation. Recovery, July 7, 1896. Natural size. (Kelly HA: Operative Gynecology. New York, D Appleton, 1898. Drawing by Max Brödel)

giving rise to a *tubal blood mole* or carneous mole (Fig. 22–4). The amount of blood reaching the cul-de-sac varies in amount, being least in cases of complete tubal abortion and greater (*pelvic hematocoele*) in incomplete tubal abortion.

Isthmic Implantation

The lumen of the isthmic portion of the tube is quite narrow and is much less distensible than the ampullary portion. Implantation in this area predisposes to early and dramatic tubal rupture (Fig. 22–5) as a result of either erosion of the trophoblast through the tubal wall or distention by the conceptus and by rapidly collecting blood. (According to Munro Kerr's clinical grouping, it is usually in isthmic pregnancy that "the woman is struck down suddenly with abdominal pain and becomes collapsed.") The site of the rupture is ordinarily toward the peritoneal cavity (Figs. 22–6 and 22–7), but in some cases rupture occurs between the leaves of the broad ligaments. In either case, bleeding is usually heavy and may be fatal if it is not dealt with promptly. Intraligamentous bleeding may diminish as the pressure builds in the broad ligament, but the anterior or posterior leaf may ultimately give way in response to recurrent hemorrhage.

Interstitial Implantation

In interstitial pregnancy, the implantation site is partially surrounded by myometrium, which can hypertrophy to an extent to accommodate the enlarging conceptus. Rupture therefore occurs later than when implantation occurs in the isthmus, being delayed usually until 12–14 weeks. When the disaster occurs, it is no less dramatic, however; indeed, rupture of the rich blood supply of the cornual area leads quickly to intraabdominal hemorrhage that can be massive, and must be dealt with at once if the patient is to survive.

CHANGES IN THE UTERUS

The response of the myometrium to the hormones of early tubal pregnancy is identical to its response to the hormones of intrauterine pregnancy. The uterus first becomes softened and then enlarges as a result of both hypertrophy and hyperplasia of the myometrial cells. If the tubal pregnancy declares itself at a very early stage, the uterine enlargement may not be clinically detectable (Table 22–1), just as it may be difficult to discern uterine enlargement before 6 weeks, in a normal intrauterine pregnancy; if a tubal pregnancy extends beyond 6 weeks, the uterus is usually found to be slightly enlarged. (In an interstitial pregnancy of 6–8 weeks' duration, an irregularity may be found at one side of the fundus. This gradually enlarges and becomes tender, making it difficult to determine whether there is a combination of degenerating fibroid and intrauterine pregnancy, or an interstitial pregnancy.)

The endometrium also responds to a tubal pregnancy as it does to an intrauterine pregnancy: the stroma is transformed to decidua, and the endometrial glands assume the feathery pattern commonly found in early pregnancy. The atypical glandular patterns that characterize the Arias–Stella reaction (see page 94) may also be found. However, in tubal pregnancy, the gestational changes usually last for only a short time, because the early death of the embryo and trophoblast results in the withdrawal of the hormones responsible for the endometrial changes. In one series of cases in which curettage was performed before lap-

FIG. 22-8. Salpingectomy. *A.* Removal of tube, including wedge of uterine cornu that contains interstitial part of tube. Dissection hugs fallopian tube to avoid ovarian blood supply. *B.* Cornu closed by figure-of-eight suture, mesosalpinx ligated by transfixation. *C.* Modified Coffey suspension of uterus; knuckle of round ligament anchored to posterior aspect of uterus to peritonealize area and suspend ovary. Anterior and posterior leaves of broad ligament attached to round ligament may now be tacked to uterus if needed to cover raw surfaces. (Wharton LR: Gynecology With a Section on Female Urology. Philadelphia, WB Saunders, 1943)

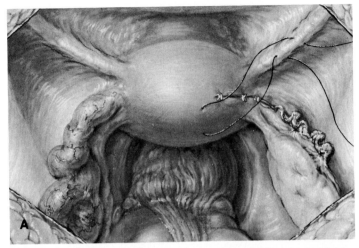

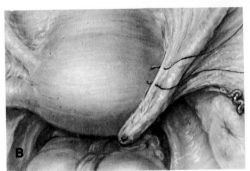
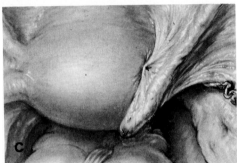

Rh-negative women who are unsensitized should receive an injection of anti-D γ-globulin after surgery.

Alternative Procedures

The most pressing problem is control of active bleeding. If the woman has been in shock, no matter how fine her condition at the moment, it is wise to complete the necessary procedure (salpingectomy) as quickly as possible and close the abdomen. If the tube is unruptured or if bleeding has been minimal, certain alternative or additional procedures can be considered.

Hysterectomy. Hysterectomy may be appropriate if the woman desires no further pregnancies, if the uterus is diseased, and if she clearly desires this to be done at the time the tubal pregnancy is dealt with (provided the physician considers the additional operation to be reasonable under the circumstances). Hysterectomy is usually the procedure of choice in ruptured interstitial pregnancy, since the cornu may be so damaged that repair is time-consuming, unsatisfactory, and accompanied by considerable blood loss.

Expression of a Tubal Blood Mole. In some cases of tubal blood mole, the contents of the tube can be easily expressed from the fimbriated end. However, the probability that the tube has been damaged by the pregnancy is great enough that this procedure should usually be reserved for women who desire further pregnancies and the contralateral tube is absent or abnormal.

Salpingostomy. In unruptured, and in some ruptured, tubal pregnancies, salpingostomy with removal of the pregnancy and conservation of the tube is feasible. There is difference of opinion as to the propriety of the procedure; 10%–20% of subsequent pregnancies will also be implanted in the tube, and there is some question whether the incidence of subsequent viable pregnancies is improved. The primary indication for an attempt at conservation is the desire for another pregnancy in a patient whose contralateral tube has previously been removed or is significantly damaged. If the opposite tube is normal, the evidence to date suggests that the probability of a subsequent viable pregnancy is just as good if the affected tube is removed.

Appendectomy. In uncomplicated gynecologic operations, appendectomy is often performed as an incidental procedure. In connection with operations for tubal pregnancy, there is no evidence to suggest that it is hazardous; but, although complications from elective appendectomy are extremely unusual, many consider it to be contraindicated if the woman desires further pregnancies because of the theoretic possibility of contamination and subsequent formation of adhesions in the region of the tube.

RARE FORMS OF ECTOPIC PREGNANCY

Ectopic pregnancies located at sites other than the fallopian tube are extremely rare, but they are encountered from time to time.

ABDOMINAL PREGNANCY

There are two types of abdominal pregnancy: 1) *primary peritoneal implantation,* which has occurred, but is so rare as to be almost a medical curiosity; and 2) *implantation secondary to tubal rupture,* in which the fetus escapes cleanly from the tube through a rupture or through the fimbriated end, leaving the chorion, and usually the amnion, attached to the tube. The chorion continues to develop, attaching itself to surrounding structures and forming a placenta which, although insecure, may be sufficient to permit subsequent development of the fetus. After the tubal rupture, the pregnancy progresses more or less normally from the patient's viewpoint, except that considerable discomfort results from the adhesions and peritoneal irritation, with flatulence, abdominal discomfort, nausea, occasional vomiting, and diarrhea and constipation. Fetal movements may be painful. As the pregnancy advances, the presenting part is found to be high; the fetus is usually felt in a transverse position lying superior to the uterus, which can often be felt lower in the abdomen. The maternal mortality is 5%–10%, and the fetal mortality is more than 90%. Congenital malformations are common. Ultrasound provides an unequivocal diagnosis.

The *treatment* is laparotomy as soon as the diagnosis is made. This is not to be undertaken lightly; although some of the operations are quite simple, others may be extremely difficult because of adhesions and because of inadvertent dislodgement of the placenta. The objective is to remove the fetus, cutting the umbilical cord close to the placenta without disturbing it. The placenta is allowed to be absorbed; if left alone, it rarely presents problems of bleeding or infection. The placenta should be removed only if it is attached to the posterior part of the tube, ovary, broad ligament and the uterus, and its blood supply can be readily ligated.

Attempts to remove the placenta from other intraabdominal organs have resulted in massive hemorrhage due to the invasive properties of the trophoblast and the lack of cleavage planes. The abdomen is closed without drainage.

Some abdominal pregnancies escape notice because the patient misinterprets the episode of tubal rupture as a miscarriage or some other minor accident. Or, as in the Clark case (Fig. 22–9), operation may have been refused when the problem was originally diagnosed. In long-neglected patients of this kind, the fetus is converted to a lithopedion, and its removal may be a very hazardous procedure.

CORNUAL PREGNANCY

In cornual pregnancy, a variant of interstitial pregnancy, implantation takes place in the cornual area at the uterine end of the interstitial portion of the tube. As it is when implantation takes place in the tube, the decidual reaction is imperfect. The implications are much the same as those of interstitial pregnancy, except that the greater mass of myometrium permits the pregnancy to advance to a somewhat later date, as late as 16 weeks in some of the cases, before rupture occurs. As noted earlier, an asymmetric pregnant uterus with a tender, enlarging mass in the cornual area may be the first sign, and the physician may first suspect an enlarging fibroid. However, it is of vital importance that an exact diagnosis be made, preferably by 10 weeks and no later than 12 weeks; when rupture occurs, the collapse that follows is so rapid and so profound that it may be fatal before it can be dealt with.

PREGNANCY IN A RUDIMENTARY UTERINE HORN

The cavity of a rudimentary horn is usually not connected with the cavity of the horn that communicates with the cervix (see Figure 5–17); in such cases, conception therefore results from external migration of the spermatozoa or the fertilized ovum. The myometrium of the rudimentary horn is usually poorly developed, and the time of rupture depends on the degree to which the myometrium can grow in response to the pregnancy (Fig. 22–10). In early pregnancy, bimanual examination may disclose what appears to be an adnexal mass lateral to the uterus. An ultrasound scan should disclose the true state of affairs, and the rudimentary horn should be promptly removed when this condition is diagnosed. If no bimanual examination is made in early pregnancy, the first sign may be intense abdominal pain and massive intraabdominal hemorrhage. Laparotomy is performed with a presumptive diagnosis of ruptured interstitial pregnancy.

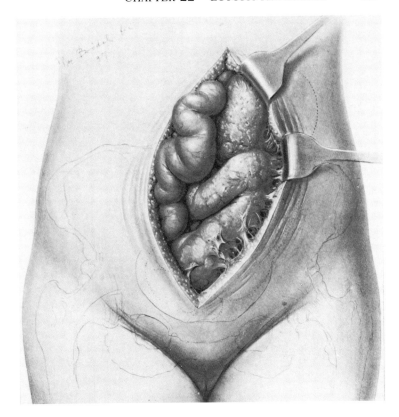

FIG. 22-9. Lithopedion lying undisturbed in the abdominal cavity. The strong adhesions holding it in place, and its position are well shown. The patient was a woman 45 years old who had had her last child when 38; 4 years before entering the clinic she became pregnant, with all the usual signs, and was taken with perfectly normal labor pains at the expected time. Dr. Barnum, who saw her 2 months later, recognized an abdominal pregnancy. The mind of the patient was unbalanced, and she would not allow any interference until after 4 years had passed. Operation by Dr. Clark. Recovery. B. H., Aug. 14, 1896. Kelly HA: Operative Gynecology. New York, D Appleton, 1898. Drawing by Max Brödel)

CERVICAL PREGNANCY

An extremely rare form of ectopic pregnancy, cervical pregnancy produces profuse vaginal bleeding without associated cramping pain. The differential diagnosis is difficult because the clinician is apt initially to suspect a cervical carcinoma or either an incomplete or septic abortion. The combination of necrotic tissue, marked vascularity, and, occasionally, secondary infection adds to the problem of differential diagnosis. Initial attempts can be made to stop the hemorrhage by local removal of the products of conception; if hemostasis is obtained, this is adequate treatment. Because of the depth of trophoblastic invasion, however, major blood vessels are often involved, and hysterectomy may be necessary. Bilateral internal iliac artery ligation has been recommended as a possible substitute, since this procedure preserves reproductive function.

The above discussion applies to pregnancies that are implanted in the cervix proper. David has recently described a variant, shown to have been implanted in the upper cervix, in which growth of the conceptus was upward into the isthmic area, such that the surrounding myometrium was able to enlarge sufficiently to retain the conceptus until delivery at term by cesarean section–hysterectomy. This report reviews 11 similar cases previously reported and suggests a new classification for the variants of cervical pregnancy.

OVARIAN PREGNANCY

The signs and symptoms of ovarian pregnancy are similar to those of tubal pregnancy. Usually, the diagnosis is not made until a laparatomy is done. The incidence of ovarian pregnancy is increasing, owing to the increased use of the IUD. The classic criteria of Spiegelberg that are needed for diagnosis of an ovarian pregnancy are: 1) the fetal sac must occupy a portion of the ovary, 2) the fallopian tube must be normal and intact on the affected side of the pelvis, 3) the ovary and sac must be connected to the uterus by the ovarian ligament, and 4) ovarian tissue must be identified in the sac. (Fig. 22–11).

Many early ovarian pregnancies grossly resemble a bleeding corpus luteum, and the diagnosis is rarely established except by histologic examination of the specimen. Treatment consists of resection of the trophoblast from the ovary, preserving as much ovarian tissue as possible. Salpingo-oophorectomy is rarely necessary.

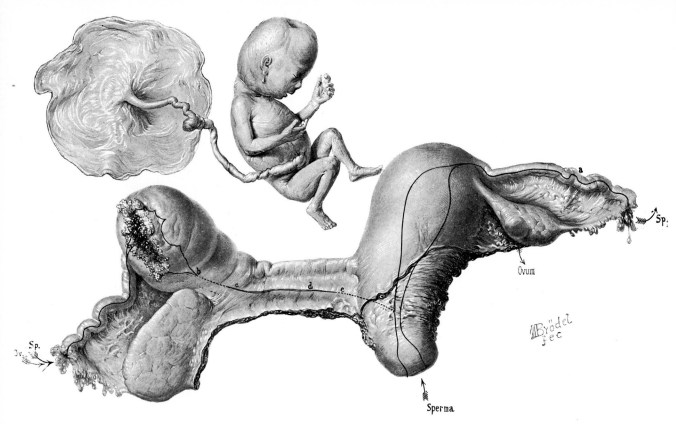

FIG. 22-10. Pregnancy in rudimentary left uterine horn: rupture and death. Viewed from behind. To *right,* a well-developed uterus. Attached to cornu is normal right tube. Ovary of usual size, and at its inner and lower portion corpus luteum of pregnancy. Springing from left side of uterus at internal os is muscular band that merges into rudimentary uterine horn, on posterior surface of which is point of rupture. Placental remains protrude through rent. Left tube passes off from outer side of rudimentary horn. Left ovary flattened. Line on well-developed uterus indicates size of uterine cavity. Line *b, c, d, e* indicates course of left Müller's duct between *c* and *d* containing a lumen; *dotted lines* consist of solid muscular cord. Above the specimen are the placenta and fetus drawn in normal size. (Kelly HA: Gynecology. New York, D Appleton, 1928. Drawing by Max Brödel)

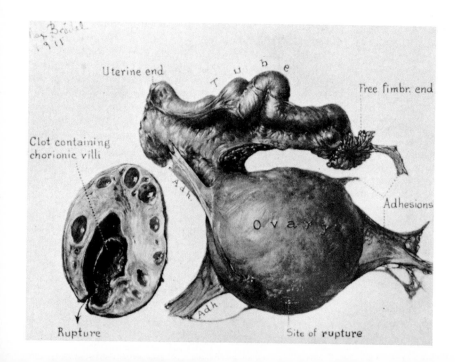

FIG. 22-11. Posterior view of the ovary and uterine tube before it was cut open. *Adh,* adhesions. Reduced one-tenth. *Left.* Transverse section through the ovary at the point of rupture of the follicle from which an extensive hemorrhage took place in life. The clot is covered with an inverted chorion and contains villi. Reduced one-tenth. (Mall FP, Cullen EK: Surg Gynecol Obstet 17:698, 1913. Drawing by Max Brödel)

ECTOPIC PREGNANCY COEXISTING WITH UNRELATED PELVIC PROBLEMS

Different kinds of ectopic pregnancy have been reported in the same patient. Ectopic pregnancy may also coexist with a normal intrauterine pregnancy, a condition known as *heterotopic pregnancy*. Rarely, an ectopic pregnancy may be the factor that unmasks some other pelvic abnormality. The prize for such an event must go to the case, which is probably unique, of a tubal pregnancy that abutted, cell to cell, against one of the rarest of pelvic cancers, adenocarcinoma of the fallopian tube.

REFERENCES AND RECOMMENDED READING

Arias-Stella J: Atypical endometrial changes associated with the presence of chorionic tissue. Arch Pathol 58:112, 1954

Beacham WD, Collins CG, Thomas EP et al: Ectopic pregnancy. JAMA 136:365, 1948

Beral V: An epidemiological study of recent trends in ectopic pregnancy. Br J Obstet Gynaecol 82:775, 1975

Beswick IP, Gregory MM: The Arias–Stella phenomenon and the diagnosis of pregnancy. J Obstet Gynaecol Br Commonw 78:143, 1971

Brady L: Report of a case of tubal pregnancy probably caused by a par-ovarian cyst. Bull Johns Hopkins Hosp 33:442, 1922

Breen JL: A 21 year survey of 654 ectopic pregnancies. Am J Obstet Gynecol 106:1004, 1970

Brenner PF, Roy S, Mishell DR, Jr: Ectopic pregnancy: A study of 300 consecutive surgically treated cases. JAMA 243:673, 1980

Bronson RA: Tubal pregnancy and infertility. Fertil Steril 28:221, 1977

Brown TW, Filly RA, Laing FC et al: Analysis of ultrasonographic criteria in the evaluation for ectopic pregnancy. Am J Roentgenol 131:967, 1978

Bukovsky I, Langer R, Herman A et al: Conservative surgery for tubal pregnancy. Obstet Gynecol 53:709, 1979

Burrows S, Moors W, Pekala B: Missed tubal abortion. Am J Obstet Gynecol 136:691, 1980

Capraro VJ, Chuang JT, Randall CL: Cul-de-sac aspiration and other diagnostic aids for ectopic pregnancy: A 22 year analysis. Int Surg 53:245, 1970

Carapeto R, Nogales FF, Jr, Matilla A: Ectopic pregnancy coexisting with a primary carcinoma of the fallopian tube: A case report. Int J Gynaecol Obstet 16:263, 1978

Carty MJ, Barr RD, Ouna N: The coagulation and fibrinolytic properties of peritoneal and venous blood in patients with ruptured ectopic pregnancy. J Obstet Gynaecol Br Commonw 80:701, 1973

Danforth WC: Referred pain in the shoulder in ruptured tubal pregnancy. Am J Obstet Gynecol 12:883, 1926

Danforth WC: Ectopic pregnancy: A study of 174 cases. J Mt Sinai Hosp (NY) 14:269, 1947

David MKP, Bergman A, Delighdish L: Cervico-isthmic pregnancy carried to term. Obstet Gynecol 56:247, 1980

DeCherney A, Kase N: The conservative management of unruptured ectopic pregnancy. Obstet Gynecol 54:451, 1979

Donald I: Practical Obstetric Problems, p 39. London, Lloyd–Luke, 1979

Fienberg R, Lloyd HED: The Arias–Stella reaction in early normal pregnancy—An involutional phenomenon. Hum Pathol 5:183, 1974

Freakley G, Norman WJ, Ennis JT et al: Diverticulosis of the fallopian tubes. Clin Radiol 25:535, 1974

Gabbe SG, Kitzmiller JL, Kosasa TS et al: Cervical pregnancy presenting as septic abortion. Am J Obstet Gynecol 123:212, 1975

Gitstein S, Ballas S, Schujman E et al: Early cervical pregnancy: Ultrasonic diagnosis and conservative treatment. Obstet Gynecol 54:758, 1979

Gray CL, Ruffolo EH: Ovarian pregnancy associated with intrauterine contraceptive devices. Am J Obstet Gynecol 132:134, 1978

Halbrecht I: Healed genital tuberculosis: A new etiological factor in ectopic pregnancy. Obstet Gynecol 10:73, 1957

Hallatt JG: Repeat ectopic pregnancy: A study of 123 consecutive cases. Am J Obstet Gynecol 122:520, 1975

Hallatt JG: Ectopic pregnancy associated with the intrauterine device: A study of seventy cases. Am J Obstet Gynecol 125:754, 1976

Halpin TF: Ectopic pregnancy: The problem of diagnosis. Am J Obstet Gynecol 106:227, 1970

Harralson JD, van Nagell JR, Jr, Roddick JW, Jr: Operative management of ruptured tubal pregnancy. Am J Obstet Gynecol 115:995, 1973

Helvacioglu A, Long M, Jr, Yang S: Ectopic pregnancy—an eight-year review. J Reprod Med 22:87, 1979

Hochberg CJ: Tubal amylase. Obstet Gynecol 43:129, 1974

Honoré LH, O'Hara KE: Failed tubal sterilization as an etiologic factor in ectopic tubal pregnancy. Fertil Steril 29:509, 1978

Jarvinen PA, Nummi S, Pietila K: Conservative operative treatment of tubal pregnancy with postoperative daily hydrotubations. Acta Obstet Gynecol Scand 51:169, 1972

Jeffcoate N: Principles of Gynaecology, 4th ed, p 214. London, Butterworths, 1975

Kallenberger DA, Ronk DA, Jimerson GK: Ectopic pregnancy: A 15-year review of 160 cases. South Med J 71:758, 1978

Katz J, Marcus RG: The risk of Rh isoimmunization in ruptured tubal pregnancy. Br Med J 3:667, 1972

Kauppila A, Rantakyla P, Huhtaniemi I et al: Trophoblastic markers in the differential diagnosis of ectopic pregnancy. Obstet Gynecol 55:560, 1980

Kelly MT, Santos-Ramos R, Duenhoelter JH: The value of sonography in suspected ectopic pregnancy. Obstet Gynecol 53:703, 1979

Kersztúry S: Examination of curettage material for the diagnosis of ectopic pregnancy. Acta Morphol Acad Sci Hung 24:359, 1976

Kumar S, Oxorn H: Ectopic pregnancy following tubal sterilization. Can Med Assoc J 22:156, 1978

Lancet M, Bin–Nun I, Kessler I: Angular and interstitial pregnancy. Int Surg 62:107, 1977

Liukko P, Erkkola R, Laakso L: Ectopic pregnancies during use of low-dose progestogens for oral contraception. Contraception 16:575, 1977

McCausland A: High rate of ectopic pregnancy following laparoscopic tubal coagulation failures. Am J Obstet Gynecol 136:97, 1980

McElin TW: Discussion of intraligamentous pregnancy, Am J Obstet Gynecol 70:182, 1955

McElin TW, Iffy L: Ectopic gestation: A consideration of new and controversial issues relating to pathogenesis and management. Obstet Gynecol 5:241, 1976

McElin TW, LaPata RE: Angular pregnancy: Report of a case. Obstet Gynecol 31:849, 1968

Mall FP, Cullen EK: An ovarian pregnancy located in the graafian follicle. Surg Gynecol Obstet 17:698, 1913

May WJ, Miller JB, Greiss FC, Jr: Maternal deaths from ectopic pregnancy in the South Atlantic region, 1960 through 1976. Am J Obstet Gynecol 132:140, 1978

Milwidsky A, Adoni A, Miodovnik M et al: Human chorionic gonadotropin (β-subunit) in the early diagnosis of ectopic pregnancy. Obstet Gynecol 51:725, 1978

Myerscough PR: Monro Kerr's Operative Obstetrics, 9th ed, p 662. Baltimore, Williams & Wilkins, 1977

Nelson RM: Bilateral internal iliac artery ligation in cervical pregnancy: Conservation of reproductive function. Am J Obstet Gynecol 134:145, 1979

Niebyl JR: Pregnancy following total hysterectomy. Am J Obstet Gynecol 119:512, 1974

Panayotou PP, Kaskarelis DB, Miettinen OS et al: Induced abortion and ectopic pregnancy. Am J Obstet Gynecol 114:507, 1972

Pauerstein CJ: From fallopius to fantasy. Fertil Steril 30:133, 1978

Pent D, Loffer FD: The natural history of an hematosalpinx. Obstet Gynecol 47:2s, 1976

Poland BJ, Dill FJ, Styblo C: Embryonic development in ectopic human pregnancy. Teratology 14:315, 1976

Pugh WE, Vogt RF, Gibson RA: Primary ovarian pregnancy and the intrauterine device. Obstet Gynecol 42:218, 1973

Rasor JL, Braunstein GD: A rapid modification of the Beta-hCG radioimmunoassay: Use as an aid in the diagnosis of ectopic pregnancy. Obstet Gynecol 50:553, 1977

Rothe DJ, Birnbaum SJ: Cervical pregnancy: Diagnosis and management. Obstet Gynecol 42:675, 1973

Saito M, Koyama T, Yaoi Y et al: Site of ovulation and ectopic pregnancy. Acta Obstet Gynecol Scand 54:227, 1975

Sanders EP: Subacute ectopic pregnancy. NZ Med J 87:41, 1978

Saxena BB, Landesman R: Diagnosis and management of pregnancy by the radioreceptorassay of human chorionic gonadotropin. Am J Obstet Gynecol 131:97, 1978

Schenker JG, Eyal F, Polishuk WZ: Fertility after tubal pregnancy. Surg Gynecol Obstet 135:74, 1972

Schneider J, Berger CJ, Cattell C: Maternal mortality due to ectopic pregnancy: A review of 102 deaths. Obstet Gynecol 49:557, 1977

Schoen JA, Nowak RJ: Repeat ectopic pregnancy: A 16-year clinical survey. Obstet Gynecol 45:542, 1975

Seppala M, Venesmaa P, Rutanen EM: Pregnancy-specific β-1 glycoprotein in ectopic pregnancy. Am J Obstet Gynecol 136:189, 1980

Spiegelberg O: Zur Casuistik der Ovarialschwangerschaft. Arch Gynaekol 13:73, 1878

Strafford JC, Ragan WD: Abdominal pregnancy: Review of current management. Obstet Gynecol 50:548, 1977

Stromme WB: Conservative surgery for ectopic pregnancy: A twenty-year review. Obstet Gynecol 41:215, 1973

Tait RL: Five cases of extra-uterine pregnancy operated upon at the time of rupture. Br Med J 1:1250, 1884

Tatum HJ, Schmidt FH: Contraceptive and sterilization practices and extrauterine pregnancy: A realistic perspective. Fertil Steril 28:407, 1977

Wharton LR: Gynecology with a Section on Female Urology. Page 693. Philadelphia, W. B. Saunders, 1943

Wolf GC, Kritzer L, DeBold C: Heterotopic pregnancy: Midtrimester management. Obstet Gynecol 54:756, 1979

Hemolytic disease of the fetus and newborn results from an immune reaction by the mother against a blood group factor on the red cells of the fetus. It occurs in approximately 1.5% of all pregnancies. The disorder arises when the fetus inherits from the father a blood group antigen that is not possessed by the mother and the mother either has or forms the corresponding antibody against that particular blood group antigen. Clinically, the most important incompatibility involves the Rh system, as when an Rh-negative mother carries an Rh-positive fetus. This situation may result in varying degrees of anemia *in utero* and in jaundice after birth. Jaundice before birth is not a problem because dangerous levels of bilirubin do not develop *in utero,* provided the fetus has access to the placenta and thence to the maternal circulation. However, anemia *in utero* may indeed be a problem; in an attempt to compensate for the anemia, the fetus manufactures blood at an accelerated rate. As a result, many immature red cells, principally erythroblasts, are prematurely passed into the fetal circulation. The presence of numerous erythroblasts on peripheral blood smears from affected infants led to the designation of this condition as *erythroblastosis fetalis.*

The Rh and ABO blood group antigens are of prime clinical importance since combined they account for approximately 98% of all cases of erythroblastosis fetalis; the remaining 2% are due to other blood group factors (K, k, Jk^a, Fy^a, hr'(c), rh''(E), rh'(C), S, M). Obstetric management and treatment are essentially the same, regardless of the responsible blood group system. Approximately 85% of Caucasians, 95% of Negroes, and almost 99% of Orientals (as well as American Indians) are Rh-positive. In one out of every seven marriages in the United States, the woman is Rh-negative and the man is Rh-positive.

Vincent J. Freda

HISTORICAL NOTE

Following the discovery of the ABO human blood group system by Landsteiner in 1900, numerous workers began to speculate that a maternal–fetal blood group incompatibility might be the cause of disease in mother or infant. Dienst, in 1908, attempted unsuccessfully to explain the preeclampsia–eclampsia syndrome on this basis. This false premise was revived by Ottenberg in 1923; he took a step in the right direction, however, when he postulated that an ABO blood group incompatibility between mother and baby might be the cause of jaundice and anemia of the newborn. In 1932, Diamond, Blackfan, and Baty presented evidence that icterus gravis, hemolytic anemia of the newborn, and hydrops fetalis were different manifestations of the same pathologic process. In 1938, Darrow postulated that the mother became sensitized to fetal hemoglobin, which, since it was chemically different from adult hemoglobin, could also be immunologically different and that the maternal antibodies passed through the placenta and attacked the fetal red cells, causing the disease. This theory was correct, except that it implicated the wrong antigen and failed to note the need for the fetus to inherit from the father an antigen that was not possessed by the mother. In 1939, Levine and Stetson postulated the correct mechanism of the disease but were unable to identify the causative agent. This identification had to await the discovery of the Rh factor by Landsteiner and Wiener in 1940. The term *Rh* was derived from the rhesus monkey, in which the factor was discovered. The necessary clinical proof to support this theory came with the confirmatory studies by Wiener and Peters, Levine and Katzn, and Burnham.

RH HEMOLYTIC DISEASE

Rh hemolytic disease of the newborn exacts a high death toll—almost 10,000 infants per year in the

United States alone. All these potentially normal infants are the victims of jaundice and anemia. While the development of exchange transfusion and other techniques has markedly reduced the occurrence of kernicterus in the live-born full-term infant, there remain the problems of preterm infants following early induction of labor and of death of the fetus *in utero*. Overall, the perinatal mortality rate from Rh hemolytic disease is 25%–30%.

It is now possible to determine the severity of Rh hemolytic disease antepartum by the use of amniocentesis and spectrophotometric analysis of the amniotic fluid, to administer blood to the fetus *in utero*, and even to prevent the disease by administration of Rh immunoglobulin.

The value of antepartum detection and management of Rh disease is well documented. Retrospective studies done in various clinics have shown that if a policy of noninterference in managing the Rh-sensitized woman is strictly adhered to, the perinatal mortality rate is approximately 30%. If a conservative policy, *e.g.*, preterm delivery in severe cases, is followed, the rate is reduced to 25%. However, with an aggressive program, including repeated amniocentesis and spectrophotometric analysis, intrauterine transfusions (when necessary), and preterm delivery (in selected cases), the rate can be lowered to about 10%. Thus, management of Rh hemolytic disease should begin antepartum and is the responsibility of the obstetrician as well as the pediatrician.

PATHOGENESIS

An interesting feature of the pathogenesis of Rh hemolytic disease is that the first Rh-positive infant almost invariably is unaffected. If a mother has not been exposed previously to the Rh factor, either by injection or transfusion of Rh-positive blood, it is extremely rare for the anti-Rh antibodies to appear during the first Rh-positive pregnancy. Similarly, if the mother has an existing circulating antibody directed against the baby's red cells, *e.g.*, anti-A antibody in a Group O, Rh-negative mother carrying a Group A, Rh-positive baby, sensitization (immunization) to the Rh factor during the first such pregnancy is uncommon.

In a retrospective study done at Presbyterian Hospital, New York, the records of 520 Rh-isoimmunized mothers were analyzed to determine the onset of immunization (*i.e.*, the first appearance of the anti-Rh antibody) in relation to the number of Rh-positive pregnancies (Table 23–1). If women who, prior to delivery of their first Rh-positive viable infant, had had an abortion or had received an incompatible transfusion or injection of blood are excluded, then of a total group of 520 Rh-isoimmunized mothers, less than 1% produced antibodies during the first Rh-positive pregnancy. The figures presented in Table 23–1 suggest

TABLE 23-1. INCIDENCE OF RH IMMUNIZATION ACCORDING TO NUMBER OF THE RH-POSITIVE PREGNANCY DURING WHICH IMMUNIZATION OF RH-NEGATIVE MOTHER FIRST OCCURRED—RETROSPECTIVE STUDY*

No. of the Rh-Positive Pregnancy	No. of Mothers	Percent of Mothers
FIRST	4	0.7
SECOND	390	75.0
THIRD	88	17.0
FOURTH OR MORE	38	7.3
TOTAL	520	100.0

* Patients with a history of blood transfusion or injection prior to the onset of immunization and patients with one or more abortions prior to the first Rh-positive pregnancy are excluded. (Freda VJ: Am J Obstet Gynecol 92:341, 1965)

(erroneously) that the risk of immunization is greatest with the second Rh-positive pregnancy, less with the third, and so on. A prospective study (Table 23–2) has shown that the incidence of immunization during the second Rh-positive pregnancy and subsequently is about the same (11%). This study confirmed the finding that less than 1% of Rh-negative women are immunized during the first Rh-positive pregnancy.

It is also evident from Table 23–2 that if the small group of women immunized during the first Rh-positive pregnancy is excluded then, of the total number of women immunized during the second, third, and fourth pregnancies (column 3) are almost identical to the corresponding percentages for the total number of nonimmunized women in each group. In this study, 407 women had more than one Rh-positive baby, 246 (60%) of these had only two Rh-positive babies; and 47 (11%) had four or more. These percentages are very similar to those for the immunized group (column 3). Thus, of the 70 women immunized after the first Rh-positive pregnancy, 45 (63%) had only two Rh-positive babies, 18 (25%) had three Rh-positive babies, and 7 (10%) had four or more Rh-positive babies.

ANTEPARTUM ASSESSMENT OF FETAL JEOPARDY

At present, the only justification for early induction of labor in an Rh-isoimmunized woman is to prevent fetal death *in utero*. At any time during gestation, the obstetrician must weigh the risk of fetal death from Rh hemolytic disease if pregnancy continues against the risk of neonatal death from preterm delivery. An individual evaluation of the condition of each immunized patient is mandatory. The assessment should be based upon the following parameters: 1) past obstetric history, including the probable zygosity of the baby's father; 2) estimated fetal maturity; 3) presence of other medical

TABLE 23–2. INCIDENCE OF RH IMMUNIZATION ACCORDING TO NUMBER OF THE RH-POSI-TIVE PREGNANCY DURING WHICH IMMUNIZATION OF RH-NEGATIVE MOTHER FIRST OCCURRED—PROSPECTIVE STUDY*

No. of the Rh-Positive Pregnancy	No. of Mothers Not Immunized at Start of Each Pregnancy‡	Mothers Who Became Immunized During Each Pregnancy†		Proportion of Mothers Having Each Pregnancy Who Became Immunized During That Pregnancy§
		No.	Percent	
FIRST	364	1	0.3	1/771 (0.1%)
SECOND	246	45	18.0	45/407 (11%)
THIRD	114	18	16.0	18/161 (11%)
FOURTH OR MORE	47	7	15.0	7/47 (15%)
TOTAL	771	71	9.0	
EXCLUDING FIRST RH-POSITIVE PREGNANCY	407	10	17.0	

* Patients with a history of injection or transfusion of blood prior to the onset of immunization and patients with one or more abortions prior to the first Rh-positive pregnancy are excluded.

† In these two columns, the same mother is not repeated as a statistic (*e.g.*, a mother with four Rh-positive pregnancies does not also appear as a statistic in the group of mothers with three Rh-positive pregnancies.)

‡ Includes mothers known to be nonimmunized at the end of a previous Rh-positive pregnancy.

§ This applies only to the group of women in this clinic; figures in this column are dependent upon the distribution of women according to the number of Rh-positive pregnancies.

(Freda VJ: Am J Obstet Gynecol 92:341, 1965)

complications, such as preeclampsia or diabetes; 4) measurement of maternal antibody titer; and 5) spectrophotometric and chemical analysis of amniotic fluid for the presence of bilirubinoid pigments.

Obstetric History

Rh hemolytic disease generally follows one of two patterns, which occur with about equal frequency: 1) the severity remains about the same from one pregnancy to the next, or 2) the severity increases with each subsequent Rh-positive pregnancy. Usually, one or the other pattern is seen in the same patient over a period of years; however, both patterns may be seen in the same patient, and it is not possible to predict the outcome of a given pregnancy on this basis alone. Significant improvement in the condition from one pregnancy to the next, although possible, is not common.

Zygosity of Father

A man is proved heterozygous for the Rh-positive factor (single genetic dose of the Rh-positive factor) if one of his parents or one of his children is Rh-negative; however, proof of homozygosity (double genetic dose of the Rh-positive factor) is seldom possible. The Rh genotype test helps determine his *probable* Rh zygosity, but such information is of only limited clinical value.

Presence of Medical Complications

The incidence of preeclampsia is no greater among even the most severely Rh-immunized mother than among nonimmunized mothers. However, if preeclampsia does complicate Rh immunization, it is an additional insult to an already endangered fetus and the prognosis for the fetus is worse. Diabetes mellitus also compounds the risk of the baby of an Rh-immunized mother.

The Role of Ultrasound and X-ray Examinations in Routine Management

An accurate determination of gestational age is extremely important in the management of women with Rh sensitization, and ultrasound is uniquely valuable for this purpose. A first scan, for crown–rump length, is done before 14 weeks' gestation (as estimated by menstrual dates and uterine size) and provides a reliable estimate of fetal age. A second scan for biparietal diameter is used at 31–32 weeks to assess whether cephalic growth falls into the large, average, or small category. A third scan at 36 weeks is taken for both biparietal diameter and trunk circumference at the level of the liver, showing the ductus venosus and giving evidence of symmetrical or asymmetrical growth. In addition, a search should be made for signs that the fetus is affected. These signs include hydramnios,

scalp edema, fetal ascites, placental enlargement, and enlargement of the liver and spleen.

Although the placenta is rarely encountered when amniocentesis is done suprapubically, as noted later, it is best to know the location of the placenta before undertaking this procedure. The placenta is localized in the course of the aforementioned scans, but if amniocentesis is to be done earlier, an additional scan may be made.

Nonstress tests of fetal heart rate and oxytocin challenge tests (see Chapter 41) can be extremely helpful in evaluating status if there is any question.

Diagnostic x-ray examinations are not utilized for fetal assessment except as an aid to intrauterine fetal transfusion, and occasionally if the fetal status is in doubt. In the latter case, 30 ml meglumine iothalamate 60% in aqueous solution (Conray) may be injected into the amniotic cavity, and an abdominal x-ray picture is taken 24 hours later. If the dye does not appear in the fetal stomach within 24 hours the fetus is considered to be in imminent danger.

Determination of Maternal Antibody Titers

Reliance solely upon determination of antibody titers in the management of Rh-negative mothers does not appreciably improve the perinatal mortality rate. If, however, measurement of antibody titers is used to detect those patients at high risk (*i.e.*, those who are sensitized), these patients can then be followed by am-

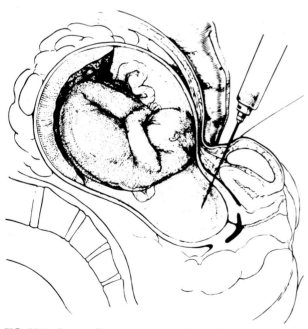

FIG. 23-1. Suprapubic puncture site for amniocentesis (Freda VJ: Hosp Pract 2 [1], 1967)

niotic fluid analysis, and perinatal mortality can be reduced. The indirect antiglobulin technique (indirect Coombs test) may be relied upon to screen the population at risk and identify mothers who have already been sensitized by a previous pregnancy or a previous blood transfusion and mothers who first exhibit such sensitization during the current pregnancy.

Titration must be carried out serially and frequently during the pregnancy. In our laboratory the critical level of antibody titer is 1:16; we have seen no intrauterine death or severely affected newborn when values are below this level. The critical level should be determined for each laboratory, however, since results in different laboratories are not comparable because of differences in technique. In a severely sensitized mother, antibody titer may be moderately high and remain at the same level throughout the pregnancy, even though the fetus is being more and more seriously affected; conversely, a mother sensitized by previous Rh-positive fetuses may exhibit a high fixed antibody titer during a pregnancy in which the fetus is Rh-negative. In such cases, determination of antibody titers is obviously useless. Nevertheless, although antibody titers cannot reliably identify the fetus that is in danger, they can consistently point out the fetus that is not. Thus, serial determinations of Rh antibody titers should be made throughout pregnancy, particularly in unsensitized or mildly sensitized mothers, since a significant rise (two tube dilutions or greater) may signal the need for amniocentesis or early delivery. It is our policy to determine titers monthly during the first and second trimesters and biweekly in the third trimester; the last measurement is made within a week of the estimated date of labor. If the titer is 1:16 or less, delivery at 38 weeks is planned, or if conditions are unfavorable for induction, spontaneous labor is awaited. If the titer is 1:32 or greater, the patient is thereafter followed by amniotic fluid analysis.

Analysis of Amniotic Fluid

Amniocentesis. At Columbia–Presbyterian Medical Center, amniocentesis is performed as an outpatient procedure. Since there is some danger of incurring a persistent high leak of amniotic fluid or, even more serious, of lacerating a large fetal vessel on the surface of the placenta, some prefer to locate the placenta by ultrasound before applying the sampling needle. However, we have found that by performing the puncture lower on the abdomen—at the suprapubic site—we can consistently avoid piercing the placenta (Fig. 23–1). Bimanual examination can locate the fetus, and elevation of the presenting part can prevent fetal trauma. We have carried out more than 7000 of these procedures with virtually no mortality or morbidity in either mother or fetus and have found them invaluable in the management of Rh pregnancies. They enable us to say, with considerable assurance, when the fetus is

FIG. 23-2. Spectrophotometric tracings of serial samples of amniotic fluid. Progressive development of abnormal hump at 450 mµ indicates fetal hemolysis. (Freda VJ: Am J Obstet Gynecol 92:341, 1965)

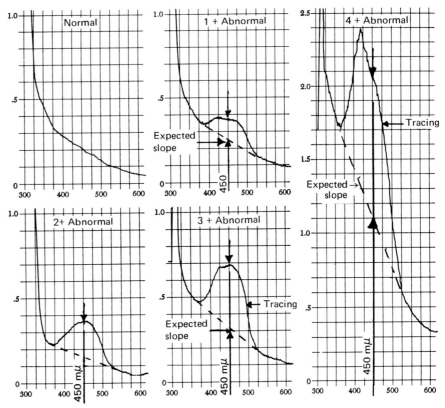

in no danger, when danger threatens but is not immediate, when hemolysis is producing significant circulatory distress, and when the threat of death is so severe as to make intervention obligatory.

The procedure is simply done. The skin over the suprapubic area is prepared and the operator elevates the fetal presenting part with one hand. Under local anesthesia, a 22-gauge, 4-in. spinal needle is passed into the amniotic cavity and 5–10 ml amniotic fluid is removed. Protected from exposure to light (which may reduce the level of bilirubinoid pigment), the fluid is centrifuged for 15 min at 4000 rpm and the supernatant subjected to spectrophotometric scanning.

Spectrophotometric Scanning of Amniotic Fluid. Since 1952, when Bevis first applied spectrophotometric scanning of amniotic fluid to the antepartum management of Rh disease, experience and information have been accumulated to show that analysis of amniotic fluid is the *sine qua non* of proper modern management of the Rh-sensitized gravida. It has been established that the quantity of bilirubin and other related products of the breakdown of hemoglobin present in amniotic fluid is an approximate index of the degree of hemolysis the fetus has suffered. The amount of these pigments present may be roughly

quantitated by scanning the amniotic fluid spectrophotometrically over the range of wavelength from 350–700 nm. Near term, amniotic fluid that contains no bilirubinlike pigments exhibits a smooth unbroken sloping line highest at the lower end of the spectrum and lowest at the higher wavelength. When pigments are present, there is typical deformation or humping of the line beginning at 375 nm, peaking at 450 nm, and returning to the normal slope at 525 nm. The difference between the expected slope and the peak of the deformation at 450 nm is proportional to the amount of pigment present, which in turn reflects the severity of fetal distress at the time of amniocentesis.

The spectrophotometric curves cannot yet be quantitated precisely. The curves are a summation of the optical densities of several colored pigments and of a turbidity that varies considerably from one specimen to another. Additional knowledge is required concerning the precise identity of the various bile pigments.

Figure 23–2 is a composite of serial tracings of amniotic fluid specimens, demonstrating the progressive development of the abnormal curve. The normal tracing is a smooth curved line that always sweeps upward in the lower wavelength range (owing to the effects of turbidity and of the vernix, uric acid, *etc.* normally present in amniotic fluid). The terms *normal* and *ab-*

TABLE 23-3. CLINICAL INTERPRETATION OF SPECTROPHOTOMETRIC AND CHEMICAL ANALYSIS OF AMNIOTIC FLUID

Classification of Abnormality	Clinical Interpretation of Fetal Status	ΔOD_{450}	Total Bilirubin (mg/dl)
1+	Normal or possibly affected	<0.20	<0.28
2+	Affected but not in jeopardy	0.20–0.34	0.28–0.46
3+	Distressed and probably in congestive heart failure	0.35–0.70	0.47–0.95
4+	Impending fetal death	>0.70	>0.95

(Gambino SR, Freda VJ: Am J Clin Pathol 46:198, 1966)

normal apply *only* to the spectrophotometric tracings, *not* to the clinical condition of the fetus. When the concentration of the related bile pigments increases, the fluid assumes a pale yellowish hue. Apparently, each of these related bile pigments (principally bilirubin plus additional breakdown products of hemoglobin) absorbs monochromatic light somewhere in the wavelength range 375–525 nm. The summation of their respective light absorptions produces a characteristic abnormality in the spectrophotometric tracing between 375 and 525 nm that is readily identified as a broad hump (an elevation above the expected slope of the curve). With increasing concentrations of these bile pigments in the amniotic fluid, the hump effect on the tracing becomes more pronounced (*i.e.*, the deviation from the expected slope of the curve increases in amplitude). The width of the abnormal hump is constant, regardless of the concentration of the bile pigments; the height of this hump *above the expected slope of the curve* increases in amplitude with increasing concentration of bile pigments in the liquor amnii. The abnormal tracings have been arbitrarily classified as 1+ to 4+, depending on the *amplitude of the abnormal hump* (*i.e., the part of the tracing that is above the expected slope of the curve at the 450-nm line*). The amplitude is an arbitrary measurement at 450 nm of a difference in optical densities between the measured and the expected curves. The amplitudes (ΔOD_{450}) corresponding to each abnormality classification are given in Table 23–3.

As shown in Figure 23–2, the 450-nm line bisects the abnormal hump in the 1+ and 2+ abnormal tracings. Also, the maximum absorption is around 450 nm (there is no actual peak effect at this early stage). However, as the 3+ abnormal tracing progresses to 4+, there is an apparent shift in the bulk of the abnormal hump toward the lower end of the wavelength scale and an associated shift in the maximum absorption from 450 to 420 nm. The author has been able to duplicate this shift by lowering the pH of the amniotic fluid (the normal pH of amniotic fluid is 7.2) and to reverse the trend by adding alkali. Figure 23–3 shows the effect on the spectrophotometric tracing of changing the pH of the amniotic fluid by the addition of first

an acid buffer and then a base. The point of maximum absorption shifts to 420 nm when the pH is lowered and returns to 450 nm with the addition of a base. The area of the hump lying to either side of the 450-nm line also shifts downward with a decreased pH, returning to its usual distribution when the pH rises to 7.4. These shifts in maximum absorption are similar to those reported for 3+ and 4+ abnormal tracings, in which fetal death is considered inevitable.

Contamination of normal amniotic fluid with hemoglobin (Fig. 23–4) or meconium (Fig. 23–5) produces characteristic changes in the tracings. The diagnostically important bile pigments (Fig. 23–6) are quite stable when the specimens are stored in the dark (and preferably in a freezer), but are unstable on prolonged exposure to light (Fig. 23–7). Note that in every abnormal tracing caused by erythroblastosis, the deviation from the normal slope of the curve *always* begins at about 525 nm, and the curve *never* resumes the normal slope until about 375 nm. This pattern holds whether or not the shift in the abnormal hump has occurred, and there has been no exception. Consequently, unless the tracing satisfies at least these basic criteria, it is never regarded as an abnormal tracing caused by erythroblastosis.

Spectrophotometric analysis of the amniotic fluid samples is essential. Visual examination is not only inherently inaccurate, but can be distorted in a false-positive direction by various contaminants. Spectrophotometry, however, can usually distinguish the color abnormalities produced by contaminant simulating hemolysis.

Clinical Interpretation of Spectrophotometric Tracings. As explained earlier, abnormal curves are classified, depending on the height of the hump above the expected (normal) slope of the curve, on an arbitrary scale ranging from 1+ to 4+ abnormal (Fig. 23–2; Table 23–3). In our laboratory, the differences in optical densities at 450 nm between the measured and the expected curves (ΔOD_{450}) are interpreted as follows (units are derived from an arithmetic scale). In most cases the L/S ratio should be determined and may serve as a guide to the timing of delivery.

$\Delta OD_{450} = 0.0$–0.20 (1+ abnormal). Tracing may revert toward normal or progress to more abnormal; fetus will not suffer intrauterine death for 2 weeks; fetus may be Rh-negative.

$\Delta OD_{450} = 0.21$–0.34 (2+ abnormal). Fetus is Rh-positive and probably affected; tracing occasionally reverts to 1+ abnormal and procedure should be repeated in 1 week. If a previous Rh-positive baby has been stillborn, a rapidly rising 2+ abnormal tracing is indication for fetal transfusion if gestation is less than 32 weeks or immediate delivery if gestation is more than 33 weeks.

$\Delta OD_{450} = 0.35$–0.70 (3+ abnormal). Fetus is Rh-positive and severely affected; may be already in congestive heart failure; should be treated by intrauterine transfusion if gestation is less than 32 weeks or immediate delivery if gestation is more than 33 weeks. A 3+ abnormal reading indicates that the fetus is in distress. We believe the rise in pigment concentration does not necessarily reflect more energetic hemolysis, but is caused by the beginning of circulatory impairment as a result of which the pigments are less effectively cleared from the blood through the placenta and tend to be excreted more copiously into the amniotic fluid by one or more pathways. A 3+ curve is also clear evidence that the fetus' condition will inevitably deteriorate. If pregnancy has reached at least the 32nd week, delivery should be undertaken with little delay, if possible by induced labor, otherwise by cesarean section.

$\Delta OD_{450} > 0.70$ (4+ abnormal). Fetus is hydropic and moribund; immediate delivery is mandatory. A 4+ abnormal value indicates that fetal death is imminent; the prognosis is poor.

Chemical Analysis of Amniotic Fluid. The chemical assays for conjugated bilirubin suggest that almost all the bilirubin in amniotic fluid, fetal urine, and cord blood is in the free state. This is not surprising since erythroblastosis fetalis is a hemolytic anemia that occurs in a fetus with immature liver and kidneys. The immature fetal kidney probably forms no barrier to the passage of free bilirubin, and the urinary bilirubin *may* be a primary source for the bilirubin in amniotic fluid. Other mechanisms are not excluded, however, and any explanation must account for the high correlation between amniotic fluid bilirubin levels and intrauterine heart failure.

When the amniotic fluid contains meconium, the chemical assay may be falsely elevated, making clinical interpretation of borderline abnormal results difficult, if not impossible. In these cases the spectrophotometric scan may also be difficult to interpret, but it is usually possible to recognize a 3+ or 4+ abnormal specimen on scan or on chemical assay.

When the amniotic fluid is blood-stained, the chemical assay must be interpreted with caution. If the blood

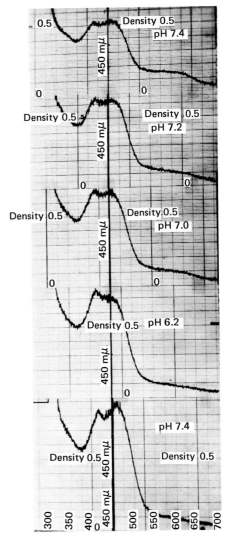

FIG. 23–3. Effect of pH of spectrophotometric tracings on amniotic fluid. To the original amniotic fluid specimen with pH of 7.4 (*bottom tracing*) acid buffer was added drop by drop until pH was 6.2; then pH was returned to 7.0, 7.2, and 7.4 by addition of alkaline buffer. Decrease in amplitude of abnormal hump is due to dilution effect of added buffer solutions. Note that at pH 7.4 the 450-mμ line bisects abnormal hump, and peak absorption is at approximately 450 mμ. However, at pH 6.2 bulk of abnormal hump lies to viewer's left of 450-mμ line and peak absorption has shifted to 420 mμ. These changes are then reversed by restoring pH to 7.4 (*top tracing*). (Freda VJ: Am J Obstet Gynecol 92:341, 1965)

is from the mother, little adverse effect is noted; if the blood is from the fetus, a false elevation of bilirubin level may be found. The presence of blood does not greatly interfere with the spectrophotometric findings, but special interpretation may be needed.

The clinical significance of varying levels of amni-

Effect of adding increasing amounts of free hemoglobin to
normal amniotic fluid

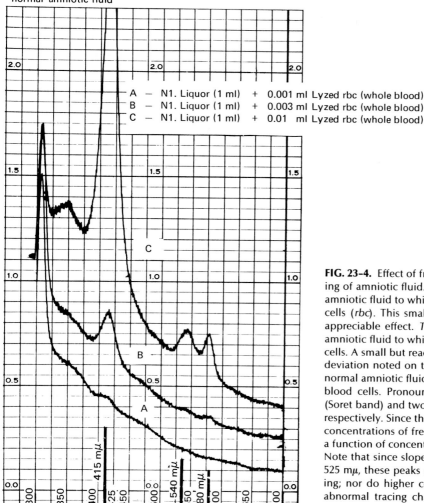

A — N1. Liquor (1 ml) + 0.001 ml Lyzed rbc (whole blood)
B — N1. Liquor (1 ml) + 0.003 ml Lyzed rbc (whole blood)
C — N1. Liquor (1 ml) + 0.01 ml Lyzed rbc (whole blood)

FIG. 23-4. Effect of free hemoglobin on spectrophotometric tracing of amniotic fluid. *Tracing A* is from 1-ml specimen of normal amniotic fluid to which has been added 0.001 ml lysed red blood cells (*rbc*). This small amount of free hemoglobin produces no appreciable effect. *Tracing B* is from same specimen of normal amniotic fluid to which has been added 0.003 ml lysed red blood cells. A small but readily identified narrow peak at 415 mμ is only deviation noted on tracing. *Tracing C* is from same specimen of normal amniotic fluid to which has been added 0.01 ml lysed red blood cells. Pronounced narrow peak can be seen at 415 mμ (Soret band) and two small companion peaks at 540 and 580 mμ, respectively. Since these latter peaks are not evident with smaller concentrations of free hemoglobin, their presence appears to be a function of concentration of free hemoglobin in amniotic fluid. Note that since slope of curve remains normal between 375 and 525 mμ, these peaks do not interfere with interpretation of tracing; nor do higher concentrations of free hemoglobin produce abnormal tracing characteristics of erythroblastosis fetalis (Fig. 23-2). (Freda VJ: Prog Hematol 5:266, 1966)

otic fluid bilirubin is shown in Table 23–3. The chemical assay of amniotic fluid bilirubin can be clinically useful when spectrophotometric scanning cannot be done, but it is not always a reliable substitute. However, unlike spectrophotometric scanning, which demands special experience both in reading the tracings and in correcting for variations in individual instruments, chemical analysis is readily available in most laboratories.

ANTEPARTUM TREATMENT
OF ERYTHROBLASTOTIC FETUS

When amniotic fluid analysis indicates that the fetus is endangered by Rh hemolytic disease, induction of

labor is not always the treatment of choice because the hazard of preterm delivery may be too great. Generally speaking, 32 weeks is the shortest gestation that produces an infant with a chance of surviving delivery, particularly if the infant must withstand exchange transfusions as well. However, this figure is being lowered each year by the increasing expertise of those involved in neonatal intensive care units.

The credit for the idea that a transfusion of blood to the fetus *in utero* might be possible belongs to Liley of New Zealand. Liley reasoned that, instead of avoiding the fetus at the time of amniocentesis, it might be possible, with x-ray assistance, to insert a needle and a catheter into the fetal peritoneal cavity. Blood could then be injected into the fetus; if absorption from the peritoneal cavity was satisfactory, the hemoglobin level

FIG. 23-5. Effect of meconium on spectrophotometric tracing of amniotic fluid. *Tracing at left* is from specimen of meconium-stained amniotic fluid from Rh-negative unaffected pregnancy (Specimen A). *Tracings at right* were obtained by adding a constant volume of Specimen A to amniotic fluid specimens of 2+, 3+, and 4+ abnormality. Meconium contamination produces a very steep curve with low linear (rather than rounded) shoulder, with only slight dip in tracing between peak absorption (at about 400 mμ) and point of return to normal slope (at 375 mμ). Although tracing abnormality occasioned by presence of meconium is different from tracing abnormalities characteristic of erythroblastosis (Fig. 23-2), it does overlap critical area for analysis (between 525 and 375 mμ), making interpretation difficult or impossible. However, meconium contamination alone does not mimic rounded shoulder effect between 450 and 525 mμ that is characteristic of severely affected infants (3+ and 4+ abnormal specimens). Thus 3+ and 4+ abnormalities are unlikely to be masked by incidental meconium, but 1+ and 2+ abnormalities may well be. (Freda VJ: Prog Hematol 5:266, 1966)

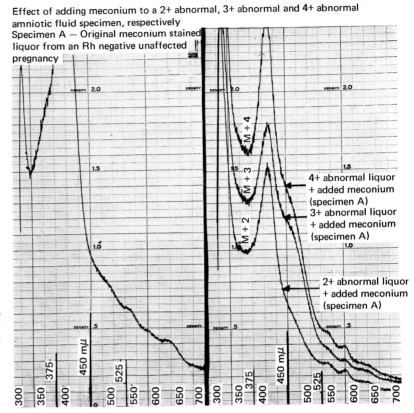

Effect of adding meconium to a 2+ abnormal, 3+ abnormal and 4+ abnormal amniotic fluid specimen, respectively
Specimen A — Original meconium stained liquor from an Rh negative unaffected pregnancy

4+ abnormal liquor + added meconium (specimen A)
3+ abnormal liquor + added meconium (specimen A)
2+ abnormal liquor + added meconium (specimen A)

would rise and the hemolytic anemia would be improved. Reports from a number of centers indicate that fetal transfusion can be a successful, indeed a lifesaving, procedure.

The transfused red cells are absorbed by way of the subdiaphragmatic lymphatics and thence through the thoracic duct to the venous circulation; the anemia is thus corrected. However, the procedure is not without risk to the fetus and requires considerable skill on the part of the operator and roentgenographer. Also, if the fetus is hydropic, a simple transfusion does not usually prevent death.

The selection of patients for fetal transfusion should be based primarily on amniotic fluid analysis and secondarily on the previous obstetric history. Neither past history nor present level of maternal antibody titers alone is sufficiently reliable to justify the hazards of the transfusion. At the present time, the exact criteria for transfusion have not been completely resolved, but it is generally agreed that a rapidly rising 2+ abnormal spectrophotometric tracing in a woman with a previous Rh-related stillbirth or a 3+ abnormal tracing, irrespective of the past history, justifies fetal transfusion. Liley's scale and the zone designations are shown in Figure 23-8, together with the corresponding Freda

designations of the degree to which the fetus is affected.

The procedure is done only after the 23rd, or before the 33rd week of gestation (Figs. 23-9 through 23-11). Amniocentesis is done 24 hours before admission to the hospital, and 30 ml radiopaque dye is instilled into the amniotic cavity. After admission, the mother is given 10 mg morphine, 90 mg sodium phenobarbital, and 25 mg promethazine, and is moved to the x-ray department where, under television fluoroscopy with an image intensifier, the pattern of ingested dye in the fetal gastrointestinal tract is localized. Under sterile conditions and local anesthesia, a 17-gauge Touhy needle is passed into the fetal peritoneal cavity, with the fetal gastrointestinal tract as a target. A polyethylene catheter is threaded through the needle, allowed to coil in the baby's abdomen, and the needle removed. From 5 to 10 ml radiopaque dye is instilled through the catheter to ensure that the catheter is in the peritoneal cavity. This can be readily ascertained by the typical appearance of the cavity on the television monitor. A volume of fresh Group O, Rh-negative, sedimented red blood cells (average hematocrit, 75%) is infused through the catheter, and the catheter is removed. The volume of cells used depends on

the gestational age of the fetus; usually 50 ml are given if the fetus is 24 weeks' gestational age, and this is increased by 20 ml at each subsequent transfusion. Repeat transfusions are done every 2 weeks until the fetus has reached sufficient maturity to tolerate labor and delivery, usually at about 33–35 weeks. During

FIG. 23–6. Spectrophotometric tracings of amniotic fluid showing 4+ abnormal curve and of pure bilirubin solution. Points on wavelength scale for takeoff and return to the baseline or expected slope of curve are approximately same on each tracing. However, tracing produced by pure bilirubin solution (bilirubin dissolved in chloroform containing 10% phenol) has narrower absorption band that tapers symmetrically to sharp peak at 450 mμ. Tracing produced by amniotic fluid specimen has wider absorption band and fairly broad (occasionally jagged) plateau at apex. Area of absorption under abnormal hump of amniotic fluid tracing, which is not accounted for by bilirubin tracing alone, presumably is due to absorption produced by other related bile pigments (various breakdown products of hemoglobin) present in amniotic fluid. (Freda VJ: Am J Obstet Gynecol 92:341, 1965)

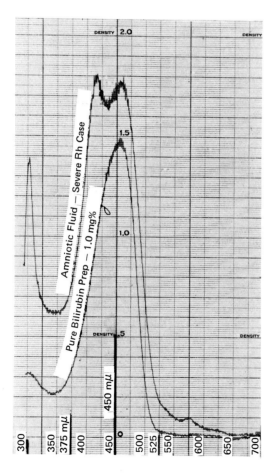

labor, fetal status is monitored by acid–base determinations, using the fetal capillary blood sampling technique, and cesarean section is done if labor does not progress well or if the fetus' condition shows evidence of worsening.

It should be stressed that a team composed of an experienced obstetrician, pediatrician, radiologist, and blood bank physician is highly desirable if good results from intrauterine transfusion are to be obtained. Experience has shown that the procedure is most rewarding when the fetus is of 24–32 weeks' gestation and least rewarding when the fetus is in jeopardy before the 24th week of gestation.

Because of technical difficulty in transfusing a fetus at 18–24 weeks, and because of the hazard of severe trauma to these very young fetuses, an open operative approach has been tried. This technique involves hysterotomy and fetal celiotomy. Initially, a complete exchange transfusion was carried out through the femoral vessel, but in subsequent (less mature) cases, an indwelling silicone catheter was implanted in the fetal peritoneal cavity under direct vision and led out through the mother's abdomen. Small amounts of fresh packed donor blood were then infused into the fetus through this catheter at frequent intervals. The danger of preterm labor is great; although pregnancy has continued for as long as 2 months following this operation and produced a live, but very premature, infant, thus far there are only a few survivors of this open approach.

POSTNATAL TREATMENT OF ERYTHROBLASTOTIC INFANT

Early and aggressive management of the severely affected newborn, including respiratory assistance, correction of acidosis, and immediate exchange transfusion, yields the best overall results in severe hemolytic disease due to Rh sensitization. One of the most important facets of the overall management of the Rh-affected baby is the close cooperation necessary between the obstetric and pediatric teams and the blood bank. The blood bank should be alerted prior to delivery of an affected infant so that donors can be available.

Donor blood is cross-matched with a maternal specimen by means of an indirect Coombs technique. At delivery, cord blood is obtained and the following determinations made: Coombs test, ABO and Rh typing, hemoglobin level, hematocrit value, white cell count, reticulocyte count, and bilirubin level. Exchange transfusion with low-titer Group O, Rh-negative donor blood is carried out immediately after birth under the following circumstances:

1. Previous kernicterus or erythroblastosis in a sibling
2. Cord blood hemoglobin level of less than 13.0 g/100 ml

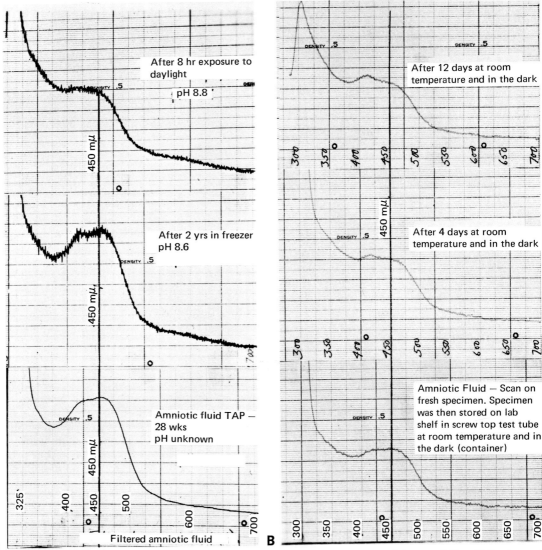

FIG. 23-7. Effect of exposure to light on stability of bile pigment in amniotic fluid. In *A, bottom tracing* is original one obtained on fresh specimen. *Middle tracing* was obtained on specimen stored for 2 years in freezer without exposure to light. *Top tracing* was obtained on same specimen after exposure to light for 8 hours. Note marked change after light exposure. *Tracings in B* demonstrate effect of storage at room temperature in dark on different specimens of amniotic fluid. Note slight but definite decrease in amplitude of abnormal hump over time. (Freda VJ: Prog Hematol 5:266, 1966)

3. Cord blood bilirubin level above 5.0 mg/100 ml
4. Obvious clinical erythroblastosis fetalis

These considerations may be extended to include high reticulocyte count (>15%) or extreme prematurity. In the face of obvious congestive heart failure, it is best to perform a small packed-cell transfusion initially and then, after stabilization of cardiac status, the routine two-volume exchange as indicated by subsequent bilirubin levels. A bilirubin level of 18–20 mg/100 ml or a rate of rise that suggests the level will exceed 20 mg/100 ml prior to the time adequate conjugation can be expected are indications for exchange transfusion. Indications for exchange may be altered in the presence of other complications, such as the respiratory distress syndrome, sepsis, preterm delivery, low serum albumin level, and decreased capacity of the serum to bind bilirubin.

The exchange should be carried out under sterile conditions through an indwelling catheter placed in an umbilical vessel. Fresh, warm, heparinized whole

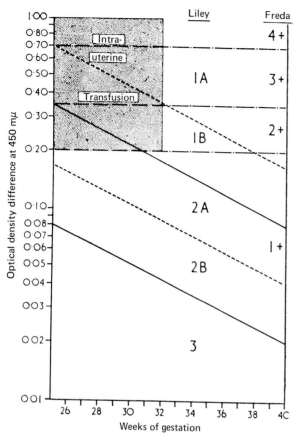

FIG. 23–8. Assessment of fetal prognosis by Liley and Freda methods. (Robertson JG: Am J Obstet Gynecol 95:120, 1966)

blood (compatible with the mother's) is used in volumes of approximately 180 ml/kg body weight to effect a two-volume exchange. Transfusion may be carried out by the continuous infusion technique or by 10- or 20-ml increments. Careful monitoring of respiration, heart rate, pulse, color, and venous pressure must be carried out during the procedure. Protamine sulfate, 22.5 mg/500 ml blood exchanged, is given to neutralize the heparin effect, and posttransfusion blood specimens are obtained for bilirubin and albumin determinations and for culture. The posttransfusion bilirubin level should be closely watched (every 4–8 hours). These infants often develop a late posttransfusion anemia that may require treatment with a packed-cell transfusion.

PREVENTION OF RH ISOIMMUNIZATION

A seemingly less dramatic development, but one of far-reaching importance, is the possibility that Rh isoimmunization as a result of pregnancy may be prevented

altogether. Levine observed that, in families with erythroblastotic infants, the father's ABO blood group was compatible with that of the mother more often than in the general population. In ABO incompatible pregnancies, it appears that the presence of anti-A and anti-B antibodies in the mother effects the removal of Group A and B Rh-positive fetal red cells from the maternal circulation without initiating an immune response to the Rh factor. Stern *et al.* have shown that it is extremely difficult to immunize Rh-negative volunteers to the Rh factor with injection of ABO-incompatible Rh-positive cells or with ABO compatible cells that have been coated *in vitro* with an excess of antibody to Rhρ.

The observation by Smith in 1909 that in the presence of passive antibody the corresponding antigen will not produce immunization has been confirmed and studied by others. From these many reports, there has emerged the immunologic principle that passive immunity strongly suppresses active immunity, but apparently a specific application of the principle to suppress the immune response was not considered.

Around 1960 it occurred to Freda, Gorman, and Pollack that mothers could be protected against Rh immunization by administration of exogenous Rh antibody shortly after delivery of the first Rh-positive child. The antibody obviously could not affect the child, yet should protect the mother against initial or primary sensitization, since it was believed that this occurred during labor and delivery rather than in earlier stages of pregnancy. Thus in 1960 they began a program to determine whether initial immunization of Rh-negative mothers by Rh factor of fetal origin could be prevented by the administration of Rh antibody immediately after childbirth. At the same time, and quite independently, Finn and his coworkers began similar experimental work, using raw plasma as their source of passive antibody.

For reasons of safety, Freda *et al.* used anti-Rh–containing γ-globulin rather than antibody-containing plasma to provide passive immunity. This led them to choose fraction II γ-globulin made from a pool of high-titer incomplete anti-Rh donor plasma. Since the original batch in 1961, many subsequent batches of this material in the form of Rh immunoglobulin have been fractionated, filtered, and provided sterile as a 16.5% solution. Since intravenous injection of γ-globulin is unsafe, Rh immunoglobulin must be administered intramuscularly. Except for its anti-Rh component, Rh immunoglobulin is not materially different from ordinary commercial fraction II γ-globulin, and freedom from side effect and hepatitis has been complete. Other workers followed this lead and began to use fraction II γ-globulin preparations in their own programs instead of anti-Rh–containing plasma.

Rh immunoglobulin was tested in male volunteers for more than 4 years. These results showed that no side effects were associated with Rh immunoglobulin

V.B.: Amniotic fluid tracing prior to each of the two fetal transfusions at 29½ and 31½ weeks respectively

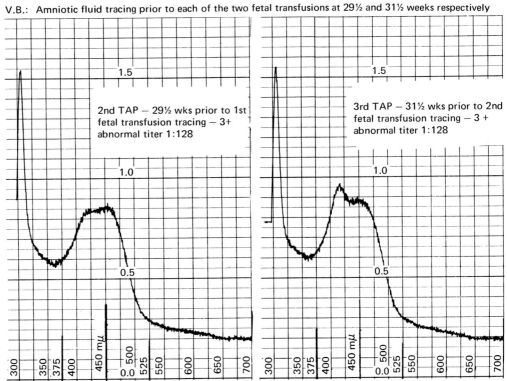

FIG. 23-9. Amniotic fluid tracings before each of two fetal transfusions at 29.5 and 31.5 weeks of gestation. Patient's first pregnancy produced a normal, unaffected infant. Her next four pregnancies produced one hydropic infant who died soon after birth and three erythroblastotic stillborn infants, the last of which was born 10 weeks before term. During her sixth pregnancy, two fetal transfusions were performed. (Freda VJ: Prog Hematol 5:266, 1966)

and that the preparation completely suppressed sensitization in subjects heavily stimulated by Rh-positive cells. It could be given as long as 72 hours after the red cells and still provide a complete effect. Because of these encouraging findings, a trial was begun in Rh-negative mothers.

The first trial in mothers was begun at Columbia–Presbyterian Medical Center in April 1964. In this trial, Rh immunoglobulin was injected intramuscularly into nonimmunized Rh-negative mothers within 72 hours of delivery of an Rh-positive infant.

Additional clinical trials with the Rh immunoglobulin preparation were then done in various centers around the world. The combined results clearly indicated that the Rh immunoglobulin preparation worked exceedingly well and was virtually completely effective in suppressing the primary Rh immune response in all the cases studied. The final proof of the complete efficacy of this preparation was obtained and confirmed when results of a significant number of subsequent Rh-positive pregnancies became known (Table 23–4).

In deciding which patients are candidates for Rh immunoglobulin, it is probably advisable to use the results of laboratory tests, primarily to rule out the need for Rh immunoglobulin rather than to rule it in. There is potential tragedy if the preparation is not given when indicated, but little or no harm if it is given when

not indicated (*e.g.*, to an already sensitized Rh-negative mother or even inadvertently to an Rh-positive mother). Consequently, every pregnancy, abortion, or ectopic pregnancy should be covered with Rh immunoglobulin unless 1) the mother is proved positive for the Rh factor, 2) the conceptus is proved negative for the Rh factor, or 3) the mother already has circulating anti-Rh antibody.

Rh immunoglobulin must be administered intramuscularly to the mother, and if possible it should be administered within 72 hours of delivery or abortion. Why is there this 72-hour time limit? When Freda, Gorman, and Pollack first planned to work with Rh-negative male volunteers at Sing–Sing Prison, they informed the warden that they planned to give Rh-positive blood to the volunteers and then return 24 hours later to give Rh immunoglobulin to half of the volunteers (*i.e.*, to the treated group but not to the controls) and that they planned to do this on a weekly, monthly, and yearly basis. The warden objected to this "obvi-

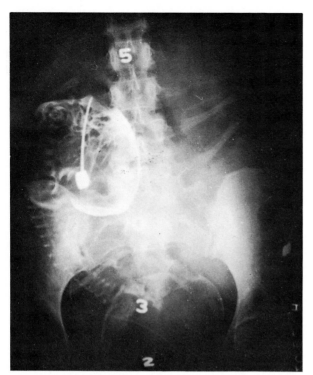

FIG. 23-10. Roentgenogram (same patient whose amniotic fluid tracings are shown in Fig. 23–9) made at 29.5 weeks' gestation, at time of first transabdominal intraperitoneal transfusion of fetus (Liley method) with 100 ml fresh packed donor blood (final hematocrit, 80%). Peritoneal cavity and diaphragm of fetus are outlined with radiopaque dye, thereby confirming correct placement of needle and catheter. Needle was allowed to remain in place to demonstrate penetration of lower abdomen of fetus by tip of needle. (Freda VJ: Prog Hematol 5:266, 1966)

ous" 24-hour scheduled revisit to the prison over a period of years. They next thought of a 48-hour interval but then realized that, when the preparation was to be given to mothers, those delivering on Friday night might be unable to receive it until 3 days later, on Monday. Therefore, it was suggested to the warden that the interval between visits (*i.e.*, between the injections of Rh-positive blood and the injection of Rh immunoglobulin) be 72 hours, and this was accepted. Since they achieved in these subjects 100% protection, it was decided to keep the 72-hour time limit for the initial studies (1964) on mothers at the Columbia–Presbyterian Medical Center. When additional clinical studies were initiated around the world, they followed this protocol, including the 72-hour time interval. Since the results from these various studies were universally favorable, when the United States Government licensed Rh immunoglobulin for produc-

tion, it stipulated that the preparation be administered within 72 hours of delivery. Probably it would be just as effective if given 96 hours, 1 week, or even 2 weeks or more following delivery. However, no study was conducted to see how long after delivery Rh immunoglobulin can be administered and still provide protection. Consequently, the occasional patient in whom the 72-hour time interval has been exceeded should still be given Rh immunoglobulin. She should be advised that, although the preparation is given belatedly, it may still protect against sensitization; even if it does not, it will certainly cause no harm.

Sometimes following delivery or abortion, results of serologic tests do not show clearly whether the mother is already sensitized to the Rh factor. In such cases, it is advisable to administer the Rh immunoglobulin, since it will cause no harm in those mothers who are already sensitized and may prove beneficial for those who are not. The rule should be to administer Rh immunoglobulin when in doubt, rather than to withhold it. In such cases, the rationale for this decision should be explained to the mother in detail.

Although it has been possible to reduce the incidence of sensitization from 14% to 1% with the routine postpartum administration of Rh immunoglobulin (Fig. 23–12), the incidence of sensitization has leveled off at about 1% and remained there. Further studies from Canada and Australia suggest that a single dose of Rh immunoglobulin during the third trimester (*e.g.*, 300μg at 28–32 weeks), in addition to the usual postpartum dose can further reduce the incidence of Rh sensitization to approximately 0.3%. Consequently, the additional antepartum dose is to be recommended.

At the Columbia–Presbyterian Medical Center, it has been the practice to administer 300μg Rh immunoglobulin routinely to all Rh-negative nonsensitized mothers who undergo amniocentesis in the second trimester for genetic studies. This dose is repeated at approximately 30 weeks and once again following delivery if the baby is Rh-positive. No ill effects have been noted among infants delivered of mothers who have received antenatal doses of Rh immunoglobulin.

Following induced or spontaneous abortion in the first trimester, a 50μg dose of Rh immunoglobulin seems to afford adequate protection in most cases. However, for any termination of pregnancy beyond the first trimester, the standard 300μg dose is recommended.

There has been a problem regarding false-positive typing of the Rh_o variant (D^u). In cases of large fetomaternal bleeds, there may be a sufficient number of Rh-positive fetal cells in the mother's circulation to yield a very weak Rh-positive result in the Rh typing. The laboratory may erroneously type these mothers as D^u-positive and the Rh immunoglobulin may be withheld—when, in fact, these are the mothers who need it

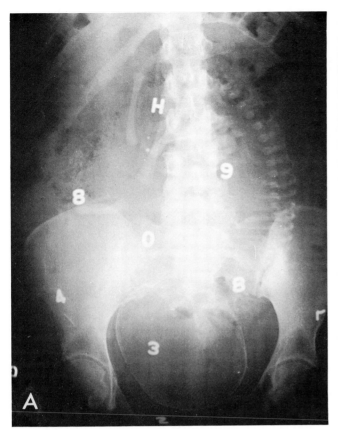
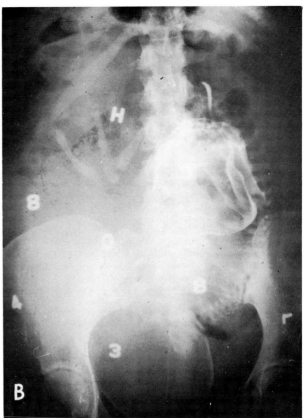
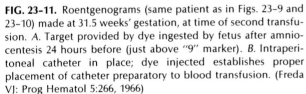

FIG. 23-11. Roentgenograms (same patient as in Figs. 23–9 and 23-10) made at 31.5 weeks' gestation, at time of second transfusion. *A.* Target provided by dye ingested by fetus after amniocentesis 24 hours before (just above "9" marker). *B.* Intraperitoneal catheter in place; dye injected establishes proper placement of catheter preparatory to blood transfusion. (Freda VJ: Prog Hematol 5:266, 1966)

the most, for they run a very high risk of becoming sensitized. In such cases, an estimation of the number of fetal cells in the maternal circulation should be carried out (*e.g.,* Kleihauer technique). The physician should be particularly aware of this possibility whenever a mother who has been previously typed as Rh-negative is reported to be D^u-positive following delivery. Again, when in doubt, it is safer to give the Rh immunoglobulin rather than to withhold it. It will cause no harm to the mother who is truly D^u-positive.

This is a prophylactic, not a therapeutic, measure and therefore is of no proved value for the mother already sensitized to the Rh factor. Thus, for the present generation of mothers who are already sensitized, physicians must still rely on amniotic fluid analysis and fetal transfusion where indicated. The ultimate conquest of any disease depends on the development of

effective prophylactic techniques. As shown in Figure 23–12, Rh immunoglubulin is an extremely effective prophylactic, and thus the conquest of Rh disease is now a reality.

ABO HEMOLYTIC DISEASE

INCIDENCE

In approximately 22% of all pregnancies in the United States, there is a naturally occurring ABO blood group incompatibility between mother and fetus (*i.e.,* the red cells of the fetus are incompatible with the mother's serum). Since only a small fraction of these pregnancies actually result in ABO hemolytic disease, it can be assumed that these infants are protected in some way against the harmful effects of the maternal antibody. Precisely how this protective mechanism operates remains unknown.

ABO hemolytic disease is clinically evident in approximately 1% of all newborn infants. The true incidence of the disease is somewhat higher, but precise

TABLE 23–4. RESULTS OF TOTAL WORLD STUDIES ON EFFICACY OF RH IM-
MUNOGLOBULIN IN PREVENTING RH SENSITIZATION

	Treated Group		Control Group	
	No. Sensitized	Total No.	No. Sensitized	Total No.
RESULTS 6 MONTHS OR MORE AFTER DELIVERY OF FIRST RH-POSITIVE IN-FANT	4	2523	160	2299
RESULTS AFTER DELIVERY OF SECOND (OR MORE) RH-POSITIVE INFANT	2	303	48	351

(Freda VJ: Karl Landsteiner Memorial Award Lecture, Presented at the 22nd Annual Meeting, American Association of Blood Banks, 1969)

statistics are difficult to arrive at for two reasons: 1) the belated appearance of jaundice in many mild cases blends into the physiologic jaundice of the 3rd–5th day of life, and 2) there is no one cord blood test that is diagnostic for ABO hemolytic disease, as a positive result on the direct Coombs test is for Rh disease.

COMPARISON OF ABO AND RH HEMOLYTIC DISEASES

Hemolytic disease due to ABO incompatibility is more common than that due to Rh sensitization; together, they account for about 98% of all hemolytic disease of the newborn. ABO disease tends to be less severe than Rh disease. Proportionately more Rh-affected babies than ABO-affected babies require exchange transfusions. Fetal death from hemolytic disease results from severe anemia and secondary heart failure. Without treatment, some 21% of Rh-affected fetuses would die *in utero,* and another 9%, although liveborn, would fail to survive an exchange transfusion. Neither of these problems occurs in ABO hemolytic disease, for it is extremely rare that this syndrome produces anemia of such degree that it causes heart failure before birth. For this reason, stillbirths due to ABO disease are rare, but neonatal death from kernicterus (brain damage from extremely high levels of serum bilirubin) may occur. Hyperbilirubinemia of this degree apparently does not occur *in utero,* but only after birth, probably because the fetus, unlike the newborn, has access to the metabolic pathways of the mother through the placenta so that critical levels of bilirubin (20 mg/dl or higher) are never reached *in utero.*

As discussed earlier, the first Rh-positive baby is usually not erythroblastotic. The first ABO incompatible baby is often affected, however. This has been explained, in part, by the observation that (except during the 1st months of life) there is regularly present, in any person's serum, those anti-A and anti-B isoantibodies that do not react with his or her own red cells (Landsteiner's rule). For reasons not entirely clear, these antibodies are harmless to the fetus except in a

small proportion of pregnancies. There is no clear-cut correlation between maternal ABO antibody titer and severity of fetal disease, so it is extremely difficult to draw a line between a safe and a dangerous ABO antibody titer. There is at this time no single maternal test that can serve in the antepartum period as an index of impending ABO hemolytic disease.

Available evidence indicates that the Rh-Hr substances are restricted to the red cells, while the ABO blood group substances are present in organ cells as well. In addition, in 80% of people (called secretors) these substances are also present in water-soluble form in the secretions and body fluids. This raises the question whether the secretory status of the fetus plays a role in the pathogenesis of ABO hemolytic disease, and indeed there is some evidence that it does.

Once severe ABO hemolytic disease occurs in a family, all future babies will be affected unless their blood is Group O or Subgroup A_2. This corresponds with the experience of families with Rh-affected children, for once an affected baby is born, all future children will be affected unless they are Rh-negative.

Finally, the ABO system has a protective action in hemolytic disease due to Rh and other blood factors. For example, when an Rh-negative mother is pregnant with an Rh-positive fetus, an additional ABO incompatibility tends to prevent the mother from becoming sensitized to the Rh factor and thereby protects the fetus against severe Rh hemolytic disease.

ANTEPARTUM DETECTION OF ABO DISEASE

As previously mentioned there is no single test that will forewarn the obstetrician of impending ABO hemolytic disease, and to perform a battery of tests on every Group O mother would be costly and impractical. Antepartum investigation is indicated

1. If the patient has had a previous baby affected with ABO hemolytic disease
2. If the patient's blood group is O and she is an elderly primigravida

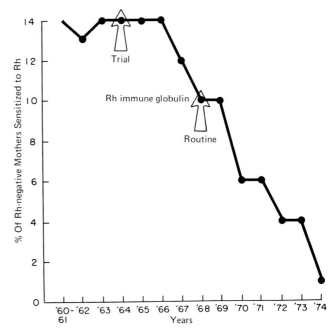

FIG. 23-12. Incidence of sensitization as a percentage of total number of Rh-negative mothers in Rh antepartum clinic of Columbia–Presbyterian Medical Center. (Freda VJ et al.: N Engl J Med 292:1014, 1975)

3. If the patient's blood group is O (with no atypical antibodies) and she has had a child with jaundice in the first 24 hours neonatally or a child with unexplained "congenital" neurologic damage
4. If the patient's blood group is O and she has experienced repeated abortions

When any of these conditions is met, the blood group of the baby's father should be determined. If it is Group O or Subgroup A_2, the infant cannot have ABO hemolytic disease, and there is no need for further testing. If the father's blood group is AB, B, or A_1, the mother's serum should be checked for anti-A or anti-B hemolysins, and the α- and β-acacia titers should be determined. This need be done only once, preferably in the last trimester, a week or two before term. A few milliliters of serum suffices for both tests.

Of primary predictive importance is the knowledge that once severe ABO hemolytic disease occurs in a family, all future babies will be affected unless their blood type is O or A_2. Some 50% of the mild and approximately 30% of the severe cases of ABO hemolytic disease occur in a first baby. Nearly all these infants have been found to be secretors. Therefore, as shown in Table 23–5, the mating that is most likely to give rise to this syndrome is one in which the mother is Group O, the father has the agglutinogen A_1 or B, and either or both are secretors. ABO hemolytic disease is not likely to occur when the mother has no anti-A or anti-B hemolysins; when it does occur, the maternal acacia titer is generally found to be higher than that of the average person. Thus, if the serologic findings in the mother are considered along with the blood groups of these matings, then it can be estimated that approximately only 5% of all matings will produce the majority of infants with ABO hemolytic disease.

In general, ABO hemolytic disease may maim (mild anemia) but will not kill the well-developed fetus. The incidence of stillbirths among the ABO-incompatible pregnancies is not significantly higher than that of the general obstetric population and can by no means be compared to the incidence of stillbirths due to Rh hemolytic disease. This fact, plus the knowledge that at the present time it is not possible to predict the outcome of any one pregnancy in which the ABO syndrome may be suspected, precludes any justification for early induction of labor on this basis alone. Nor is there any justification for performing amniocentesis in suspected ABO hemolytic disease. The ABO problem is not like the Rh problem, in which preterm delivery must sometimes be risked to avoid death *in utero*.

The chief advantage of determining antepartum that ABO disease is possible lies in the prompt institution of diagnostic and therapeutic measures after birth.

POSTNATAL DIAGNOSIS AND TREATMENT OF ABO DISEASE

When an infant whose mother's serum has no atypical antibody develops jaundice within the first 48 hours of life, ABO hemolytic disease must be suspected. Many laboratory tests facilitate this diagnosis, but no single

TABLE 23-5. SEROLOGIC PATTERN AND FINDINGS IN ABO HEMOLYTIC DISEASE

Type of Data	Father	Mother	Infant
Blood group	A_1, B, A_1B, or A_2B	O	A_1 or B
Incidence of secretor status compared with general population	Number of secretors greater than average	Distribution of secretors and nonsecretors same as in the general population	First infant almost always a secretor; subsequent infants usually secretors, but may be nonsecretors
Serologic tests and findings		1. Anti-A or anti-B hemolysins 2. Acacia titers for anti-A or anti-B usually elevated 3. Presence of $7S\gamma2$ (anti-A and anti-B) globulins that tend to resist neutralization by specific soluble blood groups substances	1. Free "incompatible" isoantibody in the serum 2. Lysis of infant's cells by mother's serum 3. Direct antiglobulin test negative or weakly positive Modified direct antiglobulin test ± positive Indirect antiglobulin test on adult red cells usually positive Direct conglutination test often positive (suspend baby's cells in Group AB serum or acacia) 4. Microspherocytosis and increased osmotic fragility 5. Reticulocytosis and often erythroblastemia
Clinical data and obstetric history		1. Incidence of repeated abortion slightly higher among Group O mothers 2. Incidence of stillbirths not significantly higher than average	1. Early onset of jaundice with or without anemia in absence of Rh incompatibility 2. Some 50% of mild cases and approximately 30% of severe cases occur in the first baby

(Freda VJ, Carter BA: Clin Obstet Gynecol 7:968, 1964)

test suffices. The diagnosis of ABO hemolytic disease depends on circumstantial evidence and the exclusion of other causes. First, the disease is always suspected when there is an early appearance of jaundice with or without anemia, especially in an Rh-compatible pregnancy in which the mother–infant blood group pattern is either O/A_1 or O/B. A negative or feebly positive result on the Coombs test helps to implicate the ABO system and tends to rule out the Rh system. The presence in the cord serum of free isoantibody that is antagonistic to the fetal blood group is also of diagnostic value. However, this finding is significant only when it is reasonably certain that the infant's subgroup is A_1 and not A_2.

Another test of diagnostic value involves incubation of the mother's serum at 37°C with the infant's red cells and with adult red cells of the same ABO group as the infant. Should the mother's serum fail to hemolyze either type of cell, the diagnosis of ABO hemolytic dis-

ease is unlikely. The infant's hemoglobin concentration can also be determined, but it is likely to be within normal limits. The reticulocyte count may be above normal limits. One fairly characteristic feature of this desease is the presence of numerous microspherocytes in the peripheral blood; these fragile red cells account for the changes in osmotic fragility. These serologic diagnostic tests are itemized in Table 23–5.

At the present time, the indications for treatment in ABO hemolytic disease are generally the same as those in Rh hemolytic disease. In either case, the infant's serum bilirubin concentration should be determined periodically during the first 72 hours, for undetected and untreated jaundice may cause brain damage in some 15% of cases. Neurologic sequelae can be prevented by prompt and adequate therapy (one or more exchange transfusions) *before* the serum bilirubin reaches the critical level of 20 mg/dl or more.

In very mildly affected infants, it has been shown

that total body exposure to fluorescent light of specified wavelength promotes breakdown of bilirubin and may indeed make transfusion unnecessary. (Such "phototherapy" is also applicable in mild physiologic hyperbilirubinemia and jaundice due to preterm delivery. It is not helpful in severely affected infants.)

REFERENCES AND RECOMMENDED READING

Allen FH Jr, Diamond LK: Erythroblastosis Fetalis. Boston, Little Brown, 1958

ACOG Technical Bulletin 13. Prenatal Antibody Screening and Use of Rho(D) Immune Globulin (Human). American College of Obstetricians and Gynecologists, June 1970

ACOG Technical Bulletin 17. Management of Erythroblastosis. American College of Obstetricians and Gynecologists, July 1972

Bevis DCA: Antenatal prediction of haemolytic disease of the newborn. Lancet 1:395, 1952

Bevis DCA: The composition of liquor amnii in haemolytic disease of the newborn. J Obstet Gynaecol Br Emp 60:244, 1953

Bevis DCA: Blood pigments in haemolytic disease of the newborn. J Obstet Gynaecol Br Emp 63:68, 1956

Bowman J: Winnipeg Antenatal Prophylaxis Trial. Scientific Symposium: Rh Antibody-Mediated Immuno-Suppression. Ortho Res Inst Med Sciences 55:1975

Burnham L: The common etiology of erythroblastosis and transfusion accidents in pregnancy. Am J Obstet Gynecol 42:389, 1941

Clarke C., Whitfield AGW: Deaths from rhesus haemolytic disease in England and Wales in 1977: Accuracy of records and assessment of anti-D prophylaxis. Br Med J 1:1665, 1979

Clarke CA, Donohoe WTA, McConnell RB et al: Further experimental studies on the prevention of Rh haemolytic disease. Br Med J 1:979, 1963

Davey MG: Antenatal Administration of anti-Rh: Australia 1969–1975. In Rh Antibody-Mediated Immuno-Suppression. Ortho Res Inst Med Sciences 59:1975

Finn R, Clarke CA, Donohoe WTA et al: Experimental studies on the prevention of Rh haemolytic disease. Br Med J 1:1486, 1961

Finn R, Harper DT, Stallings SA et al: Transplacental hemorrhage. Transfusion 3:114, 1963

Freda VJ: The Rh problem in obstetrics and a new concept of its management using amniocentesis and spectrophotometric scanning of amniotic fluid. Am J Obstet Gynecol 92:341, 1965

Freda VJ: Antepartum management of the Rh problem. Prog Hematol 5:266, 1966

Freda VJ, Adamsons K: Exchange transfusion in utero. Am J Obstet Gynecol 89:817, 1964

Freda VJ, Bowe ET: Hemolytic disease due to Rh sensitization. In Conn HF (ed): Current Therapy. Philadelphia, WB Saunders, 1969

Freda VJ, Carter B: ABO blood group system and its relationship to hemolytic disease. Clin Obstet Gynecol 7:968, 1964

Freda VJ, Gorman JG, Pollack W: Successful prevention of sensitization to Rh with an experimental anti-Rh gamma₂ globulin antibody preparation. Fed Proc 22:374, 1963

Freda VJ, Gorman JG, Pollack W: Rh factor: Prevention of isoimmunization and clinical trial on mothers. Science 151:828, 1966

Freda VJ, Gorman JG, Pollack W: Suppression of the primary Rh immune response with passive Rh IgG immunoglobulin. N Engl J Med 277:1022, 1967

Freda VJ, Gorman JG, Pollack W et al: Prevention of Rh hemolytic disease—Ten years' clinical experience with Rh immune globulin. N Engl J Med 292:1014, 1975

Freda VJ, Robertson JG: Antepartum management: Amniocentesis and experience with hysterotomy and surgery in utero. Jewish Mem Hosp Bull 10:47, 1965

Gorman JG, Freda VJ, Pollack W: Intramuscular injection of a new experimental gamma₂ globulin preparation containing high levels of anti-Rh antibody as a means of preventing sensitization to Rh. Proc IX Cong Int Soc Hematol 2:545, 1962

Gorman JG, Freda VJ, Pollack W: Prevention of rhesus haemolytic disease. Lancet 2:181, 1965

Landsteiner K, Wiener AS: An agglutinable factor in human blood recognized by immune sera for rhesus blood. Proc Soc Exp Biol Med 43:223, 1940

Levine P: The pathogenesis of erythroblastosis fetalis. J Pediatr 23:656, 1943

Levine P: The influence of the ABO system on Rh hemolytic disease. Hum Biol 30:14, 1958

Levin P, Katzin E, Burnham I: Isoimmunization in pregnancy. JAMA 116:825, 1941

Levine P, Stetson RE: An unusual case of intragroup agglutination. JAMA 113:126, 1939

Liley AW: The technique and complications of amniocentesis. NZ Med J 59:581, 1960

Liley AW: Liquor amnii analysis in the management of the pregnancy complicated by rhesus sensitization. Am J Obstet Gynecol 82:1359, 1961

Liley AW: Errors in the assessment of hemolytic disease from amniotic fluid. Am J Obstet Gynecol 86:485, 1963

Liley AW: Intrauterine transfusion of foetus in haemolytic disease. Br Med J 2:1107, 1963

Mollison PL, Mourant AE, Race RR: The Rh Blood Groups and Their Clinical Effects. Medical Research Council Memorandum 27. London, HMSO, 1952

Nevanlinna HR: Factors affecting maternal Rh immunization. Am Med Exp Biol Fenn 31 (Suppl 2), 1953

Pollack W, Gorman JG, Freda VJ: Prevention of Rh Hemolytic disease. Prog Hematol 6:121, 1969

Queenan JT: Modern Management of the Rh Problem, 2nd ed. Hagerstown, Harper & Row, 1977

Queenan JT: Intrauterine transfusions. Am J Obstet Gynecol 104:397, 1969

Robertson JG: Examination of amniotic fluid in rhesus isoimmunization. Br Med J 2:147, 1964

Robertson JG: Evaluation of the reported methods of interpreting spectrophotometric tracings of amniotic fluid in rhesus isoimmunization. Am J Obstet Gynecol 95:120, 1966

Sabbagha RE, Kipper I: The first-trimester pregnancy. In Sabbagha RE (ed): Diagnostic Ultrasound Applied to Obstetrics and Gynecology, p 59. Hagerstown, Harper & Row, 1980

Smith T: Active immunity produced by so-called balanced or neutral mixtures of diphtheria toxin and antitoxin. J Exp Med 11:241, 1909

Stern K, Davidson I, Masaitis L: Experimental studies on Rh immunization. Am J Clin Pathol 26:833, 1956

Stern K, Goodman HS, Berger M: Experimental isoimmunization to hemoantigens in man. J Immunol 87:189, 1961

Steward FH et al.: Reduced dose of Rh immune globulin following first trimester pregnancy termination. Obstet Gynecol 51 (3):318, 1978

Uhr JW, Baumann JB: Antibody formation: I. The suppression of antibody formation by passively administered antibody. J Exp Med 113:935, 1961

Uhr JW, Baumann JB: Antibody formation: II. The specific anamnestic antibody response. J Exp Med 113:959, 1961

Wiener AS: Rh-Hr Blood Types. New York, Grune & Stratton, 1954

Wiener AS, Freda VJ, Wexler I et al: Pathogenesis of ABO hemolytic disease, Am J Obstet Gynecol 79:567, 1960

Wiener AS, Wexler IB: Heredity of the Blood Groups. New York, Grune & Stratton, 1958

Wysowski DK, Flynt JW, Jr, Goldberg MF et al: Rh hemolytic disease—Epidemiologic surveillance in the United States, 1968 to 1975. JAMA 242:1376, 1979

Third trimester bleeding occurs in 2%–3% of patients. It may be due to a trivial cause (cervical polyp or "bloody show") or to a far more serious affection of the uterus (invasive carcinoma of the cervix or rupture of the uterus). The most common source of significant bleeding in late pregnancy is the placental site, as in placenta previa and premature separation of the normally implanted placenta. These two complications are potentially fatal to mother, fetus, or both. Hence, it is an obstetric maxim that all patients with third trimester bleeding be admitted to the hospital immediately and that no rectal or vaginal examination be made until all is in readiness to deal with any abnormality that may be found or any hemorrhage that the examination may provoke.

PLACENTA PREVIA

The term *placenta previa* is used to describe the condition in which the placenta is implanted in the lower pole of the uterus; usually, a portion of the placenta precedes the presenting part of the fetus. Since the relation of the placenta to the internal os of the cervix is important in the management and outcome of pregnancy, certain descriptive terms are necessary. The commonly used terminology is illustrated in Figure 24–1. In total placenta previa the entire internal cervical os is covered by placenta (Figs. 24–2 and 24–3). In partial placenta previa, only a portion of the os is covered; this is expressed as the percentage of the os covered at the time the definitive diagnosis is made. If the placenta is implanted near the internal os but does not extend beyond its edge, it is referred to as a low-lying placenta or a low implantation.

INCIDENCE

Placenta previa occurs in approximately 1/200 deliveries and is more common among women who have had more than one prior delivery. At the University of Iowa Hospitals, the incidence among 76,000 deliveries was 0.47%. The total incidence is decreasing, apparently as the result of the decline in the number of women of high parity and an increase in the number of primigravidas (Tables 24–1 and 24–2). Several factors are concerned in this alteration of patient population. The most important ones are better and more readily available means of contraception and more liberal attitudes toward surgical sterilization.

ETIOLOGY

The specific cause of placenta previa is unknown. A number of factors may affect the place of implantation in any pregnancy. Early or late fertilization, variability in the implantation potential of the blastocyst, and the receptivity and adequacy of the endometrium, which vary from cycle to cycle, may all play a role. However, it is probable that more than chance controls the site of nidation. Multiple pregnancy may predispose to placenta previa because of the increased surface area of placenta or placentas. In patients who have a scar from a uterine incision after such operations as cesarean section, hysterotomy, myomectomy, or metroplasty, it is quite common to find that subsequent placental sites include the area of the scar. There is an increased incidence of placenta previa in patients previously delivered by low cervical cesarean section, whether the uterine incision was vertical or transverse. This may result from alteration in blood supply to the area, from change in the quality and depth of the endometrium, or from change in the shape and contour of the uterine cavity. The change in size and contour of the uterine cavity after any pregnancy may account for the fact

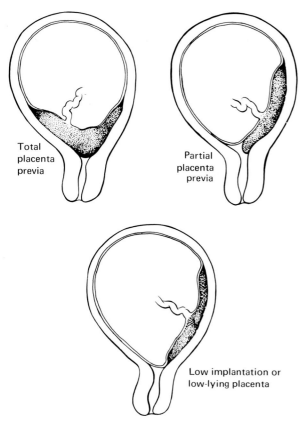

Total placenta previa

Partial placenta previa

Low implantation or low-lying placenta

FIG. 24–1. Variations of placenta previa

that placenta previa is more common in multiparas. Not only does the incidence increase with parity, but the higher the pregnancy order, the more marked the rate of increase. The vessels at the previous placental sites undergo changes that may decrease the blood supply to those regions of the endometrium. In subsequent pregnancies, therefore, more surface area may be required for placental attachment to provide adequate maternal blood flow to the intervillous space, which would increase the possibility of encroachment on the internal cervical os. The placenta from a patient with placenta previa is thinner and the maternal surface area is greater than in the normally implanted placenta.

CLINICAL COURSE

Painless bleeding is the hallmark of placenta previa. It is usually limited to the third trimester, but it can occur as early as 20 weeks.

During late pregnancy, the lower pole of the uterus becomes somewhat thinner, and the softening cervix begins to efface and dilate; if the placenta is implanted in the lower pole, the size and margins of the implan-tation site are altered by these uterine changes. Some separation at the placental margin results, and maternal bleeding occurs from the intervillous space. To a greater or lesser degree, this occurs in all types of placenta previa. The earlier in pregnancy the lower segment begins to form, and the lower the placenta, the earlier the first episode of bleeding. Unless the initial bleeding episode coincides with the onset of labor, the patient experiences no pain and the uterus remains soft. Blood loss associated with the first bleeding ranges from slight to heavy. Unless major uterine sinuses have been opened, the initial bleeding tends to stop as clots form, but may recur with renewed violence as further adjustments occur.

The bleeding may occur while the patient is resting in bed or during any type of activity. The blood is bright, like the fresh bleeding from an incision or laceration, rather than dark, like menstrual blood or that usually associated with premature separation of the normally implanted placenta.

About one-fourth of patients experience the first bleeding episode before the end of the 30th week of gestation. In slightly more than half, the initial bleeding occurs between the 34th and 40th weeks. The baby is not affected unless placental exchange is compromised by major placental detachment or maternal hypovolemia due to blood loss. Preterm delivery is the greatest threat to the infant, and the stage of pregnancy at which the first bleeding occurs may be the most important factor in fetal salvage. Rarely, asymptomatic placenta previa is found at the time of repeat cesarean section, or the patient may bleed for the first time after labor is well established.

Painless bleeding in the third trimester of pregnancy, regardless of whether it is heavy or minimal, must be considered due to placenta previa until this is ruled out.

DIAGNOSIS

History

Painless vaginal bleeding is the classic and cardinal sign of placenta previa. Its occurrence in the second half of pregnancy should instantly suggest the possibility of this complication.

Indirect Methods of Diagnosis

Only if the initial hemorrhage has stopped and if there is a clear advantage in deferring delivery until the baby is more mature are the indirect methods of diagnosis applicable. Since less than half the patients who experience painless vaginal bleeding have placenta previa, it may be of major importance either to confirm or to rule out placenta previa so that prolonged observation in the hospital will not be needed.

FIG. 24-2. Total placenta previa. *A.* Intact conceptus. Previable fetus can be seen in its amniotic sac; placenta covers entire lower uterine segment. *B.* Amniotic sac opened to show relation of fetal head to placenta. Patient (gravida 4, para 3) was admitted to delivery room in shock due to heavy vaginal bleeding and promptly expelled 6-month conceptus intact. This is unusual outcome for patients with placenta previa; without definitive treatment, exsanguination usually occurs before cervix is sufficiently dilated to permit delivery and consequent closing of uterine sinusoids by retraction of myometrium.

By far the most commonly used method of placental localization is ultrasound (standard B scan, gray scale, real time). It has the advantage of no radiation to mother or baby, and its accuracy is attested to in many reports in the literature.

It must be emphasized that these diagnostic techniques are indicated only when there is no active bleeding. If placenta previa is ruled out by ultrasound, bleeding is considered due to minor separation of a normally implanted placenta or to a local cervical lesion; occasionally, carcinoma of the cervix may be the cause and must be excluded. If placenta previa cannot be excluded, the patient must be managed as though it had been confirmed.

Definitive Diagnosis

The definitive antepartum diagnosis of placenta previa is made by palpation of the placenta at vaginal examination. Regardless of the amount of prior bleeding, this examination can provoke the most violent hemorrhage, sufficient to endanger the mother's life. Hence, it is to be performed only 1) if all is in readiness for instant cesarean section if necessary and 2) if expectant management is not appropriate.

MANAGEMENT

General Evaluation of Patient

On admission to the hospital, the patient should be placed at bedrest in an area of high-intensity care, such as the labor–delivery suite. Unless the bleeding has stopped or is minimal, an intravenous catheter should be inserted; blood drawn for typing, cross matching, and hemogram; and fluids started. The systemic manifestations of hemorrhage depend upon the amount of blood lost. The bleeding episodes usually occur during the phase of pregnancy when the circulating blood volume is increased 20%–40%; thus, the attendants may be lulled into a false sense of security if there are no major changes in pulse and blood pressure. Evidence of hypovolemia suggests that the hemorrhage has been severe unless there is some unrelated factor (*e.g.,* preeclampsia, previous hemor-

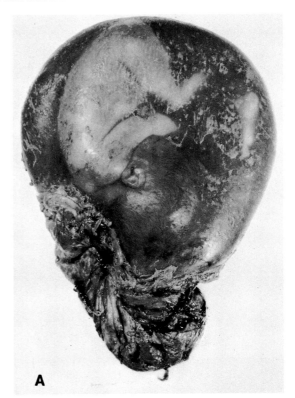

A

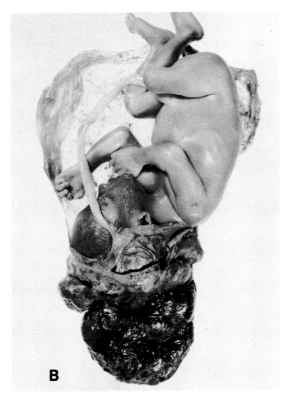

B

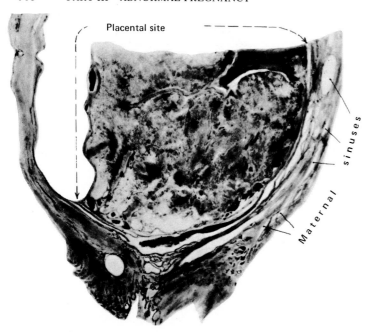
Placental site

Maternal sinuses

FIG. 24-3. Section through lower uterine segment and cervix in case of total placenta previa. Note pathologic lower uterine segment. Extensive vascularization and increased thickness of uterine wall are results of this abnormal placental location.

TABLE 24-1. OCCURRENCE OF PLACENTA PREVIA AT UNIVERSITY OF IOWA HOSPITALS, 1926–1963 AND 1964–1977

	1926–1963	1964–1977
NO. OF DELIVERIES	42,896	33,078
NO. OF PLACENTA PREVIA	224	130
FREQUENCY	1:192	1:254
INCIDENCE (%)	0.52	0.39

TABLE 24-2. DISTRIBUTION (PERCENT) OF WOMEN OF DIFFERENT PARITIES DELIVERED AT UNIVERSITY OF IOWA HOSPITALS, 1964–1976

Year	0	1–4	4
1964	31.1	56.9	11.9
1966	34.9	54.8	10.2
1968	48.6	45.1	6.3
1970	53.6	40.7	5.7
1972	56.3	39.6	4.1
1974	61.6	36.0	2.4
1976	63.7	34.8	1.5

rhage, recent use of diuretics) that has caused a decrease in blood volume.

The exact details of the episode, the history of previous bleeding, and the past obstetric and medical history should be obtained. How detailed this history must be depends on the patient's clinical and hemodynamic status. Physical examination should be complete except for vaginal and rectal examinations, which are omitted at this time. Any or all of the manifestations of hypovolemic shock may be present. Observation of the lower extremities and perineum usually reveals blood. On examination of the abdomen, the uterus is usually found to be soft, normal in tone, and not tender. With a longitudinal presentation, the fundus is usually higher than expected, since the presenting part is held high by the placenta. Breech, oblique, and transverse lies are common. Antepartum fetal death is unusual, and the fetal heart tones are usually found easily. As a rule, fetal distress or fetal death occurs only if a significant portion of the placenta is detached from the uterus or if the mother suffers hemorrhagic shock.

Concepts of Therapy

The philosophy of treatment of placenta previa has changed. Before blood was readily available and before potent antibacterial drugs were developed, immediate treatment was usually necessary to prevent the mother's death. This treatment was designed to tamponade the placenta, control bleeding, and bring about delivery, usually vaginally. The result was a maternal mortality that in some series was more than 10% and a fetal mortality that exceeded 50%. In the 1940s, it became evident that many of the maternal deaths could be prevented by immediate cesarean section, and this means of therapy was quickly accepted. The results for the baby were less salutary, however, for many of these preterm infants died.

Expectant Treatment. In 1945, Johnson and Macafee, in separate papers, introduced the current expectant treatment of selected cases of placenta previa (notably, those in which the baby is preterm and in which immediate delivery is not mandatory to stop hemorrhage). In large series of cases, they demonstrated that the first vaginal hemorrhage from placenta previa is rarely, if ever, fatal as long as no vaginal or rectal examinations are performed. The purpose of expectant treatment is to extend the period of gestation and, hence, to increase the probability of fetal survival. It has no place in the presence of persistent or recurrent bleeding and is not appropriate if pregnancy is near term.

Expectant treatment involves a period of observation in a hospital until intervention is required by the onset of labor, which is nearly always accompanied by bleeding or by recurrent or persistent hemorrhage. Should these not occur, amniocentesis for L/S ratio may be done at 36–37 weeks, and if the result is 2:1 or higher, one may undertake definitive diagnosis and elective treatment. To wait longer is to invite another episode of hemorrhage, which could unnecessarily endanger mother and fetus.

Definitive Treatment. The metreurynter (intrauterine bag), traction on a fetal foot after internal podalic version, or traction on the fetal scalp or buttocks by Willett scalp forceps were used in efforts to tamponade the placenta before the advent of blood replacement, modern anesthesia, and antibiotics. With the rarest exceptions, these practices have no place in the modern management of placenta previa. Current treatment is limited almost entirely to amniotomy for the lesser degrees of placenta previa, and cesarean section for the remainder. The decision about which of these is applicable is usually, and in almost all cases preferably, made by *double setup examination*. The following requirements should be observed:

1. The examination should be conducted in an operating room or a delivery room in which major surgery can be performed.
2. Personnel must include a scrub nurse, a circulating nurse, the physician to perform the examination and treatment, at least one physician assistant, an anesthetist or anesthesiologist, and someone to provide immediate care for the baby.
3. Instruments must be immediately ready for either vaginal or abdominal delivery, since vaginal examination may precipitate instant and massive bleeding.
4. A vein must be kept open with a large-bore catheter, and fluids should be running. If not already being administered, whole blood must be in the room.
5. The nursery and pediatric staff should have been notified to expect a high-risk infant.

When all these conditions have been met and the patient has been prepared for either vaginal or abdominal delivery, the aseptic vaginal examination is begun by visualizing the cervix. If no significant lesions are found, the vaginal fornices are palpated gently to determine whether there is anything between the fingertips and the presenting part except vaginal and uterine wall and amniotic fluid. This does not give a specific diagnosis but may provide helpful information. At this point, one finger should be carefully passed into the cervical canal. If placental tissue covers the os, there is a gritty feel to the tissue palpated. When only a portion of the internal os is covered, the placental edge is felt. The examination should be stopped immediately in either case, for even a gentle examination may precipitate the most violent hemorrhage. If no placental tissue is palpated over the os or at its margins, the membranes should be stripped away from the uterine wall and the finger inserted along the surface of the lower uterine segment. This area should be palpated as far as the examining finger can reach. Low-lying placenta is diagnosed if placental tissue is palpated during this maneuver. Since this examination may cause heavy bleeding, it must not be undertaken unless immediate diagnosis is essential or prompt delivery is planned.

The following considerations are of importance in the use of the double setup examination in patients with a history of recent bleeding unless placenta previa has been ruled out definitely by indirect methods:

1. Any patient pregnant 37 weeks or more, as determined by accurate data from early in pregnancy (dates, first examination, quickening, auscultation of fetal heart or early ultrasound) or amniotic fluid data, should have a double setup examination as soon as the maturity of the baby can be definitely ascertained. If placenta previa is found, treatment should be instituted at that time.
2. Any patient who has persistent or heavy bleeding or is in labor, regardless of the duration of pregnancy, should have an immediate double setup examination. If placenta previa is found, appropriate treatment should be carried out at that time.
3. Any patient who has a preterm fetus, is not bleeding heavily, and is not in labor should be carefully observed at bedrest for 48 hours. No vaginal or rectal examination should be performed during that time. When the bleeding has stopped, a careful speculum examination should be performed to rule out traumatic, infectious, or neoplastic lesions of the vagina and cervix. If none are found, the patient may be gradually allowed out of bed unless there is a recurrence of bleeding. If placenta previa cannot be ruled out by the indirect methods, the patient should remain under close observation until the fetus has matured. At that time an elective double setup examination is indicated. Therapy appropriate for the

diagnosis made at this examination should be instituted. Should labor begin or should persistent or heavy bleeding recur prior to the attainment of adequate fetal maturity, conservative or expectant management must be abandoned and double setup examination and appropriate therapy instituted.

Amniotomy. If at the time of double setup examination the cervix is found to be dilated 3 cm or more and the placenta covers not more than 10% of the internal os, rupture of the membranes permits the presenting part to advance against the placenta and hence to tamponade it against the bleeding maternal sinuses. If this does not control the bleeding and labor does not ensue and progress, cesarean section is indicated unless the baby is dead, in which case the presenting part may be grasped with Willett forceps and pressure maintained against the placenta by a weight attached to the handle; if the bleeding is controlled one may await progression of labor and vaginal delivery.

Cesarean Section. When the placenta completely covers the internal os, the bleeding is usually violent and rarely stops until the patient is delivered. Hence, the treatment of total placenta previa is abdominal delivery in all cases, regardless of the stage of gestation or the condition of the baby. The same is true of partial but major degrees of placenta previa.

Cesarean section without prior double setup examination is a proper procedure for the classic case in which there is bleeding of shock-producing proportions, a soft uterus, and a viable baby in good condition. With such signs, the likelihood that bleeding is due to something other than placenta previa is minuscule; vaginal examination to confirm what is already a virtual certainty only increases the bleeding, regardless of its source, and delays delivery. If placenta previa is not confirmed at cesarean section, the most scrupulous examination must be made for cervical or vaginal lesions that could produce this kind of bleeding. (Invasive carcinoma of the cervix is sometimes mentioned as such a lesion, but most obstetricians never encounter major hemorrhage from this source in pregnancy.)

Opinions differ regarding the kind of cesarean section that should be used in placenta previa (*i.e.*, classic or lower segment with vertical or transverse incision). Our preference is the lower segment operation with vertical incision, since it provides easier access to bleeding venous sinuses. In addition, if the placenta should be encountered, it is easier to find a path around it when the incision is vertical. It is possible, of course, to incise the placenta, but this may entail considerable blood loss to the baby. It is preferable to find a way around the placental edge, then to rupture the membranes, and to deliver the baby with dispatch either by the vertex or by grasping the feet and delivering as a breech. In either case, the cord should be clamped promptly after delivery.

COMPLICATIONS

Maternal morbidity and mortality may result from the placenta previa itself, from the treatment, or from a combination of both. Antepartum hemorrhage itself may be fatal or nearly so. Prolonged hypotension short of death may produce cerebral or renal damage; the latter is reversible in most instances with proper therapy. Sheehan's syndrome can occur, but it is far more likely to be associated with abruptio placentae. Clotting defects have been reported with placenta previa, but they are far less common than with abruption. Severe postpartum hemorrhage in patients with placenta previa may occur in the presence of a well-contracted uterus or atony. In the site of implantation, the lower uterine segment, the muscle content is diminished so that the natural mechanism to control bleeding—interlacing muscle bundles contracting around open vessels—may be less effective. In this event, bimanual compression of the uterus and the administration of oxytocic drugs are of little or no value. Uterine packing, which has been abandoned in most institutions, may rarely have a place in the treatment of postpartum hemorrhage from placenta previa. The other means for control of postpartum hemorrhage are bilateral hypogastric artery ligation or hysterectomy.

The anatomy and the physiologic capabilities of the endometrium of the lower uterine segment may contribute to a type of complication that may manifest itself antepartum but is not usually apparent until after delivery. The thinner endometrium, its inability to control the invasive qualities of the trophoblast, or both allow for an increase in the reported incidence of *placenta accreta, increta,* and *percreta,* any of which usually requires hysterectomy for control of postpartum hemorrhage (see Chapter 43).

Complications associated with treatment include sepsis, operative trauma to structures adjacent to the uterus, severe hemorrhage from examination or labor, blood transfusion reactions, serum hepatitis, and problems related to anesthesia. During the treatment of hemorrhage, hypovolemia must be corrected without overtransfusion or overinfusion. Continuous monitoring of central venous or pulmonary wedge pressure by intravenous catheter permits precise control of blood and fluid replacement. The maternal mortality from placenta previa in most institutions is 1% or less.

PERINATAL MORTALITY

Perinatal deaths as a result of placenta previa have decreased progressively, owing to the combination of better pediatric care, the use of expectant management, and the increasing use of cesarean section for delivery. The major problem is preterm delivery. Most reports reveal a slightly higher than usual incidence of serious congenital anomalies. Perinatal mortality in re-

TABLE 24–3. PERINATAL MORTALITY RATES FROM PLACENTA PREVIA AT UNIVERSITY OF IOWA HOSPITALS

Period	Perinatal Mortality (%)
1926–1942	42.9
1943–1952	43.5
1953–1962	20.0
1964–1972	14.7

cent years is in the range of 15%–20%. The rates for four different periods at the University of Iowa Hospitals are shown in Table 24–3.

PREMATURE SEPARATION OF PLACENTA (ABRUPTIO PLACENTAE)

Premature separation of the placenta is the term used to describe the partial or complete detachment of the placenta from a site of normal implantation in the corpus uteri at any time before delivery of the baby. It is most common in the third trimester, but may occur at any time after 20 weeks' gestation. In its various degrees it occurs in about 1% of deliveries. The detachment may be complete or partial, or only the placental margin may be concerned. The latter is sometimes referred to as *marginal sinus rupture* or *marginal sinus bleeding* (Fig. 24–4), but for practical purposes it is considered a variant of abruption. Bleeding from the placental site may dissect beneath the membranes and find its way to the outside (external, or revealed, bleeding); it may remain trapped (concealed bleeding); or it may do both, the external bleeding representing only a portion of the blood loss from the maternal circulation. As a rule, the clinical signs vary according to the degree of detachment: in the marginal type, they are usually trivial, whereas complete detachment may be quickly fatal if it cannot be dealt with at once. Hence the clinical designations of mild, moderate, or severe abruptio placentae.

ETIOLOGY

The etiology of spontaneous premature separation of the placenta is obscure. It occurs far more frequently in multiparas than in primigravid patients, and it is more common in patients over the age of 35. Preeclampsia clearly predisposes to this complication, especially in patients with underlying renovascular disease.

Trauma is concerned in some cases. A direct blow to the uterus, forceful external version, or placental site bleeding as the result of needle puncture at amniocentesis have all produced abruptio placentae, although they are indeed rare causes. The rapid reduction of

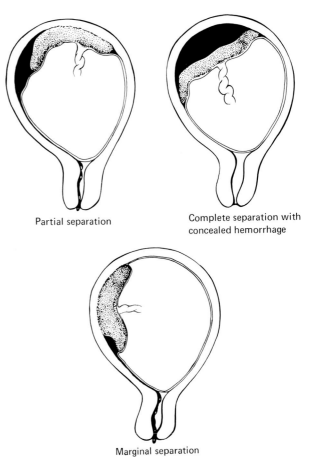

Partial separation

Complete separation with concealed hemorrhage

Marginal separation

FIG. 24–4. Various degrees of separation of normally implanted placenta.

uterine size after rupture of the membranes in hydramnios has been cited as a possible cause. Several cases of separation have been reported as the apparent result of spinal anesthesia when it is used as terminal anesthesia in the midst of an explosive second stage of labor; the precipitating factor appears to be the added uterine tone in a uterus that is already excessively irritable.

Folic acid deficiency has been suggested as an etiologic factor, but recent studies have failed to support this hypothesis.

PATHOLOGY

In patients who are predisposed to this complication, spontaneous rupture of blood vessels at the placental bed may result from lack of resiliency or other changes in the uterine vasculature. The problem is compounded by hypertension and by the fact that the uterus, being still distended, cannot contract suffi-

ciently to close off the torn vessels. Hypovolemia from the loss of blood from the maternal circulation, if sufficient, results in shock. The blood may flow beneath the placenta, shearing it off completely or in part, and may eventually separate the membranes from the uterine wall and find its way into the vagina. If there is no easy egress for the blood, its force may cause rupture through the fetal membranes into the amniotic sac, or it may extravasate between the muscle fibers of the myometrium, or both. This increases uterine tone and irritability, and uterine relaxation is incomplete. Areas of ecchymosis are common; if the extravasation is severe enough to render the uterus almost entirely blue or purple, or to prevent it from contracting normally after delivery, the condition is referred to as *uteroplacental apoplexy* or *Couvelaire uterus*. In such cases, the uterus is boardlike and tender before delivery.

As a result of myometrial damage and retroplacental clotting, large quantities of thromboplastin are released into the maternal circulation; in severe cases, this produces *disseminated intravascular clotting*. Much of this is dealt with by the circulating fibrinolysin, but the laying down of fibrin both within the blood vessels and especially in the retroplacental clot may be sufficient to deplete fibrinogen more rapidly than it can be restored. The resultant consumption coagulopathy may cause increased bleeding from the uterus, as well as from other organs.

Renal disturbance is a predictable consequence of the foregoing chain of events. Renal perfusion may be impaired by vascular spasm due to shock or by intravascular clotting. Oliguria and proteinuria may be ominous signs either of acute tubular necrosis, which may be reversible, or of acute cortical necrosis, which is not reversible.

Time seems to be an important factor in the development of both clotting defects and renal lesions. The longer the interval before delivery, the more likely and more serious these complications.

The *effects on the fetus* depend in large measure on the degree to which the uteroplacental interface is disrupted. Marginal separation may have no apparent effect. Intermediate degrees of separation may produce fetal embarrassment according to the extent to which placental exchange is lost and the degree to which uterine blood flow is impaired by continuous partial contraction of the uterine musculature. In severe cases, with complete or almost complete abruption, total anoxia and fetal death are virtually certain.

SIGNS AND SYMPTOMS

Mild Abruptio Placentae

In marginal and other minor degrees of premature separation of the placenta, there is usually no evident effect on the fetus; the heart tones remain strong and regular, and there is no excessive fetal movement. The maternal vital signs are not changed, since there is only minimal blood loss from the maternal circulation. Scant to moderate dark vaginal bleeding may occur (unless the bleeding is entirely concealed), and the uterus may fail to relax completely between contractions. Vague lower abdominal discomfort and tenderness may or may not be present. The Leopold maneuvers may be unsatisfactory because a firm uterine contraction may result from each effort to outline the baby. Although these signs are rarely enough to act upon, uterine irritability must be taken with the utmost seriousness, for it may herald a graver degree of separation.

In some cases external, usually dark, bleeding is the only sign, and the major diagnostic differentiation is from placenta previa.

Moderate Abruptio Placentae

The separation of one-fourth but less than two-thirds of the placental surface from the uterine wall is considered moderate abruptio placentae. The onset of symptoms may be gradual, beginning with the symptoms of a mild separation, or it may be abrupt, with the sudden appearance of continuous abdominal (uterine) pain that is followed promptly by dark vaginal bleeding. Although external bleeding is usually only moderate in amount, the total blood loss from the circulation may be up to 1000 ml by the time the patient is seen. There may or may not be evidence of shock (cold clammy skin, tachycardia, hypotension, oliguria), and the baby may or may not show evidence of embarrassment. The uterus is clearly tender and, of major diagnostic importance, manifests a sustained firm or partial contraction. Regardless of any prior or accompanying signs, failure of the uterus to relax between contractions must inevitably suggest the possibility of premature separation of the placenta.

Because of the sustained uterine contraction, the fetal heart may be difficult to hear with certainty. An ultrasonic fetal pulse detector may be needed to determine the baby's condition. Labor, if not already in progress, usually ensues within 2 hours. Clotting defects and renal sequelae occur in both mild and moderate forms of abruption, but they are most frequent in the severe form.

Severe Abruptio Placentae

In severe abruptio placentae, more than two-thirds of the placenta is separated from the uterus. The onset is usually abrupt, without premonitory signs or only very brief ones. The clinical picture is classic. Uterine pain is agonizing and is described as tearing, knifelike, and unremitting. The uterus is continuously boardlike and tender. External bleeding is usually only moderate, or there may be no external bleeding at all. The baby is

almost invariably dead. Shock ensues with astonishing speed; unless the condition is promptly brought under control, oliguria and consumption coagulopathy are to be expected.

TREATMENT

Mild Abruptio Placentae

When there is slight to moderate external bleeding, the uterus appears to relax well, and there is no fetal distress, abruption must be distinguished from placenta previa. If the gestation period is less than 37 weeks and external bleeding is less than moderate, the indirect diagnostic tests should be made. If placenta previa can be definitely ruled out, if external bleeding stops, and if no new signs of separation occur after a period of ambulation and observation, the patient may be sent home. However, she must be given complete and unequivocal directions as to the exact circumstances under which she must return to the hospital. If placenta previa is ruled out but moderate bleeding continues, a speculum and vaginal examination should be made. If no cervical or vaginal lesion can be found to account for the bleeding and blood loss is minimal, the physician may await the onset of labor or the appearance of new signs to suggest the need for intervention. If the patient is already in labor, the membranes should be ruptured, which usually accelerates labor and minimizes bleeding because of uterine adjustment to its smaller contents. An oxytocin infusion may help if labor is desultory or incoordinate (see Figure 35–10).

If the gestation period is more than 37 weeks, a double setup examination should be made after admission to the hospital. If placenta previa is ruled out, the membranes should be ruptured and an oxytocin infusion started if labor is not promptly effected. Electronic monitoring of the fetus is essential. Continued bleeding, failure of the uterus to relax well between contractions, or fetal distress are indications for cesarean section.

Moderate Abruptio Placentae

The immediate objectives of treatment of moderate abruptio placentae are to restore blood loss and to effect delivery. Other objectives are to maintain constant surveillance of the baby's condition and to anticipate and deal with clotting defects.

When moderate abruption with actual or impending shock is diagnosed, the following should be done at once and almost simultaneously:

1. At least 3 units of blood should be matched, and, pending their administration according to need, a vein should be kept open with a large catheter and infusion of Ringer's lactate solution or a plasma expander other than dextran.
2. A vaginal examination should be made and the membranes ruptured, regardless of whether the patient is in shock and regardless of whether abdominal or vaginal delivery is anticipated. Standard management dictates that if labor does not ensue promptly, an oxytocin infusion should be started at a rate of 2 mU/min and increased by 2 mU/min at 5-min intervals until effective labor occurs and that cesarean section should be performed a) if fetal distress occurs, as evidenced by change in fetal heart rate and pattern obtained by electronic monitor or by evidence of fetal acidemia; b) if effective labor is not established within 6 hours; or c) if delivery cannot be anticipated within 8 hours. Before operation, the exact clotting status must be known and defects corrected.
3. If shock is present or appears imminent, central venous or pulmonary wedge pressure monitoring should be started at once, provided the clotting mechanism is intact, and a Foley catheter should be inserted for accurate appraisal of urinary output. In all cases of moderate placental abruption, the baby is at high risk. Continuous electronic monitoring of the fetus is essential if abnormalities are to be noted in time for the obstetrician to deal with them.
4. Clotting defects are common even in the lesser degrees of abruptio placentae. Tests for fibrinogen and circulating fibrinolysin must be set up immediately and repeated at frequent intervals until the patient is out of danger. The tests and correction of defects are outlined in Chapter 37.

More recently, cesarean section has been used much more liberally in the treatment of both mild and moderate abruptio placentae. In Knab's study of 388 cases, 75% of the fetal deaths occurred more than 90 min after admission to the hospital, and almost 70% of all perinatal deaths involved infants who had been delivered more than 2 hours from the time of diagnosis. Among these cases, early abdominal delivery might have prevented at least some of these fatalities.

Severe Abruptio Placentae

The procedures outlined for the treatment of moderate abruptio placentae are applicable for severe separation except that 1) blood replacement is needed in a much greater amount, 2) the clotting defect is far more profound and needs much closer vigilance, and 3) with the rarest exceptions, no consideration need be given to the fetus since it is almost surely dead. Also, renal complications are more common.

The membranes should be ruptured at once, regardless of shock, and blood should be replaced as quickly as possible (2–4 liters are usually needed). The clotting status must be determined promptly and

corrected as necessary. Most patients deliver vaginally and with reasonable dispatch. Cesarean section is used only if there is a chance that the baby may still be living, if effective labor does not follow promptly, or if there is little likelihood that vaginal delivery will follow within 4–6 hours. If delivery is delayed longer, there is an increasing probability of serious maternal renal complications.

COMPLICATIONS

Maternal complications associated with moderate and severe placental separation may result either from the disease itself or from the treatment.

Postpartum hemorrhage is to be anticipated, especially in severe separation. Although the uterus may feel firm, its contractile efficiency (and hence its ability to close off bleeding sinuses) may be greatly impaired by extravasation of blood between the muscle fibers throughout the myometrium, as in the Couvelaire uterus. The problem may be compounded by persistence of a clotting defect (see Chapter 37). If conservative measures fail (correction of clotting defect, bimanual compression of the uterus, administration of oxytocic drugs), the ultimate means of controlling the bleeding is by ligation of the hypogastric arteries (see page 63 and Figure 38–2) or by hysterectomy.

Renal failure may result from ischemia, which may be caused by shock, vascular spasm, intravascular clotting, or a combination of these factors. Incompatible emergency blood transfusion may produce renal shutdown; the frequency of this complication is directly proportional to the number of units of blood transfused either because of the gravity of a condition that requires massive amounts of blood or because of the increasing statistical possibility of a mismatch. Prevention of this rare but potentially fatal complication consists mainly of the early detection and treatment of shock, the meticulous replacement of blood loss, and the proper treatment of any infection that may be present or anticipated. The evaluation and treatment of renal failure are outlined in Chapter 38. Monitoring the response of the central venous or pulmonary wedge pressure and urinary output to a provocative test may allow early detection of renal difficulty and prevention of renal failure.

Pituitary necrosis (Sheehan's syndrome), which may be a sequel of ischemia, results from the same changes that precipitate renal failure. This condition is discussed in Chapter 46. Lactation at the proper time in the puerperium suggests that the pituitary has escaped serious damage. Thyrotropic, adrenotropic, and gonadotropic pituitary function may be destroyed singly or in combination. Return of menses is adequate evidence of gonadotropic activity. Tests of thyroid and adrenal function 4–6 months after delivery

are part of the proper follow-up of patients who have suffered severe abruptio placentae.

Hepatitis may develop. It is hoped that means will soon be available for routine screening of whole blood and components so that hepatitis from these sources will cease to be a danger.

CIRCUMVALLATE PLACENTA

Another cause of bleeding in late pregnancy is circumvallate placenta although this is less common than placenta previa. The bleeding is bright, moderate in amount, and nearly always without pain. When bleeding occurs before fetal maturity, the patient may be treated expectantly. Placental localization nearly always rules out placenta previa. If bleeding is persistent or heavy, if the patient is in labor, if the fetus is known to be mature, and if placenta previa cannot be completely ruled out, double setup examination is indicated.

The treatment is nearly always induction of labor, unless there is another indication for cesarean section. At times, this complication is responsible for the spontaneous onset of preterm labor; as a result, there is an increased perinatal mortality. The diagnosis is made by inspection of the placenta following delivery.

RUPTURE OF THE UTERUS

Either spontaneous or traumatic rupture of the uterus may occur before or during labor. It is a most serious hazard to the mother, and the baby usually dies if it is extruded into the peritoneal cavity or if the maternal hypovolemia is so profound that fetal oxygenation is inadequate. The major causes are weakness of the uterine wall because of incision (previous cesarean section, hysterotomy, myomectomy, metroplasty) and difficult operative delivery (breech extraction, difficult forceps delivery, especially version and extraction). Injury, as from automobile accidents or gunshot wounds, accounts for a small percentage of cases. Improperly monitored or inappropriate use of oxytocic agents has been associated with a significant number of cases. Lower uterine segment rupture as a result of neglected obstructed labor should never occur in developed countries.

As in any ruptured viscus, pain usually, but not always, precedes the definitive tear. Severe pain and shock follow as rupture occurs, after which the pain is apt to subside. In uterine rupture, local bleeding, which may be scant or heavy, usually ensues; depending on the location of the tear, some of the blood may escape vaginally.

Rupture of a cesarean section scar is the most common type of uterine rupture. Classic vertical scars

clearly predispose to rupture; lower segment transverse scars are least apt to give way. In rupture of the classic scar, the clinical picture is of fleeting pain, often for several days before rupture; this is followed by severe pain, shock, and cessation of fetal heart tones. The pain abates after rupture, but the collapse continues and may be compounded if it is accompanied by intraabdominal hemorrhage. Immediate laparatomy is lifesaving for the mother, but of little help to the fetus, which may have already escaped into the abdominal cavity. In rupture of the lower segment scar, the picture is apt to be less dramatic, but the condition is potentially just as serious. The therapeutic procedure must be tailored to the problem. If the tear is clean and amenable to repair, the edges may be freshened and the defect sutured. If repair is not reasonable, the uterus should be removed. It is usually not absolutely necessary to remove the cervix; if the patient's condition is compromised, a supravaginal hysterectomy solves the immediate emergency more quickly and easily, and just as definitely, as a total hysterectomy.

Version and extraction, except for delivery of a second or later born baby in a multiple birth, breech extraction, and difficult midforceps deliveries are on the wane and rightly so. They should be eliminated. In addition to the possible injury to the fetus, the potential

danger of traumatic uterine rupture is ever present. Currently, delivery by cesarean section is safer for both mother and baby. The diagnosis of uterine rupture in these cases is made by manual exploration of the uterus. If uterine rupture is diagnosed, laparotomy should be undertaken immediately with due attention to vigorous appropriate management of hemorrhage and collapse. In this situation, the hysterectomy should be of the total variety because the tears often involve the lower uterine segment and extend into the cervix and vaginal fornix.

The protean lesions produced by injury cannot be categorized. Rupture has resulted from a seatbelt injury. (This is not to suggest that pregnant women should abandon seatbelts, for uterine rupture is less serious than possible death if this protection is not used.) The major signs are those of intraabdominal hemorrhage, pain, and collapse. The procedure at laparotomy depends upon the problem presented; it may be necessary to empty the uterus by hysterotomy if its bulk interferes with exposure and control of bleeding.

Oxytocin infusions can cause uterine rupture, and must be used with meticulous care, especially in parous women. Constant infusion pumps allow for safer administration, and continuous monitoring of the frequency, duration, and strength of uterine contrac-

TABLE 24-4. DIFFERENTIAL DIAGNOSIS OF BLEEDING IN LATE PREGNANCY

	Placenta Previa	Marginal Separation	Moderate Abruption	Severe Abruption	Antepartum Rupture of Scarred Uterus
EXTERNAL BLEEDING	Mild to catastrophic	Minimal to mild	None to moderate	None to moderate	None to mild
COLOR OF BLOOD	Bright	Dark	None, dark	None, dark	None, bright
BACK PAIN	None	None	None to moderate	None to moderate	None
MYOMETRIAL TONE	Normal	Normal	Hypertonicity, localized or diffuse	Hypertonicity, diffuse	Normal if baby in uterus; contracted if baby extruded
UTERINE TENDERNESS	None	Nearly always none; localized if present	Marked, usually diffuse	Marked and diffuse	None to moderate; localized if present; abdomen generally tender
FETAL STATUS AT FIRST EXAMINATION	Nearly always alive; occasionally in jeopardy	Nearly always alive; rarely in jeopardy	Frequently alive but in jeopardy	Usually dead; if alive, in jeopardy	Usually dead; if alive, in jeopardy
PRESENTATION	High incidence of breech, oblique, transverse	Normal distribution	Normal distribution	Normal distribution	Normal distribution if not extruded
STATION OF PRESENTING PART	High	High to engaged	High to engaged	High to engaged	High
SHOCK	Uncommon	None	Frequent	Very common	Frequent
COAGULOPATHY	Very rare	Very rare	Occasional	Frequent	Rare
ASSOCIATION WITH HYPERTENSIVE STATES	Normal distribution	Normal distribution	Increased	Increased	Normal distribution

tions is mandatory whether by machine or by an experienced attendant. Uterine tetany must be avoided.

Lower uterine segment rupture is a predictable consequence of neglected obstructed labor.

RUPTURED VASA PREVIA

Ruptured vasa previa is a rare complication of late pregnancy or labor that can sometimes be confused with abruptio placentae or placenta previa. If a major fetal vessel is the source of the vaginal bleeding, fetal death is virtually certain—delivery can rarely be effected quickly enough to prevent fetal exsanguination. The presence of scant vaginal bleeding may suggest bleeding from a small vessel, if the uterus is soft and there is evidence of fetal distress. The presence of nucleated red cells in a sample of expelled blood confirms the diagnosis, and delivery should be effected by the most expeditious means.

In some cases, because of a strong conviction based on the clinical picture, the physician may proceed at once to cesarean section without awaiting confirmation by a stained blood smear or chemical test for fetal hemoglobin. In a recent case, the membranes ruptured spontaneously when the cervix was 3 cm dilated. The amniotic fluid was port wine colored, which may be an important sign. Decelerative fetal heart rate patterns followed, and delivery was effected by cesarean section within 10 min. Ruptured vasa previa involving a small vessel was confirmed. The baby's condition was good, except for a hemoglobin of 12 g/dl, and the subsequent course was uneventful.

OTHER CAUSES OF LATE PREGNANCY BLEEDING

Traumatic lesions of the vagina and cervix rarely cause bleeding late in pregnancy. Lacerations of vaginal septa can occur during labor and delivery. A friable condyloma acuminatum may bleed from minor trauma and must be differentiated from other sources of bleeding. Cervical erosions and polyps rarely produce bleeding in late pregnancy. Invasive cervical carcinoma as a cause of painless vaginal bleeding in late pregnancy must be considered, although proper early prenatal care, including cervical cytology, should allow diagnosis of this entity before the second half of pregnancy.

The differential diagnosis of bleeding in late pregnancy is summarized in Table 24–4.

REFERENCES AND RECOMMENDED READING

Brenner WE, Edelman DA, Hendricks CH: Characteristics of patients with placenta previa and results of "expectant management." Am J Obstet Gynecol 132:180, 1978

Carter B: Premature separation of the normally implanted placenta: Six deaths due to gross bilateral cortical necrosis of kidneys. Obstet Gynecol 29:30, 1967

Crenshaw C, Jones DED, Parker RT: Placenta previa: A survey of twenty years experience with improved perinatal survival by expectant therapy and cesarean delivery. Obstet Gynecol Surv 28:461, 1973

Cohen WM, Chaudhuri TK, Christie JH et al: Correlation of ultrasound and radioisotope placentography. Am J Roentgenol 116:843, 1972

Golan A, Sandbank O, Rubin A: Rupture of the pregnant uterus. Obstet Gynecol 56:549, 1980

Hobbins JC, Winsberg F: Ultrasonography in Obstetrics and Gynecology, pp 49–58. Baltimore, Williams & Wilkins, 1977

Johnson HA: The conservative management of some varieties of placenta previa. Am J Obstet Gynecol 50:248, 1945

Knab DR: Abruptio placentae: An assessment of the time and method of delivery. Obstet Gynecol 52:625, 1978

Macafee CHG: Placenta previa. J Obstet Gynaecol Brit Emp 52:313, 1945

Macafee CHG, Millar WG, Harley G: Maternal and fetal mortality in placenta previa. J Obstet Gynaecol Br Commonw 69:203, 1962

Pent D: Vasa Previa. Am J Obstet Gynecol 134:151, 1979

Pritchard JA, Mason R, Carley M et al: Genesis of severe placental abruption. Am J Obstet Gynecol 108:22, 1970

Sheehan HL, Murdoch R: Postpartum necrosis of anterior pituitary: Pathological and clinical aspects. J Obstet Gynaecol Br Emp 45:456, 1938

Spaulding LB, Gallup DG: Current concepts of management of rupture of the gravid uterus. Obstet Gynecol 54:437, 1979

Preeclampsia–eclampsia, a syndrome characterized by hypertension and proteinuria and often accompanied by edema, occurs only during pregnancy or in the early puerperium. Historically, this syndrome is a classic model of conflicting and confusing hypotheses as to etiology, pathophysiology, and its effects on both mother and fetus. Repeated clinical observations and diverse laboratory procedures have failed to distinguish it from other causes of hypertension and proteinuria during pregnancy. In susceptible gravidas, the abnormalities involve many systems in varying degree. Unique facets of this syndrome are that, in its pure form, it occurs late in pregnancy and resolves completely after pregnancy without any demonstrable residual damage to the mother.

The many definitions and classifications of hypertension and proteinuria during pregnancy and the lack of specific clinical and laboratory criteria for diagnosis have led to wide discrepancies in the reported incidence of preeclampsia–eclampsia. In spite of this confusion, the syndrome of pregnancy-induced hypertension and proteinuria is undisputed as a major cause of maternal and perinatal mortality worldwide. Treatment is empiric, but early detection and good perinatal care will reduce the number of infant and maternal deaths. Undoubtedly, recommendations regarding therapy will continue to change as more is learned about the range of physiologic changes of normal pregnancy and the pathogenesis of high blood pressure and proteinuria.

DEFINITIONS AND DIAGNOSTIC CATEGORIES

Hypertension during pregnancy is defined as an elevation of systolic and diastolic pressure equal to or exceeding 140/90 mm Hg or a mean arterial pressure (*MAP*) equal to or greater than 105 mm Hg. Mean arterial pressure is equal to one-third of the pulse pressure. It may be calculated by doubling the diastolic pressure (*D*), adding the systolic pressure (*S*) to this, and dividing by 3: $MAP = \dfrac{(2 \times D) + S}{3}$. An alternative definition of hypertension is a rise in systolic pressure of 30 mm Hg or in diastolic pressure of 15 mm Hg or more. The levels cited must be present on at least two occasions 6 hours apart.

Proteinuria is the presence of urinary protein in concentrations greater than 0.3 g in a 24-hour urine collection or greater than 1 g / liter (1+ to 2+ by standard turbidimetric methods) in random urine specimens on two or more occasions at least 6 hours apart. The specimens must be clean and voided midstream, or obtained by catheterization.

More than 60 names have been applied to the hypertensive states of pregnancy. Among these are *toxemia*, *EPH* (edema, proteinuria, hypertension) *complex, gestosis, preeclampsia,* and *eclampsia.* The number of schemes for classification is even greater, which reflects the difficulty involved in accurately categorizing this disease. The definitions and classification used here are modifications of those recommended by the American College of Obstetricians and Gynecologists. Edema has been omitted as a specific diagnostic feature of preeclampsia, since it is so common in normal pregnancy and does not itself increase maternal or perinatal mortality. Basically, the classification involves determining whether hypertension or proteinuria antedate gestation, whether they occur first during pregnancy or whether these conditions are present concurrently.

Gestational hypertension is the development of hypertension during pregnancy or within the first 24 hours postpartum in a previously normotensive woman who has no evidence of hypertensive vas-

cular disease or proteinuria. The blood pressure usually returns to normotensive levels within 10 days following parturition. Some patients with gestational hypertension may in fact have preeclampsia or hypertensive vascular disease, but they do not fulfill the criteria for either of these diagnoses.

Gestational proteinuria is the presence of proteinuria during or under the influence of pregnancy without coexistent hypertension, renal infection, or known intrinsic renovascular disease.

Gestational edema is the occurrence of a general and excessive accumulation of fluid in the tissues with greater than 1+ pitting edema after 12 hours rest in bed, or of a weight gain of 2 kg or more in 1 week due to the influence of pregnancy.

Preeclampsia is the development of hypertension with proteinuria due to pregnancy or the influence of a recent pregnancy. It occurs after the 24th week of gestation, but it may develop before this time in the presence of trophoblastic disease. Preeclampsia is predominantly a disorder of primigravidas.

Eclampsia is the occurrence of one or more seizures, not attributable to cerebral conditions such as epilepsy or cerebral hemorrhage, in a patient with preeclampsia.

Superimposed preeclampsia or eclampsia is the development of preeclampsia or eclampsia in a patient with preexisting hypertensive vascular or renal disease. When the hypertension antedates the pregnancy, as established by previous blood pressure recordings, a rise in the systolic pressure of 30 mm Hg, or a rise in the diastolic pressure of 15 mm Hg, and the development of proteinuria during pregnancy are required to establish the diagnosis.

Chronic hypertensive disease is the presence of persistent hypertension of whatever cause, before pregnancy or before the 24th week of gestation, or persistent hypertension after the 42nd postpartum day.

One of the problems with this classification is that in some cases it is impossible to differentiate on clinical grounds between chronic hypertension and pregnancy-induced hypertension. If the patient's blood pressure returns to normal following pregnancy, then gestational hypertension or preeclampsia would have been the correct designation; but if the pressure remains high, chronic hypertensive disease alone or with superimposed preeclampsia may have been responsible for the elevated pressure during pregnancy. Often such categorization is retrospective. In addition, a slight accentuation in the usual third trimester rise of blood pressure may be interpreted as pregnancy-induced hypertension, when it is actually a normal physiologic change.

INCIDENCE AND RISK FACTORS

In the United States, hypertension complicates 0.5%–10% of all pregnancies. This wide variation in reported incidence reflects both differences in the criteria used for diagnosis and the populations studied. Primiparas have a higher risk of preeclampsia–eclampsia at all ages than multiparas; the ratio of primiparas to multiparas varies from 1.5:1 to 6:1 in different clinical series. In most populations studied, pregnancy-induced hypertension occurs most frequently in teenagers and in women in their late 30s and early 40s. Other conditions that predispose or are associated with the development of preeclampsia include hydatidiform mole, hydramnios, multiple pregnancy, hypertensive cardiovascular disease, chronic renal disease, and diabetes mellitus.

There is a familial tendency to the development of preeclampsia. Daughters of mothers who had preeclampsia during their first pregnancy have double the risk of developing this disorder during their own first pregnancy compared to daughters of women who did not have preeclampsia during pregnancy. Roughly one-third of women who have had preeclampsia in a previous pregnancy develop hypertension in subsequent pregnancies.

ETIOLOGY

Preeclampsia has become known as the "disease of theories." Placental, vascular, renal, metabolic, hepatic, hematologic, immunologic, and endocrine disorders all have been implicated as the cause. The more meticulous the study of the many proposed theories, the more difficult it becomes to delineate one that explains all the findings of the syndrome. The relative importance of any single predisposing factor is difficult to assess, because complex mechanisms are involved in the development of the diverse clinical, physiologic, and pathologic changes.

There are insufficient data to support geographic, racial, climatic, or nutritional factors in the etiology of preeclampsia. There is, however, an increased incidence of the syndrome in patients with underlying hypertensive disease, chronic renal disease, diabetes mellitus, and in certain socioeconomic or ethnic groups. In view of all the possible catalyzing factors peculiar to those pregnancies, it is increasingly clear that there are multiple mechanisms involved in the clinical manifestations of the syndrome.

PLACENTAL ABNORMALITIES

There is little question that preeclampsia is somehow related to the physiologic changes of pregnancy, since it does not occur in the nongravid state. A basic clini-

cal premise is that preeclampsia resolves completely and rapidly after the termination of pregnancy. This implicates the gravid uterus, fetus, or placenta as the central factor(s) in the pathogenesis of this disorder. Preeclampsia–eclampsia with characteristic histopathologic changes in the kidney, liver, and other organs has been well documented in cases of trophoblastic disease in which there is no fetus. This lends credence to the concept that abnormalities responsible for this syndrome must arise in the uteroplacental unit. Reports of preeclampsia associated with an abdominal pregnancy support the thesis that the placenta rather than the gravid uterus plays the major role in the development of preeclampsia.

Although there is no pathognomonic placental abnormality in preeclampsia, an increase in the frequency of several lesions in the placenta has been noted. These lesions include cytotrophoblast proliferation, excess syncytial knots, thickened trophoblastic basement membrane, and obliterative endarteritis. These findings are believed to be secondary to hypoxia and therefore are not the cause of the syndrome. True infarcts, retroplacental hematomas, and villus fibroid necrosis that may not be the direct result of hypoxia may also occur more often. This implies that there may be more than one mechanism by which abnormalities in the placenta are induced and that they may occur at different stages in the evolution and aging of the placenta.

Specific situations in which there is an enlargement of the placenta or rapid placental growth, *i.e.*, diabetes mellitus, multiple pregnancies, and hydatidiform mole, are associated with an increased incidence of the syndrome. It is postulated that the large placental size or other placental abnormalities may alter placental function and thereby initiate the pathophysiologic events that lead to preeclampsia.

UTEROPLACENTAL ISCHEMIA

A widely held theory is that the pathophysiologic changes in preeclampsia may be initiated by uteroplacental ischemia. The accuracy of direct and indirect methods used for computing uterine blood flow (*i.e.* cannulization of the uterine vein, injection of radioactive sodium into the uterine musculature, and simultaneous determination of maternal and fetal oxygen levels) is questioned. Although techniques for measuring uterine blood flow are indeed imperfect, comparisons of flow during normal pregnancy and during preeclampsia by several investigators indicate that there is a significant reduction of uteroplacental blood flow in preeclampsia. It is not known whether the reduction of flow precedes or follows the clinical syndrome, so ischemia as a causative factor in preeclampsia is unproved.

Experimentally produced chronic reduction of uter-

ine blood flow in dogs and baboons has resulted in a syndrome characterized by hypertension and proteinuria. Subsequent efforts by other investigators to reproduce these results have been unsuccessful in most instances. Despite this, the original experimental models support the thesis that preeclampsia may be precipitated or catalyzed by uteroplacental ischemia.

Many factors that predispose to, or aggravate preeclampsia may be associated with a compromised blood flow to the uterus. For example, hydatidiform mole is associated with rapid increase in the size of the placenta and the demand for blood may outstrip the supply. Multiple pregnancy and diabetes mellitus are conditions in which an absolute increase in the size of the placenta occurs, thereby requiring a greater vascular supply. In addition, flow may not be adequate during times of increased demand, such as labor, exercise, and other situations known to aggravate preeclampsia.

Uterine artery caliber is remarkably smaller in primiparas than in multiparas. The smaller artery size would be expected to be associated with a relatively lower rate of blood flow, which may explain why preeclampsia complicates first pregnancies so much more frequently than subsequent ones. Finally, the clinical manifestations of preeclampsia may be ameliorated by bedrest in the lateral recumbent position, a maneuver that increases uterine blood flow.

Alternative explanations and questions remain regarding these aberrations. If there is a real decrease in uteroplacental blood flow in preeclampsia, it may be due to a local vasospasm that is the result rather than the cause of the disorder. Even if decreased uterine blood flow can produce preeclampsia, the mechanism by which the reduced flow induces high blood pressure remains controversial.

DISSEMINATED INTRAVASCULAR COAGULATION

One proposed mechanism by which abnormal placental function may initiate or aggravate preeclampsia is disseminated intravascular coagulation (DIC). Although DIC may be demonstrated in severe preeclampsia–eclampsia, these changes may not be present early in the disease and therefore may be a secondary phenomena, not the cause of the disorder. It is generally agreed that DIC plays a part in the pathophysiologic changes that occur in eclampsia, but a cause and effect relationship has not been established.

IMMUNE RESPONSES

Immune disorders have been suggested as a mechanism by which placental damage may occur and initiate the changes seen in preeclampsia. It has been proposed that antigenic differences between the fetus (graft) and mother (host) may give rise to antibodies

of maternal origin that either attack and damage the trophoblasts or inhibit normal trophoblastic migration in the second trimester of pregnancy. Although normal pregnancy may require some form of controlled immunologic reaction to allow trophoblastic invasion of maternal tissues, there is considerable controversy concerning whether abnormal immune responses have any role in preeclampsia. Many investigators have failed to demonstrate abnormal amounts of antigen–antibody complexes or complement in the placental or renal basement membrane of preeclamptic patients. While an attractive theory, the role of immune mechanisms in the initiation of preeclampsia remains a matter of debate. The immunologic factors that may be concerned are discussed in Chapter 12.

PROSTAGLANDINS

Another hypothesis is that defective prostaglandin production or a loss of response to prostaglandins contributes to the development of preeclampsia. Prostaglandin E, a vasodilator, appears to exert its effect only locally, and altered synthesis of this prostaglandin in the uterine vascular bed could affect vessel caliber and thereby the blood flow through the uteroplacental unit. Observations in the monkey, dog, and rabbit indicate that angiotensin II, a potent vasopressor, increases uterine prostaglandin E production and uterine blood flow; inhibition of prostaglandin synthesis lowers uterine blood flow and raises systemic blood pressure. This suggests that in animals prostaglandin E plays a role in maintaining the resting uteroplacental vasomotor tone. If these effects are demonstrated in humans, then defective prostaglandin production may leave the pressor effects of angiotensin II unopposed and thereby could be responsible for the increased vasoreactivity of preeclampsia.

GENETIC FACTORS

Although genetic factors have been invoked in the etiology of preeclampsia, no specific chromosome abnormality or leukocyte antigen type has been identified. The increased incidence of preeclampsia in daughters of patients who manifested the syndrome during their own first pregnancy indicates that there is a familial tendency to develop pregnancy-induced hypertension and proteinuria.

MULTIPLE FACTORS

Chronic hypertension not associated with pregnancy has been described as a "disease of regulation" that is due to multiple factors. More than 25 years ago, the Mosaic Theory was proposed to explain the complex pathophysiologic and hemodynamic changes that lead to chronic hypertension. Page, after years of study, also proposed the concept that preeclampsia has multiple etiologies, numerous secondary effects, and many predisposing factors. As more is learned about the normal regulation of blood pressure in both pregnant and nonpregnant women, the explanation of the pathophysiologic changes that occur in preeclampsia becomes increasingly complex. It is probable that preeclampsia does not have a single etiology but rather that many factors contribute to the initiation and perpetuation of the pathophysiologic changes seen in this disorder. With further research, different mechanisms may be proposed.

CLINICAL COURSE

The onset of preeclampsia is sometimes abrupt, with rapid development of the classic signs and symptoms; more frequently it is gradual, in some cases sufficiently so that it is overlooked. The diagnosis is made by finding an absolute elevation or a significant rise in blood pressure in association with proteinuria. The classic clinical symptoms of preeclampsia occur late, at a time when the syndrome is irreversible. Edema may be an early sign of preeclampsia; but it is so common in normal pregnancies that unless there is a weight gain greater than 2 k in 1 week, even this characteristic feature may not suggest an abnormality. A slow rise in blood pressure or an acute rise in blood pressure frequently precedes the development of proteinuria, but there is no absolute sequence in which these findings occur. Late in the syndrome, the patient may note blurring of vision, scotomata, or photophobia. Occipital or generalized headaches and upper abdominal pain (due to swelling of the liver) are other signs of accelerated development of preeclampsia. Occasionally, with rapidly progressing disease, convulsions may be the first clinical manifestation of the disorder. Seizures in any women during third trimester of pregnancy or within a few hours of delivery, unless there is a history of a seizure disorder, should be considered eclampsia until other causes are excluded. Seizures that occur for the first time more than 8 hours postpartum are more likely to be due to some disorder other than eclampsia, such as cerebral venous thrombosis.

Preeclampsia–eclampsia occurs with increasing frequency as term is approached. It is unusual prior to the 24th week of pregnancy, or later than 12 hours after delivery. However, cases of acute hypertension and proteinuria without hydatidiform mole have been reported as early as the 16th week and as late as 2 weeks postpartum. Whether these exceptional cases have the same pathogenesis as preeclampsia that occurs late in pregnancy is open to question. In gen-

eral, about one-third of the cases of eclampsia occur antepartum, one-third intrapartum, and one-third postpartum.

BLOOD PRESSURE

In normal pregnancy, systolic and diastolic pressures are lowest during the second trimester and rise an average of 10 mm Hg between 27 and 36 weeks of gestation. A blood pressure level as low as 125/75 or a mean arterial pressure of 90 mm Hg or higher during the second trimester is associated with an increased incidence of preeclampsia in the third trimester; blood pressure elevation alone, without proteinuria or edema, is associated with an increase in perinatal mortality. The relationship of the second trimester blood pressures to the later development of preeclampsia, fetal growth retardation, and perinatal mortality is nearly linear.

An insidious rise in blood pressure may precede the development of preeclampsia by weeks. Blood pressure levels may be misleading, however, and are usually not extremely high except when the patient is severely affected or when the syndrome is superimposed on hypertensive cardiovascular disease. Marked fluctuation in blood pressure is common in severe cases, but the level of blood pressure alone does not always correlate with the severity of the other clinical manifestations. The sequence of pathophysiologic changes that contribute to a rise in blood pressure has not been resolved, but it is clear that increased peripheral vascular resistance due to vasoconstriction is the final mechanism that produces the blood pressure elevation.

PROTEINURIA

While there is no direct correlation between the amount of protein in the urine and the severity of the renal histologic changes, quantitative measurement of protein helps to evaluate the severity and progression of the clinical syndrome. Relative protein clearance measurements have characterized the nature of the proteinuria during pregnancy, but they have failed to distinguish between preeclampsia and primary renal disease. Regardless of the blood pressure level, proteinuria is associated with a higher perinatal mortality rate in the primigravida. Therefore, it is clear that proteinuria alone is a poor prognostic sign during pregnancy.

If diurnal and hourly variation of the amount of protein excreted is considerable, then an accurate appraisal of protein loss requires 24-hour quantitative determinations. Urine that is contaminated by vaginal discharge or red cells may test positively for protein, and these sources must be excluded. Very heavy pro-

teinuria, *i.e.*, in amounts exceeding 3 g/24 hours, has been well documented to be secondary to preeclampsia. Despite nephrotic levels of proteinuria, recovery postpartum is complete in most instances.

EDEMA

Varying degrees of edema are found in the majority of normal and preeclamptic pregnancies. In preeclampsia, edema has no predictive value for the ultimate outcome of the pregnancy; the mere presence of edema is of less significance than the rapidity of the weight gain. Increments of weight gain in excess of 2 kg/week, particularly in the third trimester, indicate rapid fluid retention.

Edematous women excrete more sodium in the puerperium than women without edema; the amount of sodium excretion correlates with the degree of edema and its regression. Total body exchangeable sodium is increased, and the clinical manifestations of preeclampsia have been accelerated by excessive sodium administration.

A decrease in total plasma proteins and a concomitant reduction in intravascular osmotic pressure are not a concern, since normal plasma protein levels are the rule in preeclampsia. While the amount of edema is difficult to quantitate, the following method may be used to record relative degrees of edema formation:

1+: Minimal edema of the pedal and pretibial areas
2+: Marked edema of the lower extremities
3+: Edema of the face and hands, lower abdominal walls, and sacrum
4+: Anasarca with ascites

PREMATURE SEPARATION OF THE PLACENTA

From 40%–60% of the patients with abruptio placentae have preeclampsia; among women with severe preeclampsia, abruption occurs in 10%–15% of cases. This important and sometimes disastrous complication is discussed in Chapter 24. It is a definite threat in any woman with preeclampsia, and accounts for a significant number of fetal deaths.

INTRAUTERINE DEATH

Fetal death may occur unexpectedly when a patient has the preeclampsia–eclampsia syndrome. The usual cause has been designated in the all-inclusive category of placental insufficiency. The specific entities most often responsible for perinatal death are large placental infarcts, placental growth retardation, and abruptio placentae. However, it has become increasingly ap-

parent that multiple and indirect factors may be involved.

The technologic advances in the assessment of the maternal–fetal complex have been of great value in the management of the hypertensive gravida, but it is important to emphasize that electronic and biochemical monitoring are not substitutes for careful clinical assessment. Unfortunately, many obstetricians are deluded into a false sense of security by utilizing the oxytocin challenge test, urinary estriol measurement, or some other single method of evaluation. A thorough knowledge and experience in interpretation of the results of these tests are of great importance to both perinatal survival and the future mental and physical development of infants born of preeclamptic mothers. The technical and interpretative aspects of fetal monitoring are described in Chapter 41.

MATERNAL DEATH

The most common causes of death in preeclamptic patients are congestive heart failure and cerebral hemorrhage. Factors that influence maternal mortality include age, multiple pregnancy, delayed hospitalization, failure to terminate pregnancy, physician's unawareness of the severity of the mother's disease, coexisting renal disease, and DIC. With careful selectivity, the mode of delivery (*i.e.,* cesarean section versus vaginal delivery) does not adversely affect maternal survival.

ANATOMIC PATHOLOGY AND PATHOPHYSIOLOGIC ALTERATIONS

BRAIN CHANGES

Cerebral hemorrhages or infarctions are found in 60% of eclamptic patients who die within 2 days of the onset of convulsions. The lesions include petechial hemorrhages in the cortex and subcortical region, multiple small areas of ischemic infarction, or a single massive hemorrhage into the white matter. Occasionally, a hemorrhage within the basal ganglia or the pons may rupture into the ventricular system. Varying degrees of cerebral edema have been described, especially when autopsy was performed several days after death. However, Sheehan and Lynch, reporting on 677 patients who died of eclampsia, did not find appreciable cerebral edema if the autopsy was performed soon after death.

Aseptic cerebral venous thrombosis involving the sagittal sinus and veins over the cortical region is most likely to be found in patients who develop seizures more than 6–8 hours after delivery. Massive intracerebral hemorrhage in young primiparas without antecedent hypertensive disease probably results from the intense and prolonged spasm of the cerebral vessels with subsequent loss of integrity of the vessel walls. A significant intracranial hemorrhage should be suspected if a patient continues to have seizures following delivery.

Rational explanation of the seizures is difficult, in view of the fact that eclampsia occurs in less than 5% of patients in subsequent pregnancies, even if they again develop acute hypertension and proteinuria. The cause and effect relationship of the petechial hemorrhages to convulsions is not clear; such hemorrhages may be the result of the severe or prolonged periods of cerebral hypoxia. Increased susceptibility of certain patients, *i.e.,* primigravidas, to seizures has not been explained and is especially puzzling because the hypertension and proteinuria may be less severe in the eclamptic than in the preeclamptic patient.

The rarity of eclampsia more than 12 hours postpartum suggests that whatever induces seizure activity disappears rapidly after delivery. The lack of any neurologic defect following uncomplicated eclampsia supports the concept that vasospasm or a transient metabolic disturbance are factors in the precipitation of convulsions. In contrast, when venous thrombosis is the basis for the seizures, patients apparently suffer significant cortical damage; approximately 50% have periodic seizures that persist indefinitely.

RENAL CHANGES

Renal changes in preeclampsia have been extensively studied by percutaneous renal biopsy, using light and electron microscopy. Capillary loops of the glomeruli show marked edema and narrowing of the capillary lumen. Swelling involves primarily the endothelial cells; the basement membrane and epithelial cells are altered little, if at all (Figs. 25–1 and 25–2). The cells of the mesangium may be swollen and increased in numbers. There is an increase in the number and size of the cells of the juxtaglomerular apparatus; quantitative alteration in the cytoplasmic granules is variable. Cells of the macula densa are small and atrophic. The cytoplasm of the glomerular endothelial cells shows vacuolization and deposition of amorphous material, which is a degradation product of fibrinogen, adjacent to the basement membrane.

There is no direct correlation between the degree of proteinuria and the renal histologic changes in preeclampsia. Proteinuria may occur during pregnancy without the characteristic renal glomerular lesions, but glomerular endotheliosis has not been observed without proteinuria.

Light microscopy studies of renal biopsies in teenage primigravidas show, in addition to the swollen ischemic glomeruli, a 20%–25% incidence of arterial and arteriolar sclerotic changes. These changes have

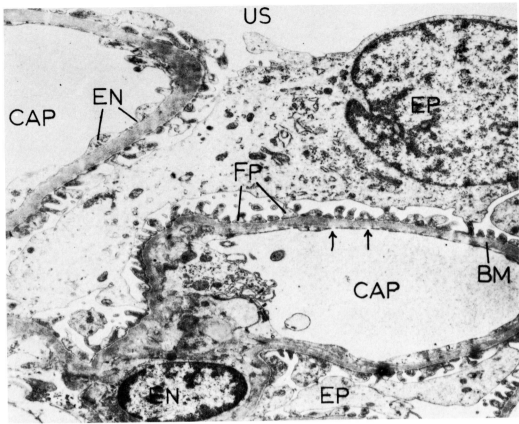

FIG. 25–1. Normal glomerular capillary from 25-year-old man, demonstrating capillary lumen (*CAP*), endothelium (*EN*), basement membrane (*BM*), foot processes (*FP*), epithelium (*EP*), and urinary space (*US*). (×10,000) (Hopper J, Farquhar MG, Yamauchi H, Moon HD, Page EW: Obstet Gynecol 17:271, 1961)

been interpreted as manifestations of vascular disease (Figs. 25–3 through 25–5). Glomerular changes characteristic of preeclampsia–eclampsia are considered reversible, but they may persist if the disease is superimposed upon hypertensive vascular disease.

In the advanced stage of preeclampsia, oliguria may be a prominent and foreboding feature. Urinary output is influenced by hemoconcentration as well as by the decrease in renal perfusion that follows arteriolar vasospasm. With bedrest, some preeclamptic patients have a significant diuresis, a decrease in edema, and a rapid weight loss, despite the persistence of the characteristic histologic findings in the glomerulus.

LIVER CHANGES

The liver is histologically normal in 20%–50% of patients who die of eclampsia. In others, the liver may have irregular, ill-defined, reddish areas of congestion and necrosis in the subcapsular area, particularly in the right lobe. Microscopically, the characteristic changes are hemorrhage and necrosis, beginning in the periportal areas and extending peripherally to involve the liver lobule (Figs. 25–6 and 25–7). Fibrin thrombi associated with extensive thrombosis are present in the capillaries and arterioles, as well as in the smaller branches of the portal vein. Such lesions may be transient. The regenerative capacity of the liver is remarkable, and patients with eclampsia who live longer than 7 days rarely have any demonstrable lesion in the liver.

A rare but catastrophic complication of preeclampsia–eclampsia is spontaneous rupture of the liver (Fig. 25–8). The initial lesion appears to be hemorrhagic necrosis in the subcapsular area; myocardial failure and passive congestion of the liver contribute to the final insult, leading to acute distention and rupture. The inconsistency in the liver lesions and the regenerative capacity of hepatic cells are responsible for the great variability in laboratory studies of hepatic function in preeclampsia.

RETINAL CHANGES

Changes in the retina vary from no demonstrable alteration to narrowing and focal constriction of the arterioles causing a decrease in the arteriovenous ratio. A retinal sheen, ostensibly due to retinal edema, is considered a differentiating feature between preeclampsia and hypertensive vascular disease. The appearance of hemorrhages and exudates in a preeclamptic patient suggests associated hypertensive vascular disease and dictates a poorer prognosis for fetal survival.

Rarely, the vasospastic phenomena and retinal edema may be so severe that the retina becomes de-tached. This is associated with either partial or complete blindness, depending on the extent of the detachment. Unless the retina is detached, visual function and acuity return completely once the preeclamptic process has subsided.

LUNG CHANGES

Pulmonary edema is often a prominent finding in preeclamptic patients, and focal areas of bronchopneumonia are not uncommon. Microscopically, there may be evidence of intravascular coagulation, fibrin

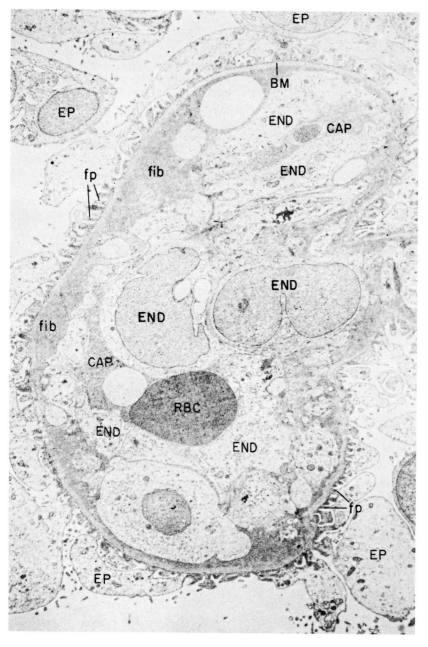

FIG. 25–2. Glomerular loop from patient with preeclampsia. Pronounced swelling has greatly restricted capillary lumen (*CAP*). Fibrinoid (*fib*) is present between endothelium (*END*) and basement membrane (*BM*) (subendothelial) and to some extent between endothelial cells (interendothelial). Epithelial foot processes (*fp*) and basement membrane appear essentially normal. *EP,* epithelium. *RBC,* red blood cell. (×11,500) (Hopper J, Farquhar MG, Yamauchi H, Moon HD, Page EW: Obstet Gynecol 17:271, 1961)

deposition, and hemorrhage into the alveolar spaces. The intravascular coagulation and alveolar hemorrhagic diathesis resemble those associated with endotoxin shock, which suggests that coagulopathy may be a significant feature in both syndromes.

Pulmonary edema may be induced in preeclampsia by overzealous intravenous infusions. Because of the contracted intravascular compartment and borderline myocardial reserve, decompensation may result from too rapid intravenous infusion of even small amounts of fluid.

CARDIAC CHANGES

Cardiac lesions in patients who have died of preeclampsia–eclampsia are usually inconspicuous. Subendocardial hemorrhages on the left side of the interventricular septum, with involvement of the papillary muscles, have been reported in two-thirds of the patients who died within the first 2 days after the onset of eclampsia. Their anatomic relation to the Purkinje fibers may contribute to conduction aberrations and cardiac decompensation.

It is difficult to correlate acute congestive heart failure with the minimal histopathologic lesions in the myocardium. With the combination of hypovolemia, decreased cardiac return, tachycardia, and the autotransfusion that occurs with evacuation of the intrauterine products, decompensation seems to be more plausible than primary cardiac failure. Digitalis is of dubious value in the prevention or treatment of cardiac failure in this situation.

ADRENAL CHANGES

Hemorrhagic necrosis of the adrenals, although pronounced when it occurs, is an inconsistent finding at necropsy. Prolonged administration of high doses of glucocorticoids may produce a similar picture. It seems likely that the stress reaction may precipitate the adrenal lesion (Figs. 25–9 and 25–10).

PLACENTAL CHANGES

The weight of the placenta in preeclampsia is not statistically different from that in normal pregnancy. There is no specific histopathologic finding, but some types of lesions are more numerous and extensive in the placentas of preeclamptic patients.

FIG. 25-3. Normal glomerulus. (PAS, ×280)

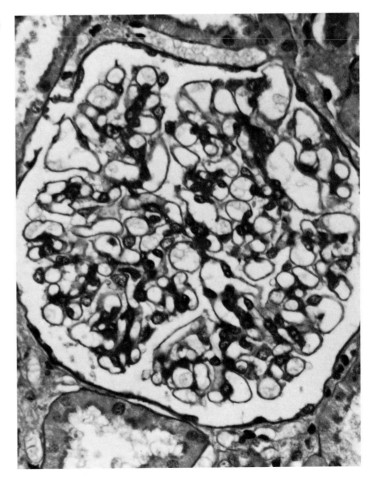

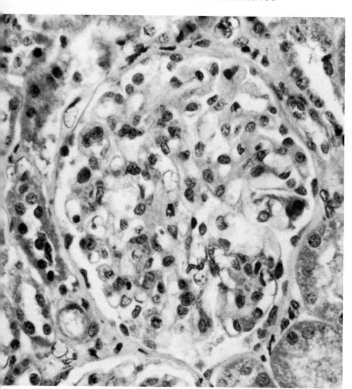

FIG. 25-4. Glomerulus from patient with preeclampsia and hydatidiform mole. Note avascularity due to swelling of endothelial cells of capillary loops. (H&E, ×280)

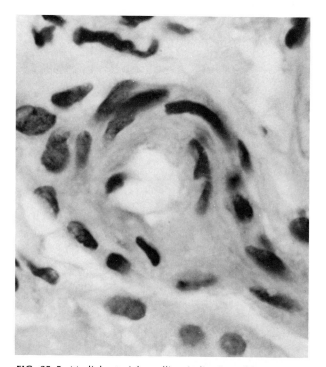

FIG. 25-5. Medial arterial swelling indicative of hypertensive vascular disease in renal tissue from teenage primipara with clinical diagnosis of preeclampsia. (H&E, ×400)

The most common and consistent abnormality in the placenta is the presence of infarcts which are red and soft in consistency, indicating recent origin, or white, a sign of long-standing compromise of the circulation. In about 60% of normal patients the placenta also shows infarcts. Red infarcts are presumed to be due to vascular obstruction with subsequent necrosis. White infarcts are associated with intervillous deposits of fibrin. Syncytial knots and retroplacental hematomas are also more common.

Microscopic studies of the preeclamptic placenta show an increase of immature trophoblasts and degenerative changes in other trophoblastic cells. There may be a loss of syncytium, thickening of the trophoblastic basement membrane, villus necrosis, and acute fibrinoid degeneration of the maternal decidual arteries. Marked congestion of the vasculature of the villus is a prominent feature. Such changes are also observed in normal placentas, however, and are probably a reflection of the normal aging process.

In normal placentation, cytotrophoblasts disrupt the normal architecture of the spiral arteries in the decidua and myometrium, and these vessels lose their musculoelastic tissue. In pregnancy-induced hypertension, the myometrial segments of the uteroplacental arterioles are not invaded by cytotrophoblasts, and these vessels retain their musculoelastic tissue. It is

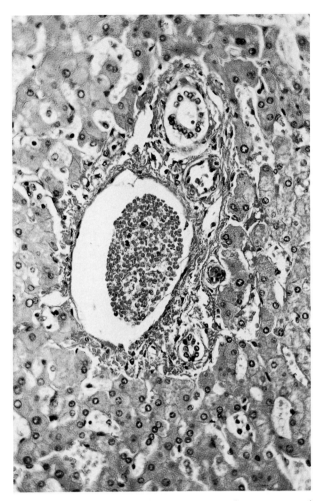

FIG. 25-6. Normal liver, demonstrating portal structures and periportal lobular architecture. (H&E, ×185)

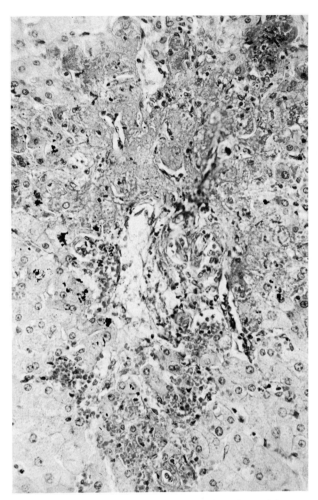

FIG. 25-7. Liver in eclampsia. Note sharply delimited hemorrhagic periportal liver cell necrosis and disruption of normal portal architecture. (H&E, ×185)

presumed they are then prone to develop a necrotizing arteriopathy. Lipid accumulation and median necrosis are early changes, whereas massive intramural fibrin deposition occurs as a secondary event. When preeclampsia is superimposed on chronic hypertension, the placental arteries show a combination of hyperplastic arteriosclerosis and acute atherosclerosis.

HORMONAL CHANGES

Plasma renin activity, and the levels of renin substrate, angiotensinogin, angiotensin II, angiotensinase, plasma aldosterone, and progesterone all increase in normotensive women during pregnancy. In preeclampsia, renin activity, aldosterone levels, and angiotensinase activity may be suppressed to levels below those of normal pregnancy. There is no difference in renin substrate levels, progesterone, cortisol, corticosterone, and antidiuretic hormone (ADH) levels between women who are normotensive and those who have preeclampsia. Urinary levels of epinephrine and norepinephrine have been found to be increased in preeclamptic patients.

The blood pressure rise that follows infusion of angiotensin II is accentuated in preeclamptic patients, and this increased response precedes the clinical manifestations of the syndrome. Angiotensin II levels are at nearly twice the prepregnant level both in normal and preeclamptic pregnancy. Since the responsiveness to angiotensin II is increased in preeclampsia, however,

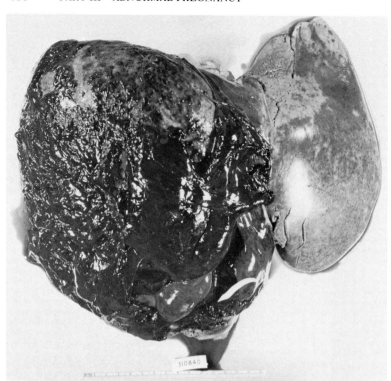

FIG. 25–8. Liver in severe preeclampsia, showing spontaneous rupture with hemorrhage.

this hormone may have a role in the vasoconstriction that is characteristic of preeclampsia.

VASCULAR REACTIVITY

It has been reported that blood from preeclamptic patients has no pressor effect when infused into normal women; but, when it is autotransfused 6 days postpartum into patients with recent preeclampsia, a rise in blood pressure results. These findings suggest that the plasma of preeclamptic women contains a pressor substance, an antagonist to a depressor substance, or a substance that activates pressor agents. The explanation of the increased vascular reactivity is speculative. Prostaglandins have been suggested as the chemical substances that counteract the effects of the angiotensin II on the vascular wall and thereby may modify vascular reactivity.

BLOOD VOLUME

A decrease in blood volume can be demonstrated in pregnant women with preeclampsia, but its hemodynamic significance is not known. It has been considered by some to have an etiologic role, and others believe it a secondary phenomenon due to contraction of the vascular bed.

INTRAVASCULAR COAGULATION

DIC is largely responsible for the glomerular endotheliosis and the widespread microscopic platelet and fibrin thrombi that are characteristic of severe preeclampsia–eclampsia. Low-grade intravascular coagulation may lead to the appearance of fibrinogen degradation products in the urine. Local deposition of fibrin is associated with the typical glomerular lesion that invariably leads to proteinuria. The platelet and fibrin thrombi produced by high-grade or accelerated DIC give rise to perivascular hemorrhage and necrosis in the brain, pituitary, kidneys, placenta, and other viscera and soft tissues.

It has been proposed that an abnormality in the placenta from whatever cause may lead to release of trophoblastic tissue into the circulation. This is a normal occurrence, but 20 times as many trophoblastic fragments are found in the uterine vessels in preeclampsia as in normal pregnancy. This tissue may be the trigger for intravascular coagulation, since trophoblasts have a higher thromboplastin content than any other tissue in the body. The more severe form of DIC occurs in complications of preeclampsia such as abruptio placentae, in which intravascular coagulation is of such magnitude that it results in a hemorrhagic diathesis that is potentially fatal.

Some degree of intravascular coagulation should be suspected in all cases of preeclampsia. As noted in

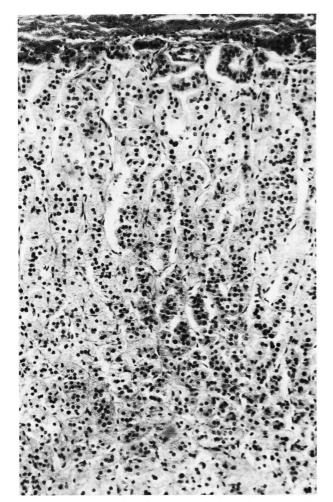

FIG. 25-9. Normal adrenal cortex, including adrenal capsule, zona glomerulosa, and zona fasciculata. (H&E, ×125)

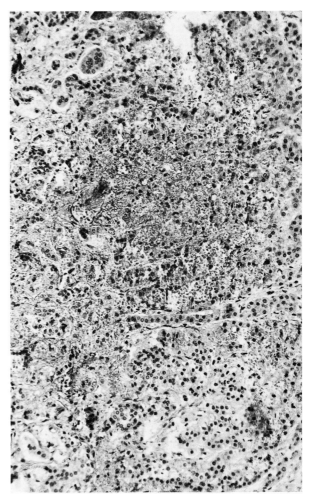

FIG. 25-10. Adrenal in eclampsia. Note focal hemorrhagic necrosis in zona glomerulosa and zona fasciculata. (H&E, ×125)

Chapter 37, routine coagulation tests are used to diagnose DIC, as well as to assess its severity and to follow its course. The activated partial thromboplastin time is one of the most sensitive screening tests for early DIC. The prothrombin time is also very useful. The degree to which these clotting tests show elevations roughly reflects the degree to which clotting factors have been consumed in DIC. The two most rapidly consumed are Factors V and VIII; however, in DIC essentially all clotting proteins decrease in concentration. The platelet count and fibrinogen levels, which also fall, correlate with the rate of DIC. As important as the absolute levels of platelets and fibrinogen is a change in their concentration over time. Fibrinogen and, possibly, platelets are increased in normal pregnancy, and a value in the normal range would actually be low for the pregnant patient. The level of fibrin degradation products is elevated in DIC, but these products may also be

detectable normally at term. In normal pregnancy, however, they are rarely higher than 40 mg/ml.

The thrombin time may be elevated because of low levels of fibrinogen, because of fibrin degradation products or because of heparin. Specific assays for fibrinogen and such degradation products should replace the thrombin time in evaluation of DIC. Factor assays support the diagnosis of DIC, but they are expensive and have limited availability.

DIAGNOSIS OF PREECLAMPSIA

SIGNS AND SYMPTOMS

Onset of hypertension and proteinuria in any patient in the third trimester of pregnancy establishes the diagnosis of preeclampsia. Usually, edema is also

found, but if the onset is acute and fulminating, there may be insufficient time for edema to develop. The additional presence of any of the following is indicative that the process is severe and that eclampsia may be imminent:

1. A sharp increase in blood pressure
2. Marked hyperreflexia and, especially, transient or sustained ankle clonus
3. Epigastric pain
4. Scotomata and other visual disturbances
5. A quantitative increase in proteinuria
6. Oliguria, with urinary output of less than 30 ml/hour
7. Drowsiness or severe headache

LABORATORY STUDIES

Laboratory studies are more helpful in assessing the severity of preeclampsia than in the diagnosis of the syndrome. The tests of interest are listed in Table 25–1.

Weight loss and diuresis indicate the mobilization of fluid, and if the syndrome is in the early stages, weight loss generally is accompanied by a decrease in blood pressure. These may be misleading signs of improvement, since the pathophysiologic changes may be irreversible and the fetus may continue to be in jeopardy. An elevated hematocrit value implies hemoconcentra-

tion, with fluid shift from the intravascular to the extracellular compartment. Such a hemoconcentration can reduce the circulating blood volume by as much as 1000 ml. A decline in hematocrit value, implying mobilization of excess extracellular fluid, suggests improvement. The level of blood urea nitrogen is rarely elevated above normal pregnancy levels (N<10 mg/dl) except in patients with intrinsic renal disease; this test may therefore be helpful in the differential diagnosis. Elevation in the uric acid level supports a diagnosis of preeclampsia. Plasma uric acid levels do not rise in patients with chronic hypertension and therefore may be useful in differentiating chronic hypertension from acute pregnancy-induced hypertension. There is a close relationship between uric acid levels and fetal outcome, regardless of the level of the blood pressure. Thiazide diuretics cause significant increases in uric acid, and the test is not helpful if these drugs have been used.

PREDICTION OF PREECLAMPSIA

Gant and associates suggested that it may be possible to predict the women who will later develop preeclampsia. In their series, more than 93% of normotensive nulliparous women who later developed pregnancy-induced hypertension showed an elevation in diastolic blood pressure of at least 20 mm Hg when turned from the lateral recumbent to the supine position between the 28th and 32nd weeks of pregnancy. Moreover, the same women showed an increased sensitivity to the infusion of angiotensin II. Conversely, 91% of those who remained normotensive had no rise in diastolic pressure with the change in position. Subsequent evaluations of the supine pressor test suggest that its accuracy may be less than originally presumed; however, positive correlations occur with sufficient frequency that the test can be helpful in identifying some of the women who are at risk.

In normotensive women, the metabolic clearance rate of dehydroepiandrosterone sulfate increases in a linear fashion throughout pregnancy. For gravidas who develop pregnancy-induced hypertension, the clearance rate decreases, beginning about 4 weeks prior to the onset of clinical symptoms. These changes support the concept that acute hypertension of pregnancy is a late consequence of multiple physiologic and metabolic alterations.

DIFFERENTIAL DIAGNOSIS

Of all patients with hypertensive vascular disease who become pregnant, approximately one-third develop superimposed preeclampsia and one-third have no change from prepregnancy blood pressure levels.

TABLE 25–1. LABORATORY DETERMINATIONS USED TO ASSESS COURSE OF PREECLAMPSIA*

Determination	Stage of Preeclampsia		
	Early	Severe	Improving
BLOOD OR SERUM			
Hematocrit	0/↑	↑	↓
Hemoglobin	0/↑	↑	↓
Na⁺ (mEq/liter)	0/↓	↓	↑
K⁺ (mEq/liter)	0	0/↓	0
Cl⁻ (mEq/liter)	0	↓	↑
CO₂ (combining power)	0	0/↓	0/↑
BUN (mg/100 ml)	0	0/↑	0/↓
Uric acid (mg/100 ml)	0	0/↑	0/↓
Total protein	0	0/↓	0/↑
Fibrinogen	0/↑	0/↑	↓
SGOT	0	0/↑	0/↓
URINE			
Volume/24 hr	0/↓	↓	↑
Protein/24 hr	0	↑	↓
Specific gravity	0	↑	↓
Na⁺/24 hr	0/↓	↓	↑
K⁺/24 hr	0/↓	↓	↑
Cl⁻/24 hr	0/↓	↓	↑
Uric acid/24hr	0	0/↓	0/↑

* Arrows indicate increase or decrease

Paradoxically, the remainder become normotensive as the pregnancy progresses beyond 3 months and remain normotensive until after delivery. It has been suggested that a midtrimester decrease indicates a favorable prognosis. Since preeclampsia is extremely rare in the first 6 months of pregnancy (except in the presence of hydatidiform mole), hypertension in the first and second trimesters is most likely essential hypertension. If the patient is first seen in the third trimester, the distinction may be difficult. In preeclampsia, the blood pressure rise usually is first noted after 32 weeks' gestation; in hypertensive vascular disease, the elevation is present earlier and the hypertension more severe. In chronic hypertension, there is little or no proteinuria, and uric acid tends to be normal; retinal changes, if present, may include vascular narrowing, hemorrhages, and exudates. After delivery, the preeclamptic syndrome abates promptly, whereas chronic hypertension persists, even though the blood pressure may decrease gradually.

Chronic Renal Disease

Patients with significant renal disease may demonstrate proteinuria with or without hypertension during their first prenatal examination. The blood urea nitrogen level may be elevated above levels characteristic for normal pregnancy whereas it tends to be normal in preeclampsia. A history of an undiagnosed or a vague disease process treated by prolonged bedrest when the patient was a child may be a clue to the diagnosis of glomerulonephritis. Lupus nephritis is a cause of proteinuria, but it is usually diagnosed prior to the onset of pregnancy and therefore seldom causes a problem in the differential diagnosis of proteinuria.

Chronic pyelonephritis, which ordinarily is not associated with significant proteinuria, should be suspected in the patient with a history of repeated cystitis or dysuria. Urine cultures should be obtained to exclude active infection. Renal disease associated with hypertensive vascular disease rarely is a cause of proteinuria and is more common in the multipara than in the primipara. It occurs more frequently in older patients and those with recurrent preeclampsia.

Other Causes of Hypertension

Coarctation of the aorta, occlusive renal artery lesions, and endocrine causes of high blood pressure are rare but may need to be differentiated from preeclampsia. *Pheochromocytoma*, an unusual cause of hypertension, is important primarily because of the high maternal and fetal mortality associated with it. Paroxysmal attacks of hypertension, severe pulsating headache, profuse sweating, elevation of body temperature, precordial or abdominal pain, palpitations, but no proteinuria suggest the possibility of this lesion.

Other Causes of Coma or Convulsions

After eclampsia, cerebral hemorrhage is the most common cause of coma and convulsions in pregnancy. Other causes to be ruled out include epilepsy, hypoglycemia secondary to insulin, and a toxic response to regional or local anesthetic agents.

TREATMENT

GENERAL PRINCIPLES

Whether or not preeclampsia may be preventable has not been documented to date by a prospective well-controlled study. If preeclampsia is recognized and treated early, it is possible to prevent eclampsia. Regardless of severity, delivery is the only definitive treatment of preeclampsia. Hence, this is the treatment of choice for any preeclamptic patient whose pregnancy is of more than 37 weeks' duration and for any patient with severe preeclampsia, regardless of the duration of pregnancy. Even if gestation is less than 37 weeks, it is futile and hazardous, unless the disease is extremely mild, to postpone delivery in the hope of allowing the baby to mature. The baby rarely gains significantly under such circumstances, and, of more importance, the single hazard of preterm delivery is far outweighed by the many and sometimes fatal dangers of preeclampsia and its sequelae.

In mild preeclampsia, bedrest in the lateral recumbent position, without other medication, produces a measurable increase in glomerular filtration, and the resulting diuresis can mobilize considerable quantities of water from the tissues. Salt restriction and diuretics, notably thiazides, were for many years regarded as the keystone of therapy for preeclampsia. Evidence has now been presented to suggest that they not only are ineffective but also may be harmful by disrupting optimal electrolyte patterns, causing the accumulation of purine metabolites, impairing placental production of estrogens, and impeding the normal expansion of the vascular volume. Sodium and water retention are part of the total picture of preeclampsia; but, according to modern thought, they should be dealt with by bedrest, especially in the lateral recumbent position, rather than by severe sodium restriction and diuretics. Salt intake of up to 6 g/day can be continued without hazard. The signs and symptoms of the syndrome may be accelerated by excessive salt intake, however, and foods that are especially high in sodium should be avoided.

Magnesium Sulfate. Magnesium sulfate is recognized as the safest and most efficacious drug in the treatment of severe preeclampsia and eclampsia. Magnesium sulfate reduces neuromuscular irritability and

acts peripherally on the vascular system to improve uterine blood supply by vasodilation. It also has tocolytic effects, but these are not to be considered when the drug is needed in the management of preeclampsia. Pritchard's protocol for its use in severe preeclampsia or eclampsia is 20 ml 20% magnesium sulfate (prepared by mixing in a syringe 8 ml 50% solution with 12 ml sterile distilled water), equivalent to 4 g, given intravenously, *slowly,* over the course of *at least* 3 minutes; this is followed immediately by 10 ml 50% magnesium sulfate in *each* buttock (total 10 g), using a 3-inch 20 gauge needle. Thereafter, 10 ml 50% solution is given deeply, intramuscularly, every 4 hours, alternating buttocks (in the conscious patient, 1 ml 2% lidocaine is drawn into the loaded syringe). It is emphasized that repeat injections are given only if the knee jerks are present, if the urine output (as measured by Foley catheter) exceeds 100 ml for the previous 4 hours, and if respirations are not depressed.

The therapeutic level of serum magnesium is 6–8 mg/dl. At levels above 10 mg/dl the knee jerks disappear, at about 16 mg/dl respirations are depressed, and at 30 mg/dl the heart stops in diastole. Urinary output should be monitored closely; if it is low, the blood concentrations can reach dangerous levels. It is of vital importance that the knee, biceps, and ankle jerks be tested before and after each injection and that calcium gluconate, which is an instant antidote, be available in ampules (10 ml 10% solution) for intravenous use.

Sedatives may be important to enforce bedrest. Phenobarbital is the standard agent, in doses of 0.06 g by mouth every 6 hours while awake. If this produces too heavy sedation, the dose may be reduced. It should be noted that phenobarbital may reduce cerebral blood flow. In eclampsia and certain cases of severe preeclampsia heavy sedation with morphine (0.015 g every 4–6 hours) may be needed; morphine, however, and also barbiturates, must be used with care if delivery is anticipated within 6 hours, for the baby will be depressed.

Antihypertensive Agents. The use of *antihypertensive agents* in the treatment of pregnancy-induced hypertension has been extensively studied both before and during labor. They were once thought to have great promise in the management of preeclampsia, but it is now clear that they do not affect the underlying mechanisms of the disease. They do not increase fetal survival and, although they may decrease the incidence of cerebral vascular accidents, antihypertensive agents are of little value in preventing maternal death. They are usually recommended if blood pressure levels are consistently high (greater than 100 mm Hg diastolic). Hydralazine hydrochloride, 5 mg, is administered intravenously and blood pressure monitored every 5 min-

utes for 20 minutes, after which 5 mg is again given if desired levels of 90–100 mm Hg diastolic are not achieved. Monitoring every 5 minutes and repeat doses every 20 minutes are continued as needed. Five to 20 mg are usually sufficient for the desired effect.

REGIMENS

The following regimens are suggested for the different stages and degrees of preeclampsia.

Mild Preeclampsia. All patients with preeclampsia should be hospitalized. For the patient with mild disease, the following therapeutic regimen is suggested:

1. Bedrest with bathroom privileges
2. Daily weighing
3. Evaluation of fetal heart tones every 4 hours
4. Phenobarbital, 30–60 mg every 6 hours while awake
5. Well-balanced diet with salt content up to 6 g/day
6. Evaluation of fetal maturity, favorability of cervix, and adequacy of maternal pelvis in anticipation of possible urgent delivery
7. Delivery by 37 weeks' gestation with or without improvement; prior to 37 weeks, need for delivery must be weighed against hazard of preterm birth

Severe Preeclampsia. For the patient with severe preeclampsia, the regimen includes the following:

1. Close observation
2. Absolute bedrest in quiet surroundings
3. Magnesium sulfate, as outlined earlier, with due attention to the listed precautions
4. Hydralazine hydrochloride, as outlined earlier, if diastolic pressure is 100 mm Hg or higher
5. Determination of fluid intake and output
6. Continuous fetal monitoring until delivery
7. Delivery after stabilization

Eclampsia. For the patient with eclampsia, the regimen is as follows:

1. Constant observation
2. Absolute quiet, in a darkened room
3. Hourly determination of urinary output and monitoring of fetal heart tones
4. Immediate availability of equipment to maintain airway and prevent trauma to tongue and lips during a seizure
5. Magnesium sulfate, as outlined earlier, with calcium gluconate available as an antidote for magnesium overdosage evidenced by loss of deep reflexes
6. Hydralazine hydrochloride, as outlined earlier, if diastolic pressure is 100 mm Hg or higher

7. Sodium diphenylhydantoin intravenously if seizures persist
8. Delivery when seizures are controlled

DELIVERY

As in other circumstances in which it is determined that delivery should be performed before the spontaneous onset of labor, the first decision to be made is *when* to deliver; the second decision is *how, i.e.,* by induction of labor or by cesarean section. Vaginal delivery is preferable, and even if the cervix is unfavorable, patients with preeclampsia–eclampsia usually respond to uterine stimulation and artificial rupture of membranes; cesarean section is necessary only rarely. Of a series of patients with eclampsia in our institution, the convulsions began during labor in one-third of the patients and immediately after delivery in another one-third. Hence, labor and delivery are extremely hazardous, and special vigilance is needed at these critical periods. Cesarean section should be elected if active labor is not established within 6 hours of the start of induction or if electronic monitoring shows evidence of fetal distress that necessitates immediate delivery. Regardless of the method of delivery, it must be remembered that hypovolemia, often of considerable proportion, is a prominent feature of this disease and that hypovolemic shock can result from degrees of blood loss that would be well tolerated without this complication.

There is little agreement regarding the anesthetic of choice for vaginal delivery or cesarean section. The expertise of those administering the anesthesia and their knowledge of the physiologic changes that occur in preeclampsia are more important than the specific agent used. Because of the unpredictable blood pressure responses that may occur when conduction anesthesia is used, other methods are generally preferred. Maintenance of adequate tissue perfusion is of prime importance, whatever method is selected.

POSTPARTUM VASOMOTOR COLLAPSE

Postpartum vasomotor collapse is a rare, dramatic, and potentially fatal reaction, that may occur 30 min to 24 hours after delivery in patients with severe preeclampsia, and should be considered in any preeclamptic patient who lapses into shock and coma within this time interval. The clinical and laboratory findings are similar to those of acute adrenal failure. Serum sodium values of 115–125 mEq/liter are common in this syndrome. If shock due to blood loss or sepsis can be excluded, treatment should consist of the immediate infusion of 300 ml 5% solution of sodium chloride within a 30-min period. Hydrocortisone 100 mg, or its equivalent, should also be given at once, intravenously, and repeated at 6-hour intervals for 24 hours. The response is usually prompt and dramatic.

PROGNOSIS

MATERNAL PROGNOSIS

Data as to the rate of recurrence of hypertension in subsequent pregnancies are conflicting and may be affected by such factors as the level of the blood pressure, the duration of preeclampsia, the parity of the patient, and the time of onset of the disorder. As a general rule, preeclampsia does not recur in later pregnancies unless there is a predisposing factor, such as essential hypertension or diabetes mellitus.

Preeclampsia and eclampsia apparently do not significantly affect the overall perinatal mortality rate in subsequent pregnancies. It has been reported that women who have had eclampsia in one pregnancy have a higher instance of intrauterine growth retardation in following pregnancies and that these pregnancies often end prior to term.

White eclamptic primiparas have no greater risk of developing hypertensive cardiovascular disease than does the general population. In contrast, black primiparas and both black and white multiparas have a higher age-adjusted mortality rate than does the general population. Thus, it appears that eclampsia does not itself cause subsequent chronic hypertension, but it may be a manifestation of a tendency toward it in the multiparous patient.

The later occurrence of diabetes in women who have had eclampsia appears to be five to ten times the expected frequency. The reason for this association is not known, especially since patients with severe preeclampsia may have lower fasting glucose levels than those of patients with uncomplicated pregnancies.

Preeclampsia is one of the leading causes of death among obstetric patients, ranking in most states immediately after sepsis. The mortality rate can be reduced dramatically by proper prenatal care and the meticulous management of preeclampsia and its complications. The prognosis therefore varies not only according to the severity of the disease, but also according to the availability and the quality of obstetric care.

It now seems clear that preeclampsia, regardless of severity, is a completely reversible disease that does not produce chronic hypertension, chronic renal disease, or any other sequela. From an extensive experience, Chesley concluded that, among patients with severe preeclampsia in whom hypertension persists at follow-up examination, hypertensive vascular disease either existed before the pregnancy or would have developed regardless of the pregnancy.

INFANT PROGNOSIS

While there has been significant reduction in maternal mortality from preeclampsia, perinatal mortality has not decreased proportionately. Of equal importance is the effect of preeclampsia on the subsequent physical and mental health of the baby who survives; there is a correlation between the severity of preeclampsia and the postnatal fate of the baby. A frequently quoted aphorism continues to be applicable even in this day and time, "There comes a time when the intrauterine passenger is safer in the nursery than in the uterus."

REFERENCES AND RECOMMENDED READING

GENERAL

Chesley LC: Historical developments. In Friedman EA (ed): Blood Pressure, Edema, and Proteinuria in Pregnancy, pp 19–66. New York, Alan R Liss, 1976
Gant NF (ed): Pregnancy-induced hypertension. Semin Perinatol, 1978
Sims EAH: Preeclampsia and related complications of pregnancy. Am J Obstet Gynecol 107:154, 1970
Studd J: Preeclampsia. Br J Hosp Med 18:52, 1977

CLASSIFICATION

Chesley L: Proposal for classification. In Friedman EA (ed): Blood Pressure, Edema, and Proteinuria in Pregnancy, pp 249–268. New York, Alan R Liss, 1976
Hughes EC (ed): Obstetric Gynecologic Terminology. Prepared by the Committee on Terminology of the American College of Obstetricians and Gynecologists. Philadelphia, Davis, 1972
Welt SI, Crenshaw MC, Jr: Concurrent hypertension and pregnancy. Clin Obstet Gynecol 21:619, 1978

INCIDENCE AND RISK FACTORS

Baird D: Epidemiological aspects of hypertensive pregnancy. In Symonds EM (ed): Clinics in Obstetrics and Gynaecology, pp 531–548. Philadelphia, WB Saunders, 1977
Davies AM: Epidemiologic aspects. In Friedman EA (ed): Blood Pressure, Edema, and Proteinuria in Pregnancy, pp 67–86. New York, Alan R Liss, 1976
National Center for Health Statistics. Monthly Vital Statistics Report, 1976. Final Mortality Statistics: 1978.
Vollman RF: Study design, population and data characteristics. In Friedman EA (ed): Blood Pressure, Edema, and Proteinuria in Pregnancy, pp 89–121. New York, Alan R Liss, 1976

ETIOLOGY

Beller FK, Schmidt EH: Local and systemic coagulation properties in hypertensive disorders in pregnancy. In Symonds EM (ed): Clinics in Obstetrics and Gynaecology, pp 563–571. Philadelphia, WB Saunders, 1977
Hodari AA, Bumpus FM, Smeby R: Renin in experimental "toxemia of pregnancy." Obstet Gynecol 30:8, 1967
Jeffcoate TNA: Pre-eclampsia and eclampsia: The disease of theories. Proc R Soc Med 59:397, 1966
Kitzmiller JL: Immunologic approaches to the study of preeclampsia. Clin Obstet Gynecol 20:717, 1977
Page EW: On the pathogenesis of preeclampsia and eclampsia. J Obstet Gynaecol Br Commonw 49:883, 1971
Scott JR, Beer AE: Immunologic aspects of pre-eclampsia. Am J Obstet Gynecol 125:418, 1976
Scott JR, Beer AE, Stastny P: Immunogenetic factors in pre-eclampsia and eclampsia: Erythrocyte, histocompatibility and y-dependent antigens. JAMA 235:402, 1976
Speroff L, Dorfman GS: Prostaglandins and pregnancy hypertension. In Symonds EM (ed): Clinics in Obstetrics and Gynaecology, pp 635–649. Philadelphia, WB Saunders, 1977
Willems J: Etiology of preeclampsia. Obstet Gynecol 50:495, 1977

CLINICAL COURSE: CORRELATION WITH PATHOPHYSIOLOGY

DeAlvarez RR: Proteinuria relationships. In Friedman EA (ed): Blood Pressure, Edema, and Proteinuria in Pregnancy, pp 169–192. New York, Alan R Liss, 1976
Ehrlich EN, Lindheimer MD: Sodium metabolism, aldosterone and the hypertensive disorders of pregnancy. J Reprod Med 8:106, 1971
Fisher KA, Ahuja S, Luger A et al: Nephrotic proteinuria with pre-eclampsia. Am J Obstet Gynecol 129:643, 1977
Friedman EA: Blood pressure relationships. In Friedman EA (ed): Blood pressure, Edema, and Proteinuria, pp 123–155. New York, Alan R Liss, 1976
Friedman EA, Neff RK: Pregnancy outcome as related to hypertension, edema and proteinuria. In Lindheimer MD, Katz AI, Zuspan FP (eds): Hypertension in Pregnancy, pp 13–22. New York, John Wiley, 1976
Kitzmiller JL, Benirschke K: Immunofluorescent study of placental bed vessels in pre-eclampsia. Am J Obstet Gynecol 115:248, 1973
Lopez–Llera M, Linares GR: Factors that influence maternal mortality in eclampsia. In Lindheimer MD, Katz AI, Zuspan FP (eds): Hypertension in Pregnancy, pp 41–50. New York, John Wiley, 1976
Naeye RL, Friedman EA: Causes of perinatal death associated with gestational hypertension and proteinuria. Am J Obstet Gynecol 133:8, 1979
Page EW, Christianson R: The impact of mean arterial pressure in the middle trimester upon the outcome of pregnancy. Am J Obstet Gynecol 125:740, 1976
Page EW, Christianson R: Influence of blood pressure changes with and without proteinuria upon outcome of pregnancy. Am J Obstet Gynecol 126:821, 1976
Pritchard JA, Cunningham FG, Mason RA: Coagulation changes in eclampsia: Their frequency and pathogenesis. Am J Obstet Gynecol 124:855, 1976
Redman CWG, Beilin LJ, Bonnar J: Variability of blood pressure in normal and abnormal pregnancy. In Lindheimer MD, Katz AI, Zuspan FP (eds): Hypertension in Pregnancy, pp 53–60. New York, John Wiley, 1976
Sellmann AH: Edema-plus-proteinuria relationships. In Friedman EA (ed): Blood Pressure, Edema, and Proteinuria in Pregnancy, pp 193–214. New York, Alan R Liss, 1976
Sullivan JM: Blood pressure elevation in pregnancy. Prog Cardiovasc Dis 16:375, 1974
Terragno NA, Terragno DA, McGiff JC: The role of prosta-

glandins in the control of uterine blood flow. In Lindheimer MD, Katz AI, Zuspan FP (eds): Hypertension in Pregnancy, pp 391–398. New York, John Wiley, 1976

Vosburgh GJ: Edema relationships. In Friedman EA (ed): Blood Pressure, Edema, and Proteinuria in Pregnancy, pp 155–168. New York, Alan R Liss, 1976

Wood SM, Burnett D, Studd J: Selectivity of proteinuria during pregnancy assessed by different methods. Perspect Nephrol Hypertens 5:75, 1976

ANATOMIC PATHOLOGY AND PATHOPHYSIOLOGIC ALTERATIONS

Assali NS, Vaughn DL: Blood volume in pre-eclampsia: Fantasy and reality. Am J Obstet Gynecol 129:355, 1977

Dennis EJ, McIver FA, Smythe CM: Renal biopsy in pregnancy. Clin Obstet Gynecol 11:473, 1968

Dennis EJ, Smythe CM, McIver FA et al: Percutaneous renal biopsy in eclampsia. Am J Obstet Gynecol 87:364, 1963

Elebute OA, Mills IH: Urinary kallikrein in normal and hypertensive pregnancies. In Lindheimer MD, Katz AI, Zuspan FP (eds): Hypertension in Pregnancy, pp 329–338. New York, John Wiley, 1976

Gant N, Chand S, Cunningham SG et al: Control of vascular reactivity to angiotensin II in human pregnancy. In Lindheimer MD, Katz AI, Zuspan FP (eds): Hypertension in Pregnancy, pp 377–390. New York, John Wiley, 1976

Gant NF, Worley RJ, MacDonald PC: The clearance rate of maternal plasma prehormones of placental estrogen formation. In Lindheimer MD, Katz AI, Zuspan FP (eds): Hypertension in Pregnancy, pp 309–314. New York, John Wiley, 1976

Howie PW: The haemostatic mechanisms in pre-eclampsia. In Symonds EM (ed): Clinics in Obstetrics and Gynaecology, pp 595–611. Philadelphia, WB Saunders, 1977

Ingersley M, Teilum G: Biopsy studies on liver in pregnancy. Acta Obstet Gynecol Scand 25:339, 1945

Kitzmiller JL, Captain JEL, Yelenosky PF et al: Hematologic assays in pre-eclampsia. Am J Obstet Gynecol 118:362, 1974

McCall ML: Circulation of the brain in toxemia. Clin Obstet Gynecol 1:333, 1958

McCartney CP: Pathological anatomy of acute hypertension of pregnancy. Circulation 30 (Suppl 2):37, 1964

Pipkin FB, Symonds EM: The renin–angiotensin system in the maternal and fetal circulation in pregnancy hypertension. In Symonds EM (ed): Clinics in Obstetrics and Gynaecology, pp 651–664. Philadelphia, WB Saunders, 1977

Robertson WB, Brosens I, Dixon G: Maternal uterine vascular lesions in the hypertensive complications of pregnancy. In Lindheimer MD, Katz AI, Zuspan FP (eds): Hypertension in Pregnancy, pp 115–127. New York, John Wiley, 1976

Robson JS: Proteinuria and the renal lesion in preeclampsia and abruptio placentae. In Lindheimer MD, Katz AI, Zuspan FP (eds): Hypertension in Pregnancy, pp 61–74. New York, John Wiley, 1976

Sheehan HL: Pathological Lesions in the Hypertensive Toxaemias of Pregnancy. In Ciba Foundation Symposium. London, Churchill, 1950

Sheehan HL, Lynch JB: Pathology of Toxaemia of Pregnancy. London, Churchill Livingstone, 1973

Smythe CM, Bradham WS, Dennis EJ et al: Renal arteriolar disease in young primiparas. J Lab Clin Med 61:562, 1964

Spargo BH, Lichtig C, Luger AM et al: The renal lesion in preeclampsia. In Lindheimer MD, Katz AI, Zuspan FP (eds): Hypertension in Pregnancy, pp 129–138. New York, John Wiley, 1976

Symonds EM, Pipkin FB: Pregnancy hypertension, parity, and the renin–angiotensin system. Am J Obstet Gynecol 132:473, 1978

Tapia HR, Johnson CE, Strong CG: Renin–angiotensin system in normal and hypertensive disease of pregnancy, Lancet 2:847, 1972

Weir RJ, Fraser R, Lever AF et al: Plasma renin, renin substrate, angiotensin II, and aldosterone in hypertensive disease of pregnancy. Lancet 1:291, 1973

Zuspan FP, Kawada C: Urine amine excretion in pregnancy-induced hypertension. In Lindheimer MD, Katz AI, Zuspan FP (eds): Hypertension in Pregnancy, pp 339–348. New York, John Wiley, 1976

DIAGNOSIS OF PREECLAMPSIA

Beller FK, Dame WR, Intorp HW, Loew H, Schiffer HP: Renal disease in pregnancy. Am J Obstet Gynecol 126:845, 1976

Gant NF, Chand S, Worley RJ et al: A clinical test useful for predicting the development of acute hypertension in pregnancy. Am J Obstet Gynecol 120:1, 1974

Gusdon JP, Anderson SG, May WJ: A clinical evaluation of the "roll-over test" for pregnancy-induced hypertension. Am J Obstet Gynecol 127:1, 1977

Lindheimer MD, Spargo BH, Katz AI: Eclampsia during the sixteenth week of gestation. JAMA 230:1006, 1974

Phelan JP, Everidge GJ, Wilder TL et al: Is the supine pressor test an adequate means of predicting acute hypertension in pregnancy? Am J Obstet Gynecol 128:173, 1977

Redman CWG, Williams GF, Jones DD et al: Plasma urate and screen deoxycytidylate deaminase measurements for the early diagnoses of preeclampsia. Br J Obstet Gynaecol 84:904, 1977

Wood SM: Assessment of renal functions in hypertensive pregnancies. In Symonds EM (ed): Clinics in Obstetrics and Gynaecology, pp 747–758. Philadelphia, WB Saunders, 1977

Zuspan FP, Talledo OE: Factors affecting delivery in eclampsia: The condition of the cervix and uterine activity. Am J Obstet Gynecol 100:672, 1968

TREATMENT

Arias F, Zamora J: Antihypertensive treatment and pregnancy outcome in patients with mild chronic hypertension. Obstet Gynecol 53:489, 1979

Chesley L: Parenteral magnesium sulfate and the distribution, plasma levels, and excretion of magnesium. Am J Obstet Gynecol 133:1, 1979

Howie PW, Prentice CRM, Forbes CD: Failure of heparin therapy to affect the clinical course of severe pre-eclampsia. Br J Obstet Gynaecol 82:711, 1975

Kelly JV: Drugs used in the management of toxemia of pregnancy. Clin Obstet Gynecol 20:395, 1977

Lawson J: Current views on the management of eclampsia. In Symonds EM (ed): Clinics in Obstetrics and Gynaecology, pp 707–715. Philadelphia, WB Saunders, 1977

Lindheimer MD, Katz AI: Sodium and diuretics in pregnancy. N Engl J Med 288:891, 1973

MacGillivray I: Sodium and water balance in pregnancy hypertension—The role of diuretics. In Symonds EM (ed): Clinics in Obstetrics and Gynaecology, pp 549–563. Philadelphia, WB Saunders, 1977

Pritchard JA: Management of severe preeclampsia and eclampsia. Semin Perinatol 2:83, 1978

Pritchard JA, Pritchard SA: Standardized treatment of 154 cases of eclampsia. Am J Obstet Gynecol 123:543, 1975

Redman CWG: The use of antihypertensive drugs in hypertension in pregnancy. In Symonds EM (ed): Clinics in Obstetrics and Gynaecology, pp 685–705. Philadelphia, WB Saunders, 1977

PROGNOSIS

Chesley LC, Annitto JE, Cosgrove RA: Long-term follow-up study of eclamptic women: Sixth periodic report. Am J Obstet Gynecol 124:446–459, 1976

Friedman EA, Neff RK: Hypertension–hypotension in pregnancy correlation with fetal outcome. JAMA 239:2249–2251, 1978

Lopez–Llera M, Horta JLH: Pregnancy after eclampsia. Am J Obstet Gynecol 119:193–198, 1974

Naeye RL, Friedman EA: Causes of perinatal death associated with gestational hypertension and proteinuria. Am J Obstet Gynecol 133:8–10, 1979

Peyser MR, Toaff R, Leiserowitz DM et al: Late follow-up in women with nephrosclerosis diagnosed at pregnancy. Am J Obstet Gynecol 132:480–484, 1978

Soffronoff EC, Kaufmann BM, Connaughton JF: Intravascular volume determination and fetal outcome in hypertensive disease of pregnancy. Am J Obstet Gynecol 127:4–9, 1977

OTHER COMPLICATIONS OF PREGNANCY

PREMATURE RUPTURE OF THE MEMBRANES

Premature rupture of the membranes is defined as the leakage of amniotic fluid prior to the onset of labor. The implications are less serious when rupture occurs at term than when the membranes rupture earlier in pregnancy.

Premature rupture of the membranes occurs in 10% of patients at term, whereas the incidence among women who deliver before term is more than 15%. About 30% of babies delivered after premature rupture of the membranes are of low birth weight.

CAUSE

The cause of premature rupture of the membranes is not known, and rupture usually occurs without warning in a woman whose pregnancy has appeared to be progressing normally.

The strength of the fetal membranes is imparted almost entirely by the connective tissue layer to which the amnion epithelial cells are attached (see Figure 16–21). Although studies of the physical properties of the membranes have revealed no notable differences between membranes of clinically normal strength and those that rupture prematurely, the question has been reopened by the studies of Skinner, Campos, and Liggins in which the collagen content (and probably also the inherent strength) of the amnion is found to decline as term is approached, and to be significantly less in prematurely ruptured membranes than in controls. They have suggested the possibility that these changes may be equivalent to the softening and increasing compliance of the cervix in late pregnancy. The suggestion has been made that premature rupture of the membranes may be enzymatically motivated, bringing to mind such substances as collagenases, which may also be involved in the cervical changes.

COMPLICATIONS

The major complications of premature rupture of the membranes are the precipitation of labor and ascending intrauterine infection. At term, spontaneous rupture of the membranes is usually followed by the onset of labor in 24–48 hours; in earlier pregnancy, however, the latent period is usually much longer, the leakage sometimes persisting without labor for several weeks.

The major cause of perinatal morbidity and mortality in premature rupture of the membranes is preterm

26

OTHER COMPLICATIONS AND DISORDERS DUE TO PREGNANCY

David N. Danforth

delivery. Also, when the membranes have ruptured, ascending intrauterine infection is a constant threat: amnionitis, omphalitis, congenital pneumonia, and, occasionally, fetal septicemia have most ominous implications; maternal septicemia and fatal septic shock have often occurred as the result of ruptured membranes. In the low-birth-weight infant, the primary risks of preterm delivery are respiratory distress syndrome (RDS), hyaline membrane disease, and intraventricular hemorrhage. In the term infant, the major risk is neonatal sepsis.

DIAGNOSIS

The diagnosis is obvious if the membranes rupture with a gush that is followed by continued and copious leakage of watery fluid from the vagina. A diagnostic problem may arise if the watery leakage is slight and

intermittent, as occurs in many women because of urinary incontinence. If it continues immediately after voiding, the membranes are probably ruptured, but the following tests can be helpful if there is doubt.

1. Examination with a vaginal speculum in place may reveal amniotic fluid draining from the cervical canal. If there is doubt, the discharge can be tested with nitrazine paper (amniotic fluid is alkaline, vaginal secretions acid). This test is often inconclusive.
2. A drop of the liquid can be mixed with 0.1% nile blue sulfate and permitted to dry on a glass slide for 5 min. The presence of *any* orange-staining fetal squames is proof-positive that the liquid is amniotic fluid.
3. The presence of anuclate fetal squames, lanugo, and the frond crystallization pattern of dried amniotic fluid that is not contaminated by blood or meconium identifies the liquid as amniotic fluid.
4. If none of the aforementioned tests is conclusive and it is imperative to determine if the membranes are ruptured, 5 ml Evans blue dye can be injected into the amniotic cavity by amniocentesis. If the membranes are ruptured, the dye should appear in the vagina in 30–40 min.

MANAGEMENT

The management of premature rupture of the membranes is determined chiefly by the time in pregnancy that it occurs. The major considerations are the potential for serious maternal or perinatal complications at the various stages of pregnancy. With regard to the fetal outlook, a liveborn baby's chance of survival is excellent after 36 weeks' gestation and good between 34 and 36 weeks' gestation. At 28 to 34 weeks the prognosis must be considered fair to poor, depending upon (1) the size and condition of the infant upon arrival in the nursery, (2) the skill of the medical team that provides the neonatal care, and (3) the physical facilities available in the nursery. In approaching the problem of premature rupture of the membranes, the clinician should be aware that under the most optimal circumstances a liveborn fetus weighing 2001 to 2500 g has a 97% chance of surviving, one born alive weighing 1501 to 2000 g has at least a 90% chance of surviving, and a liveborn fetus weighing 1001 to 1500 g has a 65% to 80% chance of surviving. Special perinatal centers are reporting survivorship of newborns weighing 750 to 1000 g. With these figures in mind the obstetrician can make a reasonable judgment of perinatal risks versus benefits of intervention in a given case.

In all cases of premature rupture of the membranes, the patient should be admitted to the hospital and an admission vaginal examination made to exclude cord prolapse and to determine the imminence of labor. (Some have advocated only a sterile speculum examination, but this does not quite supply the needed information.) Thereafter no vaginal examinations are made until labor is established or until it is decided to deliver the baby within 24 hours.

In most cases, an ultasound examination is made for cephalometry and placental localization. The lecithin/sphingomyelin (L/S) ratio should be done if there is a real question of fetal maturity; the vaginal pool may be an appropriate source of the fluid, but, if not, amniocentesis should be done. If the latter is needed, the fluid should be cultured.

After 37 Weeks

Spontaneous rupture of the membranes after 37 weeks is usually followed by the onset of labor within 48 hours, but in these patients, the risk of ascending infection is such that an oxytocin induction is usually started if labor has not begun within 24 hours. Because of both theoretic and documented risks of prolonged oxytocin administration (see page 724), the attempt should be abandoned if labor has not started within 5 hours of the infusion's initiation, and serious consideration should be given to cesarean section delivery.

Before 34 Weeks

Premature rupture of the membranes before 34 weeks may be managed either conservatively (*i.e.*, observation either until the baby is mature enough to survive without intensive care, or until infection or labor intervenes) or aggressively (*i.e.*, prompt delivery either by induction of labor or by cesarean section).

Conservative Management. The purpose of conservative management is to prolong the *in utero* existence of the fetus in an effort to minimize the serious complications of preterm delivery. It is to be remembered that during the last 2 months of pregnancy the baby grows at a rate of about half a pound a week. Also, a latent period of more than 16 hours between rupture of the membranes and preterm delivery may enhance fetal lung maturation and, hence, reduce the incidence of RDS. In the large series reported by Kappy *et al.* the latent period from rupture of membranes to spontaneous onset of labor exceeded 7 days in 19% of women whose pregnancies were of less than 37 weeks' duration and in only 4% of those beyond 37 weeks' duration. The longest latent period was 58 days.

Bedrest is an essential feature of conservative management, and it is advisable that the patient remain in the hospital as long as there is active leakage. A complete blood count and urinalysis at admission; contin-

uous external electronic record of the fetal heart rate at admission to exclude occult cord or fetal tachycardia; daily white blood count; and four times daily record of fetal heart rate (auscultation for 30 sec), temperature, pulse, and respirations are required.

If prolonged hospitalization is not feasible, the patient may be discharged home after 5 days with full explanation that this is less than optimal treatment. Home care should include bedrest with bathroom privileges; avoidance of intercourse, douches, and tampons; record of oral temperature morning, afternoon, and evening; and white blood cell count at least once and preferably twice weekly. The physician should be notified of fever, a change in the character or odor of the vaginal discharge, onset of contractions, or any change in fetal movements. If the physician cannot be assured of total compliance with all instructions, the patient should be urged to stay in the hospital, or the pregnancy should be terminated. If the leakage should stop during the hospital stay, the patient may also be discharged home, with the same instructions except that bedrest is not required. If the leakage should resume or if fever should occur, she should be readmitted immediately.

Prophylactic Antibiotics. Prophylactic antibiotics are not recommended in cases of uncomplicated premature rupture of the membranes. Their use does not influence the incidence of amnionitis or neonatal sepsis, and the growth of resistant organisms is a major threat. Moreover, such treatment will interfere with proper bacterial studies of the newborn.

Efforts to Stop Labor. The clinical use of tocolytic agents is discussed in Chapter 33. With few exceptions, they are generally contraindicated in the presence of ruptured membranes.

Prevention of Respiratory Distress Syndrome. The events in the normal maturation of the fetal lung are considered on page 319. The question is still unsettled whether a latent period of 16–24 hours between premature rupture of the membranes and preterm delivery *per se* leads to accelerated pulmonary maturation and, hence, to a reduced incidence of RDS. Current evidence suggests that such a latent period is indeed beneficial. The ability of glucocorticoids to accelerate lung maturation, as first suggested by Liggins, has been confirmed by ample clinical trials. In women whose pregnancies are 24–34 weeks' duration and in whom delivery can be delayed for at least 24 hours, the administration of betamethasone (10–12 mg/24 hours in divided intramuscular doses, continued, if possible, for 48–72 hours) significantly reduces the incidence of RDS, as well as the incidence of death from hyaline membrane disease and intraventricular hemorrhage. The most favorable cases are those of 30–32 weeks'

gestation; no benefits accrue if pregnancy is of more than 34 weeks' duration or if delivery occurs before 24 hours or after 7 days from the time of the first injection. For those who are to be managed conservatively, treatment must be repeated weekly until the L/S ratio reaches 1.8:1 to 2:1.

To date, no short-term adverse effects of preterm glucocorticoids on the infant have been demonstrated, and preliminary psychometric studies at 4+ years of age suggest no long-term detrimental effects. As Shields and Resnik note, however, extensive well-controlled clinical trials with long-term follow-up are needed to answer the question of possible long-term sequelae.

Severe preeclampsia is a specific contraindication to glucocorticoids. Possible maternal complications include increased susceptibility to, or masking of, intrauterine or other infection and, when glucocorticoids are used in conjunction with β-mimetic tocolytic agents, postpartum pulmonary edema and shock. The latter complication responds quickly to oxygen and diuretics.

Aggressive Management. In the event of amnionitis, delivery should be accomplished within 8 hours, by induction of labor if this is feasible and by cesarean section if it is not. Cervical and blood cultures are taken at once. If delivery is imminent, antibiotics are withheld until after delivery in order to facilitate bacterial studies of the newborn; if delivery will be delayed for several hours, intravenous antibiotics are started at once.

The onset of amnionitis may be difficult to pinpoint. Warning signs may include a morning temperature of 99° F, a single white blood cell count above 12,000, and fetal tachycardia above 160. The diagnosis is made without hesitancy in the presence of maternal fever, white blood cell counts above 12,000, a tender uterus, and persistent fetal tachycardia. In some cases, a fetid vaginal discharge is present.

Quantitative estimation of *C-reactive protein* (CRP) appears to have great value in the surveillance of patients who are at risk for amnionitis, since the serum value is reported to become elevated at least 12 hours before any change occurs in the other parameters (WBC, differential, temperature). The test can be performed in 20 minutes.

Between 34 and 37 Weeks

Unless there are other complications, the decision regarding management is based on the L/S ratio. A ratio of 2:1 is usually considered evidence of fetal lung maturity. In some services, 1.8:1 is used, since the minimal additional risk of RDS is considered less significant than the risk of intrauterine infection if the baby remains in the uterus. If the L/S ratio suggests immaturity of the fetal lungs, conservative management is

indicated unless there are compelling reasons to terminate the pregnancy. Glucocorticoids are not helpful at this stage of pregnancy. The L/S ratio is determined once a week; when a mature ratio is obtained, delivery is accomplished by induction of labor with oxytocin or by cesarean section if there is a malpresentation or other reason for abdominal delivery.

At the time of amniocentesis, Gram stain and aerobic and anerobic cultures are made. The presence of bacteria in the Gram stain or positive culture is indication for prompt delivery.

POSTTERM PREGNANCY

(Prolonged Pregnancy; Postmature Pregnancy; "Post-Datism")

Postterm pregnancy is variously defined by different authors. For practical purposes, delivery before 42 weeks can be considered within normal limits. If the woman is still undelivered at the end of 42 weeks (2 weeks after the projected date of labor as estimated by Nägele's rule), the possibility of postterm pregnancy should be considered and, if possible, verified. Most of the cases are accounted for by an error in menstrual dates; in others, pregnancy is actually longer than the accepted limits of normal. The data vary, but it is estimated that about 12% of women are undelivered at the end of 42 weeks' gestation. In one series, 7.3% of women delivered after 43 weeks.

ETIOLOGY

The explanation for failure to begin labor within a normal time range must lie in some defect among the myriad factors that are concerned in the normal onset of labor at term, as discussed in Chapter 29. It is usually futile to attempt to identify the particular cause of a given case of postterm pregnancy. One exception is the postterm pregnancy that occurs with an anencephalic fetus; the fetus has no hypothalamus, the pituitary is consequently hypoplastic, and the adrenals are also hypoplastic for lack of ACTH. The fetal pituitary produces no fetal oxytocin, which some investigators have implicated in the normal onset of labor, and the secretion of cortisol by the fetal adrenal is also impaired. The latter substance is clearly concerned in the onset of labor in the sheep, and it may also play some role in the human. A second exception is placental sulfatase deficiency (see page 348), which interferes with estriol formation and is accompanied by prolonged pregnancy. The diagnosis can be made when estriol excretion fails to increase after intraamniotic instillation of dehydroepiandrosterone sulfate.

HAZARDS

The risks to the mother are largely those of delivering a baby that has grown beyond its optimal size. They include such problems as dysfunctional labor, midpelvic arrest, and cephalopelvic disproportion.

Although many babies are unaffected, several reports provide evidence that the postterm fetus is at added risk of serious perinatal morbidity and perinatal death, as occurred, for example, in 13% of the postterm babies in the Knox *et al.* series. The fetal insults appear to be twofold: The first is imposed by delivery of an excessively large fetus; if the head does come through without incident one still faces the likelihood of shoulder dystocia, which in itself carries predictable neonatal morbidity and mortality. The second insult is imposed by an aging postterm placenta with failing transport mechanisms. The normal life span of the placenta is about 40 weeks; after this time, its capacity and reserve are progressively reduced in the face of increasing demands by the growing fetus. If delivery is delayed too long, intrauterine death must ultimately result. In Zwerdling's huge series, the perinatal mortality of infants born at 37–42 weeks' gestation was 1.2%; for those born after 43 weeks, it was 2.4%. Nakano's findings were similar: a perinatal mortality rate of 0.7% for babies born at term compared with a rate of 2.2% for those born after 42 weeks' gestation.

DIAGNOSIS

If labor has not started at the end of the 42nd week of pregnancy, all of the pertinent data bearing on the duration of pregnancy should be reassessed.

Menstrual dates. Complete information should have been obtained at the first visit, but, too frequently, the blank space on the record is filled in with the response to the single query: "When was your last period?" The obstetrician must also know if the period was normal, whether it began on time, and whether the customary periodicity is every 28–30 days or every 1–2 months (in the latter case, the projected date of labor may be highly unreliable). Since amenorrhea may occur after oral contraceptives have been used, it is important to know whether oral contraception was used prior to the pregnancy; if used within 3 months of the last normal menstrual period, the dates may be spurious. The obstetrician should know also whether basal body temperatures (BBT) were taken prior to the pregnancy: a persistently elevated BBT can provide a reliable indication of when the pregnancy began; coupled with an exact date of the last menstrual period, it can be used without hesitancy to calculate the duration of pregnancy.

Pregnancy Tests. The date of the first positive human chorionic gonadotropin (hCG) test can be helpful in the timing of some pregnancies. Hemagglutination inhibition tests (see Table 19–1) should be positive in almost all cases by 6 weeks' gestation, but the sensitivity of some of the tests is such that they are almost invariably negative before 5 weeks.

Pelvic Examination. The timing of pregnancy by estimation of uterine size is much more accurate at 6 or 7 weeks than it is after 3 months. Accordingly, a pelvic examination in early pregnancy is more reliable as an index of pregnancy duration than an examination after 3 months.

Auscultation of the Fetal Heart. When fetal heart tones can first be heard with the stethoscope (not Doppler instrument), the pregnancy is of at least 20 weeks' duration. This date may be useful in extrapolating the estimated date of labor.

Quickening. It is often considered that fetal movements are first felt at about 16 weeks' gestation, but this is highly unreliable and should not be used in an effort to date a pregnancy. In the author's experience, quickening may occur at any time between 3½ and 5 months; two women with normal intrauterine pregnancies insisted that they never, throughout pregnancy, felt any movements at all.

Ultrasonic Cephalometry. At some time between 20 and 26 weeks' gestation, ultrasonic cephalometry should be done if the menstrual dates are suspect, and a second scan at 31–33 weeks. As noted in Chapter 41, these 2 measurements can predict gestational age within a 5-day range. They are also useful if there is a risk of fetal growth retardation or if it seems essential to establish a term date with some accuracy.

The aforementioned factors are all used in the timing of pregnancy. In the Knox series, a diagnosis of postterm pregnancy (beyond 42 weeks) was made, according to the following criteria: *if the menstrual dates were considered to be accurate and reliable* and oral contraceptives had not been used within 3 months of the last period, then at least one of the following clinical confirmations was needed: 1) pelvic examination prior to 12 weeks, 2) auscultation of unamplified fetal heart tones for at least 22 weeks, and 3) ultrasonic cephalometry between 20 and 30 weeks' gestation. *If the menstrual history was unreliable,* at least two of these clinical confirmations were required.

EVALUATION AND TREATMENT

Beginning after 42 weeks' gestation, it is essential that fetal welfare be determined and monitored until delivery. As noted before, in many of the cases, perhaps 50%, labor will intervene before any evidence of fetal distress appears. In these cases, noninterference is recommended as long as there is nothing to suggest fetal jeopardy beyond the mere fact of postmaturity. Unfortunately, all of the applicable tests are indirect, and many have not been validated by noting the results of nonintervention when the tests are abnormal. Given the acknowledged risk of postterm pregnancy, however, significant evidence of fetal distress requires that the baby be delivered. The following tests can be helpful in making this decision.

Nonstress Testing (NST) of Fetal Heart Rate. Beginning at the end of the 42nd week, nonstressed testing of fetal heart rate should be done twice weekly. Gradually decreasing reactivity, as manifested by either a changing baseline or less frequent or smaller accelerations, should be followed promptly by a *contraction stress test* (CST), or by an *oxytocin challenge test* (OCT). Use of these tests is considered in Chapter 41. If the contraction stress test is positive, the baby should be delivered.

Estriol Excretion Studies. After the end of the 42nd week, estriol excretion studies, if they are to be used, should be made twice weekly until delivery. If the urinary excretion falls below 16 mg/24 hours or if, on successive tests, the estriol drops from normal levels by 30% or more of previous levels, the baby should be delivered. Estriol tests are used less frequently as more is learned of the prognostic significance of NST, CST, and OCT.

Human Placental Lactogen. Serum human placental lactogen (hPL) levels measured twice weekly have been reported to be helpful in assessing fetal status, a level below 4µg/ml serum suggesting serious fetal jeopardy. The value of this test has been questioned and more information is needed regarding it.

Amniocentesis. Amniocentesis has been recommended for determination of meconium-staining of the amniotic fluid; if present, this adds to the risk, but there is question whether this invasive test is needed when non-invasive methods can usually supply sufficient information. *Amnioscopy* has also been recommended for the same purpose, and there is also question whether it is needed.

METHOD OF DELIVERY

As in other cases in which pregnancy must be terminated before the onset of labor, the first decision is *when* to deliver. The next decision is *how* delivery shall be accomplished.

There is some evidence that dysfunctional labor is more common in postterm than in term labor. However, if the contraction stress test is negative and if the conditions for induction of labor are extremely favorable (cervix soft, thin, anterior, and 3 or more cm dilated; vertex presenting at station +2 to +3), the membranes should be ruptured. Most such women will start labor within 1 hour; if not, an oxytocin infusion should be started at a rate of 0.5 mU/min and increased by increments of 0.5 mU/min every 15 min either until satisfactory laborlike contractions occur or until the maximum rate (in postterm patients) of 4 mU/min is reached. If labor is not established within 6 hours of the start of the infusion, or if the continuous monitoring of fetal heart rate (an essential part of any induction) should suggest fetal distress, then cesarean section should be selected.

Cesarean section should also be selected if prior contraction stress tests were positive or if delivery is indicated and the conditions for induction are not favorable.

MISSED LABOR (DEAD FETUS SYNDROME)

Missed labor refers to intrauterine death after 20 weeks' gestation, with retention of the dead fetus within the uterus. The term *missed abortion* is applied if the fetal death occurs before the end of the 20th week of pregnancy. Although rare, the fetus occasionally remains in the uterus for many months or even years and becomes calcified.

The fetal death may be due to such factors as a knot in the umbilical cord, Rh isoimmunization, diabetes, or placental insufficiency. In many cases, there is no apparent cause. Failure of labor to start results from failure of some combination of factors normally responsible for the onset of labor at term (see Chapter 29); in missed labor, the most striking defects are lack of increasing uterine stretch, loss of fetal oxytocin and fetal cortisol, and disruption of the fetal contribution to estrogen synthesis, any of which might delay labor.

The diagnosis of missed labor is usually not difficult. As a rule, pregnancy progresses normally until suddenly, usually at some time after 28 weeks, the patient fails to perceive fetal movements. The uterus is silent, and no fetal heartbeat can be detected by real-time or time motion ultrasonography. Missed labor is diagnosed if labor fails to ensue within 48 hours of fetal death. The differential diagnosis includes abdominal pregnancy and pregnancy in a rudimentary horn.

Most women carrying a dead fetus ultimately go into labor, but the emotional impact of waiting indefinitely for this to occur is great indeed. In addition, fibrinogen levels generally begin a linear descent about 3–4 weeks after the baby dies, and severe coagulation problems, especially disseminated intravascular coagulation (see page 743), can develop in women who remain undelivered for a month or more. Current policy is to await spontaneous labor for a period not exceeding 2 weeks, unless the membranes rupture before this time, in which case induction is started promptly.

The use of prostaglandin E_2 in viscous gel, either intravaginally or intracervically, seems especially appropriate if the cervix is not favorable for induction of labor. Oxytocin may be used. Intraamniotic saline is not recommended, since the reduced amount of amniotic fluid increases the probability of hypernatremia, coagulation disorders, infection, and cardiovascular collapse.

Induction of labor is contraindicated in certain circumstances, regardless of whether the baby is living or dead. Cesarean section should be used for delivery in the presence of cephalopelvic disproportion, abnormal presentation (transverse lie is common in this syndrome), previous uterine incision, advanced maternal age, grand multiparity, and any maternal condition in which labor is contraindicated.

HYDRAMNIOS

Hydramnios refers to the accumulation of excessive amounts (2000 ml or more) of amniotic fluid. The term *polyhydramnios* is sometimes used, a redundancy equivalent to "polyhydroureter."

The factors responsible for the normal formation and exchange of amniotic fluid are discussed on page 315. Under ordinary circumstances, the sources of amniotic fluid appear to be secretion by the amnion itself, transudation from maternal serum, and fetal urine, each of which is an ongoing process that provides, at 38 weeks, a production estimated at about 500 ml/hour. This is normally balanced by the hourly removal of an equivalent volume of amniotic fluid by absorption across the fetal membranes and fetal swallowing.

The cause of hydramnios has not been explained. It might be presumed that an imbalance between fetal swallowing and voiding could be responsible, but recent studies have demonstrated that the normal ranges of swallowing (87–287 ml/day) and voiding (mean average of 23.6 ml/hour) are unchanged in cases of hydramnios. Even in the extreme cases of anencephaly and postterm pregnancy, there is no abnormal correlation between voiding, swallowing, and amniotic fluid volume. One therefore concludes that the basic derangement is in other water transport mechanisms. Among these, the complex and highly developed amnion cells overlying the placenta at once come to mind, but there are no published data regarding the possibility that these cells may be concerned.

The fact that hydramnios has always been associated with a high incidence of fetal abnormalities is not helpful in defining its etiology, since no specific eti-

TABLE 26–1. CONDITIONS FOUND WITH 100 CONSECUTIVE CASES OF CLINICAL HYDRAMNIOS

FETAL ABNORMALITY		39
Anencephaly	23	
Esophageal atresia	3	
Duodenal atresia	1	
Hydrops fetalis	3	
Tumor of chest causing pressure on esophagus	1	
Occipitocervical meningocele	1	
Hydrocephalus	3	
Achondroplasia	2	
Skin disease	1	
Spina bifida	1	
MULTIPLE PREGNANCY		9
DIABETES MELLITUS		7
NORMAL FETUS, NORMAL MOTHER		45

(Adapted from Gadd RL: In Philipp EE, Barnes J, Newton M (eds): Scientific Foundations of Obstetrics and Gynaecology, 2nd ed. London, William Heinemann, 1977)

ologic factors are found in each case. The diverse abnormalities that occurred in 100 consecutive cases of hydramnios are shown in Table 26–1. It is to be noted that there were no fetal abnormalities whatever in 61 of the cases.

DIAGNOSIS AND TREATMENT

Hydramnios is sometimes suspected at about 7 months' gestation, but the obstetrician need do nothing at this time except to be aware that if subsequent examinations confirm hydramnios, the possibility of a fetal abnormality is about 40%. As pregnancy advances, the uterus is larger than the dates would suggest, it may be difficult to hear the fetal heart or to palpate the fetal parts, and ballottement is accomplished with ease. The *diagnosis* can usually be confirmed by ultrasound scanning but regardless of the findings, an x-ray of the abdomen should be taken for diagnosis of a major abnormality or a lesser one that could be missed by ultrasound scan. If a major abnormality is found, the mother should be informed, and if she approves, steps should be taken to terminate the pregnancy. If no abnormality is found, the pediatrician should be alerted, at the time of delivery, to the presence of hydramnios during pregnancy and to the possibility of some surgical emergency, such as duodenal or esophageal atresia.

The collection of amniotic fluid can be enormous, amounting to upwards of 5 liters. In such cases, abdominal discomfort and dyspnea can be severe, often accompanied by difficulty in moving about and edema of the abdominal wall and extremities. Bedrest, salt restriction, and diuretics have been recommended but are rarely beneficial. Minor degrees of hydramnios are usually tolerated without difficulty, but, in the more

severe cases, withdrawal of amniotic fluid by amniocentesis can be extremely helpful. An intravenous catheter of the Angiocath type is inserted into the uterus (after sonography to localize the placenta so it will not be punctured) and is connected to an intravenous infusion set, the tubing of which is threaded through the infusion–withdrawal pump mechanism. The negative pressure helps to prevent clogging by particulate matter and permits even withdrawal at a rate of about 500 ml/hour. Depending on the magnitude of the hydramnios, removal of 1500–2000 ml usually suffices to relieve the symptoms. The fluid sometimes collects again rather rapidly, and the procedure may be repeated as needed. Sometimes labor intervenes. As the uterus contracts after removal of significant amounts of fluid, the obstetrician should be alert to the possibility, although rare, that the diminished intrauterine surface may result in premature separation of the placenta.

ACUTE HYDRAMNIOS

The term acute hydramnios refers to the very rapid accumulation of huge amounts of amniotic fluid over the course of a few days to 2 weeks. The condition, which appears to be associated invariably with monoamniotic twin pregnancy, is characterized by varying degrees of upper abdominal discomfort, dyspnea, and marked abdominal, vulval, and dependent edema. The condition usually occurs between 21 and 28 weeks' gestation and may terminate by premature rupture of the membranes or preterm labor. In the series of cases studied by Weir *et al.*, 14 of 16 babies were normally formed, but none survived. Transabdominal amniocentesis was not tried; since this occurs in early gestation, however, it is doubtful that amniocentesis would be of more than temporary benefit. The important differential diagnosis is placental abruption, which would be quickly clarified by ultrasound scan.

OTHER DISORDERS DUE TO PREGNANCY

Many diseases are a direct consequence of pregnancy. Some are unique to pregnancy, and others are the result of deficiencies specifically precipitated by pregnancy. Preeclampsia (see Chapter 25) is one of the most important, chiefly because of its frequency and its lethal potential for both mother and baby. The other diseases in this group, although not necessarily less important, receive less emphasis either because they are rare or because they have less serious implications.

ANEMIA

Anemia occurs commonly in association with pregnancy. It is rarely a serious complication, but its recognition, identification, and treatment are essential to proper obstetric practice. The cause may be a nutritional deficiency, chronic blood loss, a chronic infection, a metabolic disorder, or a genetic defect, acting singly or in combination. The incidence of anemia varies widely, depending upon the criteria used for its diagnosis; it occurs most frequently among population groups who are poorly nourished and receive inadequate medical care.

Hemoglobin and hematocrit values should be determined in every pregnancy at the initial visit, at about 26 weeks' gestation, and about 1–2 weeks before delivery. A venous blood sample, taken without stasis, should be used for these determinations; stasis with tourniquet or blood pressure cuff may induce hemoconcentration in the specimen, and capillary samples may be inaccurate because of dilution by tissue fluid. As a working rule, the lower limit of "normal" hemoglobin in pregnancy is of the order of 12 g/dl; the zone 11–12 g/dl should be considered suspect; and, if the hemoglobin is below 11 g/dl, even considering the hemodilution of pregnancy, the woman is probably anemic.

The most common anemia of pregnancy is iron deficiency anemia. If the hemoglobin cannot be maintained above 11 g/dl by supplemental iron therapy, some other kind of anemia should be considered, and appropriate tests should be made. If the woman is black, a sickle cell test and hemoglobin electrophoresis should be done first. Clinical judgment should dictate the order in which the other diagnostic tests are used. For mild and moderate anemia, measurements of serum iron and iron-binding capacity, mean corpuscular hemoglobin concentration, serum ferritin, and examination of a peripheral blood smear usually provide the necessary information. For more marked or unresponsive anemia, a complete hematologic survey should be obtained, including the additional tests of reticulocyte count, leukocyte and platelet count, and bone marrow aspiration. The values usually accepted as normal for pregnancy are listed in Table 26–2.

If the anemia develops rapidly near term, bone marrow aspiration may be necessary to establish or exclude megaloblastic anemia. In some instances,

TABLE 26–2. NORMAL BLOOD VALUES IN PREGNANCY

	Value	Variations
Hb (hemoglobin)	12–13.4 g/dl	
Hct (hematocrit)	37%–42%	
RBC (red blood cell count)	4–5 million/cu mm	
ESR (erythrocyte sedimentation rate)	10–60 mm/hr	Lower value in early pregnancy, gradually increasing to higher value in third trimester and first week after delivery
MCV (mean corpuscular volume)	80–96 cu μm	
MCHS (mean corpuscular Hb concentration)	32%–36%	
SERUM IRON	60μg–120μg/dl	Marked day-to-day variation
TOTAL IRON-BINDING CAPACITY	250μg–350μg/dl	
SERUM FERRITIN	10μg–200μg/liter	
WBC (white blood cell count)	10,000–30,000	Usually 10,000–15,000 in pregnancy, 20,000–30,000 in labor and 1st week after delivery
DIFFERENTIAL COUNT	Unchanged in pregnancy, left shift in labor	Increase in neutrophils (shift to left) that accounts largely for leukocytosis of labor and 1st week after delivery
BLOOD PLATELETS	230,000–400,000	Increase after delivery, to about 600,000 on 10th day after delivery
BONE MARROW	No significant change in pregnancy	

plasma hemoglobin concentration, erythrocyte fragility, and urinary and fecal urobilinogen determinations may provide useful information about the cause of the anemia.

The types of anemia due specifically to pregnancy include iron deficiency anemia, megaloblastic anemia, and refractory anemia. Other anemias can, of course, be present during pregnancy and some may be exacerbated by pregnancy; except for the aforementioned types, however, there is no specific cause-and-effect relationship. The anemias that are not pregnancy-related are discussed in Chapter 27.

IRON DEFICIENCY ANEMIA

In general, the amount of iron in the body of a normal adult woman ranges from 3000–4000 mg, of which about 2500 mg are contained within the circulating red cell mass as an integral part of the hemoglobin molecule. An amount of 700–1000 mg is stored as reserve iron in the muscles, in body cells linked to respiratory enzymes, and in the serum as transport iron. The total amount of circulating iron in the serum is about 4 mg. The serum iron, which varies in concentration from 60 μg–120 μg/dl, is in constant motion; some is used to replenish the red cell mass, some is used to replenish the iron stores, and about 1–2 mg/day is lost by excretion in the urine, sweat, and feces. The latter quantity is balanced by the daily absorption of 1–2 mg/day from food. The body conserves iron by regulating its excretion and limits the total body iron by regulating the amount that can be absorbed.

Menstruation usually draws upon the iron stores to the extent of 10–30 mg/month. If menstruation should be excessive or if the blood loss is not balanced by diminished iron excretion and increased absorption, a negative iron balance necessarily results. Few women and perhaps also too few physicians heed this continued drain upon the iron reserves, with the consequence that most women begin pregnancy with iron stores that are depleted. Ian Donald observed that in the Glasgow antepartum clinic, less than 50% of the patients entered with hemoglobin values over 10g/dl; in 30% of patients, the values were 10–12 g/dl. According to Barnes, the majority of women embark on pregnancy with their stores of iron reduced to 500 mg, 250 mg, or even less.

The amount of iron needed during pregnancy has been variously estimated, but it is clear that the demands greatly exceed the amounts available from iron stores and from an ordinary diet. Although the need for iron is much greater in the second than in the first half of pregnancy, the additional requirement over the course of an entire pregnancy can be summarized as follows: 300–400 mg are transferred to the fetus (twice this amount if there are twins); about 100 mg are lost

to the placenta, and 500 mg are needed to maintain the enlarging maternal hemoglobin and red cell mass; the blood loss at delivery accounts for an additional 180–200 mg—a total of 1000+ mg. Since the plasma volume increases at a greater rate than the enlargement of the red cell mass, the hemoglobin can be expected to decline to its lowest point at 7-½ to 8 months' gestation when the blood volume is at its maximum. Thereafter, the discrepancy lessens, with a slight, spontaneous elevation of hemoglobin as term is approached. As a rule, a decline in hemoglobin without a corresponding fall in mean corpuscular hemoglobin concentration is due to hemodilution, whereas a fall in both is due to anemia.

As noted earlier, the hemoglobin is less than 11 g/dl in iron deficiency anemia of pregnancy. The serum iron is low, and iron-binding capacity is increased. Serum ferritin, regarded as an index of iron stores, may be a more sensitive indicator of anemia than other blood tests; in iron deficiency anemia, the serum ferritin level is consistently below 12μg/liter. The most critical test is the bone marrow stain for hemosiderin; in iron deficiency anemia, no stainable iron can be found.

Effects of Iron Deficiency Anemia

The effects of mild to moderate iron deficiency anemia in pregnancy are not well documented. Unless it is adequately treated, however, moderate or even mild anemia may quickly give way to severe anemia, a condition that does have important consequences for both mother and baby. A hemoglobin level of 9 g/dl is probably the minimum level for safety; at 6.5 g/dl, the mother's life is endangered.

Effects on the Mother. Cardiac failure, the ultimate disaster, occurs with some frequency among women whose hemoglobin is of the order of 4.5–6 g/dl. Other sequelae of anemia are intolerance to even modest blood loss at delivery, predisposition to infection, and, in some of the cases, dysfunctional labor.

Effects on the Fetus. Anemia of the newborn is rarely a problem, as the transfer of iron to the fetus is not significantly impaired even when the mother is severely anemic. Late abortion and preterm labor are more common, contributing to the increased incidence of infant wastage and morbidity. Reduced estriol and evidences of fetal distress in labor are probably the result of impaired uterine and placental oxygenation with attendant fetal hypoxia. Hypoxia probably also accounts for the increased stillbirth rate when maternal anemia is severe.

Prevention and Treatment

In order to prevent iron deficiency anemia, an iron supplement must be prescribed for every pregnant pa-

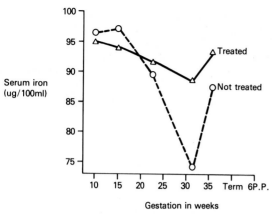

FIG. 26-1. Serum iron (50% levels) in pregnant patients treated with supplemental iron and without supplemental iron. *PP*, Postpartum. (Traft LI, Halliday JW, Russo AM et al.: Aust NZ J Obstet Gynaecol 18:226, 1978)

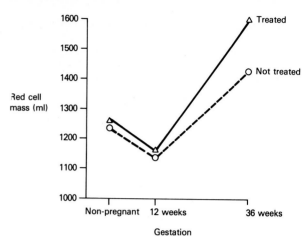

FIG. 26-3. Red cell mass in pregnancy of patients treated with iron therapy and patients not treated. (Taylor DJ, Lind T: Br J Obstet Gynaecol 86:364, 1979)

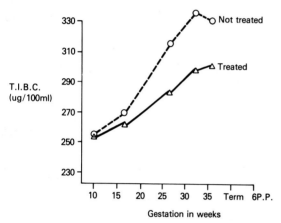

FIG. 26-2. Total iron-binding capacity (*TIBC*; 50% levels) in pregnant patients treated with supplemental iron and untreated. *PP*, Postpartum. (Taft LI, Halliday JW, Russo AM et al.: Aust NZ J Obstet Gynaecol 18:226, 1978)

tient. The effects of routine supplementation with small doses of ferrous sulfate and folic acid among normal pregnant women are shown in Figures 26-1 through 26-3, and similar effects have been demonstrated for use of ferrous sulfate alone. In normal pregnancy with hemoglobin of 12 g/dl or higher, a daily supplement of ferrous sulfate 0.3 g/day (60 mg elemental iron), together with folic acid 1 mg for prevention of megaloblastic anemia, is usually sufficient if started at the 16th week of pregnancy.

If the hemoglobin is below 12 g at the beginning of pregnancy, the equivalent of 180 mg elemental iron should be given in three divided doses with meals. The larger amount should also be given when there are multiple fetuses, when pregnancy is rapidly repeated (since iron stores are rarely replenished from the preceding pregnancy), and when the woman is large in stature. Doses in excess of 180 mg/day are inappropriate; absorption of iron is not increased, and the incidence of diarrhea and vomiting is much higher. In an anemic patient, a reticulocyte response should be noted in a week or 10 days, but a hemoglobin response may be delayed because the increase in hemoglobin mass may be hidden by the more rapidly increasing plasma volume. Treatment should be continued throughout pregnancy and for a minimum of 6 months after delivery, even though normal hematologic values have been achieved. (Iron preparations must be kept beyond the reach of children: acute iron poisoning due to ingestion of toxic doses can constitute a grave emergency.)

Parenteral iron may be needed if the anemia is first discovered late in pregnancy. When given according to recommended protocol, a rise in hemoglobin is usually first noted in about 1 week; in severely anemic women, the maximum response occurs in 4–9 weeks. *Packed red cells* therefore may be required in severe anemia if delivery is expected within 3 weeks, if an urgent operation is anticipated, or if the anemia is of sufficient degree that there is a risk of cardiac failure. A major problem in the use of packed cells in some cases of severe anemia is the possibility of circulatory overload due to the already expanded plasma volume. Techniques that have been suggested to avoid this complication are (a) the intravenous administration of a *rapid-acting* diuretic immediately before the packed cell infusion is started and (b) simultaneous phlebotomy and packed cell infusion, in which the amount of whole blood (1100–1700 ml) withdrawn is approximately equal to the volume of packed cells infused

(1000–1500 ml). Exchange transfusions are not well tolerated in labor, probably because of the repeated small autotransfusions caused by contraction of the uterus and the substantial autotransfusion that occurs when the uterus empties at delivery.

MEGALOBLASTIC ANEMIA

A rare complication of pregnancy in the United States, megaloblastic anemia is most prevalent among population groups in which malnutrition is widespread. The cause of megaloblastic anemia is a folic acid deficiency that alters the nucleic acid production necessary for normoblastic erythrocyte maturation in the bone marrow. The daily adult requirement for folic acid of approximately 50μg is increased during late pregnancy to 300μg–400μg. Megaloblastic anemia is, of course, not unique to pregnancy, but it can be specifically caused by increased folic acid demand of pregnancy and, possibly, by interference with folic acid utilization. A nutritional deficiency can compound the problem, acting as a predisposing factor.

Megaloblastic anemia should be suspected when a severe anemia occurs near term or in the puerperium. Hemoglobin concentrations between 3 and 5 g/dl are not uncommon. An accurate diagnosis can be established by bone marrow biopsy and detection of the abnormal megaloblast. The erythrocytes may be normocytic or macrocytic. The plasma iron concentration is elevated, and there is an associated leukopenia and thrombocytopenia.

Treatment of megaloblastic anemia consists of the administration of folic acid. The usual dose is 1 mg/day. Because hemoglobin synthesis is rapid, iron should be provided with the folic acid.

A routine prenatal supplement of folic acid (1 mg daily) is advised both to meet the increased demands of pregnancy and to prevent this kind of anemia. The alleged hazard of giving folic acid to all pregnant women is the possibility of masking an undiagnosed pernicious anemia or, in such a case, of permitting subacute combined degeneration of the spinal cord to progress. Addisonian anemia is *extremely* rare both in this age group and in pregnancy, and the several hazards of folic acid deficiency far outweigh this single and dubious risk.

REFRACTORY ANEMIA

The term *refractory* may be applied to any anemia that does not respond to treatment. Although uncommon, most of the cases are due to chronic infection (*e.g.*, chronic pyelonephritis) and fail to respond until the infection is controlled. In the present context, refractory anemia refers to the anemia, which may be extremely severe, that develops during pregnancy with no known cause, is resistant to all hematinics, and undergoes spontaneous remission immediately after the conclusion of pregnancy.

The diagnosis is established on the basis of refractoriness to treatment after appropriate tests have been made to exclude other types of anemia.

Refractory anemia is rare, and the problems of classification have not been solved. In many cases, the bone marrow is hypoplastic with both a relative and an absolute decrease in developing erythrocytes; in these cases, leukopenia and thrombocytopenia are also present, since all blood elements formed in the marrow are affected. In some cases, the marrow is reported as hyperplastic, suggesting selective destruction of both red cells and platelets with no measurable effect on the white cells. In some cases, the bone marrow shows an entirely normal pattern. In any case, the circulating erythrocytes are normocytic and normochromic. Normal stores of iron are demonstrated on examination of smears of the bone marrow, and the plasma iron concentration is normal or elevated.

The mechanism is obscure. It is suggested that the anemia results either from bone marrow suppression or from increased peripheral or intramedullary destruction of blood cells and platelets by some factor arising in the conceptus, probably the trophoblast.

Of the 46 cases reviewed by Perry and Harris, hemoglobin levels as low as 7 g/dl were frequently encountered; 63% of the patients died, the most prominent causes of death being hemorrhage and sepsis. Among those who survived, fetal growth was not retarded, and there were no intrauterine deaths. These authors, who managed a severe case successfully, recommend that the hemoglobin not be permitted to fall below 7 g/dl and that packed cells and platelets be administered if the hemoglobin is already below this level, if symptoms of severe anemia develop, or if abnormal bleeding should appear from any source. An infusion of packed red cells and platelets should be started when labor is imminent, and should be permitted to run slowly, with due attention to avoidance of circulatory overload, until after delivery. The objective should be a hemoglobin of higher than 7 g/dl and platelets in excess of 50,-000/cu mm. In their case, prophylactic antibiotics (ampicillin) were employed for 72 hours. Fresh whole blood, formerly thought to be essential, is evidently not required. Corticosteroids, androgens, pyridoxine, iron, folic acid, γ-globulin, and fibrinogen have all been used without benefit. Therapeutic abortion carries at least as great a risk as continuation of pregnancy, and is not recommended.

The disease recurs with sometimes greater violence in a subsequent pregnancy, and sterilization 3 months after completion of pregnancy is appropriate. In the interim, an ovulatory suppressant should be used; at least one patient died of an intraabdominal hemorrhage from a corpus luteum cyst before the anemia had resolved.

EMESIS AND HYPEREMESIS GRAVIDARUM

The symptoms of nausea and vomiting are experienced by approximately 50% of women during the first trimester of pregnancy. The symptoms vary in degree from mild morning sickness to pernicious vomiting or hyperemesis gravidarum, which can be fatal. The cause of nausea and vomiting is not known, but most probably it is related to trophoblastic activity and gonadotropin production stimulated or exaggerated by psychic stimuli. The incidence and timing of nausea and vomiting parallel the gonadotropin levels; also, nausea and vomiting are more pronounced in association with hydatidiform mole, when gonadotropin levels are high, and disappear in women destined to abort. Nausea and vomiting are usually limited to the first 10–12 weeks of pregnancy; indeed, if the symptoms persist beyond this period, a possible medical or surgical condition should be sought as the cause.

MORNING SICKNESS

The mildest form of the disorder consists of waves of nausea with or without vomiting that occur when the patient arises in the morning and may recur when the stomach is empty prior to meals. The symptoms may be precipitated by various odors and foods. Ordinarily, nutrition is not disturbed, weight loss is minimal, and the patient's daily activity is not affected. Assurance that the symptoms are limited to the early months of pregnancy, an adjustment in the patient's dietary habits, and, in some instances, the administration of a mild sedative or antinausea drug effectively control the symptoms. When the nausea and vomiting are confined to the morning hours, eating a few crackers before arising, remaining in bed for 15 min after awakening, and eating a light breakfast may be the only treatment required. If the symptoms persist throughout the day, frequent small feedings and avoidance of highly seasoned or spiced foods will reduce or eliminate the nausea and vomiting. Dairy products should be avoided and carbonated soft drinks encouraged. The foods that are best tolerated are cooked cereal with sugar but no cream, dry toast and jelly, boiled egg, baked potato, chicken, and lamb. An antiemetic (*e.g.*, Bendectin at bedtime and once during the day) may provide relief.

HYPEREMESIS GRAVIDARUM (PERNICIOUS VOMITING OF PREGNANCY)

Hyperemesis may be difficult to diagnose in its early stages, for it is preceded by a gray period of variable duration in which vomiting, although highly troublesome, does not occur after every feeding and sufficient nourishment is probably retained. This stage progresses to the point where the patient not only vomits everything she swallows, but retches between times. It is at or before this point that hospitalization is essential and that active measures must be taken to prevent the chain of events that can rapidly lead to starvation. Therapy should be prompt and energetic; almost without exception it can prevent the profound dehydration, electrolyte imbalance, and multiple vitamin deficiencies that in another era led inexorably to severe hepatic and renal damage, myelin degeneration of the peripheral nerves, scurvylike hemorrhages throughout the body, hemorrhagic and degenerative encephalopathy, and death. Therapeutic abortion was lifesaving before it became possible to monitor and correct the metabolic and nutritional abnormalities presented by hyperemesis gravidarum; at present it is rarely, if ever, required. Indeed, the patient's failure to improve significantly within 48 hours of admission to the hospital suggests organic disease.

The objectives of *management* include control of the vomiting, correction of dehydration, restoration of electrolyte balance, and provision of vitamins and calories to maintain nutrition. The patient should be placed in a quiet, well-ventilated room, preferably alone. Visitors should be restricted until marked improvement occurs. Baseline determinations of hemoglobin and hematocrit values, serum electrolyte values, carbon dioxide combining power, and blood urea nitrogen value should be obtained, and the urine tested for ketone bodies. Repeat determinations should be made daily until vomiting has ceased and used as a guide for fluid and electrolyte replacement. Since phenothiazine compounds (especially chlorpromazine) are hepatotoxic, they should be avoided if there is any suspicion that the syndrome is severe enough to have reached the stage of fatty infiltration of the liver, which is a predictable and ominous consequence of neglected or advanced hyperemesis.

During the first 24 hours, 3000 ml fluids should be given intravenously, to which ascorbic acid, vitamin B complex, and potassium chloride are added: 1000 ml 10% glucose in saline or Ringer's solution, 1000 ml 10% glucose in water, and 1000 ml protein hydrolysate solution. On subsequent days, the volume of fluid administered should be sufficient to maintain a urine output of at least 1 liter. Nothing should be given by mouth for 2–3 days and, in some instances, for a longer period if the vomiting has continued. The restoration of oral feeding must proceed slowly, beginning with dry foods such as crackers, biscuits, and toast taken frequently in small quantities. If no nausea occurs water, tea, and carbonated beverages may be added to the diet interspersed among the dry feedings. With continued control of the vomiting, bland solids may be gradually added until a full bland diet can be tolerated by the patient. Since an emotional factor

often plays an important part in pernicious vomiting, recognition of and attention to the underlying cause may help prevent a recurrence. Psychiatric treatment may be necessary.

VASCULAR DISORDERS

The pregnancy changes that predispose to vascular disorders include 1) an increase in venous pressure and a slowing of blood flow in the lower extremities and pelvis; 2) increased coagulability of the blood, as evidenced by significant increases in fibrinogen, in platelets, and in clotting factors II (prothrombin), VII (proconvertin), VIII (antihemophilic globulin), IX (plasma thromboplastin component or Christmas factor), and X (Stuart factor); 3) a considerably increased blood volume; and, of special importance, 4) a significant increase in venous distensibility apparently due to 5) specific pregnancy-related changes in the structure of the blood vessels themselves that contribute to reduced strength, reduced resiliency, and increased caliber.

VARICOSITIES

Venous varicosities are extremely common and usually involve the great saphenous vein and the veins draining into it, the veins of the hemorrhoidal plexus, the superficial veins of the vulva, or all three of these systems.

As a rule, varicosities become evident at 10–12 weeks' gestation, suggesting that much more is involved than simple obstruction to the return flow of blood by pressure of the enlarged pregnant uterus on the inferior vena cava. Varicosities reach maximum size at term and during labor, and tend to empty instantly following delivery.

Symptoms from varicose veins vary from a sensation of heaviness and vague discomfort after standing or walking to incapacitating pain that requires constant rest and elevation of the feet.

Treatment of leg varicosities should combine periods of rest and elevation of the legs with use of elastic stockings or bandages. The elastic supports should be worn from the time of arising until bedtime. Any constriction around the legs from rolled hose or garters should be avoided. Support garments that will compress vulvar varicosities and effectively reduce the discomfort are commercially available.

Surgical correction of varicosities of the legs should be deferred until the physiologic effects of the pregnancy have disappeared. The indication for surgical treatment often disappears and the results are consistently better if the ligation, stripping, or injection is postponed. Vulvar varices, regardless of their size in pregnancy, recede almost completely after delivery and virtually never require surgical correction.

TELANGIECTASIA

Areas of capillary dilation about the ankles and less commonly on the thighs are common in pregnancy. They are related to varices and are sometimes confluent, producing raised, often disfiguring, and rarely painful lesions for which there is no effective treatment except pressure bandages in extreme cases. They usually subside to an extent, but not completely, after delivery. *Cutaneous hemangiomas* and *angiectids* are probably a variant of telangiectasia, as are the cutaneous *vascular spiders* that are extremely common in pregnancy. The latter are characterized by a bright red punctate central point with branching hair-thin radials 1–2 mm in length. They are commonly found on the face, neck, arms, and upper part of the chest; usually, but not always, they vanish after delivery.

The cause of telangiectasia and its variants is unknown, except as part of the general vascular response to pregnancy. There is nothing tangible to support the repeated allegation that high estrogen levels are responsible.

ARTERIAL AND VENOUS THROMBOSIS

Phlebitis, phlebothrombosis, and thrombophlebitis of the lower extremities are rare in pregnancy, although the varicose and other pregnancy changes are predisposing conditions (see page 512).

Occlusive cerebrovascular disease due to cerebral venous thrombosis or, less frequently, to major arterial occlusion is uncommon in pregnancy; but it is less rare than in nonpregnant women of equivalent age, suggesting the probability of pregnancy predisposition. In one series, two-thirds of the cases of nonhemorrhagic hemiplegia that developed during pregnancy were due to cerebral venous thrombosis.

ANEURYSM AND VASCULAR RUPTURE

The incidence of dissecting aneurysm of the aorta and of aortic and splenic artery aneurysms is higher in pregnant than in nonpregnant women of equivalent age, and it has been estimated that 10%–20% of all maternal deaths are secondary to vascular catastrophies of one kind or another; 2%–5% of maternal deaths are due to intracranial hemorrhage. In one series of 31 cases of convulsions or coma in pregnancy, 21 were due to intracranial complications and only 6 to eclampsia.

Dissecting aneurysm of the coronary arteries is a

rare condition, but its distribution suggests that pregnancy may provide a predisposition. Among 32 such cases in women, 20 were past the childbearing age, but 12 of the patients died either during or after pregnancy. More recently, Jewett presented two additional cases of postpartum death due to this cause.

CENTRAL NERVOUS SYSTEM DISORDERS

INTRACRANIAL HEMORRHAGE

The importance of intracranial hemorrhage in pregnancy has been noted earlier and is discussed on page 522. Approximately half the cases occur in middle or late pregnancy, before the stress of labor.

GESTATIONAL POLYNEURITIS

Gestational polyneuritis, once thought to be specifically due to pregnancy, is now known to result from thiamine deficiency, precipitated by the demands of pregnancy. Thiamine is not stored in the body in large amounts and cannot be synthesized in the human body. Unless it is available in the diet, the stores are soon exhausted. In pregnancy, this condition is most often associated with intractable and inadequately or improperly treated hyperemesis gravidarum. It is characterized by paresthesia, muscle weakness, loss of deep reflexes, and vague cerebral symptoms, including confusion and disorientation. It may be fatal unless thiamine is administered promptly when symptoms develop. The pathologic findings include degenerative changes in the anterior horn cells of the spinal cord and in the peripheral nerve fibers.

CHOREA GRAVIDARUM

Like gestational polyneuritis, chorea gravidarum was for a time believed to be unique to pregnancy and to result from a specific pregnancy-related encephalitis. Most authorities now agree that it is identical with Sydenham's (rheumatic) chorea, having the same (unclear) cause, the same signs and symptoms, the same (uncertain) pathologic findings, and the same incidence of cardiac and other sequelae. Athetoid movements of one or more muscle groups and an apparent or true personality change are major characteristics.

MATERNAL OBSTETRIC PARALYSIS

Pregnancy may predispose to "maternal obstetric paralysis" because of the relaxation of the lower intervertebral joints and the muscular strain of labor; consequent prolapse of one or more lumbar intervertebral disks can result from trauma that would cause no injury in the nonpregnant state.

CARPAL TUNNEL SYNDROME (ACROPARESTHESIA)

The carpal tunnel syndrome consists of pain and paresthesias in one or both hands as the result of compression of the median nerve at the wrist beneath the tough, unyielding carpal ligament that confines the flexor tendons and, immediately superficial to them, the median nerve. The water retention of pregnancy is thought to be a predisposing factor, and the syndrome may arise *de novo* or as the result of either excessive use of the hands or tenosynovitis of the flexor sheath. Diuretics are sometimes of value; the wrist should be immobilized and work with the hands curtailed. The symptoms abate after delivery. In extreme cases, muscle atrophy may result, requiring surgical decompression by total resection of the transverse carpal ligament.

PSEUDOTUMOR CEREBRI

Pseudotumor cerebri is a condition that occurs principally in pregnancy and results from cerebral edema. The cerebrospinal fluid is normal, but the pressure is greatly increased, leading to the signs of bilateral papilledema, tinnitus, motor incoordination, headache, nausea and vomiting, and loss of visual acuity. Focal neurologic signs are absent except for the change in visual acuity, which provides one means of following the course of the disease. Cerebrospinal decompression provides relief of the headaches and may need to be repeated at intervals. Diuretics may also be helpful. The condition subsides completely after pregnancy, leaving no residual signs or symptoms. Most of the cases are associated with pregnancy, but the pseudotumor has also occurred in other conditions in which there are shifts in electrolytes and water.

OTORHINOLOGIC DISORDERS

Abnormal patency of the eustachian tube occurs frequently in pregnancy, especially during the last trimester, and produces the sensations of blockage of one or both ears and of a hollow sound to the voice. It is due to an enlargement of the eustachian tube that permits the pressure variations of breathing and phonation to be transmitted directly to the inner ear. There is no satisfactory treatment, but the symptoms abate after delivery.

The two rhinologic disorders that most commonly result specifically from pregnancy are *vasomotor rhinitis* and *epistaxis*.

During pregnancy, the nasal turbinates and septum

normally respond by greater or lesser hyperemia and congestion. If these are sufficiently marked, nasal discharge, stuffiness, and obstruction result. They may be extremely troublesome and unresponsive to local or systemic treatment. The syndrome vanishes at the conclusion of pregnancy but recurs in subsequent pregnancies. In one of the author's patients, this was an early and refractory sign in each of four pregnancies, clearing spontaneously about 1 week after each delivery.

Epistaxis is common. It is usually transient and self-limited, but on occasion it may be sufficiently violent to be life-threatening. The less troublesome variety usually results from rupture of a superficial vessel in response to irritation of an engorged area on one of the turbinates or septum, or from pregnancy-related changes in preexisting nasal polyps. If the sphenopalatine branch of the internal maxillary artery is directly involved, hemorrhage may be violent; if it is beneath the inferior or middle turbinate or far posterior it may also be inaccessible to packing and cauterization. Either carotid ligation or an approach to the internal maxillary artery through the antrum may be required to prevent exsanguination. One patient, at 6 months' gestation, required 8 pints of blood before the hemorrhage could be controlled.

DISORDERS OF THE INTEGUMENT

The normal integumentary response to pregnancy, mentioned in Chapter 17, includes the *pigmentary changes* (chloasma, linea nigra, and the increased pigmentation of normally pigmented areas) and the *striae gravidarum* (most pronounced over the abdomen, breasts, and hips). A third pregnancy response, *palmar erythema,* is also extremely common, asymptomatic, and of unknown cause; it usually vanishes after delivery. *Vascular spiders* and other *cutaneous vascular reactions* to pregnancy have been mentioned previously. In addition to these common and more or less trivial problems, certain other diseases of the skin, for the most part quite rare and in some cases extremely serious, can result directly from pregnancy.

During pregnancy there is a lengthening of the normal anagen (growing) hair phase. After delivery, the telogen follicles are converted to club (shedding) hairs; this may result in *hair loss,* especially in the frontal area, that is maximal 2–4 months after delivery; by 6 months postpartum the density of scalp hair has returned to normal. Protraction of this complaint calls for an endocrine investigation or search for a causative drug (*e.g.,* oral contraceptive).

Generalized pruritus is a troublesome, at times agonizing, but fortunately not common, affection of the skin in pregnancy; it abates after delivery, which often occurs before term. There are no objective findings, except for the excoriations that may result from scratching. Speculation about its cause has not been rewarding, with the possible exception of the finding that many of these patients have elevated serum bile acid values, and urobilin, urobilinogen, and bilirubin in the urine. These findings suggest that the pruritus is related to some hepatic disorder of pregnancy. Some suggest that this represents a mild form of intrahepatic cholestasis. A diet low in fat and high in protein and vitamins is said to be helpful, along with antihistamines and added calcium. Sedatives, antipruritic sprays, and general supportive measures are needed in severe cases.

Cutaneous tags (*molluscum fibrosum gravidarum*), either pedunculated or sessile, are quite common in pregnancy and are most frequently found on the neck and upper chest. They are not inflammatory and evidently result simply from epithelial hyperplasia. The tags are removed by ligating the base with silk or nylon thread, by cautery, or by excision.

Prurigo gestationis, an eruption peculiar to pregnancy, consists of small, highly pruritic papules usually covered by a bloody crust as a result of scratching, located especially on the extensor surfaces of the extremities, on the abdomen, and on the thorax. The condition clears spontaneously after delivery, leaving small areas of hyperpigmentation. Antipruritic sprays, oatmeal baths, antihistamines, sedatives, and general supportive measures may all be helpful. The fetus is not affected.

Papular dermatitis of pregnancy is not only incapacitating, but also has most serious implications for the baby. It is a generalized eruption of intensely pruritic papules, usually covered by a bloody crust. Its generalized distribution and the extremely high levels of urinary hCG distinguish it from the prurigo. The stillbirth rate is high. The eruption clears after delivery, to recur in subsequent pregnancies. Corticosteroids may be helpful.

Autoimmune progesterone dermatitis of pregnancy was described by Bierman in 1973. It is characterized by a severe acneiform eruption consisting of comedones, papules, pustules, and erosions with residual hyperpigmentation. Biopsies show histologic evidence of eosinophilic dermatitis and panniculitis. The disease is accompanied by profound peripheral eosinophilia (50%), hyperglobulinemia, and transient arthritis. It is reported to occur in the first trimester of pregnancy and to be associated with spontaneous abortion. Bierman suggests that the cause of this unusual disorder is related to hormone-dependent mechanisms, probably due to cell-mediated immunity against endogenous progesterone produced during pregnancy. There is some evidence to support the thesis of progesterone hypersensitivity as the cause of this disease, but several important questions remain unanswered.

Herpes gestationis is a serious and debilitating skin disease of unknown cause that is unique to pregnancy. It is characterized by generalized pruritus, followed

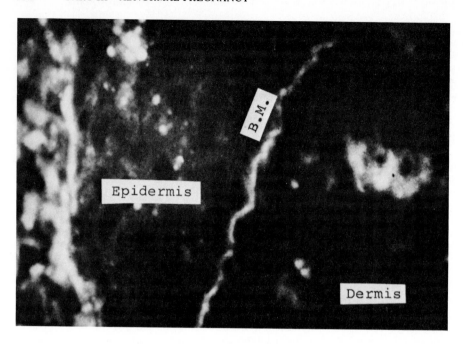

FIG. 26–4. Herpes gestationis. Fresh sera layered over normal human skin washed and stained with conjugated anti-C3. Note specific staining of basement membrane (*BM*). Nonspecific autofluorescence of reticulum fibers in dermis is also seen below BM. (×40) (Provost TT, Tomasi TB, Jr: J Clin Invest 52:1779, 1973)

shortly by the appearance of erythematous, vesicular papules about the umbilicus, spreading gradually from that point to involve the entire body. Confluence of the vesicles leads to the formation of bullae, which may contain clear fluid, pus, or blood. Severe local burning, a febrile constitutional response, and eosinophilia up to 50% are characteristic. The outlook for the mother is good, except for the areas of pigmentation that may remain after the disease terminates. The symptoms may clear within a few days of delivery or, exceptionally, may continue for extended periods. In two women who had been treated with hydrocortisone, the lesions persisted for 2 years. Exacerbation within 3 days of delivery may be an important characteristic, since it is reported to occur in the great majority of cases. The disease can now be verified by immunofluorescent demonstration of complement deposition along the basement membranes of involved areas of the skin (Fig. 26–4). *Herpes gestationis* recurs in subsequent pregnancies.

Management consists of supportive measures and local antibiotics to prevent infection. Systemic corticosteroids usually suppress the systemic manifestations, but Carruthers suggests they may prolong the disease and hence should be used with "some reluctance." Termination of pregnancy may be considered in severe cases.

There is no agreement on the outlook for the baby. Among 41 cases reported in two series, there was no increase in the rate of abortion, stillbirth, or fetal anomaly; the only fetal casualty was due to a therapeutic abortion. In other series of cases the fetus has been shown to be at substantial risk of stillbirth, preterm delivery, and congenital disease.

Impetigo herpetiformis is a rare, extremely serious inflammatory dermatitis of pregnancy that in some respects resembles pemphigus vulgaris. The disease can occur at any stage of pregnancy or the puerperium and is fatal in 70%–80% of cases. The primary lesion is a pustule from which no organisms can be cultured. The pustules, which are surrounded by a zone of erythema, coalesce to form large, oozing, crusted lesions of generalized distribution. Usually, the genitocrural areas are most seriously affected. Itching is not a prominent symptom, but the systemic reaction is profound, including prostration, fever, leukocytosis, tachycardia, vomiting, and electrolyte imbalance. No organisms can be cultured from blood samples. The cause is unknown, and there is no specific therapy. Its special severity in pregnancy suggests that the conceptus may impose an added insult or, indeed, may precipitate the disease; termination of pregnancy seems prudent if impetigo herpetiformis is diagnosed. Corticosteroids have been used, apparently with benefit in some cases, but there is nothing to suggest they have lowered the mortality rate. Antibiotics may prevent secondary infection of the open lesions. Among those who survive, the disease recurs with greater fury in subsequent pregnancies; accordingly, positive steps (*e.g.*, sterilization) should be taken to prevent further pregnancy in those who have had the disease.

Pruritic urticarial papules and plaques of pregnancy were described by Lawley *et al.* in 1979. As the authors observe, the eruption is probably more com-

mon than the seven cases in their report would suggest. It responds promptly to topical corticosteroids and has likely been encountered by many physicians who have not been impressed by its evidently specific relationship to pregnancy. The disease erupts in the last trimester of pregnancy, beginning on the abdomen and often spreading to involve the thighs. In some cases, the buttocks and arms were affected; facial lesions were never seen, and the trunk was rarely affected above the umbilicus. The question of possible fetal effects is unsettled, but the probable frequency of the disease suggests that, if there were a cause-and-effect relationship, it would have been remarked upon before. This eruption appears to be identical to that described by Spangler in 1962, and by Rahbari in 1978.

Gingivitis gravidarum, consisting of hypertrophic changes, edema, and congestion of the gingiva with blunting of the interdental papillae, is common. Bleeding, either spontaneously or on brushing, is also common. Glyoxide rinse after meals and a saline mouthwash (1 tablespoon in a glass of water) three times daily are usually helpful. In severe cases, a kind of tumor (*epulis*) may result from undue hypertrophy of one or more of the interdental papillae. The lesions are extremely vascular and may be of sufficient size to interfere with chewing and to require removal either because of their bulk or because of repeated and at times profuse bleeding. (In one such case, in which there was complete regression between pregnancies, it was decided to terminate the fifth pregnancy at 3 months' gestation because of the alarming and progressively luxuriant new growths, similar to, but larger than, those that had required surgical excision in two prior pregnancies.)

LIVER DISORDERS

The two diseases of the liver that are specifically related to pregnancy are acute fatty liver of pregnancy and recurrent jaundice of pregnancy. The former is usually fatal; the latter clears spontaneously after delivery. Since liver damage in pregnancy can be caused by tetracyclines, phenothiazine compounds (especially chlorpromazine), viral infections, and other hepatotoxic insults, these causes must be ruled out.

ACUTE FATTY LIVER OF PREGNANCY

Acute fatty liver of pregnancy, also known as *obstetric acute yellow atrophy,* was described in 1940 by Sheehan, the Liverpudlian pathologist who also described Sheehan's syndrome. The disease is reported to be extremely rare, but several recent cases suggest that it is by no means a medical curiosity. It occurs in the last

trimester of pregnancy, has no known cause, and is fatal in about 85% of cases. The clinical course consists of the sudden onset of severe epigastric pain, headache, and vomiting, followed in a few days by progressively deepening jaundice. Labor may intervene, usually resulting in delivery of a stillborn infant. Coma and death usually follow a few days later. Among those who survive, the disease appears not to recur in a subsequent pregnancy.

The liver is characteristically small and yellow. In all Sheehan's cases, microscopic examination of liver specimens "showed an identical lesion: there was gross fatty change affecting the entire lobule except a sharply defined rim of normal cells around the portal tracts. The affected cells were bloated by a fine foam of tiny fat vacuoles throughout the cytoplasm so that they resembled the cells of the suprarenal cortex. The nuclei were normal, and there was an entire absence of necrobiotic change." Pancreatitis and gastrointestinal bleeding may be associated. Failure of the damaged liver to manufacture prothrombin may account for severe hemorrhage that does not respond to vitamin K. In two of the reported cases, disseminated intravascular coagulation was a prominent feature. In three surviving patients, whose disease had been documented by liver biopsy, liver function returned to normal and the histologic appearance of the liver was normal 3 months after clinical recovery.

Laboratory findings include moderate to marked elevation of alkaline phosphatase values, slight to moderate elevation of serum glutamic oxaloacetic transaminase (SGOT) values, and leukocytosis. In addition, the coagulation profile may reveal profound prothrombin deficiency or evidence of disseminated intravascular coagulation. Computerized tomographic liver scan may reveal the low attenuation ratio that is characteristic of all types of fatty liver. The clinical and laboratory data and the differential diagnosis are documented in the fatal case presented in the Case Records of the Massachusetts General Hospital (Scully).

Definitive diagnosis requires liver biopsy. However, the implications of the disease are so threatening that it seems wise to act upon a clinical diagnosis without awaiting histologic confirmation. The probability of acute fatty liver should be suggested by the occurrence, in the last 6 weeks of pregnancy, of epigastric pain, persistent vomiting, and jaundice accompanied by elevation of alkaline phosphatase and SGOT values and leukocytosis. The presence of confusion, stupor, headache, disorientation, or hematemesis suggests that the disease is approaching its final stage. When a presumptive diagnosis is made, cross-matched blood should be available, cesarean section should be performed immediately, and vigorous supportive measures should be started. The outlook for the mother is grave, but some of the babies can be saved by prompt delivery.

RECURRENT INTRAHEPATIC CHOLESTATIC JAUNDICE OF PREGNANCY

Recurrent jaundice of pregnancy (intrahepatic cholestasis of late pregnancy, obstetric hepatosis, cholestatic hepatosis, cholangitic hepatitis) occurs also in late pregnancy and is characterized by generalized pruritus followed, usually after 2 weeks or more, by nausea, vomiting, epigastric pain, clay-colored feces, and dark urine. Mild jaundice follows several days later. There is usually no fever. Serum conjugated bilirubin and alkaline phosphatase values are elevated, but results of other liver function tests (SGOT, thymol turbidity, prothrombin index) are normal. Serum prolactin and serum cholic acid are elevated; the latter evidently has some value in predicting fetal welfare. Liver biopsy discloses no hepatocellular damage; the characteristic finding is bile stasis with dilated bile capillaries and bile thrombi. The mechanism is obscure, although Barnes suggests it may result from the effect of the pregnancy changes in steroid metabolism on the physicochemical composition of the bile. The syndrome clears promptly after delivery, but it tends to recur in subsequent pregnancies.

The condition was formerly thought to be benign, but this is not the case. Intrauterine death, low-birthweight babies, preterm labor, and postpartum hemorrhage are all significantly increased. Therefore, such patients are at high risk, and appropriate measures of surveillance must be taken.

PTYALISM

The secretion of saliva is normally not affected by pregnancy, but occasionally excessive quantities of saliva are secreted during the first trimester. The daily secretion of 1–2 liters has been reported, but this degree of excessive salivation is rare. The saliva is often bitter and may cause nausea, vomiting, and weight loss. Treatment is extremely unsatisfactory. The use of astringent mouthwashes and sucking on hard candy help disguise the bad taste of the saliva. Psychotherapy may be beneficial when it is suspected that the ptyalism has an emotional cause. Most patients fall into this category.

REFERENCES AND RECOMMENDED READING

PREMATURE RUPTURE OF MEMBRANES

Artal R, Burgeson RE, Hobel CJ et al: An in vitro model for the study of enzymatically mediated biochemical changes in the chorioamniotic membranes. Am J Obstet Gynecol 133:656, 1979

Artal R, Sokol RJ, Neunam N, et al: The mechanical properties of prematurely and non-prematurely ruptured membranes. Methods and preliminary results. Am J Obstet Gynecol 125:655, 1976

Berkowitz RL: Premature rupture of the membranes: A review and treatment plan. Contemp OB/Gyn 10:35, 1977

Danforth DN, Hull RW: Microscopic anatomy of the fetal membranes with particular reference to the detailed structure of the amnion. Am J Obstet Gynecol 75:536, 1958

Danforth DN, McElin TW, States MN: Studies on the fetal membranes: I. Bursting tension. Am J Obstet Gynecol 65:480, 1953

Depp R: Present status of the assessment of fetal maturity. Semin Perinatol 4:229, 1980

Garite TJ, Freeman RK, Linzey EM et al: The use of amniocentesis in patients with premature rupture of the membranes. Obstet Gynecol 54:226, 1979

Gibbs RS, Castillo MS, Rodgers PJ: Management of chorioamnionitis. Am J Obstet Gynecol 136:709, 1980

Kappy KA, Cetrulo CL, Knuppel RA et al: Premature rupture of the membranes: A conservative approach. Am J Obstet Gynecol 134:655, 1979

Lavery JP, Miller CP: Deformation and creep in the human chorioamniotic sac. Am J Obstet Gynecol 134:366, 1979

Liggins GC, Howie RN: A controlled trial of antepartum glucocorticoid treatment for prevention of respiratory distress syndrome in premature infants. Pediatrics 50:515, 1972

Pagageorgiou AN, Desgranges MF, Masson M et al: The antenatal use of betamethasone in the prevention of respiratory distress syndrome: A controlled double-blind study. Pediatrics 63:73, 1979

Schreiber J, Benedetti T: Conservative management of preterm premature rupture of the fetal membranes in a low socioeconomic population. Am J Obstet Gynecol 136:92, 1980

Selle J, Harris TR: Association of premature rupture of membranes with idiopathic respiratory distress syndrome. Obstet Gynecol 49:167, 1977

Shields JR, Resnik R: Fetal lung maturation and the antenatal use of glucocorticoids to prevent the respiratory distress syndrome. Obstet Gynecol Surv 34:343, 1979

Skinner SJM, Campos GA, Liggins GC: The collagen content of human amniotic membranes: Effect of gestation length and premature rupture. Obstet Gynecol 57:487, 1981

Tinga DJ, Aarnoudse JG, Rogge P et al: Letter to the Editor (regarding adverse maternal effects of combined use of terbutaline and corticosteroids). Lancet 1:1026, 1979

Young BK, Klein SA, Katz M, et al: Intravenous dexamethasone for prevention of neonatal respiratory distress: A prospective controlled study. Am J Obstet Gynecol 138:203, 1980

POSTTERM PREGNANCY

Anderson GG: Postmaturity: A review. Obstet Gynecol Surv 27:65, 1972

Andersen HF, Johnson TRB, Jr, Barclay ML, et al: Gestational age assessment. I. Analysis of individual clinical observations. Am J Obstet Gynecol 139:173, 1981

Beard R, Steer PJ: Induction of labour and perinatal mortality. Br Med J 2:516, 1977

Callenbach JC, Hall RT: Morbidity and mortality of advanced gestational age: Postterm or postmature. Obstet Gynecol 53:721, 1979

Nakano R: Postterm pregnancy: Five year review from Osaka National Hospital. Acta Obstet Gynecol Scand 51:217, 1972

Green JN, Paul RH: The value of amniocentesis in prolonged pregnancy. Obstet Gynecol 51:293, 1978

Klapholz H, Friedman EA: The incidence of intrapartum fetal distress with advancing gestational age. Am J Obstet Gynecol 127:405, 1977

Knox GE, Huddleston JF, Flowers CE, Jr: Management of prolonged pregnancy: Results of a prospective randomized trial. Am J Obstet Gynecol 134:376, 1979

Liggins GC: Fetal influences on myometrial contractility. Clin Obstet Gynecol 16, No. 3:148, 1973

Park GL: Duration of pregnancy. Lancet 2:1388, 1968

Speroff L, Glass RH, Kase NG: Clinical endocrinology and infertility, 2nd ed, p. 207. Baltimore, Williams & Wilkins, 1978

Tabei T, Heinrichs WL: Diagnosis of placental sulfatase deficiency. Am J Obstet Gynecol 124:409, 1976

Zwerdling MA: Factors pertaining to prolonged pregnancy and its outcome. Pediatrics 42:202, 1967

MISSED LABOR

Aoskan S, Portela L, Nijenson E et al: Fetal demise, an accurate diagnosis. IMJ 155:153, 1979

Mackenzie IZ, Davies AJ, Embrey MP: Fetal death in utero managed with vaginal prostaglandin E$_2$ gel. Br Med J 1:1764, 1979

Wingerup L, Anderson KE, Ulmsten U: Ripening of the uterine cervix and induction of labour at term with prostaglandin E$_2$ in viscous gel. Acta Scand Obstet Gynecol 57:403, 1978

HYDRAMNIOS

Abramovich DR, Garden A, Jandial L et al: Fetal swallowing and voiding in relation to hydramnios. Obstet Gynecol 54:15, 1979

Danforth DN, Hull RW: The microscopic anatomy of the fetal membranes with particular reference to the detailed structure of the amnion. Am J Obstet Gynecol 75:536, 1958

Gadd RL: The liquor amnii. In Philipp EE, Barnes J, Newton M (eds): Scientific Foundations of Obstetrics and Gynaecology, 2nd ed. London, William Heinemann, 1977

Weir PE, Ratten GJ, Beischer NA: Acute polyhydramnios—A complication of monozygous twin pregnancy. Br J Obstet Gynecol 86:849, 1979

ANEMIA

Barnes CG: Medical Disorders in Obstetric Practice, 4th ed, Chap. 10. Oxford, Blackwell, 1974

Cohen BJB, Gibor Y: Anemia and menstrual blood loss. Obstet Gynecol Surv 35:597, 1980

Danforth DN, Kyser FA, Boronow RC: Refractory anemia and thrombocytopenia due to pregnancy. JAMA 180:485, 1962

Donald I: Practical Obstetric Problems, Chap. 7. London, Lloyd–Luke, 1979

Fullerton WT, Turner AG: Exchange transfusion in treatment of severe anaemia in pregnancy. Lancet 1:75, 1962

Jenkins DT, Wishart MM, Schenberg C: Serum ferritin in pregnancy. Aust NZ J Obstet Gynaecol 18:223, 1978

Kelly AM, MacDonald DJ, McDougall AN: Observations on maternal and fetal ferritin concentrations at term. Br J Obstet Gynaecol 85:338, 1978

Lawson J: Tropical obstetrics. In Walker J, MacGillivray I, Macnaughton MC (eds): Combined Textbook of Obstetrics and Gynaecology, Edinburgh, Churchill Livingstone, 1976

McFee JG: Anemia: A high risk complication of pregnancy. Clin Obstet Gynecol 16:152, 1973

Messer RH: Pregnancy anemias. Clin Obstet Gynecol 17:163, 1974

Perry CP, Harris RE: Successful management of pregnancy-induced pancytopenia. Obstet Gynecol 50:732, 1977

Pitkin RM, Witte DL: Platelet and leucocyte counts in pregnancy. JAMA 242:2696, 1979

Taft LI, Halliday JW, Russo AM et al: Serum ferritin in pregnancy. The effect of iron supplementation. Aust NZ J Obstet Gynaecol 18:226, 1978

Taylor DJ, Lind T: Red cell mass during and after normal pregnancy. Br J Obstet Gynaecol 86:364, 1979

EMESIS AND HYPEREMESIS GRAVIDARUM

Kauppila A, Huhtanieme E, Ylikorkala O: Raised serum chorionic gonadotropin concentrations in hyperemesis gravidarum. Br Med J 1:1670, 1979

VASCULAR DISORDERS

Aminoff MJ: Neurological disorders in pregnancy. Am J Obstet Gynecol 132:325, 1978

Barter RH, Letterman GS, Schurter M: Hemangiomas in pregnancy. Am J Obstet Gynecol 87:625, 1963

Bryans FE: Vascular accidents in maternal mortality. Clin Obstet Gynecol 6:861, 1963

Danforth DN, Manalo-Estrella P, Buckingham JC: The effect of pregnancy and of Enovid on the rabbit vasculature. Am J Obstet Gynecol 19:715, 1964

Danforth WC: Aneurysm of the splenic artery with rupture, a rare complication of pregnancy. Am J Obstet Gynecol 50:753, 1945

Furler IM, Robertson DNS: Spontaneous rupture of the splenic artery in pregnancy. Lancet 2:588, 1962

Hume M, Krasnick G: Dissecting aneurysm in pregnancy associated with aortic insufficiency. N Engl J Med 268:174, 1963

Jennett WB, Cross JN: Influence of pregnancy and oral contraception on the incidence of strokes in women of childbearing age. Lancet 1:1019, 1967

Jewett JF: Two dissecting coronary artery aneurysms postpartum. N Engl J Med 298:1255, 1978

Manalo-Estrella P, Barker AE: Histopathologic findings in human aortic media associated with pregnancy. Arch Pathol 83:336, 1967

Minielly R, Yuzpe AA, Drake CG: Subarachnoid hemorrhage secondary to ruptured cerebral aneurysm in pregnancy. Obstet Gynecol 53:64, 1979

O'Grady JP, Day EJ, Toole AL et al: Splenic artery aneurysm rupture in pregnancy. Obstet Gynecol 50:627, 1977

Pedowitz P, Perrell A: Aneurysms complicated by pregnancy: I. Aneurysms of the aorta and its major branches. Am J Obstet Gynecol 73:720, 1957

Riva HC, Pickhardt WL, Breen JL: Rupture of splenic artery and aneurysm in pregnancy. Obstet Gynecol 10:569, 1957

Smith JC: Dissecting aneurysms of coronary arteries. Arch Pathol 99:117, 1975

DISORDERS OF THE INTEGUMENT

Bierman SM: Autoimmune progesterone dermatitis of pregnancy. Arch Dermatol 107:896, 1973

Carruthers JA: Herpes gestationis: Clinical features of immunologically proved cases. Am J Obstet Gynecol 131:865, 1978

Heikkinen J, Mäentausta O, Ylöstalo P et al: Changes in serum bile acid concentrations during pregnancy, in patients with intrahepatic cholestasis of pregnancy and in pregnant women with itching. Bri J Obstet Gynaecol 88:240, 1981

Lawley TJ, Hertz KC, Wade TR et al: Pruritic urticarial papules and plaques of pregnancy. JAMA 241:1695, 1979

Lawley J, Stingl G, Katz SI: Fetal and maternal risk factors in herpes gestationis. Arch Dermatol 14:552, 1978

Rahbari H: Pruritic papules of pregnancy. J Cutan Pathol 5:347, 1978

Rogers PE, Katz S, Jordan W et al: Dermatoses and pregnancy. Hospital Med Jan. 1972

Russell B, Thorne NA: Herpes gestationis. Br J Dermatol 69:339, 1957

Schaumburg-Lever G, Saffold OE, Orfanos CE et al: Herpes gestationis. Arch Dermatol 107:888, 1973

Spangler AS, Reddy W, Bardawill WC et al: Papular dermatitis of pregnancy. JAMA 181:577, 1962

Wade TR, Wade SL, Jones HE: Skin changes and diseases associated with pregnancy. Obstet Gynecol 52:233, 1978

LIVER DISORDERS

Breen KJ, Perkins KW, Schenker S et al: Uncomplicated subsequent pregnancy after idiopathic fatty liver of pregnancy. Obstet Gynecol 40:813, 1972

Cano RI, Delman MR, Pitchumoni CS et al: Acute fatty liver of pregnancy: Complication by disseminated intravascular coagulation. JAMA 231:159, 1975

Conaster DG, Harris RE: Fatty liver of pregnancy. JAMA 232:1125, 1975

Haemmerli UP: Jaundice during pregnancy with special emphasis on recurrent jaundice during pregnancy and its differential diagnosis. Acta Med Scand (Suppl) 179:444, 1966

Holzbach RT: Acute fatty liver of pregnancy with disseminated intravascular coagulation. Obstet Gynecol 43:740, 1974

Johnston WG, Baskett TF: Obstetric cholestasis: A 14-year review. Am J Obstet Gynecol 133:299, 1979

Laatikainen T, Ikonen E: Serum bile acids in cholestasis of pregnancy. Obstet Gynecol 50:313, 1977

Moore HC: Acute fatty liver of pregnancy. J Obstet Gynaecol Br Emp 63:189, 1956

Moore HC: Recurrent jaundice of pregnancy. Lancet 2:57, 1963

Ranta T, Unnerus HA, Rossi J: Elevated plasma prolactin concentration in cholestasis of pregnancy. Am J Obstet Gynecol 134:1, 1979

Scully RE, Galdabini JJ, McNeely BU (eds): Case records of the Massachusetts General Hospital. A case of acute fatty liver of pregnancy. N Engl J Med 304:216, 1981

Sheehan HL: The pathology of acute yellow atrophy and delayed chloroform poisoning. J Obstet Gynaecol Br Emp 47:49, 1940

Sheehan HL: Jaundice in pregnancy. Am J Obstet Gynecol 81:427, 1961

Sherlock S: Jaundice in pregnancy. Br Med Bull 24:39, 1968

Sherlock S: Diseases of the Liver and Biliary System, 5th ed. Oxford, Blackwell, 1975

Sherlock S: The liver in pregnancy. In Philipp EE, Barnes J, Newton M (eds): Scientific Foundations of Obstetrics and Gynaecology, 2nd ed. London, William Heinemann, 1977

Watson BRI, Haverkamp AD: Cholestatic jaundice of pregnancy: New perspectives. Obstet Gynecol 54:650, 1979

GENERAL AND MISCELLANEOUS

Allen GW: Abnormal patency of the eustachian tube. JAMA 200:412, 1967

Barnes CG: Medical Disorders in Obstetric Practice, 4th ed. Philadelphia, Davis, 1973

Caroscio JT, Pellmar M: Pseudotumor cerebri: Occurrence during the third trimester of pregnancy. Mt. Sinai J Med 45:539, 1978

Weir JC, Silberman SL, Cohen LA: Recurring oral pregnancy tumors. Obstet Gynecol 54:358, 1979

The obstetrician of today is expected to deal not only with parturition but also with its antecedents and sequelae. He or she is often called upon to provide women with their first continuous adult medical care and to offer guidance and supervision in medical situations that exert some direct or indirect influence upon childbearing potential. In meeting these clinical responsibilities, the obstetrician is concerned not only with the gamut of medical and surgical diseases that appear in pregnancy or coincide with it, but also with endocrine, metabolic, and emotional disturbances that interfere with reproductive physiology. The obstetrician is called upon often to be the principal consultant in premarital and genetic counseling, in determining the advisability of childbearing, in selecting the best time for pregnancy in relation to periods of optimal health, and in judging the desirability of continuing pregnancy in the presence of a serious medical disorder. These judgments are based upon an intimate knowledge of medical problems, as well as an understanding of the effects of pregnancy upon the course of the disease and *vice versa*. Naturally, gravid women are subject to all the diseases that afflict their nonpregnant sisters; however, medical disorders can alter the course of pregnancy, and the prognosis of certain diseases is influenced by the superimposition of pregnancy.

Today, liberalized abortion laws that permit interruption of pregnancy in context with the mother's total risk situation provide a basis for a wide range of appraisal and realistic reproductive counseling among the vulnerable. Nevertheless, for those who are denied this option by virtue of late registration or who choose to continue the pregnancy regardless of risk, management must offer maximum safety. Often, in these circumstances, a team of specialists from several disciplines must coordinate their efforts in establishing for the patient the planned comprehensive care she requires. To the extent possible, such intensive maternity care should be offered within a perinatal center or in a single setting that spares the patient extra visits and eliminates episodic, fragmentary, or diffused supervision.

Complete obstetric care is concerned as much with preventing fetal and newborn casualties as with promoting maternal health. The two concerns are very much interrelated, since a faulty maternal environment induced by any one of a host of significant medical disorders may be responsible for a large spectrum of unfortunate perinatal events. Thus, it is an obstetric responsibility to provide a continuum of care for all female patients prior to or during the reproductive years, with a view to promoting and maintaining a general health status optimal for childbearing. It should be recognized that emotional as well as physical handicaps have considerable influence not only upon general health and potential for future pregnancy, but also upon family planning and social adjustments. It is ap

27

COINCIDENTAL DISORDERS COMPLICATING PREGNANCY

Robert E. L. Nesbitt, Jr.
Raja W. Abdul-Karim

parent also that certain reproductive problems are caused by biochemical, molecular, and hormonal alterations, while others are related to cultural, social, emotional, and environmental influences.

Since the obstetrician–gynecologist is often the next physician to see a female patient after the pediatrician has relinquished medical supervision, it is logical to expect the obstetrician–gynecologist to assume this responsibility, to be concerned with medical problems that have persisted since childhood and adolescence, and to screen young patients for disorders that may be inimical to successful childbearing. Moreover, it is important to recognize the clinical manifestations of certain latent medical problems, such as endocrine, metabolic, emotional, and cardiac conditions, that may be induced by the stresses of pregnancy. Any physician who corrects a significant medical disorder in a woman prior to or during her childbearing era and who is able to improve her general health in the preconception pe-

TABLE 27–1. RISK OUTWEIGHS BENEFITS IN THE FIRST TRIMESTER

Drug	Effects Reported
THALIDOMIDE	Limb, auricle, eye, and visceral malformations
SEROTONIN	Increase of anomalies
PHENMETRAZINE	Skeletal and visceral malformations
TOLBUTAMIDE	Increase of anomalies
CHLORPROPAMIDE	Increase of anomalies
STREPTOMYCIN	Eighth nerve damage, micromelia, multiple skeletal anomalies
TETRACYCLINE	Inhibition of bone growth, micromelia, syndactyly, discoloration of teeth
IODIDE	Congenital goiter, hypothyroidism, mental retardation
CHLOROQUINE	Retinal damage, eighth nerve damage
METHOTREXATE (for psoriasis)	Multiple anomalies
MECLIZINE	Multiple anomalies
LSD	Chromosomal abnormalities, increase of anomalies
AMPHETAMINES	Transposition of great vessels, cleft palate
TRIMETHADIONE	Multiple anomalies
PARAMETHADIONE	Multiple anomalies
DIPHENYLHYDANTOIN	Multiple anomalies
SEX STEROIDS	VACTERL syndrome*
DIETHYLSTILBESTROL	Clear cell adenocarcinoma of vagina and cervix, genital tract anomalies
ETHANOL	Fetal alcohol syndrome
BISHYDROXYCOUMARIN	Skeletal and facial anomalies, mental retardation
SODIUM WARFARIN	Skeletal and facial anomalies, mental retardation
PODOPHYLLIN (in laxatives)	Multiple anomalies
ACETAZOLAMIDE	Limb defects

* VACTERL syndrome of defects: vertebral, anal, cardiac, tracheal, esophageal, renal or radial, and limb malformations.
(Adapted from Howard FM, Hill JM: Obstet Gynecol Surv 34:643, 1979)

TABLE 27–2. RISK VS. BENEFITS UNCERTAIN IN THE FIRST TRIMESTER

Drug	Effects Reported
GENTAMICIN	Eighth nerve damage
KANAMYCIN	Eighth nerve damage
LITHIUM	Goiter, eye anomalies, cleft palate
BENZODIAZEPINES	Cardiac defects
THIOURACIL	Goiter, hypothyroidism, mental retardation
PROPYLTHIOURACIL	Goiter, hypothyroidism, mental retardation
BARBITURATES	Increase of anomalies
CANNABIS	Increase of anomalies
QUININE	Increase of anomalies
SEPTRA OR BACTRIM	Cleft palate
DIAZOXIDE	Increase of anomalies
CYTOTOXIC DRUGS	Increase of anomalies
PYRIMETHAMINE	Increase of anomalies
METRONIDAZOLE	None
EDTA	Increase of anomalies
ATROMID S	None
BENDECTIN*	None

* Originally listed in table 27–3; moved to table 27–2 because of 1981 FDA recommendation.
(Adapted from Howard FM, Hill JM: Obstet Gynecol Surv 34:643, 1979)

riod is practicing preventive medicine in obstetrics. These efforts will make it possible to identify patients who are likely to experience reproductive problems and who have the greatest need of intensive medical care.

TERATOLOGY

Teratogens are agents that are capable of causing a deformity in the fetus. The number of such agents is legion and includes such insults as environmental pol-

lutants, cosmic radiation, and food preservatives. The teratogens with which the physician is most usually concerned are 1) the STORCH infectious diseases (syphilis, toxoplasmosis, rubella, cytomegalovirus, and herpesvirus); 2) x-ray, especially from the 2nd to the 6th week of pregnancy (a dose of more than 10 rad is probably damaging to the fetus; 1–10 rad is possibly damaging; less than 1 rad is probably not damaging); and 3) drugs.

All drugs, if taken in sufficient amount, can probably be shown to have some teratogenic potential; in each case, the physician's dilemma is to weigh the benefits of a particular drug against its potential risk, or, perhaps more to the point, to balance the risk of *not* using a particular drug against the risk of using it. Howard and Hill have prepared an excellent and comprehensive review of drug use in pregnancy. Tables 27–1 through 27–5 from that source are extremely helpful as a guide to risk versus benefit in the various stages of pregnancy and in lactating women.

AUTOIMMUNE DISEASES IN PREGNANCY

Autoimmune mechanisms have been shown to be concerned in an increasing number of disorders, many of which occur in the childbearing years and consequently are not unusual in pregnancy. Autoimmune mechanisms and their role in such disorders as systemic lupus erythematosus, rheumatoid arthritis,

myasthenia gravis, and immune thrombocytopenic purpura, as well as in renal transplantation during pregnancy are discussed in Chapter 12.

INFECTIOUS DISEASES

IMMUNIZATION IN PREGNANCY

The question of immunization often arises during pregnancy for those who either contemplate travel or are exposed to certain illnesses for which immunization is possible. Vaccination against *mumps, measles,* and *rubella* is specifically contraindicated in pregnancy. Vaccination against *typhoid fever* is permissible in pregnancy only if there is direct exposure to someone who has the disease or if there is an epidemic; even in these cases, the hazard of receiving the vaccine must be weighed against the risk of not receiving it. *Influenza vaccine* is not recommended in pregnancy, except for certain women with serious debilitating disease. *Poliomyelitis* vaccination is not recommended in pregnancy, except in the presence of an epidemic. *Cholera* vaccine is probably not harmful, and there is no special contraindication if it is needed to satisfy international travel regulations. *Yellow fever* vaccination is contraindicated in pregnancy unless there is direct exposure. *Rabies* and *tetanus* vaccination should be given to pregnant women whenever there is a specific indication.

TYPHOID FEVER

Typhoid bacilli are transmitted across the placenta to the fetus. As many as one-half to three-quarters of fetuses are lost as a consequence of abortion or preterm birth. The incidence of typhoid fever in the United States is very low because of the wide use of antityphoid vaccine. Since there may be a marked febrile response, typhoid immunization should be avoided during pregnancy except when there is an epidemic or when travel to an area of endemic infection is contemplated.

SCARLET FEVER

Following the advent of penicillin, the maternal risk associated with scarlet fever has been reduced substantially. However, since the offending organism is the hemolytic streptococcus, the risk of puerperal sepsis is great when the infection is present at the time of delivery. Thus, infected patients, as well as their infants, must be appropriately isolated and prophylactic measures instituted to minimize spread of infection. The fetal risk is ordinarily not great, although the likelihood of abortion is increased when the disease is acquired during the first trimester.

TABLE 27–3. BENEFIT OUTWEIGHS RISK IN THE FIRST TRIMESTER

Drug	Effects Reported
CLOMIPHENE	Increase of anomalies, neural tube effects, Down's syndrome
GLUCOCORTICOIDS	Cleft palate, cardiac defects
GENERAL ANESTHESIA	Increase of anomalies
TRICYCLIC ANTIDEPRESSANTS	CNS and limb malformations
HALOPERIDOL	Limb malformations
SULFONAMIDES	Cleft palate, facial and skeletal defects
RIFAMPIN	Spina bifida, cleft palate
IDOXURIDINE	Increase of anomalies
ANTACIDS	Increase of anomalies
HYDRALAZINE	Increase of anomalies
MONOAMINE OXIDASE INHIBITORS	None
SALICYLATES	CNS, visceral and skeletal malformations
ACETAMINOPHEN	None
HEPARIN	None
ISOPROTERENOL	None
TERBUTALINE	None
THEOPHYLLINE	None
PHENOTHIAZINES	None
ANTIHISTAMINES	None
INSULIN	Skeletal malformations
PENICILLINS	None
CHLORAMPHENICOL	None
ISONIAZID	Increase of anomalies
IMIPRAMINE	CNS and limb anomalies
D-PENICILLAMINE	Connective tissue defect

(Adapted from Howard FM, Hill JM: Obstet Gynecol Surv 34:643, 1979)

CHOLERA

Since travel is commonplace today among pregnant patients, there may be contact with cholera in areas where the disease is endemic, notably in Southeast Asia. Much of the current information about this disease comes from the reports of the Pakistan–SEATO Cholera Research Laboratory in Dacca, East Pakistan. In Hirschhorn's report of 160 patients, 60 of whom were pregnant, the gravity of the disease in terms of fetal loss was emphasized. Although none of the patients died, there was a 50% fetal death rate during the last trimester of pregnancy caused by the profuse diarrhea which results in marked loss of water, electrolyte imbalance, acidosis, and shock. Tetracycline therapy is usually effective in reducing the duration of severe diarrhea. Most fetal deaths occur within the first 24 hours of the onset of the illness. Prompt rehydration and correction of acidosis is lifesaving for the mother, but fetal salvage remains poor. Prevention of the disease in the mother, either by vaccination (a safe

TABLE 27-4. DRUG EFFECTS IN THE SECOND AND THIRD TRIMESTERS

Drug	Effects	Drug	Effects
AMPHETAMINES	Fetal thrombocytopenia		Increased perinatal mortality
ASPIRIN	Fetal bleeding	DIAZOXIDE	Neonatal hyperglycemia
	Premature closure of ductus arteriosus		Neonatal alopecia
	Prolonged gestation		Prolonged β-adrenergic blockage
	Increased duration of labor	PROPRANOLOL	Decreased fetal cardiac output
	Increased maternal bleeding with labor and delivery	METHYLDOPA	Neonatal meconium ileus
INDOMETHACIN	Premature closure of ductus arteriosus	RESERPINE	Increased neonatal respiratory secretions, nasal congestion, cyanosis, and anorexia
BARBITURATES	Neonatal bleeding		
	Neonatal withdrawal syndrome		Neonatal thermal instability
	(?) Decreased neonatal jaundice		Neonatal depression
DIPHENYLHYDANTOIN	Fetal or neonatal hemorrhage		Neonatal galactorrhea
PRIMIDONE	Fetal or neonatal hemorrhage	THIAZIDES	Fetal or neonatal jaundice
BENZODIAZEPINES	Neonatal withdrawal syndrome		Thrombocytopenia
CHLORAMPHENICOL	Gray baby syndrome and death	GANGLIONIC BLOCKERS	Paralytic ileus in newborn
NITROFURANTOIN	Hyperbilirubinemia	LITHIUM	Neonatal goiter
	Hemolytic anemia		Electrolyte imbalances
SULFONAMIDES	Hyperbilirubinemia	PLACIDYL	Neonatal CNS depression
TETRACYCLINES	Discoloration of infant's teeth		Neonatal withdrawal syndrome
	Depression of bone growth	NARCOTICS	Respiratory depression
CHLORPROPAMIDE	Neonatal hypoglycemia	NARCOTIC ADDICTION	Respiratory depression
			Low birth weight
CURARE	Fetal curarization		Neonatal death
LOCAL ANESTHETICS	Large doses may cause fetal methemoglobinemia	THIOURACILS	Neonatal goiter
	Hypotension as regionals		Hypothyroidism
HALOTHANE	Uterine relaxation	IODIDES	Neonatal goiter
	Decreased response to oxytocics and ergot		Hypothyroidism
		QUININE	Deafness
CYTOTOXIC DRUGS	IUGR*		Thrombocytopenia
	Hypoplastic gonads	WARFARIN	Fetal hemorrhage
	Increased susceptibility to infection		Increased stillbirth
CORTICOSTEROIDS	Placental insufficiency		Increased maternal bleeding

* IUGR = Intrauterine growth retardation
(Adapted from Howard FM, Hill JM: Obstet Gynecol Surv 34:643, 1979)

procedure in pregnancy) or by antibiotic prophylaxis in epidemic situations, seems to be the only effective way of reducing fetal loss.

ERYSIPELAS

This disease, caused by the hemolytic streptococcus, is especially serious because the organisms may invade the maternal bloodstream and give rise to fetal septicemia with resulting abortion, preterm birth, or fetal death *in utero*. In addition, there is the ever-present risk of transfer of organisms to the patient's genital tract by the attendant or by the patient herself, or to the infant if an active infection exists at the time of de-

livery. With appropriate treatment, usually penicillin, the infection is ordinarily controllable in a short time; until the lesions clear, however, strict isolation of the patient is absolutely essential.

TOXOPLASMOSIS

The etiologic agent of toxoplasmosis is the protozoan *Toxoplasma gondii*, classified as a coccidium. The disease is ordinarily innocuous in the adult. When contracted during pregnancy, however, the disease is transmitted to the fetus in nearly one-half the cases. Ninety percent of women infected during pregnancy have no symptoms or pathognomonic signs. Some de-

TABLE 27-5. DRUG EFFECTS DURING LACTATION

Drug	Effects
TETRACYCLINES	Permanent staining of teeth
	Reversible depression of bone growth
CHLORAMPHENICOL	Gray baby syndrome
SULFONAMIDES	Hyperbilirubinemia
ASPIRIN	Neonatal hemorrhage
DIAZEPAM	Neonatal sedation
LITHIUM	Electrolyte imbalance
ANTICONVULSANTS	Neonatal hemorrhage
WARFARIN	Neonatal hemorrhage
RESERPINE	Nasal obstruction, increased respiratory tract secretions
	Thermal instability
	Depression
THIAZIDES	Hypokalemia
	Thrombocytopenia
HEXAMETHONIUM	Neonatal hypotension
	Paralytic ileus
PROPRANOLOL	Bradycardia
	Decreased cardiac output
IODIDES	Hypothyroidism
THIOURACILS	Hypothyroidism
ORAL HYPOGLYCEMICS	Hypoglycemia
ERGOTAMINE	Vomiting, diarrhea in infant
ANTIHISTAMINES	Hallucinations, convulsions, excitement, and death
ANTICHOLINERGICS	Lactation inhibition
NITROFURANTOIN	Hemolytic anemia

(Adapted from Howard FM, Hill JM: Obstet Gynecol Surv 34:643, 1979)

velop a syndrome of posterior cervical lymphadenopathy, splenomegaly, fever, myalgia, malaise, and rash. Although severe typhus-like symptoms have been reported, ordinarily the course is benign, and symptoms, if present, disappear without sequelae within a few days or weeks.

The incubation period of about 10 days usually follows ingestion of the infective cysts in meat or in other food contaminated, often by the patient's own hands, by oocysts from the excrement in the pet cat's litterbox. Measures for the prevention of toxoplasmosis are outlined in Table 27–6.

The variation in virulence seems to relate to the rate of organism multiplication, and the subsequent cellular necrosis occurs during the proliferative phase. An antibody response develops quickly. Unfortunately, the clinical diagnosis is not often established, but the prevalence of this condition is indicated by the presence of immune antibodies in about 35% of the population in the United States. Prospective studies have shown that from 1 in 500 to 1 in 1300 infants is infected with *T. gondii.*

The severity of congenital toxoplasmosis in contrast to the mild maternal infection may be related to multiple factors, but the fact that large number of *T. gondii* are widely distributed in fetal tissues through the bloodstream in the destructive proliferative phase of their growth may be an important difference. In addition, of course, immature tissues are generally more susceptible to damage, and immunologic defense mechanisms to protect the fetus are relatively undeveloped. It seems likely that maternal parasitemia is the basis of transmission to the fetus, but it is not known whether transmission is possible after circulating antibodies develop in the mother.

Diagnosis depends upon serologic tests. Several excellent tests that have a high degree of specificity are available. The recommended method of study is the combined use of the Sabin–Feldman dye test or the Feldman–Lamb micromodification and the complement fixation test. Results of these tests are positive within 2 weeks after infection. The IgM fluorescent antibody titer test can also be used to diagnose active or congenital toxoplasmosis. All serologic tests for toxoplasmosis require meticulous standardization, and interpretation by trained personnel.

Affected fetuses may be born with diffuse areas of intense inflammatory reaction, focal necrosis, and calcification, centering mainly about the central nervous system but involving a variety of tissues. Important findings include macrocephaly or microcephaly, hydrocephalus, carditis, hepatitis, splenomegaly, retinochoroiditis, dermatitis, and lesions of almost any other organ in the body. In cases of severe infection, abortion, preterm birth, or fetal death *in utero* is common. When damage is less intense, neonatal or infant death may occur, or the baby may survive its defects only to succumb during childhood or within the first few decades of life. Retinochoroiditis may be the only recognizable damage in mild forms of the disease, and this affliction and also some of the other manifestations may not appear until adolescence or early adulthood.

The blood antibody titer of the neonate is as high as or higher than that of the mother. Unfortunately, weeks or months are required for observation of a sufficient decline in the infant's titer to ensure that the infant is not infected. A rather complicated screening procedure based on a test for IgM (not IgG) antibodies may obviate this problem, since IgMs are not transmitted across the placenta, but the test must be perfected before it can be used widely. The test represents an indirect IgM fluorescent toxoplasma antibody determination.

If the diagnosis can be established in the mother, usually by history and physical findings, with confirmation based on a significantly rising antibody titer and conversion of the serologic test results from negative to positive, a plan of management must be devised. Standard treatment consists of sulfadiazine in combination with pyrimethamine administered over 1 month. Intramuscular folinic acid is also given to re-

TABLE 27–6. METHODS FOR THE PREVENTION OF CONGENITAL TOXOPLASMOSIS

PREVENTION OF INFECTION IN THE PREGNANT WOMAN
Hygenic measures:
  Cook meat to ≥ 66°C, smoke it, or cure it in brine.
  Avoid touching mucous membranes of the mouth and eye while handling raw meat.
  Wash hands thoroughly after handling raw meat.
  Wash kitchen surfaces that come into contact with raw meat.
  Wash fruits and vegetables before consumption.
  Prevent access of flies, cockroaches, *etc.* to fruits and vegetables.
  Avoid contact with or wear gloves when handling materials that are potentially contaminated with cat feces (e.g., cat litter boxes) or when gardening.
  Disinfect cat litter box for five min with nearly boiling water.

PREVENTION OF INFECTION IN THE FETUS
Identification of women at risk by serologic testing.
Treatment during pregnancy—results in ≃ 50% reduction in infected infants.
Therapeutic abortion—prevents birth of infected infant only in cases of women who acquire infection in first or second trimester (<50% of cases).

(Wilson CB, Remington JS: Am J Obstet Gynecol 138:357, 1980)

duce potential intoxication. Spiramycin, which is not an antifolinic agent, has had a successful clinical trial, presumably reducing fetal infection by about 50% relative to controls, but the drug is not available in the United States at this time. Abdominal roentgenography or sonography may be helpful in establishing the presence of distortions in the fetal skull and head size. Since it is unlikely that *T. gondii* can be isolated from amniotic fluid, amniocentesis is not justified; also, no antibodies would be present. Treatment for the infant born with toxoplasmosis is similar to that for the mother and is instituted several times in the 1st year of life to minimize tissue damage and at subsequent times in an effort to arrest exacerbations.

When the maternal infection is clearly diagnosed prior to the 20th gestational week, therapeutic abortion should be strongly considered. Since there is no evidence that problems arise in subsequent pregnancies and since immunity is established after one infection, sterilization is not recommended. With respect to prevention, wider screening for toxoplasma antibodies should be employed on prospective obstetric patients. Those whose serologic test results are negative should be tested for conversion at monthly intervals during the first two trimesters of pregnancy. A suspicious first trimester maternal illness calls for the same type of serologic monitoring. All patients known to be at risk for the disease should be informed of particular hazards—cats and cat feces, sand and litterboxes, poorly cooked meats, garden soil.

COCCIDIOIDOMYCOSIS

In areas where it is endemic, coccidioidomycosis is an extremely important complication of pregnancy with dire consequences to both mother and fetus when the disease occurs in the disseminated form. It is caused by a fungus, which produces endosporulating spherules within tissues and a mass of fine septate hyphae in culture medium. *Coccidioides immitis* resides primarily in the southwestern United States. The infecting agent is always the chlamydospore, not the spherule, and infection occurs by inhalation or spread by fomites within the hospital. The primary lesion for the vast majority of victims is a self-limited pulmonary infection. In some, particularly members of the dark-skinned races, secondary infection or dissemination occurs by means of the blood or lymph. Distant lesions may be suppurative, necrotic, or granulomatous and may develop in any organ. There may be communications with the skin, including that of the face, by multiple sinuses, as well as with deeper structures, such as bone, by deeply ramifying channels.

The likelihood of dissemination is increased when the disease is contracted during pregnancy, particularly at a late stage. The placenta may become infected, but apparently it serves as a barrier, since fetal involvement is rare. Maternal mortality from the disseminated disease probably exceeds 90%. Fetal wastage is likewise extremely great from this form, especially when dissemination occurs in the early stages of gestation. The highly toxic drug amphotericin B is the therapeutic agent of choice. The side effects include hypokalemia, anemia, and renal damage. A rising value on the complement fixation test and rapid spread of the pulmonary lesion make it necessary to accept these risks of therapy, particularly in the pregnant woman who is especially vulnerable. The neonate of a surviving mother may be entirely normal.

RUBELLA (GERMAN MEASLES)

Rubella is a viral infection that represents one of the most significant common communicable diseases because it carries an ominous prognosis for the fetus if it is contracted by the mother during the early weeks of pregnancy. As a result of observations made by Gregg, an ophthalmologist, during an epidemic of German measles in Australia in 1941, it has been established that infants of women who contract the disease in the first trimester show a wide range of congenital defects, including cataracts. The offending organism is a single ribonucleic acid (RNA) virus of the paramyxovirus group, usually transmitted by droplet infection. It is estimated that, during nonepidemic periods, about 15% of pregnant women are susceptible. Clinical rubella occurs in only about 1 in 1000 pregnancies during nonepidemic periods, but the incidence rises to 22

or more per 1000 pregnancies during epidemics. Conversion of serologic test results in asymptomatic women indicates that the attack rate may be even higher. Except for transient neuritis and arthritis, or occasionally the more serious encephalitis, prompt maternal recovery can be anticipated. Depending upon the stage of pregnancy, however, the outlook for the fetus is grave. Fetal infection arising from maternal disease in the first 8 weeks of pregnancy exceeds 90%. A review of available published reports indicates that rubella in the first trimester produces serious fetal defects in approximately 25%–50% of cases. These estimates are even higher when minor impairments or late developing defects, such as hearing loss, are included.

The virus may persist in tissues for years, and the fact that growth retardation can occur even after organogenesis has been completed constitutes the basis for a concept referred to as the *expanded congenital rubella syndrome*. This includes hepatosplenomegaly, thrombocytopenic purpura, pneumonitis, hepatitis, encephalitis, lesions of the long bones and anemia.

The more classic lesions, however, affecting fetuses who acquire the infection during the time of organogenesis, are congenital heart disease, deafness, cataract, and cerebral and somatic retardation. Damage incurred at the time of primordial development between the 3rd and 7th weeks usually results in death from serious anomalies, while fetuses affected at a later date are usually less seriously damaged, and a much higher percentage may be expected to survive their disabilities. Congenital deafness is the principal defect encountered among infants born of mothers who contract rubella between the 9th and 13th weeks. After that time the likelihood of a serious congenital malformation in the infant from this cause becomes less frequent.

Perhaps the greatest hope for eliminating rubella-induced birth defects lies in prevention of the infection in pregnancy. Mass vaccination of prepubertal children with highly effective live, attenuated rubella virus vaccine offers promise, but the duration of immunity has not been established beyond 4 years. The availability of rubella antibody testing for women of childbearing age makes it possible to identify those at risk. The tests being used are hemagglutination inhibition (HAI), fluorescent antibody, and complement fixation. The hemagglutinin-inhibiting antibody is specific for rubella and does not cross-react with other viruses. A serum antibody titer of less than 1:10 is generally interpreted as indicating susceptibility. It is also compatible with a beginning infection. A second test, usually performed several weeks later, must show a fourfold increase in serum antibody titer to indicate infection clearly. It is recommended that every patient seen in premarital examination who demonstrates a negative result on the HAI test should be vaccinated. However, there must be assurance that pregnancy will not occur within 2 months of that time. A postpartal patient or any woman in the childbearing age whose HAI test result is negative may be vaccinated, but vaccination is contraindicated during pregnancy under all circumstances. The pregnant woman should avoid exposure to those who have been recently vaccinated; however, there is no conclusive evidence about the risks of transmission, and should she be so exposed, termination of pregnancy is not recommended. On the other hand, definite conversion of the serologic test result following exposure during the first trimester warrants consideration of pregnancy termination.

It seems clear that a modified form of the disease following prior vaccination carries the same fetal risks as the typical manifestation. Moreover, clinical trials have shown that γ-globulin cannot be relied upon for prevention of congenital rubella. Immune globulin should be given within 5 days of exposure to be of benefit. Its administration is not recommended for the pregnant woman who has already developed the disease. As patients and physicians consider the necessity or desirability of large doses of γ-globulin or therapeutic abortion to avert serious congenital abnormalities of the fetus, immunologic testing of the pregnant patient will become a necessary part of the diagnostic evaluation.

It should be emphasized that affected infants excrete the virus in the urine for several weeks after birth and can shed the virus from the throat for long periods of time. Thus, newborns with the congenital rubella syndrome must be considered contagious, and appropriate safeguards within the hospital must be taken to protect pregnant women from contact.

A recent paper describes an outbreak of 47 cases of rubella occurring among hospital personnel in a large medical–surgical hospital. A dietary worker was identified as the probable index case. The report notes that subclinical infection can occur in at least 10% of susceptible persons. The question is raised whether all hospital personnel having contact with pregnant women should be tested for susceptibility and the susceptible persons immunized, and also whether preemployment screening should be mandatory for prospective hospital personnel.

MEASLES (RUBEOLA)

Major congenital malformations have been reported following first trimester measles, although a clear causal relationship has not been definitely established. Abortion, preterm birth, and perinatal death appear to be more common with such maternal infections.

VARICELLA (CHICKENPOX)

Although varicella infection has no predilection for the gravid woman, there is some evidence to suggest that

the disease is more virulent during pregnancy. Greater virulence predisposes to abortion, preterm birth, or perhaps, perinatal death. Rarely, the disease takes a fulminant, fatal course. There is no clear evidence that such an infection in the mother gives rise to an increased incidence of congenital malformations. Following maternal infection, the virus is not recoverable from the infant, and there is no IgM elevation. However, following first trimester maternal infections, several infants have been born with cicatricial skin lesions, suggestive of *in utero* involvement. These infants were small for their presumed gestational age and exhibited a number of afflictions, including cortical atrophy, seizures, chorioretinitis, microphthalmia, cataracts, and limb atrophy. These defects are similar to those produced by other viruses known to be teratogenic.

If chickenpox is contracted within 2 weeks of delivery, there is high likelihood that the fetus will be infected; congenital varicella and perinatal death are quite frequent under these circumstances.

CYTOMEGALIC INCLUSION BODY DISEASE

Together with rubella and toxoplasmosis, cytomegalovirus infection is an important antecedent of congenital defects. This ubiquitous virus of the herpes group may infect the mother without producing recognizable symptoms. It is estimated that about 20% of adults show no neutralizing antibodies to the virus and may thus be considered vulnerable. The virus can be transmitted to the fetus transplacentally, and the consequences of fetal infection may be tragic— microcephaly with periventricular calcification, hepatosplenomegaly with jaundice, and thrombocytopenic purpura. There may be chorioretinitis and widespread cerebral degeneration resulting in cerebral palsy, seizures, and mental retardation among survivors. Infants with viruria or neutralizing antibodies may develop various manifestations of disease in later life. In addition to the cerebral and hepatic involvement, the lungs, eyes, kidneys, or pancreas may be affected. The virus may be recoverable from the mother's breast milk. Although rare, the uterus can apparently harbor the virus following placental infection, and fetal infection in consecutive pregnancies has been reported.

The infected tissues may contain large cells with inclusion bodies in the nuclei (owl-eye cells). These cells are found in urinary sediment. Although the typical pathologic lesion occurs in the salivary gland, the infection is generally widespread throughout the body. Generally, the fetus is infected during the viremic phase and becomes widely diseased. Apparently, the virus can persist intracellularly for years despite high antibody titers. The cervix can harbor the virus, and an ascending infection can occur in labor. Breast-fed newborns may get infections through the maternal milk.

There is evidence that cytomegalovirus infections may be much more prevalent than is generally appreciated and that the number of fetal affections from this cause may be relatively greater than those associated with such better publicized maternal diseases as rubella, herpes, and toxoplasmosis. Starr *et al.* suggest that false security has been generated by the innocuous maternal condition and the fact that the neonate may be clinically normal despite harboring and excreting the organisms. Subclinical infection in the infant is now known to be capable of producing mental retardation of variable degree, as well as auditory deficits, particularly with respect to high-frequency sound discrimination. Immunologic overstimulation and responsiveness in silent infections accompanied by chronic virus excretion cause subtle damage in the kidneys and other organs. Unfortunately, at the present time there is no specific treatment for the condition, and no vaccine is available as a preventive.

Cytomegalovirus vaccines, using live viruses, have been studied on a small scale and seem effective. Their safety is not yet established.

MUMPS

Intrauterine mumps virus infection acquired during the early stages of gestation may be associated with a high fetal death rate. Such infections have been incriminated as a possible cause of primary endocardial fibroelastosis in infants. Mumps vaccines that use live viruses should not be given during pregnancy.

SMALLPOX (VARIOLA)

The world-wide eradication of smallpox has now been accomplished, the only disease in which this goal has been achieved. Steps to prevent or deal with it are therefore no longer needed.

COXSACKIEVIRUS DISEASE

If contracted during pregnancy, coxsackievirus imposes a major risk because of its ability to infect the fetus. The fetus may succumb to myocarditis and encephalomyelitis despite a relatively minor respiratory illness in the mother. Some mothers exhibit influenza-like illness, while others have pleurodynia, pericarditis, or aseptic meningitis late in pregnancy. Infants delivered of mothers who contract the disease prior to the 8th month are usually unaffected.

Perinatal infections may occur. The teratogenic ef-

fect of these viruses is not fully clear, although coxsackievirus B *in utero* infection is implicated in congenital anomalies of the heart and urinary tract.

HERPESVIRUS INFECTION

Herpesvirus infections are discussed later in this chapter, under Diseases of the Skin.

Maternal herpes zoster is thought to be associated with an increased incidence of congenital cataracts, although a clear relationship between the two has not been established. The disease is rarely recognized in the neonate.

TUBERCULOSIS

Unsuspected pulmonary tuberculosis is discovered in about 1% of pregnant women. Since it is encountered more frequently among certain groups, notably nonwhite clinic patients, these women at least should be screened for tuberculosis, and a strong case can be made for routinely obtaining chest x-rays on all pregnant women.

When active pulmonary tuberculosis is suspected, early bacteriologic confirmation is important, because many other chronic lung diseases can mimic tuberculosis. Cytologic evaluation of sputum and bronchial secretions may be needed to rule out fungal infection or bronchogenic carcinoma. With proper shielding, oblique (20°–25° rotation) and lateral roentgenograms and planigrams of the lungs can safely be obtained. Identification of the species of acid-fast bacillus is necessary, according to Stead, because of the increasing frequency with which infections with other mycobacteria are being encountered. These include *Mycobacterium battey, Mycobacterium kansasii,* and scotochromogenic mycobacteria. While these infections require chemotherapy, communicability is not a significant threat as it is in tuberculosis. Unfortunately, in some patients with active *Mycobacterium tuberculosis* infection, organisms cannot be demonstrated even by meticulous study. In such a case, when tuberculosis is suspected and fungal infection and tumor have been excluded, it may be appropriate to give isoniazid prophylactically for 12–18 months. According to Weinstein and Murphy, prophylactic chemotherapy is most important in persons who have had active tuberculosis and who have "recovered" without receiving tuberculostatic drugs.

Pregnancy *per se,* if properly managed, has no deleterious effect upon the course of the disease, nor do labor and delivery, if these are intelligently conducted. Indeed, a patient who has been treated in a hospital throughout her pregnancy with appropriate antituberculosis drugs (usually streptomycin, isoniazid, and

para-aminosalicylic acid) may fare much better than the nonpregnant woman who has not received this specialized attention. Ethambutol is often used in place of para-aminosalicylic acid. Rifampin, although a highly effective agent, is teratogenic in animals. There is no convincing evidence that isoniazid and para-aminosalicylic acid produce any untoward effects in pregnant patients or have any teratogenicity. Streptomycin is safe for the mother, but ototoxic for the newborn. The effect is rare, but very severe when it occurs. Damage is much less common when the fetus is exposed to the drug only after the 5th month of gestation; thus, if streptomycin must be given, it should be deferred until that time.

If the patient is asymptomatic and her lesion is minimal, it may be possible to manage her at home on a supervised rest regimen, provided precautions are taken to restrict her contacts. When the pulmonary lesion is serious, the pregnant woman ordinarily is able to withstand remarkably well the surgical procedures of lobectomy, pneumonectomy, and even secondary thoracoplasty that are occasionally required. It has been clearly documented that neither the infection itself nor appropriate drug therapy exerts any harmful effect upon mother or fetus. The disease is sometimes transmitted *in utero,* but generally the infant is uninvolved. Moreover, the fetus is able to sustain itself very well despite the handicap of a seriously ill mother. The exception to this generalization is miliary tuberculosis, characterized by profound prostration and a precipitous downhill course; this is often associated with abortion, labor, or fetal death.

Although difficult vaginal delivery is to be avoided, it is usually best to minimize exertion in the second stage of labor by performing a low forceps delivery, preferably under some form of nerve block anesthesia. Deep narcosis or diminution of the cough reflex should be avoided, and certain patients benefit from supplemental oxygen administration. Abdominal delivery may be required because of the usual obstetric indications, although the timing of the intervention may be influenced to some extent by the condition of the patient, particularly in protracted labor when there is the risk of serious maternal strain and exhaustion. After delivery, it is important to continue control measures because exacerbation of the lesion can be expected if treatment is terminated prematurely. The infant should be separated from the mother until it is established that she is noninfectious. Kendig reports that up to 50% of infants born of mothers with currently or recently active pulmonary tuberculosis develop active disease in the 1st year of life if chemoprophylaxis is not carried out. Congenital tuberculosis is rare, but it may occur from hematogenous spread or aspiration of infected material before or during labor.

Since pulmonary tuberculosis is not affected by well-managed pregnancy, and treatment for the preg-

nant patient is nearly the same for comparable lesions as for the nonpregnant patient, with the same prospect of recovery, therapeutic abortion is not indicated. Adrenal tuberculosis, which once constituted a grave maternal hazard, can now be controlled satisfactorily with substitution therapy. Renal, bone, and joint tuberculosis should be treated as in the nonpregnant patient. Since genital tract tuberculosis is ordinarily associated with sterility, it is rarely encountered as a complication of pregnancy, although well-documented cases of early abortion followed by a flare-up of infection, as well as of pregnancy arising in a Fallopian tube damaged by active disease, have been reported.

LEPROSY

Although leprosy is not often encountered in the United States, the scattered reports available in the literature indicate that the outcome of pregnancy among women afflicted with active cutaneous lesions may be good, since healthy infants without evidence of the disease have been born of these mothers. The sulfone drugs have been effective.

MALARIA

The likelihood of recrudescence of malarial infections during pregnancy and the puerperium is increased, and these exacerbations are attended by an increased incidence of abortion and preterm labor. Further, the fetus may die as the result of maternal intoxication or from hypoxia. Despite the ability of the parasites to traverse the placenta, however, infection of the fetus is unusual. The mother is usually able to tolerate chloroquine and other antimalarial drugs without untoward effects, and generally the outcome of the pregnancy is satisfactory. Possible teratogenic effects of chloroquine are unknown, although normal infants have been born to mothers receiving this drug. Pyrimethamine, a folic acid antagonist, should not be used as an antimalarial during early pregnancy because of the risk of abortion or fetal malformation.

SYPHILIS

Traditionally, preterm birth and fetal death of unknown cause has aroused suspicion of maternal syphilis. Indeed, the presence of a large, pale gray placenta with the microscopic features of fibrosis, endarteritis, and clubbing of terminal villi was considered pathognomonic of fetal syphilis until relatively recently, when it was discovered that these histologic features occur as a degenerative process secondary to fetal death from any cause. Notwithstanding these misinterpretations, syphilis ranked high in the prepenicillin

era as a cause of perinatal death; in addition, many liveborn infants were left with permanent stigmas of the disease. With the advent of penicillin treatment, syphilis declined dramatically as a medical problem in obstetric patients, and fetal deaths attributable to this cause were responsible for only a small minority of perinatal losses. For almost a decade there was a steady decline in the incidence of early syphilis. However, since 1958 there has been a reversal of this trend; penicillin-resistant infections have appeared with greater regularity, and it has become necessary to renew epidemiologic controls.

Since the great majority of female patients do not have visible manifestations, it is mandatory to perform a serologic test on each pregnant woman at least once prior to delivery, preferably in both early and late pregnancy. In suspected but unsubstantiated cases of syphilis, it is desirable to follow the mother and child clinically as well as serologically after birth. Specific antitreponemal antibody tests (TPI, FTA, TPHA) are also used to establish the diagnosis.

Adequate and prompt treatment of the mother during gestation prevents the development of congenital syphilis, since penicillin traverses the placenta and achieves a therapeutic level in the fetus. If untreated syphilis in the mother is of more than 4 years' duration, the fetus may escape infection.

If the mother's blood is reactive, the cord blood also will be reactive, but this does not necessarily mean the fetus has acquired the infection. When the mother has been adequately treated at any time during gestation, the fetus is spared almost without exception. The antibody titer of the uninfected infant's blood falls progressively, and results of serologic tests usually become negative within 3 months. The cord blood may be seronegative if the mother is infected quite late in pregnancy. If the infant is infected, the blood of the infant becomes reactive, with a rising titer; usually within 3 months, signs of early syphilis develop, notably cutaneous or mucous membrane lesions, osteochondritis, and hepatosplenomegaly. If mucocutaneous lesions are present, a smear of the secretions will ordinarily reveal mycobacteria on dark-field examination.

The maintenance of a penicillin blood level ranging 0.03–0.2 units/ml over a period of 10 days is adequate treatment for any stage of syphilis. This can be accomplished by a number of schedules using any one of several penicillin preparations, notably benzathine penicillin G, PAM, and aqueous procaine penicillin G. When there is any doubt about the adequacy of previous treatment, the pregnant woman with a reactive blood test, regardless of titer, should be retreated. When a standard course of penicillin has been administered previously, it is unnecessary to repeat the treatment unless the patient has failed to achieve the normal clinical and serologic responses. Cephalosporins are the best alternatives in patients with peni-

cillin allergy, although cross allergy may occur. Erythromycin crosses the placenta poorly, and the newborn should be treated with penicillin.

LYMPHOGRANULOMA VENEREUM

A chlamydia infection, lymphogranuloma venereum has significance in pregnancy because of characteristic pelvic lesions that result in marked scarring of the rectal wall, the rectovaginal septum, and the vagina. Depending upon the extent of fibrotic changes and fixation, vaginal delivery may seriously disrupt the scar tissue, resulting in lacerations of the upper rectum and posterior cul-de-sac, particularly if the birth is traumatic. Serious hemorrhage or peritonitis may prove fatal in these circumstances. A careful pelvic examination should be performed to determine the extent and character of the disease process before a decision is made on the route of delivery. If there are extensive pelvic scarring and induration, with a thick, unyielding rectovaginal septum, abdominal delivery is much to be preferred. Chemotherapy can be used to arrest the lesion and to combat secondary infection. If colostomy has been required to divert the fecal stream in cases of rectal stricture, this should not interfere with the course of pregnancy or with delivery by either route.

GRANULOMA INGUINALE

This infection of the lower genital tract, which is caused by encapsulated organisms (Clymmatobacterium granulomatis) known as Donovan bodies, presumably of viral origin, gives rise to extensive ulcerative lesions which may involve the vagina and cervix. These lesions may be associated ultimately with extensive scarring and deformation of the birth canal. In extreme cases, soft tissue dystocia may occur because of interference with descent of the fetal head, or extensive lacerations may be produced in the course of the delivery. Depending upon the individual findings, cesarean section may be the preferred method of delivery. Ampicillin and erythromycin stearate are applicable.

RESPIRATORY DISEASES

COMMON COLD

An acute cold is significant because in a majority of instances this infection precedes the development of pneumonia. In the pregnant woman, it may complicate the choice of anesthetic or predispose to secondary bacterial invasion, notably by the streptococcus, which increases the risk of intrapartal and puerperal sepsis.

Bedrest and supportive measures should be recommended at the first sign of acute coryza to minimize these hazards.

PNEUMONIA

The significance of pneumococcal pneumonia as a maternal risk has been dramatically influenced by the advent of chemotherapy, particularly penicillin, since most infections are readily controlled by appropriate treatment. Nevertheless, the neglected case constitutes a grave hazard to the mother and fetus by virtue of cyanosis, reduced oxygen content of the maternal blood, bacteremia, and transplacental infection. In these circumstances, the likelihood of preterm birth, fetal death, or abortion is great. As a consequence of empyema, lung abscess, meningitis, and other complications, the outlook for the mother may be critical.

Every effort should be made to prevent the expectant mother from coming in contact with infections of this kind. In the event an infection does develop, she must be hospitalized and started on appropriate therapy immediately. Significant respiratory symptoms should not be treated without accurate diagnosis, nor should pulmonary infection in the pregnant woman be treated on an ambulatory basis.

INFLUENZA

The gross maternal mortality during the great influenza pandemic of 1918 was 27%; but of those whose course was complicated by pneumonia, the rate was increased to 50%. Epidemic influenza does not carry these grave risks, although the superimposition of pneumonia constitutes a serious complication. In the cases complicated by less dangerous conditions, notably laryngitis, bronchitis, and sinusitis, the prognosis for mother and fetus is good. Chemotherapeutic agents are ineffective against influenza, but they minimize the risk of pneumonia and other serious clinical sequelae. Vaccination with bivalent vaccines is recommended only for high-risk patients, i.e., those with cardiac or pulmonary disease.

Pregnant women have exhibited an increased susceptibility to Asian influenza in recent pandemics, and the disease appears to affect them with greater severity. For example, during the pandemic of 1957, some areas reported that nearly half of the women of childbearing age who died were pregnant. In all studies, it was clear that pulmonary edema, pneumonia, and secondary invasion with coagulase-positive staphylococci reduced the chance of recovery dramatically. In these cases, the fetus is always in jeopardy; in general, however, the prognosis for the infant is good. Available information indicates that this infection has no influence on the incidence of congenital anomalies.

BRONCHIECTASIS

The course of bronchiectasis is not altered by pregnancy, nor is pregnancy usually affected by the pulmonary changes. In advanced cases associated with fever, cough, foul sputum, dyspnea, and cyanosis, however, meticulous prenatal supervision is required. Postural drainage and antibiotics may be needed. In the management of labor, minimal analgesia in the first stage and conduction anesthesia for delivery are the preferred techniques of pain relief when respiratory capacity is reduced.

PULMONARY FIBROSIS

This chronic respiratory condition characterized by diffuse involvement of the lung parenchyma, may be caused by a variety of infiltrative lesions. In general, it does not interfere with successful pregnancy unless the patient is dyspneic at rest or on slight exertion. Temporary improvement is sometimes noted during pregnancy, presumably as a result of mechanical factors or, possibly, cortisone-like effects.

EMPHYSEMA

Emphysema poses a problem in pregnancy only in its advanced stages when there is insufficient oxygenation of the maternal blood. In these circumstances, pregnancy ordinarily terminates before term, and the prognosis for both mother and fetus is guarded.

KYPHOSCOLIOSIS

Marked distortion of the chest associated with pathologic lesions of the cervical and thoracic vertebrae disturbs respiratory function and cardiopulmonary circulation. Cardiac hypertrophy and dilation, as well as a substantial reduction in the vital capacity, portend poorly for the pregnancy. The fixed chest wall interferes significantly with the ventilating efficiency normally observed during pregnancy through the increased mobility of the thorax.

PULMONARY RESECTION

Pneumonectomy, pulmonary resection, and thoracoplasty are not contraindications to pregnancy if the residual functional capacity is not greatly reduced. Patients who are not dyspneic on mild exertion can be expected to go through pregnancy, labor, and vaginal delivery without difficulty, although these women should guard against any illness that would further compromise their limited respiratory capacity. Serial determinations of vital capacity or estimations of residual functional capacity furnish a useful index of the efficiency of respiration, but, from a practical viewpoint, the patient's appearance and respiratory behavior permit a fairly accurate assessment of clinical status.

ASTHMA

The symptoms of asthma may temporarily be completely relieved during pregnancy; less commonly, they are aggravated or make their appearance first at this time and disappear during the puerperium. Sensitivity to the barbiturates is not uncommon, and an overdose during labor may cause prolonged respiratory depression as well as pulmonary complications. Similarly, it is important to avoid the use of morphine because of its depressant effects. When pulmonary function is impaired, a regional anesthetic is best.

The outlook for pregnancy is good unless there is a refractory asthmatic state with emphysema, superimposed chronic bronchitis, and insufficient aeration of the maternal blood. An effort should be made to establish the cause and to eliminate the specific irritant if this can be determined. Usually, acute attacks can be controlled by intravenous aminophylline or subcutaneous epinephrine injections, and by the inhalation of bronchodilator substances. Hydration, antibiotic therapy for any associated infection in the lung, the use of expectorants, and oxygen administration are additional supportive measures. Since an emotional trigger often starts an attack, it is important to provide these patients with psychologic support. Pregnancy does not contraindicate the use of corticotropin and adrenocortical steroids in refractory cases, although severe bleeding from a duodenal ulcer has occurred during pregnancy as a consequence of this treatment. Patients under chronic glucocorticoid treatment need a larger dose when they are in labor or when any surgical procedure, *e.g.*, cesarean section, is to be performed.

CARDIOVASCULAR DISEASES

ESSENTIAL HYPERTENSION
(Hypertensive Vascular Disease)

The blood pressure limits in essential hypertension are not clearly established. In obstetric patients, the diagnosis should be considered if, before 24 weeks' gestation, a reading of 140/90 mm Hg or higher is found. Blood pressure should be taken again after 10 min of quiet rest; if still elevated, it should be taken after 1 week. If the blood pressure has remained at this level, the patient should be considered to have hypertensive vascular disease. (Routinely in such cases, the physician should feel the femoral pulse to note if it is de-

layed or of poor volume, so as not to overlook coarctation of the aorta, a rare but extremely important cause of hypertension.) In about one-third of these cases, the blood pressure remains at a stable, elevated level throughout pregnancy; in one-third, paradoxically, it drops, sometimes to normal levels, and remains so until the last weeks of pregnancy; and in one-third, preeclampsia is superimposed with elevation above the former levels.

Although essential hypertension is usually regarded as a disease of older persons, it is not rare among pregnant women. It is important in obstetrics chiefly because it predisposes to preeclampsia and fetal growth retardation and because the perinatal mortality rate is significantly elevated, increasing dramatically with the severity of the disease. Among those with labile blood pressure early in pregnancy, a significant number develop essential hypertension late in pregnancy; of those who do not, many develop the disease later in life.

If the patient is first seen in the last trimester of pregnancy, the differentiation of essential hypertension from preeclampsia may be difficult. Some of the tests that are used in the nonpregnant patient are not appropriate in the pregnant patient, *e.g.,* arteriography, renal biopsy, pyelography, and isotopic renography. Essential hypertension can usually be distinguished from preeclampsia by the absence of protein, pus, or casts in the urine and serum uric acid that is not elevated (unless the blood pressure is above 180/110 mm Hg). A family history of hypertension or a personal history of renal disease supports the likelihood of hypertensive vascular disease. If the diastolic pressure is above 100 mm Hg, the retinal changes of essential hypertension (arteriolar narrowing, arteriovenous nicking, flame-shaped or circular hemorrhages, papilledema) can often be distinguished from those of preeclampsia (segmental spasm of the retinal arterioles, no hemorrhages or exudates).

Hypertensive drug therapy is usually indicated in patients whose systolic pressure is 150 mm Hg or higher or whose diastolic is 100 mm Hg or higher. The goal is to maintain the pressure within 5 mm Hg diastolic and 10 mm Hg systolic of these levels. This may require flexibility in drugs selected and dosage. As a general rule, women who are taking medication before pregnancy should continue throughout pregnancy, with adjustment of drug and dosage as needed. Beta-adrenergic blocking agents of the propranolol type have been reported to have deleterious fetal effects, including bradycardia and neonatal hypoglycemia and respiratory depression, and in some cases premature labor. However, in the cases of Gallery *et al.,* in which a drug of this type (oxyprenolol) was used, fetal growth was evidently improved, there were no deleterious fetal or neonatal effects, and premature labor was not encountered.

Continued surveillance is needed throughout pregnancy. In the first trimester, 9 hours of rest are recommended at night; in the second trimester, 1 hour of rest is added during the day; in the third trimester, 2 hours during the day. A high-protein diet (75 gm minimum) is recommended, with salt intake to taste. Nonstress fetal monitoring, with oxytocin challenge as indicated, can provide useful information if done each week beginning at 30 weeks. Estriol excretion studies may also be helpful. The fetal growth increment should be determined by ultrasound scans at 20–26 and at 31–33 weeks' gestation. Amniocentesis for lecithin/sphingomyelin (L/S) ratio should be done at 32, 35, and 37 weeks' gestation and delivery planned as soon as this test provides evidence of fetal lung maturity. Optimal delivery time is usually 36–38 weeks' gestation, or when the fetus reaches a weight above 2500 g. However, one should not temporize if the severity of the disease dictates prompt delivery; a maternal catastrophe could be just as devastating for the fetus as for the mother.

HEART DISEASE

Incidence

Cardiac lesions that complicate pregnancy are the most significant medical hazards encountered in obstetrics, and, although heart disease is present in only 1%–2% of all pregnant women, it ranks fourth as a cause of maternal death. In the United States at large, deaths from this cause are exceeded only by deaths from hemorrhage, preeclampsia–eclampsia, and infection; in some large maternity centers, cardiovascular disease is the most common cause of maternal mortality.

From 80% to 85% of the heart disease encountered during pregnancy is of rheumatic origin; 10%–15% results from congenital defects; and 2% is the result of coronary heart disease, atherosclerotic heart disease, and thyroid heart disease. The improved survival rate of children with congenital heart disease accounts for the observed increase in the proportion of pregnant women with such defects in obstetric cardiac clinics.

Significance

Pregnancy adds a measurable burden to the heart (see Chapter 17); as long as there is not an imbalance between cardiac load and cardiac reserve, however, the outcome may be expected to be satisfactory if the patient is well managed. Certain burdens to the heart cannot be altered during pregnancy; these include a 25% increase in cardiac output, a 40%–50% increase in plasma volume, a 20%–25% increase in oxygen requirements, abnormal salt and water retention, weight gain, increased body bulk, and sudden alterations in hemodynamics at the time of delivery associated with

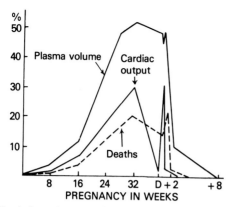

FIG. 27-1. Cardiac balance in pregnancy. (Lund CJ: Clin Obstet Gynecol 1:41, 1958)

decreased intraabdominal pressure and engorgement of the splanchnic vessels.

Available evidence indicates that cardiac output begins to increase early in pregnancy. Traditionally, a peak in cardiac output has been expected between the 32nd and 36th gestational weeks, with substantial decrease thereafter (Fig. 27-1). Ueland *et al.* suggest that these falls, observed in women who were in the supine recumbent position while under study, may have merely reflected the important effect of caval compression by the uterus on venous return. Nevertheless, the most critical periods for the pregnant woman with heart disease seem to be the first half of the third trimester and the postpartal period.

Lees *et al.* report that a maximal cardiac output of 30%–50% above the nonpregnant level may be present as early as the 4th month and is sustained throughout the latter portion of pregnancy. According to this revised concept, the pregnant cardiac patient reaches a point of near maximal stress by the 16th gestational week. If she is doing well by that time, Oparil and Swartwout consider the likelihood of continued favorable progress to be reasonably good. During labor, however, there is a further intermittent increase in cardiac output, presumably caused by increased physical activity, catecholamine release, and return of blood from the placental circulation.

Classification and Prognosis

The natural reserves depend upon the age of the patient, the duration of the cardiac lesion, and the functional capacity of the heart at the onset of pregnancy. Most physicians use the classification of the New York Heart Association, which depends upon an estimation of cardiac capacity as determined from the patient's past and present disability. It is important to remember that the classification can change rapidly during pregnancy.

Class I. Cardiac disease that does not limit acitivity. Ordinary physical activity does not cause discomfort. Patient has no symptoms of cardiac insufficiency, nor does she have anginal pain.

Class II. Cardiac disease that produces slight limitation of activity. Patient is free of symptoms while at rest, but ordinary activity is accompanied by undue fatigue, palpitation, dyspnea, or anginal pain.

Class III. Cardiac disease that produces marked limitation of activity. Less than ordinary activity is accompanied by undue fatigue, palpitation, dyspnea, or anginal pain.

Class IV. Cardiac disease that prevents patient from carrying out any activity without discomfort. Symptoms of cardiac insufficiency or anginal pain are present at rest, and any activity increases them.

An attempt should be made to assign each patient with cardiac disease to one of these categories, preferably prior to pregnancy, and to reevaluate her status at each antenatal visit. Patients belonging to Classes I and II rarely, if ever, undergo decompensation during pregnancy; however, since even the most seasoned clinician may occasionally overestimate the functional capacity of the heart, it seems best to manage all such patients as if they were potential candidates for decompensation. The great majority of patients in Classes I and II survive a well-managed pregnancy without undue risk, and the perinatal mortality rate is not significantly elevated. Fortunately, the vast majority of pregnant cardiac patients are in these two categories.

Patients in Classes III and IV make up only about 20% of the total number of obstetric patients with cardiac disease, but they account for 85% or more of the maternal deaths among this group. By and large, these patients have a poor functional capacity at the beginning of pregnancy. In addition, patients of advanced age, those with a history of cardiac decompensation, and those who exhibit a serious disorder of beat, particularly atrial fibrillation, heart block, or paroxysmal tachycardia, withstand pregnancy poorly. For those with acute valvulitis or myocarditis, the prognosis is likewise poor.

The site of the rheumatic lesion (aortic, mitral, or both) and the type of lesion are ordinarily not significantly related to the outcome of the pregnancy, although there are several notable exceptions to this generalization. A high degree of mitral stenosis results in inadequate filling of the heart because the diastolic phase is quite short. Hence, diminished cardiac output and pulmonary congestion and edema may result, and the ill effects are aggravated by tachycardia. Shunts impose the constant hazard of reversal of flow, should the peripheral circulation collapse in association with hemorrhage from any cause; septal defects and patent

ductus arteriosus are congenital lesions that may behave in this manner. Coarctation of the aorta is an unpredictable and serious anatomic defect that may terminate in rupture of the aorta. Regardless of other factors, the outlook for pregnancy is determined in large measure by the quality of antenatal supervision and care.

Chesley's data suggest that regardless of the severity of rheumatic cardiac disease in pregnancy, if the patient survives the pregnancy there is no reason to presume any delayed adverse effects or any shortening of life expectancy as the result of pregnancy *per se.*

Diagnosis During Pregnancy

The stresses of pregnancy may induce cardiac symptoms in a patient with undiagnosed heart disease, but the diagnosis of heart disease is not easy to establish during pregnancy. Functional murmurs are common, and often there are respiratory complaints (*e.g.*, dyspnea), particularly during the last few weeks of pregnancy, that confuse the clinical picture. Isolated systolic murmurs may not be significant even if they are loud. Extracardiac murmurs that arise from increased internal mammary vessel flow may be present. Other findings, such as a split first sound, a loud pulmonary second sound that moves with respiration, sinus tachycardia, edema, hyperventilation, elevated jugular venous pressure, and prominent apical impulse, may be encountered in normal pregnancy.

Certain easily detectable signs may be highly significant and constitute reliable indicators of organic heart disease. Notable among these are distended neck veins, moist basal pulmonary rales, diastolic murmurs, heart enlargement discernible on percussion and as increased cardiac shadow in chest film, cardiac dysrhythmias other than sinus or paroxysmal atrial tachycardia, central cyanosis, pericardial friction rub, pulse delay, and pulsus alternans. Diagnostic procedures such as electrocardiography, phonocardiography, and echocardiography may be used without risk to fetal welfare. Unless surgical intervention is required or the situation is urgent, cardiac catheterization should be deferred until after delivery.

Recognition of Decompensation

Cardiac decompensation is the principal cause of maternal death among pregnant patients with heart disease. Signs of failure may appear abruptly, without warning, or the onset may be gradual, beginning as persistent rales at the lung bases. The patient may complain of progressive edema, increasing dyspnea on exertion, attacks of palpitation, a sensation of smothering, and a frequent cough, sometimes associated with hemoptysis. Serial determinations of vital capacity may be helpful in determining the course. Even if there are no symptoms it is important to auscultate the lung bases at each prenatal visit.

The risk of infant mortality is also increased if maternal decompensation occurs, since uterine congestion, insufficient oxygenation, and elevation of carbon dioxide content of the blood not only compromise the fetus but also frequently give rise to preterm labor and delivery.

Management

Expert supervision and intensive care of the gravid, parturient, and puerperal woman, carried out through a team approach in a special clinic or by the cooperative efforts of an internist working with the obstetrician, are the hallmarks of successful management. The objective is to reduce the workload imposed upon the heart by elimination of physical and emotional strain; prevention of obesity, excessive weight gain, and edema; prevention or prompt control of infection, however minor; maintenance of adequate blood counts and iron stores; prevention of preeclampsia; and avoidance of hemorrhage, shock, and trauma. Rest is the single most important factor in the management of heart disease.

Antepartum Care. The patient's emotional and social state, as well as her cardiac function and obstetric situation should be carefully evaluated during the first visit. Basic cardiac function tests should be done to establish a baseline for future reference at later stages of pregnancy when reassessment is needed. Dietary instructions should be given and a program of rest decided upon once the patient's functional reserve is classified. Class I patients and most Class II patients can be satisfactorily managed while ambulatory, but office visits should be scheduled biweekly. It may be desirable to admit the patient to the hospital for periods of supervised rest, however, if the home environment is stressful. Admission is likewise indicated if signs of incipient preeclampsia appear or the patient develops an infection of any magnitude, particularly of the respiratory tract. Should anemia develop in spite of supplementary iron therapy, the cause should be investigated immediately and appropriate treatment instituted vigorously.

Generally, meticulous observations in the attempt to quantitate the patient's functional capacity are required to establish the plan of management. It must be recognized that intercurrent medical problems can trigger episodes of congestive failure. Noteworthy among these complications are respiratory infections, anemia, hypertension, and thyrotoxicosis. Volume depletion should be avoided in patients with pulmonary hypertension. The risk of subacute bacterial endocarditis, which may be greater during pregnancy and the puerperium, must be minimized by prompt treatment of all infections arising anywhere in the body. If anti-

coagulants are required, heparin offers greatest safety to the fetus, since it does not cross the placenta. The digitalis glycosides and the commonly used antiarrhythmic drugs likewise may be used as required. The same is probably true of electrical cardioversion. However, an effort should be made to avoid excessive use of diuretics, agents that increase blood pressure, and modalities capable of increasing blood volume or cardiac output.

The Class III patient requires frequent periods of rest in the hospital; if she is of advanced age or has previously experienced decompensation, supervised bedrest throughout pregnancy may be necessary. At least one-third of all Class III patients may be expected to suffer heart failure, and two-thirds of those who have previously experienced decompensation develop this serious complication. Should frank heart failure occur during pregnancy, bedrest in the hospital, where intensive care and supervision can be maintained, is obligatory for the entire course of gestation. It is unwise to attempt induction of labor, since any manipulative technique may provoke poor labor or give rise to infection. The use of oxytocin has been questioned on grounds that this preparation may contain varying amounts of vasopressor substance. If oxytocin is given as a large bolus intravenously, it can produce hypotension; when it is used according to standard protocol, however, there is no significant effect on either blood pressure or urinary output.

Intrapartum Care. Meticulous supervision during labor is mandatory; this entails careful check of the patient's pulse and respiratory rate, as well as frequent auscultation of the chest for appearance of rales. A broad spectrum antibiotic is usually administered as prophylaxis against infection, although Sugrue *et al.* have recently questioned the need for this. It is best to maintain the patient in a semirecumbent position with the head and shoulders elevated. Oxygen may be administered if there is any pulmonary embarrassment. Digitalis should be employed at the earliest signs of cardiac embarrassment but, ordinarily, not as a prophylactic measure. With frank failure, reliance is placed upon rest, oxygen, morphine, salt restriction, diuretics, and fluid restriction, as well as upon digitalis. Cardiac decompensation is strictly a medical problem, and any type of obstetric intervention tends only to aggravate the patient's condition. If she is fortuitously in a position to be delivered at this time, it is advisable to carry out a forceps delivery under local anesthesia, provided the operation can be achieved without undue stress or trauma. Nevertheless, when the patient is decompensated at the time of delivery, any procedure constitutes a grave maternal risk.

For all cardiac patients, it is desirable to minimize the duration of the second stage of labor as well as the bearing-down efforts of the patient, which bring about a significant increase in venous pressure. However, these patients also withstand trauma, hemorrhage, and shock very poorly, and it is inadvisable to leave them for long periods in the dorsal lithotomy position. Thus, shortening the second stage of labor is desirable only if it can be accomplished easily and with minimal operative interference. The ideal delivery is one that is accomplished by a simple outlet forceps procedure under some form of local or regional anesthesia. If there is cardiac embarrassment, delivery by the vaginal route is much the safest method. Cesarean section is done only for obstetric indications, never on the basis of heart disease alone.

Regional anesthesia is preferable for delivery because it does not reduce oxygenation. Continuous caudal anesthesia serves this purpose and also provides analgesia during labor, although there is a potential risk of hypotension and reduced cardiac output. Meperidine hydrochloride (Demerol) supplemented by one of the tranquilizers gives satisfactory pain relief in the first stage, and delivery can be achieved under a pudendal block, particularly in the multiparous patient. If a general anesthetic must be used, the technique should be chosen on the basis of the patient's needs, her cardiac status, and the professional talent available.

Postpartum Care. The early puerperal period may be a time of grave concern, since there is then an upswing in the incidence of decompensation, collapse, and maternal death. The cardiac output rises significantly immediately after delivery, and, in cases of mitral stenosis, the stage is set for the occurrence of pulmonary hypertension and edema. Moreover, during the several days following delivery, extravascular fluid is returned to the bloodstream for excretion, and this mobilization of fluid can place a great strain on the heart if excessive interstitial fluid has accumulated. Accordingly, except in the mildest forms of heart disease, it is best to keep the patient at rest in the hospital for at least a week following delivery, since occasionally decompensation may occur as late as the 5th day. During this period, it is advisable to continue the chemotherapy that was begun before delivery.

Congenital Heart Defects

The number of pregnant women with congenital heart disease has increased during the past two decades. The most common congenital heart lesions are septal defects and patent ductus arteriosus. Coarctation of the aorta accounts for about 10%. In addition to the prognostic significance of the functional classification, the special risks of potentially lethal reversals of blood flow (precipitated by systemic hypertension), aneurysmal or aortic rupture, and bacterial endocarditis must be considered.

The prognosis in the pregnant patient with congenital heart disease is determined to a large extent by the load on the right ventricle imposed by pulmonary hypertension. Hypotension and a low-output state in association with severe pulmonary hypertension pose a dire threat to the mother at the time of delivery or in the early puerperium. According to Jones and Howitt, the maternal mortality rate in severe primary pulmonary hypertension is 53%; in pulmonary hypertension with right-to-left shunting, 27%; in uncomplicated atrial or ventricular septal defect or patent ductus arteriosus, 1.8%. Naeye *et al.* report that precipitating factors may be a sudden decrease in venous return secondary to vena caval compression by the uterus, lower extremity venous pooling, volume loss, and reversal of intrapulmonary shunting. Moreover, elevated circulating clotting factors, depressed fibrinolysis, and thrombus formation in the arterial circulation, when augmented by the congestive failure, contribute to a high incidence of pulmonary embolization, according to Oparil and Swartwout.

The patient should be protected with appropriate antibiotics and vigorous treatment of all infections. In general, pregnancy outcome varies according to the degree of pulmonary hypertension and the degree of hypoxia. Hellegers and Neill have reported that when the hematocrit value is above 65% as a result of hypoxia, pregnancy terminates in abortion. The risk of subacute bacterial endocarditis is likewise grave, particularly when the complication develops during pregnancy. Pedowitz and Hellman report a maternal mortality rate of 3.5% for those with healed lesions and 14.2% for those in whom the complication occurred in the course of pregnancy.

For patients with septal defects, the time of delivery is fraught with danger. Measures to promote venous return are prophylactic, and it is imperative that rapid transfusion be possible. For most of the very serious defects, *e.g.,* pulmonary stenosis and Eisenmenger's complex, management is directed toward preventing failure, as in heart disease generally; if decompensation threatens or develops despite medical management, therapeutic abortion or surgical correction of the cardiac defect should be considered. Although successful pregnancies have occurred in patients with tetralogy of Fallot, signs of cardiac failure in early pregnancy may call for prompt therapeutic abortion. More recently, an improved outcome has been reported for such patients.

Other Cardiac Disorders

A special category of rare heart disease that appears postpartum and is characterized by cardiac enlargement, tachycardia, dysrhythmia, elevated diastolic pressure, and edema has been referred to as *postpartum myocarditis* or *cardiomyopathy*. The condition is refractory to usual therapy, and it carries a 20% mortality rate. Most cases have occurred among lower socioeconomic groups. The disease may appear without warning or apparent cause. In some cases immunologic relationships have been proposed, but, in others, the antecedent may be acute glomerulonephritis, preeclampsia, or beriberi. The underlying disorders must be treated appropriately.

Other Kinds of Heart Disease

In addition to hypertensive heart disease, other rarer forms include coronary, thyroidal, syphilitic, and kyphoscoliotic cardiac disease; cor pulmonale; constrictive pericarditis; heart block; and isolated myocarditis. These conditions may require specific treatment directed to the underlying problem, as well as measures to improve cardiac function; for the most part, they necessitate special consultation.

Cardiac Surgery

It has been well established that cardiac surgery can be accomplished successfully in the obstetric patient. A suitable candidate is the patient with a high degree of pure mitral stenosis and a functional capacity of Class III or IV. The disease process should be inactive, and the patient should be a reasonably satisfactory surgical risk. The optimal time for the procedure is early pregnancy, although it may be carried out at any time before the 32nd gestational week.

Among 385 patients in whom valvotomy was performed during pregnancy, the mortality rate was only 3%; a rate of 15% is usually associated with cardiac decompensation. A variety of procedures to restore cardiac structure and function, including valve replacement, mitral valvotomy, and repair of various congenital lesions, has been successfully accomplished in pregnancy. Wallace and coworkers report that the risk of morbidity or mortality due to the stresses of pregnancy in a woman with an adequate mitral valvuloplasty can be considered minimal. In their series of 248 pregnancies in 139 women, the maternal mortality rate was only 2%. There were five deaths, but three were considered probably preventable. These authors emphasize that, while most heart surgery patients can be expected to tolerate pregnancy successfully, careful management throughout gestation is required. Akbarian *et al.* warn that those subjected to placement of prosthetic valves are vulnerable to thromboembolic complications. There are additional risks in pregnancy because anticoagulation therapy is required unless the newer porcine prostheses are used, in which maternal anticoagulation is not needed.

Surgery should be performed before the childbearing years, if possible. There is a perinatal risk of 33% or more when surgery is performed during gestation,

according to Zitnik *et al.* Cardiac surgery should not be performed electively in pregnancy. Most patients who die of heart disease in pregnancy have not had the benefit of intensive care. Thus, maternal mortality is low with skilled medical care, and this fact constitutes the basis for an authoritative body of opinion opposed to cardiac surgery in gravid women except under unusual conditions.

One of these special circumstances may be coarctation of the aorta, which has been reported to carry a maternal mortality risk of 7%. The gravity of this complication may justify surgical intervention in the course of pregnancy or interruption of pregnancy if the patient's general condition does not permit surgery. When pregnancy is allowed to continue or the patient reports too late in pregnancy for cardiac surgery to be performed, it is probably best to deliver by cesarean section unless labor promises to be an easy experience.

Abortion and Sterilization

Therapeutic abortion is rarely indicated for heart disease. It may be considered for the exceptional patient who experiences heart failure at the onset of pregnancy, has previously experienced decompensation, or is of advanced age and has a long history of heart disease. Heart block associated with repeated Stokes–Adams seizures, a recent history of subacute bacterial endocarditis or coronary disease, and chronic atrial fibrillation all constitute grave maternal hazards that may sometimes justify early termination in preference to hospitalization and bedrest throughout pregnancy. It should be emphasized, however, that the latter course is nearly always preferable if the termination of pregnancy requires abdominal intervention. Thus, therapeutic abortion is a practical consideration in the management of heart disease only in the first trimester of pregnancy, since emptying the uterus by suction curettage is safely performed only during the first trimester. Instillation of hypertonic saline into the amniotic sac is an effective method of terminating pregnancy in the second trimester, but this procedure is likewise hazardous in certain patients. Potential problems relating to anesthesia, trauma, hemorrhage, sepsis, and hypernatremia, which are occasionally encountered with these techniques, constitute inordinate risks in the seriously ill cardiac patient.

In most instances, it is proper to carry out a sterilizing procedure; but, if this entails surgery, the operation should be postponed until the patient has recovered from the stresses of pregnancy and the uterine currettage. At that time, a period of rest should be provided and the procedure and anesthetic chosen after cardiac status has been reassessed and appropriate treatment and safeguards have been instituted.

ARTERIAL DISEASE

Raynaud's Disease

This disease is characterized by attacks of peripheral cyanosis that involve the upper extremities more commonly than the feet. It results from vasoconstriction, usually precipitated by cold. Although the fingers may become quite pale or cyanotic, gangrene rarely occurs. The condition does not seem to be aggravated by pregnancy. In addition to avoiding cold, dressing warmly, and provoking hyperemia by active and passive methods, some patients may require preganglionic sympathectomy. It should be borne in mind that ergot intoxication may present a similar clinical picture when this drug has been used in an attempt to induce abortion.

Dissecting Aneurysm of the Aorta

It has been said that half the cases of dissecting aneurysm of the aorta reported in women under the age of 40 have been associated with pregnancy or the puerperium. The condition is sometimes associated with coarctation of the aorta. The majority of these catastrophes occur in the third trimester at the peak of the cardiac output, and the onset is ordinarily dramatic. Death may follow the event within a very short time or may occur after a longer period in conjunction with heart failure or uremia.

DISORDERS OF VEINS

Varicose Veins

This condition is common during pregnancy. It is specifically a pregnancy-related disorder and is discussed in Chapter 26.

Venous Thrombosis

Phlebitis, thrombophlebitis, and thromboembolic disease in the obstetric patient may develop in the deep pelvic veins as well as in the femoral system. The condition may take the form either of a thrombosis associated with inflammation of the vessel wall (thrombophlebitis) or of a clot without vessel involvement (phlebothrombosis). Until the clot becomes attached to the vein wall, the latter carries the greater risk of embolization.

These diseases develop most often in the puerperium secondary to pelvic cellulitis or traumatic delivery, as discussed in Chapter 40. Other predisposing causes appear to be obesity, maternal age, estrogens (*e.g.,* to suppress lactation), increased coagulability of the blood, and stasis. In the event that the pelvic infection remains unchecked, the thrombus may become infected, necrotic, and purulent, and showers of septic

emboli may result. In some instances, thromboembolic disease may appear without any obvious provocation; without warning, fatal embolization may arise from the deep veins of the pelvis, usually 7–10 days after delivery. Fortunately, this condition occurs only once in several thousand pregnancies, probably owing to the modern practices of early ambulation, judicious use of chemotherapeutic agents, less traumatic obstetrics, and better general supportive care of patients.

The diagnosis of thromboembolic disease may be difficult in the early stages, although in the typical case there is deep pain and tenderness of the calf and thigh muscles along the course of the femoral vein, pain on dorsiflexion of the foot, difference in leg size and temperature, fever, tachycardia, and leukocytosis. Venography and ultrasound may be employed when needed. In other cases, the condition is heralded by sudden chest pain, dyspnea, pallor, cyanosis, tachycardia, and hemoptysis, indicative of pulmonary embolus. Usually within 24 hours, the chest x-ray exhibits characteristic changes. Other useful laboratory tests are measures of fibrin degradation products, arterial blood gases, lactic dehydrogenase (LDH), serum glutamic–oxaloacetic transaminase (SGOT), and bilirubin, as well as an electrocardiogram (EKG).

Heparin is ordinarily the initial treatment because of its rapid action and superior effect upon clotting mechanisms. This is monitored by thrombelastograph (normal +2 to −2; optimal hypocoagulability −4 to −6) and partial thromboplastin time (optimal hypocoagulability: 1 to 2½ times normal). If hemorrhage results during therapy, the effects can be counteracted with protamine. Fresh blood transfusions are helpful in reducing the effects of warfarin.

Several instances of extensive fetal hemorrhage resulting in death *in utero* have been attributed to the effects of warfarin administered to the mother several days prior to delivery. Moreover, since these drugs are capable of depleting fetal prothrombin activity, the risk of intracranial hemorrhage in the event of hypoxia or trauma is significant when a complication of labor and delivery is encountered. Should there be a need for anticoagulation at the time of parturition, it is best, therefore, to change back to heparin, because its action is of short duration and can be more readily counteracted.

Antibiotics should be employed if there is recognized infection, especially if septic pelvic thrombophlebitis is suspected. The use of fibrinolytic drugs may be of value as an adjunct to anticoagulation therapy. Surgical ligation of the vena cava may be considered in patients who experience repeated episodes of pulmonary embolization along with obvious extension and progression of the disease. Occasionally, it may be desirable to use a paravertebral sympathetic block in an effort to relieve vasospasm and enhance collateral circulation.

ALIMENTARY TRACT AND LIVER DISEASES

ACUTE APPENDICITIS

Although acute appendicitis complicates only about 1 in 1000–1500 pregnancies, the maternal and perinatal mortality rates associated with this event are high, and it should be regarded as one of the serious complications of gestation. The risk is greatest in the third trimester or during parturition, when the large active uterus interferes with localization of the infection.

The initial symptoms are ordinarily anorexia, nausea, vomiting, and abdominal pain. The pain is mild, dull, or crampy, in marked contrast to the severe colic associated with biliary or urinary obstruction. Either constipation or diarrhea may be present. There is a mild febrile reaction and, ordinarily, only moderate leukocytosis. Tenderness to palpation and rigidity or muscle guarding usually are present over the area where the appendix lies. In advanced pregnancy, the cecum may be displaced upward and into the right flank region by the enlarged uterus, and this fact, coupled with the loss of muscle tone in the distended abdomen, may hinder diagnosis. The gastrointestinal symptoms may be further obscured by abdominal discomfort associated with uterine contractions, especially if there are no truly localized signs, or by nausea or vomiting that may already be present, as is frequently the case during the first trimester. The disappearance of pain after several hours is not necessarily a good sign, inasmuch as it may indicate perforation of the appendix. Neglect may result in spreading peritonitis; secondary abscesses of the pelvic, perinephric, subhepatic, or subdiaphragmatic regions may occur, as may intestinal obstruction or pyelophlebitis.

Although some cases of acute appendicitis undoubtedly subside spontaneously, the mortality is high if treatment is delayed and minimal if surgery is performed promptly, even when pregnancy complicates the condition. Since the high mortality associated with acute appendicitis during pregnancy is attributable in large measure to delay in diagnosis, it is important to consider appendicitis as a possible cause for any pain in the right side. The differential diagnosis should include acute pyelonephritis, ovarian neoplasm, degenerating uterine leiomyoma, and abruptio placentae. Extrauterine pregnancy sometimes produces similar symptoms during the early gestational weeks. During the puerperium, parametritis may simulate appendicitis. Other disorders of the alimentary tract, such as acute gastroenteritis, acute diverticulitis, sigmoid volvulus, and perforated peptic ulcer, may likewise enter into the differential diagnosis. Round ligament pain often is confined to the right side and may suggest appendicitis, but there are no local or general signs of infection, and tenderness is noted in the ligament itself.

If the diagnosis is in doubt early in the disease, a few

hours of observation are permissible to watch for typical abdominal signs or laboratory evidence of a spreading infection. If appendicitis cannot be excluded after thorough evaluation, however, laparotomy should be performed regardless of the period of gestation. It is inadvisable first to empty the uterus even when the operation is performed at or near term. Adequate hydration and broad spectrum antibiotics are indicated, especially if the infection has spread beyond the appendix. Adequate sedation, as well as progesterone administered in large doses as a uterine sedative, may be employed to minimize the risk of labor. When the serosa of the uterus is acutely inflamed, these medications may not quiet the irritable uterus.

If perforation has already taken place and an abscess is present, drainage only may be feasible at the time of operation. Treatment should include continuous gastrointestinal suction, hydration, electrolyte replacement, transfusions as required, and chemotherapy to cover both gram-positive and gram-negative organisms until results of cultures and sensitivity studies are available. Appendectomy is warranted at a later date when the infection has been controlled.

DUODENAL ULCER

Peptic ulcer occurs in the portions of the gastrointestinal tract in which acid pepsin is found: the stomach, the first portion of the duodenum, and occasionally adjacent to a Meckel's diverticulum in which there is aberrant gastric mucosa. The great majority of such ulcers may be treated medically, particularly in pregnancy, when many patients experience some relief of symptoms. Care should be exercised to avoid phosphorus depletion or the milk alkali syndrome. In some instances, peptic ulcers are aggravated by pregnancy; in exceptional circumstances, the safety of mother and fetus may be seriously jeopardized. With recurrent cycles of exacerbation and healing, serious complications, such as bleeding, obstruction of the pylorus, intractable pain, and perforation, may necessitate surgical intervention even during pregnancy or the puerperium.

INTESTINAL OBSTRUCTION

Intestinal obstruction is rare during pregnancy or parturition, but its seriousness demands that it be considered in any patient who experiences abdominal pain and vomiting, particularly if there is evidence of distention. Mechanical obstruction results from extrinsic or intrinsic encroachment on the lumen of the bowel. Traction by the growing uterus on intestinal adhesions, stemming from previous abdominal surgery or pelvic inflammatory disease, is a principal cause of obstruction during pregnancy. The maternal and perinatal mortality rates are high if the diagnosis is delayed.

Although the enlarged uterus may obscure entirely the classic abdominal signs in the early stages, repeated vomiting, particularly if the vomitus is intestinal in character, should alert the clinician to the possibility of obstruction. Especially during labor, the intermittent crampy abdominal pain may not be recognized as intestinal; however, on auscultation, peristalsis is usually heard in rushes, and the note is frequently high-pitched, metallic, and tinkling. Moreover, distention is evident above the uterine fundus. An abdominal film, taken with the patient in the erect or lateral recumbent position, reveals air and fluid levels in a stepladder pattern. As a result of the repeated vomiting, the serum chlorides are low and alkalosis may be present.

Mechanical obstruction, either partial or complete should be distinguished from paralytic (adynamic) ileus, which results from reflex paralysis of the musculature of the intestinal tract without actual mechanical obstruction of the lumen. Paralytic ileus ordinarily follows intraabdominal procedures, peritonitis, hemoperitoneum, or disorders of the urinary tract, such as renal calculi. In contrast with mechanical obstruction, the peristaltic sounds are markedly hypotonic, or they may not be heard at all. There may be marked distention and repeated vomiting, but there is little pain except the general abdominal discomfort associated with marked distention.

A long intestinal tube should be passed into the small gut as an initial procedure to decompress the bowel. While continuous suction drainage is applied, water, and electrolyte replacement should be begun. In addition, it may be advisable in selected cases to administer parenteral vitamins, protein hydrolysate, and blood. A rising pulse rate or constant abdominal pain in spite of supportive therapy should suggest strangulation of the bowel, and exploration is indicated regardless of the stage of pregnancy. If there is no obvious improvement within several hours after passage of the tube, surgery should not be deferred; decompression is merely an adjuvant in the treatment of mechanical obstruction. In contrast, paralytic ileus may be satisfactorily treated solely by intubation of the gut.

The large bowel cannot be decompressed by a long intestinal tube if the ileocecal valve is competent. These closed loop obstructions require immediate surgical decompression to prevent rupture of the cecum. Even in late pregnancy, survey films of the abdomen may well demonstrate a sigmoid volvulus or other cause for the obstruction.

ULCERATIVE COLITIS

A chronic disease subject to acute exacerbations, ulcerative colitis has an unpredictable clinical course in pregnancy. Preexisting colitis may be reactivated if

quiescent or aggravated if already active, particularly during the first trimester, if the patient is fearful or anxious about the pregnancy. In some patients, however, the condition may remain unchanged or even improve. Unless the colitis is so severe that the patient suffers marked weight loss, anemia, and dehydration, there is little effect upon the pregnancy. The patient may have chronic diarrhea containing blood, pus, and mucus, as well as high fever, leukocytosis, and tachycardia. The maternal and perinatal risks in these rare circumstances are great, regardless of therapy, although the disease process may quiet down sufficiently following ileostomy to allow the pregnancy to continue.

Every effort should be exerted to control the disease by medical management, including emotional support, sedation, adequate rest, and a bland diet. Adrenal steroids may be employed in appropriate dosage without risk of producing embryonal defects. The great majority of cases are mild or moderate and can be successfully handled in this manner. Vaginal delivery is usually preferred, even when a colectomy has previously been performed; cesarean section should be reserved for purely obstetric indications.

CARCINOMA OF THE BOWEL

Carcinomas of the rectum and colon are rarely encountered in pregnancy, but these conditions will never be recognized if all rectal bleeding is attributed to hemorrhoids. Carcinoma occurring in the anal canal or the anus is a squamous lesion in contrast to the adenocarcinoma of the bowel above. Change in caliber of the feces, alternating diarrhea and constipation, passage of blood and mucus, and tenesmus suggest rectal carcinoma. These lesions mimic carcinoma of the left colon, where a constricting napkin-ring lesion may be found. The latter carcinomas are often associated with mechanical obstruction, characterized by crampy abdominal pain and distention. Contrariwise, when carcinomas arise in the right colon, where the liquid character of the fecal material diminishes the likelihood of obstruction symptoms, the presenting complaints are more commonly anemia, mild right lower quadrant pain, and marked blood loss from bulky, cauliflower-like lesions in the bowel. A mass may be palpable in the right lower quadrant of the abdomen. It should be emphasized that a high percentage of rectosigmoid lesions are accessible to the examining finger. A good many more large bowel cancers can be demonstrated and biopsied through the sigmoidoscope, while those above its reach can be diagnosed by means of a barium enema. The desirability of minimizing radiation of the fetus should not deter the clinician in the use of x-ray when carcinoma of the large gut is suspected.

Surgical treatment offers the patient the only hope of cure, the type of resection depending upon the location and characteristics of the lesion, as well as the stage of pregnancy. Ordinarily, when the pregnancy is not far advanced, it is possible to extirpate the lesion and the lymphatic glands that drain it without disturbing the uterus. Later, it may be necessary to sacrifice the uterus in accomplishing the radical procedure required to offer the patient an optimal chance of cure. O'Leary and Bepko, in a study of 100 cases of rectal and colonic cancers associated with pregnancy, concluded that these tumors are not affected by pregnancy. Thus, during the first and second trimester, a colonic or rectal carcinoma can be treated as if the patient were not pregnant. During the third trimester, cesarean section should be performed, followed by appropriate surgical extirpation either immediately or at a later date. Abortion is not therapeutic in these patients.

VIRAL HEPATITIS

Hepatitis may be caused by at least two viruses that are closely similar. Hepatitis virus A is responsible for infectious hepatitis or catarrhal jaundice, and hepatitis virus B is responsible for homologous serum jaundice. Both viruses are transmitted in blood; virus A is also transmitted in feces. The diseases have similar clinical characteristics, although in homologous serum jaundice the incubation period is longer and the onset more insidious. Many mild, unrecognized cases occur, and a carrier state appears to exist. It has been estimated that as many as 70% of the cases do not produce jaundice. The attack rate for viral hepatitis among pregnant women seems to be greatest in the later stages of gestation.

An intimate relation between Australia antigen (HAA) and the etiologic agent for most adult cases of viral hepatitis is now well established. The question of transplacental transfer enjoys great current interest because of several reports connecting various perinatal affections (e.g., neonatal hepatitis, fetal death or anomaly, and Down's syndrome in the neonate) with viral infections in the fetus. However, current evidence, reported by Holzbach, suggests that transplacental transmission of HAA from mother to fetus, if it occurs, is rare.

Hepatitis seems to show a predilection for young persons and is not infrequently encountered in pregnant women. The preicteric phase is usually characterized by fever, malaise, extreme fatigue, headaches, anorexia, nausea, vomiting, dark urine, and light feces. Jaundice appears and associated with it there may be enlargement and tenderness of the liver and right upper quadrant abdominal pain. Fever and jaundice may subside after a few days in mild cases, or they may persist for weeks, followed by a protracted convalescence characterized by extreme fatigability and weakness. In the most severe form, there may be wide-

spread degeneration of parenchymal cells of the liver, which leads to profound prostration, biochemical derangements in the blood, mahogany jaundice, coma, and death. At least two patients among reported cases have exhibited renal failure in association with hepatitis. A possible chemical or humoral mechanism has been postulated, but there is no definite evidence of a causal relationship. However, according to Douglas *et al.*, patients should be observed for signs of hepatic or renal failure or both; prompt attention, with hemodialysis if necessary, may be lifesaving.

The severe form is rarely encountered in the United States. In 378 cases of infectious hepatitis collected from the literature, the perinatal mortality rate was only 7%, and there were only 9 instances of congenital malformation. In most recent series, the maternal mortality is under 1% among well-nourished women who are given optimal medical care. In areas of the world where malnutrition and anemia are prevalent and appropriate medical care is provided only during the late stages of the illness, the maternal mortality rate may be as high as 15%–20%. In a recent study from Greece, Kehayoglou and coworkers report a maternal death rate of 7%, a preterm birth rate of 21.4%, and a fetal mortality of 14.2%. Their incidence of viral hepatitis was 0.06%, about the same frequency as in the nonpregnancy population of the same age. They conclude from their study and review of the literature that maternal outcome is rather favorable and that fetal wastage is slightly elevated. There seems a probable correlation between the severity of jaundice and the incidence of preterm birth.

Since the most important prognostic factor seems to be the patient's nutritional status when the infection occurs, basic therapy should include a diet high in protein, carbohydrates, and vitamins, along with extended rest and supervision. Plasma volume expanders, such as serum albumin or dextran, as well as cortisone in large doses, may be lifesaving in stressful situations. There should be no obstetric interference, since pregnancy has no influence on the course of the disease. Moreover, unwarranted manipulations may aggravate the condition by provoking unnecessary stress, trauma, or genital infection. If labor ensues, blood should be readily available, since these patients react unfavorably to even mild degrees of hemorrhage, shock, and anemia. The prothrombin time should be determined and one of the forms of vitamin K oxide administered. Cortisone support may be required. Immunoglobulins should be given to exposed women, although this seems more effective after exposure to the A than the B virus.

PANCREATITIS

Acute pancreatitis is rare in pregnancy. The underlying mechanisms are similar to those encountered in the nonpregnant patient, although the excessive use of alcohol is less conspicuous as a predisposing factor. In addition, acute pancreatitis in pregnant women seems to be associated more often with gallbladder disease. Most attacks commence during the third trimester of pregnancy or in the early puerperium. It has been suggested that increased intraabdominal pressure and hyperlipidemia at this time may be predisposing factors. The clinical picture, while sometimes confusing, is not greatly altered by the gravid state. Berk *et al.* believe that if more extended use of serum amylase, serum lipase, and urine amylase determinations were to be emphasized in pregnant women with dyspepsia and abdominal pain, pancreatitis might be detected with greater frequency.

Treatment is conservative and basically the same as in the nonpregnant patient. The outcome of pregnancy is ordinarily successful, and termination of the pregnancy need be considered only under exceptional circumstances.

GALLBLADDER DISEASE

Acute cholecystitis occasionally makes its appearance during pregnancy, but seems to have no special predilection for the gravid woman, despite the high incidence of digestive disturbances throughout gestation. It is true, nevertheless, that cholelithiasis is several times more common in women than in men and that almost all women who require surgical treatment because of calculi have borne children. These facts seem to implicate pregnancy as a possible causative influence and tend to suggest a possible association between the high plasma lipid content noted in pregnancy in the later development of gallstones.

Estrogens have been incriminated in the pathogenesis of the syndromes of pruritus gravidarum and cholestatic jaundice of pregnancy. Certain alterations in liver function suggest that estrogens or possibly other hormones may be metabolized abnormally or that patients exhibiting this exaggerated state of cholestasis may have an abnormal sensitivity to the effects of steroids on the hepatic transport mechanisms.

If a stone obstructs the cystic duct, an attack of acute biliary colic results, often at night following some dietary indiscretion. The pain is severe and is located in the epigastrium or the right upper quadrant. Radiation may occur to the back, the scapular region, or the right shoulder. Nausea and vomiting are common. During the attack, there are, in most cases, tenderness in the region of the gallbladder and some muscle guarding. As a rule, these attacks subside in a few hours with the aid of opiates and atropine, leaving only a residual soreness. During the intervals between attacks, there may be no symptoms, or the patient may

experience a sense of fullness, frequent eructation, and indigestion, especially after large meals or ones that include fatty foods.

Medical therapy is usually preferable to surgery during pregnancy, unless there are recurrent or persistent symptoms. If the stone in the cystic duct becomes impacted, it may give rise to suppuration or gangrene within the gallbladder, with perforation and the development of peritonitis. Usually, the clinician is alerted to this serious complication by the appearance of persistent pain, high fever, and marked leukocytosis despite treatment.

DISORDERS OF THE URINARY TRACT

A knowledge of the normal effects of pregnancy upon urinary tract structure and function (see Chapter 17) is requisite to an understanding of the pathologic conditions that involve this system in the gravid woman. Moreover, an awareness of the anatomic, biochemical, and physiologic alterations observed during pregnancy is required if the diagnostic tests and assessments of urinary tract function are to be interpreted correctly.

ACUTE GLOMERULONEPHRITIS

There is a constant association of acute glomerulonephritis with streptococcal (types 4 and 12) and, occasionally, pneumococcal infections. This makes it practically certain that these organisms, especially the former, are the usual cause, although the disease may follow almost any infection. It may also be caused by lead, mercury, or arsenic poisoning.

The characteristic history is the sudden appearance of oliguria, albuminuria, red cells and casts in the urine, moderate hypertension, and generalized edema, developing about 10–20 days after an acute infectious process such as tonsillitis, sinusitis, scarlet fever, or furuncles. The patient usually complains of malaise, headaches, nausea, and vomiting. The conspicuous changes in blood chemistry are reduction in protein content, reversal of the albumin/globulin ratio, and elevation of the blood cholesterol. Phenolsulfonphthalein excretion and blood metabolites usually are normal.

This disease is rarely encountered in pregnancy. Antibiotics have lowered the incidence of nephritis even among nonpregnant patients. When the disorder appears in the early months of pregnancy, abortion may result. Later, acute nephritis may be mistaken for preeclampsia since the conditions have in common the clinical features of hypertension, albuminuria, and edema. However, the immediate history of an infectious process, hematuria, a rising antistreptolysin titer, and low serum complement should be helpful in distinguishing the two diseases.

Treatment consists of bedrest, soft diet, restriction of salt, and antibiotics. About 2% of the patients develop chronic nephritis despite these measures.

CHRONIC GLOMERULONEPHRITIS

The chronic stage of glomerulonephritis may have its onset with an acute episode or may be preceded by a nephrotic stage in which the principal clinical features are marked albuminuria and retention of salt and water. In the chronic phase, the retention of nitrogenous waste products is disproportionate to the hypertension. The patient may complain of headaches, palpitations, dyspnea, and nocturia. In advanced cases, examination reveals hypertension, left ventricular hypertrophy, moderate anemia, and retinal hemorrhage. The urine may have a low, fixed specific gravity and contain small amounts of albumin, red blood cells, and hyaline and finely granular casts. The blood metabolites may be markedly increased. When uremia is present, the patient experiences drowsiness, headache, twitching, convulsive seizures, and finally coma, which may develop either gradually or suddenly. In these circumstances, the prognosis is exceedingly poor, whether or not the patient is pregnant. Death may occur from heart failure or apoplexy before the kidneys cease to function.

Patients with poor renal function are grave obstetric risks and should be advised against childbearing. Further deterioration of the renal reserve is to be anticipated, and fetal mortality is high. Therapeutic interruption of early pregnancy is advisable if the blood pressure is elevated and renal function is considerably reduced. Sterilization should also be performed, since the disease process is irreversible. If the pregnancy has advanced well into the second trimester when the patient is first seen, it may be best to pursue a medical regimen until the clinical situation and the need for intervention can be reassessed.

The patient with a milder form of the disease may be permitted to continue the pregnancy even when seen early, although intensive care is required to minimize the risks of the late complications. Like patients with chronic hypertension, these women are apt to give birth to undersized fetuses, owing to progressive placental dysfunction. Fetal death *in utero* may occur at or near term, and for this reason, it is often wise to terminate the pregnancy by inducing labor at about the 38th gestational week. Even in the patient whose disease is quiescent and whose renal function is normal, an acute exacerbation accompanied by hypertension and increasing proteinuria may develop as pregnancy advances. In this event, the process should be stabilized and the pregnancy terminated by the most expeditious means.

URINARY TRACT INFECTIONS

The triad of bladder trauma, stasis of urine, and bacteriuria, compounded by the paralyzing effect of anesthesia and the overdistention of the insensitive bladder in the puerperium, presents the ideal conditions for the development of urinary tract infections. Many of these infections go unrecognized because the clinical picture is not dramatic; a smoldering infection may persist in spite of therapy if there is bacterial resistance to the drug employed or if the course of treatment is terminated before the urine is sterilized. The consequences of neglect are often serious, since the patient may not experience normal involutionary changes in the urinary tract postpartum and a low-grade chronic infection may persist, causing recurrent exacerbations as well as progressive tissue damage.

Bacteriuria in pregnancy is often an indication of chronic pyelonephritis, obstructive lesions, or congenital abnormalities of the urinary tract. Asymptomatic bacteriuria in pregnancy represents, in about half the cases, a bladder infection; in the other half, bacteriuria stems from infection in one or both ureters, as well as the bladder. Kass reports that significant bacteriuria occurs in 4%–7% of pregnant women, compared with 0.5% of a group of nonpregnant college women studied. Pyelonephritis, which occurs in up to 40% of cases, is a greater risk in women with ureteric bacteriuria. Reported increases in the incidence of preterm delivery among such women may be due to underlying chronic renal pathology. The latter lesions likewise predispose to preeclampsia and fetal loss. Recent evidence suggests that antibacterial therapy, even when effective, may not eliminate these complications of pregnancy. Nevertheless, the risk of acute inflammation is minimized by appropriate therapy, and the presence of bacteria calls attention to the possibility of anatomic abnormalities or underlying pathology that requires thorough investigation.

Symptoms

Upper urinary tract infections that involve the renal pelvis, the renal parenchyma, and the ureter are noted in about 3%–4% of all pregnant women. These infections may develop suddenly, with the appearance of high spiking fever, chills, and costovertebral angle pain that extends into the flank, either unilaterally or bilaterally. The right side is almost invariably involved. Indeed, unilateral pyelonephritis limited to the left side is so unusual in pregnancy that the diagnosis should be considered suspect. The patient appears acutely ill and may complain of anorexia, malaise, and abdominal distention. The temperature may peak to 104°–106° F. Bladder symptoms may not appear in the course of the disease, although frequency, urgency, and dysuria develop subsequently as the lower tract becomes involved in the process. There may be evidence of uterine hyperirritability that simulates labor in its early stages. Edema of the renal parenchyma or partial ureteral obstruction due to swelling and blockage by inflammatory exudate may result in temporary suppression of urinary output. In these circumstances, there may be severe pain, sometimes of a colicky nature, vomiting, dehydration, and ileus of the large bowel.

The area of the involved kidney is tender to palpation, and there may be marked tenderness along the course of the ureter and over the bladder region if these organs are involved. The patient ordinarily exhibits proteinuria, and microscopic examination reveals numerous white blood cells (both singly and in clumps), red blood cells, and myriad bacteria. The blood may show a marked elevation of the white cell count; in advanced cases, there may be a mild elevation of the nonprotein and urea nitrogen values. Occasionally, grave complications may occur, taking the form of septicemia, jaundice, severe anemia, cortical or perinephric abscesses, peritonitis, and pneumonia; in these circumstances, the mother is critically ill and the likelihood of fetal death is great.

The classic case offers no diagnostic problems to the experienced clinician. There may be great variation in the clinical manifestations, however, and the atypical case may present a picture that is disturbingly similar to that of appendicitis if there is right-sided involvement, ureterolithiasis, or parametritis when the patient is puerperal.

Lower urinary tract infection (cystitis) occurs more frequently during the puerperium than before the onset of labor. It may be an exacerbation of a chronic, asymptomatic infection, or it may develop acutely during labor or in the immediate postpartal period. The local infection is usually associated with mild symptoms in conjunction with bladder function, notably urgency, frequency, dysuria, and slight suprapubic tenderness. There are no systemic complaints, and the temperature rarely rises above 101° F. Confining the infection to the lower tract is a prime objective; however, even with the prompt use of appropriate therapeutic agents, it may be difficult to prevent ascending, generalized urinary infection, particularly in the pregnant or puerperal woman. Since most offending organisms can be controlled with standard medication, it is best not to withhold therapy while the organism is being identified. Adjustments in therapy can be made later when this information is available, should the need arise. In chronic cystitis, urinary antiseptics may be employed to control local bladder symptoms, but it is usually not possible to sterilize the urine by this therapeutic approach.

Diagnosis

Culture and colony counts should be carried out repeatedly on clean-caught urine specimens when there

is the slightest suspicion of urinary tract infection. Clean-voided specimens satisfy the requirement for bacteriologic as well as microscopic examination. A first morning specimen is the preferred sample, when feasible. A count of greater than 100,000 pathogenic organisms per milliliter of urine is highly significant, although lesser numbers may be a cause of concern under certain clinical circumstances. Traditionally, the hallmark of infection has been the presence of pus cells in the urinary sediment, but it is now clear that diagnosis based solely on microscopic study of the sediment is subject to a 50% error or more. Significant urinary infections may not be accompanied by pyuria. Thus, cultures are the basic diagnostic laboratory tool. Initial infection during pregnancy is almost always caused by a gram-negative organism, usually *Escherichia coli;* however, among recurrent and particularly chronic cases, *Proteus, Aerobacter aerogenes, Klebsiella, Pseudomonas,* enterococci, and others become dominant. An infected calculus or other underlying organic uropathy or anomaly may be present in refractory cases.

In most chronic or recurrent cases, intravenous pyelography is desirable to permit visualization of the urinary tract and crude estimation of renal function. It is important to appreciate that failure to recognize obstructive lesions may lead to disorganized management, including the use of many combinations of drugs and unfortunate delays in promoting adequate drainage until one of the therapeutic agents controls the infection. If a more complete and careful study is required, it is necessary to resort to retrograde pyelography, fractional assessment of urinary function, and microscopic study of samples from the two sides. In addition, it is usually desirable to obtain clearance studies, determine the level of blood metabolites, and perform concentration tests upon the urine. It should be borne in mind that bacteremic shock may occur when instrumentation of the urinary tract is undertaken in the presence of active infection. The outcome may be acute tubular necrosis, anuria, uremia, and death, if the shock is of sufficient degree and duration.

No patient should be denied the benefits of radiography, even during pregnancy, if these studies are needed to clarify the urinary status. Radiation during pregnancy should be limited to the least amount commensurate with safe clinical practice, however, inasmuch as the fetal exposure is cumulative and potentially harmful, particularly during the period of organogenesis. The irritative effects of cystoscopy and ureteral catheterization upon the uterus limit the use of these diagnostic techniques during pregnancy. The impingement of the presenting part upon the posterior surface of the bladder during the last weeks of pregnancy may not only displace the ureteral orifices but also make inspection of the bladder difficult. Accordingly, unless these procedures are clearly indicated by the gravity of the patient's signs and symptoms, they are best deferred until the postpartum period when they can be carried out safely and with less technical and interpretive difficulty.

Treatment

Accurate bacterial identification is the cornerstone of effective therapy. The majority of acute urinary tract infections are caused by gram-negative organisms constituting normal intestinal and vaginal flora. The most important are *E. coli* and related paracolon species, *Klebsiella, Proteus,* and *Pseudomonas aeruginosa.* Enterococci, including *Streptococcus faecalis* and group D streptococci, as well as staphylococci, are less frequently encountered. Examination of unstained and Gram-stained smears of the urine sediments is invaluable in identifying the causative organisms.

Antibiotic resistance, either initially or after therapy, frequently occurs with *Proteus, Pseudomonas,* and the coliforms. Gram-positive organisms, except staphylococci, are usually effectively combated by penicillin or a broad spectrum antibiotic. A given strain of bacteria can often be eradicated from the urinary tract with an antibiotic to which it shows evidence of resistance in the usual *in vitro* sensitivity test. According to Ries and Kaye, at least 75% of symptomatic pyelonephritis during pregnancy can be prevented if patients are screened for bacteriuria during the first prenatal visit and treated if necessary.

Sulfonamides and nitrofurantoin are drugs of choice in the usual acute infection and are highly effective against *E. coli.* Nitrofurantoin is effective against *Proteus* strains as well as the coliforms. Useful alternative drugs in selected cases include ampicillin and methenamine mandelate. Other drugs that may be particularly useful in combating *Proteus mirabilis* and other *Proteus* strains are kanamycin, penicillin, and cephalothin. Polymyxin B may be the only drug effective against *B. pyocyaneus* or *Pseudomonas aeruginosa,* despite the agent's capacity for renal intoxication. Colistimethate is also a drug of choice for combating *Pseudomonas* organisms. Attention must be directed to the possibility of fetal damage in association with some of these drugs. Nevertheless, in life-threatening maternal infections, which rarely occur, the use of potent agents may be mandatory.

In acute, uncomplicated infections of the urinary tract, it is possible to eradicate the offending organism in the overwhelming majority of patients who are treated with the correct drug. The outlook for permanent cure in chronic infections is much less impressive, even though bacteria may be eliminated temporarily from the urine. After an initial satisfactory response, the common gram-negative urinary pathogens may acquire resistance rapidly, particularly in the obstetric patient, and the original sensitive strain may soon be replaced with a resistant one of the same species. In these patients, a plan of long-term therapy,

which may require a combination of drugs based on clinical experience as well as susceptibility tests, offers the best chance of cure. Without good care, there may be marked infiltration of the upper urinary tract, loss of normal peristaltic action of the ureter due to extensive fibrosis, persistence of hydroureter and hydronephrosis, and deterioration of renal function for weeks, months, or even years following childbirth. Such deterioration and functional impairment greatly reduce the ability to conceive or to sustain a pregnancy, should it occur. When the serum creatinine value is greater than 3 mg/dl or blood urea nitrogen is higher than 30 mg/dl prior to conception, there is little likelihood for a successful gestation, according to Lindheimer and Katz. Bacteriuria leads to exacerbation of pyelonephritis during pregnancy. When hypertension is present, preeclampsia often is superimposed, and there may be further deterioration in renal function. The risks of fetal death and preterm birth are quite high, and evidence of dysmaturity and fetal inanition is common.

In addition to appropriate chemotherapy, it is desirable to institute complete bedrest, ensure adequate hydration, provide satisfactory analgesia, and promote regular bowel elimination. Dramatic relief of symptoms may be achieved in some cases by promoting urinary alkalinity. If there are signs of urinary obstruction after 5–7 days of suitable therapy, it may be necessary to catheterize the involved ureter to establish adequate drainage.

The condition of all patients with known renal disease must be evaluated repeatedly during pregnancy. The essential objectives are to monitor urinary output, bacteriuria, blood pressure, serum creatinine value, and, as required, renal clearance. Stringent sodium restriction and diuretic therapy should be avoided to reduce the risks of dehydration and decreased renal perfusion. Adequate bedrest is imperative when hypertension is present. Generally, patients negotiate pregnancy fairly well unless there is significant hypertension or azotemia, despite the presence of significant nephropathy.

RENAL TUBERCULOSIS

The traditional belief that tuberculosis of the kidney rapidly pursues an unfavorable course during pregnancy, particularly in the last trimester, has been revised somewhat in recent years. Nevertheless, tuberculous lesions of the kidney that have remained dormant for many months or even years may be reactivated during pregnancy. If the parenchyma alone is involved, the urine sediment is normal; however, when the lesion breaks through into the renal pelvis, the urine contains blood, pus, and tubercle bacilli. Thus, renal tuberculosis should be suspected in the patient who exhibits pyuria and symptoms of a chronic urinary tract infection despite conventional therapy or

who develops hematuria without apparent cause. The diagnosis should likewise be considered in the patient with pyuria when the routine urine culture is negative, although it should be recognized that pyelonephritis due to secondary invaders may be superimposed on the underlying tuberculous infection. The tubercle bacilli can be demonstrated in the urine by smear, culture, or guinea pig inoculation; both intravenous urography and retrograde pyelography show distortion of the pelvis, the calyces, and the ureter, and indicate whether the lesion is basically unilateral or bilateral. Estimations of renal function are helpful in establishing the prognosis.

Streptomycin, para-aminosalicylic acid, and isoniazid should be employed to control the infection and to minimize the risk of spread when surgery is contemplated. When there is marked destruction of one kidney and there is no infection or only minimal infection in the opposite kidney, nephrectomy is the treatment of choice unless the patient is near term. Ordinarily, there is no need to terminate pregnancy, although in the presence of impaired renal function associated with bilateral disease, this may be the wisest course. Following nephrectomy for unilateral renal tuberculosis, pregnancy should not be undertaken for several years to allow time for documentation of the normality of the remaining kidney.

HEMATURIA

The appearance of gross hematuria is an urgent indication for extensive urologic investigation usually when the symptoms have subsided. The passage of clots through the ureter can mimic exactly the signs and symptoms associated with ureterolithiasis. Occasionally, the loss of blood is sufficient to cause a significant fall in the hematocrit value, even when the cause is infection. The cause of bleeding in the majority of cases is pyelonephritis, hydronephrosis, acute hemorrhagic cystitis, or rupture of a varicosity in the bladder mucosa. Less commonly, the cause is tuberculosis, stone, or tumor. Unless pathology is demonstrable, the examinations should be repeated after delivery.

URINARY CALCULI

There appears to be no close relation between the physiologic changes associated with pregnancy and the formation of calculi, despite the presence of urinary stasis and the frequent occurrence of the infection that favors their development. The young age of most gravidas and the relatively short duration of the gestational period may account for the fact that calculi complicate only about 1 in 1200 pregnancies.

When calculi appear in early pregnancy, the signs and symptoms are usually those observed in the non-

pregnant patient. A large stag-horn calculus may give rise only to a dull aching loin pain, while smaller stones in the renal pelvis or the ureter are likely to cause urinary obstruction. Nausea, vomiting, chills, and fever may be present. Acute pain in the back or colicky pain referred along the course of the ureter to the bladder and the external genitalia may be the prominent clinical feature. There are tenderness over the affected kidney and guarding in the flank muscles. Unless the ureter is completely obstructed, red blood cells and leukocytes are usually found in the urine. Chronic or recurrent infection is common, and the chief complaints may be those of pyelonephritis or cystitis, particularly urgency and dysuria.

Later in pregnancy, when there is some dilation of the renal pelvis and ureter, the pain from ureteral calculi may disappear; occasionally, the stones may be extruded as the urinary tract muscle tone diminishes and the caliber of the ureteral lumen increases. Of greatest significance, however, is the fact that infection may replace pain in the presence of calculi; unless the underlying cause is discovered, considerable renal damage may result during the course of pregnancy. Thus, protracted or recurrent urinary infection is an urgent indication for urologic investigation.

Urinary calculi may be discovered quite unexpectedly in the abdominal or pelvic x-rays obtained during pregnancy. If there are no associated symptoms or signs of infection and renal function is unimpaired, it is wiser to follow the patient expectantly until after delivery, particularly when the calculi are discovered during the third trimester. Those detected at an earlier stage of gestation may be removed with little fear of interrupting the pregnancy. When the calculi are symptomatic or are associated with infection or impairment of renal function, the need for surgical removal is more urgent. Likewise, large vesical calculi, which during labor may cause serious soft tissue damage and dystocia, should be removed during pregnancy, either transurethrally or by suprapubic cystotomy.

RENAL TUMORS, ANOMALIES, AND POLYCYSTIC DISEASE

Benign tumors of the kidney include papilloma, papillary cystadenoma, angioma, and simple or solitary cysts. The cardinal symptoms are hematuria, a flank mass, and pain. The hematuria, which may be intermittent, demands early and complete urologic investigation. Hypernephroma is the most common malignant renal tumor, but it is exceedingly rare among pregnant women; it occurs most often in the male in midlife. Other malignant tumors include papillary carcinoma and epithelioma of the renal pelvis, carcinoma, and sarcoma. Benign lesions can often be treated by local removal or partial nephrectomy without compromising the pregnancy. If there is no evidence of widespread metastases, malignant tumors are best treated by nephrectomy, if this is feasible, although the prognosis is determined by the extent of spread of the lesion and the status of the contralateral kidney.

It is not unusual to discover urinary tract anomalies in the course of urologic investigations for chronic infection and other disorders that occur during pregnancy. These may coexist with anomalies of the reproductive tract. The genitourinary defects commonly encountered are duplication of the ureters and renal pelvis, segmented ureters, and horseshoe or fused kidneys. Unless chronic infection has resulted in renal damage and impaired function, successful pregnancy can be anticipated.

Polycystic disease of the kidneys may not be recognized in a young gravida who has not yet developed the clinical signs and symptoms of the abnormality. The outcome of pregnancy depends almost entirely upon the degree of destruction of renal parenchyma and the functional reserve of the kidneys. Blood pressure elevation alone may not jeopardize the pregnancy, but renal insufficiency reduces the chances of a successful outcome commensurate with the degree of functional impairment. When there is only a small margin of kidney reserve, the pregnancy should be interrupted. Though repeated aspiration of the cysts has been tried, up to the present time no satisfactory treatment of polycystic disease has been discovered. Polycystic disease is inherited as an autosomal dominant trait, and genetic counseling is indicated.

Most patients with a single ectopic kidney do well during pregnancy, although the misplaced kidney may occasionally block the birth canal or be injured by the passage of the fetus. This condition should be suspected if a relatively immobile mass is palpated in the posterior pelvis. Since such a kidney may be mistaken for an ovarian tumor, a mass in this location is sufficient indication for intravenous pyelography, particularly if surgical excision is contemplated. Careful assessment of the renal status is indicated, since pelvic kidneys may be complicated by hydronephrosis and infection. If the kidney is fixed deep in the posterior pelvis, cesarean section is probably the preferred method of delivery.

SOLITARY KIDNEY

With the extension of surgical treatment in a variety of unilateral renal diseases, the obstetrician is called upon with increasing frequency to offer an opinion on the advisability of undertaking pregnancy or of continuing an existing pregnancy when the patient has but one kidney. The prime considerations should be the functional status of the remaining kidney, the nature of the disease process that prompted the previous surgery, and the time elapsed since nephrectomy. If the remaining organ is normal and is properly located, and

if sufficient time has elapsed since surgery to permit certainty that it is free of disease and has compensated for the loss of the other, pregnancy may be undertaken or allowed to continue with full expectation of a successful outcome. These judgments are contingent upon a thorough urologic investigation and intensive obstetric supervision and care.

DISORDERS OF THE NERVOUS SYSTEM

INTRACRANIAL HEMORRHAGE

Although intracranial hemorrhage occurs primarily in patients over 40 years of age, it is occasionally encountered in younger women, usually due to rupture of a congenital aneurysm located in the circle of Willis. Rupture of atherosclerotic vessels in association with advanced hypertensive cardiovascular disease or, rarely, hemorrhage secondary to trauma, tumor, or blood dyscrasia may likewise result in a grave intracranial lesion.

Rupture of a congenital aneurysm may occur without warning or after premonitory symptoms of headaches, faintness, or dizziness. The clinical features and prognosis depend upon the amount and duration of intracranial bleeding. During an attack, the patient is comatose, the pupils are dilated and nonreactive, the reflexes are lost, breathing is stertorous, and there is incontinence of feces and urine. there may be nuchal rigidity, increased spinal fluid pressure, and fresh blood in the fluid.

The less profound and shorter the acute phase, the better the prognosis, although focal neurologic signs may persist after relatively minor attacks. The prognosis should always be guarded, particularly during pregnancy, since recurrence is an ever-present risk. Pregnancy does not contraindicate cerebral angiography, which should be performed to determine the location and extent of the vascular lesions and to aid the surgical treatment, if this proves feasible. If hypothermia is used as a surgical adjunct, no ill effects on the gravida or her fetus should be anticipated.

There is no need to interrupt pregnancy unless there are obstetric indications. Vaginal delivery should constitute no greater hazard to the mother than cesarean section, provided labor proceeds normally, bearing-down efforts in the second stage are minimized, and the delivery is accomplished without trauma. However, since the obstetric situation may be as variable as the intracranial lesion, management of each case requires individual consideration.

POLIOMYELITIS

Although pregnancy increases susceptibility to acute anterior poliomyelitis, this infection, which is caused by a filterable virus, is rarely encountered since the advent of effective immunization practices. There seems to be no special predisposition for any particular stage of pregnancy, nor does the period of gestation influence to any predictable extent the severity and degree of paralysis. Mortality from poliomyelitis seems to be no higher among pregnant women than among nonpregnant women. Fetal mortality is about 18%, more than half resulting from spontaneous abortion. Therapeutic abortion is not recommended. Induction of labor or delivery by cesarean section are reserved for special medical or obstetric indications. Expulsive efforts in the second stage of labor may be lacking, but delivery can usually be accomplished by a low forceps operation under pudendal block anesthesia. Polio virus may cross the placenta and cause either abortion or neonatal disease. Standard support measures of the mother may be instituted, including tracheotomy and the respirator as may be required.

Routine immunization in pregnancy is not recommended. In the presence of an epidemic it is mandatory, using Salk (not Sabin) vaccine.

EPILEPSY

Although epilepsy often is diagnosed as a disease, it is primarily a syndrome that arises from one of a variety of causes. The four major clinical patterns of epilepsy are the grand mal, petit mal, psychomotor, and jacksonian types. Electroencephalography is helpful in distinguishing the type of disorder and in excluding hysteria as the basic problem. When the specific cause is unknown, the condition is termed *idiopathic epilepsy;* such cases make up more than three-quarters of the total. Since the initial seizure usually occurs before 20 years of age and practically always before age 30, the onset of epilepsy may appear first during pregnancy, and the convulsions may be mistaken for eclampsia. Since pregnancy has no predictable effect upon the course of epilepsy, therapeutic abortion is rarely indicated. During a seizure, the patient should be protected from injury and from biting her tongue. If attacks occur frequently, she should not be allowed to nurse to avoid possible injury to the infant.

Among the roughly one-third of women who have more seizures than usual during pregnancy, many have experienced convulsions at the time of their menses. A curious observation is the report that certain women convulse while carrying a male child but not a female. Patients who have frequent seizures under normal conditions are much more likely to have seizures more often during pregnancy than are those who have infrequent seizures.

Epilepsy arising for the first time during gestation is uncommon; when it does, it tends to have a focal nature. Status epilepticus is also quite rare in pregnancy. There is no major difference between epileptics and

normal women with respect to the incidence of complications during pregnancy. Epileptic mothers tend to be deficient in folic acid, but folate supplementation has been provided with caution because of the suspicion that folate may interfere with anticonvulsant medication (diphenylhydantoin) or increase the risk of convulsions. In recognizing folate deficiency anemia as a common problem among epileptics, however, certain authorities urge supplementary therapy. Blood counts must, nevertheless, be monitored carefully and drug dosage supervised with care.

Several studies suggest a higher perinatal mortality and a higher incidence of congenital anomalies among infants of epileptic women, and there is some evidence that the anticonvulsant drugs, not epilepsy *per se,* may be responsible. A combination of drugs, for example a barbiturate and diphenylhydantoin (Dilantin), appears more likely to produce an infant with defects than either drug taken separately. Infants should be watched for withdrawal symptoms and hemorrhagic tendencies. The latter condition should be treated with vitamin K.

Chronic mental deterioration has become infrequent since the use of bromides in treatment has fallen into disrepute; however, when this problem exists, it may be appropriate to recommend sterilization. The genetic status of epilepsy is unsettled, although it seems clear that the incidence of convulsions in near relatives of epileptic patients is quite low. When one parent has epilepsy of the idiopathic type, the chance of this disorder appearing in the child is only about 1 in 40. The chance is undoubtedly somewhat greater if both parents are afflicted. Hence, the presence of epilepsy should not deter marriage or childbearing, and hereditary factors alone should rarely constitute an indication for sterilization.

MULTIPLE SCLEROSIS

A disseminated disease of the central nervous system, multiple sclerosis involves both the sensory and motor systems. The characteristic clinical features are onset between 20 and 40 years of age, multiple sites of involvement, and remission and exacerbation of symptoms. The disease is chronic, and prolonged remissions are common. Although there is no specific therapy, the patient may live with the disease for many years and eventually die of debility or of another cause.

This condition rarely complicates pregnancy. According to one report, the incidence of multiple sclerosis in obstetric patients is only 0.27/1000 women. In a study of 282 patients with the disease, Leibowitz *et al.* noted that a significantly high percentage had experienced a pregnancy in the year before the onset of disease. A hazardous period in susceptible persons appears to be the 2 years just prior to the onset of clinical symptoms of multiple sclerosis. These investigators

hypothesize that there may be an incubation period or a premorbid state during which a variety of factors, including pregnancy, may precipitate central nervous system demyelination. However, there is no clear evidence that pregnancy is actually a cause. Moreover, multiple sclerosis patients whose pregnancies proceed to natural termination usually have a normal course, but there is some risk of relapse in the puerperium. Thus, there seems no reason for those afflicted with multiple sclerosis to avoid gestation, nor is this disease an indication for therapeutic abortion. Sterilization may be considered in selected patients.

HUNTINGTON'S CHOREA

The onset of Huntington's chorea ordinarily occurs between the ages of 30 and 40. This hereditary disease is transmitted through a single pair of genes; the dominant produces chorea, the recessive allele the normal condition. It is characterized by athetoid movements and mental deterioration associated with degeneration of the cerebral cortex and basal ganglia. Huntington's chorea has obstetric significance only in that the question of therapeutic abortion and sterilization often arises, since the offspring carry a 50:50 chance of developing and transmitting this dread disease.

NEURALGIA AND NEURITIS

Disorders of the peripheral nerves may appear during pregnancy from a variety of causes, the most common of which are toxic, nutritional, and traumatic. Polyneuritis is seen most frequently in association with vitamin B deficiency resulting from severe hyperemesis gravidarum or general malnutrition. Less commonly, this neurologic disorder may follow the ingestion of certain abortifacients. Traumatic nerve injuries may occur in the course of labor or delivery as a result of damage to the lumbosacral plexus or to the peripheral nerves themselves. The result may be the sudden appearance of paralysis, often preceded by a period of intense pain and paresthesia. More commonly, the injuries are less severe and result in temporary pain along the course of the sciatic nerve with accompanying muscle spasms. Mild symptoms of this type frequently appear during the later months of pregnancy, owing to pressure upon the nerve by the fetal head as it engages in the pelvis. The more serious injuries may be the result of improper placement and manipulation of obstetric forceps, incorrect positioning of the legs in stirrups for delivery, and faulty attempts at conduction anesthesia. A careful neurologic examination of the lower extremities should be a routine part of the postpartum checkup before a patient is discharged from the hospital, particularly if the delivery has been traumatic.

Facial palsy is rarely encountered in pregnant or puerperal women, but its incidence is slightly higher than in nonpregnant patients. It can be caused by a variety of conditions, including hemorrhage, tumor, otitis media, fracture, and chilling. Bilateral nerve involvement rarely is found in association with polyneuritis, sarcoidosis, myasthenia gravis, or bulbar lesions. Mostly late in pregnancy or in the early postpartum period, an idiopathic form of peripheral facial nerve paralysis known as Bell's palsy is sometimes encountered. Involvement is usually left-sided, but recently Dunn has reported a case of bilateral paresis commencing 8 days after delivery. The great majority of patients achieve complete recovery, although neural destruction occurs by the 5th–7th day in about 15%. Electrophysiologic techniques are available to establish the prognosis for recovery. Although the underlying cause of this disorder is unknown, Dunn hypothesizes that compression of the facial nerve by increased tissue pressure secondary to edema explains the relation of this condition to pregnancy. In a like manner, perineural edema of the median nerve within the carpal tunnel is thought to be the cause of the dysesthesia sometimes noted in the hand of a pregnant woman.

TUMORS

Brain tumors sometimes become clinically apparent first during pregnancy, since there may be some enlargement of the mass in association with engorgement of cerebral vessels or, as in the case of the glioma, with an increased growth rate of the neoplasm. Persistent headaches, visual disturbances, and vomiting should suggest an intracranial tumor, particularly if convulsions develop; in all such cases a careful ophthalmoscopic and visual field examination, as well as a search for localizing features should be carried out. Tomography is needed for specific localization. The results of surgery, as well as the outlook for the pregnancy, depend upon the nature of the tumor, its size and location, and the reactions of the patient during the operative procedure and in the postoperative period. If surgery is deferred, there is some risk of increased intracranial pressure during labor and delivery, although generally no ill effects are observed.

Pituitary adenomas are now diagnosed with increasing frequency. Symptomatic adenomas account for 7%–18% of intracranial tumors. The most common type is the chromophobe variety, which comprises nearly 80% of all adenomas. Such adenomas are responsible for the majority of prolactin-secreting tumors, although acidophilic adenomas sometimes produce prolactin. Tumors less than 10 mm in diameter are classified as microadenomas. Most pregnant women with microadenomas have an uncomplicated pregnancy, but careful follow-up with repeated visual field and prolactin assessments is essential. A normal course of pregnancy also occurs in most patients with treated macroadenomas; however, over one-third of pregnant women with untreated macroadenoma are at risk for complications.

PSYCHIATRIC DISORDERS

Most of the mental disorders associated with pregnancy are those in which no organic lesion is demonstrable in the brain. Of course, a woman already psychotic may become pregnant, but more often psychosis develops after the birth of the child. Mental illness complicates about 1 in 400–1000 pregnancies. Traditionally, the causes of postpartum psychosis are infectious, toxic, and idiopathic, although it is now apparent that the condition is not a distinct clinical entity and that the underlying problem is the disintegration of personality structure, usually associated with sexual maladjustment, fear, anxiety, and rejection of the pregnancy. A careful inquiry into the patient's history often shows long-standing problems in making social adjustments and in accommodating to the female role. With the birth of the infant the defensive neurotic mechanisms may be shattered, and the patient may make a complete break with reality. She may manifest aggressive, hostile behavior with destructiveness directed toward her infant; alternatively, she may threaten suicide, express ideas of great unworthiness, exhibit exaggerated changes in mood, refuse to eat, and neglect herself generally. These symptoms of puerperal psychosis are classifiable, according to the regular scheme of psychiatric diagnosis, as either manic depressive or schizophrenic. These psychotic reactions account for about 90% of the mental illness observed following childbirth. Psychotic manifestations precipitated by some toxic, infectious, metabolic, or organic disorder account for the remaining 10%. The latter patients may be confused and disoriented, manifesting fear, restlessness, and insomnia, as well as amentia. The important feature that distinguishes this condition from schizophrenia is the alternation of periods of psychosis with periods of lucidity when the patient is in contact with reality.

Psychoneurotic disorders may pose problems of significant magnitude even though the patient's ordinary defenses preserve an emotional content that is in accord with reality. A psychoneurotic patient may present multiple complaints and compromise her care by her querulous, demanding, unreasonable, autistic manner. She may reject or display open hostility to the infant or else assume an overprotective or perfectionistic attitude in caring for the baby.

The obstetrician should recognize the symptoms that warn of potential psychiatric problems. He or she should know something about the patient's personal and family history, social and marital adjustments,

psychologic maturity, and attitudes toward pregnancy and child-rearing in order to assess her probable reactions not only to the present pregnancy but also to subsequent ones. Since most women who develop psychotic disturbances during pregnancy have a history of maladjustment, immature behavioral patterns, and matrimonial difficulties, it is not surprising that 1 in 7 experiences mental illness with a subsequent gestation. Psychologic tests may be helpful in determining the stability of the patient's personality and her ability to withstand the stresses of pregnancy and motherhood, but primary reliance should be placed upon her behavioral patterns in response to gestation and other stressful situations.

Early recognition and prompt treatment reduce the duration and severity of mental illness associated with childbearing. Removing the patient to a safe and favorable environment is recommended, especially if she is suicidal. The pregnant state should not impose modifications of accepted therapeutic practices except that antidepressives should be avoided if possible. Also, if the use of lithium is essential to the patient's welfare, blood levels require careful monitoring because of the marked changes in blood volume as pregnancy advances. Electroconvulsive therapy can be administered without harm to the mother or her fetus; fractures and dislocations associated with treatment are not common. The recovery rate following appropriate therapy is the same for pregnant women as for the general population.

Although great pressures are often brought to bear upon the obstetrician to interrupt pregnancy in a patient with a psychiatric disorder, there is no clear evidence that mental illness is ameliorated by induced abortion or that abortion prevents worsening of a mild disorder. Occasionally, a genuine threat of suicide constitutes justifiable grounds. In some cases, however, termination of pregnancy may well have an adverse effect by imposing additional emotional stresses. There are psychosocial indications of sufficient magnitude to justify sterilization in many cases. Poor mothering and lack of suitable child imprinting are significant factors that impair the mental and emotional development of the offspring of these patients.

ENDOCRINE AND METABOLIC DISORDERS

DIABETES MELLITUS

Prior to the discovery of insulin, diabetes mellitus was rarely encountered as a complication of pregnancy because the great majority of patients were sterile. About one-half of these women were amenorrheic, and in the majority extreme nutritional deficiencies contributed to infertility. When pregnancy did occur in a diabetic patient, the maternal mortality rate was about 25% and fetal loss about 50%. The data indicate the potential seriousness of this complication when the disorder goes unrecognized and untreated during gestation.

There is evidence that the incidence of insulin-dependent diabetes among schoolchildren is increasing significantly, according to reports from the American Diabetes Association. In addition, better methods of managing diabetic children allow more girls with this disease to reach childbearing age. As a result, increasing numbers of women with juvenile or growth-onset diabetes may be seen at prenatal clinics in the future. Less than one-quarter of all diabetics develop the disorder before the age of 40 years; however, the condition is far more serious for this group.

Incidence

Diabetes mellitus is known to complicate pregnancy in about 1 in 100 patients, an incidence not greatly different from the rate of diabetes in the general population. These figures undoubtedly do not include many patients with latent diabetes that escapes recognition despite suggestive maternal complications and perinatal death. The incidence of diabetes is known to increase with age, and it has been estimated that 3.8% of the females in our present population will eventually become diabetic. Some prediabetics develop overt disease during gestation; others do not manifest frank diabetes until 1–25 years later. Moreover, the *dd* diabetic gene seems to have higher penetration under prevailing conditions of nutrition and medical care; it has been estimated that a doubling of the genotype for diabetes mellitus may be reached in less than ten generations. This trend has significance for the obstetrician because many of these new cases will come to light first during pregnancy. A search for defective carbohydrate metabolism is an essential part of good prenatal care and obstetric management.

Pathogenesis

Diabetes mellitus is generally regarded as a genetically determined disorder, usually inherited as a recessive trait, but occurring as a dominant trait in some families. In accordance with this genetic concept of the natural history of the disease, it is customary to consider the offspring of diabetic parents as prediabetics, even though their glucose tolerance is within normal limits. When results of glucose tolerance testing first become abnormal, without other evidence of diabetes, the state is termed *chemical diabetes*. A variety of stress situations, such as obesity, infection, and pregnancy, may be triggering mechanisms. In patients with clinical diabetes, various mechanisms underlie the insulin deficiency, and various events may precipitate frank disease. Multifactorial, as well as multigenic, considerations are implicated in the pathogenicity of diabetes, in contrast to the old, purely genetic concept.

Diabetogenic Effect of Pregnancy

A sensitive balance between glucose production and glucose utilization is maintained by the interaction of various hormones that originate from different sources and influence carbohydrate metabolism by different biochemical pathways. In addition to insulin, hormones originating in the pituitary, thyroid, and adrenal glands, including epinephrine as well as glucocorticoids, exert significant effects on carbohydrate metabolism. These actions are antagonistic to insulin (contrainsulin factors) in that they tend to elevate blood glucose levels, although the effects may be of secondary nature. These hormones, including insulin, influence fat and protein as well as carbohydrate metabolism. The anabolic processes of the growing fetus, which derive their energy from maternal resources, impose additional compensatory adjustments on available adaptive biochemical systems. Ordinarily, the increase in contrainsulin factors is counterbalanced during episodes of stress by an increase in the secretion of insulin.

There appears to be little doubt that insulin antagonism is enhanced during pregnancy. A marked increase in circulating insulin is required to maintain a normal blood glucose curve or fractional rate of glucose disposition in the face of glucose challenge. The hypoglycemic effect of exogenous insulin is likewise diminished. The fasting glucose level in the pregnant woman tends to be lower than the nonpregnancy value, while free fatty acid concentration is correspondingly elevated. This state resembles that of a nongravid subject following prolonged fasting, and a concept of "accelerated starvation" has been advanced by Freinkel. It should be noted, however, that, while there is a rise in free fatty acids, the proportional amount of fat consumed for maternal fuel remains the same or is lowered. Carbohydrates are the major source of maternal energy even during physical stress.

Normally, the gravid patient exhibits an increased plasma level of both insulin and proinsulin, but augmented protein binding of insulin during pregnancy may result in lessened physiologic activity. Moreover, a number of factors have been specifically implicated in development of a relative insensitivity to insulin. It has been suggested that hPL exerts a contrainsulin effect by reducing the biologic effectiveness of circulating insulin. In addition, it increases the mobilization of free fatty acids. Estrogens, progesterone, and corticosteroids have been noted to affect carbohydrate metabolism, and generally they are considered contrainsulin factors. However, the relation of such effects to normal gestation or a state of chemical diabetes needs further study and clarification.

Metabolic proficiency, as estimated on the basis of glucose, insulin, or tolbutamide tolerance tests, decreases directly with the length of gestation. The patient who exhibits a significant reduction in carbohydrate-metabolizing potential should be considered to possess a diabetic trait, which under the stress of gestation is capable of producing the same maternal and fetal complications observed among diabetic women. In some patients, extrapancreatic factors are principally responsible for reduced glucose tolerance and glycosuria; however, these findings may indicate a maladjustment in carbohydrate metabolism that calls for further study, careful observation, and appropriate prenatal precautions.

Pregnancy is a dynamic process involving interrelated changes in the mother, fetus, and placenta. Biochemical and hormonal processes are likewise dynamic, and fluctuations in carbohydrate metabolism, as well as variations in contrainsulin factors, during gestation are to be expected. Nevertheless, the insulin requirement generally increases progressively toward term and then declines precipitously in the immediate postpartum period. These occurrences, as well as anticipated fluctuations in glucose tolerance, have clinical significance. Because the mechanisms involved are not completely understood, it is not surprising that up to three-quarters of all gravidas whose glucose tolerance test results are abnormal show no such defects following pregnancy. However, since between one-quarter and one-third of all asymptomatic patients whose glucose tolerance test results are abnormal in pregnancy ultimately develop overt diabetes, each such woman is a subject for retesting and follow-up.

Diagnosis

Diabetes mellitus should be suspected in any patient discovered to have sugar in her urine, although it should be recognized that lactosuria is a common occurrence during the last 6 weeks of pregnancy and that the lowered renal threshold for sugar, which results from an increased filtration fraction, may be normal. When the glucose-specific paper test shows true glucose in the urine, investigation is mandatory. The response to alimentary hyperglycemia or to administration of glucose provides a truer picture of carbohydrate metabolism than does measurement of fasting blood sugar, since low values are commonly observed during pregnancy. It is generally agreed that a 2-hour postprandial blood sugar level of 140 mg/dl is indicative of diabetes mellitus and that a level of 110–140 mg/dl is suggestive of subclinical diabetes. A 3-hour glucose tolerance test is usually confirmatory.

The oral glucose tolerance test is altered in pregnancy by a slight elevation of blood glucose in the postabsorptive state and a lag in the return to normal. The oral test is more sensitive than the intravenous test, and the differences may relate in part to the alteration of gastrointestinal function during pregnancy. The upper limits of venous blood sugar as measured by the Somogyi–Nelson method for an oral glucose tolerance test during pregnancy are: fasting, 90 mg/dl; 1

hour, 165 mg/dl; 2 hours, 145 mg/dl; 3 hours, 125 mg/dl. If two or more of these values are equaled or exceeded, the result is considered abnormal. Duration of pregnancy influences the glucose curve, and the results of repeated tests in the same patient may vary. Unless the results are overtly abnormal, interpretation of the oral test may be difficult, and other assessments may be needed for diagnosis.

Clinical clues to the diagnosis should not be neglected. Women who carry the diabetic trait are often obese and tend to gain excessive weight during pregnancy. Excessive hunger, thirst, and polyuria call for investigation, although some nondiabetic gravidas complain of these symptoms. The appearance of refractory or recurrent monilial vaginitis is another clue worthy of follow-up. A family background of diabetes warns that the patient may have inherited the diabetic trait. The outcome of previous pregnancies may be suggestive; women with undiagnosed diabetes have often lost babies for unknown reasons or have given birth to malformed fetuses. They may give a history of large infants, hydramnios, or hypertensive disorders in one or more pregnancies, or their records may indicate that the placenta was large, edematous, and histologically immature. Suspicion of diabetes is intensified when examination reveals retinopathy, neurologic disorders, impairment of renal function, or unexplained vascular disturbances. Refractory or recurrent urinary tract infection or a predisposition for infections of all kinds likewise suggests metabolic disturbance.

Special attention should be paid a very rare but often fatal condition associated with diabetes. This syndrome is characterized as a hyperglycemic, hyperosmolar, nonketotic type of coma associated with hypernatremia, dehydration, and focal seizures. Prompt recognition and vigorous treatment are mandatory if these patients are to be salvaged. There is a high incidence of cerebral and vascular complications that claim the lives of almost 50% of the victims. The emphasis in therapy is on fluid replacement and massive amounts of hypotonic solutions and judicious use of insulin.

The possibility of diabetes should not be dismissed when the glucose tolerance curve reverts to normal during the postpartum period. This reversion to normal occurs sometimes even among women who have experienced diabetic coma during pregnancy. It is imperative that these patients be followed, since frank diabetes may reappear at a later age or in response to another stressful situation. In many cases, the diabetic curve can be reproduced by priming the patient with one of the glucocorticoids before the standard glucose tolerance test is performed.

Classification

An overly liberal definition of diabetes invites ill-advised obstetric intervention; however, one that does not take into account latent diabetes may be far more detrimental, since a patient with disturbed carbohydrate metabolism may be deprived of the required specialized care for herself and her infant. Fetal health relates closely to the duration of diabetes and its severity as evidenced by the degree of vascular damage. White proposed the following classification that takes these factors into account and is now in general use:

Class A. Diagnosis is made by glucose tolerance test. A typical diabetic curve may return completely to normal within several days following delivery.
Class B. Onset of diabetes occurred after the age of 20, duration of the disease is less then 10 years, and no evidence of vascular disease exists.
Class C. Onset of diabetes occurred between the ages of 10 and 20, duration of the disease is 10–19 years, and no evidence of vascular disease exists.
Class D. Onset of diabetes occurred before the age of 10, duration of the disease is more than 20 years, and vascular disease is present as evidenced by retinitis or calcification of the vessels of the legs.
Class E. Vascular disease is present as evidenced by calcification of pelvic vessels.
Class F. Nephritis is present.
Class R. Active retinitis proliferans or vitreous hemorrhage is present.

Every diabetic patient should be hospitalized when first seen in pregnancy. A detailed evaluation of the diabetes should be carried out, and the extent of vascular damage should be determined. Workup reveals evidence of microvascular disease at least in about 10% of patients, and its detection is contingent upon a careful survey of cardiovascular and renal status, as well as a radiographic search for leg and pelvic arteriosclerosis. Included are careful ophthalmologic evaluation and kidney studies with biopsies as indicated to determine whether the Kimmelstiel–Wilson syndrome or diabetic nephritis is present.

On the basis of this evaluation, therapy should be instituted. It is important that all diabetic women, regardless of the severity of their disease, be offered intensive medical supervision and expert obstetric care.

Effects of Pregnancy on Diabetes

Fluctuation in insulin requirements is one of the primary problems in the management of diabetic patients during pregnancy. Although the majority have a lowered sugar tolerance, especially in the latter half of pregnancy, some experience the reverse effect, and in others there is little change. Moreover, in the same patient the sugar tolerance may vary with the stage of gestation or in response to vomiting, infections, or other complications. In the puerperium, the involutionary processes, as well as the conversion of blood glucose into lactose in lactation, may cause wide

swings in glucose tolerance, although in most cases the result is hypoglycemia, sometimes of profound degree. Likewise, during labor, the changes in sugar tolerance are neither constant nor predictable, since the depletion of glycogen reserves may appreciably alter sugar and insulin requirements. For all these reasons, insulin dosage in pregnancy should be carefully regulated on the basis of frequent blood sugar determinations.

There seems little doubt that the pregnant woman has an increased tendency to ketosis as evidenced by the diminished carbon dioxide–combining power of the blood. Moreover, the lowered resistance to acidosis may be aggravated by the substantial elevation of the basal metabolic rate during pregnancy. The fact that minor infections and electrolyte disturbances may give rise to acidosis and even to coma gives clinical support to this contention. Ketoacidosis not only constitutes a grave maternal hazard but, even in minor degrees, is often responsible for fetal death or for serious neonatal disorders.

One of the fairly predictable occurrences in the diabetic patient is the fall in oxygen consumption that begins around the 34th–35th gestational week. This is in contrast to the situation of the normal gravida, whose oxygen consumption continues to rise until term. The diabetic patient also experiences a similar early fall in the respiratory quotient. These findings suggest that physiologic maturation of the fetus may occur several weeks earlier in the diabetic than in the normal gravida. Thus, there may be some scientific basis for early artificial termination of pregnancy in the presence of maternal diabetes.

Effects of Diabetes on Pregnancy

The degree to which diabetes is controlled during pregnancy and parturition determines in large measure the outcome for both mother and infant. With adequate care, the maternal mortality rate is essentially the same as that for nondiabetic women, since almost all deaths from diabetes complicated by pregnancy are preventable. In actual practice, however, the maternal mortality associated with this condition is increased because severe preeclampsia, ketoacidosis, uremia, cardiac decompensation, and cerebrovascular accidents in association with extreme hypertension occur in neglected cases. Infections of the skin and urinary tract, as well as neuropathies, mostly of the sensory type, may be aggravated in pregnancy. Transient seventh nerve paralysis may be encountered rarely. Vascular lesions are of greater concern among those whose diabetes had an early onset. Angina is a worrisome complaint in such patients and may herald myocardial infarction during pregnancy or the puerperal period. Increased cardiac output during pregnancy may aggravate preexisting diabetic cardiac dis-

ease characterized by an increase in myocardial connective tissue and small contramural coronary vessels.

Microaneurysms may appear in the capillaries deep in the substance of the retina along with venous stasis, congestion, and sclerosis of the retinal arteries. In advanced cases, retinal arteries may appear as silver wires, and there may be "cotton-wool" retinal exudate; such lesions may be intensified in pregnancy, and vision may be threatened. Except for retinitis proliferans, however, pregnancy does not seem to accelerate the natural course of deterioration resulting from diabetes.

Effects of Diabetes on the Baby

Perinatal salvage remains a challenge despite good medical and obstetric care, although it should be possible to achieve a satisfactory outcome in 80%–85% of cases. The primary fetal hazard is anoxia associated with either maternal preeclampsia or ketoacidosis, while the principal neonatal risk is respiratory distress with pulmonary hyaline membrane formations. The fourfold increase in the birth of infants with serious malformations, usually observed in association with hydramnios, accounts for an additional toll. Characteristically, the infants of diabetic mothers are macrosomatic, as well as edematous, and the large size of these fetuses predisposes them to trauma attributable to mechanical difficulties that necessitate operative delivery.

In general, the perinatal mortality is related directly to the degree of vascular damage. There may be rapid progression of the disease during pregnancy, resulting in increasing retinopathy, nitrogen retention, and ketoacidosis. The incidence and severity of preeclampsia correlate positively with the degree of renal vascular involvement. Preeclampsia occurs in 15%–20% of pregnant diabetic women, and while eclampsia and severe preeclampsia can usually be prevented, it is not always possible to avert milder forms of the disease, especially if there is underlying vascular damage. Preeclampsia may appear early in the third trimester, when the infant's chances for extrauterine survival are as poor as those associated with its continued subsistence *in utero,* where its welfare depends on the function of a deteriorating placenta. Moreover, the risk of placental disruption is ever present, particularly in the severely preeclamptic woman, and this complication imposes a grave hazard to both mother and fetus. Placental infarcts are more common, and the likelihood that one umbilical artery will be missing, with its associated risk of fetal anomalies, is increased.

The risk of perinatal death in the presence of significant maternal microvascular disease is at least 50% and is even higher among mothers with advanced pelvic arteriosclerosis and retinitis. Generally, ketoacidosis and superimposed preeclampsia, representing an

aggravation of vascular or renal disease, impose the greatest risk of fetal death at 32–34 weeks or earlier.

Thus, the clinical findings vary somewhat according to the class of diabetes. It has been reported that patients with mild diabetes (classes A–C) exhibit more hydramnios, excessive weight gain, preeclampsia, macrosomatic infants, large placentas, diabetic intensification, and intrapartal fetal deaths than do patients with more advanced disease (classes D–F). The latter evidence more spontaneous abortions, intrauterine fetal deaths, and neonatal deaths, but the other features are less common. Insulin requirements do not reflect severity of disease; the age of onset and duration of diabetes are more important with respect to pregnancy outcome.

Management

Antepartum Care. Diabetic patients require close supervision during pregnancy if the disease is to be controlled and major complications avoided. Biweekly visits, at which times the woman's medical status is assessed by both the obstetrician and the internist, usually suffice during the first 6 months of gestation; after that time, the patient should be seen weekly or more often, depending upon the individual circumstances. In addition, it is advisable to admit her to the hospital on several occasions to assess her diabetic status. When signs of incipient preeclampsia and infection arise or when difficulties are encountered in controlling the diabetes, hospitalization is mandatory at any time during pregnancy.

At the time of each prenatal visit, a sample of blood should be drawn for sugar, carbon dioxide, and urea nitrogen determinations. All patients should have eyeground examinations routinely. Urinalyses, complete blood counts, and renal function tests should be done regularly. Evaluation of cardiovascular status is indicated if the patient is hypertensive. Between visits, the patient should maintain a daily record of urinary sugar and acetone, and she should be instructed to report immediately any marked fluctuations. It is necessary to instruct her about diet and to impress upon her the need for absolute cooperation in carrying out medical directives. Since muscular exercise is effective in lowering the concentration of blood sugar, regularity and timing of work are important in diabetic management.

The diet should be calculated to maintain the ideal weight in the first trimester of pregnancy and to permit an average gain of no more than 3–3.5 lb/month during the last 6 months. The diet should be high in protein, usually 2g/kg body weight or a minimum of 80 g daily during the second half of pregnancy. The caloric intake depends on the nutritional and metabolic needs of the patient, but in most cases the requirement is 30–40 calories/kg. There should be an adequate carbohydrate intake, usually about 200 g daily, and enough fat to provide about 35% of the total calories. The diet is planned for three meals a day, although a bedtime supplement is required if the patient is taking insulin. Sodium intake may be slightly restricted. Chlorothiazide in daily doses of 500–1000 mg, administered in short courses of several days, and salt restriction were formerly used freely to control edema and forestall preeclampsia. There is now evidence that both these devices can be harmful and that bedrest alone is the best solution for both edema and incipient preeclampsia. These subjects are discussed in Chapter 25.

Insulin should be prescribed if dietary management alone does not correct the metabolic disorder. Oral hypoglycemic agents should not be used in pregnancy until more is known of their effects on the fetus, since, unlike insulin, they cross the placenta. Also, they may be ineffective in controlling the sharp variations in glucose tolerance that are characteristic in pregnancy. In the majority of patients, the need for insulin or for increased dosage begins in the second trimester. The need for insulin therapy in all patients with diabetes reaches a peak at the time of delivery. Some physicians who recommend insulin in chemical as well as overt diabetes report dramatic improvement in perinatal salvage when these prophylactic measures are begun in the earliest stages of gestation. The primary objective is to maintain the blood glucose level in a physiologic range, and the simplest and most convenient insulin dosage schedule that achieves this objective is the best. At present, NPH and lente insulins are popular, but the insulin program should be individualized to suit the needs of each patient. For example, the hyperlabile diabetic or the one who exhibits marked vacillation of blood sugar levels in response to infection, vomiting, parturition, or other stresses may be controlled best with repeated doses of short-acting insulin rather than fewer doses of intermediate or long-acting insulin. Unmodified insulin added to an infusion of 5% glucose in water, usually in a ratio of 1 unit insulin to 3 g glucose, should be given during labor and delivery or during surgery. The administration of fructose solutions to the mother has been used to minimize the risk of hypoglycemia in the newborn. Short-acting insulin should be continued as required for several days postpartum.

Periodic surveillance should be made according to a definite protocol such as the one shown in Figure 27-2. The problems that are sometimes encountered in interpretation of estriol excretion studies can usually be resolved by noting the estriol/creatinine ratio: intrauterine death is unusual if this ratio is rising. An L/S ratio of 2 or higher is usually evidence of fetal lung maturity, but in some diabetics, as noted in Chapter 41, the L/S ratio may be inconclusive. Under such circumstances a *"lung profile"* may greatly enhance the

	Class diabetic	Weeks gestataion																				
		20	21	22	23	24	25	26	27	28	29	30	31	32	33	34	35	36	37	38	39	40
Clinic or office visit	A–R	X		X		X		X		X	X	X	X	X	X	X	X	X	X	X	X	X
Ultrasound cephalometry	A–R			X			X			X		X		X		X		X		X		X
Amniocentesis (L/S ratio)	A–R																		X			
Predelivery hospitalization	A₁																			///	///	///
	A₂																		///	///	///	///
	B															///	///	///	///	///	///	///
	C														///	///	///	///	///	///	///	///
	D,E,F,R												///	///	///	///	///	///	///	///	///	///
Nonstress fetal heart rate monitoring Oxytocin challenge test if NST non-reactive	A₁											X	X	X	X	X	X	X	X	X	X	X
	A₂											X	X	X	X	X	X	X	X	X	X	X
	B											X	X	X	X	X	X	X	X	X	X	X
	C											X	X	X	X	X	X	X	X	X	X	X
	D,E,F,R										X	X	XX	XX	XX	XX	XX	XX	XX	XX	XX	XX
Estriol/Creatinine (24 hour excretion) (optional)	A₁													X	X	X	X	X	X	/daily///		
	A₂													X	X	X	X	X	///daily///			
	B													X	X	X	X	////daily/////				
	C													X	X	////////daily/////						
	D,E,F,R													////////////daily//////								

FIG. 27–2. Protocol prepared by R. Depp, for surveillance of the pregnant diabetic patient, Prentice Hospital, Chicago. This protocol may be modified according to local practice or special circumstance. *Class A₁,* Abnormal glucose tolerance test. *Class A₂,* Fasting blood sugar 105 mg/dl. When hypertension is present, nonstress tests (NST) should be started 2 weeks earlier, regardless of class.

accuracy of prediction. Two-dimensional thin-layer chromatography is needed to perform the profile. The necessary tests are (1) L/S ratio (2) percentage of disaturated lecithin precipitated by acetone, and (3) percentage of phosphatidyl inositol (PI) and phosphatidyl glycerol (PG). The status of fetal lung development is assessed by plotting the results of the above determinations on an appropriate grid.

The decision to deliver a patient prior to 37 weeks should be based on special indications, because fetal immaturity imposes a grave neonatal hazard. Thus, intervention prior to the 37th gestational week is justified only if pregnancy is complicated by preeclampsia, if repeated bouts of acidosis occur despite intensive medical care, if a severely edematous fetus is visualized roentgenographically or by ultrasound, or if a previous pregnancy has terminated in fetal death *in utero*

at some time prior to the 37th or 38th gestational week.

Occasionally, an asymptomatic patient whose response to the glucose tolerance test suggests diabetes but who is normal otherwise may be permitted to continue pregnancy until her condition is favorable for induction of labor, even though the length of gestation exceeds the limit prescribed for most diabetic women. In a patient of this type, the risk of fetal death *in utero* is inconsequential if past obstetric experience has been normal and if careful supervision is maintained to recognize the early signs and symptoms of complications. If glycosuria or incipient preeclampsia appears, or if excessive growth of the fetus, hydramnios, or full-term gestation is suspected, delivery should be accomplished immediately.

Great emphasis should be placed upon rest during pregnancy. For patients with microvascular disease, rest in bed in the hospital for most of the third trimester is important. The minimum should be at least 1 week in advance of the probable delivery date. Recumbency, particularly in the lateral position, has a favorable influence upon uteroplacental circulation and di-

minishing myometrial tone. Hospitalization also allows monitoring of the patient for early evidence of complications so that a decision to intervene can be made promptly and with full knowledge of circumstances. Appropriate tests can be performed on a regular, scheduled basis. Hydramnios, which may develop rapidly, can be treated by slow removal of excess amniotic fluid by transabdominal amniotomy—a procedure that occasionally extends pregnancy by several precious weeks, but more often is ineffective. Amniocentesis can be performed to test for meconium staining and to assess fetal maturity. Although L/S ratios are somewhat atypical in insulin-dependent diabetics (they fail to show a terminal rise in about one-third of the patients and demonstrate an early excessive rise in others), this parameter is a helpful adjunct in determining fetal lung maturity, according to Whitfield *et al*. Measurement of creatinine and bilirubin levels offers further evidence about fetal maturity.

Thus, hospitalization prior to anticipated delivery is important despite today's high costs for this added stay. The guidelines for management are maintenance of diabetes control with proper diet and insulin administration, early detection of maternal complications, frequent assessment of fetal status, determination of optimal time and method of delivery, and arrangements for intensive care of the newborn. If preeclampsia develops, the patient's condition should be stabilized and early delivery accomplished.

Intrapartum Care. The method of delivery should be determined by parity, size of pelvis, estimated size of fetus, presentation and position of the fetus, station, and condition of the cervix. X-ray pelvimetry should be performed if there is doubt about the capacity of the pelvis. In addition, the abdominal films may provide information about fetal size, the accumulation of excess amounts of fluid in the tissues, and calcification of pelvic vessels.

The choice between induction of labor and cesarean section should be based on the anticipated ease of labor and delivery at the time when delivery is deemed advisable. A reliable estimate of the probable effects of labor on the fetus can be obtained by fetal heart rate testing (see Chapter 41). This can be a useful guide to the choice between induction of labor or delivery by cesarean section. If induction is chosen, productive labor must ensue promptly, with full expectation of a normal course and a nontraumatic outlet forceps delivery. If these cannot be predicted or if they do not ensue, the solution is cesarean section. In the majority of patients, abdominal delivery is preferred. Conduction anesthesia, either local or regional, is usually superior to inhalation anesthesia, regardless of the approach. An infusion of 5% dextrose in water should be administered to support the patient, and one-half of her prepregnancy dose of insulin (or less, depending upon

circumstances) should be given preoperatively. Generally, premedications are withheld.

Postpartum Care. After delivery, there is characteristically a marked reduction in the insulin requirement, although in some patients glucose tolerance is highly variable before it stabilizes. The latter difficulty is likely to occur in the presence of infection. Short-acting insulin should be used for several days, the timing and dosage based on fractional urine sugar and acetone determinations. A catheter should be left in the bladder for at least the 1st day or 2 postpartum to facilitate control of the diabetes. Blood sugar and carbon dioxide analyses should be done regularly or as need arises. Ordinarily, insulin requirements gradually rise to prepregnancy levels about 7–10 days after delivery.

It is important to repeat the cardiovascular–renal workup of the diabetic patient during the postpartum period, usually after the 6-week checkup, to provide a baseline for further care. Should there be evidence of severe degenerative vascular lesions or if recent pregnancies have resulted in perinatal death despite good medical and obstetric management, sterilization may be considered.

Care of the Newborn. The newborn infant of a diabetic mother is subject to a number of special hazards, notably anoxia, physiologic immaturity despite macrosomia, respiratory distress in association with pulmonary hyaline membranes, and hypoglycemia. Increased birth weight, increased length, increased heart weight, and hyperplasia of the islets of Langerhans are common. Care of the infant at birth begins with clearance of the nasopharynx, careful resuscitation as required, postural drainage, and aspiration of stomach contents if the delivery has been abdominal. As soon as possible, the infant should be placed in an incubator with humidified compressed air for 24–48 hours, depending upon the respiratory condition. Supplemental oxygen may be required, but the concentration should not exceed 40%. Sample of cord blood should be examined at birth for glucose, pH, sodium, bicarbonate, and potassium to aid understanding and treatment of electrolyte imbalances that may arise.

All biochemical derangements should be corrected. Marked hypoglycemia should be treated with glucose administration, since available evidence indicates that glycogen stores in the brain and liver and blood glucose levels tend to potentiate the newborn's resistance to hypoxia. The administration of bicarbonate or albumin in an effort to minimize respiratory acidosis, hyperkalemia, and effusion from the pulmonary vascular bed has been recommended. Rapid digitalization may be indicated if rales appear and the liver is descending. Effective methods to prevent or treat the respiratory distress syndrome are largely controversial; since infants of diabetic mothers are particularly susceptible to

this condition, it remains a common cause of neonatal death. The matter of feeding, especially of edematous infants, is also controversial, although many pediatricians advocate the early oral administration of glucose and saline.

MATERNAL PHENYLKETONURIA

Phenylketonuria (PKU) is an inborn error of metabolism caused by an autosomal recessive trait that creates a deficiency in the enzyme phenylalanine hydroxylase and results in inability to metabolize phenylalanine to tyrosine. Johnson has shown that homozygosity for this disorder in a woman whose fetus is heterozygous produces disastrous fetal results. Elevated maternal blood phenylalanine levels during pregnancy result in fetal hyperphenylalaninemia, which is compounded by the normal tendency for amino acids to be in greater concentration on the fetal side of the placenta. Maternal risk in this disorder is not a factor; however, for the fetus, intrauterine and postnatal growth retardation, including mental retardation, is almost universal, and about one-quarter of the fetuses are malformed. Apparently, a maternal diet low in phenylalanine has questionable preventive value unless followed prior to conception. For the woman with PKU who is already pregnant, therapeutic abortion should be considered and sterilization strongly advised as a permanent measure. A simple urine test (Phenostix) is available and is usually applied routinely to every woman in early pregnancy.

DISORDERS OF THE THYROID GLAND

Hypothyroidism

A euthyroid state is required for successful pregnancy, and there is little doubt that thyroid deficiency adversely affects all stages of gestation. Extreme deficiency is usually accompanied by amenorrhea or oligomenorrhea with resultant sterility; however, less severe deficiency is compatible with pregnancy, although abortion is likely. Occasionally, the infant of a hypothyroid mother is born with congenital goiter or with true cretinism, and there seems to be an increased incidence of congenital anomalies in these infants. Thus, it seems clear that the hypothyroid patient requires exogenous thyroid not only to conceive but also to sustain normal fetal growth and development. Maternal hypothyroidism sometimes is temporarily ameliorated, possibly because of fetal thyroid hormones.

During pregnancy, there is an estrogen-mediated increase in thyroxine-binding globulin (TBG). This rise in serum concentration of TBG begins with the onset of pregnancy and reaches a level of two to three times the nonpregnant value by the 18th gestational week. A proportionate increase in the synthesis of thyroid hormone tends to saturate the increased numbers of binding sites in the serum. This increase in protein-bound thyroxine results in elevation of total serum thyroxine, butanol-extractable iodine, and protein-bound iodine. The metabolically active fraction, free thyroxine, normally remains within the nonpregnancy range. In the pregnant euthyroid woman, there is usually slight thyroid gland hyperplasia, accompanied by an increase in thyroidal iodine uptake, and the basal metabolic rate increases by 15%–20%. Hennen *et al.* suggest that these changes may be mediated in part by placental secretion of human chorionic thyrotropin. Moreover, relative iodine deficiency during pregnancy may be caused by increased renal iodide clearance and increased hormonogenesis. The fetal thyroid appears to be functionally mature by the 14th week; thus, if fetal iodine requirements are a factor, maternal sources are necessary only during the first trimester. Myxedematous women have given birth to normal infants. Thyroid hormone is known to cross the human placenta/membrane, but at a very slow rate.

The simplest and most reliable laboratory procedure for evaluating the metabolic status of the pregnant woman is determination of the free serum thyroxine concentration. Free thyroxine can be measured by equilibrium dialysis or, more simply, estimated by calculation of the free thyroxine index. Failure of the total serum thyroxine level to rise despite the increase in TBG, as in hypothyroidism, results in gross changes in the free thyroxine index. The latter is the product of the total serum thyroxine and the resin triiodothyronine (T3) uptake test divided by the resin T3 uptake of a control standard serum from a euthyroid nonpregnant patient. It should be emphasized that determination of radioactive iodine uptake is contraindicated during pregnancy, since the material is taken up avidly by the fetal thyroid.

In addition to results to these biochemical tests and suggestive history and physical signs, other clinical and laboratory findings may support the diagnosis. The biologic action of thyroid hormone can be assessed by determining the basal metabolic rate, Achilles tendon reflex time, blood cholesterol level, and glucose tolerance. A firm diffuse goiter with prominent pyramidal lobe and elevated serum titers of antithyroglobulin or antithyroid microsomal antibodies suggest Hashimoto's thyroiditis, the most common cause of hypothyroidism. It is important to remember, moreover, that thyroid deficiency may be only one feature of a multiglandular disorder.

The reserve function of the thyroid gland may be limited, and gestational hypothyroidism may develop as the gland fails to produce sufficient hormone to counterbalance the rising TBG and increased binding capacity of the serum. In the presence of iodine deficiency, both mother and fetus may develop colloid en-

largement, and a subclinical hypothyroid state may make its appearance for the first time during pregnancy. Following delivery, the secretion of thyrotropin diminishes and gland involution commences, although excessive amounts of colloid may persist.

Treatment should be instituted as soon as the diagnosis of a hypothyroid state is confirmed, because untreated gravidas experience increased fetal wastage, according to Greenman *et al.* Thyroid replacement should be complete, since Mann *et al.* have shown that incomplete restoration may adversely affect the physical and mental development of the child. The usual replacement doses are prescribed, and the free thyroxine index can be used to monitor the adequacy of the medication. In patients with endemic goiter, iodine administration is desirable as a means of reducing the risk of cretinism in the newborn. For the mother, the iodine administered in conjunction with a thyroid preparation promptly corrects the metabolic deficiency and tends to promote normal postpartal involution of the gland. The possibility of thyrotoxicosis seems to be reduced when nodular goiter is prevented and hyperplasia regresses.

Thyroid medication should not be used empirically in the hope that fetal wastage of unknown cause can be eliminated. Moreover, low levels of protein-bound or butanol-extractable iodine, or values that fail to increase during pregnancy, are common in early abortions from multiple causes. These findings usually reflect defective trophoblast and decreased elaboration of estrogen and progesterone. The TBG level fails to rise as a consequence, and the normal increase in the synthesis of thyroxine does not occur; thyroid administration at this time does not reduce the incidence of abortion. Chorionic gonadotropin and steroid excretion levels may be low well in advance of the expected rise in protein-bound iodine.

Hyperthyroidism

Pregnancy is not often superimposed upon an untreated hyperthyroid state because most women so afflicted experience severe menstrual disorders in association with gonadal failure and anovulation. Nevertheless, in a few patients, hyperthyroidism is discovered during pregnancy; in these patients, the outcome is generally good, although the risk of abortion is increased. Rarely, thyrotoxicosis has its onset during gestation, but there is no evidence that this condition is induced by the physiologic alterations in thyroid function. Symmetric enlargement of the thyroid gland, gradual and definite increase in the basal metabolic rate, and slight elevation of the protein-bound and butanol-extractable iodine levels are normal in pregnancy and are not ordinarily associated with any of the typical signs of hyperthyroidism.

The symptoms of hyperthyroidism are the same, regardless of whether toxic adenoma or diffuse hyperplasia is the fundamental pathologic lesion. Most of the symptoms are referable to increased thyroid secretion, which causes an increased metabolic rate with excessive oxidation in the tissue cells, resulting in loss of weight and weakness despite increased appetite. Tachycardia, sweating, diarrhea, tremor, nervousness, and vomiting are caused by overstimulation of the sympathetic nervous system. The disease may be complicated by exophthalmos or heart disease. Normal pregnancy may mimic some but not all of these clinical features.

The slight thyroid gland enlargement and hyperplasia observed in normal pregnancy may be due in part to placental secretion of chorionic thyrotropin, a hormone immunologically distinguishable from pituitary thyroid-stimulating hormone (TSH). Hennen *et al.* report that its secretion commences in the 1st month of gestation and persists until delivery. Interestingly, high levels produced in molar pregnancy have resulted in thyrotoxicosis that subsided upon evacuation of the mole. The long-acting thyroid stimulator (LATS), a γ-globulin with TSH-like activity, also tends to cross the placenta and may cause neonatal thyrotoxicosis. McKenzie reports that, as LATS undergoes biologic degradation during the neonatal period, the metabolic disturbance in the infant disappears. According to Galina *et al.*, iodide and antithyroid drugs also cross the placenta freely, and their improper or unmonitored use can produce neonatal goiter, hypothyroidism, or both. T_3 measurements are necessary, since T_3 thyrotoxicosis may coexist with pregnancy.

The most important simple laboratory procedure for evaluating metabolic status in pregnancy is the free serum thyroxine concentration. In thyrotoxicosis, there is an elevation in total serum thyroxine that is not commensurate with the TBG level. The presence of ophthalmopathy, pretibial myxedema, and a positive result on the LATS determination support the diagnosis of Grave's disease. Conventional thyroid scans that make use of ^{131}I, ^{125}I, or ^{99}mTc cannot be used in pregnancy because the material is stored in the fetal thyroid gland and damages it. Hoffer and Gottschalk report that a new fluorescent scanning technique using an external source of ^{241}A can be safely employed during pregnancy.

Surgery, preceded by administration of one of the antithyroid drugs until acute symptoms subside and then of Lugol's solution for at least 10 days, is a satisfactory method of treating pregnant hyperthyroid patients, particularly those with toxic adenoma. The long-continued use of antithyroid drugs, such as propylthiouracil, requires careful and close supervision. Overdose may induce thyroid deficiency, which imposes additional hazards in pregnancy. Congenital goiter has occasionally been observed in infants whose mothers were given antithyroid substances in doses in excess of physiologic needs; the dose should be reduced during the last month of pregnancy to minimize

this risk. When propylthiouracil is combined with Lugol's solution, the likelihood of injury to the fetal thyroid is remote; nevertheless, certain toxic manifestations, such as anemia and agranulocytosis, occasionally follow its administration. The routine addition of replacement doses of thyroid hormone to the antithyroid drug has been recommended after the thyrotoxicosis has been initially controlled. The combination of drugs has not resulted in a need for higher doses of antithyroid medication. Experience has shown that this approach facilitates adequate control of maternal hyperthyroidism and at the same time minimizes the occurrence of inadvertent hypothyroidism and fetal damage. However, since any maternal therapy for thyroid dysfunction may induce fetal thyroid insult, determination of free thyroxine index in cord blood of such an infant should be routine.

Malignant Disease of the Thyroid

When malignant thyroid disease is discovered during gestation it should be treated surgically rather than with radioisotopes, although it is permissible to follow with well-shielded radiation therapy. The uncertain diagnosis in many nodular enlargements of the thyroid gland requires that early surgery be considered. When the course of disease in 70 women who had one or more pregnancies subsequent to a diagnosis of thyroid cancer was compared with that in 109 women with the same diagnosis who did not later become pregnant, Hill *et al.* found no significant difference. They concluded that pregnancy subsequent to the diagnosis of thyroid cancer seemed to have no effect on the outcome of this disease.

DISORDERS OF THE PARATHYROID GLAND

Hyperparathyroidism

The incidence of hyperparathyroidism in females is three times that in males, and the peak incidence is in the fourth decade. Nevertheless, the disease is rarely encountered in pregnancy, even though gestation appears to stimulate gland activity, suggesting that many cases may go unrecognized. Since the initial report in 1938 of hyperparathyroidism in association with pregnancy (diagnosed in retrospect), only 42 cases have been reported.

The condition is characterized by excessive urinary loss of phosphorus, mobilization of calcium from the bone, hypercalcemia, calciuria, and a low serum phosphorus level. The serum alkaline phosphatase level is elevated because of the osteoclastic activity. Areas of decalcification and cyst formation are usually demonstrable in bone x-rays or biopsies. Gastrointestinal disorders, notably peptic ulcers, may have serious implications. Often, calciuria leads to renal changes,

particularly nephrolithiasis, and the outcome of pregnancy is influenced by the extent of functional impairment. In severe cases, hypertension, pyelonephritis, proteinuria, nitrogen retention, and markedly impaired renal function jeopardize the mother's life and account for most of the perinatal loss.

The disease develops as the result of adenoma or hyperplasia of one or more of the parathyroid glands. Regardless of pregnancy, the primary treatment is surgical exploration and, once the diagnosis is established, extirpation of the offending tissue. In the presence of hypercalcemic crisis, preoperative hydration is essential. Edathamil calcium disodium, a chelating agent that exchanges sodium for calcium, may be useful in preparing the patient for surgery. The increased fetal uptake of calcium (25–30 g) from the mother, which occurs largely in the last part of pregnancy, may be sufficiently protective to justify expectant management when the diagnosis is made late in the gestational period.

Hypercalcemia can be caused by many diseases and disorders. Excessive ingestion of milk and absorbable antacids can lead to the milk-alkali syndrome. Hypercalcemia also occurs in vitamin D intoxication, following thiazide therapy, and among immobilized patients. Certain endocrine disorders—hyperthyroidism, adrenal insufficiency—and malignant diseases may create the same type of calcium disorder. The presence of urolithiasis and radiographic demonstration of osteitis fibrosa support the diagnosis of primary hyperparathyroidism rather than malignant disease. In addition, the hypercalcemia of hyperparathyroidism is usually associated with hypophosphatemia, increased serum alkaline phosphatase, hyposthenuria, a decreased QoTc complex on electrocardiography, and band keratopathy.

The perinatal death rate in reported cases is 35%. Whether the deleterious effects on the fetus result from increased maternal serum calcium concentration or from parathyroid hormone remains controversial; experimental evidence suggests that both factors are operative. Some of the infants who survive gestation and the early neonatal period develop tetany when cow's milk (high phosphate content) is ingested. Rarely, infants who experience an abrupt fall in blood calcium develop tetany shortly after birth. Although the infant's parathyroid glands usually recover, permanent injury with chronic symptomatic hypoparathyroidism has been reported. Hartenstein and Gardner report that in at least eight families tetany of the newborn was associated with maternal parathyroid adenoma. Experience now shows that tetany in the newborn may be the only clue to the mother's disorder. All such cases, including those in which the mother develops a renal stone during pregnancy, should be investigated.

Patients with parathyroid adenomas seem to have an increased incidence of proliferative thyroid changes,

ranging from adenomas to carcinomas. Indeed, hyperparathyroidism is occasionally but one clinical feature of a general endocrine adenomatosis that may include functioning insulinoma, Cushing's syndrome, pheochromocytoma, or pituitary tumors of various types.

Hypoparathyroidism

Although hypoparathyroidism may be a complication of thyroidectomy, especially of radical extirpation for carcinoma, it may appear without discernible cause. Some degree of parathyroid insufficiency was reported in at least 24% of 46 patients who had been subjected to thyroidectomy on an average of 10 years prior to study.

Diarrhea in a hypocalcemic patient suggests a primary malabsorptive disorder rather than hypoparathyroidism, but it should be borne in mind that malabsorption occurs more frequently than is expected on the basis of chance in patients with proved idiopathic or pseudohypoparathyroidism. During pregnancy, the symptoms become exaggerated because of the vicissitudes of gut absorption and because the low level of ionizable calcium in the serum is further depleted by the demands of the fetus. If the patient is maintained in good calcium/phosphate balance during pregnancy, the fetus can be expected to be normal. Oral administration of supplemental calcium and dihydrotachysterol, which promotes phosphate excretion, is the current treatment of choice. The author knows of three pregnancies successfully managed in this manner. However, a case has been reported in which the infant of a hypoparathyroid primigravida was born with osteitis fibrosis cystica, lived 6.5 weeks, and was found at autopsy to have two parathyroid glands double the average adult size and striking hyperplasia of all parathyroid glands.

DISORDERS OF THE ADRENAL GLAND

Adrenal disorders complicating pregnancy have been rare in the past because untreated adrenocortical disease, either hyperfunction (Cushing's syndrome) or insufficiency (Addison's disease), are commonly associated with amenorrhea and its attendant suppression of ovulation. Diagnostic and therapeutic advances, as well as improvements in laboratory facilities and capability, have restored reproductive function to many patients who would have been deprived of motherhood heretofore.

Cushing's syndrome is discussed in Chapter 7, and congenital adrenal hyperplasia (adrenogenital syndrome) is discussed in Chapter 46. Since appropriate therapy effectively suppresses adrenocortical hyperfunction and restores normal pituitary–gonadal relations, successfully managed patients often establish ovulatory menses and regain reproductive capability. It seems probable that subclinical adrenal disorders likewise exist and that their identification and treatment should be a primary consideration in the preconception care of women who have experienced disproportionate perinatal loss. The fact that major clinical diseases, such as untreated Cushing's syndrome, are sometimes compatible with pregnancy supports this thesis.

Pheochromocytoma

For a pregnant woman who has an active pheochromocytoma, a rare but potentially fatal tumor of the adrenal medulla, the risk is 1:3 that she will die of the disease during the present pregnancy and 1:2 that she will die during subsequent pregnancies. Severe, pulsating headache, paroxysmal attacks of hypertension, profuse sweating, fever, precordial or abdominal pain and other unexpected neurologic or cardiovascular symptoms may suggest the lesion. When the clinical picture is fully developed, the patient experiences fulminating and prolonged paroxysms of hypertension and then suddenly collapses and dies with or without terminal hyperpyrexia and convulsions. Death usually occurs in the immediate puerperium. The clinician who has a high index of suspicion may promptly administer 5 mg phentolamine by infusion in an effort to lower the blood pressure sufficiently to permit surgical extirpation of the tumor. A chemical determination of the total pressor amines in the blood (epinephrine and norepinephrine), which are markedly elevated in the presence of tumor, should establish the diagnosis. These tumors are sometimes malignant; after initial resection is done, local recurrence, metastases, and death may ensue.

Adrenocortical Insufficiency

Addison's disease is characterized in its fully developed stage by asthenia, pigmentation of the skin and mucous membranes, anorexia, gastrointestinal disturbances, hypotension, and nervous symptoms. Before the introduction of adrenal replacement therapy, the maternal death rate was very high, as it is even today in the presence of unrecognized Addison's disease during pregnancy. Nevertheless, many patients with this disease actually show some clinical improvement during the second and third trimesters, presumably owing to an increase in adrenal activity as evidenced by a reduction in maintenance steroid requirement. The principal hazards arise during the first trimester in association with vomiting and during labor and the puerperium in association with stress. Adrenal crisis is particularly likely to occur immediately following delivery because of stress of labor, trauma of delivery, blood loss, infection, and electrolyte and water imbalance.

Vascular accidents of the adrenal glands in conjunction with parturition may be associated with collapse and death early in the puerperium. Although it is quite rare, venous infarction or massive hemorrhage into the adrenal gland should be considered when shock unassociated with hemorrhage occurs without warning shortly after delivery. Prompt adrenal cortical support or surgical intervention may be lifesaving, particularly when the adrenal lesion is unilateral.

Patients who have been treated with adrenal cortical hormones during the preconception period may come to labor and delivery with a relative insufficiency that requires supportive corticoid therapy. Those who have had operations for bilateral adrenal hyperplasia or who have required long-term maintenance therapy for a variety of conditions, such as adrenogenital syndrome, adrenal tuberculosis, cytotoxic atrophy, and amyloid disease, need additional steroid support at the onset of labor or before elective cesarean section. The average maintenance dose of 30 mg cortisone, or less, may need to be increased to 200 mg or more during labor. Following delivery, the daily dose of cortisone can be decreased over several days until the usual maintenance dose is reached. In the event of adrenal crisis, hydrocortisone administered by rapid infusion in a solution of 5% dextrose and saline is lifesaving. Concomitantly, cortisone should be given by mouth or by intramuscular injection during the first 24 hours or until the patient is well enough to require only her usual maintenance dose. With appropriate therapy, the patient with adrenocortical insufficiency should enjoy a reasonably good prospect of successful childbearing, but intensive medical care and close supervision are mandatory.

Potential Hazards of Adrenal Steroid Therapy

Adrenal steroids may induce serious complications or side-effects. Long-term administration in excess of optimal requirements may create iatrogenic Cushing's syndrome characterized by hypertension, diabetes, polycythemia, and easy bruising. Adrenal insufficiency, with the possibility of shock and death, attends the abrupt cessation of adrenal steroid therapy. In addition, corticosteroids affect the central nervous system, sometimes inducing euphoria. Adrenal steroids may interfere with normal collagenous tissue formation or even prevent wound healing when the dose is above the physiologic level. Thus, these potent medications are to be used only for legitimate indications and in accordance with a carefully supervised program of therapy. Although toxic doses of cortisone are capable of producing congenital defects in experimental animals, there is no clear evidence that the physiologic or pharmacologic doses of adrenal steroids employed in human beings predispose to the development of embryonal defects, even when administered in the first trimester at the time of fetal organogenesis.

DISORDERS OF THE PITUITARY GLAND

Alterations in Anterior Pituitary Function

The most common neoplasm that destroys pituitary function in adult women is the chromophobe adenoma. Since loss of menstrual function is ordinarily the first manifestation, the tumor is not often encountered in a pregnant patient. Rarely, pregnancy follows the resection of a small tumor or its shrinkage by roentgen radiation. Eosinophilic adenomas reduce gonadotropic activity by pressure of the space-occupying lesion, although in most cases acromegaloid changes appear first. Restoration of menses and the occurrence of pregnancy occasionally follow palliative x-ray or surgical treatment. An exacerbation of symptoms, including an aggravation of the acromegaloid changes, may attend gestation, presumably related to increased demands upon the pituitary by the growing fetus or to increased secretory activity of the tumor.

The most common cause of pituitary failure in women is the infarction that occurs at the time of traumatic delivery, usually in association with severe hemorrhage and shock (Sheehan's syndrome). Ovarian failure may be accompanied by hypothyroidism and adrenal failure. However, the volume of pituitary infarcted is frequently small, and these women may have sufficient functional integrity to permit reestablishment of ovulatory menses and reproductive potential. Sheehan's syndrome is discussed in Chapter 46.

Diabetes Insipidus

A rare disorder of the posterior lobe of the pituitary gland, diabetes insipidus has no predictable behavior in pregnancy, although available information suggests that the control of urine volume may be more difficult. Labor, delivery, and the puerperium are generally uncomplicated, and posterior pituitary extract can be administered throughout pregnancy without deleterious effects.

PORPHYRIA

Inherited as an autosomal dominant trait, porphyria is a rare disease characterized by an inborn error of pigment metabolism involving the porphyrins. Red porphyria pigments normally form the prosthetic group of respiratory enzymes, such as catalase, cytochrome, and peroxidase. In porphyria, there is a partial block of the biosynthesis of these enzymes. As a consequence, considerable amounts of porphyrin appear in the urine, giving it a burgundy red appearance. Of the different types of porphyria, the intermittent hereditary variety occurs predominantly in women—approximately two-thirds of the cases. The diagnosis is established when the urine contains porphobilinogen, the

colorless precursor of porphyrin. During an attack, considerable amounts of uro- and coproporphyrin color the urine red. The onset of the disease is usually between the ages of 20 and 30 years, and the prognosis is grave.

There is no specific treatment, although a variety of measures offer some symptomatic relief. The symptoms are mostly gastrointestinal, neurologic, or psychologic. Colicky or intermittent abdominal pains, vomiting, and obstipation are typical. In addition, there may be paresthesias or paralysis, including the respiratory center, labile psyche, or true psychoses. Barbiturates may initiate attacks. In some cases, hypertension and tachycardia are noted. Amenorrhea has been reported. During pregnancy, the disease has particular relevance because the abnormal amounts of porphyrin already appearing in the urine may be further increased, and exacerbations tend to occur. When the disease is suspected in a pregnant woman, appropriate tests should be performed and an attempt made to establish the type of porphyria. Hereditary features are a matter of concern. This, coupled with the unpredictable and often serious course of the disease during pregnancy, may justify abortion in early gestation; however, the beneficial effects are doubtful, and in any case abortion should not be performed during the acute stage of the disease. While some gravid women escape any real difficulties, Zilliacus and Kallio report that others develop obstetric complications such as severe preeclampsia in the late second or early third trimester.

OBESITY AND MALNUTRITION

Obesity imposes several significant handicaps on the pregnant woman: increased risk of an excessively large fetus, poor labor, and preeclampsia. The incidence of chronic hypertensive cardiovascular disease and metabolic disorders, particularly diabetes mellitus, is increased among obese women, and these conditions contribute substantially to the overall risks of pregnancy. Technical difficulties, anesthetic problems, and impaired wound healing may further complicate the course of gestation, especially should abdominal intervention be required.

The physician must be certain that excessive weight gain in pregnancy is not the result of extracellular water retention. Moreover, an endocrine basis for obesity should be suspected if the fat is unevenly deposited in a peculiar distribution. In addition to classic endocrine disorders, lesions of the hypothalamus may be responsible for both obesity and impaired ovarian function; however, these patients usually exhibit changes in personality, disturbed temperature regulation, and sometimes diabetes insipidus.

It should be borne in mind that women with nonendocrine obesity are malnourished, and often their daily intake of protein and essential vitamins is substandard. There is a positive correlation between the character of the mother's diet and the infant's length, weight, and general condition at birth. If the diet is very deficient, the incidence of preterm birth and fetal death *in utero* is increased, although probably other causative factors are likewise involved.

It has been found that superior mental development occurs in infants of above average birth weight and that development improves with maternal weight gain. Thus, monitoring of maternal weight gain is important. Eastman and Jackson, reporting on 25,154 pregnancies, noted that, except for weight loss or gain under 11 lb, a progressive increase in gain for the mother was paralleled by a rise in mean birth weight and a decrease in the incidence of low-weight infants. This was also true of a progressive increase in prepregnancy weight. These factors acted independently; small infants occurred when both were low, and average size infants when one was high and the other low. A prepregnancy weight below 120 lb with a gain of under 11 lb was associated with a high incidence of low-weight infants in white women and a very high incidence in nonwhite women. Neonatal mortality was 4.51% for low-weight white infants and 0.61% for all white infants; the respective figures for nonwhite infants were 3.65% and 0.71%. The general goal, according to these authors, should be to keep weight gain reasonably close to the average during pregnancy; women weighing under 120 lb should be permitted to eat as they wish up to the 20th week.

In the pregnant obese patient, correction of the nutritional deficiency is of prime importance and restriction of caloric intake a secondary consideration. Even though the nutritional stores may be adequate, it is unwise to prescribe a daily diet of less than 1800 calories. Moreover, the carbohydrate intake should not be curtailed below 150 g/day to spare protein and to prevent acidosis and ketosis. The obese patient will lose weight on this 1500-calorie diet (90 g protein, 150 g carbohydrate, 60 g fat), and at the same time her nutritional requirements will be met and the fetal status should be normal.

Attention has been directed to folic acid metabolism, since the formation and development of every human cell depends on an adequate supply of this nutritional factor. A deficiency is manifested by megaloblastic anemia. The importance of folic acid supplement in prophylaxis against megaloblastic anemia is definite.

DISORDERS OF THE BLOOD

SICKLE CELL DISEASE

The term *sickle cell disease*, which refers to a group of blood disorders limited to blacks, is derived from the characteristic sickle shape of the red blood cells in the

circulating blood of the affected person. Sickling can be readily demonstrated by microscopic examination of a drop of peripheral blood to which one drop of 2% sodium metabisulfite has been added. It is customary to classify sickle cell disease according to hemoglobin pattern, as determined by electrophoresis, because there are many variations of the hemoglobin molecule. The faulty mechanism in sickle cell disease lies in the single structural anomaly differentiating sickle cell hemoglobin (HbS) from normal adult hemoglobin (HbA). The abnormality has been identified in the β-chains; specifically, valine replaces glutamic acid in position 6 of the polypeptide chain. In the presence of decreased oxygenation, this abnormal molecule undergoes reversible aggregation with resultant erythrocyte distortion. The sickle-shaped cells obstruct flow within the microvasculature. Blood stasis, tissue acidosis, and aggravated oxygen deficit increase sickling and augment stasis. Sickled red cells are more susceptible to hemolysis and phagocytosis than are normal erythrocytes. The several processes occur as a vicious cycle and lead to hemolytic crisis and microinfarction within ischemic tissues.

Crisis may occur in two forms. The *hemolytic crisis* is characterized by profound, rapidly developing anemia accompanied by leukocytosis, deepening jaundice, and fever. The *painful crisis,* which results from capillary thrombosis and infarction in various organs due to sludging of the sickle cells, can be characterized by a variety of symptoms, most of them painful, including abdominal, chest, back, or long bone pain; hemoptysis; hematuria; melena; and, in some of the cases, central nervous system signs.

The normal person who inherits from each parent one normal HbA gene is characterized electrophoretically as type AA. If a person acquires an HbA gene from one parent and an HbS gene from the other, the resultant pattern is SA, the *sickle cell trait.* This hemoglobin pattern is observed in about 8% of blacks in the United States. These persons show no evidence of disease, since anemia does not develop; as a rule, there are no associated symptoms, except possibly those relating to urinary tract infections, which seem to occur in these patients with greater than usual frequency. Sickling can, however, occur at high altitudes. Also, since sickle cell trait may be associated with papillary necrosis and hematuria, these are complications that may also occur in pregnancy.

Sickle cell anemia is characterized by the homozygous genetic pattern SS. This disease, which is associated with a lifelong history of anemia, chronic illness, and recurrent abdominal and joint crises, is found in about 0.7% of American blacks. Pregnancy seems to aggravate the preexisting anemia, particularly as term approaches, and repeated transfusions are required. Transfusion reactions, infections precipitating crises, and the development of preeclampsia are bases for grave concern. The majority of the patients survive

pregnancy, but the perinatal death rate approaches 50%, since abortion, preterm birth, and fetal death *in utero* are common. Intrauterine growth retardation is a distinct feature.

Sickle cell–hemoglobin C (SC) is the most important heterozygous genetic pattern. Although it is observed in only about 0.15% of the black population, its consequences during gestation may be quite serious. The disease may be entirely quiescent in the nonpregnant state and then give rise, quite suddenly, to a variety of grave complications in pregnancy, notably hemolytic crises, particularly in the third trimester, marked bone pain in association with aggravation of erythroblastic hyperplasia, and sudden death from the embolization of minute spicules of bone with resultant pulmonary infarction. The gravity of this complication is illustrated by the report of 4 deaths among 16 pregnant women with HbSC disease.

Rarely, homozygous hemoglobin C disease (CC), sickle cell–hemoglobin F disease (SF), or sickle cell–thalassemia (STh) are encountered, but these conditions are usually mild and, in pregnancy, resemble sickle cell anemia.

Among pregnant women with sickle cell disease, anemia is a universal finding and almost invariably becomes more severe as pregnancy progresses. Acute crises occur commonly and may appear initially during the gravid state. About one-third of the patients develop preeclampsia. Susceptibility to infection is evidenced by the increased incidence of urinary tract infections, pneumonia, and puerperal endometritis in these patients. Congestive heart failure and pulmonary infarction are frequently seen. Affected patients usually appear undernourished and may have a short trunk, narrow hips, and long, spindly extremities. The skin may ulcerate around the ankles. The sclera may be icteric. There may be cardiomegaly and heart murmurs, but splenomegaly is not common in the adult. The seriousness of the disorder is emphasized by the maternal mortality rate of 25% in HbSS disease.

Management of sickle cell disease consists of close supervision, provision of adequate diet and folic acid supplement, prompt treatment of infection, and adequate blood replacement. Small daily transfusions of packed red cells are indicated during a hemolytic crisis, although it is not feasible to try to bring the hemoglobin level to normal values. Exchange transfusions have been used successfully. Adequate rest may minimize the risk of preterm birth. Hospitalization is needed promptly for complications of infection, preeclampsia, or crisis. Infusion of urea in invert sugar may be used to alleviate a crisis, provided dehydration is avoided. Oxygen administration during labor may be of some value to the fetus. Conduction anesthesia is preferred to minimize the risks of fetal hypoxia. Whenever possible, traumatic delivery should be avoided, since both mother and fetus withstand insults

poorly. Adequate blood should be held in readiness and administered at the time of delivery, as needed, to prevent shock in association with excessive blood loss. It should be remembered that shock may occur in these patients with minimal trauma and after only moderate blood loss. The administration of large quantities of blood in an effort to raise the blood pressure may provoke circulatory embarrassment and serious transfusion reactions. Hence, every effort should be exerted to make the delivery as nearly normal as possible, and the third stage of labor should be expertly managed. The selection of cesarean section for delivery should be based solely on compelling obstetric indications. Tubal ligation is justified in the seriously ill patient, particularly if she has the SC form of the disease, since pregnancy aggravates the course of the illness. This should be done at a later operation.

The grave hazards of pregnancy in patients with sickle cell disease call for effective genetic counseling. It appears that the incidence of HbSS disease in the pregnant population is the same as that found in the general population; hence, fertility rates among diseased women may not be substantially reduced, as was formerly believed. Accordingly, sterilization must be given serious consideration. Therapeutic abortion seems warranted for those already pregnant, when diagnosed early.

HEMOLYTIC ANEMIA

Anemia caused by excessive destruction of erythrocytes may be of extrinsic or intrinsic origin. Extrinsic factors are those chemicals, drugs, or toxins that cause hemolysis of normal red cells. Congenital hemolytic icterus is an intrinsic form of the disease and is characterized by erythrocytes that are unusually fragile because of their spheric shape. Acquired hemolytic anemia results from an acquired immunologic reaction that destroys the previously normal red cells. Patients who experience hemolytic crises require energetic treatment by blood transfusions. Splenectomy may be indicated, although many patients with acquired hemolytic anemia respond satisfactorily to cortisone therapy. There should be no hesitancy in employing these measures during pregnancy, since the risks of hemolytic crises, severe anemia, and repeated blood transfusions are far greater than those of surgical intervention or steroid administration.

Many drugs are capable of producing intense hemolysis when administered to patients whose red blood cells are deficient in glucose-6-phosphate dehydrogenase (G6PD). One of these, nitrofurantoin (Furadantin), a drug commonly used in treating urinary tract infections, has been reported to produce megaloblastic anemia in addition to severe hemolysis. The anemia is rapidly corrected when the nitrofurantoin therapy is stopped and folic acid is administered.

GLUCOSE-6-PHOSPHATE DEHYDROGENASE DEFICIENCY

A relatively common hereditary metabolic disorder, G6PD deficiency is found in about 10% of the black population in the United States. The condition is a red blood cell enzyme deficiency that is sex-linked and carried on the X chromosome. G6PD is important because it is the initial enzyme in the hexose monophosphate shunt. When enzyme-deficient cells are exposed to one of a host of oxidant drugs, intracellular hydrogen peroxide is formed, causing denaturation, precipitation, and splenic removal of affected cells from the circulation. G6PD-deficient red cells are unable to break down hydrogen peroxide. So-called Heinz bodies and erythrocyte basophilic stippling are seen in the peripheral blood during a hemolytic episode. The enzyme apparently has a variable biochemical activity among different populations, and the disease state is heterogenous. Persons of Mediterranean stock tend to suffer a severe form of the disorder—even more severe than that in American blacks.

Hemolysis accounts for much of the anemia encountered in these patients. Indeed, the presence of a fairly normal serum iron level during pregnancy, together with an anemic state, calls for a G6PD screening test. Anemia in these patients can be successfully treated with iron, folic acid, and adequate nutrition. Perhaps the greatest maternal risk lies in the high incidence of urinary tract infection. Perinatal risks include neonatal jaundice, fetal hydrops, and death *in utero*.

In reporting on obstetric outcome among 180 women with G6PD deficiency, Jaffe and coworkers call for wider screening, particularly among pregnant black women; repeated urine cultures, irrespective of symptoms of infection; and counseling to warn of the potential hazards of various drugs. Unfortunately, many of the drugs that can precipitate G6PD deficiency in susceptible patients are over-the-counter drugs that require no prescription: acetaminophen, phenacetin, salicylates, nitrofuran, to mention only a few. Some prescription drugs can also be a precipitating factor; for example, sulfonamides, chloramphenicol, Furadantin, nitrofurantoin macrocrystals (Macrodantin) sulfamethoxypyridazine (Kynex), salicylazosulfapyridine (Azulfidine), and dapsone. Accordingly, in these patients it may be difficult to find an appropriate agent to deal with some of the ordinary problems (*e.g.,* bacteriuria) that are encountered.

APLASTIC ANEMIA

Depression of the bone marrow with a reduction of erythrocytes, leukocytes, and platelets may result from a host of external agents such as x-ray, radioactive materials, benzene and related compounds, and many

commonly used therapeutic drugs. Aplastic anemia arises occasionally without a recognizable causative agent. The report of 9 deaths among 14 patients emphasizes the gravity of this disease when it complicates pregnancy. In depression of bone marrow associated with systemic diseases like sepsis, nephritis, and hypothyroidism, the prognosis depends upon the type and severity of the underlying illness.

MEDITERRANEAN (COOLEY'S) ANEMIA

Most patients with this disease are of Mediterranean heritage, although the admixture of races has extended the genetic base. The disease encountered during pregnancy is usually of the heterozygous type (thalassemia minor); the homozygous condition (thalassemia major) usually results in death before the reproductive years are reached. Many patients with the heterozygous form of the disease are asymptomatic until pregnancy provokes recurrent acute hemolytic crises and severe anemia. The anemia is microcytic and hypochromic in type; it is not uncommon for hemoglobin values to fall below 8 g. The diminished survival time of the erythrocytes contributes greatly to the severity of the anemia. There is a suppression of one or more of the polypeptide chains that compose the hemoglobin molecule, and the severity of each case is determined by the type and degree of this peptide chain suppression. HbF and HbA$_2$ are regularly increased, and the erythrocytes have a characteristic flattened appearance. Evidence of marked bone marrow activity is noted in the peripheral blood, and the thickened diploë of the skull, identifiable on x-ray examination, can be explained on the same basis. Multiple blood transfusions, which are required during hemolytic crises or as replacement for blood losses during delivery, should be used sparingly at other times to minimize the risk of hemochromatosis. The spleen is commonly enlarged, and it is occasionally desirable to perform splenectomy, even during pregnancy, if recurring acute hemolytic episodes impose a constant threat to mother and fetus. Increased folic acide intake is advised, but usually the anemia is unresponsive to all forms of medical therapy.

The incidence of maternal pyelonephritis, pneumonia, and pulmonary embolus seems to be increased, and the fetal mortality with β-thalassemia and α, β-thalassemia is reported to be slightly less than 15%. Patients with HbSTh disease have a much higher risk of maternal and fetal mortality.

LEUKEMIA

The classification of leukemia is based on the type of leukocyte predominantly affected. All types occur in acute, subacute, and chronic forms and may have leukemic (elevated white cell count) or aleukemic (normal or low white cell count) phases. The presence of immature cells in the bloodstream is of greater importance than an elevated leukocyte count. Acute leukemia is a fulminating, fatal disease, occurring most often in persons under 30 years of age. The onset often resembles an acute infection, but in addition, there is a marked tendency to hemorrhage. The spleen and liver may be moderately enlarged, and the cervical lymph nodes may enlarge rapidly. The characteristics of the chronic form of the disease vary somewhat with the primary offending cell type. In myelogenous leukemia, the onset is insidious, and the first symptoms are due to the greatly enlarged spleen or to anemia. Generally, there is no marked lymph node enlargement. In contrast, in the lymphatic form, a slow, painless enlargement of the cervical, axillary, and inguinal nodes is characteristic.

Treatment of the acute form of the disease may involve the use of adrenal steroids, folic acid antagonists, antimetabolites (6-mercaptopurine), or combinations of these. Blood transfusions may be given as necessary to combat anemia. In most instances, x-ray therapy is preferred in the chronic stage.

With respect to leukemias that complicate pregnancy, Stein and Dennis found only about 200 cases available for review in the literature. Analysis of these reports suggests that both acute and chronic leukemia may have adverse effects upon the outcome of pregnancy. As a general rule, however, gestation exerts no predictable effect upon the ultimate course of the disease, although exacerbation and progression have been observed. Antimetabolites administered after the first trimester have not proved harmful to the fetus, and reports of administrations even within the first 3 months of gestation have not been overly alarming. Radiation may also be employed in the chronic form of the disease without untoward effects if the fetus is shielded. The disease is not contracted by the infant, although the perinatal death rate is high, particularly when the mother's disease is acute, because of increased preterm birth rate. When the mother's disease is chronic, the fetal outlook is considerably better. Nothing is gained by interrupting pregnancy.

Rigid and close prenatal supervision is imperative. Particular attention should be paid to the correction of anemia and to the prevention of infection. Pregnancy should be allowed to continue to its natural termination; abdominal intervention should be done only for obstetric indications.

HODGKIN'S DISEASE

Slow, painless, progressive enlargement of lymph nodes and spleen; fever; cachexia; and anemia are characteristic of Hodgkin's disease. Pregnancy exerts no deleterious effect upon its course; in general, the

patient has a successful outcome, although the disease may be transmitted to the fetus. Palliative x-ray therapy can be employed during pregnancy, provided the uterine area is properly shielded. Blood transfusions are often required to combat anemia.

DISORDERS OF THE REPRODUCTIVE ORGANS

Retrodisplacement of the Uterus

Retroflexion or retroversion of the uterus is observed frequently during the early months of pregnancy, but the normal position is usually assumed by the 3rd month as the anterior wall undergoes hypertrophy and draws the organ up out of the pelvis (Fig. 27–3). Although retrodisplacement of the uterus has been implicated in spontaneous abortion, there is no clear evidence of a causal relationship.

Rarely, dense adhesions make spontaneous reduction impossible; in these circumstances, the gravid uterus increases in size until it completely fills the pelvis and becomes incarcerated beneath the promontory in the hollow of the sacrum. The cervix is drawn upward as the uterus enlarges and distorts the bladder and urethra. Rather characteristic symptoms usually make their appearance between the 13th and 17th weeks, notably lower abdominal pain, backache, urinary dribbling, cystitis, hematuria, and finally, complete urine retention. In long-neglected cases, necrosis of the bladder wall or even rupture with resultant peritonitis may develop.

Manual replacement of the retroflexed uterus with the patient in the knee–chest position should be attempted soon after the appearance of symptoms. Replacement may be facilitated by traction on the posterior lip of the cervix (Fig. 27–4). The normal position may be maintained by a pessary until there is no fear of a recurrence of the condition. If the uterus is incarcerated, the patient should be hospitalized immediately and urinary drainage established by inserting a flexible rubber catheter into the bladder. An attempt should then be made to reposition the uterus. If this effort fails, frequent knee–chest exercises and daily attempts at replacement, under anesthesia when necessary, almost always succeed in releasing the fundus. Abdominal intervention is rarely required, although after 3–4 days of unsuccessful conservative measures, laparotomy may be considered.

Occasionally, uterine prolapse may likewise lead to incarceration during the 3rd or 4th month of pregnancy if the organ is not repositioned and held in place by a pessary; spontaneous abortion is the inevitable result in neglected cases.

SACCULATION OF THE UTERUS

An extremely rare disorder of the uterus is the presence of a pouch or sac in the wall made up of very thin myometrium. A sacculation may occur at any point in the myometrium, and fetal parts can be readily palpated through it. In Danforth's case, the cranial sutures were readily palpable through the abdominal

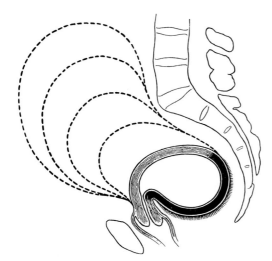

FIG. 27-3. Retrodisplacement of uterus. (Bumm E: Grundriss zum Studium der Geburtshilfe. Munich, Bergmann, 1922)

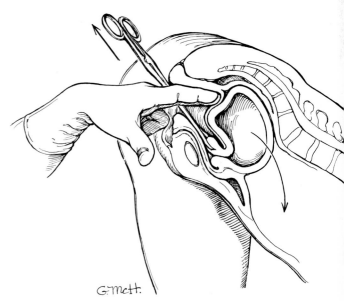

FIG. 27-4. Repositioning incarcerated retroverted uterus at 8-10 weeks' gestation. With patient in knee–chest position and tenaculum on posterior lip of cervix, pressure is exerted on posterior wall of corpus.

wall. Such sacculations are of unknown etiology and do not necessarily recur in a subsequent pregnancy. When the condition is diagnosed, it is prudent to deliver by cesarean section.

TORSION OF THE UTERUS

A relatively rare accident of pregnancy, torsion of the uterus has been reported only 108 times. A considerable literature has accumulated on this subject in veterinary obstetrics, because cornual torsion, especially in the cow, is a frequent cause of dystocia. In the human being, 80% of cases occur in association with uterine anomaly or pathologic conditions within the pelvis, notably uterus bicornis, myomas, ovarian cysts, adhesions, previous uterine suspension, or abnormalities of the spine and pelvis. The clinical picture may resemble abruptio placentae or some intraabdominal catastrophe, since the characteristic features are severe pain and shock. In early pregnancy, the treatment of symptomatic torsion of the gravid uterus is immediate laparotomy and detorsion, with adjunct surgery, if practicable, to eliminate the causative factor. When the accident occurs near term, cesarean section is the preferred treatment, especially if there is an advanced degree of torsion in association with profound symptoms. Hysterectomy should be performed when laparotomy has been long delayed, but in these cases maternal mortality is high in spite of surgery, chemotherapy, and blood administration. The outcome is influenced by the degree of torsion as well as by its duration. When it is greater than 180°, the maternal mortality rate is 50% and the perinatal loss 75%.

MYOMA UTERI

The exact incidence of myomas is impossible to determine, although they have been estimated to occur in 40% of all women at some time during their reproductive years. The great majority of these tumors are small and of little significance, and most patients' with myomas have a successful childbearing career. Nevertheless, some myomas may seriously complicate pregnancy, and gestation may cause rapid growth and degenerative changes in the tumors.

Myomas may cause sterility or diminish the chance of conception. Depending upon their number, size, and location, they may likewise increase the risk of abortion. There is little doubt that the submucous variety offers a poor endometrial environment for implantation of the fertilized ovum. These tumors may undergo necrosis and inflammatory reactions due to poor circulatory and nutritional conditions. During pregnancy, the cells of the myomas hypertrophy, and the muscle bundles may be widely separated by edema. Large tumors may undergo certain secondary changes, notably carneous, hyaline, fatty, cystic, or calcific degeneration; infection and suppuration; and, very rarely, sarcomatous transformation. These changes increase the probability of late abortion, preterm birth, and fetal death *in utero*. When extensive necrosis of the carneous type (red degeneration) occurs during pregnancy, the patient may complain of severe pain and marked tenderness over the uterus. This complication of myomas is characteristically associated with the gravid state, but it is observed occasionally in the nonpregnant uterus. Degeneration of blood vessels, local hemolysis, and resultant thrombotic processes account for the low-grade fever, peritoneal irritation, and leukocytosis. The same features may be caused by torsion of a subserous myoma that has resulted in gangrene and peritonitis.

Degenerative changes ordinarily subside after the patient has rested in bed for several days, although when the tumor is impacted in the pelvis or the mass is twisted on its pedicle, early operative intervention is imperative. Occasionally, a large uterine tumor may undergo extensive necrosis and give rise to persistent symptoms in spite of bedrest, sedation, and other control measures. If the mass is pedunculated, myomectomy can usually be performed safely without interrupting the pregnancy. In the great majority of cases, however, conservative measures are effective and surgery unnecessary.

It should be emphasized that diagnosis of the association of pregnancy and myoma is often difficult, sometimes even when the abdomen is open and the uterus is under direct vision. The presence of a myomatous uterus in conjunction with disturbances of menses may be mistaken for threatened abortion; in a patient known to have a uterine tumor, abnormal bleeding may not arouse suspicion of pregnancy until the products of conception are passed. An aborting submucous tumor gives rise to crampy pain, vaginal bleeding, and protrusion of tissue through a partially dilated cervix just as spontaneous abortion of a conceptus does. Pelvic conditions sometimes mistaken for a myomatous gravid uterus are pregnancy in one horn of a bicornuate uterus; torsion of an ovarian cyst; or the presence of a solid ovarian tumor, tuboovarian inflammatory cysts with disturbed menstrual flow, hydatidiform mole in association with theca lutein cysts, pelvic ectopic kidney, interstitial tubal or rudimentary horn pregnancy, parovarian cyst, large bladder calculi, and appendiceal abscess. The presence of a known uterine tumor is no reason to ignore the possibility of other pelvic conditions that complicate pregnancy, since many of the latter become grave problems if appropriate therapy is too long delayed.

Many patients with myomas that complicate pregnancy experience few problems until the onset of labor, although the rapid increase in size of the tumor may give rise to recurring episodes of aching pain, vague abdominal tenderness, and pressure symptoms

during the third trimester. At the onset of labor, it may be apparent that the myoma displaces the presenting fetal part or obstructs the birth canal. Moreover, the tumor may so interfere with the character and effectiveness of the uterine contraction pattern that labor is inert, dyskinetic, and prolonged. Any patient known to have a uterine myoma should have a sterile vaginal examination during the early part of the first stage of labor to determine fetal presentation and station and to rule out pelvic obstruction. Any patient who exhibits dystocia from an unknown cause should be examined carefully for the presence of a uterine tumor. If the myoma remains impacted in the pelvis and prevents descent of the presenting part, cesarean section is the preferred method of delivery. Multiple myomectomy is usually ill advised at this time, although large tumors that are likely to undergo marked degeneration and sepsis during the puerperium may necessitate hysterectomy. It is important to reserve judgment concerning the method of delivery until the onset of labor because myomas often rise out of the pelvis at term or in early parturition, especially when they arise from the anterior uterine wall.

If the birth canal is unobstructed, even though there are large tumors throughout the upper fundus, and fetal presentation is normal, vaginal delivery is usually possible. The principal hazard in delivery by this route is uterine bleeding due to a faulty third-stage mechanism and retention of part of the placenta. Inexpert attempts to remove the placenta manually may disrupt the tumor or even sever its uterine attachments. These accidents are attended by profuse hemorrhage and shock that requires repeated transfusions to maintain blood volume and prompt hysterectomy to control heavy bleeding.

Even if serious problems do not supervene during labor and delivery, all danger has not passed, since uterine tumors may undergo extensive necrosis, infection, and suppurative degeneration during the puerperium. Moreover, vigorous manipulation of the uterus, as in manual removal of the placenta or in compression and massage to maintain muscle tone and minimize blood loss, may disrupt omental or peritoneal adhesions in the region of the tumor, giving rise to subsequent intraabdominal hemorrhage. Thus, intensive supervision and care during this critical period should be routine for all patients.

OVARIAN TUMORS

Although any type of ovarian tumor may complicate pregnancy, the most common are the benign cysts, notably dermoids and serous or pseudomucinous cystadenomas. The corpus luteum of pregnancy may reach a diameter of 5–6 cm during the first trimester, but after that it gradually regresses in size. The possibility of its being confused with a true ovarian neoplasm is greatest when the structure is of maximum size, although repeated examinations usually disclose reduction of its dimensions as gestation advances. During early pregnancy, the changes in size and consistency of ovarian cysts are easily discernible, since both the tumor and the uterus can be outlined as separate masses even though their relations may be quite variable. Later, the ovarian mass may come to lie in the abdomen or in a lateral gutter of the flank and may be exceedingly difficult to locate, even when it is large.

A true ovarian neoplasm discovered during early pregnancy is best removed at about the 18th gestational week, provided the operation can be postponed until then. Oophorocystectomy performed earlier increases the chance of abortion, and removal of the cyst after the 18th week is likely to result in preterm labor. Immediate operation is required, regardless of the duration of pregnancy, when acute symptoms develop.

The decision to remove an asymptomatic ovarian tumor is based upon the seriousness of potential complications, *e.g.,* the increased probability of abortion and the likelihood of torsion, necrosis, septic degeneration, hemorrhage into the capsule, rupture followed by peritonitis, preterm birth and neonatal death, and obstruction of the birth canal that prevents normal delivery. Also, hormone-producing tumors may affect the fetus. Even after normal delivery, torsion, necrosis, and eventual sepsis of an ovarian tumor constitute serious risks in the puerperium. Thus, an ovarian cyst diagnosed late in pregnancy or after delivery is best removed in the immediate postpartum period, if the patient's general condition is satisfactory. An additional reason for removing an ovarian tumor is that its benign or malignant nature cannot be determined by pelvic examination alone.

An ovarian mass wedged below the promontory rarely rises out of the pelvis spontaneously at term or in early labor, although tumors in other pelvic or abdominal locations usually do not interfere with the descent of the presenting part. In obstructed labor, the cesarean section is the preferred method of delivery; otherwise, vaginal delivery should be accomplished and the tumor removed shortly thereafter. If the mass is found to be a dermoid cyst, the tumor can often be resected with preservation of normal ovarian tissue. The contralateral ovary should be bisected and inspected for the presence of an early tumor. If the mass is found to be a cystoma, the entire ovary should be sacrificed and the opposite ovary thoroughly examined. If the cyst is multiloculated or papillary, or if it contains areas of induration, a frozen section of suspicious tissues should be studied.

Malignant tumors of the ovary are exceedingly rare complications of pregnancy. Experience suggests that the natural course of the disease is not influenced by gestation, despite elevated steroid levels. Primary treatment should be directed toward the tumor without regard for the pregnancy, although if the lesion is

discovered late, it may be permissible to defer definitive therapy for a short time until the fetus has a reasonable chance of extrauterine survival. Delivery is best accomplished by cesarean section. The tumor-containing ovary should be extirpated, and surgery should be followed by irradiation or chemotherapy, depending upon the findings at the time of laparotomy.

CARCINOMA OF THE CERVIX

Invasive cancer of the cervix as a complication of pregnancy is uncommon but not rare; *in situ* lesions are encountered more frequently, depending upon the cancer consciousness of the physician and the extent to which cytologic screening of pregnant women is employed. Recent reports indicate that invasive cancer occurs in about 1 of 2000 obstetric patients. When searched for routinely, carcinoma in situ is discovered in 5–10 of 1000 patients. The peak incidence seems to occur at age 35. For the most part, these lesions complicate pregnancy in multigravidas, particularly those who have not had the benefit of adequate cervical care.

As a screening measure, the vaginal smear technique of Papanicolaou is about 90% reliable, and the test should be part of the first examination of every pregnant patient.

The physiologic version of the cervix during pregnancy usually makes the distal canal and squamocolumnar junction readily accessible for study. Circumferential and radial step biopsies can be taken, and representative tissues from sites where maximal cellular unrest usually occurs are easily obtainable. However, the bleeding from punch biopsy in pregnancy can be very profuse. Target lesions can be searched for with the aid of the colposcope; with this method, it is reasonable to expect not only the ectocervix but also the lower canal region to be visualized. Worrisome lesions can be biopsied or followed with increased confidence by means of this technique. When the smears suggest a lesion more serious than that demonstrated by biopsy, or when limits of a diffuse lesion extend into the canal, where inspection is not possible, conization is required. This can be accomplished without compromising the upper canal and usually without morbidity. However, the potential risks of hemorrhage, both immediate and delayed, and of infection and other complications demand strict and rational indications for this procedure. It is essential to establish not only the presence of carcinoma in situ but also the absence of invasive cancer. The histologic criteria are the same as those used in establishing the diagnosis of cervical cancer in nongravid women (see Chapter 54).

Lesions of the cervix produce the same symptoms, signs, and gross features in pregnant as in nonpregnant patients. Contact bleeding, persistent vaginal discharge, usually blood-tinged, and an ulcerative lesion on the cervix are the most notable features. In the early stages of invasion, the cancer may differ in no way from papillary erosions noted on the cervix. Visualization of the cervix is imperative whenever bleeding occurs during gestation, and biopsies may be taken from suspicious sites without fear of provoking uncontrollable bleeding or jeopardizing the pregnancy.

When there are no symptoms, routine inspection of the cervix at least twice during pregnancy and again several weeks postpartum may avert delay in recognizing carcinoma. Vaginal and cervical smears should be procured routinely during gestation and at the time of the follow-up examination after delivery. Obstetric care should not be terminated until the cervix is free of erosion, eversion, and chronic infection. Electrocauterization, antibacterial creams, and douches may be employed to advantage, provided malignancy has first been ruled out.

Carcinoma in situ may be confined to the epithelial layer of the cervix for years before it invades the underlying stroma; hence, it is safe to allow pregnancy to continue to term, provided periodic follow-up smears or biopsies are taken and the cervix is carefully inspected on each prenatal visit for the appearance of target lesions. Vaginal delivery is permitted unless there are obstetric indications for abdominal intervention; the previously coned cervix usually behaves normally in labor. After the 6th week postpartum, it is advisable to conduct a more complete histologic study of the cervix to exclude microscopic invasion. A wide, deep conization of the cervix should be performed and the remaining canal as well as the uterine cavity curetted thoroughly. If the stromal tissue has been invaded at any point, the treatment should be the same as treatment for more advanced lesions that have caused gross changes in the cervix. Noninvasive lesions should be treated by total hysterectomy and resection of a cuff of upper vagina. The remaining vagina should give a positive reaction to the Schiller stain. Occasionally, definitive treatment may be postponed because of the patient's desire for more children, but her cooperation in seeking periodic follow-up care must be assured. Expectant management is contingent upon unequivocal demonstration of continued stability of the cervical lesion.

Treatment of invasive cancer of the cervix must be decided upon according to individual circumstances, notably the duration of the pregnancy and the clinical stage of the disease. Unless the pregnancy is near term, treatment should always be directed toward the lesion without regard for fetal welfare. If the fetus is mature enough to survive in an extrauterine environment, cesarean section should be performed before radiation therapy is begun, because vaginal delivery may be attended by cervical lacerations, hemorrhage, sepsis, and spread of the disease. Deep x-ray therapy

should be started within about 10–14 days of hysterotomy and radium applied at its completion. When the diagnosis is made during the first trimester of pregnancy, or possibly as late as the early months of the second trimester, a course of deep pelvic radiation is initial therapy. Ordinarily, the fetal tissues are destroyed after a tumor dose of 2000R in 21 days has been administered, and abortion occurs during the 3rd–4th week of therapy. As soon as the uterus involutes, radium therapy is instituted. In the unusual event that abortion does not ensue during the course of pelvic irradiation, abdominal hysterotomy should be performed to avoid delay in treatment and to prevent the birth of a microcephalic infant. Radical surgery as initial therapy should be reserved for selected early cases of invasive cancer in which adequate irradiation of the tumor cannot be achieved because of technical problems or other circumstances.

The likelihood of cure is contingent upon the stage of the disease when first treated, the ability to deliver cancericidal radiation (which implies not only adequate dosage but also patient responsiveness), and, to some extent, the duration of pregnancy at the time of treatment. It is generally agreed that 5-year survival rates of patients treated during pregnancy do not differ appreciably from those of nongravidas when the clinical results are compared stage for stage. However, according to one report, the cure rates for patients treated in the last half of the third trimester and during the postpartum period were 25% for those with Stage I disease and 21% for those with Stage II disease, compared with 92% and 54%, respectively, for patients treated in the first 6 months of pregnancy. The principles of the surgical and radiation treatment of invasive cancer of the cervix are considered in Chapters 54 and 60.

CARCINOMA OF THE BREAST

Although carcinoma of the breast is reported to occur in 1 of 3500 pregnancies, this figure is probably low, since the disease often goes unrecognized until some months after delivery. The hypertrophic changes during gestation and the engorgement of the breasts during lactation make it difficult to detect small masses. Rapidly growing inflammatory cancer is often mistaken for acute mastitis, since this infection is not uncommon, especially during the puerperium. Regular examinations of the breasts are mandatory during pregnancy, and all suspicious lesions should be investigated as conscientiously as at any other time (see Chapter 59).

Pregnancy appears to increase the likelihood of rapid spread of mammary cancer, presumably because of the increased vascularity of the breasts. The lymph nodes are frequently involved early in the course of the disease. Nevertheless, stage for stage, the prognosis at the time the diagnosis is made is the same in pregnant as in nonpregnant patients and the principles of therapy are the same. Termination of pregnancy before fetal maturity does not influence the rate of growth of breast cancer. Radical surgery can be performed satisfactorily in the gravid woman, and the course of gestation is ordinarily not influenced. Postoperative radiation can be safely employed if the pelvis is adequately shielded. Moreover, x-ray therapy can be administered during pregnancy to local recurrences or to metastatic lesions in the axillae. Chemotherapy must be delayed until after delivery. Labor and delivery are conducted as in the normal patient.

Although the matter is controversial, Treves and Holleb believe that, in patients with disseminated disease, abortion, when combined with other endocrine ablation procedures, may be of some benefit. The rationale follows the general consensus that changing the hormonal environment by endocrine ablation is the most important factor in the treatment of disseminated breast cancer and that this concept holds true for the pregnant as well as the nonpregnant patient. With respect to later pregnancies following breast carcinoma, contraception is advised for 2 years because of the generally poor prognosis and intensive supervision required for all such patients. Nevertheless, the 5-year survival is unaffected by subsequent pregnancies.

MISCELLANEOUS DISORDERS

DISEASES OF THE SKIN

Pregnancy produces many changes in the skin, and some are profound although medically innocuous. Many are hormonally related, some are of vascular or pigmentary origin, and others are of unknown cause or represent a change in a preexisting condition. The disorders due to pregnancy, which are discussed in Chapter 26, include generalized pruritis; cutaneous tags; prurigo gestationis; papillary dermatitis of pregnancy; autoimmune progesterone dermatitis of pregnancy; and herpes gestationis. In addition to these distinctly pregnancy-related disorders, a host of other dermatologic problems may affect the pregnant woman.

Herpesvirus Infection

Herpesvirus hominis type II infections involving the genitalia do not seem to be influenced by pregancy in any predictable way. The greater threat is to the vulnerable fetus in its passage through the birth canal at delivery. A fatal form of neonatal infection results in hepatoadrenal necrosis and degenerative changes in many other organs. Less commonly, the infant survives only to suffer from microcephaly and microph-

TABLE 27-7. RECOMMENDATIONS FOR CESAREAN SECTION AT TERM IN WOMEN WITH PRIOR OR CONCURRENT HERPES

Genital Herpetic Lesions Present at Term	Group	Primary Genital Lesions	Recurrent Genital Lesions (or Genital Reinfection)	Status of Membranes*	Recommended Route of Delivery†	Isolation of Mother	Isolation of Newborn
YES	1	+		Intact or ruptured <4-6 hr	Cesarean section	Yes	Yes
	2	+		Ruptured >4-6 hr	Per vaginam	Yes	Yes
	3	+	or +	Baby has been delivered per vaginam		Yes	Yes
	4		+	Intact or ruptured <4-6 hr	Cesarean section	Yes	Yes
	5		+	Ruptured >4-6 hr	Per vaginam	Yes	Yes
NO, BUT CERVICOVAGINAL CULTURE OR CYTOLOGY IS POSITIVE FOR HERPES	6			Intact or ruptured <4-6 hr	Cesarean section	Yes	Yes
	7			Ruptured >4-6 hr	Per vaginam	Yes	Yes
NO, BUT THERE IS PAST HISTORY OF GENITAL HERPES, PRESENTLY INACTIVE OR STATUS UNKNOWN	8			Intact or ruptured	Per vaginam	No	No
NO, BUT NONGENITAL HERPES IS PRESENT AT TERM	9			Intact or ruptured	Per vaginam	Yes	No at birth (yes, after newborn goes out to mother)
NO, BUT THERE IS PAST HISTORY OF NONGENITAL HERPES	10			Intact or ruptured	Per vaginam	No	No

* The shorter the interval between rupture of the membranes and cesarean section, the less the risk of fetal infection. The critical period appears to be 4-6 hours.

† Dependent on evaluation of individual risks and benefits. (Kibrick S: JAMA 243:157, 1980)

thalmus. Delivery by elective cesarean section before rupture of fetal membranes and prior to the onset of labor is the preferred method (Table 27-7).

The infection is transmitted as a venereal disease and, in the female, appears as vesicles that rupture to form shallow ulcers. Smears from the lesions show rather typical eosinophilic intranuclear inclusion bodies in addition to multinucleated giant cells and dysplastic squamous cells. The organism can also be cultured from vaginal or cervical material. When the fetus is infected, these changes may be seen in desquamated cells found in the amniotic fluid. It is our policy to perform amniocentesis to obtain fluid both for culture and for cell study when the lower genital tract of the mother is infected with the herpesvirus. Rarely,

the fetus is infected by the transplacental route, despite intact membranes. It is important to distinguish between type I and type II herpesvirus serologically, because the former is not associated with genital lesions and fetal risk is thought to be minimal.

Condyloma Acuminatum

Pregnant women frequently have condylomata acuminata involving the vaginal, perineal, or perianal area. Preexisting lesions may extend and be aggravated during pregnancy as vaginal discharges increase. Local chemotherapy and meticulous hygiene constitute proper control measures. The use of podophyllin entails the risk of hypocalcemia and possible peripheral

neuropathy in the mother, as well as potential hazards to the fetus. Electrodesiccation of polypoid lesions is rarely necessary or desirable in the antepartum period.

Melanoma

During pregnancy, benign nevi may undergo malignant degeneration; yet most of the large series reported fail to suggest that pregnancy *per se* necessarily provides a stimulus for such changes. The prognosis is poor, as it is in the nonpregnant patient. Search for pigmented moles should be an integral part of prenatal care, and prophylactic excision is indicated when they appear on the genitals or feet or on the areas of the body where irritation is chronic. When the nevi increase rapidly in size, exhibit increased pigmentation, ulcerate, bleed, or become painful, their removal is imperative.

COLLAGEN DISEASES

Rheumatoid Arthritis

Common in young adults, rheumatoid arthritis occurs twice as often in females as in males. Periarthritis is the primary change; arthritis is secondary. The temperature is seldom very high, and the pain is moderate in proportion to the swelling. Striking remissions have been observed in the symptoms of rheumatoid arthritis during pregnancy, but this improvement is not a constant clinical feature. Patients being treated with cortisone prior to gestation may require smaller amounts during pregnancy; additional support is usually necessary during the puerperium when adrenal cortical activity diminishes. The reason for these differences is unclear, since transcortin binds most adrenal steroids in the plasma and the augmented blood corticoids are biologically inert. Moreover, the plasma clearance is retarded, and this factor rather than increased production may account for the elevated levels observed during pregnancy. Treatment should include careful hygiene, wholesome diet, adequate vitamins, and physiotherapy as needed.

Periarteritis Nodosa

Characterized by granulomatous nodules in the walls of small arteries that may result in aneurysm or thrombosis, periarteritis nodosa may involve almost any artery of the body. Those of the kidney, heart, and gastrointestinal system are of particular significance. The appearance of symptoms may follow sulfonamide therapy. A combination of asthma, peripheral neuritis, eosinophilia, and rising blood pressure should suggest this disorder, and the diagnosis can be confirmed by biopsy of accessible blood vessels. Improvement should not be expected during pregnancy. In the presence of renal involvement and hypertension, the outlook for both mother and fetus may be seriously compromised.

Scleroderma

This rare collagen disorder is characterized by swelling, proliferation, and fusion of the collagen fibrils of the corium. The muscles and fascia may also reveal collagen changes; occasionally, the internal organs are likewise involved. Slowly and progressively, the skin becomes dense and inflexible; the face becomes mask-like and the fingers waxy, smooth, and almost immovable. The inelasticity of the abdominal wall may restrict the enlarging uterus or interfere with the bearing-down efforts needed in the second stage of labor. Cortisone is the preferred treatment, although the clinical results are often unsatisfactory.

SARCOIDOSIS

Boeck's sarcoid is a systemic disease with granulomatous manifestations in the skin, lymph nodes, lungs, bone marrow of phalanges, liver, spleen, parotid, eyes, and other sites. It can be differentiated from tuberculosis by the lack of necrosis in the granulomatous nodules, the smaller size of multinucleated giant cells, and the grouping of the nuclei toward the center. Granulomatous lesions similar to those of Boeck's sarcoid are produced by magnesium silicate (present in talcum powder) and by beryllium (present in fluorescent bulbs) if they enter a wound. Pregnancy has been demonstrated to have a beneficial effect upon the symptoms and characteristic physical findings associated with sarcoidosis, but this advantage is lost during the puerperium when serious exacerbations may occur. The administration of cortisone in the postpartum period has been suggested as a means of avoiding this deterioration. Pregnancy is contraindicated only when marked alveolar capillary involvement results in extreme respiratory insufficiency.

LISTERIOSIS

The clinical picture of listeriosis, which is a poorly understood infection, varies from a mild, viral syndrome to severe septicemia or meningitis with high fever, leukocytosis, convulsions, and coma. The death rate may be high, particularly among infants and aged persons. The diagnosis is made by the isolation of *Listeria monocytogenes* in secretions and infected tissues or of specific antibodies in the serum. When therapy is started early, the infection can be controlled with sulfonamides, tetracycline, or penicillin.

This infection has special significance in obstetrics, because it is known to cause abortion in sheep, cattle, and rabbits. The incidence of *Listeria* in the vaginal

flora of pregnant women and the role of these organisms in the interruption of human pregnancy are yet to be determined. *Listeria* has been isolated from the genital tract, as well as from the fetus and placentas of women who have aborted. When laboratory facilities are available for isolating these organisms, it would seem advisable to screen habitual aborters for the presence of *Listeria* and to institute appropriate therapy as necessary.

HERNIA

Although intraabdominal pressure is increased during pregnancy and there is a tendency for established defects within the abdominal wall to become relaxed, the development of serious hernia is relatively uncommon. The risk of herniation is minimized by the enlarging uterus, which ordinarily displaces the intestines upward and laterally. Hernialike defects often develop at the umbilicus or at the site of a previous incision, but they rarely produce symptoms. Occasionally, when bowel or omentum is already adherent in a hernial sac, the growing fundus may produce pain or even strangulation of bowel as pregnancy advances. In exceptional circumstances, the hernia opening is large and the growing uterus may come to lie within the sac.

Although the great majority of hernias are satisfactorily managed during pregnancy by conservative measures, it is important to note any defects in the inguinal, femoral, or umbilical regions or in the underlying fascia of a previous abdominal incision, and to watch the patient closely for evidence of bowel incarceration or strangulation. An incarcerated hernia presents the symptoms of acute intestinal obstruction; a strangulated hernia, which implies interference with the blood supply of the contents of the sac, is characterized, in addition, by constant severe pain, tachycardia, and evidence of intoxication. It is imperative that the hernia be reduced immediately either by taxis or by surgery.

Hiatus hernias are far more common than previously suspected, especially among multiparous women. These defects are presumably due to a prolonged increase in intraabdominal pressure, since the majority are not demonstrable after delivery. It has been reported that, in the last trimester of pregnancy, 18.1% of multiparas and 5.1% of primigravidas have hiatus hernias. Among ten such women who were reexamined 1–18 months postpartum, hernias were observed in only three. Most patients remain asymptomatic despite these defects; occasionally, however, epigastric pain, persistent nausea and vomiting, or heartburn that is increased when the patient is lying down, presents a significant clinical problem. The hernia permits regurgitation of gastric contents into the esophagus. Symptoms may be relieved by propping up the head and shoulders at night, by eating multiple small meals, and by the use of antacid medication. Surgical correction is indicated only in the rare circumstance of bowel obstruction or strangulation.

RUPTURE OF THE SPLEEN

Traumatic rupture of the spleen results either from a fall from a height, usually with the patient landing on her feet or buttocks, or from direct injury to the region, as in an automobile accident. Spontaneous rupture is usually attributable to preexisting splenic disease, notably malaria, Banti's disease, and leukemia, although this rare complication may arise without identifiable cause. The symptoms are those of acute intraabdominal hemorrhage and shock. Prompt surgical intervention and adequate blood replacement are mandatory. The spleen should always be inspected when no other cause of intraabdominal bleeding can be found. Rarely, rupture of an aneurysm involving the splenic artery occurs during pregnancy, with catastrophic results for the mother and fetal death *in utero* secondary to severe hypoxia. Early diagnosis followed by prompt splenectomy offers the only hope of survival.

HEMATOMA OF THE ABDOMINAL WALL

Rarely, in advanced pregnancy, rupture of the main inferior epigastric artery or one of its branches gives rise to a massive hematoma within the abdominal wall. For the most part, such an accident occurs in a multipara, usually of advanced age, who has encountered some sudden abdominal muscle stress, such as a violent paroxysm of coughing or direct trauma to the area. The maternal and fetal mortality rates are high unless the condition is recognized and prompt surgical hemostasis effected. The neglected patient may develop profound shock in association with loss of large quantities of blood into the fascial planes of the abdominal wall. A small hematoma may be treated conservatively, provided the patient has stable vital signs at normal levels and is closely observed for any evidence of renewed bleeding.

RETINITIS GESTATIONIS

Retinitis gestationis is a rare, inflammatory retinitis that rarely complicates pregnancy, disappears between gestations, and is reported to recur in subsequent pregnancies. The clinical features of blurred vision, lacrimation, and increasing blindness may progress rapidly as a pregnancy advances. Reversal of the process is imperative, since the end result is scarring of the retina. The retinitis is terminated promptly by

therapeutic abortion or, in some instances, by cortisone therapy.

OTOSCLEROSIS

A defect of conduction, otosclerosis is characterized by calcific deposits in the middle ear that interfere with movement of the ossicles; it leads to progressive loss of hearing. The onset of this condition frequently occurs during the childbearing period, and there is general agreement that the process is often accelerated by pregnancy. Occasionally, the rapid development of deafness may justify interruption of pregnancy; generally, the hearing loss occurs very gradually and termination of pregnancy is unnecessary. A multiparous woman who has experienced several periods of accelerated hearing loss during her previous pregnancies may be a suitable candidate for sterilization; however, the success of the fenestration operation, which reestablishes satisfactory unaided hearing, has virtually eliminated this concern.

SCHISTOSOMAL CARCINOMA OF THE BLADDER

Primary carcinoma of the bladder in relatively young women as a result of recurrent schistosomiasis bilharzial infections of the urinary tract since childhood is sometimes encountered in pregnancy in Southeast Asia, South and Central America, and other regions, but not in the United States. Infected women excrete ova of *Schistosoma* in the urine, and apparently the long-standing local chronic bladder irritation (resulting in mucosal hyperplasia and dysplasia in response to infesting worms and ova) has a carcinogenic effect. The histologic lesion is one of squamous cell carcinoma. Apparently, pregnancy accelerates tumor growth and causes an aggravation of hematuria and pain. The cancerous bladder may obstruct labor in undiagnosed cases. If the fetus is viable at the time of diagnosis, abdominal delivery is indicated. Exenterative surgery, together with urinary diversion, provides a good chance of cure if the lesion is resectable.

RUPTURE OF THE SYMPHYSIS PUBIS

Traumatic separation or rupture of the symphysis pubis is rarely encountered today; such disruption was, in the past, associated with difficult forceps operations. The condition is characterized by symphyseal or sacroiliac pain, especially while walking or turning over in bed; occasionally, the patient is greatly incapacitated. Most patients are relieved by simple strapping and by restriction of vigorous physical activity. Usually, the symptoms subside in the postpartum period, and there is no great likelihood of recurrence in subsequent pregnancies. According to available reports, patients who have been subjected to symphysiotomy at the time of delivery enjoy a relatively comfortable postpartum course, and disorders of the symphysis are rarely encountered in subsequent pregnancies. As a matter of practical importance, it should be recognized that traumatic manipulations of the anesthetized patient, such as positioning her for delivery or moving her from the table onto a stretcher, may be the cause of serious hip and pelvic injuries.

DISORDERS OF THE SKELETON

Osteomalacia

The dietary lack of calcium and vitamin D accounts for the severe form of osteomalacia seen in some parts of the world, notably in China and Africa. The disease may also be produced by excessive urinary calcium loss, as in renal acidosis. Failure of calcium absorption from the intestinal tract and loss of vitamin D in the feces are encountered in nontropical sprue, chronic pancreatitis, extensive bowel resection, and regional ileitis.

Osteomalacia is characterized by defective calcification of newly formed bone matrix. There is general bone softening, but the most obvious defect is the marked pelvic deformity created by the upright position and weight bearing. In the extreme case, there is little space between the symphysis and the xiphoid process. The upper sacrum is displaced forward, and the sidewalls of the forepelvis are convergent, imparting a funnel shape to the pelvis.

Osteomalacia is often aggravated by pregnancy, and there may be further distortion of the skeleton due to the effect of increased body weight as well as of further depletion of calcium stores associated with fetal demands.

A balanced diet plus supplementary calcium and vitamin D are mandatory. Therapy is also directed toward the underlying cause. When an intestinal disorder is present, other deficiences, such as in vitamin K and folic acid, must be corrected. A satisfactory response to therapy can be demonstrated by x-ray evidence of increased mineralization and by an increase in blood concentration of calcium and phosphorus associated with a lowered serum alkaline phosphatase level.

X-ray pelvimetry is ordinarily required to evaluate the pelvis properly. Cesarean section is the preferred method of delivery in the presence of a significant contraction. The infant of an osteomalacic mother may have evidence of rickets, even though the concentration of calcium in the cord blood is normal; the infant is subject to tetany during the first few neonatal

otomy and radium applied at its completion. When the weeks. Appropriate calcium and vitamin D therapy usually yields good results.

Osteitis Fibrosa Cystica (Albright's Syndrome)

Idiopathic cystic disease of bone, early closure of epiphyses, irregular patches of melanin pigment in the skin overlying involved bone, and precocious sexual development characterize osteitis fibrosa cystica. Pregnancy may occur during childhood; in most instances, the outcome of a well-supervised case is good.

Chondrodystrophy

In chondrodystrophy the epiphyseal plate fails to produce adequate amounts of columnar cartilage. There is a disproportionate rate of growth between membranous and cartilaginous bone. The affected patient is a dwarf, with a large prominent forehead and flattened facial features. The trunk is normal in length, but marked lumbar lordosis causes a forward displacement of the sacral promontory and serious inlet contraction of the pelvis. Delivery by cesarean section is usually necessary.

REFERENCES AND RECOMMENDED READING

TERATOLOGY

Abdul-Karim RW (ed): Drug therapeutics. Clin Obstet Gynecol 20:229, 1977

Allen RW, Ogden B, Bentley F et al: Fetal hydantoin syndrome, neuroblastoma, and hemorrhagic disease in a neonate. JAMA 244:1462, 1980

Bossi L, Assael BM, Avanzini G et al: Plasma levels and clinical effects of antiepileptic drugs in pregnant patients and their newborns. In Johannessen SI, Morselli PL, Pippinger CE, et al (eds), Antiepileptic Therapy: Advances in Drug Treatment. New York, Raven Press, 1980

Golbus MS: Teratology for the obstetrician. Obstet Gynecol 55:269, 1980

Hill RM, Stern L: Drugs in pregnancy: Effects on the fetus and newborn. Drugs 17:182, 1979

Howard FM, Hill JM: Drugs in pregnancy. Obstet Gynecol Surv 34:643, 1979

INFECTIOUS DISEASES

Archibald HM: Influence of maternal malaria on newborn infants. Br Med J 2:1512, 1958

Bass MH: Viral and parasitic diseases of the pregnant woman affecting the fetus. Clin Obstet Gynecol 2:627, 1959

Bernirschke K, Pendelton ME: Coxsackie virus infection: An important complication in pregnancy. Obstet Gynecol 12:305, 1958

Brazin SA, Simikovich JW, Taylor-Johnson W: Herpes zoster during pregnancy. Obstet Gynecol 53:175, 1979

Brown GC, Karunas RS: Relationship of congenital anomalies and maternal infection with selected enteroviruses. Am J Epidemiol 95:207, 1972

Desmonts G, Couvreur J: Congenital toxoplasmosis: A prospective study of 378 pregnancies. N Engl J Med 290:1110, 1974

Fuchs F, Kimball AC, Kean BH: The management of toxoplasmosis in pregnancy. Clin Perinatol 1:407, 1974

Gregg NM: Congenital cataract following German measles in mother. Trans Ophthalmol Soc Aust 3:35, 1942

Hadsall FJ, Acquarelli MJ: Disseminated coccidioidomycosis presenting as facial granulomas in pregnancy: A report of two cases and a review of the literature. Laryngoscope 83:51, 1973

Hirschhorn N, Chowdhury AKMA, Lindenbaum J: Cholera in pregnant women. Lancet 1:1230, 1969

Just M, Buergin-Wolffe G, Hernandez R: Immunization trials with live attenuated cytomegalovirus. TOWNE 125. Infection 3:1975

Kendig EL: Prognosis of infants born of tuberculous mothers. Pediatrics 26:97, 1960

Kibrick S: Herpes simplex infection at term. What to do with mother, newborn, and nursery personnel. JAMA, 243:157, 1980

Kimball AC, Kean BH, Fuchs F: Congenital toxoplasmosis: A prospective study of 4048 obstetric patients. Am J Obstet Gynecol 111:211, 1971

Polk BF, White JA, DeGirolami PC et al: An outbreak of rubella among hospital personnel. N Engl J Med 303:541, 1980

Remington JS: Toxoplasmosis. In Charles D, Finland M (eds): Obstetric and Perinatal Infections: Clinical, Microbiol, Epidemiological, and Therapeutic Aspects. Philadelphia, Lea & Febiger, 1973

Schaefer G, Douglas RG, Dreishpoon IH: Extrapulmonary tuberculosis and pregnancy. Am J Obstet Gynecol 67:605, 1954

Schoenbaum SC, Weinstein L: Respiratory infection in pregnancy. Clin Obstet Gynecol 22:293, 1979

Starr JG, Bart RD, Gold E: Inapparent congenital cytomegalovirus infection: Clinical and epidemiologic characteristics in early pregnancy. N Engl J Med 282:1075, 1970

Stead WW: The new face of tuberculosis. Hosp Pract 62: 1969

Stetten DeW Jr: Eradication (of smallpox). Science 210:1203, 1980

Stray-Pedersen B: A prospective study of acquired toxoplasmosis among 8,043 pregnant women in the Oslo area. Am J Obstet Gynecol 136:399, 1980

Sutherland AM: Genital tuberculosis in women. Bull Sloane Hosp 13:127, 1967

Taylor ES: Toward an effective rubella immunity. Obstet Gynecol Surv 2:892, 1967

Tobin JO'H, Marshall WC, Peckham CS: Virus infections. Clin Obstet Gynecol 4:479, 1977

Weinstein L, Murphy T: The management of tuberculosis during pregnancy. Clin Perinatol 1:395, 1974

Wilson CB, Remington JS: What can be done to prevent congenital toxoplasmosis? Am J Obstet Gynecol 138:357, 1980

RESPIRATORY DISEASES

Austrian R, McClement JH, Renzetti D, Jr et al: Clinical and physiologic features of some types of pulmonary diseases with impairment of alveolar–capillary diffusion. Am J Med 11:667, 1951

Corner GW, Jr, Nesbitt REL, Jr: Pregnancy and pulmonary resection. Am J Obstet Gynecol 68:903, 1954

DeSwiet M: Diseases of the respiratory system. Clin Obstet Gynecol 4:287, 1977

CARDIOVASCULAR DISEASES

Akbarian M, Austen G, Yurchak PM et al: Thromboembolic complications of prosthetic valves. Circulation 37:826, 1968

Batson GA: Cyanotic congenital heart disease and pregnancy. J Obstet Gynaecol Br Commonw 81:549, 1974

Burwell CW: Special problem of rheumatic heart disease in pregnant women. Arch Intern Med 101:60, 1958

Chesley LC: Severe rheumatic cardiac disease and pregnancy: The ultimate prognosis. Am J Obstet Gynecol 136:552, 1980

Conradsson TB, Werko L: Management of heart disease in pregnancy. Prog Cardiovasc Dis 16:407, 1974

Eilen B, Kaiser IH, Becker RM et al: Aortic valve replacement in the third trimester of pregnancy: Case report and review of the literature. Obstet Gynecol 57:119, 1981

Gallery EDM, Saunders DM, Hunyor SN et al: Improvement in fetal growth with treatment of maternal hypertension in pregnancy. Clin Sci Mol Med 55:359s, 1978

Gold EM: Cardiac arrest in obstetrics. Clin Obstet Gynecol 3:114, 1960

Hellegers A, Neill C: Pregnancy after surgical correction of Fallot's tetralogy. In Eastman NS, Hellman LW (eds): Williams Obstetrics, 13th ed, pp 766–767. New York, Appleton, 1966

Jones AM, Howitt G: Eisenmenger syndrome in pregnancy. Br Med J 1:1627, 1965

Lees MM, Taylor SH, Scott DB et al: A study of cardiac output at rest throughout pregnancy. J Obstet Gynaecol Br Commonw 74:319, 1967

MacDonald HN: Pregnancy following insertion of cardiac valve prostheses: A review and further case report. Br J Obstet Gynaecol 77:603, 1970

Mendelson CL: Pregnancy and kyphoscoliotic heart disease. Am J Obstet Gynecol 56:457, 1948

Naeye R, Hagstrom JWC, Talmadge BA: Postpartum death with maternal congenital heart disease. Circulation 36:304, 1967

Oparil S, Swartwout JR: Heart disease in pregnancy. J Reprod Med 11:2, 1973

Pedowitz P, Hellman LM: Pregnancy and healed subacute bacterial endocarditis. Am J Obstet Gynecol 66:294, 1953

Petch MC: Cardiac disease in pregnancy. Postgrad Med J 55:315, 1979

Selzer A: Risks of pregnancy in women with cardiac disease. JAMA 238:892, 1977

Sugrue D, Blake S, MacDonald D: Pregnancy complicated by maternal heart disease at National Maternity Hospital, Dublin, Ireland, 1969 to 1978. Am J Obstet Gynecol 139:1, 1981

Szekely P, Snaith L: Cardiac disorders. Clin Obstet Gynecol 4:265, 1977

Szekely P, Snaith L: Heart Disease and Pregnancy. London, Churchill Livingstone, 1974

Ueland K, Metcalfe J: Heart disease in pregnancy. Clin Perinatol 1:349, 1974

Ueland K, Novy MJ, Peterson EN et al: Maternal cardiovascular dynamics. IV. The influence of gestational age on the maternal cardiovascular response to posture and exercise. Am J Obstet Gynecol 104:856, 1969

Wallace WA, Harken DE, Ellis LB: Pregnancy following closed mitral valvuloplasty: A long-term study with remarks concerning the necessity for careful cardiac management. JAMA 217:297, 1971

Welt SI, Crenshaw MC, Jr: Concurrent hypertension and pregnancy. Clin Obstet Gynecol 21:619, 1978

Zitnik RS, Brandenburg RO, Sheldon R et al: Pregnancy and open heart surgery. Circulation 39 (Suppl 1);257, 1969

ALIMENTARY TRACT AND LIVER DISEASES

Berk JE, Smith BH, Akrani MM: Pregnancy pancreatitis. Am J Gastroenterol 56:216, 1971

Blumberg BS, Sutnick AI, London WT: Australia antigen as a hepatitis virus. Am J Med 48:1, 1970

Douglas JM, Farmer RG, Vidt DG et al: Hepatitis and renal failure in pregnancy. Arch Intern Med 122:59, 1968

Fielding JF: Inflammatory bowel disease and pregnancy. Br J Hosp Med 15:345, 1976

Gorbach AC, Reid DE: Hiatus hernia in pregnancy. N Engl J Med 255:517, 1956

Gregory PB, Knauer CM, Kempson RL et al: Steroid therapy in severe viral hepatitis. N Engl J Med 294:681, 1976

Holzbach RT: Australia antigen hepatitis in pregnancy: Evidence against transplacental transmission of Australia antigen in early and late pregnancy. Arch Intern Med 130:234, 1972

Johnston JL: Peptic ulcer and pregnancy. Obstet Gynecol 2:290, 1953

Kehayoglou KA, Stravropoulos AK, Lolis DE et al: Viral hepatitis during pregnancy. Int J Obstet Gynecol 10:102, 1972

Malkasian GD, Jr, Welch JS, Hallenbeck GA: Volvulus associated with pregnancy: Review and report of three cases. Am J Obstet Gynecol 78:112, 1959

Miller JP: Diseases of the liver and alimentary tract. Clin Obstet Gynecol 4:297, 1977

Okada K, Kamiyama I, Inomata M et al: E antigen and anti-E in the serum of asymptomatic carrier mothers as indicators of positive and negative transmission of hepatitis B virus to their infants. N Engl J Med 294:746, 1976

O'Leary JA, Bepko FJ, Jr: Rectal carcinoma and pregnancy. Am J Obstet Gynecol 84:459, 1962

Rigler LG, Eneboe JB: Incidence of hiatus hernia in pregnant women and its significance. J Thorac Surg 4:262, 1935

Scholtes G: Liver function and liver diseases during pregnancy. J Perinat Med 7:55, 1979

Svanborg A, Ohlsson S: Recurrent jaundice of pregnancy. Am J Med 27:40, 1959

Tew WL, Holliday RL, Phibbs G: Perforated duodenal ulcer in pregnancy with double survival. Am J Obstet Gynecol 125:1151, 1976

Wands JR: Viral hepatitis and its effect on pregnancy. Clin Obstet Gynecol 22:301, 1979

Webb MJ, Sedlack RE: Ulcerative colitis in pregnancy. Med Clin North Am 58:823, 1974

DISORDERS OF THE URINARY TRACT

Badawy S, Karim M: Bilharzial carcinoma of the bladder with pregnancy and labor. Int Surg 56:434, 1971

Kass EH: Bacteriuria and pyelonephritis of pregnancy. Arch Intern Med 105:194, 1960

Leppert P, Tisher CC, Cheng SCS et al: Antecedent renal

disease and the outcome of pregnancy. Ann Intern Med 90:747, 1979

Lindheimer MD, Katz AI: Pregnancy and the kidney. J Reprod Med 11:14, 1973

Marchant DJ: The urinary tract in pregnancy. Clin Obstet Gynecol 21:817, 1978

Nesbitt REL, Jr, Young JE: Urinary tract infections during pregnancy and in the puerperium: Treatment with nitrofurantoin (Furadantin). Obstet Gynecol 10:89, 1957

Polk BF: Urinary tract infection in pregnancy. Clin Obstet Gynecol 22:285, 1979

Ries K, Kaye D: The current status of therapy in urinary tract infection in pregnancy. Clin Perinatol 1:423, 1974

Schewitz LJ, Seftel HC: Nephrotic syndrome in pregnancy. Med Proc 4:304, 1958

DISORDERS OF THE NERVOUS SYSTEM

Bowers VM, Jr, Danforth DN: Significance of poliomyelitis during pregnancy: An analysis of the literature and presentation of 24 new cases. Am J Obstet Gynecol 65:34, 1953

Cooper HH: Electroshock treatment of mental illness during pregnancy. S Afr Med J 26:366, 1952

Dunn JM: Bilateral Bell's palsy in the puerperium. Ob/Gyn Dig, May 1970, page 32

Fedrick J: Epilepsy and pregnancy: Report from the Oxford Record Linkage Study. Br Med J 2:442, 1973

Gomberg B: Spontaneous subarachnoid hemorrhage in pregnancy not complicated by toxemia. Am J Obstet Gynecol 77:430, 1959

Hopkins A: Neurological disorders. Clin Obstet Gynecol 4:419, 1977

Horn P: Obstetric management of poliomyelitis complicating pregnancy. Clin Obstet Gynecol 1:127, 1958

Knight AH, Rhind EG: Epilepsy and pregnancy: A study of 153 pregnancies in 59 patients. Epilepsia 16:99, 1975

Leibowitz U, Antonovsky A, Kats R et al: Pregnancy and risk of multiple sclerosis. J Neurol Neurosurg Psychiatry 30:354, 1967

Lowe CR: Congenital malformations among infants born to epileptic women. Lancet 1:9, 1973

Massey EW, Cefalo RC: Neuropathies of pregnancy. Obstet Gynecol Surv 34:489, 1979

Meadow R: The high-risk pregnancy: When the pregnant patient is epileptic. Contemp Ob/Gyn 1:40, 1973

Robinson JL, Hall CH, Sedzimir CB: Subarachnoid haemorrhage in pregnancy. J Neurosurg 36:27, 1972

Robinson JL, Hall CH, Sedzimir CB: Arteriovenous malformations, aneurysms and pregnancy. J Neurosurg ,41:63, 1974

Rolbin SH, Levinson G, Shnider SM et al: Anesthetic considerations for myasthenia gravis and pregnancy. Anesth Analg 57:441, 1978

Strauss RG, Ramsay RE, Willmore LJ et al: Epilepsy and pregnancy. Obstet Gynecol 53:344, 1979

Sweeney WJ: Pregnancy and multiple sclerosis. Clin Obstet Gynecol 1:137, 1958

PSYCHIATRIC DISORDERS

Cassidy WL, Flanagan NB, Spellman M et al: Clinical observations in manic–depressive disease. JAMA 164:1535, 1957

Kenin L, Blass NH: Mental illness associated with the postpartum state. Clin Obstet Gynecol 5:716, 1962

ENDOCRINE AND METABOLIC DISORDERS

American Diabetes Association Annual Meeting Report, Youth Committee, June 1973

Bleich HL, Boro ES: Hyperthyroidism during pregnancy. N Engl J Med 298:150, 1978

Chapman L, Silk E, Skuphy A et al: Spectrofluorimetric assay of serum cystine aminopeptidase in normal and diabetic pregnancy compared with total estrogen excretion. J Obstet Gynaecol Br Commonw 78:435, 1971

Depp R: Present status of the assessment of fetal maturity. Semin Perinatol 4:229, 1980

Eastman NJ, Jackson E: Weight relationships in pregnancy: Bearing of maternal weight gain and prepregnancy weight on birth weight in full-term pregnancies. Obstet Gynecol Surv 23:1003, 1968

Edwards OM: The management of thyroid disease in pregnancy. Postgrad Med J 55:340, 1979

Essex N: Diabetes and pregnancy. Br J Hosp Med 15:333, 1976

Freinkel N: Effects of the conceptus on maternal metabolism during pregnancy. In Leibel BS, Wrenshall GA (eds): On the Nature and Treatment of Diabetes, pp 679–691. Amsterdam Excerpta Medica, 1965

Galina MP, Avnet NL, Einhorn A: Iodides during pregnancy: An apparent cause of neonatal death. N Engl J Med 267:1124, 1962

Gemmell AA: Phaeochromocytoma and the obstetrician. J Obstet Gynaecol Br Emp 62:195, 1955

Goldsmith RS: Evaluation and treatment of hypercalcemia. Mod Med 104, Sept 22, 1969

Gordon H, Dixon HG, Cummins M et al: Simplified management of pregnancy complicated by diabetes. Br J Obstet Gynaecol 85:585, 1978

Gottesman RL, Refetoff S: Diagnosis and management of thyroid diseases in pregnancy. J Reprod Med 11:19, 1973

Greenman GW, Gabrielson MO, Howard–Flanders J et al: Thyroid dysfunction in pregnancy: Fetal loss and follow-up evaluation of surviving infants. N Engl J Med 267:426, 1962

Hartenstein H, Gardner LI: Tetany of the newborn associated with maternal parathyroid adenoma. N Engl J Med 274:266, 1966

Hennen G, Pierce JG, Freychet P: Human chorionic thyrotropin: Further characterization and study of its secretion during pregnancy. J Clin Endocrinol Metab 29:581, 1969

Hershman JM, Higgins HP: Hydatidiform mole: A cause of clinical hyperthyroidism. Report of two cases with evidence that the molar tissue secreted a thyroid stimulator. N Engl J Med 284:573, 1971

Hill CS, Jr, Clark R, Wolf M: Effect of pregnancy after thyroid carcinoma. Surg Gynecol Obstet 122:1219, 1966

Hime MC, Richardson JA: Diabetes insipidus and pregnancy. Obstet Gynecol Surv 33:375, 1978

Hoffer PB, Gottschalk A: Fluorescent thyroid scanning: Scanning without radioisotopes: Initial clinical results. Radiology 99:117, 1971

Jacobsen BB, Terslev E, Lund B et al: Neonatal hypocalcemia associated with maternal hyperparathyroidism. Arch Dis Child 53:308, 1978

Johnson CF: Phenylketonuria and the obstetrician. Obstet Gynecol 39:942, 1972

Lenke RR, Levy HL: Maternal phenylketonuria and hyperphenylalaninemia. An international survey of the outcome of untreated and treated pregnancies. N Engl J Med 303:1202, 1980

Lind T: Metabolic changes in pregnancy relevant to diabetes mellitus. Postgrad Med J 55:353, 1979

Man EB, Holden RH, Jones WS: Thyroid function in human pregnancy. VII. Development and retardation of 4-year-old progeny of euthyroid and of hypothroxinemic women. Am J Obstet Gynecol 109:12, 1971

Manger WM, Gifford RW, Jr: Pheochromocytoma. New York, Springer–Verlag, 1977

Martin DH, Montgomery DRD, Harley JMG: The occurrence of T$_3$ thyrotoxicosis in pregnancy. Ir J Med Sci 145:92, 1976

McKenzie JM: Neonatal Graves' disease. J Clin Endocrinol Metab 24:600, 1964

Merkatz IR, Adam PA (eds): Diabetes in pregnancy. Semin Perinatol 2:287, 1978

Montgomery DAD, Harley JMG: Endocrine disorders. Clin Obstet Gynecol 4:339, 1977

Posner NA, Silverstone FA: Carbohydrate metabolism in pregnancy; Management of the diabetic gravida. Obstet Gynecol Annu 6:67, 1977

Reynolds WA: Thyroid function in mother, fetus, and neonate. Obstet Gynecol Annu 7:67, 1978

Robinson RE: Clinical aspects of diabetes in pregnancy. Postgrad Med J 55:358, 1979

Sann L, David L, Frederich A et al: Congenital hyperparathyroidism and vitamin D deficiency secondary to maternal hypoparathyroidism. Acta Paediatr Scand 65:381, 1976

Schenker JG, Chowers I: Pheochromocytoma in pregnancy: A review of 89 cases. Obstet Gynecol Surv 26:739, 1971

Selenkow HA: Antithyroid–thyroid therapy of thyrotoxicosis during pregnancy. Obstet Gynecol 40:117, 1972

Selenkow HA, Robin NI, Refetoff S: Thyroid function in human pregnancy. In Senhauser DA, Anderson RR (eds): The Thyroid, Proceedings of the Fifth Midwest Conference on the Thyroid, pp 62–78. Columbia, University of Missouri Press, 1969

Towell ME, Hyman AI: Catecholamine depletion in pregnancy. J Obstet Gynaecol Br Commonw 73:431, 1966

Tricomi V, Baum H: Acute intermittent porphyria and pregnancy. Obstet Gynecol Surv 13:307, 1958

White P: Diabetes mellitus in pregnancy. Clin Perinatol 1:331, 1974

Whitfield CR, Sproule WB, Brudenelle M: The amniotic fluid lecithin sphingomyelin area ratio (LSAR) in pregnancies complicated by diabetes. J Obstet Gynaecol Br Commonw 80:918, 1973

Zaleski LA, Casey RE, Zaleski W: Maternal phenylketonuria: Dietary treatment during pregnancy. Can Med Assoc J 121:1591, 1979

Zilliacus H, Kallio H: Acute intermittent porphyria and pregnancy. Acta Obstet Gynecol Scand 41:316, 1962

DISORDERS OF THE BLOOD

Desforges JF, Warth J: The management of sickle cell disease in pregnancy. Clin Perinatol 1:385, 1974

DeSwiet M: Management of thromboembolism in pregnancy. Drugs 18:478, 1979

Fiakpui EZ, Moran EM: Pregnancy in the sickle hemoglobinopathies. J Reprod Med 11:28, 1973

Hibbard BM: The role of folic acid in pregnancy. J Obstet Gynaecol Br Commonw 71:529, 1964

Horger EO, III: Managing the patient with sickle cell disease. Comtemp Obstet Gynecol 2:55, 1973

Howie PW: Thromboembolism. Clin Obstet Gynecol 4:397, 1977

Jaffe G, Hubbard M, Clark D: Hematologic problems in

pregnancy. III. Glucose-6-phosphate dehydrogenase deficiency. J Reprod Med 12:153, 1974

Kitay DZ: Purpura: Significance and management of the ITP and TTP syndromes. Contemp Ob/Gyn 2:65, 1973

Morrison JC: Hemoglobinopathies and pregnancy. Clin Obstet Gynecol 22:819, 1979

Morrison JC, Roe PL, Stahl RL et al: Heterozygous thalassemia and pregnancy: A 25-year experience. J Reprod Med 11:35, 1973

Morrison JC, Schneider JM, Whybrew WD et al: Prophylactic transfusions in pregnant patients with sickle hemoglobinopathies: Benefit versus risk. Obstet Gynecol 56:274, 1980

O'Dell RF: Leukemia lymphoma complicating pregnancy. Clin Obstet Gynecol 22:859, 1979

Perkins RP: Thrombocytopenia in obstetric syndromes: A review. Obstet Gynecol Surv 34:101, 1979

Pritchard JA, Scott DE, Mason RA: Severe anemia with hemolysis and megaloblastic erythropoiesis. JAMA 194:457, 1965

Stein S, Dennis LH: Leukemia in pregnancy: A review. Obstet Gynecol Dig 69, 1966

DISORDERS OF THE REPRODUCTIVE ORGANS

Andrews HR: On the effect of ventral fixation of the uterus upon subsequent pregnancy and labor based on the analyses of 395 cases. J Obstet Gynaecol Br Emp 8:97, 1905

Bibbo M, Gill WB, Azizi F et al: Follow-up study of male and female offspring of DES-exposed mothers. Obstet Gynecol 49:1, 1977

Danforth DN: Discussion of paper by Fields C. Pildes RB: Sacculation of the uterus. Am J Obstet Gynecol 87:507, 1963

Donegan WL: Mammary carcinoma and pregnancy. Major Probl Clin Surg 5:448, 1979

Herbst AL: Delayed disease as a consequence of fetal exposure to radiation, infection, and exogenous hormones. Clin Perinatol 1:483, 1974

Herbst AL, Hubby MM, Blough RR et al: A comparison of pregnancy experience in DES-exposed and DES-unexposed daughters. J Reprod Med 24:62, 1980

Hubay CA, Barry FM, Marr CC: Pregnancy and breast cancer. Surg Clin North Am 58:819, 1978

Musich JR, Behrman SJ: Obstetric outcome before and after metroplasty in women with uterine anomalies. J Obstet Gynecol 52:63,

Parks J, Barter RH: Myomatous uterus complicated by pregnancy. Am J Obstet Gynecol 63:260, 1952

Sablinska R, Tarlowska L, Stelmachow J: Invasive carcinoma of the cervix associated with pregnancy: Correlation between patient age, advancement of cancer and gestation, and result of treatment. Gynecol Oncol 5:363, 1977

Schaefer G, Epstein H: Female genital tuberculosis: A review of the literature. Obstet Gynecol Surv 8:461, 1953

Studdiford WE: Pregnancy and pelvic tuberculosis. Am J Obstet Gynecol 69:379, 1955

MISCELLANEOUS DISORDERS

Ahlfors CE, Goetzman BW, Halsted CC et al: Neonatal listeriosis. Am J Dis Child 131:405, 1977

Boronow RC: Extrapelvic malignancy and pregnancy. Obstet Gynecol Surv 19:1, 1964

Dugan RJ, Black ME: Kyphoscoliosis and pregnancy. Am J Obstet Gynecol 75:89, 1957

Durfee RB: Surgical complications of the puerperium. Clin Obstet Gynecol 5:729, 1962

Hertz KC, Crawford PS, Chez RA et al: Herpes gestationis. Obstet Gynecol 49:733, 1977

Mendiones M, Solomon LM: Skin changes during pregnancy and their therapy. Ob-Gyn Dig II:19, 1974

Mersheimer WL, Wattiker BJ: Pregnancy complicated by acute abdominal emergencies. Clin Obstet Gynecol 3:98, 1960

Pearson E: Effect of pregnancy on otosclerosis. Ann West Med Surg 5:477, 1951

Reynolds AG: Placental metastasis from malignant melanoma. Obstet Gynecol 6:205, 1955

Treves N, Holleb AI: A report of 549 cases of breast cancer in women 35 years of age and younger. Surg Gynecol Obstet 107:271, 1958

Wade TR, Wade SL, Jones HE: Skin changes and diseases associated with pregnancy. Obstet Gynecol 52:233, 1978

PRINCIPLES AND EQUIPMENT

Ultrasound is a mechanical vibration of high frequency. It is totally different from electromagnetic radiation, such as visible light or x-rays. It is of the same physical nature as audible sound except that it is of much higher frequency. The frequency of ultrasound used in obstetric diagnosis is between 2.25 MHz (2.25 million cycles per second) and 5 MHz. This frequency range is used because it offers the best compromise between high resolution (sharp images) and adequate penetration of the sound to structures located deep within the abdomen. Lower frequencies allow deeper penetration, but provide less detailed images. Higher frequencies provide excellent resolution but little penetration and thus are used for studies of small organs, notably the eye.

The ultrasonic beam is produced by a transducer, the principal component of which is a piezoelectric crystal or ceramic. When an electric pulse of suitable voltage is applied to a piezoelectric substance, it vibrates and ultrasound is emitted. The frequency of ultrasound produced depends on the characteristics of the piezoelectric element, and ultrasonic vibrations of any desired frequency can be obtained by using a suitably designed transducer. Conversely, mechanical distortion of a piezoelectric substance produces a small voltage signal. In an ultrasonic scanner, the piezoelectric element is slightly distorted by the echoes returning to the transducer. These distortions produce minute voltage pulses, which are then suitably amplified and displayed. Thus, the transducer acts alternately as a transmitter and a receiver of ultrasound energy.

Medical ultrasonic scanners produce images by measuring the time taken for a sound pulse to travel from the transducer to each echoing structure and to return to the transducer. This time interval is a measure of the distance of each echoing structure from the transducer, because the velocity of sound in the body is essentially constant at approximately 1540 m/sec. This value is not precise, but it is an excellent approximation for all tissue except bone and fat, exceptions that are insignificant in obstetric diagnosis.

Ultrasonic energy is reflected at interfaces between tissues with differing acoustic properties. The greater the difference and more sudden the change, the greater the proportion of ultrasonic energy that is reflected. Even slight changes are sufficient to produce an echo that can be recorded by an ultrasonic scanner. The boundaries between the soft tissues of the fetus and the amniotic fluid, between the placenta and the uterine wall, and between the fetal brain and the falx cerebri can all be readily demonstrated ultrasonically. Differences as slight as these cannot be demonstrated

ULTRASOUND, ROENTGENOGRAPHY, AND RADIONUCLIDE IMAGING IN OBSTETRIC DIAGNOSIS

Bruce D. Doust
Vivienne L. Doust

by radiographic techniques (with the possible exception of computerized axial tomography). In ultrasonic scanning, only part of the sonic energy is reflected at any one tissue interface. Some energy passes through to deeper structures, is reflected by them, and subsequently arrives back at the transducer. The margins of trabecular bone, air in the bowel, and barium sulfate used in gastrointestinal examinations reflect the sound so strongly that it is difficult or impossible to obtain pictures from structures deep to them. Apart from the difficulties imposed by the bone of the pubic symphysis, these factors are not significant in obstetric ultrasonic diagnosis.

DISPLAY MODES

Ultrasonic information is displayed in one of four ways. In the simplest form, the *A-mode display,* the echoes

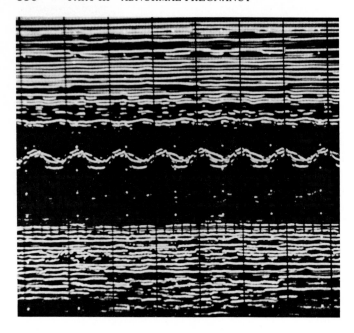

FIG. 28–1. Intrauterine fetal echocardiogram. M-mode scan taken through fetal thorax. In this type of display stationary structures trace straight lines; wavy lines represent moving structures. Sinuous trace across center of picture represents rhythmically moving structure within fetal thorax. This study is proof-positive that fetus is alive. Heart rate is 145/min and regular.

are plotted as a series of peaks along a baseline. The height of each peak relates to the strength of the echo; the position of the peak represents the depth of the echoing structure from the transducer. This form of ultrasonic display is seldom used in obstetric work.

The *M-mode display* is used for studying moving structures and is recorded on a continuously moving strip of sensitized paper. A dot representing a moving structure traces out a sinuous path; a stationary structure is represented by a straight line. This form of display is used extensively in cardiac diagnosis and is occasionally used to display fetal heart motion (Fig. 28–1).

In obstetric and gynecologic diagnosis the *compound B-mode image* is an extremely useful form of display. It is a two-dimensional display of a slice of tissue. In a B scan, the information derived from timing the echoes is combined electronically with signals that indicate the position of the transducer. The position of each echoing structure in the tissue under examination is thus determined.

The ultrasound beam is about 1 cm wide, so each scan displays a slice of tissue about 1 cm thick; it is a laminagraphic display. The appearance of the image depends not only upon the intrinsic shape of the demonstrated structures, but also on the plane of section. Thus, a B-mode scan through a fetal limb may appear as a circle or an ellipse, depending upon the plane in which the ultrasound beam sweeps across the limb. The fetal head appears as an ellipse.

Most commercially available ultrasonic B scanners have a single transducer attached to the end of a jointed arm. The transducer is placed in direct contact with the patient's skin and is moved back and forth by hand. Since this operation requires considerable skill and precision, efforts have been made to automate the procedure. At least one automatic scanner is commercially available; it contains a battery of eight large transducers immersed in a waterbath, and the patient lies prone on a membrane on top of the bath.

Modern ultrasonic scanners display their images on a television screen in 16 or 32 shades of gray. The electronic signals representing the echoes are converted to shades of gray by a device called a scan converter. The technology of scan converters has advanced considerably with the recent introduction of the digital scan converter, a device that can be compared with a computer's random access memory. This device offers greater reliability than do the older scan converters, and it facilitates electronic manipulation of the signals before the scan image is formed, thereby enhancing the visibility of organ outlines and internal structures. At present, the spatial resolution of digital scan converters is not quite as good as that of the older analog scan converters, but the difference is slight and of dubious significance.

The fourth mode of displaying ultrasonic information is the *real-time display*. Real-time devices present a sequence of images in rapid succession. These machines are the ultrasonic equivalent of a fluoroscope, *i.e.*, they produce a movie-type image. Generally, individual frames are of lower quality than the images produced by a conventional B scanner, although recent improvements have reduced the difference quite noticeably.

There are several types of real-time scanners. The

most widely available and least expensive have scanning heads that are 10–20 cm long and contain numerous transducers arranged in a row. These scanning heads are rigid and, if positioned in the sagittal plane, cannot be angled caudally. With these systems, the deeper parts of the pelvis can be examined only in a transverse plane, a minor but occasionally significant limitation. There are other real-time devices that have quite small scanning heads, but generally these are considerably more costly.

For most obstetric work, particularly measurement of the biparietal diameter of the fetal skull, real-time images are of adequate quality, and the fluoroscopic nature of the image allows most routine obstetric examinations to be completed quickly. Real-time ultrasonic examination is now the definitive method of diagnosis in suspected cases of fetal death *in utero*.

DOPPLER ULTRASOUND

When sound is reflected from a moving structure, the frequency of the returning echo is different from that of the transmitted sound. The difference is a measure of the velocity of the structure reflecting the sound. More crudely, frequency shift is evidence that somewhere within the sound beam there is a moving structure. This phenomenon is particularly useful in the assessment of blood flow in arteries and veins. In obstetric practice, the Doppler technique is used to detect fetal movement, especially fetal heart motion. It is used to confirm that a fetus is alive, and it allows monitoring of fetal heart rate during labor. The simplest and most common way of making this information available to the clinician is to feed the frequency difference to a loudspeaker. If the machine is silent, there are no moving structures within the sound beam. Any noise signifies movement. A rhythmically changing sound represents a rhythmically moving structure, *e.g.*, the fetal heart.

Recently, pulsed Doppler devices have been introduced. These devices select signals from a particular depth and ignore signals from all other parts of the sound beam. This technique allows the operator to select the precise location at which motion is measured; for example, blood flow can be determined in a single vessel or even in one part of the lumen of a vessel. At present, this technique is used in combination with a real-time scanner to evaluate blood flow, particularly in the carotid arteries. It shows promise as a means of investigating placental dysfunction by measuring blood flow in the umbilical vein, but the work is as yet experimental.

There have been recent moves toward standardizing the presentation format for ultrasonic B scans. Longitudinal scans are customarily presented with their cranial aspect to the left. In transverse scans, the anatomic right is to the left of the picture. There is still variation, however. Some authors favor a black on white presentation; others, white on black. There is little to suggest the superiority of one method over the other.

THE OBSTETRIC ULTRASOUND EXAMINATION

An obstetric ultrasonic examination involves very little patient preparation or discomfort. An examination takes 5–30 min to perform, depending on the clinical problem, the equipment available, and the experience of the operator. An examination performed with a real-time scanner takes less time than one performed with a conventional scanner. A coupling agent must be spread on the patient's skin to assist sound transmission between the transducer and the patient. Mineral oil is commonly used; aqueous preparations are also available. All obstetric and gynecologic ultrasonic examinations require that the patient's urinary bladder be moderately distended to lift the uterus above the pubic symphysis and to provide a window through which sound can travel to and from the pelvic contents.

In late pregnancy, the uterus may fall back, compressing the inferior vena cava when the patient lies supine, so that she may faint during the course of an ultrasonic examination. Incipient syncope is best treated by promptly turning the patient onto her side.

HAZARDS

The principal motive for the development of medical ultrasonic imaging was the desire to find a safe means of imaging the fetus. Unlike x-rays, ultrasound at the energy level used in diagnostic work does not ionize or produce free radicals within the tissue through which it passes. Ultrasonic energy does, however, interact with tissue in several ways that are not yet completely understood. The best understood mechanisms of interaction are the production of heat and of cavitation (formation and subsequent collapse of minute bubbles within the tissue). Cavitation can lead to direct physical disruption of tissue and to the formation of chemically active radicals. Because such interaction does occur, ultrasonic energy can be highly destructive. However, the energy required to produce tissue damage is several orders of magnitude greater than that used in diagnostic studies. In most ultrasonic instruments used in medical diagnosis, the average energy output is quite low, but the energy comes in short pulses of relatively high intensity, separated by long intervals during which the machine listens for the echoes. Although the average intensity is low, the intensity during a pulse is much higher; since the ultrasonic beam does not have an even energy distribution across its entire width, small areas of high-intensity

energy may exist for brief periods and in small volumes even when the average ultrasonic energy intensity is low. Manufacturers of medical ultrasound equipment take considerable trouble to keep the energy levels of their machines as low as possible consistent with satisfactory image quality, even though this policy makes the design of the equipment more difficult.

There have been reports of chromosomal aberrations in human leukocytes insonated with doses of ultrasound that are quite modest, but nonetheless well above those used in clinical practice. Attempts to reproduce these results have so far failed to confirm the original work; in fact, chromosomes appear to be quite resistant to ultrasonic damage. At the molecular level, ultrasonic energy has been shown to cause chemical degradation of deoxyribonucleic acid (DNA), the substance of which genetic material is composed. It has also been shown that ultrasonic insonation can decrease, at least temporarily, the number of mitoses in liver regeneration after partial hepatectomy. High-intensity ultrasonic radiation can also cause major lesions of the spinal cord, perhaps partly because it can produce stasis of the capillary blood flow. In the eye, high-energy ultrasonic radiation can result in widespread damage, but no damage has been detected at diagnostic intensities. There has also been a report of an increased incidence of fetal abnormalities in mice insonated *in utero*. These results are difficult to interpret, and it has been suggested that the effects observed may have been due to asphyxia of the mother or experimental bias rather than to ultrasound. All these experimental effects have been observed at energy levels well above those used in medical diagnosis.

The relevance of these experiments to the obstetric patient is at present dubious. There have been no confirmed reports of fetal injuries caused by ultrasonic radiation at diagnostic energy levels. This does not mean that ultrasound is harmless, but it does mean that any harmful effects are either genetic, and so may remain concealed for several generations, or somatic, but subtle or with a long latency period. Ultrasound has been used therapeutically in physical medicine and rehabilitation for many years as a means of producing heat in the depths of injured tissues. No important ill effects of this much more energetic and lower frequency form of ultrasound have been observed so far. Therefore, pulsed diagnostic ultrasound, as presently used, appears harmless. However, certainty is not likely until large-scale, long term, statistical studies have been completed.

Like any diagnostic measure, ultrasonic examination should not be undertaken unless there is a reasonable prospect that the patient will benefit from the study; but there need be no hesitancy in performing repeated studies. Doppler devices designed to measure blood flow should not be used for monitoring the fetal heart, as the energies at which they work may be considerably higher than is necessary to detect fetal heart motion. Under no circumstances should a patient be denied the benefits of an ultrasonic study for fear that, one day, a deleterious effect of ultrasound at diagnostic intensities may be discovered. Even if such an effect exists, the information obtained from ultrasonic studies is now so valuable that they are unlikely to be discontinued.

APPLICATIONS IN OBSTETRICS

DIAGNOSIS OF PREGNANCY

With some luck, it may be possible to diagnose pregnancy by ultrasonic means as early as 5 weeks after the last menstrual period. Between 6 and 7 weeks, it is usually possible to diagnose pregnancy with confidence. The gestational sac is a ringlike, strongly echoing structure that does not entirely fill the uterus.

As pregnancy advances, the fetus becomes visible within the gestational ring (Fig. 28–2). The surrounding decidual reaction results in evenly distributed echoes that are generally stronger than those coming from the myometrium of a nonpregnant uterus. The uterus enlarges, but this may be difficult to assess initially since nonpregnant uteri vary greatly in size.

At about 14 weeks, the standard hormonal pregnancy tests may again become less strongly positive or occasionally, may even be negative. If the patient is seen for the first time at this stage, ultrasound may be used to diagnose pregnancy as the cause of a pelvic mass. At 14 weeks ultrasonic diagnosis of pregnancy is straightforward, even in the most obese patient.

ESTIMATION OF GESTATIONAL AGE

Ultrasound has made it possible to estimate gestational age with high accuracy. The situations in which this precise knowledge is beneficial, and the clinical applications of the techniques, are outlined in Chapter 4.

Technique

In the first trimester, gestational age can be estimated by noting the appearance of the gestational sac. As noted earlier, the gestational sac at 6–10 weeks appears as a sharply defined, ringlike structure. The ring is somewhat asymmetric, being thicker on one side. With modern scanners, the fetus becomes visible within the ring quite early, at about 7–8 weeks after the last menstrual period.

Measurement of crown–rump length has been suggested as a means of estimating gestational age in the first trimester, and an accuracy of ± 6 days has been claimed for this method. This technique is sometimes difficult to use, because the fetus cannot always be

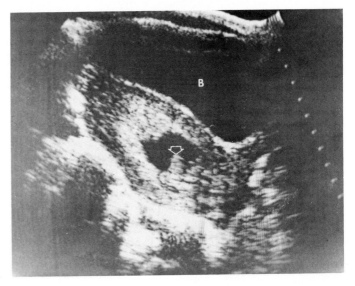

FIG. 28-2. Early pregnancy (about 7 weeks). Longitudinal midline scan shows a slightly enlarged uterus containing a gestational sac within which an embryo (*arrow*) can be seen. *B*, Bladder.

outlined satisfactorily. Between 9 and 11 weeks, the fetal head can be demonstrated; at this stage, it looks like a straight line within parentheses. Also, by this time the gestational ring fills the entire uterus, and the placenta can often be identified.

Once the fetal head can be defined, gestational age can be estimated with considerable accuracy by measuring the biparietal diameter. This is the most widely used and probably the most satisfactory technique for estimating gestational age. There have been several large series in which gestational age was correlated with biparietal diameter; all except one, in which the speed of sound was assumed to be 1600 m/sec, produced similar results. Table 28–1 has been compiled by averaging four large published series. The ultrasonically determined biparietal diameter is not the same as the external diameter of the head. The ultrasonic biparietal diameter is taken as the distance from the outside of the scalp on the near side of the head to the inside of the skull on the far side of the head. Therefore, the approximate biparietal diameter of the head can be obtained from the ultrasonic biparietal diameter by adding 5 mm to allow for the thickness of the skull and scalp on one side of the head.

The estimate of gestational age from biparietal diameter is subject to errors. For example, precise measurement of the biparietal diameter of the fetal skull requires a satisfactory horizontal section through the skull, which may not always be easy to obtain, particularly in an infant who presents by the breech. A section is deemed satisfactory if it is a regular oval, has a sharply defined outline to allow precise measurement, and shows a straight midline echo symmetrically located along the occipitofrontal diameter of the skull. Ideally, the lateral or third ventricles can also be seen (Fig. 28–3). The straight line represents the falx cerebri and other midline structures of the brain. It is wise

to take more than one section, changing the angulation of the transducer a little between pictures and seeking the largest section available on each occasion. There may be a variation of 1–4 mm between the greatest and the least values of biparietal diameter. It has been our practice to take the average of at least three, and preferably five, determinations of the biparietal diameter from images that are deemed satisfactory. Use of a single determination is likely to increase the degree of error.

Errors can also arise because the television monitors used to display the scan image are not linear. On all but the most expensive television monitors, the image of a 1-cm object varies in size according to the part of the screen on which it is displayed. This source of error can be eliminated by placing the electronically generated centimeter markers on or near the biparietal diameter so that both the markers and the image of the fetal head are magnified to the same degree.

Real-time scanners have greatly simplified the estimation of biparietal diameter and have probably improved the accuracy of the determination. There is considerable variation in the reported accuracy of ultrasonic biparietal diameter determinations. These differences of opinion probably represent differences in the time and care taken in obtaining the readings. Readings with standard deviation of ± 2 mm should be possible.

Biologic variation also causes errors in the estimation of gestational age; not all fetuses with the same biparietal diameter are the same age. A useful rule is that the age of 50% of fetuses with a given biparietal diameter is within ± 1 week of the most probable gestational age suggested by Table 28–1. For example, if the average biparietal diameter is 7 cm, the most probable gestational age is 29 weeks, but there is a 25% chance that the gestational age is less than 28 weeks

TABLE 28–1. RELATION BETWEEN BIPARIETAL DIAMETER AND GESTATIONAL AGE

Biparietal Diameter (cm)	Most Probable Gestational Age (Weeks)	Age Range Within Which 50% of Fetuses Will Fall (Weeks)
2.0	13	12–14
2.2	13.5	12.5–14.5
2.4	14	13–15
2.6	14	13–15
2.8	14.5	13.5–15.5
3.0	15	14–16
3.2	16	15–17
3.4	16.5	15.5–17.5
3.6	17	16–18
3.8	18	17–19
4.0	18.5	17.5–19.5
4.2	19	18–20
4.4	20	19–21
4.6	21	20–22
4.8	21.5	20.5–22.5
5.0	22	21–23
5.2	22.5	21.5–23.5
5.4	23	22–24
5.6	24	23–25
5.8	24.5	23.5–25.5
6.0	25	24–26
6.2	25.5	24.5–26.5
6.4	26	25–27
6.6	27	26–28
6.8	28	27–29
7.0	29	28–30
7.2	30	29–31
7.4	30.5	29.5–31.5
7.6	31	30–32
7.8	32	31–33
8.0	33	32–34
8.2	34	33–35
8.4	35	34–36
8.6	36	35–37
8.8	37	36–38
9.0*	38	37–39
9.2*	39	38–40
9.4*	40	39–41
9.6*	Over 40	
9.8*	Over 40	
10.0*	Over 40	

* Probably mature fetus.

and a 25% chance that it is greater than 30 weeks. A complete percentile chart is available in Flamme's article.

It has been suggested that each institution should compile its own tables correlating biparietal diameter with gestational age, on the grounds that the shape of the head relates to race and standard published tables may be based on an ethnic group other than the one predominating at that institution. We have found this approach unrewarding. Altitude has an effect on fetal size. Term infants born in Denver, for example, at an altitude of 1 mile are smaller than infants born at sea level. Therefore, fetal growth tables based on populations living at high altitude are probably not applicable to populations living at sea level.

Growth-Adjusted Sonographic Age (GASA)

As noted on page 809, the most sophisticated means of allowing for the effects of biologic variation in the estimation of gestational age has been developed by Sabbagha *et al.* The technique requires at least two biparietal diameter determinations. The first is performed at or before the 26th week of gestation, a time when the biparietal diameters of fetuses of the same gestational age show the least variability. Owing to the constant motion of very immature fetuses, this determination is best performed with real-time equipment. The gestational age so obtained is tentatively accepted as the most probable gestational age of the fetus. A second biparietal diameter determination is performed at 30–33 weeks when the variation between large and small fetuses of the same age is greatest.

From these two determinations it is possible to determine whether the fetal growth rate is faster than average, about average, or slower than average. A fetus that is growing faster than average has a bigger biparietal diameter than an average fetus of the same gestational age, *i.e.*, a faster growing fetus is likely to be younger than an average fetus of the same size. Similarly, a fetus that is growing more slowly than average is likely to be older than an average fetus of the same size. Once the fetus has been reclassified as large (above the 75th percentile), normal (25th–75th percentile), or small (below the 25th percentile), a more appropriate gestational age based on a more accurate appraisal of the fetus' normal growth potential can be assigned. This technique has improved the accuracy of determining gestational age and gives 95% confidence limits of 1–3 days, as opposed to 11 days for the older methods.

Other ultrasonic parameters of gestational age can be used, including estimation of the cross-sectional area of the fetal skull or thorax and estimation of uterine volume. The standard tables for these methods are not based on as large a body of data as are the tables for biparietal diameter. They are useful when a good biparietal diameter determination cannot be obtained, or when retardation of fetal growth is suspected.

FETAL GROWTH RETARDATION

When fetal nutrition is compromised, the brain has first call on the available nutrients. Thus, measurement of the biparietal diameter is an insensitive means of detecting growth retardation. There are, however,

several ways to detect fetal growth retardation. One way is to show that there is a disparity between the size of the fetal head and of the thorax, since growth of the thorax slows more markedly than growth of the fetal head. One means of estimating this disparity is to calculate the gestational age from the biparietal diameter and then, separately, from the cross-sectional area of the thorax. If the fetal head measurements suggest a substantially greater gestational age than do the thoracic measurements, then growth may be retarded. (If the thorax appears too big, there is probably either measurement error or microcephaly) Serial measurements that demonstrate a progressively increasing disparity confirm the diagnosis.

Campbell *et al.* have used the ratio of the circumference of a transverse section through the fetal skull at the level of the third ventricle to the circumference of a horizontal section through the upper abdomen at the level of the umbilical vein to detect fetal growth retardation (Fig. 28–4).

Estimation of the volume of the uterus can also be used to diagnose retarded growth. It is assumed that the uterus is a regular ellipsoid so that its volume is given by the formula:

Volume (cc) = 0.52 × Longitudinal Diameter (cm) × Transverse Diameter (cm) × AP Diameter (cm)

The longest diameter in each axis is used. Measurements are taken from the inner margin of the myometrium. Care must be taken to ensure that the three diameter measurements are taken at right angles to each other. Conditions such as hydramnios interfere with this technique. Charts showing the relationship of gestational age to uterine volume have been published by Gohari *et al.* and by Levine *et al.*

The use of ultrasound in the detection of intrauterine growth retardation is also discussed in Chapter 41.

ESTIMATION OF FETAL WEIGHT

There is a correlation between fetal biparietal diameter and fetal weight, but the standard error of the correlation is large, being ± 400–500 g. More reliable results can be obtained by using multiple regression correlations with fetal biparietal diameter, transverse thoracic diameter, abdominal circumference, and abdominal cross-sectional area, as suggested by Campogrande *et al.*

PHYSIOLOGIC EVIDENCE OF MATURATION

Real-time scanners can be used to observe fetal motion; the pattern of motion depends on the stage of gestation. In early pregnancy, fetal movement is vigorous, continuous, and apparently random. As pregnancy progresses, motion slows and becomes intermit-

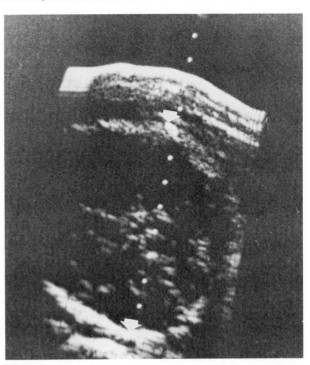

FIG. 28–3. Biparietal diameter determination. Image shows a straight midline echo, evidence that sound beam entered approximately at right angles to falx cerebri, and ventricular echoes adjacent to midline echo. Gestational age is determined from distance from inside of one side of skull to outside of other (*arrows*). External diameter of skull is greater than this distance by an amount equal to thickness of one side of skull, together with overlying scalp.

tent. Later still, coordinated, apparently purposeful movements, such as thumb sucking, develop. It has been suggested that the pattern of limb movement can be used to estimate the degree of functional maturation of the fetal central nervous system (CNS).

Fetal respiratory motion can also be observed with real-time ultrasonic instruments. First observed at about 12 weeks, breathing motion is initially irregular and infrequent. By 34 weeks, breathing is regular at a rate of 40–60 breaths/min. Fetal respiratory patterns are a sensitive index of the overall physiologic status of the fetus. Rapid, continuous respiratory motion at a rate of 120–200 breaths/min is an ominous sign, and death often ensues within 48 hours. Periods of apnea lasting more than 5 min, alternating with periods of gasping respiration, also suggest fetal distress. In general, the longer the periods of apnea, the slower the respiratory rate, and the more irregular the movements, the worse the physiologic status of the fetus. During labor, however, a 30-min period without respiratory motion is not abnormal.

Lack of all motion in the legs, together with normal

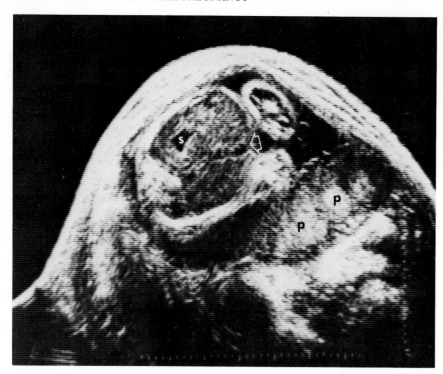

FIG. 28-4. Transverse section through pregnant uterus. Cross section of fetal abdomen shows stomach (s) and umbilical vein (*arrow*). Placenta (p) can be seen posteriorly. Fetal limb is seen in cross section, anteromedial to fetal body.

motion of the arms, has been described in a case of myelomeningocele. Unfortunately, periods of fetal limb and respiratory movement may be separated by periods of inactivity, so the examination may be quite time-consuming.

DIAGNOSIS OF MULTIPLE PREGNANCY

Multiple pregnancy is generally suspected when the uterus is larger than is appropriate for the duration of the pregnancy as estimated from the menstrual history. The suspicion of multiple pregnancy also arises if there is a family history of multiple pregnancies or if one of the fertility drugs has been used.

In early pregnancy, it may be possible to identify two separate gestational sacs (Fig. 28–5). With a real-time scanner, a vigorously moving fetus can often be seen in each sac. Later in pregnancy, the diagnosis depends on the identification of two fetal heads or two fetal hearts. It is important to demonstrate both heads in one picture (Fig. 28–6) to avoid confusion with a single fetus that changes position during the examination. Demonstration of two fetal hearts is useful, not only as confirmatory evidence of twins, but also as an indication that both are alive. The diagnosis of twins is easier and probably more reliable with real-time scanners than with conventional B scanners.

Commonly, one fetal head is a little bigger than the other. It is our practice to use the biparietal diameter of the bigger of the two fetal heads to estimate gestational age. As twins are ordinarily a little smaller than single fetuses of the same age, gestational age estimated from the larger of the two fetuses is still likely to be an underestimate of 1–2 weeks.

When only one fetal head is observed and multiple pregnancy is suspected, determination of the biparietal diameter can be used as an additional check. If the biparietal diameter suggests a gestational age less than that suggested by the menstrual history, multiple pregnancy should be considered as a possibility. Conversely, if estimates of the gestational age from menstrual history and from fetal biparietal diameter are in close agreement, multiple pregnancy is less likely. Provided reasonable care is taken in the ultrasonic examination, the diagnosis of twin pregnancy by ultrasonic means is highly reliable. It is a waste of time and a needless use of radiation to obtain roentgenographic confirmation of the ultrasonic diagnosis of twins. If three or more fetuses are thought to be present, however, x-ray films may be helpful.

PLACENTAL LOCALIZATION

Not only is the ultrasonic method of placental localization painless and accurate, it does not involve the use of ionizing radiation. The principal attraction of the ultrasonic method, however, is not its safety, but its accuracy and convenience. No other method currently

FIG. 28-5. Twins, as indicated by two separate gestational sacs within uterus. Within each gestational sac, fetus (*arrow*) can be seen. *B*, Bladder.

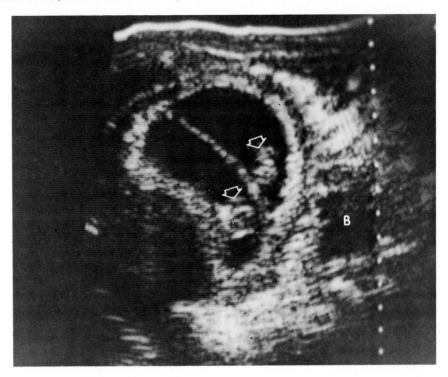

available allows such precise delineation of the placental margins. The cervix can also be delineated so that the relationship of the placental margin to the cervix can almost always be determined.

The patient is examined by transverse and longitudinal B-mode scanning with her bladder moderately distended. The degree of bladder distention is important. Inadequate bladder filling makes it difficult to demonstrate low-lying placentas, but excessive bladder distention may result in confusing appearances that resemble placenta previa. When there is doubt, additional views with a different degree of bladder distention should be obtained.

The placenta is characteristically a mural structure of crescentic shape; it is thick at its midpoint and thin at its margins. The inner aspect of the placenta is an epithelialized surface that reflects the sound strongly (Fig. 28–4). This inner margin appears as a well-defined, more or less straight line separating the body of the placenta from the remainder of the uterine contents. The placenta contains a more or less uniform cloud of minute echoing structures, which are probably placental villi. The nature of the internal placental echoes varies, depending upon the age of the placenta and the amount of calcification within it.

In early pregnancy, the internal placental echoes are similar to those of the decidua, so the location of the placental margin cannot be precisely determined. As pregnancy advances, the placenta thickens, its inner surface becomes more obvious, and the location

of the placental margin becomes progressively easier to determine. Posterior wall placentas are more difficult to delineate than anterior placentas because fetal parts interrupt the sound beam and the placenta is further away from the transducer.

Indications

There are three principal reasons for localizing the placenta:

1. When amniocentesis is contemplated, it is desirable to select a puncture site that is clear of the placenta.
2. Placental localization is useful in planning a cesarean section, since advance knowledge of an anterior placenta may be helpful.
3. Probably the most important indication for placental localization is third trimester bleeding. In general, ultrasonic examination does not indicate what other causes of bleeding could be, but it does demonstrate whether bleeding is or is not due to placenta previa (Fig. 28–7).

Placental Migration

The position of the placenta on the uterine wall may appear to change during pregnancy. This is considered due to different rates of placental growth in different parts of the uterine wall rather than to a true migration of the placenta. This phenomenon is of importance

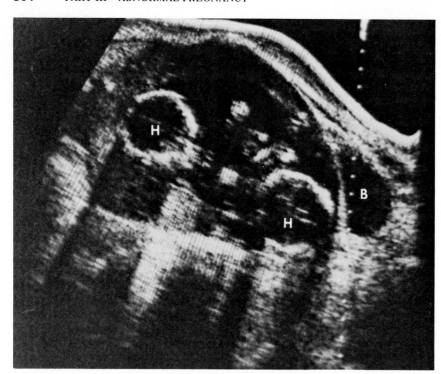

FIG. 28-6. Twins at 19 weeks. Two fetal heads (*H*) are demonstrated in single picture. *B*, Bladder.

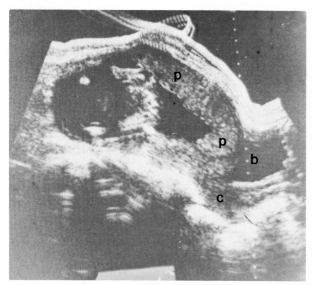

FIG. 28-7. Placenta previa. Placenta (*p*) on anterior and posterior uterine walls covers cervix (*c*). *B*, Bladder.

when a precise localization of the lower edge of a low-lying placenta is needed. Serial examinations often show progressive retreat of the placenta from the region of the cervix, and the physician should keep this migration effect in mind when assessing the prognosis of a patient in whom a low placenta is found in the late second or early third trimester. Later examination may show a more favorable placental site.

Placental Abruption

In placental abruption, the placenta separates partially from the uterine wall. It is sometimes possible to demonstrate an echo-free zone, representing blood, between the placenta and the uterine wall, which makes it possible to estimate the extent of the abruption. However, deep placental veins may have a similar appearance. Pulsed Doppler examination to detect blood flow may allow the distinction between abruptio and prominent veins. In most cases the diagnosis is apparent clinically, and such tests are not needed.

BLIGHTED OVUM

It is often possible to predict pregnancies that will abort spontaneously, although none of the various criteria of abnormality are necessarily associated with inevitable abortion. Real-time ultrasound scanners are more accurate in detecting fetal death than conventional B scanners. Lack of fetal motion after the 8th postmenstrual week strongly suggests that the pregnancy is anembryonic or otherwise grossly abnormal and likely to abort. When a real-time study suggests that abortion is likely, a repeat examination after an interval of 1 week is advisable in order to eliminate the

possibility that minor fetal movements were over-looked.

Other less reliable criteria of abnormality include 1) low implantation of the gestational sac; 2) failure of growth in the interval between two successive examinations performed at least 10 days apart; 3) an unsharp outline of the gestational sac; and 4) a thin-walled, small-for-dates, or irregular gestational sac.

HYDATIDIFORM MOLE

Hydatidiform mole is an abnormal gestation characterized by abnormal placental tissue, together with failure of the fetus to develop. A mass of trophoblastic tissue, often interspersed with blood clot, fills the uterus. A hydatidiform mole grows more rapidly than a normal conceptus so that the fundus is higher than expected for the duration of the pregnancy.

Ultrasonic examination provides a picture that is not pathognomonic, but is highly suggestive. The masses of grapelike sacs produce diffuse, chaotic echoes throughout the large uterus (Fig. 28–8). There are sometimes echo-free areas within a mole. Hydropic vesicles are echo-free and occasionally are quite large; also, areas of hemorrhage may be echo-free. The presence of bilateral multilocular cysts (theca lutein ovarian cysts) strengthens the likelihood of mole. Further evidence of hydatidiform mole is provided when a diligent search fails to demonstrate recognizable fetal parts. Conversely, identification of a well-defined fetal head or placental margin virtually rules out the diagnosis of hydatidiform mole. (The simultaneous presence of a hydatidiform mole and a fetus has been described, but it is extremely rare.)

A scan taken through a normal placenta can resemble a mole. However, other images from the same study, showing other parts of the uterus, readily allows the distinction.

Although a missed abortion may appear similar to a hydatidiform mole, it is usually possible in a missed abortion to demonstrate strongly echoing remnants of the fetal skeleton somewhere within the uterus. Occasionally, an exceptionally large hydatid vesicle is mistaken for an amniotic sac.

A submucous fibroid may have an ultrasonic appearance similar to that of a mole. This rarely causes confusion, because the clinical settings of the conditions are so dissimilar. Whenever doubt arises, a progress examination should be performed. A serum human chorionic gonadotropin level above 100,000 mIU/ml suggests mole.

Amniography (injection of radiographic contrast agent into the amniotic cavity) produces spectacular pictures in hydatidiform mole (Fig. 28–9). If it is needed, amniography can be used to distinguish missed abortion from hydatidiform mole. Contrast medium is very rapidly absorbed when injected into a hy-

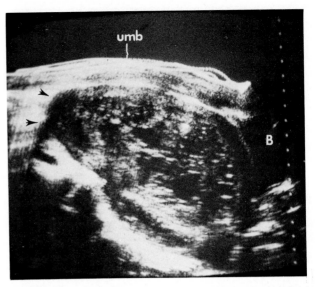

FIG. 28–8. Hydatidiform mole at 11 weeks. Midline longitudinal scan. Uterine fundus (*arrows*) extends well above umbilicus (*umb*). Uterus is much too big for normal 11-week gestation. Uterine cavity is entirely filled with mottled, structureless echoes. There is no evidence of fetal parts. This appearance strongly suggests hydatidiform mole. *B,* Maternal bladder.

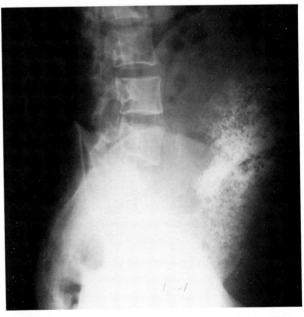

FIG. 28–9. Amniogram in hydatidiform mole. Steep oblique view (almost lateral) of lower abdomen. Contrast agent has been injected into uterine cavity. There are no fetal parts. Uterus is entirely filled with grapelike sacs typical of hydatidiform mole, outlined here by contrast medium. Amniography is no longer used to diagnose mole if ultrasound service is available.

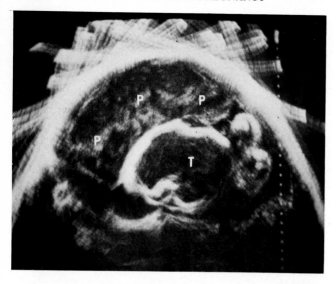

FIG. 28-10. Rh incompatibility, transverse scan 4 cm above umbilicus. Rh incompatibility is suggested by gross thickening of placenta. *T,* fetal trunk.

datidiform mole, but very slowly absorbed when injected into a missed abortion.

RH ISOIMMUNIZATION

There are several ultrasonic characteristics of Rh incompatibility: thickening of the placenta with irregularity and increased strength of the echoes coming from within the placenta (Fig. 28–10) are suggestive; edema of the scalp may cause a double skull echo; in severely affected (hydropic) fetuses, an abnormality of posture or a protuberant abdomen may be evident.

Spectroscopic analysis of amniotic fluid is the definitive method of assessing Rh disease, but ultrasound can make several contributions to the management of the affected fetus. Its most important contribution is to provide an accurate estimate of gestational age so that the optimal time for amniocentesis and delivery can be determined. Ultrasonic evidence of hydrops suggests that intrauterine transfusion is likely to be fruitless, as a hydropic fetus usually does not absorb the injected red cells from its peritoneal cavity.

FETAL DEATH

While there are ultrasonic signs of fetal death, the most reliable signs are not those of death, but of life. Real-time scanners have greatly simplified the evaluation of cases of suspected fetal death because they allow cardiac and limb motion to be readily assessed. Lack of all fetal motion during a 10-min period of care-

ful observation with a real-time scanner is strong presumptive evidence of fetal death. If the period of observation corresponds to a quiescent period and no limb motion is seen, the fetal heart must be sought. Fetal heart motion can also be recorded by an M-mode trace taken with the sound beam passing through the heart (Fig. 28–1). This technique is more cumbersome, but it can be used if a real-time scanner is not available or, if the fetus is living, if it is necessary to have documentary evidence of cardiac action at the time of the examination. Failure to demonstrate fetal heart or limb motion during a conscientious examination with a real-time scanner is strong evidence of intrauterine fetal death. However, it is evidence of a negative sort, and it is conceivable (although unlikely) that a beating fetal heart could be overlooked. A second examination, preferably by another observer, should be performed if any doubt exists. Other signs suggesting fetal death are:

1. Irregularity of the skull outline, due to collapse of the skull vault. This change, when it occurs at all, takes place about 7–10 days after death. Movement of the fetus during the scan, or inclusion of the facial bones in the plane of the scan, may also cause an irregular skull outline.
2. Loss of clarity of the fetal outline, together with a diffuse increase in the number and strength of echoes coming from within the fetus.
3. Abnormality of fetal posture, usually in the form of excessive flexion.
4. Lack of fetal growth, a sign that was much more important prior to the introduction of real-time scanners. Two serial determinations of the biparietal diameter are necessary to show that the fetus is no longer growing; if the biparietal diameter shows no growth after an interval of at least 10 days, the implication is that the baby is dead.

It must be remembered that a dead fetus may appear normal in a conventional compound B-scan examination.

HYDRAMNIOS AND ANENCEPHALY

Hydramnios, a condition characterized by an excessive amount of amniotic fluid, is associated with fetal abnormalities in about 40% of cases (see Table 26–1). The uterus is too big for the duration of the gestation. Ultrasonic examination demonstrates unusually extensive, totally echo-free areas in the uterus. The fetus may not be recognizably abnormal, but fetal parts appear isolated from one another as if floating in a vast pool of fluid. The uterine volume is excessive. When hydramnios is demonstrated, a special effort should be made to identify the fetal head. If anencephaly is suspected, a confirmatory plain x-ray of the abdomen is

FIG. 28-11. Fetal ascites (due to Rh disease). Longitudinal midline gray-scale scan. Fetal abdomen contains ascites (*a*) within which fetal intestine (*IN*) can be seen. *H*, Fetal head. *B*, Maternal bladder.

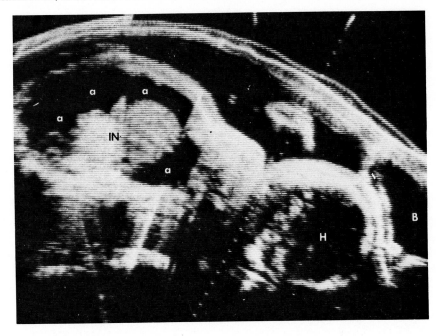

worthwhile, because the fetal head may be unusually low in the pelvis.

Very rarely, a biparietal diameter measurement may be obtained from an anencephalic fetus if the lowermost part of the skull develops despite absence of the brain and the rest of the skull. A scan in a plane immediately above the skull base shows the usual oval appearance. Failure to demonstrate the falx and ventricles may suggest anencephaly. Real-time scan usually provides better definitions of this anomaly than conventional scans.

OTHER FETAL ANOMALIES

Moderate and major hydronephrosis, and hydrocephalus can sometimes be seen. Myelomeningocele is best sought by a real-time scanner, which allows easy identification of the neural canal. Occasionally, other abnormalities can be seen ultrasonically, *e.g.*, ascites (Fig. 28-11) or a grossly distended stomach due to duodenal atresia. However, even major abnormalities cannot always be detected reliably by ultrasound, so a normal ultrasonic examination is no guarantee that the fetus is normal.

AMNIOCENTESIS

Ultrasound can be helpful in amniocentesis; when used as an integral part of the procedure it may reduce the incidence of complications by helping the physi-

cian to 1) estimate gestational age as an aid in determining the optimal time for amniocentesis; 2) localize the placenta; 3) localize the largest pool of amniotic fluid; 4) determine the depth of the amniotic fluid beneath the skin surface; and 5) determine the position of the fetal head, which should be avoided.

A detailed description of the technique of amniocentesis is provided in Chapters 23 and 41. The patient should be examined ultrasonically immediately after voiding, immediately prior to amniocentesis. It is best if the patient does not move between the ultrasonic examination and the needle puncture. Both the site and depth of the puncture should be determined. It is possible to monitor needle position with a real-time scanner. Special biopsy transducers have also been used to monitor needle position, but this technique is generally more trouble than it is worth. The distance from the puncture site to the posterior limit of the pool of amniotic fluid should be measured, and the needle should not be advanced beyond this depth; puncture of the rectum might result, leading to a disastrous bacterial contamination of the uterine contents when the needle is withdrawn.

TUBAL PREGNANCY

Ultrasonic examination in tubal pregnancy typically shows a modestly enlarged uterus that produces multiple amorphous echoes. These echoes, which are due to decidual reaction within the uterus, are not nearly as extensive or as prominent as those seen with hyda-

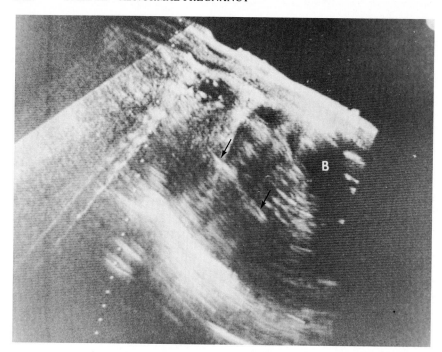

FIG. 28–12. Normal postpartum uterus. Uterus is enlarged, and uterine cavity appears as strong linear echo in long axis of uterus (*arrows*). This linear echo is good evidence that uterine cavity is empty, and there are no retained products of conception.

tidiform mole. No intrauterine gestation can be identified. In the adnexa, it may be possible to demonstrate a gestational sac, and there may be fluid (blood) in the pouch of Douglas.

About 6 weeks after the last menstrual period, the principal condition that causes confusion is a normal intrauterine pregnancy associated with a ruptured corpus luteum cyst, which may also produce blood in the cul-de-sac. At this early stage of normal intrauterine pregnancy, there may be decidual reaction and minor uterine enlargement, but no obvious gestational sac. Failure to demonstrate an adnexal mass does not exclude ruptured tubal pregnancy, so it is easy to arrive at a false diagnosis.

When the sac ruptures, its architecture becomes distorted, and it is often difficult to interpret the chaotic adnexal echo pattern. Bowel gas secondary to ileus may obscure the pelvic contents, making false-negative diagnoses more likely. If the adnexa are normal, if the pregnancy test is negative, and if an intrauterine gestation cannot be demonstrated, then tubal pregnancy is unlikely. However, there is about 70% chance of ectopic pregnancy when the uterus is empty and the pregnancy test is positive, regardless of the ultrasonic appearance of the adnexa.

The most useful contribution ultrasound can make in the assessment of suspected tubal pregnancy is to show an intrauterine gestation. Simultaneous intra- and extrauterine pregnancies have been reported, but this is so rare that the finding of an intrauterine preg-

nancy virtually eliminates tubal pregnancy as a diagnostic possibility.

EXAMINATION OF PUERPERAL UTERUS

Ultrasonic examination may be used to identify retained products of conception in the uterus (Fig. 28–12). The incidence of false-negative examinations has been reported less than 2%.

ROENTGENOGRAPHY AND RADIONUCLIDE IMAGING IN OBSTETRICS

The hazards of radiation are well known (see Chapter 60). For diagnostic purposes, a balance must be struck between over- and underutilization of x-rays. Neither course is without hazard, for underutilization of valuable diagnostic techniques results in failure or delay in diagnosis of a proportion of cases, while overutilization results in an increase in radiation-induced disease. When both the risks and the benefits of a study are imprecisely known, the task of striking a rational balance is particularly difficult. For instance, how often should an asymptomatic woman under 50 years of age

undergo screening mammography? This subject is elegantly considered in the paper by Swartz and Reichling.

For the clinician faced with a sick patient who needs prompt diagnosis, the decisions are generally simpler. The relevant facts for the clinician are that the commonly used radiologic procedures are of proved value, that radiation is not entirely harmless, that a fetus is more sensitive to radiation than is an adult, and that radiation to the gonads in those of reproductive age is likely to carry a greater hazard than radiation to other parts of the body. The clinician must ensure that any examination using ionizing radiation is the most appropriate examination for the patient, that it is performed strictly for the patient's benefit, that irradiation of pregnant patients (including the ones who do not yet realize they are pregnant) is avoided if possible, and that examinations involving irradiation of the gonads are minimized in young people. In addition, there are innumerable state and federal regulations that spell out in detail the minimum requirements for the safe use of radiation.

In radionuclide examinations, radioactive material is introduced into the body. Organs that selectively concentrate a radiopharmaceutical may receive relatively large doses of radiation. For example, ^{99m}Tc pertechnetate is taken up by both the fetal and the maternal thyroids. Thus, when organs other than the thyroid are studied, nonradioactive perchlorate should be administered to block unwanted thyroid uptake.

APPLICATIONS IN OBSTETRICS

X-RAY PELVIMETRY

The use of x-ray pelvimetry declined sharply when the genetic effects of radiation were first demonstrated. A further decline occurred in recent years due principally to (1) the declining use of midforceps delivery and, consquently, a lesser need for precise knowledge of pelvic architecture, and (2) the common use of simplified techniques that supply incomplete information. Clinical examination of the pelvis (see Chap. 30) can usually provide sufficient information.

Indications for Pelvimetry

If pelvimetry is to be used, it should be done either at term or, preferably, in early labor. The circumstances in which x-ray pelvimetry may be desirable are listed in the following. Pelvimetry is not invariably required in all these situations, nor are these the only indications.

1. Unengaged head in a primigravida in early labor. In about 25% of such cases, there is cephalopelvic disproportion at the inlet, and delivery by cesarean

section is required. In multiparas, the head may normally remain unengaged until labor is established.

2. Breech presentation if vaginal delivery is contemplated. A flat inlet and a forward lower sacrum are both unfavorable, a gynecoid pelvis is satisfactory, and a large anthropoid pelvis is best. If significant difficulty can be predicted at any level of the pelvis, or if the head is hyperextended, cesarean section must be considered. Ultrasonic cephalometry can be an important adjunct.

3. A history of difficult delivery. As a rule a second baby weighing 1.5 lb more than the first causes about the same difficulty in labor as the first baby; if the second baby is smaller than this, less difficulty should be expected.

4. Debilitating illness as a complication of pregnancy, together with a clinically small or unfavorable pelvis. If a difficult or hazardous labor can be predicted for such a patient, elective cesarean may offer the easier solution.

5. A pelvis distorted by injury or disease.

6. An irregular presenting part, the exact position and presentation of which cannot be determined clinically. A preliminary effort should be made to elucidate this problem ultrasonically.

Technique

A suitable technique for x-ray pelvimetry is described by Steer in *Moloy's Evaluation of the Pelvis in Obstetrics*. The 3 basic films that are needed are 1) a standing lateral film; 2) an inlet film, taken in such a manner as to show the shape of the inlet; and 3) a subpubic arch film, to show the splay of the sidewalls. A technique that provides less than this basic information cannot be expected to be helpful.

DETERMINATION OF FETAL ATTITUDE

A single flat film of the abdomen may be more satisfactory than ultrasound for determining fetal attitude, particularly in distinguishing brow from face presentation or anencephaly and in diagnosing hyperextension of the fetal head in breech presentation (see Figure 34–9). An x-ray film can also be useful if vaginal examination in early labor reveals an irregular presenting part. As a general rule, x-ray examination is used only if ultrasound fails to provide the necessary information.

ASSESSMENT OF FETAL MATURITY

Radiographic assessments of fetal maturity are much less precise than estimates based on ultrasonic mea-

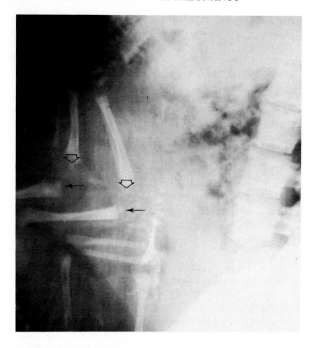

FIG. 28-13. Radiographic assessment of fetal maturity. Lateral abdominal film. Distal femoral (*black arrows*) and proximal tibial (*white arrows*) epiphyses of both knees are clearly visible. Positive identification of these epiphyses is reliable evidence of maturity. Nonvisualization may be due to immaturity or to obscuration of the epiphyses by maternal structures or inappropriate exposure factors.

surement of fetal biparietal diameter. If the x-ray films are of sufficiently good quality, lumbar vertebral bodies can sometimes be seen at 10–12 weeks, the vertebral bodies and skull at 16 weeks, the long bones at 24 weeks, the calcaneus at 25 weeks, and the talus at 27–28 weeks. The distal femoral epiphysis becomes visible at about 36 weeks, and the proximal tibial ossification center appears at 38 weeks and is well defined by 40 weeks (Fig. 28–13).

AMNIOGRAPHY AND INTRAUTERINE BLOOD TRANSFUSION

Amniography is the first step in intrauterine transfusion for hemolytic disease due to Rh incompatibility (see page 431). When water-soluble contrast agent is injected into the amniotic cavity, the fetus is outlined, floating in the opacified amniotic fluid. The fetus swallows the amniotic fluid; after a few hours, the contrast material dissipates from the amniotic cavity and concentrates in the fetal colon. The opacified colon serves as a marker during fluoroscopy so that the needle can be guided into the fetal peritoneal cavity. If the fetus is lying with its back anteriorly, the transfusion cannot

be safely performed. The fetus should be turned, or the procedure rescheduled.

Amniography may sometimes be definitive if ultrasound examination fails to diagnose a suspected fetal anomaly, or to distinguish between a missed abortion and a hydatidiform mole (Fig. 28–9).

RADIOGRAPHIC ASSESSMENT OF HYDROCEPHALUS AND OTHER FETAL ABNORMALITIES

Radiographic assessment of fetal head size is unreliable because neither the distance of the head from the film nor the angle of the head to the x-ray beam can be controlled or determined. Therefore, unless the head is markedly enlarged, a radiographic diagnosis of hydrocephalus should be regarded with caution. Ultrasonic estimates of fetal head size are far more reliable, and ultrasonic examination can usually demonstrate the lateral ventricles directly.

Other abnormalities of the fetus, such as achondroplasia and osteogenesis imperfecta, can occasionally be diagnosed radiographically *in utero*. The accuracy of these diagnoses is not known because the conditions are rare, and a negative x-ray is no guarantee of normalcy.

INTRAUTERINE FETAL DEATH

Ultrasound has virtually eliminated the need for x-ray in the diagnosis of intrauterine death. The signs that were formerly used to establish fetal death were the finding of gas in the fetal vasculature, liver, or skull (Fig. 28–14); overlapping of the skull bones (Spalding's sign; Fig. 28–15); and marked hyperflexion of the fetus, which appears as a crumpled ball due to loss of muscle tone. Of these, the only pathognomonic sign is gas in the vasculature, and this must be carefully distinguished from gas in the maternal bowel. If the fetus is found to be blurred and the maternal pelvis is not blurred, it suggests that the fetus moved during the examination and that it was living at the time the exposure was made.

ARTERIOGRAPHY AND COMPUTERIZED TOMOGRAPHY

With the exception of the assessment of choriocarcinoma, arteriography has little place in obstetric diagnosis, and even here it is rarely needed. Pelvic arteriography can define the extent of spread of choriocarcinoma. Selective hepatic angiography allows detection of vascular hepatic metastases, and response to therapy can also be monitored angiographically. The keynote of the arteriographic appearance of choriocar-

cinoma is hypervascularity. It may vary from small areas of increased vascularity to gross uterine enlargement with enlargement of arteries, early filling of enlarged veins, irregular vascular channels, stasis of contrast agent (tumor stain), and avascular areas that represent blood clot and necrotic tissue.

Arteriography is rarely performed for coincidental disease in pregnant patients and is best avoided in them, if at all possible. The radiation dose is usually large because a considerable amount of fluoroscopy is required to position the catheter for selective studies and because numerous films are required to record arterial, capillary, and venous detail. Multiple filming runs in several projections are commonly needed.

Computerized tomography (more fully discussed in Chapter 58) displays the minor differences in radiographic density between structures within the abdomen. It is particularly useful in the delineation of vascular masses. Intravenous administration of a contrast agent enhances the clarity with which vascular lesions, such as choriocarcinoma, can be demonstrated in the pelvis, the liver, the lungs, the brain, and elsewhere in the body. Computerized tomography is simpler to perform and exposes the patient to less radiation than arteriography.

RADIONUCLIDE IMAGING

Radionuclide placental localization was the only radionuclide imaging technique ever to gain popularity in obstetrics. The widespread availability of ultrasonic placental localization has rendered it obsolete, and at present it has no role in the evaluation of obstetric problems.

INVESTIGATION OF COINCIDENT DISEASE DURING PREGNANCY

The potential hazard of diagnostic radiation in pregnancy is such that certain guidelines are needed for the investigation of intercurrent disease in the presence of a known or possible pregnancy. The following rules may be of assistance in deciding when ionizing radiation should be used in the investigation of a pregnant patient:

1. Any radiographic procedure, particularly one that places the fetus in the primary x-ray beam, should be deferred until after delivery if possible. Intravenous urography, plain x-rays of the abdomen, barium enema examinations, and x-rays of the pelvis and the lumbosacral spine are examples of studies that place the fetus in the primary beam.
2. When it is necessary to irradiate the fetus directly, the amount of radiation should be kept to a minimum, primarily by taking as few films as possible

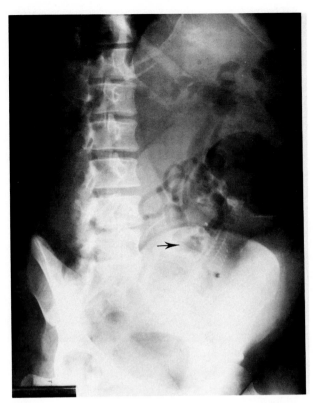

FIG. 28–14. Intrauterine fetal death. Spectacular example of gas within fetal heart (*arrow*), great vessels, and umbilical cord. Skull is filled with gas. These findings are pathognomonic of fetal death. Intrafetal gas may be much more subtle than this and may be difficult to distinguish from gas in maternal bowel. Fetal death is not necessarily accompanied by gas formation.

and minimizing fluoroscopy time. An image intensifier should be used for fluoroscopy. A camera that photographs the fluoroscopic image should be used in preference to a conventional spotfilm device. If possible, the examination should be recorded on videotape so that it can be reviewed as often as necessary without further irradiating the patient. This measure also ensures that the study is not lost if the films are destroyed by camera or processor malfunction.

3. Fluoroscopy should be conducted by an experienced radiologist. The clinician should personally consult the radiologist before the examination so that the nature of the problem and the suitability of the study are clearly understood by all concerned. Inappropriate and incomplete examinations can thus be avoided.
4. When possible, a lead apron should be used to shield the patient's abdomen.
5. Routine chest x-ray of pregnant patients is no longer recommended unless there is a clinical sus-

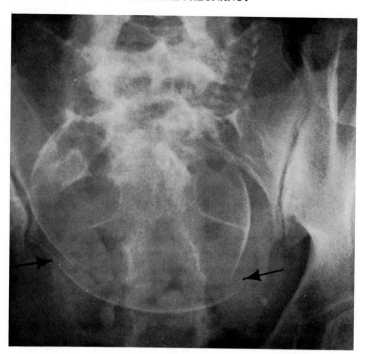

FIG. 28–15. Fetal death. Note overlapping cranial bones (*arrows*) (patient not in labor).

picion of chest disease. When the x-ray must be made prior to delivery, the examination should generally be restricted to a single posteroanterior film taken with the patient's abdomen shielded and with the x-ray beam restricted as closely as possible to the chest.

6. Examinations should be performed exclusively for the patient's benefit, not for nonmedical reasons. For example, if a previously obtained film has been mislaid, a diligent search should be instituted rather than a repeat film taken.

7. When members of different clinical services share responsibility for a patient's management, they should coordinate their efforts to ensure that duplicate x-ray requests are avoided. Most x-ray departments try to monitor requests; unfortunately, duplication errors are often detected only after a second set of films has been taken.

8. Examinations involving radionuclides should be planned sufficiently far in advance to allow adequate blocking of organs that might otherwise take up unnecessarily large amounts of radionuclide. This is true in all patients, but it is particularly important in pregnancy.

9. In the first 10–14 days after conception, a patient may not be aware that she is pregnant. Therefore, a brief menstrual history should be taken before any investigation involving irradiation of the abdomen is performed in a woman of childbearing age.

In young women, x-ray examinations involving the abdomen, pelvis, or lumbosacral spine are best restricted to the first half of the menstrual cycle, *i.e.*, to the time prior to ovulation. Some institutions routinely give a simple pregnancy test to all female patients of childbearing age prior to the performance of radiographic examinations in the belief that the test is more reliable than the history. Note should be made that the American College of Obstetricians and Gynecologists, after consultation with the American College of Radiology, the Food and Drug Administration's Bureau of Radiological Health, and the National Council on Radiation Protection and Measurement, has issued *Guidelines for X-ray Examination of Fertile Women,* in which it is stated that "there is no measurable advantage to scheduling diagnostic x-ray examinations at any particular time during a normal menstrual cycle" because 1) radiation-induced abnormalities are significantly less frequent than the natural incidence of anomalies and 2) the developing ovum is also at risk prior to ovulation. Despite this authoritative permission, most obstetricians continue to recommend that if there is no urgency, diagnostic x-ray examinations be made during the week after menstruation.

10. A careful history, a physical examination, and most biochemical tests do not involve any radiation hazard whatever.

REFERENCES AND RECOMMENDED READING

Amatuzzi R: Hazards to the human fetus from ionizing radiation at diagnostic dose levels: Review of the literature. Perinatol-Neonatol 4:23, 1980

Anderson RE, Ishida K: Malignant lymphoma in survivors of the atomic bomb in Hiroshima. Ann Intern Med 61:853, 1964

Anderson SG: Real-time sonography in obstetrics. Obstet Gynecol 51:284, 1978

Azimi F, Bryan PJ, Marangola JP: Ultrasonography in obstetrics and gynecology: Historical notes, basic principles, safety considerations and clinical applications. CRC Crit Rev Clin Radiol Nucl Med 8 (2):153, 1976

Baker ML, Dalrymple GV: Biological effects of diagnostic ultrasound: A review. Radiology 126:479, 1978

Brill AB, Masanobu T, Heyssel RM: Leukemia in man following exposure to ionizing radiation. Ann Intern Med 56:590, 1962

Brown WM, Doll R, Hill AB: Incidence of leukemia after exposure to diagnostic radiation in utero. Br Med J 2:1539, 1960

Campbell S, Newman GB: Growth of the fetal biparietal diameter during normal pregnancy. J Obstet Gynaecol Br Commonw 78:513, 1971

Campbell S, Thomas A: Ultrasound measurement of the fetal head to abdomen circumference ratio in the assessment of growth retardation. Br J Obstet Gynaecol 84 (3):165, 1977

Campogrande M, Todros T, Brizzolara M: Prediction of birth weight by ultrasound measurements of the fetus. Br J Obstet Gynaecol 84:175, 1977

Chilcote WS, Asokon S: Evaluation of first-trimester pregnancy by ultrasound. Clin Obstet Gynecol 20 (2):253, 1977

Cooperberg PL, Carpenter CW: Ultrasound as an aid in intrauterine transfusion. Am J Obstet Gynecol 128 (3):239, 1977

Ferrucci JT, Jr: Body ultrasonography. N Engl J Med 300:538, 591, 1979

Flamme P: Ultrasonic fetal cephalometry percentile curve. Br Med J 2:384, 1972

Garrett WJ, Robinson DE: Ultrasound in Clinical Obstetrics. Springfield, IL, Charles C Thomas, 1970

Ghorashi B, Gottesfeld KR: The gray scale appearance of normal pregnancy from 4 to 16 weeks of gestation. JCU 5 (3):195, 1977

Gohari P, Berkowitz RL, Hobbins JC: Prediction of intrauterine growth retardation by determination of total intrauterine volume. Am J Obstet Gynecol 127 (3):255, 1977

Haney AF: Fetal measurements. Perinatal Care 2:22, 1978

Hughey M. Sabbagha RE: Cephalometry by real-time imaging: A critical evaluation. Am J Obstet Gynecol 131:825, 1978

King DL: Placental migration demonstrated by ultrasonography. Radiology 109:167, 1973

Latourette HB, Hodges FJ: Incidence of neoplasia after irradiation of thymic region. Am J Roentgenol Radium Ther Nucl Med 82:667, 1959

Levin SC, Filley RA: Accuracy of real-time sonography in the determination of fetal viability. Obstet Gynecol 49 (4):475, 1977

Levine SC, Filley RA: Rapid B-scan (real-time) ultrasonography in the identification and evaluation of twin pregnancies. Obstet Gynecol 51:170, 1977

Phillips JF, Goodwin DW, Thomason SB, et al: The volume of the uterus in normal and abnormal pregnancy. JCU 5 (2):107, 1977

Robinson HP: Sonar measurement of fetal crown–rump length as means of assessing maturity in first trimester of pregnancy. Br Med J 4:28, 1973

Robinson HP: The diagnosis of early pregnancy failure by sonar. Br J Obstet Gynaecol 82:849, 1975

Sabbagha RE (ed): Diagnostic Ultrasound Applied to Obstetrics and Gynecology. Hagerstown, Harper & Row, 1980

Sabbagha RE, Hughey M: Standardization of sonar cephalometry and gestational age. Obstet Gynecol 52 (4):402, 1978

Sabbagha RE, Barton FB, Barton BA: Sonar biparietal diameter: I. Analysis of percentile growth differences in two normal populations using same methodology. Am J Obstet Gynecol 126 (4):479, 1976

Sabbagha RE, Barton BA, Barton FB, et al: Sonar biparietal diameter: II. Predictive of three fetal growth patterns leading to a closer assessment of gestational age and neonatal weight. Am J Obstet Gynecol 126 (4):485, 1976

Sanders RC: Letter to the Editor. JCU 1:344, 1973

Sandler MA, Sznewajs SM, Bityk LL: The effect of the distended urinary bladder on placental position and its importance in amniocentesis. Radiology 130:195, 1979

Scheer K, Nubar JC: Rapid conclusive diagnosis of intrauterine fetal death. Am J Obstet Gynecol 128 (8):907, 1977

Smith C, Gregori CA, Breen JL: Ultrasonography in threatened abortion. Obstet Gynecol 51:173, 1978

Spalding AB: A pathognomonic sign of intra-uterine death. Surg Gynecol Obstet 34:754, 1922

Steer CM: Moloy's Evaluation of the Pelvis in Obstetrics, 2nd ed. Philadelphia, WB Saunders, 1959

Stephens JD, Birnholz JC: Noninvasive verification of fetal respiratory movements in normal pregnancy. JAMA 240:35, 1978

Stewart A, Webb J, Giles D, Hewitt D: Malignant disease in childhood and diagnostic irradiation in utero. Lancet 2:447, 1956

Swartz HM: Hazards of radiation exposure for pregnant women. JAMA 239:1907, 1978

Swartz HM, Reichling BA: The risks of mammograms. JAMA 237:965, 1977

Thompson HE, Bernstine RL: Diagnostic Ultrasound in Clinical Obstetrics and Gynecology, New York, John Wiley, 1978

Wiener SN, Flynn MJ, Kennedy AW, et al: A composite curve of ultrasonic biparietal diameters for estimating gestational age. Radiology 122 (Suppl 2):781, 1977

U.S. Department of Health and Human Services: The selection of patients for x-ray examinations: The pelvimetry examination. HHS Publication (FDA) 80-8128, 1980

Wladimiroff JW: Real-Time Asssessment of Fetal Dynamics. In Bom N (ed): Echocardiology, pp 135–140. The Hague, Martinus Nighoff, 1977

PART IV

NORMAL LABOR

29

PHYSIOLOGY OF UTERINE ACTION*

David N. Danforth

The sole function of the uterus is childbearing, and its structural features, its position, its supports, and its physiologic reactions are designed to accomplish and to facilitate this single purpose. An understanding of the means by which this function is carried out requires a knowledge of the actions and reactions of the myometrium, and of the dynamics and structural changes in the uterus in pregnancy and labor.

* This chapter is a revision of the chapter prepared by D. N. Danforth and C. H. Hendricks for the third edition of this text.

THE CAUSE OF THE ONSET OF LABOR

Since the time of Hippocrates, simple causes or mechanisms have been sought to explain the onset of labor. As knowledge has increased, it has become evident that there is no simple explanation of why previously sporadic, haphazard, and wholly uncoordinated uterine contractions should suddenly, over the course of hours or days, increase in coordination and strength so that ultimately and inexorably the uterus is evacuated. In recent years, a resurgence of interest in this question has resulted in a prodigious literature bearing upon the many factors that are concerned in the regulation of uterine activity. As new data become available, it is apparent that the onset of labor results from the convergence of a number of factors, each of which, like the instruments in a symphony orchestra, must bear an optimal relationship to all of the others. Unfortunately, some investigators focus upon a single factor and declare it to be of preeminent importance as *the* cause of the onset of labor; however, all of the factors having to do with the physiology of the myometrium bear upon the onset of labor. Some of these are needed to set the stage for labor, after which others can act as direct or indirect precipitating factors.

THE PHYSIOLOGY OF THE MYOMETRIUM

The uterus possesses no intrinsic nervous mechanism akin to the Purkinje system of the heart. Hence, in the uterus the propagation of the contraction wave is after the nature of a syncytium, the contraction of one muscle cell tripping off the contraction of the adjacent one; the resulting wave spreads for variable distances over the myometrium. The ability of one muscle cell to "fire" when the adjacent one contracts and the distance the wave advances depend on many factors, including estrogen, progesterone, and prostaglandin (PG) influences; electrochemical phenomena at the cell surfaces; actomyosin and adenosine triphosphate (ATP) concentrations; electrolyte environment; stretch; and, apparently, the density of the postganglionic nerve axons, which varies according to the physiologic state of the uterus.

These factors are also responsible for the increasing reactivity of the uterus as pregnancy progresses. Oxytocin is the drug *par exellence* for stimulation of the uterus and for testing its reactivity. In early pregnancy, the uterus is exceptionally refractory to oxytocin; large doses are required to produce contractions even vaguely resembling those seen in early labor (Fig. 29–1). In the final weeks of pregnancy, the uterus becomes increasingly responsive to oxytocin, and by the time labor begins, it is exquisitely sensitive (Figs. 29–1 and 29–2). Doses of oxytocin that in early

pregnancy have little effect can, at term, produce the most violent and sustained tetany.

Much has been learned of myometrial physiology by noting the effects of administered agents and by testing the circulating blood for levels of critical constituents. In interpreting such studies, it must be remembered that the observed effects of administered agents, even if they are also produced *in vivo*, give no real information about the physiologic effects of the same agents as they are normally produced and secreted endogenously, and that blood levels of specific constituents cannot be used as a measure of endogenous production or release unless the rates of clearance and degradation are also known.

Properties of Uterine Muscle

The major properties of uterine muscle are the same as those possessed by smooth muscle in general: contraction, relaxation, coordination, and changes in length without changes in tension.

Contraction and Relaxation. Autonomous, spontaneous, rhythmic contraction and relaxation are inherent properties of all smooth muscle that clearly distinguish it from skeletal muscle. Such activity is of myogenic origin, and it occurs in completely denervated preparations and in preparations under the influence of ganglion- and nerve-blocking agents. Uterine muscle strips that have been refrigerated for 2 weeks in saline or Locke's solution quickly resume spontaneous activity when they are warmed.

Coordination. During pregnancy, prior to the onset of labor, the uterus contracts intermittently, sometimes very forcefully. These contractions, known as Braxton Hicks contractions, are totally irregular in duration, intensity, and frequency. Although they are "purposeless" from the viewpoint of evacuating the uterus, Braxton Hicks contractions do partially empty the uterus of blood and hence provide for the frequent movement of blood in the uterine sinuses and intervillous space. They also may be useful in moving the fetus about in the uterus and causing the fetus to move its muscles.

Braxton Hicks contractions are triggered from various parts of the uterus, most commonly in one or the other cornual area, and spread for variable distances over the myometrium. Some ultimately involve the entire uterus and may be just as intense as labor "pains," but most of them are propagated only for short distances.

As the time of labor approaches, the intermittent contractions become gradually more regular in frequency, duration, and intensity, and they are propagated for increasing distances over the myometrium. In labor, the most beautiful coordination is achieved;

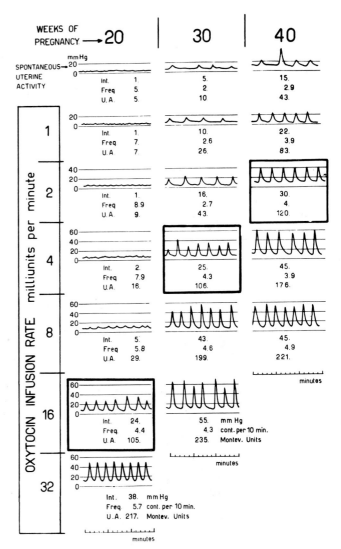

FIG. 29-1. Response to increasing doses of oxytocin adminsitered by constant pump infusion at 20, 30, and 40 weeks' gestation. Contraction pattern in heavy squares is within range usually observed in normal labor that begins spontaneously. Hypercontractility and increased tonus result from administration at excessive rate; this abnormally high activity may interfere with fetal oxygen supply and occasionally may even cause rupture of uterus. (Caldeyro–Barcia RC, Sica–Blanco Y, Posiero JJ, et al: J Pharmacol Exp Ther 121:128. Copyright © 1957, Williams & Wilkins)

the contractions are precisely regular in strength, duration, and frequency, and each contraction spreads uniformly to involve the entire myometrium. Thus, at the onset of labor the uterus is converted from an uncoordinated, protective domicile for the baby to a powerfully active and precisely coordinated unit whose

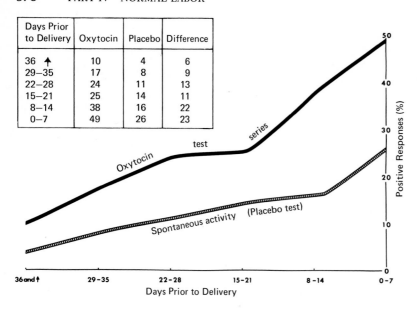

Days Prior to Delivery	Oxytocin	Placebo	Difference
36 ↑	10	4	6
29–35	17	8	9
22–28	24	11	13
15–21	25	14	11
8–14	38	16	22
0–7	49	26	23

FIG. 29-2. During final weeks before onset of labor, spontaneous uterine activity (*dotted line*) increases steadily, reaching peak in last few days before onset of labor. Response to a given dose of oxytocin (*solid line*) increases somewhat between 35th and 38th weeks; during 39th and 40th weeks, oxytocin response increases much more rapidly. (Hendrick CH, Brenner WE: Am J Obstet Gynecol 90:485, 1964)

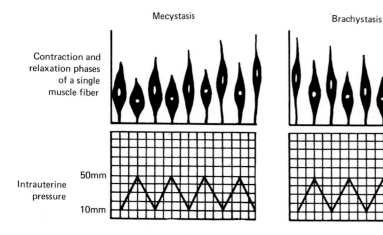

FIG. 29-3. Mecystasis and brachystasis. In mecystasis, as muscle fiber contracts, intrauterine pressure increases; with relaxation, intrauterine pressure returns to resting tone and fiber assumes longer length than before contraction. Reverse effect occurs in brachystasis.

contractions are designed to expel the conceptus. When labor is fully established, the process is inexorable: It does not stop, and it cannot be permanently stopped until the uterus is empty. (Some drugs appear to arrest labor for variable periods, but they are unpredictable and uniformly ineffective if labor has advanced to the point where the cervix is dilated 4 cm or more.)

Changes in Length Without Changes in Tension. Adjustments in length without changes in tension are essential for the orderly development of the uterus in pregnancy, as well as for the development of the lower uterine segment and ultimate evacuation of the uterus (see page 597). Such changes are by no means unique to the uterus. The stomach adjusts to accom-

modate a full meal without significant changes in intragastric pressure, and the urinary bladder can be partially emptied without significant change in intravesical pressure. These essential properties of smooth muscle are termed brachystasis and mecystasis. *Brachystasis* is a state manifested by a muscle fiber after it has assumed a relatively fixed decrease in length, at which length it resists stretch, contracts and relaxes, and manifests the same tension as before shortening. Brachystasis is the process whereby the longitudinal component of the myometrium shortens in labor, or "retracts," and accomplishes evacuation of the conceptus (Fig. 29–3). *Mecystasis* is a state manifested by a muscle fiber after it has assumed a relatively fixed increase in length, at which length it resists stretch, contracts and relaxes, and manifests the same tension

as before lengthening. Mecystasis occurs in the lower circular component of the myometrium to permit the unfolding of the lower pole of the uterus in early pregnancy and the formation of the lower uterine segment in late pregnancy and labor.

Effects of Distention and Stretch

Gillespie's classic diagram (Fig. 29–4) emphasizes the inevitability of the onset of labor. The fetus grows at a rapidly accelerating rate, more than doubling its weight in the last 2 months of pregnancy; uterine growth at this time is trivial, and the consequent stretching of the uterine wall reduces its thickness. The full import of this relation has not been enunciated, although it is certain that many of the uterine phenomena of advancing pregnancy are the direct result of myometrial stretch.

Most of the studies regarding the effects of distention have been done in the rabbit, and with a few exceptions they are considered applicable to the human. The important work of Reynolds on the effects of uterine distention can hardly be summarized in a few sentences, but some of his conclusions can be cited. Even in the castrated rabbit, uterine distention (by cylindrical paraffin pellets of known sizes) was found to constitute a specific stimulus to uterine growth. The number of cells in the myometrium increased appreciably, the cells were larger, and as many as 50 mitotic figures in metaphase were counted in the circular muscle of a single cross section of the myometrium (Fig. 29–5). When the distention–growth response was studied in animals treated with estrogens, it was clear that this hormone limited the capacity of the uterus to grow when distended. Hence, when estrogen is acting, distention is incapable of acting as a stimulus to uterine growth. Contrariwise, in progesterone-treated animals, the general effect was equivalent to that in the castrated animals; but, owing apparently to the uterine relaxation, much greater distention was required to produce equivalent effects. In sum, it seems possible to conclude, in general terms, that estrogen inhibits the growth response to distention, while progesterone enhances it. These observations have important implications when Gillespie's curves (Fig. 29–4) are considered in the light of estrogen and progesterone levels in normal pregnancy.

In addition to causing uterine growth, distention *per se* is also a direct stimulus to the mechanical activity of the uterus, causing an increase in the electrical activity and orderly propagation of the impulse (Fig. 29–6). This response has been shown to be enhanced by estrogen and depressed by progesterone, providing additional evidence for the importance of progesterone in accommodation of the fetus.

In the human, distention *per se* appears to influence the duration of pregnancy. Preterm labor is the rule in multiple pregnancy. The influence of distention is also

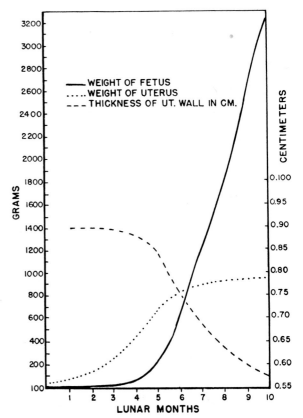

FIG. 29–4. Fetouterine relation. Note reduced uterine growth and progressive thinning of uterine wall as fetus develops most rapidly after 4th month. (Gillespie CG: Am J Obstet Gynecol 59:949, 1950)

important in the rabbit, where there is a direct relation between the degree of uterine stretch and the onset of labor. In this animal, a measure of uterine distention is obtained by comparing the total weight of the conceptus with the weight of the uterus: When this ratio reaches 1:1.5, labor begins (Fig. 29–7).

There is now good evidence that, in the estrogen-dominated uterus, the availability of prostaglandin $F_{2\alpha}$ is determined by the degree of stretch. With increasing stretch, the synthesis, myometrial concentration, and release of $PGF_{2\alpha}$ are all proportionately increased. Csapo *et al* found that the instillation of as little as 150 ml isotonic solution into the uterine cavity at term consistently produced increased uterine activity. The mechanism is presumed to be increased PG production and release as the result of stretch.

The foregoing observations indicate that uterine distention is *one* of the important forces that influence the myometrial changes of normal pregnancy and labor, although it appears not to be crucial. For example, in both the monkey and the rat removal of the fetus(es) leaving the placenta(s) in situ does not in-

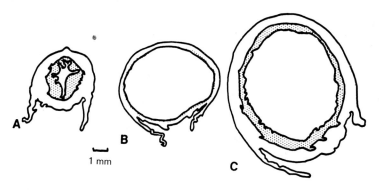

FIG. 29-5. Extent of uterine growth in untreated ovariectomized rabbit resulting from simple distention of uterus. A. Cross section of undistended part of uterus. B. Section of uterus taken immediately after distention. C. Section taken 2 weeks after distention. C is 161% greater in area than A, as measured with planimeter. (Reynolds SRM, Kaminester S: Am J Physiol 116:510, 1936)

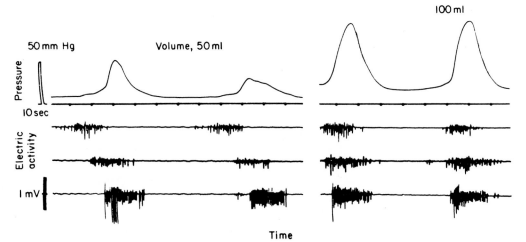

FIG. 29-6. Effect of volume changes on electric and mechanical activity of uterus. Note that, when uterine volume is 50 ml, propagation of electric activity from ovarian to cervical end is slow (~20 sec). Slow propagation results in relative asynchrony. Pressure is moderate and its development irregular. Volume increase to 100 ml facilitates propagation; uterine horn becomes active at its whole length within short period (~2 sec), resulting in synchrony. Synchrony in electric activity results in increase in pressure and regularity in shape of pressure curves. Rate of pressure rise also increases. (Csapo AI, Takeda H, Wood C: Am J Obstet Gynecol 85:813, 1963)

fluence the normal length of pregnancy; the placentas are delivered at term. Also, in extrauterine abdominal pregnancy, the empty uterus contracts at term. Perhaps, as in the case of distention and consequent stretch, some of the other factors that seem important, since they are operative in *normal* pregnancy, are not necessarily essential to the orderly structural and functional development of the uterus.

Effects of Estrogens and Progesterone

Estrogens have many myometrial effects, only a few of which can be mentioned here.

1. Estrogens are essential for the coordinated activity and reactivity of the uterus. After castration, the uterus becomes increasingly inactive, the organized pattern of myometrial motility disappears, the uterus becomes increasingly unresponsive to oxytocic agents, and atrophic changes begin. All these regressive changes are quickly reversed by estrogens. In achieving these effects, each of three classic estrogens is uniformly effective, but estradiol is most potent, estriol is least potent, and estrone is intermediate.
2. Estrogens restrict the growth response of the uterus to distention, as mentioned earlier.
3. The myometrial concentrations of the contractile protein actomyosin, its enzyme adenosine triphosphatase, and the energy source for contraction are all affected by estrogens. These relations are discussed below.
4. The resting membrane potential, which is a measure of the level of membrane polarization and, hence, of the excitability and conductive ability of the myometrial cells, is elevated by estrogens.
5. The innervation density, *i.e.*, the density of the ter-

FIG. 29–7. Relation of uterine distention to onset of labor in rabbit. With six fetuses (large litters), uterus weighs 480 g at term; with three fetuses (small litters), it weighs 280 g. Ratio of uterine weight to total conceptus weight gives measure of uterine distention. After ratio becomes 1.5:1, labor occurs. In human uterus simplex, ratio is 3:1. (Reynolds SRM: Symposium on Fertility and Sterility, Michigan State University, 1956)

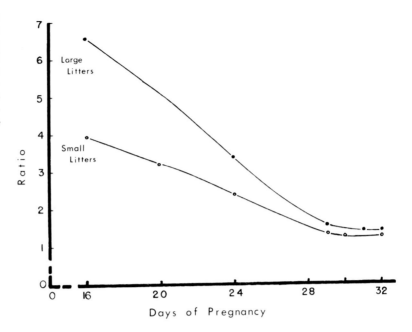

minal nerve axons, each of which makes contact with several myometrial cells, is increased by estrogens. Similarly, the concentrations of neurotransmitter substance (norepinephrine) are also increased.

6. Estrogens, notably estradiol, appear to cause the synthesis as well as release of $PGF_{2\alpha}$ from the uterus, and it has been suggested that the myometrial effects of estrogens are mediated through the action of $PGF_{2\alpha}$.

7. Under the influence of estrogens, the contraction wave is propagated in an orderly manner from one part of the uterus to the next. This is believed to result from the electrical coupling of the myometrial cells, forming a physiologic syncytium. The morphologic sites for the coupling (Fig 29–8) may be the "gap junctions" or "nexuses" where the sarcolemma of one cell is closely applied to that of the next cell, thus providing low-resistance pathways between cells. Formation of gap junctions may be initiated by rising levels of estrogens and PGs, declining levels of progesterone, or both.

The primary myometrial effect of progesterone is its interference with conduction from one cell or group of cells to another; it therefore prevents the orderly propagation of the contraction wave from one part of the uterus to the next, and tends to prevent contraction of the entire organ at the same time. This effect, termed by Csapo the "progesterone block," probably results from the sequestration of calcium in the sarcoplasmic reticulum, which suppresses both conduction and excitability. By this means, in addition to enhancing the growth response to distention, progesterone counters the stimulatory effects of both estrogens and stretch in pregnancy.

A theory that was popular for many years was that the normal onset of labor at term results from an increase in the production of estrogen and a decline in that of progesterone. Until recently, studies to clarify this relationship produced conflicting results. At present, it is generally accepted that there is no decline in serum progesterone before the onset of labor and that, although estrogen rises steadily throughout pregnancy, there is no abrupt increase in estrogen before labor.

Although there are some who dissent, most investigators consider Csapo's progesterone block theory to be valid. It is supported by recent studies in which preterm labor was effectively forestalled by prior administration of progesterone. In increasing dosage, progesterone is also believed to have been effective in preventing late abortion and preterm labor in cases of abnormal ("muscular") cervix, congenital lack of cervix, and septate uterus with a history of prior late abortion and preterm labor. More recently, Csapo has suggested that an antiprogesterone substance that blocks progesterone synthesis and is effective in inducing labor in the rat, may also be involved in the induction of preterm labor in the human. The fact that progesterone is not effective in stopping human labor is probably not pertinent. It is believed that, although small amounts of placental progesterone reach the peripheral circulation in the human, the myometrial inhibitory effect is largely achieved by direct suffusion of progesterone into the myometrium; when labor has

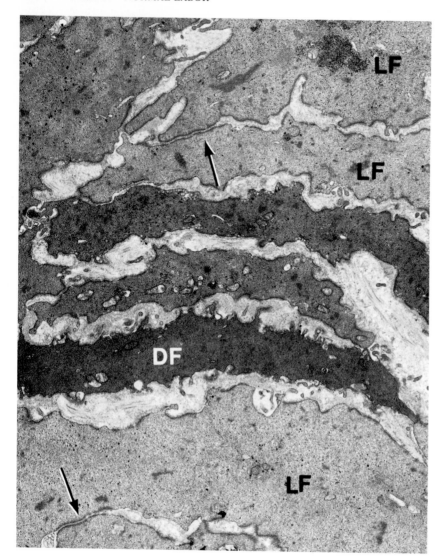

FIG. 29–8. Electron micrograph of human myometrium. *DF,* Contracted fibril. *LF,* Relaxed fibril. Thinned areas (*arrows*) probably represent nexuses or junctional gaps that provide low-resistance pathways between myometrial fibrils. (× 8000) (Dessouky DA: Am J Obstet Gynecol 125:1099, 1976)

started, systemically administered progesterone may not reach the myometrium in sufficient concentration to be effective.

Effects of Prostaglandins

PGs are synthesized in the microsomes of virtually all tissues from unsaturated fatty acids. When administered vaginally, orally, or by injection, PGs cause a variety of effects, but there is no agreement or real knowledge about whether these observed effects represent exactly the physiologic functions of normally synthesized endogenous PGs. They are widely distributed throughout the body, but are not stored to any extent and have an extremely short half-life of only a few minutes, being almost completely degraded by one circulation through the lung. They appear to act directly in the sites where they are synthesized. (One exception to this rule is luteolysis in the nonpregnant, and probably also the pregnant, animal, which results from $PGF_{2\alpha}$ that is formed in the uterus.) The release of PGs from cells has been shown to be enhanced by nervous, humoral, chemical, and physical stimuli. Indeed, mere handling of tissues can cause their release, as can the trauma of venesection or the clotting of blood, which must account for the spurious conclusions from some earlier investigations.

Administered PGs (notably of the E and F series) have been shown to enhance uterine activity and coordination, to lower the uterine threshold to oxytocin, and to produce uterine contractions that are virtually indistinguishable from oxytocin-induced contractions.

FIG. 29-9. Pathway for biosynthesis of primary prostaglandins, thromboxanes, and prostacyclins. Arachidonic acid "cascade" is shown in bold capital letters and bold arrows. Main rate-limiting step is activation of phospholipase A_2 (*top left*). Liggins GC: Br Med Bull 35:145, 1979)

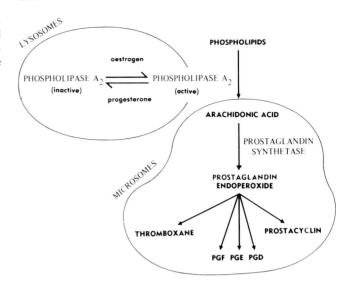

PGs of the E series have approximately ten times the potency of those in the F series. Uterine sensitivity to these substances is much greater during pregnancy, and they have been used to evacuate the uterus at all stages of pregnancy. Arachidonic acid, which is the obligatory precursor of PGs, has been used successfully to terminate pregnancy by intraamniotic instillation in the middle trimester, and it has been proposed that the release of this acid by the action of lysosomal enzymes may result in increased $PGF_{2\alpha}$ synthesis as a part of the normal sequence of events leading to labor.

Administered PGs have profound myometrial effects, but this does not answer the question whether endogenous PGs are normally concerned in the myometrial activity of pregnancy and labor. In all probability, they are, and evidence supports the several steps in the arachidonic acid "cascade" shown in Figure 29–9. However, the matter is not entirely settled; not only is arachidonic acid an obligatory precursor of PG, it is also a precursor of several other products. Its concentration in amniotic fluid increases significantly with advancing cervical dilatation in labor, but these concentrations appear to bear no relation to the concentrations of either $PGF_{2\alpha}$ or a major $PGF_{2\alpha}$ metabolite. Analyses for PG breakdown products may provide indirect evidence of PG production and utilization. Unfortunately, the data regarding serum levels of the $PGF_{2\alpha}$ metabolite, 15-keto-13, 14-dihydro-$PGF_{2\alpha}$, are conflicting, perhaps owing to differences in methodology. In one study by gas chromatographic–mass spectrometric techniques, slight increases were found before labor, marked increases during labor, and significant decreases after labor. In another study by radioimmunoassay, plasma levels of this metabolite and also an equivalent metabolite of PGE_2 revealed no minute-to-minute fluctuations, and their concentra-

tions were equivalent to those found in oxytocin-induced labor. This led to the conclusion that the rise in peripheral plasma PG metabolites is secondary to the initiation of uterine contractions of term pregnancy.

Although increases in plasma $PGF_{2\alpha}$ have not been found before labor, significant elevations have been reported during labor, with significant declines 2 hours after delivery. The maximum $PGF_{2\alpha}$ concentrations occurred between 100 and 120 sec after the peak of a uterine contraction and between 40 and 60 sec prior to the peak of the next contraction.

There is evidence that the major source of uterine PGs is the endometrium. During pregnancy, the decidual production of PGs must be balanced by an active means of PG degradation, which probably resides not only in the decidua, but also in the placenta, the myometrium, the cervix, and the fetal membranes.

The mode of action of PGs in stimulating myometrial activity and coordination has been the subject of intense investigation. As noted later, calcium ion transport is essential for uterine contraction, and there is evidence that PGs cause the release of some of the calcium that is bound in the sarcoplasmic reticulum. Indeed, the ability of PGs to alter calcium transport in smooth muscle as well as across other biologic membranes is probably the universal mechanism of PG action. It is known that stretch of the myometrial fibers causes an increased endogenous production of PGs, and it is likely that not only PG synthesis but also its cellular concentration and local release are functions of stretch.

Contractile System of the Myometrium

The basic elements of the contractile system are 1) *actin*, 2) *myosin*, 3) the high-energy phosphate com-

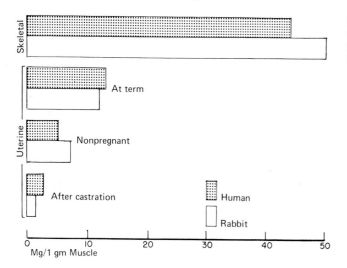

FIG. 29-10. Concentration of actomyosin in human and rabbit skeletal muscle and uterus. Note decreased quantities in nonpregnant and postcastration states. (Csapo A: Am J Physiol 162:405, 1950)

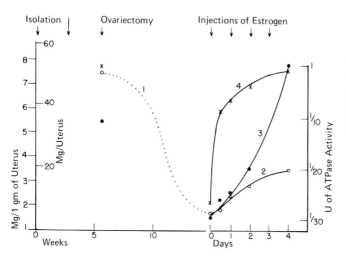

FIG. 29-11. Effect of castration and subsequent estrogen administration on contractile system of rabbit uterus. *Curve 1.* Loss of system by 2 weeks after castration. *Curve 2.* Concentration of actomyosin after estrogen administration. *Curve 3.* Actomyosin content after estrogen administration. *Curve 4.* ATPase activity after estrogen administration. Note beginning recovery in 12 hours; before this, estrogen causes hyperemia (in 30 min) and increase in water content (in 6 hours). (Csapo A: Am J Physiol 162:406, 1950)

pound *adenosine triphosphate* (ATP), and 4) the enzyme *adenosine triphosphatase* (ATPase). The myofilaments of the structural unit contain threadlike proteins; the thin filaments contain actin, and the thick filaments contain myosin. During relaxation, the actin filaments are separated from the myosin filaments; during contraction, however, the actin-containing filaments slide past and combine with the myosin-containing filaments, producing *actomyosin* (AM). AM is the contractile protein of smooth, cardiac, and skeletal muscle. ATP supplies the energy for contraction. ATPase is the enzyme that splits ATP in a manner that releases the required energy.

The working capacity of the uterus is determined by the concentration of AM, ATP, and ATPase. Uniquely among all smooth muscle, the myometrial concentration of these elements is influenced by the ovarian hormones. The concentrations are lowest in postmenopausal women and in animals after castration, but they are quickly restored to or even above their former levels by the administration of estrogens (Figs. 29–10 and 29–11). The concentrations are also increased by stretch; thus, for pregnancy, estrogens and stretch have a dual influence on the working capacity of the uterus. Through these actions, the myometrium in pregnancy is maintained in a "functional readiness" for contraction that increases as pregnancy advances.

As noted later, the contraction event is calcium-dependent, the interaction of actin and myosin occurring only in the presence of available calcium ions.

Effects of Mineral Ions

Much is known of the complex interactions of the mineral ions in the contraction and relaxation of smooth muscle. The movements of ions (notably Ca^{2+}, K^+, Na^{2+}, and Mg^{2+}) are fundamentally concerned in the regulation of membrane permeability, resting membrane potential, and membrane polarization, each of which is involved in muscle contraction and excitability. Movements of these ions have been shown to be influenced and, in the case of the uterus, controlled by estrogen and progesterone.

Calcium. The oxytocic effect of calcium was first noted by W. Blair Bell* and Hick in 1909. At that time, they stated that "we admit that we have been unable in our experiments to show definitely that labour *is* produced by the action of calcium salts in the blood, . . . [but] so far as we have gone we incline to the belief that calcium salts . . . play the most important role in this connexion." Like many of Blair Bell's prophetic observations, this statement is astonishing when considered in the light of present knowledge of the role of calcium in uterine contractility. Note, for example, a 1979 statement by Liggins, one of the leading modern students of the physiology of parturition: "Human labour is undoubtedly initiated by increased intracellular Ca^{2+} in myometrial smooth muscle, but there is less certainty of the factors causing the changes in Ca^{2+}." It has been demonstrated that available calcium is specifically necessary for uterine contraction both *in vivo* and *in vitro*, and that, without it, the uterus is not only quiescent but fails to respond to oxytocin or PGs; spontaneous activity and reactivity are restored by the presence of available calcium.

It is now well documented that calcium can be mobilized from intracellular binding sites for purposes of contraction. Chief among the binding sites is the sarcoplasmic reticulum surrounding the individual myofibrils; mitochondria and the plasma membrane and its surface vesicles are concerned to a lesser extent. The binding sites are considered intracellular compartments that alternately sequester and release Ca^{2+} to inhibit and to activate the contractile apparatus (Fig. 29–12). Calcium uptake by the sarcoplasmic reticulum is dependent on an energy source, ATP, and is mediated by an enzyme, ATPase (which is different from the actomyosin ATPase of the myofibril); as calcium accumulates, relaxation results. Fluctuations in cyclic adenosine monophosphate (cAMP) are also concerned in this process. Carsten suggests that

* In later years, William Blair Bell's name was hyphenated (Blair–Bell); his earlier articles are to be found under the name Bell and later ones, Blair–Bell. Blair Bell, the name that is now used, was cofounder, with Sir William Fletcher Shaw, of the Royal College of Obstetricians and Gynaecologists. Sir John Peel described him as a restless, ruthless, intolerant but dynamic torchbearer. He was preeminent among the obstetrician–gynecologists of the early 1900s.

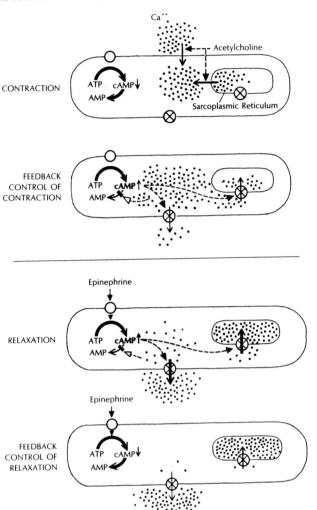

FIG. 29-12. Acetylcholine produces contraction of smooth muscle by triggering calcium influx into cytoplasm from medium and sarcoplasmic reticulum (SR). Calcium also serves as feedback control, blocking breakdown of cAMP by phosphodiesterase; increased cAMP levels then produce reaccumulation of calcium in SR. Epinephrine acts in opposite sense, triggering rise in cAMP that causes calcium reaccumulation in SR; drop in cytoplasmic calcium produces feedback control by unblocking breakdown of cAMP. (Rasmussen H: Hosp Pract 9:99, 1974)

cAMP may diminish the size of the calcium pool, leaving less calcium available for contraction and so promoting relaxation.

The contraction–relaxation event in the myometrium, like virtually all other calcium-dependent intracellular processes, appears to be modulated by *calmodulin*, the preeminent member of a newly discovered family of proteins that reversibly bind to calcium ions when the Ca^{2+} concentration increases in response to a stimulus. This induces a change in the shape of the

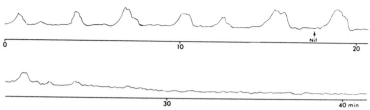

FIG. 29–13. External recording of uterine activity in a woman in 34th week of gestation. Cervix was effaced and dilated 3 cm. Nifedipine (*Nif*) was given orally in a dose of 30 mg. A transient flushing was observed after about 10 min, and there was an increase in pulse rate from 90 to 105 beats/min. Systolic blood pressure was not affected. Fetal heart rate was unchanged. Inhibiting effect on uterine activity lasted for more than 6 hours. (Andersson K–E: In Anderson A, Beard R, Brudenell JM et al [eds]: Pre-term Labour, p 101. London, Royal College of Obstetricians and Gynaecologists, 1978)

calmodulin molecule, which enables the calmodulin–calcium complex to bind to any of several enzymes, thus activating the enzyme and setting in motion the biochemical changes that produce the response to the stimulus. Marx observes that "calmodulin is hardly a household word, but in the world of cell biology it is one of the most exciting discoveries since recombinant DNA."

Progesterone enhances calcium binding in the storage depots, and this action may constitute the basis for the progesterone block. It is now apparent that oxytocin and PGs inhibit calcium binding in the sarcoplasmic reticulum. They also promote the release of previously bound calcium, and their actions as uterine stimulants are mediated through this device.

As would be expected, calcium antagonists severely depress uterine activity (Fig. 29–13). Although the several calcium antagonists seem to affect the calcium-dependent activation mechanism differently, it seems clear that they have in common the selective inhibition of the influx of calcium into the myofibril.

Effects of Nervous Mechanisms

The role of nervous influences in the control of uterine activity is poorly understood. For a time, this mechanism was entirely dismissed as unimportant because placentation, pregnancy, and labor can all proceed unhindered after transection of the spinal cord, after lumbar sympathectomy, and after section of all the extrinsic uterine nerves and removal of the uterovaginal ganglion. Indeed, Theobald refers to the report of Kurdinowsky which describes the onset of labor and coordinated activity that resulted in delivery of all pups by the totally isolated and perfused uterus of a bitch at term.

Although the foregoing observations are dramatic, there are important reasons why they cannot be interpreted to mean that nervous mechanisms play no role in the normal function of the myometrium. The first reason is the mass of clinical evidence in which the motor activity of the uterus is clearly altered by neural or reflex stimuli. For example, labor may temporarily stop when the husband or the physician first appears. Labor is rarely normally effective when the presenting part does not fit evenly into the lower uterine segment, *e.g.*, in transverse lie, occiput posterior position, or a severely asymmetric pelvis, or when the head is held up by inlet disproportion. Labor may start after administration of an enema, especially if it is large and somewhat irritating to the bowel. Stripping the membranes from their loose adhesion to the lower uterine segment can initiate labor (Fig. 29–14). The most efficient means of initiating labor is rupture of the membranes, but, since the withdrawal of 5%–10% of the amniotic fluid by transabdominal amniocentesis is not followed by labor, it is clear that much more is involved than simple adjustments of the muscle fibers and stretch responses. (It has been shown in both sheep and humans that manipulation of the cervix causes release of PGs, and that the augmentation of uterine activity as a result of such procedures as rupture or stripping of the membranes is more likely due to PG release than to the stimulation of nerve endings. Perhaps both mechanisms are concerned.)

The second reason to presume that nervous mechanisms may be important in myometrial function is that the short uterine postganglionic nerve fibers do not degenerate when the spinal cord is transected or when the preganglionic nerves are cut. Hence, intrinsic neural activity within the myometrium is retained despite section of the extrinsic nerves. Moreover, the density of this intrinsic adrenergic innervation and of the transmitter (norepinephrine) content of the individual nerves (each of which makes contact with many muscle cells) is altered by pregnancy and by the administration of estrogens and progesterone. The predominant transmitter substance is norepinephrine; little, if any, epinephrine is present. In essence, estrogens have been thought to increase both the innervation density and the norepinephrine content of the

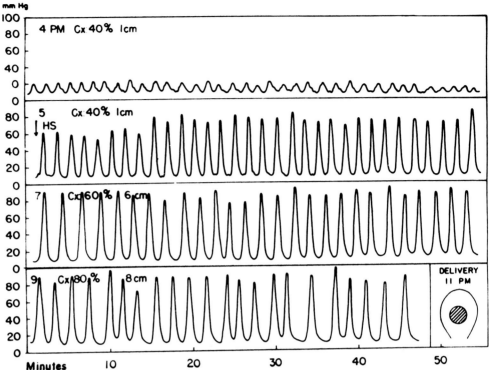

FIG. 29-14. Effect of "high sweeping" (*HS*), with rubber finger, on amniotic pressure. Original record taken from series of 50. All pressure tracings obtained through extraovular technique. Cervical progress is established by repeated vaginal examination. Placental implantation site is determined by manual exploration immediately postpartum. *Row 1.* Amniotic pressure before high sweeping. *Rows 2-4.* Amniotic pressure after high sweeping. Note increase in active pressure induced by high sweeping (in this case "active pressure area," increased by 11.6 sq cm/30 min). Labor was induced effectively by high sweeping alone, *i.e.,* without rupturing membranes and without oxytocin stimulation. (Al Csapo, H Takeda)

myometrium. The changes induced by estrogen can be reversed by progesterone. Both α- and β-adrenergic receptors are present in the myometrium, and the dominance of one over the other was convieniently thought to be determined in large measure by the hormonal status of the uterus, estrogen causing the α-receptors and progesterone the β-receptors to function predominantly. More recent work has shown that at term all fluorescent adrenergic nerves in the myometrium have disappeared and the norepinephrine concentration is reduced to almost zero. By contrast, the acetylcholine-synthesizing enzyme, choline acetyltransferase, is unchanged, suggesting both the presence of cholinergic nerves in the uterus and some possible function for them in the control of uterine activity.

There is much confusion about the uterine effects of stimulation of the hypogastric nerves and the action of adrenergic agents. The conflicting reports are due partly to species differences, which in this case are very real, and to differences in methodology. In general, the response to these stimuli appears to vary according to whether the α- or the β-receptors are predominantly concerned. In the case of the human uterus, it is generally agreed that a contractile response is initiated through the α-receptors, while a relaxation effect is mediated through the β-receptors.

Acupuncture is reported to be useful for either the induction or inhibition of labor, depending on the sites used for stimulation. If this should be confirmed, it is presumed that the nervous system must somehow be concerned.

Although the exact role of the autonomic nervous system in the uterus is not known, it is unreasonable to presume that this or any other organ would possess such a system if it did not have a real function in the control of its physiologic activity. What this role is remains to be seen.

Effects of Catecholamines

Investigators have long been interested in the effects of catecholmines on the uterus. In recent years, increasing efforts to control the activity of the human uterus in labor have led to clinical trials of the uterine response to many catecholamines and catecholamine derivatives. In general, the human uterus responds

according to whether the agents are α- or β-mimetic, as noted earlier: α-mimetic agents (*e.g.,* norepinephrine) tend to stimulate (and are sufficiently unpredictable to have no place in clinical obstetrics), while β-mimetic agents depress. Epinephrine activates both α- and β-receptors, the β-receptors predominating. The result is a depression of uterine activity; however, the uterus recovers after a time even during the infusion, suggesting later α-receptor activation. Also, a severe rebound occurs when the infusion is stopped. This fact, plus the profound cardiovascular stimulation, makes epinephrine impractical for clinical use as a uterine depressant.

The role of endogenous catecholamines in the physiologic control of uterine motility is not clear. The only direct observation has to do with the effects of stress; the blood level of epinephrine is elevated in the presence of marked anxiety, a circumstance that is reported to be associated with longer and less efficient labor.

The clinical use of β-mimetic catecholamine derivatives in the management of preterm labor is considered in Chapter 33. The β-agonists appear to act by stimulating adenyl cyclase and increasing cAMP levels, which leads to calcium binding in the sarcoplasmic reticulum, interference with propagation of the contractile impulse, and myometrial relaxation.

Effects of the Fetus

In normal pregnancy, the fetus exerts at least two influences on myometrial activity. The first of these is due to its bulk, which increases at an accelerating rate and provides the stimulus of stretch. As noted elsewhere, the factor of distention is not introduced until 12–14 weeks' gestation; after 16–18 weeks, the uterine wall becomes progressively thinner, and increasing stretch is an important factor in all of the subsequent myometrial reactions to pregnancy.

The second fetal influence is due to endocrine factors, the fetal hypothalamus, pituitary, and adrenal cortex being the organs most concerned. It has long been known that pregnancy is apt to be prolonged in the presence of anencephaly, a fetal anomaly in which there is usually no hypothalamus. The fetal pituitary is hypoplastic for lack of stimulation by the releasing hormones, as are the adrenals for the lack of adrenocorticotropic hormone (ACTH). The degree to which pregnancy is prolonged correlates with the degree of pituitary and adrenal hypoplasia. It is a reasonable conclusion that fetal cortisol is concerned in the onset of labor, and there are considerable experimental data to support this hypothesis: infusing ACTH into fetal lambs provokes enlargement of the adrenals, marked elevation of fetal cortisol levels, and the onset of preterm labor within a few days; in the fetal lamb, hypophysectomy, destruction of the fetal pituitary or hypo-

thalamus, or section of the pituitary or hypothalamus, or section of the pituitary stalk causes atrophic adrenal changes, and pregnancy is prolonged indefinitely; pregnancy is prolonged in the sheep and goat after bilateral fetal adrenalectomy. From the aforementioned studies, as well as from other data, Liggins has concluded that "the hormonal changes preceding parturition in the sheep consist of an increase of fetal cortisol, which acts on placental enzymes to cause a fall in the production of progesterone, and an increase in the production of unconjugated estrone and estradiol. This reversal of the ratio of progesterone–estrogen stimulates the formation of $PGE_{2\alpha}$ in the maternal placenta and myometrium." The myometrial consequences of the latter changes are outlined elsewhere in this chapter.

It seems likely that in women, as well as in sheep, cattle, and goats, cortisol is indeed related to the myometrial events surrounding the onset of labor, as exemplified by the clinical syndrome of prolonged pregnancy as the result of fetal anencephaly. The counterpart of this syndrome occurs in adrenal hyperplasia, and Turnbull has found that the weight of the fetal adrenal is greatly increased in cases of spontaneous, "unexplained" preterm labor compared with adrenal weights of babies born early as a result of antepartum hemorrhage, preeclampsia, or some equivalent pregnancy complication. In untreated Cushing's syndrome caused either by pituitary or adrenal neoplasms or by ACTH-secreting bronchial carcinoma, spontaneous labor occurs before the 34th week. In human labor at term, increased levels of cortisol are found in both the maternal and fetal circulation. The amniotic fluid cortisol also increases with advancing pregnancy; the steepest rise occurs after 40 weeks, suggesting that this value could be used as part of the evaluation of postterm pregnancy.

However, large doses of corticosteroids injected at or before term into pregnant women, into the amniotic cavity, or into the human fetus itself have consistently failed to initiate labor. Although the fetal adrenal appears to be concerned in the myometrial changes of labor in the sheep, its role in human labor is still not clear. If cortisol is indeed concerned, its influence appears to be mediated through its effects on progesterone secretion, with all the attendant consequences mentioned earlier.

Catecholamines, presumably of fetal origin, have been demonstrated in the amniotic fluid. The concentrations of epinephrine, norepinephrine, and especially dopamine are significantly elevated near term. It is not clear whether these changes have physiologic significance, or if they merely reflect the increasing contribution of fetal urine to the amniotic fluid volume as term is approached.

A question has also been raised as to the possible role of the fetal pineal gland in labor. Melatonin is

present in amniotic fluid in increased amounts at term, and the melatonin content of the fetal pineal gland is significantly greater during the 5 days before birth than earlier in pregnancy.

Effects of Fetal Membranes and Decidua

As noted elsewhere, arachidonic acid is the obligate precursor of PGs. Gustavii has proposed that the breakdown of lysosomes releases active phospholipase A_2, thus freeing arachidonic acid from the phospholipid stores and making it available for PG synthesis. It is also proposed that progesterone stabilizes the lysosomes of fetal membranes and decidua during most of pregnancy and that, upon breakdown, these lysosomes serve as a substantial source of arachidonic acid for PG synthesis. Liggins has suggested that this membrane mechanism may constitute a sort of "biological clock," genetically motivated, that may be part of the system determining the time of labor in different species. He also suggests that Gustavii's hypothesis may explain preterm labor in such circumstances as intrauterine infection, hemorrhage, overdistention of the uterus by hydramnios or multiple pregnancy, or rupture of the membranes, all of which could result in lysosomal disruption in the fetal membranes and decidua. Such a breakdown of decidual lysosomes could also explain the delivery of the placenta(s) at the correct time for labor after prior removal of the fetus(es).

Effects of Oxytocin

Oxytocin is a cyclic polypeptide containing eight amino acids and having a molecular weight of about 1000. It is produced in the hypothalamus and is stored in and released from the posterior pituitary.

Oxytocin is the agent *par excellence* for stimulating the uterus and for testing its reactivity. Synthetic preparations are used extensively for the induction and stimulation of labor, and the uterus becomes increasingly responsive as pregnancy advances. As noted elsewhere, oxytocin acts by causing the release of previously bound calcium from the sarcoplasmic reticulum, thus activating the contractile system. The clinical use of oxytocin in the induction and stimulation of labor is considered in Chapter 35.

Maternal Oxytocin. The hypothesis that labor is initiated as the direct result of oxytocin release from the maternal pituitary is no longer tenable. Concentrations of oxytocin in the maternal blood increase slightly as pregnancy advances, but there is no significant change at the time of the onset of labor. However, it will be recalled that the sensitivity of the uterus to oxytocin increases as pregnancy advances; increasing uterine responsiveness to unchanging oxytocin levels could have the same effect as an increase in oxytocin concentration. Late in labor, significant elevations do

occur in blood oxytocin, which lends credence to the old concept of the *Ferguson reflex* (spurt release of oxytocin in response to the stimulus of the presenting part on the cervix and upper vagina) and suggests a neurohumoral reflex that is still undefined. Further support is offered by the finding that such elevations are suppressed by spinal or pelvic regional anesthesia.

It is to be presumed that the oxytocin found in the maternal blood stream is of maternal origin, since Dawood found detectable quantities in the presence of an anencephalic fetus. With regard to the role of the posterior pituitary in normal labor, note has been made repeatedly that neither the onset nor the maintenance of labor is abnormally affected in patients with diabetes insipidus. In one case of idiopathic diabetes insipidus, a surge in plasma oxytocin similar to that of normal pregnancy was found during labor and the puerperium. In the interpretation of such data, it should be recalled that the defect causing diabetes insipidus may not involve the entire posterior lobe, or that it may be "nephrogenic" in origin, resulting from a tubular defect that interferes with water reabsorption. In cases where the entire posterior lobe is involved, oxytocin in the peripheral blood must be assumed to be either of fetal origin or to have reached the bloodstream directly from the hypothalamus. Among patients who have had total hypophysectomy, spontaneous labor is the rule, but no oxytocin studies of such patients have been reported.

Fetal Oxytocin. Evidence continues to accumulate to suggest that oxytocin from the fetal pituitary may affect uterine action, especially in labor. It was noted earlier that in anencephaly and after fetal hypophysectomy, labor is usually delayed or may be prevented. Perhaps this is due to the resulting adrenal atrophy with the loss of fetal cortisol and disruption of estrogen synthesis; or perhaps it is due to the lack of fetal oxytocin. During spontaneous labor, umbilical cord blood contains far higher concentrations of oxytocin than does maternal blood, and the concentration in umbilical artery blood is about two times that of blood in the umbilical vein. In the presence of an anencephalic fetus, oxytocin is not found in the umbilical circulation. These observations suggest a considerable production of oxytocin by the fetal pituitary and a significant flow of oxytocin from the fetus to the placenta. It is of interest that high levels of oxytocin have been reported in amniotic fluid (mean concentration 275 pg/ml before labor and 695 pg/ml during labor), in fetal urine (1800 pg/ml), and in wet meconium (80,000–175,000 pg/ml).

The placenta is an important source of enzymes that destroy oxytocin. Accordingly, fetal oxytocin would probably be suffused into the myometrium across the fetal membranes, rather than introduced into the maternal circulation through the placenta. One of these enzymes, oxytocinase, appears in the plasma of preg-

nant women. It is produced only in the placenta of the primate, with plasma levels rising throughout pregnancy to term. It rapidly inactivates oxytocin; this fact has led many workers to the belief that oxytocinase serves to protect pregnancy through prompt inactivation of any oxytocin suddenly released to the bloodstream and, consequently, to prevent excessive uterine activity. The presence of abnormally large or abnormally small amounts of the enzyme has been postulated as a possible explanation for a wide spectrum of clinical problems, such as preterm labor, inefficient labor, and failure of the uterus to respond within normal limits to exogenous oxytocin.

However, the metabolism of oxytocin is very rapid in males and in nonpregnant females, as well as in pregnant females. Oxytocin is excreted in the maternal urine and also appears to be inactivated in kidney tissues. Therefore, while oxytocinase is undeniably present in the plasma of pregnant women, its clinical importance remains undemonstrated, especially since the high concentrations of oxytocin in amniotic fluid suggest that the most direct route by which fetal oxytocin could reach the myometrium is suffusion through the fetal membranes.

THE ONSET OF LABOR

When the Gillespie curves (Fig. 29–4) are examined, it is obvious that the continuation of pregnancy beyond a given point is impossible, for the uterus must either empty or rupture. Moreover, it seems clear that nature's design for the duration of pregnancy must be unique for each species; in the evolutionary scale, as brain and head size increased, the pelvis became smaller. This, as Page has pointed out, posed a serious problem for the higher phyla, for delivery must occur before the fetal head becomes so large it cannot traverse the pelvis. In the case of *Homo sapiens*, the solution was delivery at a time when, compared with most other mammals, the fetus is approximately 1 year preterm—judged by such parameters as the development

of enzyme systems; neuromuscular coordination; ability to stand, communicate, and forage for food; and other attainments not achieved by the human until about 1 year of age. These observations lend credence to the probability that the timing of the changes leading to labor is set by a "genetic clock" that is unique for each species.

As new data become available, it is apparent that the onset of labor results from the gradual convergence of a number of factors, each of which must bear an optimal relation to all the others. According to the classic theory of Csapo, the gradually accelerating factors that tend to stimulate coordinated uterine activity are effectively counterbalanced during pregnancy by the similarly increasing production of progesterone (Fig. 29–15). The stimulatory factors include the consequences of increasing estrogens and stretch, the development of the contractile system, the increasing availability of PGs, and the continuing availability of oxytocin. The ability of progesterone to counterbalance these factors and to "block" the development of coordinated contractions appears to be twofold. Progesterone stabilizes the pools of calcium in the sarcoplasmic reticulum, making them unavailable for activation of the contractile system; also, progesterone may change the membrane potentials such that the threshold to the stimulating effects of oxytocin and PGs is raised. Oxytocin and PGs have effects that are opposite to those of progesterone, causing calcium mobilization and lowering of membrane potentials. Key words are *progesterone dominance*: as long as progesterone dominates the scene, uterine activity in pregnancy is limited to the sporadic and incoordinated Braxton Hicks contractions; when the balance shifts so the simulatory factors are dominant, labor starts.

Evidence is accumulating to support the hypothesis that the lysosomes of the fetal membranes and decidua serve as a primary source of arachidonic acid for PG synthesis. It has been proposed that progesterone receptors appear in the fetal membranes, competing with the lysosomes for progesterone. As a consequence, the lysosomes become more fragile, their con-

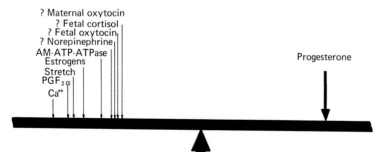

FIG. 29–15. Oversimplified summary of regulatory mechanism of pregnant uterus, illustrating balance between stimulants and suppressor. As pregnancy advances, gradual increase in progesterone balances (and effectively negates) influence of gradually increasing stimulants. At term, progesterone dominance gives way, and stimulatory factors are unopposed. *AM*, Actomyosin. (Al Csapo)

? Maternal oxytocin
? Fetal cortisol
? Fetal oxytocin
? Norepinephrine
AM-ATP-ATPase
Estrogens
Stretch
PGF$_{2\alpha}$
Ca^{++}

Progesterone

tents spill, PGs are produced in quantity, and the progesterone dominance gives way. As noted before, this thesis is attractive, since rupture of membrane and decidual lysosomes could explain the onset of labor after such insults as rupture or stripping of the membranes, intrauterine infection, the instillation of hypertonic saline for late abortion, or the trauma and hypoxia associated with preterm separation of the placenta.

The determination of the cause of the onset of labor is not merely an academic exercise, for it is through this knowledge that the most pressing clinical problem in obstetrics will be answered—the absolute control of uterine contractility, that is, the ability to start coordinated contractions at will or to stop them at will. The first may have been solved already, for oxytocin and PGs may be the ultimate agents for producing coordinated uterine contractions. The second, the ability to arrest coordinated contractions with equal precision and predictability, remains for the future. As more is learned of the factors that normally converge to produce labor, it will be possible to intervene with precision at some point in the cascade of events, and so to terminate labor that is established or to prevent it among those who are predisposed to preterm labor.

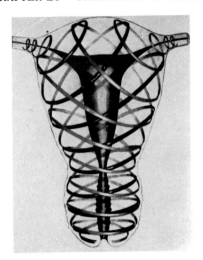

FIG. 26-16. Architecture of nonpregnant uterus. Note spiral course and bilateral symmetric arrangement of muscle fibers in planes of different inclination. Fibers cross each other at right angles in upper segment but at obtuse angles in lower segment. (Goerttler K: Gegenbaurs Morphologisches Jahrbuch 65:45, 1930)

UTERINE RESPONSES TO PREGNANCY AND LABOR

The two parts of the uterus, the corpus and the cervix, react differently to pregnancy. It is important to remember that 1) the corpus is composed basically of muscle, the cervix of connective tissue; and 2) the corpus undergoes growth and is subject to distention, while the cervix, although slightly softened, maintains its continuity as a relatively firm, more or less closed, fibrous ring until pregnancy terminates. The corpus thus functions to *contain* the products of conception, the cervix to *retain* them.

STRUCTURAL CHANGES IN PREGNANCY

The nonpregnant uterus weighs 60–80 g; the term uterus, 900–1200 g. This enormous increase is due almost entirely to proliferation of the myometrium. In early pregnancy (but not past the 3rd month), there is hyperplasia of the muscle cells, and mitotic figures are common. In the second and third trimesters, uterine growth is due almost entirely to hypertrophy, the individual muscle cells increasing in length 10–12 times, in width 2–7 times.

Uterine growth in pregnancy results from two major factors: 1) hormonal effects, which alone are operative until 12–14 weeks' gestation, and 2) distention and consequent stretching, which begins at about the 4th month of pregnancy. The proliferation of new muscle bundles is accounted for by the influence of estrogens.

The proliferatioin of new fibers comes to an end as the progesterone level increases. Further growth is primarily a hypertrophic response to distention and is enhanced by progesterone.

Architecture and Development of the Myometrium

Goerttler has clarified the architectural arrangement of the myometrium. In the unfused uterus (*e.g.*, rabbit) the muscle bundles in each uterus take a spiral course from outside in and from above downward. Similar systems are present in the fused (primate) uterus, one arising in each uterine cornu, proceeding caudad, and interdigitating as they approach the midportion of the corpus (Fig. 29–16). In the middle and upper portions of the corpus the two systems are at right angles to one another; in the lower corpus they are almost parallel. These relations are accentuated as pregnancy advances, and it seems clear that in labor a uterine contraction in the mid or upper portion of the corpus would tend to pull upward on the more transversely arranged bundles of the lower pole of the uterus. It is, therefore, convenient to refer to the *upper longitudinal component* of the myometrium, which pulls cephalad on the *lower circular or transverse component*.

In early pregnancy, the fundus becomes increasingly convex, owing to the upward pushing of the proliferating muscle. Consequently, the tubes and round ligaments insert at an increasingly lower point in the corpus as pregnancy advances. In addition, the corpus

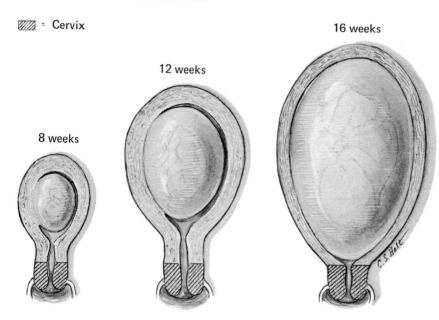

▨ = Cervix

8 weeks

12 weeks

16 weeks

FIG. 29–17. Changes in corpus relative to cervix in early pregnancy. Cervix, cross-hatched in diagram, is principally fibrous and exhibits little change in this period. Corpus, principally muscular, undergoes marked growth, and at 12 weeks, the fact that conceptus has not yet expanded to fill growing uterus results in lengthening isthmic segment. Then, with accelerating fetal growth, this space is taken up by 16th week. Unfolding normally stops at fibrous cervix, where adaptive relaxation is not possible. (Danforth DN: Am J Obstet Gynecol 53:541, 1947)

becomes globular, rather than flattened as before pregnancy, and the uterine cavity enlarges. In the first and part of the second trimesters, these changes occur almost precisely symmetrically so that the uterine appendages insert at the same level in the exact midfrontal plane of the corpus. A uterine abnormality or a uterine tumor (fibroid) in pregnancy is suggested by asymmetry of the uterus or irregularity in the attachment of its appendages.

In the first 12–14 weeks of pregnancy, the myometrium grows at a faster rate than the conceptus. On bimanual examination the corpus is felt to be softened and enlarged. *Hegar's sign* (see page 356) can usually be elicited between 5 and 10 weeks. At about 14 weeks, the conceptus begins to grow at a more rapid rate than the corpus. The reflected decidua comes in contact with the parietal decidua, and the isthmic segment "unfolds" (Fig. 29–17); because of the resulting distention, pressure is exerted upon the cervix. If the cervix is normal and is able to resist this pressure, the pregnancy continues; if it is structurally abnormal or sufficiently injured by a prior pregnancy, late abortion results.

The unfolding of the lower pole of the uterus to receive the enlarging conceptus involves mecystatic adjustments in length of the lower circular component of the myometrium that are similar to those that occur in the urinary bladder as it fills and in the stomach as a meal is eaten. As the fibers lengthen circumferentially, the thickness of the involved area is reduced, and for the remainder of pregnancy the myometrium at the lower pole of the uterus is somewhat thinner than in the midportion and the fundus. The transition is extremely gradual and does not necessarily bear any re-

lation to the site of the former anatomic internal os.

As a rule, 1) the uterus can be readily palpated abdominally at 3 months' gestation, 2) the fundus reaches the level of the umbilicus at 5 months' gestation, and 3) the uterus reaches the level of the costal margins and the xiphoid at 8+ months' gestation and drops slightly thereafter as the presenting part engages in the pelvis during the last week or so of pregnancy.

After 5 months' gestation, as the uterus grows, it gradually turns to the right. This *dextrorotation* is usually attributed to the presence of the sigmoid colon on the left and is of practical importance at the time of cesarean section, since immediately beneath a midline abdominal incision the blood vessels of the left broad ligament may be encountered.

Along with the changes in size and thickness of the myometrium, striking changes occur in the blood vessels of the corpus. The uterine arteries undergo considerable enlargement, and there is an enormous increase in the size and capacity of the ovarian vessels. Particularly in the region of the placental site, the radial arteries that traverse the myometrium enlarge considerably and form the large trunks that open into the intervillous space.

The uterus is traversed by large veins, which not only empty the placenta at its base and its margins but also carry off the large blood supply afforded the uterine muscle. Although there is some information about the gross blood flow through the uterus at term, it has not yet been possible to sort out what proportion of this goes to the intervillous space and what proportion to the uterine muscle. It is not unusual to encounter large venous sinuses in the uterine wall opposite the

location of the placenta; indeed, the blood loss from these sinuses may account for most of the bleeding at the time of cesarean section, which usually amounts to at least 500 ml.

At term, the venous blood from the uterus traverses the broad ligament in large blood vessels, many of them greater than 2 cm in diameter. Some vessels drain upward through the infundibulopelvic ligaments, but most proceed to the pelvic sidewall where they join the hypogastric vein. Although it is not improper to speak of the uerine artery, there is no such structure as the uterine vein; the veins are always multiple. These large veins are remarkably thin walled and are often located directly under the posterior peritoneum of the broad ligament. Although they are unusual, ruptures into the peritoneal cavity and fatal hemoperitoneum have been reported.

STRUCTURAL CHANGES IN LABOR

The structural changes that occur in the uterus in order to make possible its orderly evacuation at term have been the subject of much study and speculation. Unfortunately, it is not possible to watch the uterus directly as it undergoes these changes, or even to study it with contrast media and x-ray as the stomach and other hollow viscera can be studied. The methods of studying uterine contractions have provided an excellent and probably a true picture of the contraction patterns and activities of the different parts of the uterus, but the structural changes produced are more difficult to determine. One means of determining such changes is by examination of intact uteri at the different stages of labor, but such specimens are (fortunately) unusual in the human being; when they do occur, the manipulations needed for excising them distort not only the uterus itself but its relation to the pelvic landmarks. Frozen sagittal sections in the human being are even more rare, but 60–70 of them have been published, most of these near the turn of the century. The freezing techniques were slow, and the obstetric problems they portrayed were often horrendous. An example of such a specimen is shown in Figure 35–15. An alternative, which can probably be interpreted directly in terms of the structural changes in the human uterus, is the examination of frozen sagittal sections made during labor in *Macaca rhesus* or other primate having a fused uterus simplex like that of the human being. Distortion of the uterus necessarily enters here too, for the rapid freezing methods must cause significant contraction of the tissue. However, the results are informative and appear to give much insight into the structural changes of labor.

The monkey uterus is like the human uterus except for the presence of an inner lip or colliculus at the superior extremity of the cervix. This does not hamper the observations, but rather is helpful, for it can be used to mark on the intact specimen the exact upper end of the cervix. A second important feature of pregnancy in *Macaca rhesus* is that the placenta is bidiscoidal, the two disks being of about equal size, one attached to the anterior aspect of the corpus and one to the posterior. The two disks are connected by vessels that traverse one lateral aspect of the uterine cavity. A series of these frozen sections is shown in Figures 29–18 through 29–27. Although the concern here is with the uterus, these sections also show the relation of the bladder to the pelvis and uterus; the great length of the vagina in the second stage; the effectiveness of the forewaters as a dilating wedge when the membranes are intact (in Fig. 29–20 the membranes have hourglassed through and not only are of no use but may be hazardous if an edge of the placenta should be pulled off); and the placental stage of labor (in Fig. 29–26 part of the placenta can be seen in the vagina immediately after delivery).

These sections show that, during the first stage of labor, the lower pole of the uterus is gradually pulled up over the presenting part and there is no appreciable advancement of the head until the cervix is fully dilated. They demonstrate that, beginning with the first stage and continuing through labor, there is progressive shortening of the uterus. The relative rate and extent of the shortening are shown by measurements of the internal circumference of the uterus in the sagittal plane (Fig. 29–28). This progressive, ratchetlike shortening of the uterus is referred to as *retraction* or *brachystasis* (see page 578) and is one of the properties of uterine muscle. Although demonstration of brachystasis in a single fiber is not possible, this phenomenon provides the only reasonable explanation for the retractive changes that are known to occur and that eventuate, over the course of the first stage of labor, in progressive shortening and thickening of the corporeal musculature and, in the second stage, in delivery.

Retraction of the myometrium is necessary not only for expelling the baby from the uterus but also for controlling bleeding after delivery. Under normal circumstances, the uterus contracts firmly and remains well contracted after the delivery of the placenta (Fig. 29–29). By this means, the vessels and sinusoids of the uterus are closed off, and bleeding from the placental site and the adjacent denuded areas of the uterus is controlled. If the uterus fails to remain well contracted after delivery, heavy bleeding invariably results. Although postpartum hemorrhage may result from lacerations and clotting defects, its usual cause is atony of the uterus. This is the leading cause of maternal death.

Role of the Uterine Supports

Note has been made that the work of the first stage of labor is devoted to dilatation of the cervix, with little or

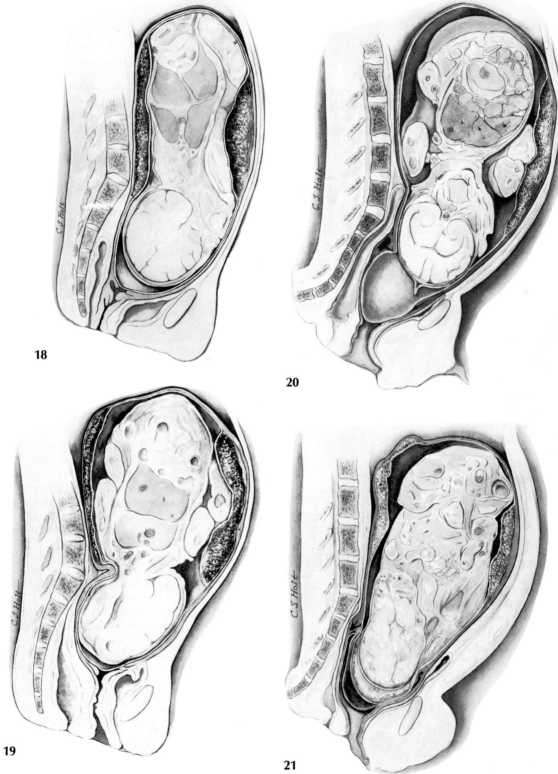

18

20

19

21

FIGS. 29-18 through 29-21. Frozen sagittal sections of *Macaca rhesus*, first stage of labor. Nembutal anesthesia. Rapid freezing by immersion in alcohol chilled to −80° C. (Danforth DN, Graham RJ, Ivy AC: Surg Gynecol Obstet 74:188, 1942)

FIGS. 29-22 through 29-24. Frozen sagittal sections of *Macaca rhesus*, early and mid–second stage of labor. (Danforth DN, Graham RJ, Ivy AC: Surg Gynecol Obstet 74:188, 1942)

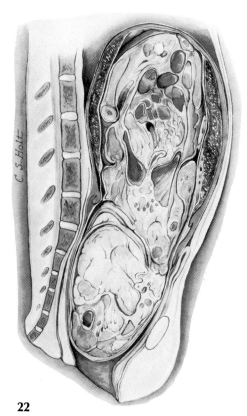

22

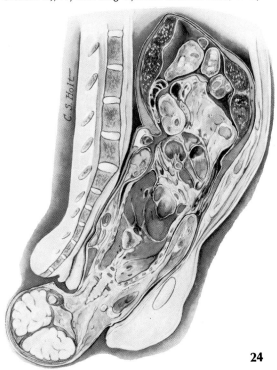

24

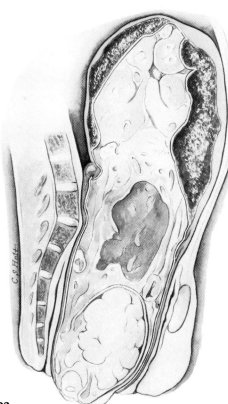

23

no advancement of the presenting part, whereas the second stage is the time of advancement of the baby and delivery. It is when the cervix is fully dilated and has completed its upward excursion that the uterine supports (notably the cardinal ligaments, the pubocervical fascia, and the uterosacral ligaments) begin their important role in uterine evacuation, for it is upon these supports that the uterus gains its purchase to expel the baby through the birth canal. In the monkey, the supports are relatively longer than in the human being; consequently, the cervix rises to a higher level before the taut supports stop its upward excursion. In the human being, x-rays of metal clips on the cervix show clearly that the supports limit the upward excursion of the cervix to the plane of the inlet (Fig. 29–30). If at this point in labor the supports were elastic, a second-stage contraction, instead of advancing the baby, would merely pull the cervix higher. The supports act as stout, unyielding guy ropes against which the uterus works during the second stage of labor (Fig. 29–31). The stress or strain upon these ligaments is proportional to the resistance to delivery offered by the bony pelvis or by the soft parts. The longer or more violent the second stage, the higher the probability of injury and ecchymosis within the structure of the ligaments.

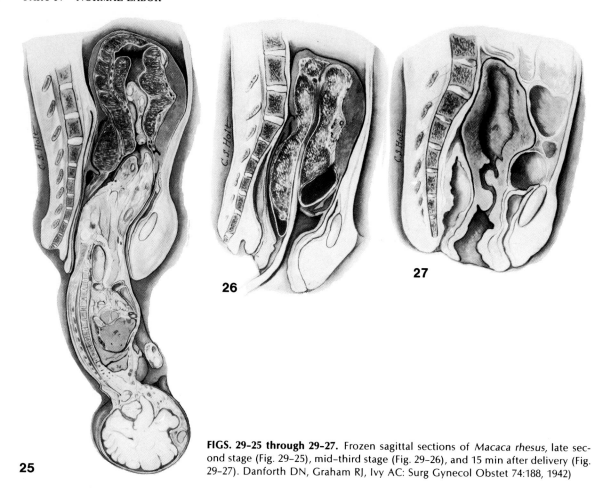

FIGS. 29-25 through 29-27. Frozen sagittal sections of *Macaca rhesus*, late second stage (Fig. 29-25), mid–third stage (Fig. 29-26), and 15 min after delivery (Fig. 29-27). Danforth DN, Graham RJ, Ivy AC: Surg Gynecol Obstet 74:188, 1942)

Historical Aspects

Controversy seethed for many years around the concept of the lower uterine segment. The term was introduced by Bandl in 1875 and engendered a huge and at times vitriolic literature because of the violent dissension about its origin and physiologic behavior. Some of the German papers are diatribes of monographic size. All agreed that, either during labor or just prior to labor, the corpus becomes divided into a thicker "upper segment" and a thinner "lower segment." The debate centered about the question whether the lower segment is active or passive and whether the cervix is or is not a part of the lower uterine segment. Aschoff's definition of the isthmus in 1905, although now shown to be inaccurate, brought order to the chaos by the simple statement that the lower uterine segment is derived not from the corpus, not from the cervix, but from the isthmus. In 1949, this comfortable concept was upset by data that showed 1) the isthmus is not a distinct and separate entity as Aschoff held, but rather is an integral part of the corpus, with properties similar

to those of the remainder of the corpus; and 2) the cervix is basically a connective tissue structure and therefore has no contractile function.

Formation of the Lower Uterine Segment

The lower uterine segment is first formed as a definitive entity during the uterine changes preparatory to labor or as the first stage of labor begins. It is well-known that, as labor advances, the entire length of the uterus shortens, the midportion and fundal areas thicken, and the lower pole becomes thinner as it is pulled upward about the presenting part. As the lower circular component of the myometrium is pulled upward about the presenting part, the transverse fibers must elongate; as they do so, the myometrial thickness must diminish. This is a mecystatic adjustment (see page 578) limited to the lower reaches of the myometrium that must dilate in order to permit the baby to pass. There is a point on the uterine wall below which circumferential dilatation must occur as the myometrium is pulled upward and above which the diameter

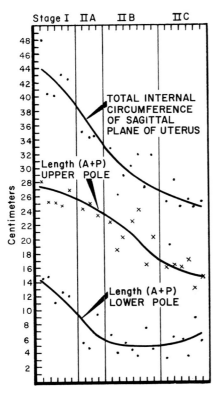

FIG. 29-28. Graph showing total internal circumference in sagittal plane of uterus during labor. Measurements made in 21 monkeys, of which 5 were sacrificed in first stage of labor (*I*), 3 in early second stage (*IIA*), 7 in mid–second stage (*IIB*), and 6 in late second stage (*IIC*). Lower edge of placenta was used in all specimens as arbitrary point for measuring length changes in lower pole of uterus and is contrasted in this graph with equivalent changes in upper part of uterus. Lines are fitted by inspection. In these specimens, first-stage shortening of uterus appears due almost entirely to retraction of lower pole of uterus as it pulls up over fetal head. Additional uterine shortening in second stage appears due almost entirely to retraction of upper pole of uterus. (Danforth DN, Graham RJ, Ivy AC: Surg Gynecol Obstet 74:188, 1942)

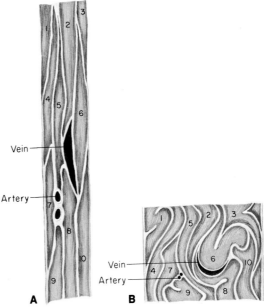

FIG. 29-29. Schematic representation of blood vessels coursing through myometrium. *A.* During pregnancy. *B.* Postpartum, occluded by myometrial retraction. Changes in individual muscle fibers shown by *numbers.* (Redrawn from Bumm E: Grundriss zum Studium der Geburtshilfe, 13th ed. Munich, Bergmann, 1921)

is already great enough so that no further dilatation need occur. The *physiologic retraction ring* necessarily appears at this point and marks the junction of the upper and the lower uterine segments. The physiologic retraction ring is evident as a ledge, thicker cephalad and thinner caudad, around the entire internal circumference of the uterus. The level at which this ring occurs in any given uterus is determined only by the relation between the size of the presenting part and its level in the uterine cavity. The *lower uterine segment* is therefore defined as the band of myometrium at the lower pole of the uterus that must undergo circumferential dilatation, and consequent thinning, as it is pulled upward about the presenting part

(Fig. 29–32). It is marked superiorly by the physiologic retraction ring and inferiorly by the fibromuscular junction of cervix and corpus.

The progressive total shortening of the uterus, the gradual thickening of the upper segment, and the upward advancement of the lower segment are the result of brachystatic adjustments in the muscle fibers of the longitudinal component of the myometrium. Brachystasis and retraction of the upper segment are progressive and do not cease until the uterus is empty; indeed, such changes are essential to supply the force needed to advance the baby and to maintain the advantage gained at each contraction.

At full dilatation, as noted earlier, the cervix is pulled upward approximately to the level of the inlet and is prevented from going higher by the stout uterine supports that are now pulled taut. Further changes in the uterus are wholly dependent upon the amount of effort expended by the uterus in overcoming the obstruction offered by the soft parts and the bony pelvis. If the obstruction is nil, as in the case of some multiparas, the uterus shortens as a whole and empties. Since the supports limit the upward excursion of the cervix, significant obstruction in the face of progressive brachystatic shortening must inevitably result in damage to the uterus, and the weakest part

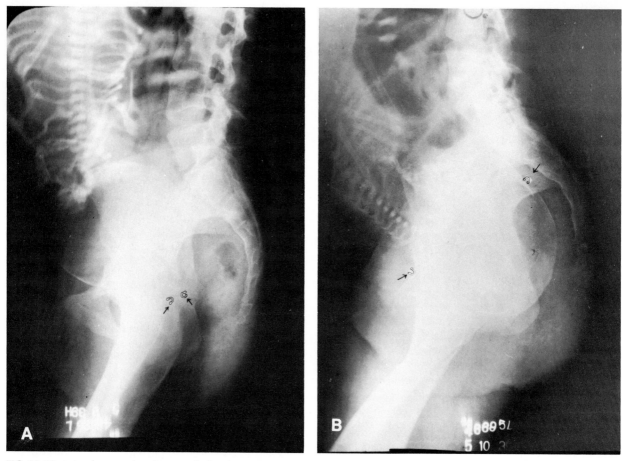

FIG. 29–30. Lateral x-rays showing metal clips (*arrows*) on anterior and posterior cervical lips. *A.* Early labor: Head not engaged, clips below spines. Clips retouched. *B.* Full dilatation: Anterior clip superior to pubic ramus, posterior clip about 2 cm below pelvic brim, head deeply engaged; delivery occurred moments after film was taken. (James Stillman)

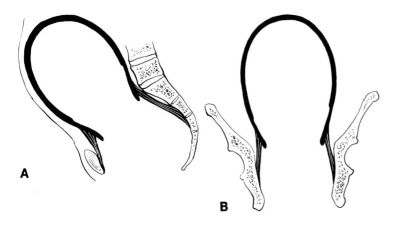

FIG. 29–31. Lateral (*A*) and coronal (*B*) diagrams showing functions of ligamentary supports of uterus in limiting upward excursion of cervix in labor. Undue tension at this time (due to obstruction to advancement of baby) may damage supports. (Danforth DN: In Davis CH, Carter B (eds): Gynecology and Obstetrics. Hagerstown, Prior, 1961)

will give way. The weakest portion of the musculature is the thinned lower uterine segment. If the obstruction is only slight or moderate, the lower segment is lengthened to a degree by the brachystatic contractions of the powerful upper uterine segment, but the baby advances slightly with each contraction. If the obstruction is absolute, however, and the baby cannot advance, the upper segment continues to thicken and the lower segment becomes excessively thinned (Fig. 29–32). The physiologic retraction ring, formerly only a small ledge, now becomes pronounced and is known as *Bandl's ring* or *pathologic contraction ring.* The formation of Bandl's ring heralds the imminent rupture of the uterus. It is sometimes evident as an indentation or transverse groove on the abdomen at a point between the symphysis and the umbilicus, giving the same general appearance as a full bladder. However, the ring rises as contractions continue, and uterine rupture through the greatly thinned lower uterine segment is inevitable unless the obstruction to delivery is immediately relieved.

UTERINE CONTRACTIONS IN PREGNANCY AND LABOR

The year 1872 marked the opening of an important new era in clinical obstetrics. It was then that Dr. John Braxton Hicks presented before the Obstetrical Society of London a paper, "On the Contractions of the Uterus Throughout Pregnancy: Their Physiological Effects and Their Value in the Diagnosis of Pregnancy." There Hicks gave evidence that the pregnant uterus contracts and relaxes from the 3rd month of pregnancy. He noted that careful palpation of the gravid uterus would allow the examiner to feel contractions, usually occurring every 5–20 min, but occasionally coming only once every 30 min. He felt that such contractile activity "is a natural condition of pregnancy" and stated that the pregnant woman is not usually conscious of these contractions, but that they may be painful on some occasions. More than 100 years after these observations were published, it is agreed that Hicks was right on all counts. The frequently used term *Braxton Hicks contractions,* which by curious happenstance incorporates the middle name of the discoverer, is a fitting tribute to Hicks' clinical acumen.

About the same time Hicks was presenting his findings in London, Schatz, in Germany, published the first tracings of uterine contractility in labor. Using an intrauterine balloon for recording, Schatz demonstrated the pattern of uterine contractility throughout labor. Among other observations, he noted the effect of postural change upon uterine contractility and demonstrated the relatively large increase in intrauterine pressure brought about by bearing down in the second stage of labor.

FIG. 29–32. Lower uterine segment. *A.* At onset of labor. *B.* Precisely at full dilatation. *C.* After full dilatation in presence of significant obstruction to advancement of baby. Bandl's ring beginning to form. (Danforth DN, Ivy AC: Am J Obstet Gynecol 57:831, 1949)

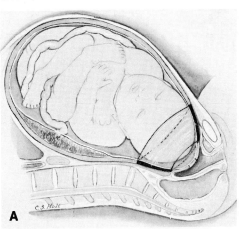

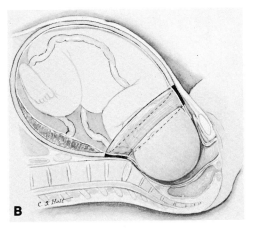

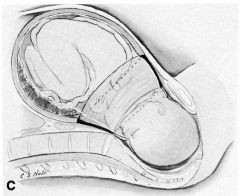

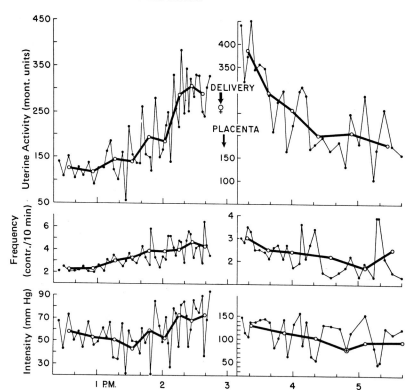

FIG. 29-33. Comparison of one subject's uterine activity in late labor (*left*) and in early puerperium (*right*). (Hendricks CH: Am J Obstet Gynecol 83:890, 1962)

These two brilliant clinicians laid the foundation for a significant portion of present day understanding of the physiology of labor. Hicks provided a part of the knowledge of prelabor and its relation to active labor. Schatz increased the understanding of the process of parturition. His pioneering technique was the all-important first step toward the now common practice of monitoring uterine activity during the course of labor.

Today, the monitoring of uterine contractility has been brought to a high degree of practical usefulness. Either external or internal measurements of uterine activity may be made. The latter provides a more accurate picture of the contractility pattern, since it permits direct documentation of changes in the intrauterine pressure. This method enables the attendant to note the general contour of the contraction, the intensity (in millimeters of mercury), the frequency of contractions, and the tonus (the "resting pressure" between contractions). The record of intrauterine pressure, properly interpreted, can help the physician identify and follow the course of normal labor. Moreover, the recording can help the clinician realize when abnormal types of uterine activity that might have a deleterious effect upon the woman or her fetus are developing.

To provide more graphic portrayal of uterine activ-

ity, Caldeyro–Barcía and Alvarez coined the term *Montevideo unit*. This is the product obtained by multiplying the frequency of the contractions (the number occurring in 10 min) by the intensity of the contractions (the average intrauterine pressure peaks of all contractions occurring in the 10-min span). The use of this device is illustrated in Figure 29–33.

DEVELOPMENT OF UTERINE ACTIVITY DURING PREGNANCY

The uterus remains relatively quiescent during the first half of pregnancy. Nevertheless, there is always some evidence of myometrial activity. There may be frequent localized (regional) contractions that may increase the intrauterine pressure only 1–5 mm Hg above the resting pressure (Fig. 29–34). The resting pressure between contractions (tonus) is relatively constant throughout pregnancy and early labor, ranging from 5–10 mm Hg. Even in early pregnancy, however, there may be bursts of greatly increased activity—much larger contractions that appear without evident cause, are not sensed by the patient, and usually subside spontaneously after a few minutes.

Toward the end of the second trimester, the regional

activity persists, but it is occasionally interrupted by the appearance of isolated contractions that in form and intensity are quite typical of the contractions observed in normal labor (Fig. 29–35). These isolated, usually painless contractions (Braxton Hicks contractions) tend to become more frequent as pregnancy advances into the last trimester, and they appear to play an important role in prelabor changes.

THE CONTRACTIONS OF PRELABOR

Prelabor is that all-important period in late pregnancy when the uterus is undergoing preparatory changes that under normal conditions help to ensure efficient labor. For the last 4 weeks before the onset of labor, the pattern of uterine contractility evolves ever closer toward that of active labor. The regional activity tends to persist into advanced prelabor, but the laborlike contractions appear with increasing frequency and tend to become better coordinated as the time for labor approaches (Fig. 29–36). Although the exact cause of cervical effacement is not known, there is some evidence that the agent responsible for the contractions of prelabor (probably PGs) may also be responsible for the effacement and slight dilatation that usually occur before the onset of true labor (Fig. 29–37).

Most Braxton Hicks contractions are painless and are noticed by the woman, if she perceives them at all, only as an intermittent tightening of the uterus. While the contractility pattern is substantially the same in women of all parities, the woman's perception of these contractions is altered considerably by previous childbearing experience. In the first pregnancy, Braxton Hick contractions are generally painless until an hour or so before the onset of true labor; but, with each succeeding pregnancy, painful contractions are apt to precede the onset of true labor by an increasingly long period. A woman in her eighth or ninth pregnancy may find painful Braxton Hicks contractions extremely troublesome as early as the 5th or 6th month.

When these painful contractions come in bursts, the woman (and her physician) may form the mistaken impression that she is in labor. The fact that it is a false labor becomes apparent only in retrospect, when the bursts of contractility have subsided and it becomes evident that the contractions are not going to progress further toward active labor. It is clinically most important not to confuse these bursts of contrac-

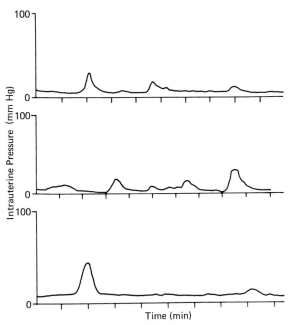

FIG. 29–35. Uterine activity in midpregnancy. *Top.* At 21 weeks, much spontaneous regional activity is present, with intermittent superimposition of poorly coordinated contractions developing 10–25 mm Hg pressure. *Middle.* At 21 weeks, in same patient as in top graph, oxytocin infused at 80 mU/min produces only minimal increment in activity. *Bottom.* At 26 weeks, regional activity persists. During 10-min period shown, there appeared one well-coordinated contraction, developing 35 mm Hg intrauterine pressure. In form and intensity, this Braxton Hicks contraction is indistinguishable from those frequently recorded in active spontaneous labor. (Hendricks)

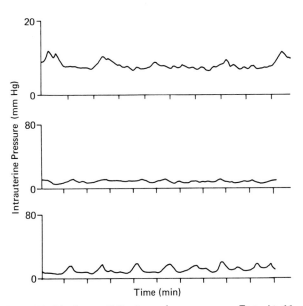

FIG. 29–34. Uterine activity in early pregnancy. *Top.* At 11 weeks, spontaneous regional type contractions develop 1–5 mm Hg intrauterine pressure above resting pressure. *Middle.* At 14 weeks, spontaneous activity is noted. *Bottom.* At 14 weeks, same patient as in middle graph shows very small response to large dose of oxytocin (100 mU/min). (Hendricks)

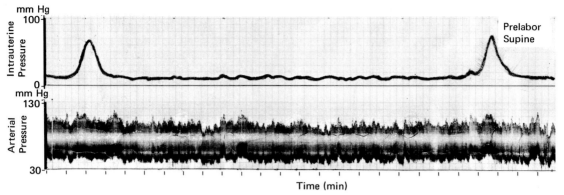

FIG. 29-36. Prelabor at term pregnancy. Note persistent regional activity with well-coordinated laborlike contractions developing more than 50 mm Hg pressure at intervals of about 20 min. (Hendricks CH: Symposium of Modern Obstetrical Practices. New York, Karger, 1970)

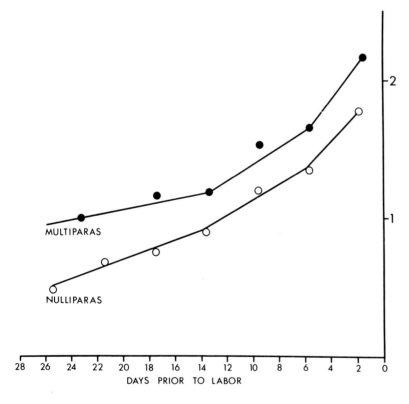

FIG. 29-37. Cervical dilatation before labor in multiparous and nulliparous women. In both, dilatation progresses steadily during last 4 weeks of gestation, but multipara's dilatation tends to exceed that of nullipara throughout this period. (Hendricks)

tions with active labor and not to treat such a woman for dystocia before there has been any real evidence of true active labor.

The Braxton Hicks contractions of late pregnancy gradually become more frequent, and their presence is announced by increasing discomfort. At the very end of pregnancy, these contractions merge by slow, imperceptible degrees into the progress of clinically recognizable active labor.

THE CONTRACTIONS OF LABOR

As a general rule, labor begins with uterine contractions occurring every 15–20 min. Before labor, the contractions often appear uncoordinated or of insufficient intensity to be recognized as effective labor contractions, although there are many exceptions.

As labor approaches, larger and larger areas of the myometrium become involved in coordinated contrac-

tile activity. The question of *pacemakers,* specialized areas from which the contractions of labor are triggered, is not entirely settled. Ivy, Hartman, and Koff observed the laboring monkey uterus directly and found that the contractions started simultaneously in the cornual areas, spreading thence to involve the entire uterus. In the human uterus, Caldeyro–Barcia found that the contractions began in one or the other cornu and only rarely on both sides simultaneously (Fig. 29–38). More recently, strain gauge studies have demonstrated one dominant pacemaker area in the uterine fundus, the exact location of which may vary in the same patient in different labors. While the notion of a pacemaker is appropriate, it appears that, under proper conditions, each myometrial cell should potentially be capable of initiating an adequate contraction that involves the entire uterus. Fortunately the anatomic arrangement of the myometrium is such that parturition is likely to be carried out successfully whether or not there is a sharply delineated pacemaker site. Because the concentration of myometrial cells is greatest at the fundus, the probability is always greater that an effective contraction will be triggered from there rather than from the lower portion of the uterus, which is less well endowed with myometrial components. Furthermore, owing to this concentration of muscular components in the fundus, the greatest contractile effort is applied at that point. Thus, as one contraction succeeds another, the lower portion of the myometrium is pulled up by the overwhelmingly greater muscular component at the top of the fundus, with the result that the lower portion is drawn thinner and thinner as labor progresses.

Thus, it is both desirable and inevitable that efficient contractions in normal labor exhibit fundal dominance, which implies that the contraction arises somewhere in the fundus of the uterus and spreads smoothly throughout the fundus and thence down over the more caudal parts of the uterus, the greatest force being developed in the fundus. The number of such contractions required to finish labor is determined in large measure by the completeness of the prelabor changes in the lowermost portions of the uterus.

During the *active phase of labor,* the contractions occur at intervals of 3–5 min and the frequency may increase to as often as one contraction every 2 min during the last half of the first stage (Figs. 29–39 and 29–40). At the outset, the contractions usually average at least 30 mm Hg intensity above the resting pressure. As labor advances, the average intensity rises to near 50 mm Hg; in some, the intensity may reach 80–100 mm Hg. The resting pressure remains within the range of 5–10 mm Hg until very late in labor, when it may rise to 12–14 mm Hg. Thus, as labor advances, both the frequency and the intensity of contractions increase. Even in the best labor, however, some contractions deviate significantly from the ideal frequency

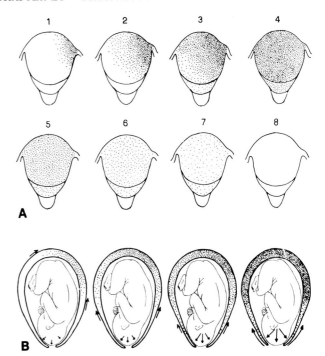

FIG. 29–38. Contractions of labor, often but not necessary arising in one or the other cornual area, propagated evenly to involve entire musculature and, as a rule, painful. *A.* Surface view. *B.* Coronal section. (R Caldeyro–Barcia)

and intensity pattern. In abnormal labor, the pattern may be seriously disturbed in form, and the contractions can lose all ability to produce further cervical dilatation (see Chapter 35).

Various attempts have been made to express the work performed by the uterine contractions during first-stage labor. A somewhat arbitrary way of comparing the course of differing types of labors is to use the peak intensities of all contractions recorded during the first stage as a rough estimate of such work. In general, it may be observed that less uterine work is required to accomplish dilatation in muliparas than in nulliparas, and in anterior than in transverse positions (Fig. 29–41).

In order for the coordinated uterine contractions in labor to be effective, there must be even and uniform fitting of the presenting part to the lower uterine segment; possibly the nerve endings mentioned earlier are concerned. Optimal fitting occurs with the head in the occiput anterior or transverse position. When the head is in the posterior position, the fitting is less favorable, and this is one of the explanations frequently given for the clinical observation that labor with the fetal head in the posterior position is longer than if the mechanism is anterior. In transverse lie, cervical dilatation may proceed normally as long as the membranes fit neatly; when the membranes rupture, further dila-

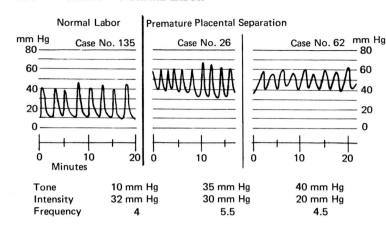

FIG. 29-39. Intrauterine pressure changes in normal labor and in premature separation of placenta. (Caldeyro–Barcia R, Alvarez H: J Obstet Gynaecol Br Emp 59:646, 1952)

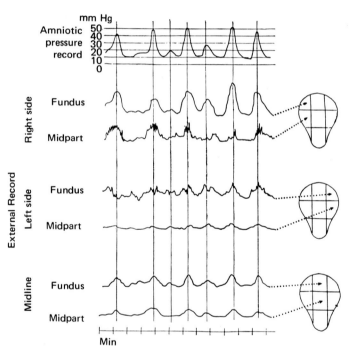

FIG. 29-40. Normal first stage of labor. Combined internal pressure recording and external recording. Note fundal dominance, especially on right side, and decreased activity toward left and midpart of uterus. Note how external contraction patterns are reflected in internal pressure variations. (Caldeyro–Barcia R, Alvarez H: J Obstet Gynaecol Br Emp 59:646, 1952)

tation of the cervix is apt to be impeded unless the shoulder or the breech comes down to replace the stimulus to the lower segment. In cases of disproportion at the inlet, when the head is prevented from entering the pelvis and fitting properly, the stimulus also may be inadequate.

As the second stage of labor is reached, the contractions occur every 1.5–2 min and last 1–1.5 min. The intensity of second-stage contractions is about the same as that in the late first stage, but the intrauterine pressure may be raised substantially by the patient's voluntary bearing-down efforts (Fig. 29–42).

Immediately after delivery of the baby, the recorded intrauterine pressure increases dramatically, producing intrauterine and intramyometrial pressures of the order of 250 mm Hg. With delivery of the baby, the uterine content is reduced by approximately seven-eighths. The delivery of the placenta brings about another sharp reduction of intrauterine volume. Thus, the continuing activity of the same contractile mass that prior to delivery produces pressures of 70–80 mm Hg, in contracting around the much smaller intrauterine volume, engenders pressures that have been recorded above 250 mm Hg. The tracings in Figures 29–33, 29–42 and 29–43 illustrate typical situations of labor, delivery, and puerperium.

FIG. 29-41. Representation of uterine work during labor expressed as cumulative sum of intensities of contractions plotted against progress in cervical dilatation (semilog). Factors tending to reduce amount of work required to complete first stage of labor are multiparity, anterior position of fetal head, and small fetal size. Slopes of lines give good indication of relative efficiency of labor. Consistent steepening of slope of dilatation after amniotomy (*broken lines*) illustrates increased efficiency resulting from this procedure. (Cibils LA, Hendricks CH: Am J Obstet Gynecol 91:391, 1965)

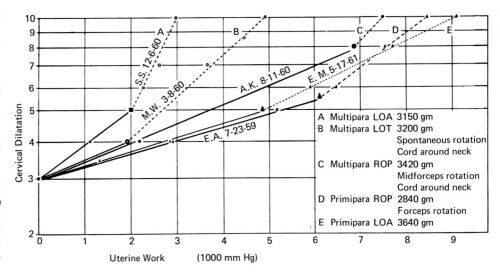

A Multipara LOA 3150 gm
B Multipara LOT 3200 gm
   Spontaneous rotation
   Cord around neck
C Multipara ROP 3420 gm
   Midforceps rotation
   Cord around neck
D Primipara ROP 2840 gm
   Forceps rotation
E Primipara LOA 3640 gm

FIG. 29-42. Continuous record of uterine activity at delivery (*D*) and postpartum. *Line A*, Intrauterine pressure. *Line B*, Intramyometrial pressure. Record is characteristic of spontaneous uterine activity, but these particular contractions resulted from oxytocin infusion started 2 hours before delivery for induction of labor and stopped at point *O* on graph. Placenta, which had been visible at introitus, was delivered at point *P* by gentle traction on cord. (Hendricks CH: Am J Obstet Gynecol 83:890, 1962)

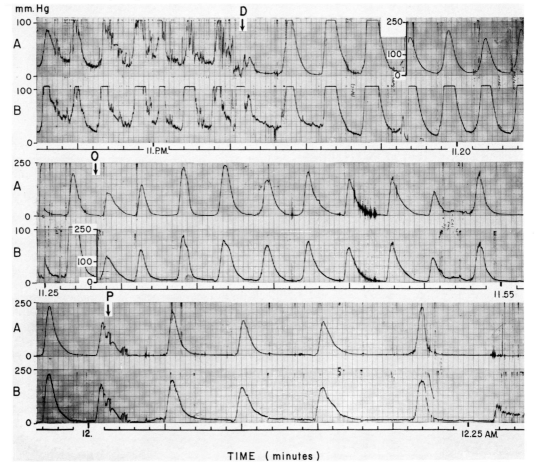

TIME (minutes)

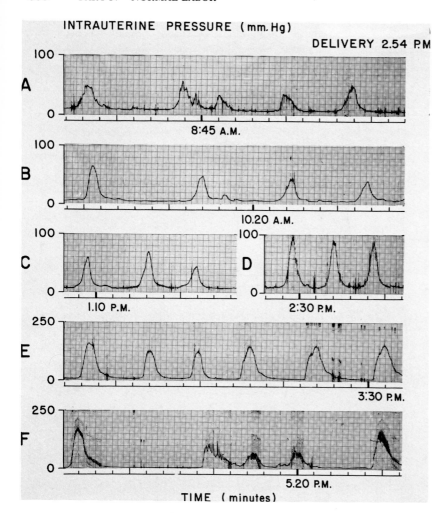

FIG. 29–43. Uterine activity as recorded through same single intrauterine catheter. *A.* Late prelabor, 6 hours antepartum (cervix 2 cm dilated, effaced 50%, station −2). *B.* Early labor, 5 hours antepartum. *C.* Active labor, 2 hours antepartum (cervix 3 cm dilated, effaced 70%, station O). *D.* Late labor, predelivery (cervix 9 cm dilated, station 0+). *E.* Spontaneous activity 0.5 hour postpartum (note change in pressure scale). *F.* Spontaneous activity 2.5 hours postpartum. (Hendricks CH: Am J Obstet Gynecol 83:890, 1962)

EFFECTS OF DRUGS ON UTERINE CONTRACTILITY

In the discussion of the physiology of the myometrium earlier in this chapter, reference was made to several agents that affect uterine motility when they are administered. Some of these have been used clinically either to stimulate or to depress uterine activity. In addition to those used in a deliberate effort to control uterine action, there is a group of agents used for other purposes that may incidentally alter the motility of the uterus.

OXYTOCICS

Oxytocin

Over the years, oxytocin has produced almost as many disasters as benefits. However, if it is *properly used*, it

is the safest and most effective pharmacologic agent for the stimulation of uterine activity. W. Blair Bell, a pioneer in so many areas of obstetrics, was the first to employ, in 1909, extracts of whole posterior lobe for the clinical stimulation of uterine activity. A few years later, B. P. Watson recommended its use for the induction of labor and in 1920 described a large series of cases in which there were no significant complications from the method. As the technique was adopted, others experienced an increasing number of uterine ruptures due to overstimulation and, of almost equal importance, severe hypertensive responses due to the presence of vasopressin in the extracts. In 1928 Kamm *et al* achieved the separation of oxytocin from the pressor–antidiuretic fraction of the posterior lobe. The next important advance was Theobald's recommendation that more precise control could be achieved by the intravenous administration of dilute solutions of oxytocin. Finally, in 1954, Du Vigneaud accomplished the

synthesis of oxytocin; this was the first successful synthesis of a biologically active peptide.

The commercial preparations of oxytocin now available (Pitocin and Syntocinon) are synthetic preparations that are virtually identical, highly uniform, and standardized in similar manner. Dosage is expressed in international units (IU) or milliunits (mU). The 1-ml ampule contains 10 IU, or 10,000 mU. A single milligram of synthetic oxytocin contains approximately 435 IU.

Oxytocin is very rapidly metabolized, its biologic half-life being in the range of 3–4 min. Administered as a constant intravenous infusion, its effect on contractility becomes evident within 2–4 min and the peak effect is attained in 10–15 min. When given intramuscularly (as may be done after, but rarely before, delivery), increased contractility of the uterus is noted within 3–5 min, the peak response appears in 15–25 min, and most of the increased activity has subsided 30–40 min after the injection.

Nonpregnant and early pregnant uteri are relatively, but not absolutely, refractory to oxytocin, and large doses beyond the ordinary pharmacologic range are required to produce even a minimal response. The same relative refractoriness occurs also at midpregnancy (Figs. 29–34 and 29–35), accounting for the ineffectiveness of oxytocin as an abortifacient. It is not useful for this purpose in the first trimester, and in the second trimester some other agents (*e.g.*, PGs, intraamniotic saline) are also required.

As pregnancy advances into the third trimester, the uterus becomes increasingly responsive to oxytocin (Figs. 29–1 and 29–2), and at term it is exquisitely sensitive to extremely small doses. It is in this group of patients that oxytocin has its greatest usefulness as a uterine stimulant.

The objective of uterine stimulation at term is to produce contractions equivalent to those that occur in spontaneous labor, *i.e.*, contractions that occur every 2–3 min, last 40–50 sec, and produce intrauterine pressures of 50–60 mm Hg. Contractions of this kind can usually be achieved by the intravenous infusion, at a constant rate, of 1–10 mU oxytocin/min. If this dose range is exceeded, or if the uterus is excessively responsive to lesser doses, the resting tone increases, the interval between contractions is reduced, and the contractions become much more forceful. Rupture of the uterus is the ultimate consequence. This is an obstetric disaster of the first order and causes oxytocin stimulation to be regarded as a major obstetric procedure to be used only by those who are fully informed of its action and who are willing to provide the constant observation that is essential. Accidents resulting from overstimulation caused the Food and Drug Administration to interdict the use of oxytocin for the elective induction of labor. This action appears to be more an indictment of improper and inappropriate use than a condemnation of the drug itself. The clinical use of oxytocin for stimulation is described in Chapter 35.

Immediately postpartum, the uterus remains sensitive to oxytocin but is somewhat less so. Many physicians administer an ampule (10 IU) intramuscularly after delivery of the placenta to ensure adequate contraction of the uterus in the early puerperium. This is especially helpful in patients who receive general anesthesia for delivery, since general anesthesia tends to diminish uterine contractility and may be associated with excessive bleeding after delivery. The *rapid* intravenous injection of even 5 IU oxytocin postpartum is contraindicated, since it may cause a transient but profound hypotension.

Ergot

From an ergot alkaloid, originally obtained from a fungus growing on rye, several useful drugs have been isolated, and several have been synthesized. *Ergonovine* and *ergometrine* are identical substances synthesized almost simultaneously by American and British investigators and named by the individual workers. Ergonovine is the American preparation. Their use is limited to the puerperium, either immediately after delivery or for the later control of bleeding due to atony. The duration and intensity of their effects in pharmacologic dose are so great that they should never be given to an undelivered patient. Impure products administered in the past over a long period produced a serious vascular disorder called *ergotism;* this is unusual with modern preparations, however, and if it occurs at all must result from very prolonged high dosage.

Ergonovine maleate (Ergotrate) may be given orally, intramuscularly, or if necessary, intravenously. The usual dose is 0.2 mg given orally, intramuscularly, or intravenously. This dose causes uterine contractions of high intensity; since the effect persists for hours (Fig. 29–44), this is a useful drug for maintaining good uterine contractility during the early postpartum period.

The extent of the uterine response is directly related to the dose and time of administration. This may be seen by comparing Figures 29–44 and 29–45. In the latter case, 0.015 mg (one-thirteenth of the usual dose) ergonovine maleate given intravenously induces only a gentle increase in contractility in the early postpartum uterus. If the usual 0.2-mg dose is given intravenously over a 10-min period rather than as a bolus (Fig. 29–45), hypercontractility and mild hypertonus may be observed, but the dramatic tetanic response shown in Figure 29–44 is lacking.

Methylergonovine tartrate (Methergine) is also in wide current use as a powerful oxytocic and has similar effects on uterine contractions.

Both drugs, when administered intravenously, have been noted to induce hypertension in some patients,

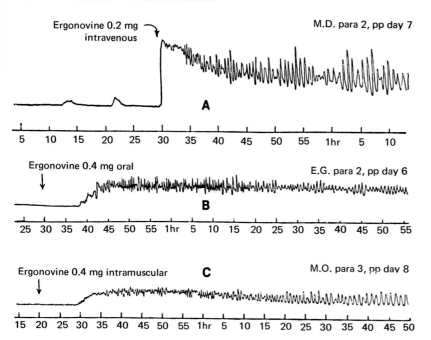

Ergonovine 0.2 mg intravenous

M.D. para 2, pp day 7

A

5 10 15 20 25 30 35 40 45 50 55 1hr 5 10

Ergonovine 0.4 mg oral

E.G. para 2, pp day 6

B

25 30 35 40 45 50 55 1hr 5 10 15 20 25 30 35 40 45 50 55

Ergonovine 0.4 mg intramuscular   **C**

M.O. para 3, pp day 8

15 20 25 30 35 40 45 50 55 1hr 5 10 15 20 25 30 35 40 45 50

FIG. 29–44. Kymographic tracings of uterine activity following administration of ergonovine 6–8 days after delivery (*A*) intravenously, (*B*) orally, and (*C*) intramuscularly. Note immediate response after intravenous administration. There is a 15- to 20-min lag after both oral and intramuscular administration, but intramuscular response is more marked. (Davis ME, Rubin R [eds.]: DeLee's Obstetrics for Nurses, 17th ed. Philadelphia, WB Saunders, 1962)

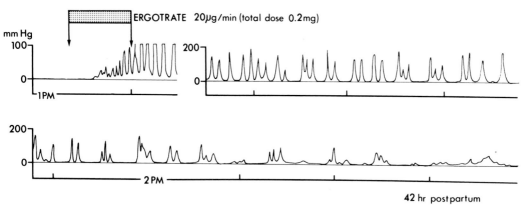

ERGOTRATE 20µg/min (total dose 0.2mg)

mm Hg

42 hr postpartum

FIG. 29–45. Effect of 0.2 mg ergonovine (Ergotrate) administered intravenously by constant infusion pump over 10-min period. Hypercontractility and transient hypertonus ensued, but no evidence of tetanic response. (Hendricks)

but methylergonovine tartrate is less likely to cause this undesirable side effect. The likelihood that hypertension will occur with either drug is minimized by using either the intramuscular or the oral route.

Prostaglandins

As noted earlier in this chapter, the effects of PGs on uterine contractility are like those of oxytocin, and their mode of action appears to be similar. Also, the uterus becomes increasingly responsive as pregnancy advances. However, the uterus is by no means refractory to PGs in early and midpregnancy, as it is to oxytocin, and PGs can produce evacuation of the uterus at any stage of pregnancy.

In the United States, use of these substances is limited by an edict of the Food and Drug Administration (FDA) to the effect that PGs may be used only if the fetus is dead or is not expected to survive; the three applicable conditions are missed abortion, induced abortion (Fig. 29–46), and intrauterine fetal death. Their use for induced abortion is discussed in Chapter 14. In countries other than the United States, PGs are widely used for the induction of labor at term and appear to have special usefulness if the cervix is "unripe."

FIG. 29-46. Effect of continuous intravenous infusion of 50μg/min $PGF_{2\alpha}$ on pregnant uterus at 18 weeks' gestation. *A.* Part of control period spontaneous activity. *B.* Sitting up to pass urine. *C.* Intact sac expelled. (Karim SMM, Hillier K: in Josimovich JB [ed]: Uterine Contraction: Side Effects of Steroidal Contraceptives. New York, John Wiley, 1973)

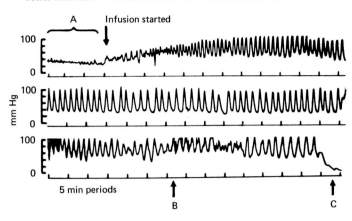

Other aspects of the physiology and pharmacology of PGs are discussed in Chapter 7.

Other Drugs with Oxytocic Properties

Several other drugs have oxytocic properties, but they are not indicated for purposes of stimulating uterine contractions and are best avoided in pregnancy. They include dimenhydrinate (Dramamine), propanolol, norephinephrine (Levophed), and acetylcholine. Disopyramide (Norpace), a cardiac antiarrhythmic agent, appears to have special usefulness for treatment of cardiac arrhythmia in nonpregnant women. In pregnancy it may induce sustained uterine contractions, and some other drug should be selected.

DRUGS THAT DEPRESS UTERINE CONTRACTILITY

The drugs that have been used clinically in an effort to terminate preterm labor are discussed in Chapter 33. They include β-mimetic catecholamines, ethanol, antiprostaglandins, calcium antagonists, and magnesium sulfate. Examples of the effects of ritodrine, ethanol, and magnesium sulfate are shown, respectively, in Figures 29–47, 29–48, and 29–49. The effect of a calcium antagonist, nifedipine, is illustrated in Figure 29–13.

Diazoxide (Hyperstat) is a nondiuretic thiazide that is used for the treatment of severe hypertensive crises. It causes immediate arteriolar dilatation and a drop in blood pressure. It also has a marked tocolytic effect, but it should not be selected as a uterine relaxant. If the drug is used in labor to treat a hypertensive crisis for which no other drug is appropriate, the uterine contractions may be expected to stop, but the other obstetric and fetal effects cannot be predicted.

Aminophylline has been reported to be an effective tocolytic agent; this effect evidently results from its ability to cause an accumulation of cAMP. The cardiovascular side effects are sufficiently severe that its use for the deliberate arrest of uterine contractions is not acceptable.

ANALGESICS, SEDATIVES, AND TRANQUILIZERS

From time to time other agents have been considered as possible suppressants of uterine activity. For many years, morphine was sometimes administered in an attempt to relax the uterus, but objective studies have demonstrated that even after large doses of morphine there is no diminution of uterine action (Fig. 29–50). Likewise, the administration of meperidine does not produce any measurable diminution in uterine contractility. To the contrary, work of Sica–Blanco and his colleagues indicates that, under certain conditions, a single intravenous dose of meperidine hydrochloride (Demerol) may initiate active labor.

As a general rule, the usual doses of analgesic, sedative, antispasmodic, and tranquilizing drugs employed in obstetric practice exert no demonstrable effect upon uterine contractility. The exceptions are aspirin and indomethacin, which are capable of blocking the synthesis of PGs. Lewis and Schulman found that a group of women taking large doses of acetylsalicylic acid for chronic disease tended to have longer labors and longer gestations than did control groups of women not taking the drug.

ANESTHETICS

General Anesthetics

Of the general anesthetic agents in common use, nitrous oxide, cyclopropane, and thiopental (Pentothal) have little effect upon uterine action as they are usually employed. With cyclopropane, some uterine relaxation can be achieved, but only under very deep anesthesia. With these agents, in analgesic doses, the woman is usually able to continue some bearing-down efforts.

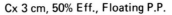

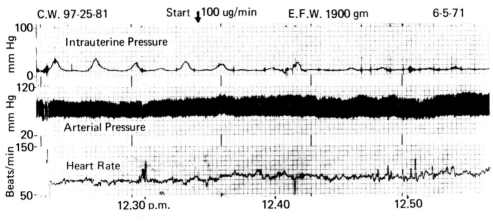

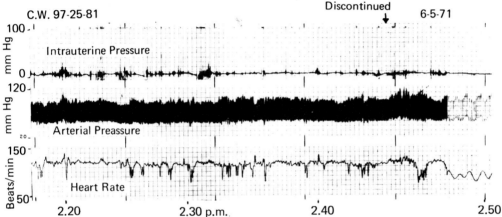

FIG. 29–47. Effect of ritodrine in a case of preterm labor. Patient G6 P2, 32 weeks' gestation, cervix 3 cm dilated, presenting part floating. Contractions on admission characteristic of true labor, diminishing very rapidly after infusion of ritodrine (100 μg/min) started. Note slight decline in diastolic blood pressure, slight increase in pulse pressure, and definite increase in pulse rate. Patient was later discharged on oral medication and readmitted 32 days later; labor was allowed to continue, and she delivered a 2675-g infant in good condition. (Cibils LA, Zuspan FP: Clin Obstet Gynecol 16:199, 1973)

Ether and halothane (Fluothane) are capable of inducing complete uterine relaxation. Ether is a specific depressant of uterine activity; uterine activity can be rapidly abolished by halothane.

It is well to remember that in addition to complete uterine relaxation, these agents also induce a deep general anesthesia that abolishes the ability of the parturient to bear down. Likewise, deep suppression of uterine contractility may be followed by postpartum hemorrhage; this danger can be partially reduced by the appropriate use of oxytocic drugs.

In modern obstetric practice, the need for inducing profound surgical planes of anesthesia to abolish uterine contractility occurs less and less often, as practices that involve major intrauterine maneuvers are replaced by less dramatic but safer alternative methods of management.

Regional Anesthetics

The major regional blocks commonly employed are caudal, lumbar epidural, and spinal anesthesia. Under optimal conditions, none of these is associated with a significant reduction in uterine contractility (Fig. 29–51). It has been noted that, when anesthetic agents containing epinephrine are used, a mild transient depression may be observed in uterine contractility, usually lasting only about 10 min and not enduring beyond 30 min postinjection. Vasicka and associates have found that spinal anesthesia is accompanied by significant reduction in uterine contractility only when the patient is severely hypotensive.

Uterine contractility, as recorded by accurate methods of tokodynamometry, is little affected by the

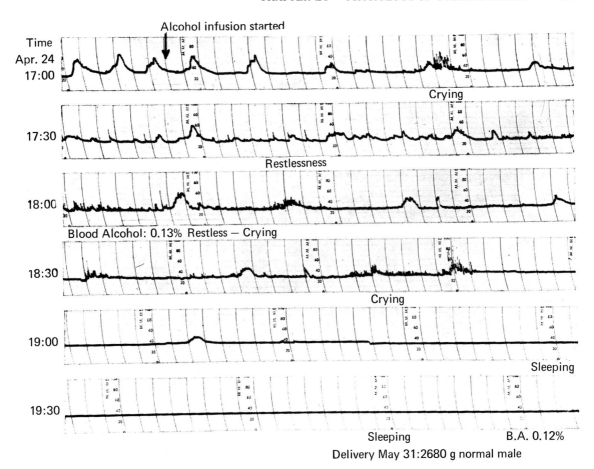

FIG. 29–48. Effect of alcohol in arresting preterm labor in patient 32 weeks pregnant, with 2 cm cervical dilatation and intact membranes (Fuchs F: J Obstet Gynaecol Br Commonw 72:1011, 1965)

induction of a major regional anesthetic block. Nevertheless, there is a widespread belief that the major blocks often slow the progress of labor. A number of possibilities suggest themselves to explain the apparent discrepancy between the uterine contractility record and the impression that labor has slowed.

1. If the block was administered so early that the patient was not yet in active labor, the block would be associated with (but not responsible for) lack of progress in cervical dilatation.
2. The contrast between the uncomfortable patient before the onset of regional anesthesia and the tranquil patient after her pain has been relieved may lead the attendants to believe that labor has been arrested.
3. In the second stage, progress may be slowed because the patient does not feel the need to push (as occurs in all major blocks) or cannot cooperate by pushing when directed to do so (as with spinal block).
4. Vaginal examination of the newly relaxed patient

just after initiation of a block sometimes results in the head being pushed to a somewhat higher level. This may disturb the finely balanced adaptation between head and cervix, making the uterine contractions less effective, even though the contractions recorded on the tracing continue and are not altered in appearance. The fetal head is particularly likely to rise to a higher station in the pelvis if the mother's legs are elevated to counteract a sudden drop in blood pressure.
5. Epinephrine administered with the blocking agent, or the release of epinephrine due to the stress of the procedure, may bring about mild reductions in uterine contractility. Such reductions may be too minor to be evident on examination of the tracing.
6. Severe hypotension, such as may occur in conduction anesthesia, actually does reduce uterine contractility.

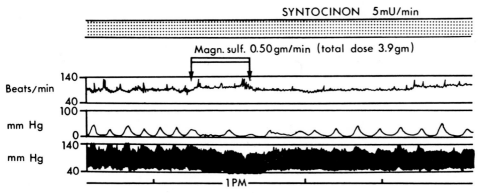

FIG. 29–49. Effect of magnesium sulfate on uterine contractility. Oxytocin induction (5 mU/min, intravenously), membranes intact. Total of 3.9 g magnesium sulfate was given intravenously at rate of 0.5 g/min. Note mild tachycardia (*top line*), transient depression of uterine contractility (*middle line*), moderate depression of arterial blood pressure (*bottom line*), and prompt recovery. (Hendricks CH: Clin Obstet Gynecol 9:535, 1966)

THE PAIN OF LABOR

Pain is apt to be most intense during the latter part of the first stage of labor, less so during the second stage, and virtually absent during and after the third stage.

The pain associated with labor has never been well explained; but, since it is clearly related to the occurrence of the uterine contractions, the words *contraction* and *pain* have come to be synonymous. The sense of pain generally begins prior to the height of a contraction. Pain is usually perceived at an intrauterine pressure of about 25 mm Hg, but this is not always the case; painful contractions have been noted at much lower intensity and painless ones at much higher. In the beginning of the first stage, the contractions last 15–30 secs. As they become more intense and longer, the pain increases. In most normal labors, it is in the suprapubic areas and laterally, both sides equally, for 6–8 cm from the midline that the distress is felt. Backache occurs most commonly in labors in which dilatation of the cervix is not proportional to the strength of the contractions; the presence of backache with the contractions suggests faulty dilatation of the cervix or improper fitting of the presenting part to the lower pole of the uterus, as may occur in certain malpositions (*e.g.,* occiput posterior) or malpresentations (*e.g.,* in certain cases of breech). Pain referred from the back down the legs is similarly explained.

When the cervix becomes fully dilated, a reflex is produced that causes the parturient to make a voluntary effort to expel the baby (*bearing down*). A trained observer can often recognize the onset of the second stage by the grunting sound made by the patient at this juncture in labor. (In the anesthetized postpartum dog, and likely other animals as well, the sudden distention of the cervix by a balloon causes the characteristic grunting, bearing-down effort.) It is reported that the more vigorous the bearing-down effort, the less the discomfort of the contractions. Whether this is true or whether the patient is distracted by the fact that she may now actually participate is a moot question. As the presenting part approaches the pelvic floor, a new distress occurs as a result of the pressure and often the actual tearing of these tissues as they are increasingly distended.

In discussing the pain of labor, note must be made of the marked variation among patients. A patient's reaction to labor cannot be predicted from her evident emotional patterns before labor; the most stoic may disintegrate emotionally, and the most apprehensive may labor with equanimity. Psychologic factors (confidence in the attendants, attitude toward the baby, proximity of relatives, and the like) are clearly concerned.

It is curious that no good explanation of the mechanism that produces the uterine pain has been offered. Uterine ischemia during contractions has been suggested; since the intrauterine pressure in certain painless Braxton Hicks contractions has been recorded as exceeding 100 mm Hg, however, this explanation leaves something to be desired. Moreover, contractions of the third stage and immediately after delivery may produce pressures of 250–300 mm Hg, but they are not painful. Additional causes of pain in labor may be stretching of the cervix; traction upon the peritoneum, adnexa, and supporting ligaments; distention of the soft parts before the advancing head; and pressure upon the urethra and bladder. All may contribute, and it is emphasized that the uterus is not necesarily the only source of the pain of labor.

A multiplicity of nerve endings in the lower pole of the uterus just superior to the cervix has been described. They appear to be receptor structures. Since they are limtied to this part of the uterus, it is possible that the stimulation of these nerve endings is responsible for the pain of labor as the lower pole of the uterus dilates before the presenting part. The fact that

FIG. 29-50. Effect on uterine activity of 8.3 mg morphine sulfate infused in 8.3 min. No effect is discernible on oxytocin-induced contractions characteristic of labor. (Eskes TKAB: Am J Obstet Gynecol 84:281, 1962)

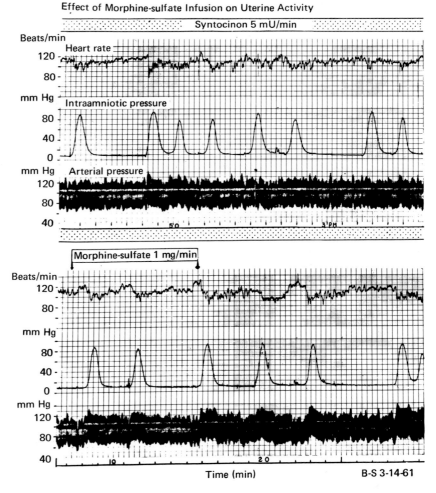

Effect of Morphine-sulfate Infusion on Uterine Activity

CHANGES IN THE CERVIX IN PREGNANCY AND LABOR

The function of the cervix is to retain the conceptus until the uterus is prepared to evacuate its contents. Figure 29–17 shows the manner in which this function is carried out, and emphasizes also that the cervix is not called upon to resist the stress of uterine distention until about the 16th week of pregnancy. Late abortion is a predictable consequence 1) if the cervix is sufficiently damaged, as by deep laceration or conization; 2) if it is congenitally abnormal, as the so-called muscular cervix or the cervix sufficiently affected by intrauterine exposure to diethylstilbestrol (DES); or 3) if it should soften sufficiently and dilate prematurely in the middle trimester.

labor pain is often relieved by local anesthesia applied to the uterosacral ligaments, to the paracervical structures, or to the area of the pudendal nerve is not helpful in explaining its causation.

PHYSICAL CHANGES

In the cervix, the physical changes caused by pregnancy are well-known, since this structure has been a focal point for all who are concerned with the conduct of pregnancy and labor.

One of the early signs of pregnancy is softening of the cervix, *Goodell's sign,* which is evident first at about 5–6 weeks' gestation and remains without significant change until the beginning of preparations for labor a month or so before term. This sign is probably due chiefly to the vascular changes characteristic of pregnancy (see Chapter 17); edema may be concerned to an extent, but the actual accumulation of water is negligible and is not sufficient to account for Goodell's sign. In addition, duskiness (cyanosis) of the cervix can be noted very early in pregnancy (*Chadwick's sign*). It is due to the increased vascularity and becomes more marked as pregnancy advances; at term, the cervix is usually light to deep purple in color.

The endocervix reacts to pregnancy by marked pro-

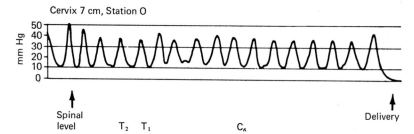

FIG. 29–51. Effect of administration of high spinal block in late labor on uterine contractility pattern. No significant effect is noted. (Bonica JJ: Principles and Practice of Obstetric Analgesia and Anesthesia. Philadelphia, FA Davis, 1972. Modified from Vasicka A, Kretchmer H: Am J Obstet Gynecol 82:600, 1961)

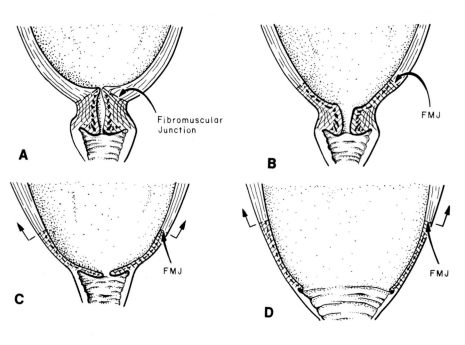

FIG. 29–52. Effacement and dilatation of cervix in primigravida. Cervical shortening generally occurs first, followed by progressive thinning and dilatation. In multipara, there is no consistent pattern, although dilatation is often well established before there is notable effacement.

liferation of the endocervical glands, which produce a tenacious mucus that acts to seal the cervical canal by the so-called mucous plug of pregnancy. The mucous plug ordinarily remains in place, especially in a primigravida, until early labor, when it may be extruded from the vagina almost intact as a blob of mucus to which a few cells of the endocervix may adhere.

Although there are no changes in the squamous epithelium of the portio vaginalis that are diagnostic of pregnancy, certain findings are present more often in the pregnant than in the nonpregnant woman. They include a higher percentage of mitotic figures in the basilar zone, a higher percentage of large so-called active nuclei in the midzone, an increased submucosal infiltration with lymphocytes and plasma cells, and the occasional presence of atypical mitotic figures, especially near the squamocolumnar junction. If present in marked degree, the normal pregnancy changes may resemble carcinoma in situ. During pregnancy, the squamocolumnar junction migrates toward and some-

times into the cervical canal, causing this area to be less accessible to colposcopic examination.

Cervical Effacement and Dilatation

Although the cervix is slightly softened to the touch, it remains thick, rigid, and closed until a few weeks before term, and the cervical canal maintains its nonpregnant length of 2–3 cm. Several weeks before the onset of labor, the cervix begins to "unfold" from above downward (Fig. 29–52) and to become perceptibly softer. This change is referred to as *effacement*. As effacement begins, the cervix also dilates slightly so that it becomes possible to introduce a finger into the cervical canal without resistance. When labor starts, the cervix is usually soft and mushy; about half of the canal has been taken up; and the external os is dilated to the extent of about 2+ cm (Fig. 29–53).

As the contractions of labor become established, further shortening occurs and the cervix becomes thin-

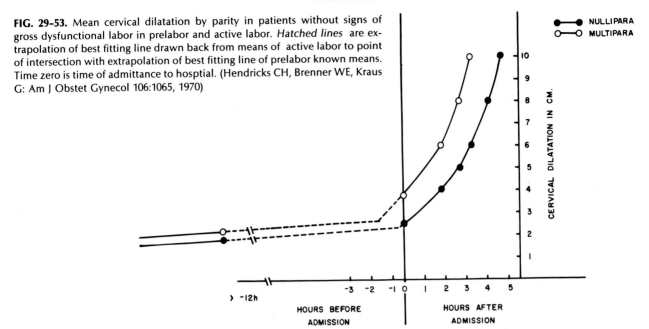

FIG. 29-53. Mean cervical dilatation by parity in patients without signs of gross dysfunctional labor in prelabor and active labor. *Hatched lines* are extrapolation of best fitting line drawn back from means of active labor to point of intersection with extrapolation of best fitting line of prelabor known means. Time zero is time of admittance to hosptial. (Hendricks CH, Brenner WE, Kraus G: Am J Obstet Gynecol 106:1065, 1970)

ner, but it cannot be forcibly dilated without injury. As a rule, when labor is well established, effacement proceeds apace, and at 6–7 cm dilatation the cervical thinning and softening are complete. When effacement is complete, the cervix is said to be "negotiable," *i.e.*, it can usually be dilated manually without significant injury. Within a month after delivery, the cervix is restored to its former rigid, undilatable state.

It is to be noted that the cervix is fundamentally a fibrous connective tissue structure. The myometrium ends at the cervix and inserts into it much as a skeletal muscle inserts into an aponeurosis. Hence, the brachystatic contractions of labor pull the cervix upward about the presenting part as labor advances. However, *the mechanical traction of labor contractions can produce full dilatation of the cervix only when effacement is complete.* Indeed, cases are recorded in which the effacement mechanisms have failed, and the force of labor contractions has resulted in annular detachment of the undilated cervix. Also, in many induced late abortions, the cervix is not prepared to dilate, and posterior cervical ruptures result.

Contrast stains show that the nonpregnant cervix is composed predominantly of tight bundles of collagen fibers. A few muscle cells are irregularly scattered at random, and, at the periphery of the cervix, there is a thin layer of attenuated smooth muscle that is continuous with the smooth muscle of the vaginal vault. With these inconsequential exceptions, the cervix is fibrous connective tissue. Reticulum fibers are present in predictable quantity, but special stains reveal no

elastic fibers in the cervix proper (elastic fibers are found in the outer third of the myometrium just superior to the fibromuscular junction, but nowhere else in the uterus). In the cervix at the time of full dilatation the collagen bundles are seen to be loosely and widely scattered and very sparse (Fig. 29–54).

BIOCHEMICAL CHANGES

Biochemical studies in which the fully dilated cervix is compared with the nonpregnant cervix have demonstrated a significant and absolute loss of collagen and glycoprotein and a proportionate increase in ground substance. Efforts to identify the ground substance changes have disclosed that, of the seven glycosaminoglycans (mucopolysaccharides) ordinarily found in mammalian connective tissue (hyaluronate, chondroitin-4 and -6 sulfate, dermatan sulfate, heparan sulfate, keratin sulfate, and heparin), all except heparin and heparan sulfate have been identified in the cervix. The total ground substance mass is substantially higher at full dilatation, apparently owing to the presence of a "new" substance, *i.e.*, not one of the aforementioned glycosaminoglycans; the nature of the "new" substance is under investigation, and at this time it seems possible that it may be a "new" glycosaminoglycan synthesized especially for the unique requirements for morphologic change in the cervix in labor. It is clear, however, that the processes of effacement and dilatation are by no means passive; rather, they are the re-

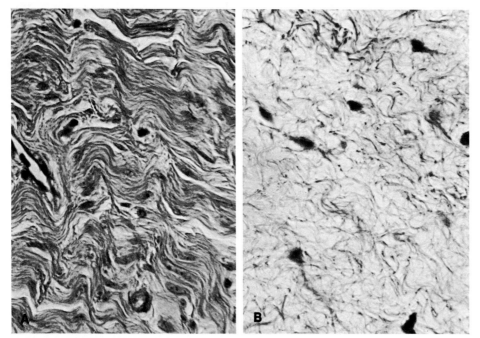

FIG. 29-54. Photomicrograph of tissue from posterior lip of cervix, approximately 1 cm above plane of external os. *A.* Nonpregnant. *B.* Immediately postpartum. These changes were originally attributed to edema and dispersion of collagen fibers, but they are now known to be due largely to actual destruction of collagen and accumulation of glycosaminoglycans. (Milligan's trichrome stain for collagen, × 835) (Danforth DN, Buckingham JC, Roddick JW, Jr: Am J Obstet Gynecol 80: 939, 1960)

sult of intensely active and dynamic changes in the structure of the cervix.

The Role of Prostaglandins

The mechanism by which PGs could cause the changes of effacement and dilatation is yet to be determined. The explanation will undoubtedly come through greater understanding of the connective tissue degradation and remodeling processes that are responsible for the marked morphologic changes. It seems clear that collagenases and proteases will be concerned, and preliminary data suggest that, like so many other phenomena of pregnancy, the effects of estrogens and progesterone will be shown to be part of the process.

The details of the remarkable phenomenon of cervical ripening are discussed in both the Liggins review and the Naftolin–Stubblefield symposium. The interested reader is referred to these sources.

Liggins has observed that no hypothesis for the initiation of human labor is complete unless it includes a satisfactory explanation of the structural changes in the cervix. He has reviewed the current status of this question; in addition, Naftolin and Stubblefield devoted a symposium to an exploration of the physiology of cervical dilatation. As noted earlier in this chapter, there is evidence that the arachidonic acid released from disturbed lysosomes in the fetal membranes is the source of substantial quantities of PGs, which are synthesized by the decidua. Although the evidence is indirect, PGs appear to have a key role in the initiation of labor. It is now apparent that these same substances can also cause effacement of the cervix (a process also known as cervical ripening or compliance). There is no direct evidence that endogenous PGs are physiologically responsible for cervical ripening, but the circumstantial evidence is impressive. PGs administered intravenously or applied locally in the form of a viscous vaginal gel suppository cause significant cervical softening. They have also been shown to be especially useful in producing cervical ripening prior to induced late abortion or induction of labor when the condition of the cervix is unfavorable. When applied *in vitro,* they greatly increase the stretch modulus of the cervix. This, plus other indirect evidence cited earlier in this chapter suggest the possibility that local release of PGs could be the trigger that leads to cervical effacement. Local release of PGs could also explain the efficacy of laminaria in producing effacement, and the severe uterine cramps and ultimate effacement, and dilatation of the cervix as a predunculated submucous fibroid moves through the lower pole of the uterus.

REFERENCES AND RECOMMENDED READING

CAUSE OF THE ONSET OF LABOR

General

Creasy RK, Liggins GC: Aetiology and management of preterm labour. In Stallworthy J, Bourne G (eds): Recent Advances in Obstetrics and Gynaecology, Vol 13, Chap 2. Edinburgh, Churchill Livingstone, 1979

Csapo AI: The regulatory interplay of progesterone and prostaglandin $F_{2\alpha}$ in the control of the pregnant uterus. In Josimovich JB (ed): Uterine Contraction—Side Effects of Steroidal Contraceptives, Chap 15, p 251. New York, John Wiley, 1973

Csapo AI: The uterus: Model experiments and clinical trials. In Bourne GH (ed): The Structure and Function of Muscle, 2nd ed, Vol II, p. 17. New York, Academic Press, 1973

Csapo AI: The "see-saw" theory of the regulatory mechanism of pregnancy. Am J Obstet Gynecol 121:578, 1975

Fuchs F: Endocrinology of labor. In Fuchs F, Klopper K (Eds): Endocrinology of Pregnancy, 2nd ed, Chap 16. New York, Harper & Row, 1977

Liggins GC, Forster CS, Grieves SA et al: Control of parturition in man. Biol Reprod 16:39, 1977

Liggins GC: Initiation of parturition. Br Med Bull 35:145, 1979

Liggins GC: What factors initiate human labor? Contemp OB/GYN 13:147, 1979

Nathanielsz PW: Endocrine mechanisms of parturition. Annu Rev Physiol 40:411, 1978

Reynolds SRM: Physiology of the Uterus, 2nd ed. New York, Hoeber, 1949. Reprint: New York, Hafner, 1965

Ryan KJ: Maintenance of pregnancy and the initiation of labor. Chap 16 in Tulchinsky D, Ryan KJ (eds) Maternal—Fetal Endocrinology. Phila, Saunders, 1980

Effects of Distention and Stretch

Csapo AI, Jaffin H, Kerenyi T et al: Volume and acitivity of the pregnant human uterus. Am J Obstet Gynecol 85:819, 1963

Effects of Estrogens and Progesterone

Boroditsky RS, Reyes FI, Winter JDS et al: Maternal serum estrogen and progesterone concentrations preceding labor. Obstet Gynecol 51:686, 1978

Csapo AI: Progesterone block. Am J Anat 98:273, 1956

Csapo AI, Pohanka O, Kaihola HL: Progesterone deficiency and premature labor. Br. Med J 1:137, 1974

Csapo AI, Resch BA: Induction of preterm labor in the rat by antiprogesterone. Am J Obstet Gynecol 134:823, 1979

Danforth DN: Cervical incompetency. In Davis CH, Carter AB (eds): Obstetrics and Gynecology, Chap 10-A. Hagerstown, WA Prior, 1962

Danforth DN, Buckingham JC: Cervical incompetence—A re-evaluation. Postgrad Med 32:4, 1962

Haning RV, Jr, Barrett DA, Alberino SP et al: Interrelationships between maternal and cord prolactin, progesterone, estradiol, 13,14-dihydro-15-keto-prostaglandin $F_{2\alpha}$ and cord cortisol at delivery with respect to initiation of parturition. Am J Obstet Gynecol 130:204, 1978

Johnson JWC, Austin KL, Jones GS et al: Efficacy of 17 α-hydroxyprogesterone caproate in the prevention of premature labor. N Engl J Med 293:675, 1975

Johnson JWC, Lee PA, Zachary AS et al: High risk prematurity—Progestin treatment and steroid studies. Obstet Gynecol 54:412, 1979

Kauppila A, Kivela A, Kontula K et al: Serum progesterone, estradiol, and estriol before and during induced labor. Am J Obstet Gynecol 137:462, 1980

Mathur RS, Landgrebe S, Williamson HO: Progesterone, 17α-hydroxyprogesterone, estradiol, and estriol in late pregnancy and labor. Am J Obstet Gynecol 136:25, 1980

Mitchell MD, Flint APF: Progesterone withdrawal: Effects on prostaglandins and parturition. Prostaglandins 14:611, 1977

Effects of Prostaglandins

Brenner WE, Hendricks CH, Braaksma JT et al: Intraamniotic administration of prostaglandin $F_{2\alpha}$ to induce therapeutic abortion. A. Efficacy and tolerance of two dosage schedules. Am J Obstet Gynecol 114:781, 1972

Challis JRG: Physiology and pharmacology of PGs in parturition. Prostaglandins, Series G, pp 47ff, 1974

Dubin NH, Johnson JWC, Calhoun S et al: Plasma prostaglandin in pregnant women with term and preterm deliveries. Obstet Gynecol 57:203, 1981

Green K, Bygdeman M, Toppozada M et al: The role of prostaglandin $F_{2\alpha}$ in human parturition. Am J Obstet Gynecol 120:25, 1974

Karim S, Hillier K: The role of prostaglandins in myometrial contractions. In Josimovich JB (ed): Uterine Contraction—Side Effects of Steroidal Contraceptives, Chap 9, p 141. New York, John Wiley, 1973

Keirse MJNC, Hicks BR, Mitchell MD et al: Increase of the prostaglandin precursor, arachidonic acid, in amniotic fluid during spontaneous labour. Br J Obstet Gynaecol 84:937, 1977

Kirton KT: Biochemical effects of prostaglandins as they might relate to uterine contraction. In Josimovich JB (ed): Uterine Contraction—Side Effects of Steroidal Contraceptives, Chap 12, p 193. New York, John Wiley, 1973

Kurzrok R, Lieb D: Biochemical studies of human semen: Action of semen on human uterus. Proc Soc Exp Biol Med 28:268, 1930

Lackritz R, Tulchinsky D, Ryan KJ et al: Plasma prostaglandin metabolites in human labor. Am J Obstet Gynecol 131:484, 1978

Levitt MJ: The chemistry of prostaglandins in relation to the female reproductive tract. In Josimovich JB (ed): Uterine Contraction—Side Effects of Steroidal Contraceptives, Chap 11, p 179. New York, John Wiley, 1973

Liggins GC, Campos GA, Roberts CM: Production rates of prostaglandin F, 6-keto-$PGF_{1\alpha}$ and thromboxane B_2 by perfused human endometrium. Prostaglandins, 19:461, 1980

MacDonald PC, Schultz, M, Duenhoelter J et al: Initiation of human parturition: I. Mechanism of action of arachidonic acid. Obstet Gynecol 44:829, 1974

Mitchell MD, Flint AFP, Bibby J et al: Rapid increases in prostaglandin concentrations after vaginal examination and amniotomy. Br Med J 2:1183, 1977

Mitchell MD, Flint AFP, Turnbull AC: Stimulation by oxytocin of prostaglandin F levels in uterine venous affluent in pregnant and puerperal sheep. Prostaglandins 9:47, 1975

Mitchell MD, Flint AFP, Turnbull AC: Increasing uterine response to vaginal distension in sheep. J Reprod Fertil 49:35, 1977

Novy MJ, Cook MJ, Manaugh L: Indomethacin block of normal onset of parturition in primates. Am J Obstet Gynecol 118:412, 1974

Novy MJ, Liggins CG: Role of prostaglandins, prostacyclin, and thromboxane in the physiologic control of the uterus in parturition. Semin Perinatol 4:45, 1980

Satoh K, Yasumizu T, Fukuoka H et al: Prostaglandin $F_{2\alpha}$ metabolite levels in plasma, amniotic fluid, and urine during pregnancy and labor. Am J Obstet Gynecol 133:886, 1979

Schulman H, Saldana L, Lin C-C et al: Mechanism of failed labor after fetal death and its treatment with prostaglandin E_2. Am J Obstet Gynecol 133:742, 1979

Southern EM (ed): The Prostaglandins: Clinical Applications in Human Reproduction. New York, Futura, 1972

Vane JR: Inhibition of prostaglandin synthesis as a mechanism of action for aspirin-like drugs. Nature (New Biol) 231:232, 1972

Waltman R, Tricomi V, Palav A: Mid-trimester hypertonic saline-induced abortion: Effect of indomethacin on induction/abortion time. Am J Obstet Gynecol 114:829, 1972

Zuckerman H, Reiss U, Atad J et al: Prostglandin $F_{2\alpha}$ in human blood during labor. Obstet Gynecol 51:311, 1978

Contractile System of the Myometrium

Perry SV, Grand RJA: Mechanisms of contraction and the specialized protein components of smooth muscle. Br Med Bull 35:219, 1979

Effects of Mineral Ions

Anderson NC, Jr: Physiologic basis of myometrial function. Semin Perinatol 2:211, 1978

Andersson K-E: Inhibition of uterine activity by the calcium antagonist nifedipine. In Anderson A, Beard R, Brudenell JM et al. (eds): Preterm Labor. Proceedings of the 5th Study Group of the Royal College of Obstetricians and Gynaecologists, London, 1977

Andersson K-E, Ingemarsson I, Ulmsten U et al: Inhibition of prostaglandin-induced uterine activity by nifedipine. Br J Obstet Gynaecol 86:175, 1979

Bell WB, Hick P: Observations on the physiology of the female genital organs. Br Med J March 27, 1909

Carsten ME: Regulation of myometrial composition, growth, and activity. In Assali NS (ed): Biology of Gestation, Vol I, p 393. New York, Academic Press, 1968

Carsten ME: Sarcoplasmic reticulum from pregnant bovine uterus: Calcium binding. Gynecol Invest 4:84, 1973

Carsten ME: Sarcoplasmic reticulum from pregnant bovine uterus: Prostaglandins and calcium. Gynecol Invest 4:95, 1973

Carsten ME: Prostaglandins and cellular calcium transport in the pregnant human uterus. Am J Obstet Gynecol 117:824, 1973

Carsten ME: Prostaglandins and oxytocin: Their effects on uterine smooth muscle. Prostaglandins 5:33, 1974

Carsten ME: Hormonal regulation of myometrial calcium transport. Gynecol Invest 5:269, 1974

Carsten ME: How does calcium control uterine contraction? Contemp OB/GYN 8:61, 1976

Carsten ME: Calcium accumulation by human uterine microsomal preparation: Effects of progesterone and oxytocin. Am J Obstet Gynecol 133:598, 1978

Carsten ME, Miller JD: Involvement of cyclic AMP in calcium accumulation by uterine sarcoplasmic reticulum. Abstracts of the 1980 meeting of the Society for Gynecologic Investigation, p 86

Cheung WY: Calmodulin plays a pivotal role in cellular regulation. Science 207:19, 1980

Danforth DN, Ivy AC: Effect of calcium on uterine activity and reactivity. Proc Soc Exp Biol Med 38:550, 1938

Danforth DN, Ivy AC: Effect of calcium on uterine contractions and on uterine response to intravenously injected oxytocics. Am J Obstet Gynecol 37:184, 1939

Danforth DN, Ivy AC: A consideration of the cause of the onset of labor. Int Abstr Surg (Surg Gynecol Obstet) 69:351, 1939

Fleckenstein A: Specific pharmacology of calcium in myocardium, cardiac pacemakers, and vascular smooth muscle. Annu Rev Pharmacol Toxicol 17:149, 1977

Kroeger EA, Marshall JM, Bianchi CP: Effect of isoproterenol and D600 (calcium antagonist) on calcium movements in rat myometrium. J Pharmacol Exp Ther 193:1, 1975

Liggins GC: Initiation of parturition. Br Med Bull 35:145, 1979

Liggins GC, Forster CS, Grieves SA et al: Control of parturition in man. Biol Reprod 16:39, 1977

Marx JL: Calmodulin: A protein for all seasons. Science 208:274, 1980

Perry SV, Grand RJA: Mechanisms of contraction and the specialized protein components of smooth muscle. Br Med Bull 35:219, 1979

Rasmussen H: Cell communication: Calcium ion and cyclic adenosine monophosphate. Science 170:404, 1970

Rasmussen H: Ions as "second messengers." Hosp Pract 9:99, 1974

Rasmussen H, Goodman DBP, Tenehouse A: The role of cyclic AMP and calcium in cell activation. CRC Crit Rev Biochem 1:95, 1972

Ulmsten U, Andersson K-E, Forman A: Relaxing effects of nifedipine on the nonpregnant uterus in vitro and in vivo. Obstet Gynecol 52:436, 1978

Effects of Nervous Mechanisms

Daniel EE, Lodge S: Electrophysiology of the myometrium. In Josimovich JB (ed): Uterine Contraction: Side Effects of Steroidal Contraceptives, p 19. New York, John Wiley, 1973

Moawad AH: The sympathetic nervous system and the uterus. In Josimovich JB (ed): Uterine Contraction—Side Effects of Steroidal Contraceptives, Chap 4, p 71. New York, John Wiley, 1973

Thorbert G, Alm P, Bjorklund AB et al: Adrenergic innervation of the human uterus: Disappearance of the transmitter and transmitter-forming enzymes during pregnancy. Am J Obstet Gynecol 135:223, 1979

Tsuei JJ, Lai Y-F, Sharma SD: The influence of acupuncture stimulation during pregnancy: The induction and inhibition of labor. Obstet Gynecol 50:479, 1977

Effects of Catecholamines

Cibils L, Pose S, Zuspan F: Effect of 1-norepinephrine infusion on uterine contractility and cardiovascular system. Am J Obstet Gynecol 84:307, 1962

Krall JF: Molecular basis of drug action on uterine smooth muscle. In Anderson A, Beard R, Brudenell JM et al. (eds): Preterm Labour. Proceedings of the 5th Study Group of the Royal College of Obstetricians and Gynaecologists, London, 1977

Kroeger EA, Marshall JM: Beta-adrenergic effects on rat myometrium: Role of cAMP. Am J Physiol 226:1298, 1974

Lederman RP, Lederman E, Work BA, Jr et al: The relation-

ship of maternal anxiety, plasma catecholamines, and plasma cortisol to progress in labor. Am J Obstet Gynecol 132:495, 1978

Phillippe M, Ryan KJ: Catecholamines in human amniotic fluid. Am J Obstet Gynecol 139:204, 1981

Pose SV, Cibils L, Zuspan F: Effect of 1-epinephrine infusion on uterine contractility and cardiovascular system. Am J Obstet Gynecol 84:297, 1962

Effects of Fetus and Fetal Membranes

Bjorkhem I, Lantto O, Lunell N-O: Total and free cortisol in amniotic fluid during late pregnancy. Br J Obstet Gynaecol 85:446, 1978

Cawson MJ, Anderson ABM, Turnbull AC et al: Cortisol, cortisone, and 11-deoxycortisol levels in human umbilical maternal plasma in relation to the onset of labor. J Obstet Gynaecol Br Commonw 81:737, 1974

Gustavii B: Studies on the mode of action of intra-amniotically and extraamniotically injected hypertonic saline in therapeutic abortion. Acta Obstet Gynecol Scan (Suppl) 25:5, 1973

Gustavii B: Release of lysosomal acid phosphatase into the cytoplasm of decidual cells before the onset of labor in humans. Br J Obstet Gynaecol 82:177, 1975

Haukkamaa M, Lahteenmaki P: Steroids of human myometrium and maternal and umbilical cord plasma before and during labor. Obstet Gynecol 53:617, 1979

Katz Z, Lancet M, Levavi E: The efficacy of intraamniotic steroids for induction of labor. Obstet Gynecol 54:31, 1979

Kauppila A, Koivisto M, Pukka M et al: Umbilical cord and neonatal cortisol levels: Effects of gestational and neonatal factors. Obstet Gynecol 52:666, 1978

Kennaway DJ, Matthews CD, Seamark RF et al: J Steroid Biochem 8:559, 1977

Liggins GC: Fetal influences on uterine contractility. In Josimovich JB (ed): Uterine Contraction: Side Effects of Steroidal Contraceptives, Chap 13, p 208. New York, John Wiley, 1973

Liggins GC: Fetal influences on myometrial contractility. Clin Obstet Gynecol 16:148, 1973

Mitchell MD, Sayers L, Heirse MJNC et al: Melatonin in amniotic fluid during human parturition. Br J Obstet Gynaecol 85:684, 1978

Okazaki T, Casey ML, MacDonald PC et al: Prostaglandin biosynthesis and degradation in human fetal membranes and uterine decidua vera. Abstracts of the 1980 meeting of the Society for Gynecologic Investigation, p 22

Page EW: The fetus as a factor in the initiation of labor. In Marshall JM (ed): Initiation of Labor, p 167. Public Health Publication 1390. Bethesda, MD, National Institute of Child Health and Human Development, Department of Health, Education and Welfare, 1963

Phillippe M, Ryan KJ: Catecholamines in human amniotic fluid. Am J Obstet Gynecol 139:204, 1981

Roopnarinesingh S, Alexis D, Lendore R et al: Fetal steroid levels at delivery. Obstet Gynecol 50:442, 1977

Schwarz BE, MacDonald PC, Johnston JM: Initiation of human parturition: XI. Lysosomal enzyme release in vitro from amnions obtained from laboring and nonlaboring women. Am J Obstet Gynecol 137:21, 1980

Effects of Oxytocin

Bell WB: The pituitary body: Therapeutic value of the infundibular extract in shock, uterine atony, and intestinal paresis. Br Med J 1609, 1909

Bell WB: Infundibulin in primary uterine inertia and in the induction of labour. Proc R Soc Med 8:71, 1915

Caldeyro-Barcía R, Heller H (eds): Oxytocin. New York, Pergamon Press, 1962

Caldeyro-Barcía R, Sica-Blanco Y, Poseiro JJ et al: A quantitative study of the action of synthetic oxytocin on the pregnant human uterus. J Pharmacol Exp Ther 121:18, 1957

Chard T, Boyd NRH, Fosling AS et al: The development of a radioimmunossay for oxytocin: The extraction of oxytocin from plasma and its measurement during parturition in human and goat blood. J Endocrinol 48:223, 1970

Dawood MY, Pociask C, Raghaven KS et al: Oxytocin levels in mother and fetus during parturition. Gynecol Invest 7:29, 1976

Dawood MY: The role of oxytocin in human labor. Res & Staff Physician 45, 1978

Dawood MY, Raghaven KS, Pociask C et al.: Oxytocin in human pregnancy and parturition. Obstet Gynecol 51:138, 1978

DuVigneaud V: Hormones of the posterior pituitary gland: Oxytocin and vasopressin. Harvey Lecture (London) 50:1, 1954–1955

Glick SM: The measurement of oxytocin by radioimmunoassay. In Josimovich JB (ed): Uterine Contraction—Side Effects of Steroidal Contraceptives, Chap 6, p 101. New York, John Wiley, 1973

Husami N, Jewelewicz R, Vande Wiele RL: Pregnancy in patients with pituitary tumors. Fertil Steril 28:920, 1977

Kamm O, Aldrich TB, Grote IW et al: The active principles of the posterior lobe of the pituitary gland. I. The demonstration of the presence of two active principles. II. The separation of the two principles and their concentration in the forms of potent solid preparations. J Am Chem Soc 50:573, 1928

Kumaresan P, Anandarangam PB, Dianzon W et al: Plasma oxytocin levels and labor as determined by radioimmunoassay. Am J Obstet Gynecol 119:215, 1974

Leake RD, Weitzman RE, Fisher DA: Pharmacokinetics of oxytocin in the human subject. Obstet Gynecol 56:701, 1980

Leake RD, Weitzman RE, Glatz TH et al: Stimulation of oxytocin secretion in the human. Abstracts of the 1979 meeting of the Society for Gynecologic Investigation, p 29

Ray BS: Some inferences from hypophysectomy in 450 human patients. Arch Neurol 3:121, 1960

Seppala M, Aho I, Tissari A et al: Radioimmunoassay of oxytocin in amniotic fluid, fetal urine and meconium in late pregnancy and delivery. Am J Obstet Gynecol 114:778, 1972

Takahashi K, Diamond F, Bieniarz J et al: Uterine contractility and oxytocin sensitivity in preterm, term, and postterm pregnancy. Am J Obstet Gynecol 136:774, 1980

Theobald GW, Graham A, Campbell J et al: The use of post-pituitary extract in physiological amounts in obstetrics. Br Med J 2:123, 1948

Vasicka A, Kumaresan P, Hans GS et al: Plasma oxytocin in initiation of labor. Am J Obstet Gynecol 130:263, 1978

Watson BP: Induction of labor: Indications and methods, with special reference to the use of pituitary extract. Transactions of the American Gynecological Society, 45:31, 1920

UTERINE RESPONSES TO PREGNANCY AND LABOR

Structural Changes in Pregnancy and Labor

Danforth DN, Chapman JCF: Incorporation of the isthmus uteri. Am J Obstet Gynecol 59:979, 1950

Danforth DN, Graham RJ, Ivy AC: Functional anatomy of

labor as revealed by frozen sagittal sections in the *Macaca rhesus* monkey. Surg Gynecol Obstet 74:188, 1942

Danforth DN, Ivy AC: The lower uterine segment: Its derivation and physiologic behavior. Am J Obstet Gynecol 57:83, 1949

Uterine Contractions

Alvarez H, Caldeyro-Barcía R: Contractility of the human uterus recorded by new methods. Surg Gynecol Obstet 91:1, 1950

Beard RW: Controlling and quantifying uterine activity. Contemp OB/GYN 13, 75, 1979

Blair-Bell W, Datnow MM, Jeffcoate TNA: The mechanism of uterine action and its disorders. J Obstet Gynaecol Br Emp 40:541, 1933

Caldeyro-Barcía R, Poseiro JJ: Physiology of the uterine contraction. Clin Obstet Gynecol 3:386, 1960

Danforth DN, Graham RJ, Ivy AC: The physiology of the uterus in labor. Quart Bull Northwestern Univ Med Sch 15:1, 1941

Hendricks CH: Uterine contractility at delivery and in the puerperium. Am J Obstet Gynecol 83:890, 1962

Hicks JB: On the contractions of the uterus throughout pregnancy: Their physiological effects and their value in the diagnosis of pregnancy. Trans Obstet Soc Lond 13:216, 1872

Duey JA, Jr, Miller FC: The evaluation of uterine activity: A comparative analysis. Am J Obstet Gynecol 135:252, 1979

Ivy AC, Hartman CG, Koff A: The contractions of the monkey uterus at term. Am J Obstet Gynecol 22:388, 1931

Jeffcoate TNA: Abnormalities of uterine action in labour. In Bowes K (ed): Modern Trends in Obstetrics and Gynaecology. New York, Hoeber, 1950

Lowenstein WR: Cellular communication by permeable membrane junctions. Hosp Pract 9:113, 1974

Marshall JM: Physiological principles of contraction in uterine muscle. In Marshall JM (ed): Initiation of Labor, pp 24, 25, 96. Public Health Publication 1390. Bethesda, MD, National Institute of Child Health and Human Development, Department of Health, Education, and Welfare, 1963

Marshall JM: Physiology of the myometrium. Norris HJ, Hertig AT, Abell MR (eds): The Uterus, p 89. Baltimore, Williams & Wilkins, 1973

Miller FC, Mueller E, Velick K: Quantitation of uterine activity: Clinical evaluation of a new method of data presentation. Obstet Gynecol 55:388, 1980

Mizrahi J, Karni Z, Polishuk WZ: Strain uterography in labour. Br J Obstet Gynaecol 84:930, 1977

Reynolds SRM: The uses of Braxton Hicks contractions. Obstet Gynecol 32:134, 1968

Richardson JA, Sutherland IA: Letter: "A cervimeter for continuous measurement of cervical dilatation" in labour—Preliminary results. Br J Obstet Gynaecol 85:975, 1978

Schatz P: Beitrage zur physiologischen Geburtskunde. Arch Gynaekol 3:58, 1872

Seitchik J, Chatkoff ML: Intrauterine pressure wave forms characteristic of successful and failed first stage labor. Gynecol Invest 8:246, 1977

Seitchik J, Chatkoff ML: Induced uterine hypercontractility pressure wave forms. Obstet Gynecol 48:436, 1977

Turnbull AC, Anderson ABM: Uterine function in human pregnancy and labour. In MacDonald RR (ed): Scientific Basis of Obstetrics and Gynaecology, 2nd ed. Edinburgh, Churchill Livingstone, 1978

Wolfs GMJA, Van Leeuwen M: Electromyographic observations on the human uterus during labour. Acta Obstet Gynecol Scand (suppl) 58:90, 1979

DRUG EFFECTS

Akamatsu TJ, Bonica JJ: Spinal and extradural analgesia–anesthesia for parturition. Clin Obstet Gynecol 17:183, 1974

Barden TP: The effect of drugs on uterine contractility. In Quilligan EJ, Kretchmer N (eds): Fetal and Maternal Medicine. New York, John Wiley, 1980

Caritis SN, Edelstone DI, Mueller–Heubach E: Pharmacologic inhibition of preterm labor. Am J Obstet Gynecol 133:557, 1979

Cibils LA, Zuspan FP: Pharmacology of the uterus. Clin Obstet Gynecol 11:34, 1968

Datta S, Kitzmiller JL, Ostheimer GW et al: Propranolol and parturition. Obstet Gynecol 51:577, 1978

Eskes TK: Effect of morphine upon uterine contractility in late pregnancy. Am J Obstet Gynecol 84:281, 1962

Fuchs F: Effect of ethyl alcohol upon spontaneous uterine activity. J Obstet Gynaecol Br Commonw 72:1011, 1965

Hendricks CH, Brenner WE: Cardiovascular effects of oxytocic drugs used postpartum. Am J Obstet Gynecol 108:751, 1970

Lewis RB, Schulman JD: Influence of acetylsalicylic acid, an inhibitor of prostaglandin synthesis, on the duration of human gestation and labor. Lancet 2:1159, 1973

Lipshitz J: Uterine and cardiovascular effects of aminophylline. Am J Obstet Gynecol 131:716, 1978

Niebyl JR, Blake DA, Johnson JWC et al: The pharmacologic inhibition of premature labor. Obstet Gynecol Surv 33:507, 1978

Pauerstein CJ: Use and abuse of oxytocic agents. Clin Obstet Gynecol 16:262, 1973

Sica–Blanco Y, Rozada H, Remedio M: Effect of meperidine on uterine contractility during pregnancy and prelabor. Am J Obstet Gynecol 97:1096, 1967

Tepperman HM, Beydoun SN, Abdul–Karim RW: Drugs affecting uterine contractility in pregnancy. Clin Obstet Gynecol 20:423, 1977

Vasicka A, Hutchinson HT, Eng MM et al: Spinal and epidural anesthesia, fetal and uterine response to acute hypo- and hypertension. Am J Obstet Gynecol 90:800, 1964

Zuckerman H, Reiss U, Rubinstein I: Inhibition of human premature labor by indomethacin. Obstet Gynecol 44:787, 1974

CHANGES IN THE CERVIX IN PREGNANCY AND LABOR

Barnes AB, Colton T, Gynderson J et al: Fertility and outcome of pregnancy in women exposed in utero to diethylstilbestrol. N Engl J Med 302:609, 1980

Beier HM: Anatomy of cervical changes at the end of pregnancy. Z Geburts Perinatol 183:83, 1979

Buckingham JC, Selden R, Danforth DN: Connective tissue changes in the cervix during pregnancy and labor. Ann NY Acad Sci 97:733, 1962

Conrad JT, Veland K: Reduction of stretch modules of human cervical tissue by prostaglandin E$_2$. Am J Obstet Gynecol 126:218, 1976

Conrad JT, Veland K: The stretch modules of human cervical tissue in spontaneous, oxytocin-induced and prostaglandin E$_2$-induced labor. Am J Obstet Gynecol 133:11, 1979

Danforth DN: Fibrous nature of the human cervix and its relation to the isthmic segment in gravid and nongravid uteri. Am J Obstet Gynecol 53:541, 1947

Danforth DN: The squamous epithelium and squamoco-

lumnar junction of the cervix during pregnancy. Am J Obstet Gynecol 60:985, 1950

Danforth DN: Distribution and functional significance of the cervical musculature. Am J Obstet Gynecol 68:1261, 1954

Danforth DN, Buckingham JC: Connective tissue mechanisms and their relation to pregnancy. Obstet Gynecol Surv 19:715, 1964

Danforth DN, Buckingham JC, Roddick JW, Jr: Connective tissue changes incident to cervical effacement. Am J Obstet Gynecol 80:939, 1960

Danforth DN, Veis A, Breen M et al: The effect of pregnancy on the human cervix: Changes in collagen, glycoproteins, and glycosaminoglycans. Am J Obstet Gynecol 120:641, 1974

Grunberger W, Husslein P: "Portio priming" in post date and low pelvic score. Geburtshilfe Frauenheilkd 39:793, 1979

Hendricks CH, Brenner WE, Kraus G: The normal cervical dilatation pattern in late pregnancy and labor. Am J Obstet Gynecol 106:1065, 1970

Herbst AL, Hubby MM, Blough RR et al: A comparison of pregnancy experience in DES-exposed and DES-unexposed daughters. J Reprod Med 24:62, 1980

Jones JM, Sweetnam P, Hibbard BM: The outcome of pregnancy after cone biopsy of the cervix: A case-controlled study. Br J Obstet Gynecol 86:913, 1979

Junqueira LCU, Zugaib M, Montes GS et al: Morphologic and histochemical evidence for the occurrence of collagenolysis and for the role of neutrophilic polymorphonuclear leukocytes during cervical dilatation. Am J Obstet Gynecol 138:273, 1980

Kleissl HP, Van der Rest M, Naftolin F et al: Collagen changes in the human uterine cervix at parturition. Am J Obstet Gynecol 130:748, 1978

Leiman G, Harrison NA, Rubin A: Pregnancy following conization of the cerix: Complications related to cone size. Am J Obstet Gynecol 136:14, 1980

Liggins GC: Ripening of the cervix. Semin Perinatol 2:261, 1978

MacKenzie IZ, Embrey MP: A comparison of PGE_2 and $PGF_{2\alpha}$ vaginal gel for ripening the cervix before induction of labour. Br J Obstet Gynaecol 86:167, 1979

MacLennan AH, Green RC: A double blind dose trial of intravaginal prostaglandin $F_{2\alpha}$ for cervical ripening and the induction of labour. N Z J Obstet Gynecol 20:80, 1980

MacLennan AH, Green RC: Cervical ripening and induction of labour with intravaginal prostaglandin $F_{2\alpha}$. Lancet 1:117, 1979

Mochizuki M, Honda T, Deguchi M et al: A study on the effect of dehydroepiandrosterone sulfate on so-called cervical ripening. Acta Scand Obstet Gynecol 57:397, 1978

Naftolin F, Stubblefield PG (eds): Dilatation of the Uterine Cervix: Connective Tissue Biology and Clinical Management. New York, Raven Press, 1980

O'Herlihy C, MacDonald HN: Influence of preinduction prostaglandin E_2 vaginal gel on cervical ripening and labor. Obstet Gynecol 54:708, 1979

Ostergard DR: The effect of pregnancy on the cervical squamocolumnar junction in patients with abnormal cervical cytology. Am J Obstet Gynecol 134:759, 1979

Roddick JW, Jr, Buckingham JC, Danforth DN: The muscular cervix—A cause of incompetency in pregnancy. Obstet Gynecol 17:562, 1961

Rossavik IKR: Total uterine impulse and cervical resistance at parturition. Am J Obstet Gynecol 136:579, 1980

Sokamato S, Sokamato M, Goldhaber P: Collagenase activity and chemical bone resorption induced by prostaglandin E_2 in tissue culture. Proc Soc Exp Biol Med 161:99, 1979

Stys SJ, Clewell WH, Meschia G: Changes in cervical compliance at parturition independent of uterine activity. Am J Obstet Gynecol 130:414, 1978

Sutherland IA, Allen DW: A cervimeter for continuous measurement of cervical dilatation in labour. Br J Obstet Gynaecol 85:178, 1978

Ulmsten U, Wingerup L, Andersson K-E: Comparison of prostaglandin E_2 and intravenous oxytocin for induction of labor. Obstet Gynecol 54:581, 1979

Weiss G, O'Bryne FM, Hochman J et al: Distribution of relaxin in women during pregnancy. Obstet Gynecol 52:569, 1978

Wilson PD: A comparison of four methods of ripening the unfavorable cervix. Br J Obstet Gynaecol 85:941, 1978

GENERAL AND MISCELLANEOUS REFERENCES

Daniel EE, Lodge S: Electrophysiology of the myometrium. In Josimovich JB (ed): In Uterine Contraction: Side Effects of Steroidal Contraceptives, Chap 3, p 19. New York, John Wiley, 1973

Garfield RE, Rabideau S, Challis JRG: Ultrastructural basis for maintenance and termination of pregnancy. Am J Obstet Gynecol 133:308, 1979

Garfield RE, Sims S, Daniel EE: Gap junctions: Their presence and necessity in myometrium during parturition. Science 198:958, 1977

Garfield RE, Sims SM, Kannan MS: Possible role of gap junctions in activation of myometrium during pregnancy. Am J Physiol 235:C168, 1978

Kirsch RE: Study on the length of gestation in the rat with notes on maintenance and termination of gestation. Am J Physiol 122:86, 1938

Peel J: The Royal College of Obstetricians and Gynaecologists, 1929 to 1979. Br J Obstet Gynaecol 86:673, 1979

Wynn RM (ed): Biology of the Uterus, 2nd ed. New York, Plenum, 1977

CHAPTER 30

MECHANISM OF NORMAL LABOR

David N. Danforth

The mechanism of labor refers to the sequence of attitudes and positions that must be assumed by the baby as it passes through the birth canal. As a general rule, the changes in position are determined by the configuration of the mother's bony pelvis; for each configuration, there is a single optimum mechanism. The physician must be aware of the normal pelvic variations in order to appreciate the details of the normal mechanism of labor.

Modern concepts of the obstetric pelvis and its influence on the mechanism of labor are based on the classic work of Caldwell and Moloy. Prior to the publication of their work, certain grossly deformed pelves were recognized as variants, but there was no understanding of the variations commonly encountered in a normal population. Caldwell and Moloy studied the human pelves in the American Museum of Natural History in New York and the large collection of T. Wingate Todd at the Western Reserve University.

On the basis of this analysis, they classified normal pelves into four major groups, according to the general shape of the pelvic inlet. They pursued their investigations at the Sloane Hospital for Women, using an instrument known as the precision stereoscope, which was developed by Moloy. This instrument resembles a standard stereoscope except that prisms are used instead of mirrors. By aligning the optical system, it is possible to place a rule on any part of the phantom image; this permits reasonably accurate direct measurement of the size of the pelvic inlet, the interspinous diameter, and the important diameters of the baby's head. Caldwell and Moloy employed this technique in the study of many hundreds of labors, and their findings form the basis of the concept of pelvic classification and the mechanism of labor that has become an integral part of the discipline of obstetrics.

THE OBSTETRIC PELVIS

ANATOMY

The bones and articulations comprising the pelvis are considered in Chapter 3. For practical purposes, the obstetrician is concerned only with the *true pelvis,* which includes the inlet, the midpelvis, and the outlet.

The *pelvic inlet* can be traced anteriorly from the iliopectineal lines along the pectineal eminence and the pubic crest to the symphysis (Fig. 30–1). Posteriorly, the inlet is bounded by the sacrum at the level of termination of the iliopectineal lines. (The sacral promontory is slightly superior to this and hence lies above the inlet.) The *plane of the inlet* is considered as a flat surface that is bounded as noted and is generally inclined at an angle of 40°–60° with the horizontal when the patient is standing. This angle is referred to as the *pelvic inclination,* and it may have much practical significance. If the angle with the horizontal is very wide, for example, so that the pelvis is inclined posteriorly, the axis of drive or force into the pelvis may be sufficiently faulty to interfere with the progress of labor.

For obstetric purposes, the plane of the pelvic inlet is considered in terms of four diameters: the anteroposterior diameter, the widest transverse diameter, and the oblique diameters. The *anteroposterior diameter* (superior strait, obstetric conjugate) extends from the posterosuperior border of the symphysis pubis to the sacrum at the level of the iliopectineal lines. For descriptive purposes, the anteroposterior diameter is divided into anterior and posterior sagittal diameters to designate the amount of space anterior and posterior to the widest transverse diameter. In the description of inlet x-rays, the anterior and posterior sagittal lengths, when considered together with the widest transverse diameter, provide instant knowledge of the general shape and capacity of the inlet. The *widest transverse*

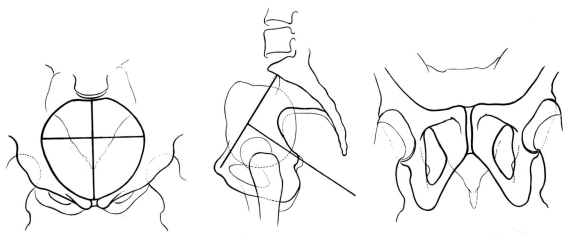

FIG. 30-1. Inlet, lateral, and front views of pelvis.

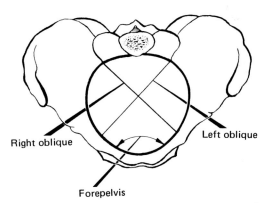

FIG. 30-2. Right and left oblique diameters of pelvic inlet and forepelvis.

diameter is invariably located posterior to the center of the pelvis and, except in asymmetric pelves, transects the anteroposterior at right angles. The *right oblique diameter* extends from the right sacroiliac joint to the left iliopectineal eminence and takes its name from the posterior landmark. The *left oblique diameter* extends from the left sacroiliac joint to the right iliopectineal eminence (Fig. 30–2).

Note should be made of two additional conjugates. The *true conjugate* (conjugata vera, CV) lies immediately superior to the obstetric conjugate and extends from the top of the pubis to the tip of the sacral promontory. It is a little longer than the obstetric conjugate, unless the promontory overhangs the inlet. The *diagonal conjugate* (DC) extends from the undermargin of the symphysis to the sacral promontory. It is said to be approximately 1.5 cm longer than the true conjugate and hence to be useful in assessing the anteroposterior diameter of the inlet. However, Eastman has shown

that, although the correlation is good in some cases, in others it is sufficiently poor to give a spurious impression of the anteroposterior diameter. Therefore, this measurement is of questionable value.

The *forepelvis* refers to the angle described by the posterior aspects of the symphysis and the pubis (Fig. 30–2). Although it is illustrated in diagrams of the inlet, this angle also affects the capacity of the midpelvis.

The *midpelvis*, for obstetric purposes, is bounded anteriorly by the posterior aspect of the symphysis and pubis, posteriorly by the sacrum at the level of S3 or S4, and laterally by the sidewalls and ischial spines.

The *sidewalls* extend from the level of the inlet at the point of the widest transverse diameter inferiorly and forward to the lower portion of the ischial tuberosities. The sidewalls are more or less straight lines; when they converge from above downward, they may limit the transverse diameter of the pelvis in the same manner that the transverse space can be limited by very prominent spines.

The *pelvic outlet* is bounded anteriorly by the inferior aspect of the symphysis (the subpubic arch), posteriorly by the tip of the sacrum (*not* the coccyx), and laterally by the ischial tuberosities.

The *axis of the pelvis* (the obstetric axis) refers to the general curve of the birth canal described by a line drawn through the center of each of the aforementioned planes (Fig. 30–3). The line curves anteriorly as the outlet is approached.

CALDWELL–MOLOY CLASSIFICATION OF PELVIC TYPES

Although the Caldwell–Moloy classification designates the four types of pelves in terms of the configuration of the inlet, certain features of the lower pelvis are also characteristic of each type. Thus, the classification is

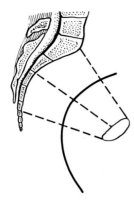

FIG. 30-3. Axis of pelvis (curve of Carus). Note that curve is more or less straight through inlet, curving anteriorly in mid-pelvis. *Dashed lines* indicate planes of inlet, midpelvis and outlet.

based upon normal variations in the following pelvic features:

Shape of inlet (width of forepelvis, ratio of widest transverse to longest anteroposterior diameter, ratio of anterior sagittal to posterior sagittal diameter)
Splay of sidewalls
Prominence of spines
Height of symphysis
Transverse diameter of outlet (bituberous)
Width of subpubic arch
Curvature and inclination of sacrum

Four basic categories are recognized which embrace all the possible normal variations in these individual features. It is emphasized that the basic types are virtually hypothetical, for it is extremely unusual to find any pelvis that conforms exactly, from front to back, from side to side, and from top to bottom, to any of them. Rather, most pelves are mixed types, showing not only combinations of the various characteristics but also much difference in size. To make an accurate assessment of the mechanism of labor, the physician must be aware both of the variations themselves and of their influence on the posture and position of the baby.

The four basic types of pelves are gynecoid, android, anthropoid, and platypelloid:

1. The *gynecoid pelvis* (Fig. 30–4) is the so-called normal type of female pelvis. The inlet is rounded, with the anteroposterior diameter very slightly shorter than the widest transverse diameter. The posterior sagittal diameter at the inlet is only slightly shorter than the anterior sagittal. The sidewalls of the pelvis are virtually straight, the spines are not prominent, the height of the symphysis is about 6 cm, the subpubic arch is wide, the transverse diameter of the

outlet is about 10 cm, and the sacrum is inclined neither anteriorly nor posteriorly, but has a gentle concavity that is midway between these two extremes.

2. The *android pelvis* (Fig. 30–5) is the so-called male type of pelvis. The inlet is wedge-shaped; the forepelvis is narrowed; and, although the anteroposterior and widest transverse diameters of the inlet may be about the same, the posterior sagittal diameter at the inlet is much shorter than the anterior sagittal. The sidewalls are typically convergent, the ischial spines are prominent, the height of the symphysis is more than 6 cm, the transverse diameter of the outlet is less than 10 cm, and the subpubic arch is narrowed. In addition, the bone structure is characteristically heavy, and the sacrum is inclined forward, especially in its lower third.

3. The *anthropoid pelvis* (Fig. 30–6) is characteristic of the ape and monkey but also occurs commonly in the human. It differs from the gynecoid in shape of the inlet, splay of the sidewalls, and position of the sacrum. The inlet is elongated anteroposteriorly, the widest transverse diameter being shorter than the anteroposterior diameter. The posterior sagittal diameter at the inlet is longer than that in the gynecoid pelvis. The forepelvis is slightly narrowed. The sidewalls are characteristically divergent, and the sacrum is inclined posteriorly. The last two characteristics account for the term "blunderbuss" pelvis.

4. The *platypelloid (flat) pelvis* (Fig. 30–7) is similar in all respects to the gynecoid, except for anteroposterior narrowing at all levels. At the inlet, therefore, the anteroposterior diameter is significantly shorter than the widest transverse, and the sacrum is forward throughout.

Table 30–1 summarizes the features of the four basic pelvic types.

CLINICAL EVALUATION

Pelvic characteristics can be determined by x-ray (see Chapter 28) or, with less exact but nonetheless sufficient detail for most purposes, by clinical examination. Definitive typing of a pelvis should usually not be attempted prior to the completion of 7.5 or 8 months' gestation. If delivery occurs before that time, the baby will be so small that the bony architecture will have no bearing upon the course of labor. Moreover, clinical evaluation of the pelvis is easier and causes far less discomfort to the patient if it is done after the soft parts have attained the relaxation and softening that reach their maximum about a month before term. Finally, when the examination is performed a month or 2 weeks before term, the presenting part has attained a considerable size, and a more accurate appraisal can be made of the capacity of the pelvis and its relation to

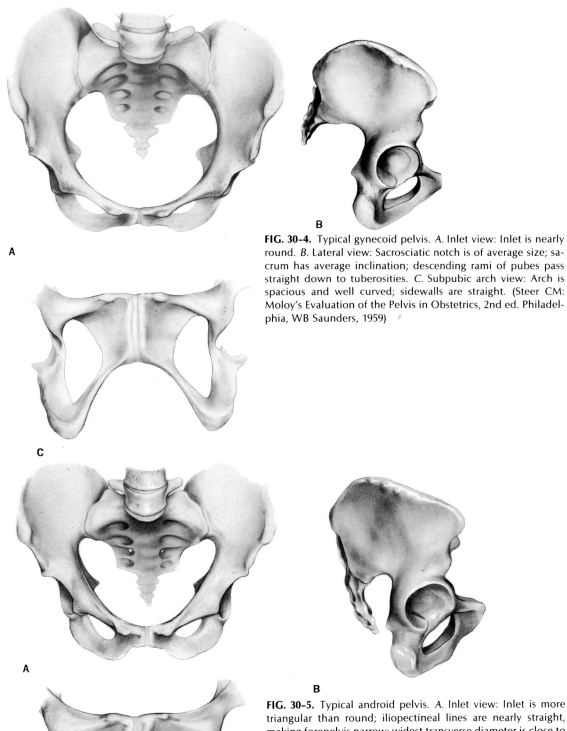

FIG. 30-4. Typical gynecoid pelvis. *A.* Inlet view: Inlet is nearly round. *B.* Lateral view: Sacrosciatic notch is of average size; sacrum has average inclination; descending rami of pubes pass straight down to tuberosities. *C.* Subpubic arch view: Arch is spacious and well curved; sidewalls are straight. (Steer CM: Moloy's Evaluation of the Pelvis in Obstetrics, 2nd ed. Philadelphia, WB Saunders, 1959)

FIG. 30-5. Typical android pelvis. *A.* Inlet view: Inlet is more triangular than round; iliopectineal lines are nearly straight, making forepelvis narrow; widest transverse diameter is close to sacrum. *B.* Lateral view. Sacrosciatic notch is narrow; sacrum has forward inclination; descending rami of pubes incline backward to tuberosities. *C.* Subpubic arch view: Descending rami arise from bottom of bodies of pubes and are straight rather than curved; sidewalls tend to converge. (Steer CM: Moloy's Evaluation of the Pelvis in Obstetrics, 2nd ed. Philadelphia, WB Saunders, 1959)

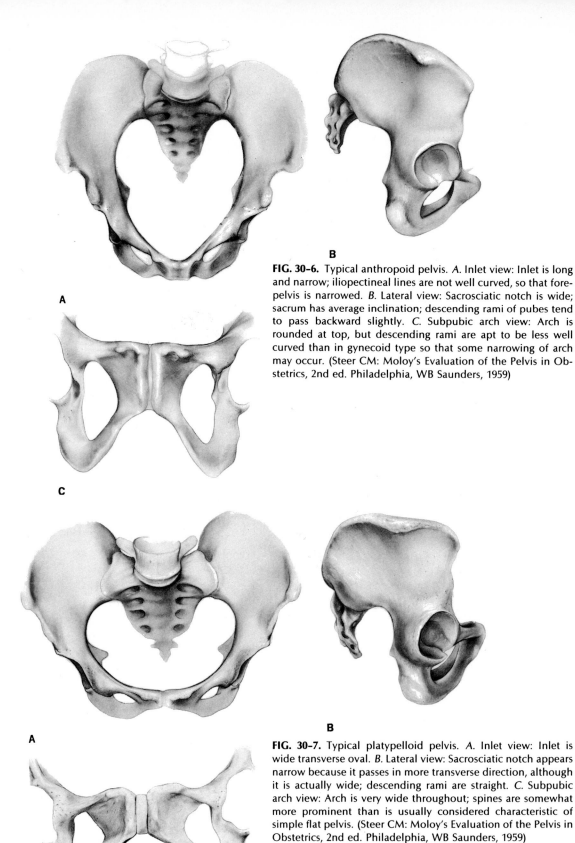

FIG. 30-6. Typical anthropoid pelvis. *A.* Inlet view: Inlet is long and narrow; iliopectineal lines are not well curved, so that fore-pelvis is narrowed. *B.* Lateral view: Sacrosciatic notch is wide; sacrum has average inclination; descending rami of pubes tend to pass backward slightly. *C.* Subpubic arch view: Arch is rounded at top, but descending rami are apt to be less well curved than in gynecoid type so that some narrowing of arch may occur. (Steer CM: Moloy's Evaluation of the Pelvis in Obstetrics, 2nd ed. Philadelphia, WB Saunders, 1959)

FIG. 30-7. Typical platypelloid pelvis. *A.* Inlet view: Inlet is wide transverse oval. *B.* Lateral view: Sacrosciatic notch appears narrow because it passes in more transverse direction, although it is actually wide; descending rami are straight. *C.* Subpubic arch view: Arch is very wide throughout; spines are somewhat more prominent than is usually considered characteristic of simple flat pelvis. (Steer CM: Moloy's Evaluation of the Pelvis in Obstetrics, 2nd ed. Philadelphia, WB Saunders, 1959)

TABLE 30-1. CHARACTERISTICS OF FOUR BASIC TYPES OF PELVES OF AVERAGE SIZE

Characteristic	Type of pelvis			
	Gynecoid	Android	Anthropoid	Platypelloid
Anteroposterior diameter of inlet	11 cm	11 cm	12+ cm	10 cm
Widest transverse diameter of inlet	12 cm	12 cm	<12 cm	12 cm
Forepelvis	Wide	Narrow	Narrow	Wide
Sidewalls	Straight	Convergent	Divergent	Straight
Ischial spines	Not prominent	Prominent	Not prominent	Not prominent
Sacrosciatic notch	Medium	Narrow	Wide	Narrow
Inclination of sacrum	Medium	Forward (lower third)	Backward	Forward
Subpubic arch	Wide	Narrow	Medium	Wide
Transverse diameter of outlet	10 cm	<10 cm	10 cm	10 cm
Bone structure	Medium	Heavy	Medium	Medium

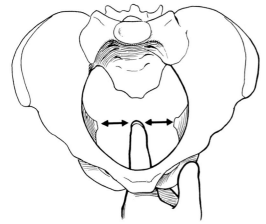

FIG. 30-8. Evaluation of transverse diameter. Lateral motion of fingers is restricted in transversely narrowed pelvis. (Steer CM: Moloy's Evaluation of the Pelvis in Obstetrics, 2nd ed. Philadelphia, WB Saunders, 1959)

the fetus. Early pelvic typing may be necessary, however, if the pelvis is grossly distorted by rickets or an old fracture or if the baby is clinically of 8 months' size despite menstrual dates that suggest a pregnancy of lesser duration.

Typing the pelvis requires a thorough knowledge of the landmarks of the pelvis and their spatial relations. This should first be obtained by study and palpation of a pelvic model. The clinical evaluation of the pelvis is illustrated in Figures 30–8 through 30–11. With practice, a satisfactory clinical appraisal can be made of most pelves; if more precise information is needed, x-ray pelvimetry should be done (see page 569). For the beginner, assessment of the ischial spines may be difficult. If the spines are prominent, they may project into the pelvis like spikes; if they are flush with the pelvic sidewalls, they may be difficult to locate except

by first identifying the sacrospinous ligament and following it forward to its anterior termination.

EXTERNAL PELVIMETRY

It was formerly believed that a reasonable appraisal of the obstetric adequacy of the pelvis could be obtained by measuring the distance between certain external pelvic landmarks. The diameters selected for measurement were the intercristal (between the iliac crests), the interspinous (between the anterosuperior iliac spines), the intertrochanteric (between the femoral trochanters), and the Baudelocque or external conjugate (from the most prominent part of the pubic bone to the dimple under the last lumbar spine). The technique of external pelvimetry is of historic interest, but the comparison of such measurements with those obtained by x-ray pelvimetry has shown conclusively that external pelvimetry is of no practical interest. The external pelvic measurements bear the same kind of relation to the internal diameters of the pelvis as the biparietal and bitemporal diameters of the head bear to the distance between the upper molar teeth.

THE FETAL HEAD

The fetal skull is composed of three major parts: the roof or vault, the face, and the base. The face and base are more or less fixed, since the bones are well fused. The vault, however, is composed of bones that are not fused; hence, this portion of the head can make the adjustments in shape that may be needed as the head passes through the narrower diameters of the pelvis. These changes in shape are referred to as *molding* (Fig. 30–12).

The bones that compose the vault are the two frontal bones, the two parietal bones, and the occipital bone. They are separated from one another by sutures and

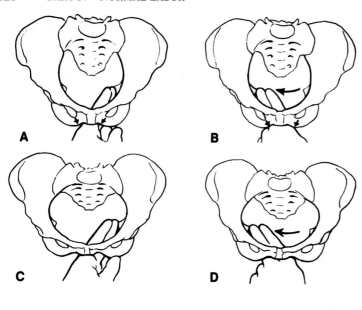

FIG. 30-9. Estimation of width of subpubic arch and inter-spinous diameter by act of pronation. *A, B.* Transversely narrowed diameters in mid- and lower pelvis. *C, D.* Wide transverse diameters in mid- and lower pelvis. (Steer CM: Moloy's Evaluation of the Pelvis in Obstetrics, 2nd ed. Philadelphia, WB Saunders, 1959)

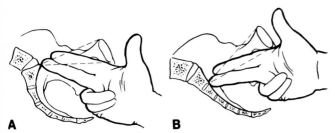

FIG. 30-10. Measurement of diagonal conjugate. When promontory is reached, index finger of opposite hand marks point of undersurface of symphysis. Distance from this point to tip of extended middle finger is length of diagonal conjugate; subtracting 1.5 cm is said to represent length of true conjugate. Promontory may be difficult to reach in early pregnancy before vagina and supports are relaxed, and in late pregnancy may be impossible to reach without disengaging presenting part. (If head is engaged, this information is not needed).

Even if accurately measured, there is great variation in its relation to the true conjugate. Since it is rarely useful and often impossible to determine, this measurement should be discarded from modern obstetric practice. (Steer CM: Moloy's Evaluation of the Pelvis in Obstetrics, 2nd ed. Philadelphia, WB Saunders, 1959)

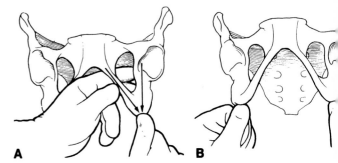

FIG. 30-11. Estimation of intertuberous diameter. *A.* Identification of ischial tuberosity at point of convergence of pubic rami and pelvic sidewalls. *B.* Measurement of intertuberous diameter. (Steer CM: Moloy's Evaluation of the Pelvis in Obstetrics, 2nd ed. Philadelphia, WB Saunders, 1959)

by the two fontanels. The sutures and fontanels are so arranged and sufficiently distinctive that palpation of these landmarks prior to delivery permits instant determination of the position of the head. This information may be of fundamental importance in following the course of labor and predicting its outcome. The relations of the sutures, fontanels, and bones of the vault are shown in Figure 30–13.

The term *fetal attitude* refers to the relation of the fetal parts to one another. In the case of the head, the

reference is to its relation to the thorax, *i.e.,* whether flexed anteroposteriorly or laterally, or extended. The atlantooccipital articulation and the flexibility of the neck permit slight lateral mobility of the head and considerable anteroposterior mobility. The lateral mobility is occasionally important. For practical purposes, the lateral diameter of the head presented to the pelvis is the biparietal diameter (Fig. 30–13); in a baby weighing about 7 lb, this diameter is about 9 cm. The presenting biparietal diameter, of course, is not influenced by the amount of flexion or extension of the head. The head usually enters the pelvis with the sagittal suture lying in the transverse plane of the mother's pelvis; when this suture lies about midway between symphysis and sacrum, the situation is referred to as *synclitism* (Fig. 30–14). When the head flexes to the right or left, and the sagittal suture approaches the

FIG. 30-12. *A.*Well-molded head of newborn child. *B.* Same head 3 days later.

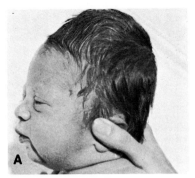
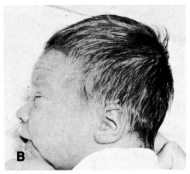

symphysis or the sacrum, the situation is referred to as *asynclitism*. Depending on the direction of flexion toward or away from the sacrum, the terms *anterior* or *posterior parietal bone presentation*, respectively, may be used (Fig. 30–15). Asynclitism may occur in normal labor as a result of a change in the axis of force (through changes in position of the uterus), or it may be a sign that the pelvis is too small to permit the head to advance into the inlet.

Although the lateral diameter that presents is not influenced by anteroposterior flexion or extension, such flexion or extension is of supreme importance in determining the anteroposterior diameter of the head that will be presented to the pelvis and, hence, in determining the amount of space required for its advancement through the pelvis. In about 95% of cases, the baby delivers headfirst; in most of these, full flexion is an automatic consequence of the fact that the occipital condyles are located near the posterior aspect of the skull, about two-thirds of the head lying anterior to this articulation (Fig. 30–16). As the head is thrust into the inlet (and is confined by the lower pole of the uterus), the longer segment of the lever yields to the pressure, and flexion results. When the head is fully flexed, with chin on the chest, the shortest anteroposterior diameter, the suboccipitobregmatic, is presented. Accordingly, the position of full flexion offers the smallest circumference of the head to the narrower planes of the pelvis. The suboccipitobregmatic diameter is a little longer than the biparietal, measuring approximately 9.5 cm in a 7-lb baby (Fig. 30–13).

In some situations, full flexion does not occur, and the result is the presentation of an anteroposterior diameter that is longer than the suboccipitobregmatic. The important variations in flexion are shown in Figure 30–17 and are named for the portion of the skull that is presented. The major attitudes when the baby presents by the head are vertex, sincipital, brow, and face.

In the sincipital presentation (the so-called military attitude), the occipitofrontal plane of the head is presented, an anteroposterior diameter of about 12 cm. In the case of brow presentation, the longest anteroposte-

rior diameter of the head, the occipitomental plane is presented. As further extension occurs, the anteroposterior diameter decreases until, in the extreme situation of face presentation, the anteroposterior diameter presented to the pelvis is only slightly longer than the suboccipitobregmatic that presents in the customary situation of full flexion.

Of the four attitudes noted, full flexion is the ideal circumstance. A military attitude gradually changes to one of flexion as the head advances into the pelvis unless mobility is impaired in the fetal neck or in the atlantooccipital articulation. A face presentation, as explained in Chapter 34, permits advancement through the pelvis, but a brow presentation does not unless the head is extremely small or the pelvis huge. A brow presentation can sometimes be converted to face or to vertex presentation. If not, delivery must be by cesarean section unless the pelvis is enormous.

PRESENTATION, POSITION, AND LIE

Certain terms are used specifically to describe the fetopelvic relations. *Lie* refers to the relation of the long axis of the fetus to the long axis of the mother (Fig. 30–18). The two possibilities are longitudinal (which is common and normal) and transverse (which is uncommon, and potentially serious). Oblique lie, a variant of the transverse lie, may also occur.

Presentation (or presenting part) refers to the part of the fetus lying over the inlet. The three major possibilities are cephalic (which occurs in about 95% of cases), breech (which occurs in perhaps 5% of labors at term), and shoulder (which is extremely rare but is ominous for both mother and baby). Cord presentation refers to the circumstance in which the umbilical cord advances into the inlet before the fetus.

Point of direction (denominator, point of reference) refers to an arbitrary, and usually the most dependent, portion of the presenting part. In cephalic presentation with well-flexed head, the occiput is the point of direction. When the fetus is in the military attitude, the occiput is also the point of direction, despite the fact

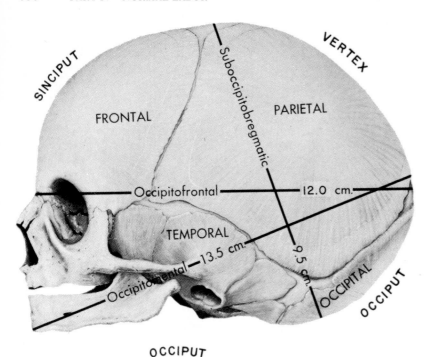

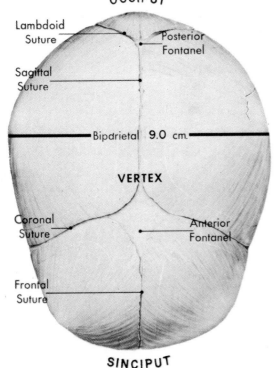

FIG. 30-13. Relation of bones, fontanels, sutures, and diameters of fetal head. (Phenomena of Normal Labor, Brochure 345, 20C. Columbus, OH, Ross Laboratories)

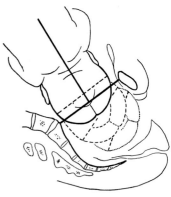

FIG. 30-14. Synclitism. Head entering pelvis with plane of biparietal diameter parallel (or synclitic) to plane of inlet. *Dotted lines* indicate changes in position as head advances. (Beck AC, Rosenthal AH: Obstetrical Practice, 6th ed. Copyright © 1955, Williams & Wilkins)

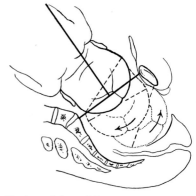

FIG. 30-15. Asynclitism. Prior to engagement, head is laterally flexed and is referred to an "anterior synclitism" or "posterior parietal bone presentation." Subsequent changes in attitude, noted by *dotted lines*, are due both to adaptation of head to pelvis and to effect of lower uterine segment and cervix. (Beck AC, Rosenthal AH: Obstetrical Practice, 6th ed. Copyright © 1955, Williams & Wilkins)

that the parietal bones may be in a more dependent position. In brow presentation, the anterior fontanel (bregma) is the point of direction; in face presentation, it is the chin (mentum); and, in breech presentation, the sacrum is the point of direction.

The head is said to be *engaged* when the biparietal diameter has passed through the plane of the inlet.

Station refers to the level of the head (or presenting part) in the pelvis. When the most dependent part of the head is at the level of the ischial spines, the station is referred to as zero. Levels 1, 2, or 3 cm above or below the level of the spines are referred to, respectively, as station −1, −2, −3, or +1, +2, +3 (Fig. 30–19). Station 0 is generally considered exact engagement, indicating that the biparietal diameter is at the level of the inlet. However, with heavy molding of

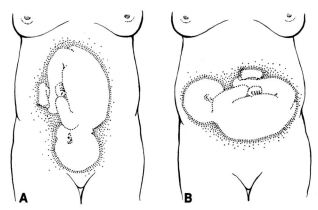

FIG. 30-18. Types of lies. *A.* Longitudinal. *B.* Transverse.

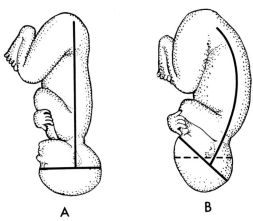

FIG. 30-16. A.Relation of head to spinal column prior to flexion. *B* Relation of head to spinal column after flexion.

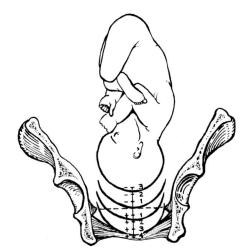

FIG. 30-19. Stations of fetal head.

FIG. 30-17. Types of cephalic presentations, according to degree of flexion or extension, and presenting diameters in each. These measurements refer to fetus of 7–7.5 lb.

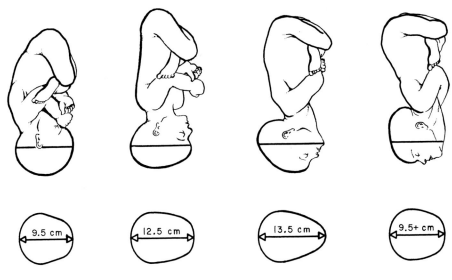

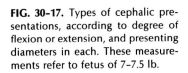

9.5 cm   12.5 cm   13.5 cm   9.5+ cm

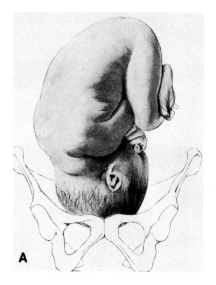

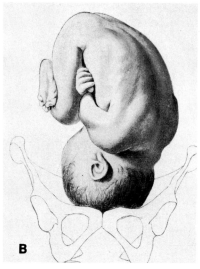

FIG. 30-20. Cephalic presentation. *A.* Right occiput anterior (ROA) position. *B.* Left occiput anterior (LOA) position. (Bumm E: Grundriss zum Studium der Geburtshilfe. Munich, Bergmann, 1922)

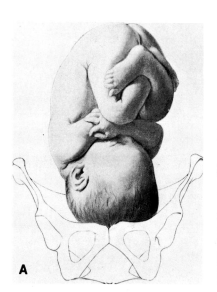

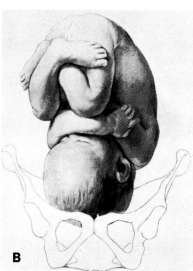

FIG. 30-21. Cephalic presentation. *A.* Right occiput posterior (ROP) position. *B.* Left occiput posterior (LOP) position. (Bumm E: Grundriss zum Studium der Geburtshilfe. Munich, Bergmann, 1922)

the head or caput succedaneum, the biparietal diameter may lie well above the inlet when the tip of the vertex reaches the interspinous diameter.

Position refers to the relation of the point of direction to one of the four quadrants or to the transverse diameter of the maternal pelvis. The point of direction may lie in either of the two posterior quadrants (right or left posterior), in either of the two anterior quadrants (right or left anterior), or in the direct transverse diameter (right or left transverse). It may also lie either directly to the front of the pelvis or directly to the back (direct anterior or direct posterior).

In defining position, the following abbreviations are used: O (occiput) in cephalic presentation, M (men-

tum or chin) in face presentation, and S (sacrum) in breech presentation. The abbreviations are further related to the appropriate part of the pelvis: ROA (right occiput anterior), LST (left sacrum transverse), LMA (left mentum anterior), and so forth. Several of the positions are illustrated in Figures 30–20 through 30–23.

THE MECHANISM OF LABOR

In considering the "normal" mechanism of labor it is customary to list five steps by which the head traverses the pelvis: descent, flexion, internal rotation, exten-

FIG. 30-22. Face presentation. *A.* Right mentum posterior (RMP) position. *B.* Left mentum anterior (LMA) position. (Bumm E: Grundriss zum Studium der Geburtshilfe. Munich, Bergmann, 1922)

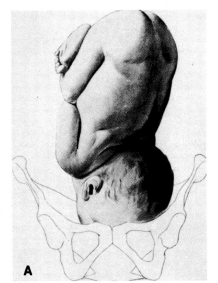
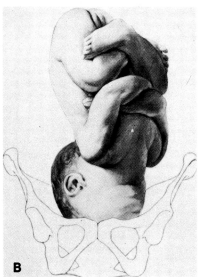

FIG. 30-23. Breech presentation. *A.* Left sacrum anterior (LSA) position. *B.* Right sacrum posterior (RSP) position. (Bumm E: Grundriss zum Studium der Geburtshilfe. Munich, Bergmann, 1922)

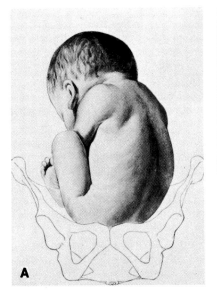
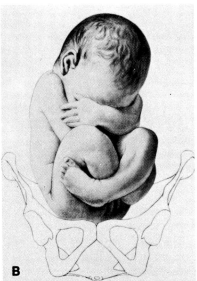

sion, and external restitution. These steps are illustrated in Figure 30–24 and are entirely accurate and appropriate for an average size gynecoid pelvis and an average size baby with the occiput the point of direction. However, no two pelves are exactly the same, just as no two faces are the same. For each pelvis there is an optimum mechanism that may be wholly different from the so-called normal mechanism described in the figure.

In most labors, which are efficient and require no intervention, the details of mechanism are of only academic interest; but a precise knowledge of mechanism may be of transcendent importance if the head arrests and must be delivered by forceps from a level above the outlet, for traction in the wrong pelvic diameter can be lethal to the baby and highly damaging to the mother. It must be remembered that 1) the bony pelvis may show great variation in individual features and 2) the birth canal is curved anteriorly (Fig. 30–3). The presenting part (for purposes of this discussion the head, with occiput the point of direction) must negotiate both the pelvic curve and any narrow areas that may be present in the pelvis.

Several other variables also influence the ease or difficulty with which the head traverses the pelvis. Among these are the quality of the uterine contrac-

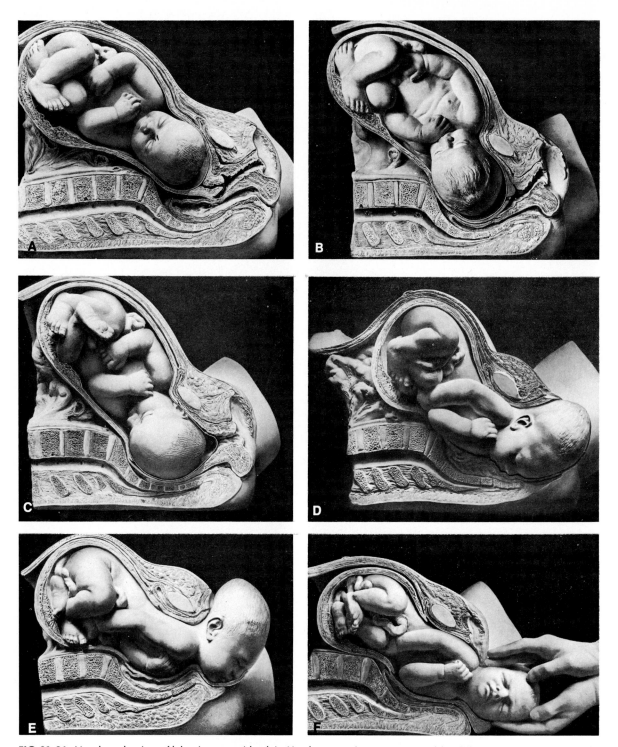

FIG. 30–24. Usual mechanism of labor in gynecoid pelvis. Head engages in transverse position (*A*), flexes a bit more and descends into midpelvis (*B*), and begins its internal rotation to occiput anterior position (*C*). As head advances, it negotiates pelvic curve by extension (*D, E*). Since shoulders traverse pelvis in oblique diameter without rotation, head undergoes external restitution toward its former transverse position immediately after it is delivered (*F*). (Reproduced with permission from Birth Atlas, 5th ed, 1960. Published by Maternity Center Association, New York)

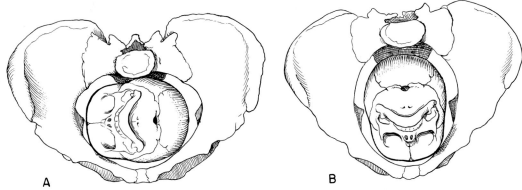

FIG. 30–25. Influence of inlet shape on engagement. Long axis of fetal head adjusts to longest inlet diameter. Transverse positions occur in platypelloid type of pelvis (*A*); posterior or anterior oblique positions occur in anthropoid type (*B*). (Steer CM: Moloy's Evaluation of the Pelvis in Obstetrics, 2nd ed. Philadelphia, WB Saunders, 1959)

tions and the ability of the head to mold; marked molding and extremely efficient uterine powers can often overcome rather high degrees of disproportion between the size of the head and the size of the pelvis. The importance of flexion of the head has already been mentioned. If the baby is small enough and the pelvis large enough, the head can advance without being influenced in the slightest by the configuration of the pelvis. As the disparity in size is reduced, a point is reached where the head must rotate one way or another to negotiate the narrow diameters and the pelvic curve. Efficient contractions, average molding, adequate flexion, and a baby large enough to use the pelvic space that is available are all required in the normal mechanism of labor. If any of these conditions are not met, the anticipated mechanism may be altered.

INFLUENCE OF INDIVIDUAL PELVIC FEATURES

Two dicta are of paramount importance in determining the changes in position that the head undergoes as it passes through the pelvis:

1. The biparietal is the narrowest presenting diameter of the head, and it must therefore go through the narrowest diameter of the pelvis at any given level.
2. The occiput generally tends to rotate to the widest or most ample portion of the pelvis at any given level.

On the basis of these maxims, the mechanism of labor can be predicted by considering first the effect of each individual pelvic feature and then the relation of each of the features to one another.

Shape of the Inlet

When the available space is used, the position of engagement is largely determined by inlet shape (Fig. 30–25). Thus, in the flat inlet, with anteroposterior narrowing, the biparietal diameter must go through this narrowed area, and engagement occurs in the occiput transverse position. In the anthropoid inlet, with transverse narrowing, engagement occurs with the sagittal suture in the sagittal plane of the pelvis. In the anthropoid pelvis, however, the forepelvis is invariably narrowed and the posterior segment deep; hence, engagement in the posterior position is the rule. In the android inlet, with narrow forepelvis and short posterior segment, the occiput rotates away from both these areas and engages in the transverse position. Transverse engagement also occurs in 70% of gynecoid pelves, since the anteroposterior diameter is slightly shorter than the widest transverse diameter.

Shape of the Forepelvis

When the forepelvis is wide, the occiput tends to rotate anteriorly, both at the inlet and in the midpelvis. When it is narrowed, the occiput tends to rotate away from the symphysis, both at the inlet and in the midpelvis.

Prominence of the Ischial Spines and Splay of the Sidewalls

The presence of prominent spines, converging sidewalls, or both has the effect of transverse narrowing in the midpelvis, and the tendency is for the biparietal diameter to descend through this narrowed area. If the interspinous diameter is wide, the head may pass this level in the direct transverse position.

Position and Configuration of the Sacrum

If the sacrum is far posterior at all levels, providing ample posterior space throughout, the head may traverse the entire pelvis in the posterior position. If the

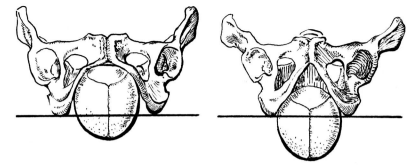

FIG. 30-26. Influence of shape of subpubic arch. *A.* Wide (gynecoid) subpubic arch, head stemming closely under symphysis. *B.* Narrow (android) arch, directing head posteriorly and requiring ample posterior segment at outlet and a wide episiotomy.

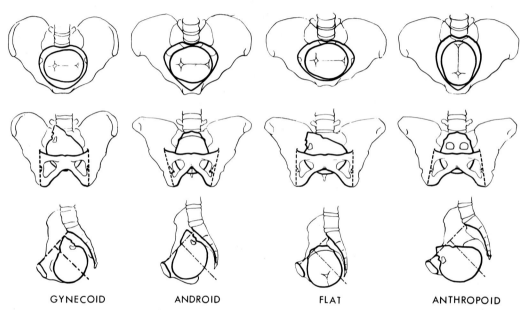

GYNECOID   ANDROID   FLAT   ANTHROPOID

FIG. 30-27 Influence of characteristic pelvic variations upon labor mechanism. (Danforth DN, Ellis AH: Am J Obstet Gynecol 86:29, 1963)

sacrum is directed somewhat anteriorly in its lower portion, the occiput tends to rotate into the more ample anterior pelvis. If the sacrum is forward throughout, as in the flat pelvis, the tendency is for the head to descend through the midpelvis in the transverse position.

Width of the Subpubic Arch and Transverse Diameter of the Outlet

When the subpubic arch is wide, the occiput may stem closely under the symphysis, using all the space (Fig. 30-26). If the arch is narrowed or if the transverse diameter of the outlet is shortened, the head is pre-

vented from stemming under the symphysis and is forced to pass more posteriorly. If the sacrum is far posterior, narrowing of the arch may have no practical significance except to require a wider episiotomy. If the sacrum is anterior, however, serious outlet disproportion may result.

Figure 30-27 shows the mechanism of labor characteristic of each of the four pure pelvic types. Since most pelves are mixed types that do not conform exactly to any one of these, the mechanism of labor may differ from the classic mechanisms shown in the diagram, in accordance with the particular pelvic features that obtain at each level of the pelvis. It is emphasized that, no matter how badly formed the pelvis may be, the head can traverse it without incident if the pelvis is large enough and the baby is small enough.

FIG. 30-28. Cephalic presentation. *A.* Occiput anterior position. *B.* Occiput posterior position. Head cannot advance as posterior unless sacrum is far back.

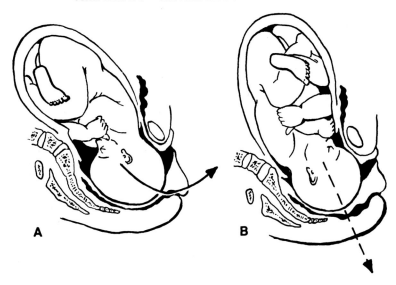

Among the most formidable conditions are those presented by the effort of an average size head to traverse an average size android, or "funnel," pelvis in which the spines are prominent, the sidewalls converge, the lower sacrum is forward, and the subpubic arch is narrow. If vaginal delivery is to be attempted, the physician must determine which pelvic diameter, the anteroposterior or the transverse, is the narrowest and try to bring the biparietal diameter through it. If traction in the occiput anterior position meets heavy resistance, the head may be rotated to the transverse and traction attempted in this position to test whether the anteroposterior diameter can accommodate the biparietal and whether the interspinous diameter is long enough to permit the head to pass this area in the transverse position. If this also offers heavy resistance, cesarean section is the proper solution, for injudicious traction either in the wrong diameter or against undue resistance may irretrievably damage the baby and seriously injure the mother.

INFLUENCE OF THE PELVIC AXIS

Under the normal circumstance of a gynecoid pelvis and a cephalic presentation in the occiput transverse position, internal rotation occurs in the midpelvis, and the pelvic curve is negotiated by extension of the head (Fig. 30–24). In the case of a face presentation with mentum anterior, the pelvic curve can also be readily negotiated by flexion of the head, with the chin instead of the occiput stemming behind and under the symphysis. A different problem is presented when the head enters the pelvis with either the occiput or the chin in the posterior position (Figs. 30–28 and 30–29). In the occiput posterior position, the head is already flexed, with chin on chest, to the maximum extent. Hence, it can advance only 1) if the sacrum is far posterior, as it is in the monkey (in which delivery face to pubes is the rule), or 2) if it can rotate to the anterior position. In the first instance, if the posterior segment of the pelvis is very wide at all levels, the head may reach the pelvic floor in the direct posterior position and, in fact, may deliver face to pubes. If the posterior segment is shorter, spontaneous rotation may occur when the occiput strikes this narrowed area; this happens in about 70% of cases. If rotation fails to occur either because prominent spines mechanically prevent rotation or because the uterine contractions fail to supply the needed force, artificial rotation is required.

A mentum posterior presentation offers much more difficulty than an occiput posterior, since it is impossible for a normal-sized head to deliver through a normal-sized pelvis in this position. In about one-half of cases in which labor starts as mentum posterior, the head rotates spontaneously to chin anterior and, as noted in Chapter 34, normal delivery usually follows. If spontaneous rotation to the anterior fails to occur, cesarean section is needed for delivery, since attempts to rotate artificially are almost uniformly unsuccessful and highly damaging.

Breech Presentation

In breech presentation, three separate mechanisms are of concern: the mechanism of the breech, the mechanism of the shoulders, and the mechanism of the after-coming head. In each case, just as in vertex

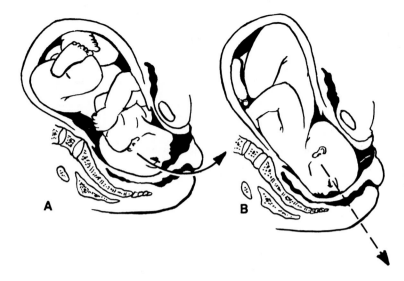

FIG. 30–29. Face presentation. *A.* Mentum anterior position. *B.* Mentum posterior position.

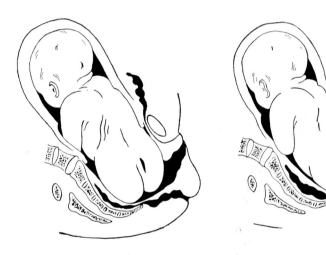

FIG. 30-30. Lateral flexion in breech presentation. (Beck AC, Rosenthal AH: Obstetrical Practice, 6th ed. Copyright © 1955, Williams & Wilkins)

presentation, the shortest diameter of the baby passes through the shortest diameter of the pelvis. At the level of the breech, the bitrochanteric diameter is the longer, and it usually (in gynecoid, android, and flat pelves) engages in the transverse position with the sacrum anterior. The breech descends in this position until the sacrum or pelvic floor is encountered and the pelvic curve must be negotiated. Since the anteroposterior mobility of the spine is very limited (especially if it is splinted by the legs), the pelvic curve must be negotiated by *lateral* flexion of the lumbar spine (Fig. 30–30). The anterior buttock then stems beneath the symphysis, the baby's back lying either to one side or in an oblique diameter. As the shoulders approach the

inlet, the longer bisacromial diameter adapts to the longer transverse diameter of the inlet, rotating to the oblique in the midpelvis, the anterior shoulder later appearing beneath the symphysis. After delivery of both shoulders, the back is usually directly anterior and the head consequently is in the direct occiput anterior position. In the anthropoid pelvis, the head can immediately enter the pelvis in the anterior position without the need for rotation; for this reason an anthropoid pelvis of large size is considered most favorable for breech delivery. Pelves of the gynecoid, android, or flat type, in which cephalopelvic relations are such that all the space must be used, are unfavorable, since the head must sometimes be rotated to the

transverse position so that the narrow biparietal diameter can pass through the narrower anteroposterior diameter of the inlet, a maneuver that can be very awkward indeed when the shoulders are already delivered. After engagement, the head negotiates the pelvic curve and is delivered by increasing flexion.

X-RAY PELVIMETRY

The use of x-ray pelvimetry and a suitable technique is discussed in Chapter 28. The latter point needs emphasis. A technique that provides information about the *entire* pelvis (see Fig. 30–1) can be of inestimable help in the cases in which it is needed. Techniques that supply lesser information are still in common use and are responsible for the increasing and unwarranted indictment of all x-ray pelvimetry.

X-ray pelvimetry is not to be used promiscuously. Its use should be limited to the cases in which it is essential for proper diagnosis or if a decision regarding the conduct of labor or method of delivery will be based upon the information it provides.

REFERENCES AND RECOMMENDED READING

Caldwell WE, Moloy HC, Swenson PC: Use of the roentgen ray in obstetrics. Am J Roentgenol Radium Ther Nucl Med 41:305, 505, 719, 1938. (These three articles are the classic summary reference to the work of Caldwell and Moloy. Dr. Caldwell was Professor of Obstetrics and Gynecology and Associate Director of the Sloane Hospital for Women, Columbia University. Dr. Moloy was Assistant Clinical Professor of Obstetrics and Gynecology in the same institution. Dr. Swenson was Assistant Attending Radiologist, Presbyterian Hospital and Vanderbilt Clinic, New York City, and was actively concerned in the development and clinical application of the Caldwell–Moloy thesis.)

Danforth DN: Clinical pelvimetry. In Sciarra JJ: Gynecology and Obstetrics, Vol 2, Chap 51. Hagerstown, Harper & Row, 1979

Danforth DN, Ellis AH: Mid-forceps delivery: A vanishing art? Am J Obstet Gynecol 86:29, 1963

Duff P: Diagnosis and management of face presentation. Obstet Gynecol 57:105, 1981

Eastman NJ: Pelvic mensuration: A study in the perpetuation of error. Obstet Gynecol Surv 3:301, 1948

Steer CM: Moloy's Evaluation of the Pelvis in Obstetrics, 3rd ed. New York, Plenum, 1975

CHAPTER **31**

CONDUCT OF NORMAL LABOR*

David N. Danforth

DEFINITIONS

Certain terms used in this and succeeding chapters must be defined. The clinical designation of *weeks' gestation* refers to the number of weeks that have elapsed since the 1st day of the last normal menstrual period, *not* the number of weeks since the date of presumed ovulation or conception. *Labor* is defined as the sequence of events by which the uterus expels the products of conception into the vagina and thence into the outer world. The term is reserved for pregnancies of more than 20 weeks' duration. Miniature labor does occur in pregnancy terminated before that time, but, if delivery occurs prior to the end of 20 weeks' gestation, the term *abortion* must be applied.

The time at which the fetus attains *viability* has

* This chapter is a revision of the chapter prepared by Richard D. Bryant and David N. Danforth for previous editions of this book.

been a point of some confusion. Historically, survival of an infant born before 28 weeks' gestation was so unusual that 28 weeks was usually considered the time of viability. Within the last decade, however, survival of infants born at 27 weeks, 26 weeks, and sometimes even earlier has become increasingly frequent. In a 1979 ruling, the U.S. Supreme Court considered the diagnosis of viability to be the individual physician's determination, not necessarily based on weight, weeks' gestation, or any other parameter. The Court stated that "viability is reached when, in the judgment of the attending physician on the particular facts of the case before him, there is reasonable likelihood of the fetus's sustained survival outside the womb, with or without artificial support."

A *preterm labor* is one that occurs after the 20th but before the end of the 37th week of pregnancy. A *term birth* is one that occurs after the 37th week of pregnancy and before the 43rd week. Delivery occurring after the beginning of the 43rd week of pregnancy is referred to as *postterm birth;* it is quite rare. Some cases of alleged postmaturity are actually term births; the confusion about dates arises because the patient's menstrual history is inaccurate or because conception was preceded by 1–2 months of amenorrhea. Similarly, some preterm births are actually term births, the pregnancy being dated not from the last normal menstrual period but rather from an episode of vaginal bleeding during the first 6 weeks of pregnancy.

A *parturient* is one who is in labor. A woman is said to be *parous* if she has given birth (regardless of whether vaginally or by cesarean section) to a baby after the 20th week of pregnancy, and her *parity* refers to the number of such deliveries she has had. A *nullipara* has had no deliveries at more than 20 weeks' gestation. A *primipara* has had one delivery at more than 20 weeks' gestation; a *multipara,* more than one. The term *gravida* followed by an arabic or Roman numeral refers to the total number of previous pregnancies (including ectopic pregnancy, hydatidiform mole, abortion, and normal intrauterine pregnancy); *para* followed by an arabic or Roman numeral refers to the number of deliveries after the 20th week of pregnancy (live birth or stillbirth, single or multiple, vaginal or cesarean section). In this context a woman who has had one spontaneous abortion, one ectopic pregnancy, and viable twins delivered by cesarean section is designated as gravida 3 para 1. A group of digits, for example, 0–3–0–2, is sometimes used to define a woman's reproductive history. The first digit refers to the number of term infants she has delivered, the second to the number of preterm infants, the third to the number of abortions, and the fourth to the number of children currently living. Although this device is intended to be more precise than the traditional designation, it can be confusing. The series of digits given in the example could refer to a woman who had had three preterm births, of whom two children are now living; it could

also refer to a woman who had had preterm triplets of whom two survived or to a woman who had had one preterm single labor and one preterm twin labor with two currently living children. The traditional designation of parity and gravidity is recommended, supplemented by additional information as needed.

A *precipitate labor* is one that lasts less than 3 hours. *Prolonged labor* used to be defined as a labor lasting more than 24 hours; the Terminology Committee of the American College of Obstetricians and Gynecologists suggests that prolonged labor is active labor that continues more than 20 hours; most obstetricians are satisfied that 18 hours is the upper limit for normal labor.

THE PRODROMES OF LABOR

There are three major prodromes of labor: lightening, Braxton Hicks contractions, and cervical effacement. In the primigravid patient, *lightening,* which refers to the settling of the presenting part into the pelvis, usually occurs 2–4 weeks before labor. If a primigravid patient goes into labor with the presenting part still unengaged, there is high probability of inlet disproportion. In the multiparous patient, however, lightening may not occur until after the beginning of labor. The disparity between primigravid and muliparous patients in this regard suggests that the phenomenon may result from differences in uterine tone, the multipara having the more relaxed uterus, but the muscular tone of the myometrium in the multipara does not differ significantly from that in the primigravida. Simple relaxation of the lower pole of the uterus as a passive phenomenon to explain the disparity is therefore untenable. It has been shown that prior to lightening the lower pole of the uterus is conical, whereas after lightening it is cup-shaped. Since intense myometrial activity is characteristic of pregnancy, the changes are best explained as a result of the active pulling up of the lower pole of the uterus around the presenting part. It is reasonable also to presume that the presenting part does not merely fall into the pelvis, but rather is pushed there by myometrial activity pulling against the pericervical axis and supports. Lightening usually occurs gradually over the course of weeks. The patient is usually aware of it by reason of the added comfort and ease of breathing that result, but these advantages are balanced by increased distress from pelvic pressure, urinary frequency, and constipation.

The rhythmic tightening of the uterus, known as *Braxton Hicks contractions* (see page 599), may be painful but is for the most part irregular in frequency, duration, and intensity. In the first pregnancy, Braxton Hicks contractions are generally painless until an hour or so before the onset of labor, but with each succeeding pregnancy such painful contractions are apt to precede the onset of true labor by an increasingly long period. A woman in her eighth or ninth pregnancy may find painful Braxton Hicks contractions extremely troublesome as early as the 5th or 6th month. Such contractions are often difficult to distinguish from true labor pains and may be referred to, usually in retrospect, as *false labor.* Despite their painful nature, careful examination usually discloses the irregularity in frequency, duration, intensity, or all three.

The softening and thinning of the cervix referred to as *cervical effacement* (see page 614) generally become evident in both primigravida and multigravida about a month before term and are usually accompanied by slight dilatation of the cervix. *Bloody show,* a discharge of pink mucus, sometimes results from the cervical changes and may precede labor by periods varying from an hour to a week or more.

In addition to the three major prodromes, certain other phenomena are common in the days or weeks preceding labor: 1) loss of 1–3 lb in weight due to water loss as the result of electrolyte shifts that in turn are produced by changes in estrogen and progesterone levels, 2) frequency of urination due to reduction in bladder capacity by pressure of the presenting part, 3) increase in vaginal secretions due to the extreme congestion of the vaginal mucous membranes, and 4) increasing backache and sacroiliac distress due to relaxation of the pelvic joints.

THE STAGES OF LABOR

Labor is divided into three stages. The *first stage* begins with the onset of regular uterine contractions accompanied by progressive dilatation of the cervix. It ends when the cervix is fully dilated. The first stage, then, is the stage of dilatation of the cervix. The exact moment of its onset may be difficult to record.

The *second stage* of labor begins when the cervix is completely dilated and ends when the baby is completely delivered. Although there is slight advancement of the presenting part in the first stage, it is not until the second stage, when the uterus gains purchase on the ligamentary supports, that uterine evacuation actually begins. The second stage, then, is the stage of delivery.

The *third stage* of labor begins when delivery of the baby is complete and ends when the placenta and membranes are delivered. This is the placental stage.

CHARACTER OF CONTRACTIONS

As noted in Chapter 29, at the onset of the first stage, contractions usually occur every 5–8 minutes, last 20–30 seconds, and achieve intrauterine pressures of 20–30 mm Hg. As the first stage advances, the contractions gradually improve in quality; by the end of the first stage, they occur every 2–4 minutes, last

30–50 seconds, and produce intrauterine pressures of about 50 mm Hg. Second-stage contractions normally occur every 2–3 minutes and last about 60 seconds, producing intrauterine pressures of about 100 mm Hg, but bearing-down efforts may cause these pressures to exceed 100 mm Hg. In the third stage, the contractions are rarely painful, although intramyometrial pressures of 250 mm Hg are common.

LENGTH OF LABOR

During the days, and occasionally weeks, before the actual onset of labor, the cervix gradually begins to soften, to become thinner, and to dilate slightly. Hence, when labor starts, the cervix is already dilated 1–3 cm in both nulliparous and multiparous patients. As a rule, the first stage of labor is completed within 8 hours in a first labor and within 4–6 hours in subsequent labors. If the first stage of labor lasts more than 12 hours, or if cervical dilatation arrests for more than 2 hours, it is considered abnormal.

The duration of the second stage depends entirely on the amount of resistance to be overcome. In a multipara with a small baby, the second stage may be only momentary, delivery occurring promptly when the cervix is fully dilated. In a primipara, or in a multipara with a large baby, considerable voluntary effort (bearing down) may be needed to advance the baby through the birth canal. The second stage of labor is considered prolonged, although not necessarily abnormal, if it lasts more than 1 hour. An active, vigorous second stage must be terminated (by vaginal delivery or cesarean section) after 2 hours because of the threat of uterine rupture, constriction ring dystocia, or fetal injury.

It is well-known that succeeding labors tend to be shorter until the fifth or sixth, after which labor is apt to lengthen. The shortening of labor is usually attributed to the somewhat more lax cervix and the progressively less resistance offered by the soft parts; the lengthening of labor after the fifth or sixth is attributed to an increase in the connective tissue of the myometrium with consequent impairment of uterine coordination.

CONDUCT OF THE FIRST AND SECOND STAGES OF LABOR

In all fields of medicine new knowledge begets new procedures and new regimens whose purpose is to improve results. In obstetrics, the new methods and new approaches have produced a decline in both maternal mortality (from 37.1 per 100,000 live births in 1960 to 9.9 per 100,000 live births in 1977) and also in perinatal mortality (from 29.3 per 1000 live births to 19.6 per 1000). Both rates continue to decline, and to the pres-

ent date perinatal mortality has dropped by 47% since 1965. These spectacular advancements are due in largest measure to an increase in the availability and quality of prenatal care, new developments in the conduct and monitoring of labor, and pediatric advances in the care of the newborn.

There is not full acceptance of the new hospital routines that have made so important a contribution. Many regard childbirth as an intensely personal experience to be shared by other members of the family, and specific criticism has been leveled at the restricted, sterile, and sometimes stark conditions of the labor and delivery rooms, the immense "gadgetry," and the increased cesarean section rate which some allege to be the direct result of fetal monitoring. Many women with these attitudes seek delivery at home, a practice that major health organizations have determined to be accompanied by unacceptably greater risk to both mother and baby. Many hospitals have responded to the criticisms by providing what is referred to as "family-centered maternity care," which has the enthusiastic approval of the organizations comprising the Interprofessional Task Force on the Health Care of Women and Infants.* The recommended practices include the presence of the husband or "supporting other" as much as possible during and after labor; a flexible rooming-in program for the newborn; special visiting dispensations for children; optional early release from the hospital; breast-feeding and handling the baby immediately after delivery; childbirth preparation classes for expectant couples; and availability of a "birthing room," a combination labor and delivery room that has a homelike atmosphere and is adjacent to the delivery room in case of emergency, but has no external evidence of the standard monitoring and support systems.

The protocol for birthing rooms varies from one hospital to another; even the same hospital may offer different options. In some, indoctrinated children are permitted to remain throughout labor. Some hospitals accede to the request for no electronic monitoring; some recommend such monitoring for 15 min every hour; some require monitoring for the first 30 min after admission (to record baseline characteristics and possible decelerative patterns) and again continuously after the cervix reaches 8 cm dilatation. Usually, labor must be conducted in a standard labor room if electronic monitoring, either optional or indicated, is to be continuous. In some birthing rooms, patients must rely entirely on Lamaze training or its equivalent for analgesia, while a partial or full range of analgesia and anesthesia is available in others. Spontaneous delivery without epistiotomy is an objective in most birthing

---

* American Academy of Pediatrics, American College of Nurse–Midwives, American College of Obstetricians and Gynecologists, American Nurses' Association, Nurses Association of the American College of Obstetricians and Gynecologists.

rooms, and such procedures as episiotomy and outlet forceps require removal to a standard delivery room; in other facilities, these procedures may be performed in the birthing room.

Obstetricians must recognize these new challenges to traditional obstetric practice. Also, they must be aware of the emotional needs and societal forces that have generated the new attitudes, as well as the data that bear on the propriety of the requested protocols. Having evaluated all of this, physicians must select the range of options that they can conscientiously offer their patients and should deviate from this only if a new service or option will offer greater safety or an improved result. The desire to let nature take its course must never be carried so far that the basic principles of good obstetric practice are neglected.

Three fundamental concepts must be kept in mind: 1) in the vast majority of cases, labor and delivery are physiologic processes and do not, in the true sense, require "management"; 2) the functions of the medical attendant are to promote the successful termination of the process and to anticipate and deal with abnormal conditions; and 3) precautions must be taken at all times to avoid endangering or injuring either the mother or the baby.

Most patients at the onset of labor are confident and adjusted to the task in store, but there is also an element of uncertainty and emotional stress, regardless of the patient's mien or her parity. This will be compounded if the medical attendant manifests hesitance, flippancy or thoughtlessness, or haste that is not occasioned by the needs of that particular patient. Reassurance and support, both emotional and physical, are keystones of the successful conduct of labor.

WHEN TO COME TO THE HOSPITAL

The woman should be advised to come to the hospital in any of the following three circumstances:

1. Uterine contractions. It is reasonably certain that labor is starting when contractions have occurred every 10 min for as long as an hour and have begun to be painful. If the pain is unremitting or severe, the patient should not wait for an hour to pass, but should come to the hospital at once.
2. Ruptured membranes. This may occur as a sudden uncontrollable gush of watery fluid or as continuous slow leakage of fluid from the vagina. The latter must be distinguished from urinary incontinence, which is not uncommon in the latter months of pregnancy; if the leakage continues after voiding, the membranes are probably ruptured and the patient should be admitted to the hospital.
3. Bleeding. Active bleeding, equivalent to a normal menstrual period, is an indication for admission to the hospital even if it is not accompanied by dis-

comfort. *Bloody show,* due to the cervical changes of early labor or prelabor, usually consists of a pink, mucoid discharge; it suggests that labor may start within hours or days, but in itself it is not an indication for admission to the hospital.

ADMISSION TO THE HOSPITAL

For all registered patients, a detailed medical, surgical, and obstetric history (see page 183), as well as the results of a complete physical examination, should be on file in the delivery room. If no information is available, it should be obtained before delivery if time permits; if not, it must be obtained after delivery.

General Evaluation and Preparation

While assisting the patient to bed, the nurse should obtain the following information and record it in the chart: the time of onset and frequency of the contractions; whether the membranes appear to be ruptured or intact; whether there has been any vaginal bleeding and, if so, its character; the time and content of the last meal; and whether the patient wears dentures or contact lenses. The nurse should also take and record the temperature, pulse, and rate of respirations; collect a urine specimen for analysis; and either take or order an admission hematocrit.

The attendant (physician or nurse–midwife, as the case may be) should then evaluate the patient's obstetric status at once, before proceeding to other matters. In order to determine whether delivery is imminent or whether there is any major obstetric problem, the attendant should

1. Take the blood pressure.
2. Listen to the fetal heart between contractions and immediately after a contraction. The heart tones should be regular, and the rate should be 120–160 beats/min. Irregularity or rate outside these limits may suggest fetal hypoxia.
3. Feel a uterine contraction to note its duration, intensity, and whether the uterus relaxes well between contractions.
4. If there is *no* history of bleeding, make a "sterile" vaginal examination to determine the station and symmetry of the presenting part; the effacement, dilatation, and position of the cervix; and the adequacy of the pelvis.

A *sterile vaginal examination* implies an antiseptic wash or spray of the introitus and adjacent skin, use of sterile gloves, and separation of the labia by the index and middle fingers of the opposite hand before the examining fingers are introduced. A sterile lubricant is desirable unless there is discharge of blood or mucus, in which case it is not needed. The index finger is usually sufficient for this examination and is consider-

ably less uncomfortable for the patient than an examination with index and middle fingers, especially in a primigravida.

Station of the presenting part and the method of recording it are discussed on page 631. As to *symmetry*, in vertex presentation, the head should be found on vaginal examination to be symmetric, firm, and rounded. If one persists, it is usually possible to feel some of the sutures in the fetal head and to determine the exact position, but the attempt at this stage of affairs only increases discomfort, prolongs the examination, and produces information that is rarely needed until labor is more advanced. Accordingly, the obstetrician should be content if the initial examination shows the head to be symmetric and well engaged (station +1 or lower) and if the head advances progressively thereafter. If the presenting part is found to be irregular (not symmetric), the possibilities of brow, face, or breech presentation, or a monstrosity, must be considered, and steps must be taken at once to make an exact diagnosis. Ultrasound scan may be helpful. An x-ray film of the abdomen is definitive.

Effacement of the cervix (see page 614) is recorded as a percentage figure: an uneffaced (0%) cervix is firm and about 2.5 cm long; 50% effacement implies that the cervix is about 1 cm thick and somewhat softer; a completely effaced cervix (100%) is soft and only a few millimeters thick. Cervical dilatation is recorded in centimeters. It is important to know the *position of the cervix*. If it is far posterior in early labor and difficult to reach, the labor may be longer than usual since the first part of it, before significant dilatation occurs, is devoted to advancing the cervix anteriorly into the axis of the vagina. If the cervix is difficult to reach it can often be made more accessible if the head is moved posteriorly by suprapubic pressure during the vaginal examination. There is no good explanation of why this maneuver may bring the cervix sufficiently anterior for the obstetrician to determine its dilatation more easily.

The method of *estimating pelvic capacity* is considered in Chapter 30, and such an estimation should be available on the prenatal record. When the patient goes into labor, however, the question of whether this particular pelvis is large enough to accommodate this particular baby must be answered. In a primigravid patient, the head should be engaged at the onset of labor (and usually a few weeks before); if it is unengaged in early labor, the possibility of inlet disproportion should be considered and kept in mind if the head fails to advance as labor progresses. If the head is already engaged, the possibility of inlet disproportion is eliminated, and attention should be directed to the ischial spines and the position of the sacrum. Excessively prominent spines may suggest transverse narrowing of the midpelvis, with the attendant problems that are considered in Chapter 30. If the head is engaged to station +2, there should be ample space to insert the index finger between the head and the sacrum; if this space is snug, it may suggest anteroposterior flattening, which may need to be taken into account when the time comes for delivery.

If delivery is not imminent, the prenatal record should be read carefully and specific questions asked to determine if there is any current or recent sore throat or upper respiratory infection, if there has been any recent illness, if any pregnancy problems have occurred that might not be entered on the prenatal record, if the patient is taking any medications or drugs, and if she is allergic to any medications. A complete history should be taken if no prenatal record is available.

The physical examination during labor is extremely important, but it need not be as detailed as the customary physical examination unless no prenatal information is available; in the latter event, a detailed examination should be made. The routine labor examination should include blood pressure, throat and teeth, heart, and lungs; the sacral and pretibial areas should be examined for edema. The principal information to be determined on examination of the abdomen is supplied by the Leopold maneuvers (see Figs. 19–8 to 19–11), in the course of which the presentation and position can be determined and the size of the baby can be estimated. It is not possible to estimate the baby's weight within a pound with any regularity, and sometimes this estimate is even farther afield. An effort should be made, however, to obtain a working opinion as to whether the baby is large, small, or of average size.

The *remainder of the admission procedure* consists of a shower (if needed and feasible), the "prep," and, usually, an enema. It was formerly thought that asepsis required shaving the pubic, vulvar, and perineal hair, but it is now agreed that this is uncomfortable and unnecessary. Accordingly, the shave is limited to the area of the intended episiotomy, and long pubic and vulvar hair is clipped with scissors. There is some difference of opinion regarding the need for an enema. Most obstetricians prefer that one be given shortly after admission unless labor is extremely active, delivery is imminent, or there is a history of recent bleeding. If there is adequate time, the enema may reflexly stimulate and improve coordination of uterine contractions (see page 721 and Figure 35–5), and it also gives reasonable assurance that the lower bowel will be empty so the fecal column will not be expelled as the head advances, contaminating the delivery field. If the patient objects to an enema, it can usually be omitted.

Determination of the State of Membranes

The membranes may rupture before the onset of labor, at any time during labor, or not until the head is being born. A damp area under the buttocks may suggest that the membranes have ruptured, but it may be due

to urine, which can be identified by odor. The management of labor depends in many cases on whether the membranes are or are not ruptured. The usual methods of determining this are 1) observation for leakage of amniotic fluid from the vaginal orifice; 2) speculum examination of the cervix (fluid from the cervical canal); 3) nitrazine test for pH of fluid in the vagina, which is notoriously inaccurate; 4) microscopic examination of the fluid. In the last test, if Nile blue staining (wet mount, 1 drop fluid, 1 drop 0.1% Nile blue sulfate) demonstrates orange-stained fat-laden fetal squames, this is proof-positive of ruptured membranes.

LABOR

Diagnosis of Onset

The onset of labor is marked by the beginning of progressive cervical dilatation in response to regular, usually painful, uterine contractions. This point may be impossible to define precisely, especially if it is preceded by a prodromal period of more or less regular, forceful, painful contractions that have no influence on the cervix. Thus, the diagnosis of prodromes of labor and false labor is usually retrospective, since a period of time must pass before it can be determined that the cervix has or has not undergone change.

In some cases, labor starts abruptly; more frequently, and especially in nulliparous women, there is a prodromal period of 1–8 or more hours during which the contractions occur at intervals of 10–15 min, cause only slight discomfort, and are quite short. The interval between contractions then shortens progressively, and the contractions gradually lengthen and become more intense. As a rule, the patient is considered to be in labor when contractions of good quality have occurred at regular intervals of 6 min or less for at least 1 hour. The probability of labor is strengthened if there is also bleeding due to the opening of small blood vessels in the cervix as effacement and dilatation begin, or if the membranes rupture. The physiology of the transition from prodromal to actual labor is described in Chapter 29.

False labor is defined as a period of more or less regular, painful contractions that are not accompanied by effacement or dilatation of the cervix and that may either stop altogether or be followed, either promptly or ultimately, by the onset of true labor. False labor is a form of disordered uterine action and is discussed further in Chapter 35.

It is important that false labor be diagnosed. By using an external monitor for uterine contractions, it is usually possible to make the distinction between true and false labor without waiting several hours to note whether cervical dilatation has begun. It has been mentioned that the contractions of true labor are abso-lutely regular and are all of the same or gradually increasing intensity and duration. Although the contractions of false labor may be forceful at times, they do not exhibit the absolute regularity of actual labor. Two or three contractions, or more, of excellent quality may occur at intervals of 2–3 min, to be followed by an 8- or 10-min interval of quiescence; or the regular intense contractions, after 10 min or more, may be followed by a few fleeting contractions of low intensity. If false labor occurs, its nature should be explained to the patient and her family so they will be aware that delivery is not imminent. In some instances, anxiety and the complaints of pain are so pronounced that sedatives and analgesics are required for their relief. These drugs must be used with caution. Morphine may be given in a single dose in an effort to terminate false labor; repeated doses should be avoided, however, for addiction is always a hazard.

Cervical dilatation is the fundamental clinical phenomenon of the first stage of labor. The cervix normally dilates just far enough to permit the passage of whatever presents itself to the cervix. The diameter of the flexed head of an average-sized fetus is between 9 and 10 cm. Full or complete dilatation, then, is considered to be about 10 cm. The body of the average fetus will easily pass through a cervix dilated enough to permit the passage of the head. Note, however, that, if the largest diameter of the presenting fetal head is only 8 cm (because of prematurity or microcephaly), from a physiologic point of view 8 cm is full dilatation.

For the first stage of labor to be considered normal, complete dilatation must be reached within 12 hours, but the average is much less than that. Multiparas usually reach full dilatation in about half the time that nulliparas do. After the fifth or sixth baby, labor tends to get longer. Dilatation does not ordinarily proceed at a constant rate. Typically, dilatation is slow until 4–5 cm dilatation is reached, then rapid until dilatation is nearly complete, then slower until full dilatation is achieved. If the cervix can be felt on vaginal examination dilatation is not complete.

One of the duties of the professional attendant during labor is to determine the amount of cervical dilatation from time to time. It will then be known how labor is progressing. The curves of the normal rate of dilatation (Fig. 35–3) should be kept in mind. Significant deviations from the normal rate of progress should alert the physician to the presence of abnormality.

The First Stage of Labor

Several matters require consideration during the first stage of labor.

Charting. A chart note is required at least every hour during the first stage. This may be either a written note or an entry in the labor sheet; if progress is not rapid, only the character of contractions and apparent

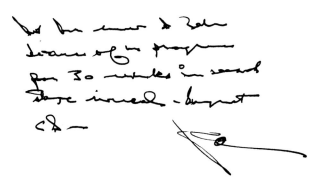

FIG. 31-1. Example of vexing narrative chart note: no date, no time, and both note and author's signature are illegible.

progress as judged by abdominal examination may be noted. Any written notes in the chart must be legible, signed, timed, and dated. The labor may need to be reconstructed a year or so hence for medical or legal reasons, and it can be immensely frustrating to try to decipher an untimed, scribbled note by one whose signature is illegible (Fig. 31-1). Use of a "partogram" (Fig. 31-2) can be very helpful in charting the course of labor. The cervix should normally dilate at the rate of 1 cm/hour.The Philpott lines (see Figure 35-4) and the Studd stencil make the evaluation of progress much more exact.

Examinations. Careful evaluation of the patient's subjective and objective symptoms and accurate interpretation of the findings on abdominal examination can suffice for following the progress of most of the labor. At least three vaginal examinations are needed: on admission, midway through the first stage when discomfort becomes more marked or medication is requested, and when the signs suggest that the cervix is fully dilated. Vaginal examination should also be done when the membranes rupture (to be sure a loop of cord has not come down), and at other times as needed to determine progress or the lack of it. Arterial pulsations are sometimes felt either inside the cervix or peripheral to it. If they are synchronous with the maternal pulse, they are produced by an artery in the rectovaginal septum or cervix. If they are synchronous with the fetal heartbeat, they are due to cord prolapse or vasa previa and are invariably of ominous portent.

Posture in Labor. When in normal labor, the patient may sit in a chair or walk about so long as the labor is not too active, the membranes are intact, and no analgesia has been administered. If she is in bed, the lateral recumbent posture, as opposed to the supine, is preferred since deviations in fetal pulse tracings are less frequent in this position, and the possibility of the supine hypotensive syndrome (see page 759) is eliminated.

Nutriment and Fluids. The emptying time of the stomach is greatly prolonged in labor; in some cases, vomitus may contain food ingested 24 hours earlier. Consequently, nothing is permitted by mouth after labor starts. Fluids are essential, however, and an infusion of 5% dextrose in water is usually started shortly after admission, to run at the rate of 1000 ml every 8 hours. This may be omitted if labor is expected to be terminated by vaginal delivery within a few hours.

Antacids. Aspiration of gastric contents is the most common cause of anesthetic death in obstetrics and is a serious threat if general anesthesia should suddenly be required. Its effects can be minimized if the acidic gastric juice is neutralized, and some have advocated administration of magnesium trisilicate or an equivalent every 2 hours in labor. Since the particulate matter of such antacids can itself cause severe and sometimes massive pneumonitis if aspirated, a clear antacid (*e.g.*, 15 ml of 0.3 M sodium citrate in 20% syrup) is preferred and is given as a single dose a few minutes before the induction of anesthesia. The preventive value of antacids is not improved by administering them at regular intervals throughout labor.

Analgesia. Obstetric analgesia is discussed in Chapter 32. In addition to its pain-relieving qualities, analgesia may also help to relax parturients who are tense and apprehensive.

Bladder. A full bladder can reflexly impede the course of labor. The woman should be asked to void every several hours during labor; if she cannot void, the bladder should be emptied by catheter whenever it can be felt abdominally. In advanced labor, catheterization can often be avoided by inserting two fingers vaginally, one on either side of the urethra, and applying suprapubic pressure during the active phase of a contraction.

Temperature, Pulse, Respirations, and Blood Pressure. Measurements of temperature, pulse, respiration rate, and blood pressure should be taken and recorded every 4 hours during labor, more often if any are abnormal.

Fetal Monitoring. There are differing opinions on whether normal women who are at lowest risk are benefited by continuous electronic monitoring of fetal heart rate and uterine contractions, (see Chapter 41), but there is no question that this practice is clearly indicated and may be lifesaving among those whose babies are at risk. Since unexpected fetal hypoxia can occur among low-risk women (due, *e.g.*, to a low-lying cord), the burden of proof appears to be on those who deliberately deprive themselves of the information to be gained from the routine monitoring of all women in labor. If continuous electronic monitoring is not being used, auscultation of the fetal heart should be

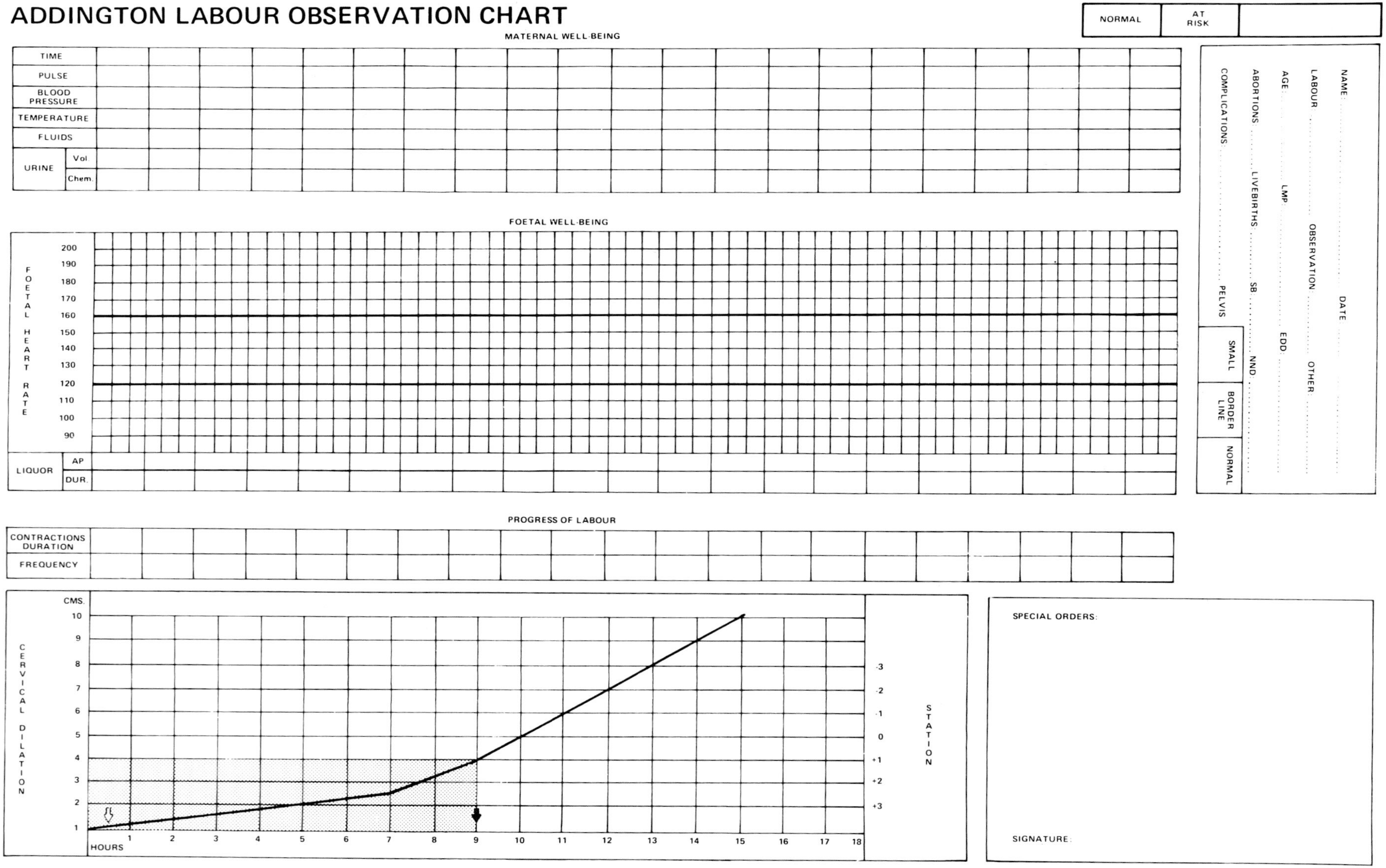

ADDINGTON LABOUR OBSERVATION CHART

FIG. 31-2. Partogram for charting course of labor. Most maternities make up own partograms to meet special needs or interests. (Notelovitz M: Am J Obstet Gynecol 132:889, 1978)

done every 15 min during the first stage of labor and every 5 min in the second stage, the latter for periods of 30 sec.

Psychologic Support. Of all the devices for the psychologic support of the patient during labor, the most important is the physical presence of another human being. The person need not be qualified to provide medical assistance; for example, the husband can be invaluable for this duty. Other psychologic aids are pleasantness, optimism, patience, gentleness, and an ability to convince the patient that she is the chief concern at the moment. The attendant should never discuss unpleasant aspects of some other patient's labor with the patient or within her hearing.

Amniotomy

The membranes usually rupture spontaneously during the first or second stage of labor. If not, they may sometimes retard progress, and artificial rupture (*amniotomy*) may be done. Some form of clamp or sharppointed instrument should be used. The patient must be prepared for vaginal examination. Sterile gloves should be worn by the examiner. If the membranes bulge far in advance of the head, and especially if the presenting part is at or above station +1, the membranes should be punctured between uterine contractions. If they are broken during a contraction, the amniotic fluid may be expelled with such force that the cord prolapses. Descent and dilatation usually accelerate after amniotomy. When labor is especially active, the possibility of amniotic fluid embolism appears to be lessened if as much fluid as possible is drained by very slightly elevating the presenting part when the first flow stops.

Summary of Danger Signs in Labor

One of the major functions of the professional attendants during labor is careful and continued observation for the detection of abnormalities. These should be looked for in every labor, because no labor can be called normal until it is completed. Some of the danger signs are listed in Table 31–1.

Signs of Full Dilatation of the Cervix

A subtle or abrupt change in the patient's mien often occurs when the cervix becomes fully dilated. Most commonly, involuntary bearing-down efforts are noted. An episode of vomiting late in the first stage may suggest full dilatation, as may a significant increase in the amount of bloody show. Sweat collects on the upper lip in many women at this time, and its sudden appearance should suggest the possibility of full dilatation. The only certain evidence of full dilatation must be obtained by vaginal examination. Perineal

bulging and gaping of the anus appear late in the second stage, when delivery is imminent.

The Second Stage of Labor

The second stage of labor should normally be completed, and the baby delivered, within 1 hour after the cervix becomes fully dilated. If progress is being made and conditions are favorable for vaginal delivery, the second stage may be permitted to last up to 2 hours; but, after 2 hours in the second stage, there is a risk of uterine rupture or constriction ring dystocia.

Bearing-down efforts are usually reflex and spontaneous. In some multiparas, and occasionally in primigravidas, two or three such efforts may suffice to advance the baby through the birth canal and to complete delivery. More frequently, and especially in the primigravida, significant voluntary effort is needed, and encouragement by the attendant can be extremely helpful. The knees should be hyperflexed toward the flanks so the force of uterine contractions (the axis of drive) is directly into the pelvic inlet. The woman should take a deep breath at the onset of the contraction and bear down exactly as though she were attempting to have a bowel movement, relaxing fully when the contraction is over. In some cases, the effectiveness of bearing down can be improved if two or three deep breaths of 50% nitrous oxide and 50% oxygen are taken at the beginning of the contraction. As a rule, the head advances slightly, but sometimes imperceptibly, with each contraction. When the perineum bulges and the scalp is visible, an episiotomy may suffice to permit spontaneous delivery; if it does not, the use of outlet forceps (a "lift-out delivery") is infinitely preferable to allowing prolonged pressure of the head against the pelvic floor in an effort to avoid forceps delivery.

PREPARATION FOR DELIVERY

Asepsis is a prime consideration in the delivery room. All personnel must wear freshly laundered clothing, cap, and mask. Clean shoe covers minimize the danger of tracking dirt from outside the labor and delivery area. The basic purpose of antisepsis is to prevent the transfer of potentially virulent organisms from patient to patient or from personnel to patient. Prevention is at least as important as antibiotics in reducing the incidence and severity of puerperal infection.

The patient should be transferred from the labor room to the delivery room in ample time to permit the usual preparations for delivery, but not so early that she will have to spend much time on the uncomfortable delivery table before she is ready to deliver. As a rule, the patient in her first labor should be moved to the delivery room 1) when the head has advanced sufficiently to cause the perineum to bulge during con-

TABLE 31-1. SUMMARY OF DANGER SIGNS IN LABOR

Observation or Finding	Possible Significance
FETAL HEART RATE RAPID, SLOW, OR IRREGULAR	Fetal distress; prolapsed or occult cord
PRESENTING PART	
Irregular	Breech, face, brow presentation; fetal monstrosity
Not palpable in pelvis	Transverse or oblique lie
Unengaged	Inlet disproportion; malpresentation (brow)
Failure to descend after cervix fully dilated	Midpelvic disproportion or error in estimate of cervical dilatation
UTERINE CONTRACTIONS	
Decrease in frequency, intensity, or duration	Uterine inertia; too much medication
Tetany or failure to relax well between contractions	Premature separation of placenta
FAILURE OF CERVIX TO DILATE PROGRESSIVELY	False labor; cervical dystocia; abnormal uterine action; excessive medication; cephalopelvic disproportion; error in estimate of cervical dilatation
VAGINAL DISCHARGE	
Active bleeding	Placenta previa; abruptio placentae; maternal laceration (cervix, uterus, vagina); clotting defect
Amniotic fluid	
Meconium-stained (vertex presentation)	Fetal distress
Port wine–colored	Ruptured vasa previa; abruptio placentae
Foul or "fruity" odor	Intrauterine infection (amnionitis)
BLOOD PRESSURE	
Elevated	Preeclampsia
Low	Shock; supine hypotensive syndrome; reaction to drug; internal bleeding
DYSPNEA, SENSE OF SUFFOCATION	Amniotic fluid embolism (may be earliest sign)
MATERNAL TACHYCARDIA	Impending shock; maternal dehydration; atropine reaction
CONTINUOUS ABDOMINAL PAIN	Premature separation of placenta; ruptured uterus; extrauterine intraabdominal surgical emergency
FEVER	Infection, either intrauterine or elsewhere
UNCONSCIOUSNESS	Postconvulsive eclampsia or epilepsy; shock; heavy sedation; amniotic fluid embolism
PROLAPSED UMBILICAL CORD	Without instant action by attendant, intrauterine fetal death

tractions, 2) if in the second stage there is evidence of fetal distress, or 3) if her bearing-down efforts would be assisted by inhalation analgesia (50% nitrous oxide, 50% oxygen) during the contractions. The multiparous patient, depending upon the speed of labor, should be moved to the delivery room when the cervix is dilated 6–8 cm.

When the patient has been moved to the delivery table, she must not be left unattended. If she has had medication for pain relief, the attendant must not turn away from her even for an instant.

For spontaneous delivery, a flat surface is usually preferred; if the woman is on a delivery table, the end should not be "broken," and she may assume whatever position is most comfortable. In England, the left lateral recumbent (Sims) posture has been preferred for many years and is probably most physiologic, since it avoids the pressure of the gravid uterus on the inferior vena cava. The supine posture is most commonly used in the United States.

For operative delivery, including delivery by outlet forceps, the lithotomy position is preferred because it improves exposure and provides easier access. The buttocks should project about 2 in. over the end of the table. The stirrups that are usually used are not without hazard, and the legs should not be put into them until delivery is immediately imminent; prolonged pressure from stirrups and straps may cause thrombosis in leg veins or damage to important nerves. A desirable alternative to the use of stirrups, if both scrub nurse and assistant are available, is to hold the legs in the manner shown in Figure 31–3. This avoids the stresses of stirrups and permits the knees to be advanced as the head crowns, thus minimizing the chance of laceration or extension of the episiotomy.

The final preparations for delivery are now made. The vulva, inner thighs, and abdomen (at least up to the umbilicus) should be thoroughly scrubbed with soap and water and rinsed. An antiseptic solution may be applied. The vagina should not be entered during this procedure. Sterile drapes should then be put on so

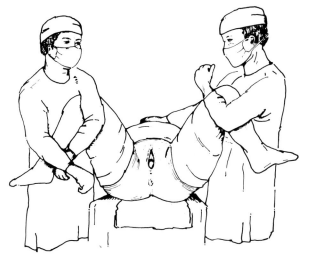

FIG. 31-3. Method of holding legs that avoids sciatic strain and pressure injury, and permits knees to be moved downward as head delivers, or, in breech delivery, as shoulders engage. (Modified from Danforth WC: Forceps. In Curtis AH (ed): Obstetrics and Gynecology, Chap 43. Philadelphia, WB Saunders, 1933)

as to cover the leg from toe to crotch, the abdomen, and at least as far up as the nipple line. The draping must be done by someone who has scrubbed and is wearing sterile gown and gloves. Breaks in technique are the joint responsibility of the attendant and all other personnel in the delivery room. Anyone whose sterile covering touches an unclean or unsterile area must drop out at once and change gloves, gown, or both.

Routine catheterization is often carried out, but there is a trend away from this procedure. The danger of introducing infection into the bladder may be greater than the danger of a full bladder.

A vaginal examination is now made to determine the presenting part, its position and station, whether the cervix is fully dilated, and whether the membranes are ruptured. If the membranes are still intact, they should be ruptured.

DELIVERY

As a general rule, if the head crowns (*i.e.*, distends the vulva, showing at the introitus a patch of scalp 3–4 cm in diameter), it can be readily delivered either spontaneously or by employing slight pressure upon the fundus (Kristeller expression). If anesthesia is used, the head may not reach the level of crowning or may recede, in which case outlet forceps should be employed if the head does not readily advance with slight fundal pressure.

Spontaneous Delivery

Most patients deliver spontaneously if simply let alone (Fig. 31–4). The physician's function is to 1) protect the perineum from excessive damage by encouraging the slow emergence of the head; 2) prevent cord complications; 3) assist with delivery of the shoulders, if necessary; 4) clear the baby's air passages; 5) encourage the baby to breathe; 6) assess the condition of the baby; 7) clamp and cut the cord; 8) supervise procedures to minimize maternal blood loss; 9) supervise the delivery of the placenta; 10) investigate or inspect the uterus, cervix, and vagina; and 11) suture as needed.

The essence of assistance during spontaneous delivery is promotion of slow distention of the perineum and dilatation of the vaginal orifice and slow delivery of the head and shoulders (the shoulders may cause tearing even when the head did not). The urge to bear down is so violent in some patients that the head or shoulders cause almost complete disintegration of the perineum. Anyone assisting at delivery should try to counteract the violent expulsive efforts by repeated instruction to the patient and should make an episiotomy in ample time if it is needed.

A special procedure to minimize perineal damage is *Ritgen's maneuver.* When the head has advanced far enough so that the chin has passed the mother's coccyx, the fetal head can be grasped by placing one hand on the scalp and the other on the chin through the postanal tissue (the fingers should be covered with several layers of sterile gauze or towel to prevent contamination of the glove). The patient should be cautioned not to bear down any more (or the anesthetic deepened enough that she cannot), and the head can then be slowly maneuvered through the vaginal orifice, always under complete control of the operator.

As soon as the head is born, the baby's neck region should be palpated. Usually, nothing abnormal is felt. In many cases, however, one to six loops of umbilical cord may be felt loosely or tightly wound around the baby's neck. If the loops are tight, circulation through

FIG. 31–4. Spontaneous delivery. Episiotomy, if needed, is ► made as head begins to crown (*A*). Pressure against perineum (*B, C*) causes head to stem closely beneath symphysis, minimizing possibility of extension of episiotomy. Soft parts may be pushed gently over head as it advances (*C, D*). By depressing head slightly (*E*) and exerting pressure upon fundus, posterior shoulder moves into hollow of sacrum, and anterior shoulder is caused to stem beneath symphysis. Anterior arm is delivered by applying pressure in antecubital fossa (*F, G*). Gentle elevation of head delivers posterior shoulder (*H*), and posterior arm is then delivered (*I*). Thorax, abdomen, and legs follow (*J, K*). Immediately after delivery of legs, baby is held up by feet (*L*) to encourage accumulated secretions to drain before baby takes first breath. (Evanston Hospital. Photos by D. Sherline)

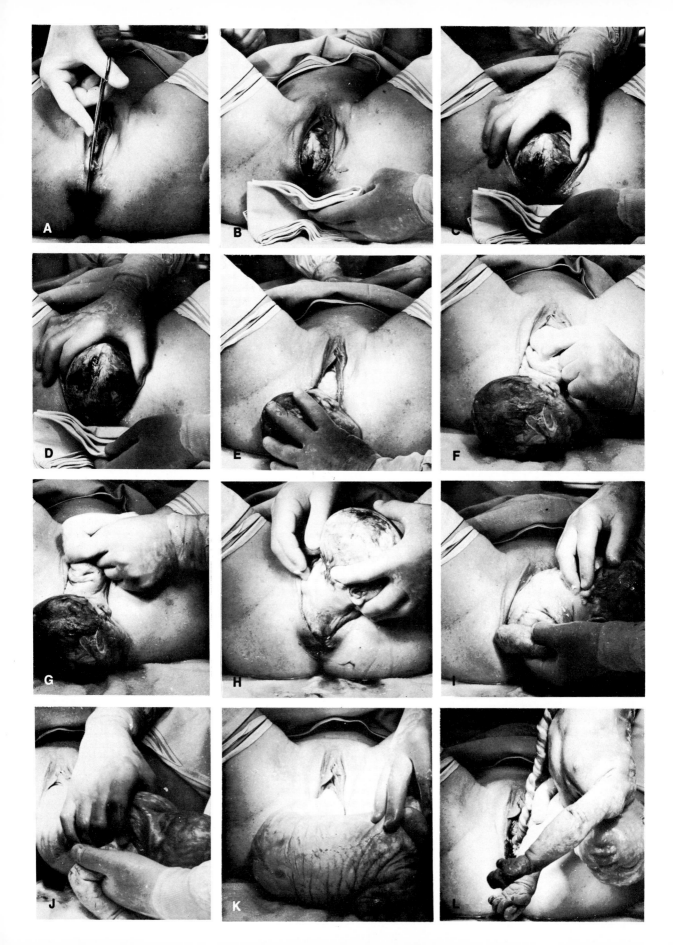

the cord may already have ceased, in which case the baby will probably try to breathe at once. Its airway should therefore be cleared promptly. Other possibilities are that the cord has ruptured; that the cord will rupture as the baby descends further; that further descent will result in separation of the placenta; or that, as delivery proceeds, the traction on the cord will cause the uterus to turn inside out, an extremely rare but serious complication. If the loops are relatively loose, they can often be relaxed or enlarged so that the baby delivers through the loops. If there are many loops or they are tight, two clamps should be placed close together on the most easily accessible bit of cord and the cord cut between the clamps. The cord can then be unwound. If either clamp slips off, that end of the cord must be reclamped at once, since it is impossible to know at that moment which end of the cord is fastened to the baby and which to the placenta.

After the head is born, in a completely unaided delivery there may be a pause. The head is no longer pressing on the perineum, and the shoulders have not descended far enough to press on it, so temporarily the patient has no urge to bear down. In addition, the amount of baby in the uterus has suddenly decreased, and it may take few moments for the uterus to adjust itself to this decreased volume. Mucus, amniotic fluid, and perhaps a slight amount of blood (maternal) can be seen running out of the baby's mouth and nose (the baby's face is usually directed downward at this time). The baby may move its head, blink its eyes, grimace, gasp, and even cry. Shortly, as the uterus resumes effective contractions, the shoulders are forced into and down through the pelvis, at the same time rotating so that one shoulder is behind the pubis and the other in the hollow of the sacrum. This rotation of the shoulders into the anteroposterior diameter of the pelvis causes the baby's head to rotate, the back of the head toward the side of the mother where the fetal back was during labor. This is the external restitution phase of the mechanism of labor. The anterior shoulder stems or pivots underneath the symphysis, and the posterior shoulder is forced outward. If the delivery is assisted, both shoulders should not be permitted to deliver at once. Just as one would negotiate a porthole, the posterior shoulder should be pushed back slightly and the anterior arm delivered by exerting pressure in the antecubital fossa (Fig. 31–4 *F* and *G*). As the posterior shoulder emerges over the perineum, the rest of the baby follows without delay or particular mechanism.

Immediately after delivery, the baby is held head down for a few seconds to permit secretions to drain (Fig. 31–4 *L*) and is then placed supine, either on the end of the delivery table or, if the obstetrician is seated, on a tray placed across his or her knees. Clearing the airway involves removing foreign material from the baby's mouth and throat. A considerable amount can be removed simply by scooping it out with the finger.

Squeezing the nose between the fingers may express small masses of thick mucus. Stroking the upper neck from the larynx toward the mandible (milking) seems to help. A soft rubber suction bulb can be used. Mechanical suction pumps (the tubing must be sterile) are sometimes employed. The gag reflex can be elicited by irritating the base of the tongue or the nasopharynx with the finger. This causes the baby to vomit, and a surprising amount of liquid may be ejected. This prophylactic procedure partially obviates the danger that the baby will vomit and aspirate gastric contents unobserved several minutes after delivery.

In vertex presentation, the presence of meconium in the amniotic fluid is not necessarily a cause for concern, but electronic fetal monitoring is indicated. If the meconium is thick, dark, and copious, and if it appears early in labor, special precautions should be taken to prevent the syndrome of *meconium aspiration*. As soon as the baby's head is delivered, before delivery of the shoulders, a DeLee suction catheter should be passed through the nares to the level of the nasopharynx and any mucus or meconium aspirated. The delivery is then completed routinely. The vocal cords should be visualized with a baby laryngoscope; the presence of meconium at the cords suggests the need for tracheal aspiration.

The official time of birth is the instant at which all of the baby is outside the mother's body. It has nothing to do with breathing, crying, cutting the cord, or any other factor. The second stage of labor terminates and the third stage starts at that moment.

The Agpar score (see page 844) is taken at 1 min and 5 min after birth. Both scores are recorded in the infant's chart.

Time of Cutting the Umbilical Cord. After delivery, the umbilical cord continues to pulsate for about 2 min. During this time, the infant receives a significant quantity of blood through the cord. The amount varies according to the level, with respect to the introitus, at which the baby is held after delivery. If the baby is held at or below the introitus, the "placental transfusion" amounts to as much as 100 ml; if held above the introitus (for example, placed on the mother's abdomen), the amount of blood received is much less. The volume of the placental transfusion is also time-related; in infants delivered by cesarean section, Ogata *et al* have shown that *after* 40 sec the direction of net blood flow reverses so that any benefits from the prior transfusion are lost. After vaginal delivery, it is therefore prudent to hold the baby at or below the level of the introitus and to delay clamping the cord for at least 20 and not more than 40 sec, time that can usually be well spent in making a preliminary evaluation of the baby's condition and thoroughly clearing the airway.

There is no full agreement on whether the placental transfusion is beneficial or harmful to the preterm in-

fant; until the matter is settled, it seems wisest in these cases to cut the cord immediately, to clear the airway as quickly as possible, and to transfer the baby forthwith to the intensive care nursery. The cord should also be cut promptly if the mother is receiving general anesthesia or if there is a maternal–fetal blood group incompatibility, an obvious cardiovascular anomaly, or severe asphyxia, in which case resuscitative measures should be taken at once.

The mechanics of cutting the cord are simple. With sterile scissors (bacteria can readily enter the umbilical circulation by this route) the cord is cut between clamps placed about 3 cm from the umbilicus.

Prevention of Ophthalmia Neonatorum. The prevention of blindness due to ophthalmia neonatorum is usually the responsibility of the obstetrician and it is essential that it be carried out within 1 hour of delivery. The classic offending organism is *N. gonorrhoeae,* but other organisms may also cause the disease by infecting the eyes of the fetus as it passes through the birth canal. Prophylaxis is usually carried out immediately after cutting the cord. For many years the standard agent for this purpose was 1% silver nitrate, 1 drop instilled in each eye and followed by saline irrigation not less than 1 minute later. More recently this has given way to ophthalmic solutions of erythromycin, tetracycline, or penicillin, which are just as effective and do not produce the intense conjunctivitis that usually follows the use of silver nitrate.

Resuscitation, Apgar scoring, and physical examination of the baby are discussed in Chapter 42.

Use of Outlet (Prophylactic) Forceps

Perhaps especially in the United States, the use of prophylactic or outlet forceps has become so much a part of normal obstetrics that it can be considered a part of normal delivery. Its purpose is to supply the final force required to deliver the head through the vaginal orifice. It is considered prophylactic because 1) the delivery is controlled by the operator, rather than being dependent upon the unpredictable voluntary effort of the patient; 2) the head, by being lifted out over the perineum, is spared an unpredictable period of stress while it presses against the perineum; and 3) injury to maternal soft parts is minimized if the procedure is combined with episiotomy.

These comments should not be construed to suggest that use of outlet forceps is preferable to a spontaneous delivery that occurs promptly either without episiotomy or immediately after episiotomy is made, as occurred in the delivery shown in Figure 31–4. However, if the head does not deliver immediately after the skull reaches the pelvic floor, the use of outlet forceps can prevent the damage to the delicate structures of the fetal brain that may result from prolonged pressure of the head against the perineum while the mother at-

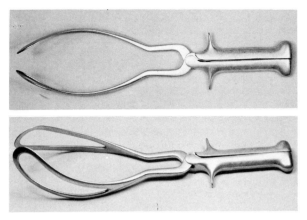

FIG. 31–5. DeLee's modification of Simpson forceps. Note smooth handles and wider crossbar for traction; lock, shank, and blade are essentially same as those of original Simpson instrument. Blades are loosely articulated to show characteristic features of English lock.

tempts to expel it. Some women insist upon spontaneous delivery, but most obstetricians believe that this is not in the best interests of the baby except when the head is expelled promptly after the skull reaches the pelvic floor. If there is delay at this point in labor, use of outlet forceps is preferable.

For the use of outlet forceps, the following conditions must obtain: 1) the scalp must be or have been visible at the introitus without separating the labia, 2) the skull must have reached the pelvic floor, 3) the sagittal suture must be in the sagittal plane of the pelvis, and 4) the membranes must be ruptured. Episiotomy is usually a part of the procedure. Anesthesia is usually required. Such methods as pudendal block, local infiltration of the perineum, saddle block, and epidural are satisfactory. These techniques of anesthesia are outlined in Chapter 32.

The obstetric forceps consists of two matched parts that articulate, or lock. Each part is composed of blade, shank, lock, and handle (Fig. 31–5). The blades possess two curves: the *cephalic curve,* which makes it possible to apply the instrument accurately to the curved lateral aspects of the baby's head, and the *pelvic curve,* which corresponds to the curved pelvic axis. The blades are referred to as *left* and *right,* according to the side of the mother's pelvis on which they lie after application. The *rule of the forceps* is "left blade, left hand, left side of the pelvis; and right blade, right hand, right side of the pelvis." According to this rule, the left blade is held in the operator's left hand and applied to the left side of the mother's pelvis (and, in occiput anterior position, to the left side of the baby's head); using the right hand, the right blade is then applied to the right side of the pelvis. When the blades are applied in this order, the right shank comes to lie

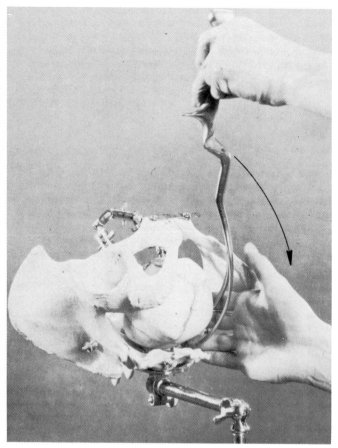

FIG. 31–6. Introduction of left blade (left blade, left hand, left side of pelvis). Handle is held with fingers and thumb, not clenched in hand. Handle is held vertically. Blade is guided with fingers of right hand. After application of blade to side of head, handle is swung downward in an arc (*arrow*) so that it protrudes as shown in Figure 31–8. (Danforth WC: In Curtis AH (ed): Obstetrics and Gynecology. Philadelphia, WB Saunders, 1933)

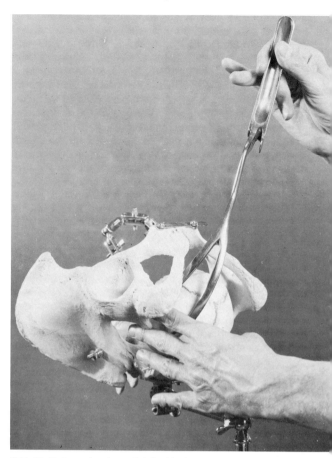

FIG. 31–7. Introduction of right blade (right blade, right hand, right side of pelvis). Left blade (already in place) not shown. Handle is grasped with fingers and thumb, not gripped in whole hand. Handle is held vertical for introduction, and swung downward as in Figure 31–6. (Danforth WC: In Curtis AH (ed): Obstetrics and Gynecology. Philadelphia, WB Saunders, 1933)

atop the left shank in such a manner that they immediately articulate, or lock.

The technique of their use in the operation of outlet forceps is illustrated in Figures 31–6 through 31–10. After delivery of the head, the remainder of the delivery is conducted as described for spontaneous delivery. The use of forceps for procedures other than outlet forceps is considered in Chapter 34.

Use of Vacuum Extractor

Instead of forceps, the vacuum extractor is being used in many parts of the world, but it has met an indifferent reaction in the United States. It consists basically of a round metal cup, 3–6 cm in diameter, to which is attached a rubber hose and a pump. The cup is pressed against the fetal scalp, and air is pumped out of the device; a partial vacuum is created, which causes the cup to adhere to the scalp. Traction on the hose can then be applied with sufficient force so that the head can be pulled through the birth canal. A huge artificial caput succedaneum is produced as the scalp is sucked into the cup. The advantages of the vacuum extractor over forceps are not clear.

Episiotomy

Episiotomy is the surgical incision of the perineum. It is made just prior to delivery, and its purposes are 1) to provide sufficient space for delivery so that the pelvic floor will not be torn as the baby delivers and 2) to provide a clean, incised wound that can be accurately repaired, with restoration of normal relationships. Some

FIG. 31–8. Both blades introduced. The two blades are brought together, or locked. If application is correct, handles lock precisely, without force. (Danforth WC: In Curtis AH (ed): Obstetrics and Gynecology. Philadelphia, WB Saunders, 1933)

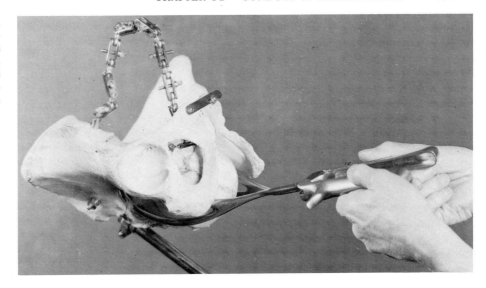

FIG. 31–9. Traction on forceps. Note grip of hands. Position of left hand as shown is used by most obstetricians. Some prefer to place fingers of right hand in crotch of instrument for facilitate traction. Either grip may be used. If heavier traction is needed, no more force should be used than can be exerted by flexed forearms. (Danforth WC: In Curtis AH (ed): Obstetrics and Gynecology. Philadelphia, WB Saunders, 1933)

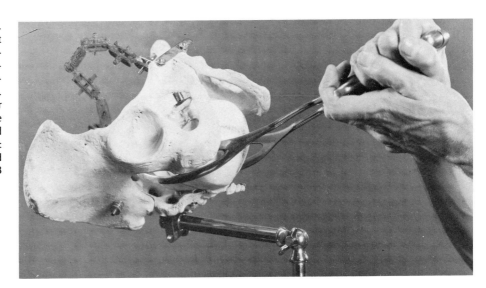

women request that delivery be conducted with no episiotomy and "no stitches." It has been estimated, however, that without episiotomy at least one in four women will sustain serious and avoidable injury to the pelvic floor. Second- and third-degree lacerations can be repaired, but the result is less satisfactory than a well-repaired episiotomy. If such lacerations are not repaired, they ultimately heal, but usually leave some distortion, loss of function, or, occasionally, real disability. The advantages of episiotomy are so great that it should be an almost routine procedure; no disadvantages of episiotomy come to mind except for the occasional woman who does not need it.

The incision begins precisely in the midline. It may be extended either directly posterior through the perineal body itself (median episiotomy), or it may extend in a mediolateral direction to right or left. The median episiotomy is preferred if the perineum is of normal length, if the subpubic arch is of average width, and if no difficulty in delivery is anticipated. Extension to or through the anal sphincter occurs in 2% to 3% of median episiotomies, but loss of function is unusual if it is recognized at once and properly repaired. The indicence of extension is reduced by advancing the legs as the head crowns (compare position of legs in Figures 31–4A and 31–4C).

The mediolateral episiotomy reduces the possibility of traumatic extension of the incision into the rectum

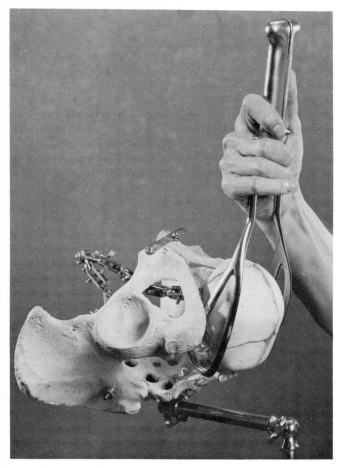

FIG. 31-10. Delivery. As head extends, handles are raised until they pass the vertical, but little force is needed. One hand suffices; other may support perineum. (Danforth WC: In Curtis AH (ed): Obstetrics and Gynecology. Philadelphia, WB Saunders, 1933)

if the perineum is short, if the subpubic arch is narrow, or if there should be difficulty in delivery. In either median or mediolateral episiotomy, the incision should be extended upward for 2–3 cm along the vaginal mucous membrane, for this clearly reduces the possibility of extension. One method of episiotomy repair is shown in Figure 31–16.

Maternal–Infant Bonding

Maternal-infant bonding appears to show significant promise as a means of eliminating many of the serious problems having to do with the psychologic development of the infant and the family unit. Indeed, Klaus and Kennell, who are largely responsible for the concept, asserted that "it is our hypothesis that the entire range of problems from mild maternal anxiety to child abuse may result largely from separation and other unusual circumstances which occur in the early newborn period as a consequence of present hospital care policies." The policies are better than they were when this was written; but the hypothesis is still relevant, and continued efforts are being made to improve family relationships from the moment of birth.

The essential components of bonding are touching, eye-to-eye contact between mother and infant, parallel facial positioning (*en face*), and the immediate presence of the husband or "supporting other." The newborn infant is suctioned, shown to the parents, dried, assessed briefly, loosely wrapped, and given to the mother for approximately 10 min, during which time breast-feeding may be attempted if it is desired. The baby is then taken to the nursery for the necessary examinations and returned to the mother, preferably in a rooming-in atmosphere, as soon as it is appropriate.

Maternal–infant bonding has received the enthusiastic approval of the American Medical Association (AMA) and the Interprofessional Task Force on the Health Care of Women and Infants, and hospitals have been urged to promote both this and other aspects of family-centered maternal and infant care.

LeBoyer's Birth Without Violence

Although his method has not received wide acceptance, LeBoyer has proposed that the baby's later growth and development are improved by reducing to the absolute minimum the stresses to which the newborn baby is ordinarily subject. Delivery room lights are extinguished except for a perineal spotlight, all extraneous noise is eliminated, and soft music is provided. Delivery is as slow, gentle, and atraumatic as possible. The baby is immediately placed on the mother's abdomen, where it can be held and gently stroked by the mother; a warm blanket is used to minimize heat loss and stimulus from the cooler room air. The cord is cut 2–3 min after delivery, and the baby is then transferred to a warm tub of water (99° F). A bath is given, and the baby remains in the water for 3–5 min. The baby is then gently dried, wrapped in a warm blanket, and transferred with the parents to the recovery room. The important points of difference from accepted practice are 1) the immediate positioning of the baby on the mother's abdomen, and the late cutting of the cord, which would reduce or eliminate the placental transfusion, and 2) the avoidance of stimuli to produce the lusty cry that is traditionally thought important in clearing the air passages and establishing pulmonary ventilation.

Most of those who read these pages will not have had the benefits attributed to LeBoyer's method, and it will be some time in the future before the salutary results, if any, can be evaluated. Preliminary data suggest that the method is not harmful to the newborn if its condition at birth is excellent.

FIG. 31-11. Uteroplacental relations in third stage of labor. *A.* Immediately after baby has been expelled from uterus and placenta has separated from its uterine attachment. Note great decrease in surface area of placental site, thickened uterine wall, and change in uterine contours. *B.* After expulsion of placenta into lower uterine segment and vagina. Corpus uteri has become globular and has risen; lower uterine segment is distended by separated placenta. (Davis ME, Boynton MW: Am J Obstet Gynecol 43:775, 1942)

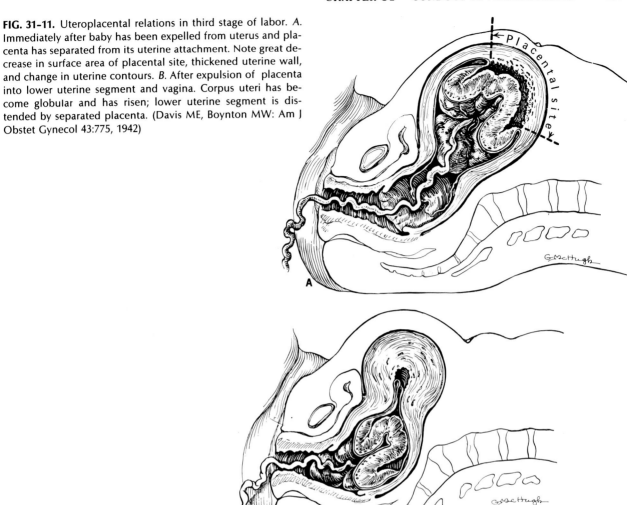

CONDUCT OF THE THIRD STAGE OF LABOR

From the standpoint of maternal risk, the third stage of labor is the most important phase of parturition. Although it occupies an insignificant period of time compared with the many hours devoted to labor, this short period involves many hazards for the mother. Postpartum hemorrhage contributes appreciably to maternal morbidity and is a leading cause of maternal death. Although the immediate blood loss is important, the manipulations necessary to control the bleeding increase the hazard of infection, which may also result in morbidity and mortality directly attributable to the third stage, although often not credited to this period.

MECHANISM OF PLACENTAL DELIVERY

The normal mechanism of the placental stage consists of two distinct phases: separation and expulsion. The physician should not initiate the latter until the former is completed. The first phase involves a slow, progressive separation of the placenta from the uterine wall and is brought about by physical changes that take place upon the evacuation of the fetus from the uterine cavity.

The placenta normally remains attached to the uterus until the expulsion of the fetus. The sudden diminution in size of the uterine cavity results in a reduction of the placenta site, the surface area of the uterine wall to which the placenta is attached. The

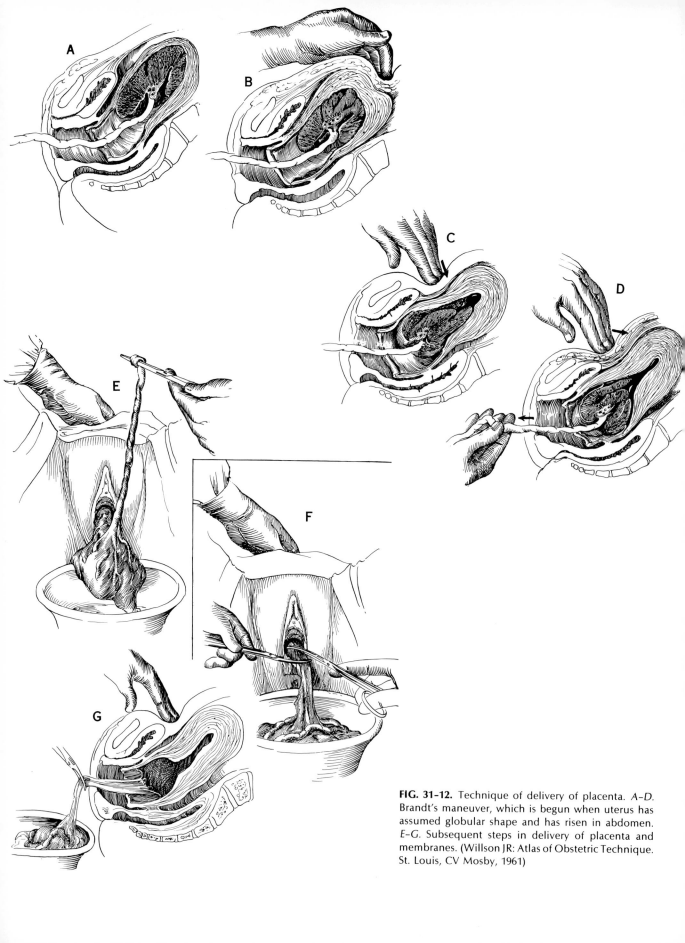

FIG. 31-12. Technique of delivery of placenta. *A–D.* Brandt's maneuver, which is begun when uterus has assumed globular shape and has risen in abdomen. *E–G.* Subsequent steps in delivery of placenta and membranes. (Willson JR: Atlas of Obstetric Technique. St. Louis, CV Mosby, 1961)

semirigid, noncontractile placenta cannot alter its surface area, and thus it partially or completely separates from its attachment (Fig. 31–11). The speed with which the uterine surface area is reduced determines the completeness of the separation.

After separation, blood accumulates behind the placenta, and the uterus rises in the abdomen. A firm uterine contraction now begins, usually within 2 min of delivery, and the uterus changes from a flattened, soft, discoid organ to one that is firm and globular. If the *Brandt maneuver* (Fig. 31–12) is started at the time of this first contraction (not before and not after), the placenta is usually delivered without incident. The Brandt maneuver consists of the following steps:

1. Firm downward pressure on the fundus (at the time of the first contraction), followed immediately by
2. Suprapubic pressure directly against the lower pole of the corpus, while, simultaneously, steady traction is made on the cord to advance the placenta into the lower uterine segment. This is followed promptly by
3. Suprapubic *upward* pressure on the corpus to move it toward the umbilicus. As the cord is held steady, the uterus is caused to move away from the placenta, which now enters the vagina and can be readily delivered by gentle cord traction.

It is emphasized that the Brandt maneuver should be started when the first contraction occurs; if this should be missed because of preoccupation with the baby or for other reasons, the maneuver should not be attempted until the uterus once more contracts firmly. It should be remembered that, whereas a rising hard uterus means that the placenta is separated and a contraction is occurring, *a rising soft uterus may mean intrauterine bleeding.* If the uterus is soft and enlarging or if fresh vaginal bleeding occurs, gentle massage of the fundus may provoke a contraction, which permits the Brandt maneuver to be attempted. If this should fail, manual removal of the placenta is indicated (Fig. 31–13).

The two major mechanisms for delivery of the placenta were described many years ago by Schulze and by Duncan (Fig. 31–14). In the Schulze mechanism, said to be the most common, the fetal surface of the placenta slips through the opening in the fetal membranes and appears at the introitus. The membranes then peel off the surface of the uterine cavity, as a rule uniformly and intact. In this case, the liquid blood and retroplacental clots are contained within the folded placenta and are not evident until the placenta is delivered and examined. In the Duncan method, one edge of the placenta first slips through the cervix and into the vagina. The remainder of the placenta follows, and the fetal membranes are peeled from the uterus as traction is made on the following edge of the placenta. The liquid blood and retroplacental clots escape from

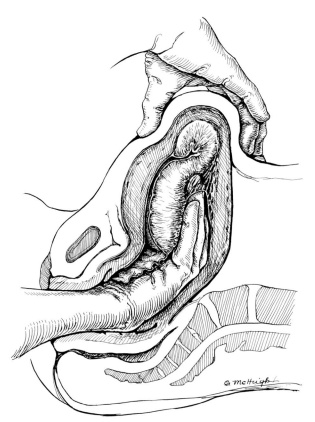

FIG. 31–13. Manual removal of placenta. Physician carefully separates attached placenta in proper plane before attempting its removal from uterus. (Davis ME, Rubin R (eds): DeLee's Obstetrics for Nurses, 17th ed. Philadelphia, WB Saunders, 1962)

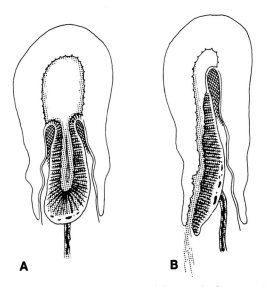

A   **B**

FIG. 31–14. Mechanism of delivery of placenta. *A.* Schulze mechanism. *B.* Duncan mechanism. (Modified from Myles MF: Textbook for Midwives. London, Livingstone, 1956)

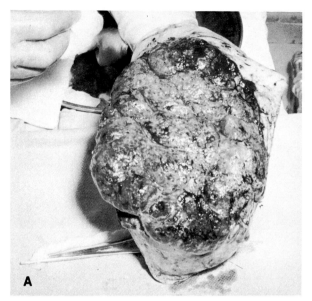

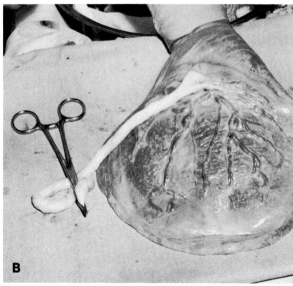

FIG. 31–15. Examination of placenta. *A.* Maternal surface is carefully sponged of clots; inspection will reveal if it is complete or if a fragment is missing. *B.* Fetal surface is then examined and note is made whether blood vessels disappear at periphery of placenta. If a patent vessel continues to edge of membranes, retained succenturiate lobe is suggested.

the uterus as the maternal surface of the placenta is delivered. The designations "shiny Schulze" and "dirty Duncan" have long been a part of obstetric parlance. In addition to the fact that it is less tidy, the Duncan mechanism is more frequently followed by retained fragments of the fetal membranes.

CONDUCT OF THE IMMEDIATE PUERPERIUM

The following steps are to be undertaken immediately after delivery of the placenta:

1. An oxytocic may be given, but there is not full agreement that oxytocics are routinely needed. The uterus normally contracts firmly after delivery of the placenta, and this is usually sufficient to maintain closure of the uterine sinuses. Despite evidence of the competence of nature to prevent excessive bleeding, many obstetricians prefer to administer an oxytocic after delivery of the placenta. This would appear to be especially prudent in women who are predisposed to postpartum hemorrhage (*i.e.,* previous twins, hydramnios, prolonged or dysfunctional labor; grand multiparity; age over 35; postpartum hemorrhage after a prior delivery; general anesthetic used for delivery).

   The customary agent is oxytocin, and the preferable route is by infusion (40 units in 1000 ml 5% dextrose in water). For undelivered women, an infusion pump is essential for accurate administration of oxytocin; for use after delivery, precision is not needed and a drip is preferable. The speed of the infusion should be adjusted according to the amount of bleeding and the tone of the uterus. It must not be run too rapidly, for an intravenous bolus of as little as 5 units of oxytocin can cause a transient but profound drop in blood pressure.

   In former years, ergonovine was a standard agent for routine use after delivery; because of occasional hypertensive responses to this drug, it is now reserved, for the most part, to cases in which the uterus remains boggy despite an oxytocin infusion. In such a case, 0.2 mg ergonovine is given intramuscularly. If bleeding and uterine atony continue, the administration of calcium gluconate (10 ml 10% solution intravenously) may have an instant and salutary oxytocic effect.

2. The placenta and membranes should be inspected (Fig. 31–15). If there is an obvious placental defect, the uterus should be digitally explored and the fragment retrieved. Despite its popularity among some obstetricians of high competence, routine exploration is not recommended; it is probably not harmful, but there is nothing to suggest that it is of any real benefit in preventing postpartum hemorrhage due to retained secundines. Exploration is recommended only if there is a missing placental fragment of sufficient size to be detected at the first inspection or if the labor or delivery was of such character that uterine rupture must be ruled out.

3. The vagina (especially in the vaginal sulci and over prominent ischial spines) and the cervix should be inspected, and lacerations immediately repaired.

4. The episiotomy (if one was made) should now be repaired. One technique of episiotomy repair is

shown in Figure 31–16. Probably no two obstetricians repair an episiotomy in exactly the same way; but most repairs accomplish the same result. The obstetrician should use the simplest and most expeditious repair that will provide a firm pelvic floor.

5. The fundus should be palpated. It should now be below the level of the umbilicus and should be firmly retracted. If the uterus is at or above the umbilicus, this may be due either to a full bladder or to the collection of blood in the uterus. The distinction is important, and intrauterine blood should be expelled by *Crede's maneuver* (a technique designed to expel the placenta, no longer used for this purpose but valuable for emptying the uterus of clots) in which the uterus is grasped anteriorly and posteriorly and squeezed.

6. The patient should be moved to the obstetric recovery room.

The obstetrician should not leave the patient until satisfied that 1) there is no active bleeding, 2) the uterus is firm and well retracted, and 3) the pulse and blood pressure are within normal limits. If general anesthesia was used for delivery, the obstetrician should not leave until the patient is fully reacted.

RECOVERY ROOM CARE

A recovery room for obstetric patients is essential to modern obstetric care. The required equipment includes suction and oxygen from a wall source and a fixed sphygmomanometer. Fluids, plasma expanders, an immediate source of blood, a tray or kit containing the drugs ordinarily used for dealing with shock and preeclampsia, central venous pressure monitoring apparatus, laryngoscope, endotracheal catheters, and a good light should be immediately available. A cart equipped with side rails is generally preferable to a bed for the patient in the obstetric recovery room. Defibrillator and electronic monitoring devices for pulse and blood pressure should be part of the standard equipment.

As a rule, obstetric patients remain on the delivery table until vital signs are stable. They are then moved to the recovery room, where they should remain under constant surveillance for at least 1 hour. At intervals of at least every 15 min the following observations should be made and recorded on an appropriate chart: pulse, blood pressure, height and consistency of the fundus, and estimate of the amount of uterine bleeding (*i.e.,* whether slight, moderate, or heavy).

The complications for which special vigilance should be maintained in the first hour after delivery include 1) excessive uterine bleeding (usually due to uterine atony, obstetric lacerations, retained placental fragments, or clotting defects); 2) hematoma forma-

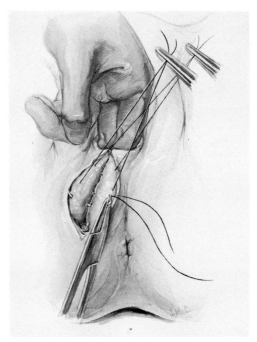

FIG. 31-16. One technique for episiotomy repair. (Right mediolateral episiotomy is shown, but same technique is applicable to median or to left mediolateral.) Vaginal mucosa has been approximated with running suture. Lifting sutures placed as shown cause perineal structures to stand out, and facilitate their approximation. Fingers in vagina push rectum away and bring vaginal sutures down so depth of incision can be readily closed. Skin is closed with interrupted sutures unless, as frequently occurs, edges fall together, in which case Allis clamps, allowed to remain in place for 10 min, suffice and usually produce less discomfort than sutures. Subcuticular sutures do not improve cosmetic result, prevent egress of any blood that may collect, and prolong procedure unnecessarily.

tion in the episiotomy site, vagina, or, rarely, in the lower portion of the broad ligament; 3) shock (due to blood loss, sepsis, anesthesia, or aspiration); 4) hypertension (due to postpartum preeclampsia or vasospasm precipitated by an oxytocic agent); and 5) convulsions (occurring as a complication of regional anesthesia, eclampsia, epilepsy, or cerebral hemorrhage). The diagnosis and management of these complications are considered elsewhere.

When hemorrhagic shock occurs in the obstetric patient, it is usually instant and precipitous. The compensatory mechanisms to resist blood loss hold up much longer than in the nonobstetric patient, and the gradual decline in blood pressure and elevation of pulse, so valuable in assessing blood loss in other surgical situations, are rarely seen. In the obstetric patient, the best guide to the imminence of hemorrhagic shock is the clinical estimate of blood loss, *not* pulse

and blood pressure, which may remain normal until moments before the collapse. When excessive bleeding occurs, measures against hemorrhagic shock should be taken at once.

REFERENCES AND RECOMMENDED READING

Abouleish E: Vomiting, regurgitation, and aspiration in obstetrics. In Abouleish E: Pain Control in Obstetrics, Chap 8, pp 138–159. Philadelphia, J. B. Lippincott, 1977

Annexton M: Parent–infant bonding. Birthing: A real family affair in California center. JAMA 240:823, 1978

Anonymous. A study of physicians' handwriting as a time waster. JAMA 242:2429, 1979

Carson BS, Losey RW, Bowes WA, Jr, Simmons MA: Combined obstetric and pediatric approach to prevent meconium aspiration syndrome. Am J Obstet Gynecol 126:712, 1976 (See also letter to editor, ibid, 133:934, 1979)

Danforth DN, Ivy AC: The effect of calcium upon uterine contractions and upon the uterine response to intravenously injected oxytocics. Am J Obstet Gynecol 37:194, 1939

Drouin P, Nasah BT, Nkounawa F: The value of the partogram in the management of labor. Obstet Gynecol 53:741, 1979

Fliegner JRH: Third stage management: How important is it? Med J Aust 2:190, 1978

Grover JW: Nonviolent birth. The Female Patient 4:62, 1979

Jeffcoate N: Medicine versus nature: The James Y Simpson memorial lecture. J R Coll Surg Edinb 21:246, 1976

Klaus MH, Kennell JH: Maternal–Infant Bonding. St. Louis, CV Mosby, 1976

McClellen MS, Cabianca WA: Effects of early mother–infant contact following cesarean birth. Obstet Gynecol 56:52, 1980

Nichols DH, Randall CL: Vaginal Surgery, pp 39–40. Baltimore, Williams & Wilkins, 1976 (Discussion of propriety of routine episiotomy.)

Notelovitz M: The single-unit delivery system—A safe alternative to home deliveries. Am J Obstet Gynecol 132:889, 1978

Ogata ES, Kitterman JA, Kleinberg F et al: The effect of time of cord clamping and maternal blood pressure on placental transfusion with cesarean section. Am J Obstet Gynecol 128:197, 1977

Pearse WH: Home birth. JAMA 241:1039, 1979

Shamsi HH, Petrie RH, Steer CM: Changing obstetric practices and amelioration of perinatal outcome in a university hospital. Am J Obstet Gynecol 133:855, 1979

Sosa R, Kennell J, Klaus M et al: The effect of a supportive companion on perinatal problems, length of labor, and mother–infant interaction. N Engl J Med 303:597, 1980

Studd J: Partograms and nomograms of cervical dilatation in management of primigravid labour. Br Med J 4:451, 1973

Taylor PM (ed): Parent–infant relationships. Semin Perinatol 3:1, 1979

Yao AC, Lind J: Placental transfusion. Am J Dis Child 127:128, 1974

Fear and anxiety, as well as pain, are known to have a marked influence on various physiologic functions. Recently, much attention has been paid to the influence of maternal psychologic stress and pain, particularly the acute stress of labor and delivery, on the maternal cardiovascular system, uteroplacental circulation, and fetal well-being. It has been shown that psychologic or painful stress to the mother during labor may cause fetal acidosis and hypoxemia, probably because uterine blood flow is reduced as a consequence of increased catecholamine release. On the other hand, many recent reports have shown that the judicious use of analgesia and anesthesia may improve maternal and fetal homeostasis, as well as the conduct of labor.

The need for relief from pain and reduction of fear and anxiety varies. Some labors are clearly easier than others. Patients who are confident, informed, well adjusted, and in good general health frequently require little medication and usually consider their labor and delivery a happy experience. Others who are apprehensive, terrified by having heard the dire experiences of others, and without confidence in their attendants may not accept childbirth with equanimity despite a relatively uncomplicated labor.

The benefits of pain relief to the parturient herself are obvious, but reduction of maternal pain may also be advantageous for the fetus and newborn. Those who care for women in labor should have a fundamental knowledge of this field, and should be prepared to utilize the appropriate methods when they are indicated, and when they will improve the safety and efficiency of labor.

CHAPTER 32

OBSTETRIC ANALGESIA AND ANESTHESIA

Hisayo O. Morishima

PHARMACOLOGY OF ANESTHETICS AND RELATED DRUGS USED IN OBSTETRICS

Many drugs and techniques are available for the relief of pain in childbirth. The basic consideration must be safety of both mother and fetus. No single drug or technique of obstetric analgesia or anesthesia is superior to all others, nor is any one applicable to all patients. Therefore, in order to select the most appropriate agent for optimal pain relief to the mother with the least risk to her and her infant, the physician must be familiar with a variety of methods and agents.

MATERNAL-FETAL TRANSFER

Physicochemical Factors

All anesthetics are highly lipid-soluble and transfer across the placenta within minutes of administration by simple diffusion, according to the concentration gradient. The distribution of anesthesia into and its ultimate removal from fetal tissues are influenced by a variety of factors. Of prime significance are the physiochemical properties of the compound. Equally important, however, are the anatomic features of the maternal circulation, the placenta, and the fetus, as well as hemodynamic and pharmacokinetic events within them. Most anesthetics are weak bases that exist in aqueous solutions partly as undissociated free bases and partly as dissociated cations.

The proportion of anesthetic in uncharged and charged forms is given by the Henderson–Hasselbalch equation:

$$pH = pKa + \log \text{ (base) / (cation)}$$

This ratio is of pharmacologic importance in local anesthetics, since the base is believed to penetrate the diffusion barriers, *e.g.*, the placenta. The cation, however, is thought to block conduction when in direct contact with nervous tissue. The pKa is that pH value at which free base and cation occur in equal proportions. Com-

monly used local anesthetics and other drugs, such as morphine and meperidine, have pKa values ranging 7.7–9.1. These values are sufficiently close to the blood pH that maternal or fetal acid–base imbalance may result in significant changes in the ratio of ionized to unionized fractions of drug. Thus, for example, in an acidotic fetus, the proportion of ionized drug is greater than that in a fetus with a normal acid–base balance. With equal blood concentrations of the unionized moiety (in equilibrium with that of the mother), the total blood concentration of a local anesthetic is also higher if the fetus is acidotic, since the local anesthetic is a weak base. This has been demonstrated clinically and experimentally. Fetal acidosis should have similar effects on other basic drugs. Molecular size is also important. Most unionized drugs with a molecular weight less than 500 cross cell boundaries readily, but most agents with a molecular weight greater than 1000 do not cross at all.

Reduction in the uterine blood flow because of maternal hypotension caused by hemorrhage, spinal or epidural block, or aortocaval compression, or because of chronic conditions such as preeclampsia and diabetes, decreases placental transfer of a drug. Change in the distribution of fetal cardiac output may change the uptake of drug by the fetal tissues. For example, when lidocaine is administered to the acidotic and hypoxemic fetal baboon, the drug uptake by vital organs, such as brain and heart, is greater than in the normal fetus. When the parturient is anesthetized with a clinical dose of thiopental given as a bolus, she may be expected to give birth to a vigorous infant because there is a rapid decrease in maternal blood concentrations of thiopental and the fetus is exposed to high maternal drug levels for only a short time. On the other hand, repeated or large doses of thiopental cause a high incidence of neonatal depression.

Inhalation agents also cross the placenta rapidly. Analgesic concentrations of these agents rarely depress the fetus or neonate, even if administered for prolonged periods. When the drugs are given in anesthetic concentrations, the incidence of neonatal depression increases. For example, cyclopropane, a potent inhalation agent, causes depression in a neonate 6 minutes after induction of anesthesia. High concentrations of nitrous oxide (70%) may depress the fetus within 10 min. Muscle relaxants such as *d*-tubocurarine or succinylcholine cross the placenta in small quantities. It was formerly believed that clinical doses of these drugs do not cross the placenta in significant amounts because of their low lipid solubility and high degree of ionization, but this has been proved to be incorrect.

All amide-linked local anesthetics have been detected in the maternal blood within minutes of administration. Mepivacaine reaches peak concentrations in maternal blood within 25–40 min following a single epidural injection. The subsequent decline is sufficiently slow to account for maternal (and fetal) accumulation after repeat or continuous injections. Absorption of local anesthetics from the paracervical area appears to be more rapid than absorption from the epidural space, owing to the greater vascularity of the area; maternal drug concentrations reach their maximum values within 9–10 min of injection. This maternal accumulation of local anesthetics may be reduced by the use of long-acting agents, such as bupivacaine or etidocaine, which require less frequent reinjection, or by the use of rapidly metabolized drugs such as 2-chloroprocaine, an ester, which is hydrolyzed by plasma pseudocholinesterase.

The relative directions of maternal and fetal blood flow within the placenta may affect the efficiency of transfer of respiratory gases, drugs, and other substances between mother and fetus. In the human placenta, these exchanges appear to be based on a "multivillous stream" vascular pattern, in which maternal blood flows successively past a large number of chorionic villi as it traverses the intervillous space. As oxygen from the maternal stream enters the fetal blood, fetal capillaries lying further downstream in the intervillous space are exposed to maternal blood of progressively decreasing oxygen tension. Comparable decline in concentration of drugs in the maternal bloodstream is also to be expected.

Anatomic and Hemodynamic Factors

Oxygen, nutrients, and drugs are carried to the fetus by the umbilical vein. Cord compression, which occurs to greater or lesser extent in at least one-third of vaginal deliveries, may diminish transfer of all of these substances to the fetus. A variable proportion of the umbilical venous blood perfuses the fetal liver and enters the inferior vena cava through the hepatic vein, while the remainder is shunted through the ductus venosus directly into the inferior vena cava. Consequently, a portion of any drug is strained through the liver before it reaches the rest of the fetus. Furthermore, the drug is diluted during its transit to the arterial side of the fetal venous blood from the gastrointestinal tract, from the lower extremities, from the head and upper extremities, and, finally, from the lungs. This unique pattern of the fetal circulation results in a delay in equilibration between fetal tissues and fetal blood, manifested by the persistent gradient in drug concentrations between the umbilical vein and the umbilical artery. This has been demonstrated with a variety of anesthetics. Distribution of fetal cardiac output may be altered by fetal hypoxemia and, even more so, by a combination of hypoxemia and acidosis. Under these conditions, blood flow to the placenta and to the fetal brain, heart, and adrenals increases substantially, while perfusion of the lungs, kidneys, spleen, and gut

diminishes. Drug distribution in fetal tissues should follow similar patterns.

Factors Affecting Fetal Tissue Uptake

Any drug transferred across the placenta is carried to fetal tissues, where its uptake depends on the tissue/blood partition coefficient of the drug and the tissue perfusion. For example, following intravenous injection of lidocaine to the mother, relatively high concentrations are found in the fetal liver, myocardium, and brain, demonstrating the rapid distribution to highly perfused fetal organs. The liver is the only organ in which lidocaine levels in the fetus exceed those in the mother. Substantial hepatic accumulation of other anesthetic drugs, such as thiopental and halothane, has been shown to occur and can be explained by the strategic situation of the fetal liver in regard to the umbilical circulation.

The importance of lipid solubility in the fetal tissue uptake of local anesthetics has recently been demonstrated in a study in which the placental transfer of several local anesthetics was compared in pregnant guinea pigs. The ratio of etidocaine or bupivacaine concentration between the fetal and maternal blood was substantially lower than that found for lidocaine. This observation was in agreement with data on the umbilical vein/maternal blood concentration ratio computed in human studies. The proportion of the injected dose recovered from fetuses over the first 60 min was remarkably similar for all three drugs studied, however. In contrast, the uptake of etidocaine or bupivacaine in the fetal myocardium, brain, and liver was substantially greater than that of lidocaine. These relatively high tissue levels of the long-acting agents in the fetus relate to the fact that bupivacaine is approximately 10 times, and etidocaine 50 times, more soluble in lipids than lidocaine. High protein binding of these agents, which in guinea pigs is similar to that in humans, failed to limit their placental transfer. The relatively low fetal blood levels of these drugs can be explained by the greater tissue uptake.

METABOLISM AND EXCRETION

Experimental data gathered over the last few years indicate that the fetus and the newborn are capable of metabolizing and excreting certain local anesthetics. For example, in plasma samples obtained from umbilical vessels at birth, 2-chloroprocaine was rapidly hydrolyzed, the half-life being approximately 43 sec. The human newborn has been shown to eliminate lidocaine and mepivacaine in its urine. Detailed pharmacokinetic study of lidocaine in fetal and newborn lambs and adult sheep indicates that the metabolic clearance in the newborn is quite similar to that in the adult and

the renal clearance is greater. Nonetheless, the elimination half-life is more prolonged in the newborn. This is due to a greater volume of distribution and tissue uptake of the drug in the newborn so that, at any given time, the neonate's kidneys are exposed to a smaller fraction of the lidocaine accumulated in the body. The renal excretion of mepivacaine in human fetuses is believed to be responsible for most of the drug in the amniotic fluid. Since the fetus swallows amniotic fluid periodically, reuptake of the drug in the fetal circulation may take place by this route.

NONPHARMACOLOGIC METHODS OF OBSTETRIC ANALGESIA

The popularity of prepared childbirth classes continues to increase. Several different methods of nonpharmacologic analgesia have been used in recent years to relieve the pain in childbirth. Among these are natural childbirth, as described by Dick–Read; psychoprophylaxis, popularized by Lamaze; the Bradley method; hypnosis; and acupuncture. Each of these techniques is useful in certain patients, and each has achieved some degree of success.

NATURAL CHILDBIRTH

The concept of conducting labor and delivery without the use of pain-relieving medication was introduced by Dick–Read in *Natural Childbirth* in 1933 and *Childbirth Without Fear* in 1944. Dick–Read tried to show that interference with the normal or natural processes of childbirth by the administration of pain-relieving drugs (or by the use of outlet forceps or other assistance in delivery) is not only needless meddling but is actually unnatural and harmful. Intensive antepartum instruction in the physiology of labor, in breathing, in muscle relaxation and contraction is part of the technique. The method relies on psychologic and physiologic principles not totally acceptable today, but the concept has some points in its favor. First, Dick–Read emphasized the desirability of antepartum instruction and advocated certain exercises that assist the patient in her reaction to the labor process. Second, he warned of the undesirable and, in fact, hazardous effects of heavy medication during labor. Finally, he pointed out that it is desirable for the patient to be conscious at the time of delivery. The less desirable aspect of the Dick–Read method lies in the fact that it becomes something of a crusade—the patient who eventually asks for analgesia may be left with a feeling of failure or guilt and inadequacy. Dick–Read's method was not wholly successful, and a new concept of psychoprophylactic preparation and delivery became increasingly popular.

PSYCHOPROPHYLAXIS: LAMAZE

The Lamaze method, discussed in Chapter 19, was introduced in the late 1950s and has since become an important part of "prepared childbirth." It is an altered form of Dick–Read's natural childbirth and, in principle, is similar to it in that intense antepartum preparation, education, and relaxation are recommended to reduce pain during labor and delivery. Unlike the earlier method, the Lamaze technique does not deny that pain is associated with the labor process. Psychoprophylaxis, skillfully employed in selected patients, may effectively decrease or even eliminate the use of medication, but it is questionable whether reducing the requirement for supplemental chemical analgesia decreases the incidence of neonatal depression. A recent study indicates that a Lamaze-trained group required less medication than untrained patients, but there was no difference in neonatal outcome between the two groups. Despite its popularity, the Lamaze method has several disadvantages. Preparation and education take a significant amount of time. Pain relief is rarely complete; indeed, complete pain relief can be obtained in only about 20% of prepared patients. Should the patient breathe incorrectly and hyperventilate, which frequently occurs, she may develop a respiratory alkalosis that can decrease uterine blood flow and consequently reduce the oxygen available to the fetus. Conversely, shallow and rapid breathing, as taught with the method, can produce respiratory acidosis that may adversely affect the fetus.

HYPNOSIS

For obstetric patients, hypnosis has never become popular, although it has been demonstrated in some women as successful and safe. The technique has been shown to be superior to pharmacologic medication in terms of infant outcome. It is, however, a time-consuming procedure; the patient must be trained from about the 5th or 6th month of pregnancy, and frequent sessions are usually required throughout the pregnancy. Like other nonpharmacologic methods, hypnosis seems to be useful for only a limited number of patients. Moreover, it has been observed that if the hypnotized patient is under only borderline control that breaks down during labor, the results may be chaotic. Hypnosis may be applicable for the amenable patient when there is no reason to anticipate a complicated labor and for the patient in whom analgesic and anesthetic drugs should be withheld. However, this technique is for the most part impractical. Only for specific indications should hypnosis be employed. It should be used only by a physician who has both experience in using the method in obstetrics and skill in managing patients under hypnosis.

ACUPUNCTURE

Although acupuncture therapy has been a part of Chinese medicine for many centuries, it is rarely employed by the Chinese today for vaginal delivery. Like hypnosis, acupuncture appears to be safe for mother and fetus, but it is effective in only a limited number of patients. Hypnotic susceptibility and successful use of acupuncture for pain relief do not appear to be related. Several United States investigators have attempted to use this method, but they found that only a small number of patients had adequate analgesia with acupuncture alone.

SYSTEMIC ANALGESIA FOR LABOR

The need for systemic analgesia in labor varies greatly from one patient to another. As a general rule, the smallest effective doses should be used. The continuous presence of a reassuring attendant and the support of the baby's father appear to be helpful in keeping the necessary dosage to a minimum.

Systemic analgesia for labor and delivery is a simple method to relieve pain and anxiety. Systemic medications frequently consist of a combination of sedatives and narcotics. All systemic analgesic agents used in obstetrics may depress the mother's vital functions and cross the placenta to depress those of the fetus. The fetal brain and heart may be affected directly by the drug itself, or the drug may impose a secondary hazard by 1) reducing maternal respiration, which may lead to maternal hypercapnia and hypoxia; 2) altering the maternal cardiovascular and hemodynamic status, thus impairing uteroplacental circulation; 3) interfering with uterine activity; or 4) interfering with the mother's voluntary efforts to bear down in the second stage.

Analgesic drugs are being used in the first stage of labor in three situations:

1. When the cervix, after 5–6 hours of painful contractions, remains firm, uneffaced, and dilated only 1–2 cm. In this circumstance, analgesia or sedation provides rest, relaxation, and perhaps sleep; when the effects of the drug subside, labor may become more effective.
2. When labor is well established, active cervical dilatation is in progress, and contractions are sufficiently painful for the patient to want relief. As a rule, this occurs in a first labor when the cervix reaches 3–4 cm dilatation and in the multipara when the cervix reaches 5–6 cm dilatation.
3. When a definite decision for cesarean section has been made. A small dose of analgesic may be administered 1–2 hours before the anticipated time of delivery in order to reduce fear and apprehension.

The major systemic drugs used for analgesia in obstetrics may be classified into the following groups: sedative–tranquilizers; narcotics; dissociative or amnesic drugs; and neuroleptanalgesia.

SEDATIVE-TRANQUILIZERS

Properly used to supplement psychologic preparation and provide emotional support, these drugs not only minimize fear and anxiety, but also induce rest and sleep. This hypnotic effect may be especially beneficial in early labor.

Barbiturates

During the early latent phase of labor, barbiturates are effective as sedative–hypnotics when delivery is not anticipated for 12–24 hours. Until recently, the most frequently used barbiturates during labor were pentobarbital (Nembutal), secobarbital (Seconal), or amobarbital (Amytal). These short- or intermediate-acting barbiturates are now rarely employed for sedation during the first stage of labor, since they do not relieve pain and may produce excitement if severe pain is present. A large dose of barbiturates, or smaller doses combined with narcotics, may produce maternal respiratory depression. Small doses of barbiturates, which do not affect maternal respiration, rapidly cross the placenta and may depress neonatal behavior for several days. There are no effective pharmacologic antagonists to the barbiturates.

Phenothiazine Derivatives and Hydroxyzine

Promethazine (Phenergan), propiomazine (Largon), chlorpromazine (Thorazine), promazine (Sparine), and prochlorperazine (Compazine), are phenothiazine derivatives that relieve anxiety during labor. The first two drugs are the most popular; the usual dosage of 25 and 20 mg, respectively, is given intravenously or intramuscularly. The tranquilizers produce tranquility and ataraxia, and reduce nausea and vomiting, which often occur during labor. The use of the more potent phenothiazines, particularly in combination with the narcotics, may result in significant maternal hypotension. Hydroxyzine (Vistaril) is not chemically related to phenothiazine, but it produces a similar ataractic effect. It should not be used intravenously, as it causes venous thrombosis and phlebitis. The tranquilizers are readily transferred across the placenta and decrease the beat-to-beat variability of the fetal heart rate, making interpretation of fetal monitoring more difficult. They also affect neonatal behavior up to 6 hours or more. Hence, they should not be repeated every time a narcotic is given.

Diazepam (Valium)

A benzodiazepine derivative, diazepam is more potent than chlordiazepoxide (Librium). In recent years, diazepam has been the tranquilizer most widely used to reduce anxiety and apprehension. This drug is a mild sedative and ataractic, but has no analgesic action. Diazepam concentrations in fetal blood that exceed maternal levels have been reported. Small doses of diazepam administered intravenously to the mother result in a marked decrease (within minutes) of beat-to-beat variability of the fetal heart rate. However, if the total antepartum maternal dose of diazepam is limited to 10 mg, the depressant effects on the full-term newborn are minimal. If large doses of diazepam are administered during labor, the newborn may be depressed, and the drug may be detected in the neonate for at least a week. Neurobehavioral examinations have shown that the newborn has decreased muscle tone for 4–24 hours after delivery when diazepam has been used. With higher doses, neonatal hypothermia may occur, probably because the drug has a depressant effect on the thermoregulatory center. Particular care should be taken to maintain a warm environment for infants of mothers who have received diazepam.

NARCOTICS AND RELATED DRUGS

Narcotics are the most effective systemic medications for relief of pain. They are used during the first stage of labor. The narcotics include morphine, meperidine (Demerol), alphaprodine (Nisentil), pentazocine (Talwin), fentanyl (Sublimaze), oxymorphone (Numorphan), and anileridine (Leritine). Numerous studies have given extensive information on narcotic effects on the fetus and neonate following administration to the mother during labor. All narcotics administered in appropriate clinical doses cross the placenta in appreciable amounts within minutes, and may produce respiratory depression and neurobehavioral alterations in the neonate.

Morphine

Potent narcotics, especially morphine, oxymorphone, and anileridine, are uniquely effective in relieving pain, but they are rarely used in current obstetric practice because of their potentially serious side effects on both mother and neonate. In the mother, respiratory depression, hypotension due to peripheral vasodilation, and vomiting are not unusual. The effects on the fetus and newborn after intramuscular injection depend on the dose and the interval before delivery. The incidence of neonatal depression increases progressively in the 2nd and 3rd hours after morphine is given to the mother. Infants born within 1 hour of

the time of injection or 6 hours afterwards usually show little, if any, narcotic effect. Comparative studies of equianalgesic doses of morphine and meperidine have shown that respiratory depression occurs more often in newborns whose mothers received meperidine.

Meperidine (Demerol)

Meperidine, one of the most widely used narcotic drugs, is administered in a dose of 50 mg intramuscularly or 25–50 mg intravenously. Although it does not eliminate pain completely, it reduces discomfort to the point where painful contractions are well tolerated. This narcotic has an excellent general relaxing effect and is sufficiently sedative to make it possible for the patient to rest between contractions. Meperidine may be found in the fetal circulation within minutes after an intravenous injection has been given to the mother. Extensive studies have shown that drug concentrations in maternal and fetal blood reach equilibrium within 6 min after the mother has been given a clinical dose intravenously. The narcotic may decrease beat-to-beat variability of the fetal heart rate. Recent studies have shown that clinical dosages of meperidine may cause fetal bradycardia or a decrease in oxygen tension (PO_2), when measured continuously with a fetal subcutaneous PO_2 electrode. Meperidine hydrochloride may also alter fetal electroencephalogram (EEG) patterns and decrease, or arrest, normal fetal respiratory movements (see Chapter 41). After delivery, the effect of the drug may continue, causing prolonged depression of neonatal respiration that may lead to respiratory acidosis and hypoxemia. Abnormal neurobehavioral scores may be found in neonates whose mothers have received meperidine hydrochloride during labor. Most of these adverse effects are related to the dose and to the time interval between administration of the drug and delivery. The incidence of neonatal depression is higher when meperidine is given 2–3 hours before delivery than when it is administered just before delivery.

Other Narcotics and Related Drugs

Alphaprodine, pentazocine, and fentanyl are more potent respiratory depressants than the narcotics that have been discussed and are not commonly used in obstetrics. The action of alphaprodine has a rapid onset and short duration; the analgesic effect occurs 1–2 min after intravenous administration and 5–10 min after subcutaneous injection. The drug's action continues 1–2 hours. Pentazocine is a synthetic analgesic, originally marketed as a nonrespiratory depressant. Analgesia occurs within 2–3 min after intravenous injection and 10–20 min after intramuscular injection. The action continues for 3–4 hours. Although pentaz-

ocine has been reported to cross the placenta in only small amounts, this analgesic offers no advantage over equianalgesic doses of meperidine. Fentanyl produces analgesia immediately after intravenous injection and lasts 20–60 min. The onset of analgesia after intramuscular administration is 7–8 min, and the drug continues to be effective for 1–2 hours.

DISSOCIATIVE OR AMNESIC DRUGS

Ketamine Hydrochloride

A phencyclidin derivative, ketamine produces complete analgesia without loss of consciousness and is widely used for obstetric anesthesia in the United States. The analgesic action occurs almost immediately after intravenous administration. It may be supplemented by nitrous oxide and oxygen for vaginal delivery, or used as an induction agent (1 mg/kg) for general anesthesia. Ketamine readily crosses the placenta, and equilibrium is rapidly established between maternal and fetal blood levels. Comparative studies of ketamine and thiopental as induction agents supplemented by nitrous oxide and oxygen for cesarean section, revealed no differences in the incidence of postoperative psychosis. The neonates had comparable Apgar scores, but results of neurobehavioral examination were more satisfactory on the 1st and 2nd days of age in the ketamine group. However, a larger dose (2 mg/kg) has been reported to produce a higher incidence of neonatal depression. Ketamine may increase uterine activity, and this effect is dose-related. Amounts larger than 1 mg/kg administered to the parturient are likely to increase uterine contractility almost to the tetanic level and to produce hypertension and a high incidence of neonatal respiratory depression. A 40% increase in uterine tone has been reported with 2 mg/kg ketamine. Consequently, large doses of this drug should not be given to obstetric patients.

Scopolamine

A belladonna derivative, scopolamine is an amnesic drug that produces mild sedation and has a tranquilizing effect. Like atropine, it decreases salivary secretions and gastric motility. Scopolamine does not produce analgesia, and large doses may cause hallucinations, delirium, agitation, and excitement. The drug is rapidly transferred to the fetus; tachycardia and loss of beat-to-beat variability of the fetal heart rate have been reported. Scopolamine was widely used in obstetrics for over 70 years; it is no longer popular, as many more effective sedatives and tranquilizers are now available. In small doses (0.4 mg), however, it is still commonly used as a premedicant agent before cesar-

ean section when the amnesic effect may be useful during light planes of general anesthesia before delivery.

NEUROLEPTANALGESIA

A drug-induced psychic and analgesic state has been termed *neuroleptanalgesia*. This method is not popular in the United States because it has profound depressant effects on the neonate. Innovar is the most commonly used drug in this group; it is a mixture of droperidol (Inapsine) 2.5 mg/ml and fentanyl 0.05 mg/ml. Droperidol, an adrenergic blocking agent, is a long-acting and potent tranquilizer with little or no effect on heart rate, cardiac output, or respiration, although it may cause peripheral vasodilatation and hypotension in the mother and prolonged depression of the newborn.

ANTAGONISTS TO SYSTEMIC ANALGESICS

Narcotic antagonists can reverse narcotic-induced respiratory depression. Nalorphine (Nalline) and levallorphan (Lorfan) are among the narcotic antagonists, but they also possess agonistic depressant actions like those of narcotics. If administered in the presence of respiratory depression from other causes, these drugs aggravate the depression. They have serious side effects and do not reduce the incidence of neonatal depression. They should not be used in obstetrics because a better and more specific antagonist, naloxone (Narcan), is now available.

Naloxone

Naloxone is by far the best narcotic antagonist and does not have agonistic action. It crosses the placenta, but has negligible effect on the neonate even when large doses are employed. The drug is administered either to the mother or to the newborn at birth, but it is more rational to administer the drug, if it is needed, to the neonate immediately following delivery than to the mother just before delivery. Reversal of maternal narcotic analgesia just before delivery (when analgesia is needed most) may result in uncontrollably difficult delivery. If the neonatal depression is narcotic-induced, injection of naloxone intravenously into the umbilical vein reverses the condition within 30–90 sec. The dose for the neonate is 10–20 µg/kg. Naloxone should be administered to the parturient if an overdose of narcotic has been given. In the adult, the recommended initial amount is 0.2–0.4 mg intravenously. Duration of the antagonistic action is relatively short—1–2 hours. It may be necessary, therefore, to give repeated injections to an overdosed neonate or mother. The routine

administration of this drug to all newborns who received narcotics transplacentally during labor is not recommended unless there is evidence of narcotism. Naloxone displaces narcotics from the opiate receptor sites in the central nervous system and blocks the normal physiologic effects of endogenous opioid substances (enkephalins and endorphins), which may dampen the stress response in newborns.

Physostigmine (Antilirium)

This agent inhibits the action of cholinesterase and thereby prolongs and potentiates the effect of neurotransmitter acetylcholine in the central nervous system. It reverses central nervous system effects, including hallucinations, delirium, disorientation, and hyperactivity caused by scopolamine and other drugs with anticholinergic activity. This drug has been used safely and effectively to reverse delirium produced by scopolamine, and it has been reported that physostigmine reverses the decreased beat-to-beat cardiac variability in the fetus caused by atropine and scopolamine. No untoward effect on neonatal outcome has been reported. Physostigmine has been claimed to reverse the sedation of diazepam, ketamine, and Innovar, but this is still debated; it is certainly not a specific pharmacologic antagonist to these drugs. The usual dose is 0.5–2 mg intravenously or intramuscularly. Intravenous administration should be slow as rapid injection may cause bradycardia and hypersalivation.

REGIONAL ANESTHESIA FOR LABOR AND VAGINAL DELIVERY

Regional methods are used more commonly than any others for pain relief during labor and delivery. These techniques relieve pain, yet the maternal upper airway reflexes remain intact, minimizing the possibility of aspiration of gastric contents. They permit the mother to remain awake, alert, and pain-free during the delivery of her child but make it possible for her to cooperate in the delivery. The preferred regional methods in obstetrics are paracervical, pudendal, spinal, caudal and lumbar epidural blocks, and infiltration of the perineum.

Labor pain is conveyed from the uterus by nerve pathways that exit from the cervix, pass along diverse routes through the pelvis, join the sympathetic chain at L2-L5, and enter the spinal cord at T10-T12 and L1 (see Chapter 3). These pathways may be interrupted at the cervix with bilateral paracervical block or by lumbar epidural block of T10-L1. Vaginal and perineal pain is mediated through the pudendal nerve, which originates from S3-S4. Pudendal block, subarachnoid block S2-S5 (saddle block), and low epidural S1-S5

(caudal block) relieve most of vaginal and perineal pain. Regional anesthesia, however, as do all anesthetic techniques, has distinct advantages and limitations. Complications must be anticipated, and an intravenous line should be placed before the block is initiated. The following must be immediately available: blood pressure monitoring apparatus, oxygen, mask, oral and nasal airways, laryngoscope, endotracheal tubes, diazepam or thiopental to treat possible convulsions, and ephedrine to treat hypotension. When complications are promptly recognized and dealt with, serious problems can usually be avoided.

METHODS OF REGIONAL ANESTHESIA

Paracervical Block

This is one of the most widely used regional techniques for pain relief during the first stage of labor because it is simple, easy to administer, and usually effective. A paracervical block is usually performed by the obstetrician when the cervix is 4–6 cm dilated in multiparous patients and 5–6 cm dilated in primiparous patients. The block is produced by infiltration of local anesthetic into the parametrium at the three o'clock and nine o'clock or 4 and 8 o'clock sites lateral to the cervix (Fig. 32–1). After careful aspiration for blood, 5 ml of a local anesthetic solution is injected. The same amount of drug is injected on the other side if no fetal bradycardia occurs within 5 min of the first injection. The duration of analgesia varies: 40–50 min with 1.5% procaine or chloroprocaine, 60–90 min with 1% lidocaine, prilocaine, or mepivacaine; and 90–150 min with 0.25% bupivacaine or etidocaine.

Following the injections, the fetal heart rate and maternal blood pressure and heart rate must be monitored closely for the next 10 min. Fetal bradycardia after maternal paracervical block is the most common and serious complication; the incidence of post–paracervical block fetal bradycardia may be as high as 50%. This usually occurs within 2–10 min and lasts 5–30 min. When fetal bradycardia occurs, it may be associated with acidosis. Some fetal deaths have been reported. When paracervical block is given to a patient whose fetus is already compromised, the incidence of bradycardia is high, its severity is compounded, and it lasts far longer. The etiology of these untoward fetal effects has not been well explained. A direct toxic effect of the local anesthetic on the fetal myocardium was once a commonly accepted explanation, but more recent evidence suggests that this type of anesthetic-induced fetal bradycardia is related to decreased oxygenation secondary to a reduction of uteroplacental perfusion caused by uterine vasoconstriction. Although the precise mechanism remains controversial, paracervical block should not be used if the uteroplacental circulation is already impaired or if the fetus is already at risk.

Pudendal Block

Bilateral blockade of the pudendal nerve is administered for pain relief during the second stage of labor and for delivery. This technique produces adequate perineal analgesia for episiotomy and repair, and for outlet forceps delivery. Supplemented with inhalation analgesia, bilateral pudendal block may be sufficient for low forceps delivery or midforceps rotation. The advantages of this technique are that it is simple to use, and adverse effects on mother and fetus are minimal. It does not affect the autonomic innervation of the uterus and does not cause maternal hypotension. This block is usually administered by the obstetrician at the beginning of the second stage of labor in the primipara and at 6–8 cm cervical dilatation in the multipara. The transvaginal approach is superior to the older transperineal technique because palpation of anatomic landmarks is easier (Fig. 32–2). All local anesthetic agents are suitable (e.g., 2% chloroprocaine or procaine, 1% lidocaine, prilocaine or mepivacaine, or 0.25% bupivacaine or etidocaine) and are injected in a volume of 10 ml on each side after careful aspiration for blood. This technique has a higher percentage of technical failure than other regional methods, and larger amounts of local anesthetic are required. However, the total recommended dose should not be exceeded.

Subarachnoid (Spinal) Block

The onset of complete analgesia after subarachnoid or spinal block is rapid; and, since only small amounts of local anesthetic are used, drug toxicity is not a problem if the block is properly administered. Even though it is easily given, the subarachnoid block is not widely used for vaginal delivery because the urge to bear down is abolished and the mother cannot cooperate. Maternal hypotension and postspinal headache are possible complications. The use of a fine needle (25 or 26 gauge) usually lowers the incidence of spinal headache. Hyperbaric local anesthetic is injected into the subarachnoid space. A small dose of drug (for example, tetracaine 3 mg or lidocaine 25 mg) is injected with the patient in the sitting position to provide S1-S5 saddle block. A larger dose (tetracaine 5 mg or lidocaine 30–35 mg) is necessary for a T10-S5 saddle block that eliminates both uterine and perineal pain. "Total spinal" anesthesia is a rare complication.

Caudal Block

Caudal blockade is another form of extradural analgesia. It may be used either as a single injection or as a continuous technique (Fig. 32–3). The single injec-

FIG. 32-1. Technique of paracervical block. Notice the position of the hand and fingers in relation to the cervix and fetal head—that no undue pressure is applied at the vaginal fornix by the fingers or the needle guide—and the shallow depth of the needle insertion. (Abouleish E: Pain control in Obstetrics, p 344. Philadelphia, JB Lippincott, 1977)

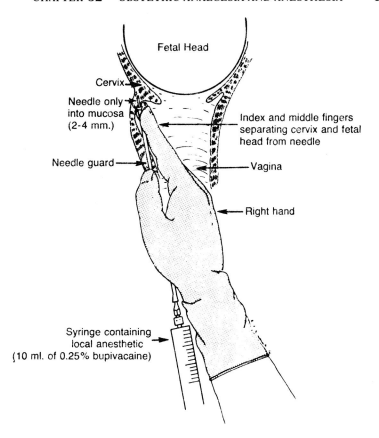

FIG. 32-2. Pudendal block, trans-vaginal approach. *Inset.* Enlargement of injection site. Note that pudendal nerve passes just posterior to junction of ischial spine and sacrospinous ligament. Needle is through sacrospinous ligament, which is used as important landmark. (From Bonica JJ: Principles and Practice of Obstetric Analgesia and Anesthesia. Philadelphia, Davis, 1967)

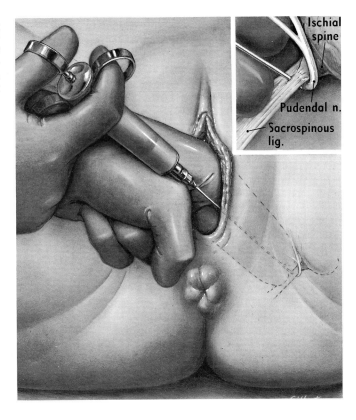

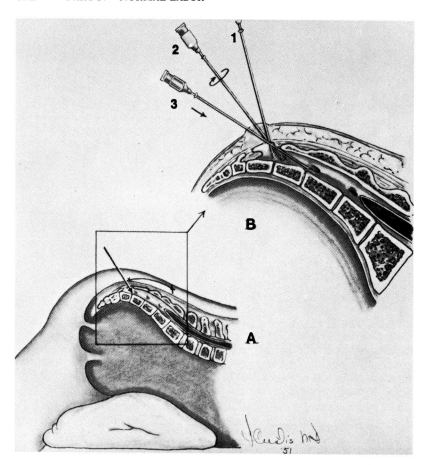

FIG. 32–3. Method of inserting caudal needle into caudal canal. In obstetric patients, either prone position with 10-in roll under pelvis or lateral decubitus position may be used. *A.* Areas of enlarged section. *B. 1:* Needle point with bevel up has pierced ligament covering opening of caudal canal. *2:* Needle lowered to approximate 50° angle with skin and advanced into caudal canal. Bevel is now rotated so it points downward. This facilitates its passage over periosteum of sacral canal. *3:* Needle is now lowered approximately 30° to 45° angle and advanced into caudal canal. (From Moore DC: Regional Block, 4th ed. Charles C Thomas, Springfield IL, 1967)

tion provides analgesia for 1–3 hours and may be repeated if needed. With the continuous technique, a plastic, pliable catheter is threaded through a needle placed in the caudal canal and remains in place after the needle is withdrawn. The anesthetic agent is injected from time to time as required. Caudal block requires more local anesthetic than lumbar epidural block and is more difficult to perform; in addition, needle placement is more painful to the patient. To provide a T10 block, a total volume of 15–25 ml 1% lidocaine, prilocaine or mepivacaine, or 0.25% of bupivacaine is required. Appropriate interval repeated doses of 15 ml maintain analgesia throughout labor and delivery.

If the needle punctures the dura, as evidenced by a flow of spinal fluid, the block must be abandoned immediately, since injection of the anesthetic solution may produce profound or even fatal spinal anesthesia. A rare but disastrous complication is puncture of the fetal head and injection of the anesthetic agent into the fetus instead of into the caudal canal. After the needle is placed in the caudal canal, and before the an-

esthetic is injected, a rectal examination must be performed to exclude the possibility of inadvertent fetal puncture.

Lumbar Epidural Block

One of the most popular methods of pain relief for the obstetric patient throughout the world in the past two decades has been lumbar epidural block. It may be used either as a single injection or as a continuous technique (Fig. 32–4). The needle is usually inserted at the level of the L2-3 or L3-4 interspace. If the pain fibers at the level of T10-L1 are blocked, the pain of first-stage uterine contractions is abolished. Larger doses of anesthetic can extend the block to the level of S5 and provide perineal analgesia; this abolishes the bearing-down reflex, although voluntary bearing down may continue effectively.

Lumbar epidural anesthesia has several advantages over caudal block. A smaller dose of anesthetic is required to produce pain relief during the first stage of labor. Lumbar epidurals are technically easier than

FIG. 32-4. Sagittal section demonstrating that needle's point rests in epidural space and fluid in syringe is released in jetlike stream pushing contents of epidural space and dura away from point of needle. (From Moore DC: Regional Block, 4th ed. Charles C Thomas, Springfield, IL, 1967)

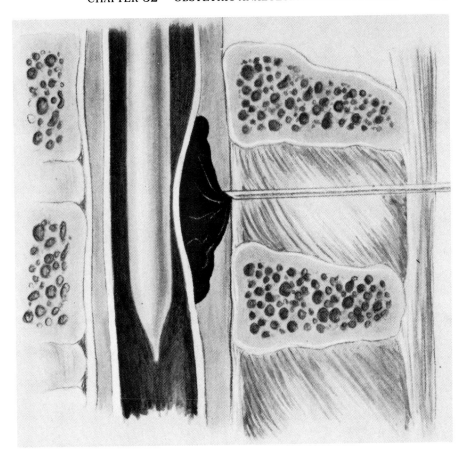

caudal blocks and have a higher success rate; they maintain the bearing-down reflex if it should be needed and, in most instances, may be extended to a level adequate for cesarean section. This block carries the least risk of direct injection of the fetus. Its disadvantages include maternal hypotension, a high incidence of accidental dural puncture with subsequent post–lumbar puncture headache, and the possibility of either subdural or intravascular injection of local anesthetic.

Single Injection Technique. When the cervix is fully dilated and the fetal head is in an acceptable position for delivery, a needle is placed in the epidural space (puncture at L3 or L4). Then, 12–14 ml of an anesthetic solution (2% chloroprocaine, 1.5% lidocaine or mepivacaine) is given in a single injection. If a longer duration of analgesia is needed, 0.25% or 0.5% bupivacaine or etidocaine may be substituted at a similar dose.

Continuous Epidural Block. Like systemic analgesia, a continuous epidural block permits uninterrupted pain relief throughout labor and delivery, but it avoids the risks of systemic analgesia. Epidural block is usually initiated during the first stage of labor when cervical dilatation reaches 4–5 cm in multiparas and 5–6 cm in primiparas. (For a detailed description of the procedure, the reader is referred to the references at the end of the chapter.) Choice of local anesthetic is based on a desire for rapid onset and long duration and, at the same time, safety for fetus and neonate. Two percent chloroprocaine hydrochloride or 1.5% lidocaine as the initial drug and, later, 0.25% bupivacaine or etidocaine produce excellent sensory analgesia with minimal motor blockade. The analgesia is achieved with 6–10 ml local anesthetic. Low concentrations should be used, whatever drug is chosen, to minimize motor block, yet maintain satisfactory analgesia. When delivery is imminent, the injection of 3% chloroprocaine produces analgesia with rapid onset and short duration. Close monitoring of maternal blood pressure and fetal heart rate is essential for at least 20 min after each injection to detect the early onset of hypotension with associated fetal bradycardia.

CONTRAINDICATIONS TO SPINAL, CAUDAL, AND LUMBAR EPIDURAL BLOCKS

The absolute contraindications to major regional blocks are patient reluctance to have spinal anesthesia, infection at the site of needle puncture, hypotension, hypovolemia resulting from hemorrhage, and coagulopathy. Relative contraindications include anatomic abnormalities of the vertebral column, preexisting neurologic disease, increased intracranial pressure, and severe fetal distress.

COMPLICATIONS OF REGIONAL ANESTHESIA AND THEIR MANAGEMENT

Hypotension

Maternal hypotension (a systolic blood pressure of 100 mm Hg or less, or a decrease of 20% below prior levels) is the most common complication of sympathetic blockade by spinal, caudal, or epidural anesthesia administered for vaginal delivery, and it is invariably associated with a proportional reduction in uterine blood flow. If maternal hypotension is not treated promptly, decreased uteroplacental perfusion may cause fetal bradycardia, asphyxia, and neonatal depression. Prevention of maternal hypotension, as well as treatment, consists of left uterine displacement, rapid intravenous infusion of a balanced salt solution—500–1000 ml before administration of the block, and injection of a vasopressor. If hypotension does occur, treatment is to place the patient in the left lateral position and to administer oxygen by loose-fitting face mask. If normal blood pressure is not restored immediately, vasopressors, such as ephedrine 10–25 mg, should be administered intravenously. The choice of vasopressor to correct maternal hypotension is somewhat limited because the agent must not cause a decrease in uteroplacental circulation by constricting the uterine vasculature. Drugs with predominantly central action (β-adrenergic), such as ephedrine or mephentermine, may be safely used. Except for fetal tachycardia, no adverse effect of ephedrine has been reported.

"Total Spinal" Anesthesia

Usually caused by an overdose of local anesthetic injected accidentally into the subarachnoid space during the performance of a block, total spinal anesthesia is the third most common anesthetic cause of maternal death; it ranks immediately behind aspiration of vomitus and cardiovascular collapse. Prompt recognition and treatment are important. Management includes endotracheal intubation; artificial ventilation; support of blood pressure with rapid infusion of fluids; intravenous ephedrine; the Trendelenburg position (or elevation of the legs); and left uterine displacement.

Headache

Post–spinal puncture headache is caused by leakage of cerebrospinal fluid through a hole made in the dura by needle puncture, either inadvertently in attempts at epidural anesthesia or deliberately as in subarachnoid block. For a mild headache, aspirin with codeine or a mild narcotic may relieve the symptoms. Also the patient should be maintained in a supine position and intravenous hydration provided. Injection of the patient's blood into the peridural space (a "blood patch") may produce prolonged relief by sealing the hole in the dura. A tight abdominal binder worn when the patient is upright is frequently of great help.

Systemic Toxic Reactions

Maternal systemic toxic reactions occur when critical concentrations of local anesthetics are exceeded in blood and tissues. High drug concentrations result from overdose, excessive systemic absorption, or inadvertent intravascular injection of local anesthetic agents. A toxic reaction may also occur when metabolism of the drug is abnormally slow. The clinical sequence includes ringing in the ears, metallic taste, headache, apprehension, excitement, dizziness, nausea, tremors, tachycardia, hypertension followed by convulsions, respiratory depression, profound hypotension, and cardiac arrest. Mild central nervous system toxicity may be treated with 100% oxygen by face mask. If severe toxic reactions or convulsions occur, the trachea must be intubated promptly and the patient ventilated artificially with oxygen. Succinylcholine may be necessary to produce paralysis. Small doses of diazepam (5 mg) or thiopental (50–75 mg) may be injected intravenously and repeated as needed. Measures to support the circulation should be established; for example, the patient's legs should be elevated, and intravenous fluids, vasopressors, and cardiac massage given as the need arises. As soon as possible, the fetal condition should be assessed. Even though maternal toxic manifestations are treated promptly and uterine blood flow is restored, recovery of the fetus may be much slower.

Accidental administration of local anesthetic to the fetus during attempts at caudal, pudendal, or paracervical block is rare, but has occurred. If the neonate is delivered intoxicated, cardiorespiratory support may be needed, together with anticonvulsive therapy. Promotion of urinary excretion of the drug appears to be more effective than gastric lavage.

INHALATION ANALGESIA AND ANESTHESIA FOR LABOR AND VAGINAL DELIVERY

Analgesia produced by subanesthetic concentrations of inhalation agents relieves pain in the first and second stages of labor. The patient remains awake, is able to cooperate, and retains her laryngeal reflexes. The analgesia does not interfere with respiration, uterine contractions, or the progress of labor. The anesthetic is usually administered with a mask, either by an anesthetist or the patient herself. The use of self-administered inhalation analgesia has never been popular in the United States, although it is widely employed elsewhere.

General anesthesia that produces unconsciousness is rarely necessary for vaginal delivery unless there are specific indications. The method is used mainly when delivery is to be by cesarean section or vacuum extraction, when a difficult forceps delivery is anticipated, or when uterine relaxation is required. It is often necessary for the mother to bear down with her contractions to propel the fetus down the birth canal in the second stage of labor, and this is obviously impossible if the mother is unconscious. Therefore, general anesthesia for vaginal delivery should not be administered until the very end of the second stage of labor. Anesthetic concentrations produce fetal and neonatal depression directly related to the depth and duration of maternal anesthesia. All parturients must be treated as if they had full stomachs. General anesthesia, or inadvertent overdose of anesthetic intended for inhalation analgesia, subjects parturients to the loss of protective laryngeal reflexes and the risk of aspiration of gastric content. Vomiting or regurgitation, airway obstruction, or asphyxia may then occur, bringing about a catastrophic situation.

It has been commonly accepted that the risk of severe aspiration pneumonitis can be lessened by routine administration of oral antacids before induction of general anesthesia. Since recent studies have shown that emulsion type antacids contain particulate matter that may produce lung damage if aspirated, a clear type antacid such as 15 ml 0.3 M sodium citrate in 20% syrup might be a better choice to raise the pH of the stomach contents. However, the efficacy of this solution remains to be ascertained in clinical practice. Because the risk of aspiration can never be completely avoided, general anesthesia is not recommended in obstetrics unless the patient's trachea is intubated immediately after consciousness is lost.

All inhalation anesthetics readily traverse the placenta and achieve equilibrium between mother and fetus. The transfer occurs rapidly because of the high rates of diffusion, lipid solubility, and low molecular weight of the anesthetics. Inhalation anesthetics are also poorly ionized and may be found in the fetus even when only analgesic concentrations are given to the mother. The concentrations for analgesia, however, do not produce any significant fetal or neonatal depression, regardless of how long they have been administered.

Several inhalation anesthetics used in obstetrics produce dose-related depression of uterine activity when given in concentrations sufficient to produce general anesthesia. Halothane (Fluothane), enflurane, methoxyflurane (Penthrane), isoflurane, ether, and chloroform cause profound myometrial relaxation. Cyclopropane and nitrous oxide are the only commonly used inhalation agents that do not significantly relax uterine muscle.

NITROUS OXIDE

For analgesia, nitrous oxide is administered in oxygen either by continuous or intermittent inhalation in various concentrations below 50%. To achieve analgesia with an intermittent method during labor, the patient must inhale 50% nitrous oxide for at least 50 sec before the onset of each contraction. Continuous administration of nitrous oxide at concentrations of 30%–40% in oxygen is more effective, and this method may be employed late in labor and continued throughout delivery of the baby and placenta. The continuous technique is especially useful in the second stage of labor when the patient must bear down to advance the presenting part to a level from which delivery may be easily and safely managed. With proper instruction and encouragement, bearing-down efforts may be far more intense and effective when the patient is given nitrous oxide analgesia than when she is given no analgesia. Continuous analgesia is also useful in the patient whose prior medication is wearing off and who needs analgesia for the 15–20 min that remain before another form of anesthesia may be administered for delivery. Continuous nitrous oxide–oxygen inhalation tides her over this short but sometimes difficult period.

METHOXYFLURANE

Analgesia by methoxyflurane in a concentration of 0.2%–0.6% has been widely used in obstetrics. It provides more satisfactory anesthesia than trichloroethylene (Trilene), popular in the past. It is best used intermittently. An effective analgesic concentration, once reached, remains relatively constant with this method. When methoxyflurane is combined with nitrous oxide, lower concentrations are required than when either of the two agents is administered alone, and the analgesia provided may be more satisfactory. No evidence of increased risk of fetal depression has

been reported for this method. High concentrations of methoxyflurane and nitrous oxide, if used for prolonged periods, may increase neonatal depression and produce high blood concentrations of inorganic fluoride ion in both mother and neonate, but they rarely affect renal function.

TRICHLOROETHYLENE

Although no longer used in the United States, trichloroethylene is used widely in Great Britain and other countries for obstetric analgesia. It is a volatile anesthetic that the patient may administer to herself during contractions. Trichloroethylene in analgesic concentrations gives effective pain relief in the first and second stages of labor. It has no toxic effects for either mother or baby, provided it is administered intermittently in analgesic concentrations by means of a nonrebreathing system in which there is no carbon dioxide absorber that can cause it to break down to the highly toxic substance, phosgene. Significant blood concentrations of trichloroethylene may linger for at least 20 min after inhalation is discontinued and, in some cases, may last as long as 2 hours.

HALOTHANE

Because of its poor analgesic characteristics, halothane is not recommended for obstetric analgesia. Halothane is a very potent agent that can cause maternal hypotension and marked relaxation of the myometrium; the latter effect predisposes to postpartum hemorrhage. Furthermore, it readily transfers to the fetus across the placenta and, in anesthetic concentration, may cause neonatal depression. It may be used to produce rapid uterine relaxation when required to facilitate intrauterine manipulations (*e.g.*, in multiple gestation, breech delivery, or the removal of a retained placenta).

ENFLURANE

Used with a continuous technique for vaginal delivery, enflurane in analgesic concentrations of 0.5%–1.25% has been shown to have no adverse effects on mother or newborn and to cause no significant myometrial depression. Like halothane, in anesthetic concentration, it causes marked uterine relaxation and may be used to facilitate intrauterine manipulation.

ISOFLUORANE

The effectiveness of isofluorane is comparable to that achieved by 40%–50% nitrous oxide in oxygen. Un-

less a high concentration of oxygen is indicated, isofluorane has very little advantage over the nitrous oxide technique. This agent also depresses myometrial activity.

OTHER AGENTS USED FOR ANALGESIA OR ANESTHESIA

Until recently, cyclopropane and chloroform were widely used in obstetrics to provide inhalation analgesia because high oxygen concentrations may be given and the speed of induction is rapid. Today, they are rarely used because cyclopropane is highly flammable and chloroform has been replaced with other safer halogenated hydrocarbons that have minimal hepatic and cardiovascular toxicity.

ANESTHESIA FOR CESAREAN SECTION

Today's increasing incidence of cesarean section (approaching 20% or more of deliveries) is in part related to the decrease in maternal risks and the benefits to the fetus when obstetric complications occur. This has been further encouraged by advances in perinatal management, greater knowledge of the pharmacology of anesthetic agents, and improved anesthetic management. Anesthesia for cesarean section most often consists of major conduction analgesia in the form of either epidural or subarachnoid block, or a light general anesthesia. The obstetrician should be well acquainted with anesthetic techniques for operative delivery and should have a basic knowledge of the effects of anesthesia on the mother and fetus.

ELECTIVE CESAREAN SECTION

Anesthesia for elective cesarean section may be either regional or general. Earlier comparisons of these techniques indicated that infants whose mothers had been given regional anesthesia, *e.g.*, lumbar epidural block or spinal anesthesia, were in better condition than those whose mothers had been given general anesthesia with potent agents such as cyclopropane. With recent advanced techniques of light, balanced general anesthesia, however, only minimal transient neurobehavioral depression is seen in newborns delivered by elective cesarean section under general anesthesia as compared with those delivered with spinal or epidural block. Improved neonatal outcome with general anesthesia is related to several factors, including prevention of maternal hypotension by left uterine displacement or uterine tilt, better maternal and fetal oxygenation because of administration of oxygen concentrations in excess of 50%, replacement of potent inhalation anesthetics like cyclopropane with analge-

sic concentrations of nitrous oxide (40%–50%), and shortening both the induction to delivery and uterine incision to delivery times.

Both regional and general anesthesia have advantages and disadvantages. When there are no contraindications, the selection of anesthesia must be based on the circumstances of each individual patient. If the patient is knowledgeable and cooperative and prefers to be awake, regional block may be used with minimal discomfort if a sensory interruption is provided to T4-T8; however, apprehensive, extremely emotional, or unstable patients may not be able to distinguish pressure and pulling sensations from surgical pain, and may become uncooperative. Language difficulties may also pose problems. Such patients may require general anesthesia.

Preanesthetic evaluation includes a discussion of anesthetic techniques with the patient. If the operation is scheduled in advance, she should be instructed to take only liquids after dinner and nothing by mouth after midnight. An antacid is given orally approximately 60 min prior to the induction of anesthesia. Since most commonly used antacids contain particulate matter that can cause lung damage if aspirated, a clear antacid (*e.g.,* 15 ml 0.3M sodium citrate in 20% syrup) is recommended. The patient may be sedated with drugs that have minimal effect on the fetus, such as meperidine 50 mg, Atropine 0.5 mg, or scopolamine 0.4 mg, particularly when general anesthesia is planned. Scopolamine is particularly useful to reduce awareness during light anesthesia.

Regional Anesthesia

Patients who undergo elective cesarean section are usually well prepared and in good condition, and either subarachnoid or lumbar epidural block may be employed effectively. Caudal anesthesia for cesarean section has no advantages over lumbar epidural block and does not reliably produce an adequate sensory block unless excessive doses of local anesthetics are used. Spinal anesthesia is frequently employed because it is a relatively simple technique and is rapidly effective. This technique has a low failure rate and produces intense sensory and motor inhibition. Only a small amount of local anesthetic is needed. Also, early maternal–infant contact is facilitated. The major disadvantage of spinal anesthesia, compared with epidural anesthesia, is the higher incidence of profound maternal hypotension. When spinal hypotension occurs, it rapidly follows the block and is often associated with maternal nausea and vomiting, as well as fetal distress. If not effectively and promptly treated, this hypotension predisposes the mother to cardiovascular collapse and pulmonary aspiration.

The techniques of spinal and epidural anesthesia have been described earlier in connection with blocks for vaginal delivery. Briefly, preparation consists of prehydration with rapid intravenous infusion of 1000 ml balanced salt solution, maternal and fetal monitoring, positioning the patient (the right lateral decubitis is most commonly used), and injecting 50 mg ephedrine intramuscularly 10–15 min before regional anesthesia is administered. (Prophylactic use of vasopressors should be avoided in patients with preexisting hypertension.) The spinal block is administered with a mixture of 1% tetracaine (6–10 mg) diluted with an equal volume of 10% dextrose, or 50–80 mg lidocaine (5%) in 10% dextrose. The lumbar epidural block method requires a 5-ml test dose followed by a full dose of local anesthetic (for example, 3% chloroprocaine, or 0.5%–0.75% bupivacaine). Left uterine displacement is maintained, and oxygen is given by face mask until the baby is delivered. Maternal blood pressure and heart rate are recorded every 1–2 min for the first 10 min, and then at least every 5 min thereafter. The level of block is tested bilaterally every minute until it is well established. Hypotension should be treated with rapid intravenous infusion of fluids, additional left uterine displacement, and administration of oxygen by face mask. If the blood pressure does not respond within a minute, ephedrine 10–25 mg should be injected intravenously. Maternal hypotension, if recognized and treated promptly, has minimal adverse effects on the neonate. If the block is not sufficiently effective, nitrous oxide analgesia may be needed until delivery, at which time the mother may receive narcotics. Should general anesthesia be required, surgery is stopped and it is induced as previously described with the placement of a cuffed endotracheal tube.

General Anesthesia

If properly administered, general anesthesia is a highly effective and safe technique for cesarean section. Advantages include rapid induction, reliable analgesia, less incidence of hypotension, and less psychologic stress. It is especially indicated in the patient with hypotension and hypovolemia due to hemorrhage since sympathetic blockade is especially dangerous in such patients. The suggested preparatory techniques are 1) approximately an hour prior to the induction of anesthesia, 15 ml clear oral antacid is given; 2) blood pressure, heart rate and electrocardiogram (EKG) are monitored; 3) an intravenous fluid infusion is started; 4) left uterine displacement is established and maintained; and 5) preoxygenation is administered with a well-fitted face mask providing 100% oxygen at high flow for 2–3 min. Preoxygenation not only increases maternal arterial oxygenation but also prevents maternal hypoxemia during endotracheal intubation. The abdominal preparation and draping are completed before the induction of anesthesia is started.

Procedure. Administration of a small dose of intravenous *d*-tubocurarine, 3 mg, about 3 min prior to in-

duction of anesthesia may prevent muscular fasciculation and reduce the increase in intragastric pressure. Intravenous induction is accomplished with either thiopental (3–4 mg/kg) or ketamine (1 mg/kg), and rapid relaxation is provided with succinylcholine (1–1.5 mg/kg). Cricoid pressure should be applied as soon as consciousness is lost and paralysis has occurred in order to facilitate rapid endotracheal intubation and to prevent regurgitation, after which the cuff is inflated. The tube is connected to the anesthetic machine, and pulmonary ventilation is begun with a mixture of nitrous oxide at 50% concentration in 50% oxygen at high flows, or nitrous oxide in a concentration of 30% in 70% oxygen plus a low concentration of a potent inhalation anesthetic agent. At this point, cricoid pressure may be released, and the surgeon may begin the abdominal incision.

Anesthesia is maintained with nitrous oxide and oxygen. A low concentration of halothane (0.5%) may be added to decrease maternal awareness. A low concentration of an inhalation anesthetic (methoxyflurane 0.5% or enflurane, up to 1%) may also be used. Succinylcholine drip is used to provide surgical relaxation up to the time of birth. Some anesthesiologists prefer to use *d*-tubocurarine or pancuronium instead of succinylcholine in a dose not exceeding 0.3 mg/kg or 0.05 mg/kg, respectively. Moderate pulmonary hyperventilation is maintained. Repeated intravenous doses of depressant agents such as thiopental or narcotics should be avoided before delivery. As soon as the umbilical cord has been clamped, anesthesia may be deepened by increasing concentrations of nitrous oxide to 60%–70% in oxygen (or adding volatile anesthetics in low concentrations) and administering small doses of thiopental, tranquilizer, or narcotics.

Toward the end of the operation, succinylcholine is discontinued or paralysis from other muscle relaxants is reversed. The patient is then given 100% oxygen. The endotracheal tube is removed when spontaneous respiration is adequate and upper airway reflexes have returned. If at all possible, the patient should become fully conscious at the time of extubation. These precautions minimize the risks of airway obstruction, laryngospasm, and pulmonary aspiration.

Complications. Major complications of general endotracheal anesthesia are 1) aspiration before endotracheal intubation and after extubation; 2) hypoxemia, hypercapnia, and hypocapnia; 3) hypotension, and 4) maternal awareness.

Pulmonary Aspiration of Gastric Contents. This is the major complication of general anesthesia in obstetrics. The majority of pulmonary aspirations occur either during induction of or recovery from anesthesia. Aspiration of vomitus or silent regurgitation of gastric contents may cause either pneumonitis from a pH of less than 2.5 or airway obstruction and suffocation due to

aspiration of particulate matter. If aspiration occurs, skillful respiratory therapy with positive and expired pressure is required, including use of a cuffed endotracheal tube for intubation and positive pressure ventilation with oxygen. Bronchodilators may be useful. The efficacy of steroids in acid aspiration is debatable. Routine administration of oral antacid before induction of anesthesia can be expected to reduce the incidence of this life-threatening complication.

Hypoxemia, Hypercapnia, and Hypocapnia. Maternal hypoxemia and hypercapnia must be avoided during general anesthesia. Such conditions may occur because of hypoventilation or airway obstruction, or because of a difficult endotracheal intubation. Should hypoxemia and hypercapnia occur, they have an immediate effect on the fetus: oxygenation is decreased and carbon dioxide is increased, resulting in combined fetal respiratory and metabolic acidosis and hypoxemia. Severe maternal hypocapnia due to marked mechanical hyperventilation may reduce uterine blood flow, which may also result in fetal hypoxemia and acidosis. Therefore, vigorous hyperventilation should be avoided.

Hypotension. Maternal hypotension immediately decreases the oxygen supply to the fetus because it reduces the uteroplacental circulation. Hypotension may be avoided or minimized by left uterine displacement to prevent aortocaval compression and rapid intravenous fluid administration. If the cause of hypotension is a deep plane of anesthesia, the plane should be lightened.

Awareness. The patient may remain aware if the plane of anesthesia is excessively light. This occurs most commonly if the nitrous oxide concentration is reduced shortly before delivery. It has been reported that paralyzed patients have experienced pain or had unpleasant memories. An extremely light plane of anesthesia increases arterial pressure by allowing sympathetic response to occur, thus releasing catecholamines. This may bring about uterine vasoconstriction and lead to a reduction in uteroplacental perfusion. The use of low concentrations of potent inhalation agents or small doses of amnesic agents such as diazepam after delivery helps to minimize awareness.

EMERGENCY CESAREAN SECTION

The choice of anesthesia for an emergency operative delivery depends on the maternal and fetal condition. A true emergency occurs when there is acute maternal hemorrhage or severe fetal distress; under these circumstances, general anesthesia, rapidly induced, is the procedure of choice. As the surgeon is preparing the abdomen, the anesthesiologist can prepare for in-

duction of anesthesia, thus minimizing delay. Regional anesthesia is not recommended for emergency cesarean section unless it was established before the emergency arose, *e.g.,* as a continuous lumbar epidural block.

Shortly before the surgeon makes the abdominal incision and during preoxygenation, the patient is given atropine 0.4 mg intravenously. Thiopental 3–4 mg/kg or ketamine 0.5–1 mg/kg intravenously is used for induction, followed by intravenous administration of succinylcholine in a minimum dose (100 mg). Cricoid pressure is applied, and the trachea is intubated. Then an analgesic concentration of nitrous oxide (50%) in oxygen, sometimes supplemented with a volatile agent (0.3%–0.5% halothane or 0.5%–0.8% enflurane) or thiopental 3–4 mg/kg, is administered. Muscle relaxation is provided with 0.1% succinylcholine drip.

After delivery, anesthesia is maintained with 60%–70% nitrous oxide in oxygen, supplemented with a small dose of diazepam, ketamine, or a short-acting narcotic.

In patients who have cephalopelvic disproportion or dysfunctional labor, when cesarean section is less urgent, continuous lumbar epidural block may be preferred to general anesthesia. In instances of severe respiratory disease or upper airway compromise, regional anesthesia may also be indicated in the interest of maternal safety.

REFERENCES AND RECOMMENDED READING

Abouleish E (ed): Pain Control in Obstetrics. Philadelphia, JB Lippincott, 1977

Albright GA: Anesthesia in Obstetrics: Maternal, Fetal and Neonatal Aspects. Menlo Park, CA, Addison–Wesley, 1978

Bonica JJ: Principles and Practice in Obstetric Analgesia and Anesthesia: Fundamental Considerations. Philadelphia, FA Davis, 1967

Crawford JS: Principles and Practice of Obstetric Anesthesia, 3rd ed. Philadelphia, FA Davis, 1972

Datta S, Alper MH: Anesthesia for cesarean section. Anesthesiology 53:142, 1980

Gutsche BB: Analgesia and anesthesia for childbirth. In Reeder SJ, Mastroianni L, Jr, Martin LL (eds): Maternity Nursing, 14th ed, pp 385–403. Philadelphia, JB Lippincott, 1980

Heardman H, Ebner M: Relaxation and Exercise for Natural Childbirth, 4th ed. New York, Churchill Livingstone, 1975

Marx GF, Bassell GM (eds): Obstetric Analgesia and Anesthesia. Amsterdam, Elsevier/North–Holland, 1980

Marx GF, Orkin LR (eds): Physiology of Obstetric Anesthesia. Springfield, IL, Charles C Thomas, 1969

Moir DD: Pain Relief in Labour. Edinburgh, Churchill Livingstone, 1971

Shnider SM, Levinson G (eds): Anesthesia for Obstetrics. Baltimore, Williams & Wilkins, 1979

PART V

ABNORMAL LABOR AND THE PUERPERIUM

33

PRETERM LABOR AND THE LOW-BIRTH-WEIGHT INFANT

Ralph C. Benson

Preterm labor is defined as labor that occurs between the end of the 20th week and the end of the 37th week of pregnancy. Infants weighing less than 2500 g at birth are classified as low-birth-weight infants. The terms *premature labor* (labor before the end of the 37th week that produces a baby weighing less than 2500 g) and *premature infant* (a baby weighing less than 2500 g and delivering before 37 weeks) have been discarded, since the infant's weight and maturity do not necessarily bear a relationship to one another or to the duration of pregnancy.

Preterm labor is the most common complication of the third trimester of pregnancy, and the delivery of an undergrown, not fully mature neonate is a clinical crisis that is invariably a threat to the life or health of the newborn and often of the mother as well. Therefore, preterm labor and delivery constitute a high-risk experience for mother and offspring. Unfortunately, abnor-

mally early labor and delivery occur in 5%–15% of all pregnancies in developed countries and are considerably more common in the developing nations and among socioeconomically deprived populations.

Babson and Benson have stated that the undersized neonate, delivered too early, poses some of the most urgent problems of modern medicine. Most of the deaths among newborn infants are associated with low birth weight, which accounts for the annual loss of more than 60,000 infants in the United States, or nearly two-thirds of all deaths during the neonatal period. The death rate of the low-weight neonate is 40 times that of the full-sized infant born at term.

The outstanding causes of morbidity and death of preterm infants are respiratory distress syndrome, hyaline membrane disease, and intracranial intraventricular hemorrhage. Also, low birth weight, especially if disproportionate to gestational age, is one of the most important risk factors for cerebral palsy. The incidence of cerebral palsy associated with low birth weight may be as high as ten times, mental deficiencies five times and lethal malformations seven times that of the full-sized infant. Emotional disturbances, social maladjustments, and visual and hearing defects are also multiplied. As if these were not enough, medical and custodial costs for these individuals are incalculable.

Pregnancy problems known to predispose to preterm labor should alert the physician to the high-risk status of mother and infant. With few exceptions, such patients should be cared for and delivered in a maternity hospital unit with consultative and support facilities capable of supplying optimal care for mother and offspring. It is reprehensible, for example, to permit a woman known to have a multiple pregnancy to deliver in a minimally equipped hospital when she could have been transferred, even in labor, to a center equipped to handle such a high-risk situation. The referral of twins or triplets to a level III infant care unit after delivery is fraught with danger. The fact that some preterm babies survive such an untimely and hazardous experience is no justification for lack of proper planning and continuity of care. The same admonitions apply to the delivery at term of a baby known in advance to be of low birth weight.

The *sex ratio* of newborn infants shows a preponderance of males at all stages of antenatal development. The male/female ratio varies from an estimated 170:100 very early in pregnancy to 106:100 at term. However, male fetuses are significantly heavier than female fetuses of equivalent age. Accordingly, among preterm infants born at the same stage of gestation, females weighing less than 2500 g outnumber males of the same weight by a ratio of approximately 110:100. Also, the prognosis for survival of undergrown infants of the same weight favors the female because of their greater chronologic age and maturity.

PRETERM LABOR

CAUSES

Preterm labor occurs in a variety of circumstances; maternal, placental, or fetal factors may be responsible. However, any of these may be purely coincidental, and mere association does not establish an etiologic role.

The multiple factors concerned in the onset of labor at term are outlined in Chapter 29. When a single factor or complication is found to precipitate labor prematurely in a significant number of cases, it must be presumed that it acts by disrupting the balance between the factors that suppress labor and those that stimulate it. In 20%–30% of the cases of preterm labor, the precipitating factor is premature rupture of the membranes. In about two-thirds of the cases, the exact cause of preterm labor can never be determined.

Factors that are known to correlate with the incidence of preterm labor include maternal age (the very young and older women are predisposed); social class (the incidence is higher in the socioeconomically deprived); weight (the malnourished are more often affected); height (women of short stature are prone); prior preterm labors; prior induced abortions; work habits (hard physical work increases the incidence); smoking; and certain pregnancy complications, *e.g.*, hypertension, bacteriuria, and antepartum hemorrhage.

Scoring systems have been devised to identify some of the women who may be at risk for preterm labor (Table 33–1). Such lists are not inclusive, but they have the virtue of directing attention to some of the important features of this problem. The following additional factors may also be concerned.

Maternal Problems

Maternal abnormalities that have a recognized relation to preterm labor include medical disorders such as serious cardiovascular or renal disease, severe anemia, cholestasis of pregnancy, marked hyperthyroidism, and poorly controlled diabetes mellitus. Abdominal surgery involving uterine displacement or manipulation (*e.g.*, large bowel resection during advanced gestation) may be inimical to continuation of pregnancy. Maternal injury (*e.g.*, a direct blow to the abdomen, a major fracture, or shock) may terminate gestation early. Preeclampsia–eclampsia may either precipitate labor or necessitate therapeutic intervention and termination of pregnancy. Uterine anomalies (*e.g.*, bicornuate or diminutive uterus) may shorten gestation. Pelvic sepsis or tumors (*e.g.*, appendicitis, large uterine fibromyomas) may cause an increase in uterine irritability. Cervical incompetence may jeopardize containment of the pregnancy. Infection, particularly when associated with hyperthermia (*e.g.*, pyelonephritis, pneumonia, malaria) or localized sepsis (*e.g.*, listeriosis) may terminate pregnancy well before the expected date of confinement.

Untreated Cushing's disease, caused either by adrenal or pituitary neoplasm, or by adrenocorticotropic hormone (ACTH)-secreting bronchial carcinoma, is associated with spontaneous labor before the 34th week of pregnancy.

Orgasm during pregnancy may be accompanied by palpable uterine contractions and even prolonged uterine spasm. Orgasmic induction of labor, perhaps in part related to the prostaglandin content of semen, has been reported. Although the data are tentative, proscription of coitus may be judicious if there is a history of early termination of pregnancy. More recently, it has been shown that vaginal examination *per se* is followed by an increase in plasma prostaglandin levels, suggesting that some cases of preterm labor may result from external stimuli, *e.g.*, vaginal examination or intercourse.

Anecdotal reference is often made to so-called psychogenic or emotionally induced abortion or early labor, *e.g.*, after fright, grief, or anxiety. Recent evidence supports this possibility, which probably was first recorded in the Bible, where note is made (1 Sam. 4:19) that the wife of Phinehas immediately went into labor when she learned of her husband's death.

Finally, the risk of preterm labor is increased by conditions that make careful supervision of pregnancy difficult, by lack of patient information, and by psychosocial stresses. However, none of these factors accounts for the total risk of preterm delivery.

Placental Abnormalities

Gross placental disorders (*e.g.*, preterm separation of the placenta, extrachorial placenta) may be directly responsible for preterm labor. Common histopathologic alternations of the placenta include stasis and edema, infarction, fibrosis, and hematoma formation. Nonetheless, these microscopic alterations may be secondary to general pathologic states associated with early labor.

Fetal Abnormalities

Multiple pregnancy or hydramnios may overdistend the uterus. Congenital adrenal hyperplasia almost always is associated with shortened gestation. Preterm labor is common (about 60%) if the fetus is affected by Potter's syndrome (renal agenesis, pulmonary hypoplasia, characteristic facies). Fetal infection (*e.g.*, rubella, toxoplasmosis) may precipitate preterm labor because of critical fetal disease. As noted before, premature rupture of the fetal membranes is one of the most common causes of preterm labor.

TABLE 33–1. EXAMPLE OF RISK SCORING FOR PRETERM LABOR

Score	Personal Data	Past History	Habits	Current Pregnancy
0	0 children at home Excellent SES*	No prior abortions > 1 year since last delivery	Light work only Minimum stress	General health good
1	2 children at home Good SES	< 1 year since last delivery	Outside work	Unusual fatigue
2	Age < 20 years or > 40 years Single parent Fair SES	2 prior induced abortions	> 10 cigarettes per day Unusual anxiety	Weight gain < 12 lbs by 32 weeks' gestation Proteinuria Bacteriuria Hypertension
3	Height < 5 feet Weight < 100 lbs Malnourished Poor SES	3 prior induced abortions	Heavy work	Breech at 32 weeks Weight loss of 5 lbs Head engaged before 34 weeks' gestation Febrile illness Uterine fibroids
4	Age < 18 years	Pyelonephritis		Bleeding after 12 weeks Cervix dilated or effaced Uterus irritable
5		Uterine anomaly 2nd trimester abortion Previous cone biopsy		Placenta previa Hydramnios
10		Prior preterm delivery Repeated 2nd trimester abortion		Multiple pregnancy Abdominal surgery

* Socioeconomic status.
(Modified from Creasy PK, Liggins CG. In Stallworthy J, Bourne G: Recent Advances in Obstetrics and Gynaecology, Vol 13. London, Churchill–Livingstone, 1979)

FREQUENCY

Year after year, about 7% of all liveborn infants in the United States are undergrown, and most are delivered after preterm labor. There are important racial differences, however, and the incidence of low birth weight is almost twice as high among nonwhites as whites. The difference between these two groups may be ascribed in part to the lower average weight of the nonwhite fetus at all stages of gestation and to the greater frequency in nonwhites of medical complications (e.g., preeclampsia–eclampsia) that predispose to preterm labor or necessitate therapeutic termination of pregnancy.

In multiple pregnancy, preterm labor is particularly common. The frequency of low birth weight is increased six times in twin gestation, which terminates, on the average, 3 weeks before the expected date of confinement.

PREVENTION

Since preterm labor occurs so commonly in socioeconomically deprived populations and among those who are at high risk, it is logical that the incidence would be sharply reduced if the factors leading to both these circumstances were corrected. These problems are largely social and only partly medical.

Preterm labor has a strong tendency to recur and may be a repetitive problem. Normal hygienic measures during pregnancy, including proper diet and rest, avoidance of overwork, and avoidance of excesses of all types (including exercise, temperature, coitus, tobacco, drugs, and alcohol) are recommended as a matter of course. For the patient with a history of repeated preterm labors, it is prudent to restrict work, travel, and exercise and to encourage rest, especially during the last trimester. Except for tobacco, which has been shown to be clearly related to preterm labor, the aforementioned factors have not been shown definitely to bear a causal relation; admonitions regarding them are intuitive rather than scientific.

Medical, gynecologic, or obstetric complications that predispose to preterm labor must be managed according to the specific requirements of each. Early diagnosis of anemia, hypertension, and other medical problems is important in any plan to achieve fetal maturity. Help at home and increased periods of bedrest should be prescribed for the patient with multiple pregnancy or early hydramnios and for the patient with a demonstrated tendency to preterm delivery. Acute infection should be treated promptly and aggressively with appropriate chemotherapeutic agents. Routine antepartum examinations, with repeated measurements of the patient's blood pressure and weight and the testing of urine for protein, permit early detection and treatment of preeclampsia; this should reduce the incidence of preterm delivery from this cause. Chronic hypertensive vascular disease is best managed with increased rest in bed. Antipressor drugs have not proved valuable for improving fetal salvage.

Medical consultation should be sought for the patient with diabetes mellitus, hyperthyroidism, cardiac disease, or other medical complication. Meticulous control of maternal diabetes mellitus, with prevention of acidosis, is of the greatest importance to fetal survival. The cardiac patient is not likely to deliver early unless cardiac failure develops, resulting in hypoxia to the fetus. Therefore, conservative management is required for maternal survival and fetal salvage. Uterine leiomyomas are best treated conservatively during pregnancy. Even if symptoms of degeneration supervene, bedrest and analgesics generally are preferable to surgical intervention, since they allow a better chance for the continuation of pregnancy and further fetal growth.

Elective major surgery or extensive dental therapy should be postponed until after delivery, if possible. In an impressive number of patients with cervical incompetence and intact membranes, the onset of premature labor has been averted or postponed by cervical cerclage, accomplished before the cervix has achieved 3-cm dilatation or 50% effacement.

A new and increasingly common cause of preterm labor is the multiple pregnancy that so often results from the use of clomiphene citrate or human menopausal gonadotropin to promote conception. The evidence that the occurrence of multiple pregnancy following administration of these agents is dose-related emphasizes that these preparations must not be used casually or by those who lack the facilities and experience to apply them with precision and to evaluate their effects.

DIAGNOSIS

Since preterm labor can sometimes be arrested by appropriate management, the diagnosis must be made as quickly as possible, before labor is so far advanced that therapy will be ineffective. A specific time of onset of preterm labor is difficult to pinpoint, however, although early rupture of the membranes may be an augury. Increasingly strong and prolonged uterine contractions every 5–10 min, 3-cm cervical dilatation, and 50% cervical effacement, particularly after leakage of amniotic fluid or the passage of blood, are strongly suggestive that labor is underway. By definition, labor is the occurrence of regular, coordinated, often painful uterine contractions that are accompanied by progressive dilatation of the cervix and that normally culminate in delivery.

The distinction between contractions of this kind and those of false labor (discussed in Chapter 29) is usually not of great moment at term, so far as fetal welfare is concerned, but before 37 weeks' gestation it may be urgent. External monitoring devices can be helpful by providing objective evidence of the character of the contractions, as well as the condition of the fetus, and they should be applied promptly in all cases in which a woman is admitted in questionable preterm labor. Over a period of time this may help the physician determine the true state of affairs.

MANAGEMENT

When preterm labor is diagnosed with certainty, it is important to decide whether an attempt should be made to stop it or whether the labor should be permitted to proceed. The following are among the situations in which attempts to arrest preterm labor may be either futile or ill-advised:

1. Advancing, active labor with the cervix dilated 4 cm or more. When labor has advanced to this point, efforts to arrest it are rarely successful.
2. Maternal complications that would be increasingly serious if pregnancy were permitted to continue. Examples are preeclampsia–eclampsia and severe cardiovascular or renal disease.
3. Fetal complications of such nature that continued intrauterine life would be hazardous. Examples are

the fetal risk associated with severe preeclampsia and severe maternal diabetes. Fetal death, serious isoimmunization, severe congenital anomalies, and marked hydramnios also weigh against attempts to stop labor. Moreover, if there is any evidence of fetal distress, detected either clinically (*e.g.*, by electronic monitoring) or by laboratory tests for fetoplacental insufficiency, there should be no attempt to stop labor. About 6% of low-birth-weight neonates display distress that would be compounded by extension of pregnancy.

4. Ruptured membranes. If this is accompanied by fever, the implication is that amnionitis may have developed, and the uterus should be emptied promptly regardless of prematurity. If there is nothing to suggest amnionitis, the risk that it may develop must be weighed against the hazard of prematurity. Moreover, clinical experience has demonstrated that attempts to stop labor are unsuccessful if the membranes are ruptured, and 20%–30% of all low-birth-weight babies are born soon after premature rupture of the membranes. Also, the cervix may be too dilated or effaced for labor to be arrested. The physiologic wheel may have turned beyond the point of reversal.

If all patients in whom attempts at the arrest of labor are either contraindicated or futile are excluded, there are only about 20% in whom the attempt may be appropriate and has some chance of success.

A final consideration in the decision whether to attempt the arrest of preterm labor is the dramatic improvement in survival, and subsequent development, of the very small newborn, as discussed later in this chapter. Under optimal conditions the outlook for these babies is such that Stewart and others have questioned whether preterm delivery is really so undesirable that heroic and sometimes hazardous measures should be taken to prevent it.

The following conditions should obtain in the woman in whom an effort is to be made to arrest labor:

1. The fetus should be alive, weigh less than 2500 g, and show no evidence of fetal distress or jeopardy.
2. The membranes should be intact.
3. There should be no obstetric or medical condition that contraindicates continued pregnancy.
4. The cervix should be dilated less than 4 cm.

Arrest of Preterm Labor

If it is decided to attempt the arrest of preterm labor, the woman should remain at bedrest. An initial pelvic examination is needed to determine the status at the time treatment is begun, but no other pelvic examinations should be made unless they are essential. Fetal heart rate and uterine contractions should be monitored externally. An ultrasound scan should be made to rule out gross malformation or abnormal presentation, since the incidence of these is higher in preterm labor, and to permit an estimate of fetal weight, which can be helpful in decisions regarding the conduct of labor and mode of delivery if the effort to arrest labor fails. Amniotic fluid should be obtained for lecithin/sphingomyelin (L/S) ratio, from the vaginal pool if the membranes are ruptured or by amniocentesis if they are intact.

Tocolytic Agents. There are no reliable data regarding the exact efficacy of tocolytic agents in the arrest of labor. In some series, simple bedrest or placebos were sometimes effective, leading to the inescapable conclusion that at least some of the women in whom labor was "successfully" arrested were not in labor. Early diagnosis is essential if tocolytic agents are to be used, for they become increasingly ineffective as cervical dilatation increases beyond 2 cm and effacement exceeds 50%. Most of the agents can suppress uterine contractions and can delay delivery for 12 to 24 hours; but in order to delay delivery for significant periods, they must be used in earliest labor, the time when the diagnosis is most difficult to make with certainty. The total incidence of preterm birth has not changed significantly since the advent of tocolytic agents, but they do appear to have a place in dealing with at least some of the cases. However, it is clear that none of the drugs introduced to date answers the imperative need for some agent that is as safe, as precise, and as predictable in stopping labor as oxytocin and prostaglandins are in starting it. At the current time, the Food and Drug Administration (FDA) is reconsidering the status of all tocolytic agents, and the status of each should be verified before it is used. The agents that have been used, with variable success, include the following:

1. Progesterone and its derivatives
2. Ethanol (alone or with adrenergic drugs)
3. β-Adrenergic (β-mimetic) drugs (isoxsuprine hydrochloride, ritodrine, salbutamol, terbutaline sulfate, fenoterol)
4. Prostaglandin synthetase inhibitors (aspirin, indomethacin, naproxen, mefenamic acid)
5. Calcium antagonists (nifedipine and verapamil)
6. Other drugs (*e.g.*, magnesium sulfate)

Progesterone Derivatives. Although prophylactic progesterone therapy of patients with a history of preterm labor has been reported to be effective in at least one series of cases, progestogens are not effective in stopping the progress of early labor. In addition, the FDA has proscribed use of these agents in pregnancy because of data suggesting that they can cause developmental anomalies.

Ethanol. Ethanol is believed to reduce the secretion of oxytocin from the posterior pituitary and may also have

a direct inhibitory effect on the myometrium. Ethanol has stopped labor for over 72 hours in certain patients and is reported effective to some degree in about half of cases of threatened preterm labor. The maximum duration of tocolytic effect is still to be determined, however. Combinations of alcohol and ritodrine have been effective in quelling labor for several weeks in a small number of cases. Nevertheless, the questions of its contribution, if any, to the fetal alcohol syndrome and its effect on the neonate's respiratory and circulatory adaptation are still unsettled. Because of these questions, plus its extremely unpleasant side effects and sequelae, the drug has been used less frequently than before.

The following protocol has been recommended by Fuchs for the use of ethanol to suppress labor:

Infusion fluid: 100 ml 95% (V/V) ethanol + 900 ml 5% dextrose water = 1000 ml 9:5% (V/V) ethanol (75.4 g/liter).

Loading dose: 15 ml/kg body weight/hour over a period of 2 hours.

Maintenance dose: 1.5 ml/kg body weight/hour for 6 hours or more.

Reloading dose: If treatment was discontinued less than 10 hours earlier, the new dose is calculated as loading dose × (number of hours/10).

When alcohol is given intravenously, inebriation and belligerence may be extremely troublesome and may also complicate the choice of anesthetic if it should be needed. Of special importance is the fact that alcohol is a potent gastric secretagogue; any patient who has received intravenous alcohol must be presumed to have significant acid stomach contents regardless of the prior duration of fasting. In one case, a near-fatal accident from aspiration of vomitus occurred during the induction of general anesthesia in a woman who had taken nothing by mouth for 24 hours but had been given alcohol intravenously.

β-Mimetic Agents. The action of the β-mimetic drugs in the suppression of labor is discussed in Chapter 29. β-Mimetic drugs have received extensive trial in the arrest of preterm labor. The cardiovascular side effects can be distressing: tachycardia occurs with some regularity, maternal hypotension is uncommon but has been reported, and right heart failure and pulmonary edema in women with no history of heart disease have also occurred. Intravenous β-mimetics regularly cause an increase in blood glucose and blood insulin levels; these are of no consequence in the normal woman, but can be important in the presence of diabetes. The two agents that have received most attention are isoxsuprine hydrochloride and ritodrine. Of the two, the cardiovascular effects of ritodrine appear to be less troublesome than those of isoxsuprine.

Hypoglycemia of the newborn, which can be observed within 90 min of birth, is a predictable consequence of the preterm use of β-mimetic agents among infants who are delivered within 5 days of the last dose of the agent; it responds promptly to specific therapy. Despite its wide and apparently safe use for more than 10 years, the Brazy–Pupkin report now raises the question of possible serious neonatal effects of isoxsuprine if delivery occurs within 72 hours of the start of the infusion: these include respiratory distress syndrome, necrotizing enterocolitis, hypotension, hypocalcemia, and death. The virtual absence of this kind of incriminating evidence among earlier reports suggests that more information is needed regarding this relationship.

The following therapeutic program with isoxsuprine has been suggested by Flowers:

Loading dose: 500 ml normal saline administered rapidly, followed by isoxsuprine HCl 50 mg diluted in 500 ml normal saline, 1 ml/min, IV for 45 min.

Maintenance dose: isoxsuprine 20 mg IM every 6 hours for 24–48 hours. If uterine contractions cease, isoxsuprine 10–20 mg orally three or four times a day may be substituted.

Contraindications: arterial bleeding or severe adverse reactions.

Adverse reactions: hypotension, tachycardia, nausea, vomiting, dizziness, abdominal pain, rash.

The protocol suggested by Bieniarz for the use of ritodrine is as follows:

Infusion fluid: 1 ampule ritodrine, 25 mg, diluted in 250 ml 5% glucose and water. This solution contains 100 µg ritodrine/ml.

Loading dose: Infusion is started at 50 µg/min, and the infusion rate is increased by 50 µ/min every 10 min until satisfactory uterine inhibition has been achieved.

Maximum intravenous dose level: 400 µg/min. Maximum dose is limited by the elevated maternal pulse rate. Intravenous administration of ritodrine is continued until at least 2 hours after contractions have ceased. In successful cases the drug is not stopped abruptly, but the dose is gradually reduced over 1 hour to prevent uterine recovery when the drug is discontinued. This may be followed by oral medication of 20–30 mg twice daily as long as needed.

Question has been raised whether serum potassium should be monitored in patients receiving β-adrenergic therapy. Gross and Sokol have observed levels in the range of 2–3 mEq/L in several patients, and are accustomed to monitor serum electrolytes and glucose before and during such therapy.

Prostaglandin Synthetase Inhibitors. There is ample evidence both in lower animals (rat, lamb, sheep) and in the human that prostaglandin synthetase inhibitors

are effective in delaying or prolonging labor. When administered to the newborn, they cause the closure of a patent ductus arteriosis, which raised the question of whether they might have similar effects on the fetus if used in an effort to arrest labor. Such effects have been demonstrated in the fetal lamb. Although only a few human cases of arterial pulmonary hypertension as a result of either indomethacin or large amounts of aspirin in late pregnancy have been reported, Rudolph concludes that "administration of prostaglandin synthetase inhibitors to the pregnant mother may produce significant circulatory effects in the fetus and may be responsible for the syndrome of persistent pulmonary hypertension of the newborn in some infants."

Calcium Antagonists. It is well known that calcium ions are needed for activation of the contractile proteins of the myometrium. Several drugs have been shown to inhibit the passage of calcium through excitable membranes, and extensive clinical use has been made of at least two of them (verapamil and nifedipine) in the treatment of ischemic heart disease. As expected, they have also been shown to reduce uterine motility (see Fig. 29–13), although doses larger than the usual range are required. Preliminary studies with nifedipine suggest it is effective in arresting preterm labor for periods varying from 3 to 17 days. In Andersson's series, the side effects were not troublesome (transient facial flushing and moderate tachycardia).

Magnesium Sulfate. Magnesium sulfate is reported to be effective as a labor suppressant, somewhat more so than ethanol. However, it is difficult to determine how many patients had a prolonged tocolytic effect. Fortunately, significant fetal or neonatal problems have not been observed after magnesium sulfate therapy. Complications appear to be unlikely if the customary admonitions for use of magnesium sulfate are observed (see page 469).

Glucocorticoid Therapy. The use of glucocorticoids to accelerate maturation of the immature fetal lung is discussed on page 477. The benefits in terms of preventing respiratory distress syndrome appear to be greatest in pregnancies of 29–32 weeks' duration. Glucocorticoids are of no benefit after 34 weeks' gestation, or if delivery occurs less than 24 hours or more than 7 days after the first injection. If delivery is delayed more than 7 days after the first injection, the treatment must be repeated. The agent used by Liggins and Howie is betamethasone (10–12 mg/24 hours in divided intramuscular injections and continued, if possible, for 48–72 hours), but they suggest that other glucocorticoids are probably no less effective.

In otherwise uncomplicated preterm pregnancy, no deleterious fetal effects have been defined, and psychometric testing of these children at 4 years of age has shown no intellectual deficits. However, theoretical questions have been raised as to the possibility of long-term effects of intrauterine exposure to high levels of glucocorticoids.

Glucocorticoids are contraindicated in the presence of severe preeclampsia because of the increased incidence of fetal death. Cases of postpartum pulmonary edema and shock (which usually respond to diuretics and oxygen) have been reported in women receiving the combination of terbutaline and glucocorticoids.

Prognosis for the Infant. Among preterm labors in which attempts to arrest labor are either unsuccessful or inappropriate, perinatal mortality has declined to levels that only a few years ago were thought to be unattainable. In the Haesslein–Goodlin series, the overall survival of newborn infants weighing 800–1350 g was 65%; in Stewart's series of cases, the mortality for newborns under 1500 g had declined to less than 40%. James observed that in a number of institutions in the United States the survival rate for babies weighing less than 1000 g is 40%–50% (see Figure 42–8). There has also been a decline in neurologic and intellectual deficits among these babies. Among Stewart's series of 259 children aged 18 months or more who had weighed 1500 g or less at birth, 91.5% had no major handicap. These astonishing advances are due to so many factors that they cannot be listed; all aspects of prenatal, paranatal, and postnatal diagnosis and care have been vastly improved, and each has contributed. If the circumstances are ideal, it is no longer appropriate to consider the tiny fetus as doomed; all whose weight is estimated at more than 600 g should be regarded as patients at risk and must receive active consideration and treatment. However, it must be emphasized that preterm delivery should be carried out in facilities that provide level III intensive perinatal care. Whenever possible the mother should be transferred to such a unit before delivery; the neonatal results are usually poor when the baby is transported after delivery.

If preterm labor starts in an area where optimal care cannot be provided for the newborn, the patient should be transferred immediately to a proper facility if there is a reasonable chance the trip can be completed before delivery. Life-threatening maternal complications must, of course, be dealt with at once, but heroic measures on behalf of a preterm baby should be taken only where intensive care for the newborn is immediately available.

The Role of Cesarean Section. There is general agreement that cesarean section is the method of choice for preterm delivery if monitoring should disclose fetal distress, if there is a breech presentation, or if there is a transverse or oblique lie. Even in the absence of such indications, there is growing conviction that cesarean section is largely responsible for the lower rates of morbidity and mortality among very low birth weight

babies (500–1500 g), and most authors consider cesarean section to be far less hazardous to the tiny newborn than vaginal delivery. Other controlled series of cases are needed to support this conclusion; but as the data accumulate the inherent maternal hazard of cesarean section must not be overlooked. For preterm cesarean section, the classical incision is usually required, which involves not only the immediate surgical risks, but also the added threat of postoperative intestinal obstruction and, in a subsequent pregnancy, uterine rupture. Cesarean section is by no means innocuous, and its risks must be taken into account in deciding the mode of delivery of the preterm baby.

Vaginal Delivery. If vaginal delivery of the preterm baby is elected, or if it is inevitable, every effort must be made to avoid trauma and to prevent hypoxia. Labor should be conducted with the mother in the recumbent lateral position, nasal oxygen should be administered during labor, continuous fetal monitoring should be started, and systemic analgesia should not be used. Lumbar epidural anesthesia is appropriate if it is needed. Although some may differ, it is recommended that the membranes be ruptured when the cervix is sufficiently dilated to permit application of an internal monitor. Reliable, efficient monitoring is essential, and the benefits far outweigh the risk of rupturing the membranes. Outlet forceps should be used unless spontaneous delivery occurs as soon as the head reaches the pelvic floor, as may be the case if the baby is very small. A deep episiotomy should be made to avoid counterpressure on the fetal head.

Oxytocin may be used for stimulation if it is needed, but special surveillance is mandatory. The infusion is started at 1 mU/min and increased every 10 min in increments of 1 mU/min until a maximum of 10 mU/min is reached or until laborlike contractions occur every 2½–3 min. Prolonged oxytocin stimulation is inadvisable in preterm labor. The infusion should be stopped if effective labor is not established in 4–6 hours.

After delivery, the baby should be placed at or below the level of the vulva. If breathing occurs quickly, the cord should be cut 30–45 sec after delivery to permit optimal placental transfusion and to allow the passage of placental and cord blood into the expanding pulmonary unit. If breathing is delayed, the cord should be cut 20–30 sec after delivery and the baby transferred immediately to a heated table for resuscitative measures.

INTRAUTERINE GROWTH RETARDATION (The Small-for-Dates Infant)

It is generally agreed that neonates whose weight is 10% below the local, normal range are undergrown. However, certain distinctions must be made. Those who are small because of a family trait usually have adequate subcutaneous tissue and well-proportioned body measurements; they are small but normal and pose no special problems. In contrast, two abnormal groups of undersized neonates may be identified:

1. Hypoplastic neonates whose size has been limited or reduced because of intrinsic impairment of cell division due to injury or genetic abnormality
2. Neonates whose undergrowth or weight loss is due to fetal nutritional failure

The hypoplastic neonate usually reveals gross anomalous features, *e.g.*, genetic disorders (Down's syndrome) or drug effects (alcohol, thalidamide). In such pregnancies, oligohydramnios, hydramnios, amnion nodosum, single umbilical artery or other placenta–cord abnormality or dysfunction may suggest the likelihood of malformation of the offspring.

Nutritional failure or chronic fetal distress usually occurs after midpregnancy and must include all the anabolic components. A gradual limitation of growth results in a proportionately small neonate who may even be in the third percentile in all growth parameters. The most vital centers usually are spared, but if the deprivation is severe, brain development may be impaired.

Subacute fetal nutritional deprivation often develops late in pregnancy. Survival may depend upon the metabolism of available tissue, which results in general wasting and reduction of fat and muscle mass. In these cases, there is also a loss of vernix and the skin is dry and fissured. While length and head size may be in the normal range, the total weight is proportionately less. Stated differently, the neonate is light for length but not necessarily small for dates. However, the metabolic deficiency often is serious.

Acute fetal distress is a relatively sudden uncompensated hypoxic crisis. Such an insult may be intolerable for an undergrown fetus. Growth retardation and asphyxia, which is intensified by labor, are a leading cause of perinatal morbidity and mortality. Hence, rescue by prompt delivery is mandatory.

CAUSES

The causes of fetal growth retardation include maternal, placental, and fetal factors.

Maternal Factors

Vargas–Lopez and coworkers have suggested that in about half the cases maternal factors can be cited as the cause of fetal growth retardation. Included are the mother's youth, short stature, first pregnancy, low socioeconomic status, urinary infection, and excessive cigarette smoking.

Teenage girls often have babies that are small for

gestational dates. About 2% of infants of adolescent mothers weigh less than 1500 g, an incidence twice that of infants born to women 25–30 years of age. This may be due to maternal immaturity or poor nutrition.

To prevent intrauterine growth retardation, it may be especially important that the woman begin her pregnancy in optimal health and nutritional state, and that her weight gain in pregnancy be within the normal range. Maternal factors generally are responsible for the availability of nutrients to the fetus, and if nutrients are insufficient, growth retardation can result. The abnormalities implicated include changes in the composition of maternal blood or circulatory dynamics that affect the intervillous space. Details are poorly understood, but limitation of uterine blood flow during pregnancy in a hypertensive gravida and poor perfusion of the placenta are examples. In multiple pregnancy, the placentas seem to be qualitatively normal and somewhat larger in size compared with single placentas in relation to fetal weight. Under these circumstances, any insufficiency of supply appears to be maternal.

Other maternal problems that are often associated with intrauterine growth retardation include hypertensive cardiovascular disease, renal disease, collagen disorders, or environmental compromise by high altitude or radiation exposure.

Placental Factors (Placental Insufficiency)

Low birth weight may result if the placenta fails as a metabolic organ because of abnormality. The weight of the placenta normally correlates well with that of the fetus. For this reason, a proportional reduction in the weight of both does not necessarily mean that the fetus is small because the small placenta did not allow the fetus to grow more rapidly. Actually, it is more likely that the close size correlation occurs because the limit of functional capacity of the placenta normally is so close to the needs of the fetus.

The functional area of the placenta often is diminished in preeclampsia and essential hypertension as well as in the small-for-dates syndrome. It is still not known whether this is a primary defect in the placenta or secondary to vascular lesions in the placental bed. For this reason, the term *uteroplacental insufficiency* has been suggested. No pathognomonic lesion has thus far been demonstrated in the placenta associated with the small-for-dates baby, despite reports of extensive true infarcts and calcification.

Gross placental abnormalities that can be responsible for intrauterine growth retardation include monozygous twinning with vascular shunt (the so-called twin-to-twin transfer syndrome) and the restricted, relatively small circumvallate placenta.

Urinary estriol levels have been reported to be low in the mother of the small-for-dates fetus, but even in a woman whose pregnancy is normal, the 24-hour estriol excretion on successive days may vary widely. Regret-tably, the lowered estriol levels cannot be correlated with early onset of labor. Chorionic gonadotropin levels in late pregnancy have been found to be raised in preeclampsia. Nonetheless, they do not always become abnormal before evidence of placental failure is apparent. Human placental lactogen assay has been found to bear no relation to the weight of the placenta or of the infant.

Enzyme tests, vaginal cytology, and placental transfer tests have been utilized to appraise the function of the placenta, but no reliable relation has been found between placental function and the early onset of labor or growth retardation.

In cases of retardation of fetal growth, three types of pathologic alterations of the placenta have been noted: 1) advanced maturity, 2) multiple microinfarcts, and 3) numerous avascular villi. These abnormalities may lead to placental insufficiency and, perhaps, to early labor and delivery.

Fetal Factors

Fetal Abnormalities. In experimental animals, genetically and experimentally induced malformations often are associated with growth retardation and slow maturation. In these instances, maldevelopment rather than inadequate supply appears responsible for small fetal size. Certain women have been known consistently to give birth to small infants, a characteristic that may be determined by heredity.

Cederqvist, in a retrospective study of the occurrence of a single umbilical artery, found that this anomaly occurred in 0.27% of cases and that other congenital anomalies were often noted also. In cases with only a single umbilical artery, the incidence of preterm delivery was not increased, but there was a suggestion of an increase in the incidence of low birth weight. If one umbilical artery and other anomalies were combined, a definite increase in early birth and a significantly low birth weight were identified.

Chronic Fetal Infection. Sepsis caused by syphilis, rubella, toxoplasmosis, or cytomegalovirus inclusion diseases often is responsible for the undergrown offspring, perhaps partially on the basis of a reduced number of cells. Although minor abnormalities may be noted in the placenta, it is unlikely that placental insufficiency is the cause of retarded growth and development in these fetuses.

IMPLICATIONS

Infants who are small for dates must be identified at birth because their unique characteristics result in liabilities quite different from those of an infant of more appropriate size for gestation. Several methods are available for classifying infants into risk categories. Table 33–2 shows a simplified grouping of newborns

TABLE 33-2. CLASSIFICATION OF NEWBORN INFANTS ON BASIS OF WEIGHT AND GESTATIONAL AGE

	Gestation (Weeks)	Weight (g)	Percent of Total Deliveries	Mortality Rate (%)	Group Characteristics	Special Problems
GROUP 1 Immature Premature	All*	<1501	1.0 ± 0.2	60–75	Thin, fragile, red skin Eyes closed Edematous	Temperature control Enzyme deficiencies (hyperbilirubinemia, hyaline membrane disease)
GROUP 2 Premature Preterm	<37	1501–2500	2.0 ± 0.3	10–15	Relatively hypotonic Weight loss 10%–20%	Susceptibility to infection Apnea and cyanosis, capillary hemorrhage Retrolental fibroplasia
GROUP 3 Small-for-dates Undergrown Malnourished Dysmature	>36	1501–2500	3.0 ± 0.5	3–5	Often malnourished with dry and peeling skin Anxious, open-eyed Increased tone and activity Minimal weight loss	Increased in congenital anomalies, intrauterine infection Perinatal asphyxia Pulmonary hemorrhage Hypoglycemia
GROUP 4 Large-for-dates	<37	>2500	3.0 ± 1.0	2–4	Often inactive Characteristics of groups 1 and 2	Problems of groups 1 and 2
GROUP 5 Normal	>36	>2500	90.0 ± 3.0	0.5	Normal Occasionally undernourished and dysmature	Generally healthy

* Less than 1% > 36 weeks
(Babson SG, Benson RC. Management of High-Risk Pregnancy and Intensive Care of the Neonate, 2nd ed. St Louis, Mosby, 1971)

by weight and gestation. Although it is recognized that neither 37 weeks' gestation nor 2500-g birth weight has any biologic significance, these points of reference are still commonly used. This method of identification draws attention to the small, term infants with their special problems (Group 3) and to the overterm babies (Group 5) of the same birth weight.

Within limits, a 37-week pregnancy is expected to yield an infant weighing about 2500 g. However, in 30% of 37-week pregnancies, the birth weight is less than 2500 g. These undergrown and often malnourished neonates differ from their "normal" preterm counterparts because their maturation is relatively advanced despite their small size; their mortality rate is consequently much lower than that of preterm infants of equivalent weight. Moreover, many preterm newborns are also undersized for their gestational age and so suffer the added disadvantage of undergrowth. A clinical appraisal of gestational age and maturity is vital to the establishment of appropriate care of the neonate. Methods and standards for making this appraisal are outlined in Chapter 42.

DIAGNOSIS AND MANAGEMENT

Intrauterine fetal growth retardation is usually first suspected clinically after 5 months' gestation when the uterine size appears to be smaller than anticipated. In about one-third of the cases, maternal weight gain and fundal growth are within the normal range, but in the remainder the maternal weight gain averages less than 2 lb/4 weeks, particularly after 30 weeks' gestation. Serial fundal measurements reveal reduced fundal growth.

The condition can be diagnosed by the tests outlined in Chapter 41. If the diagnosis is made at or near term, prompt delivery is indicated. Fetal distress is common in labor and appropriate monitoring is essential. If the diagnosis is made before term, delivery is indicated (a) when L/S ratio or phosphatidylglycerol indicates fetal lung maturity, (b) if the tests outlined in Chapter 41 give evidence of fetal deterioration, or (c) if an underlying maternal disease is becoming worse as a result of continuation of the pregnancy.

PROGNOSIS

As is true of all low-birth-weight babies, the chance of survival and normal subsequent development is much better if delivery occurs in an institution providing level III neonatal care.

Term newborns whose growth/weight ratios are two standard deviations from the mean have about eight times the perinatal mortality rate of those infants who are of similar gestational age but are of appropriate size. The former have a higher incidence of congenital anomalies and asphyxia neonatorum (often complicated by meconium aspiration). Asphyxial convulsions, hypoglycemia, and pulmonary hemorrhage are also much more frequent in the undergrown infant; prompt and proper treatment can often prevent neurologic or other permanent disability.

In one study in which small-for-dates infants were compared with infants of equivalent but appropriate weight for gestational age, the weight, length and head circumference of the former attained the tenth percentile by 6–8 months and were similar to the latter. The quarterly Bayley scores of the former were lower during the first 18 months of life, but at 24 months the two groups had similar scores.

REFERENCES AND RECOMMENDED READING

Anderson A, Beard R, Brudenell JM et al (eds): Pre-term Labour. London, Royal College of Obstetricians and Gynaecologists, 1978

Andersson KE: Inhibition of uterine activity by the calcium antagonist nifedipine. In Anderson A, Beard R, Brudenell JM, Dunn PM (eds): Pre-term Labour, p. 101. London, Royal College of Obstetricians and Gynaecologists, 1978

Avery ME: Prenatal diagnosis and prevention of hyaline membrane disease. N Engl J Med 282:157, 1975

Babson SG, Benson RC: Management of High-Risk Pregnancy and Intensive Care of the Neonate, 2nd ed, St. Louis, Mosby, 1971

Ballard PL, Ballard RA: Glucocorticoids in prevention of respiratory distress syndrome. Hosp Pract 15:81, 1980

Barden TP, Bieniarz J, Cibils LA et al: Premature labor: Its management and therapy. J Reprod Med 9:93, 1972

Barden TP, Peter JB, Merkatz IR: Ritodrine hydrochloride: a betamimetic agent for use in preterm labor. I. Pharmacology, clinical history, administration, side effects, and safety. Obstet Gynecol 56:1, 1980

Bauer CR, Stern L, Colle E: Prolonged rupture of membranes associated with a decreased incidence of respiratory distress syndrome. Pediatrics 53:7, 1974

Belizan JM et al.: Diagnosis of intrauterine growth retardation by a simple clinical method: Measurement management of uterine height. Am J Obstet Gynecol 131:643, 1978

Bieniarz J, Burd L, Motew M et al: Inhibition of uterine contractility in labor. Am J Obstet Gynecol 11:874, 1971

Bieniarz J, Motew M, Scommegna A: Uterine and cardiovascular effects of ritodrine in premature labor. Obstet Gynecol 40:65, 1972

Bieniarz J et al.: Premature labor treatment with ritodrine in multiple pregnancy with three or more fetuses. Acta Obstet Gynecol Scand 57:25, 1978

Bjerre B, Bjerre I: Significance of obstetric factors in prognosis of low birthweight children. Acta Paediatr Scand 65:577, 1976

Brazy JE, Pupkin MJ: Effects of maternal isoxsuprine administration on preterm infants. J Pediatr 94:444, 1979

Brosens I, Dixon HG, Robertson WB: Fetal growth retardation and the arteries of the placental bed. Br J Obstet Gynaecol 84:656, 1977

Caceres EM, Stewart KR, Goldsmith A: The incidence, complications and predictors of low birthweight. Int J Gynaecol Obstet 16:24, 1978

Caritis SN, Edelstone DI, Jueller–Heubach E: Pharmacologic inhibition of preterm labor. Am J Obstet Gynecol 133:577, 1979

Cederqvist L: Significance of absence of one artery in the umbilical cord. Acta Obstet Gynecol Scand 49:113, 1970

Christensen KK et al: Study of complications in preterm deliveries after prolonged premature rupture of membranes. Obstet Gynecol 48:670, 1976

Creasy RK, Liggins GC: Aetiology and management of preterm labour. In Stallworthy J, Bourne G (eds): Recent Advances in Obstetrics and Gynaecology, No. 13. London, Churchill Livingstone, 1979

Csaba JF, Sulijok E, Erth T: Relationship of maternal treatment with indomethacin to persistence of fetal circulation syndrome. J Pediatr 92:484, 1978

Csapo AI, Herczeg J: Arrest of labor by isoxsuprine. Am J Obstet Gynecol 129:482, 1977

Daikoku NH, Johnson JWC, Graf C et al: Patterns of intrauterine growth retardation. Obstet Gynecol 54:211, 1979

Diddle AW, Semmer JR, Slowey JF: Cesarean section: Changing philosophy. Postgrad Med 53:160, 1973

Doran TA, Sawyer P, MacMurray B et al: Results of a double-blind controlled study on the use of betamethasone in the prevention of respiratory distress syndrome. Am J Obstet Gynecol 136:313, 1980

Epstein MF, Nicholls E, Stubblefield PG: Neonatal hypoglycemia after betasympathomimetic tocolytic therapy. J Pediatr 94:449, 1979

Fayez JA et al: Management of premature rupture of the membranes. Obstet Gynecol 52:17, 1978

Fedrick J: Antenatal identification of women at high risk of spontaneous preterm birth. Br J Obstet Gynaecol 83:351, 1976

Fedrick J, Adelstein P: Factors associated with low birth-weight of infants delivered at term. Br J Obstet Gynaecol 85:1, 1978

Fencl M deM, Tulchinsky D: Total cortisol in amniotic fluid and fetal lung maturation. N Engl J Med 292:123, 1975

Flowers CE, Jr: The obstetric management of infants weighing 1000 to 2000 grams. J Reprod Med 20:51, 1978

Fuchs F, Fuchs AR, Poblete VF, Jr et al: The effect of alcohol on threatened premature labor. Am J Obstet Gynecol 99:627, 1967

Galbraith RS et al: The clinical prediction of intrauterine growth retardation. Am J Obstet Gynecol 133:281, 1979

Gross TL, Sokol RJ: Severe hypokalemia and acidosis: A potential complication of beta-adrenergic treatment. Am J Obstet Gynecol, 138:1225, 1980

Gruenwald P, Babson SG: Retarded fetal growth. In Davis CH (ed): Gynecology and Obstetrics, Vol 1, pp 1–16. Hagerstown, Harper & Row, 1972

Guilliams S, Held B: Contemporary management and conduct of preterm labor and delivery: A review. Obstet Gynecol Surv 34:248, 1979

Hack M, Merkatz IR, Jones PK et al: Changing trends in neonatal and postneonatal deaths in very-low-birth-weight infants. Am J Obstet Gynecol 137:797, 1980

Hemminki E, Starfield B: Prevention and treatment of premature labor by drugs: Review of controlled clinical trials. Br J Obstet Gynaecol 85:411, 1978

Haesslein HC, Goodlin RC: Delivery of the tiny newborn. Am J Obstet Gynecol 134:192, 1979

Howie RN, Liggins GC: Clinical trial of antepartum betamethasone therapy for prevention of respiratory distress in preterm infants. In Anderson A, Beard R, Brudenell JM, Dunn PM (eds): Pre-term Labour, p 281. London, Royal College of Obstetricians and Gynaecologists, 1978

James LS: In discussion of management of the fetus in preterm labour and follow-up of pre-term infant. In Anderson A, Beard R. Brudenell JM, Dunn PM (eds): Pre-term Labour, p 361. London, Royal College of Obstetricians and Gynaecologists, 1978

Kauppila A, Kaikka J, Tuimala R: Effect of fenoterol and isoxsuprine on myometrial and intervillous blood flow during late pregnancy. Obstet Gynecol 52:558, 1978

Kitzmiller JH: What are the risks of giving steroids to prevent RDS (respiratory distress syndrome). Contemp Ob/Gyn 13:5, 1979

Landesman R, Wilson KH, Continho EM et al: The relaxant action of ritodrine, a sympathomimetic amine, on the uterus during term labor. Am J Obstet Gynecol 110:111, 1971

Lauersen NH et al: Inhibition of premature labor: Multicenter comparison of ritodrine and ethanol. Am J Obstet Gynecol 127:837, 1977

Levin DL et al: Morphologic analysis of the pulmonary vascular bed in infants exposed in utero to prostaglandin synthesis inhibitors. J Pediatr 92:478, 1978

Leviton A: Neurological effects of obstetrical procedures. Surg Rounds 1:14, 1978

Liggins GC: Premature delivery of fetal lambs infused with glucocorticoids. J Endocrinol 45:515, 1969

Liggins GC: Fetal influences on myometrial contractility. Clin Obstet Gynecol 16:148, 1973

Liggins GC, Howie RN: A controlled trial of antepartum glucocorticoid treatment for prevention of respiratory distress syndrome in premature infants. Pediatrics 50:515, 1972

Liggins GC, Vaughn GS: Intravenous infusion of salbutamol in management of premature labor. J Obstet Gynaecol Br Commonw 80:28, 1973

Little RE: Moderate alcohol use during pregnancy and decreased infant birth weight. Am J Public Health 67:1154, 1977

Liu, DTY, Blackwell RJ: The value of a scoring system in predicting outcome of preterm labour and comparing the efficacy of treatment with aminophylline and salbutamol. Br J Obstet Gynaecol 85:418, 1978

Miller JM, Pupkin MJ, Crenshaw C, Jr: Premature labor and premature rupture of the membranes. Am J Obstet Gynecol 132:1, 1978

Milligan JE, Shennan AT: Perinatal management and outcome in the infant weighing 1000 to 1200 grams. Am J Obstet Gynecol 136:269, 1980

Mulvihill JJ et al: Fetal alcohol syndrome: Seven new cases. Am J Obstet Gynecol 125:937, 1976

Newcombe R, Fedrick J, Chalmers I: Antenatal identification of patients "at risk" of pre-term labour. In Anderson A, Beard R, Brudenell JM, Dunn PM (eds): Pre-term Labour, p 17. London, Royal College of Obstetricians and Gynaecologists, 1978

Newton RW, Webster PAC, Binu PS et al: Psychosocial stress in pregnancy and its influence on premature labour. Br Med J 2:411, 1979

Ouellette EM et al: Adverse effects on the offspring of maternal alcohol abuse during pregnancy. N Engl J Med 297:528, 1977

Papiernik E, Kaminski M: Multifactoral study of the risk of prematurity at 32 weeks of gestation. J Perinat Med 2:30, 1974

Penney LL, Daniell WC: Estimation of success in treatment of premature labor: Applicability of prolongation index in a double-blind, controlled, randomized trial. Am J Obstet Gynecol 138:345, 1980

Pirani BBK: Smoking during pregnancy. Obstet Gynecol Surv 33:1, 1978

Ratten GJ, Beischer NA, Fortune DW: Obstetric complications when the fetus has Potter's syndrome. I. Clinical considerations. Am J Obstet Gynecol 115:890, 1973

Richardson CJ, Pomerance JJ, Cunningham MD et al: Acceleration of fetal lung maturation following prolonged rupture of the membranes. Am J Obstet Gynecol 118:1115, 1974

Richter R, Hinselman MJ: The treatment of threatened premature labor by betamimetic drugs: A comparison of fenoterol and ritodrine. Obstet Gynecol 53:81, 1979

Rudolph AM: Effects of prostaglandins and synthetase inhibitors on the fetal circulation. In Anderson A, Beard R, Brudenell JM, Dunn PM (eds): Pre-term Labour, p 231. London, Royal College of Obstetricians and Gynaecologists, 1978

Rush RW, Davey DA: The effect of preterm delivery on perinatal mortality. Br J Obstet Gynaecol 85:806, 1978

Ryden G: The effect of salbutamol and terbutaline in the management of premature labor. Acta Obstet Gynecol Scand 56:293, 1977

Schoenbaum SC, Monson RR, Stubblefield PG: Outcome of the delivery following an induced or spontaneous abortion. Am J Obstet Gynecol 136:19, 1980

Sell EJ, Harris TR: Association of premature rupture of the membranes with idiopathic respiratory distress syndrome. Obstet Gynecol 49:167, 1977

Shennan AT, Milligan JE: The growth and development of infants weighing 1000 to 1200 grams at birth and delivered in a perinatal unit. Am J Obstet Gynecol 136:273, 1980

Shields JR, Resnik R: Fetal lung maturation and the antenatal use of glucocorticoids to prevent the respiratory distress syndrome. Obstet Gynecol Surv 34:343, 1979

Sims CK et al: A comparison of salbutamol and ethanol in the treatment of preterm labour. Br J Obstet Gynaecol 85:761, 1978

Spearing G: Alcohol, indomethacin and salbutamol. A comparative trial of their use in preterm labor. Obstet Gynecol 53:171, 1979

Spellacy WN et al: Human amniotic fluid lecithin/sphingomyelin ratio changes with estrogen or glucocorticoid treatment. Am J Obstet Gynecol 115:216, 1973

Spellacy WN et al: The acute effects of ritodrine infusion on maternal metabolism: Measurements of glucose, insulin glucagon, triglycerides, cholesterol, placental lactogen and chorionic gonadotropin. Am J Obstet Gynecol 131:637, 1977

Steer CM, Petrie RH: A comparison of magnesium sulfate and alcohol for the prevention of premature labor. Am J Obstet Gynecol 129:1, 1977

Stewart A: Follow-up of pre-term infants. In Anderson A, Beard R, Brudenell JM, Dunn PM (eds): Pre-term Labour, p 372. London, Royal College of Obstetricians and Gynaecologists, 1978

Turnbull AC: Aetiology of pre-term labour. In Anderson A, Beard R, Brudenell JM, Dunn PM (eds): Pre-term Labour, p 56. London, Royal College of Obstetricians and Gynaecologists, 1978

Vargas–Lopez E et al: Epidemiological study of premature delivery: Analysis of 19,385 cases. Ginecol Obstet Mex 27:649, 1970

Vohr BR, Oh W, Rosenfield AG et al: The preterm small-for-gestational age infant: A two-year follow-up. Am J Obstet Gynecol 133:425, 1979

Wagner NN, Butler JC, Sanders JP: Prematurity and orgasmic coitus during pregnancy: Data on a small sample. Fertil Steril 27:911, 1976

Weathersbee PS, Lodge JR: A review of ethanol's effect on the reproductive process. J Reprod Med 21:63, 1978

Yerushalmy J, van den Berg BJ, Erhardt CL et al: Birthweight and gestation as indices of "immaturity." Am J Dis Child 109:43, 1965

Zuckerman H et al: Inhibition of human premature labor by indomethacin. Obstet Gynecol 44:792, 1974

Dystocia is defined as abnormal labor. Four Ps are concerned in the efficiency of labor: the powers, the pelvis or passage, the passenger, and the psyche. The *powers* are the expulsive forces of the contracting uterus. Both normal and abnormal uterine actions are discussed elsewhere in this book. The influences and effects of the *pelvic architecture* are outlined in Chapter 30. The *passenger* (the fetus) as it passes through the pelvis in the course of labor may, by its size, its presentation, or its position, give rise to abnormalities in labor. The patient's *psyche* may have an important influence on the duration and character of labor.

None of these factors operates independently of the others, and they must all be considered when the physician attempts to determine why a particular labor does not proceed normally. If they are systematically assessed, it should be possible to determine the cause of every abnormal labor.

The position and presentation of the fetus in relation to the pelvis may produce various abnormalities of labor. The problems that arise relate basically to the fact that either the size of the fetus or the diameter of the fetus that presents to the pelvis is such that it cannot readily pass through. The uterus is often very responsive to these minor abnormalities and fails to contract efficiently. Abnormal labor is the result. Some of these problems may eventuate in spontaneous or outlet forceps delivery, and some may require cesarean section. Several must be dealt with by midforceps delivery.

FORCEPS OPERATIONS

DEFINITIONS

The various forceps operations must be defined to permit comparison of the results, not only in different institutions, but also within the same institution. The following definitions have been approved by the American College of Obstetricians and Gynecologists and are recorded in *Obstetric Gynecologic Terminology*. (Edward C. Hughes, editor, Philadelphia, Davis, 1972).

A *low forceps operation* is the application of obstetric forceps to the fetal skull when the scalp is or has been visible at the introitus without separating the labia, the skull has reached the pelvic floor, and the sagittal suture is in the anteroposterior diameter of the outlet of the pelvis.

A *midforceps operation* is the application of obstetric forceps to the fetal skull when the head is engaged, but the conditions for low forceps have not been met. In the context of this term, any forceps operation that requires artificial rotation, regardless of the station from

---

CHAPTER 34

DYSTOCIA DUE TO ABNORMAL FETOPELVIC RELATIONS*

David N. Danforth

---

which extraction is begun, is designated a "midforceps operation."†

A *high forceps operation* is the application of obstetric forceps at any time prior to the engagement of the fetal head.

The following additional terms are used: *trial for-*

---

* This chapter is a revision of the chapter prepared by Warren H. Pearse and David N. Danforth for the previous editions of this book.

† This definition of midforceps delivery has been vigorously criticized by many who aver that it distorts obstetric statistics and the study of results by lumping usually innocuous forceps deliveries (in which the skull has reached the pelvic floor but the sagittal suture is not quite in the midline) in the same category with formidable midforceps operations in which the head is barely engaged at station +1 or +2. Alternative classifications have been proposed by Danforth and Ellis (Am J Obstet Gynecol 86:29, 1963) and by Pearse (Clin Obstet Gynecol 8:813, 1965).

ceps operation, which refers to the circumstance in which the physician recognizes *in advance* that cephalopelvic relationships are not wholly favorable, but considers the possibility of safe vaginal delivery to be great enough that a tentative effort should be made. If any difficulty is encountered, the attempt is immediately abandoned in favor of cesarean section. *Failed forceps operation* is a retrospective diagnosis. The intent is to deliver vaginally; but, when undue difficulty is encountered the physician retreats and delivers by cesarean section. The subject of *outlet forceps* is considered in Chapter 31. No discussion of high forceps is included since the operation is entirely obsolete and has no place in modern obstetrics.

MIDFORCEPS DELIVERY

Today, there is a progressive and accelerating trend away from midforceps delivery, owing principally to reports of an increased perinatal mortality attributable to midforceps and, among the survivors, a significant increase in neurologic deficits and developmental abnormalities. On the basis of this experience, cesarean section is considered safer. The consequence of this trend is that in some centers, virtually the only operative deliveries are by cesarean section and outlet forceps. However, the reports that condemn midforceps cannot quite be taken at face value; they do not necessarily indict the operation *per se,* but show only that in the hands of those who performed the operations cesarean section was more successful. As for all surgical procedures, the results depend on the technical skill, judgment, and experience of the operator, qualities that cannot be acquired overnight. For the inexperienced, the use of forceps, especially midforceps, can be expected to result in a high incidence of morbidity for both mother and baby; those who have little experience in the manipulative aspects of obstetrics are wise to select cesarean section in preference to any vaginal delivery that is more complex than outlet forceps. Despite the trends, there are important reasons why obstetricians should acquire proficiency in this mode of delivery. Some midforceps deliveries, notably most rotations from the occiput posterior position, are extremely simple and atraumatic, and in skilled hands they are less hazardous to the mother and baby than cesarean section. Cesarean section is not always feasible and the physician may be forced to deliver from the midplane if the baby is to survive, *e.g.,* if there is a terminal total abruption of the placenta or a serious anesthetic problem (aspiration, anaphylactic shock, or a total spinal) that cannot be instantly solved. Finally, as an alternative to an easy midforceps delivery, cesarean section is by no means invariably innocuous; even in the most favorable cases there are factors that can affect the outcome for both mother and baby. They include difficulty in delivering the baby if the uterus is irritable or the head is deeply engaged in the pelvis; the placenta may be encountered beneath the uterine incision; it may be difficult to control bleeding from the uterine incision; and complications of anesthesia may develop. Moreover, Ledger has shown that the most seriously ill patients with hospital-acquired postpartum infections are those who have been monitored and have come to cesarean section.

Before midforceps delivery is undertaken, regardless of indication, the physician's clinical judgment must permit the unequivocal conclusion that this method of delivery offers less risk to the mother and baby than cesarean section.

Indications for Midforceps Delivery

Midforceps delivery may be indicated in the following circumstances:

1. Faults in cephalopelvic relations. These include especially malpositions of the head such as persistent occiput posterior or face positions, transverse arrest, and relatively small pelves that prevent spontaneous advancement of the head regardless of position. In the latter case, it is of vital importance to recognize true disproportion, to know the pelvic diameters in which the traction must be made, and to know the amount of traction that can be safely applied. Happily, the heavy traction of former years is no longer permissible. Cesarean section must be elected if the head cannot be readily advanced by ordinary traction.
2. Uterine inertia. Uterine inertia is not uncommon in the second stage of labor and may be sufficient to interfere with progress. Occasionally, the quality of the contractions is improved by an oxytocin infusion; but if it is not or if this is not a reasonable procedure in the circumstance, midforceps delivery is indicated, provided the conditions for its performance are favorable.
3. Conditions that threaten the life of the mother. These are unusual, and an inclusive list cannot be given. They include especially circumstances in which the second stage must be shortened, such as advanced heart disease and other cardiopulmonary conditions that produce severe dyspnea.
4. Conditions that threaten the life of the baby. The classic signs of danger are changes in the fetal heart rate (see Chapter 41, Clinical Evaluation of Fetal Status) and, in vertex presentation, the appearance of meconium where none had been present before. Provided the conditions are favorable, delivery should be accomplished without delay. When labor is unusually vigorous, partial separation of the placenta during the second stage is not unusual. It is usually manifest by failure of the uterus to relax

completely between contractions, by undue uterine pain and tenderness, and, if the membranes are ruptured, by the passage of port-wine–colored amniotic fluid. Midforceps intervention on behalf of a fetus in jeopardy may require fine clinical judgment as to whether the hazard of delivery from the midplane is greater than the danger of delay in turning to cesarean section.

Conditions for Midforceps Delivery

The conditions for midforceps delivery are as follows:

1. The cervix should be fully dilated. In an extreme emergency forceps may be applied inside a cervix dilated 8 cm (but not less than 8 cm) and Dührssen's incisions made in the cervix at the 10 o'clock and 2 o'clock positions. This is rarely necessary, however, and it is an accepted obstetric principle that full dilatation, except in extraordinary conditions, is requisite for forceps delivery.
2. The membranes must be ruptured. If left intact, the forceps will slip, and traction upon the membranes may detach an edge of the placenta. Moreover, the need for forceps delivery cannot be determined with certainty until the membranes are ruptured.
3. The head must be engaged in the pelvis, and there must be no real obstruction to further advancement. Application of forceps to a head that is movable above the pelvic brim is indefensible in modern obstetric practice. Moreover, mere engagement, although it suffices for purposes of definition, is far less favorable than location of the head at or below station +2. The higher the station at the time delivery is begun, the greater the risk to mother and baby. If molding is extreme, with large caput succedaneum, the scalp may be almost at the introitus when the biparietal diameter is still at the inlet. One should not apply forceps if the sinciput can be felt above the symphysis.
4. The child must present correctly. All vertex presentations and face presentations with chin anterior are suitable. Chin posterior and brow presentations are not suitable for the application of forceps. No attempt should be made to apply forceps to the breech.

TYPES OF OBSTETRIC FORCEPS

Two groups of obstetric forceps are available. The so-called classic forceps are those with the standard cephalic and pelvic curves already described in connection with outlet forceps (see Chapter 31). In addition to these, special forceps have been designed for dealing with certain specific problems. Since the invention of the first obstetric forceps, obstetricians have made major or minor modifications of the classic instrument to fit their individual tastes; more than 600 types have survived, each named for the physician who made the modification.

The obstetrician in training should have the opportunity to "get the feel" of each of the major modifications of the classic forceps and of the special forceps. By the time formal training is complete, he or she should have settled upon one instrument for traction in the occiput anterior position, one or two for rotating the head, and one for application to the after-coming head in the case of breech presentation. The commonly used forceps are illustrated in Figure 34–1.

APPLICATION OF FORCEPS

Two methods of forceps application are available: pelvic application and cephalic application. *Pelvic application* involves merely placing the forceps in the pelvic cavity and applying the blades to the presenting part so that they will lock, without reference to the position of the head. Mention is made of this application only for its historic interest; except in the most extraordinary circumstances, it is not permissible in modern obstetrics since it imposes stresses the head can rarely tolerate. If the forceps cannot be accurately applied to the head, cesarean section is almost invariably the proper alternative. In the *cephalic application,* the blades are applied precisely to the occipitomental diameter of the head. Provided this application is accurate and the movements are made gently, deliberately, and with knowledge of what is to be accomplished, considerable traction can be exerted and any needed rotation performed with safety. Cephalic application of forceps along the occipitomental diameter of the head is possible in several different situations, including the occiput anterior, occiput transverse, and occiput posterior positions and the face presentation (Fig. 34–2). It may also be used for the after-coming head in breech presentations.

When the forceps is applied to the head in the occiput anterior position, which is most customary, the posterior fontanel should be a fingerbreadth anterior to the plane of the shanks and equidistant from the sides of the blades; the sagittal suture should be perpendicular to the middle of the plane of the shanks in its entirety; and the fenestrations of the blades should be high enough in the pelvis that they can be barely felt or not felt at all.

CHOICE OF FORCEPS

For traction to the occiput anterior, most obstetricians in America and the United Kingdom prefer the Simpson instrument or one of its modifications. If this in-

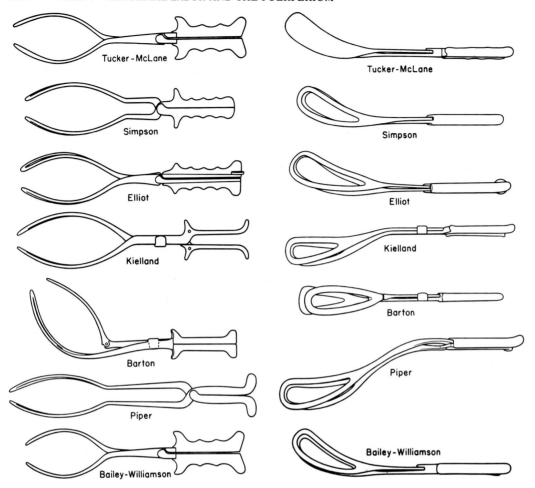

FIG. 34–1. Commonly used forceps. (Douglas RG, Stromme WB: Operative Obstetrics. New York, Appleton, 1957)

strument is accurately applied and traction is made in the proper diameters of the pelvis, considerable force may be exerted without injury to the baby. Accordingly, the Simpson or Elliot forceps is considered the safest in ordinary situations when moderate traction is needed.

For rotation from the occiput posterior to the occiput anterior position, most operators prefer the Tucker–McLane instrument, the Luikart modification of the Simpson forceps, or the Kielland forceps. If molding is marked, forceps with a round cephalic curve, such as the Tucker–McLane, may not fit the head well and may in fact cut the infant's cheek at the level of the zygomatic arch, especially if any traction is made. Hence, a forceps with a more elongated cephalic curve (*e.g.,* the Luikart–Simpson) may be preferred. Although the most frequent use of the Kielland forceps is in the occiput transverse position, it may also be used in the occiput posterior position.

For forceps rotation from the occiput transverse, either the Barton or Kielland forceps can be used. In some cases, especially when there is sufficient space posterior to the head, the Simpson forceps may be applied directly to the transverse, although this is relatively unusual in the classic transverse arrest because of flat pelvis.

For forceps delivery of the after-coming head, the Piper modification of the Simpson forceps is used in America virtually to the exclusion of all others.

In the United Kingdom the Wrigley forceps (a lightened modification of the Simpson instrument with shortened shanks and handles) is extremely popular for low and outlet forceps deliveries and for application to the after-coming head.

Although it is important to select the proper instrument, it must be emphasized that the results depend far more upon the skill and judgment of the operator than upon the selection of any particular forceps.

ABNORMAL POSITIONS THAT CAUSE DYSTOCIA

CONDUCT OF LABOR IN FETOPELVIC DYSTOCIA

In most cases of dystocia the possibility of a problem can be suspected within 6 hours of the onset of labor; the abnormality can usually be diagnosed with certainty in the next 6 hours, and it should be dealt with, usually by delivery, before 18 hours of labor have elapsed. If the problem is due to fetopelvic dystocia, it can usually be suspected, diagnosed, and dealt with in a much shorter time than if the cause is dysfunctional labor.

In fetopelvic dystocia with vertex presentation, difficulty may be suggested by either 1) excessively slow progress in the first stage (as is not unusual if the fetus is in the occiput posterior position or if the head does not fit well into the lower uterine segment because, for example, of inlet disproportion) or 2) a presenting part that remains at a relatively high station and cannot be easily impressed to deep engagement. In such cases, x-ray pelvimetry may be of special value, provided it is done by a technique that 1) includes a standing (*not* recumbent) lateral film and a film that shows inlet shape, and 2) permits the obstetrician to obtain a three-dimensional concept of the pelvis at all levels. One such technique is described in Chapter 28. Techniques that do not provide this information (*e.g.,* Colcher–Sussman) are not helpful.

If the labor is to be longer than usual, attention should be given to hydration, regular emptying of the bladder, and sedatives and analgesics as needed.

In conducting the second stage, it is emphasized that the ease and safety of midforceps delivery are much greater if maximum descent and maximum molding have been attained. Moreover, when rotation is incomplete, the lower the head, the greater the likelihood of spontaneous rotation to the anterior. Hence, unless an indication for intervention arises, the second stage should be permitted to proceed as long as progress is made, up to a maximum of 2 hours in the primigravida or 1 hour in the multipara. After a second stage of this duration, there is a risk of uterine rupture and constriction ring dystocia.

The woman's voluntary bearing-down effort may be of great importance in advancing the head to a level from which it can be safely delivered. The ability to make this effort can be impaired by heavy systemic analgesia or too early use of conduction anesthesia. It can be greatly facilitated by the thoughtful encouragement of the attendant and, in many cases, by two or three deep breaths of 50% nitrous oxide and 50% oxygen at the beginning of each second-stage contraction. Women who have had special training for childbirth are usually most effective in making this effort.

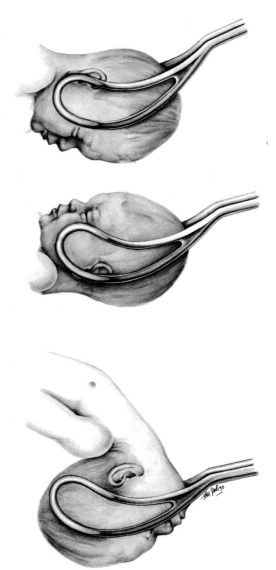

FIG. 34-2. Forceps correctly applied along occipitomental diameter in various positions of head. *A.* Occiput anterior. *B.* Occiput posterior. *C.* Mentum anterior.

OCCIPUT POSTERIOR POSITION

When the fetal occiput lies in one of the posterior quadrants of the pelvis, the position is defined as *occiput posterior.* The mechanism of labor and the role of the pelvis in persistent and arrested occiput posterior position are considered in Chapter 30. Suffice it to mention here that the anthropoid pelvis predisposes; that spontaneous rotation may be expected if the transverse diameter of the midpelvis is wide enough to permit the anteroposterior diameter of the head to ro-

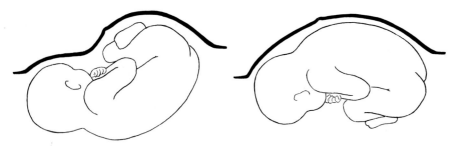

FIG. 34–3. Variation in maternal abdominal contour with fetus in occiput posterior and occiput anterior positions.

tate at this level; that transverse narrowing of the mid-pelvis because of either convergent sidewalls or prominent spines may prevent spontaneous rotation; and that in the latter case, if the lower sacrum is sufficiently forward, artificial rotation may be needed for delivery. In clinical practice, approximately 70% of fetuses in the occiput posterior position rotate spontaneously; but the rest require artificial rotation or, if the woman's sacrum is far posterior, traction as a direct occiput posterior before the head can advance.

Diagnosis

As is true of all obstetric complications, it is important that an exact diagnosis be made at the earliest possible time, for the intelligent conduct of labor depends upon it. Three major factors are concerned in the diagnosis of occiput posterior position: 1) the character of labor, 2) the abdominal contour and the findings on palpation, and 3) the findings on vaginal examination.

Character of Labor. Efficiency of the uterine contractions depends to an important extent upon the even fitting of the presenting part to the lower uterine segment. In occiput anterior position this fitting is optimal, while in occiput posterior position the fitting may be improper. Although there are exceptions to this generalization, when the child is in the occiput posterior position, labor is often desultory and relatively ineffective. Accentuated backache and, in the second stage, gaping of the anus are common. When labor does not progress at the expected rate or when the contractions are of poor quality, the first thought should be the possibility of occiput posterior position.

Abdominal Contours. When the fetus is in the occiput anterior position, the woman's lower abdomen, from umbilicus to vulva, has a gentle convexity, since the fetal head is well flexed and the depression at the nape of the neck is more or less ironed out. When the fetus is in the occiput posterior position, a considerable depression occurs between the fetal chin and the small parts, and this is reflected by a concavity above the level of the symphysis (Fig. 34–3). Although this is not an invariable finding, especially if the fetal head is deeply engaged or the maternal bladder is full, its presence should suggest the possibility of occiput posterior position.

In most instances, the fetal back and small parts can be felt on abdominal examination. Particularly if the fetal back is on the right, occiput posterior position should be considered.

Findings on Vaginal Examination. If the cervix is fully dilated or is so situated and sufficiently pliable that the examiner can readily sweep the examining finger anteriorly over the head from left to right, and if the fetus is in the occiput posterior position, the four suture lines that enter the anterior fontanel will be encountered. (One can rarely reach the posterior fontanel.) This confirms the diagnosis of occiput posterior position. In early labor, or if the cervix is posterior so that this examination would be difficult or painful, the definitive diagnosis may be left for later. If the first two factors are present, however, the physician should make the tentative diagnosis of occiput posterior position and should conduct the labor accordingly. Prior knowledge, either by x-ray or clinical examination, of an anthropoid pelvis strengthens the probability of occiput posterior position.

Management of Labor

Since labor is apt to be longer, full attention should be given to fetal monitoring, judicious use of sedatives and analgesics, attention to hydration, and, in some cases, stimulation of labor by oxytocics.

Anterior rotation may be encouraged during either the first or second stage of labor by allowing the fetal spine to fall toward the anterior abdominal wall of the mother. This can be achieved either by placing the mother in the Sims position on the side opposite that to which the fetal occiput is directed or, somewhat more effectively, by placing the mother in the knee–chest position through from two to four uterine contractions.

Unless intervention becomes necessary, a full second stage should be permitted to achieve maximum molding and maximum descent of the head.

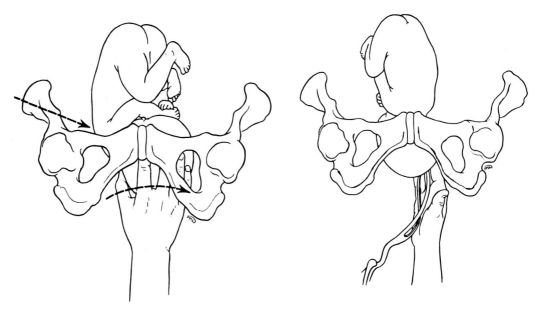

FIG. 34–4. Manual rotation of head in right occiput posterior (ROP) position. *A.* Head grasped by whole hand and rotated to anterior position; assistant pushes shoulder toward patient's left. *B.* Rotation complete; right hand maintains head in position while left blade of forceps is applied. Right hand is used for rotation, regardless of whether from ROP or LOP, and left blade of forceps is always introduced first. (Danforth WC: Am J Obstet Gynecol 23:360, 1932)

Management of Delivery

As noted earlier, approximately 70% of fetuses in the occiput posterior position rotate to the anterior spontaneously; delivery in such cases offers no unusual problem. Nor does a special problem arise in those that are normally destined to deliver face to pubes without rotation. In the monkey, the posterior mechanism and spontaneous delivery face to pubes are the rule. In a woman with a classic anthropoid pelvis and a sacrum directed far posterior, a similar outcome of labor may be expected, and no intervention is required. With such a pelvis, if uterine inertia results in the arrest of the head in the occiput posterior position very deep in the pelvis, the head may be gently delivered in the direct posterior by outlet forceps. In either case, a wide episiotomy is usually required.

Artificial rotation is needed if occiput posterior position persists because of 1) a forward lower sacrum that impedes progress or 2) transverse narrowing of the midpelvis that prevents spontaneous rotation. Two techniques are available: manual rotation and forceps rotation.

It is emphasized that the resident in training should master a technique for rotation from the occiput posterior and should use it with confidence when the circumstances are appropriate. The present trend away from the deliberate performance of a difficult vaginal delivery is entirely correct. However, the trend toward cesarean section in all cases in which the head cannot be readily advanced in the posterior is clearly not in the best interests of either mother or baby. In most cases, rotation from the posterior is not a difficult procedure,

and it can usually be accomplished much more quickly and safely than cesarean section.

Manual Rotation. Manual rotation is preferred by some obstetricians. Many techniques have been described, one of which is shown in Figure 34–4. Basically, the head is grasped with the whole hand, fingers widely spread, and is elevated above the point of arrest. An assistant pushes the anterior fetal shoulder across the maternal abdomen. The rotation is then accomplished, and forceps are applied for delivery. This technique is especially favored by those who have a small hand. The operator whose hand is large will probably prefer forceps rotation. Both techniques are acceptable and widely used, but the obstetrician should master one and should use it exclusively unless unusual circumstances require a variant.

Forceps Rotation. Forceps rotation may be carried out 1) after elevating the head above the level of arrest, 2) at the level of arrest, or 3) by spiral advancement of the head. Spiral advancement of the head is to be eschewed except in the most extraordinary circumstances; it requires much force and is attended by a high probability of both fetal and maternal damage. Rotation at the level of arrest, as in Bill's rotation, is

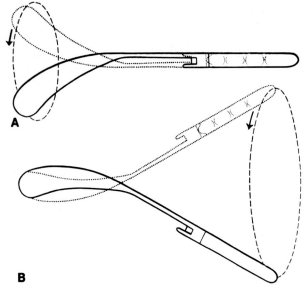

FIG. 34–5. Forceps rotation of head in occiput posterior position. *A.* Incorrect technique. *B.* Correct technique. If handles are rotated in same axis, blades describe wide arc and surely tear vagina. Handles must be swung widely and tips of blades kept at approximately same point. (Douglas RG, Stromme WB: Operative Obstetrics. New York, Appleton, 1957)

satisfactory if the spines are not prominent and if there is ample transverse space in the midpelvis; but in most circumstances rotation is easiest if the head is elevated above the level of arrest so that adequate transverse space is ensured. In the standard forceps rotation, classic forceps (preferably the Luikart–Simpson or Tucker–McLane) is applied to the posterior, then the head is elevated slightly and flexed. By swinging the handles of the forceps in a wide arc so the tips of the blades remain in the same axis, rotation is accomplished in a single sweep or preferably intermittently through short arcs, but in either case with the utmost gentleness (Figs. 34–5 and 34–6). When the rotation to the anterior position has been accomplished, one blade of the forceps is removed, while the other blade is left in place to prevent the head from spinning back to its former position. One blade of a second pair of forceps is applied opposite the splinting blade, the handles are rearranged to lock, the second blade is now inserted, and delivery is accomplished as though the position had originally been anterior.

If Kielland forceps is chosen, rotation may be carried out in the axis of the forceps, since this instrument has substantially no pelvic curve. When the rotation is accomplished, classic forceps may be substituted for the Kielland, since the lack of pelvic curve may prevent the use of the proper traction.

BROW PRESENTATION

With partial extension of the head, the brow of the infant may become the presenting part. The large (13.5 cm) occipitomental diameter of the head then presents to the pelvis as one diameter, the biparietal remaining as the other. Unless the pelvis is exceptionally large or the baby very small, spontaneous delivery with the head remaining in this position is unlikely; however, it is in these two situations that brow presentation is most frequently encountered. While loops of cord around the neck or some other anterior neck mass, such as a cystic hygroma, should be looked for as possible causes, they are seldom found.

Diagnosis

Diagnosis is difficult on abdominal examination, although the bony prominence of the occiput may be felt high during palpation downward along the fetal back. Vaginal and rectal examinations are often confusing, but the physician may be alerted to the possibility of brow presentation by the very high station. X-ray may be needed for diagnosis.

Management

Unless the head is markedly smaller than the pelvis, spontaneous delivery is not to be expected if the head remains in the brow presentation. It may correct spontaneously, converting either to a face presentation by further extension or to an occipital presentation by further flexion. Manual correction may be attempted but should be undertaken only with the membranes intact or at the time of their rupture, and with due awareness that the cord may prolapse before the head. Any such attempt should be quickly abandoned if it is not immediately successful. If conditions appear unfavorable for manual correction and active labor is in progress, it is entirely appropriate to perform cesarean section at once.

FACE PRESENTATION

With full extension of the head, the face of the infant may become the presenting part. The diameter that is perpendicular to the biparietal is, in this instance, the distance from beneath the chin to the bregma, a diameter very little greater than the 9.0–9.5 cm of the suboccipitobregmatic. In general, the prognosis for vaginal delivery in face presentation is relatively good insofar as diameters of the head are concerned. It is only when the chin (commonly used as the point of reference in face presentation) and fetal chest point posteriorly that difficulties arise. When the head reaches the upper midpelvis, it is already extended to

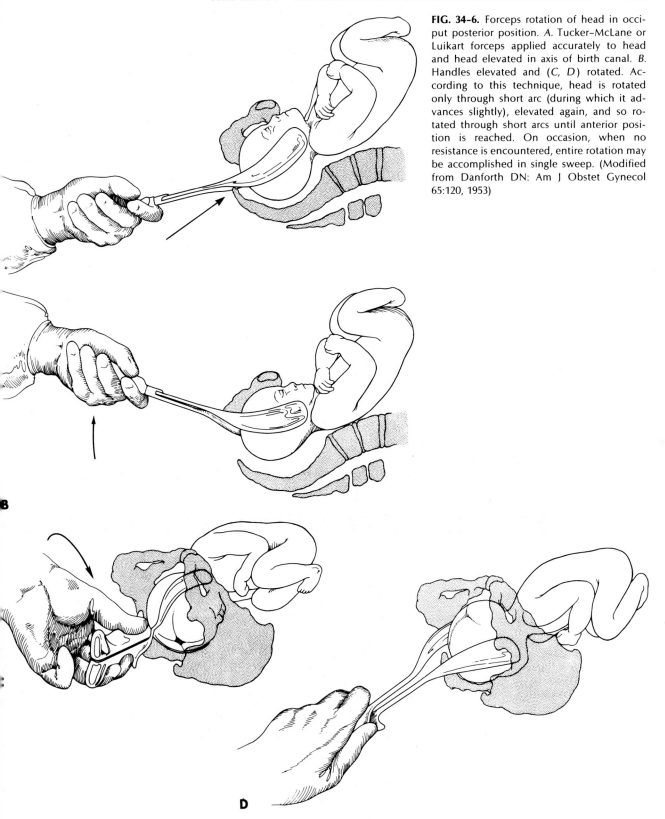

FIG. 34–6. Forceps rotation of head in occiput posterior position. *A.* Tucker–McLane or Luikart forceps applied accurately to head and head elevated in axis of birth canal. *B.* Handles elevated and (*C, D*) rotated. According to this technique, head is rotated only through short arc (during which it advances slightly), elevated again, and so rotated through short arcs until anterior position is reached. On occasion, when no resistance is encountered, entire rotation may be accomplished in single sweep. (Modified from Danforth DN: Am J Obstet Gynecol 65:120, 1953)

the maximum degree and cannot negotiate the pelvic curve (see Fig. 30–30).

Etiology

In many instances, face presentation is the end result of a brow presentation that has undergone further extension. Thus, face presentation is often seen under the same circumstances—a small infant in a large pelvis. In addition, any factors that prevent adequate flexion of the head may result in face presentation; thus, large size of the infant or some relative pelvic disproportion, particularly at the inlet, may favor its development. Abnormalities of the neck, while often mentioned as causes, are seldom found.

Diagnosis

The diagnosis can rarely be made on abdominal examination. Vaginal or rectal examination discloses an irregular presenting part, which at once suggests the following possibilities: 1) face presentation, 2) breech presentation (especially footling or full breech), 3) compound presentation, or 4) severe congenital anomaly (especially anencephaly). It is usually necessary to resolve these doubts by x-ray examination, particularly if the baby is large or there is some clinical evidence of relative disproportion.

Management

Since the diameters of the fetal head presenting are not significantly greater than normal, spontaneous delivery or delivery by outlet forceps can be anticipated if the chin is anterior. Attempts at conversion to an occiput presentation are not advised; when the chin remains posterior, forceps or manual rotation is rarely either safe or feasible. A mentum posterior position that persists after labor is established is best managed by cesarean section, regardless of parity or size of the baby.

TRANSVERSE ARREST

The term *transverse arrest* refers to the arrest of the fetal head in the transverse position, usually in the midpelvis, rarely at the outlet, with failure of progress for at least 30 min. The two major causes are 1) anteroposterior flattening in the midpelvis or lower pelvis, as occurs in the platypelloid or android pelvis, and 2) uterine inertia. The head ordinarily engages in the transverse position, the sagittal suture lying transversely across the pelvis. If there is anteroposterior narrowing in the midpelvis and outlet, the head tends to traverse these levels in the direct transverse position, without anterior rotation. In the gynecoid pelvis, anterior rotation tends to occur in the lower midpelvis.

In the latter case, if uterine inertia occurs prior to the time of internal rotation, progress may cease, the head remaining in the transverse position.

Management

The management of transverse arrest depends upon its cause.

If the pelvis is of normal configuration and adequate size, if the arrest occurs at a relatively low level, and if it is believed to have resulted only from desultory second-stage contractions, an oxytocin infusion, administered at a rate that will provide contractions every 2.0–2.5 min lasting 30–50 sec, often suffices to induce further descent, anterior rotation, and subsequent delivery either spontaneously or by outlet forceps. As an alternative, if the patient is fatigued, if there has been no progress for 30 min, if the head is at a low level, and if the obstetrician is certain the baby can be safely delivered, or if there is an indication for immediate delivery, classic forceps may be applied to the transverse position (or manual rotation may be done at the level of arrest) and the head rotated and delivered.

If the arrest is due to anteroposterior narrowing of the pelvis (a flat or platypelloid pelvis), its management depends on the depth of engagement, the need for prompt vaginal delivery, and the skill and experience of the operator. If progress ceases for 30 min or if elapsed time in the second stage requires termination of labor, cesarean section should be elected if the head is not deeply engaged (to or beyond station +3) or if there is any question of the adequacy of the pelvis below the point of arrest. If the head is deeply engaged, if the pelvis is considered adequate, and if the operator's skill and experience permit him to approach this kind of problem with confidence, a trial forceps may be appropriate. The attempt should be promptly abandoned if there is undue resistance.

In transverse arrest due to flat pelvis, the head must be advanced in the transverse position until the level for rotation on the pelvic floor is reached. Two techniques are available: one with Kielland forceps and one with Barton forceps. The Kielland forceps was designed originally for application to the head in deep transverse arrest. It has a sliding lock that facilitates application. Knobs are located on the handles; these should point toward the occiput, and before application the physician should face the perineum holding the articulated forceps as it will be applied to the head, with the knobs facing the occiput. In the classic application of the forceps, the anterior blade is introduced anteriorly with the concavity of the cephalic curve looking upward. The blade is then rotated 180°, away from the occiput and toward the knobs, and applies itself to the anterior parietal bone. In modern usage, it is more usual to introduce the anterior blade posteriorly or laterally and to "wander" it around the head until it lies next to the anterior parietal bone. The posterior

FIG. 34–7. Forceps advancement of head in transverse position. *A.* Introduction of anterior blade of Barton forceps in midline posteriorly. *B.* Anterior blade "wandered" to position in front of head; advantage of hinged blade is apparent. *C.* Posterior blade introduced, forceps locked, axis traction handle attached. (Barton LJ, Caldwell WE, Studdiford WE: Am J Obstet Gynecol 15:16, 1928)

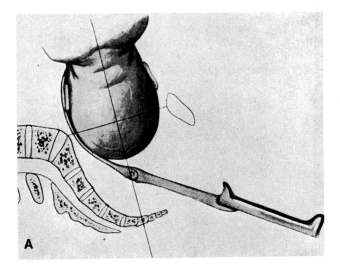

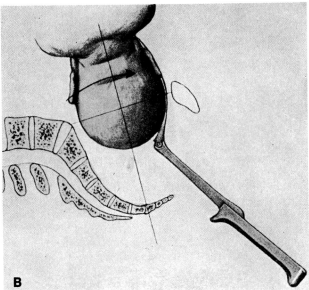

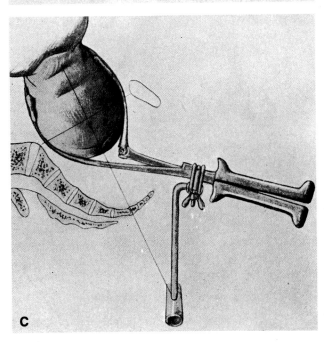

blade is then introduced and the forceps articulated. Traction is made as an occiput transverse until the head passes the area of anteroposterior narrowing. After anterior rotation, traction with the Kielland forceps must be made with great care because there is no pelvic curve on the forceps. Many operators prefer to substitute classic forceps at this point.

The Barton forceps was originally designed for application to a transversely arrested head at the pelvic inlet. In such instances today cesarean section delivery is the method of choice for mother and baby, but the Barton forceps may be used for delivery of a head in the occiput transverse position lower in the pelvis (Fig. 34–7). The hinged anterior blade is introduced posterior to the head and is "wandered" over the occiput or face until it lies over the anterior parietal bone. The posterior blade is introduced directly behind the head, and the blades are articulated, again assisted by a sliding lock. The head may be readily advanced in the transverse position, rotated, and classic forceps substituted for delivery. Both instruments are satisfactory for this midforceps operation, and each has its strong supporters. In skilled hands, the use of either instrument can be both easy and atraumatic. However, they can be highly damaging if undue force is required to accomplish delivery.

ABNORMAL PRESENTATIONS THAT CAUSE DYSTOCIA

TRANSVERSE LIE

When the infant lies in the transverse or one of the oblique diameters of the uterus, rather than presenting either by the breech or by the head, the situation is described as a *transverse lie.* Accurately, this might be described as a transverse presentation, but since the latter term has always given confusion with transverse positions of the vertex, the term transverse lie is preferable and is generally used.

Labor in transverse lie is fairly efficient so long as the membranes are intact and fit well into the lower pole of the uterus. When they rupture, the needed stimulus is lost, dysfunctional labor results, and full dilatation of the cervix is rarely achieved. Moreover, when the membranes rupture cord prolapse commonly follows; if it cannot be dealt with at once, the baby is doomed.

Etiology

An important cause of transverse lie is the presence of anything in the lower portion of the uterus that prevents engagement of the fetus in longitudinal lie. This is commonly the placenta. Indeed, if the fetus is found to be lying transversely or obliquely, placenta previa or some other lower uterine segment mass, such as a myoma, should be considered. However, most transverse lies are seen in multiparas with lax abdominal walls in which the uterus falls well forward, and the fetus simply fails to assume a longitudinal lie.

Diagnosis

Leopold's maneuvers (see page 365) should suggest the diagnosis, for the fetal ovoid lies transversely across the abdomen; neither head nor buttocks occupies the fundal portion of the uterus, and no presenting part can be palpated above the pelvic inlet. The diagnosis is confirmed when vaginal or rectal examination discloses the pelvis to be empty of fetal parts. Similar findings might be offered by a monster of the acardiac type, but this is so rare that the possibility should rest only fleetingly in the examiner's mind. If there should be any doubt, x-ray of the abdomen gives final information. The most common diagnostic error is to make only a casual abdominal examination and to note that on pelvic examination "the presenting part is not reached." Whenever the presenting part cannot be reached on vaginal or rectal examination, the most searching effort to make an exact diagnosis must be undertaken immediately. In the majority of such cases, the baby is found to be in the transverse lie or in an oblique lie (the head or breech being in the iliac fossa). The latter condition must be approached exactly as though the lie were transverse.

Management

Prior to 36 weeks' gestation, nothing need be done, since the presentation commonly corrects itself to a longitudinal lie. After 36 weeks, but before the onset of labor, weekly vaginal examinations should be done to detect the imminence of labor. If the cervix becomes soft, thin, and partially dilated, the patient should be admitted to the hospital and treated as though labor had begun. If the membranes rupture, the baby may be lost because of cord prolapse. Accordingly, if labor is thought to be imminent or has started, cesarean section should be performed immediately. There are only two possible exceptions.

External Version. If labor is just beginning, membranes are intact, and the uterus is not unduly irritable, it may be possible to push the head over the pelvic inlet and down into the pelvis. If the head can be caused to engage easily, the membranes can be ruptured; as the uterus gains tone, the head will maintain the new position. Management is then the same as in vertex presentation. No anesthesia should be employed for the external version, and fetal heart tones should be monitored constantly to ensure that cord complications do not occur. If there is any difficulty in accomplishing external version, immediate cesarean section should be elected.

Internal Podalic Version. Internal podalic version is no longer an acceptable method for delivery in transverse lie, regardless of how favorable the conditions may appear to be. In some of the older articles on this kind of management, an infant mortality of 40% and maternal deaths in excess of 5% are reported. If the baby is already dead, the physician may be tempted to deliver by this method to avoid an unproductive cesarean section. However, the maternal risk is so great that most obstetricians elect cesarean sections regardless of the condition of the baby.

BREECH PRESENTATION

When the fetus presents with the buttocks toward the pelvis, it is a *breech presentation*. The mortality from vaginal delivery of all infants presenting by the breech, preterm infants included, is about 5.5 times that of infants presenting by the vertex. If pre-term infants are excluded, the perinatal mortality in breech presentations is still 3.5 times higher in many large-scale studies, although accurate diagnosis, careful selection, and good management should reduce this to 1% or less. The majority of perinatal deaths in term breech births is accounted for by cord prolapse and other cord complications or by tentorial tears and cerebral hemorrhage during delivery of the after-coming head. Molding, of course, must occur in a matter of moments rather than hours, and the sudden stresses may be highly damaging to the delicate and vital supporting structures.

The fetal morbidity and mortality ascribable to breech delivery are so great that cesarean section is usually preferred, and in at least one hospital the specific approval of the department chairman is required in all cases in which it is intended to deliver a breech vaginally. In the term infant, the primary hazards are those mentioned in the preceding paragraph. In the preterm infant, the head is usually larger than the breech, and there is the danger of the after-coming head being trapped by the cervix and lower uterine segment that are dilated only enough to permit passage of the breech.

In breech presentation, the posture of the lower extremities affects the prognosis of labor. Three major possibilities (Fig. 34–8) are described as follows:

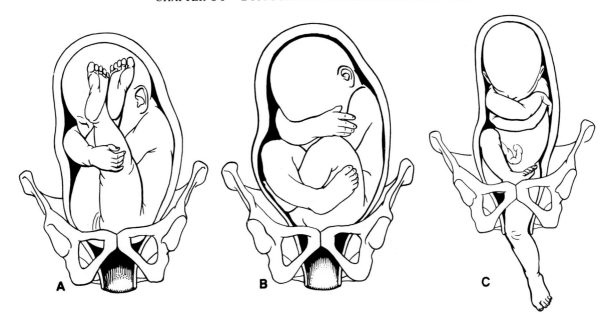

FIG. 34-8. Types of breech presentations. *A.* Frank breech. *B.* Complete or full breech. *C.* Incomplete breech (single footling). (Nursing Education Service, Ross Laboratories)

1. *Frank breech* means that the thighs are flexed on the abdomen and the legs are extended; thus, the infant's feet are at the chin.
2. *Complete breech* (full breech) means that the thighs are flexed on the abdomen and the legs are flexed on the thighs so that the infant is sitting tailor fashion and the feet present at the level of the buttocks.
3. *Incomplete breech* (footling breech) means that one or both thighs are extended so that the feet and legs present below the level of the breech. If one leg is completely extended and the other flexed, the presentation is described as a *single footling;* if both legs are extended below the level of the buttocks, it is described as a *double footling.*

Etiology

When the fetus is small in relation to the overall size of the uterine cavity, it tends to move about freely and may assume any presentation. It is only in the latter stages of pregnancy, particularly beyond 32 weeks' gestation, that the fetus accommodates itself to the shape of the uterus. Since the upper portion of the uterus is wider and the lower portion of the uterus and the lower uterine segment are narrower, the wider pole of the fetus tends to accommodate to the larger part of the uterus, and the smaller pole to the less roomy portions. In the preterm fetus, the head is the larger pole and tends to occupy the fundus. At term, however, the breech is the larger and occupies the fundus unless this space should be compromised by

such factors as a fundal septum, the placenta, or a large fundal fibroid. The incidence of breech presentation at various fetal weights is shown in Table 34–1.

Diagnosis

The Leopold maneuvers for abdominal examination usually, but not always, identify the fetal head in the uterine fundus and the breech in the pelvis. The fetal heart tones are generally best heard above the umbilicus, but this is not a reliable sign. On vaginal examination, the presenting part is usually irregular and may be confused with a face or compound (head and arm) presentation, or a cranial abnormality. If there is doubt when the patient is admitted in labor, the diagnosis should be made by x-ray of the abdomen. The course of labor and complications to be anticipated depend to a considerable extent on the position of the legs, and ef-

TABLE 34-1. INCIDENCE OF BREECH PRESENTATION ACCORDING TO FETAL WEIGHT

Fetal Weight (g)	Incidence (%)
1000	23
1500	12
2000	8
> 3000	3

forts should be made to determine whether the breech is frank, complete, or incomplete.

If a breech presentation is diagnosed during pregnancy, external version (see page 366) has been advocated to substitute the more favorable vertex presentation for the less favorable breech. However, as term approaches, spontaneous conversion to the vertex is likely to occur.

Decision as to Method of Delivery

At the time of admission to the hospital, an abdominal x-ray should be taken to confirm the presentation and to determine the attitude of the baby. A tentative decision should then be made whether vaginal delivery is appropriate or whether cesarean section should be elected. The factors important in making this decision have been summarized by Zatuchni and Andros in a "breech scoring index" that can serve as a useful guide. According to this index, 0, 1, or 2 points are assigned for factors of increasing parity, prior breech delivery, cervical dilatation, station, decreasing gestational age, and estimated fetal weight. The authors suggest that those whose score is 3 or less at the onset of labor be delivered by cesarean section; those with a score of 4 are carefully reevaluated; those with a score of 5 or more may be expected to deliver vaginally without difficulty. Like other recipes for the solution of clinical problems, the index may be helpful, but it should not be considered a substitute for the keen clinical judgment that is required in the evaluation of every breech presentation. Moreover, the index does not quite take into account all the factors the obstetrician must consider in making such an evaluation. If the evaluation is confined to the points listed in the index, some other factor of preeminent importance may be overlooked.

In general, *the factors that are favorable for vaginal delivery* include:

1. Gestational age of more than 36 and less than 38 weeks (If the pregnancy is of *less* than 36 weeks' duration and the baby less than 6 lb, the head is apt to be larger than the breech and may be trapped in the cervix, which is dilated sufficiently for the breech to pass, but not the head.)
2. Estimated fetal weight of more than 6 lb and less than 7 lb
3. Presenting part at or below station 0 at the onset of labor
4. Cervix soft, effaced, and dilated 3 cm or more
5. Ample gynecoid or anthropoid pelvis (in which the after-coming head can be expected to enter the pelvis in the direct occiput anterior position)
6. History of prior breech delivery of baby weighing more than 7 lb or prior vertex delivery of baby weighing more than 8 lb
7. Frank breech presentation

In general, *the factors that are unfavorable for vaginal delivery* include:

1. Gestational age of less than 36 or more than 38 weeks
2. Estimated fetal weight of less than 6 lb or more than 7 lb
3. Presenting part at or above −1 station
4. Cervix firm, incompletely effaced, less than 3 cm dilated
5. History of difficult prior vaginal delivery or no prior vaginal delivery
6. Android or flat pelvis (In breech, the head approaches the pelvis in the occiput anterior position; in android and flat pelves, the head may be required to rotate to the transverse position in order to pass through the inlet, thus causing difficulty in engagement.)
7. Footling or full breech presentation
8. Hyperextension of fetal head (demonstrated by x-ray—see below)

None of the aforementioned factors, unless extreme, should necessarily determine the desirability of vaginal delivery or the need for cesarean section. All must be assessed and the decision made in terms of the entire picture.

The inherent hazard of breech presentation is such that some obstetricians prefer to deliver all breeches by cesarean section. However, several recent studies suggest that vaginal delivery is entirely appropriate in certain carefully selected cases of breech presentation, and it has the special advantage of avoiding the risks of cesarean section. This trend is becoming increasingly apparent, but the importance of the careful selection of cases and the obstetrician's proficiency in breech delivery must be emphasized. The need for proficiency is illustrated not only by the cases in which there is a choice between vaginal or abdominal delivery, but also by those in which delivery must be vaginal because the breech is already crowning or through the introitus when the patient is admitted, or because fetal distress or some major maternal complication toward the end of labor makes instant delivery mandatory.

In evaluating fetopelvic relations and the operations necessary for delivery, the physician must be aware of the normal mechanism of labor for breech delivery as outlined in Chapter 30. Each of the three distinct mechanisms (breech, shoulders, and head) must be specifically anticipated with awareness that the longest fetal diameter (the bitrochanteric, the bisacromial, the suboccipitobregmatic) should traverse the widest part of the pelvis at any given level. Accordingly, the performance of a breech delivery requires not only knowledge that the baby can traverse the pelvis, but also knowledge of the pelvic architecture so the optimal diameters can be utilized.

In summary, the physician should decide at the

onset of labor if the circumstances are favorable and the size of the fetus will permit its ready vaginal delivery through this maternal pelvis. If not, delivery should be by cesarean section.

It is sometimes said that there can be no trial of labor in breech presentation, but the statement must be qualified. Of the four Ps concerned in the efficiency of labor, the early consideration of the pelvis and passenger have already been emphasized. The influence of the powers and the psyche can be assessed as labor progresses. If there is no fetopelvic disproportion, cervical dilatation and descent of the breech should occur progressively. If contractions are inefficient or the presenting part remains unengaged, this may signal unrecognized disproportion. Oxytocin stimulation in breech presentation after arrest of progress in the active phase of labor has led to poor fetal outcomes and should rarely be used, since lack of progress often reflects fetopelvic abnormalities. In these contexts, trial of labor does have a place in the management of breech presentation.

Influence of Fetal Leg Position. The position of the fetal legs considerably influences the course and outcome of labor. In frank breech, the body is splinted by the legs reaching up underneath the chin. Lateral flexion of the fetus may be inhibited, and the breech in this position does not always descend satisfactorily in the pelvis, particularly if the anteroposterior diameters are reduced. It should be noted that the frank breech presentation is more common in the primigravida, while complete and incomplete breech presentations are more common in the multipara. Thus, failure of lateral flexion is more common in the first delivery. Dysfunctional labor occurs more often in complete than in frank breech, since the breech does not fit evenly into the cervix and lower uterine segment.

The completely flexed extremities usually occupy the pelvic cavity satisfactorily enough to exclude prolapse of the cord, but this must be determined when the membranes rupture. The incomplete (single or double footling) breech presents a real risk of cord prolapse, since the presenting part tends to fill the pelvis poorly. Such a presentation is more common when the fetus is preterm, compounding the problems of such a delivery.

Influence of Attitude of the Fetal Head. Hyperextension attitudes of the fetal head (Fig. 34–9) are unusual, but they can be an ominous sign in breech presentation. If the abdominal x-ray taken on admission reveals hyperextension of 90° or more (the angle between the cervical vertebrae and a line constructed as an upward extension of the main axis of the upper thoracic vertebrae), delivery by cesarean section should be elected. If the angle is less than 90° and all other conditions are favorable for vaginal delivery, this may be pursued; however, a repeat film should be taken later in labor to be sure the extension has not increased. The cause of hyperextension is not known. Behrman considers most of the cases to be due to spasm or hypertonus of the neck muscles. Some of the cases appear to be related to Down's syndrome. In others, a cord around the neck has been implicated.

The keys to management of labor in the breech presentation are 1) early determination of fetopelvic relations and prediction of whether they will permit vaginal delivery, 2) determination of the exact position of the extremities, and 3) observation for prolapse of the umbilical cord. Electronic fetal monitoring should be continuous throughout labor.

Management of Delivery

In another era, before cesarean section was used so commonly in breech presentation, it was essential that the obstetrician be qualified to deal not only with the "easy" breech delivery, but also with the very serious problems that can occur at each step of the delivery. The earlier references appended to this chapter describe such problems and the means of dealing with them. In addition, this is one area of obstetrics in which the manikin or bony pelvis and fetal doll are by no means obsolete. Those who seek proficiency in vaginal breech delivery will not encounter enough patients so delivered to acquire confidence in their approach to even the most favorable cases. Assiduous practice with a mounted bony pelvis and fetal doll can be immensely helpful. Before a breech delivery this device can also be valuable in demonstrating to an assistant exactly what he or she is expected to do during delivery of the breech, the shoulders, and the head, so there will be no hesitancy or need for instruction as the delivery unfolds. There are three basic modes of delivery of the breech: spontaneous delivery, assisted breech delivery, and breech extraction. With either of the latter two, the after-coming head may be delivered by manual maneuvers or by forceps.

Spontaneous Breech Delivery. The greatest risk to the fetus occurs in spontaneous breech delivery. The spontaneous and often unattended delivery is commonly preterm, and this plus precipitous delivery, often with sudden changes in intracranial pressure in the infant, contributes to the high mortality among these babies. Precipitous delivery should be avoided whenever possible by careful observation of the patient, and attempts should be made, even if the mother is exerting strong expulsive force, to guide, control, and prevent too rapid delivery of the head.

Assisted Breech Delivery of Body. The ideal mode of delivery is assisted breech delivery. The buttocks, or buttocks and feet, of the infant should be crowning, distending the vulva with each contraction. At this point, a generous episiotomy should be made, even if

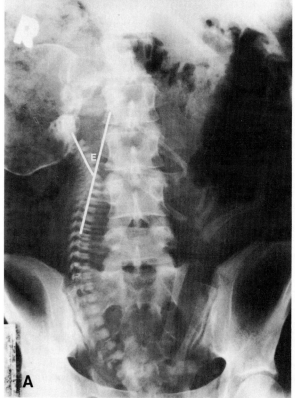
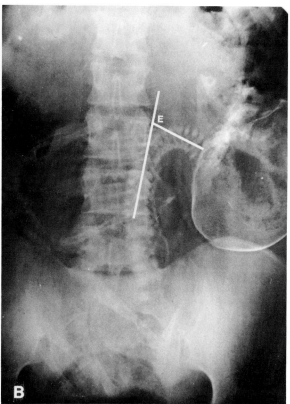
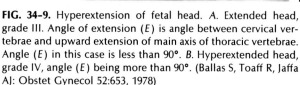

FIG. 34–9. Hyperextension of fetal head. *A.* Extended head, grade III. Angle of extension (*E*) is angle between cervical vertebrae and upward extension of main axis of thoracic vertebrae. Angle (*E*) in this case is less than 90°. *B.* Hyperextended head, grade IV, angle (*E*) being more than 90°. (Ballas S, Toaff R, Jaffa AJ: Obstet Gynecol 52:653, 1978)

the baby is relatively small, so that extra room is available for any manipulation that may be needed. If episiotomy is deferred until it is really needed, it may be too late. With the next contraction the patient should be urged to bear down and should spontaneously deliver the baby to the umbilicus. While anesthesia is not a point of discussion here, it should be stated that regardless of what mode of anesthesia is employed, the delivery is facilitated if the patient maintains voluntary abdominal powers until the baby is delivered to the umbilicus. Thus, local or pudendal block or low spinal or epidural anesthesia serve satisfactorily among the regional anesthesias; if a general anesthesia is to be employed, it should ordinarily not be instituted until this point.

In complete breech the legs are already extended. In frank breech it may be necessary to bring down each leg carefully, taking care to sweep them across the fetal flank and gently extract them one at a time.

After delivery of the buttocks, the fetal back *must* be facing the anterior; if the abdomen is permitted to turn anteriorly, the difficulties can be insurmountable unless the position can be readily corrected by the method described by Piper and Bachman. The Prague maneuver, designed to deliver the baby with abdomen anterior and illustrated in many texts, is highly lethal; few babies survive the suggested manipulations.

The mother, if able, should again be urged to bear down, and gentle downward traction (at a 45° angle toward the floor) should be made with the baby held with one hand encircling either hip, the fingers on the abdomen, and the thumbs over the fetal sacrum (Fig. 34–10). This traction is facilitated if a sterile towel is wrapped about the body of the infant. A few inches of the umbilical cord should be pulled downward at this time to obviate undue traction on the cord.

Delivery of the baby should continue in a downward direction, and no attempt should be made to deliver the arms until the tip of one scapula can be seen. Continued downward traction may spontaneously deliver the arms and shoulders, but if it does not, the infant whose back is anterior or in one of the anterior quadrants, should be supported by the obstetrician or by an assistant and the posterior arm delivered first (Fig. 34–11). If the arm has not spontaneously dropped into the hollow of the sacrum, the physician should place

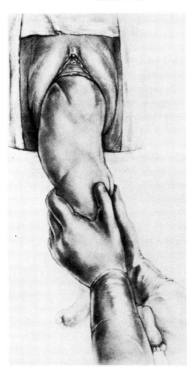

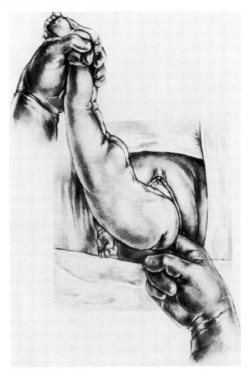

FIG. 34-10. Assisted breech delivery, downward traction on body. (Willson JR: The Management of Obstetric Difficulties, 6th ed. St. Louis, Mosby, 1961)

FIG. 34-11. Assisted breech delivery; delivery of posterior arm. (Willson JR: The Management of Obstetric Difficulties, 6th ed. St. Louis, Mosby, 1961)

two fingers along the humerus as a splint and gently wipe the arm downward over the chest. At this point, the anterior shoulder may drop beneath the symphysis so that the anterior arm will deliver. If it does not, the physician should gently rotate the back through 90°–180° so that the opposite shoulder becomes posterior and the second arm can be delivered. Throughout this time an assistant should be applying gentle downward pressure on the uterine fundus to be certain that the fetal head maintains flexion and satisfactorily follows the shoulders into the pelvis. For ease of delivery it is wise to form a sling of a second sterile towel around the baby's chest and hold the arms to the sides.

Delivery of After-Coming Head. At this point, it is generally found that the fetal head has maintained good flexion and descended readily into the pelvis so that the chin is near the infant's chest and the face is visible at the perineum. Delivery may be accomplished manually at this point in two classic fashions or a combination thereof. With the infant astride the physician's arm, the index and middle fingers are applied to the malar eminences on the infant's face and pressure is exerted toward the chest so as to maintain flexion of the head. The finger should not be inserted into the

infant's mouth, however, as serious injury can result. Gentle downward traction is then made by the opposite hand with the index finger hooked over one shoulder and the middle finger over the other (Mauriceau–Smellie–Veit maneuver; Fig. 34–12). Alternatively, the infant may be supported on the obstetrician's arm and flexion of the head maintained as before, while the obstetrician applies pressure from above downward on the uterine fundus and the fetal head through the mother's abdomen (Wigand–Martin maneuver). This careful downward pressure may also be maintained by an assistant.

If there is any delay in proper flexion or descent of the head, it is wise to apply *forceps to the aftercoming head* and effect a controlled delivery. The Piper forceps is commonly used in the United States. It has a standard cephalic curve and fenestrated blades, but the shank is joined to the blades at such an angle that the blades remain horizontal beneath the infant's body when properly applied rather than extending at an upward angle as do standard forceps applied to the aftercoming head (Fig. 34–13). In applying the Piper forceps, the physician must remember that the fetal head is tightly held against the vaginal tissues by muscle pressure and surface tension, and inserting a finger laterally will release the head somewhat. If the forceps

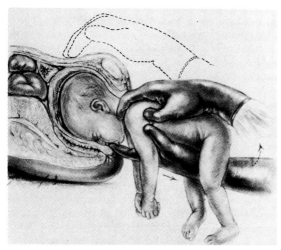

FIG. 34–12. Assisted breech delivery; Mauriceau-Smellie-Veit maneuver. (Willson JR: The Management of Obstetric Difficulties, 6th ed. St. Louis, Mosby, 1961)

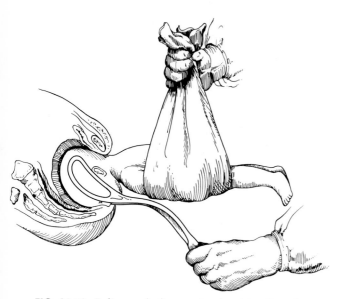

FIG. 34–13. Delivery of after-coming head by Piper forceps. Arms and body of infant are held in a towel sling as recommended by Savage. Assistant grasps towel or infant's feet or both. Operator delivers head by flexion, keeping handles below horizontal. (Modified from Dennen EH: Forceps Delivery. Philadelphia, Davis, 1964)

is to be inserted, it is wise to place four fingers of the opposite hand between the vaginal wall and the fetal head to guide the forceps into place. Because of the angle the shank makes with the blade, the forceps should be inserted with the shank and handles almost horizontal. When the blades are locked, traction can

be made and the head delivered by flexion as the physician gradually lifts the handles upward.

Breech Extraction. Breech extraction is the maneuver in which the physician intervenes before the buttocks have completely passed through the introitus. The procedure is permissible for a second twin that presents by the breech or requires internal podalic version because of a transverse lie.

In singleton pregnancy, full and footling breech usually offer no difficulty; the feet are readily accessible and the legs and buttocks can usually be delivered without incident. Breech extraction in frank breech is another matter. Not only is it one of the most difficult of obstetric maneuvers, but also it imposes great risk on both mother and baby; cesarean section is preferred if this is a reasonable alternative. In modern obstetrics the operation is usually reserved for 1) delivery of a second twin, 2) cases in which the physician is already committed (for whatever reason) to vaginal delivery and the breech cannot be delivered by the mother's voluntary effort, or 3) cases in which instant vaginal delivery is made mandatory by severe fetal distress or some maternal problem in which cesarean section is not feasible.

Breech extraction should not be attempted under regional or local anesthesia. Deep inhalation anesthesia, usually with halothane, is necessary to provide the required uterine relaxation. When the uterus is sufficiently relaxed, the appropriate hand (the left if the fetal back is to the mother's left) is introduced along the posterior aspect of the fetal legs. If the umbilical cord is found between the legs, it should be disentangled before the extraction is begun. Heavy digital pressure in the popliteal fossa (Pinard's maneuver) causes the knee to flex, making it possible to trigger the fingers over the ankle, to grasp the foot between index and middle fingers, and to deliver it into and through the vagina by downward traction. It is usually desirable that both feet be so delivered at once; but if this is not feasible, traction on the delivered leg toward the mother's thigh causes the buttocks to advance so they are "sitting" on the perineum sacrum posterior. With the help of a finger in the opposite groin, the physician now moves the delivered leg toward the mother's opposite leg, thus bringing the sacrum to the anterior position and permitting delivery of the other leg by upward pressure in the popliteal fossa, then sweeping the leg out across the baby's flank. The remainder of the delivery is conducted as noted in preceding paragraphs.

Importance of Physician Assistant. A key factor in management of breech delivery is skilled assistance. Hospitals that have made it mandatory for two qualified physicians to be present at every breech delivery have demonstrated a marked reduction in perinatal mortality associated with breech deliveries. The pres-

ence of a second physician for consultation and assistance may be expected to decrease the risk if breech delivery is elected.

SHOULDER PRESENTATION

Regardless of whether or not the arm is prolapsed, shoulder presentation is a major complication that must be recognized as early in labor as possible. The shoulder fits quite well into the lower pole of the uterus, and labor usually proceeds apace. This may result in neglect, which inevitably leads to rupture of the uterus. Many such cases are recorded in the earlier literature, and at least 10 of the 90-odd frozen sagittal sections published near the turn of the century were of women who died from this complication. If shoulder presentation is diagnosed before labor, nothing needs to be done, since the problem will likely resolve spontaneously. If diagnosed in early labor, it should be dealt with at once by cesarean section.

If the diagnosis is made late in labor the problem is much more serious because of the threat of uterine rupture and the other hazards of prolonged, obstructed labor. If the baby is living, cesarean section must be performed immediately, despite the risk of infection. If the baby is dead and there is a possibility that the uterus has ruptured, delivery must also be by cesarean section; the uterine defect should be repaired if this is feasible or the uterus removed if it is not.

If the baby is dead, the cervix fully dilated, and the uterus intact, the physician must choose between a destructive operation and vaginal delivery, or cesarean section. Those who work in developing countries and have much experience in dealing with obstructed labor are satisfied that, in their hands, the safest and most expeditious means of dealing with such a case is to tie a tape to the prolapsed wrist (so the arm will not be lost), and to decapitate with the Blond–Heidler saw (*not* a Braun hook or other instrument); the thorax and trunk are readily delivered by traction on the arm, and the head is retrieved by traction in the mouth or by a blunt hook in the formen magnum. As discussed in Chapter 39, destructive operations of this kind can be extremely difficult, and for the uninitiated cesarean section may offer the safer alternative.

COMPOUND PRESENTATION

Compound presentation refers to prolapse of the fetal hand alongside the presenting breech or vertex, or the foot alongside the head. The combination of hand and vertex is usually least troublesome; as the head advances, the hand tends to remain in place so that it is ultimately out of the way. The combination of hand and breech also tends to resolve spontaneously, but it must be verified that it is the hand and not the foot

that is prolapsed (the hand has no heel, and fingers can be readily moved in any direction).

The combination of foot and head may be more serious, and it also tends to be complicated by cord prolapse. If the foot cannot be pushed upward as labor advances, cesarean section is the wisest choice. Version and extraction may be tempting, but this operation carries the same great risks that obtain when it is used for the delivery of an infant in transverse lie.

CEPHALOPELVIC DISPROPORTION THAT CAUSES DYSTOCIA

Cephalopelvic disproportion can produce dystocia in two ways. If the head is too large to pass through the pelvis, it cannot advance beyond the level of obstruction. If this is at the inlet, the problem can usually be recognized early, since the head fails to engage. If the narrowed pelvic diameters are at the midpelvis or outlet, the cephalopelvic relations may be difficult to assess until the head reaches the level in question; often it is wise to wait until full dilatation to note whether sufficient molding may be achieved to permit the head to advance.

Test of labor is a retrospective term, used when the patient has made a good voluntary effort for 2 hours in the second stage, and the membranes have ruptured, but it is apparent that the baby cannot be safely delivered from below; cesarean section is elected. In this context, the test of labor is rarely applicable in modern obstetrics, for it is usually possible to diagnose absolute disproportion before 2 hours of the second stage have elapsed. A 2-hour second stage is not always to be avoided, however. As noted before, in certain cases of occiput posterior in which the obstruction to advancement is due only to the inability of the head to negotiate the pelvic curve in the occiput posterior position, a full second stage may be clearly desirable. Manual or forceps rotation is greatly facilitated if maximum descent and maximum molding have occurred before intervention is undertaken, and delivery may be very simple indeed if one waits until these two effects are achieved.

Cephalopelvic disproportion also may prevent the proper and even fitting of the presenting part into the lower uterine segment and cervix, one of the requisites for effective contractions in labor. If the head is held up by bony disproportion, it may fit improperly, resulting in irregular or ineffective uterine contractions. This sequence of events occurs most commonly in four situations: 1) in inlet disproportion, in which the head is prevented both from engaging into the pelvis and from settling evenly into the lower pole of the uterus; 2) in the pelvis that is inclined far posteriorly, the symphysis being located almost on a plumb line caudad to the sacral promontory (in this situation the head overrides the symphysis and cannot settle into

the lower pole of the uterus; 3) in a severely asymmetric pelvis where the uterine supports are irregularly placed so that even without true disproportion the fitting of the head may be uneven; and 4) in occiput posterior and similar positions in which the cephalopelvic relations are such that symmetric fitting is prevented. Asynclitism (see page 628) can produce the same effect. Instead of converting itself, the asynclitism may become permanent during the balance of the labor if a large enough caput succedaneum develops to hold the head in that position.

In all the aforementioned situations uterine inertia is the result. Some can be dealt with by stimulation with oxytocics; but if true cephalopelvic disproportion is the cause, it must be recognized at the earliest opportunity and cesarean section performed at once.

A developing caput on the fetal head may be some indication of the strength of contractions and the degree of disproportion. The station of the head is also a helpful sign, since a well-flexed occiput anterior position with the head at the level of the ischial spines indicates that the largest diameter of the fetal head has already entered the inlet. If the head is not at station 0, fundal or suprapubic pressure should be exerted in a downward direction in an attempt to determine whether the head will enter the pelvic inlet. History of previous deliveries may be unreliable, since a baby only slightly larger than those previously delivered may not be capable of passing through the pelvis. If progress is unsatisfactory and evaluation determines this to be due to disproportion, cesarean section delivery gives a lower perinatal mortality than a difficult operative vaginal delivery. Maternal morbidity is also lower.

There is little to be gained by allowing a patient to labor more than 2 hours in the second stage; indeed, there is great hazard. When, because of inlet contraction, the head fails to engage after 1 hour in the second stage, cesarean section should be elected.

SHOULDER DYSTOCIA

Shoulder dystocia is an extremely serious complication of labor that can be highly damaging, or even fatal. In Swartz's series of 31 cases, 16% of the babies died; only 18 escaped without injury. It occurs when the shoulders are too large to enter the inlet or when they present in an unfavorable diameter. It is to be remembered that the bisacromial diameter is the long diameter and that, when space is at a premium, this longest diameter must adapt to the long diameter of the inlet. As a rule, the shoulders present to the inlet with the bisacromial diameter either in the anteroposterior diameter of the pelvis or in one of the oblique diameters. If the shoulders are large and the anteroposterior diameter of the pelvis is relatively short, the anterior shoulder overhangs the symphysis and fails to engage. The problem is relatively unusual in the anthropoid pelvis, in which the anteroposterior diameter is long; it is more common in the flat pelvis.

Shoulder dystocia may be anticipated if the baby is large or if the inlet is small. It is suspected when, immediately after delivery of the head, the chin is observed to pull tightly back against the perineum, giving the face the appearance of double chin and chubby cheeks. It is diagnosed when slight downward pressure on the head fails to cause the anterior shoulder to stem under the symphysis. In dealing with this problem, it must be remembered that the cervical nerve roots can be seriously damaged by injudicious downward traction to the head in an effort to deliver the anterior shoulder; whenever such traction is made, it must be made gently and should be only of sufficient force to cause the advancement of the anterior shoulder that is *already* beneath the symphysis and approaching the subpubic arch.

When shoulder dystocia is diagnosed, the following steps must be taken at once:

1. The middle finger of one hand (the right hand if the baby's back is to the patient's left) is placed in the posterior axilla and the heaviest possible traction is made in an effort to advance the posterior shoulder into the hollow of the sacrum, thus providing more room for the anterior shoulder to stem beneath the symphysis. Simultaneously, an assistant exerts heavy suprapubic pressure (in an effort to cause the anterior shoulder to engage) and fundal pressure (to cause it to advance). If this fails,
2. Using the same hand as before, and the same abdominal pressure by an assistant, the obstetrician moves the posterior shoulder across the midline so as to bring the bisacromial diameter into an oblique diameter of the pelvis, which may permit the shoulder girdle to advance. If this fails,
3. The posterior shoulder is moved in an arc of 180° so that it now becomes anterior and the previously impacted anterior shoulder is now posterior, but at a lower level so that it may be delivered. This maneuver, the Woods screw principle, is a modification of Lövset's maneuver for the delivery of the shoulders in breech presentation. If this fails,
4. The appropriate hand is introduced posteriorly along the baby's thorax, the posterior forearm is grasped, and the posterior arm is delivered; the anterior shoulder and arm follow without difficulty. This step is almost invariably successful, but it produces uterine rupture in many of the cases. It should therefore be omitted if the baby is dead, and the physician should proceed immediately to
5. Cleidotomy, the ultimate solution. Deliberate fracture of the clavicle, although advocated in many texts, is rarely possible; the bone must be cut by

heavy embryotomy scissors, preferably through an incision made with the Simpson perforator.

DWARFISM

Dwarfism is not often encountered in obstetric practice, but the problems it poses can be considerable. Among obstetric patients of short stature, the pelvic inclination and configuration are commonly abnormal. Breech presentation is more common than it is in persons of normal stature. If the head does engage in late pregnancy, respiratory difficulty may be so severe as to preclude vaginal delivery or continuation of pregnancy. Some women of abnormally short stature can and do deliver vaginally, but cesarean section is customary because of either respiratory distress or poor fetopelvic relationships.

REFERENCES AND RECOMMENDED READING

GENERAL

Donald I: Practical Obstetric Problems, 5th ed. London, Lloyd–Duke, 1979

Douglas RG, Stromm WB: Operative Obstetrics, 3rd ed. New York, Appleton–Century–Crofts, 1976

Myerscough PR: Monro Kerr's Operative Obstetrics, 9th ed. Baltimore, Williams & Wilkins, 1977

FORCEPS DELIVERY

Bachman C: The Barton obstetric forceps: A review of its use in 55 cases. Surg Gynecol Obstet 45:805, 1927

Barton LJ, Caldwell WE, Studdiford WE: A new obstetric forceps. Am J Obstet Gynecol 15:16, 1928

Danforth DN: A method of forceps rotation in persistent occiput posterior. Am J Obstet Gynecol 65:120, 1953

Danforth DN, Ellis AC: Midforceps delivery—A vanishing art? Am J Obstet Gynecol 86:29, 1963

Danforth WC: The treatment of occiput posterior with special reference to manual rotation. Am J Obstet Gynecol 23:360, 1932

Danforth WC: Forceps. In Curtis AH (ed): Obstetrics and Gynecology, Vol II. Philadelphia, Saunders, 1933

Das K: Obstetric Forceps: Its History and Evaluation. St. Louis, Mosby, 1929

DeLee JB: The prophylactic forceps operation. Am J Obstet Gynecol 1:34, 1920

Dennen EH: Forceps Deliveries, 2nd ed. Philadelphia, Davis, 1964

Hughey MJ, McElin TW: Forceps operations in perspective. II. Failed operations. J Reprod Med 21:177, 1978

Hughey MJ, McElin TW, Lussky R: Forceps operations in perspective I. Midforceps rotation operations. J Reprod Med 20:253, 1978

Laufe LE: Obstetric Forceps. New York, Hoeber, 1968

Livnat EJ, Fejgin M, Scommegna A et al: Neonatal acid-base balance in spontaneous and instrumental vaginal deliveries. Obstet Gynecol 52:549, 1978

Marin RD: A review of the use of Barton's forceps for the rotation of the fetal head from the transverse position. Aust NZ J Obstet Gynaecol 18:234, 1978

McBride WG, Black BP, Brown CJ et al: Method of delivery and developmental outcome at five years of age. Med J Aust 1:301, 1979

BREECH PRESENTATION

Ballas S, Toaff R: Hyperextension of the fetal head in breech presentation: Radiological evaluation and significance. Br J Obstet Gynaecol 83:201, 1976

Ballas S, Toaff R, Jaffa AJ: Deflexion of the fetal head in breech presentation. Incidence, management and outcome. Obstet Gynecol 52:653, 1978

Behrman SJ: Fetal cervical hyperextension. Clin Obstet Gynecol 5:1018, 1962

Bird CC, McElin TW: A six-year prospective study of term breech deliveries utilizing the Zatuchni–Andros prognostic scoring index. Am J Obstet Gynecol 121:551, 1975

Bowes WA, Jr, Taylor ES, O'Brien M et al: Breech delivery: Evaluation of the method of delivery on perinatal results and maternal morbidity. Am J Obstet Gynecol 135:965, 1979

Brenner WE, Bruce RD, Hendricks CH: The characteristics and perils of breech presentation. Am J Obstet Gynecol 118:700, 1974

Caldwell WE, Studdiford WE: A review of breech deliveries during a five year period at the Sloane Hospital for Women. Am J Obstet Gynecol 18:623; 720, 1929

Collea JV, Rabin SC, Weghorst GR et al: The randomized management of term frank breech presentation: Vaginal delivery vs cesarean section. Am J Obstet Gynecol 131:186, 1978

Cruikshank DP, Pitkin RM: Delivery of the premature breech. Obstet Gynecol 50:367, 1977

DeCrespigny LJC, Pepperell RJ: Perinatal mortality and morbidity in breech presentation. Obstet Gynecol 53:141, 1979

Gimovsky ML, Petrie RH, Todd D: Neonatal performance of the selected term vaginal breech delivery. Obstet Gynecol 56:687, 1980

Karp LE, Doney JR, McCarthy T et al: The premature breech: Trial of labor or cesarean section? Obstet Gynecol 53:88, 1979

Lewis BV, Seniviratne HR: Vaginal breech delivery or cesarean section. Am J Obstet Gynecol 134:615, 1979

Løvset J: Shoulder delivery by breech presentation. J Obstet Gynaecol Br Emp 44:696, 1937

Mann LI, Gallant JM: Modern management of breech delivery. Am J Obstet Gynecol 134:611, 1979

Morley GW: Breech presentation: A 15 year review. Obstet Gynecol 30:745, 1967

O'Leary JA: Vaginal delivery of the term breech. A preliminary report. Obstet Gynecol 53:341, 1979

Piper EB, Bachman C: The prevention of fetal injuries in breech delivery. JAMA 92:217, 1929

Savage JE: Management of the fetal arms in breech extraction: A method to facilitate application of Piper forceps. Obstet Gynecol 3:55, 1954

Woods JR, Jr: Effect of low-birth-weight breech delivery on neonatal mortality. Obstet Gynecol 53:735, 1979

Zatuchni GI, Andros GJ: Prognostic index for vaginal delivery in breech presentation at term. Am J Obstet Gynecol 98:854, 1967

COMPOUND PRESENTATION

Ang LT: Compound presentation following external version. Aust NZ J Obstet Gynaecol 18:213, 1978

SHOULDER DYSTOCIA

Benedetti TJ, Gabbe SG: Shoulder dystocia. A complication of fetal macrosomia and prolonged second stage of labor with midpelvic delivery. Obstet Gynecol 52:526, 1978

Golditch IM, Kirkman K: The large fetus. Obstet Gynecol 52:26, 1978

Morris WIC: Shoulder dystocia. J Obstet Gynaecol Br Emp 62:302, 1955

Swartz DP: Shoulder girdle dystocia in vertex delivery. Obstet Gynecol 17:194, 1960

Woods CE: A principle of physics as applicable to shoulder delivery. Am J Obstet Gynecol 45:796, 1959

DWARFISM

Tyson JE, Barnes AC, McKusick VA et al: Obstetric and gynecologic considerations of dwarfism. Am J Obstet Gynecol 180:688, 1970

Dystocia due to abnormal uterine action implies *improper function of the motor component of the uterus* (the myometrium) *when there is no unusual resistance* on the part of the bony pelvis, the presenting part (maladaptation or abnormal size), the soft tissues, or, more rarely, the cervix itself. It is often termed *dysfunctional labor.*

Most cases of dystocia due to abnormal uterine action involve *secondary uterine inertia;* labor starts but then slows substantially or actually comes to a halt. This may occur in either the nullipara or the multipara, although serious uterine dysfunction is identified more frequently in the nullipara. Far less common is *primary uterine inertia.* This is a special form of dysfunctional labor, usually occurring in a first labor, in which painful contractions continue to occur even though there is no evidence of progression into the active phase of labor. *Uterine rings* may also produce dystocia.

DYSTOCIA DUE TO SECONDARY UTERINE INERTIA

Secondary uterine inertia should be suspected sooner than it can be diagnosed. It should be diagnosed within 2 hours of its appearance. A reasonable goal in management is to effect delivery by the most appropriate method within 2–6 hours after onset of the dysfunction. Once treatment is instituted, progress may still be somewhat slow, but it should be constant.

CAUSES

When there is no mechanical barrier to the progress of active labor, the explanation for the development of dysfunctional labor may be obscure. It has been observed that, after 12 hours, labors become steadily more dysfunctional. This raises the question of "fatigue" in the contractile system. There is not the slightest evidence, however, that the myometrium becomes fatigued as a result of the contractions of labor.

It has also been observed that the labor process tends to be less efficient in the face of various systemic abnormalities. For example, there is a strong association between dysfunctional labor and dehydration or food and electrolyte deprivation in the laboring woman. The patient who approaches labor with an excessively fearful attitude may be a candidate for dysfunctional labor. Uterine conditions may also affect the efficiency of the contractile process. For example, intrauterine infection may be associated with inefficient labor, and, rarely, premature separation of the normally implanted placenta leads to an abnormal contraction pattern and consequent failure of labor to progress.

It has been suggested that drug administration too

CHAPTER

35

DYSTOCIA DUE TO ABNORMAL UTERINE ACTION

Charles H. Hendricks

early in labor may slow cervical dilatation; yet, in most instances, accurate recordings of uterine contractility fail to show that therapeutic doses of analgesic, sedative, or tranquilizing drugs reduce contractility. Magnesium sulfate, sometimes given during labor as an anticonvulsant in severe preeclampsia, may slow the speed of cervical dilatation either when labor begins spontaneously or when contractions are being enhanced by oxytocin. This is not surprising, since magnesium sulfate is used by some to suppress pre-term labor (see Chapter 33).

Spinal, caudal, or epidural block is associated in some instances with the slowing of labor, although tracings of uterine contractions usually fail to indicate any significant reduction in uterine contractility after the initiation of such regional blocks. Some clinicians are convinced that vaginal examination of patients who are under such a major block tends to dislodge the

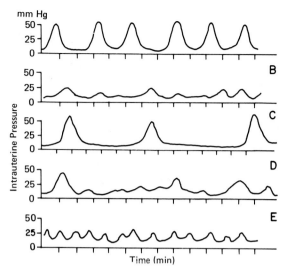

FIG. 35-1. Uterine contractility patterns in labor. *A.* Typical normal labor *B.* Subnormal intensity, with frequency greater than needed for optimal performance. *C.* Normal contractions, but too infrequent for efficient labor. *D.* Incoordinate activity. *E.* Hypercontractility.

presenting part, pushing it upward in the pelvis, and thus eliminating the beneficial effect upon labor of a fetal part that is well fitted into the lower uterine segment and closely applied to the cervix.

Although there is no uniformly acceptable explanation of dysfunctional labor, the syndrome can, nevertheless, be recognized and satisfactorily treated.

GENERAL CONSIDERATIONS

Dystocia due to decreased or incoordinate uterine contractility can be readily identified and managed if the clinician can 1) determine the time of onset of labor, 2) recognize the limits of normal labor, 3) rule out mechanical dysfunction, and 4) recognize and bear in mind the condition of the fetus.

Establishing the Time of Onset of Labor

In order to judge the significance of subsequent events, the physician must determine the probable time of onset of clinically active labor, *i.e.*, the time after which normal clinical progress should be anticipated. This time, determinable only in retrospect, begins when the contractions have become painful, when they occur quite regularly over a period of time at intervals no greater than 5 min apart, and after which there is evidence of progress in cervical dilatation.

Recognizing Characteristics of Normal Labor

The clinician should have clear expectations of the course of labor, based upon a knowledge of the prime features of normal labor:

1. Normal labor usually begins with the cervix already dilated approximately 2 cm. Ideally, in a first labor, the presenting part is already at or below the spines; in the parous parturient, this is less often true. In either case, normally progressing labor is almost always associated with a presenting part that fits snugly and evenly into the lower portion of the uterus and is closely applied to the upper rim of the cervix.
2. Normal labor is associated with progressively more painful contractions that come at increasingly close intervals. The contractions usually occur at regular intervals, develop at least 40 mm Hg intrauterine pressure, and are well coordinated in form (Fig. 35–1*A*). Between contractions, the intrauterine pressure usually ranges from 6–12 mm Hg. The intensity of uterine contractions can be estimated quite satisfactorily by palpating the uterus at a point not over the body of the fetus. At the height of a good contraction, moderate pressure does not indent the uterus. Between contractions, the uterus should be relaxed, nontender, and easily indented by only slight pressure. When the uterus is contracting effectively, vaginal examination discloses the cervix to be tightly applied to the fetal presenting part. It should be emphasized that a series of five or six consecutive contractions must be assessed to determine adequately the contraction pattern because of the variability in both the frequency and the intensity of contractions in early labor.
3. Once begun, normal labor is a constantly advancing process, and the course of cervical dilatation normally forms a progressively accelerating curve, without evidence of deceleration (Fig. 35–2).
4. In normal and efficient labor, the time required for the active phase is seldom long. About 60% of normal nulliparas complete the first stage within 6 hours, while 80% of multiparas complete the first stage within this span of time. Nearly all the rest complete the first stage within 12 hours from the onset of active labor.

Ruling Out Other Causes of Dystocia

The clinician must determine that bony resistance, soft tissue resistance, or excessive or premature pain-relieving medication is not making a major contribution to the dystocia. Furthermore, these factors should be reassessed as often as necessary, always asking the question, "Is vaginal delivery feasible in this case?"

Recognizing the Condition of the Fetus

At any point in labor when the fetus appears to be in jeopardy, the well-being of the fetus becomes of paramount concern in the further management of labor.

CLINICAL CHARACTERISTICS

Altered Contractility Patterns

The development of dysfunctional labor is usually accompanied by one or more of the following: 1) contractions that seem less intense to the obstetrician and often are less painful to the patient (Fig. 35–1B), 2) contractions that come at less frequent intervals (Fig. 35–1C), and 3) contractions that have a poorly coordinated pattern (Fig. 35–1D). Clinically, abnormal contractility may be indicated not only by an alteration in the frequency and evident intensity of contractions, but also by the fact that during the peak of a contraction the cervix is not under good tension but tends to hang loosely around the presenting part.

Cervical Dilatation Patterns

A most helpful method of detecting and estimating the severity of dysfunctional labor is to plot the course of cervical dilatation against time. According to Friedman's classic analysis of cervical dilatation in labor, normal labor begins with a latent phase (which others consider to be the very end of the weeks of prelabor) of a few hours, followed by the active phase of labor. The active phase includes a brief period of acceleration, followed closely by a "phase of maximum slope," which is followed in turn by a deceleration phase, *i.e.,* a slowing at the very end of the cervical dilatation phase (Fig. 35–3). Significant slowing of any phase of the process constitutes evidence of dysfunctional uterine activity.

When painful contractions occur over a long period without evidence of cervical dilatation, *i.e.,* a prolonged latent phase (Fig. 35–3A), either labor is about to begin or the contractions represent false labor. These frequent, small, painful contractions (Fig. 35–1E) are examples of primary uterine inertia. Whatever the cause, adequate treatment restores the labor curve to a normal contour.

Another evidence of dysfunction is very slow progress in the active phase (Fig. 35–3B). While this type of dysfunction may ultimately resolve itself, active intervention may be indicated to avoid an unduly prolonged labor in the interest of mother and fetus.

The most common type of dysfunction is arrest of labor after part of the active phase has been completed (Fig. 35–3C). Intervention is usually necessary to bring about a successful outcome within a reasonable period of time. Prompt and appropriate treatment can

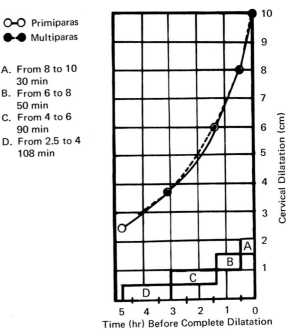

FIG. 35–2. Normal curve of cervical dilatation, with constant acceleration in rate of progress. (Adapted from Hendricks CH, Brenner WE, Kraus G: Am J Obstet Gynecol 106:1065, 1970)

restore the remainder of the dilatation curve to approximately the contour it would have had if labor had not been arrested.

The work of Philpott and Castle on the management of dysfunctional labor has great potential for improving the management of secondary uterine inertia. Their concept is built upon the observation that cervical dilatation during the active phase should advance at the rate of at least 1 cm/hour. An "alert line" is constructed on the time graph (Fig. 35–4), beginning at 1 cm of dilatation at the time the patient is hospitalized in labor and advancing 1 cm for each succeeding hour. The progress of a woman hospitalized in labor with 2 cm cervical dilatation, whose dilatation proceeds at the rate of at least 1 cm/hour, remains within zone 1 on the chart, which is the normal zone. If progress lags significantly, however, the curve of cervical dilatation eventually crosses the alert line into zone 2, indicating dysfunctional labor. The physician may either institute treatment for dysfunctional labor at this point or elect to follow the course of cervical dilatation one step further. If an additional lag develops, the cervical dilatation line eventually crosses the "action line" into zone 3, where intervention is strongly indicated. In general and under almost all conditions, labor that advances more slowly than 1 cm/hour warrants thoughtful investigation with a view to more active management.

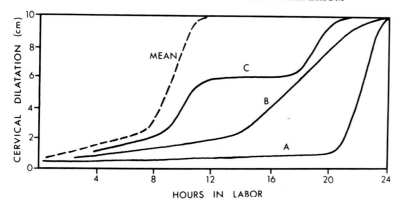

FIG. 35-3. Cervical dilatation abnormalities compared with mean normal dilatation curve. *A.* Prolonged latent phase. Failure of clinically active labor to begin over 20-hour period. *B.* Dysfunction represented by slow progress in all phases of cervical dilatation curve. *C.* Secondary arrest in active phase of cervical dilatation. (Adapted from Friedman EA: Labor: Clinical Evaluation and Management. New York, Appleton, 1967)

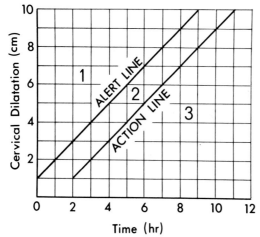

FIG. 35-4. Chart for gauging dysfunctional labor. See text for explanation. (Adapted from Philpott RH, Castle WM: J Obstet Gynaecol Br Commonw 79:592, 1972)

RELATIONSHIP OF DYSFUNCTIONAL LABOR TO CEPHALOPELVIC DIFFICULTIES

By definition, dysfunctional labor is not concerned with cephalopelvic disproportion or other mechanical factors that impede the progress of the fetus through the birth canal. Nevertheless, the lines between mechanical obstruction and myometrial dysfunction often become blurred. It is a fact that the myometrium seldom makes its maximum contractile effort during the course of normal labor. It is also true that mild degrees of mechanical obstruction to the progress of labor may slow cervical dilatation. Such mild degrees of obstruction can often be overcome by proper management.

A slowing in the rate of cervical dilatation in a labor that has previously been progressing normally is often an indication of the presence of some mechanical factor that significantly affects the woman's chances of completing labor efficiently and safely. A good case in point is the labor that advances normally until about 8 cm dilatation, after which progress stops altogether. Investigation often reveals the presence of a mechanical problem—a large head, an arrested transverse position, some degree of asynclitism, or combinations of these.

Successful management in such a case requires the physician to exercise a fine balance of judgment. First, the degree to which any mechanical defect is causing the labor to be ineffective must be assessed. Second, it must be determined that there is no insuperable mechanical obstacle to successful vaginal delivery. Third, if oxytocin is to be used, it must be used physiologically, skillfully, conservatively, and realistically. Fourth, the physician must recognize the limits of time and stimulation that may be properly applied.

MANAGEMENT

In determining the proper course of treatment, the obstetrician should consider 1) the patient's general condition, 2) whether simple corrective measures may be sufficient, 3) whether amniotomy or oxytocin administration is indicated, and 4) whether cesarean section is indicated.

General Supportive Measures

Care should have been taken during the patient's prior hours of labor to keep her from becoming exhausted, to keep her well hydrated, and to provide moderate sedation as needed. Consideration of these factors should continue throughout labor. Labor should not be long enough to produce excessive fatigue; fluid intake should be maintained at a satisfactory level throughout labor; and sedation, if needed, should be given primarily for discomfort rather than as "treatment" for anxiety. In well-conducted labor for which the woman has been well prepared and during which she is supported and reassured by the medical atten-

dants, medication is seldom needed simply because of anxiety.

Simple Corrective Measures

Sometimes the simplest of measures increases the effectiveness of labor. For example, emptying an overdistended bladder late in the first stage often speeds the completion of cervical dilatation and appears to encourage further descent of the presenting part. This usually can be done without catheterization.

An enema may enhance uterine contractions. Laboratory studies have shown that this procedure does indeed increase uterine contractility, thus confirming the time-honored clinical impression of its effectiveness. The potential value of an enema is shown in Figure 35–5.

A change in the patient's posture may also improve contractions. In general, contractions come less frequently when the parturient is lying on her side than when she is supine; but, with the patient on her side, contractions tend to be better coordinated and more intense (Fig. 35–6). A good rule is to permit the patient to labor in the position she finds most comfortable. Occasionally, labor resumes with increased vigor if the woman is permitted to walk in the hall or sit up in a comfortable chair. (*Caution:* The patient should not be allowed out of bed if the membranes have ruptured and the fetal head is not yet deeply engaged.)

The obstetrician should not rely entirely upon such simple maneuvers, nor should their employment delay overlong the initiation of more definitive treatment. Depending upon the urgency of the situation, it may be appropriate to consider amniotomy, the use of oxytocin, or cesarean section.

Amniotomy

Artificial rupture of the membranes (amniotomy) is the most effective single maneuver for facilitating the progress of labor. When used in dysfunctional labor, it must be done with full recognition that amniotomy is an absolute commitment by the physician to deliver the baby within a reasonable time, usually within a few hours. Furthermore, when the fetal head is above station 0, amniotomy may be followed by cord prolapse; accordingly, the membranes should be ruptured in this situation only by an experienced physician, for a good clinical indication, and in a well-equipped obstetric unit. Depending upon the circumstances, amniotomy may be done before, after, or in conjunction with the use of oxytocin.

The effectiveness of amniotomy in the enhancement of inefficient labor is illustrated by Figure 35–7, which shows the cervical dilatation patterns of three successive labors of the same woman. In each case, as judged by cervical dilatation, there was some evidence

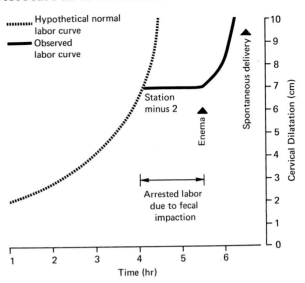

FIG. 35–5. Cervical dilatation curve in labor arrested by mechanical obstruction (large fecal impaction). Enema given at point indicated was followed promptly by resumption of normal dilatation. (Holt WA, Hendricks CH: Obstet Gynecol 34:505, 1969)

of inefficient uterine action. In each case, after treatment consisting solely of amniotomy, the cervical dilatation curve became normal, and the first stage was completed within a relatively short time.

Oxytocin

Physiologic Basis for Oxytocin Use. For the stimulation of uterine contractility in late pregnancy, oxytocin is still the *sine qua non*. Oxytocin is a polypeptide hormone normally produced in the human. As outlined in Chapter 29, after the active principle was first recognized in 1909 by Blair Bell, extracts of the posterior pituitary gland were used with varying degrees of success for more than four decades. Later, the oxytocic fraction was separated from the vasopressor fraction, and management of labor with oxytocin became common. Both of the commonly used oxytocic preparations, Syntocinon and Pitocin, are now prepared by synthesis, and are similarly standardized.

Oxytocin is usually supplied in 1-ml ampules that contain 10 IU (10,000 mU). It is rapidly eliminated or inactivated by either the pregnant or nonpregnant human, its half-life being no longer than 2–3 minutes. Properly administered, and in the physiologic dose range (1–20 mU/min), oxytocin is capable of inducing uterine contractions that are indistinguishable from those observed during normal human pregnancy and labor (Fig. 35–8). During late pregnancy, uterine sensitivity to oxytocin increases progressively, reaching a maximum shortly before term. The maximum

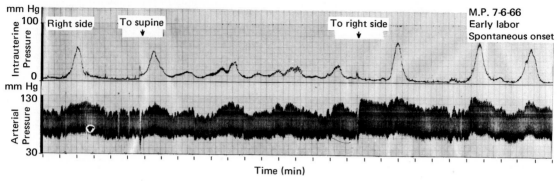

FIG. 35-6. Effect of change in position on uterine activity. Severely incoordinate uterine activity became well coordinated when patient turned supine to lateral position.

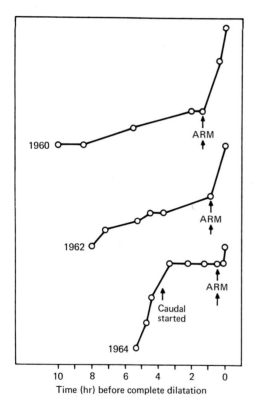

FIG. 35-7. Effect of artificial rupture of membranes (*ARM*) in three successive labors in same patient. No treatment other than amniotomy was used. *Top.* After 6.5 hours in first stage, dilatation had progressed only from 3 to 5 cm. After artificial rupture of membranes, final 5 cm of dilatation was completed in 80 min. *Middle.* After 7 hours of desultory labor, dilatation had progressed only from 4 to 7 cm. After artificial rupture of membranes, dilatation was complete within 50 min. *Bottom.* Normal labor was arrested at 9 cm cervical dilatation after caudal analgesia was started. Dilatation was completed promptly after artificial rupture of membranes. (Hendricks CH: Symposium on Modern Obstetrical Practice. New York, Karger, 1970)

sensitivity varies from patient to patient, but it is always within a reasonable physiologic range.

The threshold level for an initial response may be as little as 0.5 mU/min at the very end of pregnancy. Within the physiologic dose range, oxytocin produces great increases in uterine activity, which may be plotted as an exponential curve. Above the physiologic range the response becomes less efficient and notably less safe. The inadvertent administration of oxytocin in doses beyond the safe range is responsible for some of the risks sometimes attributed to oxytocin. Such unfortunate results are usually brought about by failure to understand the nature of the drug, its great potency, and how it should be used. Oxytocin is most efficient when it is given in modest amounts and at a constant rate. Such a constant and precise rate of administration can be ensured only by the intravenous route.

The ability to use intravenous oxytocin solutions within safe physiologic limits has become an important asset of the modern obstetrician. The physician who assumes responsibility for the use of oxytocin should know the dose, control the dose, and be prepared to adjust the dose as conditions change during labor. The average intravenous dose needed to stimulate uterine contractility ranges from 1–10 mU/min. In the occasional patient, 20 mU/min may be indicated; very rarely, a higher dose is necessary.

Prerequisites to Oxytocin Use. Certain conditions should be met before oxytocin is used in the management of dysfunctional labor:

1. There must be clear evidence that the progress of labor is slowing down. Administration of oxytocin simply to speed a normally advancing labor is unwarranted, unphysiologic, and potentially dangerous.
2. There must be no identifiable mechanical impediment to successful progress in labor.
3. The head should be the presenting part, and it should be well applied to the cervix and the lower

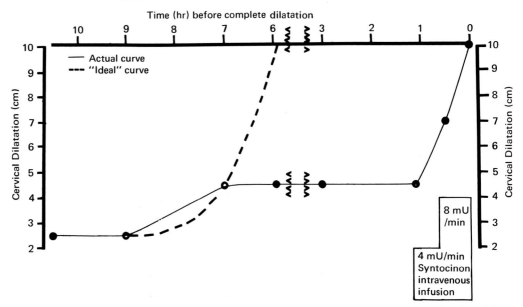

FIG. 35–8. Effect of oxytocin administration on desultory labor. Spontaneous labor in a multipara was arrested at 4 cm cervical dilatation. After 5 hours without progress, dilute solution of oxytocin was administered intravenously. Cervical dilatation was completed within 1 hour in approximately same pattern (*dashed line*) that would have been anticipated had progress in cervical dilatation not been interrupted. (Hendricks CH: Symposium on Modern Obstetrical Practice. New York, Karger, 1970)

segment of the uterus. Oxytocin stimulation of inertial labor in breech presentation is inefficient and may be actually perilous for the fetus. Its use in compound presentation or transverse lie is flatly contraindicated.

4. The fetus should be in good condition.
5. The uterus should not be scarred by a previous operative procedure.
6. The woman should not be a grand multipara (para 6 or above). The grand multipara whose uterus is stimulated by oxytocin has a disproportionately high risk of uterine rupture. In such a woman, oxytocin should be used only upon the most urgent indications, in an extremely small dose, for the shortest possible time, and with constant monitoring of uterine activity and fetal heart rate pattern.

Technique of Oxytocin Administration. Optimally, oxytocin should be given by a constant infusion pump. This method has the advantage of safety, since the pump cannot inject the oxytocin at a speed that is faster than its speed setting. It also permits the administration of a desired amount of oxytocin in a very small volume of fluid, virtually eliminating the possibility of water intoxication, which sometimes occurs after intravenous administration of large doses of oxytocin with large amounts of hypotonic fluid. Alternatively, 5 IU oxytocin can be placed in 1 liter 5% glucose in normal saline. In this solution, there is thus 5 mU oxytocin/ml solution. If the infusion equipment delivers the solution as 20 drops/ml, 1 mU oxytocin is contained in 4 drops.

The infusion should be started at 2 mU/min, either by setting the pump to deliver that amount or, in the case of the infusion solution described, by starting at 8 drops/min. The infusion speed should *not* be increased immediately. If there is no appreciable increase in uterine activity after 15 minutes, it is reasonable to advance the infusion speed to 5 mU/min (either the 5-mU speed indicated on the pump or as 20 drops/min of the solution). If the contractions are still inadequate after a further 20–30 min, the infusion speed may be increased to 10 mU/min. In a few cases, there may be some advantage in later increasing the speed to 20 mU/min, but it is rarely necessary to exceed the dose of 20 mU/min in the enhancement of labor or induction at term. Before the infusion speed is increased beyond 20 mU/min, it is wise to reassess pelvic adequacy and previous progress of the labor.

When oxytocin is being infused during labor, the infusion should be continued throughout labor and delivery in order to provide optimal control over uterine contractility during delivery and immediately postpartum.

In many well-equipped hospitals, there is a growing tendency to recommend that oxytocin be used only when uterine activity and fetal heart rate patterns are being electronically monitored. Whether or not elec-

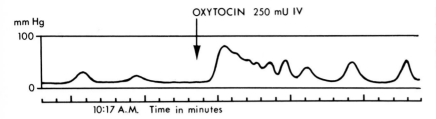

FIG. 35-9. How *not* to use oxytocin. Intravenous injection of one-fourth ampule (250 mU) elicited hypercontractility associated with hypertonus, which lasted for about 5 min.

tronic monitoring equipment is available, it is mandatory that, when oxytocin is being employed, the physician immediately responsible for the patient's care be in attendance in the labor suite.

Dangers, Complications, and Limitations of Oxytocin Use. The administration of oxytocin may produce three dangerous complications: excessive uterine contractility, uterine rupture, water intoxication. Also, hyperbilirubinemia may occur in the infant.

Excessive uterine contractility is almost always the result of excessive dose. For example, the intravenous administration of one-fortieth ampule (250 mU) may result in a period of hypercontractility that persists in some degree for as long as 5 min (Fig. 35–9). Such episodes of hypercontractility may encroach upon the fetal oxygen supply, since the maternal arterial input becomes progressively more diminished after the intrauterine pressure exceeds about 28 mm Hg.

Rupture of the uterus is an avoidable complication. Almost always, it occurs in multipara and is particularly apt to occur in the grand multipara or the woman with a scarred uterus. It also may occur when oxytocin is used in doses beyond the physiologic range or when the drug is used to stimulate uterine activity in cases of unrecognized cephalopelvic disproportion.

Water intoxication occurs when large doses of oxytocin are administered with large volumes of electrolyte-free fluid over a prolonged period so that the patient becomes waterlogged. This happens because oxytocin administered in excess of 50 mU/min may act as an antidiuretic. This catastrophic situation should never occur in the woman at term, since in such a patient there is never a need either for such a large dose of oxytocin or for a large volume of electrolyte-free fluid.

Hyperbilirubinemia appears more frequently in infants who have had substantial exposure to oxytocin *in utero*. The incidence and severity of the condition have been shown to be both time- and dose-related, being especially marked when doses as high as 32 mU/min have been employed over relatively long periods. This problem reemphasizes the general guidelines that oxytocin is optimally used at a dosage no higher than 20 mU/min and that every effort should be made to confine the entire management of secondary uterine inertia to the shortest practicable time, usually no more than 6 hours.

Cesarean Section

For severe dystocia due to abnormal uterine action, cesarean section is an important alternative delivery method that should be considered as soon as the diagnosis is made. It is no longer a last resort treatment of dysfunctional labor. Abdominal delivery only after 25 hours of dysfunctional labor is more indicative of neglect than of conservative management. The following findings in case of dysfunctional labor should make the physician incline toward abdominal delivery:

1. A persistently flat dilatation curve despite active treatment. This is an ominous sign and must not be ignored.
2. A previously well–thinned out cervix that subsequently becomes progressively thicker, edematous, and cyanotic. This condition is usually more evident in the anterior cervical lip, but, on occasion, the posterior cervix also may be involved.
3. Inadequate response to modest doses of oxytocin.
4. Thick, greenish yellow amniotic fluid or persistent fetal bradycardia.
5. Maternal preeclampsia, tachycardia, or low-grade fever.

It is no longer an important goal to bring about delivery *per vaginam*, seemingly almost without regard as to how radical may be the methods needed to avoid cesarean section. Certainly, cesarean section done under modern hospital conditions is vastly preferable to the outmoded and hazardous podalic version and extraction, Dührssen's (cervical) incisions, or difficult forceps delivery. Nevertheless, the obstetrician should not lose sight of the fact that fetal passage through the birth canal is the only truly physiologic mechanism for parturition. In some communities, the appearance of almost any challenge during the course of labor leads to a virtually automatic decision to deliver by cesarean section. No matter how sophisticated the medical facilities available for the care of a woman in labor, cesarean section delivery *per se* should not become the "norm." The treatment of secondary uterine inertia

FIG. 35-10. Effect of oxytocin in correcting uterine incoordination. Grossly incoordinate activity, characterized by excessive frequency causing hypertonus (*top*), was converted to normal labor (*bottom*) by infusion of oxytocin, 4 mU/min. (Caldeyro–Barcia RC: Int Congr Gynaecol Obstet 1:65, 1959)

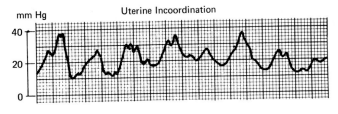

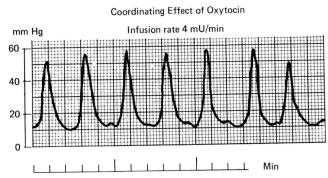

should be directed actively, thoughtfully, safely, and with fine clinical discrimination toward the prospect of vaginal delivery. Cesarean section should be reserved for those situations in which there is sufficient reason to believe that the maternal or fetal immediate and long-range interest is best served by abdominal delivery.

DYSTOCIA DUE TO UTERINE HYPERCONTRACTILITY

Sometimes termed *primary uterine inertia* or *hypertonic uterine inertia*, uterine hypercontractility is paradoxic, puzzling, and relatively rare. It is paradoxic because it usually occurs before active, progressive labor has been established. Its etiology is unknown, but it is observed almost exclusively in anxious nulliparas at term or beyond. The patient experiences frequent contractions that are painful out of all proportion to their clinical effect. She may also complain of some tenderness on uterine palpation between contractions. Recordings of intrauterine pressure usually show frequent, well-coordinated contractions, with the uterus never entirely relaxing between contractions.

Such a patient is sometimes benefited by being moved to a quiet room away from the labor suite, by moderately heavy sedation, and by strong reassurance from the medical attendants. Turning her to the lateral position often corrects the most bizarre aspects of the abnormal uterine activity. Oxytocin in a physiologic dose may be effective in stopping the hypercontractility and in bringing about a uterine activity pattern in-

distinguishable from that of normal spontaneous labor (Fig. 35–10).

PROLONGED LABOR

THE MODERN CONCEPT

Prolonged labor used to be defined as true, clinically evident labor lasting more than 24 hours, but under modern obstetric conditions, neither the mother nor the fetus should be subjected to a labor of this length. It is more appropriate to set the upper time limit for normal labor at 18 hours. Prolongation in either the first or second stage may contribute to this time. The approximate further length of labor may be anticipated by making a projection based on the development of cervical dilatation in the first half of labor.

If labor does not follow the expected course in terms of time and progress in the first stage, the physician should begin to plan further action, remembering that dysfunctional labor should be suspected during the first 6 hours of labor, that the diagnosis should be made and treatment instituted before the patient has been in labor for 12 hours, and that, with few exceptions, delivery should be effected within 18 hours after the onset of labor. For the management of dystocia due to inefficient uterine activity, the obstetrician's goal may be stated simply: safe delivery of the patient by the least traumatic possible means within 2–6 hours after the diagnosis is made. In dysfunctional labor under adequate treatment, cervical dilatation may remain slow, but it should be progressive.

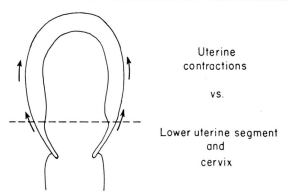

Uterine
contractions

vs.

Lower uterine segment
and
cervix

FIG. 35–11. Major factors involved in first stage of labor.

CAUSES

Prolongation of labor may not be due solely to inadequacy of myometrial function. The first stage of labor may be looked upon as the effort of the motive forces, uterine contractions, to overcome the resisting forces, the lower uterine segment and the cervix (Fig. 35–11). The lower uterine segment and the cervix are acted upon together during the normal first stage of labor, and these portions of the uterus are relatively passive. Some descent of the fetus usually occurs during the first stage of labor. Descent during this stage is desirable, but, particularly in the multipara, it is not a necessary component of normal first-stage labor.

Palpation of the cervix is most useful in assessing the response of the passive portions of the uterus to labor. Normally, just prior to the onset of active labor, the cervix softens considerably; on palpation, it has a consistency like that of the relaxed lip. It is thinned by 25%–80% of its normal thickness. The internal os may be palpated as a softly elastic ring that is usually dilated about 2 cm during the last week or two prior to the onset of labor. This is the *ripe* cervix. When labor begins before these preparatory changes have occurred, the cervix is termed *unripe*. In such instances, prolongation of the first stage may be anticipated, owing to the increased forces of resistance that must be overcome (Fig. 35–11).

The term *cervical dystocia* has been given to the circumstance in which the uterine contractions of labor appear to be adequate but the cervix fails to soften and dilate at the expected rate. In many of the cases so diagnosed, the problem is not in the cervix but rather in the clinical appraisal of the effectiveness of the uterine contractions; as noted before, both false labor and dysfunctional labor may be difficult to distinguish from true labor. However, the cervix itself is indeed sometimes the source of the difficulty, and the effacement mechanisms ordinarily triggered in the latter part of pregnancy, prior to labor, are not activated (see Chapter 29). The nature of the triggering stimulus

and the detail of the changes themselves are unknown. In normal circumstances, the cervix, composed almost entirely of dense fibrous connective tissue, is firm and unyielding until the last weeks of pregnancy, when softening and effacement are first noted. These and the further normal changes of labor are accompanied by a loosening and dissociation of the collagen fibrils that make up the larger fibers and bundles, and by an absolute loss of collagen from the cervix. Failure of these processes to occur can result in cervical dystocia. Amniotomy and, if clinically appropriate, an oxytocin infusion may solve the problem. If not, cesarean section may be the best means of delivery.

DANGERS OF PROLONGED LABOR

Much more is involved in prolonged labor than annoyance and inconvenience to the obstetrician and to the patient. Survival is also at issue. After 15 hours of first-stage labor, the fetal death rate increases sharply with each hour that passes before complete dilatation of the cervix; the fetal death rate also increases with each minute that the second stage is prolonged beyond 2 hours. Many factors are concerned, but the end result is a higher infant mortality the longer the labor proceeds beyond its normal limits (Fig. 35–12).

The most dire effects upon the mother are those that occur when the second stage of labor is prolonged, when uterine rupture is the ultimate disaster. Other consequences of prolonged labor are an increased incidence of infection, serious dehydration, and postpartum hemorrhage due to atony and lacerations that sometimes accompany a difficult vaginal delivery. Also of no small moment is the patient's emotional response to a long, tedious, difficult labor, which may color her attitude toward the whole subject of human reproduction.

DYSTOCIA DUE TO UTERINE RINGS

Three kinds of rings have been described in the uterus: the physiologic retraction ring, the pathologic retraction ring (Bandl's ring), and the constriction ring.

The *physiologic retraction ring* occurs precisely at the junction of upper and lower uterine segments. It is a normal and necessary result of the circumferential dilatation and consequent thinning of the lower pole of the uterus that occur either preparatory to labor or during early labor. These uterine changes are discussed in Chapter 29. The ring can be visualized by a high classic cesarean section incision that begins in the lower uterine segment and extends upward past the abrupt thickening in the myometrium that characterizes the upper uterine segment. The ring can be readily palpated through a lower segment cesarean

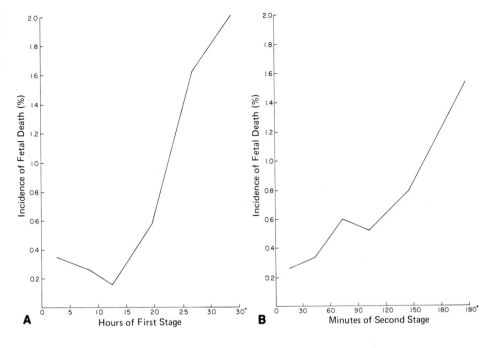

FIG. 35-12. Effect of duration of first (*A*) and second (*B*) stages of labor on infant mortality. (Adapted from Hellman LM, Prystowsky H: Am J Obstet Gynecol 63:1223, 1952)

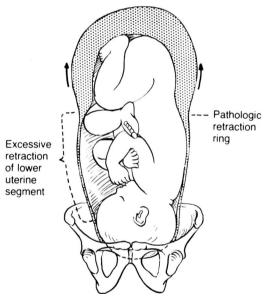

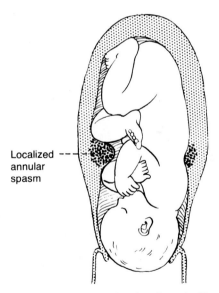

FIG. 35-13. Pathologic retraction ring (Bandl's ring) occurring at junction of upper and lower uterine segments as a result of obstructed labor.

FIG. 35-14. Constriction ring dystocia. Ring conforms to a fetal depression.

section incision by following the uterine wall upward.

The *pathologic retraction ring* (Fig. 35–13) is an accentuation of the physiologic retraction ring; it also occurs at the junction of upper and lower uterine segments, but in a neglected, mechanically obstructed second stage of labor (see Figure 29–32 and accompanying text). The ring can be felt by abdominal palpation, and it moves cephalad as the neglect continues. Uterine rupture through the lower uterine segment is inevitable unless the obstruction is relieved or the patient is delivered by cesarean section.

Constriction ring (Figs. 35–14 and 35–15) is a

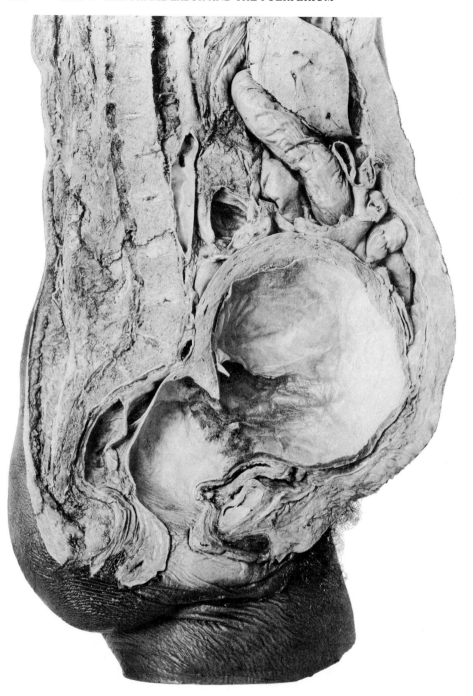

FIG. 35–15. Constriction ring. Frozen sagittal section. Fetus in occiput anterior position. Death resulted from eclampsia in second stage of labor. Uterus lay obliquely slightly to right of midline, causing left section of corpus to appear smaller than its actual 8+-month size. Constriction ring projects anteriorly into fetal depression between chin and thorax. (Canton E, Gonzalez JB: Atlas de Anatomia y de Clinica Obstetrica Normal y Patologica. Buenos Aires, Pueser, 1910, plate XXXV, p 105)

complication rarely encountered in ordinary obstetric practice. Its mechanics are not well understood. Characteristically, it occurs in prolonged labor with ruptured membranes. Because of the intense incoordination believed to result from "exhaustion," the uterus relaxes poorly and applies itself to the contours of the baby. The "rings," therefore, do not go all the way around the uterus, as do the physiologic and pathologic retraction rings, but rather conform to a depression in the baby, such as the neck or abdomen. A cardinal sign is said to be that the presenting part recedes during a contraction. The treatment is cesarean section, using an anesthetic that relaxes the uterus for delivery.

The physiologic retraction ring is a normal, desirable, and almost inevitable anatomic development during the course of normal labor. In contrast, both the pathologic retraction ring and the constriction ring denote severe obstetric pathology; these two rings have in common the fact that they tend to develop only after labor has continued too long against some sort of mechanical obstruction. Fortunately, with earlier recognition and active management of inertial labor, pathologic retraction and constriction rings are becoming a rarity.

REFERENCES AND RECOMMENDED READING

D'Souza SW, Black P, Macfarlane T: The effect of oxytocin in induced labour on neonatal jaundice. Br J Obstet Gynaecol 86:133, 1979

Friedman EA: Aberrant Labor Patterns in Labor: Clinical Evaluation and Management. New York, Appleton, 1967

O'Driscoll K, Jackson RJA, Gallagher JT: Prevention of prolonged labour. Br Med J 2:477, 1969

O'Driscoll K, Jackson RJA, Gallagher JT: Active management of labour and cephalopelvic disproportion. J Obstet Gynaecol Br Commonw 77:385, 1970

O'Driscoll K, Stronge JM, Minogue M: Active management of labour. Br Med J 3:1017, 1973

Philpott RH, Castle WM: Cervicographs in the management of labour in primigravidae: I. The alert line for detecting abnormal labour. J Obstet Gynaecol Br Commonw 79:592, 1972

Philpott RH, Castle WM: Cervicographs in the management of labour in primigravidae: II. The action line and treatment of abnormal labour. J Obstet Gynaecol Br Commonw 79:599, 1972

Schulman H: Prolonged and abnormal labor. Am J Obstet Gynecol 95:732, 1966

CHAPTER 36

OTHER COMPLICATIONS OF LABOR

Michael Newton

SOFT TISSUE OBSTRUCTION

Abnormalities of the bony pelvis are the most common causes of obstruction in labor. Occasionally, tumors in the pelvis may be responsible. These may arise from the uterus, the ovary, or the retroperitoneal area. The most common are leiomyomas of the uterus. Although leiomyomas usually enlarge during pregnancy, they almost always rise out of the pelvis as the uterus increases in size. Thus, labor is not obstructed unless the leiomyoma is cervical in origin and enlarges within the true pelvis or arises from a long pedicle; both conditions are rare. Ovarian tumors also frequently rise out of the pelvis during pregnancy, although they are less likely to do so than leiomyomas. Cystic teratomas seem particularly likely to remain in the pelvis and to produce obstruction. For this reason (and because of the possibility of malignancy), ovarian tumors more

than 6 cm in diameter should be removed during pregnancy.

Retroperitoneal tumors, such as neurofibroma and sarcoma, and pelvic kidney are very rare and do not ordinarily obstruct labor. However, they may be noted for the first time during the pelvic appraisal in early labor. They are typically firm, bossed, and fixed to the anterior aspect of the sacrum either in the midline or slightly to one side.

The possibility of obstructed labor from a pelvic tumor should be suspected on the basis of pelvic examination during pregnancy. Characteristically, a soft, round mass, located posteriorly, is first encountered by the examining finger; the cervix is high and anterior, and the presenting part is unengaged. If the patient is in labor, cesarean section is usually the treatment of choice, for the mass can rarely be dislodged. If the patient is within 6 weeks of term but not in labor, it is acceptable to await the onset of labor, since the obstructing mass may dislodge spontaneously, permitting vaginal delivery and later evaluation and management of the lesion.

Soft tissue obstruction may also arise from the cervix, which may fail to dilate despite adequate uterine contractions either because of intrinsic properties or because of scarring from previous operations or trachelorrhaphy.

Soft tissue obstruction in the lower genital tract usually results from unduly rigid perineal tissues or previous plastic operations. The diagnosis is usually made *post facto* when a laceration occurs. An unusual form of lower genital tract obstruction occurs in the Middle East; the customs of female circumcision, infibulation, and inserting rock salt into the vagina after delivery often cause serious vaginal stenosis and obstruction to subsequent delivery.

CORD ACCIDENTS

Cord accidents are the most acute threat to the life of the fetus prior to delivery. They include knots, coils around the fetus's neck or body, and prolapse of the cord. The majority of these difficulties become manifest during labor, but they occasionally occur during pregnancy. The chief problem resulting from a cord accident is occlusion of the cord with resulting fetal asphyxia. A short cord may very rarely produce separation of the placenta by traction when the fetus moves or descends in the birth canal.

CORD KNOTS AND COILS

The length of the cord is usually about 60 cm, although it ranges from 30–120 cm. The length is not well correlated with the weight of the fetus or the placenta. True knots are present in 1%, coils around the

neck in 25%, and coils around the body in 2%. A long cord is more likely to be associated with knots and coils. Knots are often observed after delivery and are usually so loose that umbilical circulation is not impaired, although less tension is required to occlude a thin than a thick cord. If a knot sets before delivery and remains set, fetal death follows at once. This may be suspected if, before labor, there are no apparent obstetric complications but the patient reports that she feels no fetal movement whatever and examination shows no evidence that the baby is alive.

Cord entanglement is occasionally detected before labor. When there is no cephalopelvic disproportion, a persistently abnormal position of the fetal head (usually in a cephalic presentation) or unexplained failure of the head to descend into the pelvis suggests cord around the neck. It is confirmed if pressure on the fetal head consistently produces slowing or irregularity of the fetal heart. A positive response to a nonstress or oxytocin challenge test (see Chapter 41) also suggests cord entanglement. Rarely, roentgenography shows the head held at an unusual angle. If the diagnosis of a knot or coil can be made with reasonable certainty before labor, cesarean section is indicated.

During labor, knots or coils may produce signs of cord compression and fetal anoxia; if routine electronic monitoring is being used, these effects are immediately apparent. If not, the diagnosis may be both difficult and delayed. Such accidents are rare, but their occasional occurrence is one reason for recommending the continuous monitoring of all women in labor. The subject of electronic monitoring is discussed in Chapter 41.

When the cord is found around the neck at the time of delivery of the head, it should be loosened or, if necessary, cut to permit delivery of the baby's body.

CORD PROLAPSE

Prolapse of the cord is a special form of cord accident. The cord descends into the birth canal in front of the presenting part (Fig. 36–1). In the most obvious clinical situation, the membranes have ruptured and the cord is found in the vagina or protruding from the introitus. Other varieties of prolapse include presence of the cord below the presenting part within the intact membranes (cord presentation) or presence of the cord beside but not below the presenting part (occult prolapse).

Incidence and Importance

Cord prolapse occurs more frequently when the presenting part does not properly fill the lower uterine segment and is not fully applied to the cervix. Thus, the incidence is greater with preterm than with full-

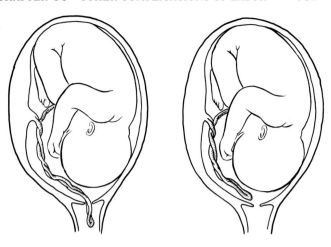

FIG. 36–1. Cord prolapse (*left*) and occult cord prolapse (*right*).

term fetuses. It is highest with a compound presentation and more common with a transverse than with a longitudinal lie; in the latter, it is more common with a breech than with a cephalic presentation. Among breech presentations, it is more common when the presenting part is a single footling, followed in frequency by double footling, complete breech, and frank breech, in that order. In the last instance, it is little more common than with a cephalic presentation (1/1000).

Other conditions that predispose to cord prolapse are hydramnios and multiple pregnancy. Situations in which the fetal head may not fit well into the pelvis include disproportion and premature rupture of the membranes, either spontaneous or artificial.

The danger of cord prolapse lies in the compression of the cord between the hard presenting part and the cervix or other part of the birth canal. This is more likely to happen when the presenting part is bony (such as the fetal skull or sacrum), when the membranes have ruptured, or when uterine contractions occur. Thus, compression may be intermittent, but it may also occur suddenly and with lethal results for the fetus.

Diagnosis

A prolapsed cord may be seen at the vulva or felt vaginally. Even if it is not prolapsed through the cervix, cord compression may result, leading to fetal anoxia, fetal distress, and fetal death. The first clinical manifestations of these are alterations in the fetal heart rate.

The only other clinical sign indicative of fetal distress is the presence of meconium in the amniotic fluid. This may be apparent externally if the membranes have ruptured. The passage of meconium is

common and of little concern in breech presentation, but it may be a grave sign in cephalic presentation.

Management

The woman in whom predisposing factors for cord prolapse are noted (*e.g.,* footling breech presentation, unengaged head) should be considered a high-risk patient. An attendant should remain with her constantly during labor, and a qualified obstetric–gynecologic consultant should be immediately available at all times. The progress of labor should be followed carefully by vaginal examinations. It is essential that such an examination be made promptly when the membranes rupture, since the cord is particularly likely to descend at this time. If equipment is available to monitor the fetal heart, this should be used throughout labor. If the fetal heart rate can only be determined by the stethoscope, this should be done at least every 10 min during the first stage of labor and after each contraction during the second stage. The amount of analgesia and anesthesia given to the mother should be minimized so that, if the fetus's blood supply is compromised, depression added by drugs will be lessened. All possible methods of emotional and physical support during labor should be used.

Discovery of a prolapsed cord either outside the introitus or below the presenting part on vaginal examination necessitates immediate action. Vaginal examination should be performed to determine the presence of pulsations in the cord, the amount of cervical dilatation, and the station of the presenting part. If the cord is pulsating and the fetus is alive and viable (estimated weight, 750–1000 g or more), treatment consists of lessening pressure on the cord and effecting delivery as quickly as possible.

The immediate pressure on the cord may be relieved by displacing the presenting part upward and lowering the patient's head or elevating her hips with a pillow. The knee–chest position may be used in some instances. Decreasing the pressure on the fetal head during contractions usually requires that the examiner keep a hand within the vagina to protect the cord until delivery can be accomplished. Oxygen should be administered to the mother (by nasal catheter or mask) in order to decrease fetal anoxia. The pulsations in the cord should be checked constantly. No attempt should be made to replace the cord in the uterus, although excess coils may be replaced in the vagina to protect the cord.

Prompt delivery usually requires cesarean section. When the cervix is not completely dilated, there is no question that this should be performed. When the cervix is fully dilated, judgment is needed to determine the quickest method of delivery. If all the conditions for immediate vaginal delivery are favorable (no disproportion, presenting part deeply engaged, cervix fully dilated), this method should be chosen. If conditions are not favorable for vaginal delivery, cesarean section is indicated.

The advantages of immediate cesarean section in almost all instances of cord prolapse demonstrate that every hospital offering obstetric care should have its delivery suite equipped to permit this operation to be performed with little or no delay at all times of the day and night. Internal podalic version used to be considered appropriate for the management of cord prolapse, but the associated infant morbidity is so high that this is no longer acceptable as standard management.

Even if the situation is an emergency, it is essential to explain as much as possible to the patient. A quiet simple statement of the problem and what is being done will do more than anything else to lessen her apprehension.

If the cord is not pulsating, or if it is pulsating and the fetus is not viable, there is no urgency, for the baby is either already dead or doomed. Labor can be allowed to proceed to vaginal delivery. Stimulation of labor with intravenous oxytocin may be appropriate, if needed.

If prolapse of the cord occurs in a situation in which immediate delivery cannot be performed (*e.g.,* at home), the patient should be transported as soon as possible to a properly equipped hospital. Her head should be kept lower than her hips and the cord covered with a moist towel to protect it. If feasible, an effort should be made to keep the presenting part elevated. If oxygen is available, it should be given in transit.

INFECTIONS

INTRAPARTUM INFECTION

Acute generalized maternal infection may be present during labor and can be transmitted to the fetus through the membranes. These disorders include acute virus infections (influenza, herpes, or chickenpox), acute bacterial infections (pyelonephritis or pneumonia), and chronic infections (syphilis or tuberculosis). These conditions may be instrumental in starting labor or may be present coincidentally in the patient who goes into labor. In any case, the maternal disease should be treated appropriately. Isolation from other patients may be necessary during labor. The baby should be specially examined for signs of the same disease and managed according to the findings.

Overwhelming intrapartum infection occasionally results in septic shock (see page 756). Measures are then needed to monitor and restore circulating blood volume and to deal with the complications that may result.

CHORIOAMNIONITIS

An important problem related to labor and delivery is the specific infection of the membranes, amniotic fluid, and fetus included in the general term *chorioamnionitis*. Although bacteria are found in the amniotic fluid in about 8% of cases even with intact membranes, infection most commonly follows rupture of the membranes. The longer the interval after rupture, the more likely that chorioamnionitis will occur. The subject of premature rupture of the membranes is discussed in Chapter 26.

Electronic monitoring techniques that involve invasion of the amniotic cavity may be associated with an increase in maternal infection, regardless of the duration of monitoring.

Diagnosis

A patient who has ruptured membranes and who is developing intrauterine infection usually has no specific symptoms. Signs include 1) a rise in pulse and temperature, 2) a change in the nature of the draining amniotic fluid from clear to cloudy or purulent, and 3) increased uterine irritability. Fetal tachycardia, distress, and even intrapartum death may result. The primary laboratory test is culture of a sample of amniotic fluid. This specimen should be obtained, but treatment should be started concomitantly.

Pathology

Evidence of chorioamnionitis may be found on histologic examination of the membranes, cord, and placenta. It consists primarily of collections of inflammatory cells, usually polymorphonuclear leukocytes. However, small collections of cells, particularly lymphocytes and plasma cells, may be found even when there is no clinical infection.

Treatment

Prompt administration of antibiotics is essential whenever intrauterine infection is suspected. Ampicillin (500 mg every 6 hours) or cephalothin (0.5–1 g every 4–6 hours) is most appropriate, since the bacteria commonly found are *Escherichia coli, Streptococcus faecalis,* and *Proteus.* In the interest of the fetus, the delivery should be expedited, either by stimulation of labor with oxytocin or by cesarean section if necessary. Intrapartum infection used to be considered an indication for extraperitoneal cesarean section. With effective antibiotics, this operation, often tedious and complicated in the hands of those unaccustomed to performing it, is no longer necessary. Once delivered, the baby should be considered at high risk and should receive special care.

Prevention

Infection may be introduced into the amniotic sac by amniocentesis or by artificial rupture of the membranes. In both cases, the chance of infection can be minimized by observing strict indications for the procedure and by using proper aseptic technique. Vaginal examinations should be performed with appropriate aseptic precautions and only as frequently as is absolutely necessary. A specific time limit should be set within which delivery should occur.

MULTIPLE PREGNANCY

The physiology of twinning is considered in Chapter 43. Special problems of labor and delivery arise when the uterus contains two or more fetuses. These include preterm labor, abnormal presentations, abnormal labor and delivery, and postpartum uterine atony. Multiple pregnancy is usually first suspected when the uterus is found to be larger than expected according to the dates. It can be diagnosed with certainty by an ultrasound scan or, if this is not available, by x-ray of the abdomen.

Once the diagnosis is made, the babies should be considered at high risk, Arrangements should be made for consultation by a qualified obstetrician–gynecologist and for delivery in a hospital that is adequately equipped to deal with the complications of labor and delivery and to provide optimal care for infants of low birth weight. During pregnancy, extra rest and a high-protein diet with adequate vitamin and iron supplements are essential. The patient should be examined at more frequent intervals than is a patient with a normal single pregnancy. Bedrest, for 1–2 weeks, if labor threatens or in any case at some time between the 32nd and 36th weeks may lessen the chance of preterm labor. Such bedrest can occasionally be arranged at home, but hospitalization may be required. During the last few weeks of pregnancy, preparations must be made and kept ready 24 hours a day for labor and delivery and for the care of the number of infants expected.

When twins are present, labor usually begins early, at 37–38 weeks' gestation; about 30% of twins are delivered before 37 weeks. The mean length of gestation for triplets and quadruplets is even shorter (35 and 34 weeks, respectively). Distention of the uterus undoubtedly contributes to this, but it is not the only factor. Preterm labor increases the likelihood of babies of low birth weight. Also, malpresentation, which is likely to complicate labor in any multiple pregnancy, is more frequent when labor starts before term.

Good antepartum care may lessen the chance that labor will start before the fetuses are large enough to survive. Of first importance is early diagnosis. Although twins are not common (and triplets or higher

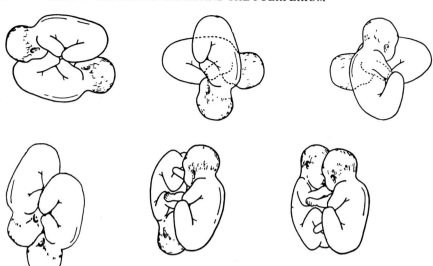

FIG. 36–2. Combinations of presentations of twins (Beck AC, Rosenthal AH: Obstetrical Practice. Baltimore, Williams & Wilkins, 1955)

numbers of fetuses are even less common), their incidence is increased in certain circumstances. Since hereditary factors may be important in dizygotic twins, a history of fraternal twins in the family is helpful. Black women are more likely to have twins than white or oriental women. Also, a high incidence of two or more fetuses has been noted after the use of clomiphene citrate and related drugs to induce ovulation. In this case the likelihood of multiple fetuses, and also the number of fetuses, appears to be dose-related.

ABNORMAL PRESENTATIONS AND POSITIONS

Abnormal presentation is more likely with twins than with a single fetus. Thus, the first twin may be expected to present by the vertex in only about 70% of cases; the second twin, in only about 50% of cases. Combinations of presentations (Fig. 36–2) occur with the following approximate frequency:

	Percent
Cephalic–cephalic	39
Cephalic–breech	37
Breech–breech	10
Cephalic–transverse	8
Breech–transverse	5
Transverse–transverse	1

In addition to these, various combinations of oblique lies are occasionally found.

A rare complication of labor and delivery in twin pregnancy is fetal entanglement or locking. This has been reported to occur once in 817 twin deliveries and once in 87 twin deliveries with vertex–breech combinations. The most common type can be termed *interlocking* (Fig. 36–3). This occurs at or below the pelvic

inlet, characteristically when the first twin presents by the breech. In this condition, the neck of the baby is elongated and its head is locked above the head of the second twin, which has descended into the pelvis. Other types of entanglement may occur above the pelvic brim and can be termed *collisions*. For example, the two heads may descend simultaneously so that neither one can enter the pelvis, or the arm of one twin may be around the neck of the other. Conjoined twins may present a similar difficulty in labor and delivery and are preferably dealt with by cesarean section.

The possibility of entanglement should always be kept in mind when twins are present. Rarely, collided or conjoined twins may be suspected when the twins are found in the same position relative to each other on repeated examinations. Sometimes this suspicion may be reinforced by roentgenography. During labor, the same findings may be accompanied by failure of any presenting part to descend into the pelvis. Once collision is diagnosed with reasonable certainty, cesarean section is indicated.

MANAGEMENT OF LABOR AND DELIVERY

Monitoring techniques are appropriate, but can usually be applied only to the presenting fetus. Because the babies are likely to be small, all possible emotional and physical support should be given to the mother during labor, and analgesia should be held to a minimum. Preparations must be made for the reception of the infants; for this purpose, it is usually wise to have a second qualified physician present, in addition to the one conducting the delivery.

Provided no complications occur, the management of the first stage of labor in multiple pregnancy does

not differ from that in single pregnancy with the same presentation. The forces of labor are similar, and cephalopelvic disproportion is less likely because the babies are usually small.

It is important to have an anesthesiologist (or anesthetist) present in the delivery room. Regional anesthesia (spinal, epidural, or caudal) is generally contraindicated because the persistently high uterine tone may hinder the intrauterine manipulations that may be necessary for the delivery of the second baby. Generally, local anesthesia in the form of perineal infiltration or pudendal block is preferable, with intermittent inhalation analgesia during contractions if needed. Deep general anesthesia may be needed at any time if intrauterine manipulations are indicated.

Since the perinatal loss is considerably higher with the second twin, the management of its delivery is crucial. The sudden emptying of the uterus after the delivery of the first twin results in a decrease in uterine contractions. These, however, resume quickly. Too rapid delivery of the second baby may result in increased uterine atony with possible postpartum hemorrhage. On the other hand, delay increases the duration of reduced placental circulation to the second twin, possibly leading to greater hypoxia. The increased chance of malpresentation, prolapsed cord, or premature placental separation adds to the danger.

An appropriate plan of management for the second twin is to attempt to direct the head into the inlet. If this can be readily accomplished, fetal monitoring should be continued, and the head should be expected to advance as labor continues. The optimal time for delivery of the second twin is 5–20 min after delivery of the first twin, and the objective is to accomplish this without difficult operative procedures. Midforceps delivery of a second twin, version and extraction, and breech delivery used to be considered appropriate means of dealing with the second twin. However, the demonstrated hazards to the second twin are such that, if any major operative maneuvers are anticipated for delivery of the second twin, cesarean section after delivery of the first twin is now preferred.

When interlocking occurs, *i.e.*, when the head of the first baby cannot be delivered and the head of the second baby is entering or has entered the pelvis, the loss of the first baby is almost certain. With the patient under deep anesthesia, an attempt must be made to displace the second head upward, deliver the first baby, and then deliver the second baby as soon as possible. This is not easy, and failure may necessitate decapitation of the first twin in order to deliver the second twin alive. Lister has described such a case.

POSTPARTUM UTERINE ATONY

Distention of the uterus by twins may make postpartum contractions of the uterus less effective and pre-

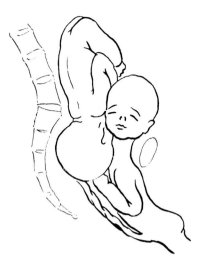

FIG. 36–3. Fetal interlocking. (Clyne DGW: Textbook of Gynaecology and Obstetrics. London, Longmans, 1963)

dispose to atony and hemorrhage. For this reason, intravenous oxytocin (at least 30 units in 1000 ml 5% dextrose in water) should be given after the delivery of twins. Observation of the patient for at least 2 hours postpartum is especially important.

SOFT TISSUE LACERATIONS

The possibility of a laceration of the birth canal must be kept in mind at every delivery. Special predisposing factors include rapid labor, induction or stimulation with oxytocin, abnormal presentation or position, a large baby, rigid tissue, or instrumental delivery. In these situations, examination of the birth canal immediately after delivery is very important. If vaginal bleeding develops later and is not clearly due to uterine atony, the birth canal should be promptly reexamined for lacerations, even if previous examination showed no lacerations.

CERVICAL LACERATIONS

Cervical lacerations are usually not preventable except in two circumstances: 1) when, in order to expedite delivery, the almost fully dilated cervix is manually pushed back over the fetal head, and 2) in the rare circumstance when traction is applied to forceps introduced inside the cervix before full dilatation. Spontaneous cervical lacerations can sometimes be predicted in the driving, vigorous labor in which vaginal examination suddenly discloses that the cervix is not palpable on one side, whereas on the other a thick, heavy rim is present.

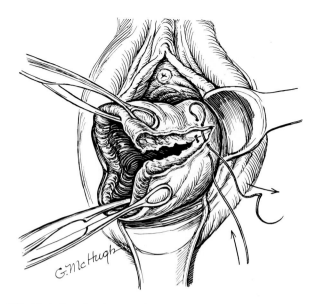

FIG. 36–4. Repair of cervical tear. Either vertical mattress sutures (as shown here) or through-and-through sutures may be used. Sutures may be interrupted or continuous.

Except for those that result from manual or instrumental trauma, cervical lacerations occur almost invariably at the lateral angles. They are of varying depth, from a trivial mucosal tear to one that extends as high as the broad ligament.

The cervix should be examined for tears immediately after delivery. This can usually be done easily and quickly by palpation between the first two fingers of the examining hand. If a laceration more than 2.5 cm in length is felt or suspected, the cervix should be inspected visually. The standard obstetric instrument tray must contain retractors and sponge forceps suitable for this purpose as well as for the repair of any laceration that may be found (Fig. 36–4). Lacerations of the cervix and upper vagina should be repaired before the episiotomy is closed. If they extend too high for ready visualization, the physician should place a suture in the uppermost point that is accessible and apply traction on this and successive sutures until the top of the tear is reached. Several techniques are available for the repair of cervical lacerations. The author prefers the use of a continuous 2–0 chromic suture that extends from the upper limit of the laceration to the rim of the cervix. The suture must pass deeply into the substance of the cervix; if it is too close to the edge, there will be only a bridge of mucous membrane across the site of the laceration after it heals. Tears less than 2.5 cm long ordinarily heal without repair and without evidence that they have occurred; those that are longer and any lacerations that bleed, regardless of length, must be repaired.

VAGINAL AND PERINEAL LACERATIONS

Rigidity and thickness of the vaginal and perineal tissues vary among patients. Previous perineal operations, either episiotomy or repair at earlier deliveries or plastic procedures, present fibrous obstruction and predispose to lacerations. Explosive descent of the head through the vagina and especially through the introitus is also a predisposing factor. A comfortable, relaxed, properly instructed, cooperative patient can often control the bearing-down effort sufficiently to permit delivery without lacerations.

Vaginal lacerations are especially apt to occur over very prominent spines in difficult forceps deliveries. They may also occur as "sulcus tears" in the vaginal sulci, either *de novo* or as an extension of the episiotomy incision. They are usually diagnosed by palpation and confirmed by direct inspection. They should be repaired before the episiotomy or any perineal laceration, usually by interrupted or continuous 2–0 chromic sutures.

Perineal lacerations are classified as first, second, or third degree. In a first-degree laceration, only the skin is torn; in a second-degree laceration, the skin and underlying structures are involved; and in a third-degree laceration, the anal sphincter is torn. A third-degree laceration may extend through the sphincter and through the anal and rectal mucous membrane. The latter is sometimes termed a fourth-degree laceration.

First-degree perineal lacerations may require no repair, since they usually heal promptly without discomfort. An exception to this may be periurethral laceration, which tends to bleed more. The most common type of laceration, the second degree, is repaired in two steps. The repair is quite similar to that of an episiotomy (see Fig. 31–16), except that special care must be taken to identify the irregular edges and to effect a proper anatomic restoration.

It is important to determine whether the anal sphincter or the rectal or anal mucosa is involved in a perineal laceration, since failure to repair any of these may result in fecal incontinence. If the anal or rectal mucosa is torn, repair should be made with a continuous suture that inverts the edges into the lumen. The ends of the cut anal sphincter should be identified and approximated with interrupted sutures. The remainder of the repair of a third-degree laceration is similar to that of a second-degree tear.

The site of repair should always be carefully examined to see that no bleeding is occurring and that no hematoma is forming beneath the surface. If hemostasis is uncertain, a gauze pressure pack may be inserted in the vagina for 12 hours. Postoperatively, pain may be the major problem; as for an episiotomy, it may be alleviated by anesthetic sprays, a heat lamp to the perineum, or Sitz baths.

HEMATOMAS OF THE GENITAL TRACT

Rupture of a blood vessel in the genital tract and development of a hematoma may occur during and after delivery. Predisposing causes include those listed for soft tissue lacerations. A hematoma may involve only the vulva or vagina, or it may extend to or primarily involve the broad ligament.

HEMATOMAS OF THE VULVA AND VAGINA

Additional causes for a hematoma in the vulvar or vaginal area include inadvertent damage to a blood vessel during injection of a local anesthetic or unexpected extension of an episiotomy. When the bleeding starts in the perineum or beside the vagina, it may extend along tissue planes downward into the vulva, laterally into the paravaginal area, and upward beneath the broad ligament (especially if it starts high in the vagina).

A hematoma in the lower genital tract may be detected while the patient is on the delivery table. Management then consists of ligating the bleeding vessel(s) and, if necessary, inserting a vaginal pack. More commonly, the hematoma develops slowly in the hours following delivery. The patient complains of pain in the perineal area, much more than would normally be expected. Pressure on the bladder or rectum may produce a constant urge to urinate or defecate. On examination, bluish discoloration or bruising of the vulva and perineum may be seen and rectal examination may disclose a large tender paravaginal mass. If blood loss has been great and has continued for some time, a fall in blood pressure, a rise in pulse, and symptoms of shock may be present.

Ideal treatment of a vulvar or vaginal hematoma consists of evacuating the clot under anesthesia and ligating the bleeding vessel(s). This may be quite difficult, however, and treatment may have to be limited to insertion of a pressure pack into the cavity or the vagina—to be removed after 12 hours. Blood transfusions should be given as necessary, and antibiotics are advisable.

BROAD LIGAMENT HEMATOMAS

Bleeding into the broad ligament or a broad ligament hematoma may result from dissection upward of blood arising from a vaginal laceration. However, it is much more likely to follow rupture of the uterus or of a vessel (often varicose) in the broad ligament. A hematoma of the broad ligament may extend widely into the retroperitoneal area or occasionally break through into the peritoneal cavity.

Diagnosis of a broad ligament hematoma may be difficult. Often, examination of the lower genital tract and even of the uterine cavity immediately after delivery fails to disclose the bleeding, and there is frequently little external bleeding. Later, however, the patient develops lower abdominal pain, symptoms of pressure on the bladder and rectum, and, if the hematoma is large, shock. A tender mass may be felt on abdominal and pelvic examination. Signs of peritoneal irritation, tenderness, rigidity, and rebound tenderness may be present, particularly if the blood has entered the peritoneal cavity. If bleeding has continued for a long time, anemia may be detected. Aspiration of blood from the peritoneal cavity or from an expanding mass may confirm the diagnosis.

Management depends first on adequate replacement of blood. Next, the uterine cavity and upper vagina should be reexamined to ascertain whether the uterus is ruptured. If it is not, and the patient's condition remains stable, expectant treatment may be continued. If the hematoma continues to expand or the uterus is ruptured, laparotomy is indicated. Then, if possible, the hematoma should be evacuated and bleeding vessel(s) ligated. This may not be easy. If attempts to control bleeding are unsuccessful, hysterectomy, bilateral ligation of the hypogastric arteries, or packing the pelvis may be necessary.

PLACENTA ACCRETA

Placenta accreta, an unusual complication of the third stage of labor, is the abnormal adherence of the placenta to the uterine wall. The decidua is deficient, and the chorionic villi penetrate the endometrium. They are in contact with the myometrium and may even enter it. The physiologic line of cleavage, the spongy layer of the decidua, is missing. Complete placenta accreta is extraordinary, but small areas of adherence may be more common than is generally realized. It is not uncommon to find placenta accreta at the site of the scar from a prior cesarean section. When the villi extend through the myometrium, the condition is known as *placenta increta;* when they reach or even penetrate the serosa, it is called *placenta percreta* (Fig. 36–5). An association between placenta accreta and placenta previa has been noted occasionally.

Under normal circumstances, the placenta separates from the uterine wall within 5–10 min after delivery of the baby and is then delivered spontaneously or with the aid of pressure and cord traction. Manual removal of the placenta is indicated if separation does not occur within 15 min or if excessive bleeding occurs prior to that time.

The most common causes of delayed delivery of the placenta are retention within the uterine cavity or failure of a portion of the normally attached placenta to separate from the uterine wall. In these cases, manual

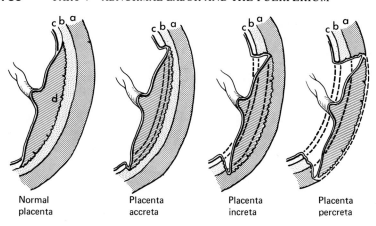

FIG. 36-5. Placenta accreta, increta, and percreta. *a*, Myometrium. *b*, Decidua basalis. *c*, Decidua spongiosa. *d*, Placenta with chorionic villi.

Normal placenta · Placenta accreta · Placenta increta · Placenta percreta

removal is usually accomplished easily. This is done, after appropriate aseptic preparation (and anesthesia, if necessary), by inserting the fingers into the uterus, finding the plane of cleavage between the placenta and the uterine wall, and peeling out the placenta (see Figure 31–13).

Placenta accreta must be suspected when no plane of cleavage can be found (complete placenta accreta) or when a small area of placenta cannot be detached (partial placenta accreta). In either case, the attempt to remove the placenta is usually accompanied by severe bleeding. When only a small part of the placenta is adherent, that portion can often be removed by extra manipulation and bleeding controlled with massage and intravenous administration of oxytocin. If efforts to detach the placenta are obviously unsuccessful and bleeding continues, prompt blood replacement is necessary. Conservative measures such as uterine packing or waiting to repeat the attempt at removal later are ill advised. Immediate laparotomy and hysterectomy should be performed.

INVERSION OF THE UTERUS

Inversion of the uterus is a rare complication of the end of labor. The uterus is turned inside out so that the top of the endometrial cavity protrudes through the cervix into the vagina and even outside the introitus (Fig. 36–6). Although inversion is usually complete, partial inversion may occur. Inversion may be acute, subacute, or chronic, depending on the time when it is recognized. Inversion occurs rarely after abortion.

The causes of inversion are said to be multiparity with consequent laxness of the uterine wall or faulty management of the third stage of labor with excessive fundal pressure or traction on the cord or placenta. However, over half the cases in several reported series have occurred in primiparas, and, in many instances, the condition seems to arise spontaneously or with

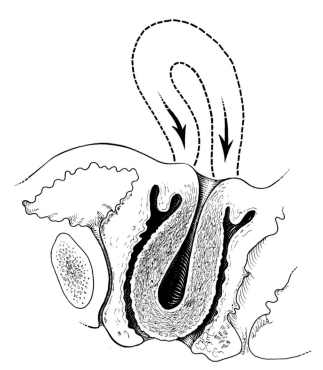

FIG. 36-6. Inversion of the uterus.

minimal manipulation of the uterus in the third stage of labor. Thus, it is difficult to assign any consistent cause.

Diagnosis

Acute inversion is diagnosed when an unusual hard mass is felt in the vagina or such a mass is seen protruding from the introitus at the end of labor. If the placenta is still attached to the fundus, it may be felt in the lower vagina with the inverted uterus above it. In addition, the patient usually experiences shock out of

proportion to the blood loss, which is not usually excessive, at least initially. Further bimanual examination reveals that the fundus of the uterus is not in its usual place and only an indentation is felt at this site.

Management

Immediate replacement of the uterus is the procedure of choice as soon as the diagnosis is made. This should be done while blood is being obtained and given to the patient. It should not be delayed until shock is overcome; this may never happen. Anesthesia should be given, if necessary. With the hand in the vagina, the uterus is lifted up out of the pelvis, thus putting tension on the uterine ligaments. Then it may be possible, by gentle manipulation, to restore the uterus to its normal position. After the inversion is treated, the uterus should be massaged and oxytocics given. Recurrence is unlikely. If manual replacement of the acutely inverted uterus fails, operative repair may be necessary. A cervical incision at 6 o'clock may permit vaginal replacement. If this fails, laparotomy may be performed and traction made on the fundus and round ligaments (which are inverted into the cup) with instruments, aided by a vertical incision in the posterior part of the constricting ring (Haultain's operation).

In subacute or chronic inversion, the condition is not discovered until hours or days later. In these instances, replacement from below is not usually possible. Operative repair should be performed abdominally (Haultain's operation) or vaginally (Spinelli's operation). In the latter, the anterior wall of the inverted cup portion of the uterus and cervix is incised throughout its length, the uterus replaced, and the defect in the uterine wall sutured.

REFERENCES AND RECOMMENDED READING

Charles D, Finland M: Obstetric and Perineal Infections. Philadelphia, Lea & Febiger, 1973

Cohen M, Kohl SG, Rosenthal AH: Fetal interlocking complicating twin gestation. Am J Obstet Gynecol 91:407, 1965

Daw E: Triplet Pregnancy. Br J Obstet Gynaecol 85:505, 1978

Evrard JR, Gold EM: Cesarean section for delivery of the second twin. Obstet Gynecol 57:581, 1981

Fox H: Placenta accreta, 1945–1969. Obstet Gynecol Surv 27:475, 1972

Freeman RK: Intrapartum fetal evaluation. Clin Obstet Gynecol 17:83, 1974

Gordon H, Pipe N: Induction of labor after intrauterine death: A comparison between prostaglandin E_2 and oxytocin. Obstet Gynecol 45:44, 1974

Gunn, GC, Mishell DR, Morton DG: Premature rupture of the membrane: A review. Am J Obstet Gynecol 107:469, 1970

Keith L, Ellis R, Berger GS et al: The Northwestern University multihospital twin study. I. A description of 588 twin pregnancies and associated pregnancy loss, 1971 to 1975. Am J Obstet Gynecol 138:781, 1980

Koh KS, Chan FH, Monfared AH, Ledger WR, Paul RH: The changing perinatal and maternal outcome in chorioamnionitis. Obstet Gynecol 53:730, 1979

Lee WK, Baggish MS, Lashgari M: Acute inversion of the uterus. Obstet Gynecol 51:144, 1978

McCaffrey RM, O'Leary JA: Rudimentary horn pregnancy simulating missed labor. Obstet Gynecol 25:130, 1965

MacVicar J: Chorioamnionitis. Clin Obstet Gynecol 13:272, 1970

Migliorini GD, Pepperell RJ: Prolapse of the umbilical cord: A study of 69 cases. Med J Aust 2:522, 1977

Minogue M: A review of twin pregnancies: National Maternity Hospital (1967–1971). J Ir Med Assoc 67:181, 1974

Persson P, Grennert L, Gennser G et al.: On improved outcome of twin pregnancy. Acta Obstet Gynecol Scand 58:3, 1979

Rayburn WF, Beyney A, Brinkman DL: Umbilical cord length and intrapartum complications. Obstet Gynecol 57:450, 1981

Read JA, Cotton DB, Miller FC: Placenta accreta: Changing clinical aspects and outcome. Obstet Gynecol 56:31, 1980

Spellacy WN, Gravem H, Fisch RO: The umbilical cord complications of true knots, nuchal coils and cords around the body. Am J Obstet Gynecol 94:1136, 1966

Vaughn TC, Powell LC: The obstetrical management of conjoined twins. Obstet Gynecol 53:67S, 1979

Watson P, Besch N, Bowes WA, Jr: Management of acute and subacute puerperal inversion of the uterus. Obstet Gynecol 55:12, 1980

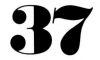

CHAPTER 37

COAGULATION DEFECTS

Ashley T. Coopland

Hemorrhage is a common cause of maternal morbidity and is still a leading cause of maternal death. A mechanical dysfunction is usually implicated as the cause, but there remains a small percentage of cases in which failure of the body's hemostatic mechanism is a significant factor. Fortunately, enough is known about the conditions that predispose to these disorders and the means of dealing with them that hemostatic defects can frequently be anticipated and managed effectively.

The old concept of "obstetric hypofibrinogenemia" has gradually faded into obscurity. As more is learned of the intricate mechanism of hemostasis, it is evident that bleeding defects encountered in obstetric patients are not due simply to fibrinogen depletion, but rather to much more complex factors. Their pathophysiology is similar to that of many disturbances in hemostasis encountered in other fields of medicine.

PHYSIOLOGY OF HEMOSTASIS

Hemostasis is a highly complex phenomenon that basically involves three interdependent mechanisms: vascular retraction, platelet function, and plasma coagulation. The entire process is not completely understood, although there have been significant advances in knowledge of the individual processes involved.

Simply stated, hemostasis is achieved in the following manner. When a blood vessel is cut, platelets rapidly accumulate at the site, adhere to the cut edges of the wound (presumably to exposed collagen in the vessel wall), and subsequently adhere to each other. Coincidentally, the vessel undergoes retraction, a process that is enhanced by vasoactive substances released by the accumulating platelets. Almost simultaneously, the plasma coagulation system produces a fibrin network that is a more permanent seal for the loss of vascular integrity than is the temporary platelet plug. Finally, the fibrinolytic system is activated to remove excess fibrin and to restore the patency of the vessel. A patient may tolerate a minor impairment in one of these processes, but defects in any two are likely to produce a significant bleeding diathesis. These mechanisms are, to a great extent, interdependent.

PLATELETS

Platelets, which circulate in the blood within well-defined numeric limits, play a basic role in hemostasis. It has been suggested that they have an endothelial support function and in some way maintain endothelial integrity. Of greater importance, they provide the initial hemostatic plug when vascular integrity is lost and, in conjunction with vascular retraction, are vital to the primary hemostatic defense. In addition, platelets are known to contain serotonin, as well as enzymes that convert endoperoxidases, normally located in the intima of blood vessels, into a prostaglandinlike substance, thromboxane, that causes platelets to clump and vessels to constrict.

Platelets are also known to contain adenosine diphosphate (ADP), platelet factor III (phospholipid from the platelet membrane), and catecholamines. Serotonin and the catecholamines are powerful potentiators of ADP, which is probably responsible for the profound physical and chemical changes observed in the platelets at the site of vascular trauma.

Platelet problems occur in two general situations: 1) When platelets are decreased in number (*thrombocytopenia*) and 2) when they have functional defects (*thrombocytopathia*). Thrombocytopenia may be primary (idiopathic thrombocytopenic purpura [ITP]) or secondary (a condition due to a variety of drugs or to a number of diseases). Bleeding manifestations are usually seen only when the platelet count is signifi-

cantly low, *i.e.*, less than 25,000/cu mm. Functional platelet inadequacy may be seen in certain congenital conditions (*e.g.*, Glanzmann's thrombasthenia, von Willebrand's disease) and in certain acquired lesions (*e.g.*, drug effects, toxic effects of fibrin breakdown products). In such cases, the platelet count is likely to be normal or only moderately reduced, but the bleeding is similar in character to that encountered in thrombocytopenia. Clinically, impaired platelet function may be manifested by bleeding from the gums, cutaneous petechiae and ecchymosis, persistent bleeding from venipuncture and intramuscular injection sites, as well as continuous oozing from surgical incisions.

TABLE 37–1. COAGULATION FACTORS

	Nonpregnant	Pregnant
PLATELETS	175,000–400,000/cu ml	
FIBRINOGEN	200–400 mg/dl	300–700 mg/dl
FACTOR V	75%–125%	200%–400%
FACTOR VII	75%–125%	
FACTOR VIII	75%–150%	200%–600%
FACTOR IX	75%–150%	200%–400%
FACTOR X	75%–125%	200%–400%
FACTOR XI	70%–130%	
FACTOR XII	70%–130%	
FACTOR XIII	9.4 units/ml	4.6 units/ml

MECHANISM OF BLOOD COAGULATION

The plasma coagulation factors are soluble proteins and are subject to constant turnover, but they are maintained at relatively steady concentrations. These are listed in Table 37–1, which shows approximately normal values for nonpregnant and pregnant patients. The increases in coagulation protein concentrations that occur during pregnancy are usually attributed to the overall alteration in protein metabolism that accompanies gestation.

The culmination of the several reactions that constitute the blood clotting process is the conversion of the soluble protein fibrinogen to the insoluble protein fibrin, which is the substance of the definitive clot. The end result is arrived at by one of two pathways that are termed intrinsic or extrinsic according to whether the changes are initiated within or outside the vasculature. This series of reactions is depicted in simplified form in Figure 37–1.

The fibrinogen-to-fibrin conversion deserves special comment. As a result of the prior sequential reactions involving many of the other coagulation proteins, the proteolytic enzyme thrombin is formed. This acts on the fibrinogen molecule and splits two arginyl–glycyl bonds, producing fibrin and two small molecular fragments, fibrinopeptides A and B. Initially, the fibrin formed is in the monomeric form, which is still soluble, but it spontaneously polymerizes to form an insoluble fibrin polymer, the visible clot. The process is not complete at this point, however, because fibrin stabilization, a considerably slower reaction, has yet to take place. This reaction is mediated by factor XIII, the activity of which is initiated by thrombin. Fibrin is stabilized by the formation of cross linkages between the strands of fibrin polymer, which produces both tensile strength, and resistance to fibrinolytic dissolution. Unlike that of other coagulation factors, the activity of factor XIII is thought to be reduced during normal pregnancy, although this reduction appears to have no functional significance.

The coagulation system is continuously controlled by several serine antiproteinases, of which antithrombin III is one of the most important. This enzyme neutralizes such substances as thrombin, plasmin, and the activated forms of some of the clotting factors. The inhibitory effect of antithrombin III is greatly enhanced by heparin.

THE FIBRINOLYTIC SYSTEM

Fibrinolysis depends on the circulating enzyme precursor *plasminogen* and a delicately balanced system of activators and inhibitors (Fig. 37–2). Clinically, the most important initiating factor is the activation of coagulation factor XII; thus, the onset of coagulation sets in motion the fibrinolytic system. Many other stimuli can also activate the fibrinolytic system, including exercise, anoxia, electroconvulsive therapy, and certain drugs.

When a clot is formed, plasminogen is adsorbed onto the fibrin strands; this "gel"-phase plasminogen is distinct from "sol"-phase plasminogen, which normally circulates in the plasma. *Plasminogen activator* appears to have a greater affinity for gel-phase than for sol-phase plasminogen. Consequently, when plasminogen activator is released into the circulation, it preferentially activates gel-phase plasminogen in the clot, producing *plasmin*, the enzymatic principle of the fibrinolytic system. Plasmin then digests fibrin, lysing the thrombus from within. Although the release of excessive quantities of plasminogen activator may activate sol-phase plasminogen as well, *hyperplasminemia* develops only when the circulating inhibitors are overwhelmed, at which time circulating free plasmin can digest fibrinogen and other coagulation proteins. Such a situation is rare, however, because the plasmin inhibitors normally circulate in high concentration.

The lysis of fibrin produces *fibrin breakdown products* (FBP), molecular fragments that have immunologic identity with fibrin. These products are thought to have three major antihemostatic functions: 1) anti-

Intrinsic System

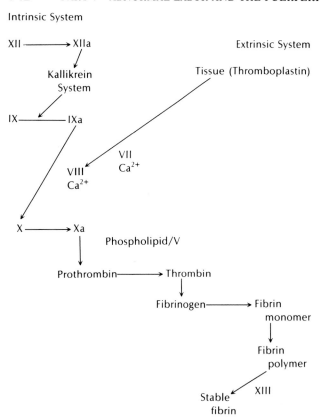

FIG. 37–1. Coagulation sequence.

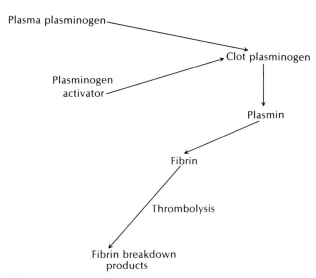

FIG. 37–2. Sequence of events in fibrinolysis and production of fibrin breakdown products.

platelet, 2) antithrombin, and 3) antipolymerization. It was noted earlier that platelets provide one of the first lines of defense against bleeding. Experimental and clinical evidence suggests that FBP can interfere with platelet function and produce a hemorrhagic diathesis that is characterized by prolonged bleeding from small vessels. Some authors believe that FBP also have an antithrombin effect, but this has been questioned. Although the addition of FBP to normal plasma significantly prolongs the time required for coagulation in several tests, the effect is probably due to inhibition of fibrin polymerization. FBP do not affect the action of thrombin on synthetic substrates.

The primary means by which FBP affect hemostasis is probably by interfering with fibrin polymerization. A clot formed in the presence of FBP is defective, both structurally and functionally. In addition, such a clot is more susceptible to lysis by plasmin; this lysis not only breaks down the clot, but also produces increased quantities of FBP. Fletcher and colleagues have studied many patients with acquired hemorrhagic diathesis and have shown that this antipolymerization effect is the principal mechanism by which "pathological plasma proteolysis" produces abnormal bleeding.

LABORATORY TESTS

TEST FOR COAGULATION DISORDERS

It is possible to test either specifically or indirectly for most of the components concerned in the clotting of blood and to define the specific deficiency in most cases. Some of the tests are ordinary laboratory procedures, while others require special facilities and the expertise of highly trained personnel. No single test can adequately screen patients for bleeding disorders, nor can any single test elucidate the cause of defective hemostasis in a particular patient. Several tests are necessary (Table 37–2) and they should be chosen to assess the various phases of hemostatic function:

1. *Platelet-vascular evaluation.* The integrity of the platelet-vascular phase can be measured easily by the Ivy bleeding time test. The platelets can be evaluated numerically by direct counting, either by the use of phase-contrast microscopy or, more commonly, by automatic counter methods. An adequate estimate of the number of platelets may be gained from the examination of the Wright-stained blood film. Platelet studies should be carried out on edetate (EDTA) anticoagulated blood. Functional activity of platelets is assessed by more sophisticated methods, including the study of platelet aggregation and adhesiveness.
2. *Screening tests of coagulation.* Determination of the standard clotting time is not a sensitive test of coagulation function. More sensitive, more accurate, and more reproducible are the determinations of

TABLE 37-2. TESTS OF HEMOSTATIC FUNCTION

Time	Test
IMMEDIATE	Bleeding time
	Platelet count
	Partial thromboplastin time
	Prothrombin time
LATER	Fibrin breakdown products
	Factor assays, especially fibrinogen
	Fibrinolytic tests: euglobulin lysis time, plasminogen concentration, thrombin time

partial thromboplastin time (PTT) and the *prothrombin time* (PT). The PTT test measures the activities of factors VIII, IX, XI, and XII (of the intrinsic system) and factors I, II, IV, and X (common to both systems). The PT test measures the activity of factor VII (peculiar to the extrinsic system) and factors I, II, V, and X (common to both systems). Neither of these tests is absolute because the end point in each, the formation of a visible clot, is open to subjective variation.

3. *Specific assays.* Individual assays can be carried out for most of the coagulation factors, although many are of academic interest only. In obstetric practice, one of the most frequently employed is the determination of plasma *fibrinogen concentration,* preferably by a method that measures fibrinogen directly. The clot observation test, long used as an index of the ability of blood to clot, is not recommended since a small, rapidly retracting clot can give the impression of no clot at all. The PTT can be done at least as rapidly in almost every hospital.

TESTS OF THE FIBRINOLYTIC SYSTEM

In addition to its former use to determine ability of blood to clot, the classic clot observation test has also been used as a measure of fibrinolytic activity: if a clot forms and subsequently dissolves rapidly, the test is interpreted to suggest that fibrinolysis is excessive. This test is difficult to standardize because there may be much subjective variation in interpretation. Also, it is performed at room temperature, whereas all tests of coagulation and fibrinolytic function should be carried out at body temperature. Moreover, scrupulously clean glassware, so necessary for such studies, is usually not available in a labor suite. Finally, although an adequate clot may form with a small concentration of fibrinogen, the subsequent clot retraction may suggest that the clot has dissolved, giving the erroneous impression of pathologic fibrinolysis. *The most useful method for determining the presence and degree of fi-* *brinolysis is the measurement of fibrin breakdown products.* This may be done by several methods. The hemagglutination method is fairly exact, but reasonably time-consuming. The latex agglutination test is much more rapid. The staphylococcus clumping test, which is highly accurate, is also available. Most experienced hematologic laboratories can carry out one or more of these determinations.

As mentioned earlier, the fibrinogen-to-fibrin conversion reaction is extremely sensitive to the presence of FBP. Determination of the thrombin time, carried out according to the method of Fletcher *et al.,* is an extremely sensitive test of the third stage of coagulation and gives an indication as to the degree of FBP activity.

CLASSIFICATION OF DISORDERS OF HEMOSTASIS

Hemostatic disorders may be either hereditary or acquired. *Hereditary hemostatic disorders* are unusual in obstetric patients. Von Willebrand's disease, the most common hereditary bleeding disorder in women, is characterized by a factor VIII abnormality, associated with a defect in platelet function. The platelet disorder is probably due to the lack of a plasma factor, since such patients' platelets function normally in the presence of plasma from normal or even hemophilic patients. Patients with many congenital bleeding disorders may improve during pregnancy, but a significant bleeding diathesis sometimes develops in the puerperium. For a review of these uncommon hemostatic disorders the reader should consult the classic review by Quick.

The *acquired disorders of hemostasis* include disseminated intravascular coagulation (DIC), circulating factor VIII inhibitors, and acquired thrombocytopenias. Of these, the most important in the obstetric patient is DIC.

DISSEMINATED INTRAVASCULAR COAGULATION

An intermediary mechanism of disease, DIC complicates a large number of obstetric, medical, and surgical situations. The bleeding diathesis in the patient with abruptio placentae or the "dead fetus syndrome" is virtually identical to that encountered in the patient with widely disseminated malignancy, heat stroke, or the Kasabach–Merritt syndrome of multiple giant hemangiomas. The obstetric situations in which DIC is most apt to be encountered are

Abruptio placentae
Dead fetus syndrome
Amniotic fluid embolism

Gram-negative septicemia
Preeclampsia–eclampsia
Miscellaneous conditions associated with pregnancy
    Kasabach–Merritt syndrome
    Acute pancreatitis
    Disseminated lupus erythematosus
    Hematologic malignancies

Abruptio placentae is the most common associated cause, but DIC is frequently encountered in prolonged retention of a dead fetus and in gram-negative septicemia.

PATHOPHYSIOLOGY

DIC is the response of the body to the entry into the circulation of a coagulation-promoting material, although this procoagulant moiety is frequently not identified. In abruptio placentae and in amniotic fluid infusion, the inciting material appears to be elements of decidual tissue or amniotic fluid, whereas in gram-negative septicemia, it seems to be an endotoxin that combines with some formed element in the blood, presumably the leukocyte, to produce a thromboplastic principle. In response to these stimuli, platelets aggregate and fibrinogen forms. Fibrinogen is rapidly converted into fibrin and deposited in the microcirculation. The site and speed of fibrin deposition depends on many factors, *e.g.*, the portal of entry of the agent, the state of the vascular tree at the time of fibrin deposition, the adequacy of the reticuloendothelial system, and the efficiency of the fibrinolytic system. In addition, some organs are more susceptible than others; the adrenals, pituitary, and the kidneys are especially vulnerable.

As soon as fibrin is deposited, the fibrinolytic system is activated in an effort to clear the blocked circulation. The process of fibrinolysis produces FBP, which impair hemostasis. The resulting bleeding defect, which is characterized by prolongation of bleeding from small vessels, can be gauged clinically by the bleeding time. In addition, the PTT and PT are both prolonged, and the platelet count is decreased, although not to levels that would suggest thrombocytopenia as the cause of the bleeding.

Several authors have compared DIC to the *generalized Shwartzman reaction,* which has been experimentally produced in the rabbit by two appropriately spaced injections of endotoxin. After the second injection, the animal develops bilateral renal cortical necrosis and, frequently, hemorrhagic manifestations identical to those seen in DIC. Although the rabbit appears to be unusually susceptible to this reaction, it has been produced in other animals as well. Significantly, in the pregnant rabbit, a single dose of endotoxin elicits the reaction; in a sense, therefore, pregnancy may "prepare" the animal for the generalized Shwartzman reaction. Similarly, the animal may be "prepared" by induction of reticuloendothelial blockade, by pretreatment with adrenocorticosteroids, by inhibition of the fibrinolytic system, and by pretreatment with agents that produce vasoconstriction. Alternatively, the reaction may be prevented by heparinization, by pretreatment with agents that produce generalized vasodilatation, and by those agents that induce fibrinolysis.

TREATMENT

In obstetric situations, the most urgent consideration is correction of the disorder giving rise to the DIC; in most cases, this alone suffices to correct the coagulation defect. The clinical management of these obstetric problems is considered in the discussions of the specific disorders. In mild or even moderate cases, specific therapy of the DIC is usually not needed if the inciting cause can be dealt with immediately. In severe cases, additional treatment is needed.

If hypovolemia is present it should be dealt with by administration of whole blood. Additional objectives are 1) to restore the reduced levels of coagulation factors and platelets, and 2) to clear the circulation of FBP. The first need can be met by administration of fresh blood, if it is available, or, if it is not, fresh-frozen plasma (2–3 units), cryoprecipitate (16–20 bags), and platelet concentrates, if necessary. In severe cases, heparin may also be needed. This is usually started as an intravenous bolus of 5000 units, followed by a continuous infusion of about 1000 units/hour, adjusted according to the response.

It is emphasized that the use of heparin in cases of this kind is a major form of therapy. If improperly used, it can have most serious consequences. Heparin should be used only when it is absolutely necessary and only by those who are thoroughly familiar with this form of therapy. If any major part of the vascular system is disrupted, as by lacerated uterine vessels, heparin may greatly increase the bleeding.

Abruptio Placentae

The initial escape of blood beneath the placenta in abruptio placentae results in local tissue injury and necrosis. Thromboplastin is liberated, which activates the extrinsic system. DIC sometimes occurs quite early, even when there is only minimal placental separation. If abruptio placentae is suspected, tests should be made for FBP, PTT, and PT. If the tests suggest DIC, the patient should be delivered promptly.

Blood loss in abruptio placentae is often underestimated, and hypovolemia may be present even when arterial pressure is normal. Central venous pressure monitoring is therefore important and, together with urinary output, should be used as a guide to the correction of depleted blood volume. As noted earlier,

fresh blood is preferable, since it restores the depleted coagulation factors, antithrombin III, and platelets; banked blood restores volume but compounds the depletion of platelets and also of coagulation factors V and VIII. If fresh blood is not available, fresh-frozen plasma, cryoprecipitate, and, if necessary, platelet concentrates should be administered as noted.

The longer the patient with a coagulation defect remains undelivered, the more profound the defect becomes. In a serious and progressing hemostatic defect, the administration of heparin may interrupt the DIC and facilitate clearing of FBP, thus minimizing the possibility of renal damage due to glomerular fibrin deposition and other sequelae.

Two forms of therapy that were formerly thought to be important are now known to be either unnecessary or potentially harmful. Specific attempts to correct the depleted levels of fibrinogen are no longer recommended. Fibrinogen is only one of the coagulation factors that is missing, and the capacity of the liver to restore fibrinogen is virtually unlimited. There is also no place for the use of fibrinolytic inhibitors. Fibrinolysis is a physiologic reaction to the presence of excessive amounts of fibrin within the microcirculation, and it is vital to the functional integrity of the organs involved that the circulation be cleared as rapidly as possible.

Intrauterine Death

The coagulopathy of the *dead fetus syndrome* develops slowly and is due to the escape of thromboplastic substances from the degenerating products of conception into the maternal circulation. The syndrome rarely occurs within 4 weeks of fetal death, but it can be expected in about 35% of women undelivered after 5 weeks. Accordingly, it can usually be prevented by delivery within 4 weeks. Periodic coagulation studies are usually started 2 weeks after intrauterine death, and special vigilance is begun after 3 weeks. If DIC is present, heparin should be administered for 24–48 hours before any operative intervention. This allows time for clearance of FBP and the spontaneous restoration of the coagulation factors that are continuously consumed in the course of continuing DIC.

Amniotic Fluid Embolism

Amniotic fluid embolism is usually a cataclysmic episode characterized by the sudden onset (during labor in the presence of ruptured membranes) of dyspnea, chest pain, pulmonary edema, shock, and, sometimes within minutes, death. Not all cases are immediately fatal. In those who survive the initial insult, DIC results from the activating effect of the infused amniotic fluid on the coagulation sequence. In addition to the vigorous supportive measures that are usually required, heparin may also be of signal value.

Gram-negative Endotoxemia

In the experimental animal, heparin prevents the development of the generalized Schwartzman reaction. In the human, DIC frequently complicates *septic shock*, which is the human counterpart of the generalized Schwartzman reaction. In such cases, the probable inciting cause for DIC is endothelial damage by the circulating endotoxin; the contact of the circulating blood with exposed collagen activates the intrinsic coagulation system. Antibiotics, blood transfusion, intensive supportive therapy, and removal of the focus of infection are cornerstones of the treatment of this serious condition. In some of the cases, heparin may be lifesaving.

Preeclampsia–Eclampsia

The association of preeclampsia–eclampsia with coagulation disorders is well-known. In this case, DIC may be triggered by endothelial damage resulting from the intense segmental vasospasm. The coagulopathy should be dealt with by vigorous treatment of the inciting cause. Heparin is not indicated; in several series of cases, it has been found not to be helpful. Also, there is a serious question of the wisdom of deliberate anticoagulation in a disorder that of itself may predispose to intracranial hemorrhage.

FACTOR VIII INHIBITORS

Rarely, acquired inhibitors to coagulation factor VIII may cause a significant hemorrhagic diathesis in the pregnant woman. In a classic article in 1961, Margolius *et al.* described 40 patients with acquired factor VIII inhibitors who fell into three broad groups:

1. Lupus erythematosus
2. Hemophiliacs repeatedly transfused
3. Patients in the puerperium

Acquired factor VIII inhibitors are important in obstetrics because their presence is almost invariably missed until the patient has bled excessively and frequently has received inappropriate therapy. Such cases are uncommon, but they have been known to occur.

THROMBOCYTOPENIA

A numeric deficiency of platelets is one of the least common underlying hemostatic defects encountered in the pregnant patient. A variety of drugs has been implicated, but of particular interest in obstetric situations is that thrombocytopenia occurs in association with thiazide diuretics. In such cases, both mother and fetus may develop thrombocytopenia.

Autoimmune thrombocytopenic purpura, discussed

in Chapter 12, is a disease in which the maternal circulation contains antibodies to platelets. The antibodies may be passively transferred to the fetus so that the baby, when born, may exhibit transient thrombocytopenia.

Thrombocytopenia in pregnancy should be managed by the hematologic specialist.

REFERENCES AND RECOMMENDED READING

Coopland AT: Blood clotting abnormalities in relation to pre-eclampsia. Can Med Assoc J 100:121, 1969

Coopland AT, Alkjaersig R, Fletcher AP: Reduction in a plasma factor XIII (fibrin stabilizing factor) concentration during pregnancy. J Lab Clin Med 73:144, 1969

Coopland AT, Israels ED, Zipursky A, Israels LG: The pathogenesis of defective hemostasis in abruptio placentae. Am J Obstet Gynecol 10:311, 1968

Coopland AT, Livingstone RAL: Heparin treatment of abruptio placentae. Can Med Assoc J 103:337, 1970

Davie EW, Ratnoff OD: Waterfall sequence for intrinsic blood clotting. Science 145:1310, 1964

Dieckmann WJ: Blood chemistry and renal function in abruptio placentae. Am J Obstet Gynecol 31:734, 1936

Ellis EF, Belz O, Roberts LJ, Payne RA, Sweetman BJ, Nies AS, Oates JA: Coronary arterial smooth muscle contraction by a substance released from platelets: Evidence that it is thromboxane A_2. Science 193:1135, 1976

Fletcher AP, Alkjaersig R, Sherry S: The maintenance of a sustained thrombolytic stake in man: 1. Induction and effects. J Clin Invest 38:1096, 1959

Goodnight SH, Jr: Cryoprecipitate and fibrinogen. JAMA 241:1716, 1979

Hathaway WE, Bonnar J: Perinatal Coagulation. Monographs in Neonatology. New York, Grune & Stratton, 1978.

Howie PW, Prentice CRM, McNicol GP: Coagulation, fibrinolysis and platelet function in pre-eclampsia, essential hypertension and placental insufficiency. J Obstet Gynaecol Br Commonw 78:992, 1971

Kowalski E, Budzynski AZ, Kopec M, Latallo ZS, Lipinski B, Wegrzynowicz Z: Studies on the molecular pathology and pathogenesis of bleeding in severe fibrinolytic status in dogs. Thromb Diath Haemorrh 12:69, 1964

Macfarlane RG: An enzyme cascade in the blood clotting mechanism and its function as a biochemical amplifier. Nature 202:498, 1964

McKay DG: Progress in disseminated intravascular coagulation. Calif Med 186:279, 1969

Margolis A, Jr, Jackson DP, Ratnoff OD: Circulating anticoagulants: A study of 40 cases and a review of the literature. Medicine 40:145, 1961

Ness PM, Perkins HA: Cryoprecipitate as a reliable source of fibrinogen replacement. JAMA 241:1690, 1979

Pritchard JA, Cunningham FG, Mason RA: Coagulation changes in eclampsia: Their frequency and pathogenesis. Am J Obstet Gynecol 124:855, 1976

Quick AJ: Menstruation in hereditary bleeding disorders. Obstet Gynecol 28:37, 1966

Ratnoff OD: The coagulation cascade revisited. Ann R Col Phy Surg Can 11:196, 1978

Rebuck JW: Blood platelets. Transfusion 3:1, 1963

Sher G: Pathogenesis and management of uterine inertia complicating abruptio placentae with consumption coagulopathy. Am J Obstet Gynecol 129:164, 1977

Talbert LM, Blatt PM: Disseminated intravascular coagulation in obstetrics. Clin Obstet Gynecol 22:889, 1979

Triantaphyllopoulos DC: Nature of the thrombin inhibiting effect of incubated fibrinogen. Am J Physiol 197:575, 1959

Wodzicki AM, Coopland AT: Coagulation and the hypertensive diseases of pregnancy. Am J Obstet Gynecol 129:393, 1977

TRANSFUSIONS

David H. Vroon

Blood is a complex substance containing multiple cellular and soluble elements. The transfer of this complex material between unrelated humans is a type of tissue transplantation that, unlike many other surgical procedures, cannot be readily undone. While much has been learned about blood compatibility testing, there remain significant gaps in knowledge. Furthermore, hazards associated with transfusion extend beyond those related to immune phenomena. Transfusion of blood products always presents a risk that must be measured against the possible benefits to the patient. Human blood is also a vital and limited natural resource that cannot be manufactured; demand frequently exceeds supply. The prescribing physician must be aware of the need to economize in the use of this valuable resource and is responsible for actively encouraging volunteer replacement of blood. Unnecessary administration of blood is wasteful and detrimental to patient care.

Indications for blood transfusion generally fall into three categories: 1) to facilitate the delivery of oxygen to tissues, 2) to correct hypovolemia, and 3) to restore adequate circulating levels of cellular or soluble constituents, including hemostatic factors. Since these needs seldom occur simultaneously, routine administration of all components present in fresh whole blood is not appropriate. Infusion of separate cellular or noncellular constituents selected to correct a specific deficiency is always preferable. Component transfusion more effectively corrects the specific deficiency, minimizes untoward reactions associated with unneeded blood constituents, and promotes conservation of a valuable natural resource (since fractionation of a single donor unit of blood serves the needs of several patients).

High-speed differential refrigerated centrifugation and a closed system of plastic bags allow fractionation and storage of blood components without danger of bacterial contamination and enable preparation of cellular and noncellular blood fractions in hospital and community blood banks. In addition, the number of noncellular plasma derivatives prepared and distributed commercially is increasing (Fig. 38–1). Each blood component has a specific use, produces a specific type of reaction, and has its own life cycle both *in vivo* and in the collection container. Effective and judicious use of blood must be based on a thorough knowledge of these characteristics.

CHAPTER 38

TRANSFUSIONS, SHOCK, AND ACUTE RENAL FAILURE

David H. Vroon
David N. Danforth
Manuel R. Comas
Robert E. Cuddihee
Denis Cavanagh

ERYTHROCYTE AND VOLUME REPLACEMENT

Red cells are readily stored *in vitro;* they have a shelf life of 21 days at $1°–6°$ C when collected in acid-citrate-dextrose (ACD) or citrate-phosphate-dextrose (CPD) anticoagulants and probably more than 5 years when stored at ultralow temperatures. Posttransfusion recovery exceeds 70% for refrigerated and 90% for frozen red blood cells, and the potential posttransfusion life span is essentially normal for stored red blood cells. Nevertheless, specific physicochemical and functional changes incidental to refrigerated storage may at times be significant considerations in the recipient. These are specifically discussed below with regard to massive red cell transfusions.

Erythrocytes can be replaced by infusion of whole

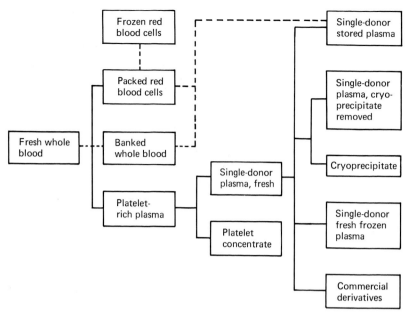

FIG. 38-1. Derivation of blood components.

TABLE 38-1. CHARACTERISTICS OF VARIOUS RED CELL PREPARATIONS

Unit	Volume (ml)	Hematocrit (%)	Red Cell Mass (ml)	Other Cellular and Soluble Elements	Total Protien (g)	Hepatitis Risk
WHOLE BLOOD	520	40	200	Leukocyte, platelet, and protein antigens maximal	49	Present
PACKED RED BLOOD CELLS	300	60–70	200	Cellular and soluble plasma elements significantly reduced	36	Present
FROZEN RED BLOOD CELLS⅞	300 in saline	60–70	200	Nonerythrocyte cellular and plasma elements absent	30	Present

blood, packed red blood cells, or frozen red blood cells. Characteristics of these preparations are summarized in Table 38–1. The need to restore or maintain oxygen-carrying capacity—the most common circumstance requiring transfusion—is satisfied only by infusion of red blood cells.

ANEMIA

Transfusion to correct chronic anemia is indicated primarily for those conditions not amenable to medical therapy, *e.g.,* congenital hemolytic or aplastic disorders. Patients with anemia secondary to nutritional deficiencies or chronic blood loss are candidates for transfusion only when underlying conditions predispose to heart failure or oxygen deprivation in the presence of a decreased red cell mass. Occasionally, a need for immediate general anesthesia and impending labor

requires transfusion; however, every effort should be made to detect anemia in advance of hospitalization and to correct it with appropriate hematinics.

The majority of patients with anemia do not have a plasma volume deficit; usually, there is a plasma volume excess. Infusion of packed cells is, therefore, almost always preferable to administration of whole blood in the patient with chronic subacute anemia. Packed red cells supply twice as much hemoglobin per unit of volume transfused as does whole blood; their use, therefore, provides a greater increment in hemoglobin concentration or oxygen-carrying capacity with less danger of circulatory overload. In addition, use of packed red cells minimizes nonspecific reactions due to extraneous cellular and soluble elements that do not contribute to oxygen-carrying capacity; and, when frozen red cells are used, the risk of hepatitis is greatly reduced.

In all cases, the decision to transfuse and the

amount of the transfusion should be based on clinical judgment rather than solely on arbitrarily selected hemoglobin or hematocrit values. Cause and duration of anemia, as well as activity and cardiopulmonary status of the recipient, are major considerations. Infusion of 1 unit of packed red blood cells produces, on the average, a 3% increment in recipient hematocrit. Since risk is compounded with multiple-unit transfusions, every effort should be made to limit the number of units used. The accreditation agency practice of citing frequency of single-unit transfusions as an index of careless transfusion procedure should be condemned. There are certainly valid indications for administration of a single unit of packed cells, and no physician should be tempted to administer a second unit to avoid criticism.

BLOOD LOSS

Before a transfusion is given to correct acute blood loss of traumatic, surgical, or spontaneous origin, red cell mass and volume replacement must be considered. While infusion of whole blood has been accepted as therapy of choice for acute blood loss, there is growing evidence that the use of salt solutions alone or with packed red blood cells is often advantageous. Massive acute hypovolemia due to blood loss requires replacement with whole blood. However, acute blood loss, particularly during a surgical procedure, is usually not massive and often does not exceed 1000 ml. Replacement in these patients must be governed by several considerations.

First, the major hazard of acute blood loss is failure to maintain adequate tissue oxygenation. While maintenance of blood pressure is germane to tissue oxygenation, an adult can sustain rapid loss of 1000–2000 ml blood or up to 40% of blood volume without developing irreversible shock. Both blood pressure and renal blood flow can be sustained by infusion of saline fluids without the hazards of transfusion. Rapid loss of 450 ml blood is insignificant; billions of blood donors experience such a loss every year.

Second, acute blood loss rarely mandates replacement of nonerythrocyte cellular and noncellular blood elements. Leukocyte and platelet extravascular reserves are moderately large, and hemorrhage is regularly associated with leukocytosis and thrombocytosis. Erythrocyte extravascular reserves, on the other hand, are minimal and are returned to the circulation over a period of weeks. The concept that plasma protein must be replaced in order to maintain blood volume, promote healing, and reduce the risk of infection, particularly in surgical patients, is not based on fact. Plasma proteins are readily replaced; indeed, repeated removal of 1000 ml plasma weekly from healthy donors for plasmapheresis has no significant effect. In health, albumin synthesis is as high as 16 g/day. Furthermore,

albumin distribution throughout the body is such that only 40% exists in the intravascular compartment; loss of as much as 2000 ml blood in an adult results in only a 15% depletion of total body albumin. The total protein present in whole blood is not significantly different from that in packed cells (Table 38–1). The amount of protein in 1 unit of plasma can be supplied by an average serving of meat.

Mild to moderate acute blood loss is well tolerated and usually requires only red blood cell replacement when oxygen-carrying capacity is significantly compromised. Administration of a balanced salt solution augmented by packed red blood cells should therefore be considered treatment of choice. Whole blood transfusion is indicated to combat extensive hemorrhage and impending hypovolemic shock.

MASSIVE TRANSFUSIONS

Transfusion of sufficient blood to constitute total volume replacement within 12–24 hours presents special problems. In the adult, the amount needed is usually 8–10 units of whole blood. Banked or stored whole blood undergoes physical and functional alterations, and its administration in large amounts may produce potentially deleterious changes in hemoglobin affinity for oxygen, clotting mechanisms, and acid–base balance.

Refrigerated storage is associated with a decrease in red cell organic phosphate, particularly 2,3-diphosphoglyceric acid (2,3-DPG), which controls liberation of oxygen in tissue. Depletion of intracellular 2,3-DPG increases hemoglobin affinity for oxygen and therefore diminishes the erythrocytes' capacity to deliver oxygen to tissues. Loss of 2,3-DPG occurs somewhat more slowly in CPD-treated blood than in ACD-treated blood; significant decreases are noted after 7–10 days of storage. Restoration of organic phosphates and normal oxygen affinity may require 24–72 hours after transfusion of stored cells. Transient changes in recipient oxygen dissociation curves have been demonstrated, although deleterious clinical effects are not well documented. On theoretic grounds, therefore, massive transfusions are associated with significant risk of temporary anoxia. This can be averted by making sure that most of the units given have been stored for less than 1 week.

Clotting complications due to rapid deterioration of factors V and VIII and platelets in stored blood are commonly encountered following massive transfusions. All other clotting factors are stable in refrigerated blood. To counteract the effects of depletion of factors V and VIII, 2 units of fresh-frozen plasma should be given after the infusion of the first 8–10 units of banked blood; thereafter, 1 unit of fresh-frozen plasma should be given for every 4 units of blood infused. Clotting complications due to platelet depletion

are less common; replacement with platelet concentrates should be based on platelet counts.

The problems associated with increased hemoglobin affinity for oxygen and clotting defects can be prevented by the use of fresh whole blood. However, since blood stored for less than 24 hours is usually not obtainable in emergency situations, specific component therapy is often the best alternative.

The addition of acid preservative solution to stored blood presents the recipient of multiple units with a large acid load. Significant acidosis may occur, particularly in the presence of shock or compromised respiratory or renal function. The acid–base response to multiple transfusions is variable, and administration of sodium bicarbonate may effect an undesirable leftward shift of the oxygen dissociation curve. Bicarbonate administration should be guided by arterial blood gas and pH determinations. Additional storage-related changes, such as increased plasma potassium, reduced ionized calcium, and increased citrate content are usually significant only in transfusion of children or of adults with hepatic or renal disease. Plasma constituents can be greatly reduced if packed cells rather than whole blood are given.

Because infusion of multiple units of blood at refrigerated temperatures has been associated with cardiac arrhythmias and even cardiac arrest, blood should be warmed as it is transfused. The use of warm blood also enhances the sensitivity of blood pressure measurement. The heat-exchanging equipment must be carefully monitored, however, since overheating the blood may trigger hemolysis with consequent disastrous effects. The practice of warming the entire container of blood at room temperature or in a water bath should be condemned on grounds of inadequate heat exchange and danger of bacterial growth.

EMERGENCY TRANSFUSIONS

Clinical circumstances sometimes mandate blood replacement before the usual compatibility testing has been completed. Communication with the blood bank in these situations must be clear and rational. The risk of a fatal transfusion reaction must be carefully weighed against the risk of irreversible shock or exsanguination. ABO groupings and Rh typing of the patient's blood, selecting donor blood of the same ABO and Rh type, and complete cross matching require approximately 90 min. A dire emergency may warrant abbreviation of this process, and transfusion must never be delayed unnecessarily. Even in an emergency, however, the safest and most expedient compromises must be employed.

Group- and type-specific blood should be administered when time permits analysis of the patient's blood. Previous records must not be accepted as evidence of blood group. When time does not permit

grouping and typing of the recipient's blood, group O Rh-negative blood may be administered; however, in such cases, at least 70% of the plasma should be removed before transfusion to avoid subjecting the patient to dangerous levels of antibodies, specifically anti-A and anti-B. In emergency situations, it is preferable to employ packed cells (type-specific if there is time for typing; group O, preferably Rh-negative, if there is not) and to accomplish additional volume expansion with albumin or plasma protein fraction preparations that are free of antibodies. In all cases, routine compatibility testing should be initiated in the blood bank. Significant incompatibility can often be detected by the time blood is transported to the patient's side. The attending physician should be notified immediately if there is such an incompatibility.

PLATELET TRANSFUSIONS

Platelets function in hemostasis by plugging injured vessels and by releasing a phospholipid, platelet factor 3, which contributes to the coagulation process. The causes of thrombocytopenia are numerous. In obstetric and gynecologic practice, significant acute thrombocytopenia is most often associated with syndromes of disseminated intravascular coagulation and the infusion of massive quantities of blood. Platelet replacement should be guided by the platelet count. Active bleeding with a platelet count of less than 70,000/cu mm is a clear indication for replacement.

Blood platelets retain little hemostatic function after 24–48 hours of refrigerated storage. Platelets must be harvested from freshly collected blood. When stored with agitation at room temperature, they remain viable and functional for up to 72 hours. Fresh blood, platelet-rich fresh plasma, and platelet concentrates are sources of functional platelets. Of these, platelet concentrates offer the advantage of providing large numbers of platelets (70%–80% of fresh whole blood) in a small volume of plasma (less than 50 ml). After infusion, platelets are hemostatically effective for not more than 5 days. In a previously sensitized recipient, the presence of platelet antibodies may reduce the beneficial effect to a matter of hours. An increment of 50,000 platelets/cu mm can be expected from the transfusion of 1 unit of platelet concentrate per 7 kg of body weight. The increment is significantly less in a patient with sepsis, fever, or active bleeding; however, hemostasis may be achieved in a bleeding patient without a significant increase in platelet count. In general, when platelet replacement is indicated in an adult, infusion of platelets harvested from 8–10 units of fresh donor blood is required. Volume considerations usually dictate the choice of platelet concentrates rather than fresh whole blood. Since platelets are suspended in plasma and contain small numbers of red blood cells, ABO and Rh compatibility is desirable but not always

TABLE 38-2. BLOOD PLASMA FRACTIONS AVAILABLE FOR REPLACEMENT OF NONCELLULAR ELEMENTS

Plasma Fraction	Functional Constituents (% of Fresh Whole Blood)	Unit Volume (ml)	Therapeutic Indications	Advantages	Disadvantages
SINGLE-DONOR PLASMA	All plasma proteins except labile clotting factors	240	Volume expansion Plasma replacement	Relatively low cost	Hepatitis risk Antibodies and all other plasma protein antigens included
SINGLE-DONOR PLASMA, FRESH-FROZEN	All plasma proteins	240	Clotting defects due to multiple or unknown factor deficiencies	Relatively low cost	Same as single-donor plasma Large volume required
PLASMA PROTEIN FACTOR	Albumin α-Globulin β-Globulin	250 or 500	Volume expansion Plasma replacement	Lack of antibody No hepatitis risk Room temperature storage	Relatively high cost
CRYOPRECIPITATE	Factor VIII (60%) Fibrinogen (23% average of 250 mg/unit)	< 10	Classic hemophilia von Willebrand's disease Fibrinogen replacement	Less than 3% plasma protein Low volume required Minimal immune reactions Relatively low cost	Few red cell antigens present Hepatitis risk Unassayed factor VIII and fibrinogen
ALBUMIN, 5% IN BUFFERED SALINE	Albumin (5 g/100 ml)	250 or 500	Volume expansion Plasma replacement	Same as plasma protein fraction	Same as plasma protein fraction
ALBUMIN, 25% SALT-POOR	Albumin (25 g/100 ml)	50 or 100	Volume expansion Protein replacement Neonatal hyperbilirubinemia Cerebral edema	Same as plasma protein fraction Significant serum albumin increments attainable	Risk of circulatory overload due to oncotic pressure Relatively high cost
FACTOR II-VII-IX-X COMPLEX	Clotting factors II, VII, IX, X	40	Vitamin K–dependent factor replacement Specific factor replacement hemophilia B	Minimal total protein Low volume required	Increased hepatitis risk

possible, owing to urgency of need and deficiency of supply. In an Rh-negative woman of childbearing age, infusion of a platelet preparation from Rh-positive donors may result in isosensitization.

TRANSFUSION OF NONCELLULAR PLASMA COMPONENTS

Blood plasma fractions commonly available for replacement of noncellular elements are summarized in Table 38-2. Some of these products are routinely prepared in blood banks; others are available as commercial derivatives. Effective use depends on a thorough knowledge of their specific constituents, indications, advantages, and disadvantages.

The immediate goal in treatment of acute hemorrhagic shock is volume replacement to sustain blood pressure and circulation. Fluid replacement with buffered salt or protein solutions is effective and appropriate while blood is being readied. Although plasma is an effective volume expander, its possible content of anti-A and anti-B antibodies, aggregated and denatured protein, and the hepatitis virus are significant disadvantages. Plasma derivatives such as 5% albumin and plasma protein fraction in combination with buffered salt solutions are the plasma volume expanders of choice since they contain no antibodies and are heat-treated to kill hepatitis virus. Disadvantages are higher cost and limited supply of these commercial plasma protein derivatives. There is some evidence that albumin is overused for purposes of volume expansion. The expense of this agent is a matter of concern, and efforts are being made to find less costly substitutes that are equally effective. Although there are still unanswered questions regarding it, hetastarch (Hespan) may be one such agent.

Indications for treating hypoproteinemia by infusion

of protein solutions are unclear. The widespread practice of treating all degrees of hypoproteinemia is probably without merit. The benefit is not sufficiently defined in many cases to justify infusion of plasma with its associated risk of hepatitis transmission. Protein solutions treated to kill hepatitis virus are available. Significant elevation of plasma proteins is obtainable only when 25% albumin is infused.

Clotting disorders due to a deficiency of soluble clotting factors can be alleviated by infusion of fresh-frozen plasma, cryoprecipitate, factor VIII concentrate, or prothrombin complex concentrate. All carry some risk of hepatitis. The latter two are associated with the highest risk, since they are prepared from plasma pools. Administration of these products should be guided by the results of the basic clotting tests described in Chapter 37.

Congenital deficiencies of individual clotting factors are, for practical purposes, limited to lack of factors VIII, IX, and XI—uncommonly encountered in obstetric and gynecologic practice. Acquired hemostatic defects are usually due to multiple factor deficiencies. Liver disease, ingestion of oral anticoagulants, and hemorrhagic disease of the newborn involve the vitamin K–dependent factors II, VII, IX, and X. Clotting defects associated with massive transfusion of banked blood involve primarily platelets and labile factors V and VIII. Deficiencies secondary to disseminated intravascular coagulation involve primarily platelets, factors V and VIII, fibrinogen, and prothrombin. Administration of fresh-frozen plasma in combination with platelet concentrates is effective in all these conditions when replacement therapy is warranted.

Commercial preparations of fibrinogen prepared from plasma pools are no longer available for clinical use because of the unacceptably high incidence of posttransfusion hepatitis. Fibrinogen replacement is rarely needed, but if there should be an indication, adequate fibrinogen levels can be obtained by infusion of cryoprecipitate with significantly less risk of hepatitis transmission. Each bag of cryoprecipitate contains an average of 250 mg fibrinogen; 16–20 bags are usually required for replacement therapy. Disadvantages of cryoprecipitate are the variability in plasma fibrinogen response and the large volume that must be infused. Acute hemolytic reactions and hemolytic anemia from anti-A or anti-B antibodies are readily avoided by using blood type–specific cryoprecipitate.

HAZARDS OF BLOOD TRANSFUSION

The transfusion of blood or its components can produce several types of adverse reactions. Some of these reactions are life threatening; others are inconsequential. Some are avoidable; others are inherent risks of transfusion. Some adverse reactions occur immediately and are readily recognized; others are delayed and often not recognized, or are blamed on a previous transfusion. It is estimated that untoward reactions occur in more than 5% of transfusions.

IMMEDIATE TRANSFUSION REACTIONS

Immediate adverse effects of transfusion are circulatory overload, air embolism, septicemia, hypothermia, chemical intoxication, and antigen–antibody reactions. Hypothermia and chemical intoxication are discussed under Massive Transfusions. Circulatory overload is by far the most common immediate complication; the importance of minimizing infused volume is a major reason for the use of packed red blood cells rather than whole blood.

Types of Immediate Reactions

Septicemia due to infusion of contaminated blood may be associaed with chills, fever, and profound shock that requires emergency measures. Most often gram-negative bacilli capable of growing at 4° C are responsible, and they may produce deadly endotoxins. Prevention of transfusion septicemia depends on careful collection and storage of blood. Since a rise in temperature accelerates the growth of any contaminant, storage at room temperature and prolonged infusion must be avoided. Any unit of blood exposed to temperatures that exceed 10° C should be considered unusable.

Reactions may occur between donor cellular or protein antigen and recipient antibodies. Less common reactions result from infusion of donor antibodies. Reactions that activate complement and lyse cells are most severe. Vasoactive substances, generated by complement activation and cell destruction, result in release of hemoglobin and other intracellular proteins, some of which have thromboplastinlike activity. These substances account for the anaphylactic shock, renal failure, and bleeding diathesis observed in severe transfusion reactions.

Immune intravascular destruction of erythrocytes is the most feared complication of transfusion therapy. Shock, bleeding diathesis, and renal failure may occur precipitously and threaten life. Present day serologic techniques effectively protect against this hazard, but human error is ever-present; clerical errors related to misidentification of donor units and recipient account for the majority of acute hemolytic reactions to transfusion. Great care must be taken to ensure that the proper specimen is sent to the laboratory for cross matching and that the proper unit is administered to the intended recipient.

Immune reactions to leukocytes, platelets, and plasma factors are common causes of less severe transfusion reactions. Since complement activation is minimal, there are no anaphylactic symptoms. Fever

and chills are predominant. Leukocyte and platelet antibodies are common in multiparous women and in recipients of multiple transfusions. Modern serologic techniques neither detect incompatibilities nor prevent sensitization to these cellular elements. Reactions are minimized by infusion of packed cells rather than whole blood. However, with the exception of frozen red cells, sufficient plasma and cellular antigens remain in packed cells to effect sensitization. Reactions to plasma proteins are less well documented. Allergic reactions are common and are manifested by itching, erythema, and urticaria. Respiratory symptoms are rare. These reactions tend to occur in patients with an allergic history, and the patient with a previous allergic transfusion reaction is likely to experience another. Reactions with anaphylactoid symptoms have been rarely observed in patients with antibodies to IgA immunoglobin.

A recipient's immune reaction caused by infusion of donor antibodies is usually less severe or even unnoticed, owing to immediate dilution of the antibody in the recipient. However, such a reaction should not be ignored. Infusion of blood or plasma containing platelet or leukocyte antibodies may induce thrombocytopenia or leukopenia in the recipient. Group O blood, platelet concentrates, and cryoprecipitate prepared from pooled blood all contain significant amounts of anti-A and anti-B antibodies. These products, given to a recipient with group A, B, or AB blood, may precipitate immediate systemic reactions or spherocytic hemolytic anemia. Neutralization by the addition of specific soluble substances A and B is unreliable. For this reason, emergency transfusion of group O blood should employ packed cells rather than whole blood. When a large amount of platelets of cryoprecipitate prepared from pooled blood is to be infused, group-compatible units should be selected, if possible.

Investigation and Management of Immediate Transfusion Reactions

Immune reactions to transfusion are almost always associated with chills and fever. Initial manifestations of serious reactions may be indistinguishable from those of inconsequential reactions. Therefore, onset of these symptoms is always reason to stop the transfusion and investigate their cause. Additional transfusions should be avoided until the reaction is defined. All transfusion reactions should be reported to the blood bank and investigated to the extent considered appropriate in consultation with the blood bank director.

The occurrence of chills, fever, back pain, or a drop in blood pressure with oozing of blood suggests a hemolytic reaction. Elevated plasma hemoglobin value, hemoglobinuria, or a positive result in the direct antiglobulin test is confirmatory. All specimens, including blood containers, should be returned to the blood bank for serologic testing. Clerical records should be immediately checked to exclude mistaken identity of either donor blood or recipient. The donor blood should be examined by gram staining and cultured to exclude bacterial contamination.

Immune, coagulation, and renal disorders associated with acute hemolytic transfusion reactions are life threatening and require vigorous therapy. Mannitol, initially 25 g for adults and up to 150 g/24 hours, and saline solutions with sodium bicarbonate should be administered immediately to maintain urinary output of 1–3 ml/min. Inability to maintain urine flow is presumptive evidence of acute tubular necrosis, and fluids should then be restricted and the possible need for dialysis kept in mind. When anaphylactic shock is life threatening, vasopressors are indicated. However, vasoconstriction may contribute to renal damage. Bleeding disorders suggest defibrination has occurred, and this should be confirmed by laboratory tests, as discussed in Chapter 37. Intravenous administration of heparin may inhibit intravascular clotting. When replacement therapy is required to control bleeding, platelet concentrates, fresh-frozen plasma, or cryoprecipitate may be employed. Erythrocytes may be transfused as packed cells or whole blood after cross matching with a fresh specimen from the patient. When ABO incompatibility is the cause of the hemolytic reaction, group O packed cells should be given.

DELAYED COMPLICATIONS OF TRANSFUSION

Delayed adverse effects of transfusion include sensitization, delayed antigen–antibody reactions, and disease transmission.The frequency and significance of many delayed reactions are not known; more often than not they proceed unrecognized. Occasionally, red blood cell incompatibility occurs with antibody titers too low to be serologically detectable or to cause an immediate reaction. Transfusion of donor cells containing the appropriate antigen may elicit an anamnestic response, with an antigen–antibody reaction occurring several days after transfusion. Systemic manifestations are only occasionally observed; destruction of transfused cells goes unnoticed or masquerades as an autoimmune hemolytic process. A similar situation may occur with platelet antigens; infusion of donor platelets may elicit an immune response that results in thrombocytopenia.

The selection of blood with the same ABO and and Rh characteristics as the patient's does not guarantee that recipient isosensitization to one of numerous other red cell antigens will not occur. Fortunately, most red cell antigens (except in the ABO, Rh, Kell, and Duffy systems) do not readily elicit an antibody response. Nevertheless, isoimmunization has been estimated to occur in as many as 1% of single-unit transfusions. Transfusion that is free of immediate ill effects may still produce immunization that may inter-

fere with future pregnancies or transfusions. Chances of eliciting antiplatelet and antileukocyte antibodies are even greater, and their production may interfere with future transfusions or organ transplants.

Infectious diseases transmissible by blood include bartonellosis, brucellosis, trypanosomiasis, cytomegalic viral disease, infectious mononucleosis, hepatitis, malaria, and syphilis. Present methods of donor screening and blood processing have eliminated all but hepatitis as serious clinical problems. The frequency of posttransfusion hepatitis is approximately 7%. Type B hepatitis accounts for about 10%–15% of the cases, and the remainder are comprised of non–A and non–B hepatitis. Risk has been shown to correlate with (1) the presence of hepatitis B surface antigen (HB_sA_g) in donor blood; (2) the proportion of commercial donors; and (3) the number of donor units included in the transfusion volume. Morbidity and mortality from icteric hepatitis in adults are significant; the percentage of blood recipients with anicteric infections who suffer chronic liver damage is unknown.

Elimination of HB_sA_g-positive donor units cannot totally eliminate posttransfusion hepatitis, but it can help considerably. Further reduction is possible through judicious use of transfusion in general and through selection of component units that carry a lower risk of hepatitis. Presently, the only available blood products that have no risk of hepatitis transmission are immune serum globulin, plasma protein fraction, and albumin preparations. Derivatives prepared from plasma pools, such as factor VIII and IX concentrates, carry the greatest risk.

REFERENCES AND RECOMMENDED READING

Alexander MR, Ambre JJ, Liskow BI: Therapeutic use of albumin. JAMA 241:2527, 1979

American Association of Blood Banks: Blood Component Therapy. Chicago, Twentieth Century Press, 1969

American Medical Association: General Principles of Blood Transfusion. Chicago, AMA, 1973

Blumberg N, Bove JR: Un-crossed matched blood for emergency transfusion: One year's experience in a civilian setting. JAMA 240:2057, 1978

Chaplin H, Jr: Packed red blood cells (current concepts). N Eng J Med 281:364, 1969

Goodnight SH, Jr: Cryoprecipitate and fibrinogen. JAMA 241:1716, 1979

Myhre BA: Fatalities from blood transfusion. JAMA 244:1333, 1980

Ness PM, Perkins HA: Cryoprecipitate as a reliable source of fibrinogen replacement. JAMA 241:1690, 1979

Solowag HB, Bereynak CE: Plasma fibrinogen levels following cryoprecipitate infusion. Transfusion 10:326, 1970

Thompson WL: Blood Substitutes and Plasma Expanders. New York, Alan R Liss, 1978

SHOCK*

David N. Danforth

Shock is a clinical syndrome caused by a critical reduction in the perfusion of tissues by blood, resulting in a deficiency of oxygen, electrolytes, hormones, and other essential cell requirements. The clinical problems of shock result from a decrease in blood flow rather than a decrease in blood pressure. Shock may be produced by any one of a number of unrelated causes, such as hypovolemia (following hemorrhage or dehydration), cardiac failure, hypersensitivity (anaphylactic or allergic), infection, neurogenic disturbance, and blood flow impediment. In obstetrics, shock and shocklike states are usually the result of profound maternal disturbances. In the antepartum period, the fetus is also in jeopardy, for maintenance of adequate perfusion of maternal tissues by blood is essential for fetal survival.

HEMORRHAGIC SHOCK

The causes of major hemorrhage in obstetric patients include especially postpartum hemorrhage, incomplete abortion, ruptured ectopic pregnancy, and all the causes of bleeding in late pregnancy. The degree of hemorrhage that may result in shock in a particular patient varies greatly, depending on such factors as the initial hematrocrit and hemoglobin values, the rapidity of blood loss, the duration of bleeding, the presence of infection, and the effects of anesthetic and other drug administration.

Hemorrhagic shock is the shock of hypovolemia. As a result of hemorrhage, the circulating blood volume is reduced, venous return to the heart is impaired, and cardiac output is lowered. An immediate compensatory response is the reflex activation of adrenergic receptors and the release of increased amounts of catecholamines into the circulation; tachycardia and vasoconstriction result. In addition, fluids pass from the extravascular space into the vascular system in an effort to maintain the circulating blood volume. These compensatory reactions may temporarily maintain the blood pressure and provide adequate tissue perfusion; but, if the blood loss is not quickly replaced, the tissues become increasingly hypoxic, metabolic acidosis occurs, and widespread capillary and tissue damage results.

The clinical picture of hemorrhagic-shock is well-

---

* This section is a revision of the material prepared by Keith P. Russell for previous editions of this book.

TABLE 38-3. CORRELATION OF CLINICAL FINDINGS AND MAGNITUDE OF VOLUME DEFICIT IN HEMORRHAGIC SHOCK*

Severity of Shock	Clinical Findings	Reduction in Blood Volume
NONE	None (normal blood donation)	Up to 20% (500 ml)†
MILD	Minimal tachycardia	15%–25% (750–1250 ml)
	Slight decrease in blood pressure	
	Mild evidence of peripheral vasoconstriction with cool hands and feet	
MODERATE	Tachycardia, 100–120	25%–35% (1250–1750ml)
	Decrease in pulse pressure	
	Systolic blood pressure 90–100 mg Hg	
	Restlessness	
	Increased sweating	
	Pallor	
	Oliguria	
SEVERE	Tachycardia, over 120	Up to 50% (2500 ml)
	Systolic blood pressure below 60 mm Hg and frequently unobtainable by cuff	
	Mental stupor	
	Extreme pallor, cold extremities	
	Anuria	

* Blood volume changes based on clinical observations of Beecher HK, Simeone FA, Burnett CH et al.: Surgery 22:672, 1947.

† Based on blood volume of 7% in 70-kg male of medium build.

(Smith I.I., Weil MH: In Weil MH, Shubin H (eds): Diagnosis and Treatment of Shock, Baltimore, Williams & Wilkins, 1967)

known and may correlate well with the magnitude of the volume deficit (Table 38-3). However, in the obstetric patient, the signs of mild shock are less reliable since the compensatory mechanisms appear to hold up longer and do not give way gradually as in the nonobstetric patient. When moderate shock appears, it often does so abruptly, with little warning. Accordingly, in obstetric hemorrhage, the decision to begin intravenous fluids and blood replacement is based upon estimated blood loss rather than upon the customary premonitory signs of a gradually rising pulse rate and a gradually declining blood pressure.

The immediate *treatment of hemorrhagic shock* includes elevation of the legs to an angle of about 30° (the Trendelenburg position may interfere with cerebral circulation and respiratory exchange), the administration of oxygen by a loose-fitting mask, and infusion of lactated Ringer's solution through a large-gauge needle or catheter. Blood is drawn for typing and cross matching, and the lactated Ringer's solution is then run in *rapidly*, between 1 and 2 liters being administered during the 1st hour. As a result of this therapy alone, pulse and blood pressure usually return to normal; if blood loss has not been excessive, they tend to remain stable. If the total blood loss has been extreme or if bleeding continues, the improvement is transient, and accurately matched blood, which should be available by this time, should be given. In addition

to providing time for accurate matching of blood, lactated Ringer's therapy appears also to reduce the amount of blood required.

Urine output provides an excellent measure of organ perfusion, and a Foley catheter should be inserted. Hourly urine output of 50 ml or more suggests good renal perfusion. Output below 25 ml/hour implies inadequate renal perfusion; tubular ischemia and necrosis can result.

In addition to other vital signs, determination of central venous pressure (CVP) and, in some patients, pulmonary wedge pressure can provide important information regarding fluid requirements. CVP should be measured in all cases of shock. CVP does not necessarily reflect blood volume, but it does indicate the ability of the heart to accept and expel the blood returned to it and, therefore, is an excellent guide to the need for fluids and an aid in the prevention of circulatory overload. The catheter used for monitoring CVP can also be used to withdraw blood samples and administer required fluids. Medications, with the possible exception of heparin, should be given by another route. The insertion of the CVP catheter is not wholly without hazard; such complications as cardiac tamponade and perforation have been reported. However, CVP has become standard practice for the monitoring of most shock syndromes, and those who deal with these problems should become proficient in its use. The CVP

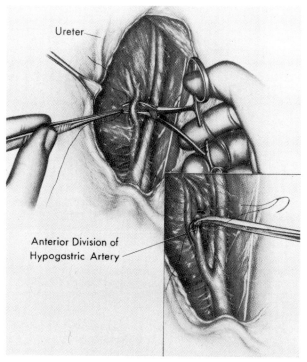

FIG. 38-2. Ligation of right hypogastric artery. Peritoneum is opened lateral to bifurcation of common iliac artery, and ureter is reflected medially with peritoneal flap. There is much variation in length and point of division of hypogastric artery into anterior and posterior branches. If possible, anterior branch should be selected for ligation and silk suture placed around it. *Inset* shows anterior division of hypogastric artery ligated and excised, and transfixion ligature placed distal to initial silk tie. (TeLinde RW, Mattingly RF: Operative Gynecology, 4th ed. Philadelphia, JB Lippincott, 1970)

catheter is first attached to a manometer, and the system is filled with saline. The catheter is threaded through the median basilic or subclavian vein for a distance that conforms to the circuit to the right atrium. Normal CVP is 5–8 cm H_2O; in the presence of significant hemorrhage, CVP is below 5 cm H_2O, and such a value is an indication for the transfusion of whole blood until the CVP reaches 8–12 cm H_2O. An elevated CVP (above 15 cm H_2O) occurs in the presence of such complications as fluid overload, pulmonary embolus, and left heart failure. If there is doubt about the possibility of overload, the CVP response to the rapid loading of the circulation may be tested with 100–200 ml saline over the course of 5–10 min. Circulatory overload is considered imminent if the CVP rises by as much as 5 cm H_2O and remains elevated for more than 5 min, or if it fails to decrease halfway to preexisting levels within 15 min.

Pulmonary wedge pressure supplies a more accurate assessment of cardiopulmonary embarrassment than CVP, but its measurement requires special expertise and equipment. The Swan–Ganz catheter, equipped with an inflatable balloon tip, is threaded into the right atrium under pressure monitoring. The balloon is then inflated with 0.8 ml air and is propelled by blood flow through the right ventricle, ultimately wedging into one of the smaller radicles of the pulmonary artery. Pressure determinations can be made and samples of blood collected from these compartments, permitting more exact diagnosis of cardiopulmonary disturbance. Measurement of pulmonary wedge pressure may be required to distinguish between the aforementioned causes of elevated CVP or to evaluate more complicated forms of shock that do not respond to the measures outlined here.

It is essential to determine the source of the bleeding and to control it. Bleeding often stops as shock develops, but it can be expected to resume as the circulation is restored. If a major surgical procedure is needed, fine judgment may be required to determine whether to operate before shock is entirely relieved; in most cases, the procedure should be deferred until the vital signs and blood volume are stabilized, or at least until appropriate fluids are being administered. Hysterectomy is usually indicated for uncontrollable uterine bleeding. Ligation of the hypogastric (internal iliac) arteries (Fig. 38–2) is appropriate if hysterectomy is not feasible because of technical problems imposed, for example, by a broad ligament hematoma, or because a quicker and less traumatic solution is needed.

SEPTIC SHOCK

Septic shock (bacterial shock, bacteremic shock, endotoxin shock) is a clinical syndrome of acute circulatory failure associated with bacteremia. In obstetrics, the clinical insults that lead most frequently to septic shock are infected (septic) abortion and chorioamnionitis secondary to premature rupture of the membranes. Pyelonephritis is an occasional cause. There are no recent estimates of mortality, but it is clear that the prognosis is improved if the problem is recognized early and is treated in an informed and aggressive manner. In the late 1950s, when less was known of the condition, the mortality ranged 70%–90%.

The causative organisms are usually, but not always, gram-negative bacteria: *Escherichia coli* predominates; others less frequently concerned are *Klebsiella, Proteus, Pseudomonas,* and *Meningococcus.* In one series of cases, 13% were due to *Bacteroides fragilis.* Clostridia cause 0.5% of cases of septic shock. Staphylococci and nonhemolytic anaerobic streptococci can also produce the syndrome. In the case of gram-negative organisms, the vascular effects are pro-

duced by endotoxin released from the disintegrating bacteria in the necrotic nidus of infection. In gram-positive septic shock, the identity of the precipitating agent is less clear, bu the clinical syndrome and its treatment are the same.

Many efforts have been made to clarify the primary events that lead to shock, and many theories have been advanced, but the matter is still unsettled. Secondary events are clearer; blood pools in the microcirculation, which results in decreased venous return to the heart, diminished cardiac output, hypotension, and inadequate tissue perfusion, which in turn produce hypoxic tissue damage, accumulation of lactic acid, and metabolic acidosis. Disseminated intravascular coagulation appears to be the result of endothelial damage, platelet destruction, and leakage of fluid from the vascular to the extravascular space. Renal cortical ischemia and necrosis are predictable consequences in refractory cases, and similar damage may occur in the pituitary, adrenal, liver, and spleen.

Septic shock must be considered in any febrile patient with chills and hypotension. Cavanagh and Rao divide the natural history of septic shock into three phases:

1. The early or warm hypotensive phase is characterized by fever of 101°–105° F (38.4°–40.6° C), warm moist skin and flushed face, tachycardia, chills, and hypotension of 85–95 mm Hg systolic. The sensorium shows no impairment, and urine output is more than 30 ml/hour. This phase may last for several hours, depending on the severity of the infection.
2. The late or cold hypotensive phase, which clinically resembles shock due to hemorrhage, is characterized by cold, clammy skin, hypotension on the order of 70 mm Hg systolic or less, cyanosis of the nail beds, subnormal temperature, rapid thready pulse, impaired sensorium, and oliguria.
3. Irreversible shock, the final phase, is characterized by severe metabolic acidosis with sharply elevated levels of blood lactic acid, anuria, cardiac failure, respiratory distress, and coma.

Phases 1 and 2 are usually responsive to aggressive therapy; in Phase 3, treatment is a measure of desperation and is usually futile.

The crucial features of *management* are 1) the monitoring and replacement of intravascular volume, 2) the improvement of tissue perfusion, and 3) the immediate control of infection by appropriate antibioitics and surgical intervention either for drainage of pus or for removal of the nidus of infection. CVP monitoring should be started at once. A Foley catheter should be inserted to monitor urine output, which is an excellent gauge of organ perfusion. Blood samples should be drawn for culture, electrolyte determination, urea nitrogen measurement, complete blood and platelet counts, hematocrit determination, and coagulation profile. Material from vagina and uterus should be cultured and smears examined for predominant organisms. Blood cultures should be repeated at least every 24 hours and also at times of chills or temperature spikes. In septic abortion when uterine perforation seems possible, roentgenography should be done with the patient in the upright or lateral recumbent position to determine the presence of free air or a foreign body in the abdominal cavity. Serial electrocardiograms (EKGs) can often provide important information. The hematocrit should be determined every 3–4 hours. In severe cases, an arterial blood sample may be taken for lactic acid determination; mortality is exceptionally high in association with a lactic acid value greater than 2 mM/1000 ml.

Antibiotics should be started intravenously with the infusion fluid immediately after samples for culture are obtained. The Gram-stained smear can be helpful in preliminary selection of the agent (see Chapter 13). Many drugs have been used successfully, the most popular being penicillin, 5–10 million units every 4 hours; this has the disadvantage of providing 1.6 mEq potassium for every million units, however, and another agent should be substituted if urine output is less than 30 ml/hour or if EKG suggests hyperkalemia. Ampicillin (which causes sodium accumulation and is hazardous if there is circulatory overload), 1 g every 4 hours, is considered by some to be the agent of choice for *E. coli* and *Proteus* infections. Other agents that can be used alone, concomitantly with penicillin or ampicillin, or in combination are cephalothin and (with due attention to urine output) gentamicin and kanamycin.

Septic shock is a form of hypovolemic shock, and the guides to be used for volume replacement are CVP, blood pressure, and hourly urine output. In most cases, CVP is low (2–4 cm H_2O), sometimes extremely low, due to hypovolemia resulting from splanchnic pooling. Complete blood count, hematocrit, and electrolyte determinations can be helpful in deciding the nature of the fluids to be administered. The CVP should be maintained above 4 cm H_2O, preferably between 6 and 10 cm H_2O. Elevation above 12 cm H_2O brings the danger of overload and pulmonary edema.

Some patients respond purely to volume expansion. Whole blood should be administered as needed. In some cases, fresh-frozen plasma or albumin are suitable. Because of the almost prohibitive cost of albumin, less expensive equivalent agents are being sought. One such drug that appears to show high promise is 6% hetastarch (Hespan), a drug whose colloidal properties are comparable to those of albumin.

Dopamine (Intropin; a naturally occurring catecholamine that is the immediate precursor of norepineph-

rine) is proving to be of signal value in the treatment of septic shock. It increases both cardiac output and blood pressure. At low doses ($2\mu g$–$5\mu g/kg/min$) cardiac output begins to increase with little or no effect on peripheral resistance. At doses greater than $20\mu g/kg/min$, generalized pressor effects usually occur. In addition, it is unique among catecholamines in producing dilation of the renal vasculature, increase of renal blood flow, and increase in urinary output. Side effects (ventricular arrhythmias, nausea and vomiting, angina pectoris) are unusual when smaller doses are used. The effectiveness of dopamine appears to be much greater if it is started soon after the onset of shock, that is, as soon as hypotension and diminished urine output are evident. Blood volume deficits, as evidenced by CVP levels below 10 cm H_2O, should first be corrected. In cases of moderate shock, the drug is started as an intravenous infusion at the rate of $2\mu g$–$5\mu g/kg/min$ and is gradually increased until there is response in blood pressure and urinary output. In more severe cases, it may be necessary to start with higher doses and to increase the rate more rapidly. Most patients respond to infusion rates below $20\mu g/kg/min$, but some have required more than $50\mu g/kg/min$. When a satisfactory response in blood pressure and urinary output has occurred, the infusion should be continued at the smallest dose that will maintain these effects. The duration of the infusion varies, according to the need, from 30 min to several days.

The increased urinary output with dopamine therapy provides immediate need for increased intravenous fluids. CVP and urinary output can be used to monitor the fluid requirements.

Dopamine usually suffices; but, in some cases, other vasoactive agents are required. Isoproterenol (Isuprel) may be used in conjunction with dopamine if it is necessary to increase the cardiac inotropic effect and to decrease pulmonary resistance. If there is intense peripheral vasoconstriction, as in the cold hypotensive phase, isoproterenol or isoproterenol with dopamine may be more effective than dopamine alone. Levarterenol (1-norepinephrine; Levophed) may be used if dopamine is insufficient to maintain the arterial pressure; however, both this drug and metaraminol bitartrate (Aramine) have intense vasoconstrictive action and may compromise tissue perfusion. They are not indicated for routine treatment. It is emphasized that all of the aforementioned agents are potent drugs. For those who use them only occasionally, the prescribing information can be of valuable assistance. The use of combinations of these drugs requires special expertise in the measurement and interpretation of their hemodynamic effects.

There is increasing agreement that glucocorticoids are useful and should be given. An example is methylprednisolone sodium succinate (Solu-Medrol), given intravenously initially as a bolus of 30 mg/kg body weight and then as a continuous infusion of 15–30 mg/kg/24 hours.

After 6–8 hours of antibiotic therapy and treatment of hypovolemia, attention must turn to the nidus of infection. If it can be removed surgically, this should be done. Some cases of septic abortion can be cured by curettage, but if only negligible amounts of tissue are obtained or if there is no clear improvement within 3 hours, hysterectomy with bilateral salpingo-oophorectomy and high ligation of the pedicles of the ovarian veins is indicated. Because of the possibility of septic pulmonary embolization, the inferior vena cava should be plicated or, according to Collins' recommendation, ligated. Hemodialysis should be started promptly if oliguria persists after operation (see Acute Renal Failure). Antimicrobial therapy should be continued for 1 week after the signs and symptoms of infection have disappeared.

AMNIOTIC FLUID EMBOLISM

Amniotic fluid embolism is usually a cataclysmic event characterized by the sudden onset of dyspnea, chest pain, pulmonary edema, shock, and, sometimes within minutes, death. Most often, it occurs in a multigravid patient late in the first stage of labor, when the membranes have ruptured and the fetal head fits snugly into the lower uterine segment. Oxytocin may have been used for the induction or stimulation of labor. Under the pressure of uterine contractions, the amniotic fluid flows under the placental margin or to the site of a uterine, cervical, or vaginal laceration, where it gains access to the maternal venous channels; the resulting pulmonary embolization may be massive. The release of thromboplastin into the maternal circulation culminates, within minutes or hours, in activation of the extrinsic clotting pathway and consequent widespread disseminated intravascular coagulation. An exact diagnosis can be made only by the demonstration of particulate matter of the amniotic fluid (sloughed squamous cells, lanugo hair, meconium, vernix) in the pulmonary vasculature. Not all cases can be so documented; but, among those that are diagnosed, it is estimated that death occurs in at least 80% of the cases.

The typical clinical picture is catastrophic, with instant collapse and death. A spectrum of lesser consequences may result from the infusion of smaller quantities of amniotic fluid. Dyspnea, often slight, may be the first sign; if it appears in any patient who is in hypertonic labor after the membranes have ruptured, it should immediately suggest embolism. Subsequent symptoms may be distress, malaise, a sense of suffocation, agitation, and unexplained cough. Among the cases reviewed by Cornu *et al.*, vomiting, chills, and

fever occurred in some patients. Cyanosis, tachycardia of the order of 140+ beats/min, and a respiratory rate of 40+/min occur relatively early, followed by collapse after a variable period. Fibrin breakdown products can usually be demonstrated, the number of platelets is reduced, prothrombin time and thrombin–fibrinogen time are increased. Oxygen, heparin, intravenous hydrocortisone, and whole blood transfusions are urgently needed. Monitoring of hemodynamics and urinary output must be undertaken at once. In at least one surviving patient, the definitive diagnosis was made by the finding of characteristic particulate matter in blood from the right side of the heart; in at least two cases, pulmonary artery blood obtained through a Swan–Ganz catheter provided the diagnosis. Peritoneal dialysis or hemodialysis may be needed if the process is sufficiently severe to cause tubular necrosis and anuria.

The only preventive possibilities are avoidance of measures that would tend to produce a tumultuous, driving labor (*e.g.*, injudicious administration of oxytocin or other stimulating agents to a patient whose labor is progressing satisfactorily). Also, it is reasonable to presume that after spontaneous or artificial rupture of the membranes, as much amniotic fluid as possible should be allowed to escape vaginally to minimize the likelihood of the fluid being forced back into the maternal circulation.

SUPINE HYPOTENSIVE SYNDROME

The supine hypotensive syndrome is a shocklike state that can occur in a pregnant woman at or near term as a result of partial occlusion of the vena cava by the pressure of the large gravid uterus. Venous return to the heart is impaired, producing the clinical syndrome of hypotension, tachycardia, sweating, nausea, weakness, and air hunger. Recovery is immediate when the woman is turned on her side. The syndrome, first described by McRoberts in 1951, is ample reason for urging women to rest on the side rather than supine after the 7th month of pregnancy. The knowledge, gained from fetal monitoring, that the baby fares better if labor is conducted in the lateral rather than the supine recumbent position suggests that subclinical degrees of this syndrome also occur.

POSTPARTUM VASOMOTOR COLLAPSE

Although shock most commonly occurs as a result of acute blood loss and other reduction in the oxygen-transporting mechanism of the blood, changes in electrolyte and steroid metabolism may result in shocklike states, especially in the postpartum period when there are profound adjustments and alterations in the electrolyte and steroid systems. *Adrenal cortical insufficiency* can result in shock, Addison's disease representing a typical clinical example. Although most patients with Addison's disease can be carried through pregnancy on replacement therapy, the increased stresses of pregnancy, especially when complications such as infection, preeclampsia, or blood loss occur, result in a greater need for hormone substances. Vasomotor collapse and shock can follow a reduction in these substances, and adrenal crises can occur.

Preeclampsia can also result in shock and shocklike states. Such collapse is frequently associated with marked reduction in the concentration of sodium and chloride in the serum. In most cases, following delivery, mobilization of the extravascular fluid restores sodium concentration to near normal levels. This syndrome is discussed on page 471.

Anesthesia should be mentioned as a cause of postpartum vasomotor collapse. Spinal anesthesia ("spinal shock") as well as overdoses of toxic gases such as cyclopropane have been incriminated. All these hypotensive reactions are aggravated when anemia or blood loss, chronic or acute, further complicates the picture. In addition, the pregnant patient is much more likely than the nonpregnant patient to develop severe degrees of systemic hypotension as an immediate result of anesthesia. For these reasons, the doses of anesthetic agents given most pregnant patients must be considerably less than those administered to the nonpregnant patient.

The manifestations of *amniotic fluid embolism* may first appear after delivery, especially in the presence of extensive lacerations of the uterus, cervix, or vagina.

In all cases of postpartum obstetric shock, there is the possibility that Sheehan's disease (pituitary infarction resulting from collapse of the pituitary portal system) may follow. In one case, the pituitary ischemia was found to be selective, limited to the posterior lobe; diabetes insipidus was the result.

OTHER CAUSES OF SHOCK

Other potential causes of shock in the pregnant patient include myocardial infarction and cardiac dysrhythmias. Anaphylactoid reactions due to hypersensitivity to various drugs may give rise to shocklike conditions. Cardiovascular abnormalities associated with congenital cardiac defects, coarctation of the aorta, and similiar conditions may result in circulatory insufficiency. All such potential causes of shock and shocklike states in pregnancy must be considered and evaluated by the physician both at the time of the patient's initial physical examination and during the course of her prenatal care.

REFERENCES AND RECOMMENDED READING

Alexander MR, Ambre JJ, Liskow BI: Therapeutic use of albumin. JAMA 241:2527, 1979

Arnar-Stone Laboratories, Inc: Proceedings of a symposium. (A) Use of dopamine in shock. I. Septic shock. (B) Dopamine in clinical use. Princeton, Excerpta Medica, 1976

Blanchard K, Dandavino A, Nuwayhid B et al.: Systemic and uterine hemodynamic responses to dopamine in pregnant and nonpregnant sheep. Am J Obstet Gynecol 130:669, 1978

Cavanagh D, Rao PS: Septic shock (endotoxin shock). Clin Obstet Gynecol 16 (2):25, 1973

Collins CG: Suppurative thrombophlebitis of the pelvis. Am J Obstet Gynecol 180:681, 1970

Collins ML, O'Brien P, Cline A: Diabetes insipidus following obstetric shock. Obstet Gynecol 53:16S, 1979

Cotton DB, Benedetti TJ: Use of the Swan-Ganz catheter in obstetrics and gynecology. Obstet Gynecol 56:641, 1979

Courtney LD: Amniotic fluid embolism. Obstet Gynecol Surv 29:169, 1974

Deane RM, Russell KP: Enterobacillary septicemia and bacterial shock in septic abortion. Am J Obstet Gynecol 79:528, 1960

Grimes DA, Cates W, Jr: Fatal amniotic fluid embolism during induced abortion. South Med J 70:1325, 1977

Lumley J, Owen R, Morgan M: Amniotic fluid embolism. Anaesthesia 34:33, 1979

McRoberts WA, Jr: Postural shock in pregnancy. Am J Obstet Gynecol 62:627, 1951

Masson RG, Ruggieri J, Siddiqui MM: Amniotic fluid embolism: Definitive diagnosis in a survivor. Am Rev Respir Dis 120:187, 1979

Pomerance W: Chorioamnionitis and maternal sepsis. In Monif GRW (ed): Infectious Diseases in Obstetrics and Gynecology, Hagerstown, MD, Harper & Row, 1974

Reid PR, Thompson WL: The clinical use of dopamine in the treatment of shock. Johns Hopkins Med J 137:276, 1975

Russell KP: Septic shock and acute renal failure. In Reid DE, Barton TC (eds): Controversy in Obstetrics and Gynecology. Philadelphia, WB Saunders, 1969

Santamarina BAG: Septic abortion and septic shock. In Charles D, Finland M (eds): Obstetric and Perinatal Infections. Philadelphia, Lea & Febiger, 1973

Schumer W: Hypovolemic shock. JAMA 241:615, 1979

Schwarz RH: Shock Associated with Septic Abortion. ACOG Technical Bulletin No 9, July 1968

Sheehan HL: Tissue effects of shock. Clin Obstet Gynecol 4:932, 1961

Sheehan HL, Moore HC: Renal Cortical Necrosis and the Kidney of Concealed Accidental Hemorrhage. Springfield, IL, Charles C Thomas, 1953

Shires TG, Canizaro PC, Carrico J: Shock. In Schwartz SI (ed): Principles of Surgery. New York, McGraw-Hill, 1979

Smith LL, Weil MH: Shock due to blood loss. In Weil MH, Shukin H (eds): Diagnosis and Treatment of Shock. Baltimore, Williams & Wilkins, 1967

Studdiford WE, Douglas GW: Placental bacteremia: A significant finding in septic abortion accompanied by vascular collapse. Am J Obstet Gynecol 71:842, 1956

Swan HJC, Ganz W, Forrester J, Marcus H, Diamond G, Chonette D: Catheterization of the heart in man with use of a flow-directed balloon-tipped catheter. N Engl J Med 283:447, 1970

Weil MH: Endotoxin shock. Clin Obstet Gynecol 4:971, 1961

ACUTE RENAL FAILURE

Manuel R. Comas
Robert E. Cuddihee
Denis Cavanagh

Acute renal failure is the sudden reduction of renal function over the course of hours or days. It is manifested by oliguria (less than 400 ml urine excreted in 24 hours) or anuria, and increasing azotemia. The decrease in urine volume may result from a reduction in the glomerular filtration rate or from increased reabsorption or "back-leak" of the filtrate. There often is no apparent structural alteration in the kidney on light or electron-microscopic examination. Acute renal failure may result from primary alteration in the kidney itself, or it may follow dysfunction of other organ systems. The consequence of decreased renal function from whatever cause is an accumulation of waste products, metabolites, electrolytes, and substances normally removed from the circulating blood by the kidney.

CLASSIFICATION

Clinically it is useful to divide acute renal failure into three types, according to the site of origin: 1) prerenal, 2) intrinsic renal, and 3) postrenal. This differentiation is sometimes difficult to establish, but early distinction between these three types helps determine the proper therapeutic approach.

Prerenal Failure

In prerenal failure, the primary defect is reduced kidney perfusion as a result of poor circulatory dynamics. This type of failure occurs in patients with hypovolemia due to blood loss or dehydration, hypoproteinemia as in the nephrotic syndrome, or poor cardiac function as in heart failure. The renal failure is usually reversible if kidney perfusion is improved promptly. Prerenal failure usually does not produce permanent changes in renal morphology.

INTRINSIC RENAL FAILURE

A true renal parenchymal failure, intrinsic renal failure is subdivided into two categories, according to morphologic alterations: renal cortical necrosis and acute tubular necrosis. *Renal cortical necrosis* is seen in patients who have suffered prolonged renal ischemia or those in whom intravascular coagulation has complicated the picture. Morphologically, there is ex-

tensive destruction of glomeruli and tubules; cell nuclei and cellular boundries disappear, and capillary and tubular lumina are obliterated. If the cortical necrosis is bilateral and total, this condition is irreversible. However, in a few cases, the necrosis may be patchy in distribution and the remaining nephrons may hypertrophy sufficiently to allow the patient to survive, although usually with severely impaired renal function.

In *acute tubular necrosis,* the blood vessels and glomeruli do not show significant morphologic changes, but the tubules do. The tubular epithelial cells may appear swollen or necrotic. Some tubules are dilated and the epithelium is flattened. The lumina may be filled with granular or hyaline casts. Interstitial edema and a nonspecific inflammatory cell infiltrate may be seen. Acute tubular necrosis is usually reversible after an oliguric period lasting 10–14 days.

POSTRENAL FAILURE

Postrenal azotemia is most often due to obstruction of the urinary tract at or below the level of the renal pelvis. Obstruction of the ureters or urethra is rare in pregnancy, but it is the cause of more than 10% of all cases of renal failure seen in a general hospital. From whatever cause, the blockage results in an increased intraluminal pressure throughout the nephron, which causes a fall in the glomerular filtration rate. Pyelonephritis, a frequent complication, further increases the parenchymal damage. Microscopic examination shows the tubules to be dilated and to contain colloid casts. There may be foci of interstitial inflammation throughout the medulla and cortex. This condition is potentially reversible, but the prognosis depends on the duration and severity of obstruction before corrective treatment.

ETIOLOGY

In general, renal failure in obstetric patients occurs as the result of complications of pregnancy; persistent physiologic effects of pregnancy after delivery; medications administered; infection; or shock. Purely obstetric diseases associated with renal failure include abruptio placentae, severe preeclampsia, eclampsia, extensive obstetric soft tissue trauma, amniotic fluid embolism, abortion, and sensitivity to specific obstetric or abortifacient drugs. Complications characterized by coagulopathy, circulating fibrinolysins, hemorrhagic shock, endotoxic shock, and water and electrolyte depletion predispose the patient to renal failure.

Infection *per se* does not usually produce renal failure unless associated with endotoxin shock, as in septic abortion or chorioamnionitis due to *Escherichia coli, Aerobacter, Pseudomonas,* and other gram-negative bacilli. Infections by organisms that produce an exotoxin, such as *Clostridium perfringens,* are also capable of producing renal failure. Other infectious processes during pregnancy that may produce renal failure are acute pyelonephritis and sepsis associated with acute pancreatitis or acute torsion of pelvic viscera.

When dealing with infection, the physician must keep in mind that many antibiotics are nephrotoxic and can cause renal failure, mainly through renal tubular damage. The nephrotoxic antibiotics include amphotericin B, colistin, and the aminoglycosides (streptomycin, kanamycin, gentamicin, tobramycin, and amikacin).

Other factors that contribute to acute renal failure are acute adrenocortical failure, prolonged administration of steroids without reinforcement during pregnancy or after delivery, prolonged use of diuretics, incompatible blood transfusions resulting in hemoglobinuria, and cardiac failure. In addition, the possibility of an acute exacerbation of subclinical borderline chronic renal failure must be kept in mind. There is also a possibility of obstructive uropathy secondary to cervical malignancy, leiomyomas, and ovarian neoplasms. If the patient has had a cesarean section or a cesarean–hysterectomy, the possibility of retroperitoneal hematoma or ligated ureters must be considered.

In the syndrome of *acute postpartum renal failure,* bilateral renal cortical necrosis and disseminated intravascular coagulation (DIC) occur within the first 6 weeks following an uncomplicated pregnancy and delivery. The etiology of this syndrome is obscure, but suggested factors include drug sensitivity (ergot) and a primary immunologic mechanism.

PREVENTION

Acute renal failure among obstetric and gynecologic patients is often preventable. An effective program of prevention should include

1. Prompt replacement of blood in the event of severe hemorrhage
2. Careful observation for early signs of septic shock in patients with septic abortion, pelvic infection, chorioamnionitis, or pyelonephritis
3. Early detection of infection by C. perfringens and prompt hysterectomy when uterine infections have been caused by this microorganism or when soap or Lysol has been used to induce abortion
4. Avoidance of elective abortion induced by hypertonic saline injection
5. Careful monitoring of patients being treated with nephrotoxic drugs, with frequent determination of blood urea nitrogen (BUN) and serum creatinine levels
6. Prompt detection and correction of intravascular volume depletion
7. Meticulous care to avoid the administration of in-

compatible blood, and observation for transfusion reactions

8. Early delivery in cases of abruptio placentae and severe preeclampsia and eclampsia
9. Heparinization in selected patients with DIC, particularly when DIC occurs after delivery or hysterectomy
10. Pelvic examination with cytologic evaluation of the cervix on a yearly basis for all women to rule out pelvic neoplasms that may cause obstructive uropathy

DIAGNOSIS

Clinical experience has shown that renal failure is most likely to occur in certain groups of patients or after certain incidents in the course of pregnancy. Knapp and Burden have emphasized that patients with the following conditions are considered at high risk for renal failure:

Those with preexisting renal disorders
    Structural damage: glomerulonephritis or pyelonephritis
    Hypoalbuminemic states: nephrotic syndrome or chronic liver disease
    Chronic hypertensive disease
Those with previously normal kidneys, but with
    Severe preeclampsia or eclampsia
    Antepartum hemorrhage, especially abruptio placentae
    Postpartum hemorrhage
    Amniotic fluid infusion
    Septicemia, especially if associated with abortion or chorioamnionitis
    Nephrotoxins, especially antibiotics such as aminoglycosides or cephaloridine, particularly if diuretics have been given
    Incompatible blood transfusion

However, many patients who display features of the high-risk category maintain normal renal function during pregnancy and delivery, while others with few or no risk factors may develop severe renal problems. As noted by the same authors, renal failure should be suspected when certain observations are made:

Features suggesting renal involvement
    Proteinuria
    Hematuria
    Cylindruria (urinary casts) or other abnormality of sediment
    Hypertension
    Sodium retention or edema
    Signs of DIC
Features suggesting renal failure
    Oliguria, anuria
    Inappropriate retention of electrolytes or water

Azotemia and increased serum creatinine
Decreased creatinine clearance

It is essential that prerenal and postrenal failure be differentiated from intrinsic renal failure, although this is sometimes difficult. However, prompt differentiation of these conditions is necessary because their management is quite different.

DIAGNOSIS OF PRERENAL FAILURE

The diagnosis of prerenal failure implies that, if the perfusion of the kidney were to be improved, renal function would return to normal. Blood transfusion may be needed if blood has been lost, saline or water replacement if dehydration has occurred, albumin infusion if there is hypoproteinemia, or improvement in cardiac function if the patient has suffered heart failure.

In obstetric patients, the customary causes of prerenal oliguria are hypovolemia and hypotension. In hypovolemia, the skin is of poor turgor, mucous membranes are dry, there is poor filling of the neck veins when the patient is in the supine position, and postural hypotension may be present. A low central venous pressure (CVP) (0–5 cm H_2O) confirms the diagnosis of extracellular fluid volume depletion. The CVP is also helpful in monitoring the replacement of the fluid deficit.

The *differentiation between prerenal failure and acute tubular necrosis* may be facilitated by an analysis of the blood and urine chemistry (Table 38–4). This analysis requires only a random urine specimen of 5–10 ml and a 10-ml sample of blood. The differential points are valid only if the kidneys were functionally normal before the insult, and they may not be present if the patient has recently received a potent diuretic. Moreover, congestive heart failure can produce prerenal failure with the same findings on urinalysis as volume depletion. However, congestive heart failure and volume depletion can be differentiated on the basis of physical findings.

If the physical findings and the blood and urine chemistries suggest that hypovolemia is the cause of the oliguria, then a *therapeutic trial of volume expansion* may be indicated (Table 38–5). For this therapeutic test to be effective, the patient's blood pressure must be adequate for glomerular filtration (mean blood pressure at least 60 mm Hg), and the serum albumin concentration must be sufficient to maintain intravascular volume. If there is no response after the second dose of saline and furosemide, and the patient's blood pressure and CVP are normal, the oliguria most probably is due to intrinsic renal failure rather than prerenal failure. A therapeutic trial of volume replacement must always be supervised carefully for signs of volume overload. There is no satisfactory alternative to

TABLE 38–4. DIFFERENTIATION OF PRERENAL AZOTEMIA FROM ACUTE TUBULAR NECROSIS

	Prerenal Azotemia (mEq/liter)	Acute Tubular Necrosis (mEq/liter)
URINE SODIUM CONCENTRATION	< 20	> 50
URINE CREATININE/SERUM CREATININE	> 40	< 10
BUN/SERUM CREATININE	< 20	< 10
URINE OSMOLALITY/SERUM OSMOLALITY	> 1.5	< 1.1
FeNa $\left(\dfrac{\text{URINE SODIUM/SERUM SODIUM}}{\text{URINE CREATININE/SERUM CREATININE}} \right)$	< 1	> 3

TABLE 38–5. PROGRAM FOR THERAPEUTIC TRIAL OF VOLUME EXPANSION FOR OLIGURIA DUE TO HYPOPERFUSION

Immediate Management
If CVP is not elevated and there are no signs of congestive heart failure:
Give normal saline, 500 ml intravenously, in 45 min; then give mannitol, 25 g and furosemide, 120 mg, intravenously.
If urine flow is at least 40 ml/hour:
Replace estimated extracellular fluid volume deficit with 0.9% NaCl and replace measured urine loss with 0.45% NaCl.

Further Management
If no response occurs in 2 hours and CVP is not elevated:
Give normal saline, 500 ml intravenously in 45 min and furosemide, 240 mg, intravenously.

frequent clinical examination for such signs as tachycardia, gallop rhythm, or basilar rales. The CVP or pulmonary capillary wedge pressure (PCWP), as measured by Swan–Ganz catheter, should be monitored during the infusion. If physical signs of heart failure occur, if the CVP rises to more than 15 cm H_2O, or if the PCWP rises to more than 12 mm Hg, then the infusion should be discontinued.

DIAGNOSIS OF POSTRENAL FAILURE

In the nonpregnant woman, the diagnosis of postrenal failure is made by high-dose intravenous pyelography and tomography. In addition to ruling out urinary tract obstruction, these tests may provide other helpful information. In a few cases, further studies with antegrade (by needling of the renal pelvis) or retrograde pyelography are needed.

In pregnancy, there must be a strong indication of obstruction before radiologic investigation is requested. The possible hazards of fetal radiation must be balanced against the need to establish the cause of renal failure. If obstruction still seems likely after clinical examination, bladder catheterization, and cystoscopy, an intravenous pyelogram limited to three films will give no more radiation than pelvimetry. When evaluating pyelography in pregnancy, the physician should always remember that unilateral or bilateral hydroureter and hydronephrosis may be physiologic. Ultrasonic examination of the kidney is an alternative method that may prove especially appropriate in pregnancy, since it may permit the diagnosis of obstruction to be made without exposing the fetus to radiation. It may also be useful in localizing the kidney for biopsy.

DIAGNOSIS OF INTRINSIC RENAL FAILURE

Only after prerenal and postrenal factors have been carefully searched for and corrected should a diagnosis of intrinsic renal failure be made. A careful review of the history and physical findings may suggest other than purely obstetric causes of renal failure. Careful selection of laboratory investigations may aid in diagnosis. For example, hypocomplementemia may be seen in lupus erythematosus with severe renal involvement, in mesangiocapillary glomerulonephritis, and in acute poststreptococcal glomerulonephritis.

If DIC is or has been present, the strong possibility of bilateral renal cortical necrosis must be considered. A coagulation profile should be obtained and a smear of the peripheral blood examined. Thrombocytopenia, the presence of schistocytes, prolonged prothrombin and partial thromboplastin times, a decreased fibrinogen level, and an elevated level of fibrin breakdown products strongly suggest a consumption coagulopathy. In those patients in whom the diagnosis is in doubt, a renal biopsy may be the only way to establish a definite diagnosis. In deciding whether to recommend this procedure, the physician must consider the extent to which results obtained will influence predelivery treatment. The patient may well receive the same treatment, regardless of the histologic findings; in that case, the biopsy with its attendant risks can be avoided.

DIC, red blood cells or red cell casts in the urine,

and anuria that persists are seen more frequently with renal cortical necrosis than with acute tubular necrosis. Renal biopsy that shows necrosis of cortical glomeruli and destruction of other cortical structures may establish the diagnosis. It must be remembered that the necrosis may be patchy in distribution.

CLINICAL COURSE OF INTRINSIC RENAL FAILURE

The clinical course of acute tubular necrosis is usually divided into three distinct stages: the oliguric, the diuretic, and the recovery phase. They are related in time to the initial insult and to the process of repair.

In the *oliguric phase,* the urine output is usually less than 400 ml/24 hours. This phase lasts from a few days to several weeks and is characterized by increasing azotemia and hyperkalemia. The excreted urine is dilute and has a specific gravity close to that of plasma ultrafiltrate (1.010).

The *diuretic phase* is manifested by an increasing and sometimes excessive urine output, which may reach 6–7 liters/day. The urine is still dilute, and renal function may remain severely impaired. Azotemia is still present, and there may be marked electrolyte imbalance due to great loss of electrolytes in the urine. Almost 25% of fatalities from acute tubular necrosis occur during the diuretic phase.

The *recovery phase* is manifested by a return to normal urine volume and a gradually improving renal function. Most patients who reach the recovery phase eventually regain normal glomerular filtration rates.

MANAGEMENT OF ACUTE RENAL FAILURE

The major areas to be considered in the management of acute renal failure are water balance, nutrition, acid–base balance, infection, cardiovascular complications, anemia, and coagulopathies.

WATER BALANCE

Fluid intake in the afebrile patient should be limited to the volume of measured fluid output, such as urine or gastrointestinal drainage, plus 400 ml/day to replace insensible water loss. If the patient is febrile, 100 ml additional fluid is allowed for each 1 ° C of temperature elevation. Accurate recording of the patient's fluid intake and output, and daily measurement of her weight are essential in managing water balance. If fluid balance is maintained properly, the patient should lose 0.2–0.3 kg/day. If the patient's weight remains stable or increases, she is in positive fluid balance, and fluid intake should be restricted further.

NUTRITION

The traditional management of nutrition in acute renal failure has been to minimize protein intake and to provide at least 100 g/day carbohydrate to reduce endogenous protein catabolism. Several oral preparations that provide high concentrations of glucose in a small volume are available commercially. A mixture of equal parts of Karo syrup and gingerale also provides a high concentration of glucose, and it is well accepted when chilled and flavored with lemon juice. According to this regimen, if the patient cannot tolerate oral feedings, glucose must be administered intravenously. This is best accomplished by the administration of 20%–50% glucose through a central venous catheter that has been passed into the vena cava. One thousand units of aqueous heparin is added to each liter of intravenous fluid to prevent clotting of the catheter. Because of the high incidence of septicemia associated with central venous catheters, scrupulous care must be taken in their insertion and maintenance. Anabolic steroids, such as nandrolone decanoate (Deca-Durabolin), may decrease the endogenous protein breakdown and slow the progression of azotemia. Multivitamins should be administered daily.

Recently, the aforementioned traditional regimen has given way to an alternative method that has several advantages. In this method, the emphasis is on adequate protein and caloric intake (3500–4000 Cal) rather than protein restriction. Early and repeated dialysis, together with the intake of protein (1 g/kg body weight), is preferred to protein restriction. This regimen produces less protein depletion and promotes wound healing. Nasogastric drip feedings over 24 hours by means of soft, narrow bore tubes have been used to overcome the problems of anorexia that may prevent adequate nutrition despite the correct dietary prescription. High-calorie tube feeding may cause diarrhea, but codeine phosphate, 30 mg orally with each diarrheic movement, usually controls this problem.

ACID–BASE AND ELECTROLYTE BALANCE

Acute renal failure results in metabolic acidosis and hyperkalemia. The course of the acidosis is best followed by monitoring arterial blood gases and serum bicarbonate levels. Although the metabolic acidosis may cause tachypnea, it is usually well tolerated until the serum bicarbonate falls below 15 mEq/liter. The acidosis is treated by the intravenous injection of sodium bicarbonate. However, repeated injections of sodium bicarbonate may lead to overexpansion of the extracellular fluid volume as a result of the large amounts of sodium administered. For this reason, the management of persistent or severe metabolic acidosis may require dialysis.

Hyperkalemia

Potassium excess, a common and serious problem in the management of acute renal failure, can cause cardiac arrest unless it is promptly diagnosed and treated. All patients in acute renal failure are at risk of developing hyperkalemia, even if their potassium intake is restricted. A catabolic state due to shock, trauma, sepsis, or inadequate caloric intake can cause elevation of the serum potassium. Acidosis causes hyperkalemia by producing a shift of potassium from the intracellular to the extracellular compartment. Some frequently unconsidered sources of exogenous potassium are stored whole blood (10–30 mEq K+ per 1000 ml serum) and potassium salts of penicillin (1.2 mEq K+ per million units penicillin).

The serum potassium concentration should not be allowed to rise above 6 mEq/liter; when the level reaches 7 mEq/liter, serious cardiac arrhythmias or asystole may occur. Hyperkalemia may cause muscle weakness, decreased tendon reflexes, acroparesthesias, and an irregular pulse. However, cardiac toxicity may occur before any symptoms of hyperkalemia are apparent. *Frequent electrocardiographic monitoring is essential in these patients.* The electrocardiographic abnormalities seen progressively with increasing hyperkalemia are tall, symmetrically peaked T waves, especially in leads V_3 to V_5; lengthening of the P–R interval; widening of the QRS complex; disappearance of P waves; and formation of a sine wave configuration of the QRS complex (Fig. 38–3). If the serum potassium concentration is 7 mEq/liter or higher, or if the electrocardiogram shows signs of hyperkalemia, one or more of the following measures should be taken immediately:

1. Give 10 ml 10% calcium gluconate intravenously over 3 min. Calcium counteracts the effect of potassium on the heart. Calcium salts should not be administered in the same container or through the same tubing as sodium bicarbonate, however, because this causes precipitation of calcium carbonate. Intravenous calcium should not be given to patients who are receiving digitalis, because this combination may produce cardiac arrhythmias.
2. Give 1 ampule (44.6 mEq) sodium bicarbonate intravenously over 5 min. The relative alkalosis produced by the sodium bicarbonate drives the potassium from the extracellular space back into the cells, thereby lowering the serum potassium level. This may be repeated if necessary after the serum potassium concentration is rechecked. However, the danger of congestive heart failure from administration of the sodium must be kept in mind.
3. Administer 300 ml 20% glucose with 30 units regular insulin at a rate of 200–300 ml/hour. As the glucose enters the cells and is deposited as glycogen, potassium also enters the cell. This method reduces

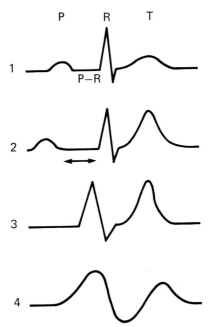

FIG. 38–3. EKG changes of hyperkalemia. *1.* Normal EKG. *2.* T wave "tented" and P–R interval lengthened. *3.* Disappearance of P wave and widening of QRS complex. *4.* Sine wave pattern.

the serum potassium level as long as the infusion is continued, but potassium may again leave the cells and enter the extracellular space after the infusion is stopped, causing a rebound hyperkalemia.

All three of these emergency measures for lowering the serum potassium have their onset of action within 5–15 min, but their effect rapidly disappears as soon as they are discontinued. At the same time as these measures are employed, a cation-exchange resin should be administered to decrease total body potassium, or dialysis should be initiated.

Polystyrene sulfonate resin (Kayexalate) is a cation-exchange resin that binds potassium ions and removes them from the body. It exchanges potassium ions for sodium ions on a one-for-one basis and therefore can be responsible for a large sodium load. Because its onset of action is about 1 hour after administration, the use of Kayexalate is not suitable when the serum potassium must be lowered rapidly in patients with severe hyperkalemia. It is usually given as a retention enema in a suspension containing 50 g Kayexalate in 200 ml 10% dextrose in water, or in 100 ml 70% sorbitol and 100 ml water. The enema should be retained for 1 hour, and it may be repeated as often as necessary to lower the serum potassium concentration to the desired level. Kayexalate may also be administered orally as 30 g (2 heaping teaspoonfuls) sus-

pended in a few ounces of water or gingerale. The administration of 1 oz 70% sorbitol at the same time facilitates transit of the resin through the gastrointestinal tract and reduces the chance of impaction of the Kayexalate. Each gram of Kayexalate binds approximately 1 mEq potassium. In the adult patient, the average fall in potassium after a 50-g dose is about 1 mEq/liter. After severe hyperkalemia has been controlled, Kayexalate can be administered in doses of 20–50 g/day to prevent subsequent rise of serum potassium. However, the risk of vascular overload from the sodium administered (1 mEq sodium gained from each mEq potassium lost) must be considered.

If these measures do not reduce the toxic levels of potassium, then peritoneal dialysis or hemodialysis must be performed as an emergency measure to lower the serum potassium concentration.

Hyponatremia

Although hyponatremia is often seen in acute renal failure, it is not an indication for the administration of sodium. In association with acute renal failure, hyponatremia almost always indicates excess water (dilutional hyponatremia) rather than deficit of sodium. Further restriction of water intake is then indicated.

Hyperphosphatemia

The hyperphosphatemia that usually accompanies acute renal failure can be controlled by the oral administration of aluminum hydroxide gel, 30 ml, three times daily with meals.

INFECTION

The most common cause of death in patients with acute renal failure is sepsis. Not only are these patients more susceptible to infection, but also an established infection is much more difficult to deal with in a patient with renal failure. Furthermore, the diagnosis of infection may be difficult to make in these patients, since the usual febrile response to infection may be suppressed in uremia.

Prophylactic antibiotics should not be used. However, as soon as the presence of an infection is confirmed, treatment with appropriate antibiotics should be initiated. The dose of most antibiotics must be reduced in patients with acute renal failure, because of the risk of drug accumulation and intoxication (Table 38–6). If it becomes necessary to use nephrotoxic antibiotics, serum concentrations of the drug should be monitored to prevent toxicity and to ensure therapeutic blood levels.

The common practice of leaving an indwelling catheter in the bladder of the patient with acute renal failure should be avoided. In most cases, catheterization of the bladder is not necessary, and it only leads to urinary tract infection.

CARDIOVASCULAR COMPLICATIONS

Congestive heart failure is common in patients with acute renal failure. When the patient has no preexisting organic heart disease, the failure is usually due to salt and water overloading, with resultant overexpansion of extracellular fluid volume. This situation should be managed by dialysis to remove the excess fluid volume. Digitalization is seldom indicated because it often leads to digitalis toxicity, and the congestive heart failure cannot be relieved until the volume overload is corrected.

Hypertension occurs in about 25% of patients with acute renal failure. It is usually mild and requires no specific treatment. Since it is due in part to increased extracellular fluid volume, it can often be corrected by dialysis. If antihypertensive medication is required, α-methyldopa (Aldomet) in a dosage of 750–3000 mg daily is usually effective.

Fibrinous pericarditis occurs in about 20% of patients with acute renal failure. Cardiac tamponade can follow if a serious effusion occurs or if hemorrhage into the pericardial sac results from heparinization during hemodialysis. Once the diagnosis of cardiac tamponade is established, emergency pericardiocentesis is indicated. If the tamponade recurs, pericardiectomy may be necessary.

GASTROINTESTINAL COMPLICATIONS

Anorexia, nausea, and vomiting are common symptoms of uremia. They are usually corrected by dialysis and seem to be improved by a reduction in protein intake. Bleeding may occur from anywhere in the gastrointestinal tract, either from ulcers or from diffuse gastroenteritis. When ulcers occur, bleeding is aggravated by the coagulation defects associated with uremia. Acute pancreatitis may occur, but diagnosis may be difficult because of the elevated serum amylase levels that are usually present with renal failure.

OTHER COMPLICATIONS

Anemia usually occurs with acute renal failure and may appear as early as the first week. It is a normocytic, normochromic anemia and is caused by a combination of shortened erythrocyte life span and impaired erythrocyte production. The anemia should be monitored closely and transfusions of packed red cells administered if the hematocrit falls below 25%. Defects in coagulation are also commonly encountered in renal failure. Most clearly defined is a decrease in platelet

TABLE 38-6. MODIFICATION OF ANTIBIOTIC DOSAGE IN ACUTE RENAL FAILURE

Antibiotic	Nephrotoxicity	Average Maintenance Dose	Interval
PENICILLINS			
Ampicillin	No*	0.5 g	12 hr
Carbenicillin	No	2.0 g	12 hr
Methicillin	No*	1.0 g	8 hr
Oxacillin	No	0.5 g	6 hr
Penicillin G	No	1 million units	12 hr
Ticarcillin	No	2.0 g	12 hr
CEPHALOSPORINS			
Cephalexin	?	0.25 g	24 hr
Cephaloridine	Yes	Do not use.	Do not use.
Cephalothin	Probably	0.5 g	8 hr
Cephazolin	?	0.2 g	24 hr
TETRACYCLINES			
Doxycycline	No	100 mg	24 hr
Tetracycline	No†	Do not use.	Do not use.
AMINOGLYCOSIDES			
Amikacin	Yes	7.5 mg/kg	72 hr (scr × 9)§
Gentamicin‡	Yes	1 mg/kg	48 hr (scr × 8)§
Kanamycin†	Yes	7.5 mg/kg	72 hr (scr × 9)§
Tobramycin‡	Yes	1 mg/kg	48 hr (scr × 6)§
MISCELLANEOUS			
Chloramphenicol	No	12 mg/kg	6 hr
Clindamycin	No	300 mg	12 hr
Colistimethate	Yes	150 mg	36 hr
Erythromycin	No	400 mg	6 hr

* Can cause acute allergic interstitial nephritis.

† Does not cause renal damage, but causes elevated BUN by antianabolic effect.

‡ The aminoglycoside antibiotics are ototoxic as well as nephrotoxic.

§ The interval between doses, in hours, can be calculated by multiplying the patient's serum creatinine concentration (scr) by the factor indicated.

adhesiveness and adenosine diphosphate–induced aggregation. Patients with active bleeding may require transfusion with platelet packs or fresh whole blood to establish normal hemostasis.

DIALYSIS

The increasing availability of hemodialysis and peritoneal dialysis has facilitated the management of patients with acute renal failure, but the overall survival rate has not improved significantly except when dialysis is used very early. Patients who are dialyzed before uremic symptoms appear and before the BUN exceeds 100 mg/100 ml have a higher rate of survival than do those who are not dialyzed until they are symptomatic or until the BUN exceeds 150 mg/100 ml. Early and frequent dialysis not only seems to reduce the incidence of uremic complications, but also allows the patient a more generous intake of fluid, calories, and protein, which hastens recovery, particularly following surgery.

The generally accepted indications for dialysis are as follows:

1. Symptomatic circulatory overload manifested by congestive heart failure, edema, or serous effusions
2. Hyperkalemia with a serum potassium level over 6.5 mEq/liter that does not respond to conservative measures
3. The presence of uremic symptoms, such as anorexia and nausea, neuromuscular irritability, confusion, or a pericardial friction rub
4. A BUN over 120 mg/100 ml or daily increases of 30 mg/100 ml in patients with severe sepsis or tissue necrosis
5. Severe metabolic acidosis that cannot be controlled with the administration of bicarbonate
6. The presence of a dialyzable poison or drug

The choice between peritoneal dialysis and hemodialysis is determined by availability of these modalities and the condition of the patient. Peritoneal dialysis has greater simplicity, results in fewer complications,

and is available in any hospital, regardless of whether a dialysis unit is at hand. Peritoneal dialysis can be performed in the presence of an enlarged, nonpregnant uterus, and in the presence of peritonitis. Conditions that contraindicate peritoneal dialysis are late pregnancy, previous abdominal surgery with adhesions, and the presence of intraabdominal drains.

Hemodialysis is more efficient than peritoneal dialysis and therefore corrects imbalances of fluid and electrolytes more rapidly. However, it requires the surgical insertion of an arteriovenous shunt and the administration of heparin. Also, rapid changes of circulating blood volume often result, which may be poorly tolerated by an unstable patient. Although the use of regional heparinization minimizes the risk of distant bleeding, peritoneal dialysis is the preferred method of treatment in patients with conditions that predispose to bleeding, such as peptic ulcer or pericarditis.

Following the oliguric phase, which lasts about 10–14 days, the patient enters the diuretic phase of acute renal failure. The onset of this phase is heralded by a progressively increasing volume of urine. Large amounts of water and electrolytes are excreted during this period, and the patient's survival demands adequate replacement of the excessive losses. Accurate recording of fluid intake and output, and daily weights, as well as daily determinations of BUN, serum creatinine, and urine and serum electrolytes are important in managing the patient in this phase. If the patient can tolerate oral feeding, it is best to replace fluid and electrolyte losses orally. However, if the daily urine output reaches 5–6 liters, intravenous replacement may be necessary. Half-strength Ringer's lactate or 0.45% chloride solution can be used to prevent a fall of serum potassium below 3.5 mEq/liter. The measurement of the urinary loss of potassium is helpful in determining the amount of potassium supplementation needed.

Even with the onset of the diuretic phase, the azotemia may not improve immediately; the patient may require dialysis for 4–5 more days. If the urine volume does not spontaneously decrease after 5–7 days of diuresis, it may be necessary to reduce gradually the replacement of fluid loss in order to determine whether the diuresis is being prolonged by excessive administration of fluids. This is best done by limiting fluid replacement to only 75% of measured losses until the urine volume decreases to normal. The state of hydration must be carefully assessed during this period, because, if the patient has lost the capacity to concentrate urine, she may become severely dehydrated when fluid replacement is curtailed.

In the recovery phase, the urine volume decreases to normal, and the glomerular filtration rate slowly approaches normal, although many patients never recover completely normal renal function. The ability to concentrate the urine returns to normal much more slowly than does the glomerular filtration rate; this capacity is restored only after several years in some patients and never in others.

REFERENCES AND RECOMMENDED READING

Body WN, Burden RP, Aber GM: Intrarenal vascular changes in patients receiving oestrogen-containing compounds. Q J Med 44:415, 1975

DeAlvarez RR: Preeclampsia–eclampsia and renal diseases in pregnancy. Clin Obstet Gynecol 21:881, 1978

Dhar SK, Chandrasckhar M, Smith EC: Renosonogram in diagnosis of renal failure. Clin Nephrol 7:15, 1977

Donadio JW, Jr, Holley KE: Pospartum acute renal failure: Recovery after heparin therapy. Am J Obstet Gynecol 118:510, 1974

Espinel CH: The FE$_{Na}$ test: Use in the differential diagnosis of acute renal failure. JAMA 236:579, 1976

Farber M: Pregnancy and reanl transplantation. Clin Obstet Gynecol 21:931, 1978

Felding C: Pregnancy following renal diseases. Clin Obstet Gynecol 11:579, 1968

Harkins JL, Wilson DR, Muggah HF: Acute renal failure in obstetrics. Am J Obstet Gynecol 118:331, 1974

Harrington JT, Cohen JJ: Acute oliguria. N Engl J Med 292:89, 1975

Hawkins DF, Sevitt LH, Fairbrother PF et al.: Management of septic chemical abortion with renal failure: Use of conservative regimen. N Engl J Med 292:722, 1975

Kleinknecht D, Jungers P, Chanard J et al.: Uremic and non-uremic complications of acute renal failure: Evaluation of early and frequent dialysis on prognosis. Kidney Int 1:190, 1972

Kleinknecht D, Grunfeld J, Gomez PC et al.: Diagnostic procedure and long-term prognosis in bilateral renal cortical necrosis. Kidney Int 4:390, 1973

Knapp MS, Burden RP: The recognition and managment of renal failure in pregnancy. Clin Obstet Gynecol 4:717, 1977

McGeown MG: Renal disorders and renal failure. Clin Obstet Gynecol 4:319, 1977

Marchant DJ: Alterations in anatomy and function of the urinary tract during pregnancy. Clin Obstet Gynecol 21:855, 1978

Mookerjee BK, Bilefsky R, Kenall AG, et al.: Generalized Schwartzman reaction due to gram negative septicemia after abortion. Recovery after bilateral cortical necrosis. Can Med Assoc J 98:578, 1968

Penn I, Makowski E, Droegemueller W: Parenthood in renal homograft recipients. JAMA 216:1755, 1971

Price HV, Salaman JR, Laurence KM et al.: Immunosuppressive drugs and the fetus. Transplantation 21:294, 1976

Robson JS, Martin AM, Buckley VA, McDonald MK: Q J Med 37:423, 1975

Rosenmann E, Kanter A, Bacani RA et al.: Fatal late postpartum intravascular coagulation with acute renal failure. Am J Med Sci 257:259, 1969

Schrier RW: Acute renal failure. Kidney Int 15:205, 1979

Sun NC, Johnson WJ, Sung DT et al.: Idiopathic postpartum actue renal failure: Review and case report of a successful renal transplantation. Mayo Clin Proc 50:395, 1975

Walls J, Schorr WJ, Kerr DNS: Prolonged oliguria with survival in acute bilateral cortical necrosis. Br Med J 4:220, 1968

Yoshikawa T, Tanaka KR, Guze LB: Infection and disseminated intravascular coagulation. Medicine 50:237, 1971

Zacur HA, Mitch WE: Renal disease in pregnancy. Med Clin North Am 61:89, 1977

CHAPTER

39

CESAREAN SECTION AND OTHER OBSTETRIC OPERATIONS

Leo J. Dunn

The terms *cesarean section, laparotrachelotomy,* and *abdominal delivery* all refer to the delivery of a fetus weighing 500 g or more by abdominal surgery that requires an incision through the wall of the uterus. They do not refer to surgery for an abdominal pregnancy, hysterotomy for abortion, or vaginal hysterotomy for delivery. On the basis of history (see Chapter 1) and practical value, cesarean section continues to be one of the most important operations performed in obstetrics and gynecology. Its lifesaving value to both mother and fetus has increased rather than declined over the decades, although specific indications for its use have changed. The initial purposes of preserving the life of a mother with obstructed labor or delivering a viable infant from a dying mother have gradually expanded to include the rescue of the fetus from more subtle dangers. Four major forces have led to reduced maternal risk from cesarean section: 1) improvement in surgical techniques, 2) improvement in anesthetic techniques, 3) development of safe blood transfusion, and 4) the discovery of antibiotics.

There has been a progressive increase in the incidence of cesarean section in relation to total deliveries. Whereas in the previous decade cesarean section accounted for about 5% of all deliveries, in many hospitals it is now used in nearly 20%. The reasons for this change include an increase in the number of fetal problems believed better managed by cesarean delivery, the tendency to perform repeat cesarean section in patients previously delivered by this method, and the rise in the ratio of primigravid to multiparous parturients, since primary cesarean section is approximately nine times more common in primigravidas than in multiparas.

INDICATIONS

Cesarean section is indicated 1) when labor is considered unsafe for either mother or fetus, 2) when delivery is necessary but labor cannot be induced, 3) when dystocia precludes vaginal delivery, and 4) when an emergency mandates immediate delivery and the vaginal route is not possible or not suitable.

LABOR CONTRAINDICATED

Under certain conditions, forceful uterine contractions, as in normal labor, constitute a real or potential hazard to mother, fetus, or both. Conditions in which the forces of labor increase the risk to the mother include central placenta previa, previous cesarean section (especially of the classic type), previous myomectomy, previous uterine reconstruction, or previous repair of a vaginal fistula. In such circumstances, normal labor and vaginal delivery may result in uterine rupture, hemorrhage, or serious lacerations of the birth canal, endangering the life or future health of the mother.

Conditions that threaten the fetus and that may be worsened by labor include placenta previa, velamentous insertion of the cord or other forms of vasa previa, and cord presentation. During the past decade, electronic fetal monitoring and fetal scalp pH determinations have been adopted as methods of detecting more subtle dangers involving a relative insufficiency in maternal–fetal exchange that may result in fetal compromise or death. This subject is discussed in Chapter 41.

DELIVERY NECESSARY BUT LABOR NOT INDUCIBLE

In conditions such as isoimmunization, diabetes mellitus, and hypertensive disorders, poor intrauterine environment constitutes an ever-increasing threat to the fetus so that preterm delivery may be desirable. If attempts to induce labor are unsuccessful, cesarean section is the alternative. Similarly, when preeclampsia–eclampsia or premature rupture of the membranes with amnionitis threatens maternal well-being and induction of labor is not successful, cesarean section is used. Safe and more effective methods of inducing labor earlier for preterm delivery would reduce the need for cesarean section.

The need for early delivery accounts for approximately 52% of all cesarean sections, mainly because the operation is repeated in subsequent pregnancies of patients previously delivered by this method. The need for early delivery accounts for only 2% of primary cesarean sections.

DYSTOCIA

The historical indications for cesarean section include fetopelvic disproportion, abnormal fetal presentations, dysfunctional myometrial activity, and tumor previa. They represent the mechanical problems of uterus, fetus, or birth canal that prevent the successful or safe progress of labor and vaginal delivery. Breech presentation, particularly in preterm infants, has assumed increased importance in this category. Cesarean section is being used increasingly for delivery of a second twin if malposition, malpresentation, or a tight cervix or lower uterine segment is encountered.

Dystocia is the stated indication for approximately 26% of all cesarean sections and 54% of all primary cesarean sections.

MATERNAL OR FETAL EMERGENCY

Certain maternal or fetal conditions require immediate delivery of the fetus when vaginal delivery is either not possible or not suitable. Such circumstances include significant abruption of the placenta, hemorrhage from placenta previa, prolapse of the umbilical cord, or impending maternal death. These conditions account for 19% of all cesarean sections and 38% of all primary cesarean sections.

COMPLICATIONS

Cesarean section is not an innocuous procedure free of significant maternal or fetal risks. A variety of complications—including unexplained fever, endometritis, wound infection, hemorrhage, aspiration, atelectasis, urinary tract infection, thrombophlebitis, and pulmonary embolism—occurs in 25%–50% of patients. The frequency of maternal death related to cesarean section varies with the institution and with the condition necessitating the procedure. Accepted maternal death rates are from 1/1000 to 2/1000 operations. As many as 25% of these deaths are related to anesthetic complications.

Abdominal delivery is advantageous only to a fetus who is subject to definite risk from labor or vaginal delivery. Comparison of survival rates and neurologic follow-up of infants delivered by elective cesarean section and infants delivered vaginally shows approximately a twofold increase in death rates and neurologic abnormalities in the former group. Given ideal circumstances for vaginal delivery and for cesarean section, vaginal delivery is more advantageous to both mother and infant.

Late complications of cesarean section include intestinal obstruction from adhesions and dehiscence of the uterine incision in subsequent pregnancies. Both these complications are more common when the classic incision is used. An incision in the lower uterine segment may dehisce prior to labor, but more commonly the scar thins to a transparent "window" that holds during pregnancy but may rupture with uterine contractions. A classic incision ruptures in 1%–3% of later pregnancies and, compared with a lower uterine segment incision, causes three times as many symptomatic ruptures and most of the maternal deaths from rupture.

A rare complication not generally appreciated is the lethal combination of uterine infection and classic incision. Invasion of the incision by the infecting organism quickly leads to dehiscence, and the uterine infection then drains freely into the peritoneal cavity. Only prompt surgical intervention with hysterectomy and vigorous antibiotic therapy can salvage the patient.

Although attitudes toward cesarean section have changed radically and indications have become more liberally interpreted, wide variations in the use of cesarean section within the practices of physicians sometimes reflect the status of their knowledge and judgment rather than the nature of their practices. Periodic review of all primary cesarean sections is a useful and desirable function in any hospital providing maternity care and can identify physicians whose level of information and competence results in a use of the procedure that is either too liberal or too restricted.

MANAGEMENT OF PATIENT WITH PREVIOUS CESAREAN SECTION

The progressive rise in the incidence of cesarean section in the United States must be viewed against the background of an increasing public interest in approx-

imating the most natural circumstances for childbearing that are possible within the limits of safety. These two trends suggest that, in the future, women previously delivered by cesarean section will express interest in vaginal delivery. The debate as to the safety of vaginal delivery following previous cesarean section is not new, and there continues to be a divergence of opinion. Some dogmatic statements may help define the choice:

1. Any patient in whom the indication for the primary cesarean section persists must be delivered by repeat cesarean section. The most common example is the small pelvis resulting in fetopelvic disproportion.
2. Any patient previously delivered by cesarean section should subsequently be cared for, if vaginal delivery is intended, only in a facility fully equipped and prepared for uterine rupture and by a physician trained in the management of such a serious complication.
3. The classic uterine incision scar is subject to dramatic rupture both spontaneously before term and at any time during labor and constitutes a greater hazard to mother and fetus than does a lower segment incision.
4. Not all patients previously delivered by cesarean section need be delivered by that method in subsequent pregnancies. The risk of rupture of a lower uterine segment scar, as previously noted, is relatively low with normal labor. Common practice at this time, however, is to perform the repeat operation electively. Although policies can be established, flexibility is important. It is unreasonable, for example, to insist upon repeat cesarean section in a multiparous patient whose previous cesarean delivery was necessitated by placental abruption, when she is admitted to the hospital in labor with advanced cervical dilatation, the head deeply engaged, and no demonstrable abnormality.

It is the obligation of the physician who electively repeats the cesarean section to procure evidence of fetal maturity. Conversely, it is the obligation of the physician who delivers such a patient vaginally to explore the uterine cavity carefully after delivery to rule out uterine rupture and to be adequately prepared for treatment if rupture occurs.

The dictum that sterilization is absolutely indicated with the third cesarean section has been disproved. However, the integrity of the uterine scar must be evaluated at the time of repeat cesarean section. Physician and patient should have a clear understanding regarding the possible indications for sterilization before the performance of each repeat cesarean section. In practice, however, considering current concepts of family size, repeated incisions in the uterus, and repetitive anesthetic risks, it is the unusual patient who wishes to undergo more than three cesarean sections.

TYPES OF CESAREAN SECTIONS

Types of cesarean sections are differentiated by the location and direction of the uterine incision. (The type of incision used to open the abdomen is not used in categorizing the cesarean section.) Uterine incisions are divided into two major types:

1. Incisions in the upper segment of the uterine corpus (Fig. 39–1). The vertical incision in this location is usually referred to as the *classic incision.* The transverse incision, rarely used in the United States, was originally referred to as the *Kehrer incision.*
2. Incisions in the lower uterine segment (Fig. 39–2). These incisions are in the lower portion of the uterus and require that the bladder be displaced downward in order to expose the appropriate area. The most frequently used is the *transverse (Kerr) incision.* A vertical incision may also be made in this

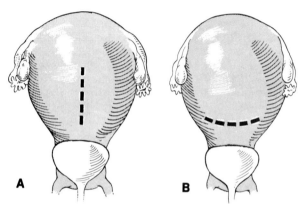

FIG. 39–1. Incisions in upper segment of uterus. *A.* Classic incision. *B.* Kehrer incision.

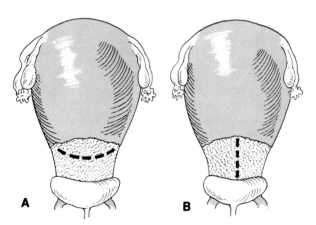

FIG. 39–2. Incisions in lower uterine segment. *A.* Kerr incision. *B.* Sellheim incision.

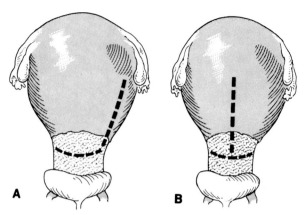

FIG. 39–3. Undesirable variations of uterine incisions. *A.* J-shaped incision. *B.* T-shaped incision.

area, but such an incision will involve the upper uterine segment unless the lower segment is quite elongated by labor; this is known as the *Sellheim incision*.

Occasionally, a variation is used, usually because of unanticipated difficulty during cesarean section. Two of these are worth mentioning (Fig. 39–3). They are undesirable and can be avoided by careful assessment and planning of the uterine incision.

The *J-shaped incision* is generally the result of an attempt to perform a transverse lower uterine segment incision when the lower uterine segment is too narrow. The inadequacy of the incision is not realized until delivery is attempted, and then a vertical extension is made surgically from one end to avoid spontaneous extension into the broad ligament. In subsequent pregnancies this incision should be regarded as bearing the risks of a classic incision.

The *T-shaped incision* may be made for the same reasons or in the hasty management of the unexpected finding of placental implantation beneath the area of incision. The operator, having made an inadequate transverse incision, now performs a vertical incision beginning in the center. This incision does not heal well and is even more likely to rupture in subsequent pregnancies than is the classic incision.

Transperitoneal versus extraperitoneal cesarean section refers to the techniques used to reach the uterine wall. The rationale for the extraperitoneal approach was based upon the belief that it would reduce the chance of death from peritonitis in a patient with an infected uterus. It has been discarded, however, as it has not proved superior to the less complicated transabdominal lower uterine segment operation. Vaginal cesarean section and vaginal hysterotomy are also of historical interest only.

Other procedures for "peritoneal exclusion," which were originally developed by Frank and Sellheim, are from time to time "rediscovered." The operator first enters the peritoneal cavity and then "excludes" the abdominal cavity by sewing the cephalad edge of parietal peritoneum to the visceral peritoneum and serosa of the uterus after the bladder has been displaced from the lower uterine segment but before the uterus is incised. These procedures are rarely used in contemporary obstetrics.

ANESTHESIA

The choice of anesthetic technique and agents is dictated by a number of factors (see Chapter 32). In summary, a patient with signs of fetal distress, hemorrhage, or shock; with previous injury or surgery to the spine; or with cutaneous infections of the lower back is obviously not a candidate for spinal or epidural anesthetic techniques. Similarly, a patient with active pulmonary disease, such as pneumonia or tuberculosis, is not a candidate for inhalation anesthesia. Under conditions of severe maternal disease, local infiltration might present less maternal risk than either inhalation or regional block.

In the majority of cases, however, there are no clear-cut indications or contraindications, and the choice lies with the technique itself and the skills of the anesthetist. Under such circumstances, the relative advantages and disadvantages of regional block and inhalation anesthesia are so similar that, if the anesthetist is clearly more skilled in one than the other, the most familiar technique should be chosen.

Maternal and fetal hemodynamics are markedly affected by maternal position. The dorsal recumbent position, usually used for cesarean section, is disadvantageous to both mother and fetus, primarily because the inferior vena cava is compressed. This decreases venous return and maternal cardiac output, causing hypotension and reduced uterine perfusion referred to as the *inferior vena cava syndrome*. In this syndrome, the weight of the pregnant uterus may have a progressively greater compressive effect upon the aorta as the mean arterial pressure falls, thus reducing blood flow to the pelvis. Obviously, hypotension produced by regional anesthetic techniques compounds this problem. Techniques such as using attachments to the operating table that mechanically displace the uterus laterally, placing inflatable wedges under the patient, or tilting the table to use the effect of gravity to displace the uterus laterally have been reported effective but are not widely used. Manual displacement of the uterus to the patient's left is the most frequently used technique in current practice. Rapid intravenous infusion of 1 liter physiologic solution containing sodium immediately before the initiation of regional anesthesia has reduced the incidence of hypotension.

Considerable data support the presumption that the status of the fetus worsens as the time of exposure to

anesthesia lengthens. Progressive fetal depression, evidenced by lower Apgar scores, as the induction-to-delivery time is prolonged makes it important to avoid unnecessary delay during the operative procedure. For example, the abdomen should be fully prepared, draped, and ready for the incision before general anesthesia is induced. On the other hand, reckless surgical techniques for rapid delivery of the fetus should be condemned. An induction-to-delivery time of 5–15 min is reasonable if maternal oxygenation, blood pressure, and displacement of the uterus are monitored and maintained with care.

Anesthetic agents that produce marked relaxation of the myometrium (*e.g.,* halothane) may result in excessive postpartum bleeding.

PROCEDURE

Cesarean section requires the same preoperative care needed for any major surgery, plus additional consideration for the status of the fetus. A patient who has been in labor for a long period may show signs of dehydration or acidosis, and these should be corrected. Since anemia is relatively common in pregnancy, determination of hemoglobin or hematocrit value is important prior to surgery. Blood should be available for immediate transfusion because of the ever-present risk of hemorrhage. Since the bladder will be in the operative field, it is necessary to catheterize the patient prior to the procedure and leave the catheter indwelling. The patient should receive an explanation of the procedure, including risks and the reason it is necessary. The appropriate permission forms should be on record for the procedure, the anesthetic, the administration of blood, and hysterectomy, if that proves necessary.

In a repeat cesarean section, where timing of the procedure is determined electively, evidence of fetal maturity is important. Death or damage from unrecognized low birth weight is always a hazard to the fetus in the elective repeat cesarean section. In the past, a patient was allowed to begin labor before the repeat cesarean section was done in order to reduce the hazard of preterm delivery to a minimum. Today procedures such as diagnostic ultrasound and determination of amniotic fluid lecithin/sphingomyelin (L/S) ratio are reliable indicators of fetal maturity and have reduced fetal death from preterm delivery in repeat cesarean section. The prudent physician uses the best means available to demonstrate fetal maturity before performing an elective cesarean section.

PREPARATION

Preparation of the abdomen includes shaving the skin of the abdomen and mons pubis, scrubbing the area with an antiseptic soap, and preparing the skin with

some antiseptic agent such as nonorganic iodide. The abdomen is draped so that the area between the umbilicus and the mons pubis is exposed.

The use of prophylactic antibiotics (see page 245) is an issue on which opinion is divided. Patients with prolonged rupture of membranes, especially those with associated unsuccessful labor, have a high incidence of post–cesarean section infections. In this instance, cesarean section should be regarded as are other operative procedures in which gross contamination of the operative wound occurs. Use of antibiotics in these patients is indicated and is not prophylactic in the true sense. Those patients undergoing repeat cesarean section without known complication are more clearly the issue. Gall has shown in a prospective study that preoperative antibiotics can be shown to benefit these patients as well as those that were in labor. The problems of cost and risk versus benefit are important additional considerations; serious infections are often not prevented by this treatment.

CHOICE OF UTERINE AND ABDOMINAL INCISIONS

The transverse incision in the lower uterine segment is the preferred method and the one on which the technique described in the following is based. There is no doubt that the classic incision is associated with more immediate and remote morbidity than incision in the lower uterine segment. Although in subsequent pregnancies a lower segment incision may stretch and become a thin window or even separate, it generally causes few clinical problems until term or until exposed to the forces of labor. There is no apparent difference in morbidity or subsequent risk between the transverse and vertical incisions in the lower uterine segment if the upper segment of the corpus is not incised. The classic incision, however, may rupture dramatically at any time from the midpoint of gestation to term and tolerates the forces of labor less well. The risk to the mother and fetus from this incision is clearly greater. Other considerations regarding choice of incision are discussed under Variations.

The usual abdominal incision is in the midline, although both paramedian and Pfannenstiel's incisions are commonly used in some institutions. Use of the Pfannenstiel incision increases the induction-to-delivery time both in the primary procedure and in subsequent cesarean sections. Furthermore, repetition of this incision in subsequent pregnancies results in a higher incidence of bladder injuries.

TECHNIQUE

The abdomen is opened in layers in a relatively rapid fashion; any large vessels encountered are clamped, but no attempt is made to achieve meticulous hemo-

stasis that might delay delivery of the fetus. During this portion of the procedure, the anesthesiologist must pay careful attention to the patient's blood pressure lest the inferior vena cava syndrome, previously discussed, cause a relative uteroplacental insufficiency and compromise the fetus. If such occurs, the anesthesiologist or an assistant must move the uterus to the patient's left to improve venous return. The abdominal cavity should be briefly inspected to note the direction and degree of rotation of the uterus. Folded, moistened laparotomy pads are placed on either side of the uterus to reduce peritoneal soilage from amniotic fluid, but are not essential. Retractors placed in the abdominal wound and drawn laterally expose the anterior surface of the uterus and the bladder covering the lower uterine segment. With smooth forceps, the operator identifies the fold of peritoneum between the serosa of the uterus and the serosa of the bladder (Fig. 39–4A). This loose portion of peritoneum is elevated in the midline and incised, allowing entrance into the space between the bladder and the lower uterine segment (Fig. 39–4B). The closed scissors are then bluntly inserted in a lateral direction through this opening beneath the peritoneum, further separating the bladder from the overlying peritoneum. The area of peritoneum over the line of blunt dissection is incised laterally; underlying veins in the broad and cardinal ligaments must be carefully avoided. The operator should now be able to reflect the bladder from the lower uterine segment (Fig. 39–4C, D) using either digital pressure or a folded sponge on a sponge clamp. A small margin of peritoneum can be freed from the serosa of the uterus in the superior portion of the incision to aid in closure of the peritoneum following the delivery of the fetus. If such a peritoneal flap cannot be easily developed at the time, this step should be postponed to avoid unnecessarily delaying delivery of the fetus.

The operator should now be looking directly upon the fascia covering the lower uterine segment. In the midline, a few centimeters below the peritoneal incision, a small incision in the transverse direction can now be made with a scalpel (Fig. 39–4E). If care is taken in making this incision, the fetal membranes will bulge into the incision without being ruptured. The operator then inserts a finger between the fetal membranes and the overlying wall of the uterus. Using this finger as a guide, the operator inserts the lower blade of bandage scissors into the wound and extends the incision laterally in a gentle upward curve (Fig. 39–4F). The assistant should retract the abdominal wall firmly on the side toward which the operator is dissecting. Under direct vision, the operator should make this half of the incision as far laterally as possible without entering the broad ligament. When this half of the incision has been completed, attention is directed to the opposite side and the procedure repeated. Once this has been completed, a crescent-shaped or curvi-

linear incision has been formed in the lower uterine segment and the fetal membranes are bulging into the incision.

An alternative method of opening the uterus is to make a shallow curvilinear incision through the pubocervical fascia the full length of the desired opening. The incision is extended through to the fetal membranes in a small area in the center of the wound. Inserting both index fingers into the opening, the operator draws them apart and, with lateral pressure, bluntly opens the uterus. This method, which works best in a patient with a thin lower uterus segment following labor, has the advantage of reduced bleeding from the incision.

The operator now inserts one hand beneath the lower edge of the uterine wound and over the fetal membranes in order to feel the presenting fetal part. In the case of vertex presentation, the occiput is identified and gently pressed, resulting in increased flexion of the fetal head. The operator's fingers are gradually insinuated between the uterine wall and the fetal head, and, with pressure by this hand, the head can be brought toward the uterine incision (Fig. 39–4G). The membranes can be ruptured and stripped away from the fetal head. The head is then brought into the incision, and the assistant or operator can exert fundal pressure on the fetal buttocks to gently push the fetal head through the incision. Once the head has been delivered, the mouth and the nares may be rapidly suctioned with a bulb suction device by the assistant as the operator completes the delivery (Fig. 39–5). The fetal shoulders are delivered with gentle traction on the fetal head in a manner similar to that used for vaginal delivery. Specially designed forceps or a vectis may be used instead of the operator's hand in delivering the head through the uterine incision.

Following delivery of the shoulders, the fetus is extracted and should be held in a head-down position to improve drainage of the mouth and nares and to reduce the chance of aspiration. The mouth and nares may again be suctioned, the cord is clamped and divided, and the fetus may now be resuscitated by an assistant, preferably outside the operative field.

The operator now manually removes the placenta, separating it bluntly from the uterine wall with the fingers held extended in a rigid manner and the back of the hand toward the uterine wall to prevent injury to

FIG. 39–4. Cesarean section. *A.* Reflection of peritoneum from ► serosa of uterus to bladder is identified. *B.* Peritoneal reflection between uterus and bladder is elevated and incised. *C.* Bladder is displaced away from lower uterine segment. *D.* Bladder is retracted and incision is planned to be 2–3 cm below peritoneal incision. *E.* Small incision is made through uterine wall to fetal membranes. *F.* Uterine incision is made in a curvilinear shape, using bandage scissors. *G.* Fetal head is elevated through uterine wound by operator's hand.

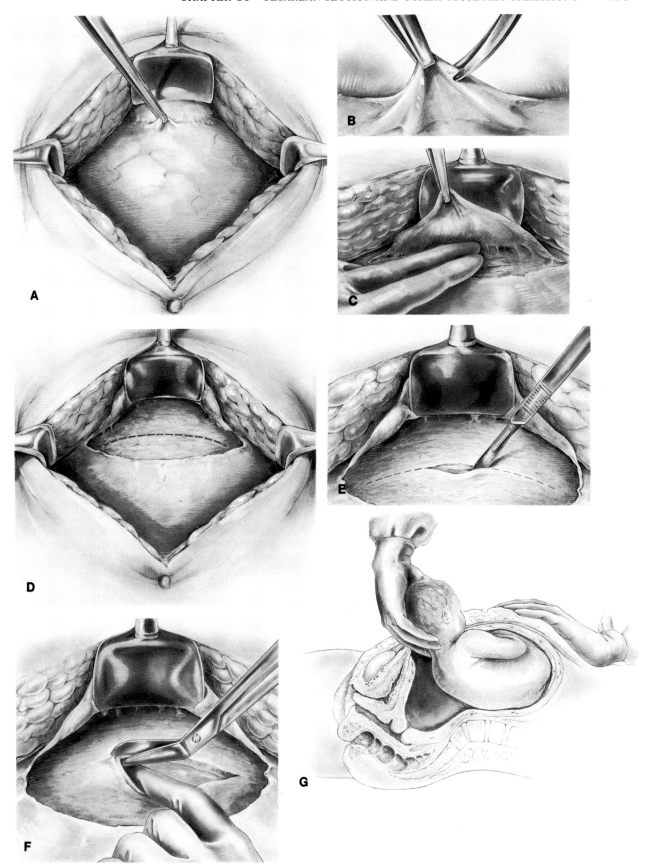

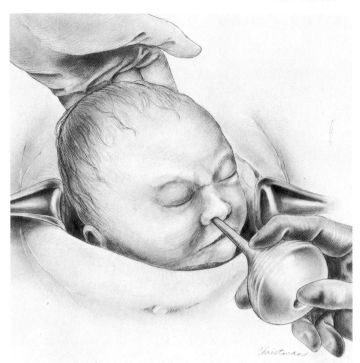

FIG. 39-5. Mouth and nares of infant are suctioned as soon as possible.

the wall by flexed fingertips. Oxytocin, 10 IU, added to the patient's intravenous infusion helps uterine contractions to reduce the amount of bleeding. Some physicians inject the oxytocin directly into the uterine wall, but this is dangerous; if oxytocin enters the circulation as a bolus, hypotension or cardiac arrythmias may result. For the same reason, deliberate intravenous injection of an undiluted bolus of oxytocin is hazardous.

The uterine cavity should be inspected for any structural abnormality or retained placental tissue. The surface should then be wiped with a dry laparotomy pad to remove any adherent segments of membranes.

Digital dilatation of the endocervical canal from above is not necessary and should not be done unless some unusual circumstance suggests nonpatency of the canal.

The cut edges of the uterine wall can now be grasped with Allis clamps, Allis–Adair clamps, T clamps, or other clamps that are noncrushing. These clamps hold the edges for traction and compress bleeding venous sinuses. Crushing clamps should be avoided, as they result in devitalized tissue in the uterine incision. It is preferable not to elevate the uterus outside the abdominal cavity for the repair of the incision, as this exposes fallopian tubes to unnecessary trauma.

The first layer of closure (Fig.39–6A) should be of O-chromic catgut in a continuous, locked stitch anchored securely at the angle of the incision. The continuous locked suture should be held with firm tension by the assistant throughout the closure. Although the operator should avoid including large segments of the endometrium in the closure, inclusion of a narrow band gives satisfactory results and eliminates the risk of sinuses that may cause postoperative hemorrhage. The second layer of closure (Fig. 39–6B) imbricates the first; O chromic catgut is used in either interrupted stitches in figures-of-eight, Lembert stitches, or a continuous suture placed in such a manner as to cover completely the first layer of closure. The peritoneum is then reapproximated with a continuous layer of 2-0 plain or chromic catgut (Fig. 39–6C). If, during the closure, any areas of bleeding are still noted in the incision line, separate interrupted sutures of O chromic catgut in figures-of-eight should be placed in the bleeding area to secure hemostasis.

The uterus and visceral peritoneum having been reapproximated, the packs are removed from the abdominal cavity and any residual blood or amniotic fluid removed by suction. If meconium soilage or exposure to infected amniotic fluid has occurred, the pelvic cavity should be lavaged with normal saline. The ovaries and tubes should be inspected, as should the remainder of the abdominal cavity. Prophylactic appendectomy is offered to patients routinely in some institutions, and the complication rate from this additional procedure is relatively small. The abdomen is then

closed in layers. Postoperative management of the patient should be similar to that of any patient who has undergone major surgery.

The operator should be aware that a postpartum patient who has undergone major trauma, including cesarean section, is at high risk for the development of thrombophlebitis and thromboembolism. For that reason, meticulous care of the patient's legs in the operating room is of importance, as is spontaneous movement of the legs and early ambulation following cesarean section. The urinary catheter may be removed on the 1st postoperative day. The patient is usually able to tolerate a clear liquid diet by the 2nd postoperative day and can be expected to recover rapidly through the 2nd–5th postoperative days. Discharge from the hospital can be considered for the average patient any time on the 5th–7th day, preferably the latter, depending upon the patient's condition and the availability of continued care in her home.

CLOSURE OF THE CLASSIC INCISION

The thickness of the uterine wall may require a three-layer closure to and including the serosa. Continuous suture techniques may be used, but interrupted sutures frequently give a more exact closure. The first layer should include roughly half the thickness of the wall; stitches should be closely spaced and may be simple sutures or figures-of-eight. The second-layer sutures should be placed so as to avoid leaving a space between the layers and should come close to but not penetrate the serosa. The third layer should close the serosa in a manner that minimizes the raw surface to which the abdominal cavity will be exposed. The closure should be continuous, not locked, with 2-0 chromic material. Each bite with the needle should begin on the raw surface of the wound and exit through the serosa a few millimeters from the cut edge. By this technique, the cut edge is infolded and the serosal surfaces are brought over to cover. This is sometimes referred to as a "baseball stitch."

VARIATIONS

Under unusual circumstances, the operator may wish to use some variations of the cesarean section technique described.

Following prolonged obstructed labor, the operator occasionally encounters a fetal head deeply impacted in the midpelvis and a greatly elongated and thinned lower uterine segment. Under these circumstances, it may be necessary for an assistant to dislodge the fetal head from the midpelvis with a hand in the vagina either immediately before or during the cesarean section. The manipulations necessary during the delivery of this fetal head, combined with the thinning of the

FIG. 39-6. Wound closure. *A.* First layer of closure. *B.* Second layer of closure. *C.* Closure of visceral peritoneum.

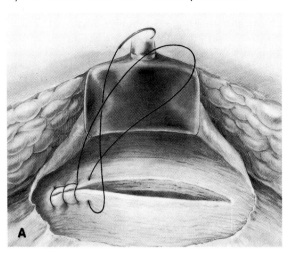

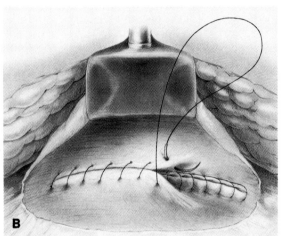

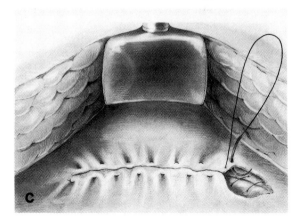

lower uterine segment, may result in a lateral extension of a transverse incision and laceration of the uterine vessels. Under these circumstances, therefore, a vertical incision in the lower uterine segment should be considered. The incision is usually comparable in length to the transverse incision because of the elongated nature of the lower uterine segment, and extension of the vertical is less hazardous to the patient than extension of the transverse incision.

Occasionally, *e.g.,* in the presence of a posterior placenta previa or preterm delivery, the lower uterine segment is so narrow that a transverse incision is inadequate. Under these circumstances a vertical incision in the lower segment is necessary, even if it extends into the upper segment of the uterus. A classic incision may even be necessary under such circumstances. For similar reasons, in the presence of an extremely large fetus, the classic incision may be the best choice to avoid extension into the uterine vessels.

Breech presentation after labor usually can be safely managed through a transverse incision in the lower uterine segment, but the operator should be careful to make the incision as wide as possible at first so that delivery of the head is not delayed by the need to extend an inadequate uterine incision.

Transverse lie with fetal back down or shoulder presentation is usually an indication for a classic incision in the uterus. Attempts to deliver such a fetus through a transverse lower segment incision may well result in extension of the uterine incision into the uterine vessels. Transverse lie with fetal back up (umbrella position) need not be managed by a classic incision and can be considered similar to a breech presentation.

Occasionally, the operator encounters the maternal surface of the placenta when opening the uterus. This can produce considerable anxiety or panic on the part of the operator because of the profuse hemorrhage. Several points become important: 1) good suction must be available so that the operative field can be kept reasonably clear for visualization, 2) the operator must move quickly to extend the incision to the full opening believed necessary for delivery of the fetus, and 3) the placenta should not be cut or fractured because disruption of the vessels on the chorionic plate may result in serious fetal hemorrhage. Instead, the placenta should be separated from the uterine wall (as previously described for removal of the placenta) in order to allow access to the fetal membranes. The membranes should be punctured and the fetus delivered through this opening and through the uterine incision. It may be possible to deliver the fetus by the vertex in this situation, but the operator may find it necessary to grasp the feet and deliver the fetus by version and extraction instead. Fetal depression and breathing difficulty, owing to aspiration, should be anticipated.

Amnionitis has been considered an indication for the extraperitoneal technique of cesarean section. Experience has shown so little difference in the subsequent maternal morbidity between the transperitoneal lower uterine segment incision and the extraperitoneal lower uterine segment incision that the extraperitoneal approach has now become passé. Furthermore, in view of the increase in fetal depression with prolonged anesthesia of any type, it seems best not to prolong the induction-to-delivery time by using the extraperitoneal approach.

POSTMORTEM CESAREAN SECTION

The occurrence of circumstances that lead to cesarean birth following the death of the mother is fortunately so rare that most obstetricians never perform such an operation. The principles are relatively simple. Maternal death must be quickly established—on clinical grounds if necessary, but preferably by electrocardiographic or electroencephalographic findings if the patient is being monitored. Aseptic precautions are ignored, and the abdomen and uterus are opened rapidly with vertical and classic incisions, respectively. The fetus is quickly delivered, given immediate resuscitation, and moved to an intensive care nursery as soon as possible. The placenta should be removed manually and the uterus and abdomen closed. Experience suggests that efforts to auscultate fetal heartbeat before deciding upon cesarean section may give erroneous information. The time from apparent fetal death to actual fetal death or serious damage is unknown. The prognostic factors of importance are the length of gestation, the cardiovascular status of the mother prior to death (*e.g.,* prolonged marginal status with septic shock versus excellent status prior to accidental death), and the interval from maternal death to delivery. At best, the prognosis for the baby is dubious; survival can probably be expected if delivery is accomplished within 10 min of apparent maternal death, but the severity of brain damage from cerebral hypoxia is less easy to predict. It has been suggested that, if modern life support systems are in use, the outlook for the baby may be improved if the cesarean section can be done before the mother's actual death.

OTHER OBSTETRIC OPERATIONS

INDUCTION OF LABOR

Induction of labor is the deliberate initiation of labor prior to its spontaneous onset. The procedure may be either elective or indicated.

Elective induction of labor is defined by the Food

TABLE 39-1. METHOD FOR PREDICTING SUCCESS OF INDUCTION OF LABOR

Physical Findings	Rating			
	0	1	2	3
CERVIX				
Position	Posterior	Midposition	Anterior	
Consistency	Firm	Medium	Soft	
Effacement (%)	0–30	40–50	60–70	80 >
Dilatation (cm)	0	1–2	3–4	5 >
FETAL HEAD				
Station	−3	−2	−1	+1 >

(Modified from Bishop EH: Obstet Gynecol 24:266, 1964)

and Drug Administration (FDA) as "the initiation of labor for the convenience of an individual with a term pregnancy who is free of medical indications." The most obvious hazard of elective induction is the iatrogenic delivery of a preterm infant. Accordingly, all possible steps must be taken to be certain, regardless of menstrual dates (which are not always accurate), that the fetus is at term and that labor is imminent. Determination of the L/S ratio and prior ultrasound scans can be helpful; in some cases, they are essential. The imminence of labor and the likelihood of successful induction can usually be predicted by the findings on pelvic examination.

Indicated induction refers to the initiation of labor after 20 weeks' gestation when the benefits of delivery to the fetus or the mother exceed the benefits of continuing the pregnancy. Some of the circumstances for which induction of labor may be indicated are premature rupture of the membranes, abruptio placentae, preeclampsia–eclampsia, amnionitis, maternal isoimmunization, certain cases of fetal jeopardy (*e.g.,* fetal growth retardation, postterm pregnancy), certain cases of maternal disease (*e.g.,* diabetes mellitus, hypertensive vascular disease), intrauterine fetal death, and certain other maternal medical problems.

CONTRAINDICATIONS TO INDUCTION OF LABOR

Induction of labor is contraindicated in certain situations, such as cephalopelvic disproportion, abnormal presentation, most cases of previous uterine incision (*e.g.,* cesarean section, myomectomy), advanced maternal age, grand multiparity (more than five), multiple pregnancy, certain cases of fetal jeopardy (*e.g.,* abnormal oxytocin challenge test), and any maternal condition in which labor is contraindicated.

DANGERS OF INDUCTION OF LABOR

Regardless of whether oxytocin is used, induced labors tend to be shorter and more vigorous than spontaneous labor, possibly because most candidates for induc-

tion have physical signs that are extremely favorable for short labor.

For the fetus, the preeminent risk is prematurity if adequate steps have not been taken to eliminate this possibility. Other risks are those of either precipitate or prolonged labor; hypoxia due to hypercontractility of the uterus; and, as a consequence of rupture of the membranes, infection and cord prolapse. Hyperbilirubinemia of the newborn has been found to result from prolonged oxytocin infusion, and other fetal consequences have also been postulated. When due attention is given to selection of patients and technique of induction, however, Niswander, Friedman, and their coworkers found that there is no significant increase in adverse infant outcome from induction of labor.

For the mother, the dangers include such problems as the consequences of tumultuous labor (*e.g.,* rupture of the uterus, premature separation of the placenta, cervical laceration); precipitate or prolonged labor; failure of induction, perhaps necessitating either cesarean section or instrumental delivery; intrauterine infection; postpartum hemorrhage; and amniotic fluid embolism.

SELECTION OF PATIENTS FOR INDUCTION

The findings on vaginal examination largely determine whether the conditions for induction are favorable, equivocal, or unfavorable. Bishop has emphasized the important factors in making this decision by a scoring system (Table 39-1) in which a score of 0, 1, 2, or 3 is given for each of four designated qualities of the cervix and for station of the fetal head. A total score of 9 or above indicates that labor may be induced with only a small chance of failure. The *most favorable* case is one in which the head is engaged to station +1 or lower and the cervix is soft, more than 50% effaced, directly in the axis of the vagina, and dilated at least 3 cm. The *least favorable* case is one in which the head is not engaged and the cervix is firm, posterior, uneffaced, and dilated less than 2 cm. When conditions are favorable, labor should be expected to begin promptly after the

induction is started and to proceed apace. When they are unfavorable, the attempt at induction may or may not be successful; if labor does ensue, it can be expected to be protracted and difficult.

METHODS

Continuous electronic monitoring of fetal heart rate and uterine contractions should be part of any method for the induction of labor. It should be started 15 minutes before the induction is begun in order to establish baseline characteristics.

Artificial Rupture of the Membranes

Most obstetricians consider amniotomy to be an essential part of any procedure for the induction of labor. If the conditions for induction are especially favorable, rupture of the membranes and drainage of a small amount of amniotic fluid suffice to start labor in about half the cases. According to one technique, preferred by many obstetricians, the patient is admitted to the hospital early in the morning without breakfast. An enema is given, and the membranes are ruptured artificially. Oxytocin is used only if labor has not started within 1 hour.

Oxytocin Induction

It is important that the physician understand clearly the indications, contraindications, prerequisites, and techniques of oxytocin use before deciding to induce labor by means of oxytocin. The clinical use of oxytocin in dysfunctional labor is discussed in Chapter 35. The same admonitions apply to its use for induction.

Oxytocin can be of great benefit for the induction or stimulation of labor. Its misuse, however, creates major maternal and fetal hazards, and the FDA has now proscribed its use in elective induction of labor. Moreover, in medically indicated induction, the FDA stipulates that the drug be given intravenously and that the initial dose be limited to "no more than 1–2 mU/min. This dose may be gradually increased in increments of no more than 1–2 mU/min until the patient experiences a contraction pattern similar to normal labor," *i.e.,* contractions of good intensity lasting 40–50 sec and occurring every 2–3 min. The uterus should relax to normal baseline tone between contractions, and the maximum rate of the infusion should not exceed 20 mU/min. If satisfactory effects are not achieved with a flow rate of 20 mU/min, higher doses are also unlikely to be effective and can be hazardous. The necessary precision in rate of flow may be obtained with a drip technique, but an infusion pump is preferable. Most of the problems encountered with oxytocin use result from high infusion rates over long

periods. When labor is established, the infusion should be slowed and ultimately discontinued.

Some obstetricians prefer to begin induction with an oxytocin infusion, rupturing the membranes only when labor is established. This method avoids the commitment of ruptured membranes, but induction failures are apt to be more common than when the membranes are ruptured as a first step; also, the labors are somewhat longer, and the total oxytocin dose is usually greater.

There is increasing doubt of the propriety of attempted induction when conditions are not favorable and a long induction-to-delivery time can be anticipated. In one such technique, sometimes used in an effort to avoid cesarean section when delivery is indicated, an oxytocin infusion is run for 6–8 hours with the objective of softening and partially dilating the cervix. This is followed by 8–10 hours of rest, and the infusion is then resumed in the hope that delivery can be accomplished vaginally at some time during the second infusion period. Note has already been made that hyperbilirubinemia may occur in the newborn after prolonged exposure to oxytocin, and the question has been raised whether there may also be long-term deleterious effects on the surviving infant. When the conditions for induction are not favorable and delivery is indicated, cesarean section is usually preferable if the baby is living.

The physician must be aware that oxytocin has definite antidiuretic activity. Urinary output is demonstrably reduced at an infusion level of 20 mU/min and may be markedly reduced at higher rates. Prolonged or excessive oxytocin administration, coupled with intravenous glucose infusion, has led to water intoxication and maternal death.

Induction by Prostaglandin Administration

At the present time, the uses of prostaglandins E_2 and $F_{2\alpha}$ being investigated continue to include induction of labor. More data must be obtained before their value or lack of value can be clearly established. It is certain that they induce labor at term with an effectiveness not radically different from that of oxytocin. The prerequisites for their use are similar to those described for oxytocin. These substances are not entirely without maternal risk, however, as documented by occasional maternal deaths reported to be associated with their use for abortions. The risk of overstimulation and the development of hypertonus also exists. The gastrointestinal side effects of prostaglandins occur with induction of labor as with the induction of abortion. Direct effects on the fetus, not attributable to the process of labor, have not been established.

Since prostaglandins appear to have a direct effect on cervical ripening (see page 616), they may have special usefulness in cases of indicated induc-

tion when the conditions are unfavorable. Several routes have been used to administer them for induction of labor: intravenous, oral, buccal, extraamniotic, and vaginal or rectal. The Friedman *et al.* protocol is the oral administration of prostaglandin E_2 in dose of 0.5 or 1 mg hourly until "strong clinical labor" occurs.

The risks of this method of induction are not entirely known, and the FDA has not approved their use if the baby is living. However, they have been used extensively for this purpose outside the United States, and most reports are favorable. Some concern has been expressed regarding the fact that hypercontractility and abnormal fetal heart rate patterns sometimes occur, although residual effects in the offspring have not been demonstrated. More recently, the intravaginal use of prostaglandin E_2 in viscous gel (0.2 mg in 10 ml hydroxyethylcellulose gel) has been proposed as an effective agent for softening an unripe cervix in preparation for induction. Among 95 primigravidas in the O'Herlihy–MacDonald series, there were no untoward fetal or maternal effects. In 47% of the 95 patients, labor followed "spontaneously;" in the remainder, subsequent labors were normal, and the incidence of cesarean section was significantly lower than that in a control group.

Other Methods of Induction

Introducing a gloved finger inside the cervix and separating the membranes in a 360° sweep is a technique described as *stripping the membranes.* It is an old method that is not very effective unless the patient is near the onset of spontaneous labor. The time interval from procedure to onset of labor is quite variable and unpredictable. The frequency with which this technique is used is difficult to assess, as many physicians use it casually during an office examination and do not record it as an attempt at induction. It is not a significant method of induction and, although believed to produce no complications, may be followed by premature rupture of membranes or a dysfunctional latent phase.

Electrical induction of labor remains in the experimental stage. The method is possible, but its practicality as a routine procedure has not been demonstrated in the United States.

Acupuncture is reportedly an effective method of inducing labor. As is true of other uses of acupuncture, carefully performed studies that would yield objective evidence are lacking.

If the fetus is dead and uterine enlargement is consistent with a gestation of 16 weeks or more, labor can be induced by the introduction of various substances, such as hypertonic saline, urea, or prostaglandins, into the amniotic sac. Specific techniques are discussed in Chapter 14. (See also Missed Labor, Chapter 26.)

SURGICAL SEXUAL STERILIZATION

Although failure rates of surgical sterilization appear higher when the operations are performed at the time of cesarean section or following vaginal delivery, they should not be delayed for that reason. Tubal ligation adds little time or morbidity to cesarean section and is a much less complicated procedure than hysterectomy. The Pomeroy technique is the most simple and gives satisfactory results, although the Irving procedure is associated with fewer failures.

Tubal ligation following vaginal delivery can be easily performed through a small transverse infra- or intraumbilical incision. The procedure takes only minutes to perform, has few complications, and does not significantly prolong postpartum recovery.

VERSION AND EXTRACTION

Once a subject for considerable debate and advocated for a variety of obstetric problems, the version and extraction procedure has now been replaced by cesarean section. The major obstetric problem for which version and extraction is sometimes appropriate is for delivery of a second twin, but even in this circumstance it is permissible only if the conditions are extremely favorable, that is, a baby no larger than the first twin, an ample pelvis, and an anesthetist who is capable of administering an anesthetic that will provide full uterine relaxation. Internal podalic version is a formidable obstetric operation, and even in the most favorable circumstances many modern obstetricians prefer to employ cesarean section for delivery of a second twin in preference to version and extraction, or, indeed, if the head of the second twin does not engage in the pelvis promptly after delivery of the first.

If version and extraction is elected for delivery of the second twin, the following principles should be followed:

1. The procedure should not be done if the membranes have been ruptured for some time and the uterus is firmly contracted around the fetus.
2. The membranes should not be ruptured until a fetal foot or both feet are clearly in the operator's control.
3. Deep anesthesia must be induced, preferably with an agent that has a marked relaxing influence upon the myometrium (*e.g.*, halothane).
4. The fetal head must be displaced to a level above the iliac fossa.
5. Traction should be gentle but sufficient to result in continuous progress in turning and extracting the infant (Fig. 39–7).
6. After delivery, the uterus and birth canal must be carefully inspected for injuries, as these are a prime hazard to the mother following this procedure.

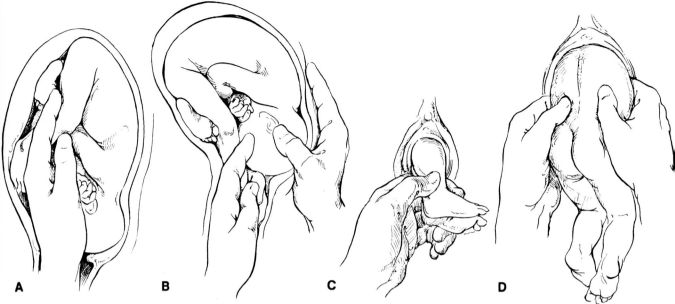

FIG. 39-7. Version and extraction. *A.* Feet are grasped. *B.* Baby is turned; hand on abdomen pushes head toward uterine fundus. *C.* Feet are extracted. *D.* Torso is delivered. From this point onward, procedure is same as for uncomplicated breech delivery.

7. As is true for all other operative obstetric procedures, the patient should be prepared in advance for immediate blood transfusion.

The inexperienced operator will find it difficult to distinguish a foot from a hand during this maneuver. This is a critical point, since an error will result in a prolapsed arm with a shoulder presentation. For practice, the physician should feel the hand and foot of a newborn infant and note that when the appendage is straightened into the axis of the leg or arm the heel becomes a definite prominence that has no analogous structure in the hand. A few benign practice sessions can save considerable anxiety at a critical moment.

The technique of breech delivery that completes this procedure is described in Chapter 34.

HYSTERECTOMY IMMEDIATELY FOLLOWING DELIVERY

INDICATIONS

Occasionally, hysterectomy must be performed immediately following cesarean or vaginal delivery. A useful classification is based on emergency indications (uterine rupture, uncontrollable uterine hemorrhage, placenta accreta, uterine infection) and nonemergency indications (sexual sterilization, carcinoma *in situ,* uterine leiomyomas).

Emergency Indications

Uterine rupture, especially when it is the dehiscence of a previous cesarean section scar, usually (but not always) mandates immediate hysterectomy. The tear may be repaired if the patient strongly wishes to retain fertility, if her condition is not jeopardized by continued hemorrhage, and if competent repair is technically possible. The wound edge should be debrided before the edges are reapproximated. Suturing techniques are similar to those used for cesarean section repair.

Uncontrollable uterine hemorrhage may result from uterine rupture, uterine atony, placenta accreta, placental site sinusoids following placenta previa, or a coagulation defect. When surgery is indicated to control hemorrhage of uterine origin, the operator must assess the patient's desire to preserve childbearing capacity, as well as the present danger. Nonsurgical management is indicated in such circumstances as uterine atony or coagulation defect.

To staunch bleeding, it is emphasized that bimanual uterine massage, oxytocin administration, and replacement therapy, including administration of fresh blood, should be employed before surgical intervention is considered. Hemorrhage from sinusoids in the lower uterine segment associated with placenta previa may be controlled with mattress sutures or figures-of-eight using 2-0 or 0 chromic catgut placed with an atraumatic needle. If uterine atony is the cause of bleeding and future childbearing is strongly desired, surgical

interruption of the arterial flow to the uterus may be tried as the first measure of control. The operator may proceed to bilateral ligation of the hypogastric arteries or the uterine arteries. If this proves efficacious, the problem is solved and the patient's fertility maintained. If not, hysterectomy can be performed.

The lifesaving value of hysterectomy for the treatment of severe uterine infection should be emphasized. The patient who has experienced a second trimester septic abortion with septic shock, peritonitis, or uterine perforation may be saved by prompt hysterectomy. Clostridial infection, dehiscence of a classic incision with uterine infection, or severe uterine infection unresponsive to antibiotics should also be treated by hysterectomy.

Nonemergency Indications

Weighing risk versus benefit of hysterectomy for nonemergency indications is much less certain than for emergency conditions. Hysterectomy performed at term is associated with hemorrhage, infection, thromboembolism, and injury to contiguous organs. Haynes and Martin have shown that the use of hysterectomy has declined, in spite of an increase in the incidence of cesarean section. This reflects the generally accepted conservative approach in which elective indications for hysterectomy are relatively few, primarily because the complication rate may exceed 50%.

When a less complicated operation is adequate or a safer time can be chosen, the patient's best interest is served by a conservative approach. Tubal ligation is a less dangerous operation at term than hysterectomy. When carcinoma *in situ* must be treated, removal of the entire cervix is much more certain and technically less complicated in the nonpregnant state. These decisions require good judgment based upon existing skills, facilities, and the needs of the individual patient.

PROCEDURE

The technique of hysterectomy is described in Chapter 61. Some points are especially pertinent to its performance immediately following cesarean or vaginal delivery, however.

In general, blood is conserved if the cesarean section uterine wound is rapidly closed prior to beginning the hysterectomy. The ovaries should be preserved, if normal, and the operator should be aware that the relative shortening of the uteroovarian ligament at term necessitates extra care in the placement of clamps and sutures in this area. Since the vascular system of the uterus is greatly distended, especially the venous system, considerable care should be taken in the proper placement of clamps and sutures so that a minimum of adjustments need be made.

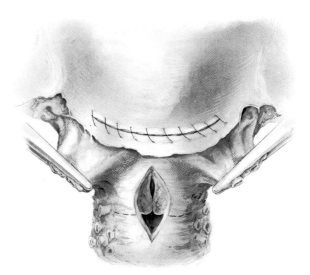

FIG. 39–8. Demonstration of uterine cervix.

The state of the uterus at term makes it difficult for the operator to determine by palpation the location of the portio of the cervix when performing a hysterectomy. Because of this difficulty, portions of the cervix are sometimes left behind even though the operator's intention is to remove it completely. Figure 39–8 illustrates a method of overcoming this difficulty. While the operator is deciding at what point the specimen is to be transected for removal, a vertical incision can be made in the lower uterine segment and extended caudad until the limits of the cervix can be identified. This incision is essentially bloodless when performed at the proper time. Drainage of the pelvic cavity may be necessary, depending on the adequacy of hemostasis.

In emergent situations that would be solved by supravaginal hysterectomy, this operation, which is much simpler and quicker, should be selected in preference to total hysterectomy unless there is a compelling reason to remove the cervix.

DÜHRSSEN'S INCISION OF THE CERVIX

Operations originally devised to avoid the hazards of cesarean section at a time when that procedure was attended by high mortality have gradually disappeared. Deliberate incision to open an undilating cervix for the purpose of delivery is almost never done in modern obstetric practice. However, the rare emergency may occur where knowledge of the procedure can solve a critical problem.

The incisions are usually made when the cervix is well effaced and more than 5 cm dilated. The area to be incised is grasped with two empty sponge forceps, and

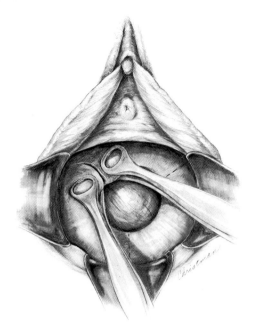

FIG. 39–9. Dührssen's incision at 10, 2, and 6 o'clock positions.

the incisions are made at the 10, 2, and 6 o'clock positions with a pair of sterile bandage scissors (Fig. 39–9).

Incising an incompletely dilated cervix to free the head during the delivery of a preterm fetus in breech presentation may be lifesaving. In this circumstance, visualization and use of ring forceps may not be possible, and the operator must carefully perform the procedure with tactile guidance only.

Following the procedure, careful examination should be undertaken to rule out extension of any of the incisions. Repair should be performed under direct vision, with absorbable suture material.

DESTRUCTIVE OPERATIONS

The need for destructive procedures upon a dead fetus that cannot be otherwise delivered *per vaginam* is so rare that most present day obstetricians are totally unfamiliar with such procedures. With proper medical care and proper hospital management of labor, the mechanical problem of delivering vaginally a dead fetus whose size or presentation has resulted in a long, obstructed labor is rarely encountered; the fetus who cannot be delivered vaginally is delivered by cesarean section. In developing countries, however, a significant segment of a hospital's clientele often consists of women who are admitted, many of them *in extremis,* with unresolved and very seriously obstructed labor. In such cases, a skillfully performed destructive operation may be far safer and simpler than cesarean section.

Every obstetrician should be familiar with the procedures for managing such cases; those who work in areas where they are apt to be encountered should study the papers of Lawson, Lister, and others, who describe such cases in detail and the best means of dealing with them. The following discussion is a brief summary of the solution of some of the clinical problems in which destructive procedures may be appropriate.

VERTEX PRESENTATION WITH CEPHALOPELVIC DISPROPORTION

When hydrocephalus is the basis for cephalopelvic disproportion, and the fetus presents by the vertex, needle aspiration of fetal cerebrospinal fluid can be readily performed before cervical dilatation is advanced. Transvaginal needle or trochar puncture of the fetal head through a partially dilated cervix decompresses the head enough to allow vaginal delivery.

When the fetal head is of normal size, cephalopelvic disproportion may result from an abnormally small pelvic inlet or an unusually large fetus. In either case, the vertex is firmly lodged in the inlet but not engaged. In the usual case, the patient has reached the second stage of labor, and the cervix is fully dilated and retracted. The physician should determine that the fetus is dead and should note any traumatic injury to the vagina from previous attempts at delivery, since a traumatic vesicovaginal fistula sometimes develops. The vagina should also be examined for uterine bleeding and the abdomen for signs of uterine rupture; evidence of uterine rupture mandates immediate laparotomy.

Techniques that involve crushing the fetal skull by means of the cranioclast and cephalotribe have been abandoned by Lister and Lawson, who have had extensive experience with the problem. Instead, a Simpson perforator is pushed through the skull. The operator's other hand should steady the point of the instrument to prevent maternal injury from the instrument's sliding off the skull when the thrust is made. After the skull is perforated, the instrument's blades are separated widely, turned 90°, and again opened widely. The instrument is advanced to the center of the skull, where the septa are destroyed by rotating and opening the instrument. When the skull contents have been evacuated, the edges of the hole are grasped with four Ochsner clamps and the head delivered by traction.

This technique is apparently quite successful and avoids the use of instruments that are awkward and unfamiliar to the average physician. In spite of this improvement, it is still necessary and important to explore the uterus carefully for evidence of rupture or laceration. Late complications such as fistula into bladder or rectum may still occur from necrosis.

BREECH PRESENTATION AND FETOPELVIC DISPROPORTION

When a hydrocephalic fetus presents by the breech, the cerebrospinal fluid can be drained by passing a needle into the fetal head through the maternal abdomen in a manner similar to that used for amniocentesis. As an alternative, the breech and shoulders can be delivered as in the usual breech delivery, and the hydrocephalic head fixed at the inlet by traction on the breech. If a suture is accessible, a needle can be inserted to drain the fluid. If not, a knife laminectomy is performed on the highest accessible vertebrae, and a uterine dressing forceps is pushed through the spinal canal into the head to allow drainage of the cerebrospinal fluid. As the head collapses, it passes into the pelvis and is easily delivered.

When the after-coming head of a normally formed dead fetus is impacted at the inlet, the head is fixed by traction on the trunk, the skull is perforated through any accessible area, the tentoria are destroyed, and the partially collapsed head usually delivers without incident. If it is needed, a blunt hook can be inserted through the opening in the head, with the point of the instrument directed toward the foramen magnum.

TRANSVERSE LIE

In the series of neglected cases involving transverse lie, described by Lister, decapitation by the use of the Blond Heidler saw was superior to the use of hooks or scissors. The Blond Heidler saw is similar to other wire saws, except that the outer two thirds is protected by rubber sheaths, leaving only the center third exposed for cutting. This minimizes the maternal risk during use.

COMPLICATIONS

The patient who faces a destructive procedure is likely to be in poor general condition and subject to both immediate and delayed risks. Dehydration, acidosis, infection, and exhaustion are commonly present. Administration of intravenous fluids, electrolytes, and antibiotics should be immediately considered. Antibiotic coverage should be broad and of maximum dose. Blood should be cross-matched and made available for immediate use.

The most serious immediate complication of both the obstetric process and the destructive operation is uterine rupture. In every patient who has delivered vaginally, a thorough manual exploration of the uterine cavity should be done to rule out uterine rupture. If bleeding occurs postpartum, the patient should be reexamined, as rupture can be missed with a single examination. Since such women are usually in poor con-

dition, if a rupture is found, it should be dealt with by the simplest and most expeditious means. Hysterectomy is reserved for the cases in which suture of the defect is not feasible or will not control bleeding.

Vesicovaginal or rectovaginal fistulas may be produced by immediate intrapartum injury or may develop later from avascular necrosis. The crushing of the pelvic organs between the presenting fetal part and the bony pelvis produces an injury that may result in a later slough. Constant drainage of the urinary bladder for 10 days after delivery is recommended to minimize the stress of bladder distention and to allow healing. If a fistula forms, 3 months should be allowed before repair is attempted. Some control of urinary leakage can be obtained in the interim by the use of the Tassette cup with drainage bag attached to the leg.

REFERENCES AND RECOMMENDED READING

CESAREAN SECTION

Arthur RK: Postmortem cesarean section. Am J Obstet Gynecol 132:175, 1978

Benson RC et al: Fetal compromise during elective cesarean section. Am J Obstet Gynecol 105:579, 1969

Bottoms SF, Rosen M, Sokol RJ: The increase in the cesarean birth rate. N Engl J Med 302:559, 1980

Browne ADH, Hynes T: Multiple repeat cesarean section. J Obstet Gynaecol Br Commonw 72:693, 1965

Case BD: Cesarean section and its place in modern obstetric practice. J Obstet Gynaecol Br Commonw 78:203, 1971

Clemetson GA et al: Tilt-bend cesarean section. Obstet Gynecol 42:290, 1973

Crawford JS et al: Time and lateral tilt at cesarean section. Br J Anaesth 44:477, 1972

DeLee JB: An illustrated history of low or cervical cesarean section. Am J Obstet Gynecol 10:503, 1925

DePalma RT, Leveno KJ, Cunningham FG, et al: Identification and management of women at high risk for pelvic infection following cesarean section. Obstet Gynecol 55:185s, 1980

Evrard JR, Gold EM: Cesarean section and maternal mortality in Rhode Island—Incidence and risk factors 1965–1975. Obstet Gynecol 50:594, 1977

Farrell SJ, Andersen HF, Work BA Jr: Cesarean section: Indications and postoperative morbidity. Obstet Gynecol 56:696, 1980

Fothergill RJ et al: Neonatal acidemia related to procrastination at cesarean section. J Obstet Gynaecol Br Commonw 78:1010, 1971

Fox GS, Houle GL: Acid–base studies in elective cesarean sections during epidural and general anesthesia. Can Anaesth Soc J 18:60, 1971

Fox GS et al: Anesthesia for cesarean section: Further studies. Am J Obstet Gynecol 133:15, 1979

Gall SA: The efficacy of prophylactic antibiotics in cesarean section. Am J Obstet Gynecol 134:506, 1979

Goodlin RC: Aortocaval compression during cesarean section. Obstet Gynecol 37:702, 1971

Haesslein HC, Goodlin RC: Extraperitoneal cesarean section revisited. Obstet Gynecol 55:181, 1980

Haynes DM, Martin BJ, Jr: Cesarean hysterectomy: A twenty-five year review. Am J Obstet Gynecol 134:393, 1979

Hellegers AE, Eastman NJ: The problem of prematurity in gravidas with cesarean section scars. Am J Obstet Gynecol 82:679, 1961

Kalappa R et al: Maternal acid–base status during cesarean section under thiopental, N$_2$O, and succinylcholine anesthesia. Am J Obstet Gynecol 109:411, 1971

Lane FR, Reid DE: Dehiscence of previous uterine incision at repeat cesarean section. Obstet Gynecol 2:54, 1953

Loosen PT, Prange AJ Jr: Extraperitoneal cesarean sections in the People's Republic of China. Letter to the editor, N Engl J Med 303:226, 1980

Marshall CM: Cesarean section: Lower segment operation. Baltimore, Williams & Wilkins, 1939

Merrill BS, Gibbs CE: Planned vaginal delivery following cesarean section. Obstet Gynecol 52:50, 1978

Pedowitz P, Schwartz RM: The true incidence of silent ruptures of cesarean section. Am J Obstet Gynecol 74:1071, 1957

Petitti D, Olson RO, Williams RL: Cesarean section in California—1960 through 1975. Am J Obstet Gynecol 133:391, 1979

Phelan JP, Pruyn SC: Prophylactic antibiotics in cesarean section: A double-blind study of cephazolin. Am J Obstet Gynecol 133:474, 1979

Piver MS, Johnston RA: The safety of multiple cesarean sections. Obstet Gynecol 34:690, 1969

Redick LF: An inflatable wedge for prevention of aortocaval compression during pregnancy. Am J Obstet Gynecol 133:458, 1979

Saldana LR, Schulman H, Reuss L: Management of pregnancy after cesarean section. Am J Obstet Gynecol 135:555, 1979

Shamsi HH et al: Changing obstetric practices and amelioration of perinatal outcome in a university hospital. Am J Obstet Gynecol 133:855, 1979

Stevenson CS et al: Maternal death from puerperal sepsis following cesarean section. Obstet Gynecol 29:181, 1967

Weber CE: Postmortem cesarean section: Review of the literature and case reports. Am J Obstet Gynecol 110:158, 1971

INDUCTION OF LABOR

American College of Obstetricians and Gynecologists: Induction of labor. ACOG Tech Bull No. 49, May, 1978

Bishop EH: Pelvic scoring for elective induction. Obstet Gynecol 24:266, 1964

Cates W, Jr, Hordaan HVF: Sudden collapse and death of women obtaining abortions induced with prostaglandin F$_{2\alpha}$. Am J Obstet Gynecol 133:398, 1979

Clinch J: Induction of labor: A six-year review. Br J Obstet Gynaecol 86:340, 1979

Department of Health, Education, and Welfare: Food and Drug Administration Bulletin: New restrictions on oxytocin use. Vol 8 No. 5, Oct–Nov, 1978

Flaksman RJ, Vollman JH, Benfield GD: Iatrogenic prematurity due to elective termination of the uncomplicated pregnancy: A major perinatal health problem. Am J Obstet Gynecol 132:885, 1978

Friedman EA, Sachtleben MR, Wallace AK: Infant outcome following labor induction. Am J Obstet Gynecol 133:718, 1979

Hertz RH, Sokol RJ, Knoke JD: Clinical estimation of gesta-

tional age: Rules for avoiding preterm delivery. Am J Obstet Gynecol 131:395, 1978

Johnson A, Hyatt D, Newton J: Experience with prostaglandin F$_{2a}$ (free acid) for the induction of labor. Prostaglandins 7:487, 1974

Karim SMM, Amy JJ: Prostaglandins and human reproduction. In MacDonald RR (ed): Scientific Basis of Obstetrics and Gynaecology. Edinburgh, Churchill Livingstone, 1978

Niswander KR, Turoff BB, Romans J: Developmental status of children delivered through elective induction of labor. Obstet Gynecol 27:15, 1966

O'Herlihy C, MacDonald HN: Influence of prostaglandin E$_2$ vaginal gel on cervical ripening and labor. Obstet Gynecol 54:708, 1979

Patterson SP, White JH, Reaves EM: A maternal death associated with prostaglandin E$_2$. Obstet Gynecol 54:123, 1979

Tylleskar J, Finnstrom O. Leijon I, et al: Spontaneous labor and elective induction—a prospective randomized study. I. Effects on mother and a fetus. Acta Obstet Gynecol Scand 58:513, 1979

Wingerup L, Andersson K-E, Ulmsten U: Ripening of the uterine cervix and induction of labour at term with prostaglandin E$_2$ in viscous gel. Acta Obstet Gynecol Scand 57:403, 1978

DESTRUCTIVE OPERATIONS

Borno RP, Bon Tempo NC, Kirkendall HL, Jr, et al: Vaginal frank breech delivery of a hydrocephalic fetus after transabdominal encephalocentesis. Am J Obstet Gynecol 132:336, 1978

Danforth DN: A method of delivery for hydrocephalus associated with breech presentation. Am J Obstet Gynecol 53:541, 1947

Lawson JB: Obstructed Labor. J Obstet Gynaecol Br Commonw 72:877, 1965

Lister UG: Obstructed labor: A series of 320 cases occurring in 4 years in a hospital in southern Nigeria. J Obstet Gynaecol Br Commonw 67:188, 1960

GENERAL AND MISCELLANEOUS

Baggish MS, Hooper S: Aspiration as a cause of maternal death. Obstet Gynecol 43:327, 1974

Banta HD, Thacker SB: Costs and benefits of electronic fetal monitoring. Washington, DC, National Center for Health Sciences Research, 1978

Bonica JJ: Principles and Practice of Obstetrical Analgesia and Anesthesia, Vol I, Fundamental Considerations. Philadelphia, Davis, 1967

Bonica JJ: Principles and Practice of Obstetrical Analgesia and Anesthesia, Vol II, Clinical Considerations. Philadelphia, Davis, 1969

Evard JR, Gold EM: Cesarean section for delivery of the second twin. Obstet Gynecol 57:581, 1981

Hill DJ, Beischer NA: Hysterectomy in obstetric practice. Aust NZ Obstet Gynaecol 20:151, 1980

Hobbins JC et al: The fetal monitoring debate. Obstet Gynecol 54:103, 1979

Krebs HB et al: Intrapartum fetal heart rate monitoring: I and II. Am J Obstet Gynecol 133:762; 773, 1979

CHAPTER 40

THE PUERPERIUM

William E. Easterling, Jr.
William N. P. Herbert

The puerperium is that variable period, usually 6–8 weeks, beginning with the delivery of the placenta and ending with the resumption of ovulatory menstrual cycles. The puerperium is less pecisely defined in the nursing mother; but, in general, it consists of at least 4–6 weeks of involutional changes that result in the so-called nonpregnant parous state.

Traditionally, both mother and infant have been discharged from the hospital on the 3rd postpartum day; but, with escalating hospital costs and the desire of many women to return home as soon as possible, they are frequently discharged sooner. Normal activities also are resumed earlier than in the past. Ambulation usually begins the day of delivery. Gradually increasing exercise is encouraged, with limitations best judged by the woman herself. Abstinence from intercourse is dictated by perineal tenderness, which generally ceases within 3–4 weeks. Women planning to begin or resume careers commonly do so 6–8 weeks after delivery.

The complete postpartum examination is routinely scheduled 6 weeks following delivery, since many of the puerperal changes have been completed or nearly completed by then. Communication prior to that time may be necessary and should be encouraged. The postpartum visit serves several purposes. It provides an opportunity to discuss contraception, lactation, menses, exercise, and other pertinent topics. A thorough physical examination ensures that the physiologic changes are occuring normally and detects any abnormalities.

PHYSIOLOGY OF THE PUERPERIUM AND CLINICAL MANAGEMENT

UTERUS

Involution and Contractions

Following delivery of the placenta and membranes, the uterus comes to lie at a level below the umbilicus, the fundus resting on the sacral promontory. It is approximately 14 cm long, 12 cm wide, and 10 cm thick (about its size at 15–16 weeks' gestation), and weighs about 1000 g. Although the uterus may take a somewhat discoid form as it relaxes, it resumes a globular shape as it intermittently contracts. In the ensuing days, the uterus undergoes a remarkable decrease in size (involution) so that it weighs only about 500 g at the end of the 1st week, when it once again lies entirely within the true pelvis. As the increase in myometrium during pregnancy results largely from an increase in the size rather than the number of myometrial cells, involution is associated with a substantial decrease in the amount of cytoplasm and size of the individual cells. Uterine contractions, as measured by intrauterine pressure, increase dramatically in intensity immediately after delivery, presumably owing to the greatly decreased intrauterine volume around which the myometrium is contracting. Hendricks *et al.* reported that high levels of uterine activity diminish smoothly and progressively, becoming stable after the first 1–2 hours postpartum. Thereafter, contractions become increasingly incoordinate with the passage of time, but coordination can be restored by administration of oxytocin or by the application of an apparent oxytocin-releasing stimulus (*e.g.,* suckling). This increased myometrial activity contributes to uterine hemotasis by compressing the intramural vessels, which allows thrombosis to occur. The intense uterine contractions persist throughout the early puerperium, causing the so-called *afterpains*. Analgesia may be required, particularly for the more severe pain sometimes experienced by the multipara. For unknown reasons, afterpains are not usually experienced after the birth of the first child.

Placental Site

Immediately postpartum, the placental site is an elevated, irregular area consisting of mostly thrombosed vascular sinusoids. According to Williams' classic description, the area undergoes an exfoliation because the placental site is undermined by an ingrowth of endometrial tissue. The shedding of this mass of organized thrombi and obliterated arteries prevents scar formation and preserves an intact, normal expanse of endometrial tissue. The superficial layer of decidua surrounding the placental site becomes necrotic during the first few days, and the postpartum vaginal discharge consists of this sloughed tissue with an admixture of serum and leukocytes. The cells of the endometrial glands in the remaining decidua rapidly grow across the denuded surface, completing regeneration by the end of the 3rd week.

Cervix

The cervix up to the lower segment persists as an edematous yet thin, fragile tissue for several days. Immediately following delivery, the ectocervix appears ragged, with numerous small but clinically insignificant bleeding points. The tissue appears devitalized and is indeed an optimum site for the development of infection. The lateral margins are often lacerated, and changes in these areas eventually may lead to the typical fish mouth appearance of the parous cervix. The cervical os, which admits two fingers for the first 4–6 days of the puerperium, thereafter constricts until it will admit only the smallest curet by the end of the 2nd week. The striking changes that occur in the cervix during the days and weeks after delivery are among the most dramatic of all connective tissue remodeling processes, equivalent in degree to the cervical changes of labor that permit effacement and dilatation to occur without significant injury. As described in Chapter 29, there is much new interest in these processes, which remain unexplained.

Lochia

The uterine discharge following delivery is termed lochia. It is at first bright red, changing in a few days to reddish brown, the *lochia rubra;* this consists mainly of blood, and decidual and trophoblastic debris. After 6–8 days, the lochia becomes more serous, the *lochia serosa*, and consists of old blood, serum, leukocytes, and tissue debris. This is followed in several days by the *lochia alba,* a whitish yellow discharge containing serum, leukocytes, decidua, epithelial cells, mucus, and bacteria, which may continue until about 2 weeks after delivery. Lochia rubra that is unabated after 2 weeks suggests retained secundines or formation of a so-called *placental polyp,* an organized fragment of retained placental tissue. This bleeding sometimes responds to ergonovine (0.2 mg orally every 4 hours while awake for 2 days), but curettage is often needed. Clots and frank red vaginal bleeding are not lochia and must be considered in the category of postpartum hemorrhage.

VAGINA AND INTROITUS

After delivery, the vagina is a spacious, smooth-walled cavity; it decreases to its nonpregnant size by the end of the 6th–8th week. Rugae typically appear by the end of the 4th week, but they are never again as prominent as in the nulliparous woman. The vaginal introitus initially appears erythematous and edematous, particularly in the area of the episiotomy or laceration repairs. Careful episiotomy repair should ultimately result in an introitus barely distinguishable from that of the nulliparous woman. Care of the perineum consists mostly of good hygiene during the initial 2 weeks; soap-and-water cleansing, particularly after bowel movements, should be sufficient. Hot baths help to diminish perineal tenderness and promote healing of the episiotomy.

The uterus and lower genital tract require special observation, particularly during the initial hours of the puerperium. Hemorrhage from retained placenta or from uterine atony (suggested by a fundus that refuses to contract in response to gentle massage) and perineal or paravaginal hematomas may develop insidiously.

URINARY TRACT

Trauma to the urethra and bladder associated with the passage of the infant through the pelvis leads to predictable changes. The bladder wall is edematous and hyperemic, and there may be small areas of hemorrhage in the muscularis that are not of clinical significance. Secondary to the trauma and enhanced by analgesia, particularly by conduction anesthesia, the bladder may be relatively insensitive to intravesical pressures that ordinarily initiate the urge to urinate. As a result, urinary retention may develop. Frequent palpation of the bladder in the suprapubic region and insistence that the patient void within the first 4–5 hours after delivery should prevent overdistention. If the patient is unable to void, the bladder should be catheterized; if the problem persists or if more than 600 ml urine are removed by catheter, an indwelling catheter may be required for the first 24 hours. Following removal of the indwelling catheter, careful checks for residual urine should be made until the volume is less than 100 ml on two occasions.

The glomerular filtration rate remains elevated during the 1st week after delivery; the urinary output greatly exceeds the fluid intake, often reaching 3

liters/24 hours. This, along with insensible perspiration, accounts largely for the weight loss of about 12 lb during this period. Proteinuria and, less frequently, glycosuria may appear during the 1st week; but, if they are of the physiologic kind, they disappear within a few days. The pregnancy dilatation of the ureters and renal pelves subsides to normal within 6 weeks.

ABDOMINAL WALL

The abdominal wall is quite lax during the first 1–2 weeks after delivery, a fact that may be of great clinical importance in the interpretation of acute surgical disorders that sometimes occur at this time. For example, the abdominal rigidity and guarding, so important in the diagnosis of such diseases as acute appendicitis, do not occur during the early puerperium, and the diagnosis must be made without the assistance of this customary sign. In the average woman, the abdominal wall returns to a nearly nonparous state in about 6–7 weeks. During this time, the skin regains its elasticity, although some striae may persist. With proper exercise, the muscles regain significant tonus. Infrequently, with or without an unusually distended uterus, such as in multiple pregnancy, the rectus abdominis muscles remain separated from the median line, a condition termed *diastasis recti abdominis*. Although this defect may be disturbing, surgical correction is seldom necessary, and the separation becomes less evident with the passage of time.

GASTROINTESTINAL TRACT

The typical decreased motility of the gastrointestinal tract in the puerperium persists for only a short time, although a return to normal motility may be delayed by excess analgesia or anesthesia. Women with otherwise normal gastrointestinal function may benefit from laxative assistance once or twice during the first few days. Should a third- or fourth-degree laceration of the perineum occur, feces softeners or mild laxatives are indicated.

CIRCULATION

Ueland and Hansen have shown that the *cardiac output,* which continues to increase in the first and second stages of labor, peaks during the early puerperium. Although the mean values are somewhat lower, the same changes occur in patients delivered under conduction anesthesia. This particular study demonstrated peak increases of 60%–80% above prelabor levels, a value somewhat higher than that reported by others. After the first few minutes postpartum, cardiac output decreases to values about 40%–50% above prelabor levels, returning to nonpregnant levels in the ensuing 2–3 weeks. These changes are primarily due to appreciable alterations in stroke volume. There is little alteration in blood pressure, and bradycardia occurs fairly consistently regardless of the type of anesthesia employed for delivery. The decrease in heart rate probably accounts in part for the decline in cardiac output. Evacuation of the uterus, with the associated descent of the diaphragm, restores the normal cardiac axis and leads to the normalization of other electrocardiographic features during the early puerperium.

Varicosities of the lower extremities and hemorrhoidal plexus, not uncommon during pregnancy, regress promptly after delivery. Varices of the vulva, which are less common, can be seen to empty immediately after delivery. At times, local treatment of hemorrhoids with heat and analgesic creams is necessary, but a decision on surgical correction of all varicosities should be delayed several months, since regression is usually complete or nearly so by that time.

Puerperal alterations in *blood volume* depend on several variable factors, including blood loss at delivery, and mobilization and subsequent excretion of extravascular water. Blood loss leads to an immediate but limited decrease in total blood volume. Thereafter, the normal shifts in body water result in a slow decline that ultimately reaches about 10% at the end of the first 3 days. Subsequently, there is a more gradual decline to nonpregnant levels. During the first 72 hours, there is a disproportionately greater decrease in plasma volume than in cellular components, resulting in a slight net increase in hematocrit over the immediate postpartum value.

Puerperal changes in the *blood constituents* may be clinically confusing unless the physician is aware of them. The leukocytosis of pregnancy is usually on the order of 12,000/cu mm; during the first 10 days or 2 weeks of the puerperium, counts of 20,000 or 25,000/cu mm are not unusual, owing largely to an increase in neutrophils with consequent shift to the left. This, plus a normal increase in the erythrocyte sedimentation rate to 50 or even 60 mm/hour, may confuse the interpretation of acute infections during this time. The red blood count and hematocrit are usually elevated, probably because of the increased red cell mass of pregnancy, which is constricted as the blood volume declines with fluid loss. The coagulation factors I, II, VIII, IX, and X decline within a few days to prepregnant levels. Fibrin split products are elevated during the 1st week or 10 days, probably as the result of their release from the placental site. The total proteins, normally low in pregnancy, return to normal levels during the puerperium, and serum electrolyte concentrations follow a similar course. The plasma lipids, elevated in pregnancy, also decline to normal levels.

WEIGHT CHANGE

Approximately half of the average 25-lb weight gain of pregnancy is lost at delivery. During the initial days of the puerperium, largely as a result of diuresis, an additional 6–8-lb weight loss can be expected. Most women lose the remaining weight gained at pregnancy over the ensuing weeks, returning to the prepregnant weight within several months. Parity alone has very little effect on weight.

GENERAL

Shaking chills are not unusual in the first hours after delivery and are usually of no concern. Their exact cause is not known, but they are usually attributed to heat loss resulting from delivery of the baby and placenta, and loss of amniotic fluid. A warm blanket can minimize the discomfort.

Fatigue is customary during the first few days after delivery; extra rest and longer periods of sleep are invariably needed. This is easy to arrange in a hospital setting, but special plans should be made if early discharge is contemplated.

Ambulation is encouraged soon after delivery if neither conduction nor general anesthesia was used, or promptly after the effects of anesthesia have subsided. Early ambulation is largely responsible for reducing the incidence of thrombophlebitis (the "milk leg" or "phlegmasia alba dolens" of another era) to almost zero, and it also improves bladder and bowel function.

Diet requirements for nursing mothers are slightly higher than those for nonpregnant women. There should be special emphasis on protein (an additional 20 g/day) and calories (an additional 500 cal/day). For those not nursing, the recommendations are the same as those for the nonpregnant woman, as outlined in Chapter 11.

ENDOCRINOLOGY OF THE PUERPERIUM

LACTATION

During pregnancy, the breasts are exposed to high concentrations of estrogen and progesterone. The prolactin level also increases markedly, secondary to estrogen stimulation of lactotroph hyperplasia, reaching the highest point just prior to delivery. Increased levels of insulin and human placental lactogen (hPL) stimulate further breast growth during gestation. It is generally held that while all the hormonal elements (estrogen, progesterone, thyroid, insulin, and free cortisol) necessary for breast growth and milk production are present in elevated concentrations during pregnancy, the high levels of estrogen inhibit active alveolar secretion by blocking the binding of prolactin to breast tissue, thus inhibiting the milk producing effect of prolactin on the target epithelium.

Following delivery, estrogen, progesterone, hPL, and insulin blood levels decrease rapidly, followed by diminishing concentrations of prolactin. Milk production and associated breast engorgement begin about 3 days after delivery with the fall in estrogen, and they are enhanced by suckling, with the attendant brisk increase in prolactin secretion.

Once lactation has been established, suckling is the single most important stimulus for the maintenance of milk production. The conventional concept is that tactile nerve endings in the areola transmit a stimulus to the nuclei of the hypothalamus, resulting in an increase in synthesis and transport of oxytocin to the posterior pituitary and then its release into the circulation; oxytocin then stimulates contraction of the myoepithelial cells surrounding the alveoli, causing milk to be moved into the larger reservoirs beneath the nipple. This may be accompanied by ejection of milk from the breast and is commonly called the *let-down reflex*. Although the concept is well established, the recent studies of Lucas and coworkers have cast some doubt on the belief that oxytocin release is necessarily essential for satisfactory milk flow during breast feeding. It does seem clear that prolactin is important in the maintenance of lactation, afferent stimuli from the nipple reaching the hypothalamus and initiating a complex response that results in prolactin release. This response is probably mediated through the prolactin inhibiting factor (dopamine), but prolactin-releasing factors may also be concerned. These relationships are considered in more detail in the section on inappropriate lactation in Chapter 46. The net result is a temporary increase in prolactin secretion that stimulates the milk-producing epithelium of the alveoli. The amounts of prolactin released gradually decrease during the first weeks of nursing. The factors that maintain milk production after the 3rd–4th month, when the prolactin level reaches its normal nonpregnant level and there are no episodic increases in response to suckling, are poorly understood at this time.

Suppression of Lactation

A mother wishing to stop breast-feeding need only discontinue suckling. Because the release of oxytocin is interrupted, milk accumulates in the alveoli and major ducts, leading to a cessation of milk formation that is probably secondary to the increase in intraalveolar and intraductal pressure. The time-honored practice of breast-binding to terminate lactation probably acts by the same mechanism.

When a mother does not wish to nurse, simple breast-binding or a number of different short-acting and long-acting steroid preparations may be used to suppress lactation. These preparations include estro-

gen, which is thought to inhibit the prolactin effect on the target breast tissue. One effective agent for preventing lactation is Deladumone (a combination of estradiol valerate and testosterone enanthate) administered intramuscularly in single dose of 4 ml at the time of delivery. Bromocriptine has been used extensively in Europe for the inhibition of both normal and inappropriate lactation by direct suppression of prolactin secretion, and is now approved in the United States for this purpose.

Desirability of Breast-feeding

In recent years, the practice of breast-feeding has increased in the United States. Many comparisons have been made between breast-feeding and bottle-feeding with either cow's milk or commercial infant formula. From a nutritional standpoint, a simple comparison of the specific components within the milk or milk product is not informative, since it fails to point out differences in absorption rates and suitability of the various components for the infant. Breast milk has less protein than cow's milk, but the amino acid composition is more tailored to the metabolism of neonates. Although breast milk and cow's milk have about the same content of iron, the percentage of absorption is greater with breast milk, probably because of different protein-binding properties. The immunologic advantage afforded by breast milk is not found, of course, in other milk products. Immunoglobulins (especially secretory IgA, but also IgG and IgM), lactoferrin, lysozyme, the bifidus factor, and cellular elements protect the neonate against a variety of infections. Breast-feeding may also be more hygienic.

Another significant consideration of breast-feeding is the psychologic aspect. Although close interaction is certainly possible without nursing, the intimacy of nursing can strengthen the bond between mother and infant. On the other hand, social pressure to breast-feed may cause the mother undue anxiety and guilt, making the experience unpleasant to the point of interfering with the normal process of lactation.

Other aspects of comparison between breast milk and other milk products involve economic and contraceptive considerations. Breast-feeding is significantly less expensive than bottle-feeding, and lactation interferes in varying degrees with ovulation, affording some protection against pregnancy. This contraceptive impact is more significant in regard to populations than to individual cases, however; mothers who choose to breast-feed should not rely upon lactation to provide complete contraception.

In many ways, breast milk seems superior to other milk products. Therefore, breast-feeding should be encouraged. However, the woman who elects not to breast-feed or who, for some reason, is unable to nurse her child successfully should not be made to feel guilty or anxious.

As a general rule, it should be assumed that any drug ingested by a nursing mother may be present in her breast milk, but the concentrations are usually low compared with blood levels in the mother. Factors concerned in the transfer of drugs from blood to breast milk include plasma concentration, molecular size, degree of acidity, protein binding, and lipid solubility of the specific agent. Metabolism of a drug by the neonate depends also on the neonate's age and development at the time the drug is administered. Current literature should be reviewed regarding any given drug; however, medications thought contraindicated for the nursing mother include chloramphenicol, streptomycin, metronidazole, sulfa, antithyroid and some anticancer agents, some diuretics, and, of course, radioactive agents. Although there is no definitive information on the use of hormone preparations (*e.g.*, oral contraceptives) by nursing mothers, these agents are currently suspect because of the possibility of long-term or delayed effects on the infant. A more complete list of drug effects during lactation is shown in Table 27–5.

It was formerly thought that the incidence of breast cancer was lower among women who had nursed their babies, but it now seems clear that this is not the case.

HYPOTHALAMIC–PITUITARY–OVARIAN FUNCTION

The physiology of the hypothalamus, the pituitary, and the ovaries during the puerperium is not well understood. Much information is available concerning the length of postpartum amenorrhea in both nonlactating and lactating women. The observations, summarized by Vorherr, indicate that 40% of nonnursing mothers resume menstruation within 6 weeks after delivery, 65% within 12 weeks, and 90% within 24 weeks. About 50% of the first cycles are ovulatory. In nursing mothers, menstruation returns within 6 weeks in only 15% and within 12 weeks in only 45% In about 80% of these women, the first ovulatory cycle is preceded by one or more anovulatory cycles.

It has long been held that increased prolactin levels inhibit release of gonadotropins, thereby reducing ovarian steroid production and accounting for the physiologic puerperal amenorrhea. This inhibitory effect may be more pronounced on the release of luteinizing hormone (LH) than on that of follicle-stimulating hormone (FSH). Jaffe and others have shown that FSH and LH levels are very low in the early weeks postpartum and that the level of FSH increases gradually, followed by an increase in the LH level. Investigating this phenomenon and using synthetic luteinizing hormone-releasing hormone (LHRH), LeMaire *et al.* have demonstrated a temporary pituitary insensitivity to LHRH both in lactating and nonlactating women studied within the first 3 weeks postpartum. However, the nursing and nonnursing mothers responded in a

similar manner to LHRH at 6 weeks after delivery. Keye and Jaffe have reported that administration of gonadotropin-releasing hormone to nonnursing puerperas resulted in a return of FSH response to early follicular phase levels by the 3rd week and a return of LH response by the 4th week postpartum. It is of interest that this response was followed by a period of FSH and LH hyperresponsiveness throughout the remainder of the 8-week study period. This excess reaction to the releasing hormone remains unexplained.

Studying the pituitary–ovarian axis, Zarrate *et al.* observed that exogenous gonadotropins (human menopausal gonadotropins) administered in the immediate puerperium had no effect on estrogen, pregnanediol, and pregnanetriol excretion in lactating women. More recently, Andreassen and Tyson reported a significant ovarian output of estradiol in response to LHRH in both nursing and nonnursing women after the 28th day postpartum; no response was noted in either group between days 4 and 21, suggesting a temporary refractive state in the ovaries. Thus, the genital hypoplasia and infertility characteristic of the lactating mother may be due to pituitary, ovarian, and perhaps hypothalamic suppression, but the exact nature of this changing endocrine milieu is unclear at this time.

ABNORMALITIES OF THE PUERPERIUM

As the new mother enters the puerperium and faces the previously unencountered threats to her health, all those responsible for her welfare must exercise careful observation and provide expert care. Although many abnormalities may occur during the puerperium, only a few are serious or life-threatening. For many years, postpartum hemorrhage was the leading cause of maternal mortality; but, with the increased availability of blood in the past two decades, infection has come to the forefront as the leading cause of death. Eclampsia remains third. It should be remembered, however, that illness unrelated to pregnancy may affect a woman in the puerperium.

INFECTION

Puerperal infection is defined as infection of the genital tract, sometimes secondarily extending to other organ systems. To assist clinicians and to establish conformity in reported studies, the Joint Committee on Maternal Welfare defined *febrile morbidity* as "a temperature of 100.4° F (38° C) or higher, the temperature to occur on any 2 of the first 10 days postpartum exclusive of the first 24 hours and to be taken by mouth by a standard technique at least four times daily." Extragenital infections such as cystitis, pyelonephritis, or pneumonitis must be excluded. The defi-

nition was designed to exclude, as nearly as possible, noninfectious causes of fever. When the definition was prepared, the first 24 hours were excluded because the febrile response to most infections introduced during labor occurs after the 1st day, whereas fever on the 1st day suggests an infection that was present before labor. However, this is not always the case; in a recent series, most patients with temperature elevations in the first 24 hours postpartum were found to have genital tract infections. The onset of fever after the 10th postpartum day usually signifies infection of a nonobstetric nature.

Because of the ready availability of antibiotics, puerperal and related infections have come to be treated with less respect by some health care personnel. This may be an ominous development; laxity in aseptic technique is often found to be the explanation for episodic increases in the incidence of maternal infections. This fact, along with the growing number of organisms that are resistant to antibiotics, warns against relaxing any of the well-established standards of asepsis. Particular attention must be given to asepsis in the presence of conditions that predispose to infection, such as premature and prolonged rupture of the membranes, soft tissue trauma and the residual devitalized tissue, prolonged labor, and hemorrhage. The poorly nourished and anemic patient is also much more vulnerable to infection.

The physician's task in the selection of antimicrobial agents increases almost daily because of the ever-increasing number of organisms that are drug-resistant and because of the proliferation of new drugs. The scene changes quickly, but the obstetrician–gynecologist is obligated to maintain an up-to-date working knowledge of the agents themselves, their field of usefulness, their similarities and antagonisms, and their toxic effects. Current monographs can be helpful, and the package inserts are a reliable source of prescribing information. (See also Chapter 13.) The final selection of an antimicrobial agent is based on clinical consideration and identification of the organism and its sensitivities. Until this identification is available, a Gram stain of the infected material may provide an important clue to the responsible organism and may greatly narrow the choice of antimicrobial agents.

Microorganisms

Anaerobic streptococci are the most common cause of puerperal infections, but identification of the organism or organisms specifically responsible for a given infection is difficult, since the vagina normally harbors many types of bacteria. Cultures may be helpful when correlated with Gram stain and clinical judgment. In addition to anaerobic streptococci, *Bacteroides* and *Clostridium perfringens* (*welchii*) are common inhabitants of the normal genital and intestinal tracts, but they rarely cause trouble in the normal woman. How-

ever, extremely serious infections can result when these organisms have access to devitalized necrotic tissue and blood clots. Clostridial infection can produce gas gangrene, hemolysis, septic shock, and, in some cases, death. *Bacteroides* cause a less dramatic infection, usually in conjunction with other anaerobes. When they flourish in fresh wounds, marked local necrosis follows quickly, and large abscesses can develop in 1–2 days. If the bloodstream is invaded, pelvic thrombophlebitis and distant metastatic abscesses can result in prolonged and debilitating illness. Under conditions appropriate for anaerobic growth, such as when placental fragments have been retained or tissue has been traumatized and devitalized, endometritis is the initial infection, producing fever and foul-smelling lochia. If the infection is not controlled, the result may be widespread thrombophlebitis of the iliac veins, vena cava, and left renal vein. Septicemia may be followed by the implantation of bacteria on damaged heart valves or by abscess formation in the liver or lungs.

Puerperal staphylococcal infections are especially difficult to control. These potentially pathogenic organisms are found everywhere, both in the community and in the hospital, and lapses in aseptic technique invite infection by these organisms. In addition to their ubiquity, many staphylococcal strains are resistant to antimicrobials so that, once established, infection can be difficult to eradicate.

The noninvasive types of staphylococcal infection may lead to the formation of abscesses, which are best treated by local application of heat, incision, and drainage. If a systemic reaction (fever, chills, and malaise) develops, antibiotics should be administered according to the sensitivity of the isolated strain. The organism must be assumed to be penicillin-resistant until results of sensitivity studies are available. The β-hemolytic streptococcus, once the leading cause of puerperal infection, is now an unusual cause of infection, but it cannot be entirely ignored. Untreated, such an infection (with either Group A or Group B organisms) can be devastating if it invades the parametrium and peritoneal cavity. The virulence of the organism demands prompt treatment when it is identified as the pathogen.

The past several years have seen a rising incidence of gram-negative enteric bacterial infections. *Escherichia coli* is the most common offender, followed by *Klebsiella, Enterobacter,* and *Proteus* species. Infections by enterococci and *Pseudomonas aeruginosa* have increased in frequency. In some hospitals, these organisms are the leading causes of puerperal infection. The more virulent strains produce sepsis, which, if uncontrolled, may result in septicemia and endotoxic shock. An extremely disturbing characteristic of these bacteria, especially the strains found in hospitals, is their demonstrated ability to develop antibiotic resistance.

Clinical Manifestations

Postpartum infections of the genital tract are usually insidious in onset; in the early stage, they present the clinician with the uncomfortable and challenging problem of diagnosis by exclusion. Endometritis, the most common form of puerperal infection, may occur without any localizing signs or symptoms. The earliest indication of puerperal sepsis usually occurs 2–5 days postpartum; but, if the membranes were ruptured for some time before delivery, the infectious process may have begun earlier and become manifest sooner. The early indications of infection are malaise, anorexia, and fever. Differential diagnosis must always include urinary tract infections, particularly after operative delivery or catheterization. Operative delivery under general anesthesia must always engender a high degree of suspicion for respiratory complications. The obstetrician must also be on guard for the early symptoms of mastitis, manifest by tender, indurated, and erythematous areas in the breast. Thrombophlebitis with its attendant deep vein tenderness, and lower genital tract infection with its associated perineal and perirectal pain, complete the list of common puerperal infections. It should be emphasized that a febrile course during the puerperium may be a manifestation of any one of a multitude of systemic disorders that may exacerbate during this time of stress.

Types of Infections

Metritis. *Endometritis* is more properly termed deciduitis, since the superficial layer of the endometrium is involved; this area is the most common site of puerperal infection. In the simplest form, inflammatory changes occur in the superficial layers, with leukocytic infiltration limited to this area, and producing the "fruity" odor that is typical of normal lochia. In more severe forms, the infectious process may spread to the adjacent myometrium and, if untreated, may eventually progress to the parametria.

Infection involving the broad ligament adjacent to the uterus is termed *parametritis*. In its mildest form, it may be limited to this region; more often, the tubes, ovaries, and pelvic peritoneum are involved. Isolated parametritis may follow cesarean section, but it is usually associated with endometritis. When the infection is low grade or has been neglected, there may be considerable inflammation, induration, and even abscess formation. With appropriate treatment, severe induration and even small abscesses may resolve to the point of being undetectable on later pelvic examination, and they may not impair subsequent fertility; the outcome, however, is by no means always so favorable.

Evidence of any of these pelvic infections usually does not appear before 24 hours postpartum and is signaled by sustained temperature greater than 100.4° F (38° C). The patient may complain of mild malaise

and anorexia, but report no localizing symptoms. Except in cases of fulminating sepsis, the early signs of infection may be no more than a temperature of 101°–102° F (38.3°–38.9° C) with a white blood cell count still within the normal range for the early puerperium (10,000–15,000/cu mm). Untreated, the minimum changes may persist for 24–48 hours, depending on the virulence of the offending organism and the host's resistance. On the other hand, the most severe infections may be associated with chills, extreme lethargy, lower abdominal pain, and fever that spikes to 103°–104° F (39.4°–40° C) in the early stages. In such instances, there is almost invariably some parametrial involvement, although localized infection with episodic bacteremia may present a similar picture.

The *diagnosis of metritis* should be made only after a complete physical examination, including a careful search for deep vein tenderness and examination of the lungs, abdomen, urinary tract, and pelvis. In women delivered by cesarean section, abdominal tenderness due to the incision must be distinguished from that due to infection. Even in more severe infections of the endometrium, no significant uterine tenderness may be elicited by abdominal or vaginal palpation. The diagnosis of parametritis is usually obvious. In addition to a clinical picture of severe infection, there is usually significant tenderness lateral to the uterus on both abdominal and pelvic examinations. Moving the uterus to one side or the other also produces pain. If there is associated pelvic peritonitis, signs of peritoneal irritation may be detected low in the abdomen. A sample of intrauterine material may be obtained for culture, but the wide variety of microorganisms that comprise the normal flora of the genital tract frequently obscures the precise etiology of infection; therefore, a Gram stain of the material may give the best preliminary guidance to the choice of antibiotic. Blood cultures are also indicated when the patient appears disturbingly ill or has an extremely high fever. It is generally the accepted practice to obtain urine for examination of the sediment and for culture prior to instituting treatment, since a urinary tract infection without typical symptoms may be the cause of the fever or may coexist with a uterine infection.

The *management of metritis* is primarily the administration of antibiotics. The choice of agents is largely empirical, since the final results of transcervical cultures may be misleading, as noted earlier. Fortunately, most microorganisms that cause pelvic infection are sensitive to many of the common antibiotics. The selection of antibiotics and route of administration are largely dictated by the severity of the infection. Penicillin, ampicillin, or a cephalosporin is frequently used, alone or in combination with an aminoglycoside (streptomycin, kanamycin, gentamicin), depending on the severity of the clinical manifestations.

Response to antibiotics is usually prompt; but, even

so, treatment should be continued for 10 days. Lack of response within 36–48 hours or worsening of the clinical manifestations requires reevaluation and additional or different antibiotics based on experience and culture results. In addition, pelvic thrombophlebitis should be considered.

Curettage is indicated when retention of placental fragments is suggested by vaginal bleeding, a widely patent cervical os, or passage of tissue resembling the placenta. If curettage is necessary in the acutely ill patient, antibiotics should be given intravenously, preferably 2–4 hours before surgery. In the most severe cases, when all medical management fails, removal of the infected uterus, tubes, and ovaries may be lifesaving. It is impossible to distinguish clearly between indications for continued conservative management and indications for the more radical surgical approach. Such a judgment is dependent on the careful assessment of each case.

Generalized Peritonitis. A rare complication of the puerperium, generalized peritonitis, when it does occur, is usually associated with endoparametritis following operative delivery. As in most cases of peritonitis, there is usually diffuse direct and rebound tenderness and an associated paralytic ileus, sometimes with vomiting and abdominal distention. Except when a parametrial abscess ruptures, making emergency surgical intervention mandatory, puerperal peritonitis should be managed conservatively with antibiotics and supportive measures.

Perineal Infections. Localized infection of a repaired episiotomy or perineal laceration is one of the more common infections of the puerperium. These areas are particularly prone to infection in the presence of small, unnoticed hematomas. In most instances, the patient complains of unusual discomfort. Examination of the perineum reveals an edematous, erythematous lesion, usually with purulent drainage, and a tender area of induration in the involved site. Except when associated with hematoma, these infections usually do not produce fluctuant areas early in their course. Significant fluctuance within the first 24–48 hours strongly suggests hematoma.

Management of these localized infections, often caused by staphylococci, includes removal of the sutures to enhance drainage. When there is any degree of fluctuance, the wound should be carefully probed with either a large Kelly clamp or a uterine dressing forceps to open any areas of loculation; if a cavity of more than 2–3 cm is identified, drainage can be better assured by packing the space loosely with a material such as iodoform-treated gauze to maintain a drainage tract. Sitz baths not only encourage drainage and healing, but also relieve perineal pain. Systemic reaction to the infection (evidenced by fever and leukocytosis)

should be treated with antibiotics following culture and sensitivity studies.

Mastitis. As a result of shorter postpartum hospitalization, mastitis is seldom seen during the period of inpatient care. Indeed, early discharge has probably led to a decreased incidence of this complication, since the patient in her home is less likely to be exposed to pathogens. Mastitis is usually caused by coagulase-positive *Staphylococcus aureus*. The route of infection is sometimes through a fissure of the nipple, but more often the route is not apparent. The source of the pathogen may be the mother's own hand, although it is more commonly the infant. Since the infection usually involves the parenchyma, ducts, and glands, the offending bacteria are present in the milk. The most important preventive measures include frequent soap-and-water cleansing of the breasts and precautions to keep the infant free of bacteria.

The clinical manifestations are usually obvious. Fever, malaise, and breast tenderness are commonly present. Examination of the involved breast reveals erythema, induration, and marked tenderness to palpation. In the early phase, the induration is relatively brawny; but, if the process is left untreated, areas of loculation and abscesses may develop. Management includes culture of milk, material from the nipple, and sometimes material from the infant's mouth, followed by administration of antibiotics and local application of heat. Penicillin remains the antibiotic of choice; but, when the patient is hypersensitive or when a penicillin-resistant organism is suspected, erythromycin or another broad spectrum antibiotic should be used. Abscesses require incision and drainage.

Nursing from the involved breast need be discontinued only until after the acute phase. A breast pump may be used periodically, but some women find it less traumatic to express the milk manually.

Urinary Tract Infections. The relatively high incidence of urinary tract infections in the puerperium is usually attributed to trauma-induced hypotonicity of the bladder and frequent catheterization.

Cystitis, usually characterized by frequency and burning on urination, is rarely accompanied by significant fever. Pyelonephritis, which is much more dramatic, is frequently accompanied by shaking chills, spiking fever of 104° F (40° C), and flank pain. The *Murphy punch,* a sharp blow over the costovertebral angle, reveals deep-seated tenderness and muscular rigidity. Almost invariably, either the right side only or both sides are involved; unilateral left-sided puerperal pyelonephritis is so unusual that a positive reaction to the Murphy punch on the left side only should prompt the physician to reconsider the diagnosis. The organism responsible is usually Escherichia coli. As in other infections, culture and sensitivity studies are essential. Bactericidal agents (penicillins, cephalosporins, aminoglycosides) are usually effective.

THROMBOPHLEBITIS AND THROMBOEMBOLIC DISEASE

Thrombophlebitis and thromboembolic disease occur in fewer than 1% of all puerperas. Nevertheless, they occur significantly more often in the puerpera than in the nonpregnant woman. Incidence data suggest that these disorders may be less common than they were 25 years ago; however, the older data were based on clinical diagnosis only and may have been erroneous. The apparent decline in incidence may also be attributed partly to early ambulation, general improvement in patients' overall health, and fewer instances of traumatic operative delivery. The decrease in the occurrence of pulmonary emboli is attributed not only to the aforementioned factors but also, more importantly, to current early recognition and treatment of deep vein thrombophlebitis. It is extremely important to recognize deep vein thrombophlebitis in its earliest phases. The obstetrician should maintain a continuing high level of suspicion and should make a daily check of the calves and femoral triangles of every patient.

Deep vein disorders in the puerpera have been variously attributed to sluggish circulation in the large sinuses, trauma to pelvic veins secondary to pressure from the fetal head, and estrogen-induced hypercoagulability, perhaps mediated by increased concentration of antithrombin III. Lastly, pelvic infection may initiate changes that lead to thrombophlebitis in the adjacent veins.

Superficial thrombophlebitis usually involves the saphenous system and is easily diagnosed by the physical finding of tenderness along the course of the vein, often with areas of palpable thrombosis. Skin temperature is usually increased in the involved regions of the lower extremities, but there may be little or no erythema or peripheral edema. Before concluding that the process is limited to the superficial system, the physician must carefully check the deep veins, including examination by Doppler ultrasonography. It must be noted, however, that the Doppler ultrasound technique is more useful above the knee than below it. Limited superficial disease can be managed by bedrest, analgesics, the use of elastic stockings, and a footboard.

Fever, deep vein tenderness, Homans' sign, and venous obstruction as evidenced by swelling of the extremity usually make the diagnosis of *deep vein thrombophlebitis* apparent. However, it must be strongly emphasized that deep vein disease is clinically unsuspected in a high percentage of cases. Venography is the most reliable diagnostic procedure, but the technique is not a practical approach in all institutions.

The Doppler ultrasound technique, which is safer and simpler, can be highly accurate in the hands of those who have acquired the necessary skill in its use.

In deep vein disease, anticoagulation, preferably with intravenous heparin, should be initiated immediately. An initial dose of 5,000–7,000 units should be followed by doses of 5,000–10,000 units every 4 hours until the whole blood clotting time (measured by the method of Lee and White) has doubled or tripled or until the activated partial thromboplastin time has increased by a factor of 1.5–2. In the past several years, there have been a number of reports supporting the use of continuous intravenous administration of heparin. Many of these studies indicate that this method is safer than intermittent injection with or without laboratory control and is no less effective for prevention of thromboembolism. Constant infusion prevents undesirable fluctuations in anticoagulation. Either activated partial thromboplastin time or whole blood clotting time should be used to adjust the initial dose (24,000 plus or minus 6,400 units/day). Most authorities favor conversion to sodium warfarin (Coumadin) 10–14 days after acute symptoms have subsided and recommend continuing this form of anticoagulation for a 6-week postsymptomatic period of treatment. Strict bedrest and physical therapy are important adjuncts in the management of thrombophlebitis.

The diagnosis of *massive pulmonary embolism* is sometimes clear-cut, with the sudden onset of pleuritic type chest pain, cough with or without hemoptysis, fever, apprehension, and tachycardia, all warning signs of impending catastrophe. Friction rub and signs of pleural effusion and atelectasis may be present. In the most severe cases, there may be associated hypotension, diaphoresis, electrocardiographic signs of right heart strain, and increasing central venous pressure. Any of these signs are indications for immediate diagnostic procedures. Unfortunately, most pulmonary emboli are not suspected; therefore, the physician must maintain a keen and continuing suspicion of this disorder. If there is a possibility of a pulmonary embolus, a lung scan should be obtained as soon as possible. If the scan is entirely negative, a pulmonary embolism has been excluded. If the results are equivocal, pulmonary angiography should be done. With a scan or angiogram diagnosis of embolus, immediate anticoagulation, preferable by constant intravenous infusion, results in recovery of the vast majority of these patients. However, recurrent embolization should prompt serious consideration of vena caval and ovarian vein ligation.

Suppurative thrombophlebitis should be managed as described previously, but every effort should be made to identify the responsible microorganism; the patient should be treated with vigorous intravenous administration of the appropriate antibiotics.

Thrombophlebitis may occur in the ovarian veins and other pelvic vessels. When it does, it is termed *right ovarian vein syndrome* or pelvic thrombophlebitis. Patients with this syndrome usually complain of abdominal pain, and it may be difficult to distinguish this pain from pain due to metritis. Fever is common. A sausage-shaped tender mass may be palpated in the midabdomen, usually on the right side. Pelvic thrombophlebitis should be suspected when patients fail to respond to appropriate antibiotic administration in the first 72 hours after a diagnosis of pelvic infection. Anticoagulation with heparin leads to dramatic improvement in such patients.

POSTPARTUM HEMORRHAGE

Hemorrhage is a leading cause of maternal death in the United States. Postpartum hemorrhage, particularly that due to uterine atony, is the most frequently encountered hemorrhagic complication of pregnancy. It usually occurs during the 1st hour after delivery of the placenta, but serious blood loss may occur as late as 2–3 weeks after delivery. Hemorrhage has traditionally been defined as acute blood loss in excess of 500 ml, but since the average blood loss approximates this amount it has been suggested that postpartum hemorrhage be defined as blood loss in excess of 1000 ml.

Postpartum hemorrhage can in many cases be prevented by meticulous obstetric technique. Avoidance of trauma during labor and delivery, avoidance of unnecessarily prolonged anesthesia, and continuous observation of the tonus of the emptied uterus, perhaps with the prophylactic use of oxytocin, are among the important factors. Following the end of the third stage, it is common practice to inspect the cervix for lacerations and to explore the uterine cavity manually for tears or retained placental fragments. At the same time, the amount of bleeding can be assessed and vaginal lacerations identified and sutured. Episiotomy repair should be completed with dispatch. (The repair of a routine and uncomplicated episiotomy should require 10 minutes at most. Simple, rapid techniques often provide much better support than elaborate, time-consuming repairs.)

Uterine Atony

The most common cause of serious postpartum hemorrhage is failure of the uterus to contract satisfactorily. Overdistention secondary to hydramnios, large or multiple infants, high parity, prolonged labor, and many general anesthetic agents predispose to the development of uterine atony. Atony as the primary cause of hemorrhage should be diagnosed only after other causes of blood loss have been ruled out, since acute blood loss in itself may precipitate atony.

Management of uterine atony consists of fundal massage (with care not to displace the uterus inferiorly because such a displacement may have a tour-

should be treated with antibiotics following culture and sensitivity studies.

Mastitis. As a result of shorter postpartum hospitalization, mastitis is seldom seen during the period of inpatient care. Indeed, early discharge has probably led to a decreased incidence of this complication, since the patient in her home is less likely to be exposed to pathogens. Mastitis is usually caused by coagulase-positive *Staphylococcus aureus*. The route of infection is sometimes through a fissure of the nipple, but more often the route is not apparent. The source of the pathogen may be the mother's own hand, although it is more commonly the infant. Since the infection usually involves the parenchyma, ducts, and glands, the offending bacteria are present in the milk. The most important preventive measures include frequent soap-and-water cleansing of the breasts and precautions to keep the infant free of bacteria.

The clinical manifestations are usually obvious. Fever, malaise, and breast tenderness are commonly present. Examination of the involved breast reveals erythema, induration, and marked tenderness to palpation. In the early phase, the induration is relatively brawny; but, if the process is left untreated, areas of loculation and abscesses may develop. Management includes culture of milk, material from the nipple, and sometimes material from the infant's mouth, followed by administration of antibiotics and local application of heat. Penicillin remains the antibiotic of choice; but, when the patient is hypersensitive or when a penicillin-resistant organism is suspected, erythromycin or another broad spectrum antibiotic should be used. Abscesses require incision and drainage.

Nursing from the involved breast need be discontinued only until after the acute phase. A breast pump may be used periodically, but some women find it less traumatic to express the milk manually.

Urinary Tract Infections. The relatively high incidence of urinary tract infections in the puerperium is usually attributed to trauma-induced hypotonicity of the bladder and frequent catheterization.

Cystitis, usually characterized by frequency and burning on urination, is rarely accompanied by significant fever. Pyelonephritis, which is much more dramatic, is frequently accompanied by shaking chills, spiking fever of 104° F (40° C), and flank pain. The *Murphy punch,* a sharp blow over the costovertebral angle, reveals deep-seated tenderness and muscular rigidity. Almost invariably, either the right side only or both sides are involved; unilateral left-sided puerperal pyelonephritis is so unusual that a positive reaction to the Murphy punch on the left side only should prompt the physician to reconsider the diagnosis. The organism responsible is usually Escherichia coli. As in other infections, culture and sensitivity studies are essential. Bactericidal agents (penicillins, cephalosporins, aminoglycosides) are usually effective.

THROMBOPHLEBITIS AND THROMBOEMBOLIC DISEASE

Thrombophlebitis and thromboembolic disease occur in fewer than 1% of all puerperas. Nevertheless, they occur significantly more often in the puerpera than in the nonpregnant woman. Incidence data suggest that these disorders may be less common than they were 25 years ago; however, the older data were based on clinical diagnosis only and may have been erroneous. The apparent decline in incidence may also be attributed partly to early ambulation, general improvement in patients' overall health, and fewer instances of traumatic operative delivery. The decrease in the occurrence of pulmonary emboli is attributed not only to the aforementioned factors but also, more importantly, to current early recognition and treatment of deep vein thrombophlebitis. It is extremely important to recognize deep vein thrombophlebitis in its earliest phases. The obstetrician should maintain a continuing high level of suspicion and should make a daily check of the calves and femoral triangles of every patient.

Deep vein disorders in the puerpera have been variously attributed to sluggish circulation in the large sinuses, trauma to pelvic veins secondary to pressure from the fetal head, and estrogen-induced hypercoagulability, perhaps mediated by increased concentration of antithrombin III. Lastly, pelvic infection may initiate changes that lead to thrombophlebitis in the adjacent veins.

Superficial thrombophlebitis usually involves the saphenous system and is easily diagnosed by the physical finding of tenderness along the course of the vein, often with areas of palpable thrombosis. Skin temperature is usually increased in the involved regions of the lower extremities, but there may be little or no erythema or peripheral edema. Before concluding that the process is limited to the superficial system, the physician must carefully check the deep veins, including examination by Doppler ultrasonography. It must be noted, however, that the Doppler ultrasound technique is more useful above the knee than below it. Limited superficial disease can be managed by bedrest, analgesics, the use of elastic stockings, and a footboard.

Fever, deep vein tenderness, Homans' sign, and venous obstruction as evidenced by swelling of the extremity usually make the diagnosis of *deep vein thrombophlebitis* apparent. However, it must be strongly emphasized that deep vein disease is clinically unsuspected in a high percentage of cases. Venography is the most reliable diagnostic procedure, but the technique is not a practical approach in all institutions.

The Doppler ultrasound technique, which is safer and simpler, can be highly accurate in the hands of those who have acquired the necessary skill in its use.

In deep vein disease, anticoagulation, preferably with intravenous heparin, should be initiated immediately. An initial dose of 5,000–7,000 units should be followed by doses of 5,000–10,000 units every 4 hours until the whole blood clotting time (measured by the method of Lee and White) has doubled or tripled or until the activated partial thromboplastin time has increased by a factor of 1.5–2. In the past several years, there have been a number of reports supporting the use of continuous intravenous administration of heparin. Many of these studies indicate that this method is safer than intermittent injection with or without laboratory control and is no less effective for prevention of thromboembolism. Constant infusion prevents undesirable fluctuations in anticoagulation. Either activated partial thromboplastin time or whole blood clotting time should be used to adjust the initial dose (24,000 plus or minus 6,400 units/day). Most authorities favor conversion to sodium warfarin (Coumadin) 10–14 days after acute symptoms have subsided and recommend continuing this form of anticoagulation for a 6-week postsymptomatic period of treatment. Strict bedrest and physical therapy are important adjuncts in the management of thrombophlebitis.

The diagnosis of *massive pulmonary embolism* is sometimes clear-cut, with the sudden onset of pleuritic type chest pain, cough with or without hemoptysis, fever, apprehension, and tachycardia, all warning signs of impending catastrophe. Friction rub and signs of pleural effusion and atelectasis may be present. In the most severe cases, there may be associated hypotension, diaphoresis, electrocardiographic signs of right heart strain, and increasing central venous pressure. Any of these signs are indications for immediate diagnostic procedures. Unfortunately, most pulmonary emboli are not suspected; therefore, the physician must maintain a keen and continuing suspicion of this disorder. If there is a possibility of a pulmonary embolus, a lung scan should be obtained as soon as possible. If the scan is entirely negative, a pulmonary embolism has been excluded. If the results are equivocal, pulmonary angiography should be done. With a scan or angiogram diagnosis of embolus, immediate anticoagulation, preferable by constant intravenous infusion, results in recovery of the vast majority of these patients. However, recurrent embolization should prompt serious consideration of vena caval and ovarian vein ligation.

Suppurative thrombophlebitis should be managed as described previously, but every effort should be made to identify the responsible microorganism; the patient should be treated with vigorous intravenous administration of the appropriate antibiotics.

Thrombophlebitis may occur in the ovarian veins and other pelvic vessels. When it does, it is termed *right ovarian vein syndrome* or pelvic thrombophlebitis. Patients with this syndrome usually complain of abdominal pain, and it may be difficult to distinguish this pain from pain due to metritis. Fever is common. A sausage-shaped tender mass may be palpated in the midabdomen, usually on the right side. Pelvic thrombophlebitis should be suspected when patients fail to respond to appropriate antibiotic administration in the first 72 hours after a diagnosis of pelvic infection. Anticoagulation with heparin leads to dramatic improvement in such patients.

POSTPARTUM HEMORRHAGE

Hemorrhage is a leading cause of maternal death in the United States. Postpartum hemorrhage, particularly that due to uterine atony, is the most frequently encountered hemorrhagic complication of pregnancy. It usually occurs during the 1st hour after delivery of the placenta, but serious blood loss may occur as late as 2–3 weeks after delivery. Hemorrhage has traditionally been defined as acute blood loss in excess of 500 ml, but since the average blood loss approximates this amount it has been suggested that postpartum hemorrhage be defined as blood loss in excess of 1000 ml.

Postpartum hemorrhage can in many cases be prevented by meticulous obstetric technique. Avoidance of trauma during labor and delivery, avoidance of unnecessarily prolonged anesthesia, and continuous observation of the tonus of the emptied uterus, perhaps with the prophylactic use of oxytocin, are among the important factors. Following the end of the third stage, it is common practice to inspect the cervix for lacerations and to explore the uterine cavity manually for tears or retained placental fragments. At the same time, the amount of bleeding can be assessed and vaginal lacerations identified and sutured. Episiotomy repair should be completed with dispatch. (The repair of a routine and uncomplicated episiotomy should require 10 minutes at most. Simple, rapid techniques often provide much better support than elaborate, time-consuming repairs.)

Uterine Atony

The most common cause of serious postpartum hemorrhage is failure of the uterus to contract satisfactorily. Overdistention secondary to hydramnios, large or multiple infants, high parity, prolonged labor, and many general anesthetic agents predispose to the development of uterine atony. Atony as the primary cause of hemorrhage should be diagnosed only after other causes of blood loss have been ruled out, since acute blood loss in itself may precipitate atony.

Management of uterine atony consists of fundal massage (with care not to displace the uterus inferiorly because such a displacement may have a tour-

niquet effect on the uterine veins and provoke further blood loss) and the administration of oxytocin. If the uterus does not respond, reexamination of the cavity and curettage with a sharp, large (Hunter) curet should be the next step. In rare instances, hysterectomy or hypogastric artery ligation may be required. Intrauterine packing has no place in present day management of uterine bleeding.

Lacerations

If not recognized and repaired immediately, lacerations of the uterus, cervix, vagina, and perineum may lead to significant blood loss. Repair is usually accomplished with ease if adequate exposure is maintained. Long, wide retractors and one or two assistants may be needed. Sulcus extension of the episiotomy (usually mediolateral) is also easily managed, but care should be taken to ensure hemostasis by beginning the repair above the uppermost level of the tear. If hemorrhage occurs after the woman has left the delivery room, she should be returned there for reexamination and repair of any lacerations overlooked at the initial postdelivery inspection.

Hematomas

Hematomas that occur postpartum are usually located in areas of laceration or episiotomy repair. The perineal pain and obvious mass noted on examination make the diagnosis easy in most instances. Occasionally, a hematoma develops unassociated with interruption of the mucosa, presumably secondary to traumatic rupture of a deep vessel. In such a case, diagnosis may be more difficult and blood loss more serious. The latter is particularly true when the hematoma tends to dissect superiorly into the broad ligament.

Management of hematomas includes exploration with incision, drainage, and ligation of the bleeding vessel. If the hematoma is evacuated within the first few hours after delivery and good hemostasis is accomplished, the cavity may be closed with figure-of-eight sutures. Otherwise, a drain should be left in the defect. Management of larger pelvic hematomas may require laparotomy and, in the rare case of a tear that extends into the broad ligament, hysterectomy.

Other Causes of Postpartum Hemorrhage

When some degree of placenta accreta occurs, all efforts at conservative management, including curettage, may be unsuccessful. Hysterectomy is required in many such cases. Uterine rupture, whether spontaneous or secondary to operative trauma, is a serious complication that necessitates laparotomy either for repairing the defect, if feasible, or for removing the uterus. Preoperative diagnosis of both placenta accreta and uterine rupture is difficult, but these conditions must be suspected when there is no obvious cause for continued uterine bleeding.

Delayed Hemorrhage (Late Postpartum Hemorrhage)

Delayed hemorrhage, defined as excessive blood loss occurring more than 24 hours after delivery, is usually caused by retained placental fragments. If a placental fragment is retained for a week or so, necrosis and some degree of organization occur, resulting in the so-called placental polyp. Treatment consists of curettage.

Subinvolution of the placental site is an indistinct clinical entity that is frequently diagnosed when delayed hemorrhage occurs, and curettage yields only decidua and organized thrombi. When there is no hemorrhage, *subinvolution of the uterus* is a nondescript diagnosis, usually made at the routine 6-week examination when the uterus has not returned to "normal size." Subinvolution probably represents the extreme of normal variation.

PUERPERAL PSYCHIATRIC DISORDERS

All manner of psychiatric problems may be encountered in the puerperium, but serious disorders are extremely rare. During the 1st week, and usually on the 3rd day postpartum, 70%–80% of women encounter a transient depression, often accompanied by tearfulness. When asked what the problem is, the woman usually responds, "I don't know. I just feel like crying." The condition is self-limited and usually vanishes within a few hours or a day. All that is needed is understanding and reassurance. The condition is not easily explained, and its etiology probably varies to an extent from one woman to another. The major physiologic stresses of the puerperium, including the huge mobilization of water and the endocrine upheaval, may be concerned. In many cases, it seems clear the mother suddenly realizes that she has indeed survived pregnancy and delivered a healthy baby, and that she can no longer use this important, if subconscious, worry as a substitute for dealing with the day-to-day problems that must now be faced.

In occasional cases, the postpartum depression may have more significant implications. When the patient shows no tearfulness, a lack of interest in the baby, and undue concern about the problems that will be encountered after she returns home, the obstetrician should consider the possibility of a problem that is more serious than the "baby blues." If it persists for more than 24 hours, the opinion of a psychiatrist may be needed.

In former years, anxiety was common in new mothers during the 1st weeks at home. This occurred principally among women who had little or no contact with

their baby during the hospital stay, who had no first-hand knowledge of the baby's needs or routine care, who were totally dependent on other persons for the decisions and techniques required of them, and who considered themselves to be trapped in an untenable position they had not planned and for which they were wholly unprepared. In the modern era, most women carry a baby to term because they really want a baby, and they desire to learn as much about infant care as possible. The educational programs available both during pregnancy and in the hospital are such that most mothers are confident and well prepared, and they do not encounter the profound sense of inadequacy and dependence that was so common 20 and 30 years ago. In addition, the several facets of "family-centered" obstetric care (see Chapter 31) appear to be of special importance in achieving a satisfying and lasting family adjustment.

Between the simple, virtually physiologic, mild 3rd day depression and the true psychoses there is a gamut of neuroses that can occur in the puerperium. Some are trivial and self-limited, and do not require special care; in others, the patient is greatly benefited by referral to a psychiatrist. A useful yardstick for the obstetrician in determining the need for psychiatric assistance in these cases is the answer to the question of whether the neurotic manifestations are of sufficient magnitude to interfere with the patient's effectiveness and her ability to cope with the ordinary day-to-day tasks and activities with which she is faced. True psychoses usually occur when the stage for psychosis was set prior to pregnancy; the stress of pregnancy and delivery are precipitating and nonspecific factors.

DISCHARGE INSTRUCTIONS

Activity. Some women regain their full strength and vigor more quickly after delivery than others. Periods of rest as needed during the day are desirable, and most women should be advised to avoid, if possible, a return to full employment or a full schedule of household activity for at least 1 month.

Sitz baths may be helpful if the episiotomy or repaired lacerations are painful. There is no contraindication to tub baths.

Sexual intercourse is permitted as soon as it is comfortable. The 6-week period of abstinence formerly recommended is no longer thought to be important.

Contraception. Oral contraceptives are to be avoided if the mother is nursing; if she is not nursing, they may be started at once. Intrauterine devices, diaphragms, and foams are not recommended until after the puerperium. If the mother is nursing and contraception is desired, condoms are most suitable until the postpartum office visit, when other methods may be considered.

Exercises are probably not needed to restore the tone of the abdominal muscles, for the ordinary activity of the puerperium and the normal regression of the pregnancy changes are usually sufficient to accomplish this. However, the process may be hastened to an extent by leg-raising and other excercises that place the rectus abdominis muscles at stress.

POSTPARTUM EXAMINATION

The postpartum examination is usually scheduled for 6 weeks after delivery, a time when most of the systemic pregnancy changes have receded, the uterus is involuted, the cervix has resumed its nonpregnant contour and appearance, the episiotomy and any perineal lacerations have healed, and the breasts (unless the woman is nursing) have softened to permit easy examination. This is an extremely important visit, not only for evaluation of the woman's physical status, but also to permit the physician to determine whether there are problems requiring additional therapy. Medical or other disorders that complicated pregnancy or delivery and were not of sufficient severity to require earlier follow-up should be specifically evaluated at this time.

In the woman who has experienced an entirely normal pregnancy, labor, and puerperium, the evaluation should consist of a pelvic examination, with specific attention to involution of the uterus and vagina, the pelvic supports, and the cervix; cytologic evaluation of the cervix; investigation of the tone of the abdominal wall; examination of the breasts; estimation of hemoglobin or hematocrit; urinalysis; blood pressure determination; and weight determination.

Specific inquiry should be made as to whether the woman wishes to begin another pregnancy at once, and if she does not, what measures she wishes to take to prevent it. The various methods of contraception should be discussed (see Chapter 14), and she and her physician should select the one that appears most appropriate for her.

REFERENCES AND RECOMMENDED READING

Andreassen B, Tyson JE: Role of the hypothalamic–pituitary–ovarian axis in puerperal infertility. J Clin Endocrinol Metab 42:1114, 1976

Billewicz WZ, Thompson AM: Body weight in parous women. Br J Prev Soc Med 24:97, 1970

Bowes WA, Jr (ed): The puerperium. Clin Obstet Gynecol 23:971, 1980

Brown TK, Munsick RA: Puerperal ovarian vein thrombophlebitis: A syndrome. Am J Obstet Gynecol 109:263, 1971

Filker RS, Monif GRG: Postpartum septicemia due to group G streptococci. Obstet Gynecol 53:28S, 1979

Hendricks CH, Eskes TKAB, Saameli K: Uterine contractability at delivery and in the puerperium. Am J Obstet Gynecol 83:890, 1972

Jaffe RB, Lee PA: Serum gonadotrophins before, at the inception of, and following human pregnancy. J Clin Endocrinol Metab 29:1281, 1969

Jelliffee DB, Jelliffee EFP: Current concepts in nutrition. Breast is best: Modern meanings. N Engl J Med 297:912, 1977

Josey WE, Staggers SR: Heparin therapy in septic pelvic thrombophlebitis: A study of 46 cases. Am J Obstet Gynecol 120:338, 1974

Keye, WR, Jaffe RB: Changing patterns of FSH and LH response to gonadtrophin-releasing hormone in the puerperium. J Clin Endocrinol Metab 42:1113, 1976

Kletzky OA, Marrs RP, Howard WF, et al: Prolactin synthesis and release during pregnancy and puerperium. Am J Obstet Gynecol 136:545, 1980

Le Maire WJ, Shipiro AG, Riggal F et al: Temporary pituitary insensitivity to stimulation by synthetic LRF during the postpartum period. J Clin Endocrinol Metab 38:916, 1974

Lucas A, Drewett RB, Mitchell MD: Breast-feeding and plasma oxytocin concentrations. Br Med J 281:834, 1980

Monif GRG: Infectious Diseases in Obstetrics and Gynecology. Hagerstown, MD, Harper & Row, 1974

Munsick RA, Gillanders LA: A review of the syndrome of puerperal ovarian vein thrombophlebitis with some original observations on ovarian venous blood flow postpartum. Obstet Gynecol Surv (in press)

Reynolds SRM: Right ovarian vein syndrome. Obstet Gynecol 37:308, 1971

Salzman EW, Deykin D, Shapiro RM et al: Management of heparin therapy: Controlled prospective trial. N Engl J Med 292:1046, 1975

Stirrat GM: Prescribing problems in the second half of pregnancy and during lactation. Obstet Gynecol Surv 31:1, 1976

Ueland K, Hansen JM: Maternal and cardiovascular dynamics: III. Labor and delivery under local and caudal anesthesia. Am J Obstet Gynecol 103:8, 1969

Vorherr H: The Breast. New York, Academic Press, 1974

Vorherr H (ed): Human lactation. Semin Perinatol 3: 191, 1979

Welsh JK, May JT: Anti-infective properties of breast milk. J Pediatr 94:1, 1979

Williams JW: Regeneration of the uterine mucosa after delivery with special reference to the placental site. Am J Obstet Gynecol 22:664, 1931

Winikoff B, Baer EC: Translating "breast is best" from theory to practice. Am J Obstet Gynecol 138:105, 1980

Zarate A, Canales ES, Soria J et al: Ovarian refractoriness during lactation in women: Effect of gonadotrophin stimulation. Am J Obstet Gynecol 112:1130, 1972

PART VI

THE FETUS, PLACENTA, MEMBRANES, AND THE NEWBORN

CLINICAL EVALUATION OF FETAL STATUS

Richard Depp

Epidemiologically, it is useful to classify perinatal morbidity and mortality by a number of schemes. The most obvious and frequently used schemes correlate morbidity and mortality either with gestational age, which has the strongest relationship to morbidity and mortality, or with birth weight, which is also an indirect means of estimating gestational age. Most morbidity and mortality, *e.g.,* respiratory distress syndrome (RDS), hyperbilirubinemia, and intraventricular hemorrhage, result from preterm delivery. Intrauterine growth retardation, congenital anomalies, and chromosomal aberrations are also significant factors. A lesser contributions is made by maternal disease, such as preeclampsia and diabetes.

Although correlations of perinatal mortality with gestational age and maternal disease are useful for comparison, they do not allow evaluation of the impact of changing technology in obstetrics and neonatology. More importantly, simple correlations do not allow comparison of populations with different risk characteristics. To accomplish this end, it is useful to classify morbidity and mortality according to preventability; as technology improves, the incidence of "unpreventable" insults should decrease. Much of the morbidity and mortality associated with such events as spontaneous preterm labor, placental abruption, cord accidents, and maternal disease is now considered unpreventable, but new therapeutic protocols may improve the outcomes. Some of the perinatal deaths that are now unpreventable include those associated with congenital anomalies, severe chromosomal abnormalities, and fetal–neonatal developmental abnormalities. The remaining deaths are either potentially or absolutely preventable; many are iatrogenic. In the potentially preventable category, death results from failure either to implement adequate surveillance or to heed ominous warnings; except in retrospect, most are only potentially preventable, given the constraints of current practice. Preventable and iatrogenic morbidity and mortality are a continuum that ranges from a neonatal death secondary to RDS in an infant of a diabetic mother who had only marginal indications for delivery to frankly iatrogenic neonatal death following elective induction of labor or repeat cesarean section where fetal maturity was not confirmed. It is estimated that 8%–15% of RDS is iatrogenic.

Objective clinical evaluation of fetal health status is a primary goal of obstetric care. Prior to the late 1960s, the management of pregnancies thought to be associated with increased risk for fetal mortality was empiric. Pregnancies were frequently terminated by induction or cesarean section at a gestational age selected according to published data that compared the risk of intrauterine demise to the risk of neonatal death at each week of gestation. For example, all pregnancies complicated by diabetes were interrupted at 37 weeks, the point in gestation at which the cumulative risk of intrauterine and neonatal death was the lowest. Large numbers of otherwise normally developing fetuses were thus delivered prior to full maturation. The benefit was a reduction in fetal mortality in the subset of high-risk patients with true uteroplacental insufficiency; the cost unfortunately was often unnecessary neonatal morbidity or mortality in patients who were indeed at risk, but in whom the uteroplacental function was sufficiently intact that intrauterine death would not have occurred. Management of pregnancy complicated by isoimmune disease is another example. Inability to assess the specific status of the fetus at risk for erythroblastosis fetalis other than by historical data and antibody titers often resulted in the unnecessary preterm delivery of an Rh-negative fetus in cases in which the father was heterozygous for the D antigen.

The development of amniocentesis to evaluate the pregnancy at risk for isoimmune disease in the early 1960s revolutionized obstetric practice and initiated

interest in the development of other techniques to evaluate fetal status. Since that time, techniques to determine fetal gestational age and growth, amniotic fluid content, endocrine products of the fetoplacental unit, and fetal heart rate (FHR) antenatally or in labor and to obtain fetal scalp blood samples have become available to the practicing clinician. Most techniques, if properly applied antenatally, allow the physician to delay intervention until maturity is attained. Proper use of instantaneous FHR determinations and scalp blood sampling should promote more selective use of cesarean delivery for fetal distress. As a result of the availability of new diagnostic tools and superb neonatal care, the measure of clinical success is no longer perinatal mortality, which has been reduced dramatically in many centers, but rather perinatal morbidity.

Perinatal mortality is primarily the result of the triad of preterm delivery, intrauterine growth retardation, and lethal congenital anomalies. The relative contribution of the first two entities can be reduced only by early patient risk assessment and identification, accurate assignment of gestational age, evaluation of fetoplacental function, and, most importantly, assessment of fetal organ maturity. All data collected must then be interpreted in proper context with the risk of maternal disease. The ability to make selective decisions that minimize unnecessary intervention, iatrogenic conditions caused by preterm delivery, and preventable fetal demise is largely responsible for recent improvements in perinatal morbidity and mortality.

RISK SCORING

When the mother's condition is stable, therapeutic decisions regarding intervention in pregnancy should be based on the issue of benefit (reduced mortality) versus risk (morbidity and mortality of preterm delivery). Ideally, intervention should occur when the risk of intrauterine demise (detected by some objective technique) outweighs that of neonatal demise, usually from RDS. Since neonatal mortality is clearly linked to gestational age, proper interpretation of clinical data and assessment of risk is often limited by the obstetrician's ability to assign gestation age. The risk of fetal death or neonatal morbidity may be falsely magnified or reduced if the true gestational age is inappropriately reduced or increased by age assignment error. Diagnostic ultrasound provides the most reliable prediction of fetal gestational age; however, its accuracy decreases rapidly after 26–28 weeks' gestation. It is thus clear that patient risk identification and management must be undertaken prior to this time. Ideally, a systematic approach should be implemented in the first trimester, when uterine size correlates best with gestational age. A risk identification scheme must be relatively simple and more importantly must allow identification of the population of patients who are re-

sponsible for the vast majority of cases of perinatal morbidity and mortality. It is also essential that the population so identified be of a managable size, and the percentage of normal outcomes in this group must not be so large that the use of expensive antenatal assessment tools is economically unjustifiable.

Several semiobjective scoring systems have been developed to identify the patient at risk. Such systems usually consider the impact of five factors: 1) maternal disease that coexists with pregnancy but is not related to it; 2) maternal disease or complications related to pregnancy; 3) socioeconomic status as measured by such factors as income, husband's occupation or education, and race; 4) genetic factors; and 5) maternal biologic factors such as height, weight, and age. Recently, objective risk indicators observed in labor have been added to the scoring systems. These systems have the theoretic advantage of 1) assessing the risk of synergistic antenatal, intrapartum, and neonatal factors that predict perinatal morbidity and mortality; and 2) identifying the patient who requires specialized care.

Unfortunately, the interaction of the risk factors is not simple; they may have either cumulative or opposing effects in terms of modifying perinatal outcome. The use of more sophisticated statistical techniques, *e.g.*, covariant or multiple regression techniques, may be necessary. The interaction of such risk factors as nonwhite, lower socioeconomic class, minimal education, out-of-wedlock or teenage pregnancy, poor nutrition, extremes of maternal height and weight, stress, fatigue, need to work, and decreased use of contraception is complex and difficult to assess.

Nesbitt and Aubry have developed a semiobjective scoring system that assigns a relative score of 0, 5, 10, 15, 20, or 30 to each of a number of risk factors. The total score is determined by subtracting the weighted risk of each identified factor from a perfect score of 100. A score of less than 70 indicates considerable risk. Risk factors with a value of 30 or more points are

Abortions (three or more)
Fetal death (two or more)
Neonatal death (two or more)
Syphilis at term
Diabetes (all)
Hypertension: severe, chronic
Hypertension: nephritis
Heart disease, Classes III and IV
Adrenal, pituitary, thyroid disorder
Rh sensitization
Severe obesity
Prior cesarean section
Submucous fibroid
Contracted pelvic plane

The actual outcome of pregnancies in the low-risk versus high-risk groups is depicted in Figure 41–1.

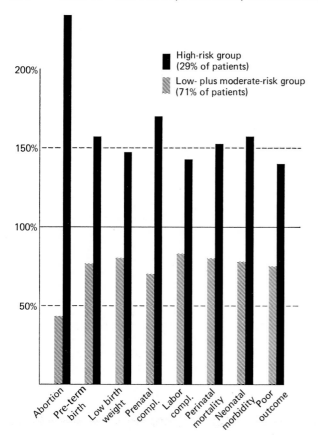

FIG. 41-1. Pregnancy outcome according to estimate of vulnerability based on index score; 100% is average incidence for total group in each category. (Modified from Nesbitt REL, Aubry RH: Am J Obstet Gynecol 103:972,1969)

Hobel *et al.* have also devised an expanded scoring system that includes two risk scores. The first, the antenatal score, focuses on problems detected in the history or antenatal period. This score can be continuously updated or recalculated at 32 weeks. The second, the intrapartum score, overlaps with the antenatal score but focuses largely on problems encountered in late pregnancy or labor, as well as on placental factors, such as placenta previa or abruption, and fetal factors, such as preterm labor, fetal monitor abnormality, or abnormal presentation. Assessment of risk in both the antenatal and intrapartum periods yields four possible risk groups (low-low, low-high, high-low, and high-high). Perinatal mortality in one series of patients classified according to this system are shown in Table 41–1. The total score is useful to determine the level of care and supervision that is appropriate for the patient under consideration.

Although a scoring system does identify a population subset that requires special attention, a critical review of available data shows that predictive ability is limited until the onset of labor. Of total neonatal morbidity and perinatal mortality (Table 41–2) 50% and 39%, respectively, arise from the population who were assessed as low-risk during pregnancy. If risk status is reassessed at the onset labor, the percent of fetal morbidity and mortality contributed by the low-risk population drops to 30% and 9%, respectively.

The importance of implementing a risk assessment system has been emphasized in a systematic review of 973 perinatal deaths. In that series, 25% of deaths were considered preventable. Avoidable factors were found in 20% of the unpreventable deaths, and multiple errors in management were found in 25% of the cases. Inaccurate assessment of gestational age, fail-

TABLE 41-1. RISK GROUP CHARACTERISTICS FOR 1,417 PATIENTS STUDIED PROSPECTIVELY BETWEEN 1969 AND 1972

Risk Groups				High-Risk Neonatal Mortality		Perinatal Mortality	
Prenatal	Intrapartal	N*	%	N*	% of Group	N*	% of Group
I. Low	Low	642	45	39	6.1	1	0.2
II. High	Low	233	16	29	12.5	3	1.3
III. Low	High	320	23	72	23.2	17	5.3
IV. High	High	222	16	83	39.9	25	11.3
		1417	100	223	16% of 1417 births	46	3.2% of 1417 births

* N, Number of cases.

(Hobel CJ: In Spellacy WN [ed]: Management of the High-Risk Pregnancy. Baltimore, University Park Press, 1976)

TABLE 41–2. LOW RISK VS. HIGH RISK: RELATIVE CONTRIBUTION (RETROSPECTIVE) TO TOTAL NEONATAL MORBIDITY AND PERINATAL MORTALITY*

Period	Risk	No.	Neonatal Morbidity (% Total)		Perinatal Mortality (% Total)	
PRENATAL	Low	962	111	(50)	18	(39)
	High	455	112	(50)	28	(61)
INTRAPARTUM	Low	875	68	(30)	4	(9)
	High	542	155	(70)	42	(91)
TOTAL		1417	223		46	

*Derived from Table 41-1
(Data derived from Hobel CJ: In Spellacy WN [ed]: Management of High-Risk Pregnancy. Baltimore, University Park Press, 1976).

ure to detect poor fetal growth, and limited antenatal fetal evaluation of fetal pulmonary maturity and uteroplacental function were common features in the series.

Since most preventable deaths are associated with preterm delivery or intrauterine growth retardation, early identification of patients at risk for either is important. Such identification allows the physician to emphasize prophylactic measures such as bedrest or adequate diet; to gather baseline data (ultrasound) for later comparison; to advise the patient to report immediately the first warning signs of preterm labor (low back pain, cramps, increased vaginal discharge, spotting), which might make it possible to inhibit preterm labor; or to begin early evaluation of fetal health status (serial cephalometry, abdominal circumference, nonstress testing). Table 41–3 summarizes selected weighted risk factors associated with preterm labor and intrauterine growth retardation according to the time of detection, the risk of poor outcome, and their usefulness as early or late predictors of preterm labor or intrauterine growth retardation. Scores of 1, 5, and 10 indicate slight, moderate, and severe risk. A total score of less than 10 implies low risk; a score of 10 or above, high risk.

DETERMINATION OF GESTATIONAL AGE

Decisions to intervene or not to intervene in high-risk pregnancy usually hinge on evaluation of maternal and fetal health. When intervention is necessary, it is usually for fetal indications; severe preeclampsia is a notable exception in which deterioration of maternal status is a primary consideration. In all cases, evaluation of gestational age, lung maturity (also indirectly estimated by gestational age), and integrity of the fetoplacental unit are the key variables. Intervention prior to fetal lung maturity should occur only when there is documented evidence of uteroplacental insufficiency or significant maternal health deterioration.

Accurate prediction of gestational age is the cornerstone of high-risk pregnancy management. The incidence of patients with suspect dates ranges from 22%–40%. There may be significant differences in neonatal morbidity and mortality between a fetus estimated to be at 29–30 weeks and a fetus estimated to be at 32–33 weeks' gestation. Such differences are particularly important in the management of preterm labor and rupture of the membranes prior to 32–34 weeks. Failure to assign gestational age accurately in cases considered for elective repeat cesarean section at term may result in iatrogenic preterm delivery. The incidence of postterm pregnancy may also be artificially increased by inaccurate menstrual dates; in such instances, the result is often unnecessary antenatal testing for the uncompromised fetus and prolonged and difficult oxytocin inductions. Unfortunately, in many cases, a cesarean section is required after an unsuccessful induction in the presence of an "unripe" cervix.

CLINICAL ESTIMATION

Clinically, a history of regular menses with minimal variation in flow duration or quantity is reassuring regarding the reliability of menstrual data. Close correlation of fundal height with gestational age prior to 28 weeks, maternal recognition of fetal movement (quickening) at 18–19 weeks' menstrual age, and detection of fetal heart sounds at 18–20 weeks by fetoscope are useful supporting data (Table 41–4). Lack of correlation suggests an incorrect age assignment. Total reliance on these clinical estimators is hazardous in the management of high-risk pregnancy, however. Even when a menstrual history is designated "reliable," one cannot be certain of gestational age. In addition, the detection of fetal heart sounds as a measure of gestational age has limited value unless the patient is seen weekly; otherwise the critical observation point may pass unobserved.

TABLE 41–3. COMMON CLINICAL PROBLEMS WITH RELATIVE RISK FOR GROWTH RETARDATION, PRETERM DELIVERY, OR POOR OUTCOME

Variables Predictive of Poor Outcome	Score	Intrauterine Growth Retardation	Preterm Delivery
HISTORICAL: MEDICAL PROBLEMS			
Age ≤ 15; age ≥ 35	5		
Diabetes, insulin-dependent	10	E*	E
Diabetes, Class A	10		
Heart disease, Class III, IV	10	E	E
Hypertension, chronic	10	E	E
Renal disease, moderate or severe	10	E	E
Family history: diabetes, genetic factors, hypertension, SS hemoglobin	5		
HISTORICAL: PREVIOUS PREGNANCIES			
Stillborn	10	E	E
Preterm delivery	10		E
Neonatal death	10		E
Habitual abortion	10		
Cervical incompetence	10		E
Fetal anomaly	5		
Preeclampsia	5		
Eclampsia	10		
Cesarean section	10		E
Hemolytic disease, Rh	10		E
Multiparity ≥ 5	5		E
DEVELOPING PROBLEMS, FIRST TRIMESTER			
Infections: TORCH	10	E	
Drug abuse	10	E	
Vaginal spotting	10	E	
Smoking	5	E	E

* E, Risk can be predicted relatively early in pregnancy.
(Modified from Hobel CJ: In Spellacy WN [ed]: Management of High-Risk Pregnancy. Baltimore, University Park Press, 1976)

ULTRASOUND

The increasing use of diagnostic ultrasound has dramatically improved the accuracy of fetal gestational age determinations. The technical aspects of the various tests are discussed in Chapter 28. Table 41–5 summarizes the predictive range and confidence limits of crown–rump and biparietal diameter measurements (BPD) at various gestational ages. In normal gestation, the rate of growth is probably a function of genetic predisposition. As shown in Figure 41–2, the variance about the mean of BPD measurements increases with advancing gestational age. The fact that fetuses growing in upper percentile limits have more rapid growth rates than those growing in the lower percentile ranks must be considered in the interpretation of all cephalometry data. Unless it is possible to assign a reliable specific percentile growth pattern, it is necessary to predict gestational age by matching a single BPD to a point on an established growth curve at the 50th percentile. Cephalometry probably should not
be used to assign gestational age if the first scan is after 28 weeks' gestation because of the ± 3-week variance.

In some cases, gestational age is established by basal body temperatures, prediction of ovulation timing, a crown–rump length measurement, or a second trimester BPD that correlates well with menstrual age. Although it is often acceptable to predict gestational age within a ± 11-day interval, as may be accom-

plished by a single scan prior to 27 weeks, management of many high-risk problems requires a more accurate estimation. Since there appears to be significant advantage to early examination by ultrasound, the clinician must develop a selective plan of management that includes ultrasonic estimation of gestational age prior to 26 weeks in pregnancies at high risk for gestational age inaccuracy, preterm delivery, and intrauterine growth retardation. The indications for cephalometry prior to 26 weeks in each case are

Those at risk for inaccuracy in assignment of gestational age
Irregular menses
Recent discontinuance of oral contraception
Fundal height versus LMP age discrepancy
Late appearance of fetal movement
Late appearance of fetal heart sounds
Obesity
Maternal age greater than 35 years

Those at risk for preterm delivery (second scan at 31–33 weeks may also be desirable)
Prior cesarean section
Candidate for elective induction of labor
Candidate for "indicated" induction
Prior preterm labor
At risk for altered fetal growth
At risk for twins

Family history
Ovulation induction
Those at risk for altered fetal growth (paired scans at 20–26 and 31–33 weeks, plus probable serial third trimester scans, should be done)
Prior newborn small for gestational age or intrauterine growth retardation
First trimester bleeding
First trimester viral infection
Essential hypertension
Diabetes
Family history of hypertension or diabetes

Unfortunately, this scheme does not include patients who first develop high-risk characteristics in the third trimester that require assessment of gestational age or fetal growth:

Preterm labor
Premature rupture of membranes
Hydramnios/oligohydramnios
Poor maternal weight gain
Poor fundal height growth
Essential hypertension or preeclampsia

Other useful indications for ultrasound (see Chapter 28) include

Confirm normal pregnancy
Gestational sac (5–6 weeks)
Fetal viability (7th week)
Fetal echoes (8th week)
Prior to amniocentesis
Locate placenta, umbilical cord, fetal structures
Confirm viability
Follow-up of abnormal α-fetoprotein
Detect fetal anomalies
Cephalic
Spina bifida
Renal
Limb reduction

TABLE 41-4. CLINICAL PREDICTION OF MATURITY: TIME REQUIRED FOR 90% CONFIDENCE THAT PREGNANCY IS *AT LEAST* 38 WEEKS' GESTATION

Indicator	Weeks
Reliable last menstrual period	42
Unreliable last menstrual period	45
First fetal heart sounds	21
Quickening, nulliparas	25
Quickening, multiparas	25

TABLE 41-5. PREDICTION OF GESTATIONAL AGE BY ULTRASONIC DETERMINATION OF CROWN–RUMP LENGTH AND BIPARIETAL DIAMETER

Author	Time of Examination	Predictive Range in Determining EDL*	Confidence Limits (%)
Campbell	2nd trimester	± 9 days	84
Varma	2nd trimester	± 9 days	91
Sabbagha	20–26 weeks	± 11 days	90
	27–28 weeks	± 14 days	90
	≥ 29 weeks	± 21 days	90
Sabbagha *et al.*	GASA†	± 1–3 days	95
Robinson and Flemming	Crown–rump, 7–14 weeks	± 1–4 days	95

* *EDL,* Estimated date of labor.
† *GASA,* Growth-adjusted sonographic age. Paired scans: first at 20–26 weeks, second at 31–33 weeks.

Percentile chart—sonar BPD at intervals of one week.

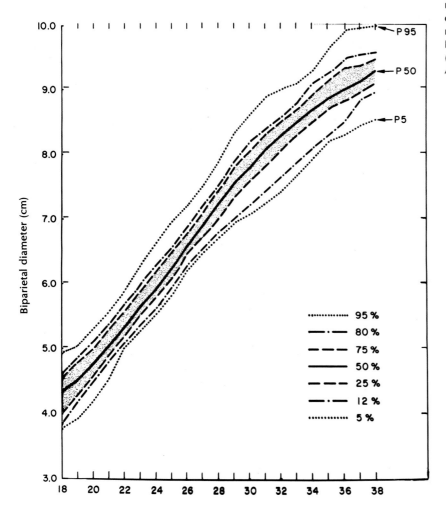

FIG. 41-2. Gestational age as X-coordinate of graph depicting normal growth of the biparietal diameter (*BPD*); maximum separation of large versus small BPDs between 30–33 weeks' gestation. (Sabbagha RE, Barton FB, Barton BA: Am J Obstet Gynecol 126:479, 1976)

GROWTH-ADJUSTED SONOGRAPHIC AGE

Sabbagha has demonstrated that the normal fetus tends to maintain an apparently predetermined cephalic growth pattern throughout pregnancy. On the basis of this concept, it is possible to assign a growth-adjusted sonographic age (GASA) that predicts gestational age within a ± 5-day range; it also allows division of cephalic growth curves into three basic ranks: 1) BPDs greater than the 75th percentile, 2) BPDs between the 25th–75th percentile, and 3) BPDs less than the 25th percentile. Variation in the external environment. (uteroplacental insufficiency) may alter the projected course somewhat; however, since cephalic growth is spared until the late phase in most cases of placental insufficiency, this predictable pattern is disrupted in only a few instances prior to 33 weeks.

To estimate the GASA, the clinician must order two cephalic measurements, the first at 20–26 weeks and the second at 31–33 weeks. Should the slope of cephalic growth be in excess of the 75th percentile, the fetal BPD is assumed to have been consistently large for gestation. In such a case, the gestational age assigned at the time of the first scan is reassigned to a gestational age consistent with a BPD at the 75th percentile (*i.e.*, earlier gestation) at the time of the original scan; to accomplish this, gestational age is reduced 7 days. In contrast, the fetus whose head growth slope is less than the 25th percentile is assumed to have had a BPD at the 25th or lower percentile at the time of the initial scan, and thus the gestational age is increased by 7 days. The original assignment is maintained if an average BPD growth slope (25th–75th percentile) is observed.

DETECTION OF ABNORMALITIES IN FETAL GROWTH

Intrauterine growth retardation (IUGR) may be a function of either intrinsic (chromosomal abnormalities, congenital anomalies, first trimester TORCH complex viral infections, or idiopathic) or extrinsic (uteroplacental insufficiency) factors. Although there are exceptions, growth retardation of the intrinsic type tends to be symmetrical, *i.e.,* both cephalic and chest–abdominal measurements are two or more standard deviations below the mean for gestational age. In contrast, the extrinsic growth retardation tends to be asymmetrically small, *i.e.,* cephalic head size is proportionately larger.

The *prenatal diagnosis of IUGR* is difficult. A high clinical index of suspicion is essential, particularly if ultrasound is to be used to maximum benefit. Maternal failure to gain 2 lb/month in the third trimester and markedly retarded fundal height growth in a patient with established dates are clinical warning signs. Maternal vascular disease is the most commonly associated clinical problem, accounting for approximately 20%–30% of cases. Unfortunately, most of the remaining 70%–80% of cases are idiopathic or are associated with congenital infections (20%).

CEPHALOMETRY

Although it is clinically useful to detect slowing of cephalic growth, total reliance on serial cephalometry can be misleading. Measurements of the abdominal circumference or total intrauterine volume may provide additional information. While serial scanning is theoretically ideal, clinical application may be difficult for a number of reasons. The precision of the serial determinations may vary; clinical problems may not become apparent until after 26 weeks' gestation; slowing of cephalic growth may be a late manifestation of IUGR; and the pattern of fetal growth retardation may vary.

If risk factors for impaired fetal growth do not appear until the third trimester and an early BPD measurement is not available, the clinician must accept the $\pm$ 14–21 day range of prediction for a single scan at 27 or more weeks' gestation. In addition, subsequent evaluation of cephalic growth is limited. Since gestational age is uncertain, growth evaluation is limited to a comparison with the mean population growth rate. Growth should average at least 2 mm/week up to 34 weeks and at least 1 mm/week measured over a 2–3 week interval, even in the lowest percentile ranking.

Serial cephalometry, although helpful, has a false-abnormal diagnosis rate of 18% (Table 41–6); fetuses with retarded cephalic growth but normal birth weight are thought to be normal. In contrast, approximately 9% of cases have normal cephalic measurements in the presence of birth weights below the normal range for gestation. These false-normal cases represent "cephalic sparing"; such fetuses are probably at greater risk for intrauterine death as a result of uteroplacental insufficiency.

GROWTH-ADJUSTED SONOGRAPHIC AGE, PERCENTILES

It may be possible to reduce the number of false-normal and false-abnormal results by using GASA in conjunction with abdominal circumference mesurements. GASA allows the physician to compare predicted with observed cephalic growth rather than simply comparing observed growth with a population mean growth rate. In addition, birth weight of less than 3000 g can be predicted in 5% of fetuses in the greater than 75th,

TABLE 41–6. DIAGNOSIS OF SMALL-FOR-GESTATIONAL AGE FETUS BY SERIAL ULTRASONIC CEPHALOMETRY

Weight	Cephalic Growth Patterns			
	Normal No. (%)*	Borderline† No. (%)*	Retarded‡ No. (%)*	Total
Appropriate for gestational age	220 (83)	18 (69)	21 (18)	259
Borderline or small for gestational age	22 (8)	4 (15)	16 (14)	42
Small for gestational age	24 (9)§	4 (15)	77 (68)	105
Total	266 (100)	26 (100)	114 (100)	406

* % is percent of column.
† Distribution of birth weights appears close to that of normal growth rate category.
‡ Difference between birth weights of normal versus retarded categories is highly significant ($P < 0.001$).
§ 9% false-normal secondary to cephalic sparing in a population with asymmetric retardation pattern.
(Modified from Campbell S., Dewhurst CJ: Lancet 2:1002, 1971)

in 15% of those in the 25th–75th, and in 55% of those in the less than 25th pecentile. Clearly, special evaluation efforts should be focused on the cases with cephalic growth patterns at less than the 25th percentile. IUGR associated with significant uteroplacental insufficiency is usually asymmetric. There is subcutaneous and organ (especially liver) wasting in the presence of cephalic sparing. A single BPD may fall within normal gestation-dependent limits for the population but may deviate at 31–33 weeks from that expected if GASA was determined.

ABDOMINAL CIRCUMFERENCE

Recently, it has become feasible to measure the fetal abdominal circumference at the level of the ductus venosus. Under normal circumstances, the ratio of the cephalic/abdominal circumferences is greater than 1:1 up to the 35th–36th week. If gestational age is precisely established, continued cephalic growth in the presence of poor abdominal growth suggests asymmetric retardation; in contrast, persistent cephalic and abdominal growth 2 or more standard deviations below the mean for gestation suggests symmetric retardation. Reexamination of the original series by Campbell and Dewhurst (Table 41–6) in which cephalic measurements, but not abdominal circumference measurements, were available suggests that approximately three-fourths (77/101) of fetuses with intrauterine growth retardation demonstrate a symmetric pattern with a low weight percentile and retarded cephalic growth. In future studies, it will be important to determine if these fetuses also have a low abdominal circumference percentile. Measurement of abdominal circumference at the level of the ductus venosus will clarify this issue in the future, particularly when cephalic growth is at less than the 25th percentile or when cephalic growth subsequent to GASA assignment is less than predicted.

TOTAL UTERINE VOLUME

Oligohydramnios accompanies most cases of significant IUGR. As a result, assessment of uterine volume (fetal and placental mass plus amniotic fluid) by measuring transverse and longitudinal diameters of the uterus has recently been advocated as a useful measure in diagnosis of this problem. A value more than 1.5 standard deviations below the mean for gestational age is highly suggestive of IUGR; a value of 1–1.5 standard deviations below the mean for gestation is a grey zone where the diagnosis is less secure. Recently, clinicians have begun to assess amniotic fluid pockets with real-time ultrasound. A pocket of fluid greater than 1 cm in diameter is helpful in ruling out growth retardation. For this more simplified approach, it is not necessary to know the precise gestational age as is required for total intrauterine volume comparisons.

SIGNIFICANCE OF MECONIUM IN AMNIOTIC FLUID

ANTENATAL MECONIUM

For many years, detection of amniotic fluid meconium was thought to be helpful in assessing antenatal fetal status. However, recent evidence suggests that the discovery of amniotic fluid meconium before early labor is usually not associated with poor fetal outcome. In fact, ten perinatal deaths occurred in a series of 392 patients with prolonged pregnancies, although all had clear amniotic fluid at the time of amniocentesis done within 7 days of delivery. Furthermore, a finding of meconium in the amniotic fluid cannot be used to distinguish acute and subsequently corrected fetal distress state from either a chronic ongoing one or simply the physiologic passage of meconium. Since antenatal detection of meconium requires amniocentesis or amnioscopy, the potential for complications, such as rupture of membranes, hemorrhage, and infection, that might be encountered at the time of amniocentesis or amnioscopy probably outweighs any potential benefit. The availability of more efffective noninvasive tools to assess fetal health has reduced the clinical significance of amniotic fluid meconium detected in the antenatal period.

INTRAPARTUM MECONIUM

It is generally accepted that the presence of meconium during labor when the fetus is in the vertex presentation is simply an indication that the fetus' condition should be more carefully evaluated. The passage of meconium was formerly considered a sign of great significance, but the recent trend is not to rely on it as an indication for intervention; rather, clinicians have begun to consider more specific indicators of fetal health such as intrapartum electronic monitoring and, where necessary, scalp blood sampling.

Meconium, when there are no other indictors of fetal distress, has been reported to be associated with perinatal mortality ranges up to 4.5%–8.8%. However, as early as 1962, Fenton and Steer noted that neonatal outcome is good in a great porportion of cases associated with meconium passage and suggested that more specific indicators be developed both to determine the significance of meconium and to diagnose fetal distress.

Three explanations for the passage of meconium have been proposed: 1) a normal event that occurs with progressive fetal maturation; 2) hypoxia-induced

peristalsis and sphincter relaxation; and 3) umbilical cord compression–induced vagal stimulation in mature fetuses. There does appear to be a link between gestational age and meconium passage. Meconium passage is infrequent prior to 32–34 weeks, and there is a significant increase in its passage after 38 weeks. The cause of the meconium passage may vary from patient to patient; in some cases it may result from a combination of causes. This may be the reason that no clear relationship has been demonstrated between its passage and fetal outcome.

Currently, the approach to management in the presence of meconium involves consideration of three variables: 1) the consistency of the meconium (old and thin versus new and particulate), 2) the time of its appearance (early labor versus late labor), and 3) its relationship to specific monitor patterns. Thick, particulate (fresh) meconium passed for the first time in late labor in association with nonremediable severe variable or late FHR decelerations is clearly ominous; but the presence of meconium alone is not a sign of fetal distress, nor is it predictive of outcome. More specific indicators of fetal asphyxia include nonremediable severe variable decelerations, late decelerations (particularly with poor baseline variability), or acidosis confirmed by scalp blood sampling.

INTRAPARTUM FETAL MONITORING

Definition of the term *fetal distress* was unclear until the early 1970s. In previous years, the presence of bradycardia, tachycardia, FHR irregularity, passage of meconium in vertex presentations, and falling or low estriol levels were accepted as evidence of fetal distress. Although all are associated with an increased incidence in fetal morbidity and mortality, they are nonspecific indicators; many babies born in the presence of these indictors demonstrate no abnormality (false-positive), while many asphyxiated babies are born with no meconium or stethoscopically detected FHR alterations.

INDICATIONS FOR FETAL MONITORING

The indications for fetal monitoring vary with the attitudes and experience of both the patient and the medical attendant. Since traditional auscultatory techniques are not reliable in evaluating or predicting fetal status, one could logically insist that all patients in labor be monitored routinely. The need for monitoring among the high-risk group is obvious, and is generally accepted. Among the low-risk group, fetal compromise is unusual, but it is also unexpected; fetal monitoring would appear to have special importance in permitting instant diagnosis when it does occur. In both groups of patients, continuous monitoring not only can demonstrate intrauterine conditions that are ominous, but also, when the tracing pattern is normal, can prevent intervention because of presumed problems that do not actually exist. In addition, routine monitoring has other distinct advantages. It eliminates the need for high nurse/patient ratios to maintain continuous surveillance of fetal cardiovascular status; interruption of progress in labor can be reviewed retrospectively as soon as it is noted so that uterine activity can be evaluated immediately when progress is found to be abnormal; a permanent record is available for educational purposes, for peer review, or for review at a later date. Of greatest practical benefit, the technique detects important pathologic patterns that cannot be revealed by traditional methods.

Despite the aforementioned benefits of routine fetal monitoring, acceptance is not universal. Many patients and physicians insist that routine monitoring cannot be justified because fetal complications are considered unusual in the low-risk population and, furthermore, that the technique disrupts the "natural labor processes" and increases the likelihood of intervention, including cesarean section, for presumed fetal distress. Two studies by Haverkamp support these contentions, since it was concluded that electronic monitoring provides no benefit over traditional stethoscopic methods. Both studies involving patients primarily at 30–34 weeks have certain drawbacks that limit the clinical application of the conclusions. Although there were no differences in Apgar scores or in neonatal morbidity and mortality, the studies were conducted with a ratio of nurses to patients so high that it is virtually impossible to duplicate in most institutions; the incidence of ominous FHR patterns was higher in the monitored group than in the "blinded" or control group, implying higher initial risk in the monitored women, but the validity of the monitoring diagnoses was supported by subsequent low Apgar scores in these newborns; in the monitored group, there were more cesarean sections for indications other than fetal distress, but the monitor can hardly be considered responsible. Banta and Thacker reached conclusions similar to those of Haverkamp. Their study, too, has been seriously challenged; Neutra, in an extensive appraisal, found that continuous monitoring does reduce neonatal mortality. It is concluded that continuous monitoring would prevent one death for every 1000 births at term. The major reduction in intrapartum mortality as a consequence of monitoring is in preterm labors.

INSTRUMENTATION

FHR and uterine activity may be monitored by either external (indirect) or internal (direct) methods (Fig. 41–3). The external method provides less information, but it is noninvasive and has wider clinical application.

FIG. 41-3. Methods of monitoring fetal heart rate and uterine contractions. *A.* Indirect method (ultrasonocardiography). Signals derive from external transducers attached to maternal abdomen. *B.* Direct method. Recordings are made from electrode applied directly to fetus. A transcervical intrauterine pressure transducer is used. Data obtained by direct method are the most precise. (Richard H. Paul)

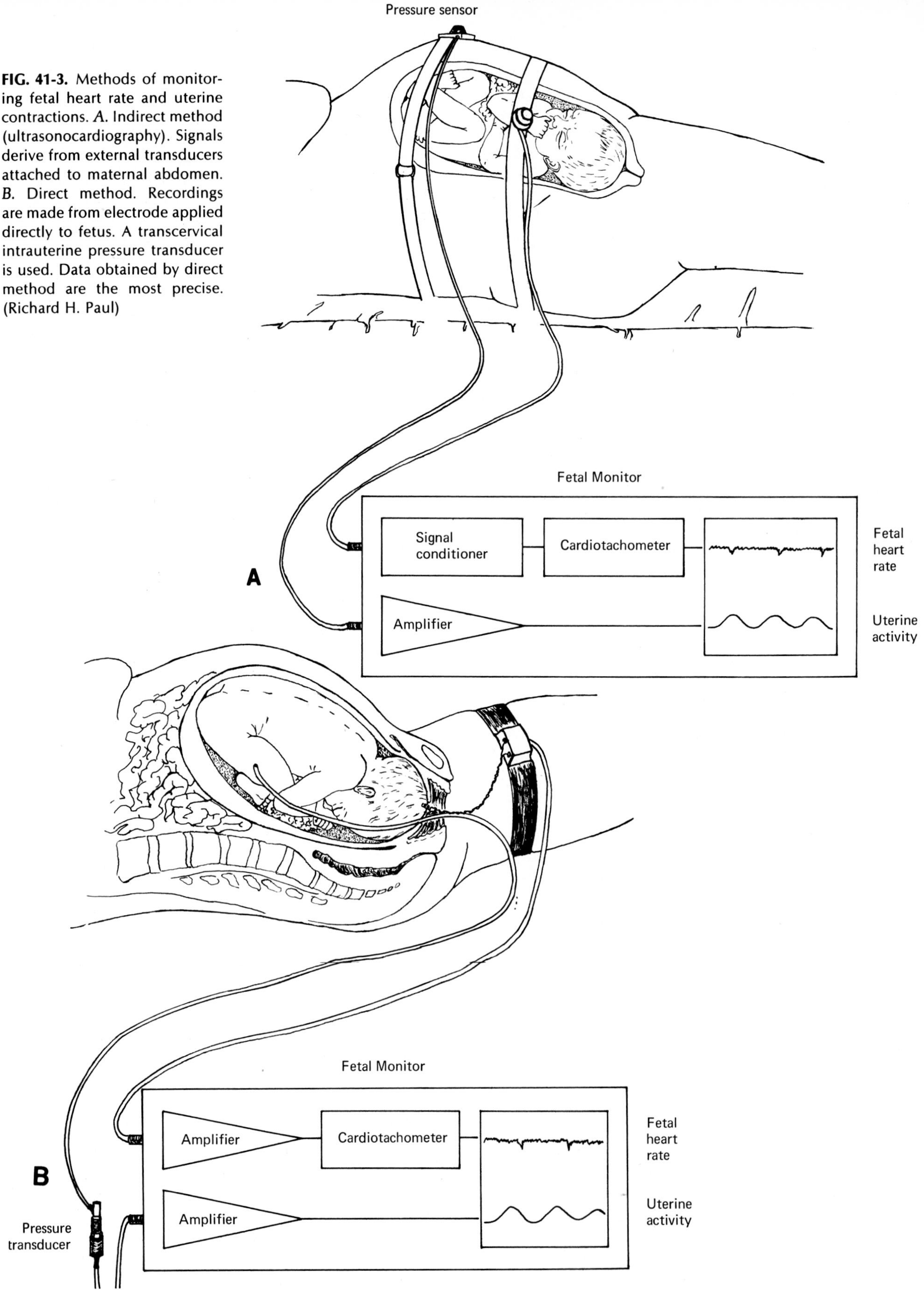

FIG. 41-4. Fetal heart rate recorded (*top*) from electrode applied directly to fetus and (*bottom*) by indirect ultrasound method. Records were made simultaneously. Precision and accuracy of interval measurement are much greater when direct method is used. (Richard H. Paul)

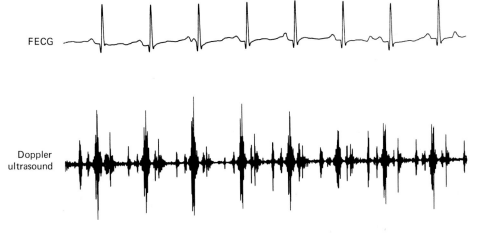

FECG

Doppler ultrasound

Internal monitoring requires that the membranes be ruptured and that the cervix be sufficiently dilated to permit insertion of the intrauterine catheter and application of the fetal scalp electrode. Also, internal monitoring has resulted in such complications as uterine perforation and fetal injury. Amnionitis and postpartum endometritis are both more frequent following internal monitoring, but much of the increased risk results from the indication for internal monitoring (*e.g.,* prolonged rupture of membranes, prolonged induction of labor) rather than from the invasive procedure *per se.*

For *external monitoring,* the techniques available for FHR assessment include phonocardiography, abdominal fetal electrocardiography, and ultrasonocardiography; uterine contractions are detected by tocodynamometry. Instruments are applied to the abdominal wall and are held in place by belts. Unfortunately, many patients are inappropriately kept in the supine posture in the belief that the recordings are improved; however, excellent records can be obtained if the patient is tilted to one side. The Trendelenburg position, as may be needed in cases of cord prolapse or compression, can make it difficult to obtain adequate external records, and internal monitoring may be mandatory. External monitoring may be impractical when the patient is markedly obese or agitated.

Internal monitoring provides more detailed and more accurate records that are more readily interpreted and are not affected by the patient's position. Uterine activity is measured by means of an open-ended fluid-filled polyethylene catheter inserted through the cervix into the uterine cavity, and connected to a strain gauge transducer. This is not always needed, but it can be especially valuable for monitoring uterine activity when labor is augmented or induced, or if the patient is obese or agitated, or if the external record is not clear or appears to be spu-

rious. Fetal scalp electrodes of the spiral or clip type are commonly used to record FHR. They have the same advantages and disadvantages as the intrauterine pressure catheter. Their most important advantage is the clarity with which FHR variability is recorded, an evaluation that is rarely possible by external FHR monitoring (Figs. 41–4 and 41–5). In clinical practice, the combination of a fetal scalp electrode and external tocotransducer is commonly employed.

CONTINUOUS FHR MONITORING

Traditional auscultatory techniques to evaluate fetal cardiovascular status are no longer acceptable; few actual measurements are recorded, and the predictive correlation with outcome appears to be poor. In a review of 24,863 labors, Benson *et al.* concluded that there is no single auscultatory indicator of fetal distress, except in the most extreme circumstances.

The technique of continuous electronic FHR monitoring has been developed independently by a number of investigators. The classification proposed by Hon is most universally accepted in the United States. It is most applicable to intrapartum monitoring; however, it can also be applied to antenatal FHR monitoring, most notably in the oxytocin challenge test (OCT) or contraction stress test (CST).

Instantaneous Measurement of FHR

In the nonstressed state, the FHR reflects the interplay of cardioaccelerator and cardiodecelerator reflexes (Fig. 41–6). Analysis of the FHR involves evaluation of two elements (Fig. 41–7): 1) baseline FHR, which is the portion of the FHR that occurs between uterine contractions or periodic changes in the FHR; and 2) periodic FHR changes, which are short-term (less than 10 min) alterations in FHR that are asso-

ciated with uterine contractions or occur in association with fetal movement.

Baseline FHR. There are two major elements, rate and variability, in the baseline FHR. The baseline rate is established by the predominant rate, independent of decelerations or accelerations, in a 10-min interval; a new baseline is established only if a change persists longer than 10 min. The normal FHR ranges 120–160. Tachycardia is FHR in excess of 160, bradycardia, FHR less than 120.

Of the three elements, baseline rate, baseline variability, and periodic change, baseline FHR is the least predictive. The differential diagnosis of fetal tachycardia includes

Immaturity
Prematurity

Maternal fever
Minimal fetal hypoxia
Uterine tachysystole
Drugs (*e.g.,* atropine, scopolamine)
Arrhythmias
Hyperthyroidism
β-mimetic tocolysis

Tachycardia may be an early manifestation of distress but of itself is not an indicator for intervention. Bradycardia may be seen normally in postdate pregnancies and occasionally with fetal heart block; with few exceptions, it is not a cause for intervention, particularly in the presence of good baseline variability.

Current fetal monitors record an FHR point on the monitor graph for each cardiac R–R interval, using the formula 60/R–R interval; an R–R interval of 500 msec corresponds to an FHR of 120. In the normal resting state, the duration of each interval varies, which is termed *short-term* or *beat-to-beat variability*. In addition to short-term or beat-to-beat variability, there is

FIG. 41-5. Manner in which fetal heart rate is depicted on monitor chart when recorded by direct (*top*) and indirect (*bottom*) methods. (Richard H. Paul)

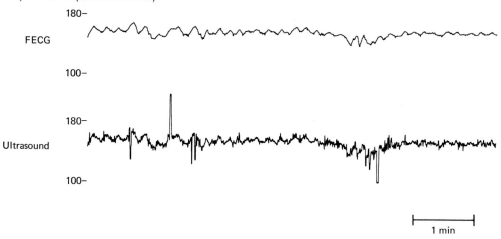

FIG. 41-6. Nervous control mechanisms affecting fetal heart rate (*FHR*). Normal rate at right results from interplay of stimuli from autonomic nervous system. Loss of controlling mechanisms may result from hypoxia and central nervous system damage. (Richard H. Paul)

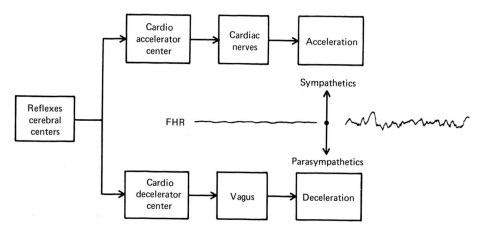

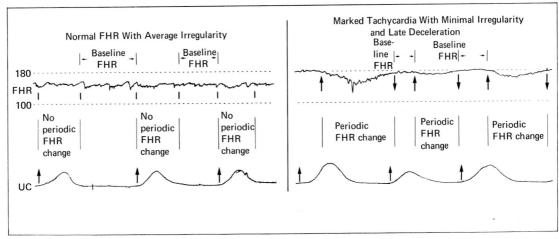

FIG. 41-7. Evaluation of fetal heart rate (*FHR*) is subdivided into control (nonstressed or baseline) and stress (periodic) portions. Baseline rate may correspond to time between contractions (UC), as shown at *left*, or may be only a short interval, as shown at *right*. (Hon EH: An Atlas of Fetal Heart Rate Patterns. New Haven, Harty Press, 1968)

long-term variability, which occurs as reasonably predictable periodic oscillations or irregularities of the FHR with a frequency of 2–6 cycles/min. The magnitude of long-term variability is usually measured by the vertical distance in beats/min between peak and nadir of the 2–6 cycle oscillations. Normal values for short-term and long-term variability are ±2–3 beats/min and 6–15 beats/min, respectively. The following is the differential diagnosis of decreased variability when the long-term variability is less than 6 beats/min:

Hypoxia (early)
Drugs
  Tranquilizers (diazepam)
  Narcotics
  Atropine, scopolamine
  Barbiturates
  Local anesthetics
  Magnesium sulfate
Prematurity, immaturity
Tachycardia
Physiologic sleep
Uterine tachysystole (prolonged)
Cardiac and central nervous system anomalies
Arrhythmias, especially of nodal type

Periodic FHR Changes. Accelerations and decelerations are included under the general heading, periodic change. They are of short duration (less than 10 min) and must be distinguished from tachycardia and bradycardia, respectively. Periodic changes usually occur repetitively in association with contractions or in association with fetal movement. In contrast, tachycardia and bradycardia persist for greater than 10 min and bear no apparent relationship to contractions or fetal activity.

Accelerations. Commonly seen in response to fetal movement, periodic accelerations are graphically represented by short-term increases in the heart rate above baseline. Accelerations preceding or following decelerations are frequently called "shoulders."

Decelerations. In contrast to accelerations, decelerations are represented by periodic slowing of the FHR in association with uterine contractions. The classification of decelerations (Fig. 41–8) is based upon evaluation of the uniformity of shape, magnitude, and timing of a series of decelerations versus the shape, magnitude, and timing of a group of uterine contractions. Decelerations are a cardiovascular response to stress or insult.

Uniform decelerations are of two types, early and late. In both kinds, there is a definite and recurring relationship between the wave form of the uterine contraction and that of the FHR deceleration. The FHR wave form is relatively symmetric, and the onset and offset of the deceleration have a uniform temporal relationship to the onset and offset of the uterine contraction. The descending limb of the FHR curve drops at a rate similar to (or less than) the ascending limb of the associated uterine contraction curve. In general, the magnitude of the deceleration is related to the magnitude of the associated contraction.

Uniform decelerations are subdivided into late and early deceleration categories according to their temporal relationship to the uterine contraction. Deceleration uniformity is more significant in assigning a group of decelerations to a particular category than is the temporal relationship between the peak of the uterine contraction and the nadir or low point of the decelera-

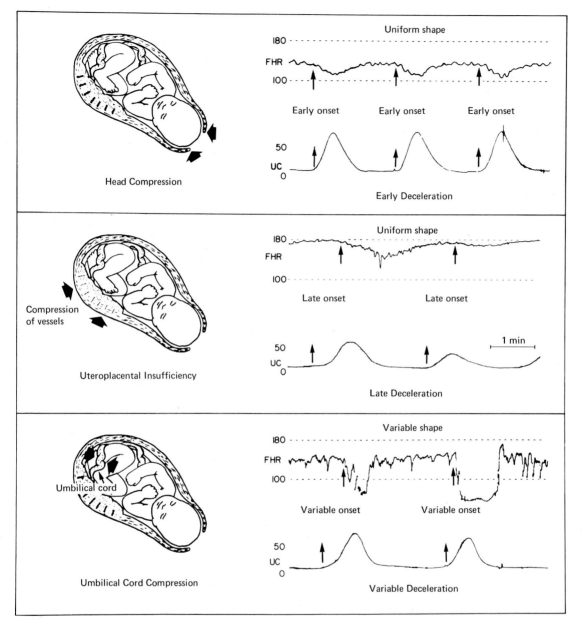

FIG. 41-8. Deceleration patterns of fetal heart rate (*FHR*) and their implied causative mechanisms. Intrauterine pressure (*UC*) is measured in millimeters of mercury. (Hon EH: An Atlas of Fetal Heart Rate Patterns. New Haven, Harty Press, 1968)

tion. Variable decelerations may bear a late temporal relationship to uterine contractions, but, as the name implies, there are differences in shape, magnitude, or temporal relationship, or in all three.

Early decelerations are uniform decelerations whose shape and characteristics reflect or mirror the shape

and intensity of associated uterine contraction curves. This pattern, which is most commonly observed during the latter half of the first stage of labor, is due to vagal stimulation associated with fetal head compression (Cushing's reflex); the effect is reduced or blocked by administration of atropine. Early decelerations are not common clinically, but they must be distinguished from late decelerations.

Late decelerations are uniform decelerations whose shape and characteristics, as determined by evaluation

TABLE 41-7. CHARACTERISTICS OF EARLY, LATE, AND VARIABLE DECELERATIONS

Early Decelerations	Late Decelerations	Variable Decelerations
Onset is early (usually first 15 sec) in contracting phase.	Onset is late (20–30 sec lag) in contracting phase.	Onset bears a variable time relationship to beginning of the associated contraction; onset may be early or late; however, most are early.
Offset almost coincides with offset of uterine contraction.	Offset is delayed after offset of contraction (latent period).	Offset may be coincidental or delayed with respect to offset of associated contraction.
Duration is usually less than 90 sec.	Duration is usually less than 90 sec.	Duration varies from a few seconds to minutes
FHR and variability are usually normal.	Baseline FHR is usually in normal or moderate tachycardia range; in terminal phases of asphyxia, baseline may be in bradycardia range.	Baseline FHR is usually in normal range, unless repeated and severe.
FHR usually does not fall below 100 beats/min (variable or combined pattern should be suspected if rate falls to less than 100)		FHR usually falls below 100 beats/min; decelerations to as low as 50–60 beats/min are not uncommon.
Magnitude of drop in FHR should reflect (mirror image) relative intensity of associated contractions when decelerations are viewed as a group.	Magnitude of drop in FHR should, particularly in early stages of appearance, reflect relative intensity of associated contractions when declerations are viewed as a group.	Magnitude of deceleration does not necessarily reflect relative intensity of associated contractions when decelerations are viewed as a group.
		"Take-off" accelerations frequently precede variable declerations; a similar "overcompensation shoulder" acceleration frequently marks their conclusion.
		Note: Although decelerations seen in the second stage of labor undoubtedly are associated with head compression, their wave form dictates that they be called variable decelerations.

of a group of decelerations, reflect the shape and intensity of uterine contraction curves. They begin at or after the peaks of contractions, some 20–30 seconds after onset of contractions. Failure to adhere to this rigid definition results in overdiagnosis. The presumed etiology is uteroplacental insufficiency.

Variable (nonuniform) decelerations are characterized by a wave form that does not reflect the shape or intensity of associated uterine contraction curves. They may be sporadic, varying in time of onset relative to uterine contractions, and tend to be angular and saw-toothed in appearance; the descending limb of the deceleration falls faster than the ascending limb of the associated uterine contraction rises. Variable decelerations are presumably the result of umbilical cord compression. Since they are vagally mediated, much of the deceleration may be abolished by the administration of atropine; this is, however, not recommended.

The characteristics of early, late, and variable decelerations are noted in Table 41–7.

Clinical Application

The clinical evaluation of a fetal monitor tracing should begin with an evaluation of uterine activity. Uterine contractions serve as useful reference points for the analysis of FHR response because of their repetitive and stressful nature. Contractions reduce the exchange of carbon dioxide and oxygen between the maternal and fetal compartments, and either physically compress the fetal head or compress the umbilical cord between the presenting part and maternal pelvis. In most instances, a fetus can easily tolerate the respiratory stress of three to four contractions per 10-minute interval. The monitor can also provide reassuring signs, which include the following:

Normal baseline rate 100–150
Normal baseline variability
Accelerations with fetal movement
Prompt return to baseline with no evidence of de-

creasing baseline variability or increasing baseline rate when decelerations are variable

Uterine tachysystole is a form of excessive uterine activity in which contractions occur at a frequency of five or more per 10-min interval. Elevation of resting uterine tonus also imposes fetal respiratory stress. Usually, the resting tonus (measured by intrauterine pressure catheter) is less than 10–15 mm Hg. Methods that may reduce "relative" or absolute excess uterine activity are listed in Table 41–8.

Variable decelerations also cause fetal respiratory stress; during the deceleration, carbon dioxide tension rises while oxygen tension decreases. Some decelerations are quite dramatic, dropping 50 or more beats below the baseline. In term pregnancies, such decelerations are of minimal significance unless they repeatedly fall below 70 beats/min (probable complete cord compression) and last longer than 1 min. A scheme to evaluate the severity of variable decelerations is summarized in Table 41–9. Reassurance that the fetus is compensating well is provided by serial observations of good baseline variability and the lack of a relative increase in baseline rate. Uterine tachysystole may act in a cumulative manner to aggravate the respiratory insult of variable decelerations. The management scheme frequently employed to modify the occurrence or severity of variable decelerations is outlined in Table 41–10.

Late decelerations are the most ominous of all deceleration wave forms. This pattern suggests fetal hypoxia, which may be chronic or subacute. Late decelerations associated with chronic uteroplacental insufficiency (maternal diabetes, preeclampsia, or intrauterine growth retardation) are commonly associated with a lack of baseline variability. In contrast, acute and usually remediable uteroplacental insufficiency may be observed following prolonged spontaneous or oxytocin-induced uterine tachysystole. Acute uteroplacental insufficiency may also be noted in association with maternal supine hypotension or dehydration. In such instances, the late decelerations are commonly associated with normal baseline variability. Table 41–11 summarizes clinical observations commonly associated with late decelerations with good variability versus those with poor baseline variability.

Therapy for late decelerations is largely related to prevention. Since most occur as the result of postural hypotension, excessive use of oxytocin, or the administration of epidural anesthesia without intravenous volume loading, implementation of protocols to minimize these complications is extremely important (Table 41–12).

Intervention for fetal distress is usually motivated by repetitive, nonremediable, severe variable decelerations or late decelerations that do not respond to classic therapeutic maneuvers. In general, the clinician has 30 min in which to modify the observed pattern. Observations that should hasten intervention include prolongation of decelerations or rapidly disappearing baseline variability. In some instances, reassuring signs, such as persistent normal baseline variability, lack of a relative increase in baseline rate, and rapid ascent from the deceleration nadir, may allow delay in intervention, particularly in association with variable decelerations. In contrast, preterm labor or intrauterine growth retardation may hasten intervention, since the fetus has limited reserves.

In considering intervention for late decelerations, the clinician must differentiate late decelerations that are associated with baseline variability (frequently remediable) from those in which there is no variability (nonremediable and usually chronic). In the former instance, position change, hydration, oxygen, and, where possible, reduction of oxytocin infusion is effective. Associated scalp blood pH values may be surprisingly high, but this should not lull the physician into a

TABLE 41–8. MANAGEMENT SCHEME FOR EXCESS UTERINE ACTIVITY

Possible Cause	Therapy
Oxytocin (excess)	Lower dose; infusion pumps for precision in dose.
Lumbar epidural	Fluid preload; avoid supine hypotension
Paracervical block	Low dose and concentration; avoid in fetal acidosis
Contraction coupling and tripling	Lateral position, fluids; if severe, consider β-mimetic or magnesium sulfate

TABLE 41–9. SCHEME TO ASSIST IN EVALUATING SEVERITY OF VARIABLE DECELERATIONS

	Duration of Deceleration		
Nadir of Deceleration	<30 Sec	30–60 Sec	>60 Sec
>80 beats/min	Mild	Mild	Moderate*
70–80 beats/min	Mild	Moderate*	Moderate–severe*
<70 beats/min	Moderate	Moderate–severe*	Severe

* Frequency of less than two such decelerations in 30 min reduces severity one grade.
(Modified from Kubli FW, Hon EH, Khazin AF et al.: Am J Obstet Gynecol 104:1190, 1969)

sense of false security. Without appropriate management, baseline variability will disappear. The presence of late decelerations associated with little or no variability (Fig. 41–9) increases the likelihood of fetal metabolic acidosis.

FETAL SCALP BLOOD SAMPLING

Although the value of continuous fetal monitoring in predicting outcome is generally accepted, there is justifiable concern regarding the rising incidence of cesarean section for fetal distress that has followed the widespread use of electronic monitoring. A relationship between FHR and scalp blood acid–base values has been recognized, but it may be difficult to predict the pH of a fetus who develops an abnormal FHR pattern. This consideration is perhaps most valid in the presence of late decelerations, ordinarily thought to reflect fetal hypoxemia but found to be associated with normal scalp blood pH values in approximately 50%–60% of cases. In some instances, physician response to seemingly dramatic variable decelerations is inappropriately aggressive. It has thus been proposed that fetal scalp blood pH determinations be used to complement electronic fetal monitoring and assess fetal status more accurately when a monitor pattern suggests fetal distress; a reassuring pH value may prevent unnecessary intervention.

The clinical use of scalp blood sampling is based on the assumption that most cases of fetal acidosis are due to asphyxia. In the fetus, pH determination is a better clinical predictor of asphyxia than is fetal oxygen assessment. The normal fetal scalp blood pH in the first stage of labor is 7.25–7.45. A value of 7.20–7.24 is considered intermediate, whereas a value of less than 7.2 is considered abnormal. In most cases, a scalp pH of less than 7.16 results in an abnormal Apgar score.

Clinically, a value of 7.25 is normal. A repeat sample need not be collected unless the FHR pattern deteriorates. A value of 7.20–7.24 requires repeated sampling at 15- to 20-min intervals, depending on the severity of distress indicated by the FHR pattern and the trend of the pattern. Decreasing serial pH values are an indication for delivery. A value less than 7.20 is also an indication for delivery unless the FHR pattern is improving. If maternal acidosis is likely, maternal blood pH should be measured to rule out maternal contribution to a low fetal pH. A high or low maternal pCO_2 may modify the fetal scalp blood pH. In contrast, accumulation of fixed acids in the maternal compartment has a less dramatic effect, since charged particles (H^+) cross the placenta more slowly than does highly soluble CO_2.

Fetal scalp blood sampling is potentially important when fetal distress is suspected, mild late decelerations are observed, or there is no baseline variability.

TABLE 41–10. MANAGEMENT SCHEME FOR VARIABLE DECELERATION

Therapy	Objective
Change maternal position	Reduce cord compression
Decrease uterine activity by decreasing oxytocin, or administering β-mimetic, or magnesium sulfate	Increase uteroplacental flow; increase recovery time for oxygen and carbon dioxide exchange
Administer maternal oxygen	Increase maternal–fetal oxygen gradient
Prepare for intervention	Reduce interval from decision to delivery
Elevate presenting part if all else fails	Reduce cord compression temporarily

TABLE 41–11. CLINICAL IMPLICATIONS OF GOOD VS. POOR BASELINE VARIABILITY WITH LATE DECELERATIONS

Good Baseline Variability	Poor Baseline Variability
Probably normal fetus	Chronic insufficiency, e.g., preeclampsia, diabetes
Demonstrable insult (CLE, PCB, hypotension, hyperstimulation)	Aggravated by added stress of labor
Usually remediable	Usually not remediable

CLE, Continuous lumbar epidural anesthesia. *PCB*, Paracervical block.

TABLE 41–12. MANAGEMENT SCHEME FOR FETUS WITH LATE DECELERATIONS

Therapy	Objective
Decrease uterine activity	Improve recovery time for oxygen and carbon dioxide exchange
Place mother in lateral decubitus position	Increase uteroplacental blood flow
Provide oxygen, 5–7 liters/min	Increase maternal–fetal oxygen gradient
Maternal blood volume expander	Correct hypotension; increased uteroplacental blood flow
Prepare for operative delivery	Reduce decision–delivery interval

In some instances, the fetal pH is unexpectedly low. However, the issue is not always clear. Fetal blood sampling is not possible in all cases. A number of conditions must be met: the membranes must be ruptured, the cervix must be at least 2 cm dilated, and the head must be engaged in the maternal pelvis. It may be difficult to procure an adequate sample, particularly

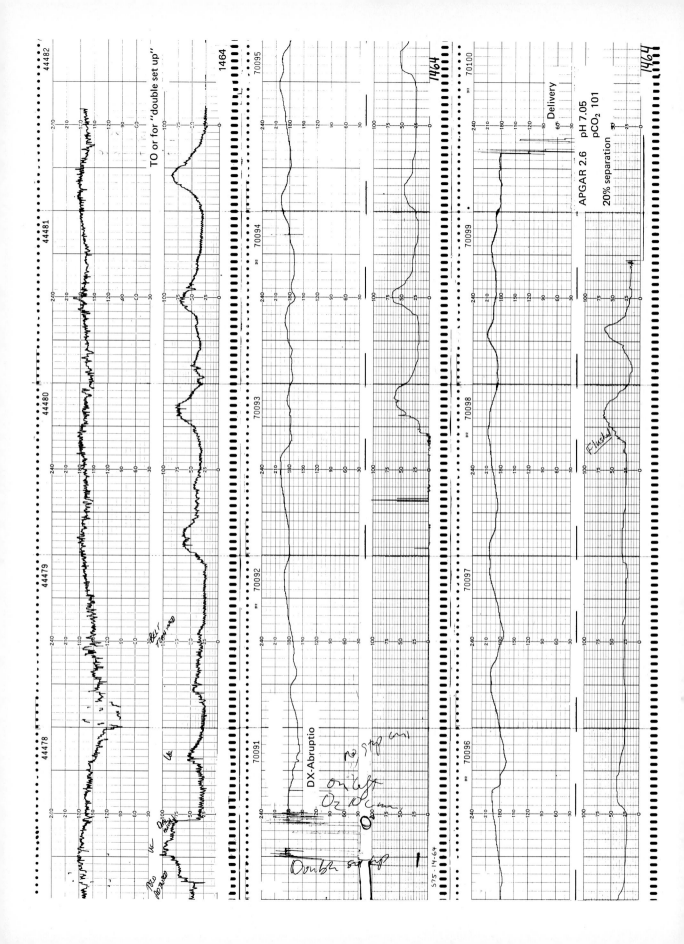

◄ **FIG. 41-9.** Fetal heart rate and uterine contraction data in a patient with placental abruption. Records in *top panel* were obtained by an external method; those in *lower two panels* by direct technique. Cesarean delivery. Newborn's condition is indicated at bottom right. (Richard H. Paul)

when fetal scalp hair is thick. Decisions usually require serial determinations unless a single value is significantly abnormal. Spurious results may occur in association with maternal acidosis or alkalosis, or in the presence of scalp vasoconstriction or molding. Finally, there is the issue of "monitoring the inevitable." Clearly, electronic monitoring, if properly interpreted, is highly predictive of the blood gas status of the fetus. The correlation of repetitive severe variable or late deceleration patterns with fetal acid–base balance is well established, especially when baseline variability is poor. Abnormal monitor patterns may precede acidosis by significant intervals. Although a normal scalp blood gas level may allow the clinician to delay a short period of time, the presence of persistent nonremediable severe variable or late decelerations or any magnitude almost uniformly predicts the eventual development of acidosis.

The clinician must consider the expected interval to delivery, the degree of distress shown by the pattern, and the presence of unusual risk (preterm labor or intrauterine growth retardation) in making decisions. When there is doubt, measurement of scalp blood gases may be of value. However, as proficiency in evaluating FHR tracings increases, the frequency of cesarean section for fetal distress decreases. The primary cesarean section rate for fetal distress at Prentice Women's Hospital and Maternity Center of the Northwestern University Medical Center is 1.5%. This is consistent with published rates in centers using scalp blood gases to complement the electronic fetal monitoring assessment.

ANTENATAL FETOPLACENTAL EVALUATION

Fetoplacental status may be assessed in the third trimester by biochemical (estriol or placental lactogen) or biophysical (nonstress test [NST], CST, or OCT) means. Usually, the result is reassurance that pregnancy can be safely continued. Most reassuring results are associated with favorable outcomes (low false-negative rate); the incidence of false-positive test results (no evidence of fetal or placental disease at delivery following an abnormal test result) ranges from 40%–60%. Intervention on the basis of a single abnormal result, particularly in the presence of uncertain fetal pulmonary status, should be unusual unless the maternal status deteriorates.

Fetal assessment tests should be ordered when there is a risk of uteroplacental insufficiency. By de-

sign, these tests provide little or no useful information in the evaluation of pregnancies in which perinatal morbidity and mortality subsequently result from trauma, congenital anomalies, or cord accidents. Since most assays and procedures are expensive, the clinician should ensure that the test to be ordered provides useful information that cannot be gained by other means. Historically, biochemical assay of urinary estriol has been the most commonly used test. In recent years, biophysical assessments of fetoplacental respiratory function (NST, CST, or tests of fetal activity) have largely replaced biochemical assays. In general, the NST and CST are considered reliable, can be performed at less frequent intervals, and are less expensive than currently available biochemical measures of fetoplacental function.

CONTRACTION STRESS TEST (OXYTOCIN CHALLENGE TEST)

Since uterine contractions are associated with a reduction in uteroplacental blood flow, spontaneous or oxytocin-induced contractions with a frequency of three in 10 min may be used clinically as a standard test of fetoplacental respiratory function. Stress of this magnitude has been proved clinically to be useful in separating the occasional fetus with suboptimal oxygen reserve from the vast majority of those with normal reserve, and it does not significantly compromise the normal fetus with adequate reserves. In contrast, a fetus who has chronic deprivation (uteroplacental insufficiency, *e.g.*, as a result of advanced diabetes, preeclampsia, or intrauterine growth retardation) presumably has diminished fetal reserve, which is manifest by repetitive late decelerations associated with most contractions of any frequency.

The CST or OCT is indicated in the following circumstances:

> Nonreactive NST
> Diabetes mellitus
> Preeclampsia
> Chronic hypertension
> Intrauterine growth retardation
> Postterm pregnancy (42+ weeks)
> History of previous stillbirth
> Narcotic addiction
> Sickle cell hemoglobinopathy
> Chronic pulmonary disease
> Organic heart disease
> Rh isoimmune disease
> Meconium-stained amniotic fluid

Testing is ordinarily initiated in pregnancies at high risk for uteroplacental insufficiency at 36–37 weeks, but it may begin as early as 28–30 weeks if intrauterine growth retardation is suspected or if maternal cardiovascular status is compromised.

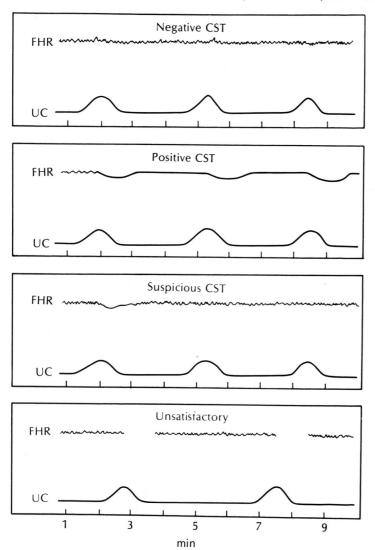

FIG. 41-10. Representation of possible contraction stress test (*CST*) outcomes. Upper channel of each strip is fetal heart rate (*FHR*); lower channel reflects uterine contractions (*UC*) in a 10-min time interval. (Depp R: In Sabbagha RE [ed]: Diagnostic Ultrasound Applied to Obstetrics and Gynecology. Hagerstown, MD, Harper & Row, 1980)

Oxytocin is not required if spontaneous uterine activity is sufficient; usually, it is necessary to induce uterine activity with intravenous oxytocin, and an infusion pump should be used for this purpose. FHR is recorded for a baseline (nonstress) period of 15–20 minutes. If three contractions per 10 min are observed within this time interval, oxytocin need not be administered. If three contractions are not observed, oxytocin is administered at an initial rate of 0.5 mU/min and increased by 2-mU increments until three contractions occur in a 10-minute interval. It is rarely necessary to exceed 20 mU/min.

The test results are negative (normal) if there are no late decelerations associated with at least three contractions within a 10-minute "window" (Figs. 41–10 and 41–11). Such a result is reassuring; it is associated with a 1–2/1000 false-normal rate. The proce-

dure is usually repeated weekly, but more frequent testing may be indicated for insulin-dependent diabetics, in moderate to severe preeclampsia, or in postdate pregnancies associated with oligohydramnios.

The presence of consistent and persistent late decelerations with most uterine contractions, regardless of their frequency, constitutes a positive CST result (Fig. 41–12). This is often associated with decreased baseline variability and a lack of FHR accelerations with fetal movement. Since positive results on a CST indicate uteroplacental insufficiency, delivery should be accomplished within a relatively short interval if the fetal lungs are mature. It should be remembered, however, that approximately 30%–60% of such test results are actually false-positive (false-abnormal); if allowed to labor subsequently, these patients may demonstrate no further late decelerations. For this

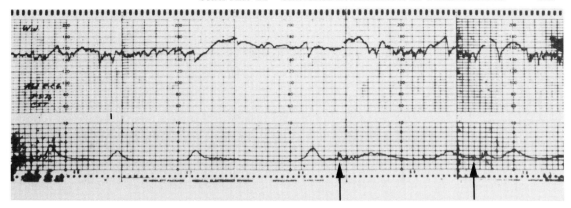

FIG. 41-11. Reactive (negative) result of contraction stress test using abdominal EKG as source. Lower channel reflects uterine contractions of 40- to 60-sec duration. Small superimposed peaks represent fetal movement. Fetal heart rate (FHR) baseline (upper channel) is 145–150. Note accelerations of FHR in response to fetal movement (*arrows*) on lower channel. The estimated magnitude of accelerations is 25–30 beats/min. (Depp R: In Sabbagha RE [ed]: Diagnostic Ultrasound Applied to Obstetrics and Gynecology. Hagerstown, MD, Harper & Row, 1980)

reason, it may be safe to attempt vaginal delivery if it is possible to rupture the membranes, apply a direct scalp electrode, and allow the patient to labor in a lateral decubitus position. If not, cesarean section should be considered.

If the lungs are immature, fetal status can also be evaluated by daily determinations of plasma or urinary estriol levels; the pregnancy may be allowed to continue as long as the estriol is stable or rising. Although a positive CST result is less predictive (30%–60% false-positive) than a negative one (99% true-negative), the probability of a true-positive diagnosis is improved if the FHR fails to accelerate with fetal movement. Most women who exhibit a positive OCT result accompanied by accelerations with a magnitude of at least 15 beats/min in response to fetal movement can tolerate labor or some delay until delivery. If there are no accelerations and little or no baseline variability, it is unlikely that the supplemental use of serial estriol measurements will be helpful in allowing the pregnancy to continue until fetal maturity is reached; it is also unlikely that labor will be tolerated without further evidence of late decelerations.

NONSTRESS TEST

Although the CST and OCT are highly predictive and their results have a very low false-negative rate, they are time-consuming, require intravenous fluids and oxytocin, and are best performed in a labor unit. These procedures are therefore costly. Since it is unusual to find a positive CST or OCT result if a prior NST result is negative, a negative NST usually suffices for predictive purposes.

A reactive (negative) NST result is characterized by the presence of two or more accelerations of the FHR in 20 min or less. The accelerations must be at least 15 beats/min above the baseline; apparently, it does not matter if the accelerations follow spontaneous movement or are in response to manual stimulation. A

nonreactive (positive) NST result is characterized by fewer than two 15 beats/min accelerations in a 40-min time interval. If the fetus is not reactive within the first 20 min, the fetus should be stimulated artificially and observed for an additional 20 min before being designated nonreactive. This minimizes the possibility of lack of activity associated with fetal sleep cycles.

A reactive result on an NST is very reassuring. The false-negative rate approximates that of a CST; most series report a false-negative rate of 1–3/1000. There has been some concern that a necessary intervention may be delayed if the clinician waits for a nonreactive NST result. This concern does not seem realistic for several reasons. First, the NST appears to be a very conservative indicator of fetal status in that the abnormal rate is 35% for the NST versus 3% for the CST. This tenfold increase in the population judged to be at risk identifies a subset population that may be better served by the CST with the associated lower false-abnormal rate of its results. Second, there appears to be a gradation of nonreaction (decreasing acceleration magnitude, more obvious loss of baseline variability); clearly, the flatter the baseline, the less favorable the outcome. Since these changes are generally observed over time, a CST can be ordered to evaluate fetal status at a very early time in development of the nonreactive state. Third, most CSTs with false-positive results are characterized by a baseline that is reactive. Fourth, there does not appear to be an increase in perinatal mortality when patients who have a reactive NST result are compared with those who have a nonreactive

"36 wks"
fundus 27 cm
Oxytocin 1.2 mμ

42 y.o. G-5 P-2

IUGR

◄ **FIG. 41-12.** Positive response to contraction stress testing, indicating abnormality of fetal heart rate. Rate is unduly smooth, there is no acceleration associated with fetal movement (*FM*), and late decelerations are clearly evident in *lower panel.* (Richard H. Paul)

NST result followed by a negative CST result. Finally, from a practical standpoint, the diminished cost and the patient convenience of the NST allows the clinician to assess certain high-risk pregnancies more frequently and less expensively than is realistically possible if the CST is used as the primary test procedure.

The NST is usually used as a screening test. When results are reactive, tests may safely be repeated at weekly intervals; some clinicians repeat them more frequently in insulin-dependent diabetics, preeclamptics, and cases at high risk for intrauterine growth retardation. Approximately one-third of the test results are nonreactive, and such cases require a CST. Ninety percent of subsequent CSTs show negative results. Even the few who subsequently have a positive CST result have a good outcome. Most deaths are associated with preterm delivery.

FETAL ACTIVITY

Assessment of fetal activity has been used subjectively by clinicians for many years. Recently, it has been reconfirmed that fetal movements are an expression of fetal well-being. A sudden increase (cord compression or placental abruption) or a decrease (chronic uteroplacental insufficiency) in activity may precede fetal demise. Some have suggested that antepartum surveillance of patients with decreased fetal movement would be more beneficial in reducing perinatal morbidity than simply monitoring all classically high-risk patients. Total reliance on such a scheme is unlikely, however, since patients tend to observe a decrease in fetal movement as gestation progresses; patient reliability also varies.

ESTRIOL

Third trimester biochemical assessment of the fetoplacental unit is most commonly done by measuring either urinary or plasma estriol. Since estriol is the product of fetal and placental compartments, its assay had great theoretic potential. Prior to the early 1970s, serial urinary estriol assays were the only technique commonly used to evaluate fetal health. There are potential limitations, however, since factors not strictly related to fetal health may be associated with abnormal values.

As noted in Figure 18–5, estriol synthesis is complex. Each site in the synthesis pathway has the potential for disruption. Maternal precursors, largely pregnenolone (21-carbon steroid), serve as a substrate for the fetal adrenal synthesis of the 19-carbon steroid dehydroepiandrosterone sulfate (DHEAS). Fetal adrenal function is dependent on interaction between the fetal adrenal and the fetal hypothalamus–pituitary axis and, on occasion, suppression by exogenous steroids. Chronic low-for-gestational-age estriol values may be seen in association with anencephaly (presumed failure of central stimulation) or aplasia of the fetal adrenal.

DHEAS undergoes 16-α-hydroxylation largely in the fetal liver. This rate-limiting step accounts for approximately 90% of urinary estriol. 16-α-Hydroxy DHEAS then undergoes hydrolysis by placental sulfatase to 16-α-DHEA and is subsequently aromatized (introduction of three double bonds in ring A) to form estriol. Free estriol is conjugated to either the glucuronide or sulfate form in the maternal liver or kidney. Approximately one-half of the estriol conjugate is excreted into the enterohepatic circulation by means of bile. Intestinal bacteria hydrolyze the estriol conjugate to free estriol, which is then reabsorbed. As a result, liver or biliary disease or disturbance of gut flora (*e.g.*, by oral antibiotics) may reduce estriol levels detected in the maternal urine.

The analysis of urinary estriol is complex and time-consuming. The first step in analysis is acid or enzyme hydrolysis. Significant reduction of recovery occurs in the presence of the urinary antiseptic methenamine. Many laboratories correct for these recovery losses by using an internal standard of radioactive estriol-16-glucuronide; this policy, however, is not widespread.

Clinically, serial estriol determinations are most commonly employed in the management of pregnancy complicated by diabetes, hypertension, suspected intrauterine growth retardation, or postmaturity. Specimens are usually collected on a daily basis with diabetes and two to three times per week with the latter three conditions. Serial determinations are essential; a single value should virtually never be used for assessment or management. In most instances, serial values are compared to a standard curve. Abnormal patterns may be manifest in one of three patterns: 1) progressive downward slope; 2) rapid fall (35%–40% of baseline established by average of values for preceding 3 days); and 3) persistent low values. The clinician must be hesitant in acting immediately on the basis of low values, which can result from failure to collect a true 24-hour specimen, renal function impairment, or overestimation of gestational age. A high level of urinary glucose or methenamine therapy for cystitis may also be associated with false-abnormal values. Assay of 24-hour urinary creatinine excretion in parallel with estriol provides a reasonable internal standard to de-

termine if 24-hour collection is complete. Assessment of gestational age and renal function is also helpful.

Some clinicians have favored the calculation of an estriol/creatinine ratio from serial short-term urine collections. However, in those institutions still measuring estriols, the recent trend is toward plasma estriol assay. Plasma estriols may be assayed as 1) unconjugated (free) estriol, which comprises 8%–10% of total estriol; 2) total estriol; and 3) immunoreactive estriol. Patient unreliability in collecting a true 24-hour urinary specimen and convenience have provided the impetus for the use of plasma estriol assessment. Plasma estriol collection is rapid, simple, and complete. Rising or stable values within normal limits are reassuring. Unfortunately, false-positive results are common.

Plasma unconjugated estriol levels are primarily dependent upon fetoplacental production and secretion rates; they are therefore less affected by disorders of maternal liver or kidney. Distler *et al.* feel that plasma free estriol is the most useful of the plasma tests in the management of the pregnant diabetic. Total plasma estriol includes both the unconjugated and conjugated (glucuronides and sulfates) fractions. The assay includes solvent extraction or enzyme hydrolysis prior to radioimmunoassay. Assay time is 6–8 hours.

Some advocate the use of immunoreactive estriol, which reflects approximately 40% of total estriol. This assay has the advantage of eliminating the extraction process; thus, the assay time is considerably less than that for either total or unconjugated estriol. At the present time, clinical use of plasma estriol determinations is not widespread.

HUMAN PLACENTAL LACTOGEN

Human placental lactogen (hPL) is a single-chain polypeptide hormone (isolated by Higashi in 1961 and Josimovich and MacLaren in 1962) with a molecular weight of approximately 21,000 and a half-life of approximately 25 min. It is produced by the syncytiotrophoblast. Although the precise function of this hormone has not been determined, it does have inherent somatotrophic, lactogenic, mammotropic, and luteotropic activities. As a result, it has also been called *human chorionic somatomammotropin* (see Chapter 18). It is immunologically similar to human growth hormone.

The clinical significance of hPL is controversial. The level of hPL correlates best with placental weight; however, this is not consistent. The value of hPL in assessing placental integrity is limited. It was originally thought that hPL levels might be useful in predicting the outcome in patients with threatened abortion. However, many patients with low hPL values do not abort; the low values may result from clinical overassessment of gestational age. Real-time ultrasound is probably more accurate in predicting eventual outcome than is hPL; presence of an intact fetal sac or fetal heart motion is much more specific.

Levels of hPL have also been used to assess fetoplacental function in hypertensive diseases of pregnancy, diabetes, and postterm pregnancy, as well as to predict intrauterine growth retardation. There is a high false-positive and false-negative rate when hPL is used to assess these conditions. Furthermore, hPL levels do not necessarily fall prior to or immediately after intrauterine fetal death.

FETAL MATURITY ASSESSMENT

In 8%–15% of newborns who develop RDS, no prior effort was made to assess fetal pulmonary maturity or to assess gestational age correctly. Spontaneous preterm labor, premature rupture of the membranes, and high-risk pregnancies requiring preterm intervention for maternal–fetal indications account for most newborns delivered prior to functional pulmonary maturity.

AMNIOCENTESIS

Amniocentesis was first applied to clinical obstetrics as a means to evaluate fetal status in Rh isoimmune disease. It has subsequently been employed for a wide range of fetal evaluation procedures and is sometimes performed as early as 14–15 weeks' gestation. Midtrimester amniocentesis to detect the presence of inherited disorders is an increasingly common procedure (see Chapter 2). Evaluation of fetal cells contained in the amniotic fluid in the midtrimester allows the clinician to determine fetal sex and chromosome complement. Amniotic fluid may also be assayed for α-fetoprotein levels, which are particularly useful in the detection of open neural tube defects.

Later in pregnancy, usually after 22–24 weeks, amniocentesis is commonly employed to evaluate the severity of fetal involvement with Rh isoimmune disease (ΔOD_{450}) as discussed in Chapter 23, to assess fetal maturity (creatinine, ΔOD_{450}, osmolality, percent amniotic fluid cells stained orange by Nile blue), and, most recently, to predict fetal lung maturity (lecithin/sphingomyelin [L/S] ratio, shake test, lung profile) accurately.

Spectrophotometric analysis of amniotic fluid for an absorption peak at 450 mμ (bilirubin) is most typically used to determine the degree of fetal hemolysis associated with Rh isoimmune disease (see Chapter 23). The ΔOD_{450} in unaffected pregnancies is commonly 0 by 36–37 weeks; as a result, a value of 0 was accepted in the past as an indication of fetal maturity. This technique is no longer employed for this purpose, since the level may reflect maternal plasma bilirubin levels

rather than fetal hemolysis; also, the values do not correlate uniformly with fetal lung maturation.

Amniotic fluid creatinine level has also been used to estimate fetal maturity, a value of 2 mg/dl suggesting maturation. Most likely, rising levels reflect increasing maturation of fetal kidney and muscle mass. This determination suffers similar drawbacks to those of ΔOD_{450}.

Amniotic fluid osmolality has also been used. Values decrease approximately 1 mOsm/week after 20 weeks, as the contribution of hypotonic fetal urine to amniotic fluid increases. Like amniotic fluid creatinine, amniotic fluid osmolality levels decrease too slowly and too sporadically to provide an accurate assessment of gestational age or maturity.

Amniotic fluid cells stained with Nile blue are of two types: blue staining indicates epithelial cells; orange staining is most characteristic of fetal sebaceous gland debris. The presence of orange bodies in excess of 10% is usually associated with a fetal age of 35 or more weeks. Greater than 30% orange staining indicates the fetus is probably 36 or more weeks. Unfortunately, the test is limited by the tendency of cells to clump. Also, low values do not necessarily predict immaturity.

At present, the most commonly used indicators of fetal maturity are amniotic fluid L/S, shake test, or lung profile. It is more important clinically to predict functional pulmonary maturity than to predict gestational age at 36–37 weeks, as predicted by the previously mentioned determinations.

Amniocentesis Technique

In most institutions, amniocentesis is performed either with ultrasonic guidance to a fluid "pocket" or after a report that indicates the location of a "window" where the placenta will not be damaged by the amniocentesis needle.

The patient is instructed to empty her bladder. The abdomen is then prepared and draped. Local anesthetic is injected in the skin in the anterior abdominal wall at the most appropriate site. Amniotic fluid is aspirated under sterile conditions (Fig. 41–13) through a 20- to 22-gauge needle. Up to 30 ml is withdrawn and centrifuged to separate the fluid into supernatant and cell-rich fractions.

Complications of Amniocentesis

Complications are infrequent, and the benefits usually far outweigh the slight risk of maternal or fetal damage. Fetal complications include direct fetal trauma, cord hematoma, hemorrhage and preterm labor, and premature rupture of the membranes. Maternal complications include amnionitis, fetomaternal transfusion, and amniotic fluid embolism. Some investigators advocate the administration of anti–Rh_0 globulin to nonsensitized Rh-negative women at the time of am-

niocentesis; this seems appropriate, especially if the placenta is located on the anterior uterine wall. If the amniotic fluid obtained is significantly bloody, the specimen should be tested to determine if the blood is of fetal or maternal origin. If fetal, the FHR should be evaluated. Prompt delivery may be necessary if distress is noted at a point in gestation when fetal survival is likely.

LUNG MATURATION

The changes leading to maturation of the fetal lung are outlined on page 319. *Surfactant,* released by the lamellar bodies into the amniotic fluid, is a complex mixture of substances that act as a detergent to lower the alveolar surface tension, and so reduce the tendency of the alveoli to collapse. If delivery occurs before the fetal lungs are properly protected by surfactant, the neonate almost inevitably develops RDS (a clinical state of respiratory distress) or hyaline membrane disease (an autopsy finding of a hyaline membrane lining the pulmonary alveoli). The constituents of surfactant can be measured and show characteristic changes in concentration with advancing pregnancy. Eighty to 90% (by weight) of the lipid is phospholipid, of which lecithin is the major phospholipid (70%–80%). Protein (10%–20%) and carbohydrate (1%–2%) comprise the remainder of surfactant. Saturated dipalmitoyl lecithin (DPL) accounts for 50% of the total lecithin. Phosphatidylglycerol (PG*), phosphatidylinositol (PI), and phosphatidylcholine (PC) are acidic phospholipids that are critically important in stabilizing lecithin in the surfactant layer. Of these, PG seems to be most active; it first appears in the amniotic fluid at 35–36 weeks' gestation, and rapidly increases thereafter. Acetone-precipitated disaturated lecithin gradually increases as pregnancy advances; PI also increases up to 35–36 weeks when it peaks, declining thereafter.

L/S Ratio

Under ordinary circumstances, surface-active lecithin begins to appear in the amniotic fluid at approximately 24–26 weeks. Sphingomyelin appears earlier, and its concentrations are higher early in the third trimester. Since sphingomyelin concentrations change very little with advancing pregnancy, they can be used as an internal standard for lecithin by calculating the L/S ratio. Prior to 30–32 weeks in uncomplicated pregnancies, the ratio is generally less than 1.5. At 34–35 weeks, there is a fourfold rise in lecithin, while sphin-

---

* It is unfortunate that PG, long established as the acronym for prostaglandins, is now selected also to refer to phosphatidylglycerol. One would think that PGL, as used in Fig. 41–14, would be more suitable, but there appears to be no enthusiasm for deviating from the use of PG to designate both substances (Editor).

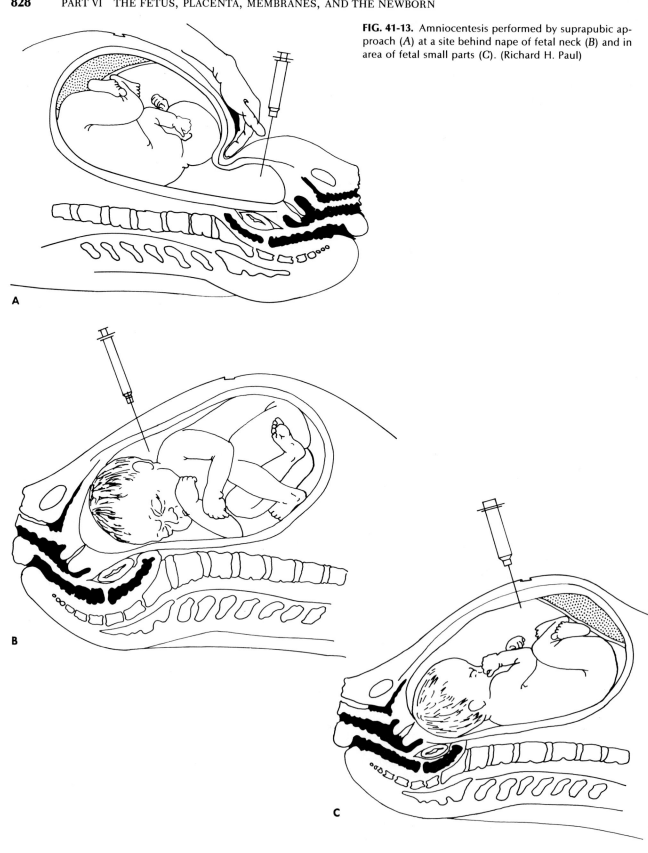

FIG. 41-13. Amniocentesis performed by suprapubic approach (A) at a site behind nape of fetal neck (B) and in area of fetal small parts (C). (Richard H. Paul)

gomyelin remains relatively stable or may decrease at the time of the lecithin surge. An L/S of 2, ordinarily obtained at 35–36 weeks' gestation, is clinically accepted as a reliable indicator of functional pulmonary maturity.

The timing of lung maturation may be altered in certain fetal or maternal diseases, and, in some cases, the factors that alter surfactant appearance become apparent only after delivery. Class A diabetes and intrauterine growth retardation are two such factors. It is thus not surprising that, in unselected patient series, the L/S ratio may bear no relation to gestational age or birth weight. Hence, the clinician can never reliably predict pulmonary maturity, even when sure of dates. Assessment of surfactant activity is therefore important, regardless of dates, whenever intervention for maternal or fetal indications, or inhibition of preterm labor is considered. This may be especially important early in the third trimester, since mature lung function is sometimes found as early as 28–30 weeks. Approximately 19% of women at risk for preterm delivery prior to 33 weeks, and 35% of those who are at risk to deliver between 33–36 weeks, demonstrate an L/S ratio in excess of 2.

An L/S ratio in excess of 2 correctly predicts pulmonary maturity in approximately 98% of cases; only 2% of cases with such a ratio develop RDS (false-mature/false-normal). Most false-mature results are associated with perinatal asphyxia, maternal diabetes, or Rh isoimmune disease. In contrast, an L/S ratio less than 2 is not as predictive; only 37%–46% of infants born within 72 hours of an L/S ratio less than 2 actually develop RDS (true-abnormal).

Lung Profile

Predictive reliance can usually be placed on the L/S ratio if the value is more than 2. In cases in which the L/S ratio is low or intermediate or in which the L/S ratio may give a spurious implication of lung maturity (gestational or class A to C diabetes, Rh disease, perinatal asphyxia), the lung profile, as suggested by Gluck's group, may be extremely helpful in predicting RDS. The profile consists of the L/S ratio and assay of the percentages of disaturated lecithin, PI, and PG. Of these, PG appears to be most important: if it is absent from amniotic fluid, RDS appears to be inevitable; regardless of a low or intermediate L/S ratio, if it is present in concentration of 3% or more, the fetal lung can be considered mature. Disaturated lecithin and PI are added parameters that complete the profile; all may be plotted on a grid (Fig. 41–14) and consistency of the values permits reasonable prediction of lung maturity that is much more reliable than L/S ratio alone in borderline or questionable cases. In a series of cases in which the L/S ratio was less than 2, the profile correctly predicted lung maturity in 14 of 18 cases, thus increasing the prediction of true outcome from 68% to 93%.

Surfactant Assessment in High-risk Pregnancy

The timing of functional maturation (L/S ratio greater than 2) of the fetal lung may vary according to maternal or fetoplacental disease states. Functional maturation evidenced by PG in excess of 3% ordinarily occurs at 35 weeks. It may occur as early as 28 weeks in association with class F and R diabetes, pregnancy complicated by severe hypertension–proteinuria syndromes, and prolonged rupture of the membranes. In contrast, maturation is often delayed in class A diabetics.

The issue of surfactant assessment in pregnancies complicated by maternal diabetes is both controversial and worrisome. Currently, the infant of the diabetic mother has a sixfold increase in risk for developing RDS. It is generally accepted that traditional assessment of surfactant by means of the L/S ratio has a false-mature rate of 5%–6% in diabetics versus an expected rate of 2% in the normal population. A higher incidence of cesarean section, asphyxia, and preterm delivery, all of which increase the risk of RDS, may influence the difference in predictability. Furthermore, errors in assignment of gestational age are common in diabetic patients. It appears that the presence of PG in excess of 3% gives better evidence of pulmonary maturity in these patients than does an L/S ratio of 2 or more.

Pregnancy complicated by hypertensive disease, particularly when it is severe and is associated with significant proteinuria or placental infarction, may be associated with accelerated pulmonary maturity, which is manifest by early elevation of the L/S ratio. In some cases, even though the L/S ratio is less than 2, PG may be elevated to a mature 3% level as early as 29–30 weeks. Maturation is generally not accelerated if the hypertension is mild, or is of acute onset during pregnancy.

Prolonged rupture of the membranes may be associated with early pulmonary maturation. There is some controversy regarding this issue, since most studies are retrospective and do not control for other factors that may influence surfactant induction. However, when membranes have been ruptured longer than 24 hours and the lung profile has been corrected for gestational age, it has been noted that PG appears earlier (by 1.5 weeks), mean L/S ratios are higher, and a mature L/S ratio is reached earlier.

Shake Test (Rapid Test for Surfactant)

Although the L/S ratio has gained widespread acceptance as a predictor of pulmonary maturity, the assay is slow, complicated, costly, and subject to some errors of precision in the ordinary community hospital. In

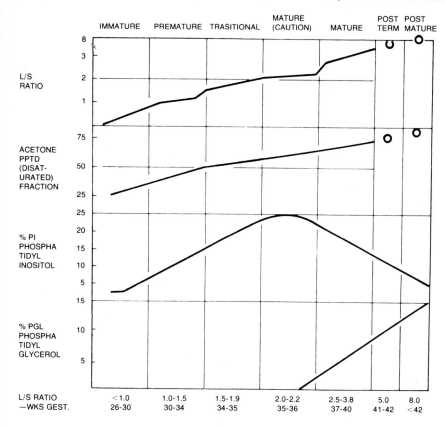

FIG. 41-14. Form used to report lung profile. L/S ratio, acetone-precipitated disaturated lecithin, phosphatidylinositol, and phosphitydylglycerol are recorded at points on curves. Values usually fall within a given grid and lung maturity may be read off at *top* of form. (Kulovich MV, Hallman MB, Gluck L: Am J Obstet Gynecol 135:57, 1979. Copyright © by the Regents of the University of California, 1977)

most institutions, procedures to determine the L/S ratio are performed only during certain hours and thus surfactant assessment is not always possible when acute conditions require immediate management decisions. As a result, Clements *et al.* have developed the "shake" or "foam stability" test. The procedure requires mixing amniotic fluid with 0.9% saline in various proportions until there is a volume of 1 ml, then adding 1 ml 95% ethanol. The resultant mixture is shaken for 15 sec and allowed to stand for 15 min. A complete ring of stable bubbles in the meniscus of the 1:1 and the 1:2 dilution is a positive result, a stable form in the 1:1 but not the 1:2 dilution is an intermediate positive result, and a lack of foam in the 1:1 dilution is clearly negative. Although there has been some hesitancy to accept the shake test as a valid measure of pulmonary maturity, the concern appears not to be justified, since the reported false-mature (false-positive) rate is similar to that of the L/S ratio. Positive results reliably predict functional pulmonary maturity; intermediate and negative results indicate increasing risk for RDS.

Clinically, it is equally as important to predict pulmonary immaturity as it is to predict pulmonary maturity. False-negative (false-immature) results are common with both the L/S ratio and shake test, even when done within 24 hours of delivery. The usefulness of an intermediate L/S ratio (1.5–2) in predicting the subsequent development of RDS appears to be greater than that of an intermediate shake result (positive in the 1:1 but not 1:2).

The result of the shake test may be positive in the presence of an immature L/S ratio (false-negative) with subsequent normal neonatal outcome. The shake test therefore complements the L/S ratio, particularly when the L/S ratio is immature. The shake test may actually be able to detect accelerated lung maturity in the presence of an L/S ratio in the 1.5–1.9 range. Certainly, a lung profile may show maturity in the presence of an L/S ratio less than 2.

NEW DEVELOPMENTS

FETAL BREATHING MOVEMENT

Fetal chest wall movements were detected as early as 1888. However, it was not until 1970 that Dawes *et al.* were able to document the presence of negative fluctuations of thoracic pressure independent of amniotic fluid pressure changes in fetal lambs by implanting intratracheal catheters. It was subsequently suggested

that antenatal assessment of fetal breathing movement (FBM) would eventually prove to be a useful clinical tool. More recently, efforts have been made to assess the physiologic and pathophysiologic variables that influence FBM and to develop the technical tools required to assess this activity reliably and easily. The availability of real-time ultrasound now makes evaluation of FBM a realistic clinical consideration.

Physiology

Although control of FBM is similar to the control of neonatal respiratory activity, there does appear to be some difference from respiratory control in adults; this may be a function of the maturation of the respiratory control system that occurs after the neonatal period. The most notable exception is the poor responsiveness of the fetal carotid body to hypoxemia and hypercapnia.

Two predominant breathing patterns have been demonstrated in the fetal lamb: 1) a rapid, shallow, regular pattern that accounts for approximately 90% of FBM and 2) a more sporadic pattern characterized by deeper and slower respiratory movements at a rate of 1–4/min that accounts for approximately 5% of FBM. The rapid pattern appears to be correlated with rapid eye movement sleep; the slow pattern appears not to be associated with any particular state of wakefulness or sleep. Additional intermittent positive pressure fluctuations have been observed in fetal lambs with intratracheal pressure catheters; these movements are thought to be secondary to coughing, gasping, or hiccups.

FBM is probably secondary to diaphragmatic rather than chest wall muscle activity. Control seems to be central, generated within medullary respiratory centers and transmitted to the diaphragm by means of the phrenic nerve. Physiologic variables that modify FBM in animals also appear to be active in the human fetus. The most significant of these are blood sugar levels, pCO_2, pO_2, labor activity, fetal presentation, and fetal sleep. Temperature is of lesser significance, although FBM decreases when temperature is reduced and increases to a panting pattern when temperature is increased. FBM also appears to have a diurnal variation that is independent of blood sugar levels.

Blood Sugar. In the fetal lamb, maternal hypoglycemia diminishes both the amplitude and frequency of FBM. An increase in FBM follows meals. This may be a direct effect of glucose. However, some authors have speculated that the variation in respiratory activity is the result of local excesses of carbon dioxide produced by increased glucose oxidation that stimulates medullary chemosensitive areas and produces FBM.

Carbon Dioxide and Oxygen. FBM also seems to be influenced by changes in maternal gas mixtures. An increase in carbon dioxide or a decrease in oxygen content doubles the proportion of time during which FBM is present; tracheal fluid flow and depth of respiratory movement also increase. FBM is arrested when the fetal lamb is rendered hypoxic by a drop in P_aO_2 from 23 mm Hg to 16 mm Hg. The effect is long-lasting; the fetus does not recover from a 1-hour hypoxic episode for several hours.

Labor. Especially when the fetus is in the vertex presentation, labor activity is associated with a higher incidence of apnea and periodic breathing. In fact, FBM decreases several days prior to the onset of labor. It may be that the descent of the fetal head against the maternal pelvic wall increases intracranial pressure, thereby exerting an inhibitory action on FBM. As labor progresses, the mean percentage of time during which FBM occurs decreases significantly even without hypoxemia and acidemia. Apnea may develop in well-established labor. This may also be the result of maternal hyperventilation and associated fetal hypocapnia. Some authors have speculated that a very subtle decrease in oxygen saturation, when there is no metabolic acidosis, may also be a factor in the decrease in FBM. It is interesting to note that FHR variability increases in association with an increase in FBM and fetal activity during labor.

Tracheal Fluid Efflux. Respiratory tidal volume of the neonatal lamb is 80 ml fluid compared to 1–2 ml tracheal fluid prior to delivery. Although there is some agreement regarding net outflow of fluid, there is uncertainty regarding the volume of amniotic fluid that is actually drawn into the tracheobronchial tree. ^{51}Cr-labeled red cells injected into the human amniotic sac of abnormal human pregnancies reach the lung periphery in significant volume. In contrast, experiments in fetal lambs indicate that the net outflow of fluid is of the same magnitude as that inspired. The latter studies used fetal intratracheal catheters and thus measured net flow as opposed to the red cell studies, which measured uptake volume independent of efflux. Such studies are of potential clinical importance. If intrauterine amniotic fluid uptake is large, intrapartal meconium aspiration prior to delivery may be more common than thought; surgical intervention solely to prevent meconium aspiration in a patient with meconium-stained fluid would then appear to be unnecessary.

Observation of FBM in Humans

It is sometimes possible to detect FBM on the uterine activity channel of fetal monitor recordings, but the records may be difficult to evaluate. Real-time ultrasound can provide reasonably precise assessment of chest wall movement, including both number of movements per unit of time and nature of each movement.

Simultaneous videotape recordings have also increased the feasibility of this technique.

Normal Characteristics. FBM may be observed as early as 11 weeks. It is reliably identifiable at 13–14 weeks' gestation. Movements are irregular in early fetal life but become more regular with advancing gestation. Under normal circumstances, FBM can be seen over 30%–90% of observation time. Breathing activity rarely occurs continuously for more than 10 min; apneic periods of up to 108 min have been observed in normal fetuses. The most frequent movements are rapid and of small amplitude. The usual frequency of movements is 30–70/min.

Pharmacologic Agents That Affect FBM. Animal studies have delineated physical, environmental, and psychologic FBM variables as a result of drug effects. This has not been possible in human pregnancies. It appears that, in general, central nervous system (CNS) stimulants increase FBM, while CNS depressants reduce it; drug dose:response is not consistent. It has also become apparent that the human fetal CNS is not as sensitive to stimulant or depressant drugs as once thought. The FBM of the uncompromised fetus appears to be modulated to a greater extent by maternal plasma glucose levels than by drugs. Agents that inhibit FBM include methyldopa, nicotine, and alcohol. Although CNS stimulants such as caffeine, epinephrine, isoproterenol, doxapram hydrochloride, and pilocarpine have been found to stimulate FBM in animals, the effects have not been as uniform in the human. The effects of β_2-receptor stimulants are inconsistent; terbutaline sulfate increases FBM, whereas salbutamol appears to have no such effect.

Clinical Application

At the present time, FBM assessment is predominantly a research tool. Although the usefulness of FBM for antepartum and intrapartum assessment is not well established, preliminary results are promising. Clinical studies to date indicate that FBM assessment is as predictive as the NST. In addition, it appears to be as practical as the NST; most tests require 10–30 min.

Fetal Distress and Perinatal Mortality. Most studies indicate that if FBM is seen during more than 50% of an observation period, the mortality is almost zero, whereas the presence of prolonged apnea or only isolated deep breaths is followed by a mortality of almost 100%.

Some have correlated FBM changes with pathologic monitor patterns. When FBM occurred during less than 50% of observation time, 15 of 17 fetuses subsequently experienced late decelerations in FHR during labor. Late decelerations were frequently accompanied by gasping activity. Most recently, it has been suggested that the percent breathing time is of lesser importance than the quality of FBM.

Small-for-gestational-age Fetus. FBM tends to occur for less than 50% of an observation period in the small-for-gestational-age fetus, whereas it occurs approximately 60%–90% of the observation period in the fetus whose size is appropriate for gestational age. If acidosis and birth asphyxia further complicate the case, it is not unusual to observe persistent and prolonged apnea with isolated, slow chest wall movements.

Prediction of Normal Outcome. Real-time scanning has made FBM assessment feasible, but the question of normal criteria has not been totally resolved. Although early studies suggested a cutoff point for high-risk at movement during more than 50% of an observation period, several investigators using real-time ultrasound have reported normal outcome with mean FBM incidences of less than 50% in the third trimester. Recent investigators propose that FBM be assessed in a 30-min interval; the only criterion for normalcy is normal FBM observed in this interval; percent movement time is considered to be of much less importance. If this concept is substantiated, the need to assess the percent duration of FBM activity will be eliminated, which will simplify the procedure and reduce the performance time. Manning and Platt have used this technique to predict an Apgar score ≥ 7 in 99% of cases (true-negative) and to predict an abnormal Apgar score of <7 in 90% of cases (true-positive). These prediction rates are similar to those of the NST.

FBM and Nonstress Testing. More recently, Manning and associates have studied the simultaneous application of the NST and determination of FBM. If both are used, the false-negative rate for predicting good outcome for the NST (3.6%) and FBM (3.6%) is reduced to 3%. More important, the false-positive prediction of an Apgar score of <7 is reduced from 20.2% for the NST and 12.1% for FBM, to 5.9% if both tests are used.

FBM and Stress Testing. As described previously, the CST and OCT have a false-positive rate that varies from 30%–60%. The presence of a "reactive" baseline reduces the false-positive incidence by approximately 50%. FBM also seems to be of value in identifying the false-positive subset. A recent study of 14 patients with a positive CST result yielded a false-positive rate for FBM of 0% versus 58.3% for the CST. No data are available to determine how many false-positive OCTs also had reactive baselines. The false-negative rate was 20% for FBM and 0% for the CST in that particular subset. It thus appears that FBM may be useful to select the patient who will be able to tolerate labor in spite of a positive CST result.

BIOPHYSICAL PROFILE

The assessment of five fetal biophysical measurements has been combined into a "profile" in an effort to identify the fetus at risk with greater precision. The evidence suggests it is more reliable than any single indicator in reducing false-positive results. The profile includes assessment of FBM plus four other biophysical variables: 1) NST results, 2) fetal tone, 3) fetal movement, and 4) amniotic fluid volume. The false-negative rate is low, and the false-positive rate is high, for any single test. Incorporation of the five tests into an overall profile improves the already low false-negative rate; but, more importantly, it significantly reduces the false-positive rate. The use of such a biophysical profile clearly deserves further research. If future studies support these initial impressions, this profile may be the test of the future. Equally important, the profile may be performed in an average of 10 min if the NST is excluded from the profile. This performance interval compares favorably with that of the NST, which requires 20–30 min.

REFERENCES AND RECOMMENDED READING

RISK SCORING

Harper RG, Sokal MM, Sokal J et al: The high risk perinatal registry: A systematic approach for reducing perinatal mortality. Obstet Gynecol 50:264, 1977

Hobel CJ: Recognition of the high risk pregnant woman. In Spellacy WN (ed): Management of the High-risk Pregnancy. Baltimore, University Park Press, 1976

Hobel CJ, Hyvarinen MA, Okada DM, Oh W: Prenatal and intrapartum high-risk screening. Am J Obstet Gynecol 117:1, 1973

Nesbitt REL, Aubry RH: High risk obstetrics. Am J Obstet Gynecol 103:972, 1969

FETAL GESTATIONAL AGE AND GROWTH ASSESSMENT

Battaglia FC, Lubchenco LO: A practical classification of newborn infants by weight and gestational age. J Pediatr 71:159, 1967

Campbell S: The assessment of fetal development by diagnostic ultrasound. Clin Perinatol 1:507, 1974

Campbell S, Dewhurst CJ: Diagnosis of the small for dates fetus by serial ultrasonic cephalometry. Lancet 2:10002, 1971

Campbell S, Newman GB: Growth of the fetal biparietal diameter during normal pregnancy. Br J Obstet Gynaecol 78:513, 1971

Depp R, Dynamics of fetal growth. In Sabbagha RE (ed): Diagnostic Ultrasound Applied to Obstetrics and Gynecology. Hagerstown, MD, Harper & Row, 1980

Gohari P, Berkowitz RL, Hobbins JC: Prediction of intrauterine growth retardation by determination of total intrauterine volume. Am J Obstet Gynecol 127:255, 1977

Hertz T, Sokal R, Knoke J et al: Clinical estimation of gestational age: Rules for avoiding preterm delivery. Am J Obstet Gynecol 131:395, 1978

Robinson HP, Flemming JEE: A critical evaluation of sonor "crown–rump length" measurements. Br J Obstet Gynaecol 82:702, 1975

Sabbagha RE: Intrauterine growth retardation: Antenatal diagnosis by ultrasound. Obstet Gynecol 52:252, 1978

Sabbagha RE: Intrauterine growth retardation. In Sabbagha RE (ed): Diagnostic Ultrasound Applied to Obstetrics and Gynecology. Hagerstown, MD, Harper & Row, 1980

Sabbagha RE, Barton BA, Barton FB et al: Sonar biparietal diameter: II. Predictive of three fetal growth patterns leading to a closer assessment of gestational age and neonatal weight. Am J Obstet Gynecol 51:383, 1978

Usher R, McClean F, Scott KE: Judgment of fetal age: II. Clinical significance of gestational age and an objective method for its assessment. Pediatr Clin North Am 13:835, 1966

MECONIUM

Abramovici H, Brandes JM: Meconium during delivery: A sign of compensated fetal distress. Am J Obstet Gynecol 118:251, 1974

Fenton AN, Steer CM: Fetal distress. Am J Obstet Gynecol 83:354, 1962

Green J, Paul R: The value of amniocentesis in prolonged pregnancy. Obstet Gynecol 51:293, 1978

Meis PJ, Hall M, III, Marshall JR, Hobel CJ: Meconium passage: A new classification for risk assessment during labor. Am J Obstet Gynecol 131:509, 1978

Miller FC, Sacks DA, Yeh SY et al: Significance of meconium during labor. Am J Obstet Gynecol 122:573, 1975

INTRAPATRUM MONITORING

Continuous Electronic

Banta HD, Thacker SB: Policies toward medical technology: The case of electronic fetal monitoring. Am J Public Health 69:941, 1979

Benson RC, Shubeck F, Deutschberger L et al: Fetal heart rate as a predictor of fetal distress. Obstet Gynecol 32:259, 1968

Haverkamp AD, Orleans M, Langendoerfer S et al: A controlled trial of the differential effects of intrapartum fetal monitoring. Am J Obstet Gynecol 134:399, 1979

Haverkamp AD, Thompaon HE, McFee JG et al: The evaluation of continuous fetal heart rate monitoring in high-risk pregnancy. Am J Obstet Gynecol 125:310, 1976

Hobbins JC, Freeman R, Queenan JT: The fetal monitoring debate. Obstet Gynecol 54:103, 1979

Hon EH: An Atlas of Fetal Heart Rate Patterns. New Haven, Harry Press, 1968

Hon EH, Quilligan EJ: The classification of fetal heart rate: II. A revised working classification. Conn Med 31:779, 1967

Neutra RR: Effect of fetal monitoring on neonatal death rates. N Engl J Med 299:324, 1978

Painter MJ, Depp R, O'Donoghue PD: Fetal heart rate patterns and development in the first year of life. Am J Obstet Gynecol 132:271, 1978

Paul RH, Hon EH: Clinical fetal monitoring v. effect in perinatal outcome. Am J Obstet Gynecol 118:529, 1974

Paul RH, Khazin SA, Yeh S et al: Clinical fetal monitoring: VII. The evaluation and significance of intrapartum baseline FHR variability. Am J Obstet Gynecol 123:206, 1975

Schifrin BS, Dame L: Fetal heart rate patterns: Prediction of Apgar score. JAMA 219:1372, 1972

Continuous Electronic Monitoring Plus Scalp Blood

Kubli FW, Hon EH, Khazin AF et al: Observations on heart rate and pH in the human fetus during labor. Am J Obstet Gynecol 104:1190, 1969

Wood C, Lumley J, Renou P: Clinical assessment of fetal diagnostic methods. J Obstet Gynaecol Br Commonw 74:823, 1967

Wood C, Newman W, Lumley J et al: Classification of fetal heart rate in relationship to fetal scalp blood measurements and Apgar score. Am J Obstet Gynecol 105:942, 1969

Scalp Blood Gases

Adamsons K, Beard RW, Meyers RE: Comparison of the composition of arterial, venous and capillary blood of the fetal monkey during labor. Am J Obstet Gynecol 107:435, 1970

Beard RW, Morris ED, Clayton SG et al: Foetal capillary pH as an indicator of the condition of the foetus. J Obstet Gynaecol Br Commonw 74:812, 1967

Saling E, Schneider D: Biochemical supervision of the fetus during labor. J Obstet Gynaecol Br Commonw 74:799, 1967

ANTENATAL EVALUATION

Contraction Stress Test

Braly P, Freeman RK: The significance of fetal heart rate re-activity with a positive oxytocin challenge test. Obstet Gynecol 50:689, 1977

Freeman RK: The use of the oxytocin challenge test for antepartum clinical evaluation of uteroplacental respiratory function. Am J Obstet Gynecol 121:481, 1975

Freeman RK, Goebelsman U, Nochimson D et al: An evaluation of the significance of a positive oxytocin challenge test. Obstet Gynecol 47:8, 1975

Pose SV, Castillo JB, Mora–Rojas EO et al: Test of fetal tolerance to induced uterine contractions with a diagnosis of chronic distress. In Perinatal Factors Affecting Human Development, pp 96–103. Washington, DC, Pan-American Health Organization, 1969

Ray M, Freeman RK, Pine S et al: Clinical experience with the oxytocin challenge test. Am J Obstet Gynecol 114:1, 1972

Trienweiler MW, Freeman RK, James J: Baseline fetal heart rate characteristics as an indicator of fetal status during the antepartum pariod. Am J Obstet Gynecol 125:618, 1976

NST and Fetal Movement Activity

Evertson LR, Gauthier RJ, Schifrin BS et al: Antepartum fetal heart rate testing: I. Evolution of the nonstress test. Am J Obstet Gynecol 133:29, 1979

Kubli F, Rutgers H: Semiquantitative evaluation of antepartum fetal heart rate. Int J Gynaecol Obstet 10:180, 1972

Lee CY, Diloretto PC, Logrand B: Fetal activity acceleration determination for evaluation of fetal reserve. Obstet Gynecol 48:19, 1976

Nochimson DJ, Twibeville JS, Terry JE et al: The non-stress test. Obstet Gynecol 51:419, 1978

Pratt D, Diamond F, Yen H et al: Fetal stress and nonstress tests: An analysis and comparison of their ability to identify fetal outcome. Obstet Gynecol 54:419, 1979

Rochard F, Schifrin BS, Goupil F et al: Nonstressed fetal heart rate monitoring in the antepartum period. Am J Obstet Gynecol 126:698, 1976

Sadovsky E, Yaffe H, Polishuk WZ: Fetal movement monitoring in normal and pathologic pregnancy. Int J Gynaecol Obstet 12:75, 1974

Estriol

Diczfalusy E, Mancuso S: Oestrogen metabolism in pregnancy. In Klopper A, Diczfalusy E (eds): Foetus and Placenta. Oxford, Blackwell, 1969

Distler W, Gabbe SG, Freeman RK et al: Estriol in pregnancy: V. Unconjugated and total plasma estriol in the management of diabetic pregnancies. Am J Obstet Gynecol 130:424, 1978

Duenhoelter JH, Whalley PI, MacDonald PC: An analysis of the utility of plasma immunoreactive estrogen measurements in determining delivery time of gravidas with a fetus considered at high-risk. Am J Obstet Gynecol 125:889, 1976

Goebelsmann U, Freeman RK, Mestman JH et al: Estriol in pregnancy: II. Daily urinary estriols in the management of the pregnant diabetic woman. Am J Obstet Gynecol 115:795, 1973

Human Placental Lactogen

Higashi K: Studies on the prolactin-like substance in human placenta. Endocrinol Jap 8:288, 1961

Josimovich JB, Kosov B, Mintz DH: Roles of placental lactogen in foetal–maternal relations. In Wolstenholme GEW, O'Connor M (eds): Foetal Anatomy, Ciba Foundation Symposium. London, Churchill, 1969

Josimovich JB, MacLaren JA: Presence in the human placenta and term serum of a highly lactogenic substance immunologically related to pituitary growth hormone. Endocrinology 71:209, 1962

Spellacy WN, Teoh ES, Buhi WC et al: Value of human chorionic somatomammotropin in managing high risk pregnancies. Am J Obstet Gynecol 109:588, 1971

FETAL MATURITY

Bishop EH, Carson S: Estimation of fetal maturity by cytologic examination of the amniotic fluid. Am J Obstet Gynecol 102:654, 1968

Cher B, Statland BE, Freer DE: Clinical evaluation of the qualitative foam stability index test. Obstet Gynecol 55:617, 1980

Clements JA, Platzker ACG, Tierney DF et al: Association of the risk of the respiratory distress syndrome by a rapid test for surfactant in amniotic fluid. N Engl J Med 286:1077, 1972

Farrell PM, Wood RN: Epidemiology of hyaline membrane disease in the United States: Analysis of national mortality statistics. Pediatrics 58:167, 1976

Gluck L, Kulovich MV: Lecithin/sphingomyelin ratios in amniotic fluid in normal and abnormal pregnancy. Am J Obstet Gynecol 115:539, 1973

Gluck L, Kulovich MV, Borer RC et al: Diagnosis of respiratory distress syndrome by amniocentesis. Am J Obstet Gynecol 109:440, 1971

Gluck L, Kulovich MV, Borer RC et al: The interpretation and significance of the lecithin/sphingomyelin ratio in amniotic fluid. Am J Obstet Gynecol 120:143, 1974

Goldenberg RL, Nelson K: Iatrogenic respiratory distress syndrome: An analysis of obstetric events preceding delivery of infants who develop respiratory distress syndrome. Am J Obstet Gynecol 123:617, 1975

Kulovich MV, Gluck L: The lung profile: II. Complicated pregnancy. Am J Obstet Gynecol 135:64, 1979

Kulovich MV, Hallman MB, Gluck I: The lung profile: I. Normal pregnancy. Am J Obstet Gynecol 135:57, 1979

O'Brien WF, Cefalo RC: Clinical applicability of amniotic fluid tests for fetal pulmonary maturity. Am J Obstet Gynecol 136:135, 1980

Pitkin RM: Amniotic fluid in estimating fetal maturity. Contemp Obstet Gynecol 4:13, 1974

Schleuter MA, Phibbs RH, Creasy RK et al: Antenatal prediction of graduated risk of hyaline membrane disease by amniotic fluid foam test for surfactant. Am J Obstet Gynecol 134:761, 1979

NEW DEVELOPMENTS

Boddy K, Robinson JS: External method for detection of fetal breathing in utero. Lancet 2:1231, 1971

Boddy F, Dawes GS: Fetal breathing. Br Med Bul 31:3, 1975

Boddy K, Dawes GS, Robinson JS: In Comline RS, Cross KW, Dawes GS, Nathanielsz PW (eds): Foetal and Neonatal Physiology, pp 63–66. Proceedings of the Sir Joseph Bancroft Centenary Symposium held at Cambridge, 1972. London, Cambridge University Press.

Dawes GS, Fox HE, Leduc BM et al: Respiratory movements and paradoxical sleep in the foetal lamb. J Physiol 210:47P, 1970

Dawes GS, Fox HE, Leduc BM et al: Respiratory movements and rapid eye movement sleep in the foetal sheep. J Physiol 220:119, 1972

Duenhoelter JH, Pritchard JA: Human fetal respiration. Obstet Gynecol 42:746, 1973

Duenhoelter JG, Pritchard JA: Human fetal respiration: II. Fate of intra-amniotic hypaque and ^{51}Cr-labeled red cells. Obstet Gynecol 43:878, 1974

Manning FA: Fetal breathing as a reflection of fetal status. Postgrad Med 61:116, 1976

Manning FA, Platt LD: Fetal breathing movements and the abnormal contraction stress test. Am J Obstet Gynecol 133:590, 1979

Manning FA, Platt LD: Fetal breathing movements and the non-stress test in high-risk pregnancies. Am J Obstet Gynecol 135:511, 1979

Manning FA, Platt LD, Sipos L: Antepartum fetal evaluation: Development of a fetal biophysical profile. Am J Obstet Gynecol 136:787, 1980

Patrick J, Natale R, Richardson B: Patterns of human fetal breathing activity at 34–35 weeks' gestational age. Am J Obstet Gynecol 132:507, 1978

Patrick J (ed): Fetal breathing movements. Semin Perinatol 4:249, 1980

42

THE NEWBORN INFANT

L. Stanley James
Karlis Adamsons

Survival of the newborn infant depends primarily upon prompt expansion of the lungs and the establishment of gaseous exchange. In addition, the infant must regulate body temperatue and produce energy from materials obtained from the environment. Most organ systems concerned with homeostasis reach functional maturity prior to term, and several of them, notably the cardiovascular, renal, and skeletomuscular systems, are exercised to some extent during fetal life; those concerned with thermoregulation, on the other hand, are not challenged until after birth.

During the first minutes, hours, and days of life many alterations in morphology and function take place, perhaps the most dramatic being in the heart and lungs. Although animal experimentation has contributed greatly to our knowledge, our understanding of the many profound changes occurring in the early moments of life is still incomplete.

PHYSIOLOGY OF THE FETUS

DEVELOPMENT OF LUNG AND ALVEOLAR DIFFERENTIATION

During fetal life, the lung has a glandular appearance. Development commences about the 24th day as an outpouching of the gut that branches into the surrounding mesenchyme. Cartilage deposition begins at about the 10th week and continues until the 24th.

The potential air spaces are initially lined by cuboidal epithelium that begins to flatten between the 16th and 20th weeks, coinciding with capillary ingrowth to establish contact with the epithelium. During this time, the epithelial cells begin to differentiate into two distinct types (Type 1 and Type 2 cells). Type 1 are vacuolated alveolar cells with some lipoid material; Type 2 are nonvacuolated, look more like connective tissue cells, and have lamellar inclusions (see Fig. 16-28).

PRODUCTION OF FLUID BY LUNG

There is a considerable quantity of fluid in the fetal lung prior to delivery. This fluid appears to be an ultrafiltrate of plasma with selective reabsorption or secretion; it is more acidic and has a higher chloride content than plasma. With the onset of respiration, reabsorption of this fluid must be quite rapid. Its low protein concentration, together with the fall in pulmonary artery pressure that occurs when the lung expands, would facilitate this process.

RESPIRATORY MOVEMENTS

Rhythmic movements of the chest wall and of the diaphragm have been demonstrated to occur in mammalian fetuses at the completion of the first third of gestation. They are associated with relatively large variations in fetal blood flow in the descending aorta and in heart rate. In the well-oxygenated primate fetus near term, these respiratory movements occur 30%–40% of the time. Respiratory movements are depressed by anesthetic and analgesic agents and by asphyxia. They are reinitiated as gasps in the presence of marked oxygen deprivation. Inhalation of nicotine leads to prolonged suppression of fetal respiratory movements in the human. Present evidence strongly supports the contention that bronchial and amniotic fluid is not inhaled during regular breathing but only during the deep gasping of asphyxia.

SURFACE TENSION PHENOMENON AND LUNG FUNCTION

The normal mature lung contains a surface tension–reducing substance that confers stability during

deflation and is responsible for the fine foam formed during acute pulmonary edema. This substance has been identified as a phospholipid together with a specific protein. It can usually be demonstrated by 18–20 weeks' gestation, when the fetal lung can be expanded, and its presence coincides with the appearance of lamellar inclusions in the Type 2 alveolar cell. The presence of surface-active agent is important in reducing the work required for initial lung expansion and maintaining the stability of the expanded alveolus.

CIRCULATION

Current knowledge of the fetal circulation has been gained principally through studying lambs delivered by hysterotomy. In this species, the uterus does not contract once the fetus is removed, and the placenta remains attached to the uterine wall. Providing the lamb is kept warm and the cord circulation is not interrupted, the fetus will not breathe and the heart can be catheterized, blood samples withdrawn, and radio-opaque substances injected.

These studies have shown that arterialized blood from the placenta flows into the fetus through the umbilical vein and passes rapidly through the liver into the inferior vena cava; from there, it flows through the foramen ovale into the left atrium, soon to appear in the aorta and arteries of the head (Fig. 42–1). A portion bypasses the liver through the ductus venosus. Venous blood from the lower extremities and head passes predominantly into the right atrium, the right ventricle, and then into the descending aorta through the pulmonary artery and ductus arteriosus. Thus, the foramen ovale and the ductus arteriosus act as bypass channels, allowing a large part of the combined cardiac output to return to the placenta without flowing through the lungs. Approximately 55% of the combined ventricular output flows to the placenta, while 35% perfuses body tissues, the remaining 10% flowing through the lungs.

The pulmonary arteries and arterioles of the fetus, like those of the systemic circulation, are characterized by a high ratio of wall thickness to the lumen. Pulmonary blood flow is not constant and can be increased up to fivefold by injection of acetylcholine or histamine in microgram quantities into the pulmonary artery. The degree of fetal oxygenation influences pulmonary vascular resistance, pulmonary arterial flow increasing if the mother is given 100% oxygen to breathe. Acute asphyxia of the fetus produces intense pulmonary vasoconstriction, which markedly reduces pulmonary blood flow.

The crista dividens, a structure projecting from the posterosuperior border of the foramen ovale, separates the inferior vena caval flow into two streams before the atria are reached, the stream from the ductus venosus being guided largely into the left atrium. It is improbable that the ductus venosus has any important function in the latter part of fetal life. In the piglet, lamb, and monkey, it is a minute channel at term, and in the foal it is occluded before birth.

THERMOREGULATION IN THE FETUS

Under normal conditions, the body temperature of the human fetus is approximately 0.5° C higher than that of the mother. This gradient is determined by the ratio of the heat output of the fetus to the rate of placental perfusion and the direction of flows through the villous capillaries and the intervillous space. The amount of heat dissipated from the body surface into the amniotic fluid is small in comparison with that exchanged across the placenta. Under conditions of hypo- or hyperthermia, the temperature of the fetus parallels that of the mother, although the thermal gradient between fetus and mother increases with the rise in maternal temperature. Oxygenation of the fetus appears to be relatively unaffected as long as fetal temperature does not exceed 41.5° C. When this limit is exceeded, the fetal circulatory system deteriorates rapidly. In contrast, lowering of fetal body temperature does not interfere with fetal oxygenation even though there is a linear fall in fetal heart rate and blood pressure as fetal body temperature is reduced.

RESPIRATORY GAS EXCHANGE ACROSS PLACENTA

Some of the controversy concerning the environment in which the fetus develops has been resolved following the development of techniques for implanting catheters into fetal and maternal vessels for prolonged periods without interrupting pregnancy. These techniques have been successfully employed in sheep, goats, and, more recently, in the rhesus monkey. They have enabled serial sampling of arterial and venous blood from the unanesthetized mother and fetus.

As the fetus grows, the functional capacity of the placenta appears to increase to keep pace with the fetus' needs. There are species variations with regard to the relative increase in weight of the fetus and placenta as development proceeds, but the human placenta continues to grow and increase in weight to term. The gradients for hydrogen ion and carbon dioxide tension across the placenta are small (approximately 0.05 pH units and 8 mm Hg, respectively) so that the fetus is neither acidotic nor hypercapnic under normal conditions. Although oxygen tension of fetal arterial blood is low by adult standards, oxygen consumption of the fetal lamb and goat is similar to basal values obtained after birth and appears to remain constant during the third trimester. Hemoglobin concentration and oxygen-carrying capacity of fetal blood during the third trimester are similar to those of the

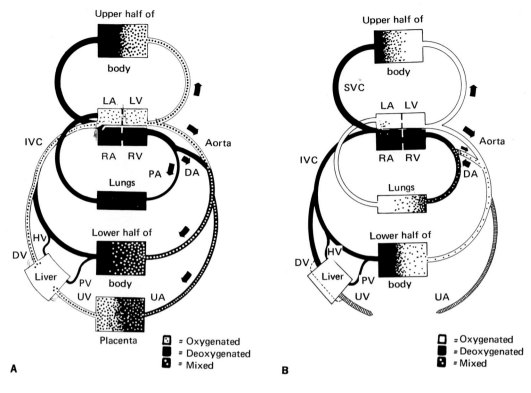

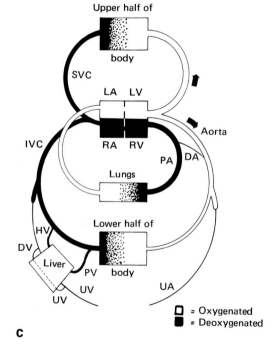

FIG. 42–1. Schematic representations of fetal (*A*), neonatal (*B*), and adult (*C*)circulation. LA, LV, RA, RV refer to four chambers of heart. *DA,* Ductus arteriosus. *PA,* Pulmonary artery. *UA,* Umbilical artery. *UV,* Umbilical vein. *PV,* Portal vein. *HV,* Hepatic vein. *DV,* Ductus venosus; *IVC,* Inferior vena cava. *SVC,* Superior vena cava. Arrows indicate direction of blood flow.

adult animal and do not change as pregnancy advances, unless the animal is subject to stress, such as operative procedure for blood sampling. Adequate oxygenation of the tissues is probably maintained in the face of a relatively low arterial oxygen tension because of an umbilical vein saturation of 80%–85% together with a high cardiac output.

Thus, the evidence responsible for the belief that the fetus has a limited control over its oxygen supply and lives under conditions of oxygen deprivation as term approaches can largely be discounted.

PHYSIOLOGY OF THE NEWBORN

BIRTH ASPHYXIA

Oxygen levels in the umbilical arterial blood at birth range from 0 to nearly 70% saturation even in the most vigorous and healthy infants. The average value is 22%; in nearly one-quarter, it is less than 10%. The relatively low oxygen levels are accompanied by varying degrees of hypercapnia and acidosis, the average carbon dioxide pressure being 58 mm Hg and the average pH 7.28 (compared with 40 mm Hg and pH 7.4 in the adult); lower pH and higher carbon dioxide pressure are associated with lower oxygen levels.

These observations suggest that during the final stages of labor and delivery, the exchange of oxygen and carbon dioxide across the placenta is reduced, leading to various degrees of asphyxia at birth. Direct proof of this concept has been provided by the animal experiments described earlier. More recently, sampling of blood from the fetal scalp has shown that, as labor progresses, the fetus gradually becomes acidotic. This latter technique is a most important advance in monitoring the condition of the fetus and is finding increasing clinical application (see Chapter 41).

Several factors can disturb the normal functional relation between fetal and maternal circulations and cause fetal acidosis. Blood flow through the intervillous space is reduced or may stop during strong uterine contractions; it is also reduced if the mother becomes hypotensive as a result of compression of the inferior vena cava or aorta by the uterus. Maternal hyperventilation leading to alkalosis also appears to lead to a reduction in intervillous flow and to fetal acidosis. In addition to these factors, changes in maternal acid–base balance as a result of excessive muscular activity or dehydration during prolonged labor or as a result of respiratory depression from drugs and anesthesia are reflected in the fetus. On the fetal side, cord compression occurs in approximately one-third of all deliveries and probably is the most common mechanism to interfere with transplacental exchange.

The composition of cord blood at birth is therefore the result of a disturbance in the functional relation between mother and fetus during labor and delivery, whether this be *per vaginam* or by cesarean section, and does not reflect adaptation to a hypoxic environment *in utero*. Since these changes occur inevitably, considerable limitations are imposed upon the interpretation of data relating to the composition of cord blood. This applies not only to respiratory gases but also to all substances that are continuously exchanged between mother and fetus.

RECOVERY FROM BIRTH ASPHYXIA

During the first minutes after birth, pH continues to fall while lactate levels rise. This occurs as a result of the unloading of acid products from areas that have been underperfused during asphyxia. By 1–3 hours of age, pH and lactate levels in the healthy infant are near normal for the adult; however, they remain acidotic for considerably longer in the depressed infant.

Following lung expansion, arterial oxygen tension rises and carbon dioxide tension falls rapidly. Recovery is accomplished initially by pulmonary elimination of carbon dioxide and not by renal excretion of hydrogen ion. By 24 hours, the healthy newborn has reached the same acid–base balance as the mother prior to labor.

A number of factors slow the rate of recovery from birth asphyxia. The most important are preterm delivery, and analgesic and anesthetic drugs given prior to delivery. Delay in recovery is also seen in the more asphyxiated infants, probably because of circulatory impairment and central nervous system depression. This group includes infants who have aspirated meconium prior to delivery.

An additional factor that delays recovery is a sustained increase in metabolic rate as a result of exposure of the naked newborn to room temperature (Fig. 42–2). Under these conditions, metabolic acidosis persists, although the vigorous infant achieves a normal pH by increasing carbon dioxide elimination. In the depressed infant, cooling after birth causes a fall in pH and a greater increase in metabolic acidosis. The time at which the cord is clamped following delivery does not appear to influence the newborn's acid–base readjustment.

Several explanations have been offered for the low arterial carbon dioxide pressure (about 32 mm Hg) observed in healthy infants once normal acid–base balance has been achieved. These include hyperventilation due to anoxia or increased levels of organic acids, the influence of progesterone on the respiratory center, the presence of shunts through the fetal channels during the neonatal period, and the respiratory response to mild cold stress noted earlier. At present, it is not known which, if any, of these factors plays the major role.

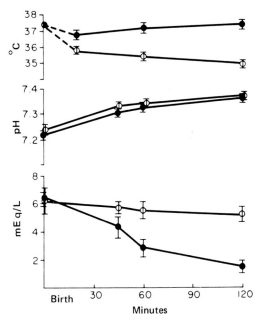

FIG. 42–2. Deep body temperatures (colonic), pH, and excess acid during first 2 hours of life in two groups of healthy infants. In one group (•) body temperature was maintained by infrared lamp; in other (o), body temperature was allowed to fall while infant was exposed to environmental temperature of 25° C (room temperature).

RESPIRATION

Onset of Breathing

The first breath is in part a continuation of the fetal respiratory movements before birth. However, a number of additional factors appear to be important for the initial effort to expand the lungs and for the subsequent maintenance of rhythmic breathing.

Among the stimuli implicated, asphyxia holds a favored position as the principal driving force. There is little doubt that a fall in arterial oxygen tension and pH, accompanied by a rise in carbon dioxide tension, produces gasping *in utero* as well as after birth. Rhythmic breathing may follow an improvement in oxygenation and normalization of acid–base state. The respiratory drive during asphyxia depends upon the presence of carotid and aortic chemoreceptors, which are known to be functional in the newborn. However, neither hypoxia nor hypercapnia alone initiates breathing in the experimental animal. This suggests that either the chemoreceptors of the fetus do not respond to hypoxia in the presence of normal pH and carbon dioxide tension or that the state of activity of the respiratory neurons is such that the afferent stimuli from the carotid and aortic chemoreceptors do not lead to a sufficient efferent discharge.

The short time interval between birth and the first breath suggests that the respiratory centers are activated by impulses from peripheral receptors initiated by stimuli other than the relatively slow changes in blood composition. Thermal stimuli immediately after birth must be intense. Calculations based on the rate of fall of skin temperature in the 1st minutes of extrauterine life indicate that at room temperature the newborn human infant loses about 600 cal/min.

While thermal stimuli appear to be of particular importance, tactile stimuli do not. Strong stimulation of the fetal lamb by surgical incision produces a gasp, but rhythmic breathing is not initiated. Occlusion of the umbilical cord causes a prompt but transient rise in blood pressure and occasional gasping; however, breathing can occur in the presence of intact umbilical circulation both *in utero* and after delivery.

The First Breath

Most infants make respiratory efforts within a few seconds of being born, and after the first few breaths the lungs are almost completely expanded. This was not the case earlier in the century, when heavy maternal medication and general anesthesia were widely employed for delivery. The onset of breathing was frequently delayed for several minutes, during which tactile and thermal stimuli were applied, often combined with the administration of analeptics.

The first inspiration is usually followed by a cry as the infant expires against a partially closed glottis, creating a positive intrathoracic pressure of up to 40 cm H_2O. Within a few minutes, functional residual capacity reaches about three-quarters of final aeration.

Although the intrathoracic pressures recorded during the first breaths are high, it is surprising how often initial lung expansion appears to require little effort. The work for initial lung expansion is undeniably greater than that for quiet breathing, but it is not greater than that performed many times a day during vigorous crying.

Dimensions and Operational Factors of Lung in Postnatal Period

Following lung expansion, the functional residual capacity is about 70 ml in the term infant and changes little over the first 6 days of life. The respiratory rate is approximately 30/min in the mature infant and 40/min in the preterm infant. Tidal and minute volumes are approximately 20 and 600 ml, respectively, for the mature infant and 10 and 400 ml for the preterm. There is a significant direct relation between minute volume and weight of the infant, the volume of air breathed being greater by approximately 120 ml/kg body weight in the larger infant.

Basal oxygen consumption values range 4–5 ml/kg body weight/min and are approximately 30% higher than those of the adult man. The difference is due to

the infant's having a greater proportion of tissues with high metabolic rates in relation to total body weight. The respiratory quotient has limited meaning in the early neonatal period because of disparity between production and output of carbon dioxide. Immediately after birth, the baby is recovering from a metabolic and respiratory acidosis, and if the baby is exposed to room temperature (25° C), this problem can be very considerably compounded.

The sensitivity of the respiratory center of the newborn to carbon dioxide is similar to that of the adult. Ventilation increases at least 100% in the vigorous infant when alveolar carbon dioxide tension changes from 40 to 50 mm Hg. Ventilation is depressed if the alveolar carbon dioxide tension rises above 80 mm Hg.

The ventilatory response to breathing a gas mixture of low oxygen content is not as pronounced in the newborn infant as in the adult; hyperpnea may not appear, or it may last only a few minutes. Animal experiments indicate that this diminished response can result from cool environmental conditions. If 100% oxygen is substituted for air, there is a temporary decrease in ventilation in the healthy infant but no change in oxygen consumption. On the other hand, administration of higher oxygen mixtures increases ventilation in infants with the respiratory distress syndrome and restores oxygen consumption to normal levels in infants depressed at birth.

Respiratory Responses During and Following Asphyxia

The cardiovascular, respiratory, and biochemical changes that occur during asphyxia under controlled conditions are predictable. Information on this subject is most complete in the newborn monkey. During the initial phase of asphyxia of the unanesthetized newborn animal, respiratory efforts increase in depth and frequency for up to 3 min. This period, called primary hyperpnea, is followed by primary apnea lasting for approximately 1 min. Rhythmic gasping then begins and is maintained at a fairly constant rate of about 6 gasps/min for several minutes. The gasps finally become weaker and slower. Their cessation marks the beginning of secondary apnea.

There is some variation of the duration of gasping (time to the last gasp) in different species, depending on the initial acid–base state, drugs given to the mother, environmental temperature, and degree of maturity of the species at birth. At a given environmental temperature, the principal determinant of duration of gasping in the nonanesthetized animal is the initial arterial pH. Narcotics and systemic anesthetic agents administered to the mother can abolish the period of primary hyperpnea and prolong primary apnea; large doses can suppress all respiratory efforts. Gasping is always prolonged at lower body temperatures.

During primary apnea, a variety of stimuli, such as

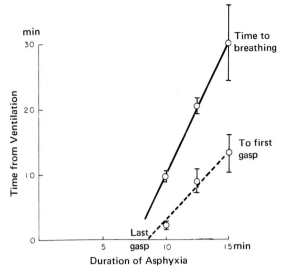

FIG. 42–3. Time from ventilation to first gasp and to rhythmic breathing in newborn monkeys asphyxiated for 10, 12.5, and 15 min at 30° C. Mean time from onset of asphyxia until last gasp was 8.42 ± 0.24 (SE) min. (Adamsons K, Jr, Behrman R, Dawes GS, James LS, Koford C: J Pediatr 65:807, 1964)

pain, cold, and analeptics, can initiate gasping. Once the stage of secondary apnea has been reached, these stimuli are without effect. Gasping can, however, be reinitiated by artificial ventilation or correction of acidosis by administration of base. There is a linear relation between the duration of asphyxia and recovery of respiratory function after resuscitation. In newborn monkeys, for each minute after the last gasp that artificial ventilation is delayed, there is a further delay of 2 min before gasping begins again and of 4 min before rhythmic breathing is established (Fig. 42–3). This indicates that the longer artificial ventilation is delayed during secondary apnea, the longer it will take to resuscitate the infant.

CHANGES IN CIRCULATION AFTER BIRTH

With the onset of respiration and lung expansion, pulmonary vascular resistance falls. This appears to be due largely to the direct effect of oxygen and carbon dioxide on the blood vessels; resistance decreases as oxygen tension rises and carbon dioxide tension falls. Lung expansion *per se* contributes to lowering the pulmonary vascular resistance. There then follows a gradual transition from the fetal to the adult type of circulation, the foramen ovale and ductus arteriosus remaining open for varying lengths of time.

Pressure in the left atrium falls in the first few hours of life to levels below those in the normal adult; by 24 hours, it may be less than 1 mm Hg above that in the

right atrium. This small pressure difference probably accounts for the persistence of a right-to-left shunt through the foramen ovale for 24 hours or longer.

Pulmonary arterial pressure remains relatively high for several hours. As the pulmonary vascular resistance falls, the direction of blood flow through the ductus arteriosus reverses. In the first hours of extrauterine life, the flow is bidirectional, but the shunt eventually becomes entirely left to right and by 15 hours of age is functionally insignificant.

The ductus arteriosus constricts in response to an increase in arterial oxygen tension. Sympathomimetic amines also cause it to constrict. Hypoxemia can cause a constricted ductus to reopen and at the same time may reestablish the fetal pattern of circulation by increasing the pulmonary vascular resistance. This response of the ductus arteriosus to oxygen or hypoxia is thus opposite to that of the pulmonary arterioles, enabling the right ventricle to contribute a variable fraction of its output to placental perfusion during fetal life. The different reactivity of these vessels during hypoxia, although an asset to the fetus, becomes a liability for the newborn infant. Hypoxic episodes in early neonatal life can lead to a rise in pulmonary vascular resistance and opening of the ductus arteriosus, increasing any residual right-to-left shunt. The reasons for the different responses of these vessels to hypoxia have not so far been determined.

THERMOREGULATION IN THE NEWBORN

Measurements of metabolic rate in the immediate neonatal period have established that newborn human babies, like most warm-blooded mammals, increase their metabolic rate in response to cold; their low thermal stability is due to excessive heat loss rather than to impaired heat production.

The difference in rate of thermal energy dissipation between the newborn and the adult can be explained largely by differences in physical characteristics. At birth, the body mass of the human baby is about 5% that of the adult, while surface area amounts to nearly 15%. The high ratio between body surface and body mass, together with increased curvature of body surfaces, facilitates thermal exchange by convection and radiation. Thickness of skin and subcutaneous fat insulating deeper body structures is significantly less at birth, resulting in greater thermal conductance and a higher skin temperature at low environmental temperatures. As a result of these differences, heat loss per unit of body weight in the term infant is approximately four times that in the adult. This value increases further for the preterm infant or the infant of small body size.

In the immediate neonatal period, the body temperature of the human newborn may fall as much as $2°-3°C$ (Fig. 42–2). It has been calculated that heat losses in the initial minutes following birth may amount to as much as 200 cal/kg/min under normal delivery room conditions. Several factors are responsible for the high rate of heat loss. At the time of delivery, the deep body temperature of the newborn is about $0.5°C$ and the skin temperature about $2.5°C$ higher than that encountered during extrauterine life; there is virtually no thermal gradient between peripheral tissues and deeper structures. Evaporation of amniotic fluid from the skin also contributes to heat loss. Excess heat stored in the peripheral and deeper tissues of the fetus minimizes the impact of the new environment. For the fetus at term, the overall reserve could be as much as 4000 cal.

It remains to be elucidated whether the transient fall in peripheral and deep body temperature that occurs immediately after birth favors or hinders adaptation to extrauterine life. Thermal stimuli might be important in the initiation and establishment of breathing by increasing the state of activity of the reticular system. Cold perception induces cutaneous vasoconstriction and raises systemic vascular resistance, which might be important in the reduction of right-to-left shunting through the patent ductus arteriosus. Prolonged exposure of the naked infant to room temperature, on the other hand, has been shown to lead to progressive metabolic acidosis, particularly in the depressed infant or the infant with impaired pulmonary function.

In homeothermic species, the first line of defense in reducing heat loss consists of cutaneous vasoconstriction, which diminishes the temperature gradient between body surface and environment. Vasoconstriction in response to cold stimuli is present not only in the term infant but also in the preterm infant from the time of birth. Further reduction in heat loss can be achieved by postural changes that decrease the body surface available for thermal exchange. Increase in metabolic rate in response to cold also serves to maintain body temperature, and the naked newborn responds in this way. Although measurements have not yet been made in the 1st minutes of life, infants only 15 min old are able to double or even triple their oxygen consumption. A similar response has been documented in preterm infants.

Oxygen consumption in the cold environment is predominantly a function of the temperature gradient between body surface and environment, not of the absolute values of deep body, skin, or environmental temperatures. Basal metabolic rates are observed in healthy mature newborns with varying deep body or skin temperatures as long as the temperature gradient between skin and environment is less than $1.5°C$. Once this limit is exceeded, oxygen consumption begins to rise at a rate of approximately 0.6 ml/°C, reaching values up to 15 ml/kg/min. This compares favorably with maximal heat production of the adult under severe cold stress. From a teleologic point of

view, dependence on the thermal gradient rather than the absolute temperature is advantageous because it enables the newborn to reduce oxygen consumption to basal levels as soon as thermal conditions are favorable, allowing a gradual rise in body temperature to normal levels without additional expenditure of energy.

Increased muscular activity probably plays a major role in heat production. However, the metabolic rate can rise without shivering or increased muscular tone, as shown in animal experiments during paralysis of the neuromuscular junction. The brown adipose tissue of the newborn appears also to be a source of heat production. The brown fat deposits in the interscapular region, axillae, perirenal areas, and around large vessels in the chest are rich in blood and nerve supply and have a high mitochondrial content and a high metabolic rate *in vitro*. Although thermal output of brown fat could make an important contribution to total heat production in certain newborn animals, it cannot be essential for temperature regulation in all homeothermic species, since the newborn piglet, which has virtually no adipose tissue, either white or brown, shows an excellent metabolic response to cold. It is not known to what extent other organs, such as liver and brain, contribute to the increase in total body metabolism during cooling.

The physiologic mediator that links perception of cold with increased metabolic activity and thus increased heat production is still unknown. Sympathomimetic amines can increase heat production in the adult, and this response is pronounced in the cold-adapted and in the newborn animal. Increase in oxygen consumption has been observed during intravenous infusion of norepinephrine in the human newborn. On the other hand, adrenergic blockade does not alter the increase in oxygen consumption upon exposure to cold, although it does obliterate the response to exogenous noradrenalin.

A variety of factors can interfere with normal homeothermal responses in the newborn. Hypoxia is of particular importance, although the sensitivity to oxygen lack varies among species. The newborn human fails to respond to cold when breathing gas mixtures of 15% oxygen. If respiration and adequate oxygenation are not promptly established after birth, the effects of birth asphyxia upon thermoregulation can be rather long-lasting. Differences in deep body temperature between asphyxiated and vigorous infants have been detected for up to 20 hours after birth.

Few data are available about the effects of hypnotics, analgesics, anesthetics, and neuromuscular autonomic blocking agents upon thermoregulation of the newborn. Administration of meperidine hydrochloride to the mother during labor leads to greater fall in the infant's body temperature in the neonatal period. In the experimental animal, administration of reserpine, a drug known to deplete the body of catecholamine stores, has produced thermal instability of the newborn by interfering with heat conservation. If the depression of the newborn is due to excessive maternal medication, it is important to recognize that a fall in body temperature not only potentiates but also prolongs the effect of most analgesic and anesthetic drugs.

RESUSCITATION

The delivery room must be prepared for adequate and prompt treatment of severe asphyxia at birth, whether it is expected or not. All members of the delivery room team should be trained in methods of resuscitation, for both mother and baby may be in difficulty at the same time. Indecision or ineffective therapy may lose the few moments during which the baby can be helped.

Every piece of apparatus necessary for emergency resuscitation should be carefully checked before each delivery. There should be suction apparatus, a plastic oropharyngeal airway, a laryngoscope equipped with a pencil handle and a blade, and a plastic endotracheal tube with a stylet. Oxygen should be available. All examinations and needed resuscitation should be conducted on an appropriate table or resuscitator equipped with an overhead source of heat to maintain the baby's body temperature.

INITIAL TREATMENT AND APPRAISAL OF INFANT

The fetal heart rate should be determined after every contraction during the final stages of labor or, preferably, monitored continuously. The growing use of electronic monitoring of fetal heart rate and biochemical monitoring of fetal acid–base state has enabled earlier recognition of warning signs of fetal distress and allows the obstetrician to take appropriate measures before the infant becomes severely asphyxiated.

Immediately after delivery, the baby should be held head down while the cord is clamped and cut. The infant should then be placed supine on a table, the head kept low with a slight lateral tilt. A nurse or assistant should listen to the heartbeat immediately, indicating the rate by finger movement. If help is not available, the rate can be detected from pulsation of the umbilical cord. A strong beat with a rate of over 100/min indicates that there is no immediate emergency. Distant heart sounds or a slow rate indicates severe depression, calling for resuscitative measures. While the nurse is listening to the heart, the physician should aspirate the mouth, the pharynx, and the nose with a catheter. This suction should be brief. From birth to completion of suctioning should take about 1 min. Slapping the soles lightly frequently aids in initiating a deep breath and crying. More severe methods of stimulation, such as dilating the anal sphincter, hot and cold

TABLE 42–1. CLINICAL EVALUATION OF NEWBORN INFANT IN DELIVERY ROOM BY APGAR SCORING METHOD

Sign	0	1	2
Heart rate	None	Slow (below 100)	Over 100
Respiratory effort	None	Weak cry; hypoventilation	Good; strong cry
Muscle tone	Limp	Some flexion of extremities	Active motion; extremities well flexed
Reflex irritability (response to stimulation of sole of foot)	No response	Grimace	Cry
Color	Pale	Blue	Completely pink

tubbing, or vigorous back-slapping, are traumatic, ineffectual, and a waste of time.

The initial appraisal of the newborn should start at the moment of birth, with particular attention to the first few breaths and the evenness and ease of respiration. A congenital laryngeal web or choanal atresia can cause complete airway obstruction; both require immediate treatment. A diaphragmatic hernia with abdominal viscera in the chest, abdominal distention from ascites, congenital cystic lungs, or intrauterine pneumonia may all cause respiratory difficulty and may even prevent lung expansion.

The scoring system introduced by Apgar in 1952 is a useful method to quantitate the clinical evaluation of the baby (Table 42–1). The score is based on heart rate, respiratory effort, muscle tone, reflex irritability, and color. A score of 0 is given for no heartbeat, no respiratory effort, no muscle tone, no reflex response to a glancing slap on the soles of the feet, and a pale color. A score of 1 is given for a slow heartbeat, slow or irregular respiratory effort, some flexion of the extremities, a grimace in response to a glancing slap on the soles of the feet, and a blue coloration. A score of 2 is given for a heart rate over 100, a good respiratory effort accompanied by crying, a cry in response to the slap on the feet, and a completely healthy coloration. At 60 sec after complete birth of the infant, the five objective signs are evaluated and scored as 0, 1, or 2. A score of 10 indicates an infant in the best possible condition. The majority of infants are vigorous, with a score of 7–10, and cough or cry within seconds of delivery. No further resuscitative procedures are necessary for them. Mildly to moderately depressed infants form the largest group requiring some form of resuscitation at birth. These infants are pale or blue at 1 min after delivery; they have not established sustained respirations and may be nearly flaccid. However, heart rate and reflex irritability are good. Their score may be 4, 5, or 6. The severely depressed infant is flaccid, unresponsive, and pale; its Apgar score is 0, 1, or 2.

Immediately after the cord is cut and breathing is established, a drop of 1% silver nitrate is instilled in each eye as prophylaxis against gonorrheal ophthalmia. In some states, it is stipulated that silver nitrate be used in each case; in others the use of less irritating agents, such as penicillin or tetracycline ointment, is permitted.

TREATMENT OF MODERATELY DEPRESSED INFANT

The time required for recovery, and also the completeness of recovery, are direct functions of the duration of asphyxia (Fig. 42–3). If initial resuscitative measures have produced no response by 1.5 min after delivery, the progressing asphyxia usually leads to diminished muscular tone and a fall in the heart rate. A small plastic oropharyngeal airway should then be inserted into the mouth and oxygen applied under pressure of 16–20 cm H_2O for 1–2 sec. Although this pressure is sufficient to expand the alveoli, some oxygen will reach the respiratory bronchioles. The rise in intrabronchial pressure stimulates pulmonary stretch receptors. This stimulus, added to that of the chemoreceptors, initiates a gasp in about 85% of the cases.

If there is no respiratory effort and the heart rate continues to fall, the infant becoming completely flaccid, the larynx should be visualized with the laryngoscope. This is not a difficult procedure, but skill should be obtained by practice on the stillborn. An ideal method of teaching and learning this technique is the use of an adult cat anesthetized with ketamine hydrochloride.

Intubation is best accomplished with the infant lying supine on a flat surface. A folded towel under the head and slight extension of the neck places the infant in a position resembling a sniffing posture. The head should be steadied with the right hand and kept in line with the body. The laryngoscope is held in the left hand, and the blade is introduced at the right corner of the mouth and advanced between tongue and palate for about 2 cm. As it is advanced, the blade is swung to the midline. This moves the tongue to the left of the blade. The operator looks along the blade for the rim of the epiglottis. The laryngoscope is gently advanced into the space between the base of the tongue and the epiglottis (Fig. 42–4). Slight elevation of the tip of the blade exposes the glottis as a vertical dark slit bordered posteriorly by pink arytenoid cartilages.

If foreign material such as small blood clots, meco-

nium-stained mucus, or vernix obstructs the larynx, quick brief suction is indicated. When the glottis is seen to be patent, a curved endotracheal tube is introduced at the right corner of the mouth and inserted through the cords until the flange of the tube rests at the glottis. Care must be taken not to intubate the esophagus. The laryngoscope is then withdrawn. Rarely, the glottis is obstructed by a laryngeal web. If this is partial or thin, it may be perforated with a stylet, or the opening may be enlarged with an endotracheal tube. The presence of a thick membrane requires immediate tracheostomy.

If stimuli from these procedures have not initiated a spontaneous gasp, positive pressure should be applied to the endotracheal tube. Brief puffs of air blown through the tube with enough force to cause the lower chest to rise gently usually starts spontaneous respiration. If the stomach rises, however, the esophagus has been intubated instead of the trachea, and the position of the tube must be corrected. Pressures between 25 and 35 cm H_2O are necessary to expand the alveoli initially and can be applied safely for 1–2 sec. Experience in applying this pressure should be gained by puffing into a spring manometer. Oxygen-enriched gas may be delivered to the infant by placing a tube carrying oxygen in the operator's mouth.

If the endotracheal tube is fitted with appropriate-sized adapters, it can be connected to a rubber bag of oxygen or oxygen-enriched gas mixture, or to one of the mechanical devices for applying positive pressure.

Artificial expansion of the lungs can initiate a spontaneous gasp. With the first or second application of positive pressure, the infant usually makes an effort to breathe. The endotracheal tube may be withdrawn after the infant has taken five or six breaths.

TREATMENT OF SEVERELY DEPRESSED INFANT

No time should be lost in establishing ventilation. The glottis should be inspected immediately with the laryngoscope. If meconium or thick meconium-stained mucus has been aspirated into the trachea, it must be suctioned out at once prior to inflation of the lungs. It is usually possible to accomplish this within 1 min after delivery. These severely depressed infants may require 3–8 min of artificial ventilation before a spontaneous gasp is taken. The endotracheal tube can be removed as soon as quiet and sustained respiration is established.

Under some circumstances, lung expansion is impossible in spite of proper intubation. There are four conditions in which this occurs: 1) massive aspiration of meconium that cannot be removed by suctioning, 2) intrauterine pneumonia with organization of exudate, 3) large bilateral diaphragmatic hernias with hypoplastic lungs, and 4) congenital adenomatous cysts

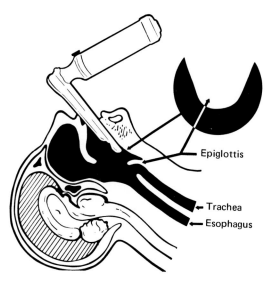

FIG. 42–4. Sagittal view of mouth and pharynx showing relation of laryngoscope blade to epiglottis.

of the lung. Infants with the first two conditions are usually severely depressed at birth. However, those with hypoplastic lungs may be initially vigorous, scoring as high as 7 at 1 min of age, and may make strenuous but ineffective respiratory efforts. At present, there is no available treatment for this condition. Congenital adenomatous cysts of the lung are associated with hydrops fetalis, and the condition is usually fatal.

USE OF CARDIAC MASSAGE

Blood pressure and heart rate fall during prolonged asphyxia. If the blood pressure is unduly low at the beginning of resuscitation, positive pressure ventilation is unlikely to be successful unless the heart is massaged. Cardiac massage has been successfully applied through the intact chest wall in human infants.

External manual compression of the heart between the chest wall and vertebral column forces blood into the aorta. Relaxation of pressure allows the heart to fill with venous blood. When combined with proper ventilation, external manual heart compression often maintains blood pressure and adequate oxygenation until spontaneous cardiac activity returns.

The technique consists of intermittent compression of the middle and lower third of the sternum 100–120 times per minute with the index and middle fingers. Massage is interrupted every 5 sec to permit two or three inflations of the lung. It should be employed only after the lungs have been well expanded when a heartbeat cannot be detected or the heart rate does not rise promptly. Cardiopulmonary resuscitation is most

successful when there has been no evidence of fetal distress.

USE OF ANALEPTICS AND DRUG ANTAGONISTS

Analeptics such as nikethamide serve no useful purpose in resuscitation of the newborn. Although they may shorten primary apnea, they are ineffective in secondary apnea (see earlier discussion) and may cause hypotension and convulsions, even if given in the clinically recommended dose.

N-allylnormorphine has been found useful when the depression of respiration in the newborn is due to transplacentally acquired opiates and related compounds. The recommended dose is 0.2 mg/kg body weight. The drug should be given after expansion of lungs and the establishment of adequate oxygenation. Although crying and restlessness often follow the administration of N-allylnormorphine, they are frequently of brief duration and may be followed by even more profound depression of the central nervous system due to the intrinsic depressant properties of the compound.

The role of epinephrine in the resuscitation of the severely asphyxiated fetus or newborn remains to be determined. Studies with fetal monkeys have demonstrated that large doses of epinephrine (1–5 mμ/kg) administered either intravenously or intraarterially initiate heart action and restore blood pressure and heart rate to normal in the severely asphyxiated fetus. However, because epinephrine increases pulmonary arterial pressure considerably above normal, there is a distinct risk of increasing filtration of plasma into the alveolar spaces with the resultant clinical picture of pulmonary edema.

RAPID CORRECTION OF pH

In experimental animals, maintenance of normal pH during asphyxia by rapid intravenous infusion of alkali, together with glucose, prolongs gasping and delays cardiovascular collapse. Resuscitation is also facilitated if alkali and glucose are infused at the same time artificial ventilation is started. It has been proposed that the beneficial effects of pH correction are derived from prolongation and acceleration of anaerobic glycolysis, restitution of oxygen-carrying capacity of hemoglobin and responsiveness of cardiovascular muscle to sympathomimetic amines, and fall in pulmonary vascular resistance.

Administration of alkali to the asphyxiated newborn has been shown to increase the rate of recovery and responsiveness of the infant. However, the demonstration that alkali administration is associated with intracranial hemorrhage and hypernatremia has caused much concern. These adverse effects of alkali appear to be due to injudicious use, particularly in the presence of impaired carbon dioxide elimination. If given in too high a concentration, in too great a quantity, and in the presence of severely impaired ventilation, the adverse effects undoubtedly outweigh the benefits.

The most severely asphyxiated infants—those with an arterial pH below 7.0—have a base deficit of 26 mEq/liter or greater, in addition to a marked elevation in carbon dioxide tension. By means of artificial ventilation alone, the base deficit can be reduced by approximately 10 mEq/liter in 5–10 min, provided good alveolar ventilation is achieved and circulatory collapse does not persist. It is advisable initially to attempt to correct one-half of the residual metabolic component of the mixed acidosis. Thus a 3-kg infant would receive 8 mEq base. This calculation assumes that the extracellular volume is one-third the body weight.

In infants who are so severely asphyxiated that the heart rate does not return after good lung expansion and several episodes of cardiac massage, infusion of alkali or further resuscitation efforts are not recommended.

USE OF HYPOTHERMIA

There are several reasons why hypothermia might be a valuable adjunct in the resuscitation of the asphyxiated newborn. Metabolic rate could be lowered; increased peripheral vasoconstriction could help to maintain blood pressure; carbon dioxide tension could be lowered, owing to increased solubility of carbon dioxide at lower temperature; and pH could be elevated, owing to changes in the dissociation constants of water and the other acids. However, the rate of cooling is slow, particularly in the presence of a collapsed circulation, and the rise in pH and fall in carbon dioxide tension are small compared with the changes that accompany ventilation.

Experiments in which cooling starts at the same time as asphyxia have no bearing on asphyxia before birth when the fetus is at a warmer temperature than the mother. Hypothermia as a resuscitative procedure has been tried under controlled experimental conditions in newborn monkeys asphyxiated prior to cooling; respiration was not reinitiated and brain damage not prevented.

PHYSICAL EXAMINATION IN DELIVERY ROOM

As soon as respiration is well established, the newborn baby should be carefully examined to determine the presence of abnormalities, such as tracheoesophageal fistula, duodenal atresia, imperforate anus, or arteriovenous fistula, that require prompt attention. It is also important that the less serious defects and birth in-

juries be discovered first by the physician so that necessary explanations can be made to the mother. The sequence in which various systems of the infant are examined differs somewhat from that customarily employed in the adult.

SKIN

The color is normally pale pink, save for the hands and feet, which may remain cyanotic for more than an hour, even in vigorous infants. Some differential cyanosis of the lower part of the body due to persistence of right-to-left shunting through the ductus arteriosus is often present for the first 30 min of life. This is demonstrated more clearly if the infant is given high concentrations of oxygen for 5–10 sec. Persistence of differential cyanosis indicates failure of ductus closure, high pulmonary vascular resistance, or a preductal coarctation. These changes are less apparent in infants with pigmented skins. Generalized cyanosis, even with gross cardiac anomalies, after the onset of respiration is rare. Presumably, it is caused by cutaneous vasoconstriction. It is seen in the first few minutes of life in infants who experience difficulties in establishing ventilation.

Generalized pallor indicates either intense vasoconstriction or anemia. The former is present in more asphyxiated infants. The latter should be suspected in the presence of erythroblastosis, placenta previa, or multiple pregnancy, but it can also occur as a result of intraplacental shunts between fetus and mother and, occasionally, with a nuchal cord.

Yellow appearance of the skin and umbilical cord is usually the result of meconium staining and is accompanied by golden coloring of the vernix and meconium in the amniotic fluid. It is also seen in erythroblastotic infants who are severely anemic at birth. Since retention of bilirubin is a late phenomenon in erythroblastosis fetalis, jaundice at birth is rather rare, it may be seen at birth, however, with severe intrauterine infection and hepatitis.

The skin of a normal infant is smooth and elastic. Subcutaneous fat varies in thickness from a fraction of a millimeter in the region of the thorax and scalp to a few millimeters over the abdomen, back, and buttocks. Vernix is usually seen, particularly in the skin folds, and lanugo is present over the back. Diminution of elasticity and subcutaneous fat, together with peeling and wrinkling of the skin indicate intrauterine malnutrition. In the mature infant, such changes are accompanied by meconium staining. They occur more frequently in the presence of prolonged gestation, or maternal hypertension or preeclampsia. The birth weight of these infants is usually less than expected for the gestational age, and they are prone to hypoglycemia in the neonatal period.

Thickening of subcutaneous tissue can be due to edema or fat. The latter is common in infants of diabetic or prediabetic mothers.

Petechiae over the head and neck are seen when there has been a tight nuchal cord or delay in delivery of the body due to shoulder impaction. The presence of pigmented nevi or hemangiomas should be recorded and hemangiomas carefully examined for bruit or pulsation that would indicate an arteriovenous fistula.

Rashes, which are rare, result from viral (varicella, rubella, and cytomegalic inclusion disease) or protozoal (syphilis) infection *in utero*.

HEAD AND NECK

There is considerable variation in the shape of the head as the result of molding during labor and delivery, particularly in the infants of primiparas and in those presenting with the occiput posterior. The head is spheric in infants delivered by the breech or by cesarean section. Excessive elongation should be noted because of the possibility of tentorial tears. Edema of the subcutaneous tissue of the leading parts (usually occiput) is common. Cephalhematoma differs from scalp edema (with or without subcutaneous extravasation of blood) by being confined within the area of one of the cranial bones. Vacuum extractors create a sharply demarcated circular edema that may reach up to 2 cm in thickness. It disappears more slowly than the naturally occurring edema. Forceps marks consisting of depressions or edema with erythema and sometimes abrasions frequently signify a traumatic delivery and may be associated with cranial nerve injuries or skull fractures. These should be suspected, particularly in cases of improper application of forceps (face–mastoid). Fortunately, in modern obstetrics, the elimination of most complicated vaginal deliveries in favor of cesarean section has considerably reduced the incidence of these complications.

The anterior fontanel is open and should be palpated for size and tension. Bulging is diagnostic of increased intracranial pressure and may indicate hydrocephalus or intracranial hemorrhage. The posterior fontanel is closed and is frequently difficult to outline due to scalp edema. If open, hydrocephalus should be suspected. A small or closed anterior fontanel occurs in a condition known as craniosynostosis and is not infrequently accompanied by microcephaly or an abnormally shaped head. Soft spots in the skull (craniotabes) are present in about one-third of all newborn infants, preferentially located in the parietal area. Rarely, a cranial bone may be missing, indicating osteogenesis imperfecta.

The eyes are usually closed but may be open in postterm infants; in severe asphyxia they may be wide open and staring. The pupil's size and reactivity to light and the color of the sclera should be noted. Fixed

dilated pupils, or anisocoria, indicates severe asphyxia or brain damage. Subconjunctival hemorrhage is occasionally seen following difficult breech or impacted shoulders delivery.

Examination of the position and shape of the external ear is important because malformations are associated with renal anomalies. If the ears are low-set or the configuration is deformed, the umbilical cord should be examined to determine if it lacks one umbilical artery, and the infant should be closely observed for the passage of urine.

Saddle deformity of the nose, a pathognomonic sign of congenital syphilis, has virtually disappeared with the advent of antibiotics and the improvement in antenatal care.

Since infants are obligatory nose-breathers, occlusion of the upper airway can cause respiratory difficulties; choanal atresia has resulted in death from asphyxia in infants with no other abnormality of the respiratory tract. Testing for nasal patency is best achieved by occluding one nostril and the mouth, rather than passing a catheter, which can be injurious. Microglossia or underdevelopment of the lower jaw (micrognathia) can also cause obstruction of the airway and can be responsible for difficulties encountered during resuscitation. Slight recession of the mandible is not uncommon in normal infants. Masses in the neck, notably by enlarged thyroid, can cause tracheal compression that may necessitate tracheotomy. The palate should be inspected with the laryngoscope or palpated. However, even careful palpation is likely to miss posterior defects.

THORAX

The chest must be observed and auscultated for evenness of aeration. By 5 min of age, adventitious sounds normally remain only over the precordial area. Sternal or intercostal retraction in term infants is abnormal and indicates airway obstruction or incomplete lung expansion. In preterm infants, some retraction is expected because of the softness of the chest wall and less compliant lung. Prolongation of expiration with or without an audible grunt is also abnormal and frequently is the first sign of incipient respiratory distress syndrome.

Diminished or absent breath sounds on one side, are indicative of pneumothorax or diaphragmatic hernia with abdominal viscera in the chest. Percussion usually differentiates the two. Soft or distant heart sounds associated with an increase in heart rate are found with pneumomediastinum. If any of these conditions is suspected, the chest should be x-rayed. (Pneumomediastinum can always be managed conservatively and pneumothorax usually so; however, if a tension pneumothorax develops, this should be promptly treated by inserting a blunt needle into the intrapleural space and instituting underwater drainage. Diaphragmatic hernia requires prompt consultation and operative correction.)

The clavicles and ribs should be palpated for fractures, which can be associated with vascular or nerve injuries. This is particularly important if pneumothorax or pneumomediastinum is present. Occasionally, fracture of a rib leads to emphysema of the chest wall, causing crepitus.

The heart is nearly in the midline, and there is frequently marked precordial activity during the first 30 min of life, when bidirectional shunting through the ductus arteriosus is maximal. The heart rate following delivery is 160–170 beats/min, which is 15% higher than the rate during labor. By 20–30 min of age, the rate returns to the previous level. Although the reason for this transient acceleration of heart rate is not known, it probably represents a response to high levels of catecholamines, as well as various tactile, auditory, and thermal stimuli. Furthermore, increased total cardiac output in the presence of bidirectional shunting is necessary if the rate of tissue perfusion is to remain constant.

A pansystolic crescendo murmur is present in approximately 15% of all infants during the first 2 hours of life. It is more common in preterm infants and in those recovering from severe asphyxia. Its cause has not yet been determined. Two likely possibilities are shunting through the ductus arteriosus and regurgitation through the mitral or tricuspid valve. Only one-third of infants with cardiac malformation have detectable murmurs in the neonatal period.

ABDOMEN

Before the abdomen is palpated for abnormal masses, the catheter used for oropharyngeal suction during resuscitation should be passed through the mouth and esophagus into the stomach. When the catheter tip is in the proper position, there is usually a bulge in the left upper abdominal quadrant. Even if this is not seen, suction should be applied to the tube and the stomach emptied. Should no secretions be obtained, the position of the catheter should be verified by injecting air through it while auscultating the epigastrium. Esophageal atresia or tracheoesophageal fistula must be suspected if difficulties are encountered in the passage of a catheter. The stomach of the newborn infant contains 4–8 ml fluid, the volume tending to be greater in those born by elective cesarean section. Duodenal atresia or other types of upper gastrointestinal tract obstructions are likely to be present if larger quantities of fluid are obtained.

Emptying the stomach is essentially a diagnostic procedure, but it may be therapeutic if the volume of

fluid in the stomach is large enough to interfere with movement of the diaphragm. If a soft rubber or plastic catheter is used, there is virtually no danger of visceral injury. Perforation of the stomach in the newborn may occur spontaneously as a result of muscular defects or ulcers.

The liver and kidneys can readily be felt at this time; the liver is relatively large, extending about 3 cm below the costal margin in the midclavicular line.

The anal region should be inspected and the patency of the lower large bowel tested by insertion of the previously used rubber catheter for 8 cm. If anal atresia is present, the bladder should be catheterized and the urine examined for particulate matter, since a rectovesical fistula is frequently associated with this condition.

GENITALIA

Examination of the female genitalia is limited to inspection of the labia and clitoris, which is normally hypertrophied. Opaque viscous mucus normally covers the introitus. The urethral meatus is not identified, but patency of the urinary tract can be verified by observing passage of urine.

In the male infant, the prepuce is usually adherent and should not be retracted. The position of the testicles should be noted. They are normally in the scrotum, although during the examination they may be retracted toward the inguinal ligament by high tone of the cremaster muscle.

BACK AND EXTREMITIES

The sacrum should be examined for pigmentation and abnormal hair, which is not uncommonly associated with occult spina bifida. Limb position and movement should be observed. Normally, the limbs are flexed and exhibit irregular movement when the infant is stimulated to cry or exposed to cold. Flaccid extension of a limb suggests a nerve injury, which most commonly involves the arm as a result of brachial plexus damage. The extremities should be palpated for fractures. Since these are frequently incomplete, they are not readily detected; if there is a reasonable index of suspicion, the limb should be x-rayed. The digits should be counted and examined for webbing.

NEUROLOGIC EXAMINATION

Usually limited to the testing of the grasp and Moro reflexes, neurologic examination is brief. If the infant has had a low Apgar score and remains limp after res-

piration is established, there is an increased possibility of neurologic impairment. When the infant is asphyxiated at birth, the examiner should evaluate the anterior fontanels and look for signs of brain swelling, such as separation of the cranial sutures. Examination of eyegrounds reveals retinal hemorrhages in most such cases. Because brain swelling secondary to partial or prolonged oxygen deprivation *in utero* requires several hours to develop, its failure to appear immediately after delivery does not exclude the development of this serious complication.

Diagnosis of systemic congenital anomalies such as mongolism may be possible at this time. However, unless the diagnosis is unequivocal, signs should be interpeted with caution because they may result from birth trauma.

SMALL-FOR-GESTATIONAL-AGE INFANT

Infants weighing less than 2500 g may be either truly immature or small for gestational age as a result of impaired intrauterine growth. The use of the graph developed by Lubchenko *et al.* (Fig. 42–5) is helpful in identifying babies whose weights are inappropriate for gestational age. About one-third of low-birth-weight infants fit into the category of small for gestational age. In the remainder, the low weight is appropriate for the preterm delivery. A number of clinical signs are useful in separating the truly immature infant from the one who is small for gestational age. The scalp hair of the truly immature infant is fine and fuzzy, and individual strands are hard to distinguish; in the mature infant, scalp hair is coarse and silky and appears as individual strands. The earlobe of the preterm infant is pliable and has no cartilage. In the infant between 36 and 38 weeks old, there is some cartilage and a brisk rebound. The pigmented area of the breast is approximately 5 mm at 35 weeks' gestation; the breast nodule is not palpable or is lacking in the truly preterm infant, measures 2 mm at 36 weeks, 4 mm at 38 weeks, and 7 mm at term. Sole creases are minimal in the preterm infant; usually only the anterior transverse crease is present. From 34 to 38 weeks, there is an increase in creases over the anterior two-thirds of the sole, and at term the sole is covered with creases. In the immature male, the testes are low in the inguinal canal, and the scrotum is small with few rugae. In the term infant, the tests are in the scrotum, which is pendulous and has extensive rugae.

PLACENTA AND MEMBRANES

The placenta should be inspected for completeness, and its dimensions should be recorded. Increase in placental mass, particularly in its thickness, suggests

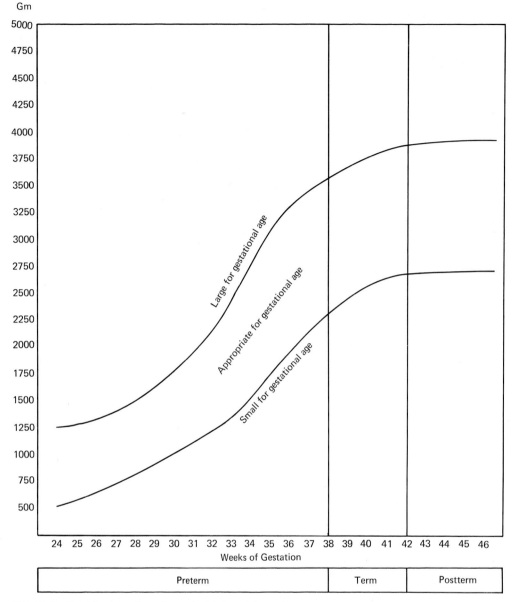

FIG. 42–5. Classification of newborns by birth weight and gestational age. (Lubchenko LO, Hansmann C, Boyd E: Pediatrics 37:717, 1966)

fetal hyperinsulinemia secondary to intermittent maternal hyperglycemia. Other causes of abnormal placental enlargement are hemolytic diseases of the fetus and fetal syphilis. The maternal surface of the placenta should be inspected for infarcts or attached blood clots. Infarcts often indicate maternal vascular disorder that has resulted in occlusion or thrombosis of the spiral arteriole. An attached blood clot may be diagnostic of a hitherto unsuspected premature separation of the placenta with its implications regarding coagulation disorders.

Brown or green discoloration of the amniotic surface indicates a prolonged exposure of the tissue to meconium. Vesicle formation is pathognomonic of renal agenesis. In the presence of multiple pregnancy, the placenta and membranes should be examined with special care, noting the number of chorionic sacs, vascular anastomoses from one placenta to the other, and the possibility of twin-to-twin transfusion, as de-

scribed in Chapter 43. Also, zygosity should be determined.

LABORATORY PROCEDURES

In all cases of blood incompatibility, blood should be removed from the umbilical cord for typing by the Coombs method and for hematocrit determination. If the infant appears pale, a capillary blood sample should be taken from a heel prick after warming the limb, and a microhematocrit determination should be done. When the membranes have been ruptured for longer than 12 hours, a section of the cord and surface of the placenta should be removed for microscopic examination, and material for culture should be taken from the amniotic surface of the placenta as well as from the nose and throat of the infant; a sample of the infant's blood should also be cultured. If facilities are available, a blood sample, either from the umbilical vessels or a heel prick, should be obtained in severely asphyxiated infants with a persistent low Apgar score and examined for pH and carbon dioxide pressure. This provides a measure of the degree of the asphyxia before birth and during resuscitation and serves as a guide for therapy. As stated earlier, correction of acidosis facilitates recovery of the asphyxiated experimental animal.

RESPIRATORY DISTRESS SYNDROME

This syndrome, also known as hyaline membrane disease, is one of the most common causes of death in the neonatal period in communities where obstetric care is of a high standard and infection of the newborn is no longer a major problem. It appears to be a failure of cardiopulmonary system to adapt to extrauterine conditions. The cause is unknown, but the syndrome is more common in preterm infants and in those subjected to severe asphyxia during labor and delivery. Prenatal tests of amniotic fluid can determine pulmonary maturity with high accuracy, thus permitting, in cases where the information is needed, a prediction about the probability that the infant will develop respiratory distress syndrome (see Chapter 41).

Careful observation reveals that these infants are not normal at birth. The onset of respiration is irregular or delayed, some degree of intercostal retraction is usually present, and expiration is accompanied by phonation in the form of a grunt or cry. Reduced muscle tone and cyanosis are also usually present.

Mildly affected infants gradually recover over the first 6–12 hours of life with appropriate warmth and oxygen. In others, cyanosis deepens, respiratory rate rises, and breathing becomes more labored with marked retractions of the soft tissues around the rib cage and sternal indrawing. These signs reflect the decreasing compliance of the lungs due to a combination of atelectasis and congestion. Blood gas analysis reveals low oxygen tension, elevated and rising carbon dioxide tension, and acidosis, partly respiratory and partly metabolic.

Differential diagnosis includes congenital heart disease, aspiration of meconium, diaphragmatic hernia, and pneumothorax. These causes are, by comparison rare.

The possibility of preventing this syndrome by accelerating lung maturation by the administration of glucocorticoids appears to offer great promise. The beneficial effects of accelerated maturation have been demonstrated both in the fetal lamb and in a large controlled trial in humans. While questions remain as to the complete safety of this therapy, at present there appear to be no adverse effects on the preterm infant in the neonatal and early infant period.

Approximately half of the infants with moderate to severe symptoms in the first 6 hours of life recover spontaneously. In those who die, respiration and circulation gradually fail. At autopsy, the lungs are solid and airless, having the consistency of liver. Microscopic examination shows widespread atelectasis, with irregular dilatation of bronchial ducts giving the appearance of Swiss cheese. In addition, a pink material, the hyaline membrane, lines the alveolar ducts. Autopsy studies demonstrate that hyaline membranes are rarely present in infants weighing less than 1000 g.

The surface tension of extracts from lungs of infants who have died from the respiratory distress syndrome is higher than expected, indicating that the syndrome is associated with lack or diminution in the amount of surface-active material. The smallest human fetus in which the presence of surface-active material has been demonstrated weighed only 300 g. This stage of development coincides with the appearance of lamellar inclusions. From animal experiments, it appears that an adequate pulmonary circulation is necessary if the integrity of the Type 2 alveolar cells, which produce the surface-active material, is to be maintained.

Since there is no specific therapy, treatment is essentially supportive: assisting ventilation, maintaining oxygenation, and providing adequate fluid and calories. With technical advances in care, the mortality from this condition has fallen dramatically in recent years.

SURVIVAL AND BRAIN DAMAGE AFTER ASPHYXIA

It is widely believed that the newborn human infant can withstand complete oxygen lack for prolonged periods without serious sequel. This impression stems from reports of infants being delivered alive some time

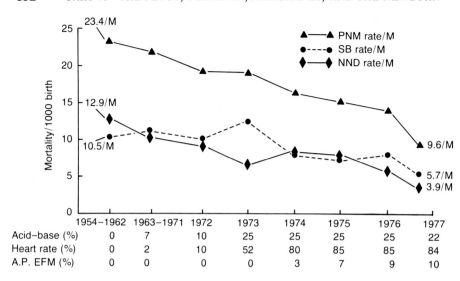

	1954–1962	1963–1971	1972	1973	1974	1975	1976	1977
Acid–base (%)	0	7	10	25	25	25	25	22
Heart rate (%)	0	2	10	52	80	85	85	84
A.P. EFM (%)	0	0	0	0	3	7	9	10

FIG. 42–6. Trends in perinatal mortality (*PNM*), stillbirth (SB), and neonatal death rates (*NND*) of infants over 1000 g 1954–1977 in relation to fetal heart rate and acid-base monitoring during labor and antepartum stress tests. (Statistics from Columbia Presbyterian Medical Center, New York)

after the mother's death and of successful resuscitation following prolonged apnea at birth. However, reports of difficult resuscitation are rarely, if ever, accompanied by details of long-term follow-up, and a considerable number of liveborn infants in whom the period of asphyxia at birth has not been remarkable demonstrate neurologic impairment at a later age.

Additional support for this contention has been obtained from experiments with small mammals indicating that the tolerance to asphyxia is greater in the newborn than in the adult. Several factors could account for this difference in tolerance to asphyxia. The foremost is the state of development of the central nervous system. Although the degee of maturity at the time of birth varies considerably among species, there is little doubt that metabolic activity of the brain tissue of most newborns is low compared with that of adults. As a result, the time interval to reach a state incompatible with cell survival is longer in the newborn, provided other variables, notably temperature, availability of suitable substrates, and disposition of end products are identical. A second factor favoring the newborn relates to substrate stores in tissues where energy requirements for maintenance of functional integrity are high. At birth, the glycogen stores in the myocardium are considerably greater than those in the adult, permitting the circulation of the newborn to be better maintained during asphyxia. Metabolic end products, particularly hydrogen ion, can therefore be distributed between sites of high and low metabolic activity for a longer period. Finally, the fall in body temperature in the newborn after birth may offer additional protection because the energy available is expended over a longer time interval.

The only factor not favoring the newborn is the high proportion of total body mass occupied by tissues of high basal metabolic activity. In the term infant, there

is about five times as much brain tissue per unit of body weight as in the adult. Thus, the compartment available for distribution of products formed during anaerobic glycolysis is relatively smaller, resulting in a proportionately greater change in the composition of the internal environment for a given quantity of energy transformed.

The net effect of these four variables determines whether tolerance to asphyxia is greater in the newborn than in the adult.

How long can resuscitation be delayed with safety in the apneic newborn human infant? Asphyxiated newborn monkeys that are resuscitated before the last gasp show little or no permanent cerebral damage. On the other hand, prolongation of asphyxia for 4 min beyond the last gasp is accompanied by widespread tissue damage and abnormal behavior in the surviving animals. Thus, for the newborn monkey, the "safe" period of anoxia is short if functional integrity is to be maintained. The same may be true for the human newborn. For this reason, and because the duration of asphyxia to which the fetus has been subjected prior to delivery is not known, no time should be lost in resuscitation of the apneic newborn.

During the last decade there has been a marked decrease in perinatal mortality (Fig. 42–6) and morbidity (Fig. 42–7) in many of the tertiary centers for high-risk patients. This is especially striking in cases involving very low birth weight infants (Fig. 42–8). A number of factors have contributed to this improvement. There has been greater attention to both antepartum and intrapartum surveillance of the fetus by electronic and biochemical monitoring, especially in the low-birth-weight infant. Transitional nurseries have been established in the delivery suites, enabling the newest methods of newborn intensive care to be applied with no delay. Improved understanding has

FIG. 42-7. Trends in perinatal morbidity 1960–1977 as assessed by 1- and 5-min Apgar score ∠ 6 in relation to fetal acid–base and heart rate monitoring. (Statistics from Columbia Prsesbyterian Medical Center, New York)

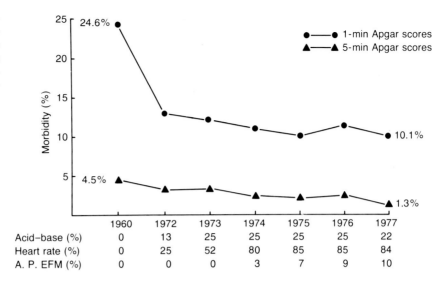

	1960	1972	1973	1974	1975	1976	1977
Acid–base (%)	0	13	25	25	25	25	22
Heart rate (%)	0	25	52	80	85	85	84
A. P. EFM (%)	0	0	0	3	7	9	10

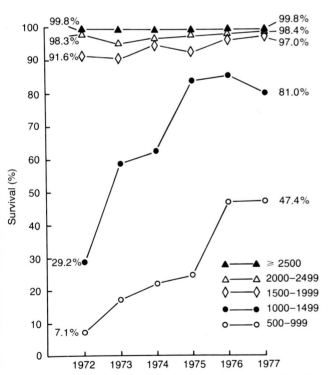

FIG. 42-8. Neonatal survival rate by birth weight. (Statistics from Columbia Presbyterian Medical Center, New York)

lead to important advances in the technology of respiratory support and intravenous nutrition. However, it is not known what the relative role of each of these factors has been. The improved survival rate does not so far appear to be associated with an increase in the number of infants with neurologic deficits, but more detailed long-term follow-up observations are necessary before the final outcome can be truly assessed.

REFERENCES AND RECOMMENDED READING

Adamsons K, Jr, Towell ME: Thermal homeostasis in the fetus and newborn. Anesthesiology 26:5321, 1965

Baum JD, Robertson NRC: Immediate effects of alkaline infusion in infants with respiratory distress syndrome. J Pediatr 87:255, 1975

Bland RD, Clarke TI, Horden LB: Rapid infusion of sodium bicarbonate and albumin into high-risk premature infants soon after birth: A controlled, prospective trial. Am J Obstet Gynecol 124:263, 1976

Dawes GS: Revolutions and cyclical rhythms in prenatal life: Fetal respiratory movements rediscovered. Pediatrics 51:965, 1973

Farrell PM, Avery ME: Hyaline membrane disease. Am Rev Respir Dis 3:657, 1975

Gluck L, Kulovich M, Borer R et al: The interpretation and significance of the lecithin/sphingomyelin ratio in amniotic fluid. Am J Obstet Gynecol 120:142, 1974

Granberg P, Ballard RA, Ballard PL et al: Effect of antenatal beta methasone in preterm infants. Pediatr Res 9:396, 1975

Gruenwald P: Chronic fetal distress and placental insufficiency. Biol Neonate 5:215, 1963

James LS: Physiology of respiration in newborn infants and in respiratory distress syndrome. Pediatrics 24:1069, 1959

James LS: Effect of pain relief for labor and delivery on fetus and newborn. Anesthesiology 21:405, 1960

James LS: Perinatal events and respiratory distress syndrome. N Engl J Med 292:1291, 1975

Johnson JD, Malachowski NC, Grobstein R et al: Prognosis of children surviving with the aid of mechanical ventilation in the newborn period. J Pediatr 84:272, 1974

Karlberg P: Adaptive changes in immediate postnatal period, with particular reference to respiration. J Pediatr 56:585, 1960

Liggins GC, Howie RN: A controlled trial of antepartum

glucocorticoid treatment for prevention of the respiratory distress syndrome in premature infants. Pediatrics 50:515, 1972

Liggins GC, Howie RN: Prevention of RDS by maternal steroid therapy. In Gluck L (ed): Modern Perinatal Medicine, p 415. Chicago, Yearbook, 1974

Lubchenko LO, Hansmann C, Boyd E: Intrauterine growth in length and head circumference as estimated from live births at gestational ages from 26 to 42 weeks. Pediatrics 37:403, 1966

Purvis MJ: Onset of respiration at birth. Arch Dis Child 49:333, 1974

Rey HR, Rootenberg J, Hugh S et al: An on-line data base system and file structure for perinatology. Int J Systems Sci 10:11, 1979

Reynolds EOR, Taghizadeh A: Improved prognosis of infants mechanically ventilated for hyaline membrane disease. Arch Dis Child 49:505, 1974

Simmons MA, Adcock EW, Bard H et al: Hypernatremia and intracranial hemorrhage in neonates. N Engl J Med 291:6, 1974

Stewart A: Follow-up of pre-term infants. In Pre-Term Labour, Proceedings of the Fifth Study Group of the Royal College of Obstetricians and Gynaecologists, 1977

Windle WF: Asphyxial brain damage at birth with reference to the minimally affected child. In Greenhill JP (ed): Year Book of Obstetrics and Gynecology, p 238. Chicago, Year Book, 1970

Wolstenholme GEW (ed): Somatic Stability of the Newly Born. Ciba Foundation Symposium. London, Churchill, 1961

Thirty and more years ago, it was standard practice to weigh and measure the placenta, to measure the cord, and to take one or more placental biopsies at virtually all deliveries. This practice was discontinued in most institutions because no discernible benefits, either practical or experimental, were derived from the masses of information. More recently, however, interest among anatomic pathologists has been renewed, because it has been shown that a host of placental abnormalities give much insight into many of the clinical problems of pregnancy and the newborn.

In 1961, Benirschke outlined important steps in examination of the placenta, membranes, and cord. This paper is still the definitive treatise on the subject. The obstetrician's examination should include inspection of the maternal surface of the placenta after adherent clots have been wiped away, inspection of the fetal surface of the placenta; inspection of the umbilical cord and determination of its approximate length, number of vessels, and site of insertion; and examination of the membranes. If an immediate diagnosis is needed, *e.g.*, when an intrauterine infection is suspected, a segment of placenta and umbilical cord should be submitted for frozen section examination. This enables an immediate histopathologic diagnosis of chorioamnionitis and may also reveal severe cases of villous infection. When there is no urgency, paraffin-embedded sections provide the best material for histopathologic study. Light microscopic diagnoses can be made from placentas that have been refrigerated at 4° C for several days. Placentas should not be stored in freezers, because this produces artifacts that distort the microscopic picture.

Indications for pathologic examination include a maternal history of recurrent reproductive failure (low birth weight or spontaneous abortion in more than one pregnancy), clinically suspected acute or chronic intrauterine infection, growth retardation, dysmorphia, diabetes, multiple births, and erythroblastosis. Gross surgical pathology evaluation in such cases should include inspection of slices made every 2 cm throughout the placenta. At least six blocks of tissue are taken. A minimum of four sections are taken from the placenta proper, including one piece from the area near the insertion of the umbilical cord and one from the lateral aspect, towards the site of rupture of the membranes or any site of apparent hemorrhage or abruption. A sample of membrane roll is taken, as well as a section of the umbilical cord. The inspection to determine the number of vessels in the umbilical cord should be made at least 3 cm distal to the placenta; the normal anastomoses that occur within 3 cm may give a spurious representation of the number of vessels in the cord. Special procedures, outlined by Benirschke, are needed for multiple pregnancy.

43

ABNORMALITIES OF THE PLACENTA, MEMBRANES, AND UMBILICAL CORD

Geoffrey Altshuler

GROSS ABNORMALITIES OF THE PLACENTA

Normally, the placenta is round or oval, 15–20 cm in diameter and 1.5–3 cm thick. In normal pregnancy, its weight varies with the fetal weight in a ratio of approximately 1:6, thus averaging about 500 g. The shape of the placenta is extremely variable. For example, there may be two or more lobes connected by an isthmus of placental tissue (Fig. 43–1). These minor variations in placental shape are thought to be caused by differences in decidual nutritional potential at various endometrial sites during placentation. They are seldom of clinical significance.

Placenta Succenturiata. An accessory placental lobe may be found a variable distance from the main placental mass; the two are linked by vessels coursing

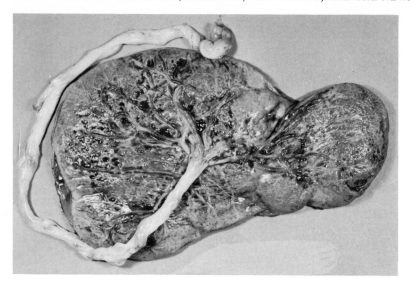

FIG. 43-1. Bilobed placenta. Normal pregnancy, labor, and delivery.

over the fetal surface of the membranes. The accessory lobe may be retained in the uterus following delivery, increasing the hazard of postpartum hemorrhage and infection. If a defect is found in the membranes, with abrupt termination of fetal vessels at its margin, the uterus should be explored manually to locate and remove a retained accessory lobe.

Placenta Circumvallata. A complete or incomplete ring, situated at a variable distance from the point of insertion of the umbilical cord, may be present on the fetal surface of the placenta. This ring demarcates the peripheral extent of the chorionic plate and the terminal point for fetal vessels that course outward from the cord. The ring consists of a double fold in the amnion and chorion. The first fold involves those structures that course toward the center of the placenta, while the second and superior fold sends amnion and chorion coursing upward and outward toward the uterine wall. Decidua vera separates the two folds of membranes, and villi extend beyond the margin of the chorionic plate into the decidua vera.

This placental abnormality has been linked to a variety of clinical sequelae. The incidence of abortion is said to be increased. Bleeding in the second and third trimesters of pregnancy may be associated with placenta circumvallata and erroneously suggest placenta previa. Intermittent hydrorrhea and preterm labor may also occur. However, opinions differ about both the clinical significance and the pathogenesis of placenta circumvallata. The 1927 paper by Williams is of special interest, and his illustrations (Fig. 43–2) are still the classic representation of this relatively unusual placenta.

Placenta Membranacea. On rare occasions, a thin membranous placenta is attached to the entire interior uterine surface rather than to a localized area. Bleeding may occur in late pregnancy as the development of the lower uterine segment and effacement of the cervix cause the villi to separate from decidua in the vicinity of the cervix. During the third stage of labor, spontaneous separation of a membranous placenta may not be complete, and manual removal may be difficult. Blood loss in the third stage may be excessive.

Placenta Accreta. On occasion, because decidua is lacking or faulty, placental villi develop a contiguous relation with myometrium (placenta accreta). In more extreme cases, villi may invade the myometrium (placenta increta) or penetrate the myometrium to the serosal surface of the uterus (placenta percreta). These are discussed in Chapter 36.

Infarcts and Placental Ischemia. True placental infarcts occur after occlusion of a maternal artery in the decidual plate or after decidual hemorrhage from a maternal vessel deprives a section of villi of its blood supply. Under such conditions, chorionic tissue becomes necrotic, since it depends upon maternal blood for nourishment. Fresh infarcts appear red; older lesions are yellow or white. The infarct is generally well circumscribed and surrounded by normal villi. Such lesions are common and are not necessarily associated with maternal or fetal abnormality (Figs. 43–3 and 43–4).

Diffuse perivillous entrapment of degenerate villi, with proliferation of X cells, can compromise the local circulation. Areas of shrunken villi and condensed, knotlike syncytiotrophoblast are also a manifestation of

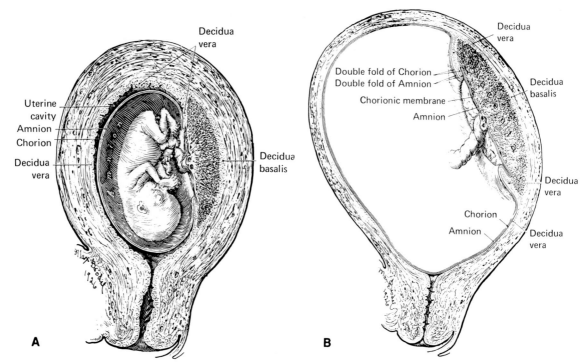

FIG. 43-2. Placenta circumvallata. *A.* At 12 weeks' pregnancy, maternal surface of placenta is in contact with decidua basalis. Fetal surface is composed of central chorionic membrane and, at periphery, extrachorionic zone covered by decidua. Fetal membranes are reflected at margin of central portion, giving rise to circumvallate ring. *B.* In late pregnancy, well-developed annulus can be seen. Note relations of chorionic membrane, extrachorionic decidua, and duplication of membranes. (Williams JW: Am J Obstet Gynecol 13:1, 1927)

placental ischemia. *X-cells* (Fig 43–5) are of trophoblastic origin, and although their significance is unknown, they are especially frequent in degenerating placentas of infants that are small for gestational age.

Placentomegaly. In single pregnancy, a placental weight above 600 g (after removal of cord, membranes, and adherent clots) should be considered pathologic. Although the cause is unknown, abnormally large placentas are usually associated with diabetes, hydropic manifestations of fetal heart failure, hydrops of immunohemolytic anemia, severe maternal anemia, and chronic intrauterine infections. Increased placental weight has also been correlated with increasing maternal age and parity.

Placental Cysts. Cysts that vary in size from microscopic to 5 cm in diameter may be found across the fetal surface of an otherwise apparently normal placenta. They are generally filled with a curdy yellow or brown fluid and are considered to be of chorionic origin. Smaller cysts are sometimes found deeper in the placenta and may result from liquefaction in areas of excessive fibrin deposition. These placental cysts are lined by X cells.

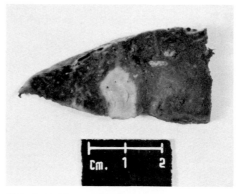

FIG. 43-3. Placental infarct. Cross section of segment of placenta after fixation in formalin. Fetal surface is at top, maternal surface at bottom. A thrombus in a maternal arteriole was demonstrated.

Placental Calcification. Calcification occurs commonly in normal placentas, and calcium deposits increase as pregnancy advances. In some instances, calcium deposits can be detected only by microscopic examination; in others, deposits are sufficiently extensive to impart a gritty feel to the maternal surface.

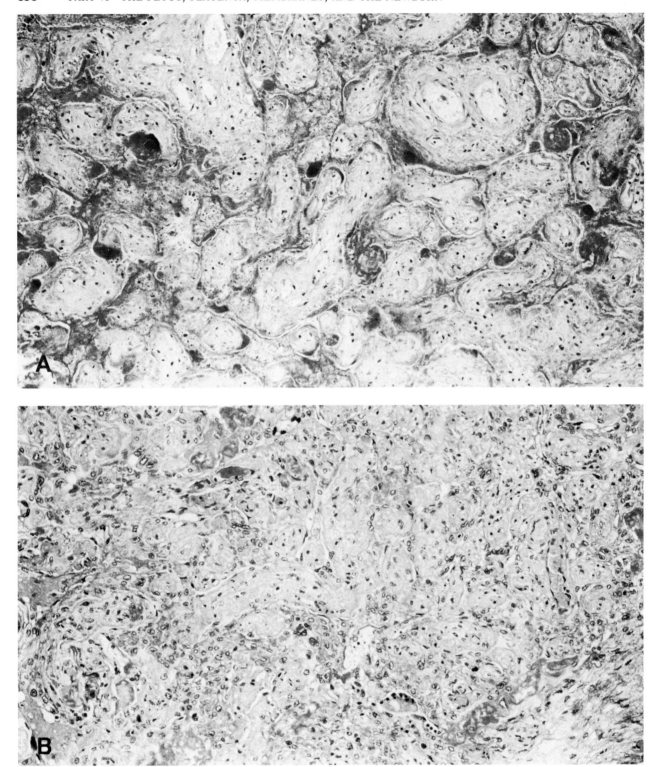

FIG. 43-4. *A.* Acute placental infarction. Note ghost-like retention of villous architecture and syncytiotrophoblast knots. (H & E, × 180) *B.* Chronic placental infarction. Placental villi are replaced by X cells and fibrinoid material. (H & E, × 180)

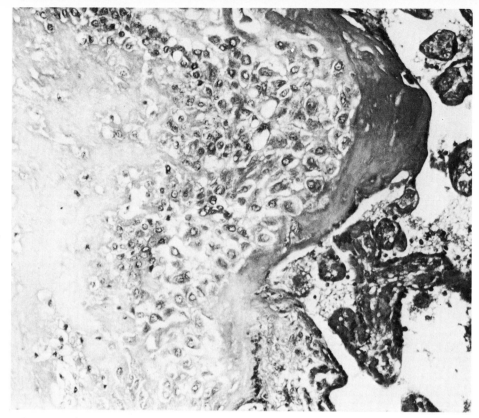

FIG. 43-5. Light microscopy features of placental cyst. Numerous X cells produce a homogeneous cyst content. (H & E, × 180)

MICROSCOPIC ABNORMALITIES OF THE PLACENTA

The number of microscopic abnormalities that can be found in the placenta is legion. The normal life span of a placenta is 40 weeks. The normal changes of increasing senescence that characterize the term placenta are outlined in Chapter 16. In recent years, intense interest in placental histology has resulted in the categorization of microscopic abnormalities and the recognition of certain lesions that may be of clinical significance. Most, but not all, of the changes can be found in isolated areas of "normal" placentas; their presence in profusion may be evidence of a pathologic process.

Decidual Arteriopathy. Atherosclerosis and fibrinoid degeneration of decidual arterioles are especially prevalent in cases of maternal hypertension, preeclampsia, chronic renal insufficiency, and diabetes. Widespread luminal obliteration and fibrinoid necrosis may lead to such complications as preterm delivery, stillbirth, and intrauterine growth retardation. Immunofluorescent studies suggest that these lesions are the result of an immunopathologic process that can lead to impaired placental perfusion.

Maternal Floor Infarction. Occasional placentas have a 3- to 6-mm band of fibrinoid tissue across the maternal surface. When this tissue covers more than 50% of the surface, the placenta may be compromised by severe placental ischemia. Intrauterine fetal growth retardation may result, and the placenta shows this abnormality in about 5% of such cases. The pathogenesis of this lesion is not known.

Fetal Vasculopathy. Studies of the fetal placental vasculature have revealed three major groups of lesions (Fig. 43–6).

1. Vascular collapse and obliterative sclerosis. These changes are associated with stillbirth and situations in which villous blood flow is severely reduced or nonexistent.
2. Thrombotic lesions. Placental intravascular coagulation can result from hypoxia, acidosis, or infection. The lesions are characterized by the same features as are those of intravascular coagulation in other organs: fibrin deposition, organized thrombi, and recanalized thrombi are common findings, especially in cases of fetal death. These lesions can also be associated with preeclampsia and fetal growth retardation, or with cases in which the umbilical cord circulation is impaired by a cord knot or by compression.
3. Endovasculitis. Endothelial inflammatory processes may be proliferative, or they may show fibrinoid ne-

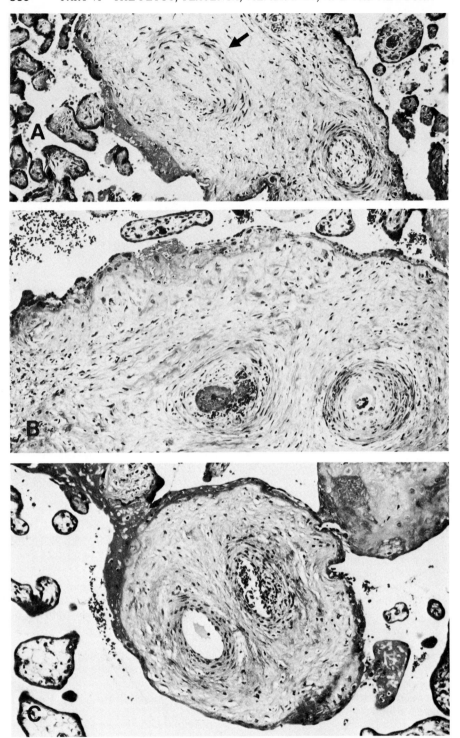

FIG. 43-6. Placental villi, fetal vasculopathy. *A.* Note vascular collapse in three vessels at lower right aspect. Obliterative sclerosis (*arrow*) possibly includes old thrombosis. (H & E, × 180) *B.* Placenta of spontaneous abortion. Presence of fibrin in central vessel indicates that fetal intravascular coagulation preceded fetal death. (H & E, × 180) *C.* Endovasculitis of fetal septal vessel. Inflammatory cell vascular infiltrates are obvious in central vessel. (H & E, × 180)

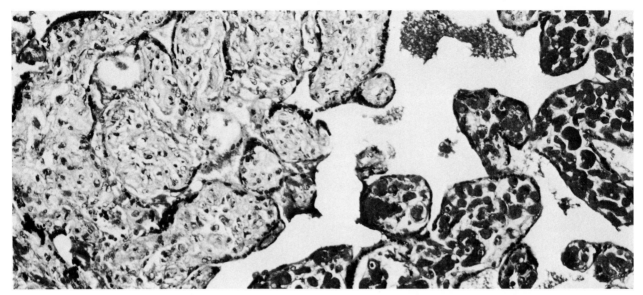

FIG. 43-7. Chorangiosis and villitis. Each villus toward right includes more than ten vascular channels (chorangiosis). Villitis is present in villi toward the left. (H & E, × 180)

crosis or endovascular sclerosis. These lesions are an important feature of infections that are particularly likely to involve endothelial cells, *e.g.,* herpes simplex virus, cytomegalovirus, rubella virus, and syphilis.

Chorangiosis. In a normal third trimester placenta, it is rare to find more than four vascular channels in a single chorionic villus, even allowing for the probability that the same vessel has been sectioned more than once. In chorangiosis, the villi are filled by blood vessels, and the diagnosis is made by the finding of more than ten vascular channels within one villus (Fig. 43–7) in each of ten samples taken from different areas of the placenta. Chorangiosis is a common finding in placentas of women with preeclampsia and diabetes; the presumed cause for the vascular proliferation is chronic tissue hypoxia as a result of persistent, low-grade uteroplacental ischemia. The lesion is also common in infections that cause villitis. When chorangiosis is especially widespread, it may function as an arteriovenous shunt that can lead to intrauterine cardiac failure.

Dysmaturity of Chorionic Villi. The steps in the maturation of the placenta are outlined in Chapter 16. The normal placenta develops in three stages that correspond to the gestational trimesters. In the first trimester, the placenta is characterized by large hydropic chorionic villi bordered by cytotrophoblast and syncytiotrophoblast; in the second trimester, there is proliferation of the Hofbauer or stromal cells; in the third trimester, there is progressive reduction in villous size,

leading to small terminal villi that contain no more than four vascular channels and are bordered by occasional knots of syncytiotrophoblast.

In some third trimester and term placentas, there is a persistent and increased proliferation of Hofbauer cells, associated with a lack of syncytiotrophoblastic knots (Fig. 43–8). These findings constitute a pathologic marker of placental dysmaturity. They have been found to correlate with chronic fetal–placental infection. Such evidence of relative placental immaturity is also found with fetal immunohemolytic anemia and, rarely, chronic fetal–maternal transfusion.

NEOPLASMS OF THE PLACENTA

Although the placenta contains abundant varieties of tissue that commonly give rise to neoplasms in other organs, placental tumors are quite rare. The most common of these, gestational trophoblastic neoplasia, is considered in Chapter 21. The other two primary tumors that have been described are hemangioma and teratoma.

Hemangiomas (Fig. 43–9) large enough to be evident grossly occur in from 1/8,000 to 1/50,000 cases; with diligent search, microscopic hemangiomas are found in approximately 1/100 placentas. Hydramnios is a common occurrence in cases of placental hemangioma, its incidence being approximately 50% with the larger tumors and 10% with smaller ones. Congenital fetal malformations of various kinds occur with some frequency, perhaps 15%–20% of cases.

Teratoma of the placenta has been described, but

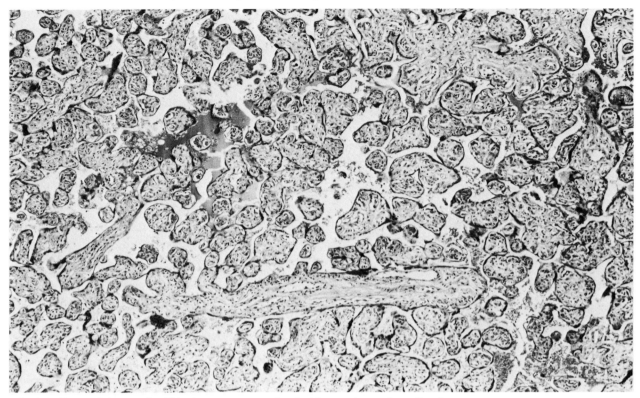

FIG. 43-8. Placental dysmaturity. This placenta was associated with a newborn who suffered neo-natal hepatitis after a 40 weeks' gestation. Villi show stromal cell hypercellularity and a relative lack of syncytiotrophoblastic knots. (H & E, × 75)

some do not accept this diagnosis for the tumors that have been reported. If there is such a tumor, it is sufficiently rare to be a pathologic curiosity with no known clinical significance.

Metastatic malignant tumors are extremely rare. The lesions are an unusual manifestation of widespread blood-borne disease. Reports include cases of melanoma, leukemia, lymphoma, and carcinoma of the breast and gastrointestinal tract.

INFLAMMATION OF THE PLACENTA, MEMBRANES, AND CORD

Bacteria and viruses can reach the contents of the uterus either by the maternal bloodstream or by ascent from the vagina and cervix. *Intervillositis* is the name given to the inflammatory reaction surrounding the chorionic villi; it is characteristic of maternal blood-borne infection, and there may be no sign of ascending infection. *Villitis* (Fig. 43–10) is the term used to describe inflammatory cell proliferation with the placental villus itself. It is morphologic evidence of transplacental infection; the causative maternal blood-borne infective agent produces the inflammation within the fetal placental villi. *Chorioamnionitis* indicates ascending intrauterine infection. In the last trimester, the umbilical cord is often additionally involved in the ascending inflammatory process, and histologic examination of frozen sections of the cord can provide a rapid means of diagnosis. Inflammation within the umbilical cord indicates fetal infection and may justify active therapy prior to the actual appearance of clinical signs in the neonate.

Chorioamnionitis is almost invariably present in spontaneous abortion before 28 weeks, but the umbilical cord is almost always clear of infection in these cases; after 28 weeks, funisitis is commonly associated with chorioamnionitis. This striking discrepancy has not been explained. In the search for the causative organism of chorioamnionitis, investigation should not be confined to aerobic bacteria; anaerobic bacteria, mycoplasma, chlamydia, cytomegalovirus, herpes simplex, and other viruses may also be causative.

TORCH INFECTIONS

Toxoplasmosis, rubella, cytomegalovirus, and herpes simplex (TORCH infections), as well as syphilis, pro-

duce characteristic placental lesions. In three of these (toxoplasmosis, cytomegalovirus, and syphilis), the causative organisms can be positively identified by light microscopy. For the identification of cytomegalovirus, indirect fluorescent antibody kits are now commercially available.

Characteristically, the placenta in TORCH infections shows placental dysmaturity and focal villitis. The inflammatory lesions may be proliferative, necrotizing, or granulomatous, and the cell infiltrates, in addition to neutrophils, may include plasma cells and lymphocytes. As noted before, endovasculitis involving the terminal villi, either of the acute inflammatory or chronic sclerosing kind, is a common result of placental infections with cytomegalovirus, rubella, herpes simplex, and syphilis. Deposits of hemosiderin may mark the sites of previous endovascular infection and perivascular hemorrhage. In some of the TORCH infections, nucleated red cells and erythroblasts may be found in the placental vasculature in such profusion as to suggest Rh isoimmunization.

Purulent lesions are commonly found in *Escherichia coli* and *Listeria monocytogenes* infections, and the bacteria may be readily identified even in routine hematoxylin and eosin sections.

VILLITIS OF UNKNOWN ETIOLOGY

In random examination of placentas, at least 5% show focal villitis for which the specific infectious cause is neither morphologically nor clinically apparent. The placentas of as many as 25% of newborns who are small for gestational age show these lesions. Other important correlations include spontaneous abortion, stillbirth, preterm delivery, recurrent reproductive failure, hepatitis, and various congenital anomalies. It is possible that viruses, mycoplasma, chlamydia, and anaerobic organisms have an etiologic role in these events, since these organisms commonly reside in the genital tract.

ABNORMALITIES OF THE MEMBRANES

Stratified Squamous Metaplasia of the Amnion. Placentas often show umbilicated amniotic lesions with a diameter of less than 5 mm. These lesions, which are called stratified squamous metaplasia, are of importance only because of their gross similarity to amnion nodosum. The multilayered epithelial structure of stratified squamous metaplasia is easily identifiable by light microscopy, but it has no known clinical significance.

Amnion Nodosum. Elevated amniotic nodules less than 5 mm in diameter are characteristic of amnion nodosum. By light microscopy, these lesions show

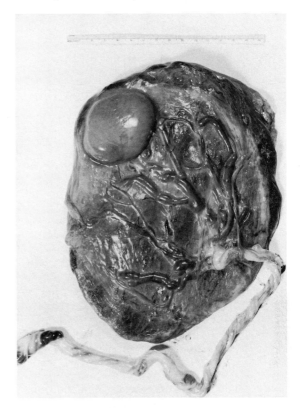

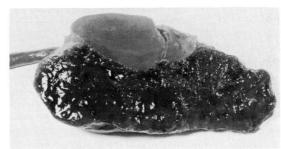

FIG. 43-9. Hemangioma of placenta. Lesion was firm and rubbery in consistency and yellow gray on cut surface. In this case, there were no associated fetal abnormalities.

conglutinated vernix caseosa that makes them easily identifiable even if they are not grossly apparent. Amnion nodosum is pathognomonic of oligohydramnios. Because of oligohydramnios, sustained compression about the fetal thorax leads to lung hypoplasia. Dyspneic newborns who have low-set ears and so-called Potter's facies may be difficult to ventilate because of lung hypoplasia; in this context, the observation of amnion nodosum raises strong question of nonfunctioning kidney syndrome, such as renal agenesis or renal dysplasia. The alternate cause of amnion nodosum is oligohydramnios of prolonged amniotic leakage.

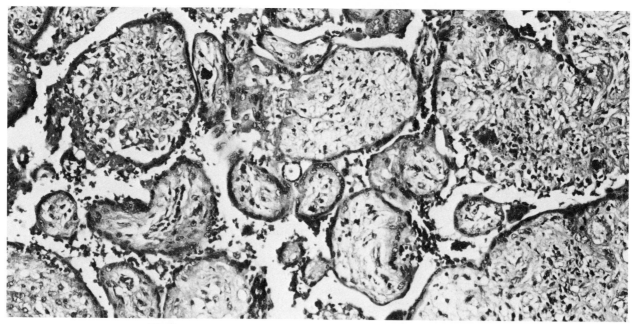

FIG. 43-10. Placenta, 13 weeks'-gestation. Cytomegalovirus was present in placenta and macerated organs of fetus. Note severity of villitis. (H & E, × 180)

Meconium Staining of the Membranes. Meconium staining of amniotic fluid and membranes is associated with fetal stress that has resulted in evacuation of the lower bowel. Most babies are unaffected by this, although passage of meconium may produce meconium aspiration pneumonia if the meconium discharge is longstanding. Microscopic examination of the amnion may establish temporal relationships. Acute meconium staining may produce amniotic epithelial necrosis within 3 hours, but staining in excess of 3 hours is required to produce chronic features of meconium staining, such as ballooning of the amniotic epithelium and meconium pigment in macrophages within the deep subepithelial amniotic connective tissue.

Amnion Bands. Amniotic bands coursing across a part of the uterine cavity have long been known to be responsible for fetal anomalies such as digital constriction rings, syndactyly, craniofacial defects, and club feet. Their cause is presumed to be separation of amnion from chorion, with repair by mesoblastic proliferation. Placental amniotic bands may not be immediately evident, and careful inspection of the placental surface may be needed to find them.

ABNORMALITIES OF THE UMBILICAL CORD

Variations in Length. The average length of the umbilical cord at term is 55 cm; however, wide variations may

be encountered. A very short cord may cause complications in labor if it interferes with the descent of the fetus during the second stage; when the cord length is insufficient, the fetal presenting part advances with each contraction but retreats with myometrial relaxation. Marked irregularity and slowing of the fetal heart rate are associated with contractions. Causes of these arrhythmias include hypoxia and increased fetal vagotonia secondary to a cord stretch reflex. Shortness of the umbilical cord may cause cord rupture, premature separation of the placenta, or even inversion of the uterus.

A cord of greater than average length is likely to coil about fetal parts. One or more loops of cord are coiled about the fetal neck in one-fifth of term deliveries. This occurs too frequently to be considered a complication of labor, and seldom can fetal injury be attributed to looping of the cord. Determination of cord-related fetal injury requires a demonstration of pathologic change, such as cervical edema associated with cord about the neck.

Infection (Funisitis). As noted earlier, funisitis is part of the picture of chorioamnionitis, placentitis, and fetal infection. In suspected cases, frozen section may provide a rapid diagnosis. Fig. 43–11 illustrates such a section, showing characteristic chemotaxis.

Knots. Occasionally, true knots are noted in the umbilical cord. Generally, these are loose and consequently harmless to the fetus. If drawn tight, fetal circulation

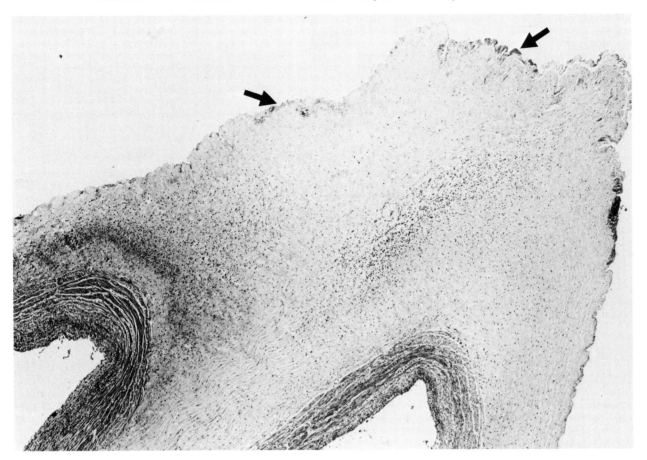

FIG. 43-11. Funisitis, umbilical cord chemotaxis. Bands of polymorphonuclear leukocytes appear selectively attracted toward bacteria (*arrows*) at surface of cord. (H & E, × 50)

may be obstructed, and hypoxia may result. These complications are evidenced by cord diameter and color differences on either side of a knot and thromboses within the adjacent umbilical cord and contiguous placental vessels.

Torsion. Marked torsion of the umbilical cord may be encountered. In most instances, it is associated with fetal death. It is often the result, rather than the cause of death, since it may be due to excessive agonal fetal movement.

Abnormal Insertion. In most instances, the cord is joined to the placenta in a more or less central location, although connection near the periphery is not unusual. The term *battledore placenta* is applied when the cord is inserted at the margin of the placenta; no particular clinical significance is attached to this variation. Velamentous insertion of the cord may have serious implications for the fetus, however. With this type of insertion, fetal vessels travel a variable distance from the placenta to the point of cord insertion (Fig. 43–12) and may cross the membranes beneath the presenting part of the fetus and adjacent to the cervical canal (vasa previa). This is a most serious complication; for, if the vessels should rupture during labor, the baby may exsanguinate before delivery. The diagnosis and management of vasa previa are discussed in Chapter 24. Velamentous insertion of the umbilical cord is twice as common in twin pregnancies as in single pregnancies, which supports the hypothesis that the etiology of the condition is trophotropism, a phenomenon of preferential growth. When the uterus is occupied by another developing placenta (or by a fibroid or some other abnormality of the myometrium or the endometrium), the villous tissue grows away from the offending structure rather than uniformly away from the insertion of the umbilical cord.

Single Umbilical Artery. The incidence of true single umbilical artery is reported to be 0.25%–1%. Of these cases, 25%–50% are associated with fetal malforma-

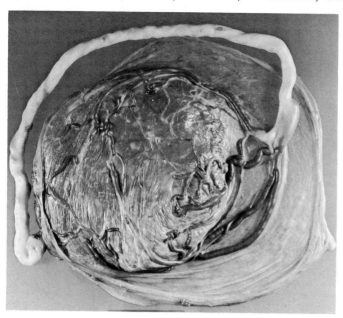

FIG. 43-12. Velamentous insertion of umbilical cord. Fetal vessels traverse membranes to reach placental disk.

tions of one kind or another, but there is no predilection for any particular type of anomaly. Infants who survive the neonatal period do not later show an increased incidence of anomalies, but there is evidence that they have an increased risk of inguinal hernia.

Edema of the Umbilical Cord. In about 5% of deliveries, the umbilical cord is found to be edematous, with a diameter of 2 cm or more. Most of the babies are unaffected, but some investigators have noted a correlation with preterm delivery and respiratory distress syndrome. Links to the latter are low amniotic pressure, increased water content in the fetoplacental unit, and a low red cell mass in the newborn.

Miscellaneous Cord Abnormalities. Varices have been reported. Hematomas are found occasionally, with extravasation of blood into the Wharton's jelly and rarely, leakage of blood into the amniotic fluid; the high perinatal death rate associated with these lesions (40%–50%) has not been explained. Other cord abnormalities include stricture, calcification, hemangioma, angiomyxoma, myxosarcoma, and teratoma.

TWINNING

The incidence of twins varies greatly among nations, from a maximum of 1 multiple birth for every 51 single births in Chile to 1 multiple birth for every 294 single births in Venezuela. In the United States, the Collaborative Perinatal Study found an incidence of 252

twin births among 21,591 deliveries (1:86) in whites and 317 twin births among 24,126 deliveries (1:76) in blacks.

In animal models, one of the etiologic factors in twinning has been shown to be overripeness of the ovum due to delayed ovulation. In humans, the cause is not clear. For dizygotic twins, it is suggested that the differences in rate of twinning for different countries may be due to differences in pituitary gonadotropin production. The high rate of twinning among women who receive "fertility drugs" is cited as evidence of this possibility.

Twins are either *monozygotic* (identical), resulting from the early division of a single ovum fertilized by a single sperm, or *dizygotic* (fraternal), resulting from fertilization of two ova by separate spermatozoa at the same ovulation (Fig. 43–13). The determination of zygosity is important, and the parents should be given this information as soon as it is available.

EXAMINATION OF THE PLACENTA

Twin placentas are either *monochorionic* or *dichorionic,* terms that are used to refer, respectively, to the presence of a single chorionic mass and, consequently, a single placenta for both twins, or two placentas, one for each twin. Many of the latter are fused to some extent, some sufficiently so that the placenta may appear to be monochorionic. In such cases, the placenta and the septum dividing the twins must be

FIG. 43-13. Placentation and incidence data of twins. Monochorionic twins are always monozygous. Dichorionic twins may also be monozygous.

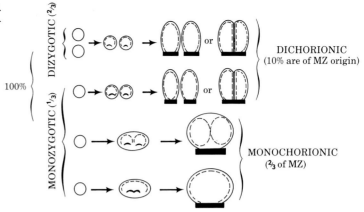

DICHORIONIC
(10% are of MZ origin)

MONOCHORIONIC
(2/3 of MZ)

carefully examined. If there is no septum between the twins, the placenta is monoamnionic and monochorionic; the twins are identical. If a septum divides the twins, but it is comprised only of two layers of amnion with no intervening chorion, the placenta is diamnionic and monochorionic; the twins are identical. Sometimes a septum comprised of only two amnions can be recognized immediately by its great transparency, in contrast to the relative opacity of a septum in which chorionic tissue intervenes. Also, since amniotic tissue contains no blood vessels, the presence of any vascular and other chorionic tissue in the septum indicates dichorionic placentation. However, regardless of the gross impression, a microscopic section should be made both for confirmation and for permanent record.

The fetal surface of the placenta should be carefully examined, preferably by means of injection techniques, to note whether the vessels from one side anastomose with those from the other side. In monochorionic placentas, there is free anastomosis of vessels from one side with those of the other; in fused dichorionic placentas, there is no communication between the vessels of the two sides.

The distinction between a mono- and a dichorionic placenta is important. Monochorionic placentation is always diagnostic of monozygosity, which occurs in two-thirds of the cases of identical twins. In one-third of monozygous twins, splitting of the fertilized ovum occurs very early, and there are two separate (dichorionic) placentas; in 10% of the cases of dichorionic placentas, the twins are monozygotic (Fig. 43–13).

When dichorionic placentas are associated with twins of different sex, no further tests are needed, since the twins are clearly fraternal. If they are of the same sex, zygosity can often be determined by studies of blood groups; if the blood groups are different, the twins are fraternal. If the blood groups are the same, the physician may proceed through the blood types, *e.g.,* Rh, Duffy, Kell, M, N. If all are the same, it is likely the twins are identical. Rarely is it necessary to proceed further, but if ultimate proof were needed HLA typing and some of the esoteric genetic studies would provide the best evidence currently available. If all turn out the same, it is safe to conclude that the twins are identical.

TWIN TRANSFUSION SYNDROME

Twin-to-twin transfusion refers to the transfer of blood from one twin to the other through the interplacental anastomoses of the monochorionic placenta. The donor twin is anemic, pale, and usually smaller and lighter; in addition, this twin's organs may be smaller, as evidenced by a smaller liver and, roentgenographically, a smaller heart. The recipient twin is plethoric, polycythemic, and usually larger. Diamnionic–monochorionic placentas usually have artery-to-artery anastomoses or combinations of artery-to-artery and artery-to-vein anastomoses. Depending on the kinds and degree of anastomoses, there may be virtually no exchange of blood from one twin to the other, or the transfusion may be of such magnitude as to be fatal to both twins.

Hydramnios is frequently associated with the twin transfusion syndrome. When it occurs, the customary causes of hydramnios (see Chapter 26) are to be considered. If it occurs in multiple pregnancy, some thought should be given to the possibility of twin-to-twin transfusion.

Considerable disparity is sometimes found between twins having dichorionic placentas. In such cases, some cause other than twin-to-twin transfusion must be sought, since there is no anastomosis of vessels from one side to the other in this type of placenta.

REFERENCES AND RECOMMENDED READING

Altshuler G, Russell P: The human placental villitides: A review of chronic intrauterine infection. Curr Top Pathol 60: 64, 1975

Benirschke K: Examination of the placenta. Obstet Gynecol 18:309, 1961

Benirschke K: Accurate recording of twin placentation. Obstet Gynecol 18:334, 1961

Benirschke K, Driscoll SG: The Pathology of the Human Placenta. New York, Springer–Verlag, 1967

Fox H: Pathology of the Placenta. Philadelphia, WB Saunders, 1978

Freese UE: Diseases and anomalies of the placenta, membranes, and umbilical cord. In Sciarra JJ (ed): Gynecology and Obstetrics, Vol 2. Hagerstown, MD, Harper & Row, 1979

Ornoy A, Crone K, Altshuler G: Pathological features of the placenta in fetal death. Arch Pathol Lab Med 100:367, 1976

Russell P: Inflammatory lesions of the human placenta: II. Villitis of unknown etiology in perspective. Am J Diag Gynecol Obstet 1:339, 1979

Sander CH: Hemorrhagic endovasculitis and hemorrhagic villitis of the placenta. Arch Pathol Lab Med 104:371, 1980

Some abnormalities that occur in the fetus and newborn are iatrogenic; some are of genetic origin; some result from infection; and some are due directly or indirectly to incidental complications of pregnancy. In some cases, the causes are unknown. Malformations that can be attributed to multifactorial inheritance are listed in Table 44–1.

Among babies who survive the insult, it may be difficult or even impossible to determine the cause. Among those who do not survive, the causes may be elusive, and the frequency with which they are found is directly related to the diligence with which they are sought and the expertise of the pathologist who makes the search. In all cases of abnormality in which the cause is not immediately apparent, the placenta, membranes, and cord should be examined with care as outlined in Chapter 43. In all cases of perinatal death, an autopsy should be performed, and it should include careful examination of the brain and its supporting structures, and examination of the spinal canal. The results of 46 consecutive neonatal autopsies are shown in Table 44–2. Even in cases of severe maceration, it should be possible to determine such abnormalities as situs inversus, lack of genitourinary tract structures, and cardiovascular anomalies that may indicate genetic factors of which the family should be aware. Not all baby autopsies are fruitful, but the attempt should be made; a pathologist's report stating only "macerated stillbirth" should not be acceptable.

ANOMALIES OF TWINNING

Discordancy of Monozygotic Twins. As noted in Chapter 43, monozygous twins are "identical" in that they arise from the same ovum. However, in some cases they may be very different. A major difference in monozygous twins can result from artery-to-artery and artery-to-vein anastomoses; a marked predominance of the latter can produce the critical and sometimes fatal hemodynamic differences that occur in the twin-to-twin transfusion syndrome. It is also possible for such abnormalities as cleft palate, hypothyroidism, diabetes, skin diseases, coronary heart disease, hypertension, amyotrophic lateral sclerosis, and psychologic and psychiatric disorders to appear in only one monozygotic twin. Genetic aberrations can also occur in only one of monozygotic twins; approximately 15 cases of heterokaryon monozygous twinning have been reported, in which chromosomal nondisjunction complicates the twinning process. A twin with Turner's syndrome thus may be partner to a normal twin or to a twin with Down's syndrome.

Acardiac Monster. An unusual variant of twinning is an acardiac monster (Fig. 44–1), wherein there is circulatory reversal through an assortment of interplacental anastomoses in the diamnionic–monochorionic placenta. Many kinds of acardiac monsters have been described, varying from severe malformations with normal skeletal and cerebral structures, to a complete lack of head and limbs. The umbilical artery is usually single. The sex of the two twins is invariably the same, but karyotypic differences have been reported.

Conjoined Twins. For at least 300 years, numerous kinds of conjoined twins have been reported. More than three-quarters of them were of thoracopagus type. The reported incidence varies from 1/2,800 to 1/200,000, a wide range that probably results from variations in the acquisition of vital statistics rather than from epidemics. Failure of the yolk sac to split is the most likely cause.

Fetus Compressus and Papyraceus. When a fetus dies, progressive compression produces a condition called fetus compressus. Eventually, a fossillike form war-

TABLE 44–1. MALFORMATIONS ATTRIBUTED TO MULTIFAC-TORIAL INHERITANCE

Congenital Malformations	Incidence in General Population (%)	Recurrence Rate Among Relatives (%)*			
		Siblings	Offspring	Parents	Monozygotic Twin
Cardiac defects					
Atrial septal defect	0.1	3.3	2.5	3.5	
Patent ductus arteriosus	0.06	2.3	2.8		
Tetralogy of Fallot	0.03	2.0	4.2		
Cleft lip & palate:					
Whites	0.08	3.9	3.5		31
Blacks	0.04				
Navajos	0.20				
Japanese	0.17				
Cleft palate					
Whites	0.05	3.0	6.2		40
Blacks	0.04				
Navajos	0.03				
Club foot (talipes equinovarus)	0.1	2.9			33
Dislocation of hip, congenital	0.07	4.3			35
Hypospadias					
Whites	0.6	7.0		6.0†	
Blacks	0.2				
Legg-Perthes disease	0.08	3.9			
Meningo-myelocele, anencephaly, encephalocele		5.2	2.3		21
Whites	0.4†				
	0.14‡				
Jews	0.08				
Blacks	0.06				
Pyloric stenosis	0.2	3.2	16.2¶		22
			4.6‖		

* Data collected from many sources in different countries. It should be noted that recurrence rates vary in different countries.
† South Wales (U.K.)
‡ Boston
§ Fathers
¶ If mother affected
‖ If father affected
(Holmes LB: N Engl J Med 295:204, 1976)

TABLE 44–2. AUTOPSY FINDINGS IN 46 CONSECUTIVE NEONATAL AUTOPSIES, OKLAHOMA CHILDREN'S MEMORIAL HOSPITAL

Finding	No.
Hyaline membrane disease	34
Intraventricular hemorrhage	26
Infection: pneumonia, sepsis, or meningitis	21
Necrotizing enterocolitis	16
Multiple anomalies	8
Meconium aspiration	3
Birth injury	1
Hemolytic disease of the newborn	0

rants the designation of fetus papyraceus. This occurs most commonly in association with diamnionic–monochorionic placentation, probably as a consequence of fatal twin-to-twin transfusion syndrome.

Mosaicism and Chimerism. A *mosaic* is a person who has cell populations of more than one genotype or karyotype; these are usually derived from a single zygote through somatic mutation, crossing over, or mitotic nondisjunction. A *chimera* is a person who has a mixture of genotypes or karyotypes that results from chorionic vascular anastomoses, transplantation, or double fertilization and subsequent participation of both fertilized meiotic products into one developing embryo. Whenever the clinician diagnoses hermaphroditism, whole body chimerism should be evaluated by complete blood grouping and karyotype studies of several tissues. Whole body chimeras have more than one blood group and more than one karyotype.

TERATOGENIC ABNORMALITIES

There are at least two means by which malformations of embryos and fetuses can result from exposure to teratogenic agents. Such agents may cause cell necrosis, or they may destroy cell function by biochemical paralysis. In the presence of fetal infection, inflammatory reparative sequelae may produce severe malformation. Even by the 13th week of gestation, the fetus is immunologically competent and capable of a severe inflammatory reaction. Coxsackievirus can cause fetal myocarditis, endocarditis, and valvulitis, so it is not surprising that congenital cardiac malformations correlate with maternal coxsackievirus infection. Many other infectious agents can damage other organ systems, the teratogenic effects resulting from fetal inflammation and repair. Several years ago, elevation of umbilical cord serum IgM was considered indicative of infection by the TORCH agents, *i.e.*, toxoplasmosis, rubella virus, cytomegalovirus (Fig. 44–2), and herpes

simplex virus, and by syphilis. Subsequent studies have shown this test to be unreliable, since more than 50% of newborns with proved cytomegalovirus and rubella virus infection do not show an elevation of umbilical cord serum IgM. Conversely, elevated serum IgM in noninfected newborns may result from antibody production against maternal IgG antibody rather than against the infectious agent itself. Placental light microscopic examination may therefore provide a more reliable diagnosis than indirect serologic studies.

In 1961 and 1962 a sedative–tranquilizer, thalidomide, was widely used by pregnant women in West Germany and Australia. At least 5000 severely malformed babies were born as a result. The thalidomide disaster is the classic prototype of the heinous effects that can follow the use of untried drugs in pregnancy, and it gave new impetus to the most searching scrutiny of all drugs and other agents that may have teratogenic effects. This subject is discussed in Chapter 27.

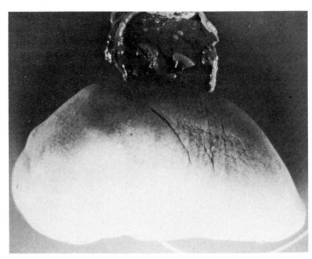

FIG. 44-1. Acardiac monster.

CENTRAL NERVOUS SYSTEM MALFORMATIONS

Anencephaly. In anencephaly, a failure of neural tube closure leads to deficiency of the skull vault (Fig. 44–3). The fetus usually has no hypothalamus but does have a pituitary gland. Deficient hypothalamic fetal hormone results in fetal adrenal atrophy. Lack of this and other trophic hormones may explain why many anencephalic fetuses have prolonged gestation. About 75% of anencephalics are stillborn; the remainder usually die within a few days of birth.

The incidence of this anomaly is highest in Ireland, where it occurs without known cause in 5.9/1000 births. Potato blight was considered to correlate with anencephaly, but this hypothesis has been disproved. Anencephaly and spina bifida often occur together in singletons, but this concordance is rare in twins. There is a high prevalence but low concordance of anencephaly among like-sexed twin pairs.

Although the etiology of anencephaly is unknown, a cranial defect (cranioschisis) is presumed to be the primary factor. Brain exposure (exencephaly) results, giving rise to the progressive cerebral deterioration that characterizes anencephaly.

Arnold–Chiari Malformations. Types I, II, and III Arnold–Chiari anomalies resemble one another; a conical deformity of the posterior midline cerebellum and the elongated brain stem extend to or below the foramen magnum. In the type IV deformity, the cerebellum and brain stem are located within the posterior fossa. A common variant of type IV is the *Dandy–Walker malformation* in which a defect in the inferior vermis of the cerebellum is contiguous with a large fourth ventricle ventriculocele. Type II anomalies are character-

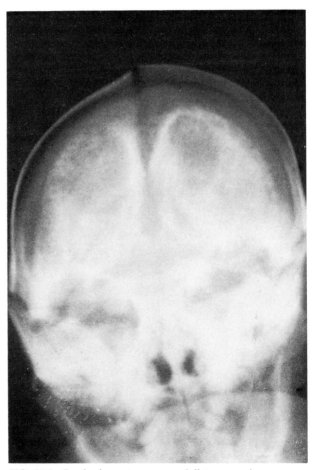

FIG. 44-2. Cerebral roentgenogram, full-term newborn; severe periventricular calcification due to congenital cytomegalovirus infection.

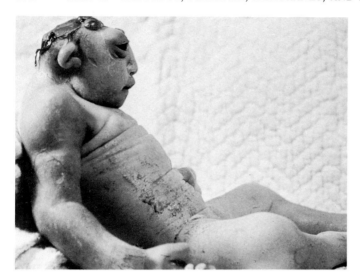

FIG. 44-3. Anencephalic infant shortly after delivery. Note nondevelopment of calvaria. (RA Stander)

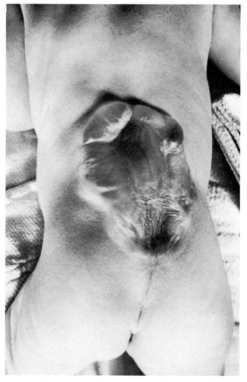

FIG. 44-4. Spina bifida with myelomeningocele. (RA Stander)

istically associated with myelomeningocele (Fig. 44–4) and hydrocephalus.

The Dandy–Walker and Arnold–Chiari malformations may have different causes because they develop at different times in the embryonic period. Alternatively, a spectrum of host responses to a single cause could be operative. In suckling hamsters, it has been shown that inoculation of reovirus type I can produce Arnold–Chiari malformations.

Hydrocephalus. Reovirus type I inoculation, by both extraneural and intracerebral routes, can produce aqueductal stenosis and hydrocephalus in neonatal hamsters, ferrets, rats, and mice. The following viruses have also been shown to produce hydrocephalus in various animal models: mumps virus, arboviruses, influenza and parainfluenza viruses, adenoviruses, papoviruses and Rous sarcoma virus. The pathogenesis of human hydrocephalus may involve cicatricial aqueductal stenosis or inflammatory sequelae elsewhere within the ventricular system. Genetically transmitted hydrocephalus in humans has also been occasionally reported. Additional anomalies are sometimes associated (Fig. 44–5).

CONGENITAL HEART DISEASE

Although cardiac anomalies usually occur as isolated defects, at least 15% of all anomaly syndromes include a cardiac malformation. Such anomalies do not cause spontaneous abortion except for the rare instances in which closure of the ductus arteriosus results in fetal death. Prostaglandin synthetase antagonists such as acetylsalicylic acid and indomethacin, when given to the mother, may cause the ductus arteriosus to close and, for this reason, are contraindicated as tocolytic agents. Hypoplastic left heart syndrome and transposition of the great vessels are common causes of perinatal death whenever the ductus arteriosus closes. Examples of the former include aortic atresia or stenosis, mitral atresia or stenosis, and certain cases of coarctation or interruption of the aortic arch.

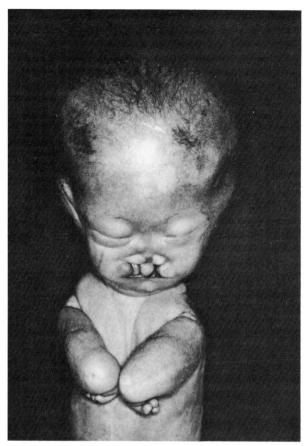

FIG. 44-5. Hydrocephalus, bilateral cleft lip and palate, and phocomelia.

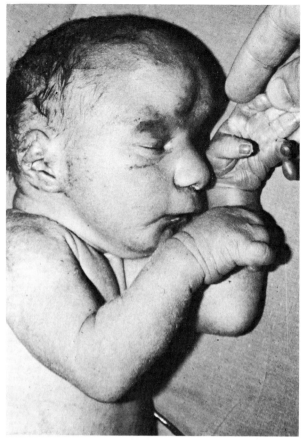

FIG. 44-6. Trisomy 18 (E). Characteristic features include dolichocephaly and micrognathia.

GENETIC DEFECTS

Genetic aberrations account for a significant number of malformations. The physician may first be alerted to the possibility of genetic abnormality by a baby who has low-set ears and is small for gestational age, features common to many such disorders. Autosomal trisomy syndromes, perhaps especially Down's syndrome, trisomy 13–15 (D), and trisomy 18 (Figs. 44–6 and 44–7) are not uncommon (see Chap. 2). Many types of osteochondrodysplasia are known to be genetically transmitted.

OSTEOCHONDRODYSPLASIA

In 1977, an international nomenclature of constitutional disease of bone was developed under the aegis of the European Society for Pediatric Radiology and the National Foundation—March of Dimes. Twenty-one types of osteochondrodysplasia were classified as being

identifiable at birth. Of these, the following are associated with high fetal and neonatal mortality and are likely (unless otherwise indicated) to be genetically transmitted by autosomal recessive means.

Achondrogenesis. Type I (Parenti–Fraccaro) and type II (Langer–Saldino) achondrogenesis are invariably lethal. They may be diagnosed *in utero* when hydramnios necessitates fetal roentgenography. Diagnostic features include severe dwarfism, deficient vertebral ossification, and a commonly associated generalized edema. In type II achondrogenesis, the head is disproportionately large in relation to the trunk, but ossification of the cranial bones is normal. Although there are histopathologic differences between the two conditions, both types show a severe disturbance of enchondral ossification.

Thanatophoric Dysplasia. As implied by the Greek word *thanatophoros* ("death bearing"), thanatophoric dwarfism is invariably lethal. Hydramnios and

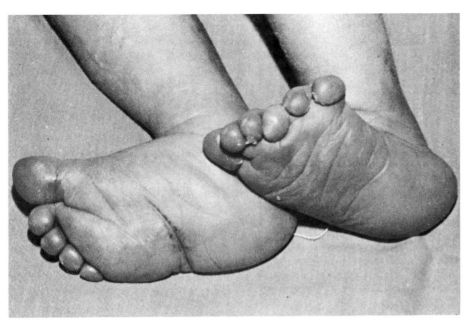

FIG. 44-7. Rocker-bottom feet in trisomy 18 (D).

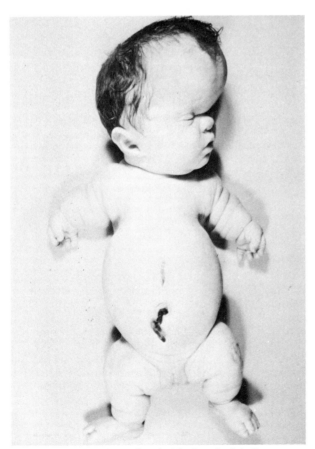

FIG. 44-8. Thanatophoric dwarf with cloverleaf skull.

breech presentation are commonly associated. There are two variants; one has a cloverleaf skull deformity (Fig. 44–8), the other does not. Both have a trunk of normal length, a large head, a small chest, and roentgenographic vertebral features of platyspondylisis with severely widened disk spaces. The histopathology of both types includes markedly reduced enchondral ossification, resulting from minimal proliferation, hypertrophy, and structural alignment of epiphyseal cartilage.

Lethal Osteochondrodysplasia with Small Thorax and Polydactyly. Jeune's syndrome (asphyxiating thoracic dysplasia), the Ellis–van Creveld syndrome (chondroectodermal dysplasia), and the Majewski and Saldino–Noonan syndromes (short-rib polydactyly) are uncommonly encountered entities of lethal dwarfism.

Homozygous Achondroplasia. The frequently recognized entity of achondroplasia is genetically transmitted in an autosomal dominant manner. Homozygous offspring of achondroplastic parents resemble thanatophoric dwarfs and die in early infancy.

Campomelic Syndrome. Of all the osteochondrodysplasias, the campomelic syndrome is the only one with associated malformations so complex as to include the heart, kidneys, central nervous system, and even cleft palate and tracheomalacia. Skeletal anomalies include bowing of the lower limbs, mesomelic dwarfism, joint dislocations, foot deformities, a bell-shaped thorax, dolichocephaly, and small facial bones.

Osteogenesis Imperfecta. The triad of bone fragility, blue sclerae, and otosclerotic deafness characterizes osteogenesis imperfecta. The condition results from hypoplasia of bone mesenchyme, biochemically evidenced in some cases by alteration of the lysine and hydroxylysine content of collagen. There are at least four syndromes of this disease, of which the fatal congenital variety with blue sclerae is transmitted in an autosomal recessive manner. The fetus suffers fractures and, if not stillborn, dies during or shortly after delivery (Fig. 44–9). Normal parents who have had one infant affected with osteogenesis imperfecta congenita are unlikely to give birth to a second affected child.

ABNORMALITIES OF THE EXTREMITIES

Defects of the limbs may occur as isolated minor malformations, or they may be accompanied by major anomalies that are not overtly apparent. Examples include talipes, polydactyly, and syndactyly. For most of these malformations, cytogenetic studies show no chromosomal anomalies. Examination of the associated placenta can be helpful. A newborn with talipes may additionally suffer lung hypoplasia and kidney agenesis or dysplasia; placental amnion nodosum (see Chapter 43) is a characteristic feature of this complex. Amniotic bands, also described in Chapter 43, are an occasional cause of amputation stumps, constriction rings, and other abnormalities of the extremities.

ABNORMALITIES OF THE GASTROINTESTINAL TRACT

Tracheoesophageal Fistula and Esophageal Atresia. Several kinds of congenital anomalies of the esophagus occur in a reported incidence that varies from 1/800 to 1/5000. At least 90% of these anomalies consist of esophageal atresia associated with a fistulous tract from the proximal end of the lower portion of the esophagus to the trachea just above the tracheal bifurcation. The affected newborn regurgitates excessively and a transnasal or oral catheter cannot be passed. Prompt operative correction produces excellent results.

Neonatal Intestinal Obstruction of Miscellaneous Cause. Bile-stained vomitus is an early sign of acute abdominal obstruction. Causes include malrotation with midgut volvulus, duodenal atresia, intestinal duplications, and meconium ileus. The latter may be a manifestation of cystic fibrosis. Other causes include Hirschsprung's disease and imperforate anus.

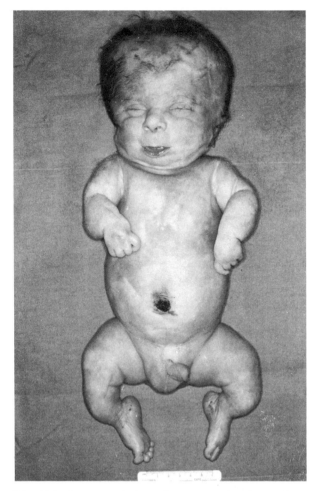

FIG. 44-9. Osteogenesis imperfecta congenita. X-ray shows multiple fractures of ribs, skull, and extremities.

ABNORMALITIES OF THE ABDOMINAL WALL AND GENITOURINARY SYSTEM

Omphalocele. Whereas umbilical hernias are common and usually require no operative treatment, omphaloceles often require two-stage surgical repair. These abnormalities are characterized by a total deficiency of the peritoneal, muscular, and connective tissue layers of the central anterior abdomen.

Cloacal Exstrophy (Vesicointestinal Fissure). Exstrophy of the lower abdomen is characterized by bladder exstrophy, including external intestine within the exposed areas of bladder; bifurcation of the penis or clitoris; imperforate anus; and a short colon. Myelocystocele and omphalocele are often associated, as are malformations of the ureters and kidneys.

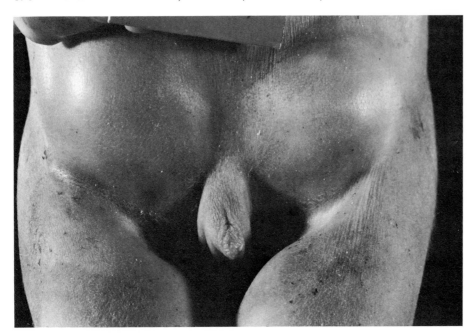

FIG. 44-10. Prune belly syndrome. Cryptorchidism and hypospadias are associated with protuberant abdominal content. Latter results from cystic kidneys and deficient musculature in anterior abdominal wall.

Prune Belly Syndrome. The lack of abdominal musculature, when combined with genitourinary anomalies and cryptorchidism, is known as the prune belly syndrome (Fig. 44–10). Talipes, hip dislocation, and various musculoskeletal abnormalities often occur in this syndrome. When severe urinary tract malformations are present, resultant oligohydramnios often leads to fatal lung hypoplasia.

BIRTH INJURIES

In occasional cases, birth injuries are sustained in uneventful spontaneous delivery, but they occur most commonly in breech delivery, in midforceps delivery, in preterm delivery, and in cases of shoulder dystocia. As obstetric care improves, the frequency of birth injury declines.

FACIAL ABRASIONS

The most common birth injury is an abrasion of the face that results from the pressure of obstetric forceps. Traction need not be heavy to produce such abrasions; pressure of the blades against the face as the head is advanced may suffice. Abrasions occur more frequently if the forceps are applied inadvertently to an oblique diameter of the head. When Tucker–McLane forceps are used to apply even slight traction, abrasions almost inevitably are found at the level of the zygomatic arches; accordingly, these forceps are not suited for traction and should be used only for outlet forceps. The abrasions usually heal without incident, but in some a scar remains.

CRANIAL INJURY

The most frequent cranial injury is *caput succedaneum,* a localized edema of and beneath the scalp that results from impaired venous return in the scalp veins as a consequence of pressure as the head advances through the pelvis (Fig. 44–11). Caput succedaneum is common in prolonged labor. The swelling extends beyond the cranial sutures, and usually subsides spontaneously within a few days. *Cephalhematoma* (Fig. 44–12) is an organized hemotoma separating the periosteum from the underlying bone, either because of continued pressure or, more often, because of the trauma of obstetric forceps. The swelling, which may be bilateral, usually overlies the parietal bone and is sharply limited to the area of the bone, which distinguishes this lesion from caput succedaneum. The swelling may enlarge during the first 2 days of life, thereafter remaining unchanged for 2–3 weeks. As a rule, it subsides very slowly in subsequent months. Treatment is expectant; incision or aspiration is not recommended. Some cephalhematomas become calcified and converted to bone, the bump remaining until it is obscured as the skull thickens and enlarges.

Skull Fracture

Linear fractures, usually beneath a cephalhematoma, are ordinarily quite short and occur in the cleavage lines of the parietal bone at right angles to the sagittal suture. No treatment is required, and no damage to the central nervous system results. Depressed frac-

tures (Fig. 44–13) are usually not true fractures, but rather are depressions of the parietal bone that result from prolonged compression against the maternal symphysis pubis or sacral promontory. Normal skull contours are usually regained spontaneously, and no treatment is needed unless there is evidence of intracranial bleeding.

FIG. 44-11. Caput succedaneum over vertex. (Potter EL: Pathology of the Fetus and the Infant, 2nd ed. Chicago, Year Book, 1961)

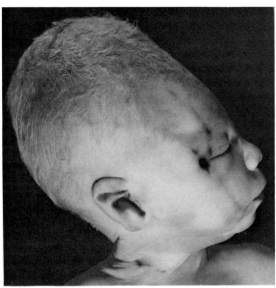

Intracranial Hemorrhage

Subdural hemorrhage is traumatic in origin. It was a frequent result of the difficult obstetric maneuvers that are no longer used in ordinary practice, and it can result from excessive molding. Rupture of the large venous sinuses in the tentorium or falx cerebri causes massive bleeding into the subdural space. The baby is either depressed or stillborn. If the former, the symptoms develop slowly and are characterized by increasing irritability, a bulging fontanel, and, in some cases, convulsions. Some babies recover completely; some apparently recover and develop long-term sequelae; others have a progressive downhill course terminating in neonatal death.

Intraventricular hemorrhage is most commonly associated with preterm delivery, in which the prolonged or recurrent episodes of hypoxia produce congestion and ultimately rupture of the small subependymal veins, with rupture into the ventricle or into the brain substance. Unless there is evidence to the contrary, subependymal and intraventricular hemorrhage should not be attributed to trauma or to obstetric mismanagement.

FIG. 44-12. Cephalhemotoma over left parietal bone. (Potter EL: Pathology of the Fetus and Infant, 2nd ed. Chicago, Year Book, 1961)

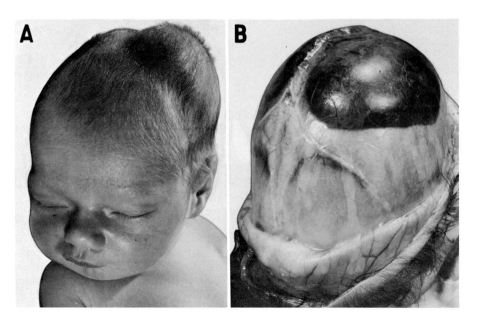

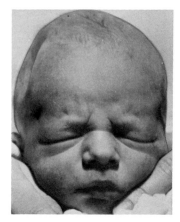

FIG. 44-13. Depressed fracture of skull in region of right parietal bone. (Potter EL: Pathology of the Fetus and Infant, 2nd ed. Chicago, Year Book, 1961)

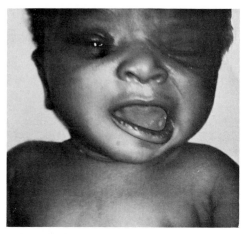

FIG. 44-14. Paralysis of right side of face from injury to right facial nerve. (Potter EL: Pathology of the Fetus and Infant, 2nd ed. Chicago, Year Book, 1961)

Cerebral Palsy

For many years, it was presumed that all cases of cerebral palsy were traumatic in origin; such terms as *brain-damaged child* and *minimal brain damage* immediately implied inept and probably traumatic delivery. Eastman was among the first to emphasize the fallacy of this position, suggesting lack of oxygen as a critical factor. Later studies have shown that, among pregnancies that result in a child with cerebral palsy, prenatal maternal bleeding is from three to six times as frequent as in controls; chronic fetal hypoxia, as may occur in threatened abortion, placenta previa, partial separation of the placenta, preeclampsia, and placental

insufficiency, appears to be concerned in at least half the cases. Mechanical injury and dystocia appear less prominently among the causes.

NERVE INJURY

Facial (Bell's) Palsy. Paresis or paralysis of the facial muscles with inability to close the eye on the affected side (Fig. 44–14) can occur in spontaneous delivery, but it is usually attributed to pressure by the tip of the forceps blade on the facial nerve. Complete recovery usually occurs spontaneously within 2–3 weeks; no treatment is needed except protection of the eye to prevent corneal damage.

Brachial Plexus Palsy. The brachial plexus, especially the fifth and sixth cervical roots, can be damaged when there is difficulty in delivering the after-coming head in breech delivery or by extreme lateral flexion of the head in an effort to deal with shoulder dystocia. This condition is known as *Erb's* or *Duchenne's palsy* (Fig. 44–15). The arm is limp, rotated medially at the shoulder, and held in extension and abduction. If the seventh and eighth cervical and first thoracic nerves are also injured, the entire arm is affected. In *Klumpke's palsy* only the seventh and eighth cervical nerves are affected, resulting in wrist drop and paralysis of the muscles of the hand. Usually, the injury consists of laceration of the nerve sheath with edema and hemorrhage. If the nerves are not actually severed, the outlook is excellent, recovery following in 1 month to 2 years.

It is important that brachial plexus injury be promptly diagnosed. The arm should be held in abduction, the elbow flexed and the wrist extended. Suitable measures are to tie the arm to the head of the bassinet, to pin a tie to the mattress above the infant's head, or to apply a small airplane splint. Physiotherapy, consisting of light massage and passive movements, is started after a few weeks and is continued for the duration of the disability.

Since the phrenic nerve is derived in part from the brachial plexus, phrenic nerve palsy may occur in conjunction with Erb's palsy. This produces paralysis of one side of the diaphragm, recurrent cyanosis, and dyspnea. Recovery is usually spontaneous, but it may be slow and can be complicated by pulmonary infection.

Spinal Cord Injury. The direct and contributory causes of spinal cord injury and their effects are summarized in Tables 44–3 and 44–4. An example of this type of injury is shown in Figure 44–16. It is emphasized that examination of the cervical and thoracic spinal cord is an integral part of the autopsy of babies who die during labor or in the neonatal period. This simple

procedure is so often omitted that there is no real knowledge of the frequency of this lesion.

FRACTURES

In breech delivery, the femur may be fractured during attempts to deliver extended legs, or the humerus may be fractured during delivery of the arm. Fracture of the clavicle may be either spontaneous or deliberate in shoulder dystocia. Most such fractures are of the greenstick type, and they heal without incident if appropriate splints are applied.

MUSCLE INJURY

The most frequent, and potentially serious, muscle injury is to the sternocleidomastoid, which can be damaged by excessive traction after delivery of the head in vertex delivery or after delivery of the shoulders in breech delivery. A palpable hematoma develops in the affected muscle (Fig. 44–17). Treatment consists of passive stretching of the muscle several times daily. If untreated, the mass may organize, with consequent shortening of the muscle and torticollis. (Most cases of torticollis are due not to this injury, but to congenital maldevelopment of the muscle and are often accompanied by other congenital abnormalities.)

NEONATAL CRISES

PERINATAL BRAIN DAMAGE

Manifestations of brain damage may be precipitated by postnatal factors, but preterm delivery and compromising fetal experiences are usually the primary cause. Intraventricular hemorrhage, the most common lesion, has been reported in as many as 6% of stillborns and 60% of neonatal autopsies. Koehl and Altshuler reviewed the 1970 Cincinnati Children's Hospital autopsies of newborns who died of hyaline membrane disease within the first 3 days of life; their perinatal brain damage findings were similar to those of other observers. Two-thirds suffered intraventricular hemorrhage, usually associated with germinal matrix hemorrhage about the caudate nucleus of a lateral ventricle. Cerebellar hemorrhage occurred in 18% of the newborns. The cause of some instances of cerebellar hemorrhage may be tight binding of ventilator face masks.

Two or more lesions are often found in one brain studied in neonatal autopsies. Anoxic–ischemic neuronal necrosis may result from a range of insults, *e.g.,* blood loss, septic shock, hypoglycemia, and acidosis. Severe hypoxemia and reduced cerebral perfusion,

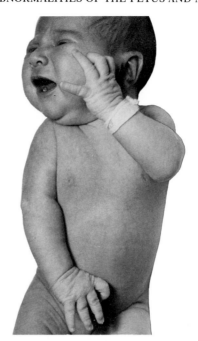

FIG. 44-15. Erb's palsy resulting from injury of fifth and sixth cervical roots of brachial plexus. (Potter EL: Pathology of the Fetus and Infant, 2nd ed. Chicago, Year Book, 1961)

TABLE 44–3. CAUSES OF SPINAL CORD INJURY AT BIRTH

DIRECT CAUSES
  Injurious force at delivery
    Traction on spinal axis of fetus, causing stretch injury of vertebral column, cord, and brain stem structures
    Flexion of spinal column, excessive in degree, causing stretch injury and compression
    Torsion of spinal column causing stretch injury
CONTRIBUTING FACTORS
  Intrauterine fetal malposition: brow, face, breech presentation
  Dystocia
  Preterm delivery
  Primiparity
  Precipitous delivery
  Intraspinal vascular occlusive phenomena in fetus
  Vertebral and foramen magnum malformations in fetus

(Modified from Towbin A: Arch Pathol 77:620, 1964)

however, are the final common pathways by which neuronal necrosis occurs. Affected sites most frequently include the hippocampus, brain stem, thalamus, basal ganglia, and boundary zone cortex between major arterial vascularization sites. Periventricular leukomalacia, which may be complicated by hemorrhage, is often associated with perinatal infections; it is frequently a consequence of endotoxemia.

TABLE 44-4. CLINICAL EFFECTS OF NEONATAL SPINAL CORD AND BRAIN STEM INJURY

SUDDEN DEATH OF FETUS DURING LABOR (STILLBIRTH) OR DIRECTLY AFTER
SHORT SURVIVAL OF INFANT
    Respiratory depression at birth; shallow respiration; apnea
    Neurologic symptoms; "spinal shock"; limp and pale appearance
    Pulmonary complications of hyaline membrane disease; pneumonia
LONG-TERM SURVIVAL OF INFANT
    Spinal cord injury; neurologic sequelae
        Transient paralysis
        Permanent paralysis (paraplegia, tetraplegia)
        Spasticity (clinically mild or latent)
    Spinal nerve root injuries; neurologic sequelae
    Brain stem injury
        Cranial nerve deficits
    Cerebral hypoxic devastation (secondary)
        Motor defects of cerebral palsy
        Mentation deficits
        Epilepsy

(Towbin A: Arch Pathol 77:620, 1969)

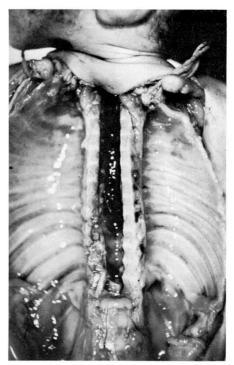

FIG. 44-16. Spinal epidural hemorrhage of cervical and thoracic regions mainly, in preterm infant (7 months' gestation). Respiratory depression was present after delivery; infant lived 36 hours. (Towbin A: Arch Pathol 77:620, 1964)

FIG. 44-17. Mass in right sternocleidomastoid muscle in infant 2 months of age. (Potter EL: Pathology of the Fetus and Infant, 2nd ed. Chicago, Year Book, 1961)

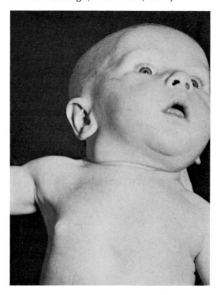

HYALINE MEMBRANE DISEASE

The term *hyaline membrane disease* is used to describe the pathologic changes that are responsible for the respiratory distress syndrome, which is inevitable when babies are born before their lungs have reached functional maturity. It is the leading cause of neonatal death. The lungs are heavy, atelectatic, airless, and sink in water. The alveoli and terminal bronchioles are lined by an intensely eosinophilic hyalinelike membrane, and the peripheral air spaces are collapsed. The membrane appears about 6 hours after birth, but the signs begin within the first few hours, being characterized especially by expiratory grunts and severe intercostal retraction. As noted in Chapter 16, the basic defect is a lack of surfactant production from the alveolar type II cells.

PERINATAL BACTERIAL INFECTION

Group B hemolytic *Streptococcus* is now the most common cause of perinatal bacterial sepsis, compared with *Escherichia coli*, which was the most common cause 10–15 years ago. Group B hemolytic *Streptococcus* can be isolated from cervical cultures of 5%–30% of asymptomatic pregnant women and also from their sexual partners. There are two neonatal clinical pictures. An acute septicemic form occurs in the first few hours or days of life, typically with features of pneumonia. A delayed meningitic manifestation appears anywhere from the 2nd to the 12th week of life.

E. coli accounts for about 75% of gram-negative perinatal infections. Staphylococci and *Listeria monocytogenes* may uncommonly cause pneumonia, meningitis, and sepsis, as may many other organisms.

NECROTIZING ENTEROCOLITIS

The most common surgical emergency in newborns is necrotizing enterocolitis. Its incidence has risen dramatically in the last 10 years, probably because improved obstetric care has permitted survival of many fetuses who otherwise would have been stillborn. Clinical signs of the disease include abdominal distention, vomiting, and gastrointestinal bleeding. The precipitating cause is intestinal ischemia secondary to shock. Despite the name, inflammation is not a feature of necrotizing enterocolitis. The intestine shows infarction, most commonly in the ileocecal area. Perforation, peritonitis, and cicatricial stenotic repair are common sequelae. The fundamental cause of the disease is unknown, but infectious agents and hyperosmolar feedings may be implicated. Breast milk, which contains secretory IgA and leukocytes, may have a partially protective effect, but the disease has developed in infants whose only diet was breast milk.

REFERENCES AND RECOMMENDED READING

Ambani LM, Joshi NJ, Vaidya RA et al. Are hormonal contraceptives teratogenic? Fertil Steril 28:791, 1977

Averback P, Wiglesworth FW: Congenital absence of the heart: Observation of human funiculopagous twinning with insertio funiculi furcata, fusion, forking and interpositio velamentosa. Teratology 17:143, 1978

Benirschke K, Kim CK: Multiple pregnancy. N Engl J Med 288:1276; 1329, 1973

Bhettay E, Nelson MM, Beighton P: Epidemic of conjoined twins in Southern Africa? Lancet 2:741, 1975

Caviness VS, Jr: The Chiari malformations of the posterior fossa and their relation to hydrocephalus. Dev Med Child Neurol 18:103, 1976

Chefetz MD: Etiology of cerebral palsy: Role of reproductive insufficiency and multiplicity of factors. Obstet Gynecol 25:635, 1965

Crosby WM: Trauma during pregnancy: Maternal and fetal injury. Obstet Gynecol Surv 29:683, 1974

Eastman NJ: Mount Everest in utero. Am J Obstet Gynecol 67:701, 1954

Eastman NJ: Editor's note regarding cerebral palsy. Obstet Gynecol Surv 11:381, 1956

Fuldner RV: Cerebral palsy: Where next? Arch Neurol Psychiatr 74:267, 1955

Heinonen OP, Slone D, Shapiro S et al.: Birth defects and drugs in pregnancy. Littleton, MA, Publishing Sciences Group, 1977

Holmes LB: Current concepts in genetics: Congenital Malformations. N Engl J Med 295:204, 1977

Illingsworth RS: Why blame the obstetrician? A review. Br Med J 1:797, 1979

James WH: A note on the epidemiology of acardiac monsters. Teratology 16:211, 1977

Johnson RT: Hydrocephalus and viral infections. Dev Med Child Neurol 17:807, 1975

Kaufman MH, O'Shea KS: Induction of monozygotic twinning in the mouse. Nature 276:707, 1978

Kjessler B, Johnansson GSO: Alpha-fetoprotein (AFP) in early pregnancy. Acta Obstet Gynecol Scand, Suppl 69:1977

Kosloske AM: Necrotizing enterocolitis in the neonate. Surg Gynecol Obstet 148:259, 1979

Krous HF, Turbeville DF, Altshuler GP: Campomelic syndrome—Possible role of intrauterine viral infection. Teratology 19:9, 1979

Latham D, Anderson GW, Eastman NJ: Obstetric factors in cerebral palsy. Am J Obstet Gynecol 68:91, 1954

Lenz W: Thalidomide and congenital abnormalities. Lancet 2:1358, 1961

McBride WG: Thalidomide embryopathy. Teratology 16:79, 1977

Mulvihill JJ, Yeager AM: Fetal alcohol syndrome. Teratology 13:345, 1976

Nakano KK: Anencephaly: A review. Dev Med Child Neurol 15:383, 1973

Niswander KR: The obstetrician, fetal asphyxia, and cerebral palsy. Am J Obstet Gynecol 133:358, 1979

Norman MG: Perinatal brain damage. In Rosenberg HS, Bolande RP (eds): Perspectives in Pediatric Pathology, Vol 4, p 41. Chicago, Year Book, 1978

Pramanik AK, Altshuler G, Light IJ et al. Prune-belly syndrome associated with Potter (renal nonfunction) syndrome. Am J Dis Child 131:672, 1977

Reimer CB, Black CM, Phillips DJ et al.: The specificity of fetal IgM: Antibody or antiantibody? Ann NY Acad Sci 254:77, 1975

Remington JS, Klein JO: Infectious diseases of the fetus and newborn infant. Philadelphia, WB Saunders, 1976

Rimoin DL International nomenclature of constitutional disease of bone. J Pediatr 93:614, 1978

Shapiro S, Slone D, Hartz SC et al.: Are hydantoins (phenytoins) human teratogens? J Pediatr 90:673, 1977

Shoenfeld Y, Fried A, Ehrenfeld NE: Osteogenesis imperfecta. Am J Dis Child 129:679, 1975

Sillence DO, Rimoin DL, Lachman R: Neonatal dwarfism. Pediatr Clin North Am 25:453, 1978

Smith DW: Teratogenicity of anticonvulsive medications. Am J Dis Child 131:1337, 1977

Warkany J: Congenital Malformations. Chicago, Year Book, 1971

Yang SS, Heidelberger KP, Brough AJ et al.: Lethal short-limbed chondrodysplasia in early infancy. In Rosenberg HS and Bolande RP (eds): Perspectives in Pediatric Pathology, Vol 3, p 1. Chicago, Year Book, 1976

PART VII

GYNECOLOGIC DISORDERS

45

PEDIATRIC GYNECOLOGY

Vincent J. Capraro

In the past, pediatric gynecology was a "no man's land." The pediatrician avoided pelvic examination and had little to offer with regard to treatment of either the ordinary problems or the range of congenital anomalies. The gynecologist, on the other hand, rarely saw children and adolescents and lacked instruments to perform the examination. Today, gynecologic problems among this group are recognized and successfully treated. Such problems, however, require a unique approach, special methods of examination, specialized instruments, and familiarity with pelvic pathology in children.

GYNECOLOGIC EXAMINATION OF THE CHILD

The attitude of the physician is the determining factor in the success of gynecologic examination of children. The clinician must reexamine personal beliefs con-

cerning sexuality if the patient is to receive the best of care. Most errors of pediatric gynecology are those of omission rather than commission; they result from performing either no examination whatever or an incomplete one. The Victorian notion that the young virgin will be deflorated is all too prevalent among modern practitioners. When the child is examined properly with pediatric instruments, it is usually possible to open the hymenal orifice without tearing the hymen. It is vital that the physician explain to the mother that the hymen will not be damaged by the examination and why. In experienced hands, a female child may be examined at any age, provided the proper equipment and technique are used.

SEDATION AND ANESTHESIA

Most infants and children can be examined without resorting to anesthesia. With patience and tact, a complete examination can be accomplished without traumatizing the child physically or psychologically. Once a child has been hurt as a result of a poorly performed examination, however, she will resist further attempts at examination.

Mild sedation may be required in certain cases. An analgesic frequently employed ("CM3") consists of a solution of 1 ml meperidine hydrochloride 50 mg, 1 ml chlorpromazine hydrochloride 12.5 mg, and 1 ml promethazine hydrochloride 12.5 mg. The usual dose is 1 ml of the solution IM/20 lbs of body weight up to a maximum of 2 ml. Sick children receive half the usual dose. In addition, application of a local anesthetic (lidocaine [Xylocaine] 5% ointment) to the hymenal ring sometimes minimizes discomfort. Rarely, when analgesia alone is insufficient, anesthesia is required for examination. It is better to perform a complete examination under general anesthesia than to walk away from a painful examination with incomplete findings.

HELPFUL HINTS FOR EXAMINATION

In examining a child, several measures can be used to obtain her cooperation and minimize her fear of future examinations. It is helpful, for example, if the examiner wears street clothes. A specially trained nurse who has empathy for children and is skilled in therapeutic communication is an invaluable asset. In dealing with congenital anomalies, the nurse can help parents to ventilate their fears and to dispel the guilt that many feel after the birth of a defective child.

The mother can be an asset or a detriment. In examining a younger child, the mother provides the patient with a sense of security, and it is best to keep her in the room. The mother sits on the table's edge and holds her baby in the dorsal lithotomy position. The physician sits on a chair directly in front of the mother in order to perform the examination. Gynecologic stir-

FIG. 45-1. Mother or nurse assistant in street clothes distracts patient's attention from examination of genital area. Teg lithotomy block positions patient properly and comfortably.

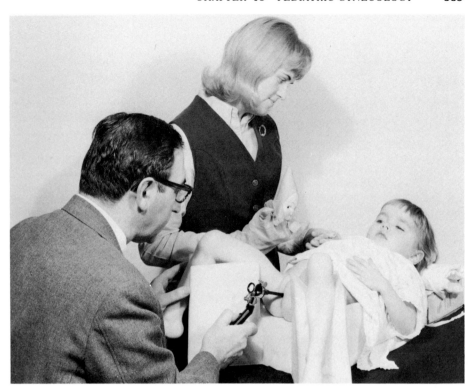

rups are generally too large for young children and the Teg lithotomy block is far more comfortable and more convenient for the examiner (Fig. 45–1).

With a pubescent girl, it is usually best to keep the mother out of the examining room. If a question is raised, there may be a confrontation between the adolescent and her mother, with the result that the physician may lose effectiveness in dealing with the patient.

Asking the patient to help with the examination is of definite value, since it makes the examination seem less assaultive. Using the patient's fingers, the labia can be separated and the hymen and urethra exposed. This also permits the use of the physician's fingers without the patient realizing it (Fig. 45–2). Subsequent steps are shown in Figure 45–3. By means of this technique, it is often possible to examine children without the use of any anesthesia.

Many children retain a tense abdomen either because they are afraid or because they are ticklish. Placing the patient's hand in the palm of the examiner's hand and asking her to help palpate often relaxes the abdominal musculature sufficiently to allow the physician to make an adequate examination.

EXAMINATION OF INFANTS AND CHILDREN

The gynecologic examination of infants and children can be divided into four parts: 1) inspection and palpa-

tion of the vulvar structures, 2) visualization of the vagina and cervix, 3) bimanual abdominopelvic examination (rectal in small children, vaginal in teenagers), and 4) examination of the extrapelvic sex areas.

Inspection and Palpation of the Vulva

While inspecting and palpating the vulva and groin, the physician should seek answers to the following questions for each structure: Is it there? Is the location normal? Does the structure look normal? Does it appear that it will function normally?

The *mons pubis* is palpated for abnormal structures. Pubic hair is normally not present until the child approaches menarche. Its presence in a premenarchel child suggests an excess of androgen, which could be the result of adrenogenital syndrome, or sexual precocity due to constitutional precocious puberty, premature pubarche, or exogenous androgen.

The *groin* is palpated for masses that, if noted, may indicate lymphadenopathy or herniation of the peritoneal sac. In patients with hernia, masses within the hernia may be gonads. Occasionally, an overzealous surgeon removes one of the masses only to find that a normal ovary has been excised.

Pubic hair usually develops at about the same time as the breasts. The normal female escutcheon is a triangle pointing downward and sharply cut off at the level of the pubic symphysis. The male hair pattern is

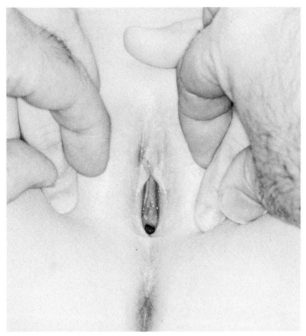

FIG. 45-2. Child helps examiner by separating labia. This not only assures her that she will not be hurt but also distracts her, thus permitting examiner to use fingers without her realizing it.

diamond in shape and extends up toward the umbilicus. The male pattern in a female may be pathologic, due to androgen stimulation, or simply a family trait.

The *clitoris* is inspected for size. It is relatively prominent at birth, especially in preterm infants. Since it does not grow as fast as the rest of the vulva, it appears less prominent as the child becomes older. However, an absolute increase in size suggests androgen stimulation. It is often difficult to determine whether a clitoris is normal or enlarged, because the normal size varies considerably (0.6–2 cm in length, 0.3–0.9 cm in width). The best way to follow patients with clitoral hypertrophy is to take serial photographs over time; this is especially helpful in borderline cases.

The *labia majora* are normally smooth. If rugae are present or if there is labial fusion, the physician must seek a source of androgen to which the child may have been exposed. The labia majora are palpated for masses. If present, they may be gonads—either ovaries in females or testes in patients with hermaphroditism. It must be remembered that the labia majora are not as well developed in the young child as in the adult.

The *labia minora* are prominent and quite edematous at birth due to maternal estrogenic hormones. This subsides within a few weeks. Normally, the labia minora are easily separated and do not obscure the view of the hymen and urethra. In some cases, how-

ever, they are adherent (labial synechia); until they are separated by local estrogen cream, the examiner cannot visualize the hymen, vagina, or urethra. Labial adhesions also occur secondary to inflammation.

The *hymen* is also quite edematous and prominent at birth due to maternal estrogen stimulation. It is exposed by placing the fingers lateral to the vaginal orifice, separating the structures laterally, and then depressing downward toward the coccyx. This maneuver usually exposes the hymen and its orifice, permitting partial visualization of the vagina. The child can be asked to take a deep breath or to cough, since this changes the intraabdominal pressure and sometimes opens the hymenal orifice. Another technique may be used to visualize the vagina; by pulling the labia out toward the examiner, the vaginal canal may become visible (Fig. 45–4). If, after this step, the presence of a vagina cannot be verified, a well-lubricated probe or rubber catheter should be introduced to confirm the presence of a vagina.

The *urethra* must be specifically identified. Children with ambiguous genitalia or other congenital anomalies frequently lack a urethral orifice in the normal location.

Visualization of the Vagina and Cervix

The standard Graves speculum and even the so-called infant Graves speculum are too large for examining the small child. Other instruments have been devised for visualization of the pediatric vagina and cervix. The Killian nasal speculum is a handy instrument that is readily available in any hospital or clinic. The physician can make an atraumatic examination with this instrument, but it is usually not long enough to expose the upper vagina and cervix. In the smaller child, we use a vaginoscope that we devised from an otoscope made by Cameron Miller (Fig. 45–1 and 45–3). In older children, specula of various sizes may be used. The Huffman vaginal speculum, devised by Dr. John Huffman in Chicago, is excellent for examining the adolescent patient (Fig. 45–5).

Vagina. At birth, the vaginal mucosa is thick and moist. Within a few weeks, it becomes thin, atrophic, and reddish, and it remains so until estrogen is produced at puberty. At this time, the mucosa becomes thicker, moister, and paler. Many of the principles of therapy in children depend on the vaginal mucosa, of which there are two types: childhood, or anestrogenic, and adult, or estrogenic (Table 45–1).

Cervix. In the young, it is difficult at times to distinguish the surface of the cervix from the vaginal mucosa, because the cervical epithelium is pleated and rugose until puberty. The distinction can sometimes be made by color: the cervix is usually much redder than the vaginal walls.

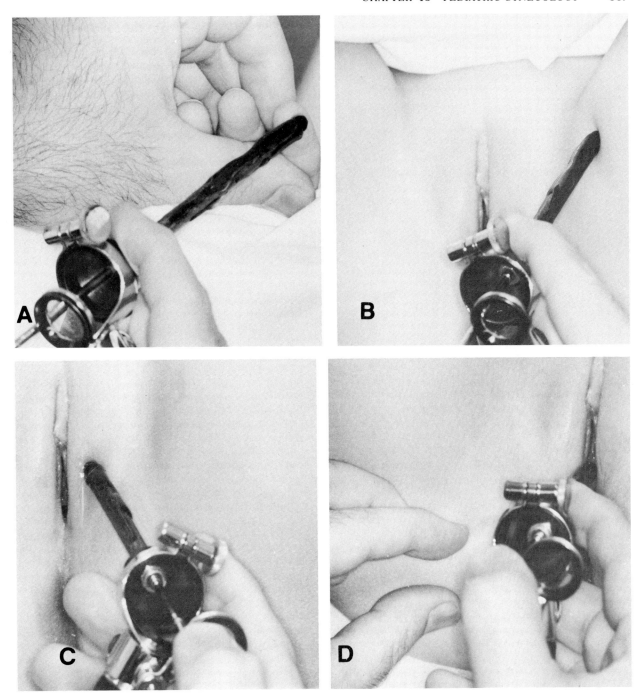

FIG. 45–3. Vaginoscopic examination. *A.* Child touches well-lubricated vaginoscope with her index finger; examiner points out that it feels funny, slippery, and cool. *B.* Speculum is then placed against inner left thigh, and examiner repeats that it feels slippery and cool. *C.* Speculum next touches left labium majus, while examiner makes same remarks. *D.* When speculum is passed through hymenal opening, patient does not jump because previous three steps have conditioned her to feel of speculum. Note that examiner's left hand simultaneously presses patient's right buttock firmly to distract her from speculum as it is passing painlessly through hymenal orifice.

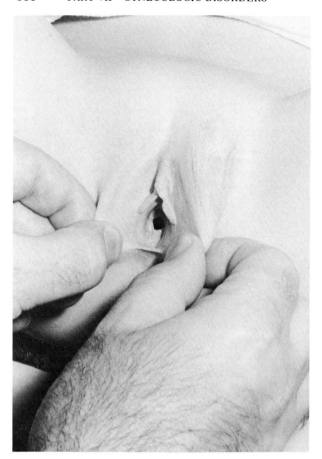

FIG. 45-4. Pulling labia gently laterally and toward examiner reveals hymenal opening and permits visualization of vaginal canal.

Bimanual Abdominopelvic Examination

A digital rectal examination combined with abdominal palpation is possible even in young children. In some children, it may be possible to do a one-finger vaginal examination with the index finger; if not, the fifth digit can be used. In very small children, the rectal examination usually reveals no palpable masses. The small mass occasionally palpable in the midline is more often the cervix than the body of the uterus. The size ratio of corpus uteri to cervix in children is 1:2. In the adolescent, the rectal examination can be done with the index finger. Usually, the cervix and uterus can be palpated easily. At this time, the ratio of uterus to cervix is about 1:1. Normal ovaries or tubes cannot be palpated during adolescence, and palpable adnexal masses in this age group are usually pathologic. It is prudent to do the less traumatic rectal examination first and then to attempt a one-finger vaginal examination. In some adolescents, a vaginal examination may be impossible.

Examination of Extrapelvic Sex Areas

Breasts. The breasts are enlarged at birth in both sexes, and a nodule that measures approximately 1 cm is usually present beneath the areola. This is due to stimulation of the breast tissue by maternal hormones. In some newborns, a clear discharge is present ("witch's milk").

The breasts develop early in puberty. Estrogen promotes the development of the nipple and duct structures, and it induces pigmentation of the areola. Progesterone is responsible for lobular acinar budding. The physician should keep in mind that the development of breasts is related to age (see Figure 8–5). Accurate measurement of breast size may be important in later evaluation of breast development.

In the early developing breasts, a little "button" that is the source of future breast development is present beneath the areola. Unfortunately, we have seen patients who have had this bud excised because it was thought to be a tumor, thus dooming the young girl to life without breast development.

Development of breast tissue prematurely may be due to premature sexual development or to exogenous estrogen. In some premenarcheal children whose breasts appear to be developing, the growth is due entirely to adipose tissue. It is therefore important to distinguish fat from breast tissue during palpation. Failure of the breasts to develop at puberty is suggestive of delayed puberty or one of the intersex problems.

Breast development is frequently asymmetric, one breast developing faster than the other. Over time, the disparity in size usually decreases so that the breasts later appear equal in size. However, if they are measured, a difference can still be noted.

Axillary Hair. The patient at puberty should have axillary hair. Its premature appearance should lead the physician to search for a source of androgen. Lack of axillary hair suggests testicular feminization syndrome, pituitary deficiency, or gonadal dysgenesis.

Skin. The presence of acne on the face or body suggests androgen secretion. This may be normal or abnormal, depending on the age of the child.

Height, Weight, and General Body Contours. The gynecologist whose horizon lies at the umbilicus is short-sighted and misses many diagnoses in the child with gynecologic problems. The patient's height, weight, and general body contours, as well as their relationship to the patient's age, must also be considered. If growth is advanced, the physician must consider exposure to an anabolic steroid, which may come from the ovary, adrenals, or exogenous sources. If growth is retarded, she may be suffering from endocrine problems, such as hypothyroidism or panhypopituitarism, or she may have a genetic defect, such as Turner's syndrome. As

FIG. 45-5. Huffman vaginal speculum, with a blade 1 cm wide and 11 cm long.

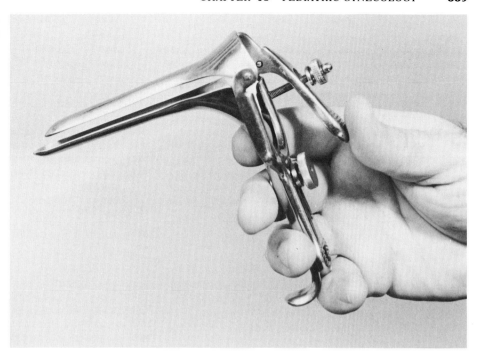

TABLE 45-1. CHARACTER OF VAGINA IN CHILDREN

	Childhood or Anestrogenic	Adult or Estrogenic
EPITHELIAL CELLS	Thin layer of noncornified, round or oval cells, with vesicular nuclei; nucleus to cytoplasm ratio of 2:3	Thick, succulent, cornified cells that are polygonal with dark pyknotic nuclei; nucleus to cytoplasm ratio of 1:15
PH	Neutral, no lactobacilli	Acidic, lactobacilli present

noted in Chapter 8, an optimal height-weight ratio is necessary for the onset of menstruation.

The body contours also give some indication of maturity. If the child has not been exposed to estrogen, she shows straight body lines. As ovarian estrogen secretions begin, the pubertal child develops padding in the hips, thus demonstrating the normal female body contour.

INFECTIONS OF THE FEMALE GENITAL ORGANS IN CHILDREN AND ADOLESCENTS

The most common childhood gynecologic infection is vulvovaginitis. (Infections of the cervix, tubes, and ovaries occur in older, sexually active females.) There are a number of reasons why children are prone to vulvovaginal infection. The vaginal orifice is not well protected in the child because she has no pubic hair and no padding of the mons and labia. In addition, be-cause of the closer proximity of the anus, the child's vagina is more prone to fecal contamination. Poor perineal hygiene is also more common in children, as are skin, upper respiratory tract, and parasitic infections, all of which are etiologic factors in vulvovaginitis.

Symptoms of vulvovaginitis may vary from slight discomfort to pruritis and burning with discharge. Nonspecific vaginitis rarely involves more than the lower one-third of the vagina, whereas specific infections often extend to the entire vagina and cervix.

Table 45-2 is a comprehensive list of etiologic factors. By far the most common are the first five categories.

In order to treat this disease properly, certain minimal diagnostic procedures are necessary to determine etiology. Unless the etiology is known, attempts at therapy are often futile and recurrences are frequent. The definitive diagnosis of vaginitis is made by examination of vaginal secretions, which requires invasion of the vagina. Passing a dry cotton-tip applicator through

TABLE 45–2. FACTORS ASSOCIATED WITH VULVOVAGINITIS IN CHILDREN

I. Mixed, nonspecific, bacterial infections of the vagina
II. Single, specific, bacterial infections of the vagina
   A. Nongonorrheal
      1. *Escherichia coli, Bacillus proteus,* staphylococcus
      2. Hemolytic streptococcus
      3. Pneumococcus
      4. Typhoid, shigella
      5. Diphtheria
   B. Gonorrhea
III. Infections with other microorganisms
   A. Monilia
   B. Trichomonad
IV. Pinworm infestation
V. Local physical factors
   A. Foreign body in vagina
   B. Trauma
      1. Physical
      2. Chemical
      3. Thermal
      4. Self-induced—masturbation, neurodermatitis
   C. Gynecologic neoplasms, polyps, labial agglutination
   D. Urologic problems
      1. Urethral prolapse
      2. Anomalous ureter exit into vagina
   E. Rectal problems
      1. Anomalous anal opening into vestibule or vagina
      2. Anal fissure, pruritus
VI. Allergic manifestations
VII. Systemic illnesses with vaginal manifestations
   A. Measles
   B. Scarlet fever and hemolytic streptococcus infections
   C. Smallpox
   D. Typhoid, dysentery
   E. Blood dyscrasias
   F. Draining pelvic abscesses
VII. Skin diseases with vulvar manifestations
   A. Condyloma acuminatum
   B. Herpes simplex, herpes zoster

(Modified from Altcheck A: Surg Clin North Am 40:1071, 1960)

the sensitive hymen to obtain specimens is traumatic, especially when multiple specimens are required. In order to avoid this, a simple technique to aspirate vaginal secretions was devised (Fig. 45–6). As many tests as desired can be performed with a single aspirate. Complete studies include 1) bacterial smears and cultures; 2) monilial culture; 3) Papanicolaou smear to detect pus cells, red blood cells, malignant cells, and for estrogen effect; 4) wet smear (saline suspension); 5) wet mount (20% potassium hydroxide; 6) vaginoscopy; 7) Scotch tape swab of the anus for pinworm (Graham test); and 8) laboratory tests, *e.g.,* complete blood count and urinalysis.

A PRACTICAL APPROACH TO VULVOVAGINITIS IN CHILDREN

Since most children with vulvovaginitis are seen as outpatients, it may be difficult and expensive to perform detailed studies. Many patients respond to simple treatment, and a step-by-step approach that leaves the more difficult and expensive steps for patients who do not respond to simple treatment.

The following steps are not always taken in order. If, for example, a foreign body is suspected, the physician would proceed directly to step 6, vaginoscopy. If gonorrhea is suspected, the physician would start with step 5, smears and cultures.

Step 1: Local Treatment to Vulva

Sitz baths with plain water are ordered once or twice daily. If perineal hygiene is poor, the mother is asked to add two tablespoonfuls of baking soda or Epsom salts. This implies a medicinal rather than a cleansing bath and may encourage compliance. A bland dusting powder is applied to the vulva after each bath. White cotton panties are worn instead of synthetic nylon panties for several reasons. First, the colored dye used in some underclothing may irritate the vulva. Second, cotton absorbs moisture, thereby keeping the perineum dry. Synthetic materials do not absorb moisture, and local secretions and vaginal discharges that remain on the vulva may cause maceration. The mother is also instructed to teach the child to wipe herself from "front to back." This avoids the contamination that occurs when the child wipes herself in such a manner as to bring bacteria from the anal area to the vulva.

Step 2: Systemic Treatment

In patients who have vulvovaginitis associated with infections elsewhere, such as upper respiratory tract and urinary infections, systemic antibiotics are used. When such infections are related, the response to systemic antibiotics is gratifying.

Step 3: Local Therapy in the Vagina

In the premenarcheal child with the anestrogenic vagina, Furacin E urethral inserts may be used. These are made to fit the adult urethra and easily slide into the vagina of a child. They contain nitrofurazone, an antibacterial agent, and estrogen in the form of diethylstilbestrol (DES) 0.1 mg. The mother is instructed to break one in half lengthwise and to insert half of one stick into the vagina each night for a fortnight. This alters pH and converts the immature anestrogenic vagina to the mature type, which is capable of combating the infection. Oral estrogen is not needed to convert an anestrogenic vagina, and it also has the obvious disad-

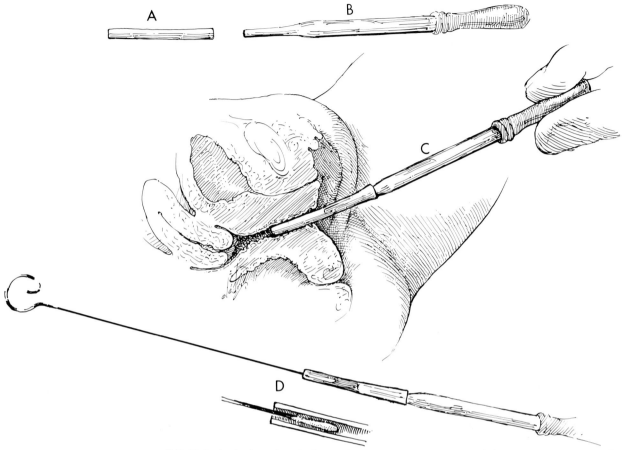

FIG. 45-6. Aspiration of vaginal secretions. *A.* 4 to 5 cm segment of plastic intravenous tubing. *B.* Ordinary medicine dropper. *C.* Sagittal view of aspirator being introduced painlessly through opening in hymen. Secretions are easily aspirated with a single invasion of vagina. *D.* Small cotton-tip applicator to obtain specimen of vaginal secretions. Such sampling can be repeated as often as necessary.

vantage of systemic estrogen stimulation that can produce breast hypertrophy or uterine bleeding.

Step 4: Wet Mount Studies

A wet mount using saline is prepared in addition to a wet mount using 20% potassium hydroxide. They are examined for pus cells, red blood cells, *Trichomonas vaginalis, Candida albicans,* bacteria, parasitic ova, and sperm. On the basis of this information, specific therapy is often possible.

Step 5: Smears and Cultures

If there is a recurrence, smears and cultures of the vaginal secretions are made. These are expensive, and they must be taken properly and delivered promptly to the laboratory.

Step 6: Vaginoscopy

If there is still no response after step 5, vaginoscopy is performed to rule out the presence of foreign bodies. Foreign bodies, such as tiny bits of toilet paper, do not come out of the vagina spontaneously and usually produce recurring episodes of infection until they are removed.

Step 7: Scotch Tape Test for Pinworms

Pinworm eggs are not normally found in the stool; instead, the female worm migrates, usually at night, to the perianal region to deposit eggs. If Scotch tape is placed with its sticky side outward on a tongue depressor, the sticky surface may be pressed against the anal region. It is then placed firmly against a microscopic slide and removed, leaving some of the material at-

TABLE 45-3. 500 CASES OF VULVOVAGINITIS; ETIOLOGY AND AGE DISTRIBUTION

Etiology	Number	Age in Years (Average)
Nonspecific (mixed)	213	8.8
Monilia (Candida)	63	12.5
Foreign body	55	7.2
Streptococcus	45	10.4
Physiologic	33	11.5
Staphylococcus	30	6.9
Gonococcus	24	9.9
Trichomonas	15	11.9
Pinworms	8	6.3
Congenital anomalies	6	6.2
Escherichia coli	5	4.6
Other	2	5.0
4° tear	1	14.0

tached to the slide. The application of toluene clears everything but the eggs and adult worms, which can now be detected with a low-power microscope objective. Diagnostic tapes for easy use are available commercially.

EXPERIENCE WITH 500 CASES OF VULVOVAGINITIS

A study was made of 500 children with vulvovaginitis seen by the Buffalo Pediatric Gynecology Service. The youngest patient was 5 months old; the oldest, 16 years old. The largest numbers of patients were aged 6, 7, and 8. The etiologic factors and the average age according to etiologic factors are shown in Table 45–3.

Mixed Bacterial Vulvovaginitis (Nonspecific)

By far the largest number of patients have nonspecific vulvovaginitis, and quite often a multitude of organisms is found. It may be difficult to determine which organisms are normal, which are pathogenic, and which are contaminants. The treatment of choice is local, as outlined in step 3. Huffman recommends the use of vaginal suppositories of 9-aminoacridine monohydrochloride in the treatment of nonspecific vulvovaginitis caused by members of the *Proteus* group, anaerobic bacteria, or gram-positive bacilli.

In the older child with an estrogenic vagina, local application of triple sulfa cream (Sultrin) each night frequently suffices. Vaginal suppositories such as Furacin or Trichofuron may also be used with satisfactory results. Unfortunately, mixed bacterial vulvovaginitis frequently recurs after an apparent cure, and it may be difficult to differentiate recurrence from reinfection. Many treatment failures may be traced to poor hygiene or parasitic intestinal infections.

Vulvovaginitis is frequently associated with urinary tract infection. Huffman found that pyuria does not usually lead to vaginitis in children who have no congenital anomalies (*e.g.*, microperforate hymen, ectopic ureter). This is surprising, since the reflux of urine into the vagina is commonplace in young girls. However, vulvovaginitis is often of great importance in the etiology of lower urinary tract infection in children. Apparently, the short urethra allows infection to reach the urinary tract from the vagina. In addition, dysuria may be caused by vulvovaginitis alone, secondary to sterile but acidic urine flowing over an inflamed vulva.

Vulvovaginitis Due to Foreign Body

Foreign bodies were found in the vagina with surprising frequency, and the discharge was recorded as bloody in almost all cases. Indeed, foreign bodies, not tumors, are the most frequent cause of bloody vaginal discharge in children. Visualization by vaginoscopy should be undertaken in all patients complaining of such a discharge. Cure follows removal of the foreign body (Fig. 45–7).

Use of x-rays is not recommended because of 1) expense, 2) hazards of pelvic radiation, and 3) the fact that the foreign body can be visualized only if it is radiopaque.

Physiologic Leukorrhea

Physiologic leukorrhea may occur at two times in the life of the female. It occurs first in the newborn, when the vaginal mucosa is thickened because of the high maternal estrogen levels. Desquamation of the superficial cells results in a clear discharge. This physiologic leukorrhea of the newborn subsides within a few weeks, when the maternal estrogen influence abates.

Physiologic leukorrhea may also occur at puberty. For some time prior to the menarche, the vagina is stimulated by rising estrogen levels. The vaginal epithelium thickens, and desquamation causes discharge. Additional discharge is due to clear mucus secreted from the recently activated endocervical glands. It is important to recognize this clinical entity and to differentiate it from pathologic vulvovaginitis, since unwarranted treatment may lead to dermatitis medicamentosa. The diagnosis is rather simple. The lack of pus cells and red blood cells in the discharge signifies that there is no inflammatory lesion. In addition, there are no trichomonads or monilia organisms, and bacterial cultures are negative.

Although the average age of patients in the study with this kind of physiologic leukorrhea was approximately 11.5 years, which corresponds to the age of the menarche, it can occur as early as age 8. In looking at vaginal smears in young children, evidence of estrogen stimulation often appears as early as age 6 or 7. It appears that estrogen secretion starts considerably before the time of menarche, even though it produces no breast development or menses until later.

reassuring the patient and her parents may suffice. If there is an abnormality in which one could predict failure of breast development or menses that would be corrected by hormone therapy, then the plan for treatment is outlined to the patient and her family. Knowledge that something can be done is comforting. Junior bras with prostheses are very helpful in some cases.

A functioning vagina is necessary for the adolescent girl's self-image. However, surgery should be performed on the child who does not have a functioning vagina only when she reaches full body size; an artificial vagina obviously will not grow as a small girl grows. In addition, the patient must want the corrective surgery and must be motivated to cooperate in using vaginal molds or dilators during the postoperative period. Otherwise, the neovagina may become stenotic and obliterated.

The sterile patient is never told she cannot have children. She is told that she CAN have children; but, like one of every six married couples, she must adopt hers. This positive approach is much less traumatic emotionally than a negative one.

Most patients can be cared for by the gynecologist and pediatrician or family physician working together, especially if the girl's parents are stable and responsible. In some cases, additional professional help is needed. The clinician should not hesitate to use a clinical psychologist or psychiatrist to help the patient and her family over emotional hurdles.

TYPES OF CONGENITAL ANOMALIES OF THE GENITALIA

Congenital abnormalities of the female genitalia may conveniently be classified into three groups: 1) those associated with other anomalies in distant areas of the body, such as the heart, kidney, or central nervous system; 2) those associated with local bowel or bladder lesions; and 3) those limited to the genitalia.

The Clitoris

The clitoris can become enlarged from androgen stimulation, whether the androgen is of endogenous or exogenous origin. Endogenous sources may be the 1) adrenal gland (adrenogenital syndrome or adrenal tumor) or 2) the gonad (tumor, intersexuality, polycystic ovaries disease). Patients with intersex problems generally have an enlarged clitoris from birth; at adolescence, androgen causes growth of the clitoris along with other signs of virilization.

When the clitoris appears to be enlarged, it is necessary to distinguish which structures are enlarged. Enlargement may be due to hypertrophy of the soft tissue around the clitoris, the clitoris itself (glans and corpora), or both. If only the soft tissue is involved, excision with preservation of the glans and corpora is all

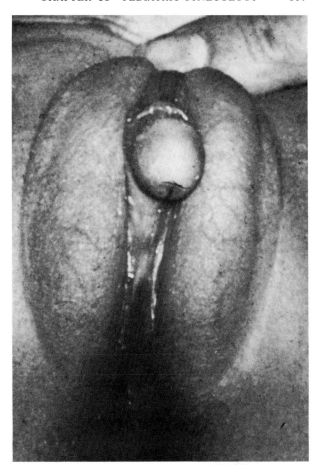

FIG. 45–9. Enlarged phallus in female, age 4 years.

that is necessary. When the corpora and glans are truly enlarged, the clitoris must be amputated at the attachment to the pubic symphysis, or the stump may continue to grow. Painful erections would require further surgery (Fig. 45–9).

The baby with a slight enlargement of the clitoris resulting from intrauterine exposure to androgens or progestational drugs during pregnancy is kept under observation; since the exposure stops at birth, the clitoral growth also stops. The baby "grows around" the slightly enlarged clitoris, and, in time, the vulva appears normal.

The Labia

Labioscrotal Fusion. In the male, the labioscrotal folds normally fuse during intrauterine life in response to androgen; if the female fetus is similarly exposed to androgen, a similar midline fusion results. In severe cases, the vagina and urethral orifices are covered and

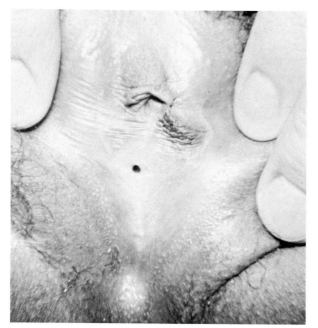

FIG. 45–10. Adhesions of labia minora in a 13-year-old girl. Urethral and vaginal orifices are obliterated from view. Note tiny opening that permitted passage of urine.

a urogenital sinus forms. If corrective plastic surgery is deferred until adolescence, two problems must be considered: 1) an adequate channel must be provided for escape of menstrual blood, and 2) the vaginal orifice must be exposed surgically to permit normal sexual function. If the caliber of the vagina is inadequate, graduated vaginal dilators can be used with good results.

Hypertrophy of Labia Minora. In some instances, adolescent patients are seen with marked hypertrophy of the labia minora. The patient or her mother may be concerned about the abnormality. Generally, reassurance that this is simply a variant of normal, such as big feet, is all that is necessary. If the hypertrophy is very marked or embarrassing to the patient, or if the labia are vulnerable to irritation, an excision and plastic repair may be done. The question of whether some cases of large labia minor result from masturbation is a moot one. More likely, hypertrophy is a simple variant of normal, and masturbation is probably not concerned.

Labial Synechia. Labial adhesions are usually seen in the preadolescent female. The labia minora adhere in the midline, obliterating urethral and vaginal orifices and giving the impression of anatomic abnormality. The adhesions should not be separated forcefully; local application of estrogen cream is recommended. After the labia separate, they can be seen to be anatomically

normal. Occasionally, this lesion is seen in adolescents, secondary to vaginitis. Figure 45–10 shows adhesions of the labia minora in a 13-year-old girl. She has normal secondary sexual characteristics and responded well to local applications of estrogen cream.

The Ureters

Ectopic ureters are usually diagnosed before adolescence. In some instances, these children are erroneously believed to be incontinent or to have enuresis or chronic vaginitis. A case in point was a 12-year-old girl who complained of incontinence of small amounts of urine since early childhood and gave a history of several episodes of vaginitis. Cystoscopy revealed nothing unusual. A vaginogram showed retrograde filling of a left ectopic ureter (Fig. 45–11). More detailed inspection of the vulva revealed a small opening just beneath the urethral orifice. When dye was injected into this opening, retrograde filling of a right ectopic ureter was

FIG. 45–11. Vaginogram with retrograde filling of left ectopic ureter.

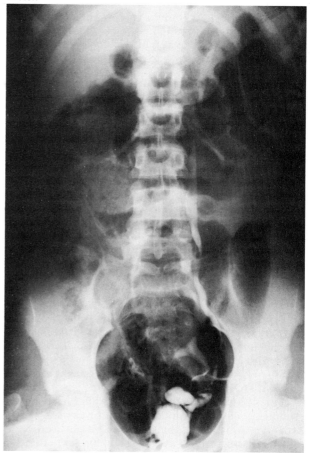

seen. This patient was successfully treated by transecting the ectopic ureters at their insertion and implanting the proximal segments into the bladder.

The Hymen

Imperforate Hymen. The presenting complaint in the patient with imperforate hymen is usually an acute episode of pain. The standard textbook description is cyclic pain recurring monthly, finally followed by hematocolpos and hematometra that cause an acute episode of severe pain. In our experience, however, most patients do not have recurring cyclic pain. Physical examination reveals a tender lower abdominal mass (hematometra) and, on rectal examination, a bulging mass caused by hematocolpos. The hymen is intact, bulging outward. Treatment should be limited to excision of a portion of hymen to establish adequate drainage. Vaginal examination should *not* be done, since it may cause infection by introducing bacteria into the blood-filled vagina and uterus. Prophylactic antibiotics are recommended.

Microperforate Hymen. Some patients appear at first glance to have an imperforate hymen. Pressure with the examining finger at 6 o'clock may reveal a tiny opening just below the urethra (Fig. 45–12). Microperforation of the hymen is a congenital anatomic deviation similar to imperforate hymen, but the clinical manifestations are quite different. Microperforation is associated with a high incidence of repeated urinary tract infection and vulvovaginitis. These conditions usually occur during childhood and are caused by urine trapped in the vagina. Microperforate hymen is treated by enlarging the opening by an incision from 12 o'clock to 6 o'clock and repairing the incison from 9 o'clock to 3 o'clock.

Rigid Hymen. Usually the hymen has an adequate opening that can be distended easily, and penetration at the first coitus presents no serious problem. However, if the hymen is thick and rigid, it may be necessary to dilate the hymenal opening forcefully, with the patient under anethesia. In some instances, it may be best to excise the thick, rigid segment.

The Vagina

Congenital Lack of Vagina. Symptoms and physical findings in the patient who has no vagina depend on whether or not the patient has a functioning uterus. The entire vagina, the lower vagina alone, or the upper vagina alone may be lacking. Each of these variations may be accompanied by a functioning or a nonfunctioning uterus, although most patients without a vagina have no functioning uterus. Their presenting complaint is usually delayed menarche.

An artificial vagina can be created at any time after

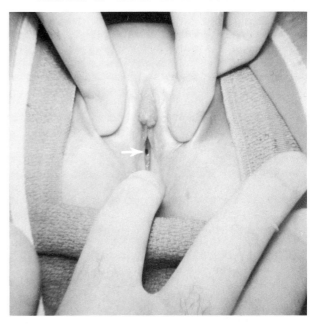

FIG. 45–12. Separation of labia and pressure on perineum toward floor reveals microperforate hymen (*arrow*) in a young patient who had sustained recurrent urinary tract infections.

the patient reaches full body size. Various corrective techniques have been devised. With the Frank nonoperative technique, the patient uses dilators to create a vagina forcefully over a period of time. In the Wharton technique, a canal is dissected between the bladder and rectum, and a vaginal mold is worn until epithelialization slowly takes place. The McIndoe technique is similar except that a split-thickness skin graft is placed over the mold to achieve immediate epithelialization. In the Pratt technique, a segment of sigmoid colon is used to line the newly created vaginal canal. A simpler technique is the vulvovaginoplasty described by Williams, in which the labial tissues are used to form a vaginal canal. Our recent experience with this procedure seems to be satisfactory, but further observation is necessary to evaluate long-term results.

Some patients simply have a stenotic vagina or vagina of inadequate depth that will respond to the use of dilator therapy without surgery.

Septate Vagina. The patient with a septate vagina does not require treatment unless she experiences dyspareunia. The longitudinal septum may run the entire length of the vagina, or it may be partial. If required because of dyspareunia, incision of the septum increases the caliber of the vagina.

Blind Vaginal Pouch. All variations of blind uterine horns and blind vaginal pouches can occur. The problem is the same in all cases; menstrual blood fills the

cavities, causing a confusing array of symptoms and pelvic findings. Recently, a 13-year-old girl was examined because she had a history of amenorrhea for 1 month. Normal monthly menses had occurred since she was age 11. A large, cystic mass was found filling the upper vagina and right adnexa. Vaginogram revealed distortion of the upper right side of the vagina by a space-filling lesions, and a uterus deviated to the left. Dilatation and curettage were impossible due to the mass in the upper vagina. Laparotomy showed a uterus didelphys. The left side was normal and drained through its cervix into a normal vaginal canal. The right uterus was filled with old blood, as determined by needle puncture, and was connected to a blind vaginal pouch that caused the large palpable mass. Adequate drainage was established by creating a window in the medial side of the right blind vaginal canal so that it drained into the left vaginal canal to the outside. The patient has been symptom-free since surgery.

Transverse Annular Septum of Vagina. The transverse annular septum can occur at various levels in the vagina and probably results from nonperforation where the urogenital sinus of the vagina joins the upper müllerian duct. The septum may be complete (imperforate) or incomplete (perforate). Symptomatology and physical findings vary according to the level at which the septum is located and according to whether the septum is perforate or imperforate. A complete septum causes hematocolpos and hemtometra, and dystocia may result. Dyspareunia is noted, especially if the septum is low in the vagina. Surgical excision is the treatment of choice, but care must be taken to excise the entire fibromuscular ring.

The Breast

Anomalies of the breast that may occur are supernumerary breasts (polymastia) or nipples (polythelia), or lack of breasts (amastia) or nipples (athelia). These lesions may be unilateral or bilateral. It is necessary to recognize these defects early and to offer an explanation and emotional support to the patient. Reassurance that corrective surgery is sometimes possible is important. When amastia occurs, it is usually associated with abnormalities of the chest wall.

Prolapsed Urethral Mucosa

In some children, a vulvar tumor appears to be prolapsed from the vagina; on examination, however, the physician finds that the tumor does not emanate from the vagina. The hymen and the vaginal canal can be identified. The mass is caused by prolapse of the urethral mucosa. This is not a rare lesion, and the diagnosis is confirmed by introducing a catheter through the dimple in the center of the mass and ob-

taining urine. The treatment is surgical excision and reapproximation of the mucosal surfaces. These children do well.

AMBIGUOUS SEXUAL DEVELOPMENT

Ambiguity of genitalia results from any one or a combination of the following: 1) virilization, 2) lack of development, 3) duplication of development, 4) abnormal development, or 5) genetic influences. These factors may be operative antenatally or postnatally. The diagnostic measures leading to diagnosis and management of sexual ambiguity are shown in Figure 45–13. Ambiguity due to antenatal factors may continue after birth if the disease is inherent in the child, such as the adrenogenital syndrome. If the genital abnormality was caused by exogenous factors in pregnancy, such as androgens or gestagens administered to the mother or a functioning ovarian tumor in the mother, the condition does not progress after birth (Fig. 45–14). Some types of genital ambiguity are found to have familial incidence, in particular, certain forms of male hermaphroditism and adrenogenital syndrome.

Regardless of etiology or classification, the first crucial problem is determination of in which sex the child is to be reared. This decision must be made early in order to provide the best opportunity for normal psychosexual development; preferably, it is made in the first few weeks of life.

Once the sex that the individual should be assigned and reared as has been determined, it is of utmost importance that the physician keep track of the patient and family. Problems of gender identity are common, and long-term psychologic support and guidance should be anticipated from the outset.

The term *pseudohermaphroditism* often causes confusion; for this reason, the simpler terms *male hermaphroditism* (male intersexuality), *female hermaphroditism* (female intersexuality), and *true hermaphroditism* are preferable. The practical classification of Jones and Scott is useful:

1. Gonadal aplasia and dysplasia
2. Male intersexuality (nonfamilial and masculinizing)
3. Male intersexuality (familial, feminizing, masculinizing, or mixed)
4. Klinefelter's syndrome
5. Other syndromes of male intersexuality
6. Female intersexuality associated with adrenal hyperplasia
7. Female intersexuality not resulting from adrenal hyperplasia
8. Other syndromes of female intersexuality
9. True hermaphroditism

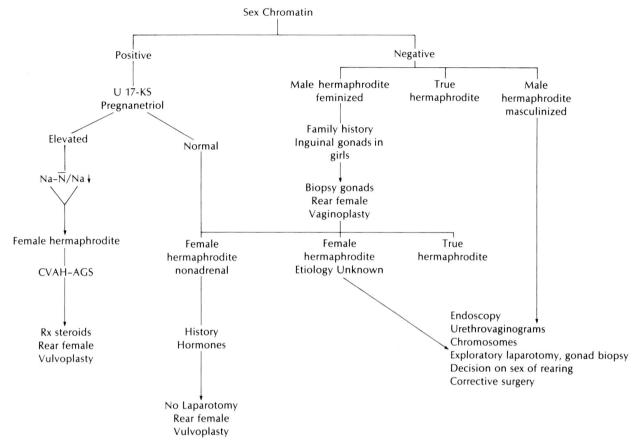

FIG. 45-13. Pattern of diagnostic studies to arrive at correct diagnosis and management of newborn with ambiguous genitalia. *CVAH–AGS,* Congenital virilizing adrenal hyperplasia–adrenogenital syndrome.

TYPES OF INTERSEXUALITY

Inherited enzyme deficiencies along the pathways of testosterone or cortisol production can lead to both male and female intersex problems. The classic example of this is congenital virilizing adrenal hyperplasia (CVAH), in which an enzyme defect leads to a decrease in cortisol production. This, in turn, stimulates the anterior pituitary to secrete excess adrenocorticotropic hormone (ACTH) leading to adrenal hyperplasia and excess production of adrenal testosterone. The genitalia are masculinized and these females often appear to be males with cryptorchidism (Fig. 45–15).

The most common enzyme deficiency leading to CVAH is 21-hydroxylase deficiency. There are two forms: one with salt wasting and one without. A less common form is 11-β hydroxylase deficiency, which results not only in CVAH but also in the production of steroids that promote sodium retention. As a result, hypervolemia and hypertension may be present.

Lack of the enzyme 5-α reductase prevents the conversion of testosterone to dihydrotestosterone (DHT). DHT is responsible for male genital development in the embryo, whereas testosterone appears to be responsible for virilization at puberty. Patients with this syndrome have a 46, XY genotype and ambiguous genitalia (often female-appearing) at birth. The phallus is often hypoplastic, and there is labioscrotal fusion with a blind vaginal pouch. Müllerian derivatives are lacking. At puberty, these patients develop male secondary sexual characteristics, *e.g.,* beard and deep voice. Except for the genitalia, they appear phenotypically male. Deficiency of 5-α reductase belongs to a larger group of conditions known as pseudovaginal perineoscrotal hypospadias (PPSH) that have an identical clinical presentation but in which enzyme deficiency cannot always be found.

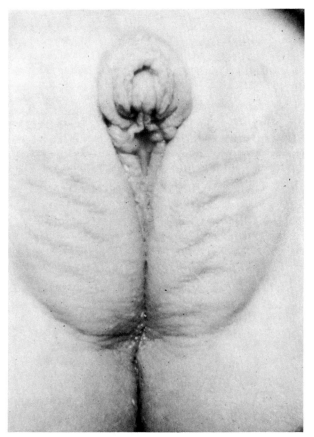

FIG. 45-14. Female hermaphrodite, nonadrenal type. This 2-year-old child had erections when bladder was full. Mother had received medroxyprogesterone acetate during pregnancy.

Errors in adrenal or testicular hormone biosynthesis may also result in male hermaphroditism. Plasma testosterone is decreased in all of these disorders. Complete testicular feminization (see pages 40 and 913) is a syndrome in which androgen insensitivity is a result of either a decreased amount of androgen cytosol receptor or inability of the receptor to bind androgen. This results in female external genitalia with a blind vaginal pouch. Müllerian derivatives are lacking. At puberty, these genotypic males appear as phenotypic females but lack axillary and pubic hair. There are also incomplete forms of this syndrome.

True hermaphrodites have both ovarian and testicular tissue. They may have separate ovarian tissue and separate testicular tissue, but more often they have one or more ovotestes. The internal duct system usually follows the gonad of the same side if they are separate. The external genitalia are usually either ambiguous or essentially male. However, a well-developed vagina and uterus may be present. Some of these pa-

tients exhibit chimerism (46, XX / 46, XY); some are 46, XY; but most have a 46, XX genotype. A possible explanation for the presence of testicular tissue when there is no Y chromosome may be the translocation of a testicular determinant from the Y chromosome to the X chromosome or to an autosome. Proof of such a determinant (the H–Y antigen) has been found. This antigen is postulated to be the gene product of, or closely linked to, the Y testicular determinant.

Female anatomic deviations from the normal that are not really problems of intersexuality, but cause confusion by altering the appearance of the vulva include 1) polyps of the hymen, 2) cysts of the hymen, 3) ectopic ureter, 4) imperforate hymen, 5) microperforate hymen, and 6) vaginal septa. Once recognized, these lesions can be easily treated.

PROBLEMS INVOLVING THE PARENTS

The parents of a child with ambiguity of the genitalia are usually greatly concerned. Many feel they are being punished because of their own sexual practices, and it is important to eradicate such myths at the start. The physician may suggest that the child be given an ambiguous name; since name changing can cause considerable upheaval within the family and community, giving the child a name that is applicable to both genders, such as Francis (ces), precludes the need to change the name if the appropriate sex of rearing is later found to differ from that implied by the original name.

The term *sex chromatin* should not be used in discussions with parents or patients. A statement that the female patient is sex chromatin–negative may be misinterpreted as a lack of some part of normal female sexuality. On the other hand, a patient can be labeled Barr body–positive or Barr body–negative without any implication of sexuality.

The physician should also use terms that are easily understood by lay persons and are not likely to cause anxiety. For example, if the clitoris is enlarged, it should not be referred to as a penislike structure, but rather as an "overdeveloped" clitoris. If the ovaries are not producing hormones properly or if mixed gonads are present, the physician should not refer to the patient as being without ovaries, but rather as having "underdeveloped" gonads. If there is no normal ovary or if the patient is to be reared as a female, the term *gonad* should be used instead of the term *testis*. The mother and father must be convinced they are dealing with a girl or a boy, as the case may be. An attitude of uncertainty is detrimental to the child's future gender identity. In general, it has worked out well for the pediatrician, the endocrinologist, and the gynecologist to work as a team and for one of these specialists to speak for the group.

SEX OF REARING

The sex of rearing does not depend exclusively on gonads or sex chromatin. It depends primarily on whether this child can best function sexually as a male or female. In general, it is preferable to assign the gender within the baby's own chromosomal sex. However, if the appropriate structures of the external genitalia are not present, sex conversion must be considered.

In the case of the male hermaphrodite with inadequate development of the genitalia, the size of the phallus is the determining factor in deciding the sex of rearing. If the child does not have an adequate phallus that will function sexually as a male organ, a sex conversion operation should be performed, and the patient should be reared as a female.

It is difficult to predict how much penile growth will occur over the first few weeks of life. A therapeutic trial with testosterone cream may help to determine whether or not the penis will grow (Table 45–4).

Females born with genital virilization due to congenital adrenal hyperplasia are reared as females, regardless of the degree of masculinization of the external genitalia. The internal genitalia in these patients are normal for a female and require no treatment; if necessary, the external genitalia can be corrected surgically.

Male hermaphrodites with androgen insensitivity (testicular feminization syndrome) are reared as females. The body contour at puberty is female.

DIAGNOSTIC APPROACH

The diagnostic workup of children with ambiguous genitalia requires a logical planned approach, as outlined in Figure 45–13.

History and Physical Examination

A family history is obtained. A female born with virilization may have congenital virilizing adrenal hyperplasia, and knowing that the family has a history of this disorder will aid in making a diagnosis. In obtaining the family history of a patient with the testicular feminization syndrome, it may be found that other relatives have had abnormalities of the "ovaries" and have had them removed. Some cases of male hermaphroditism of the masculinizing type may have a familial pattern.

In the older patient, the history of menstruation or the lack of it is important in arriving at the diagnosis. Also, the development of the other secondary sex characteristics should be investigated thoroughly in both the patient and members of her family.

Exposure to androgenic or gestagenic hormones

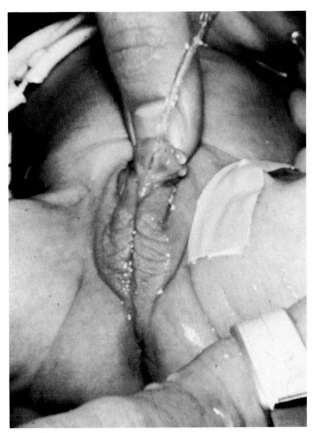

FIG. 45–15. Congenital virilizing adrenal hyperplasia, salt-losing type. Newborn female appears to be a cryptorchid male with hypospadias. Note enlarged clitoris and fusion of labial folds. Complete urogenital sinus is present.

must be investigated. If the infant is born with evidence of virilization, the physician must check the prenatal record to be sure that the mother had not received hormone therapy that could produce fetal virilization. The physician must also rule out a functioning ovarian tumor or an adrenal tumor in the mother that may have produced androgens, causing virilization in the baby. An older child who exhibits virilization may have been exposed to exogenous androgen, administered in error or in contaminated medication.

Vaginoscopy and Cystoscopy

Vaginoscopy should be performed whenever the genitalia are ambiguous. In order to be sure a cervix is present, the structure must be visualized directly.

Any patient with abnormalities in the development of the müllerian duct system may also have abnormalities of the urinary system. It is often useful to work

TABLE 45-4. SEX ASSIGNMENT IN CASES OF MICROPENIS

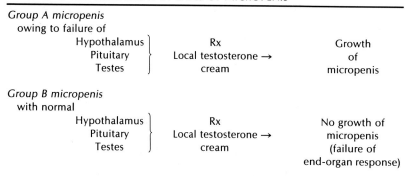

Group A: Rear as male. Phallus responds to androgen. Treat with androgen at puberty.

Group B: Rear as female with necessary sex conversion surgery early in life. Phallus does not respond to androgen, and therapy at puberty will be futile.

with the urologist and perform vaginoscopy in conjunction with the urologic studies so that anesthesia is required only once.

Buccal Smear

The buccal smear shows whether the patient has Barr bodies (sex chromatin), and may give preliminary information before the karyotype is available. The normal female has Barr bodies in 20%–40% of the cells, whereas the male has none. Question has been raised whether this test is accurate in the first few days of life, since a greater percentage of Barr bodies is found a few days later. However, enough are present early that the test can be considered reliable. The mean Barr body count on the 1st day of life in normal females is about 7%; on the 2nd day about 8%; and on the 4th and subsequent days, about 10+ %, gradually increasing thereafter.

Chromosome Karyotype

Although expensive and time-consuming, chromosome karyotyping should be done in patients with ambiguous genitalia. Some patients are mosaic showing more than one type of genetic cell line. In addition to blood samples, it may be necessary to study other tissues, such as skin or gonads, in these patients.

X-rays

X-ray examinations can be helpful in arriving at a diagnosis. Bone age should be determined; an advanced bone age may be the result of excessive steroids, as in adrenogenital syndrome. X-ray examinations can also be used to follow such patients. If the bone age advances too rapidly, the adrenal activity is not being adequately suppressed.

Vaginograms and hysterograms are helpful when the labioscrotal folds are fused. In the adrenogenital syndrome, for example, it can be assumed that the patient has a normal vagina and uterus, but the only way to confirm this is to visualize the vagina either directly by vaginoscopy or by x-ray. If the degree of labioscrotal fusion is severe, it is easier to perform radiographic studies (see Chap. 58). If a urogenital sinus is present, a urethrovaginogram can precisely define the structures behind the fused perineum. Gynecography can also be used to outline the pelvic organs.

Endocrine Studies

In the patient with congenital virilizing adrenal hyperplasia, the 24-hour urinary excretion of 17-ketosteroids and pregnanetriol is elevated. The administration of cortisone to the child causes a drop in both these values, thereby confirming the diagnosis. In the forms of this disease associated with sodium loss, the resulting hyponatremia, if not diagnosed, can cause death. The administration of deoxycorticosterone acetate (DOCA) corrects the salt loss. In early life, DOCA is given by injection. It may later be administered yearly in subcutaneous DOCA pellet implants.

In some instances, it may be necessary to know if estrogen is being produced. This can be studied in 24-hour urinary excretion specimens. If the patient has a vagina, vaginal cytology reflects estrogen production, as do cells in the urinary sediment. Preliminary research suggests that axillary pH may also reflect estrogen production.

In gonadal dysgenesis, the estrogen levels are low, and pituitary gonadotropin excretion levels are high.

Laparoscopy and Laparotomy

Laparoscopy is rarely satisfactory in children with ambiguous genitalia. Even with the wide exposure of an abdominal incision, it may be difficult to determine whether the oviducts, round ligaments, uterus, and gonads are normal or abnormal. Sometimes the gonadal vasculature must be followed to determine if gonads are present. If the physician is concerned about intersexuality and accepts the risk of administering anesthesia to the child, an exploratory laparotomy is preferable.

In the patient who has clinically clear-cut gonadal dysgenesis, laparoscopy with biopsy of the streaks suffices to make the diagnosis. However, with the other types of intersexuality, it is necessary to perform a biopsy and examine frozen sections in order to determine the patient's conditions. In general, laparotomy to rule out true hermaphroditism is performed if all of the findings cannot be explained in terms of the anatomic abnormality, the genetic component, or the hormonal deviations. The phenotypic female with XY sex chromosomes requires laparotomy to remove dysgenetic gonads because of the high incidence of malignancy. In general, if the patient has intraperitoneal gonads that are not normal ovaries, gonadectomy should be performed.

NONSURGICAL TREATMENT FOR GENITAL ABNORMALITIES

Physical therapy in the form of dilatation is indicated in patients with inadequate or stenotic vagina. Patients with adrenogenital syndrome who have stenosis of the vagina respond well to the use of graduated dilators. Other patients may develop a vagina of adequate depth by the use of dilators.

Medical therapy is indicated in many patients. In addition to the various modes of endocrine therapy described previously, patients whose gonads do not produce estrogen (gonadal dysgenesis and male hermaphrodism) are given estrogens.

Surgery is required in some patients. This must be done with care, and it must be properly timed.

SURGERY OF THE AMBIGUOUS GENITALIA

The aim of surgery and, indeed, all therapy in patients with ambiguous genitalia is to

1. Restore anatomic and sexual function
2. Make the patient socially acceptable among her peers
3. Make the appearance of the genitalia psychologically acceptable to the patient and her family

The surgery itself may be reconstructive (vaginoplasty), ablative (gonadectomy or phallectomy), or curative (adrenalectomy, gonadectomy).

The age of the patient and the nature of the problem influence the extent and type of surgery. Given a severely virilized patient with a complete urogenital sinus, labioscrotal fusion, and enlarged clitoris, clitoridectomy is performed in infancy for cosmetic reasons; at the same time, the urogenital sinus opening is enlarged sufficiently to permit free flow of urine. Consideration of the vagina should be deferred. In addition to the cosmetic need for a normal-appearing vulva and the anatomic need for free flow of urine, the genitalia must be prepared in the prepubertal period to permit the free egress of menstrual flow. In the sexually mature patient, the physician must be concerned not only with the cosmetic apearance, the free flow of urine, and the menstrual flow, but also with the adequacy of the vaginal depth and caliber for coitus.

REFERENCES AND RECOMMENDED READING

GYNECOLOGIC EXAMINATION OF THE CHILD

Capraro VJ: Pediatric gynecology. J. St. Barnabas Medical Center 2:223, 1965

Capraro VJ: Sexual assault of female children. Ann NY Acad Sci 142:817, 1967

Capraro VJ: Gynecologic examination in children and adolescents. Pediatr Clin North Am 19:511, 1972

Capraro VJ, Capraro EJ: Vaginal aspirate studies in children. Obstet Gynecol 37:462, 1971

INFECTIONS OF THE FEMALE GENITAL ORGANS IN CHILDREN AND ADOLESCENTS

Altcheck A: Vulvovaginal irritation and discharge in children. Surg Clin North Am 40:1071, 1960

Capraro VJ: Vulvovaginitis and other local lesions of the vulva. Clin Obstet Gynaecol 1:533, 1974

Capraro VJ, Gallego MB: Vulvovaginitis in children. Pediatr Ann 1974

Hare MJ, Mowla A: Genital herpesvirus infection in a prepubertal girl. Br J Obstet Gynaecol 84:141, 1977

Huffman JW: Principles of pediatric gynecology. In Wynn H (ed): Obstetric and Gynecologic Annual, 1974. New York, Appleton–Century–Crofts, 1974

Huffman JW: Premenarchal vulvovaginitis. Clin Obstet Gynecol 20:581, 1977

Shore WB: Nonvenereal transmission of gonococcal infections in children. J Pediatr 79:661, 1971

Tunnessen W, Jr, Jastremski M: Prepubescent gonococcal vulvovaginitis. Clin Pediatr 13:675, 1974

Wersserbacher G: Chronic urinary tract infections and vulvitis in girls with high posterior commissures. Paediatr Paedol 9:60, 1974

DES EXPOSURE

Anderson B, Watring WG, Edinger DD et al: Development of DES-associated clear-cell carcinoma: The importance of regular screening. Obstet Gynecol 53:293, 1979

Antonioli DA, Burke L, Friedman EA: Natural history of diethylstilbestrol induced genital tract lesions: Cervical ectopy and cervicovaginal hood. Am J Obstet Gynecol 137:847, 1980

Barnes AB: Menstrual history of young women exposed *in utero* to diethylstilbestrol. Fertil Steril 32:148, 1979

Burke L, Antonioli D: Vaginal adenosis. Factors influencing detection in a colposcopic evaluation. Obstet Gynecol 48:413, 1976

Capraro VJ: Danger of diethylstilbestrol. NY State J Med 73:853, 1973

Cogrove MD, Benton B, Henderson BE: Male genitourinary abnormalities and maternal diethylstilbestrol. J Urol 117:220, 1977

Gill WB, Schumacher GFB, Bibbo M: Pathological semen and anatomical abnormalities of the genital tract in human male subjects exposed to diethylstilbestrol *in utero.* J Urol 117:477, 1977

Glebatis DM, Janerich DT: A statewide approach to diethylstilbestrol—the New York program. N Engl J Med 304:47, 1981

Hajj SN, Herbst AL: Evaluation and management of diethylstilbestrol-exposed offspring. Surg Clin North Am 58:87, 1978

Herbst AL, Cole P: Age incidence and risk of diethylstilbestrol-related clear cell adenocarcinoma of the vagina and cervix. Am J Obstet Gynecol 128:43, 1977

Herbst AL, Ulfelder H, Poskanzer DC: Adenocarcinoma of the vagina: Association of maternal stilbestrol therapy with tumor appearance in young women. N Engl J Med 284:878, 1971

Ng AB, Reagan JW, Nadjii M, Greening S: Natural history of vaginal adenosis in women exposed to diethylstilbestrol *in utero.* J Reprod Med 18:1, 1977

O'Brien PC, Noller KL, Robboy SJ et al: Vaginal epithelial changes in young women enrolled in the National Cooperative Diethylstilbestrol Adenosis (DESAD) Project. Obstet Gynecol, 53:300, 1978

Sandberg EC, Hebard JC: Examination of young women exposed to stilbestrol *in utero.* Am J Obstet Gynecol 128:364, 1977

Stafl A, Mattingly RF: Vaginal adenosis: A precancerous lesion? Am J Obstet Gynecol 120:666, 1974

CONGENITAL ANOMALIES

Capraro VJ: Congenital anomalies. Clin Obstet Gynecol 14:988, 1971

Capraro VJ, Bayonet NP, Aceto T, Macgillivary M: Premature thelarche. Obstet Gynecol Surv 26:2, 1971

Caparo VJ, Bayonet-Rivera NP, Magoss I: Vulvar tumor in children due to prolapse of urethral mucosa. Am J Obstet Gynecol 108:572, 1970

Capraro VJ, Dewhurst CJ: Breast disorders in childhood and adolescence. Clin Obstet Gynecol 18:25, 1975

Capraro VJ, Dillon WP, Gallego MB: Microperforate hymen: A distinct clinical entity. Obstet Gynecol 44:903, 1974

Capraro VJ, Gallego MB: Breast disorders in adolescents. Pediatr Ann 4:82, 1975

Capraro VJ, Greenburg H: Adhesions of the labia minora: A study of 50 patients. Obstet Gynecol 39:65, 1972

Mandell J, Stevens PS, Lucey DT: Diagnosis and management of hydrometrocolpos in infancy. J. Urol 120:262, 1978

McIndoe AH, Banister JB: Operation for cure of congenital absence of vagina. J Obstet Gynaecol Br Emp 45:490, 1938

Pratt JH, Smith GR: Vaginal reconstruction with a sigmoid loop. Am J Obstet Gynecol 96:31, 1965

Williams EA: Congenital absence of the vagina: A simple operation for its relief. J Obstet Gynaecol Br Commonw 71:511, 1964

AMBIGUOUS SEXUAL DEVELOPMENT

Capraro VJ: Diagnosis and management of ambiguous sexual development. In Reid DE (ed): Controversy in Obstetrics and Gynecology II, pp 691–705. Philadelphia, WB Saunders, 1974

Dewhurst CJ, Gordon RR: The Intersexual Disorders. Baltimore, Williams & Wilkins, 1969

Jeffcoate TNA, Fliegner JRH, Russell SH et al.: Diagnosis of the adrenogenital syndrome before birth. Lancet 2:553, 1965

Jones HW Jr, Park IJ, Rock JA: Technique of surgical reassignment for micropenis and allied conditions. Am J Obstet Gynecol 132:870, 1978

Jones HW Jr, Scott WW: Hermaphroditism, Genital Anomalies, and Related Endocrine Disorders. 2nd ed. Baltimore, Williams & Wilkins, 1971

Silvers WK, Wachtel SS: H–Y antigen: Behavior and function. Science 195:956, 1977

Simpson JL: Disorders of Sexual Differentiation: Etiology and Clinical Delineation. New York, Academic Press, 1976

Simpson JL: Diagnosis and management of the infant with genital ambiguity. Am J Obstet Gynecol 128:137, 1977

Simpson JL, New MI, Peterson RE et al.: Pseudovaginal perineoscrotal hypospadias (PPSH) in sibs. Birth Defects 7:140, 1971

Wachtel SS, Koo GC, Breg WR et al.: Serologic detection of a Y-linked gene in XX males and XX true hermaphrodites. N Engl J Med 295:750, 1976

Walsh PC: The differential diagnosis of ambiguous genitalia in the newborn. Urol Clin North Am 5:213, 1978

GENERAL

Huffman JW: The Gynecology of Childhood and Adolescence. Philadelphia, WB Saunders, 1968

Jones HW Jr, Heller RH: Pediatric and Adolescent Gynecology. Baltimore, Williams and Wilkins, 1966

Ulfelder H, Robboy SJ: The embryologic development of the human vagina. Am J Obstet Gynecol 126:769, 1976

The menstrual abnormalities and gynecologic endocrine disorders discussed in this chapter are derangements of the normal processes considered elsewhere in this book. Special attention is directed to Chapters 6 and 7, which deal with normal endocrine physiology.

ABNORMALITIES OF MENSTRUATION

Patients with abnormal vaginal bleeding constitute a major portion of gynecologic practice. The characteristics of normal menstruation are described in Chapter 8. The terms *menstrual periods, menses,* or *periods* should be used to indicate regular cyclic sloughing of the endometrium following the hormonal changes associated with ovulation. Bleeding that does not fit this definition is not menstruation. It should be described in relation to amount, duration, and interval, and should be referred to only as bleeding.

ABNORMAL UTERINE BLEEDING

The terms to describe abnormal bleeding are not entirely satisfactory because they do not indicate the cause of the abnormality. The accepted standard terms are *oligomenorrhea* (menstrual bleeding that occurs less frequently than normal), *polymenorrhea* (bleeding that occurs more frequently than usual and may or may not be associated with ovulation), *menorrhagia* (increased amount or duration of menstrual bleeding), and *amenorrhea* (no vaginal bleeding). The most common types of abnormal bleeding and their causes are

1. Midcycle staining—caused by the midcycle estradiol rise and fall associated with ovulation
2. Delayed menses with excessive bleeding—associated with threatened abortion or anovulation
3. Frequent bleeding—associated with anovulation, chronic pelvic inflammatory disease, or, rarely, hypothyroidism
4. Profuse cyclic bleeding—associated with submucous leiomyomas, adenomyosis, and endometrial polyps
5. Irregular or intermenstrual bleeding—associated with oral contraceptive treatment, endometrial polyps, or cancer of the uterus or cervix
6. Postmenopausal bleeding (sometimes mucoid in nature)—associated with cancer of the endometrium, endometrial hyperplasia, or estrogen therapy

It is important to recognize that patients with abnormal uterine bleeding have histologic evidence of endometrial disease only 45% of the time when no gross pelvic disease is present, and only 35% of the time when pelvic disease is grossly demonstrable, *i.e.,* an enlarged pelvic organ or a palpable mass (Table 46–1).

CHAPTER 46

ABNORMALITIES OF MENSTRUATION AND GYNECOLOGIC ENDOCRINE DISORDERS

A. Brian Little
James Goldfarb

The remaining 65% of patients with abnormal bleeding and grossly demonstrable disease have no apparent endometrial abnormality.

Abnormal bleeding is related to age. Curettage for abnormal bleeding is most often done on women aged 40–50 years, and malignancy, hyperplasia, and endometrial atrophy are most common in women over 40. Although Sutherland's original series included a small but significant number of patients with tuberculosis, this disease is rare in the United States. However, tuberculosis should be considered a possible cause of abnormal bleeding in women who have lived in the British Isles, Mediterranean countries, Asia, Africa, or South America.

The presence of secretory endometrium almost always denotes a normal ovulatory cycle; the presence of proliferative endometrium may or may not indicate anovulation, since, if the examination had been deferred for a week, secretory endometrium might have been

TABLE 46–1. ENDOMETRIAL HISTOLOGY IN 1000 WOMEN WITH ABNORMAL UTERINE BLEEDING AND GROSS PELVIC DISEASE AND 1000 WOMEN WITH ABNORMAL UTERINE BLEEDING BUT WITHOUT GROSS PELVIC DISEASE

Histologic Diagnosis	Without Pelvic Disease* (%)	With Pelvic Disease* (%)
Atrophy	1	5
Irregular shedding	1	0
Malignant disease	1	2
Tuberculosis	1	1
Uterine polyps	1	2
Irregular ripening	2	1
Chronic endometritis	11	4
Hyperplasia	27	20
No abnormality	55	65

* Disease includes fibroids (8.3%), chronic salpingitis or salpingo-oophoritis (14%), adenomyosis of the uterus (3%), chronic parametritis (3%), ovarian neoplasms (2%). Multiple diseases are included, so figures do not add to 100%.

(Adapted from Sutherland AM: In Meigs JV, Sturgis SH (eds): Gynecology, Vol III, p. 167. New York, Grune & Stratton, 1957)

present. If proliferative endometrium is diagnosed in the secretory phase time period as determined by the subsequent "menstrual" flow, then it is diagnostic of anovulation. The presence of normal proliferative endometrium more than 1 year after the menopause is abnormal.

DYSFUNCTIONAL UTERINE BLEEDING

Dysfunctional uterine bleeding is abnormal bleeding that occurs when there is neither a pregnancy nor any demonstrable pathologic condition, including infection and neoplasm. It is usually a result of anovulation, but it may reflect defects in the follicular or luteal phase of an ovulatory cycle. In older patients, abnormal bleeding should be investigated by histologic examination of the endometrium. In younger patients, the diagnosis can usually be made on clinical grounds; but, if abnormal bleeding persists, the endometrium must be examined. The various causes of dysfunctional uterine bleeding are summarized in Figure 46–4.

Bleeding depends on the response of the endometrium to the hormonal variations and the endocrine state that exists when hormonal stimulus occurs. An example is the effect of oral contraceptives. These drugs produce changes in the endometrium that are histologically different from those associated with normal endogenous estrogen and progesterone secretion. Since the bleeding resulting from administration of contraceptives clinically resembles that occurring at various stages of the normal menstrual cycle, treatment that leads to additional bleeding is often insti-

tuted, and dilatation and curettage may ultimately be required for control of this bleeding. Curettage relieves immediate bleeding, but does not solve the problem. Whether bleeding results from inappropriate estrogen–progestin stimulus or from disease must be determined before additional hormonal support is given. Persistent bleeding uncontrolled by a change in oral contraceptive dosage must be investigated by biopsy, curettage, or both.

BLEEDING ASSOCIATED WITH FOLLICULAR PHASE DEFECTS

Premature maturation of the ovarian follicle may result from pituitary hyperstimulation. This produces a cycle that is less than 22 days but has a normal ovulation and a normal luteal phase. If the proliferative phase of the endometrium develops normally, the luteal phase is characterized by normal secretory endometrium. If the endometrium is inadequately prepared, less than optimal ovulation is followed by abnormal secretory endometrium and infertility.

Premature maturation of the ovarian follicle occurs most commonly in the perimenopausal years. As early as age 40, follicle-stimulating hormone (FSH) levels begin to rise, even in regularly ovulating women, owing to altered ovarian response or to diminished production of *inhibin,* a protein hormone produced by ovarian follicles that inhibits FSH but not luteinizing hormone (LH). Associated with the rise in FSH levels in ovulating perimenopausal women is a normal or slightly elevated estradiol level and a progressively shortened proliferative phase. Perhaps the relative infertility of women at this age relates to dysmaturity of the ovum itself.

A prolonged proliferative phase, most commonly occurring in young women, leads to oligomenorrhea; most of these women have a normal luteal phase and normal fertility, but ovulation, and consequently the times at which conception is possible, are less frequent. Occasionally, such "oligoovulation" may be associated with later premature ovarian failure.

Dysfunctional uterine bleeding with an ovulatory pattern and follicular phase defects (Fig. 46–1) is usually associated with a cycle shorter than 22 days or longer than 34 days.

BLEEDING ASSOCIATED WITH LUTEAL PHASE DEFECTS

Profuse and prolonged flow in an ovulatory cycle may be caused by delayed involution of the corpus luteum and is referred to as *irregular shedding* (Fig. 46–2A). This usually results in a prolonged flow, but no reduction in fertility, and may occur only intermittently. Persistence of the corpus luteum or corpus luteum

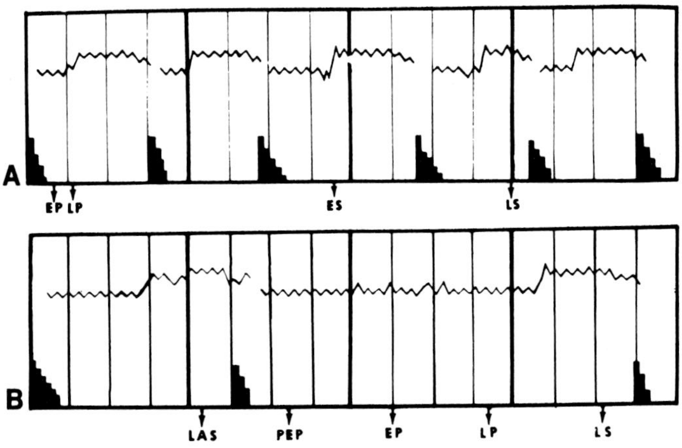

FIG. 46-1. Dysfunctional uterine bleeding associated with ovulatory patterns and follicular phase defects. Each part shows four 28-day periods, each divided into four segments of 7 days each. *Upper curve,* basal body temperature; *blocks,* uterine bleeding. *A.* Premature follicle maturation, cycles shorter than 22 days. *B.* Prolonged cycle (over 34 days) with delayed follicle maturation. *EP,* Early proliferative phase. *LP,* Late proliferative phase. *ES,* Early secretory phase. *LS,* Late secretory phase. *LAS,* Late or atypical secretory phase. *PEP,* Poor early proliferation. (Arronet GH, Arrata WSM: Obstet Gynecol 29:97, 1967)

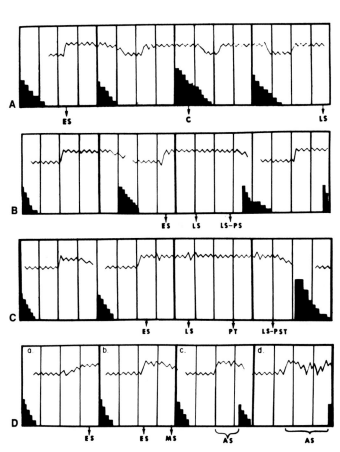

FIG. 46-2. Dysfunctional uterine bleeding associated with ovulatory patterns and luteal phase defects. Each part shows four 28-day periods, each divided into four segments of 7 days each. *Upper curve,* basal body temperature; *blocks,* uterine bleeding. *A.* Delayed involution of corpus luteum, with irregular shedding of endometrium and profuse and prolonged menstrual flow. *B.* Short-term persistence of corpus luteum, with variable delay in onset of next menses. *C.* Long-term persistence of corpus luteum (pseudocyesis), with undue delay in onset of menses. *D.* Luteal phase inadequacy, with unduly shortened luteal phase (c) and variations in basal body temperature: gradual rise at ovulation (a), unsustained down-slanting postovulatory phase (b), and drop to preovulatory level in at least two recordings in luteal phase (d). *ES,* Early secretory phase. *C,* Combined early proliferative and late secretory phases, premenstrual. *LS,* Late secretory phase. *LS-PS,* Late secretory phase with marked pseudodecidua. *PT,* Pregnancy test negative. *LS-PTS,* late secretory phase with marked pseudodecidua and thrombosed necrotic tissue. *MS,* Midsecretory phase. *AS,* Atypical secretory phase. (Arronet GH, Arrata WSM: Obstet Gynecol 29:97, 1967)

cyst may lead to a delay in subsequent menses often accompanied by premenstrual spotting (Fig. 46–2*B*). The corpus luteum can often be felt on examination and must be distinguished from ectopic pregnancy. Long-term persistence of the corpus luteum may result in pseudocyesis (Fig. 46–2*C*).

Luteal phase inadequacy (Fig. 46–2*D*) has received much attention as a cause of infertility and early spontaneous abortion. However, it may also be the cause of dysfunctional uterine bleeding, manifested by either premenstrual spotting or polymenorrhea. Luteal phase inadequacy can be diagnosed by basal body tempera-

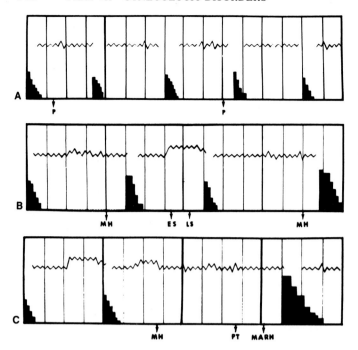

FIG. 46-3. Dysfunctional uterine bleeding associated with anovulatory patterns and abnormal persistence of unruptured follicles. Each part shows four 28-day periods, each divided into four segments of 7 days each. *Upper curve*, basal body temperature; *blocks*, uterine bleeding. *A.* Follicle persistence, an ovulatory cycle lacking progestational changes. *B.* Short-term follicle persistence. *C.* Long-term follicle persistence. *P,* Proliferative phase. *MH,* Mild hyperplasia. *ES,* Early secretory phase. *LS,* Late secretory phase. *MARH,* Marked hyperplasia (gland cystic). (Arronet GH, Arrata WSM: Obstet Gynecol 29:97, 1967)

tures that show a short (less than 10 days) luteal phase or by endometrial biopsies from two cycles that show maturation of the endometrium more than 2 days later than expected for a particular cycle. In this syndrome, FSH and estradiol levels are often below normal in the follicular phase. This is thought to be both cause and effect of the inadequate development of the dominant follicle that is destined to ovulate. Low LH levels in the luteal phase and inadequate midcycle surges of LH have also been suggested as possible causes of luteal phase inadequacy. Another common finding in these patients that is not understood is the disparity in time between the midcycle LH and FSH peaks, which normally coincide. *Luteal phase inadequacy* can also be demonstrated by a gradual instead of a sharp rise of the basal body temperature at ovulation, a shortened luteal phase, or a dwindling of the corpus luteum effect with a decline in basal body temperature (classic corpus luteum defect). The discrepancy in the dating of the secretory endometrium that usually ensues results in infertility; although ovulation occurs, the endometrium or the inadequate corpus luteum cannot support implantation and an early occult abortion follows.

BLEEDING ASSOCIATED WITH ANOVULATION

Ovulation may occur infrequently, sporadically, or not at all (Fig. 46–3). In anovulation, either amenorrhea or intermittent excessive flow ensues, depending on

the effective stimulation of the endometrium. Some of the complexities of the menstrual cycle and the associated bleeding have been clarified by Vande Wiele and associates. They wove 34 known variables of the normal menstrual cycle into a computer program and, by perturbing the system, demonstrated that extreme variations in the patterns of normal endocrine and ovulatory function result in occasional cycles of anovulation and abnormal bleeding.

DIAGNOSIS OF MENSTRUAL DISORDERS

The physician's first obligation is to obtain a data base; and, in this instance, description of the abnormal bleeding is most important. The pattern of bleeding should then be related to ovulation. This can be done tentatively on the basis of history and confirmed by laboratory tests. Clinical history of *mittelschmerz* (pain in the groin at midcycle), wet mucoid vaginal secretion at midcycle, and menstrual cramps and other molimina (discomfort or sense of tension preceding or accompanying menstruation) may all suggest an ovulatory cycle. Tests that confirm ovulation include 1) endometrial biopsy demonstrating secretory or menstrual endometrium, 2) biphasic basal body temperature curves, 3) cytologic examination of consecutive vaginal smears showing shift from estrogen- to progesterone-dominated smears, 4) examination of cervical mucus over several days during which ferning appears and then disappears, and 5) presence of serum pro-

gesterone or urinary progesterone metabolites in levels consistent with the progestational phase of the menstrual cycle.

Of these tests, the endometrial biopsy (see Fig. 47–8) is probably the most important and simplest method of evaluating abnormal bleeding. If the specimen is taken immediately before an expected period, immediately after the onset of bleeding, or, in women whose bleeding is totally irregular, during a bleeding episode, its examination indicates immediately whether ovulation has occurred. Also, it can demonstrate distinct pathologic disorders (*e.g.*, chronic endometritis or atypical hyperplasia of the endometrium) that rule out dysfunctional uterine bleeding (see Fig. 47–9).

If normal ovulation is confirmed by the finding of normal secretory endometrium, the cause of the menstrual disorder can confidently be sought below the level of the ovaries, in the uterus (*e.g.*, adenomyosis), or in the endometrium (*e.g.*, endometrial polyps). Depending on the circumstances and the woman's age, dilatation and curettage may be indicated.

If ovulation does not occur, the cause should be determined. In such cases, the excessive bleeding is usually the result of unopposed estrogen stimulus followed by breakthrough bleeding which may be secondary to dysfunction at the level of the hypothalamus–pituitary, the thyroid, the adrenal, or the ovary; all should be investigated by appropriate tests. Sometimes psychiatric disturbances with hypothalamic mediation are at fault; sometimes pelvic disease, such as submucous fibroids or inflammatory disease, is contributory. Rarely, blood dyscrasias (*e.g.*, platelet or specific factor deficiencies) are responsible for the bleeding.

MANAGEMENT OF DYSFUNCTIONAL UTERINE BLEEDING

Management depends in large measure on the patient's age.

In the adolescent, dysfunctional bleeding is almost invariably of the anovulatory type, possibly due to a decrease in hypothalamic sensitivity to positive estrogen feedback; serious pathologic problems are rare. Anovulatory bleeding in the adolescent is usually adequately managed by reassurance unless the bleeding is sufficient to cause anemia or hygienic problems, in which case it can usually be controlled by a trial of progestin on cycle days 15–25. Examples are medroxyprogesterone (10 mg) or norethindrone (1–5 mg). If this fails or if the excessive bleeding recurs, examination under anesthesia and dilatation and curettage are indicated. However, dysfunctional bleeding in the adolescent is usually self-limited and ceases when ovulatory menstruation begins. If it persists for more than 1 year, an endocrine profile should be prepared and treatment directed to the endocrine disorder.

In the woman of childbearing age, an endometrial biopsy may suffice for preliminary diagnosis and preliminary management; if the bleeding abnormality is not resolved within a few months, however, dilatation and curettage are necessary. When no pathology is found, this procedure alone is usually followed by normal menstruation; but, in 25%–30% of cases, the excessive bleeding recurs after several months. However, it is emphasized that any salutary clinical effects of curettage are incidental. The preeminent reason for the procedure is to rule out such causes of bleeding as polyp, chronic endometritis, and carcinoma of the endometrium.

When the patient is anovulatory but demonstrates normal secretion of estrogen (as judged by examination of vaginal smear or cervical mucus) and infertility is not a concern, progesterone or progestin (*e.g.*, medroxyprogesterone) may be given on a cyclic basis. Medroxyprogesterone, 10–30 mg daily for 5 days from day 20 to day 25 is usually sufficient. The first cycle of such treatment (following a period of anovulation during which the endometrium may have become hyperplastic) may produce excessive bleeding that begins 2–3 days after treatment. In subsequent cycles, bleeding is usually less severe until a menstrual flow that is normal or even a little less than usual is achieved. If the anovulatory bleeding is excessive, intravenous administration of conjugated estrogens (Premarin, 20 mg) may be tried, followed by high oral doses of a combination estrogen–progestin; however, such doses must be higher than those used for contraception (*e.g.*, 5 mg Enovid or 2–10 mg Ortho-Novum).* The heavy flow that results from a hyperplastic endometrium can usually be controlled by these methods until the patient's blood status can be evaluated and she is sufficiently reassured to understand and tolerate the flow that follows the administration of progesterone. She is then cycled normally. If abnormal bleeding still occurs, organic disease must be sought. Adequate instruction of the patient is a very necessary part of such management. Once the initial bleeding episode is controlled, the problem can be managed subsequently with cyclic progestin therapy (recognizing that ovulation is not likely taking place) or by the use of a combination oral contraceptive preparation.

For some women whose families are complete and for whom continued oral contraception is undesirable, *e.g.*, because of age, hysterectomy may be a reasonable solution.

When infertility and excessive bleeding is due either to an inadequate luteal phase or to anovulation, clomiphene citrate can be used to solve both problems. The regimen for use of this agent is discussed in Chapter 47.

---

* Premarin: conjugated estrogens; Enovid 5 mg: 100µg mestranol plus 5 mg norethynodrel; Ortho-Novum 2–10 mg: 100µg mestranol plus 2 or 10 mg norethindrone.

FIG. 46–4. Summary of follicular and luteal phase defects that result in dysfunctional uterine bleeding. (GH Arronet)

NORMAL (FUNCTIONAL) UTERINE BLEEDING

	Follicle Maturation Early/Late	Ovulation	Luteal Phase Early/Late	Endometrium	Menstrual Pattern	Functional Diagnosis
1	Normal	Normal	Normal	Normal biphasic changes	Eumenorrhea	Normal ovulatory cycle Perfect biphasic cycle
2	Normal & short	Normal	Normal	Normal biphasic changes	Eumenorrhea	Short normal ovulatory cycle not shorter than 22 days
3	Normal & prolonged	Normal	Normal	Normal biphasic changes	Eumenorrhea	Long normal ovulatroy cycle not longer than 34 days

DYSFUNCTIONAL UTERINE BLEEDING

I Ovulatory Group

4	Short	Normal	Normal	Accelerated proliferation Normal secretory changes	Polymenorrhea	Premature follicle maturation cycles shorter than 22 days "Polyovulation"
5	Prolonged	Normal	Normal	Retarded proliferation Normal secretory changes	Oligomenorrhea	Delayed follicle maturation cycles longer than 34 days "Oligovulation"
6	Normal	Normal	Normal/ slightly delayed	Combined secretory & proliferative changes in early follicle phase	Menorrhagia after regular interval	Delayed involution of corpus luteum
7	Normal	Normal	Normal/ delayed	Prolonged secretory changes	Menorrhagia after slightly prolonged interval	Short-term corpus luteum persistence
8	Normal	Normal	Normal/ missing	More prolonged secretory changes with marked pseudodecidual reaction	Severe menorrhagia after more prolonged interval	Long-term corpus luteum persistence (pseudocyesis)
9	Normal	Normal	Inadequate	Inconsistent, atypical changes throughout luteal phase	Eumenorrhea with or without interval variations	Luteal phase inadequacy "imperfect biphasic cycle"

II Subovulatory Group

10	Normal or prolonged	Normal or missing	Normal or missing	Normal biphasic changes or proliferation only	Eumenorrhea alternating with oligo- or hypomenorrhea	Ovulation alternating with anovulation

III Anovulatory Group

11	Normal	Missing	Missing	Proliferation only	Menorrhea with normal or shortened interval	Anovulation "Perfect Monophasic Cycle"
12	Normal/ slightly delayed	Missing	Missing	Proliferation only with mild hyperplasia	Metrorrhagia with prolonged interval	Short-term follicle persistence
13	Normal/ delayed	Missing	Missing	Proliferation only with variable degrees of marked hyperplasia	Severe metrorrhagia following more prolonged interval	Long-term follicle persistence
14	Deficient	Missing	Missing	Poor proliferation only	Oligohypomenorrhea	Deficiency of follicle maturation "Imperfect Monophasic Cycle"
15	Deficient/ deficient missing	Missing	Missing	Early proliferation gradually changing to atrophy	Secondary amenorrhea first degree	Ceasing follicle maturation
16	Missing	Missing	Missing	Nonfunctioning, atrophy	Secondary amenorrhea second degree	Ceased follicle maturation, no cycle

AMENORRHEA

It has been traditional to divide amenorrhea into primary and secondary types. According to this classification, *primary amenorrhea* refers to failure to menstruate before the age of 18, and *secondary amenorrhea* refers to the cessation of menses for 3 months or more after they have once become established. These are useful designations. However, classifying amenorrhea according to the specific portions of the reproductive system that may be at fault has the advantages of grouping cases with a common cause and allowing an orderly approach to the solution of the problem.

The terms *cryptomenorrhea* (hidden menstruation)

and *false amenorrhea* denote the failure of an otherwise normal menstrual flow to appear externally; cyclic ovarian activity and endometrial response are normal, but egress of the blood is blocked, as by an imperforate hymen.

PHYSIOLOGIC AMENORRHEA

The most common causes of amenorrhea are pregnancy and the menopause. In the former, amenorrhea is due to suppression of pituitary gonadotropins by the increasing quantities of estrogen produced during pregnancy; in the latter, amenorrhea reflects exhaustion of the ova and consequent failure of the ovary to respond to gonadotropins. Physiologic amenorrhea can also occur in adolescence during the 1st year after the menarche; it is then not unusual for bleeding episodes to occur only at infrequent intervals. This is due principally to the irregular gonadotropin release that sometimes occurs in girls at this age; the problem usually solves itself within a year and requires neither investigation nor treatment.

AMENORRHEA DUE TO GENETIC DEFECTS

There are two major genetic defects (testicular feminization and Turner's syndrome) in which amenorrhea is a primary characteristic and is often the symptom that causes the patient to consult the physician. These entities and their variants are also discussed in Chapter 2.

Testicular Feminization

In testicular feminization (the feminizing testis syndrome), the patient usually has a blind vaginal pouch, but no uterus, cervix, or ovaries. Undeveloped testicles are usually found in the abdomen or the inguinal areas; in the latter case, they may be mistaken for bilateral inguinal hernias. Such testes are cryptorchid in type, with immature germ and Sertoli cells and no evidence of spermatogenesis. The habitus is that of the phenotypic female. The breasts are well developed, often remarkably so (Fig. 46–5), and the external genitalia appear normally female except that pubic (as well as axillary) hair is usually lacking. Libido is usually well developed, and an initial inquiry from the patient, in addition to amenorrhea, may concern the short vagina. LH values are elevated. FSH values are normal unless the gonads are removed, in which case they increase to postmenopausal levels. This may result from loss of gonadal inhibin. Normal male values of serum testosterone are present, implying androgen insensitivity of the target organs, and recent work has indeed demonstrated that some of the tissues of such patients are deficient or lacking in testosterone-binding protein. This explains the lack of axillary and pubic

hair. Development of the secondary sex characteristics is also presumed due to the androgen insensitivity, which permits these structures to respond to the biologically active estrogens that are normally produced in small amounts by the testis. Peripheral conversion of androgens to estrogens may also contribute to this development.

At later ages, other characteristics may be observed in patients with testicular feminization, such as the tendency to tall stature, long arms, large feet, and large hands. The breasts, although large, have little glandular tissue; the nipples are small and the areolae pale.

It is recommended that the primitive gonads in such patients be removed after puberty because of their propensity for malignant change. In Morris and Mahesh's series of 50 patients, the testes were malignant in 12 and showed neoplasia in 26. After removal of the testes, sufficient estrogen should be prescribed to maintain the feminine identity.

It is important that there be no challenge to the feminine gender of such a person, and it is imprudent to divulge to the patient, her parents, or her husband the details of the disorder except to indicate that pregnancy is not possible. Such patients can and do function normally as females; if they are informed that testicles have been removed and they are really males, the resulting crisis in gender identity can be disastrous, often leading to major and virtually insoluble psychiatric illness.

Turner's Syndrome

Pure gonadal dysgenesis (Turner's syndrome) is a genetic disorder characterized by a karyotype of 45, XO, failure of normal development of the gonad, and other malformations. Classically, the syndrome is described as sexual infantilism, with short stature, primary amenorrhea, webbing of the neck, wide carrying angle, and shield-shaped chest. Coarctation of the aorta and congenital malformations of the renal collecting system also occur. The presence of hypergonadotropic, hypoestrogenic amenorrhea, along with the other signs, suggests the diagnosis. Karyotyping should be done to confirm the diagnosis, since there are variants, particularly mosaics, in which the management or the prognosis (*e.g.*, for fertility) may be modified.

Dysgenesis of the gonad is associated with failure of follicle development, failure of ovulation, and, therefore, sterility. In addition, estrogen secretion is lacking or minimal (arising only from the adrenal), and, for this reason, the patient should be given estrogens. Carcinoma of the endometrium has been reported to occur in some patients with this syndrome, presumably as a result of prolonged unrelieved estrogen therapy. Exogenous estrogen administration should be started after the growth potential has been attained, to supplement the low output of estrogen from the adre-

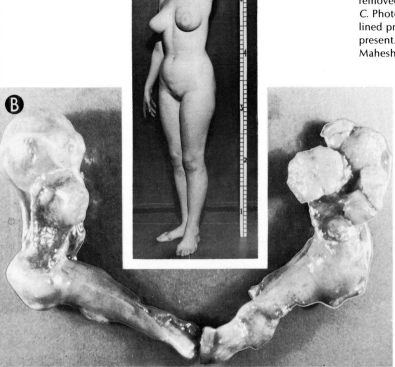

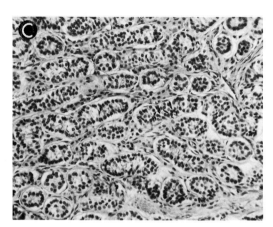

FIG. 46–5. *A.* Testicular feminization in 18-year-old apparent female with primary amenorrhea, minimal sexual hair, large breasts and areolae, but small nipples. FSH before surgery: over 13, less than 52 mouse uterine units; 17-ketosteroids, 21 mg/24 hours; 17-ketogenic steroids, 5.5 mg/24 hours; pregnanetriol, 1.2 mg/24 hours. *B.* Gonads and rudimentary uterine structures removed from patient in *A.* Note nodular appearance of gonad. *C.* Photomicrograph of gonad. Immature testicular tubules are lined principally by primitive germ cells with some Sertoli cells present. Note marked resemblance to fetal testis. (Morris JM, Mahesh VB: Am J Obstet Gynecol 87:731, 1963)

nal. The results in terms of development of the external genitalia and breasts can be striking. Either cyclic estrogen or estrogen plus 10 days of progestin at the end of the cycle is the preferred treatment.

Mosaicism is not uncommon and can be identified by karyotype. Identification of the Y chromosome makes an important difference, since gonadoblastomas (said to occur exclusively in patients with gonadal dysgenesis) are found primarily in those with mosaicism for the Y chromosome. It is recommended that laparotomy and gonadectomy be performed in such patients. Alternatively, gonadal biopsy can be done and the gonad removed if the Y chromosome is present in the gonadal tissue. The patient with typical Turner's syndrome, with XO karyotype, is unlikely to have a neoplasm of the streak gonad.

PATHOLOGIC AMENORRHEA

The pathologic causes of amenorrhea can be divided into four major groups according to the part of the reproductive system that is basically at fault: 1) the

uterus and vagina, 2) the ovaries, 3) the pituitary, and 4) the hypothalamus and central nervous system.

Primary Disorders of the Uterus, Vagina, or Hymen

Defects in the uterus, vagina, or hymen may be such that either menstrual blood is not produced or its egress from the uterus or through the vagina is prevented.

Failure of the uterus to produce menstrual blood is usually secondary to failure at the level of the ovaries, pituitary, or hypothalamus. However, amenorrhea may be the direct result of such uterine disorders as tuberculous endometritis or endometrial synechiae. The latter, *Asherman's syndrome*, is a scarring of the uterine cavity that results from curettage, usually performed for postpartum hemorrhage or abortion, with the formation of adhesions of the endometrial surfaces. Treatment consists of breaking the adhesions, inserting an intrauterine device, and administering estrogens until the endometrium has regenerated.

Imperforate hymen and failure of proper develop-

ment of the müllerian duct system may account for failure to menstruate. An intact hymen can be diagnosed by visualization of the fourchette and the vaginal opening and treated by simple incision. Imperfect development of the müllerian duct system may allow menstrual blood to accumulate in blind pouches of the uterus (particularly extra horns), cervix, or vagina. This may cause cramps without the appropriate menstrual flow. Examination of these patients, generally young girls, discloses a dilated vagina or uterus, which can be identified as enlarged and tender on rectal examination. Such findings mandate a genetic evaluation as well as a search for adjacent congenital malformations, such as those of the kidney and its collecting system. If possible, hematometra or hematocolpos (blood contained in the uterine cavity or vagina) should be drained through the perineum or vagina. If its true nature is not recognized and such a mass is removed abdominally, the patient's future reproductive potential is destroyed. Rarely, lack of müllerian duct development is accompanied by cramps and the lower abdominal pain associated with ovulation (mittelschmerz). The patient has neither a uterus nor a cervix; she may have no vagina or only a very short one. Normal ovaries are usually present. Once karyotyping has demonstrated that the patient is a normal female, she can be taught to use glass vaginal dilators to increase the length of the vagina. In some cases, split-thickness skin grafts can be used to create a vagina. A great deal of understanding and support must be offered such a patient to enable her to form a functional vagina and carry on as a normal woman, albeit sterile.

Primary Ovarian Failure

Primary failure at the level of the ovary is an unusual cause of amenorrhea except at menopause, when the supply of ova is exhausted. Gonadal agenesis and dysgenesis as a cause of amenorrhea have been discussed earlier. Sometimes dysgenesis is not apparent until the patient reaches her middle or late 30s, when the clinical features of the menopause appear. For amenorrheic patients in this age group, pregnancy must, of course, be excluded first. When the patient is not pregnant, serum FSH and LH levels should be determined; if they are elevated, the diagnosis is premature menopause.

Autoimmune disease of the ovary may result in insensitivity to gonadotropins and, consequently, primary ovarian failure with amenorrhea, which may be either primary or secondary. In such cases, gonadotropin levels are elevated, and the ovary has many normal resting follicles. Diagnosis requires minilaparotomy and an adequate ovarian biopsy, a procedure that some consider important for all women with premature menopause. If many primary follicles are found in the ovary, the diagnosis is *ovarian insensitivity,* and such

patients may be at risk for other autoimmune disorders. Although immunosuppressive therapy has not been adequately explored, there is reason to presume that it could be helpful. If pregnancy is desired, it is theoretically possible that ovulation might follow gonadotropin suppression with estrogens, an effect that has been observed in a few cases. If no follicles are found in the ovarian tissue, the diagnosis is ovarian dysgenesis, and karyotype is indicated; if a Y chromosome is present, gonadectomy should be performed to prevent the possible development of gonadoblastoma and later virilism.

Destruction of the ova by such factors as radiation, infection, cancer, or chemotherapy are unusual causes of amenorrhea.

Primary Pituitary Failure

Primary pituitary failure, evidenced by little or no gonadotropin in the serum, may be either anatomic or functional. The usual causes of pituitary dysfunction are tumor, infarction, inflammation, and irradiation; all are relatively rare.

Tumor. In the case of tumor, amenorrhea may be the first symptom. Such tumors include prolactin-secreting tumor, chromophobe adenoma, and craniopharyngioma. The patient may demonstrate panhypopituitarism in which all pituitary tropic hormones are variously affected, but the general result is abnormally low responses of target organs, *i.e.,* poor adrenal response to stress, ovarian atrophy, and hypothyroidism. The tumor may develop slowly, and amenorrhea may not result for many years. Alternatively, amenorrhea may appear many years before the classic signs of erosion of the sella turcica can be observed. The measurement of glycoprotein pituitary hormones by radioimmunoassay permits early identification of a hormone-producing pituitary tumor when the symptoms suggest this possibility. Visual field plots and tomography are helpful in delineating a pituitary tumor. Pituitary microsurgery has been developed to the extent that pituitary adenomas can usually be removed without destruction of the whole pituitary gland. Serum prolactin measurements are useful in identifying such tumors, since 25% of all pituitary tumors are accompanied by elevated levels of prolactin.

Infarction. Infarction of the pituitary gland can occur following pregnancy, as the result of either puerperal infection with septic thromboemboli or hemorrhage with shock and consequent collapse of the pituitary blood flow. The former was discovered by Simmonds, the latter by Sheehan, and their names are associated with the syndromes. The term *Simmonds' disease* has been used interchangeably with hypopituitary cachexia, although it was originally described as a specific postpartum disease. *Sheehan's disease* has been

more rigorously defined pathologically, and pituitary infarction of varying degrees has been identified in postpartum patients who have experienced hemorrhage late in pregnancy with varying periods of associated shock. Either hemorrhage *per se* or the microthrombi associated with infarction (as in Simmonds' disease) are thought to be the cause of the pituitary ischemia and infarction.

The symptoms and signs of Simmonds' and Sheehan's diseases are those resulting from loss of endocrine function of the glands stimulated by the specific pituitary tropic hormones: FSH, thyroid-stimulating hormone (TSH), adrenocorticotropic hormone (ACTH), and human growth hormone (hGH). Amenorrhea may be the first symptom, and both hypothyroidism and Addison's disease may accompany pituitary infarction or hypofunction. Instead of the usual clinical picture (lethargy, apathy, loss of weight, low blood pressure, myxedema, and general cachexia), disease may be occult, in which case failure of the adrenal to respond to stress may cause death or severe illness as the result of such insults as surgery or intercurrent disease. Sheehan's and Simmonds' diseases are rarely encountered today, as obstetric care has improved and blood for replacement is generally available during delivery; but minimal infarction of the pituitary still occurs, producing characteristic variations from normal, but no clear-cut cachectic syndrome.

Functional Disorders. The functional pituitary disturbances associated with amenorrhea can result from intrinsic causes (*e.g.*, congenital defects of the pituitary and specific gonadotropin biosynthetic enzyme deficiencies) or from causes outside the pituitary. The latter include lactation, immaturity, pregnancy, estrogen-secreting tumors, and psychologic influences.

Hypothalamic Disorders

The hypothalamic disorders that result in amenorrhea are occasionally produced by neoplasms. More commonly, they are caused by emotional problems, starvation, and selective suppression of gonadotropin-releasing factors by oral contraceptive agents.

Emotional Problems. The role of emotional problems in the causation of amenorrhea is well-known. A classic example is the amenorrhea so common among women confined to concentration camps in World War II. Less severe stresses, as occur frequently among students and young career women, can produce a similar response.

Anorexia Nervosa. This problem is a frequent cause of adolescent amenorrhea. Its seriousness is attested by reported death rates of 2%–10%. The amenorrhea associated with anorexia nervosa is due not only to starvation, but also to the psychologic disturbance at the root of the refusal to eat. Amenorrhea is an early symptom, occurring before significant emaciation develops. Weight loss of 25–30 lb and more can be sufficient to constitute a medical emergency. The hypothalamic effect appears to be selective, since serum TSH and ACTH levels remain normal, despite the fact that levels of FSH, LH, and estrogens decrease to levels normally found before puberty. On remission, they revert to normal cycling levels.

Sometimes anorexia nervosa is difficult to differentiate clinically from Simmonds' or Sheehan's disease. Radioimmunoassay for the aforementioned hormones enables the distinction. It has been documented that the onset of menses in adolescence requires a minimal weight for height; weight loss leads to amenorrhea, and weight gain restores the menstrual cycle (see Chap. 8, Fig. 8–4). The role of undernutrition in a given case of adolescent amenorrhea can sometimes be determined by the index of fatness compared with that expected at 18 years of age. Girls become relatively and absolutely fatter between the ages of 16 and 18. More weight gain is required for the restoration of menses at 18 years than for the initial onset of menses at an earlier age.

Because of the psychiatric overtones in anorexia nervosa, it is usually prudent to have a knowledgeable psychiatrist collaborate in therapy.

Suppression by Oral Contraceptives (Post-Pill Amenorrhea). A primary effect of oral contraceptive agents in the deliberate production of infertility is suppression of the hypothalamic gonadotropin-releasing factors. Cyclic activity in the pituitary and, consequently, in the ovary is thereby eliminated. In most women, cyclic hypothalamic–pituitary–ovarian activity, with resultant menstruation, resumes within 3 months after oral contraception is discontinued. If 6 months elapse before the appearance of menstruation, post-pill amenorrhea is diagnosed. In such women, both estrogen and gonadotropin values are usually low, but adrenal function, as determined by 17-ketosteroid and 17-hydroxycorticosteroid levels, is normal. The amenorrhea is usually due to sustained hypothalamic suppression and in about half the patients is relieved by clomiphene citrate. Those who respond to clomiphene citrate are usually women who have elevated serum estrogen levels and a normal response to LH-releasing hormone (LHRH). However, other causes of amenorrhea must be ruled out before therapy is initiated. Post-pill amenorrhea and the amenorrhea resulting from such long-lasting agents as depo-medroxyprogesterone acetate are considered in Chapter 14.

In some cases of post-pill amenorrhea, serum prolactin levels are elevated. As noted later in this chapter (see Galactorrhea–Amenorrhea Syndrome), it can be postulated that many of these cases are due to suppression of the hypothalamic prolactin-inhibiting factor; in some, a pituitary tumor may be found.

AMENORRHEA RESULTING FROM SYSTEMIC ILLNESS

Amenorrhea is characteristically associated with debilitating illnesses such as chronic nephritis and multiple sclerosis, as well as with some severe psychiatric disorders. Pulmonary tuberculosis is sometimes accompanied by amenorrhea, probably because of the general debilitation that attends this disease; if the tuberculosis has spread to and destroyed the endometrium, amenorrhea is a necessary consequence. Starvation as a cause of failure of menstruation has been mentioned previously; its opposite, gluttony, can also produce amenorrhea. Amenorrhea is often associated with severe thyrotoxicosis and sometimes with hypothyroidism, evidently because of alteration in the metabolism of both estrogens and androgens. In cirrhosis of the liver, the normal metabolism of estrogens is impaired, with consequent elevation of circulating estrogen levels; usually amenorrhea, but sometimes totally irregular bleeding, is the result. In their developed stages, most of these associated problems are immediately evident on examination. However, even in their early stages, they may produce menstrual failure, and subclinical disorders of this kind should be considered when the diagnosis is not apparent as a result of routine inquiries.

DIAGNOSIS OF AMENORRHEA

When amenorrhea occurs in a woman of childbearing age, the first step in diagnosis is to rule out pregnancy. If the patient is not pregnant and there are no obvious anomalies and obstructive lesions of the uterovaginal canal, the initial history and physical examination will suggest areas for further investigation. Leads that suggest systemic illness should be pursued. In primary amenorrhea, a karyotype is often needed to rule out gonadal dysgenesis, testicular feminization syndrome, and mosaicism. Laparoscopy may be helpful in the diagnosis of variants and as a guide to management.

When there are no obvious abnormalities, the following tests can narrow the list of possible explanations for the amenorrhea. First, 100 mg progesterone is administered intramuscularly, in a single dose or 10 mg medroxyprogesterone acetate (Provera) can be given by mouth daily for 5–7 days. If no bleeding results, conjugated estrogen, 1.25 mg daily, is given for 21 days followed by 100 mg progesterone intramuscularly in a single dose or 10 mg medroxyprogesterone acetate by mouth daily for 5 days. If bleeding does not follow progesterone alone but does follow the estrogen–progesterone combination, serum FSH values should be determined. These tests are interpreted as follows:

1. Since progesterone produces uterine bleeding only if the endometrium has been primed by estrogen, the occurrence of bleeding following progesterone alone indicates that the endometrium is intact and has been acted on by estrogens. The diagnosis is anovulation. If no withdrawal bleeding follows progesterone, it can be presumed either that estrogen is available but the endometrium is incapable of response or that the endometrium has not been primed by estrogen. The latter may be due either to primary ovarian failure or to failure at the hypothalamic–pituitary level.

2. Administration of estrogen plus progesterone tests the capacity of the endometrium to respond. If no bleeding occurs, the source of the amenorrhea is at the uterine level (*e.g.*, endometrial synechiae, which can be diagnosed by hysterosalpingography, or destruction of the endometrium by tuberculosis) or results from obstruction (*e.g.*, vaginal atresia, imperforate hymen, or cervical stenosis). If bleeding follows administration of estrogen plus progesterone, the problem can be further clarified by determining serum FSH levels.

3. High FSH levels suggest ovarian failure, which can result from total attrition of ova (as in menopause), ovarian destruction by infection or cancer, or ovarian dysgenesis. Lack of FSH or low levels of FSH suggest that the pituitary is at fault, and such possibilities as tumor, infarction, or infection should be investigated by sellar roentgenography plotting of visual fields and tests for other tropic hormones.

In the presence of an estrogen-primed endometrium, as evidenced by bleeding after administration of progesterone, investigation of the cause of the ovulatory failure can be a complex undertaking because of the multiplicity of factors that can affect the sequence of events required for normal ovulation. Basically, ovulation is triggered by the LH surge that occurs in response to increasing levels of estradiol, and any interference with either of these factors can result in anovulation. The possibility of hypopituitarism (either total or selective) has been mentioned earlier.

Below the level of the pituitary, failure or blunting of the LH surge can result from the circulation of constant or only gradually increasing levels of progesterone, estrogen, or androgen. In the first case, progesterone dominance, pregnancy is the prototype, but equivalent failure of the LH surge can occur in the presence of persistent corpus luteum cyst and pseudocyesis. Estrogen dominance, the so-called constant estrus, is associated with feminizing or estrogen-producing ovarian tumors (theca cell tumor, granulosa cell tumor), polycystic ovarian disease (Stein–Leventhal syndrome), the adrenogenital syndrome, thyroid dysfunction, and obesity. The androgen-dominant type of anovulation, usually accompanied by hirsutism, is associated with arrhenoblastoma of the ovary, androgen-secreting adrenal tumors, and other situations in which excess androgens are secreted.

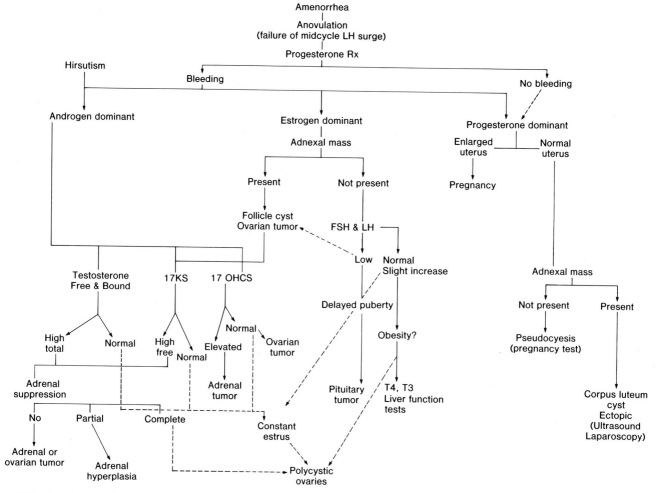

FIG. 46–6. Schema for amenorrhea. (Modified from Rothchild IM: Functional amenorrhea. In Maeck HC, Sherman AI [eds]: The Neuroendocrinology of Reproduction. Springfield, IL, CC Thomas, 1971)

Figure 46–6 presents a flow sheet summarizing the initial diagnostic approach to anovulatory amenorrhea. It should be remembered that 1) the clinical designation of progesterone dominance, estrogen dominance, or androgen dominance can usually narrow the investigation; 2) pituitary function often requires detailed investigation; 3) because of the frequent association of adrenal and thyroid disorders with amenorrhea, function of these structures may have to be appraised according to the measures outlined in Chapter 7; and 4) in cases not readily explained by standard investigation, subclinical systemic disease may be the root of the problem.

TOXIC SHOCK SYNDROME

The toxic shock syndrome is a bizarre, sometimes fatal illness that appears to be related both to menstruation and to the use of tampons. The syndrome is new in the sense that national attention was not directed to it until the spring of 1980. The incidence appears to be about 1 case of toxic shock syndrome per 20,000 menstruating women.

The disease is characterized by the sudden onset, usually during menstruation, of profuse, watery diarrhea and vomiting, fever above 102° F, profound lethargy, confusion, and hypotension that sometimes progresses to shock. A sunburn-like rash that desquamates a few days later is present. The vaginal, buccal, pharyngeal, and conjunctival mucous membranes are intensely hyperemic. In about 8% of cases the shock syndrome leads to death.

About 95% of the reported cases occurred during menstruation. More than 95% of the women regularly used tampons during menstruation; all sizes and types of tampons are represented. In about 75% of the cases *Staphylococcus aureus* was cultured from the cervix or vagina prior to treatment. In about 30% of cases the syndrome recurred at subsequent menstruation, but

the recurrence rate was lower among patients who were treated with beta-lactamase-resistant antibiotics such as cephalosporins or pencillinase-resistant penicillins during their first episode.

Treatment depends on prompt recognition of the syndrome, volume repletion, and antistaphyloccal antibiotics. Corticosteroids may also be useful.

Although both menstruation and tampons are factors in most cases, the toxic shock syndrome has also been reported in children, in men, in nonmenstruating women, and in women who have not used tampons. Because, in most cases, the portal of entry is the vagina, the total absence of pelvic manifestations is striking. These discrepancies will be clarified as more is learned about this curious syndrome. In the meantime, although tampon use has not been interdicted, women are cautioned that it may be wise to use napkin protection at night and to change tampons during the day at intervals no longer than 6 hours.

GYNECOLOGIC ENDOCRINE DISORDERS

POLYCYSTIC OVARIAN DISEASE

Polycystic ovarian disease (sclerocystic ovarian disease, Stein–Leventhal syndrome) is an endocrinologically bizarre condition that has provoked intense differences of opinion regarding the metabolic deviations concerned and, indeed, the manifestations of the disorder. The combination of amenorrhea, hirsutism, and infertility in the presence of polycystic ovaries was originally described by Stein and Leventhal in 1935, and both the classic syndrome and its many variants continue to be discussed as the Stein–Leventhal syndrome. Stein originally performed laparotomy to obtain wedge biopsies of the enlarged ovaries. The ovaries were gray white, enlarged to 3–5 cm in diameter, and smooth in contour. On the cut surface, the cortex was much thickened and crowded with multiple clear cysts 2–6 mm in diameter (see Fig. 57–9). Theca interna activity was increased; corpora albicantia and, rarely, corpora lutea were found. Of 60 patients, 45 resumed normal menstruation after removal of the wedge of tissue, and 9 began to menstruate somewhat irregularly; among those whose ovaries were shown to be polycystic, 72% became pregnant. Stein suggested that the disorder is "probably due to hypersecretion of the gonadotrophic hormones of the anterior pituitary lobe."

At the time it was described, the syndrome was believed to be a rather rigidly defined entity, and the possibility of related variants was not seriously considered. In the intervening years, insight into this disorder has been gained through increased knowledge of the synthesis and metabolism of steroid hormones and the hormonal control of pituitary, ovarian, and adrenal function. It is now known that polycystic ovarian disease embraces a large and diffuse group of related problems; their common denominator, as the now accepted designation implies, is *bilateral* polycystic ovaries.

SIGNS AND SYMPTOMS

As noted in the early reports, obesity, amenorrhea, infertility, and hirsutism are indeed present in many of the patients; but they are not always present, and other symptoms may also occur. Table 46–2 presents the signs and symptoms reported in 1079 published cases reviewed by Goldzieher and Green.

CAUSE

The biochemical and endocrinologic data that bear on the cause of polycystic ovarian disease are voluminous. This is an extremely complex disorder, and variants occur with sufficient frequency that all statements regarding cause must be qualified.

A fundamental part of the picture is a "steady state" of hypothalamus and pituitary, with failure of the normal cyclic phenomena and continuous release of constant levels of gonadotropins. A second important part of the picture is the continued growth of new follicles and distortion of some of the normal pathways of ovarian steroidogenesis. The exact nature of the defect in ovarian steroidogenesis is unsettled, but it is suggested that enzyme deficiencies, probably resulting from constant gonadotropin effects, are responsible for increased production of androstenedione (which is converted peripherally to both estrone and testosterone) and 17-hydroxyprogesterone (a precursor of testosterone); the increased androgen production leads to hirsutism and, in some cases, other evidence of virilization. The increased estrogen production at a constant

TABLE 46–2. FREQUENCY OF SYMPTOMS IN 1079 PUBLISHED CASES OF OVARIAN POLYCYSTIC DISEASE*

Symptom	Frequency (%)	
	Mean	Range
Biphasic basal temperature	15	12–40
Virilization	21	0–28
Corpus luteum at operation	22	0–71
Dysmenorrhea	23	
Functional bleeding	29	6–65
Obesity	41	16–49
Amenorrhea	51	15–77
Hirsutism	69	17–83
Infertility	74	35–94

* Based on 187 references.

(Goldzieher JW, Green JA: J Clin Endocrinol Metab 22:325, 1962)

level has the dual effect of hypothalamic inhibition (with failure of the LH surge) and endometrial stimulation, unopposed by progesterone, with the consequence, in some cases, of endometrial hyperplasia or even carcinoma of the endometrium. A vicious cycle results; the failure of estradiol to rise sharply at midcycle leads to failure of the LH surge and to anovulation. FSH and LH (and estrogen and androgen) then assume persistent, nonfluctuating circulating concentrations. The mean LH level is usually higher than in normal women, while the FSH level is low or low-normal. Thus, in some cases the hypothalamus or pituitary may be fundamentally at fault; in others, the ovary.

The adrenal may also be concerned. Testosterone itself and other androgens, as well as androgen precursors, can be formed in the adrenal, and they can profoundly influence the course of events in the polycystic ovary. Also, the abnormal steroidogenesis of the polycystic ovary can affect adrenal steroidogenesis. Thus, in some cases, the adrenal may be primarily at fault; in others, the adrenal aberrations may be secondary.

DIAGNOSIS

In most cases, a tentative diagnosis is reached on the basis of clinical history, physical examination, and, frequently, endoscopic examination; the classic tests of gynecologic endocrine function are then performed. However, because of the multiplicity of biochemical and biologic systems involved in both the classic disorder and its many variants, no single laboratory test can be used to diagnose polycystic ovarian disease unequivocally. The combination of high LH and normal FSH levels can be suggestive.

At the outset, primary disease of the adrenal must be ruled out, and for this purpose urinary 17-ketosteroids (17-KS) and 17-hydroxycorticosteroids (17-OHCS) or plasma cortisol are measured; in the presence of significant aberration, the tests outlined in Chapter 7 may be required for diagnosis. A serum testosterone level, free and bound, is indicated, particularly if there is significant hirsutism. Thyroid function should be tested if thyroid dysfunction is suspected. Since, generally, the diagnosis of polycystic ovarian disease is clinically apparent, no further tests may be needed. If the patient is not amenorrheic, determination of FSH, LH, and prolactin levels are not necessary. Furthermore, the amenorrheic patient who has withdrawal bleeding after the administration of progesterone does not need to incur the expense of pituitary hormone determinations, with the exception of a prolactin determination, which may clarify the problem if the clinical signs and symptoms are ambiguous.

In some, but not all, cases the source of the androgens composing the 17-KS (*i.e.*, adrenal or ovary) can be clarified by comparing the 17-KS values that follow

adrenal suppression by dexamethasone with those that follow ovarian stimulation by human chorionic gonadotropin (hCG). If dexamethasone fails to suppress the 17-KS value below 5 mg/day and if elevated 17-KS excretion follows stimulation by hCG, the implication is that ovarian androgens are being secreted in excess. These tests are generally sufficient to allow a provisional diagnosis and initiation of therapy.

Determination of blood levels of androstenedione, testosterone, and dehydroepiandrosterone can also clarify the major source of androgen secretion as ovary, adrenal, or both. Measurement of the production rates of these hormones, and of estrone, would be extremely helpful, but the tests are not readily available for clinical use. Adrenal and ovarian vein catheterization for steroid concentration measurements has also been done, but this procedure is still investigational.

TREATMENT

The modes of therapy available are adrenal suppression, administration of clomiphene citrate, and wedge resection of the ovaries.

When the 17-KS values are slightly elevated and a significant adrenal component cannot be excluded, it is appropriate to determine whether ovulation will result from adrenal suppression by either dexamethasone or prednisone, adjusting the dose so that the 17-KS excretion rates remain between 7 and 10 mg/24 hours. In some cases, ovulation, menstruation, or even pregnancy may follow; adrenal suppression should be discontinued if ovulation does not occur within 3 months.

The regimen for administration of clomiphene citrate is outlined in Chapter 47. The exact mode of action of clomiphene citrate is not entirely understood, but the drug has certain antiestrogenic properties; in the constant estrus of polycystic ovarian disease, it causes a mild increase in the release of FSH and LH over the 5 days during which it is administered. This is followed by a fall and subsequent rise of FSH (which provides a new stimulus for follicular growth), a sharp increase in estrogen, release of a surge of LH, and, 6–12 days after completion of the 5-day course, ovulation. Polycystic ovaries are especially sensitive to the effects of clomiphene citrate, and the overstimulation syndrome (acute enlargement of the ovaries, ascites, fluid shifts from the circulating blood to the extravascular spaces) occurs more quickly and with smaller doses than it does with normal ovaries. In polycystic ovarian disease, the starting dose is 50 mg daily for 5 days, and special attention is given to the "chair syndrome" (pain on sitting down in a chair) and to pelvic examination before the next course is started. The effectiveness of clomiphene citrate is somewhat self-limiting; the drug is much less effective after four to six cycles. In some cases, increasing the dose gradually

from 50 mg daily for 5 days to a maximum, in the fourth or fifth treatment cycle, of 100 mg twice daily for 5 days may produce ovulation when smaller doses failed.

Wedge resection of the ovaries brings on ovulation by altering ovarian steroidogenesis and producing a fall in C-19 (androgenic) and C-18 (estrogenic) steroids. A rise in FSH follows, producing maturation of a new group of follicles, a sharp elevation of estradiol, and a surge of LH with subsequent ovulation. In one group of patients, there was no change in gonadotropin levels after wedge resection until the midcycle surges occurred, suggesting that the mechanism for ovulation after wedge resection in some cases may be local (intraovarian) rather than central. When the ovaries are enlarged and polycystic, as in Stein's classic cases, wedge resection is followed by normal cycles in about 80% of cases and by pregnancy in about 65% of formerly infertile women. Hirsutism is decreased in only about 15% of cases.

Wedge resection of the ovaries should be considered only in those patients who have documented polycystic ovaries and who fail to ovulate after adrenal suppression and an adequate trial of maximal doses of clomiphene citrate (including hCG augmentation). Even in these patients, it may be preferable to try a course of therapy with human menopausal gonadotropins (see page 945) before resorting to wedge resection.

CUSHING'S SYNDROME

Cushing's syndrome is classified among gynecologic endocrine disorders chiefly because of the frequent occurrence of amenorrhea (in some cases the presenting complaint) and hirsutism. The term *Cushing's disease* is reserved for cases that conform to Cushing's original description, made in 1932—patients with basophilic adenoma of the pituitary who exhibit truncal obesity, hypertension, weakness and fatigability, amenorrhea, hirsutism, abdominal striae, edema, glycosuria, and osteoporosis. The signs and symptoms of Cushing's disease are due to an excess of glucocorticoids, which can result not only from adrenal stimulation by a basophilic adenoma of the pituitary, but also from primary adrenal disorders (hyperplasia or adenoma) or from the prolonged administration of ACTH or glucocorticoid. The entire complex, regardless of primary cause, is referred to as *Cushing's syndrome.*

The pathophysiology, diagnosis, and treatment of Cushing's syndrome are discussed in Chapter 7.

CONGENITAL ADRENAL HYPERPLASIA

Classically described as female pseudohermaphroditism, congenital adrenal hyperplasia (*adrenogenital syndrome*) is a genetically transmitted disorder that may be first identified at any time before birth to adulthood. It has been diagnosed in the first half of pregnancy by determination of amniotic fluid levels of 17α-hydroxyprogesterone or androstenedione and also by HLA typing of cells obtained from the amniotic fluid.

The most notable features of this syndrome are the virilization and deep pigmentation of the external genitalia, precocious development (virilism), short stature, and failure of menstruation. According to Wilkins, congenital adrenal hyperplasia accounts for most cases of female pseudohermaphroditism and half of the patients with ambiguous genitalia. There are all variations, ranging from complete virilization of the external genitalia to normal. In later childhood and adolescence, breast development without normal onset of menses may be a suspicious clinical event. However, breasts may fail to develop, and pubic and axillary hair may be sparse.

The adrenogenital syndrome is produced by a clinically identifiable enzyme defect that interrupts the pathway leading to cortisol synthesis. The result is a cortisol deficiency, which, by negative feedback, leads to secretion of excessive amounts of ACTH and, consequently, excessive stimulation of the adrenal, adrenal hypertrophy and hyperplasia, and the secretion of excessive quantities of adrenal androgens that are responsible for the virilization of affected patients. The enzyme defect can occur at any of several points along the pathway of cortisol synthesis, which accounts for the several variants of the disorder that have been described.

Congenital adrenal hyperplasia is managed by replacement with cortisol. With replacement doses of cortisol, Wilkins demonstrated that, when this syndrome is diagnosed early, normal female development takes place, the onset of puberty occurs as expected, and even normal pregnancy and childbirth are possible. Adequacy of adrenal suppression by replacement therapy can be assessed by measurement of 24-hour urinary 17-KS excretion. Serum levels of testosterone or androstenedione have also been suggested as a convenient index of the adequacy of treatment, because determination of these levels does not require 24-hour urinary collections.

The influence of this disorder on the outcome of pregnancy is of particular interest, as there is increasing concern about the effect of prepartum administration of androgens on the physical and behavioral outcome of the offspring. Both the children of mothers who received androgens prepartum and children with congenital adrenal hyperplasia at birth have been studied. The former had abnormal external genitalia (virilization of females); the latter were considered to have tomboy attributes in adolescence. Before cortisol became available for replacement, it was necesary to rear extremely virilized children as males (and may still be so in neglected cases).

GALACTORRHEA–AMENORRHEA SYNDROME

The spontaneous secretion of a milky fluid from the breasts at times other than following pregnancy or while nursing is termed *inappropriate lactation* or *galactorrhea*. Although organic lesions of the breast usually produce a bloody or green secretion from one breast only, it is nevertheless important to rule out such disease before considering other possibilities. A careful breast examination and, in women over 35, X-ray mammography should be done.

If a local breast lesion has been ruled out, a pituitary neoplasm must then be excluded as the cause of the disorder. Chromophobe adenoma, growth hormone-producing tumors resulting in acromegaly, and benign prolactin-secreting tumors (Forbes–Albright syndrome) can result in galactorrhea. Unfortunately, blood prolactin levels are not always helpful in making the diagnosis, for they may not reflect the patient's clinical status with regard to breast secretion. Primary hypothyroidism should also be considered among the possible causes. Although the problems are undoubtedly related, eponyms have been attached to the galactorrhea–amenorrhea syndrome according to whether it immediately follows pregnancy or occurs in the nulliparous woman; the former is known as the Chiari–Frommel syndrome, the latter, as the Ahumada–del Castillo syndrome.

Thyroid and prolactin studies and roentgenographic evaluation of the sella turcica (including polytomograms) should be done in most patients with the galactorrhea–amenorrhea syndrome. The major causes of hyperprolactinemia and galactorrhea are listed in Table 46–3. The physiology of normal lactation is outlined in Chapter 40. Most cases of galactorrhea–amenorrhea are due to the inappropriate release of prolactin from the anterior lobe of the pituitary. The galactorrhea results from stimulation of the mammary glands by prolactin. The cause of the amenorrhea is less obvious, but two factors appear to be concerned: 1) elevated prolactin levels (above 15 mg/ml serum) interfere with the secretion of hypothalamic gonadotropin-releasing hormones, preventing the release of LH and FSH and, thus, resulting in failure of both ovulation and menstruation; and 2) elevated prolactin levels may directly affect the ovary, having an adverse effect on the action of gonadotropin.

It has long been known that the release of prolactin from the pituitary is normally held in check by a hypothalamic prolactin-inhibiting factor (PIF); prolactin secretion is enhanced when PIF is withdrawn or counterbalanced. To date, PIF has not been identified chemically. However, it has been postulated that PIF is actually dopamine, a compound that results from decarboxylation of dihydrophenylalanine and is the immediate precursor of norepinephrine in the biosynthetic pathway of catecholamines. Dopamine is present in high concentration in the hypothalamus; when it is released, it is an intense inhibitor of the release, and probably also the synthesis, of prolactin by the lactotrope cells of the pituitary.

Many, perhaps most, of the cases of inappropriate lactation are fundamentally due to failure of PIF, either because of a defect in synthesis or a defect in receptor binding. Thyrotropin-releasing hormone (TRH) and LHRH (designated by some as *luliberin*) produce elevated prolactin levels, probably mediated through PIF abnormalities. Prolactin levels in chronic renal failure are significantly elevated, most likely as a result of defects in PIF synthesis or use.

Drugs that are dopamine antagonists (*e.g.*, chlorpromazine and similar antipsychotics) can cause prolactin release and consequent lactation. Dopamine agonists would be expected to have the opposite effect. One such drug, 2-bromo-α-ergocryptine (bromocriptine) has had extensive clinical trial and is now clinically available as bromocriptine mesylate (Parlodel). Like dopamine, bromocriptine activates the dopamine receptors of the lactotrope cells, suppressing prolactin release, lowering serum prolactin levels, and, in galactorrhea–amenorrhea, leading to resumption of ovulation and menstruation. The mechanism of the latter effect is not clear; the likely explanation is that the decrease in prolactin levels removes the impediment to secretion of gonadotropin-releasing factors by the hypothalamus, permits resumption of cyclic fluctuations in pituitary gonadotropins, and relieves the block to gonadotropin action on the ovary.

At present, the Food and Drug Administration (FDA) stipulates that bromocriptine may be used for 1) suppression of postpartum lactation and 2) for treatment of the galactorrhea–amenorrhea syndrome, but *only* a) if the duration of treatment does not ex-

TABLE 46-3. MAIN CAUSES OF HYPERPROLACTINEMIA AND GALACTORRHEA

Physiologic Causes	Pathologic Causes
Pregnancy	Drugs
Childbirth	Dopamine-receptor antagonists—*e.g.,* chlorpromazine, metoclopramide
Mechanical breast stimulation	Dopamine-depleting drugs—*e.g.* reserpine
Stress	α-Methyldopa
Neonatal	Hypothalamic–pituitary disease—*e.g.* pituitary adenomas, craniopharyngiomas, and cysts
	Myxedema (excess thyrotropin-releasing hormone)
	Chronic renal disease, particularly with hemodialysis

(Modified from Parker D: N Engl J Med 301:873, 1979)

ceed 6 months, b) if the patient does not have a pro-lactin-secreting pituitary tumor, and c) if the patient uses mechanical (not oral) contraceptives for the duration of treatment. Mechanical contraception is necessary because bromocriptine can induce ovulation even if oral contraception is being used and because it may have teratogenic effects.

PITUITARY TUMORS

Pituitary tumors are an important cause of galactorrhea–amenorrhea, and they account for a considerable number of cases of infertility. Most, but not all, of the pituitary tumors that give rise to elevated prolactin levels involve the lactotrope cells and are designated by some as prolactinomas.

The diagnosis requires first that other causes of galactorrhea–amenorrhea–hyperprolactinemia be ruled out, primarily, hypothyroidism and drug ingestion. After this has been done, the possibility of tumor should be considered. In the presence of tumor, the normal circadian variation in the serum prolactin level (lowest at noon, highest after sleep) is lost, as is the normal prolactin response to TRH. In about 65% of pituitary tumors, the serum prolactin is elevated. In one series, all levels above 300 ng/ml were associated with tumor; among women with galactorrhea, 57% of those with serum prolactin higher than 100 ng/ml had demonstrable pituitary tumors. Pituitary polytomograms are usually definitive in making the diagnosis.

Three modalities are available for the treatment of prolactin-secreting pituitary adenomas: radiation, surgery, and bromocriptine (in Europe and Canada). Radiation is rarely used at present; gland size may not diminish for as long as 6 months (an important consideration if encroachment of the tumor on the optic chiasm has caused visual field defects), and secretion of other pituitary hormones may be damaged. Surgery, usually by the microsurgical transsphenoidal approach, has gained wide acceptance as a safe and effective means of removing pituitary tumors, and, until the advent of bromocriptine, this was the treatment of choice for all such tumors. In the countries where bromocriptine may be used for this purpose, it has been shown to have a prompt and profound effect in reducing the size of pituitary tumors. Although the drug is clearly effective, an exact protocol for its use has not yet been defined. Some have advocated this drug for all prolactinomas (and growth hormone–producing tumors). Some recommend its use only for microadenomas (tumors less than 1 cm in diameter) and employ surgery for all macroadenomas and tumors that produce visual field defects. Some prefer to shrink the larger tumors with bromocriptine prior to surgical removal. The exact mechanism by which these dramatic effects are achieved is not known.

HIRSUTISM AND VIRILISM

Hirsutism in the female refers to an abnormal and sometimes sudden growth of hair in purportedly unusual areas—chin, upper lip, rhomboid of Michaelis, inner aspects of the thighs, around the areolae, and on the lower abdomen, producing a male escutcheon. It is emphasized that the mere presence of hair in these areas does not constitute hirsutism, since hair growth of this kind is often a familial or racial characteristic. Rather, the term refers to the sudden appearance of hair where none had been present before or an unusual acceleration of growth. *Virilism* refers to actual masculinization, usually characterized by hirsutism, voice changes, receding temporal hairline, assumption of male habitus and muscle distribution, and enlargement of the clitoris. Virilism invariably results from excess androgen; hirsutism can result either from excess androgen or from nonendocrine causes (Table 46–4). In each patient, all the factors should be given at least passing consideration. Virilism of special interest to the gynecologist is that resulting from endogenous androgen excess.

Since androgens are precursors in the biosynthetic pathway for both estrogen and cortisol, distortion or interruption of either pathway can result in androgen excess. Such precursor substances as dehydroepiandrosterone and androstenedione are formed in both the ovary and the adrenal. Both are themselves weak androgens, but, in sufficient amounts, they can produce hirsutism or even virilism. Moreover, both can be metabolized to testosterone by such peripheral tissues as skin, liver, and kidney. In this connection, it should be remembered that very large amounts of the androgenic precursors are required to produce the same masculinizing effects that can result from a minute excess of testosterone. Accordingly, virilism resulting from such substances as androstenedione or dehydroepiandrosterone produces significant elevations of urinary 17-KS, whereas, if testosterone is at fault, the elevation of 17-KS may be trivial or may not appear at all.

The history, with special note of any menstrual deviations, and physical examination may disclose stigmas that suggest likely areas for investigation. Masculinizing ovarian tumors are extremely rare, and often such a tumor is so small that the ovary is not significantly enlarged; however, an enlarged ovary requires investigation. In the presence of acquired hirsutism, laparotomy is usually required. If the hirsutism is clearly not a familial or ethnic trait, and if drugs, central nervous system disease, and pituitary disease can be confidently ruled out, an effort should be made to determine whether androgen is indeed present in excessive amounts and, if so, its source. First, 24-hour urinary excretion of 17-KS and 17-OHCS should be determined, and plasma testosterone values should be obtained. Depending on these find-

TABLE 46-4. CAUSES OF HIRSUTISM

A. Heredity
1. Familial hypertrichosis
2. Hair follicle sensitivity to normal endogenous androgens (or increased peripheral presence of dihydrotestosterone)
3. Precocious pubarche or adrenarche
4. Male with hermaphroditism raised as a female (at puberty)
B. Cerebral cortex and hypothalamus
1. Encephalitis
2. Multiple sclerosis
3. Hyperostosis frontalis interna
C. Pituitary
1. Acromegaly
2. Achard–Thiers syndrome (bearded diabetes)
3. Cushing's disease (pituitary basophilism)
D. Thyroid
1. Juvenile hypothyroidism
E. Adrenal cortex
1. Adrenogenital syndrome
2. Cushing's syndrome
F. Ovary
1. Menopause
2. Stein–Leventhal syndrome
3. Hyperthecosis
4. Stromal luteinization
5. Hilar cell hyperplasia
6. Ovarian tumors
   a. Hilar cell adenoma
   b. Luteoma
   c. Arrhenoblastoma
   d. Adrenal rest tumor
   e. Mixed tumors (gynandroblastoma)
G. Miscellaneous
1. Exogenous medications
   a. Androgens
   b. Dilantin
   c. Some synthetic progestins
   d. Cortisone and related steroids
2. Pregnancy
3. Anorexia nervosa
4. Some acute stressful situations
5. Local irritation
6. Idiopathic

(Gold JJ (ed): Gynecologic Endocrinology, 2nd ed. Hagerstown, MD, Harper & Row, 1975)

ings, the effects of adrenal and ovarian suppression and stimulation can be measured in an effort to determine the nature of the abnormality. Adrenal and ovarian vein catheterizations have proved helpful in locating the source of androgen production in some cases, although the results are sometimes equivocal and, occasionally, even misleading.

In many cases of hirsutism, all test results are normal. Conditions that may be identified in such an investigation include polycystic ovarian disease, adrenogenital syndrome, Cushing's syndrome, and masculinizing ovarian tumor. In each of these cases, effective treatment may or may not arrest the hirsutism; usually, new hair growth is stopped, but the hair already present does not disappear. After menopause, many women note an increase in body hair. This is most likely due to the higher testosterone/estrogen ratio that appears after the menopause.

Depilatories and electrolysis should be prescribed as needed. Shaving is an appropriate means of dealing with excessive hair growth; contrary to popular belief, it neither accelerates hair growth nor stimulates new growth.

Some cases of hirsutism are believed to result from excessive sensitivity of the hair follicles to normal amounts of circulating endogenous androgen; others may result from steroid biosynthetic derangements not detectable by conventional laboratory methods. For example, in premenopausal women with idiopathic hirsutism, it has been shown that the metabolism of Δ 5-pregnene may be abnormal. It is likely that many of these problems will be clarified as more is learned about the rates of production and metabolism of the responsible steroid hormones. In the meantime, preliminary data suggest that both spironolactone, an aldosterone antagonist, and cimetidine, an agent that blocks androgen action at the hair follicle, may be helpful in dealing with the problem of hirsutism.

REFERENCES AND RECOMMENDED READING

GENERAL

Gold JJ, Josimovich JB (eds): Gynecologic Endocrinology, 3rd ed. Hagerstown, MD, Harper & Row, 1980

Speroff L, Glass RH, Kase NG: Clinical Gynecologic Endocrinology and Infertility, 2nd ed. Baltimore, William & Wilkins, 1978

Wilkins L: Diagnosis and Treatment of Endocrine Disorders in Childhood and Adolescence, 2nd ed. Springfield, IL, Charles C Thomas, 1967

Yen SSC, Jaffe RB: Reproductive Endocrinology. Philadelphia, WB Saunders, 1978

ABNORMAL UTERINE BLEEDING

Arronet GH, Arrata WSM: Dysfunctional uterine bleeding. Obstet Gynecol 29:97, 1967

Claessens EA, Cowell CA: Acute adolescent menorrhagia. Am J Obstet Gynecol 139:277, 1081

Jones GS: Luteal phase defects. In Behrman SJ, Kistner RW (eds): Progress in Infertility, 2nd ed, pp 299–325. Boston, Little Brown, 1978

Sherman BM, Korenman SG: Measurement of serum LH, FSH, estradiol and progesterone in disorders of the human menstrual cycle: The inadequate luteal phase. J Clin Endocrinol Metab 39:145, 1974

INFERTILITY

Kamran S. Moghissi
Tommy N. Evans

Barren marriages have played an important historical role, affecting the fate of nations and empires. Most women have a strong desire to bear children. Failure to do so may be tragic for some women and can result in unhappiness, marital discord, and ill health. Approximately 10%–15% of married couples in the United States are infertile.

The terms *sterility* and *infertility* are often used interchangeably. However, *sterility* is better applied to describe the woman who can never become pregnant because of a congenital anomaly, disease, or operation. *Infertility* is used to describe the presumably normal patient who is unable to conceive during a specific period of time, usually 1 year. Primary infertility exists when there has been no prior conception. Secondary infertility may follow one or more previous pregnancies.

In determining the cause of infertility and in treating it, the physician must consider the couple to-gether. Although it is usually the woman who initiates an infertility investigation, simultaneous investigation of the husband is important. Approximately 40% of barren marriages are due to some defect in the husband, a fact that is often difficult for a husband to accept.

Diagnosis of infertility should not be based on an arbitrary period of inability to conceive. Over 60% of fertile couples initiate a pregnancy within 3 months of trying to do so and almost 85% within the first 12 months. Approximately 80% of the couples in the United States practice contraception at some period during their marriages. Contraception *per se* probably does not increase infertility, but the incidence of infertility shows a distinct progression with advancing age. The peak of fertility is between 20 and 25 years of age; fertility decreases after 30 in women and after 40 in men. Older couples, although married only briefly, deserve early investigation. Instruction and reassurance may be all that is required. Spermatozoa are in the fallopian tubes during midcycle in healthy young women who experience coitus three times or more weekly without contraception.

Among couples who seek medical aid because of infertility, about 40% subsequently conceive. In another 40%, the cause of sterility is found but cannot be corrected, so pregnancy is impossible. In the remaining 20%, no pregnancy occurs even though there is no detectable cause of infertility.

CAUSES OF INFERTILITY IN THE FEMALE

Female fertility depends upon 1) normal ovarian function, 2) endocrine preparation of a normal uterus for implantation, 3) cervical mucus favorable for sperm transport, 4) normal anatomic development permitting coitus, 5) lack of obstruction, and 6) normal tubal function (Fig. 47–1). Physiologic infertility occurs during that period of the cycle remote from the time of ovulation, during pregnancy, after menopause, and, frequently, during lactation.

VAGINAL ABNORMALITIES

Vaginal obstruction to intromission may result from a rigid hymen or a small hymenal orifice. Less commonly, it is due to an intact hymen or congenital absence of the vagina. Psychogenic vaginismus may also occur. Pregnancy is rarely achieved when the ejaculate is deposited at the vaginal introitus without intromission.

Adequacy of vaginal secretions may be important. Normal vaginal fluid is acid (pH 3–5) and inactivates spermatozoa in a short time. Seminal fluid is alkaline and, together with cervical mucus, provides a buffering system that renders the pH of the upper vagina

Treloar AE, Boynton RE, Behn BG: Variation of the human menstrual cycle through reproductive life. Int J Fertil 12(1):77, 1967

Vandekerckhove D, Dhont M: The relationship between serum LH levels, as determined by radioimmunoassay, and the life span of the corpus luteum. Ann Endocrinol (Paris) 33:205, 1972

Vande Wiele RL, Bogumil RJ, Dyrenfurth I et al.: Regulation of the menstrual cycle in women. Recent Prog Horm Res 26:63, 1970

Van Look PFA, Lothian H, Hunter WM et al.: Hypothalamic–pituitary–ovarian function in perimenopausal women. Clin Endocrinol (Oxf) 7(1):13, 1977

Vigersky RA, Mehlman I, Glass AR et al.: Treatment of hirsute women with cimetidine. N Engl J Med 303:1042, 1980

Wu CH: Estrogen–androgen balance in hirsutism. Fertil Steril 32:269, 1979

Yen SSC, Vandenberg C, Rebar R et al.: Variations of pituitary responsiveness to synthetic LRF during different phases of the menstrual cycle. J Clin Endocrinol Metab 35:931, 1972

Yen SSC, Vicic WJ: Serum follicle stimulating hormone levels and puberty. Am J Obstet Gynecol 106:134, 1970

Yen SSC, Vicic WJ, Kearchner DV: Gonadotropin levels in puberty: I. Serum luteinizing hormone. J Clin Endocrinol Metab 29:382, 1968

releasing hormone testing. Am J Obstet Gynecol 135:651, 1979

Stein IF, Leventhal ML: Amenorrhea associated with bilateral polycystic ovaries. Am J Obstet Gynecol 29:818, 1935

Tolis G: Prolactin: Physiology and pathology. Hosp Pract 15:85, 1980

Tulandi T, Kinch RAH: Premature ovarian failure. Obstet Gynecol Surv 36:521, 1981

Tyson JE, Zacur RA: Diagnosis and treatment of abnormal lactation. Clin Obstet Gynecol 18:65, 1975

Utian WH, Begg G, Vinik AI et al.: Effect of bromocryptine and chlorotrianisene on inhibition of lactation and serum prolactin: A comparative double blind study. Br J Obstet Gynaecol 82:755, 1975

Vaughn TC, Haney AF, Wiebe RH et al.: Spontaneous regression of prolactin-producing pituitary adenomas. Am J Obstet Gynecol 136:980, 1980

Wass JAH, Moult PJA, Thorner MO et al.: Reduction of pituitary-tumour size in patients with prolactinomas and acromegaly treated with bromocriptine with or without radiotherapy. Lancet 2:66, 1979

Weiland AJ, Bookstein JJ, Cleary RE et al.: Preoperative localization of virilizing tumors by selective venous sampling. Am J Obstet Gynecol 131:797, 1978

Wentz AC, Jones GS: Prognosis in primary amenorrhea. Fertil Steril 29:614, 1978

Wiebe RH, Hammond CH, Handwerger S: Prolactin-secreting pituitary microadenoma: Detection and evaluation. Fertil Steril 29:282, 1978

Wolf AS, Musch K, Lauritzen C: Hyperprolactinemia in anovulatory women: Incidence and endocrine features. J Endocrinol Invest. 2:5, 1979

Yen SSC, Tsai CC, Vandenberg G et al.: Gonadotropin dynamics in patients with gonadal dysgenesis: A model for the study of gonadotropin regulation. J Clin Endocrinol Metab 35:897, 1972

Younglai EV, Richmond H, Atyeo R et al.: Arrhenoblastoma in vivo and in vitro studies. Am J Obstet Gynecol 116:401, 1973

Zervas NT, Martin JB: Management of hormone-secreting pituitary adenomas. N Engl J Med 302:210, 1980

TOXIC SHOCK SYNDROME

Davis JP, Chesney J, Wand PJ et al.: Toxic shock syndrome. Epidemiologic features, recurrence, risk factors, and prevention. N Engl J Med 303:1429, 1980

Shands KN, Schmid GP, Dan BB et al.: Toxic shock syndrome in menstruating women. Association with tampon use and *Staphylococcus aureus* and clinical features in 52 cases. N Engl J Med 303:1436, 1980

Tofte RW, Crossley KB: Clinical experience with toxic shock syndromes. Letter to the Editor. N Engl J Med 303:1417, 1980

MISCELLANEOUS

Astwood EB: Estrogens and progestins. In Goodman LS, Gilman A (eds): The Pharmacologic Basis of Therapeutics, 4th ed, pp 1538–1564. New York, Macmillan, 1970

Bogumil RJ, Ferin M, Rootenberg J et al.: Mathematical studies of the human menstrual cycle: I. Formulation of a mathematical model. J Clin Endocrinol Metab 35:126, 1972

Bogumil RJ, Ferin M, Vande Wiele RL: Mathematical studies of the human menstrual cycle: II. Stimulation performance of a model of the human menstrual cycle. J Clin Endocrinol Metab 35:144, 1972

Boiselle A, Tremblay RR: New therapeutic approach to hirsute patient. Fertil Steril 32:276, 1979

Chari S, Hopkinson CRN, Duane E et al.: Purification of "inhibin" from human follicular fluid. Acta Endocrinol 90:157, 1979

Cruikshank DP, Chapler FK, Yannone ME: Differential adrenal and ovarian suppression. Obstet Gynecol 38:724, 1971

Cumming DC, Yang JC, Rebar RW et al.: Treatment of hirsutism with spironolactone. Abstr of 1981 meeting of Society for Gynecologic Investigation.

Cushing H: The basophil adenomas of the pituitary body and their clinical manifestations. Bull Johns Hopkins Hosp 50:137, 1932

Dinnerstein AJ, O'Leary JA: Granulosa-theca cell tumors. Obstet Gynecol 31:654, 1968

Dunnihoo DR, Grieme DL, Woolf RB: Hilar cell tumors of the ovary. Obstet Gynecol 27:703, 1966

Goldston WR, Johnston WW, Fetter BF et al.: Clinicopathologic studies in feminizing tumors of the ovary. Am J Obstet Gynecol 112:422, 1972

Keye WR Jr, Chang J, Wilson CB et al.: Prolactin-secreting pituitary adenomas. III. Frequency and diagnosis in amenorrhea-galactorrhea. JAMA 244:1329, 1980

Liddle GW: The adrenal cortex. In Williams RH (ed): Textbook of Endocrinology, 5th ed, pp 233–322. Philadelphia, WB Saunders, 1974

Novak ER, Kutchmeshgi J, Mupas RS et al.: Feminizing gonadal stromal tumors. Obstet Gynecol 38:701, 1971

Noyes RW, Hertig AT, Rock J: Dating the endometrial biopsy. Fertil Steril 1:3, 1950

Rock J, Garcia CR, Pincus G: Synthetic progestins in the normal human menstrual cycle. Recent Prog Horm Res 13:323, 1957

Ross GT, Cargille CM, Lipsett MB et al.: Pituitary and gonadal hormones in women during spontaneous and induced ovulatory cycles. Recent Prog Horm Res 26:1, 1970

Ross GT, Vande Wiele RL: The ovaries. In Williams RH (ed): Textbook of Endocrinology, 5th ed, pp 368–422. Philadelphia, WB Saunders, 1974

Rothchild IM: Functional amenorrhea. In Mack HC, Sherman AI (eds): The Neuroendocrinology of Human Reproduction, pp 171–182. Springfield, IL, Charles C Thomas, 1971

Sherman BM, Korenman SG: Hormonal characteristics of the human menstrual cycle throughout reproductive life. J Clin Invest 55:699, 1975

Sherman BM, West JH, Korenman SG: The menopausal transition: Analysis of LH, FSH, estradiol, and progesterone concentrations during menstrual cycle of older women. J Clin Endocrinol Metab 42:629, 1976

Steinberger A, Steinberger E: Secretion of an FSH inhibiting factor in cultured Sertoli cells. Endocrinology 99:918, 1976

Strauss S, Pochi PE: The hormonal control of human sebaceous glands: Observations in certain endocrine disorders. In Astwood EB, Cassidy CE (eds): Clinical Endocrinology II, pp 798–808. New York, Grune & Stratton, 1968

Swerdloff RS, Odell WD: Serum luteinizing and follicle stimulating hormone levels during sequential and nonsequential contraception of eugonadal women. J Clin Endocrinol Metab 29:157, 1969

Tramont CB: Cyclic hormone therapy: A report of 305 cases. Geriatrics 21:212, 1966

Van Look PFA, Hunter WM, Fraser IS et al.: Impaired estrogen-induced luteinizing hormone release in young women with anovulatory dysfunctional uterine bleeding. J Clin Endocrinol Metab 46:816, 1978

Wallach EE (ed): Dysfunctional uterine bleeding. Clin Obstet Gynecol 13:363, 1970

Yen SSC: Chronic anovulation. In Yen SSC, Jaffe RB (eds): Reproductive Endocrinology, pp 324–340. Philadelphia, WB Saunders, 1978

AMENORRHEA AND RELATED CONDITIONS

Archer DF, Nankin HR, Gabos PF et al.: Serum prolactin in patients with inappropriate lactation. Am J Obstet Gynecol 119:466, 1974

Bardin CW, Lipsett MB: Testosterone and androstenedione blood production rates in normal women and women with idiopathic hirsutism or polycystic ovaries. J Clin Invest 46:891, 1967

Board JA, Redwine FO, Moncure CW et al.: Identification of differing etiologies of clinically diagnosed premature menopause. Am J Obstet Gynecol 134:936, 1979

Boyd AE, Reichlin S: Galactorrhea–amenorrhea, bromergocrytine and the dopamine receptor. N Engl J Med 293:451, 1975

Burry KA, Schiller HS, Mills R et al.: Acute visual loss during pregnancy after bromocriptine-induced ovulation: The elusive tumor. Obstet Gynecol 52:19s, 1978

Coulam CB, Ryan RJ: Premature menopause I: Etiology. Am J Obstet Gynecol 133:639, 1979

DeClercq JA, van de Calseyde JF: Polycystic ovarian disease: Diagnosis, frequency and symptoms in a general gynaecological practice. Br J Obstet Gynaecol 84:380, 1977

DiZerega G, Kletsky OA, Mishell DR: Diagnosis of Sheehan's syndrome using a sequential pituitary stimulation test. Am J Obstet Gynecol 132:348, 1978

Domingue JN, Richmond IL, Wilson CB: Results of surgery in 114 patients with prolactin-secreting pituitary adenomas. Am J Obstet Gynecol 137:102, 1980

Frantz AG: Prolactin. N Engl J Med 298:201, 1978

Frisch RE, McArthur JW: Menstrual cycles: Fatness as a determinant of minimum weight for height necessary for their maintenance or onset. Science 185:949, 1974

Frisch RE, Wyshak G, Vincent L: Delayed menarche and amenorrhea in ballet dancers. N Engl J Med 303:17, 1980

Goldenberg RL, Grodin JM, Rodbard D et al.: Gonadotropins in women with amenorrhea. Am J Obstet Gynecol 116:1003, 1973

Goldzieher J: Polycystic ovarian disease. Clin Obstet Gynecol 16:82, 1973

Gonzalez ER: Hyperprolactinemia: Still perplexing but eminently treatable. JAMA 242:401, 1979

Greenblatt RB, Mahesh VB: Some new thoughts on the Stein–Leventhal syndrome. J Reprod Med 13:85, 1974

Greenblatt RB, Mahesh VB, Gambrell RD: Arrhenoblastoma. Obstet Gynecol 39:567, 1972

Griffin JE, Wilson JD: The syndromes of androgen resistance. N Engl J Med 302:198, 1980

Groll M: Gonadotropic patterns in psychogenic amenorrhea. Int J Gynaecol Obstet 16:53, 1978

Hsu LKG, Crisp AH, Harding B: Outcome of anorexia nervosa. Lancet 1:61, 1979

Jewelewicz R, Zimmerman EA: Current management of the amenorrhea–galactorrhea syndrome. Fertil Steril 29:597, 1978

Judd HL, Rigg LE, Anderson DC et al.: The effects of ovarian wedge resection on circulating gonadotropin and ovarian steroid levels in patients with polycystic ovary syndrome. J Clin Endocrinol Metab 43:347, 1976

Katz M, Carr PJ, Cohen BM et al.: Hormonal effects of wedge resection of polycystic ovaries. Obstet Gynecol 51:437, 1978

Kirschner MA, Bardin CW: Androgen production and metabolism in normal and virilized women. Metabolism 21:667, 1972

Korth-Schutz S, Virdis R, Saenger P et al.: Serum androgens as a continuing index of adequacy of treatment of congenital adrenal hyperplasia. J Clin Endocrinol Metab 46:452, 1978

Larsen JW, Warsof SL, Kent SG et al.: Prenatal diagnosis of congenital adrenal hyperplasia (CAH) in twin females by measurement of amniotic fluid androstenedione (Δ_4A) and 17α-hydroxyprogesterone (17-OHP) concentrations. Abstracts of 1979 Meeting of the Society for Gynecologic Investigation

McGregor AM, Hall K, Scanlon MF et al.: Reduction in size of a pituitary tumor by bromocriptine therapy. N Engl J Med 300:291, 1979 (See also letter to editor, idem, ibid 300:1392, 1979.)

McKenna TJ, Miller RB, Liddle GW: Plasma pregnenolone and 17-OH-pregnenolone in patients with adrenal tumors, ACTH excess, or idiopathic hirsutism. J Clin Endocrinol Metab 44:231, 1977

Morris JM, Mahesh VG: Further observation on the syndrome "testicular feminization." Am J Obstet Gynecol 87:731, 1963

Murray FT, Osterman J, Sulewski J et al.: Pituitary function following surgery for prolactinomas. Obstet Gynecol 54:65, 1979

Nader S, Kjeld JM, Blair CM et al.: A study of the effects of bromocryptine on serum oestradiol, prolactin, and follicle stimulating hormone levels in puerperal women. Br J Obstet Gynaecol 82:750, 1975

Parkes D: Drug therapy: Bromocryptine. N Engl J Med 301:873, 1979

Perez-Lopez FR: Hypothalamic pituitary disorders expressed by galactorrhea. Obstet Gynecol 46:621, 1975

Post K, Biller BJ, Adelman LS et al.: Selective transsphenoidal adenomectomy in women with galactorrhea–amenorrhea. JAMA 242:158, 1979

Raj SG, Thompson IE, Berger MJ et al.: Clinical aspects of the polycystic ovary syndrome. Obstet Gynecol 49:552, 1977

Raj SG, Thompson IE, Berger MJ et al.: Diagnostic value of androgen measurement in polycystic ovary syndrome. Obstet Gynecol 52:169, 1978

Rebar RW, Harman SM, Vaitukaitis JL: Differential responsiveness of LRF after estrogen therapy in women with hypothalamic amenorrhea. J Clin Endocrinol Metab 46:48, 1978

Rowe TC, Shearman RP, Fraser IS: Antecedent factors and outcome in amenorrhea–galactorrhea. Obstet Gynecol 54:535, 1979

Shearman RP, Smith ID: Statistical analysis of relationship between oral contraceptives, secondary amenorrhea and galactorrhea. J Obstet Gynaecol Br Commonw 79:654, 1972

Sheehan HL: The incidence of postpartum hypopituitarism. Am J Obstet Gynecol 68:202, 1954

Shewchuk AB, Adamson GD, Lessard P et al.: The effect of pregnancy on suspected pituitary adenomas after conservative management of ovulation defects associated with galactorrhea. Am J Obstet Gynecol 136:659, 1980

Soules MR, Jelovsek FR, Wiebe RH et al.: Amenorrhea: Observations based on the analysis of luteinizing hormone-

TABLE 46-4. CAUSES OF HIRSUTISM

A. Heredity
  1. Familial hypertrichosis
  2. Hair follicle sensitivity to normal endogenous androgens (or increased peripheral presence of dihydrotestosterone)
  3. Precocious pubarche or adrenarche
  4. Male with hermaphroditism raised as a female (at puberty)
B. Cerebral cortex and hypothalamus
  1. Encephalitis
  2. Multiple sclerosis
  3. Hyperostosis frontalis interna
C. Pituitary
  1. Acromegaly
  2. Achard–Thiers syndrome (bearded diabetes)
  3. Cushing's disease (pituitary basophilism)
D. Thyroid
  1. Juvenile hypothyroidism
E. Adrenal cortex
  1. Adrenogenital syndrome
  2. Cushing's syndrome
F. Ovary
  1. Menopause
  2. Stein–Leventhal syndrome
  3. Hyperthecosis
  4. Stromal luteinization
  5. Hilar cell hyperplasia
  6. Ovarian tumors
     a. Hilar cell adenoma
     b. Luteoma
     c. Arrhenoblastoma
     d. Adrenal rest tumor
     e. Mixed tumors (gynandroblastoma)
G. Miscellaneous
  1. Exogenous medications
     a. Androgens
     b. Dilantin
     c. Some synthetic progestins
     d. Cortisone and related steroids
  2. Pregnancy
  3. Anorexia nervosa
  4. Some acute stressful situations
  5. Local irritation
  6. Idiopathic

(Gold JJ (ed): Gynecologic Endocrinology, 2nd ed. Hagerstown, MD, Harper & Row, 1975)

ings, the effects of adrenal and ovarian suppression and stimulation can be measured in an effort to determine the nature of the abnormality. Adrenal and ovarian vein catheterizations have proved helpful in locating the source of androgen production in some cases, although the results are sometimes equivocal and, occasionally, even misleading.

In many cases of hirsutism, all test results are normal. Conditions that may be identified in such an investigation include polycystic ovarian disease, adrenogenital syndrome, Cushing's syndrome, and masculinizing ovarian tumor. In each of these cases, effective treatment may or may not arrest the hirsutism; usually, new hair growth is stopped, but the hair already present does not disappear. After menopause, many women note an increase in body hair. This is most likely due to the higher testosterone/estrogen ratio that appears after the menopause.

Depilatories and electrolysis should be prescribed as needed. Shaving is an appropriate means of dealing with excessive hair growth; contrary to popular belief, it neither accelerates hair growth nor stimulates new growth.

Some cases of hirsutism are believed to result from excessive sensitivity of the hair follicles to normal amounts of circulating endogenous androgen; others may result from steroid biosynthetic derangements not detectable by conventional laboratory methods. For example, in premenopausal women with idiopathic hirsutism, it has been shown that the metabolism of Δ 5-pregnene may be abnormal. It is likely that many of these problems will be clarified as more is learned about the rates of production and metabolism of the responsible steroid hormones. In the meantime, preliminary data suggest that both spironolactone, an aldosterone antagonist, and cimetidine, an agent that blocks androgen action at the hair follicle, may be helpful in dealing with the problem of hirsutism.

REFERENCES AND RECOMMENDED READING

GENERAL

Gold JJ, Josimovich JB (eds): Gynecologic Endocrinology, 3rd ed. Hagerstown, MD, Harper & Row, 1980
Speroff L, Glass RH, Kase NG: Clinical Gynecologic Endocrinology and Infertility, 2nd ed. Baltimore, William & Wilkins, 1978
Wilkins L: Diagnosis and Treatment of Endocrine Disorders in Childhood and Adolescence, 2nd ed. Springfield, IL, Charles C Thomas, 1967
Yen SSC, Jaffe RB: Reproductive Endocrinology. Philadelphia, WB Saunders, 1978

ABNORMAL UTERINE BLEEDING

Arronet GH, Arrata WSM: Dysfunctional uterine bleeding. Obstet Gynecol 29:97, 1967
Claessens EA, Cowell CA: Acute adolescent menorrhagia. Am J Obstet Gynecol 139:277, 1081
Jones GS: Luteal phase defects. In Behrman SJ, Kistner RW (eds): Progress in Infertility, 2nd ed, pp 299–325. Boston, Little Brown, 1978
Sherman BM, Korenman SG: Measurement of serum LH, FSH, estradiol and progesterone in disorders of the human menstrual cycle: The inadequate luteal phase. J Clin Endocrinol Metab 39:145, 1974

ceed 6 months, b) if the patient does not have a pro-lactin-secreting pituitary tumor, and c) if the patient uses mechanical (not oral) contraceptives for the duration of treatment. Mechanical contraception is necessary because bromocriptine can induce ovulation even if oral contraception is being used and because it may have teratogenic effects.

PITUITARY TUMORS

Pituitary tumors are an important cause of galactorrhea–amenorrhea, and they account for a considerable number of cases of infertility. Most, but not all, of the pituitary tumors that give rise to elevated prolactin levels involve the lactotrope cells and are designated by some as prolactinomas.

The diagnosis requires first that other causes of galactorrhea–amenorrhea–hyperprolactinemia be ruled out, primarily, hypothyroidism and drug ingestion. After this has been done, the possibility of tumor should be considered. In the presence of tumor, the normal circadian variation in the serum prolactin level (lowest at noon, highest after sleep) is lost, as is the normal prolactin response to TRH. In about 65% of pituitary tumors, the serum prolactin is elevated. In one series, all levels above 300 ng/ml were associated with tumor; among women with galactorrhea, 57% of those with serum prolactin higher than 100 ng/ml had demonstrable pituitary tumors. Pituitary polytomograms are usually definitive in making the diagnosis.

Three modalities are available for the treatment of prolactin-secreting pituitary adenomas: radiation, surgery, and bromocriptine (in Europe and Canada). Radiation is rarely used at present; gland size may not diminish for as long as 6 months (an important consideration if encroachment of the tumor on the optic chiasm has caused visual field defects), and secretion of other pituitary hormones may be damaged. Surgery, usually by the microsurgical transsphenoidal approach, has gained wide acceptance as a safe and effective means of removing pituitary tumors, and, until the advent of bromocriptine, this was the treatment of choice for all such tumors. In the countries where bromocriptine may be used for this purpose, it has been shown to have a prompt and profound effect in reducing the size of pituitary tumors. Although the drug is clearly effective, an exact protocol for its use has not yet been defined. Some have advocated this drug for all prolactinomas (and growth hormone–producing tumors). Some recommend its use only for microadenomas (tumors less than 1 cm in diameter) and employ surgery for all macroadenomas and tumors that produce visual field defects. Some prefer to shrink the larger tumors with bromocriptine prior to surgical removal. The exact mechanism by which these dramatic effects are achieved is not known.

HIRSUTISM AND VIRILISM

Hirsutism in the female refers to an abnormal and sometimes sudden growth of hair in purportedly unusual areas—chin, upper lip, rhomboid of Michaelis, inner aspects of the thighs, around the areolae, and on the lower abdomen, producing a male escutcheon. It is emphasized that the mere presence of hair in these areas does not constitute hirsutism, since hair growth of this kind is often a familial or racial characteristic. Rather, the term refers to the sudden appearance of hair where none had been present before or an unusual acceleration of growth. *Virilism* refers to actual masculinization, usually characterized by hirsutism, voice changes, receding temporal hairline, assumption of male habitus and muscle distribution, and enlargement of the clitoris. Virilism invariably results from excess androgen; hirsutism can result either from excess androgen or from nonendocrine causes (Table 46–4). In each patient, all the factors should be given at least passing consideration. Virilism of special interest to the gynecologist is that resulting from endogenous androgen excess.

Since androgens are precursors in the biosynthetic pathway for both estrogen and cortisol, distortion or interruption of either pathway can result in androgen excess. Such precursor substances as dehydroepiandrosterone and androstenedione are formed in both the ovary and the adrenal. Both are themselves weak androgens, but, in sufficient amounts, they can produce hirsutism or even virilism. Moreover, both can be metabolized to testosterone by such peripheral tissues as skin, liver, and kidney. In this connection, it should be remembered that very large amounts of the androgenic precursors are required to produce the same masculinizing effects that can result from a minute excess of testosterone. Accordingly, virilism resulting from such substances as androstenedione or dehydroepiandrosterone produces significant elevations of urinary 17-KS, whereas, if testosterone is at fault, the elevation of 17-KS may be trivial or may not appear at all.

The history, with special note of any menstrual deviations, and physical examination may disclose stigmas that suggest likely areas for investigation. Masculinizing ovarian tumors are extremely rare, and often such a tumor is so small that the ovary is not significantly enlarged; however, an enlarged ovary requires investigation. In the presence of acquired hirsutism, laparotomy is usually required. If the hirsutism is clearly not a familial or ethnic trait, and if drugs, central nervous system disease, and pituitary disease can be confidently ruled out, an effort should be made to determine whether androgen is indeed present in excessive amounts and, if so, its source. First, 24-hour urinary excretion of 17-KS and 17-OHCS should be determined, and plasma testosterone values should be obtained. Depending on these find-

FIG. 47-1. Causes of infertility. *a.* Defective or inadequate sperm. *b.* Cervical abnormality. *c.* Uterine abnormality. *d.* Tubal abnormality. *e.* Ovarian abnormality (anovulation).

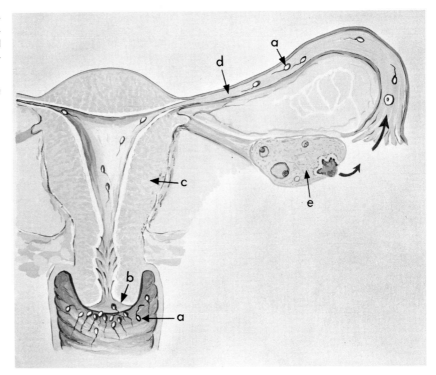

more alkaline. Such a medium seems to be essential for normal sperm transport. Vaginitis may cause dyspareunia and reduce fertility. However, conception can occur despite severe vaginal infection.

CERVICAL ABNORMALITIES

The uterine cervix and its secretions have an important function in reproduction. Cervical mucus is receptive to spermatozoa at or near the time of ovulation and impedes their penetration at other times. The mucus also acts as a sperm reservoir, protects the sperm cells from the hostile environment in the vagina, filters out abnormal and unsuitable spermatozoa, protects sperm from phagocytes, and may play a role in sperm capacitation. Nutrients found in cervical mucus supplement the energy requirements of spermatozoa.

Cervical mucus is a complex secretion produced by the secretory cells of the endocervix. It contains 92%–98% water. The principal constituent of cervical mucus is a carbohydrate-rich glycoprotein of the mucin type. Other constituents include serum type proteins, lipids, enzymes, and inorganic salts.

Secretion of cervical mucus is regulated by the ovarian hormones; estrogens stimulate production of copious amounts of watery mucus, while progesterone inhibits and alters the secretory activity of cervical epithelial cells. Many cyclic changes occur in cervical mucus (Fig. 47–2). At midcycle, near the time of ovulation, cervical mucus becomes more profuse, thinner, alkaline, and acellular; it also exhibits a good spinnbarkheit (Fig. 47–3) or stretchability (5 cm or more). Mucus collected near the time of ovulation and dried reveals a characteristic crystallization pattern or ferning on microscopic examination (Fig. 47–4). Progestational agents and pregnancy changes prevent ferning and abolish spinnbarkheit. A viscous plug of inspissated mucus effectively obstructs sperm penetration. Chronic infection of the endocervix may also impair penetration. However, conception can occur, and frequently does, in patients with extensive cervical erosions and chronic cervicitis. Obstetric and surgical injuries of the cervix (*e.g.,* lacerations, trachelorrhaphy, or amputation) may interfere with conception. Hostile cervical mucus may be demonstrated by placing a drop of midcycle mucus on a coverslip with a drop of normal semen adjacent to it (Miller–Kurzrok test). Failure of penetration of the mucus by spermatozoa suggests unfavorable cervical mucus.

Malpositions, such as elongation and anterior placement of the cervix with retrodisplacement of the uterus, advanced uterine descensus, and a pinhole cervical os, may also interfere with conception. Retroversion of the uterus alone is rarely a cause of infertility. Occasionally, the epithelium of the endocervix is totally destroyed as a result of deep conization, exten-

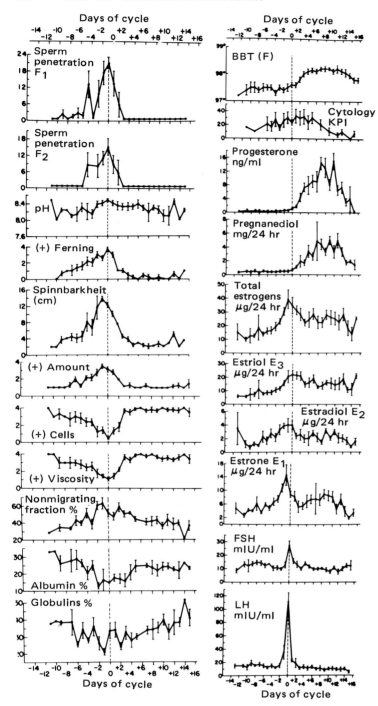

FIG. 47–2. Composite of serum gonadotropin and progesterone levels, urinary estrogen and pregnanediol values, basal body temperature (*BBT*), karyopyknotic index (*KPI*) of vaginal cytology, and cervical mucus properties throughout menstrual cycle in 10 normal women. Day 0 is day of luteotropic hormone (*LH*) peak (*dotted line*). Vertical bars represent 1 standard error of the mean. F_1 and F_2 indicate number of sperm in first and second microscopic fields (×200) from interface, 15 min after start of *in vitro* test of cervical mucus penetration by sperm. (Moghissi KS et al.: Am J Obstet Gynecol 114:405, 1972)

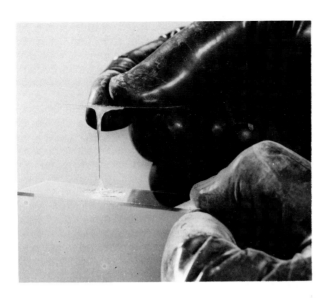

FIG. 47-3. Technique for determining spinnbarkheit (fibrosity) of cervical mucus.

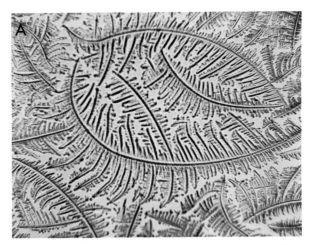

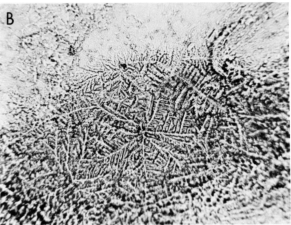

FIG. 47-4. *A.* Typical ferning of cervical mucus at midcycle. *B.* Incomplete (atypical) ferning during early secretory phase of cycle.

sive or repeated cauterization, or cervical amputation. The resultant dry cervix is not compatible with normal function and may cause infertility.

UTERINE ABNORMALITIES

Hypoplasia of the uterus may reflect endocrine disturbance. Prognoses regarding future pregnancy based on uterine size are often in error. With correction of an underlying endocrine imbalance, normal maturation of the uterus may occur.

Inadequate progestational stimulation or inadequate secretory response of the endometrium may prevent nidation of the ovum.

Endometritis, particularly the chronic granulomatous type (*e.g.,* tuberculosis), may affect sperm transport as well as implantation of the fertilized ovum. Amenorrhea and intrauterine synechiae (Asherman's syndrome) may result from inflammatory destruction of the endometrium or, more frequently, from uterine curettage during the postpartum period or after incomplete abortion.

Uterine tumors, especially polyps and fibroids, may cause infertility by distorting the uterine cavity and producing obstruction. Usually, submucous fibroids or large intramural tumors are involved. Interference with vascularity and nutrition of the endometrium may explain infertility associated with fibroids even when there is no significant anatomic displacement. Pregnancy may occur after myomectomy unless there is a demonstrable distortion of the uterine cavity or fallopian tubes. However, fibroids are often of secondary

importance in infertility, since they in turn may be associated with anovulation, hyper- and polymenorrhea, and endometrial hyperplasia. Fibroids are not common in young women. They are usually found after the age of 35, a period of declining fertility.

Congenital malformations of the uterus may be associated with infertility, abortion, and preterm labor.

Prostaglandins are substances found in large amounts in semen, in both male and female generative tracts, and in many other human tissues. They alter uterotubal activity, but their precise role in sperm transport and fertilization is not yet defined.

TUBAL AND PERITONEAL ABNORMALITIES

Peritubal and periovarian adhesions following peritonitis from appendicitis or from postabortal or puerperal

sepsis may interfere with ovum pickup by the fimbriae of the fallopian tube or obstruct entrance of the ovum into the fimbriated end of the tube. Inflammatory damage may interfere with tubal motility, secretions, and ciliogenesis of the endosalpinx, blocking or interfering with sperm migration and ovum transport. Probably 20%–40% of female infertility is due to tubal obstruction. This often follows previous salpingitis but may occur secondary to transient tubal spasm or endometriosis. Endometriosis is more common among infertile women. Both ovarian and parovarian tumors can obstruct the fallopian tube and affect ovulation and entry of the ovum into the tube. Rarely, marked elongation and other congenital defects involving the fallopian tubes are responsible for infertility.

OVARIAN ABNORMALITIES

Anovulatory cycles are common during the first few years after menarche and for several years prior to menopause. Otherwise, ovulation usually occurs in women who are menstruating normally and regularly. Approximately 15% of infertile women have ovulatory defects. Oligomenorrhea and amenorrhea are frequently associated with oligoovulation (infrequent ovulation) or anovulation (lack of ovulation), usually secondary to hypothalamic, pituitary, or ovarian deficits. Less commonly, ovarian tumors, hyper- and hypothyroidism, adrenal dysfunction, and systemic disease prevent ovulation. Even with evidence of continuing ovulation, severely debilitating diseases can lower fertility.

Recent investigations have emphasized the importance of the intraovarian steroid milieu in the regulation of ovulation. The antral fluid of the preovulatory follicle contains relatively large amounts of estradiol and progesterone, low physiologic levels of prolactin, low levels of androgens, and concentrations of LH and FSH that approach 30% and 60%, respectively, of those found in the plasma. Disturbances of the intrafollicular hormonal environment, such as a decrease in estrogen concentration or an increase in the androgen or prolactin level, may lead to anovulation. Hyperprolactinemia (with or without amenorrhea) and galactorrhea may be associated with anovulation or luteal phase defects. In cases of galactorrhea–amenorrhea, particularly when associated with hyperprolactinemia, pituitary adenoma must be suspected and investigated. Other causes of ovulatory defects may be faulty nutrition, metabolic dysfunction, and psychogenic disturbances.

A variant of the abnormal ovulatory process that leads to infertility is a luteal phase defect. There are several types of luteal phase abnormalities: a) an inadequate luteal phase that is associated with deficient corpus luteum function and inadequate progesterone production, b) a short luteal phase defined as a luteal phase of less than 12 days, and c) a luteal phase in which the luteal deficiency is so severe that it may be confused with anovulation. Luteal phase defects may be due to abnormal stimulation of the graffian follicle or to a defective intraovarian milieu, e.g., hyperandrogen states or increased prolactin levels.

PSYCHOGENIC SEXUAL DISTURBANCES

Vaginismus, dyspareunia, and frigidity in the female, and impotence in the male, nearly always are psychogenic. Misapprehension and guilt reactions to normal sexual urges occur. Frequent coitus, masturbation, nocturnal orgasms, and continence have no demonstrable physical ill effects except those secondary to the patient's psychologic reaction. Some patients attribute infertility to lack of libido or orgasm. Although normal sexual response may promote conception, pregnancy does occur without orgasm. Some women who have borne many children deny that they have ever had an orgasm. Dyspareunia and frigidity may be incidental factors when there is no genital disease. Both may reduce fertility by reducing the frequency of coitus. Escape of seminal fluid after coitus probably is of little consequence; only a small amount of seminal fluid in the proper place is required. Furthermore, large numbers of sperm are known to penetrate cervical mucus shortly after ejaculation. Infrequently, apareunia and dyspareunia associated with anxiety and apprehension may be associated with tubal spasm and infertility.

Coitus at 24- to 48-hour intervals during the period of fertility is desirable for conception. Too frequent coitus occasionally impairs fertility, but prolonged abstinence does not necessarily increase fertility.

CAUSES OF INFERTILITY IN THE MALE

Developmental abnormalities such as testicular hypoplasia, cryptorchidism or late descent of the testicles, and testicular dysfunction may cause infertility in the male.

Pituitary gonadotropin stimulates the germinal cells lining the seminiferous tubules to produce spermatozoa and the interstitial cells to secrete androgens. Failure of these functions can result from hypopituitarism and hypothalamic disorders. Spermatogenesis may be deficient or lacking (azospermia) in an otherwise normal male. Virility and libido are regulated by androgens produced by Leydig cells, are unrelated to sperm production, and are usually unaffected even in azospermic men. While male fertility often declines after 40, it may persist into old age. Orchitis due to mumps, tuberculosis, syphilis, or other inflammatory disease may alter spermatogenesis. Inflammatory disease of the epididymis and ductus deferens can result in ob-

structive infertility. Infection of the seminal vesicles and the prostate may alter the quality, volume, and pH of seminal fluid, which serves as a vehicle for spermatozoa and serves other protective and nutritive functions. Gonadal damage resulting from trauma, surgery, or radiation may cause oligospermia or azospermia. Exposure of the testicle to heat reduces spermatogenesis. Varicocele is not a common abnormality, but it may be associated with infertility. Fertility is sometimes restored after ligation of the spermatic vein. In some cases, tight "jockey shorts" can raise scrotal temperatures sufficiently to impair sperm production.

As in the female, systemic debility and stress in the male may reduce fertility. Occupations may be a contributing factor. Fertility appears to be higher among rural than urban people and among manual laborers than those whose work involves intellectual pursuits. Probably, the difference in age at the time of marriage is more important than the social class distribution. Relative frequency of intercourse may also be a factor. Nutritional status of the male is probably not of major importance except when it is prolonged or associated with some endocrine disturbance, such as hypopituitarism or Fröhlich's syndrome. Certain drugs (alkylating agents, sex steroids, alcohol) depress spermatogenesis, and others (*Rauwolfia* derivatives) can depress libido.

In its contribution to infertility, Klinefelter's syndrome (usually sex chromatin–positive) is comparable to Turner's syndrome or ovarian dysgenesis (sex chromatin–negative) in the female. Degenerative changes in the seminiferous tubules may result from torsion of the testes, herniorrhaphy, or a large varicocele or hydrocele. Strictures involving the ejaculatory apparatus may contribute to infertility. The penile urethra and accessory glands concerned with ejaculation may be underdeveloped. Usually, such underdevelopment is associated with generalized hypogonadism. Hypospadias or the much less common epispadias not only can prevent proper deposition of the seminal fluid but also can dissipate the ejaculatory force.

INVESTIGATION OF THE INFERTILE COUPLE

Any couple who seeks medical aid to accomplish pregnancy deserves attention, regardless of the duration or apparent extent of the problem. Not all such couples require full-scale investigation. Anxiety about imagined rather than real infertility may be the only problem. As a general rule, formal infertility study may be deferred until after about 1 year of ordinary effort to achieve pregnancy. Both husband and wife should undergo tests at approximately the same time, and neither should be subjected to extensive investigation without being aware that comparable information is being obtained about the spouse as the investigation

progresses. Early in the investigation, the couple should be apprised of anticipated procedures, duration of investigation, and cost involved. At least 10 months may be required for investigation, therapy, and evaluation of results.

Detailed medical histories and general physical examinations aid in the exclusion of medical and gynecologic disease associated with infertility. *The medical history of the woman* should include information about 1) the patient's age and duration of infertility; 2) duration of marriage and previous marital and sexual history, including pregnancies; 3) pubertal development; 4) previous inflammatory disease and all prior medical treatment; 5) previous surgery, particularly involving the genitourinary system; 6) previous infertility studies and results; 7) marriage compatibility (elicited by indirect questioning); 8) constitutional and metabolic disease; and 9) duration of contraception and methods employed. *The history of the man* should include information about 1) age; 2) pubertal onset and development; 3) general physical status; 4) previous endocrine disease, gonadal trauma, or exposure to radiation; 5) delay in descent of testicles; 6) previous orchitis or prostatitis; 7) previous genital surgery; and 8) past severe illnesses. Separate questioning of the couple is desirable to permit corroboration and to encourage confidential disclosures. Questioning can also provide information regarding the frequency and technique of coitus and the couple's awareness of the fertile time in the menstrual cycle.

During the interviews, the physician can acquire some idea about the motivation of the couple, as well as their fitness, for parenthood. Physical examination of the wife should include a careful pelvic examination, and that of the husband should include examination of the genitalia for the presence of developmental or organic anomalies. Examination may reveal systemic disease that would contraindicate pregnancy. Consciously or subconsciously, the physician's investigation and treatment may be influenced by such judgments. After the first few office visits, enough information may have been obtained to warrant recommending psychiatric evaluation.

Preliminary tests should include urinalysis, complete blood count, and screening tests for venereal disease, *e.g.*, culture for gonorrhea and serologic test for syphilis, on both wife and husband. Additional laboratory tests such as thyroid function tests (for suspected hypo- or hyperthyroidism); measurement of urinary 17-ketosteroids, 17-hydroxysteroids, and pregnanetriol (for suspected adrenal disorders); assay of serum androgens; determination of gonadotropin and prolactin values (for amenorrhea); and buccal smear and chromosomal studies (for genetic disorders) may be performed when indicated.

Successful diagnosis of the cause of infertility and its proper management depend to a large extent on a well-organized and logical workup of the infertile cou-

ple. For the male, the basic infertility survey includes history, physical examination, laboratory tests, and semen analysis. For the female, it involves history; physical examination; laboratory tests; evaluation of the cervix, uterus, tubes, and peritoneum; detection of ovulation; assessment of immunologic compatibility; and evaluation of psychogenic factors. Procedures commonly used in the evaluation of female infertility are

Evaluation of cervix
　Assessment of quantity and quality of cervical mucus
　Postcoital test of interaction between sperm and cervical mucus
　In vitro test of cervical mucus penetration by sperm
Evaluation of uterus
　Hysterosalpingography
　Endometrial biopsy
　Hysteroscopy
Assessment of tubal patency
　Rubin test
　Hysterosalpingography
　Pelvic endoscopy (culdoscopy, laparoscopy)
Assessment of peritoneum
　Culdoscopy
　Laparoscopy
Detection of ovulation
　Recording basal body temperature
　Assessment of quantity and quality of cervical mucus
　Cytologic examination of material from vaginal smear
　Determination of serum progesterone level
　Determination of urinary pregnanediol level
　Endometrial biopsy
Evaluation of immunologic compatibility
　Franklin–Dukes test
　Sperm agglutination tests
　Sperm immobilization tests

Many of these procedures must be performed at a specific time of the menstrual cycle. Some of the studies may be combined, and the order in which they are performed can be altered for the convenience of the patient or to suit specific circumstances.

SEMEN ANALYSIS

Even in a sophisticated laboratory, semen analysis provides only a rough measure of the functional ability of sperm. When infertility is persistent, semen analysis should always be repeated. The usual procedure is to obtain at least two or three semen analyses at 2- to 3-week intervals in order to establish a pattern for various semen characteristics. A specimen obtained shortly after intercourse may be deceptively low in sperm count. Semen collected in a clean wide-mouth

TABLE 47–1. STANDARD SEMEN ANALYSIS

Parameter	Average Values
CONSISTENCY	Fluid (after liquefaction)
COLOR	Opaque
LIQUEFACTION TIME	≤ 20 min
pH	7.2–7.8
VOLUME	2–6 ml
MOTILITY (GRADE 0–4)	$\geq 50\%$
COUNT (MILLIONS/ML)	20–100
VIABILITY (EOSIN)	$\geq 50\%$
MORPHOLOGY (CYTOLOGY) CELL TYPES	$\geq 60\%$ normal oval
CELLS (WHITE BLOOD CELLS, OTHERS)	None to occasional
AGGLUTINATION	None
BIOCHEMICAL STUDIES (*E.G.,* FRUCTOSE, PROSTAGLANDINS, ZINC), IF DESIRED	

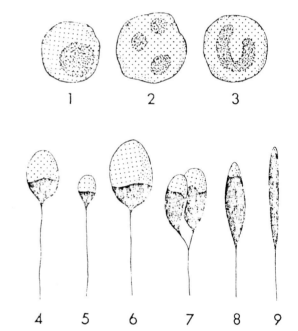

FIG. 47–5. Morphologic variations of spermatozoa. *1, 2,* Immature cells. *3,* White blood cell (for comparison with immature cells). *4,* Oval sperm (normal). *5,* Small (microcytic) sperm. *6,* Large (macrocytic) sperm. *7,* Double-headed (bicephalic) sperm. *8, 9,* Tapering forms.

container either by masturbation or coitus interruptus after 2–5 days continence usually permits an accurate evaluation. A condom should not be used for semen collection since most condoms are treated with spermicidal chemicals that interfere with sperm viability.

The specimen should be kept at room temperature and examined within 1 hour. Table 47–1 shows the information that is usually contained in a semen analysis report. The morphologic variations in spermatozoa are shown in Figure 47–5.

There is no general agreement on a standard quality of semen consistent with fertility. Obviously, a high sperm count, good motility, and a large percentage of normal sperm in an ejaculate that liquefies promptly and is devoid of exogenous cells, debris, immature sperm cells, and agglutination all increase the likelihood of subsequent pregnancy. It is difficult to evaluate the fertility potential of a specimen in which one or several parameters are below average, however. Even with counts below 10 million, provided other semen characteristics (motility and morphology) are not grossly abnormal, pregnancy may occur.

To assess more accurately the fertility potential of sperm, attempts have been made to assay certain sperm acrosomal enzymes, such as acrosin, that are concerned in the fertilization process and to study sperm fertilizing capacity. In the latter technique, the ability of spermatozoa to initiate *in vitro* fertilization of zona-free hamster eggs is used as an index of their fertilizing potential. These experimental methods, although not yet clinically available, indicate the need for more refined techniques to assess male fertility potential.

Volume of less than 1 ml and a total count of less than 50 million are usually associated with infertility, but neither excludes the possibility of impregnation. Except in rare instances, aspermia is uncorrectable. Sometimes a surgically removable obstructive lesion coexists with normal spermatogenesis, but this is not true aspermia. Testicular biopsy aids in the diagnosis of normal spermatogenesis associated with obstructive azospermatosis. Seminal deficiency may be attributed to nutritional deficiency, debilitating illness, metabolic disease, trauma, radiation, gonadotropic inadequacy, obstructive lesions of the epididymis and the vas deferens, and congenital defects such as Klinefelter's syndrome. Determination of 17-ketosteroid excretion rate, serum testosterone value, gonadotropin assays, and testicular biopsy may be required individually or collectively to arrive at the cause of male infertility.

EVALUATION OF THE CERVIX

Survival of spermatozoa within the reproductive tract of the female depends on their prompt penetration of the cervical mucus. Interaction between cervical mucus and sperm is determined by the Sims–Huhner (postcoital) test, which consists of examination of mucus aspirated from the cervical canal 2–8 hours following coitus near the time of ovulation. The quantity and quality of cervical mucus (spinnbarkheit, ferning,

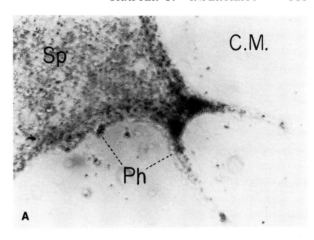

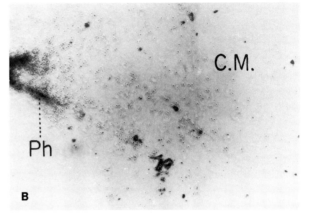

FIG. 47–6. *In vitro* test of cervical mucus penetration by sperm. Phalanx (*Ph*) formation. Spermatozoa (*Sp*) fanning out from apex of phalanges and penetrating cervical mucus (*CM*). (Moghissi KS et al.: Fertil Steril 15:15, 1964)

viscosity, cellularity, and pH) are evaluated. When cervical mucus is suitable and the semen of good quality, there should be at least 10–15 sperm per high-power field in a specimen of endocervical mucus 6–8 hours after coitus. This finding (a positive result) suggests normal cervical mucus with adequate estrogenic response, a fertile husband, and satisfactory coital technique. Presence of less than 5 active sperm per high-power field (a negative result) is indicative of oligospermia, unsuitable cervical mucus, or faulty coital practices. In the latter instance, a repeat test after a shorter interval following intercourse is recommended.

A postcoital test alone is not sufficient to assess male fertility and should not replace semen analysis. Occasionally, vaginitis and cervicitis cause an erroneous interpretation of this test. A negative result on the Sims–Huhner test should be followed by an *in vitro* test of cervical mucus penetration by sperm. (Fig. 47–6).

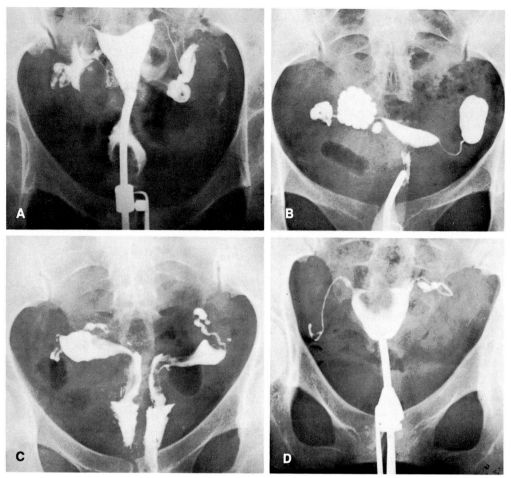

FIG. 47–7. Hysterosalpingograms. *A.* Normal uterus and fallopian tubes with peritoneal spill. Note outline of ovarian beds and leakage into proximal part of vagina. *B.* Loculation of contrast material in inflammatory pockets at distal ends of tubes. *C.* Uterus didelphys with double vagina. *D.* Large filling defect in uterine cavity due to submucous fibroid. Note incomplete tubal filling and no peritoneal spill.

On rare occasions, the presence of antisperm antibodies in cervical mucus may cause immobilization of sperm in cervical mucus.

A dry cervix with no evidence of mucorrhea at midcycle and cervical stenosis is usually associated with a history of trauma (conization, cauterization, or amputation). The diagnosis is easily made by inspection of the cervix. Cryptomenorrhea and hematometra may be associated with severe cervical stenosis.

EVALUATION OF THE UTERUS

Anatomic abnormalities of the uterus are usually recognized by pelvic examination. For a precise diagnosis, hysterography is often required. Polyps, submucous myomas, uterine synechiae, and congenital deformities are recognized by hysterography (Fig. 47–7). Hysteroscopy using fiberoptic equipment may be useful in the recognition of intrauterine disorders.

Examination of an endometrial biopsy (Fig. 47–8) obtained at midluteal phase (day 21 of a 28-day cycle) or later in the cycle is an integral part of an infertility survey. Its purpose is not only to confirm ovulation, but also to assist evaluation of corpus luteum function. Morphologic dating of endometrium should coincide with the day of the cycle on which the specimen was obtained (Fig. 47–9). An immature or out-of-phase endometrium is incompatible with normal fertility and indicates inadequacy of corpus luteum function or improper end-organ response.

ASSESSMENT OF TUBAL PATENCY

Tubal patency can be assessed by the passage of gas or contrast material through the cervix, uterine cavity, and fallopian tubes. Another method is direct endoscopic visualization of indigo carmine solution escaping from the fallopian tubes after injection through a uterine cannula. Simultaneous observation of the pelvic structures by means of culdoscopy, colpotomy, or laparoscopy can be of adjunctive value. Probably the safest time to carry out a tubal patency test is following menstruation and before ovulation, since at this time there is no risk that a fertilized ovum will be displaced.

Rubin Test

The Rubin test (Fig. 47–10) involves insufflation of the uterus and tubes with carbon dioxide under pressure after a tightly fitting cannula has been inserted into the cervical os. This is an office procedure, easily carried out with any one of the several commercially available apparatuses. Pressure should not exceed 200 mm Hg because of the danger of tubal rupture. Carbon dioxide instilled under pressure indicates tubal patency on the basis of 1) a kymographic tracing showing characteristic pressure changes (Fig. 47–11), 2) abdominal auscultation of gas escaping from the tubal fimbriae, and 3) referred phrenic shoulder pain when the patient sits up following insufflation. The patient's perception of pain during insufflation can sometimes give a clue to the location of tubal obstruction. Lack of both pain and evidence of tubal patency suggests bilateral obstruction of the cornual or interstitial portions of the fallopian tubes. Obstruction lateral to these points often produces pain as the obstructed tube dilates under pressure. Occasionally, tubal spasm falsely suggests bilateral tubal obstruction. Repeat examination after the administration of atropine and a sedative may yield normal results after initial failure.

Hysterosalpingography

Hysterosalpingography is more revealing than the Rubin test, as congenital malformations of the uterus and distortions produced by submucous myomas and endometrial polyps can be visualized simultaneously by this technique. Also, the exact points of obstruction can be identified and the feasibility of tubal reconstruction assessed. Radiopaque contrast material, such as iodized oil or a water-soluble material, is injected and its dispersion visualized by roentgenography. An abnormal diffusion pattern suggests previous pelvic inflammatory disease with residual peritubal and periovarian adhesions.

Hysterosalpingography may be of therapeutic as well as diagnostic value. The reason for this is uncertain. Pregnancy following hysterosalpingography has been attributed to a therapeutic effect of the iodine in the contrast material, to the penetration of filamentous tubal adhesions, and to the stimulating effect of x-radiation. Abnormalities detected by hysterosalpingography should be further investigated by pelvic endoscopy in cases of intractable infertility.

Hazards of Tubal Patency Tests

Extreme pain and patient anxiety may necessitate carrying out tubal patency tests under anesthesia, but this is seldom necessary and, indeed, should probably be the signal to discontinue the test. Carbon dioxide gas rather than air should be used for the Rubin test, as fatal air embolism has been reported when air was used. Embolism with contrast material may also occur but seldom is associated with morbidity. Both the Rubin test and hysterosalpingography can ignite a subacute pelvic inflammatory process. Specific anaphylactic reactions to contrast material (e.g., iodine sensitization) may occur. After the use of iodized oil, penetration of uterotubal vessels with subsequent microembolization in the lungs and granulomas in the fallopian tubes and endometrium have been reported. Abortion can result from a tubal patency test during pregnancy; however, many pregnancies have survived such procedures. A tubal patency test is probably contraindicated within 24 hours of the end of the menstrual period, immediately after uterine curettage, following recent pelvic inflammatory disease, and during pregnancy.

Pelvic Endoscopy

Although pelvic endoscopy was established at the turn of the century, widespread use of procedures for visualizing the pelvic and abdominal viscera did not become popular until sophisticated endoscopic devices were developed. Modern optical systems, such as high-intensity fiberoptic light sources, have greatly enhanced the safety and popularity of pelvic endoscopy for detection of causes of infertility and other pathologic conditions.

Pelvic endoscopy is indicated when hysterosalpingography suggests tubal or peritoneal abnormality and the patient fails to become pregnant, when ovarian disease or endometriosis is suspected, and when a complete infertility survey reveals no abnormality. In a significant proportion of patients in the latter category, endoscopy reveals unsuspected tubal or ovarian disease, such as endometriosis and peritubal adhesions. Pelvic endoscopy is mandatory before certain surgical operations such as tuboplasty, conservative operations for suspected endometriosis, or wedge resection of ovaries

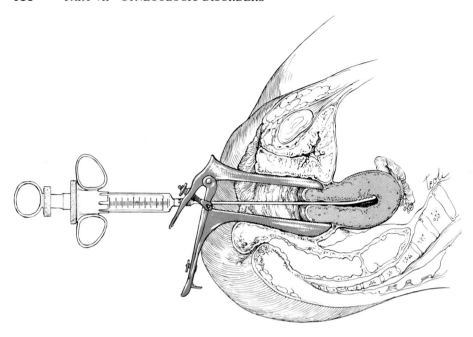

FIG. 47–8. Technique of endometrial biopsy with Novak suction curet.

for polycystic ovarian disease (Stein–Leventhal syndrome). Wedge resection is now rarely required, since ovulation usually can be induced with clomiphene citrate or sequential gonadotropins.

Culdoscopy. After the report by Decker and Cherry in 1944, culdoscopy became popular in the United States. The patient is given heavy analgesia and is placed in the knee–chest position. The posterior cul-de-sac is infiltrated with local anesthetic and entered with a metallic trocar. Creation of a pneumoperitoneum is facilitated by the negative intraperitoneal pressure and the patient's position, and culdoscopic examination of pelvic structures is by direct visualization (Fig. 47–12). Indigo carmine or similar dyes may be injected through a cannula inserted into the cervix, and the patency of the fallopian tubes can be evaluated. Culdoscopy provides only limited visibility of the proximal portion of the fallopian tubes and no access to the anterior aspect of the uterus and bladder. Because of these limitations, the procedure has lost much of its former popularity.

Laparoscopy. Laparoscopy has been used in Europe for many years and has almost completely replaced culdoscopy in the United States.

The technique is described in Chapter 61. The procedure is usually performed with the patient in the modified lithotomy position and under general anesthesia. An insufflation cannula is placed in the cervix to be used for uterine manipulation and for the subsequent injection of indigo carmine dye to test tubal patency. After a special needle has been inserted through an infraumbilical incision, the peritoneal cavity is distended with several liters of carbon dioxide or nitrous oxide. A trocar is then introduced, and a fiberoptic laparoscope placed through the trocar shield. This permits a detailed examination of pelvic as well as other abdominal structures (Figs. 47–13 and 47–14). Introduction of a probe through a second incision facilitates manipulation of the uterus, ovaries, and fallopian tubes in a manner not customarily achieved with culdoscopy. Patency of the fallopian tubes can be evaluated and any area of obstruction identified. The procedure also enables the operator to sever adhesions, obtain ovarian biopsies, and perform other minor procedures.

DETECTION OF OVULATION

Development of new techniques of hormone assay has led to more accurate methods of ovulation detection and prediction. The only direct proof of ovulation is pregnancy or recovery of an ovum from the fallopian tube. All other tests are either indirect or presumptive (Fig. 47–2). The most practical methods for assessing ovulation are 1) basal body temperature (BBT) recordings (Fig. 47–15); 2) examination of daily vaginal smears; 3) demonstration of characteristic changes in the cervical mucus (increase in volume and spinnbarkheit; decrease in viscosity with fern formation near ovulation, followed by decrease in amount, disappearance of ferning, and spinnbarkheit;

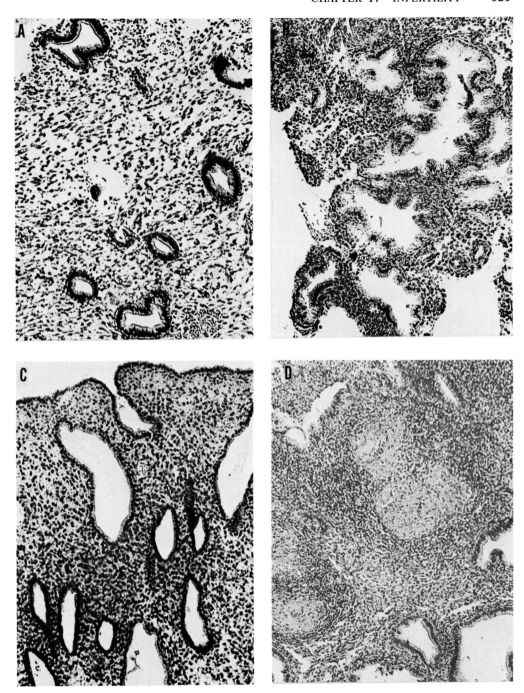

FIG. 47-9. Endometrial biopsies. *A.* Proliferative phase with low gland epithelium and central nuclei. *B.* Secretory phase with compact stroma, round cell infiltration, and convoluted or sawtooth glands with basal nuclei. *C.* Proliferative pattern in biopsy obtained during anovulatory cycle 3 days before menstruation. *D.* Tuberculous endometritis in infertile patient with epithelioid tubercles with Langhans giant cells and round cell infiltration. (JR Gosling)

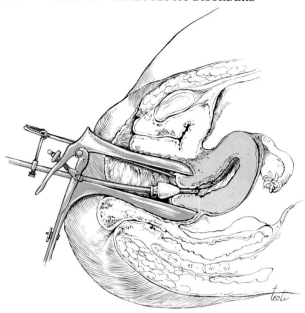

FIG. 47-10. Cannula inserted into cervix for either Rubin test (carbon dioxide insufflation) or hysterosalpingography.

and increase in viscosity and cellularity during the luteal phase); and 4) evidence of secretory change in endometrial biopsies obtained during the latter part of the luteal phase. Mittelschmerz and midcycle spotting are only presumptive evidence of ovulation and are not reliable.

Vaginal smears show a high maturation or karyopyknotic index coinciding with the time of ovulation. Occasionally, vaginal cytology can be difficult to interpret because similar changes are associated with anovulatory follicular maturation.

Radioimmunoassay demonstrates a surge of serum luteinizing hormone (LH) in midcycle, and ovulation is believed to occur usually within 24 hours after the LH peak. Serum and urinary estradiol values reach a peak 1 day prior to the LH surge. Both serum progesterone and urinary pregnanediol (a metabolite of progesterone) levels begin to rise with ovulation and reach a peak about 1 week later (Fig. 47–2). These hormone analyses reliably reflect ovulatory events but are of little practical value because of the cost and time required to perform them. A single assay of serum progesterone or urinary pregnanediol performed during the midluteal phase may provide presumptive evi-

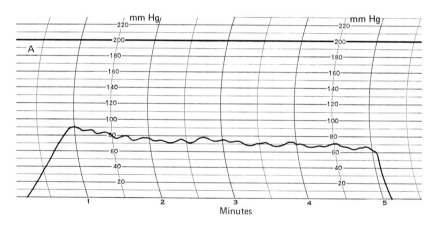

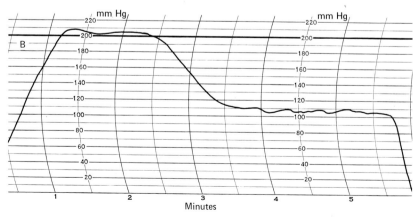

FIG. 47-11. Kymographic tracings recorded during Rubin tests indicating (A) normal pattern and (B) release after initial obstruction.

FIG. 47-12. Insertion of culdoscope through posterior vaginal vault; patient in knee–chest position.

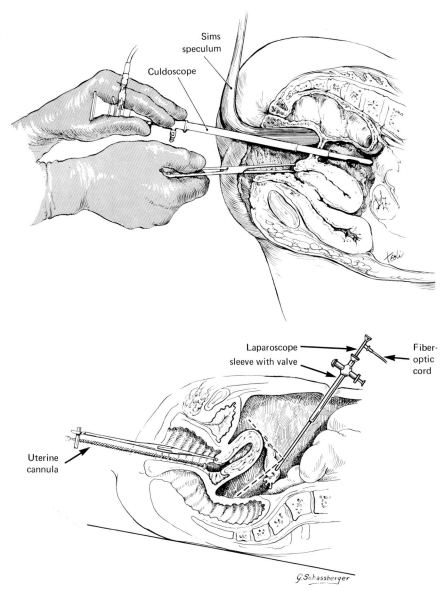

FIG. 47-13. Technique of laparoscopic examination of the pelvic cavity; patient in modified lithotomy position.

dence of ovulation without indicating the actual time it occurred.

Endometrial biopsy is an office procedure that usually can be performed with minimal or no algesia just before or at the onset of menstruation. Typical secretory change in an endometrial biopsy obtained just before or at the onset of menstruation is presumptive evidence of ovulation (Fig. 47–9). Endometrial histology can be misleading if the patient has ingested a progestogen which produces secretory changes comparable to those associated with ovulation.

IMMUNOLOGIC INCOMPATIBILITY

The possibility that immune mechanisms may be responsible for some cases of infertility has provoked intense study in recent years. These relationships are considered in Chapter 12. Relevance of the microagglutination test to immunologic infertility has been questioned, since it has been shown that the active serum protein fraction causing head-to-head agglutination in this test system may be a steroid-binding β-lipoprotein (see Fig. 47–15).

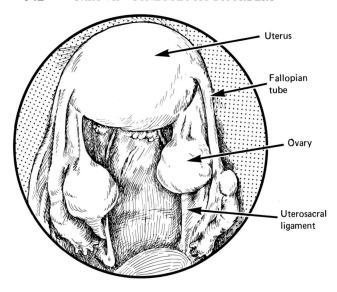

FIG. 47-14. Schematic view of pelvic structures as observed through laparoscope.

TREATMENT

After the investigation of both husband and wife has been completed, a specific therapeutic program can be outlined. If no abnormalities have been found, the couple may need only information with respect to the probable time of ovulation and appropriate coital technique and frequency. When abnormalities have been detected, treatment should be directed toward the correction of specific disorders. Improvement of general health, correction of obesity, and avoidance of stress, extreme fatigue, excessive smoking, and alcohol consumption should be emphasized.

TREATMENT OF THE MALE

Genetic and anatomic disorders may lead to severe oligo- or azospermia. The prognosis is poor if spermatogenesis does not occur or is inadequate. Deficient sperm in the seminal plasma secondary to obstruction of the vas deferens or epididymis can often be corrected surgically. Prevention of male infertility is abetted by early surgical or endocrine treatment of cryptorchidism and appropriate prophylaxis or treatment of orchitis. In recent years, several therapeutic modalities have evolved to correct disorders of spermatogenesis caused by hypothalamic–pituitary malfunction with occasional success. These include 1) administration of testosterone (100–200 mg weekly for 3–4 months), which usually results in a decrease in sperm count fol-

lowed in some instances by rebound or subsequent increase; 2) administration of clomiphene citrate, to which a patient with a reduced or low-normal output of gonadotropic hormone may show a favorable response; 3) administration of human chorionic gonadotropin (hCG) to stimulate endogenous testosterone production; 4) administration of human menopausal gonadotropin (hMG) and hCG as a source of follicle-stimulating hormone (FSH) and LH when clomiphene citrate therapy has been unsuccessful or when a selective gonadotropin deficiency is demonstrated; 5) administration of the amino acid arginine, which has given good results in some.

The single most important advance in the field of male infertility during the last decade has been recognition of varicocele as a cause of oligospermia and asthenospermia. High ligation of the internal spermatic vein in a patient with varicocele and a sperm count consistent with the condition may be followed by improvement in sperm motility and other parameters of semen quality. In patients with varicocele, recent studies suggest that, within an average of 8 months after the operation, a pregnancy rate of approximately 40% may be expected.

Glucocorticoid therapy for male infertility is justified only in those patients with a frank endocrinopathy, such as adrenal hyperplasia. Thyroid preparations administered to a euthyroid male are of no value.

TREATMENT OF THE FEMALE

Treatment of Cervical Abnormalities

When a properly timed postcoital test produces a negative result, penetrability of cervical mucus should be investigated by placing ovulatory mucus on a glass slide adjacent to a specimen of semen and examining the mucus–sperm interaction under the microscope (Miller–Kurzrok test). Alternatively, sperm migration may be observed in a capillary test tube. To determine whether cervical mucus or sperm is abnormal, sperm of known fertility and donor ovulatory mucus may be used in cross testing.

Lack of sperm in cervical mucus in an otherwise normal couple may be due to dyspareunia, apareunia, or, occasionally, severe cervical prolapse. Appropriate management of these conditions should restore fertility.

Chronic endocervicitis is best treated with systemic administration of antibiotics after cultures have identified the responsible organism.

Hostile cervical mucus may reflect inadequate estrogenic stimulation, inadequate response of the cervical epithelium, or anovulation. Cervical mucus in these instances remains viscous and somewhat cellu-

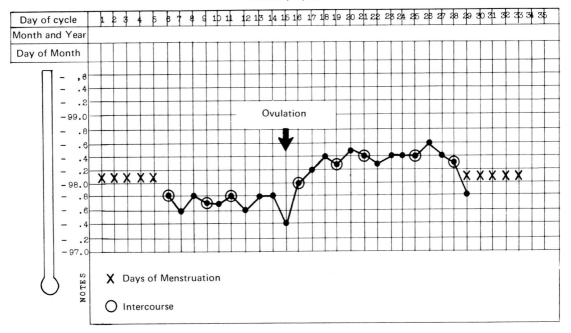

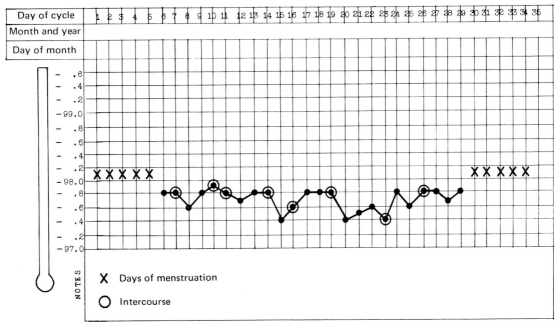

FIG. 47–15. Basal body temperature records suggesting (*A*) ovulatory and (*B*) anovulatory cycles. As a rule, intercourse on day 16 (*A*) would be expected to be fruitful; but, as is shown here, this is not always the case.

lar with low spinnbarkheit and atypical ferning. A mildly acid pH may persist throughout the cycle. These abnormalities can usually be overcome by the administration of 0.1 mg stilbestrol or 10–20 µg ethinyl estradiol daily from day 7 through day 15 of the cycle. Efforts to make the vaginal environment more favorable for spermatozoa by precoital alkaline douching are of dubious value.

Treatment of Uterine Abnormalities

Congenital anomalies of the uterus, such as bicornuate or septate uterus that are associated with infertility or repeated abortion may be treated surgically by means of a unification procedure. Endometrial polyps can easily be removed by dilatation of the cervix and curettage. Uterine synechiae (Asherman's syndrome) are best treated by surgical debridement, insertion of an intrauterine device, and estrogen therapy. Myomectomy may be warranted when hysterosalpingography or hysteroscopy demonstrates tumor encroachment on the uterine cavity or fallopian tube ostia, provided other causes of infertility have been excluded.

Inadequate luteal endometrial phase or inadequate progestational preparation of the endometrium may be improved by postovulatory cyclic progesterone therapy.

Chronic endometritis due to tuberculosis or other infections requires appropriate antibiotic and chemotherapeutic management.

Anterior displacement of the retroverted uterus with a Smith–Hodge pessary may rarely be effective when the elongated cervix of a retroposed uterus is far removed from the seminal pool or when the male semen volume is small.

Treatment of Fallopian Tube Disease

Unilateral or bilateral tuboplasty to remedy obstruction may be indicated when other causes of infertility have been ruled out. Endoscopic examination of the tubes and other pelvic structures to evaluate the nature and extent of tubal disease should precede tuboplasty.

At the time of operation for tubal obstruction, salpingolysis may be indicated if peritubal adhesions are present. During the past few years, considerable progress has been made in tubal surgery. Improved operative techniques, including the use of inert material such as polyglycolic sutures, and microscopic or other magnifying devices, have significantly increased the success rate of reconstructive tubal operations. With the use of microsurgical techniques for salpingoplasty, pregnancies have been reported in as many as 60% of patients. In the presence of advanced tubal pathology, however, even these techniques yield poor results. Patient selection is of critical importance in successful tubal surgery.

Salpingostomy is reserved for fimbrial occlusion. If the obstruction is medial and the fimbriae normal, surgical correction by reimplantation of the patent portion of the tubes into the uterus or by an end-to-end anastomosis may be feasible. Implantation of the ovary into the uterus (Estes' operation) is probably ill-advised; it is associated with an increased risk of uterine rupture, and the few pregnancies that have occurred after such an operation have rarely gone to term.

In the presence of minimal tubal abnormality (*e.g.*, fimbrial stenosis), hydrotubation (repeated intrauterine instillation of a hydrocortisone solution during the follicular phase of the cycle) has been suggested but is of doubtful value. This procedure consists of insertion of an insufflation cannula into the cervix and perfusion of the uterus and tubes with a solution of saline containing hydrocortisone (50 mg in 15–20 ml saline). Some investigators have added various antibiotics and proteolytic enzymes to this solution. The procedure is performed once or twice each week for several months during the follicular phase.

Recently, the technique of *extracorporeal (in vitro) fertilization* has been advocated as a last resort for patients whose fallopian tubes have been completely destroyed or removed but who have a normal uterus and at least one functioning ovary. The technique is rather involved and consists of 1) harvesting ova at the time of ovulation by laparoscopy, 2) *in vitro* fertilization in a special culture medium, 3) culture of the fertilized egg until the blastula reaches the 8- to 16-cell stage, and 4) transcervical implantation of the embryo into the uterine cavity. Steptoe and Edwards and several other groups of scientists have reported normal term pregnancy achieved by this technique. The procedure is highly experimental, and many technical, scientific, and ethical problems remain to be resolved before it can be widely used. However, it does open new avenues for research and patient management in this rapidly advancing field.

Treatment of Anovulation

In the presence of anovulatory cycles with or without amenorrhea, the diagnostic approaches outlined in Chapter 46 are applicable to the management of infertility. Judicious management of ovulation failure requires the establishment of the precise cause of anovulation by means of hormone assays, pelvic endoscopy, and other diagnostic procedures.

Clomiphene Citrate. A synthetic compound related to chlorotrianisene (TACE), clomiphene citrate is a weak estrogen. It is indicated for the treatment of ovulatory failure when there is evidence of follicular function with adequate endogenous estrogen production but no cyclic stimulation by pituitary gonadotropin. Clomiphene is a potentiator of gonadotropin, which causes an increase in ovarian secretion of estrogen. Peripherally, this compound has antiestrogenic proper-

ties. An intact hypothalamic–pituitary–ovarian axis, even though functionally inadequate, is necessary for the drug to act.

In properly selected cases, clomiphene citrate is successful in inducing ovulation in approximately 70% followed by pregnancy in 40%. It is the drug of choice for the treatment of anovulation due to polycystic ovarian disease (Stein–Leventhal syndrome), oligoovulation, post-pill amenorrhea, and in some cases of amenorrhea–galactorrhea. Patients with premature menopause, ovarian dysgenesis, or pituitary destruction are not responsive to clomiphene citrate.

A usual course of clomiphene citrate (Clomid) consists of a dose of 50 mg once or twice daily for 5 days (a total of 250–500 mg) starting on the 5th day of the cycle. (Larger doses of clomiphene have been used when there are specific indications and when the usual regimen has failed to induce ovulation.) In the presence of amenorrhea and a normal level of estrogen, endometrial bleeding is provoked by progesterone, 100 mg intramuscularly on two successive days, or medroxyprogesterone acetate (Provera), 10 mg daily for 7 days. Clomiphene citrate is then started on the 5th day after the bleeding starts. During the administration of clomiphene, there is at first a transient rise in circulating gonadotropins, followed quickly by a return to normal. Approximately 1 week following the conclusion of the 5-day course of treatment, there is a dynamic burst in circulating gonadotropins to levels characteristic of ovulation. Hence, the optimum time for intercourse is 5–10 days after completion of the 5-day course. Up to six courses may be required.

The gonadotropin burst that attends the use of clomiphene citrate acts as a marked stimulus to the ovaries, and significant ovarian enlargement and multiple ovulations may result. Ovarian enlargement is rarely troublesome; but, in a sensitive patient, it can be sufficient to cause pain, ovarian hemorrhage, tortion, or rupture. It is therefore important that a pelvic examination be performed before every course of clomiphene citrate, and immediately if abdominal pain occurs. If the ovaries are found to be enlarged, clomiphene citrate, should be discontinued until there is complete regression; subsequent doses should be smaller than those that produced the enlargement. If marked ovarian enlargement occurs, large doses of an oral contraceptive will cause rapid regression.

Side effects of clomiphene citrate occur with sufficient frequency that the patient should be warned of them. She should be instructed to call the physician immediately if she experiences abdominal pain, severe bloating or fullness, or the "chair syndrome" (pain on sitting down in a chair). Other bothersome, but usually less serious, side effects include hot flashes, depression, transient photophobia and blurring of vision, breast discharge, and mastalgia.

If ovulation has not occurred after six courses of clomiphene citrate, several other devices may be tried: 1) the LH surge resulting from clomiphene citrate may be supplemented by administration of hCG (a single intramuscular dose of APL, 5000–10,000 IU, on the 7th day after completion of 5 days of clomiphene citrate); 2) if the pretreatment endogenous estrogen level is judged subnormal, a salutary effect may be achieved by administration of conjugated estrogens (1.25 mg daily) for 10 days before a 5-day clomiphene citrate course and hCG 7 days after the course of clomiphene citrate is completed; 3) if this fails after three courses, and no untoward effects have been observed up to this time, the clomiphene citrate dose may be increased to a maximum of 50 mg four times daily for 5 days (1000 mg) followed 7 days later by a single injection of hCG; 4) if no pregnancy follows, clomiphene citrate may be abandoned and the use of hMG considered.

Human Menopausal Gonadotropin. HMG (Pergonal) is a potent preparation that causes intense stimulation of the ovaries. Its use is not without hazard; hyperstimulation and multiple ovulations may result, and special precautions and special facilities for the appraisal of its effects are mandatory. The only indication for the use of hMG as primary treatment without prior trial of clomiphene citrate is pituitary failure or ablation confirmed by the lack of endogenous gonadotropins.

Contraindications to the use of hMG include 1) a high level of endogenous gonadotropins, indicating primary ovarian failure; 2) overt thyroid or adrenal dysfunction; 3) an intracranial tumor, e.g., pituitary tumor; 4) abnormal uterine bleeding of undetermined cause; and 5) any cause of infertility other than anovulation.

Women vary widely in their sensitivity to hMG. Even the same woman may demonstrate variable sensitivity during different treatment cycles. The therapeutic objective is to stimulate the ovary so that follicular maturation occurs and to produce estrogens in amounts equivalent to those normally present in the immediate preovulatory phase. Exactly at this point (not before, not after), the administration of 10,000 IU hCG as a single injection or in divided doses over 2–3 days usually results in ovulation. HCG is derived from the urine of pregnant women and produces an effect similar to the midcycle LH surge in the normal cycle.

Because of the variable response, the time at which the appropriate level of estrogen production will occur cannot be anticipated. Frequent, preferably daily, tests must be made to determine estrogen levels. Cervical mucus ferning, spinnbarkheit, and the nature of the vaginal smear can provide adequate evidence of response in early phases of the induction, but they are not sufficiently precise for evaluation of the hMG response in the late follicular phase. An acceptable method is to monitor the patient's response until 4+ ferning of the cervical mucus is achieved. Thereafter, daily assay of total urinary estrogens or serum estradiol levels is required. In the normal 28-day ovulatory

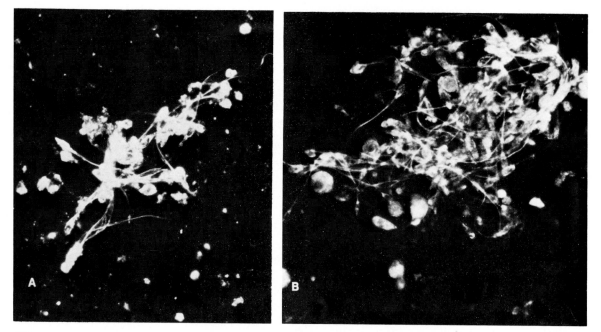

FIG. 47-16. Sperm agglutination. *A.* In rabbit serum containing antibodies to human sperm. *B.* In human serum containing sperm-agglutinating and sperm-immobilizing antibodies.

cycle, the value for total urinary estrogens averages 60µg–70µg/24 hours, with normal variations from 20µg–100µg.* HCG is administered immediately when the total urinary estrogen value reaches 100µg/24 hours. Ovulation usually follows 1–2 days after the hCG injection. Serum estradiol assays may be used in lieu of urinary estrogens to monitor the hMG effect.

HMG is supplied in ampules containing 75 IU FSH and an equal amount of LH. A workable schedule is to administer one ampule each day for 3 successive days; if the urinary estrogen level is less than 50µg/24 hours, two ampules each day may be given for the next 3 days, and the amount similarly increased every 3 days until the urinary estrogen level is 50µg–100µg/24 hours (or serum estradiol reaches 800–1000µg/ml). Then (or earlier if the total urinary estrogen level reaches 100µg/24 hours) hMG is discontinued and hCG administered. It is hazardous and usually futile to persist if pregnancy has not been achieved after three such courses.

In addition to daily assessment of total urinary estrogen level, vaginal examinations should be performed daily and cervical mucus or vaginal cytology studied. Moderate enlargement of the ovaries occurs in 7%–10% of patients. Most cases of significant enlargement of the ovaries, sometimes with ascites, and

most cases of multiple pregnancy occur when the total urinary estrogen level rises to 100µg–200µg/24 hours. Rapid enlargement of the ovaries sometimes begins during hMG treatment, but maximum ovarian stimulation occurs 7–10 days after ovulation (hCG administration). If the ovaries are palpably enlarged during treatment, hMG should be stopped; if they are palpably enlarged at the end of the hMG course, hCG should not be given (Fig. 47–17).

Bromocriptine. Bromocriptine (Parlodel^R) is a dopamine receptor agonist and activates postsynaptic dopamine receptors. The drug is a semisynthetic peptide alkaloid and is believed to act by stimulating the release of prolactin-inhibiting factor from the hypothalamus, thus regulating the release of prolactin from the anterior pituitary. Bromocriptine itself is also a potent inhibitor of the synthesis and release of prolactin by the pituitary gland, although it has little or no effect on other pituitary hormones. Bromocriptine is indicated for the treatment of anovulation associated with hyperprolactinemia with or without the galactorrhea–amenorrhea syndrome (Fig. 47–18). It may also be effective in patients who have luteal phase deficiency resulting from hyperprolactinemia. When there is no demonstrable pituitary tumor, bromocriptine therapy initiates ovulatory menstrual cycles and suppresses galactorrhea in about 75% of anovulatory patients with galactorrhea–amenorrhea.

Although bromocriptine is a potent drug for induc-

---

* The level of urinary estrogens varies with the methods used and from one laboratory to another. Each laboratory should establish its own norms.

FIG. 47-17. Induction of ovulation with hMG and hCG, leading to single fetus pregnancy and normal term delivery. This patient had primary amenorrhea and did not respond to clomiphene citrate. Induction cycle was monitored by urinary estrogen assay.

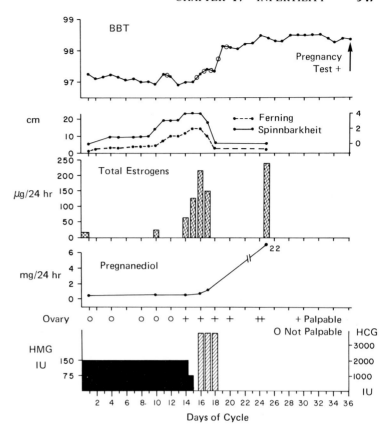

ing ovulation in patients with hyperprolactinemia, the drug has so far been approved in the United States only for the treatment of amenorrhea and galactorrhea. It has not been conclusively demonstrated that the use of this drug is safe in pregnancy; preliminary reports on the outcome of over 400 pregnancies after bromocriptine therapy immediately before and during pregnancy have revealed no deleterious effects on the fetus, mother, or the course of pregnancy, however (Fig. 47–19).

Patients selected for bromocriptine therapy should be screened carefully for pituitary adenoma. Only those found to have a normal pituitary and elevated prolactin levels (above 20 ng/ml) should be considered for treatment. The usual dosage is 2.5–7.5 mg/day taken with meals in divided doses until normal ovulatory menstrual cycles are established. Duration of treatment should not exceed 6 months. It is recommended that treatment be initiated with 2.5 mg daily and be increased to therapeutic doses within the 1st week. Adverse reactions in decreasing order of frequency include nausea, headache, dizziness, fatigue, abdominal cramps, nasal congestion, and constipation.

Wedge Resection of Ovaries. Bilateral ovarian wedge resection is reserved for the rare patient with polycystic ovarian disease who does not respond to clomiphene citrate or gonadotropin therapy.

Other Modes of Treatment. Both hyper- and hypothyroidism may be associated with anovulatory cycles. Correction of thyroid dysfunction usually produces ovulation unless the disorder has been of long duration.

Hydrocortisone and its derivatives induce ovulation in women with hyperfunction of the adrenal cortex or those with a deficiency of enzymes involved in adrenal steroidogenesis (*e.g.,* a 21-hydroxylase defect).

X-ray stimulation of the pituitary or ovaries has been used with occasional success, but its possible mutagenic effects have made it obsolete.

TREATMENT OF IMMUNOLOGIC INFERTILITY

The only available treatment for infertility caused by sperm-agglutinating or sperm-immobilizing antibodies consists of an attempt to reduce the antibody titer in the woman's reproductive tract by use of condoms for 6–12 months. Pregnancy may occur when use of condoms is discontinued. The effectiveness of this treatment has not been critically evaluated. (See Chap. 12)

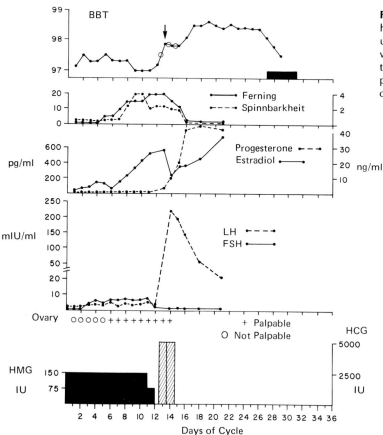

FIG. 47–18. Induction of ovulation with hMG and hCG. This patient had primary amenorrhea and was unresponsive to clomiphene citrate. Induction cycle was monitored by radioimmunoassay of serum estradiol levels. Note biphasic BBT and rise of serum progesterone after hCG administration, indicating ovulation.

ARTIFICIAL INSEMINATION

Artificial insemination may be accomplished using either the husband's sperm (AIH, homologous insemination) or semen from a donor (AID heterologous insemination).

Homologous insemination is rarely successful when the cause of infertility cannot be determined or when there is sperm deficiency. Artificial techniques are hardly an improvement over normal coitus unless there is some developmental anomaly preventing intromission or normal ejaculation. Hypospadias and epispadias may be indications. Other rare indications include a displaced cervix far from the seminal pool in the posterior vaginal fornix, small seminal volume (less than 1 ml), and retrograde ejaculation.

A special technique that has produced relatively encouraging results is that of split-ejaculate insemination. The husband is instructed to supply a semen sample, after 2 days abstention, by masturbation into two separate containers. The first portion of the ejaculate usually contains 75% of all spermatozoa and may be used for insemination. The procedure is particularly useful in patients who have a large semen volume, liquefaction defects, or sperm motility disorders.

Insemination with donor semen is still controversial. There are many religious and legal implications. Both husband and wife should unequivocally support heterologous insemination before it is considered by the physician. If either has reservations about it, such a procedure is contraindicated. It is preferable that the initial proposal come from the couple rather than the physician. Arguments against artificial insemination with donor semen are 1) reactions of the couple to a child thus produced are not predictable, 2) the legal status of the child is uncertain, 3) it sometimes is difficult to be certain that the husband is and will remain sterile, 4) it contravenes some religious precepts, and 5) the child may be disinherited at the whim of the husband. Nevertheless, artificial insemination with donor semen is rapidly becoming more common, and pioneering efforts are being made in some states to legalize artificial insemination and to legitimize the status of the babies conceived in this manner.

Before insemination, the following should be determined: 1) the probable time of ovulation, 2) tubal pa-

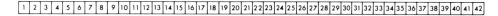

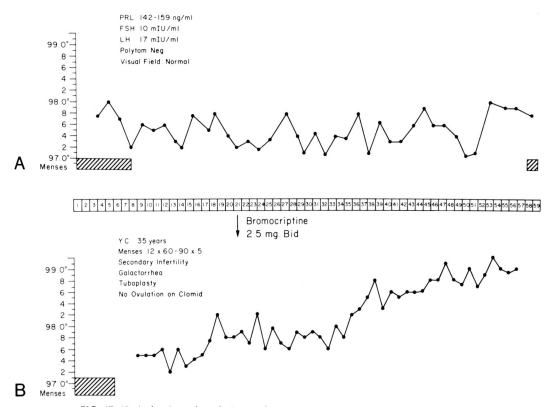

PRL 142-159 ng/ml
FSH 10 mIU/ml
LH 17 mIU/ml
Polytom Neg
Visual Field : Normal

A
Menses

Bromocriptine
2 5 mg. Bid

Y C   35 years
Menses 12 x 60 - 90 x 5
Secondary Infertility
Galactorrhea
Tuboplasty
No Ovulation on Clomid

B
Menses

FIG. 47–19. Induction of ovulation and pregnancy with bromocriptine in an anovulatory woman with hyperprolactinemia. *A.* Anovulatory cycle characterized by monophasic basal body temperature. *B.* Ovulation and pregnancy (elevation and sustained rise of basal body temperature resulting from bromocriptine therapy).

tency, 3) lack of a medical contraindication to pregnancy, and 4) evidence that the patient is not already pregnant. Within 1 hour of collection, a few milliliters of semen are drawn into a sterile syringe, and 0.5–1 ml instilled within the cervical canal. The remainder of the specimen is sprayed over the cervix and into the proximal vagina. Insemination within the uterine cavity may precipitate uterine contractions and expulsion of the semen. The donor should be carefully selected with respect to race, blood type compatibility, physical appearance, general health, and genetic background. Anonymity must be preserved.

PSYCHOTHERAPY

Psychotherapy helps some infertile couples. Occasionally, serious psychogenic problems are not apparent on the surface and can be fathomed only after repeated consultation. The couple's motivation is important.

Becoming pregnant may be obsessional from the time it is first suspected that pregnancy is not possible. Need for ego support and proof of sexual identification may underlie the desire for pregnancy. After intensive infertility investigation and treatment followed by a single pregnancy, some women practice contraception indefinitely or even request sterilization.

PROGNOSIS

Some patients become pregnant in spite of, not because of, the investigation and treatment employed. This fact dictates caution in interpretation of the efficacy of specific therapeutic procedures. Prolonged and piecemeal therapy can produce considerable emotional harm, create serious tensions, and even disrupt the marriage. Tact is needed when informing a couple about the prognosis for future pregnancy. Unless the husband is a castrate or the wife has undergone hys-

terectomy, it is probably ill-advised to tell any couple that a successful pregnancy is impossible.

ADOPTION

When pregnancy seems improbable, adoption may be proposed by the couple. It should be suggested only indirectly by the physician. The suitability of the couple for parenthood with respect to physical and economic status, as well as emotional stability must be considered. Women are generally more enthusiastic about adoption than are their husbands. Contrary to general belief, adoption of a baby probably does not enhance fertility.

REFERENCES AND RECOMMENDED READING

Behrman SJ: Artificial insemination. Clin Obstet Gynecol 22:245, 1979

Belsey MA, Eliasson R, Gallegos AJ et al: Laboratory Manual for Examination of Human Semen and Semen–Cervical Mucus Interaction. Geneva, World Health Organization, 1980

Biggers JD: In vitro fertilization and embryo transfer in human beings. N Engl J Med 304:336, 1981

Cohen MR: Laparoscopy, Culdoscopy and Gynecography. Philadelphia, WB Saunders, 1970

Decker AW, Cherry T: Culdoscopy: New methods in diagnosis of pelvic disease—preliminary report. Am J Surg 64:40, 1944

Fullenlove TM: Experience with over 2000 uterosalpingographies. Am J Roentgenol Radium Ther Nucl Med 106:463, 1969

Hafez ESE, Evans TN (eds): Human Reproduction—Conception and Contraception, 2nd ed. Hagerstown, Harper & Row, 1980

Horwitz ST: Laparoscopy in gynecology. Obstet Gynecol Surv 27:1, 1972

Jones GS: Luteal phase insufficiency. Clin Obstet Gynecol 16:255, 1973

Kitner RW: Use of clomiphene citrate, human chorionic gonadotropin, and human menopausal gonadotropin for induction of ovulation in the human female. Fertil Steril 17:569, 1966

MacLeod J: Human male infertility. Obstet Gynecol Surv 26:335, 1971

Moghissi KS: The function of the cervix in fertility. Fertil Steril 23:295, 1972

Moghissi KS (ed): Current concepts in infertility. Clin Obstet Gynecol 22:9, 1979

Moghissi KS, Syner FN, Evans TN: A composite picture of the menstrual cycle. Am J Obstet Gynecol 114:405, 1972

Roland M: Management of the Infertile Couple, Springfield, IL, Charles C. Thomas, 1968

Shulman S: Immunologic barrier to fertility. Obstet Gynecol Surv 27:553, 1972

Soupart P: Fertilization. In Hafez ESE (ed): Human Reproduction—Conception and Contraception, 2nd ed. Hagerstown, Harper & Row, 1980

Steptoe PC, Edwards RG: Birth after reimplantation of a human embryo. Lancet 2:366, 1978

Sweeney WJ: Pitfalls in present day methods of evaluating tubal function: 1. Tubal insufflation. Fertil Steril 13:113, 1962

Sweeney WJ: Pitfalls in present day methods of evaluating tubal function: II. Hysterosalpingography. Fertil Steril 13:124, 1962

Taymor ML: Evaluation of anovulatory cycles and induction of ovulation. Clin Obstet Gynecol 22:145, 1979

Tredway DR, Settlage DSF, Nakamura RM, Motoshima M, Umezaki CU, Mishell DR: Significance of timing for the postcoital evaluation of cervical mucus. Am J Obstet Gynecol 121:387, 1975

Wallach EE: Evaluation and management of uterine causes of infertility. Clin Obstet Gynecol 22:43, 1979

White MM, Green Armytage VG: The Management of Impaired Fertility. New York, Oxford, 1962

Wu CH: Monitoring of ovulation induction. Fertil Steril 30:617, 1978

CONGENITAL ANOMALIES

Congenital anomalies of the female reproductive tract are considered in detail in Chapter 5. They are myriad in type, depending upon the degree and kind of involvement, and occur at any level from the fimbriated end of the fallopian tube to the vaginal introitus and external genitalia. They may take the form of agenesis, imperfect development with consequent narrowing (atresia), or duplication of any part of the uterus or vagina, owing to a failure of fusion of the müllerian duct system. Occasionally, an embryonic state persists, as in certain cases of fused labia minora and imperforate hymen.

Fused labia minora may result from maternal ingestion of androgenic hormones during pregnancy or from failure to keep the infant's perineal area properly clean (see Fig. 45–12). The condition may interfere with normal urination or obstruct coitus later in life. Daily application of an estrogenic cream frequently suffices to separate the labia and restore the normal relations of the external genitalia.

The hymen, which separates the internal from the external genitalia, may constitute a complete wall of mucous membrane (imperforate) or may be lacking. The hymenal opening varies in size and shape; it may be crescentic, fringed, biperforate, or cribriform. The imperforate hymen presents a clinical problem only after menarche, when the accumulation of menstrual blood may result successively in hematocolpos, hematometra, and hematosalpinx. The patient gives a history of menstrual molimina and periodic pelvic pain without external bleeding. Examination reveals a thin, fluctuant, bluish black, bulging septum, frequently under great tension. A radial or cruciate incision and removal of one or more segments of the membrane allows the thick, chocolate-colored liquid to escape slowly.

When a congenital defect is found, particularly of the internal genitalia, a thorough investigation of both the genital and urinary tracts should be made, since other anomalies of the müllerian (paramesonephric) and wolffian (mesonephric) systems are apt to coexist. Knowledge of these defects may be of great clinical importance in the management of a subsequent pregnancy or in the evaluation of a gynecologic disorder.

ACUTE INJURIES

Most acute injuries and lacerations of the vulva, vagina, and uterus occur at parturition, and their management is an obstetric problem. Nonacute injuries incurred during childbirth to the supporting structures of the uterus and vagina may become gynecologic problems later in life.

Nonobstetric acute injuries include those resulting from falls, coitus, sexual assault, and a variety of miscellaneous traumas. They vary in extent from a simple bruise of the vulva or perineal area or a small abrasion of the vestibular mucous membrane to an enormous hematoma involving half or more of the perineal area (Fig. 48–1) and horrendous lacerations of the vulva, pelvic floor, and vagina. In managing an acute injury, the physician must observe the following order of procedure:

1. An accurate history of precisely how the injury occurred should be carefully recorded. There is a medicolegal component in any case of genital tract injury, irrespective of the patient's protestations. (The procedure to be followed in the case of alleged rape is outlined in Chapter 9.)
2. The vulva and vestibule should be carefully inspected under a good light, with the patient in the lithotomy position—if possible, on a gynecologic examination table with her legs in the stirrups. A pho-

STRUCTURAL DEFECTS OF THE FEMALE REPRODUCTIVE TRACT

Harold M. M. Tovell
David N. Danforth

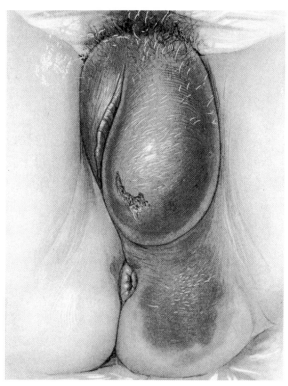

FIG. 48-1. Hematoma of vulva occupying left labium majus and extending downward out of perineum. Vaginal outlet is discolored and all surrounding parts distorted and infiltrated with blood. Below is abrasion of skin. Patient fell astride a chair. (Kelly HA: Operative Gynecology. New York, Appleton, 1898. Drawing by Max Brödel)

tographic record of the injury might be considered with the patient's permission.

3. A gentle, single-digit vaginal examination should be performed to search for any vaginal wall hematoma or laceration or for a foreign body. Speculum examination, if feasible, should also be performed to confirm the findings or to determine if there is any injury above the introitus.

4. A rectal examination should be made to determine any injury to the sphincter or rectal wall or the presence and extent of a perineal hematoma.

Superficial abrasions and lacerations will granulate and heal well and require no sutures. Arterial bleeding, however, may require ligation of the offending vessel; gentle pressure suffices to control oozing. Irrigation and lavage with an aqueous antiseptic solution are essential.

Large, painful hematomas may develop and be extremely frightening to the patient. They absorb slowly, seldom become infected, and are best managed by hot compresses or sitz baths.

Extensive injuries, including large lacerations of the vulvar appendages, vagina, and perineum, require prompt repair, usually in an operating room. Good exposure and assistance with blood replacement and general anesthesia may be required. The possibility of injury to the urethra, bladder, or both, and to the anal sphincter and canal or rectum, should always be considered. An indwelling bladder catheter should be placed for 1–2 days, longer if the urethra or bladder has been injured. Usually no permanent damage results from acute injuries to the vulva, vagina, or perineum if their repair is based on sound surgical principles and management. Subsequent weakness and prolapse may develop, however, if the pelvic diaphragm (levator muscles and fascia) is torn. Depending on the nature of the injury, prophylactic use of an antibiotic and antitetanus vaccine should be considered.

VAGINAL ATRESIA DUE TO INJURY

The most common causes of acquired vaginal atresia are childbirth injury, overzealous vaginal plastic operation, and the intravaginal application of radium.

Atresia following childbirth injury may occur at any level in the vagina, usually along a lateral wall in the upper third. It is felt as a sharp, annular, constricting band of tissue and may result from a faulty repair of a laceration or failure to perform a needed repair. No treatment is necessary except in the presence of dyspareunia. Some annular bands can be released by simple incision in one or more places. Graduated obturators may be used to dilate a constricting band in the lower third of the vagina.

Not infrequently, vaginal atresia occurs following anterior and posterior colporrhaphy, with resulting dyspareunia or complete inability to have intercourse. Removal of too much redundant anterior or posterior vaginal wall skin or excessive tightening of the levator ani muscles during the posterior wall repair and perineorrhaphy contributes to this distressing and potentially medicolegal problem. The gynecologist should be constantly aware of this danger when performing vaginal plastic procedures.

Vaginal atresia often follows radium treatment for cervical cancer unless preventive measures are taken. The vault narrows within a month after removal of the radium; the anterior and posterior walls become adherent within 2 months, making intercourse either unsatisfactory or impossible and the cervix completely inaccessible for follow-up examination. To prevent this distortion, the patient may be instructed in the regular use of a vaginal obturator, commencing shortly after removal of the radium, or the gynecologist or radiotherapist may digitally break any adhesions and expose the cervix at weekly intervals until the vaginal walls have healed or until intercourse is resumed.

CERVICAL INJURIES

The great majority of cervical injuries are obstetric in nature and occur when the cervix is retracting over the advancing fetal head in the terminal phase of the first stage of labor. Less obvious or concealed injuries to the cervix are usually functional in nature and may be iatrogenically produced at the time of dilatation and curettage in a young, nulliparous girl with a congenitally atretic or stenotic cervical canal (Fig. 48–2).

Obstetrically acquired cervical lacerations usually occur at the lateral angles of the external os and may extend to or beyond the vaginal vault and into the lower uterine segment. They should be repaired immediately upon completion of the third stage of labor.

Uncomplicated lacerations that are not repaired result in the so-called fish-mouth type of cervix in which one or both lateral angles of the external os have a deep cleft. Old, stellate lacerations are sometimes seen. They are usually shallow lacerations that result from multiple tears around the circumference of the cervix during labor and delivery.

Uncomplicated cervical lacerations that are properly repaired at the time of delivery are of no clinical importance. If they are not repaired and heal poorly, however, two important disorders may result. First, the columnar epithelium of the cervical canal grows on the ectocervix, forming an ectropion from which severe chronic cervicitis and leukorrhea may result. Although the exact relation of ectropion to carcinoma is not clear, it has been suggested that, within the abnormally located columnar epithelium, atypical squamous metaplasia or intraepithelial neoplastic changes may occur which, if not treated, can ultimately progress to carcinoma of the cervix.

The second important disorder results from a laceration that occurs high in the canal. Poor healing and scar tissue interrupt the continuity of the fibrous cervical ring so that it cannot withstand the stresses of the second trimester of a subsequent pregnancy and a late abortion inevitably occurs. Such concealed lacerations in the upper cervix, whether produced at childbirth or at the time of dilatation and curettage, are responsible for the syndrome of cervical incompetence.

RELAXATION OF PELVIC SUPPORTS

The term *relaxation* describes the weakening effects of the lengthening and attenuation of the fascial supports of the urethra, bladder, uterus, upper posterior wall of the vagina, and rectum. Although relaxations may occur in both young and old virginal women, the great majority are the delayed but direct result of childbirth. If injury to the supports is extensive, evidence of relaxation may appear soon after delivery. More often, the symptoms and signs of pelvic relaxation appear in the menopausal and postmenopausal

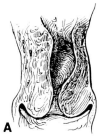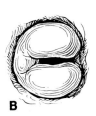

FIG. 48–2. *A.* Concealed cervical injury. Cervix feels normal, and speculum examination does not disclose defect. *B.* Deep left cervical laceration seen on a speculum examination. (Danforth DN: In Davis CH, Carter B (eds): Obstetrics and Gynecology. Hagerstown, MD, Prior, 1953)

era, when the tonic effect of the ovarian hormones on the pelvic tissues is lost and atrophic changes in the fascial supports begin. Pelvic relaxation should be regarded in the same way as a hernia elsewhere is regarded. Both are produced by a weakness of the supporting tissues and are progressive in nature; no amount of exercise or rest will correct the abnormality or restore the normal anatomic relations.

ANATOMIC CONSIDERATIONS

Proper understanding of the clinical manifestations and surgical management of pelvic relaxations is based upon a detailed knowledge of the functional anatomy of the bony, ligamentous, and fascial supports of the pelvic organs. The student is urged to review the appropriate sections in Chapter 3.

Pelvic Diaphragm

The pelvic diaphragm, formed by the bilaterally situated, fan-shaped levator ani muscles extending in the central pelvis between the peripheral anterior and posterior bony segments and lateral pelvic walls, effectively supports the pelvic structures directly over the pelvic outlet. As depicted in Figure 3–12, the muscles blend together in the midline, where they surround and support the three openings in the pelvic floor through which pass the terminal portions of the urinary, reproductive, and intestinal tracts. Sometimes called the levator sling, the thick, striated muscle and its overlying fascia are capable of providing the necessary support for the pelvic viscera and yet allow considerable expansion to meet the functional demands of a normal vaginal delivery and bowel evacuation. Any congenital or acquired weakness eventually results in widening of the opening and subsequent herniation of the pelvic viscera through the floor of the pelvis.

Perineal Musculature

The more superficially located muscles of the perineum are depicted in Figures 3–25 and 3–27. They are the paired ischiocavernosus, bulbocavernosus, deep and superficial transverse perineal muscles, together with the external anal sphincter and musculofascial tissues of the urogenital diaphragm. Together, they form a second layer of support, but are seldom, if ever, effective in preventing the eventual downward displacement of the bladder, vagina, or rectum once the levator muscles have been seriously weakened.

Endopelvic Fascia

The fibroareolar connective tissue that fills the space below the pelvic peritoneum and above the upper fascial sheaths of the levator ani muscle is the endopelvic fascia. With varying degrees of thickness, depending on functional requirements for support, it covers the bladder, vagina, cervix, uterus, rectosigmoid, and anal canal, and forms fascial sheaths for vessels and nerves passing through the pelvis. A diagrammatic representation of the fibroareolar connective tissue lining and pelvic walls and viscera is depicted in Figure 3–10. Note that the tissue is loosely arranged in areas where no stress is encountered, as in the paravesical and pararectal spaces. In other areas, where greater support is required to withstand the stresses incurred during the functional activity of the organ involved, the loose meshwork of fascial tissue is condensed into thick, fibrous bands, forming the vesicouterine, cardinal, and uterosacral ligaments and the fascial sheaths that surround the pelvic organs.

In essence, the function of the endopelvic fascia is to provide both ligamentous and fascial supports for all pelvic viscera, nerves, and blood vessels, and to fill the empty spaces between the viscera and the pelvic sidewalls below the peritoneum and above the levator ani muscles.

Supporting Structures of the Reproductive Tract

The following major supports of the uterus and vagina are of concern in the surgical repair of pelvic relaxations:

1. The cardinal ligaments (transverse cervical or Mackenrodt's ligaments), passing medially from the lateral pelvic wall to the paracervical fascia on the lateral aspect of the cervix, are the primary supports of the uterus and upper vagina. They contain the blood vessels, lymphatic channels, and nerves for the central pelvic viscera and are sometimes referred to as the lateral parametrium.
2. The uterosacral ligaments extend from the presacral or perirectal fascia to the paracervical and upper paravaginal fascia, where they incorporate with the cervical and vaginal attachments of the cardinal lig-

aments. Their primary function is to maintain the uterus in anteversion and the cervix at a right angle to the vaginal axis, and to assist in suspension of the upper part of the vagina. They also carry blood vessels, lymphatic channels, and nerves to the central pelvic viscera and are sometimes referred to as the posterior parametrium.
3. The pubocervical fascia includes the pubovesical and vesicouterine components of the endopelvic fascia. It extends from the posterior aspect of the symphysis pubis, passes beneath the bladder, and incorporates with the paracervical fascia anteriorly and laterally, where it blends into the cervical attachments of the cardinal ligaments. The pubocervical fascia is the primary support of the anterior vaginal wall and the bladder.
4. The paravaginal and perirectal fasciae maintain the integrity of the posterior two-thirds of the vagina. This endopelvic fascial sheath surrounds the vagina and rectum and is fused in the lower half or two-thirds of the vagina, below the peritoneum, in the deepest point of the pouch of Douglas and above the hymenal ring at the vaginal introitus. Further support in this area is supplied by the strong bellies of the levator muscles and their overlying fascia.

SYMPTOMS OF PELVIC RELAXATION

Symptoms of pelvic relaxation generally relate to the particular structure or structures involved—urethra, bladder, uterus, cul-de-sac, or rectum. The patient may refer to these symptoms as a swelling, protrusion, pulling or dragging sensation, fatigue, or sense of pressure. Low backache, though frequently associated with pelvic relaxations, is probably secondary, if related at all, to the postural adjustments made by the patient in an attempt to alleviate the primary symptoms, since an unaccustomed postural attitude produces back strain. Symptoms that suggest a structural defect, uterine displacement, or both, include urinary incontinence with stress, pelvic pain or pressure, or a feeling of fullness in the pelvis, particularly after prolonged periods of standing or deep penetration during coitus. Finally, the longer the structural defects have been present, the more pronounced the symptoms become.

TYPES OF PELVIC RELAXATIONS

Weakness in the supports of the reproductive tract is like any hernia, referred to in terms of the anatomic site or organ involved. Urethrocele, cystocele, rectocele, and uterine prolapse are commonly used to describe pelvic hernias or pelvic relaxations. In addition, perineal lacerations and uterine displacement are encountered in clinical practice.

Urethrocele

Herniation of the paravaginal fascia under the urethra may permit the structure to bulge into the vaginal canal, producing a urethrocele. The patient may be asymptomatic or may complain of a vaginal mass or protrusion and incontinence of urine on stress if the weakness involves the fascial supports in the region of the posterior urethrovesical angle. A bulge in this area may be mistaken for a urethral diverticulum or redundant vaginal skin and should be carefully distinguished at the time of examination.

Cystocele

A cystocele is a bulging of the anterior vaginal wall beneath the floor of the bladder (Fig. 48–3). It results from loss of support in the area that is normally maintained by the pubocervical or paravaginal fascia and the permanent stretching of the oblique tunnel of the levator sling through which the vagina passes. The patient may complain of a bearing-down sensation, a vaginal protrusion, and urinary stress incontinence if there is a coexisting urethrocele. The weakness in the anterior vaginal wall can be readily palpated, or the bulging can be accentuated with stress such as is produced by coughing, straining, or bearing down. If the posterior wall of the vagina is depressed with a Sims speculum, the bulging of the anterior vaginal wall below the bladder can be readily observed. If a significant portion of the bladder lies below the urethrovesi-

cal junction, residual urine may remain after voiding; this predisposes to recurrent episodes of urinary frequency, urgency, and cystitis; ascending urinary tract infection may also develop.

Uterine Prolapse

When the primary supporting ligaments of the uterus (the cardinal ligaments) are attenuated or injured, the uterus is permitted to drop (Fig. 48–4). For clinical staging and descriptive purposes, three degrees of uterine prolapse are recognized: 1) in first-degree prolapse some descent of the uterus has occurred, but the cervix has not reached the vaginal introitus; 2) in second-degree prolapse the cervix, alone or with part of the uterus, passes through the vaginal introitus; 3) in third-degree prolapse or procidentia (Fig. 48–5) the entire uterus protrudes beyond the vaginal introitus, and the examining fingers can be brought together at the introitus, above the uterine fundus. Because the bladder is normally adherent to the cervix above the vaginal vault, it is brought down with the uterus (Fig. 48–6). The peritoneal pouch of Douglas is also elongated in marked uterine prolapse. Accordingly, in advanced uterine prolapse, cystocele and enterocele are either potential or real and require attention at the time of surgical repair.

The symptoms of uterine prolapse result from the discomfort and inconvenience of the protruding mass

FIG. 48–3. Cystocele. *A.* Exposed by Sims speculum. *B.* Sagittal view.

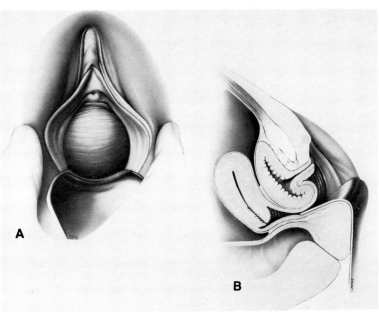

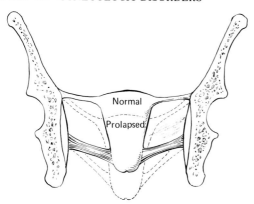

FIG. 48-4. Uterine prolapse or descensus. Schematic representation showing supporting influence of transverse cervical ligaments. When these are attentuated or lengthened, gravity and intraabdominal pressure bring uterus to lower level in pelvis. (Modified from Kelly HA: Gynecology. New York, Appleton, 1928)

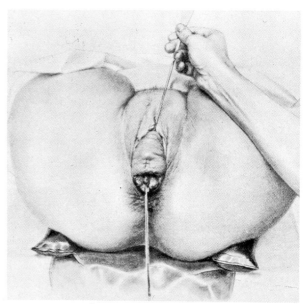

FIG. 48-6. Partial prolapse of uterus and vagina. Sound is introduced into bladder to show altered direction of urethra. Light spot on anterior vaginal wall plainly shows position of end of sound in bladder. (Kelly HA: Operative Gynecology. New York, Appleton, 1898. Drawing by Max Brödel)

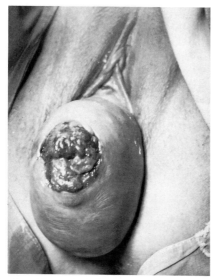

FIG. 48-5. Procidentia with marked decubitus ulceration and granular erosion of cervix. Bladder is on anterior aspect of mass. Pouch below cervix contains loops of small bowel.

as well as from irritation of the exposed cervix and vaginal epithelium. Frequently the cervix is markedly elongated and eroded, producing bleeding and discharge.

Procidentia is a most complex anatomic distortion. Anteriorly, the bladder has advanced with the uterus, and with it the trigone. Not only are the ureters exposed to easy surgical injury, but kinking or edema may already have given rise to chronic obstruction and hydroureter; hence, renal damage may be associated. Posteriorly, advancement of the pouch of Douglas with

consequent enterocele places loops of small bowel within easy reach of the surgeon's knife. It should be evident that repair of a third-degree prolapse and maintenance of a functional vagina is no easy task and requires meticulous knowledge of the relations that are present (Fig. 48-7) as well as the most careful attention to the restoration of the pelvic supports.

If the condition is of long standing, such severe edema may have developed in the prolapsed structures that they cannot be easily repositioned. Firm and sometimes prolonged circumferential pressure, beginning with the most dependent portion, often reduces the size of the prolapsed structures so that replacement can be accomplished. If this is not effective, keeping the patient at bedrest for 24 hours, with the hips, and particularly the prolapsed structures, elevated, generally lessens the edema sufficiently to permit easy repositioning.

Enterocele

An enterocele is a herniation of the investing fascia of the posterior part of the vagina at the level of the pouch of Douglas between the uterosacral ligaments and below the cervix (Fig. 48-8). It may be caused by a congenital weakness of the fascial supports in this area that produces a narrow-necked peritoneal sac associated with a deep cul-de-sac. More frequently it is acquired through obstetric trauma, and the sac is

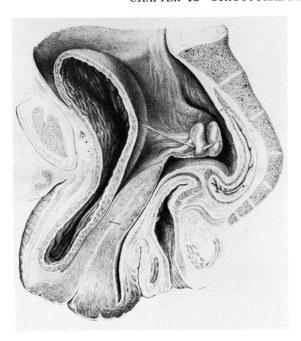

FIG. 48-7. Parasagittal section showing approximate relations of procidentia illustrated in Figure 48-5. (Halban J, Tandler J: Anatomie und Ätiologie der Genitalprolapse beim Weibe. Vienna, Braumüller, 1907)

FIG. 48-8. Sagittal section demonstrating relative position of enterocele and rectocele. (Telinde RW, Mattingly RF: Operative Gynecology, 4th ed. Philadelphia, JB Lippincott, 1970)

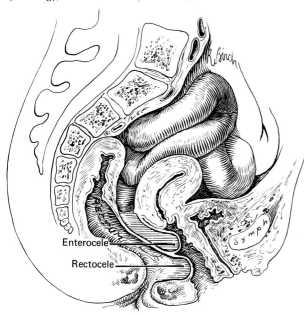

wider but shorter. Since it lies above the rectovaginal septum, the sacculation contains loops of small bowel and occasionally omentum, but not rectum. Depending on its size and extent, there may be no symptoms or a dull dragging sensation, low backache, and, rarely, deep pelvic pain. If an enterocele is large enough, protrusion can be very troublesome.

A common error in gynecologic surgery is failure to recognize and correct either a potential or an existing enterocele. All too often, the bulge in the posterior vaginal wall is interpreted as a large or high rectocele. Examination for enterocele is best performed with an anterior vaginal wall retractor held in place and a finger in the rectum. If the upper portion of the vaginal sacculation fails to admit the examining finger, an enterocele most likely exists. In any operation undertaken to correct prolapse of the uterus or rectocele, an enterocele should be looked for and, if present, corrected. No rectocele repair has ever repaired an enterocele, and failure to repair an enterocele at the time of surgery for symptomatic uterine prolapse may fail to cure the patient's complaints.

Rectocele

A rectocele is a herniation of the anterior rectal wall through the relaxed or ruptured vaginal fascia and rectovaginal septum (Fig. 48-9). The supports are weakened or torn by childbirth and further weakened with straining at defecation. The defect is accentuated when the patient bears down.

A slight to moderate rectocele is asymptomatic, but as the hernia increases in size, the fecal column tends to be pushed into the sacculation protruding into the vaginal canal. A fairly common complaint is that defecation can only be accomplished with digital pressure applied vaginally against the sacculation.

Prolapse of the Vagina

Prolapse of the vagina is an uncommon but very distressing condition that occurs after removal of the uterus, either abdominally or vaginally. It is invariably associated with enterocele and often with cystocele. The condition can arise *de novo* a number of years after hysterectomy, or it can result from failure to recognize and correct a potential or existing enterocele at the time of the hysterectomy. Also, failure to reattach the vaginal vault to the uterosacral and cardinal ligaments and pubocervical fascia following removal of the uterus can be a contributing factor.

Chronic Perineal Lacerations

Old or chronic laceration of the perineum results from either failure to repair or improper repair of acute second- or third-degree perineal lacerations, the majority of which occur at childbirth.

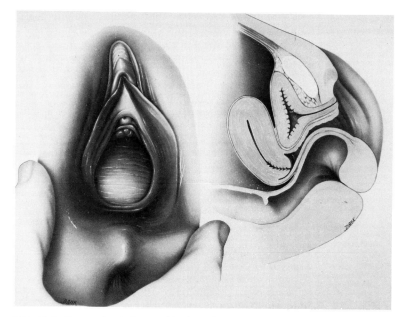

FIG. 48-9. Rectocele. **A.** Exposed by lateral traction. **B.** Sagittal view.

Old second-degree lacerations involve only the substance of the perineal body and not the sphincter ani. The thickness of the perineum between the distal portion of the vagina and the vestibule and the anal canal is greatly reduced so that the introitus gapes. A rectocele is usually present. The symptoms are usually negligible, but occasionally there is a complaint of loss of sexual sensation for both partners at the time of intercourse. In some cases, surgical repair may be indicated.

In an old third-degree laceration, the sphincter ani is divided and retracted sufficiently to cause incontinence of both feces and flatus (Fig. 48-10). The perineal body and lower 1-2 in. of the midportion of the posterior vaginal wall may be missing and the introitus widely gaping. Surgical repair is essential to relieve the patient's distressing and often embarrassing symptoms.

TREATMENT OF PELVIC RELAXATIONS

Pelvic relaxations of varying types and degrees are found in all women who have delivered children vaginally. Although symptom-producing pelvic relaxations may occur in any age group, they are most common after the climacteric. They should always be treated surgically, preferably when the patient has completed her family, unless there are strong contraindications to the anesthesia required for the surgical repair, such as chronic debility, severe cardiopulmonary disease, extreme age, or disability.

The more common indications for treatment are in the case of anterior vaginal wall relaxations, sensation of a protruding mass, recurrent cystitis, and urinary stress incontinence; in the case of posterior vaginal wall relaxations, difficulty with defecation, vaginal protrusion, and loss of sensation during intercourse; in the case of uterine descensus, protrusion, pelvic discomfort, sensations of pressure or bearing down, and lack of sensation at time of coitus.

Surgical Therapy

The operative procedures used to correct symptomatic relaxations are described in Chapter 61. The only point to emphasize here is that the successful repair of any vaginal wall weakness or uterine prolapse depends on the ability of the gynecologic surgeon to dissect the various supports, to reconstruct the normal relations of the vaginal and uterine supporting structures, and to reestablish a functional vagina. Such palliative procedures as colpocleisis or vaginectomy are performed only in those rare instances in which all other methods of gaining support have failed and the maintenance of vaginal function is of no importance.

Nonsurgical Therapy

Various types of pessaries are illustrated in Figure 48-11. When properly selected, they are useful in the patient with symptomatic pelvic relaxation, who, for one reason or another, is unable to undergo surgical repair. A pessary can be effective when the uterus prolapses with the bladder, but it is useless if there is so much relaxation at the vaginal outlet that it is promptly expelled with any increase in intra-

abdominal pressure, such as during coughing or defecation.

The choice of pessary must be individualized for the patient's needs. A ring pessary is effective for prolapse of the uterus, but is of little use for a cystocele. A rubber or plastic doughnut-shaped pessary with a collapsible ring, or the Smith–Hodge pessary (Fig. 48–12), is useful when a cystocele exists (Fig. 48–13). A soft, pure gum rubber, cube-shaped pessary with concave surfaces on all sides is beneficial in an appropriately selected patient (Fig. 48–14).

Any physician who inserts a pessary assumes responsibility for its care. The patient must be advised that the pessary should not be painful or uncomfortable and that if it is, it probably has become displaced and should be checked and another size or a different type inserted. If the patient is unable to remove the pessary herself at bedtime and reinsert it each morning, she should be examined at 2- or 3-month intervals for vaginal irritation. All postmenopausal patients in whom a pessary is placed should be given oral or topical estrogen therapy to improve the tone and resistance of the vaginal epithelium.

DISPLACEMENT OF THE UTERUS

The term *displacement of the uterus* usually indicates a displacement in the coronal plane of the pelvis. Thus, the uterus may be in a position of anteflexion, misposition, or retroflexion. Normally, the uterus is located in a position of moderate anteversion in the anterior pelvis with its long axis approximately at a right angle to the axis of the vaginal canal, as shown in Figure 3–6. Other terms used to describe the position of the uterus refer to the direction of the long axis of the uterus in relation to that of the vaginal canal. There may be lateral displacement, anteversion, retroversion, or retrocession.

Many positional differences are simple anatomic variations, which are asymptomatic and of no clinical consequence. By far the most common simple displacement of the uterus is retroversion, which may be congenital or acquired following childbirth or as a result of cul-de-sac disease. The latter is usually part of a disease process and may therefore be of clinical significance. Lateral displacement of the uterus may occur in association with adnexal disease, when the uterus is either pushed aside by a large ovarian tumor on the opposite side or pulled to the side of the disease process by inflammatory adhesions or scars.

CONGENITAL RETROVERSION OF THE UTERUS

Congenital retroversion of the uterus by itself is seldom of any clinical import. Although a variety of pelvic symptoms has been attributed to a congenitally retroverted uterus (dysmenorrhea, dyspareunia, infertility,

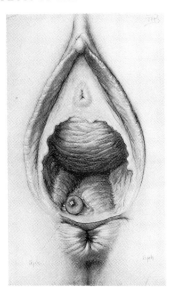

FIG. 48-10. Complete tear of perineum. Note well-defined sphincter pits and retraction and thickening of muscle, with deep dimple behind it. Vaginal cyst due to inclusion of vaginal mucosa in healing process is seen in right sulcus in scar area. (Kelly HA: Operative Gynecology. New York, Appleton, 1898. Drawing by Max Brödel)

back pain, menorrhagia), the position of the uterus in the pelvis as the sole cause of these symptoms has never been substantiated. The uterus is invariably freely mobile and can be manually anteverted during pelvic examination or tilted forward if the patient assumes the knee-chest position.

A movable, symptom-producing retroverted uterus can be held in an anteverted position with a Smith–Hodge pessary. The only indications for using the pessary to antevert a congenitally retroverted uterus are 1) to assist the uterus to rise out of the pelvis more easily in early pregnancy and thus possibly relieve back pain; 2) occasionally, when no other cause can be found for infertility, to achieve a more favorable relation between the external cervical os and the seminal pool deposited in the posterior fornix; and 3) to relieve deep pelvic dyspareunia or dysmenorrhea unresponsive to other therapeutic procedures. If the symptoms are completely relieved for 3 months while the pessary has maintained the uterus in an anteverted position and if they recur after removal of the pessary, a uterine suspension procedure might be considered.

ACQUIRED RETROVERSION OF THE UTERUS

Acquired retroversion of the uterus most often follows childbirth and results from an attenuation during

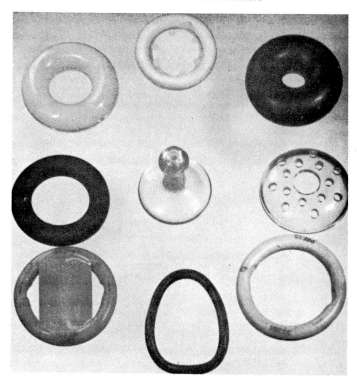

FIG. 48–11. Types of pessaries. Clockwise, beginning at 12 o'clock position: round solid plastic ring, rubber doughnut, plastic disk with perforation, collapsible ring, Smith–Hodge pessary, Gellhorn pessary (center), collapsible ring with central support, solid rubber ring, inflatable rubber doughnut. (Parsons L, Sommers S: Gynecology. Philadelphia, WB Saunders, 1962)

pregnancy of the two sets of ligaments most responsible for maintaining the uterus in anteversion—the uterosacral and round ligaments. In most women, the uterus returns to an anterior position within 2 months following delivery; in approximately one-third, it remains retroverted.

Fixed retroversion results from traction on the corpus from adherent pelvic and especially adnexal lesions, notably those due to chronic salpingo-oophoritis and endometriosis. Large myomas of the uterus may also cause uterine retroversion. Pelvic symptoms are due to the underlying disease. In the course of corrective surgery aimed at preserving or improving fertility, mobilization of the uterus and adnexa and their maintenance in an anterior position, away from old and potential new sites of adherence, is probably the most valid single indication for a uterine suspension operation.

Uncomplicated acquired uterine retroversion is rarely symptomatic. Occasionally, a patient may have difficulty in conceiving because the cervix points toward the anterior vaginal wall, away from the seminal pool left in the posterior fornix after coitus in the supine position.

Backache is not a symptom of uncomplicated uterine retroversion. More often, low back pain is caused by spasms of the small muscles of the back, often associated with an abnormality of the bony spine. Faulty posture, poor general health, and obesity may be contributing factors, but not the retroverted uterus.

Chronic pelvic congestion syndrome, a condition usually associated with a retroverted uterus, has been described as a cause of deep pelvic and low back pain. Viewed at operation, the pelvic veins seem to be enlarged, tortuous, and engorged, and a congested uterus is found in the retroverted position. The ovaries are frequently enlarged and prolapsed and often contain many follicular cysts. The woman may have menstrual abnormalities, and frequently the clinical picture associated with premenstrual tension is exaggerated. The clinical syndrome, more frequently seen in white women, may also be associated with chronic cystic mastitis. Heavy psychologic overtones are often present, and the diagnosis of congestion syndrome must be made with caution.

Symptoms associated with fixed uterine retroversion are, as mentioned before, due to the associated condition maintaining the uterus in the retroverted position. Deep pelvic pain and low backache, dysmenorrhea, dyspareunia, and menstrual irregulari-

ties are among the more commonly encountered complaints.

INVERSION OF THE UTERUS

Inversion of the uterus is the circumstance in which the uterus turns inside out so that the endometrium lining the fundus extends through the dilated cervix; if inversion is complete, the entire structure is prolapsed through the cervix into the vagina. The adnexa are usually carried into the inversion cup with the fundus.

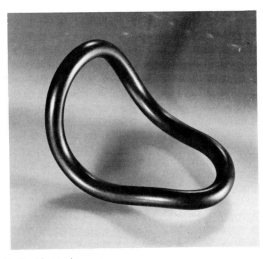

FIG. 48-12. Smith–Hodge pessary.

Although inversion is rare, it must be recognized at once when it is encountered. It results either from delivery or from the presence of uterine tumor.

Polypoid submucous fibroids that arise from the fundus by a wide stalk may, if they are large enough to distend the lower pole of the uterus, give rise to uterine contractions that ultimately cause the tumor to be extruded through the external os; the fundus follows. Inversion may also be produced by heavy traction on a polypoid tumor that presents at the external os. Occasionally, vaginal hysterectomy may be necessary, and the physician should be prepared to undertake this operation when large polypoid submucous fibroids are to be removed vaginally, either by excision or avulsion.

The inversion that follows labor may be spontaneous or may result from the combination of excessive fundal pressure and traction upon the umbilical cord in an effort to expel the placenta attached in the fundus. The management of this condition in its acute stage is an obstetric problem and is considered in Chapter 36.

In chronic uterine inversion, infection and edema of the exposed endometrium are the rule. Excessive bleeding is also common, owing to failure of the endometrial hemostatic mechanisms. In addition, the adnexa, which are within the inversion cup, are usually congested and adherent both to one another and to the uterine serosa. A pulling, abdominal discomfort may be present because of the adnexal congestion as well as the prolonged tension upon the infundibulopelvic ligaments and round ligaments.

FIG. 48-13. Sagittal view of Smith–Hodge pessary in place. Observe how uterus is held in normal position. (Parsons L, Sommers S: Gynecology. Philadelphia, WB Saunders, 1962)

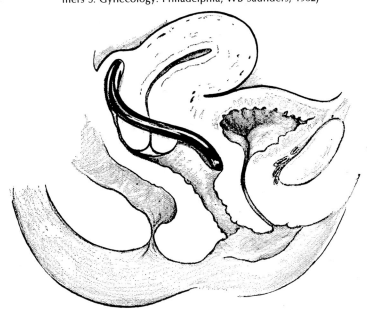

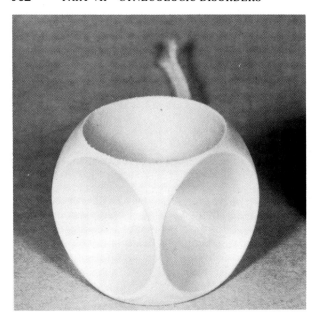

FIG. 48–14. Pure gum rubber cube pessary, which comes in various sizes. Support is provided by suction action of six concave surfaces. Pessary is self-positioning upon insertion and provides effective support in vaginal prolapse. (Milex Products, Chicago)

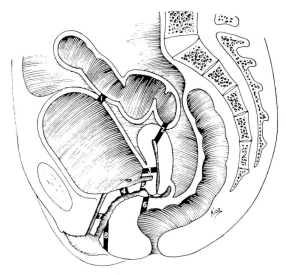

FIG. 48–15. Common sites for fistulas. *1,* Vesicocolic. *2,* Uterocolic. *3,* Vesicouterine or vesicocervical. *4,* Vesicovaginal. *5,* ureterovaginal. *6,* Rectovaginal. *7,* Urethrovagina. *8,* Vaginoperineal. (Jeffcoate TNA: Principles of Gynaecology, 3rd ed. London, Butterworth, 1967)

Uterine inversion of long standing should be treated surgically. Unless an effort must be made to preserve childbearing potential, hysterectomy is the definitive procedure. The prolapsed structure should be treated by antiseptic vaginal douches before operation. The approach should be abdominal. The condition is corrected by making an incision through the posterior aspect of the cervix and extending into the posterior vaginal vault and having an assistant push the fundus upward from below. When normal relations are restored, the defect is repaired and hysterectomy performed.

FISTULAS

A fistula is an abnormal or unnatural communication from one hollow viscus to another or from a hollow viscus to the outside. In the female reproductive tract, fistula may result from congenital anomaly, gynecologic surgery, obstetric injury, cancer, radiation therapy, trauma, or infection. The most common sites for fistulas are shown in Figure 48–15.

Enterovesical, enterouterine, and enterovaginal fistulas generally involve the sigmoid colon or rectum. In the first two, the condition is usually primary in the bowel, resulting from malignant disease, diverticulitis, pelvic abscess, or tuberculosis. In the last-named, the customary causes are surgical injury (the result of colpoperineorrhaphy) and obstetric injury with perforation of the rectum or suture of the rectum. Fistulas that result from injury or infection are usually amenable to surgical closure, but those associated with malignant disease are not.

Fistulous openings from the urinary tract into the vagina are commonly urethrovaginal, vesicovaginal, or ureterovaginal. A urethrovaginal fistula is almost invariably the result of an inept attempt at vaginal delivery with forceps; fortunately, such injuries have become rare indeed. Vesicovaginal fistulas result commonly from obstetric injury, but may also result from pelvic fracture if bone spicules perforate the bladder, from cancer, and from injury during gynecologic surgery. Ureterovaginal fistulas are almost invariably the result of injury at the time of hysterectomy, either simple or radical.

In the case of surgical injuries of either ureter or bladder, the defect is usually not evident until the local edema begins to subside and the sutures give way, 7–10 days after the operation; at this time, urinary incontinence becomes evident. Examination of the patient in the knee–chest position, using a Sims speculum to hold the posterior vaginal wall away, may permit diagnosis of a urinary tract fistula. If not, three large pledgets of cotton may be placed in the vagina, one above the other, and methylene blue solution run into the bladder. If only the lowest pledget stains, the fistula is urethral; if the middle or upper pledget stains, the fistula is vesical; if none stains but the upper one is wet, the fistula is ureteral.

It is of special importance that the exact nature of a urinary tract fistula be determined. A small vesicovaginal fistula may close spontaneously without incident. The outlook for a ureterovaginal fistula is more dismal,

for even if the drainage stops, closure of the fistula is generally accompanied by stenosis of the ureter; hydronephrosis and ultimate loss of the kidney are to be expected if the lesion is not dealt with in time.

In addition to the foregoing, postoperative urinary or fecal drainage may occur through an abdominal incision. An abdominal wall urinary fistula results almost invariably from inadvertent suture of the bladder at closure of the abdominal incision or unrecognized incision into the bladder when the abdominal cavity is entered. Such fistulas rarely close spontaneously. Recognition of such injuries at the time they are made is of utmost importance. If 5 ml indigo carmine is instilled into the bladder before operation, there is instant spill of blue dye, and thus instant diagnosis, if the bladder is injured. This simple, harmless device should be routine in all operations associated with even a remote possibility of bladder injury.

Fistulas involving small intestine and draining either vaginally or through an abdominal incision are rare; they usually occur when there has been much dissection of adherent adnexal masses (extensive endometriosis, residues of pelvic inflammatory disease, carcinoma of the ovary), with denudation of the serosa of bowel and pelvis. Small bowel fistulas rarely close spontaneously, and their repair is usually no small undertaking.

REFERENCES AND RECOMMENDED READING

HYMEN AND LABIA

Capraro VJ, Greenberg H: Adhesions of the labia minora: A study of 50 patients. Obstet Gynecol 39:65, 1972

PELVIC SUPPORTS

Goff BH: The surgical anatomy of cystocele and urethrocele with special reference to the pubocervical fascia. Surg Gynecol Obstet 87:725, 1948
Green TH, Jr: Gynecology, 2nd ed. Boston, Little Brown, 1971
Porges RF, Porges JC, Blinick G: Mechanisms of uterine support and the pathogenesis of uterine prolapse. Obstet Gynecol 15:711, 1960
Ulfelder H: The mechanism of pelvic supports in women: Deductions from a study of the comparative anatomy and physiology of the structures involved. Am J Obstet Gynecol 72:856, 1956

ENTEROCELE

Kinzel GE: A study of 265 cases. Am J Obstet Gynecol 81:1166, 1961
Meigs JV: Enterocele. In Meigs JV, Sturgis SH (eds): Progress in Gynecology, Vol II. New York, Grune & Stratton, 1950

PERINEAL TEARS

Watson BP: Complete tear of perineum. In Meigs JV, Sturgis SH (eds): Progress in Gynecology, Vol I. New York, Grune & Stratton, 1946

PELVIC PAIN

Allen WA: Chronic pelvic pain. Am J Obstet Gynecol 109:198, 1971
Taylor HC, Jr: Chronic pelvic congestion. Am J Obstet Gynecol 57:211; 637; 654, 1949

49

THE URINARY TRACT AS RELATED TO GYNECOLOGY

**George W. Mitchell, Jr.
Martin Farber**

The related embryologic development of the urinary and reproductive tracts in the human female, their close anatomic proximity, and their joint susceptibility to the injury induced by various pathologic conditions have, of necessity, led to continuing attention by physicians whose sphere of interest is the female pelvis. The trend toward consolidation of obstetrics and gynecology as a single discipline and the emergence of urology as a specialty in its own right have modified the scope of urologic practice by gynecologists to those situations in which urologic dysfunction is directly attributable to gynecologic disease or its treatment. Such situations are numerous, and the student as well as the physician will do well to bear constantly in mind the close interrelation.

The portions of the urinary tract which are of specific interest to the gynecologist are the ureters, the bladder, and the urethra. The kidney is, indeed, an important structure and it may be secondarily affected by

gynecologic disease, *e.g.,* by ureteral obstruction from an extrinsic pelvic tumor, by ascending infection, or by intrinsic damage as a consequence of septic shock or transfusion reaction. The gynecologist must have direct knowledge of such conditions, but with these exceptions most renal problems are within the province of either the urologist or the nephrologist.

Symptoms referable to the pelvis may originate from any one or all of the pelvic viscera, and the patient, in giving her history, is often unable to identify correctly the source of the difficulty. Persistent lower quadrant or lower midline pain in the absence of demonstrable gynecologic disease should lead the examiner to investigate the urinary tract. Bleeding from the vagina is often first noticed at the time of voiding and interpreted as hematuria; conversely, hemorrhage from either urethra or rectum may be misidentified as being of uterine origin because of the patient's familiarity with the vicissitudes of menstruation. Pelvic pressure, urinary frequency, burning on urination, and nocturia may be associated with either intrinsic genital or urinary tract disease or a combination of both. On physical examination, a distended bladder may resemble an ovarian cyst or, by back pressure on the uterus, may lead to a diagnosis of retroversion. Tumors and calculi in the bladder or ureters are palpable as pelvis masses, and infiltrating carcinomas of the bladder spread through the lateral lymphatics in much the same manner as carcinomas of the cervix. So many such examples can be adduced that overlapping of the two fields seems to be the rule rather than the exception.

The most significant factor in urology is urinary stasis. When absolute stasis exists, life is immediately threatened. Partial stasis is more insidious but, if allowed to persist, carries implications almost as serious in the long run. Obstruction may occur at any point from the kidney to the urethral meatus and may be of simple mechanical or dysfunctional neuromuscular type. Gynecologic disease is responsible for much urinary stasis in the female and thus triggers a sequence of events which has protean clinical manifestations.

THE URETHRA

At the lower end of the urinary tract, the female urethra lies in an exposed position and is subject to more disorders than its small size would indicate. Descending from the bladder neck a distance of approximately 4 cm to its meatus in the vestibule of the vagina, the urethra gradually narrows from its proximal towards its distal end. Along its entire length the superior surface is in apposition with the symphysis pubis, and below it is supported by the submucosal smooth muscle of the vagina and by its own covering of connective tissue, the attenuated endopelvic fascia. It first perforates the interdigitating fibers of the pubococcygeus

muscle and, at its midportion, the fascia of the urogenital diaphragm.

The urethra is lined at its proximal end by transitional epithelium and at its lower third by squamous epithelium, which responds cyclically to the action of ovarian hormones. Cytologic examination of smears from the distal urethra provides an accurate assay of ovarian function.

The muscular wall is continuous with that of the bladder and consists of inner and outer longitudinal layers separated by an oblique layer. These oblique and longitudinal layers exert a paradoxic influence and are important in the physiology of micturition. A small, circular, striated muscle, the external urethral sphincter, is looped around the outer longitudinal layer of the main urethral wall. This muscle is relatively weak in the female and its constricting function can even be lost without causing symptoms.

A series of compound racemose glands, the glands of Skene, are situated close to the posterolateral wall of the distal urethra, with openings into the urethral floor and into the vagina close to the external meatus.

DISEASES

Complete obstruction of the female urethra as a result of either intrinsic or extrinsic disease is most uncommon. The descent of a large submucous myoma into the cervix or vagina or the impaction of an ovarian or uterine tumor in the posterior pelvis occasionally pushes the urethra against the pubis with force sufficient to occlude it, and in these cases anuria usually develops quite suddenly. A poorly fitted pessary or contraceptive device in the vagina may have the same effect. Blood clots and bladder calculi may also descend into the vesical neck and cause total retention; the remote possibility of a foreign body having been deliberately inserted into the urethra by an emotionally disturbed individual must not be overlooked.

Relative obstruction of the urethra is often unrecognized. Fibrosis as the end result of severe infection is seldom seen today, but constricting scars due to operative procedures may require repeated dilitation in order to prevent urinary reflux which can flow backward as far as the renal pelves. Congenital obstructions at the bladder neck in female children and adults have received considerable attention in the urologic literature and have been traditionally treated by transurethral resection. Such obstructions have been labeled "female prostates," but usually consist of folds of mucosa which have a valvular action. A cervix pointing anteriorly as a result of marked uterine retroversion may simulate such a lesion at the time of cystoscopy.

The appearance at the urethral meatus of *prolapsed mucous membrane* as a result of varices, injury, or the atrophy of supporting tissues may suggest an erroneous diagnosis of neoplasm, especially when the ever-

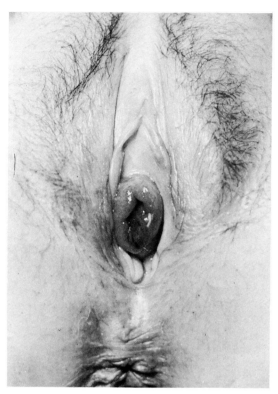

FIG. 49-1. Urethral prolapse. (From Haines M, Taylor CW: *Gynaecological Pathology.* London, Churchill, 1962)

sion takes the form of a rosette around the full circumference of the orifice (Fig. 49–1). When varices are present, thrombosis may lead to extreme sensitivity or pain in the area. Granulations forming around the everted tissue are called *caruncles.* They have a bright red, polypoid appearance and cause contact bleeding, often difficult to distinguish from vaginal bleeding. Though usually relatively innocuous in themselves, their treatment, whether by resection, fulguration, or radical cauterization, may produce permanent stricture, a very difficult therapeutic problem. Conservative management is usually indicated; careful surgery is justified only when symptoms warrant.

True *polyps* and *papillomas* occur in the proximal urethra and are more likely to cause bleeding than obstruction. They can be seen only by endoscopic visualization.

Malignant neoplasms of the urethra are rare but, when they do occur, usually take an exophytic form and are difficult to distinguish from carcinomas of the vulva even by histologic examination of biopsies. In the late stages the presenting complaint may be urinary retention.

Urethroceles and *urethral diverticula* are important in the development of urinary infections and, occasionally, of incontinence, but seldom cause retention.

The *acute urethral syndrome,* characterized by dysuria and frequency, is described in Chapter 50.

THE BLADDER

The urinary bladder is a hollow muscular organ situated between the uterus and vagina posteriorly and the abdominal wall and pubis anteriorly. It is attached to the uterus and vagina by connective tissue that increases in density from above downward, but is separated from the pubis by the space of Retzius.

A powerful smooth muscle, the detrusor, forms the wall of the bladder. Composed of both longitudinal and oblique layers, this muscle is responsible for the involuntary completion of micturition once it has begun. The detrusor becomes thicker from the bladder dome downward, and there is a marked condensation of fibers near the base, or trigone, where contractions originate.

The junction of the bladder and urethra, the vesical neck, has received much attention as the site of the internal sphincter and is thought to play a prominent role in preserving urinary continence. Histologically and anatomically, no separate sphincter muscle exists, but the overlapping oblique and longitudinal fibers surrounding the urethra and bladder suggest a specially adapted and stronger muscle component at this point.

The bladder is principally supported on the arch formed by the levator ani muscle group, especially the pubococcygeus. The levator fascia blends with the endopelvic fascia, which invests the bladder to form a dense layer beneath its dependent portion and provide a line of defense against prolapse. This layer lies directly under the submucosal smooth muscle of the vagina, which also supports bladder and urethra until it loses its elasticity with old age or succumbs to childbirth injury. When disrupted, these structures may be reapproximated and tightened by various surgical procedures.

The bladder is lined by transitional epithelium that contains sensory nerve endings responding to heat, cold, touch, and pain. It is paler over the trigone than it is over the dome and is crossed by small superficial blood vessels.

The principal nerve supply of the bladder is autonomic (Fig. 49–2). The parasympathetic division is derived from the second, third, and fourth sacral segments, which traverse the lateral pelvic walls beneath the great vessels to ganglia within the bladder adventitia. These nerves are both efferent and afferent and are chiefly responsible for maintaining bladder tone, promoting detrusor contraction, and mediating the stretch reflex. The sympathetic division is a continuation of the lumbar ganglionic chains and the intermesenteric plexus combined to form the hypogastric nerve, which traverses the presacral area to a plexus anterior to the rectum. The fibers penetrate the base of the broad ligament and enter the bladder in the region of the trigone. These are also both efferent and afferent, probably assisting in initiating detrusor action, in closing ureteral orifices against reflux, and in intensifying bladder sensation. Section of the hypogastric nerve, however, produces no demonstrable effect on bladder function.

The somatic muscle that envelops the urethra is supplied by a branch of the external pudendal nerve. The levator ani muscles concerned with the voluntary initiation and cessation of micturition are supplied by the pudic nerve from the second and third sacral nerves.

The parasympathetic reflex arc has its center in the sacral cord and is connected through the lateral gray columns with higher centers in the lumbar cord and in subcortical and cortical areas. A break in this long network of nerve tissue at the cord level severs the reflex arc from central control, while injury to the parasympathetic reflex itself makes the bladder completely autonomous. Owing to its rich intrinsic system of ganglia and nerve fibers, some tone and function may remain even in such difficult circumstances.

Cinefluoroscopic studies of the dye-filled bladder

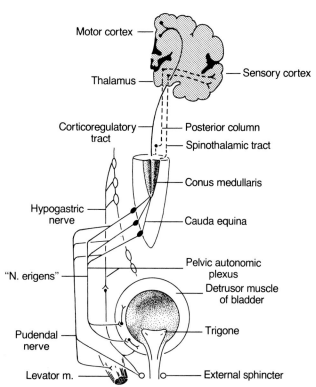

FIG. 49–2. Nerve supply of bladder. Interruption of nerve pathways at any level results in varying degrees of bladder disability.

and urethra provide a continuous record of their appearance at different stages of normal function and under pathologic conditions. In the collapsed state the silhouette is that of a Y, whether viewed anteriorly or laterally. The superior margin of the bladder is indented and the degree of indentation is exaggerated by the pressure of an anteverted uterus (Fig. 49–3). The lateral view demonstrates the acute angle between the bladder base and urethra and shows the beginning projection of the dome across the pubic symphysis.

As the bladder fills, it assumes a globular shape, slightly asymmetric as a result of the relative fixation of the bladder base, which serves as a pivot. Distention causes posterior rotation of the uterine fundus and overdistention causes bulging of the lower anterior abdominal wall. The exposed position of the expanding bladder within the pelvis, its proximity to the rectus muscles and to the uterus, and its compressibility make its internal pressure gradient liable to sudden change from variations in external stress.

DISEASES

Cystitis, the commonest of all bladder diseases, is subsequently considered in connection with urinary tract infections.

Because of its capacity, the bladder is subject to *mechanical obstruction* only where it joins the urethra and ureters. If denervated, however, its loss of contracting power causes functional obstruction. Failure of the ureterovesical valves allows reflux of urine from the contracting bladder up the ureters, with resultant high stasis. Severe, long-standing infections, such as that caused by tuberculosis, or the rigid, contracted bladder of encrusted cystitis, may produce an obstructive effect.

Endometriosis is rare in the bladder. It is a cause of hematuria at the time of menses but is never sufficiently extensive to produce urinary stasis. The characteristic small bluish cysts show up well at cystoscopy.

Large *cystoceles,* especially those associated with marked prolapse of the uterus, produce enough angulation of the proximal urethra and vesical neck to cause gradual dilatation of the bladder and trabeculation of its muscular wall. This is most pronounced when the urethral tube is relatively well supported, and the result, when the bladder can no longer compensate, may be acute urinary retention. Such a denouement occurs most often in an elderly woman and may cause her, for the first time, to seek medical assistance. Although many patients with cystoceles are asymptomatic and others can manage their problem temporarily either by manual replacement to facilitate voiding or by the intravaginal use of pessaries, surgery is usually indicated to prevent long-term urinary tract complications.

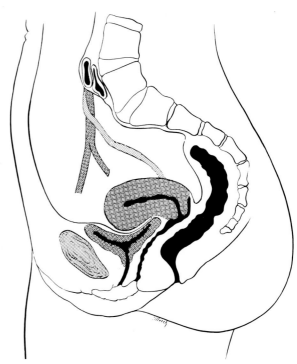

FIG. 49–3. Lateral view of pelvic viscera. Anteverted uterine fundus indents collapsed bladder, causing filling defect that may be noted in cystograms and at cystoscopy.

THE URETERS

The ureters are muscular tubular structures lined by transitional epithelium and carrying a rich vascular and nerve supply. The caliber is variable, and several natural areas of constriction are the sites at which calculi or clots usually lodge. The smallest diameter is in the isthmic portion, which runs for about 1 cm through the bladder wall to the ureteral orifice. In general, the diameter averages about 2 mm in the uncontracted state. As a lifeline, the ureter must not only remain patent but must also preserve its peristaltic activity.

The pelvic ureter passes along the posterior peritoneum of the broad ligament to the parametrium, then forward toward the cervix, inclining medially to enter the wall of the bladder base at an oblique angle. It is separated from the cervix by about 12 mm at the closest point and is situated about 1 cm from the lateral vaginal fornix. The uterine vessels cross over the ureter in the parametrium, and the terminal ureter is enveloped in plexuses of small arteries and veins that aid its recuperative power after injury.

The ureter is vulnerable to extrinsic pressure from gynecologic disease at two main points: (1) at the junction of the upper and lower halves at the pelvic

brim as the ureter passes over the common iliac arteries, and (2) in the terminal portion where it traverses the lower broad ligament and enters the bladder in close apposition to the anterolateral margin of the uterine cervix. Late metasteses from pelvic malignancies to the lumbar and preaortic lymphatics occasionally block the ureter as high as the ureteropelvic junction, but this is an exception. Nearly any pathologic process in the pelvis, whether inflammatory or neoplastic, has the potential to obstruct the distal half of the ureter over its 15 cm length.

EFFECTS OF PREGNANCY

Hydroureter and hydronephrosis are frequently, but not invariably, associated with the late stages of normal intrauterine pregnancy. This is probably due to the pressure exerted by the enlarging uterus, particularly the fetal head, but the inhibiting action of the high levels of progesterone on ureteral musculature, with the resultant decrease in the frequency and amplitude of contractions, may play a part. Occasionally the dilatation is seen only on one side, more often the right. The administration of large doses of progestational agents may also decrease ureteral peristalsis, but has not been shown to produce hydronephrosis.

OBSTRUCTION

The lymphatic pathways from the cervix follow the course of the uterine vessels as they pass over the terminal ureter and provide channels for the early spread of *carcinoma of the cervix* through the parametrium.

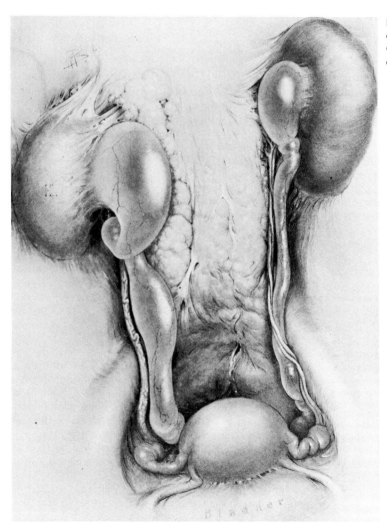

FIG. 49–4. Bilateral hydronephrosis and hydroureter due to carcinoma of cervix. (Kelly HA: Operative Gynecology, Vol 2. New York, Appleton, 1899; drawing by Max Brödel)

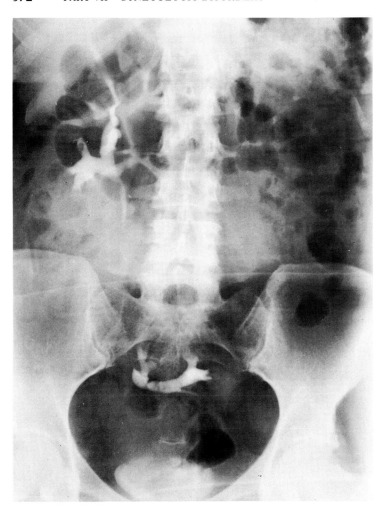

FIG. 49–6. Pelvic kidney demonstrated by intravenous pyelography in patient admitted to hospital for removal of easily palpable pelvic mass.

certain knowledge of adequate function of another kidney.

Final location of the adult kidney on the side contralateral to its ureteral origins and usually fused to the lower pole of the orthotopic kidney is designated *crossed renal ectopia*. A further variation is observed if the kidneys are joined, usually at their lower poles, across the midline by an isthmus of renal parenchyma, thereby producing a horseshoe configuration. When symptomatic, these anomalies cause pain and fever due to stasis of urine and infection.

INFECTIONS OF THE URINARY TRACT

The inevitable result of urinary stasis is infection, but not all urinary tract infections are associated with stasis. Because of its frequency and potential seriousness, infection is a source of interest to investigators and clinicians. The symptoms, microbiology, course, and study of urinary tract infections in pregnancy, as noted in Chapter 27, are also applicable to the gynecologic patient.

The vulva, vagina, and cervix customarily harbor bacteria and other parasites, many of which are pathogenic. As a result of variations in host resistance, they may, at any time, give rise to local inflammation. The chief symptom of such disease is usually a persistent discharge, one of the most common complaints of the gynecologic patient. The short female urethra, its meatus bathed by vaginal discharge, is vulnerable to ascending infection, especially if the junctional epithelium has become everted as a result of childbirth trauma or has been violated by catheters, sounds, or cystoscopes. The fact that the urethra and bladder base share with the vagina some of the same lymphatics and blood vessels exposes them to invasion through these channels. Every woman who has a history of fre-

Anomalies of Renal Mass

The symptom complex of *bilateral renal agenesis,* pulmonary hypoplasia, and the typical facies including hypertelorism, prominent epicanthal folds that sweep inferiorly and laterally under the lower lid, flattening and broadening of the nose, low-set ears with sparse cartilage formation, and a prominent depression between the lower lip and chin, together with genital malformations, constitutes *Potter's syndrome.* Although maternal estriol excretion is normal during the affected pregnancy, in 50% of cases the fetus is small for dates, tends to deliver prematurely, and frequently presents by the breech. The incidence of this syndrome is reported to be about 1:3500 births. It may be suspected antenatally if oligohydramnios is present. Intrauterine death is common.

Unilateral renal agenesis is clinically diagnosed in 1:1500 patients. Commonly, the solitary kidney is affected by hydronephrosis, calculus, or pyelonephritis due to vesicoureteral reflux or ureteral stricture at the ureteropelvic junction. In the asymptomatic state it should be strongly suspected if there is asymmetric, anomalous development of the müllerian ducts such as unicornuate uterus, or double uterus and single cervix with rudimentary noncommunicating uterine horn, or double uterus and cervix with unilaterally imperforate vagina. Fifteen percent of patients with Rokitansky–Küster–Hauser syndrome have unilateral renal agenesis and, conversely, 90% of patients with unilateral renal agenesis will be found to have a significant anomaly of the müllerian ducts.

Renal hypoplasia should be considered in the differential diagnosis of hypertension in young women or children. It is diagnosed if there is a generalized decrease in renal mass to less than two-thirds' normal size or a segmental reduction in renal mass due to localized renal tubular atrophy and glomerular myelinization. In the latter situation (*Ask–Upmark kidney*) the increased renin activity in venous effluent from the affected kidney is believed to be secreted by the hyperplastic juxtaglomerular apparatus of the adjoining renal parenchyma.

Anomalies of Renal Duplication

Ureteral duplication without renal duplication is the most common anomaly of the urinary tract and occurs in 0.6% of patients. In two-thirds of cases the duplication is incomplete and generally asymptomatic. The ureteral bifurcation is present in the upper 4 cm in 25% of cases, within 8 cm of the bladder in another 25%, and in between in the rest. Unusually asynchronous ureteral peristalsis causes regurgitation of urine from one limb of the bifid ureter to the other (saddle reflux), causing chronic infection. One limb of the bifid ureter may end blindly, either not associated with any renal parenchyma or causing chronic pyelo-

nephritis, which can often be alleviated by excision of the blind limb with or without the involved renal segment.

In the remaining cases in which ureteral duplication is complete but the kidney is not duplicated, the ureter serving the upper renal pole almost invariably passes under its duplicate at the level of the linea terminalis of the pelvis and ends inferior to the termination of the ureter serving the lower pole. Although most patients are asymptomatic, vesicoureteral reflux involving the lower-pole ureters may lead to hydronephrosis and pyelonephritis because of the short intravesical course of the lower-pole ureter, which obviates the sphincteric action of the bladder musculature and renders the ureteral orifice incompetent. Incontinence of urine alternating with normal voiding results when the upper-pole ureter ends ectopically in the vestibule, urethra, vagina, cervix, uterus, or rectum. Alternatively, distal obstruction of the ectopic ureter may cause hydronephrosis or chronic infection.

Rarely, duplication of the urinary tract results in the formation of a supernumerary kidney with no parenchymal attachment to the ipsilateral kidney. Although commonly asymptomatic, stasis and infection may develop and ultimately lead to the correct diagnosis.

Anomalies of Renal Position

Abnormalities of renal position, with or without fusion, are categorically the least common of the renal anomalies. Concomitant with variable failure of ascent to the normal adult position, the affected kidneys may be malrotated, medially displaced, show fetal lobulations on their external surfaces, be associated with anomalous vasculature, or they may be fused. Simple renal ectopia involving the kidney unilaterally is the most common variety (autopsy incidence, 1:3000), resulting in a pelvic location in 60% of cases. Pelvic fixation and fusion of the kidneys producing an amorphous renal mass (lump, discoid, or cake kidney) occurs in 1:17,000 autopsy cases. These anomalies may be diagnosed in the asymptomatic patient because of their association with anomalies of the müllerian ducts. When symptomatic, they may cause acute or chronic infection due to hydronephrosis or the affected patient may present with dyspareunia. *They must always be included in the differential diagnosis of a pelvic mass.* Labor is obstructed in 37% of cases, leading to delivery by cesarean section.

An ectopic kidney may be situated low in the midline of the abdomen or in the pelvis, either in the midline or to the right or left. In the latter case it is easily confused with an ovarian tumor and unless a preoperative urogram has been made it may first be diagnosed at the time of laparotomy (Fig. 49–6). A *pelvic kidney* is probably the most common retroperitoneal "tumor" in women, and it must not be removed unless there is

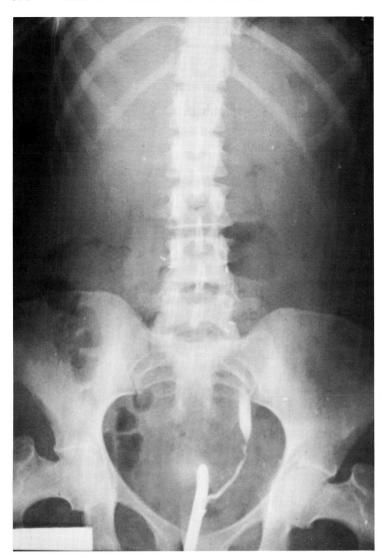

FIG. 49–5. Left ureteral obstruction in patient who developed left pyelonephritis 5 weeks after pelvic surgery. Retrograde pyelogram demonstrates 2-cm strictured area with typical pencil-shaped dilatation of ureter proximal to it.

which suggests that the urinary tract should be radiographically defined in all women with pelvic masses or preoperative incontinence of urine.

ANOMALIES OF THE BLADDER AND URETHRA

Anomalies of the bladder and urethra are the least common of the urinary tract malformations. Congenital absence of the bladder, which is caused by complete failure of formation of the superior portion of the ventral cloaca, results in infection or incontinence when the ureters terminate in the vestibule or the vagina. The bladder and the urethra may be completely or partially duplicated, or complete sagittal or frontal septa may be formed. These unusual anomalies are commonly accompanied by vertebral, anal, rectal, and genital malformations. Urachal anomalies are caused by failure of complete embryonic obliteration of the distal ventral cloaca. The urachus may be completely patent from the vertex of the bladder to the umbilicus or partially patent, resulting in a urachal cyst, sinus, or diverticulum.

ANOMALIES OF THE KIDNEYS AND URETERS

Congenital anomalies of the kidneys and ureters are the most common malformations found in women and may be categorized as (1) anomalies of renal mass, (2) anomalies of renal duplication, and (3) anomalies of renal position (with or without fusion).

The ureter may be compressed by enlarged lymph nodes surprisingly early in the course of the disease, and its own wall and lymphatics may be directly involved (Fig. 49–4). More often this is a late manifestation. Hydroureter and hydronephrosis associated with cervical malignancy are ominous signs, and a nonfunctioning kidney is of even more serious significance, since it indicates obstruction of long duration.

Because of the urinary tract implications, a thorough urologic investigation is indicated in all cases of carcinoma of the cervix, both before and after therapy. This should include intravenous pyelography or, in cases of hypersensitivity to intravenous radiopaque material, retrograde pyelography. The latter is also essential to delineate the point of obstruction when deficient renal function leads to poor visualization of the dye. Cystoscopy should be routine and determinations of blood urea nitrogen and creatinine are standard tests of renal reserve.

Accepted techniques of radiation therapy for carcinoma of the cervix are designed to deliver the maximal dose to the primary tumor and lymphatic spread while sparing the bladder as much as possible. Theoretically, the bladder can tolerate as much as 6,000 gamma rads with recovery, but the lower urinary tract is invariably damaged to a greater or lesser degree by the treatment. In the bladder the *radiation-induced lesions* vary from an acute inflammatory reaction (radiation cystitis) to ulceration and fistula formation. The ureters are encased in dense fibrous tissue that may constrict as surely as the malignant process. These changes can occur months or many years after therapy and sometimes cannot be differentiated from persistent or recurrent carcinoma; however, recurrence is statistically more likely to be the cause of later obstruction. When severe renal impairment results from obstruction, either primary or secondary, temporary urinary diversion may be necessary while the patient is being evaluated for definitive treatment. In most cases this can be accomplished by percutaneous nephrostomy.

Pelvic surgery, especially hysterectomy, is an important cause of ureteral injury or obstruction. Persistent postoperative urinary tract symptoms or flank pain and, in some cases, unexplained fever should be investigated by intravenous urography (Fig. 49–5). Radical surgery for carcinoma of the cervix constitutes a serious hazard to the lower ureters and bladder. In addition to direct injury at the time of operation, the stripping of the nerve supply produces long-lasting atony and the ligation of blood vessels causes strictures and fistulae in about 4% of patients. Some patients have temporary and usually bilateral hydroureter and hydronephrosis as a result of the operation.

Late carcinoma of the vulva and vagina may involve the bladder and ureters in a manner similar to carcinoma of the cervix. *Adenocarcinoma of the corpus uteri* usually extends to higher lymphatic pathways, but when it spreads downward to the cervix, it can mimic cervical malignancy. *Ovarian carcinoma,* although it more often obstructs the intestines than the ureter, can, in the late stages, compress the ureters in three areas. If it is large enough to rise out of the pelvis, its weight may impinge upon the ureters at the brim of the pelvis; invasion along the infundibulopelvic ligament may involve a slightly lower segment and peritoneal metastases in the posterior pelvis may involve the ureter at its entrance into the broad ligament.

Retroperitoneal malignancies are sometimes low enough to be palpable by bimanual examination. Obstruction of the ureters from these tumors may occur at any level.

Retroperitoneal fibrosis, a benign disease of unknown cause, but occasionally associated with previous therapeutic abortion, may shut off one or both ureters, but relocation or reanastomosis around the obstruction is curative.

The possibility of obstruction must be considered when *large tumors of either uterine or adnexal origin* are present and pyelography should be requested prior to therapy. The subacute and chronic forms of pelvic inflammatory disease, whether postabortal or stemming from salpingitis, are of great concern, since the ureteral wall may be directly involved by infection and may become atonic. Pyelography is important, especially when large abscesses are present. The oliguria or anuria due to mechanical obstruction in postabortal sepsis must be carefully distinguished from the renal shutdown that occurs with septic shock. Ureteral obstruction due to endometriosis has been reported but is uncommon. The treatment of these conditions is both medical and surgical, the latter approach being technically complicated by dislocation of the ureters and bladder as a result of reaction in the local tissues. Ureteral injury due to simple hysterectomy is not uncommon. Prolapse of the uterus may cause angulation of the ureters and upper urinary tract dilatation. Congenital or other benign strictures of the lower ureters which have been said to occur in females in the absence of other demonstrable disease are extremely rare or nonexistent.

CONGENITAL ANOMALIES OF THE URINARY TRACT

Developmental malformations of the müllerian ducts are frequently accompanied by anomalies of the urinary tract. All women with such duct malformations should be cystoscoped and the upper urinary tract should be defined by intravenous pyelography. Although they may cause symptoms as diverse as dyspareunia, hypertension, flank or abdominal pain, dysuria, frequency of urination, or leukorrhea, congenital anomalies of the urinary tract are often asymptomatic,

brim as the ureter passes over the common iliac arteries, and (2) in the terminal portion where it traverses the lower broad ligament and enters the bladder in close apposition to the anterolateral margin of the uterine cervix. Late metastases from pelvic malignancies to the lumbar and preaortic lymphatics occasionally block the ureter as high as the ureteropelvic junction, but this is an exception. Nearly any pathologic process in the pelvis, whether inflammatory or neoplastic, has the potential to obstruct the distal half of the ureter over its 15 cm length.

EFFECTS OF PREGNANCY

Hydroureter and hydronephrosis are frequently, but not invariably, associated with the late stages of normal intrauterine pregnancy. This is probably due to the pressure exerted by the enlarging uterus, particularly the fetal head, but the inhibiting action of the high levels of progesterone on ureteral musculature, with the resultant decrease in the frequency and amplitude of contractions, may play a part. Occasionally the dilatation is seen only on one side, more often the right. The administration of large doses of progestational agents may also decrease ureteral peristalsis, but has not been shown to produce hydronephrosis.

OBSTRUCTION

The lymphatic pathways from the cervix follow the course of the uterine vessels as they pass over the terminal ureter and provide channels for the early spread of *carcinoma of the cervix* through the parametrium.

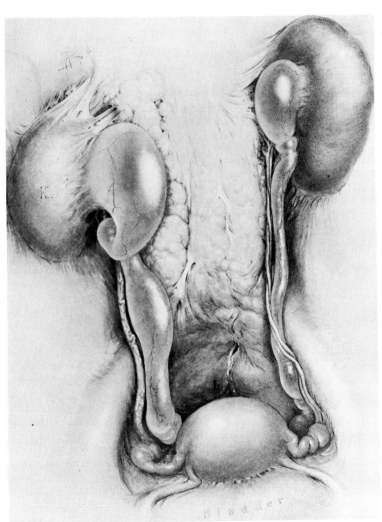

FIG. 49–4. Bilateral hydronephrosis and hydroureter due to carcinoma of cervix. (Kelly HA: Operative Gynecology, Vol 2. New York, Appleton, 1899; drawing by Max Brödel)

and urethra provide a continuous record of their appearance at different stages of normal function and under pathologic conditions. In the collapsed state the silhouette is that of a Y, whether viewed anteriorly or laterally. The superior margin of the bladder is indented and the degree of indentation is exaggerated by the pressure of an anteverted uterus (Fig. 49–3). The lateral view demonstrates the acute angle between the bladder base and urethra and shows the beginning projection of the dome across the pubic symphysis.

As the bladder fills, it assumes a globular shape, slightly asymmetric as a result of the relative fixation of the bladder base, which serves as a pivot. Distention causes posterior rotation of the uterine fundus and overdistention causes bulging of the lower anterior abdominal wall. The exposed position of the expanding bladder within the pelvis, its proximity to the rectus muscles and to the uterus, and its compressibility make its internal pressure gradient liable to sudden change from variations in external stress.

DISEASES

Cystitis, the commonest of all bladder diseases, is subsequently considered in connection with urinary tract infections.

Because of its capacity, the bladder is subject to *mechanical obstruction* only where it joins the urethra and ureters. If denervated, however, its loss of contracting power causes functional obstruction. Failure of the ureterovesical valves allows reflux of urine from the contracting bladder up the ureters, with resultant high stasis. Severe, long-standing infections, such as that caused by tuberculosis, or the rigid, contracted bladder of encrusted cystitis, may produce an obstructive effect.

Endometriosis is rare in the bladder. It is a cause of hematuria at the time of menses but is never sufficiently extensive to produce urinary stasis. The characteristic small bluish cysts show up well at cystoscopy.

Large *cystoceles,* especially those associated with marked prolapse of the uterus, produce enough angulation of the proximal urethra and vesical neck to cause gradual dilatation of the bladder and trabeculation of its muscular wall. This is most pronounced when the urethral tube is relatively well supported, and the result, when the bladder can no longer compensate, may be acute urinary retention. Such a denouement occurs most often in an elderly woman and may cause her, for the first time, to seek medical assistance. Although many patients with cystoceles are asymptomatic and others can manage their problem temporarily either by manual replacement to facilitate voiding or by the intravaginal use of pessaries, surgery is usually indicated to prevent long-term urinary tract complications.

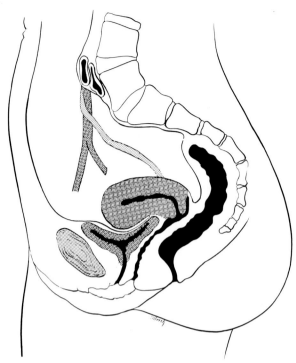

FIG. 49–3. Lateral view of pelvic viscera. Anteverted uterine fundus indents collapsed bladder, causing filling defect that may be noted in cystograms and at cystoscopy.

THE URETERS

The ureters are muscular tubular structures lined by transitional epithelium and carrying a rich vascular and nerve supply. The caliber is variable, and several natural areas of constriction are the sites at which calculi or clots usually lodge. The smallest diameter is in the isthmic portion, which runs for about 1 cm through the bladder wall to the ureteral orifice. In general, the diameter averages about 2 mm in the uncontracted state. As a lifeline, the ureter must not only remain patent but must also preserve its peristaltic activity.

The pelvic ureter passes along the posterior peritoneum of the broad ligament to the parametrium, then forward toward the cervix, inclining medially to enter the wall of the bladder base at an oblique angle. It is separated from the cervix by about 12 mm at the closest point and is situated about 1 cm from the lateral vaginal fornix. The uterine vessels cross over the ureter in the parametrium, and the terminal ureter is enveloped in plexuses of small arteries and veins that aid its recuperative power after injury.

The ureter is vulnerable to extrinsic pressure from gynecologic disease at two main points: (1) at the junction of the upper and lower halves at the pelvic

quency, urgency, dysuria, nocturia, or hematuria, or who, in the absence of specific symptoms, repeatedly shows positive urine cultures should have an examination of the genital tract, including direct visualization and bacteriologic cultures. In addition to taking a careful urologic history on all patients with complaints that are primarily gynecologic, particularly in the case of genital bleeding for which no obvious cause can be found, it is necessary to examine the urinary sediment and culture a urine sample. When quantitative analysis by a bacterial colony count is available, urine for culture should be taken by the *clean-catch technique*. This method consists of cleansing of the inner labia and urethral meatus, spreading the labia, and collecting a midstream-voided sample of urine in a sterile tube or pan. The fresh specimen should than be implanted on a culture medium within the hour. Colony counts of more than 100,000 organisms per ml are considered significant, and counts of this magnitude on two separate specimens assure an accuracy of 95%. If a catheter must be used, care should be exercised to assure the best sterile techniques and the procedure should be performed by experienced or carefully supervised personnel. When a bacteriology laboratory is not immediately available, slide and dipstick tests packaged for office use have an accuracy of approximately 85%. The most common pathogens in the vagina are seldom found in the urine, but they may give rise to severe urinary symptoms as a result of local hyperemia, edema, and secondary infection.

Because of a relative lack of estrogen, the prepubertal child and the postmenopausal woman are susceptible to vaginal and, hence, lower urinary tract infections. The probable mechanism is an elevation of the vaginal pH that, in the normal female of reproductive age, ranges from 3.8 to 4.2. Since the epithelium of the female urethra is affected by estrogen deprivation, varying degrees of urethritis are almost universal in older women. In the prepubertal child, lack of genital cleanliness, agglutination of the vulva, foreign bodies in the vagina, and sexual manipulation should be suspected as possibly contributing to persistent urinary symptoms.

Cystocele is seldom the cause of urinary tract infection. Women with large cystoceles are usually able to empty their bladders almost completely. For this reason repair of cystoceles to eliminate recurrent urinary infections is not advisable and the presence of an indwelling catheter postoperatively is likely to exacerbate the difficulty.

The *diagnosis of urinary infection,* apart from the history, is made by examination of the urine and by direct visualization of urethra and bladder using either water or carbon dioxide cystourethroscopes. Urinary sediment usually contains red and white blood cells and occasionally granular, hyaline, and pus cell casts, indicating renal involvement. The detection of antibody-coated bacteria—complexes that form only in the upper urinary tract—in urinary sediment by immunofluorescence has made it possible to differentiate between renal and vesical infection. At cystoscopy, erythema, edema, vascular dilatation, and exudate formation may be noted in the absence of a positive urine culture or abnormal urinary sediment. Bacteriuria does not necessarily imply infection of bladder mucosa and, conversely, significant infection of the bladder submucosa may exist in the presence of urine negative for bacteria. Many organisms capable of producing cystitis are not diagnosed by routine culture techniques: these include strains of mycoplasma, virus, and *Chlamydia trachomatis*. The latter has been implicated in up to 20% of cases of nongonococcal urethritis in males. Since it is thought to be venereally contracted, its presence in the female genitourinary tract seems highly probable. *Interstitial cystitis,* a disease of unknown cause marked by pelvic pain, dysuria, and the appearance of localized areas of hyperemia or ulceration of the bladder mucosa has no known etiology and is not associated with positive routine cultures.

A less serious example of inflammation of the bladder mucosa without bacteriuria is *urethrotrigonitis,* a condition marked by hyperemia and, in the advanced state, by a membranous exudate and granularity confined to the local area. Urethrotrigonitis is a common finding in parous and postmenopausal women, causing frequency, urgency and, when of marked degree, urgency incontinence. Its frequent association with the condition described as *detrusor dyssynergia,* a dysfunction causing the patient to void involuntarily, suggests a possible cause-and-effect relationship.

Residual infection in the glands of Skene is difficult to eradicate and constantly feeds bacteria into the urinary stream. Paraurethral cysts or abscesses in the anterior vagina may develop as a result of the blockage of one or more of the ducts of the infected gland system. A more serious complication is paraurethral cellulitis from a chronic inflammation originating in these glands. Milking of the urethra from the proximal portion downward may produce a purulent exudate and the small, reddened duct openings may be visualized by urethroscopic examination. Urethral diverticula may contain residual urine, which breeds infection.

Trauma may initiate infections in the lower urinary tract, especially when there is stasis. The milking of the urethra previously described can cause bacteriuria. Prolonged or frequent coitus may cause enough damage to the vesicovaginal wall to produce cystitis; a common example is "honeymoon cystitis," in which the urine is often grossly hemorrhagic.

Gynecologic and urologic operations, especially those that necessitate the use of an indwelling catheter for several days, traumatize the bladder. Experience has shown that the incidence of infection is directly proportional to the length of time the catheter remains in the bladder, and after 3 days the incidence

approaches 100%. Multiple individual catheterizations cause less difficulty but do not remove the danger. Even without the catheter the risk of urinary infection following hysterectomy is great. The gentlest dissection of the bladder from the anterior aspect of the uterus causes injury, and postoperative cystoscopic observation will show marked edema, redness, and infolding and roughening of the mucosa. Postoperative retention of urine with bacteriuria is a common and sometimes troublesome occurrence.

High-pressure douches, irritating vaginal and urethral suppositories, lacerations and fractures of pelvic supports or viscera, and foreign bodies are included in the list of possible causes of trauma. Among the foreign bodies are numerous therapeutic and sanitary devices such as contraceptive diaphragms, pessaries, and tampons, any of which, if retained for a long period of time, gives rise to infection.

Infections at the endometrial and tubal levels also contribute to the development of cystitis and occasionally to renal involvement. Salpingitis and postabortal parametritis and their sequellae make up the majority of such infections. Appendicitis, diverticulitis, and infected uterine, ovarian, or rectal tumors, have a similar impact on the urinary tract.

TREATMENT

The management of bacteriuria or more serious infections of the urinary tract associated with gynecologic disease must combine appropriate urinary antisepsis with treatment of the pelvic disorder. In 95% of lower urinary tract infections in women the offending organism is *Escherichia coli*. The presence of other oganisms suggests an obstructive uropathy or inadequate therapy, resulting in the emergence of resistant strains. When urinary tract infections recur despite attempts to eliminate predisposing factors and after appropriate antibacterial therapy, a thorough evaluation is indicated. After two recurrences, the patient should have intravenous pyelography, cystoscopy, and cystometric studies. When upper urinary tract infection is suspected, renal function studies such as serum creatinine, creatinine clearance, and blood urea nitrogen should be done. Ultrasonograms are helpful in diagnosing dilatation of the upper urinary tract and the presence of residual urine in the bladder after voiding.

In vitro sensitivity studies need not be done for the first episode of lower urinary tract infection, and the patient should be treated immediately on the basis of symptoms after the culture has been taken. *E. coli* is sensitive to many antibacterial drugs of which the most commonly used are sulfasoxazole and ampicillin. Either drug should be given for a minimum of 10 days to 2 weeks, and during this time the patient should force fluids and void frequently. Recurrent or persistent infection should be treated with the appropriate drug after sensitivity studies have been done. Because of rapid bacterial adaptation to sulfonamides, another drug such as nitrofurantoin should be used for repeated infections, even if the organism remains *E. coli*. Individuals whose problem seems related to coitus should take the drug prophylactically in low dosage for 24 hours immediately before or following coitus, and should make it a practice to void after intercourse. Long-term acidification of the urine by diet and the use of cranberry juice is helpful as an adjunct measure. Postoperative patients who have had indwelling catheters should be treated after the catheter has been removed and cultured, again for a period of approximately 2 weeks. Follow-up cultures at the time of return visits are highly advisable, although in most instances normal voiding will wash out the bacteria, even without the benefit of drugs. Patients with known upper urinary tract infections must be treated vigorously for long periods of time and in some cases indefinitely.

There is no specific treatment of urethrotrigonitis other than to eliminate local infections and improve local hygiene. The use of estrogenic creams in the vagina is helpful in postmenopausal women. Instrumentation and operations are counterproductive. The use of tetracycline empirically on the chance that mycoplasma or Chlamydia may be present may be considered but, on a theoretic basis, this is unlikely to be effective in more than 20% of cases. Since the symptoms are subject to spontaneous remissions (and relapse), the patient may at least be given reassurance that they will not last forever.

PHYSIOLOGY OF MICTURITION

Interest in female urology has centered on the problem of stress urinary incontinence for which no uniformly satisfactory treatment has been devised. Carefully conducted anatomic studies and clinical experiments designed to demonstrate the faulty mechanism underlying this symptom have shed considerable light on the physiology of micturition, previously poorly understood, and have emphasized the need for a thorough understanding of the basic disorder before treatment is instituted. Refined techniques for the radiographic study of the bladder and the urethra in the quiescent state during filling and in the act of voiding have contributed much to present knowledge, and these studies have been correlated with precise measurements of intravesical and intraurethral pressures, constantly recorded by electronic apparatus.

The bladder musculature remains inert when the lumen is empty and as filling begins. From a zero baseline, the pressure gradient rises very slowly, with the exception of abrupt, temporary excursions upward in response to external stimuli, until near capacity. Increases in intra-abdominal pressure, even those due to

normal inspiration, markedly affect the intravesical pressure. At about 150 ml the first desire to void is experienced, even though no dramatic rise is noted on the cystometrogram. During early filling there is sufficient tone in the overlapping oblique detrusor fibers of the bladder and urethra to keep the vesical neck closed. As the bladder is increasingly distended, proprioceptive nerve endings in the bladder wall transmit the sensation to the sacral spinal cord if there is no cortical control (e.g., the newborn infant, the very old, and those who suffer from spinal cord or brain injury), and the reciprocal motor impulse travels directly back through the reflex arc, initiating spontaneous involuntary detrusor contraction, or enuresis. Under normal conditions the impulses pass upward through the posterior columns of the spinal cord to centers in the thalamus and cerebral cortex. The perception of fullness passes to the corticoregulatory centers in the motor cortex which have an inhibitory control over the reflex arc of the bladder. When the individual wishes to void, the reflex arc can be relieved of this inhibition and detrusor action begins. Sensations of pain and temperature are also conducted through the parasympathetic system to the sacral cord and pass upward through the spinothalamic tracts to related centers in the thalamus and sensory cortex. It is possible that the sympathetic nervous system through the hypogastric nerve also plays a part in mediating the intensity of this reaction. If the individual decides not to void, inhibition can be maintained and the bladder can adapt to further filling.

By a more direct voluntary action beginning in the motor cortex and traveling to the levator ani muscles through the pudendal nerves, the muscular supports of the pelvic diaphragm are relaxed, allowing the bladder neck to drop. The same impulse contracts the external urethral sphincter, which shortens the urethra and pulls open its proximal portion. Simultaneously, the diaphragm is set by a short inspiration and the rectus muscles are tightened to increase intra-abdominal pressure. The involuntary detrusor impulse begins in the region of the trigone and passes upward over the dome of the bladder and downward to the midportion of the urethra. The result is a powerful contraction of the entire detrusor, which then reduces bladder volume and propels urine toward the outlet while opening the urethrovesical junction and the proximal urethra. This converts the lower bladder and proximal urethra into a funnel shape, promoting bladder emptying. If the individual desires to stop the process at this point, inhibition is reinstated, the levator muscles are contracted, and the urine that has entered the proximal urethra is drawn back into the bladder. If normal micturition proceeds, the bladder rotates on its axis forward toward the pubis to be finally located directly over the funnel, assuring optimal contracting force against minimal resistance. The force of the contraction subsides as the bladder empties and normal rest-

ing relationships are reinstated. Stretching of the bladder beyond the normal capacity of 400 to 500 ml initially causes a drop in both pressure and sensation but, if continued, produces dysfunction of the entire reflex arc, prolonged loss of sensation, atony of the detrusor, and damage to the intrinsic innervation.

The complexity of this physiologic process increases its susceptibility to trauma and disease, causing dysfunction that may result either in inability to void or in incontinence.

INCONTINENCE

Urinary incontinence is the involuntary loss of urine, a symptom that may have several different aspects and may occur under a variety of normal and pathologic conditions. It is important to recognize that this is a common symptom, not necessarily a complaint, and that the majority of the women who have it do not need treatment. Small amounts of urine are lost from time to time by the normal individual under emotional strain, when wearing a tight girdle, in a cold climate, or as a result of sudden movement. At the opposite extreme is the plight of the woman whose urinary incontinence has rendered her a social outcast. This is true especially of vesicovaginal fistula, which is rare in modern times and is usually amenable to surgical correction. Before the historic work of J. Marion Sims it was one of the most dreaded of gynecologic disorders (p. 20).

Persistent urinary incontinence, regardless of volume, is a symptom that merits attention. Its cause should always be ascertained and appropriate corrective measures instituted when they are indicated.

DIAGNOSIS

Many different types of incontinence are recognized and careful differential diagnosis is necessary.

History. The history is of the utmost importance. It should include a detailed description of the incontinence: duration, severity, progression, degree of wetting, relation to stress, frequency of occurrence, remissions, and dribbling. Attention should also be directed toward associated symptoms: frequency, urgency, incomplete emptying, nocturia, hematuria, pyuria, dysuria, pelvic and costovertebral angle pain, incontinence of feces, and vaginal discharge. Information should be elicited concerning urinary dysfunction in childhood, urinary infections, pelvic diseases, operations, childbirth injuries, neurologic disorders, diabetes, psychiatric illness, and psychosexual difficulties. Table 49–1 lists three groups of questions that are helpful in determining the nature of the incontinence.

TABLE 49-1. DETAILED HISTORY TO BE TAKEN FROM PATIENTS WITH URINARY INCONTINENCE

QUESTION GROUP A

1. Have you had treatment for urinary tract disease, such as stones, kidney disease, infections, tumors, injuries?	Yes	No
2. Have you had repeated kidney infections?	Yes	No
3. Is your urine ever bloody?	Yes	No
4. Is the volume of urine you usually pass (check one): Large _____ Average _____ Small _____ Very small _____		
5. When you lose your urine accidentally, are you ever not aware that it is passing?	Yes	No
6. Do you always have a severe sense of urgency before you lose your urine?	Yes	No
7. Do you lose urine as a constant drip from the vagina?	Yes	No
8. Did you have difficulty holding urine as a child?	Yes	No
9. Is it usually painful or difficult to pass your urine?	Yes	No

QUESTION GROUP B

1. As a child did you wet the bed?	Yes	No
2. Do you wet the bed now?	Yes	No
3. Have you ever had paralysis, polio, multiple sclerosis, a serious injury to your back, cyst or tumor on your spine, a stroke, tuberculosis, syphilis, diabetes, pernicious anemia?	Yes	No
4. Does the sound, sight, or feel of running water cause you to lose urine?	Yes	No
5. Is your loss of urine a continual drip so that you are constantly wet?	Yes	No
6. Are you ever not aware that you are losing, or are about to lose, control of your urine?	Yes	No
7. Is your clothing (check one): Slightly damp _____ Wet _____ Soaking wet _____ Do you leave puddles on the floor _____		
8. Have you had an operation on your spine, brain, or bladder?	Yes	No
9. Do you find it frequently necessary to have your urine removed by means of a catheter because you are unable to pass it?	Yes	No

QUESTION GROUP C

1. Do you lose urine by spurts during coughing, sneezing, laughing, lifting?	Yes	No
2. Do you lose urine when you are lying down?	Yes	No
3. Do you lose urine when you are sitting or standing erect?	Yes	No
4. When you are urinating, can you usually stop the flow?	Yes	No
5. Did your urinary difficulty start after delivery of an infant?	Yes	No
6. Did it follow an operation?	Yes	No
7. Was your operation (check one): Hysterectomy, abdominal incision _____ Hysterectomy, removed through the vagina _____ Removal of a tumor, abdominal incision _____ Vaginal repair operation _____ Suspension of the uterus _____ Cesarean section _____		
8. If your menstrual periods have stopped, did the menopause make your condition more severe?	Yes	No
9. Is your control of urine good unless you cough, sneeze, laugh, lift, or strain?	Yes	No
10. Do you have difficulty holding urine if you suddenly stand erect from a sitting or lying-down position?	Yes	No
11. Do you find it necessary to wear protection because you get wet?	Yes	No

"Yes" answers to Question Group A suggest intrinsic urinary tract disease. "Yes" answers to Question Group B suggest neurogenic dysfunction. "Yes" answers to questions *1–4* of Question Group C suggest stress incontinence; questions *5–8* aim to elicit the cause, and questions *9* and *10* indicate the severity of the condition.

(Adapted from Hodgkinson CP: Clin Obstet Gynecol 6:163, 1963)

Physical Examination. A complete examination, including neurologic examination, should be performed. The pelvic examination should include a search for infections, tumors, scarring, or atrophy in the external genitalia, vagina, and cervix. The muscular tone of the perineum, levators, and anal sphincters should be evaluated. The degree of anterior vaginal wall relaxation and the position of the urethrovesical junction should be noted. The internal genitalia should be palpated to determine their size, position, mobility, and relation to the bladder.

Laboratory Tests. In addition to complete blood count, urinalysis, and urine culture, laboratory tests should

include serologic test for syphylis, glucose tolerance test, and blood urea nitrogen and creatinine determinations.

Special Tests. Many diagnostic procedures are available to complete the evaluation. All have application in special situations and the degree of reliance to be placed on any one of them is determined, to some extent, by the experience and personal preference of the examiner. These tests include (1) demonstration of stress incontinence by having the patient, with her bladder partially filled, cough and strain in both erect and lithotomy positions, (2) control of incontinence by elevation of the bladder neck manually or with a clamp in order to show the probable effect of surgical correction, (3) cystometry (Fig. 49–7) when neurologic deficit is suspected, (4) cystoscopy when disease of urethral or bladder mucous membrane is suspected, (5) intravenous pyelography in severe displacements of bladder or uterus, with intrapelvic disease, in proved urinary infection, and when congenital anomaly is suspected, (6) urethrocystography to show urethrovesical relations and degree of support, and (7) cinefluoroscopy to demonstrate disorders of function in obscure problems.

TYPES OF INCONTINENCE

Enuresis. The primary enuresis that occurs in children is bedwetting for which no pathologic or psychiatric cause can be found. It is due to the persistence of the automatic bladder action of infancy when the reflex arc is free of the control of higher centers. The continuation of this condition beyond the fifth year in the absence of anomaly or disease is cause for concern that serious emotional problems may be involved.

Neurogenic Incontinence. Normal control of voiding depends upon a fine balance in the reciprocal relations between several muscle groups, and precise nervous control is necessary to execute these functions. The gynecologist must be able to differentiate incontinence due to failure of nervous control from that caused by other factors. A simple water manometer may be used to determine the bladder's reaction to varying degrees of internal stress (Fig. 49–7). Pressure gradients thus obtained, combined with careful observation of sensory responses during filling, offer an approximation of the level of the neurologic deficit, although they give no clue to the nature of the responsible lesion.

Neurogenic incontinence can be classified on the

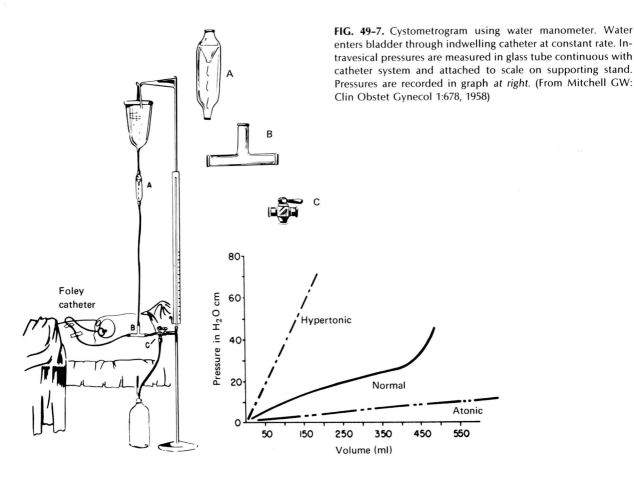

FIG. 49-7. Cystometrogram using water manometer. Water enters bladder through indwelling catheter at constant rate. Intravesical pressures are measured in glass tube continuous with catheter system and attached to scale on supporting stand. Pressures are recorded in graph *at right.* (From Mitchell GW: Clin Obstet Gynecol 1:678, 1958)

basis of the anatomic level of the lesion if it is recognized that there is a broad spectrum of clinical possibilities based upon the severity of the lesion and that the situation is seldom static and must frequently be re-evaluated.

When the neural damage is above the reflex arc (automatic bladder, normal cord bladder, hypertonic bladder), the bladder empties automatically, freed from the inhibitory control of higher centers, as is normally the case in newborn infants. The reflex is often hypertonic and precipitate voiding ensues. This situation is common following head injuries, brain tumors, cerebrovascular accidents, spina bifida, and diseases of the spinal cord above the sacral centers, but is rare in gynecologic practice. If the central lesion is not progressive, there is a tendency toward improvement, especially if some sensory perception has been preserved; the condition may be further aided by continuous tidal drainage. Neurogenic incontinence resulting from hypertonic bladder must be distinguished from incontinence resulting from increased irritability due to local causes such as infections or interstitial cystitis and from the spasticity sometimes engendered by acute anxiety.

When there is neural damage of bladder reflex centers or of the peripheral nerves of the reflex arc (autonomous bladder, hypotonic bladder), the bladder, completely deprived of its extrinsic nerve supply, must depend upon the local action of the myoneural plexus and its own smooth muscle contractility. Lack of tone allows increased capacity and a large residual urine volume leads to overflow incontinence and chronic infection. This condition is not uncommon in gynecologic practice, since it may be associated with disruption of the pelvic (parasympathetic) nerves by radical surgery. Injuries and tumors of the sacral cord or cauda equina, myelomeningocele, combined degeneration of the cord, and diabetic neuropathy may also be responsible. Diabetes, in particular, has been associated with neurogenic vesical dysfunction, even in the absence of other evidence of neuropathy. Management includes scheduled voiding reinforced by abdominal contraction and suprapubic pressure and prevention of infection. This type of neurologic deficit must be distinguished from bladder hypotonicity produced by obstructions in the urethra and bladder neck, from postoperative and postpartum states, and from hysteria and other psychiatric causes of prolonged urinary retention.

Sensory paralysis of the bladder in the absence of motor deficit is encountered in tabes dorsalis and in combined degeneration and other spinal cord diseases. The result is the same as when both sensory and motor centers are involved except that scheduled voiding, begun early, offers a better chance for satisfactory function.

Motor paralysis of the bladder in the absence of sensory deficit occurs in about 10% of patients who have had acute poliomyelitis with skeletal muscle paralysis.

The urinary dysfunction is usually reversible over a considerable time and treatment consists of keeping the bladder decompressed.

Faulty intrinsic innervation of the bladder (megalobladder), a congenital deficiency of ganglia and nerves in the bladder wall, is usually discovered in infancy or childhood after retention, overflow incontinence, and infection have appeared as sequelae. Some type of constant drainage must usually be instituted. Similar irreversible damage to intrinsic nerve components may occur with prolonged overdistention of the bladder.

Overflow (Paradoxic) Incontinence. Constant or intermittent dribbling of urine is representative of many conditions causing overdistention of the bladder. The hypotonic bladder wall is unable to cope adequately with the large volume of residual urine, and small amounts are forced out from time to time by gradually accumulating hydrostatic pressure within the bladder and by movements increasing intra-abdominal pressure. Because the loss of urine may be exaggerated by stress, it is occasionally confused with pure stress incontinence. Partial mechanical obstruction to the normal outflow of urine characteristically causes chronic urinary retention and the degree of obstruction and the length of time it exists determine the rapidity with which overflow incontinence appears. The early phases may pass unknown to the victim. When detrusor hypertrophy and the straining of the abdominal muscles can no longer compensate, a vicious circle is set up, with prolonged distention gradually producing more severe intrinsic nerve damage.

All causes of partial retention may lead eventually to overflow incontinence. Some of the potent drugs used as tranquilizers and central nervous system depressants may contribute to detrusor inhibition and should be avoided when there is a question of bladder competence. If obstruction is present, it must be relieved surgically, if possible, and thereafter long-term catheter drainage combined with the prophylactic use of a urinary antiseptic must be instituted in an attempt to restore bladder tone. Cholinergic drugs and the direct instillation of agents irritating to the bladder are of little more than temporary assistance.

Urgency Incontinence. Urgency incontinence (precipitous micturition) denotes bladder irritability associated with exaggeration of pressure sensation and voiding response. The patient experiences an imperative desire to void, even when filling is minimal, and if facilities are not immediately available, she loses small amounts of urine. In the severe case, the bladder may empty completely before control can be established. In addition, voiding may not alleviate the symptom, and an unpleasant sensation of incomplete emptying may remain in the absence of any residual. Such irritability may be present in the early stages of urinary retention and may also be due to the local action of certain drugs

and chemicals, but the majority of cases are caused primarily by infection.

Urgency is the characteristic symptom of urethrotrigonitis. It often occurs without wetting, but the sensory response closely mimics actual micturition and the patient may think she is really incontinent. Anxiety, cold weather, and cyclic variations related to menstruation may affect the degree of urgency and tend to make it an intermittent condition, with apparently spontaneous remissions and exacerbations.

Urgency incontinence is easily confused with stress incontinence unless a careful history is taken. The two frequently coexist and compound the patient's discomfort.

Treatment is nonoperative and consists of reassurance, eradicating local infections, and attention to regular voiding habits.

Incontinence Caused by Urethral Diverticula.

Small suburethral pouches constitute reservoirs of infection and contribute to higher infections, urgency, and more severe dysfunction. They may also retain enough urine to cause leakage after micturition is completed; postvoiding dribbling is pathognomonic of this lesion. Since their openings into the urethra are difficult to find, the forceful introduction of radiopaque material by means of a special catheter with two inflatable bulbs to block outflow from both proximal and distal ends of the urethra may be necessary for visualization of the defect.

Excision of diverticula is curative, but recurrences are common, due, in many instances, to inadvertent subtotal removal.

Incontinence Caused by Fistulas.

Fistulas between the vagina and the ureter, bladder, or urethra usually cause constant leakage of urine; in the occasional case, the loss may be intermittent and the pathologic condition obscure. A history of pelvic surgery, radiation therapy, or obstetric laceration suggests the cause of the incontinence and the injection of colored dye directly into the urethra demonstrates a urinary tract connecting, at the lower level, with the vagina. A similar dye used intravenously shows ureteral fistulas quite clearly unless renal function on the affected side is too poor to excrete the material.

Psychiatric Incontinence.

Minor neuroses predispose to the development of urinary incontinence and reduce the incidence of cure. In incontinence due to other specific factors, neuroses are often associated with further deterioration in the patient's condition.

Psychotic individuals may be partially or completely incontinent because of their mental illness. The incontinence may consist of random voiding as a result of loss of social consciousness. Overflow incontinence may be associated with depressive states because of a failure to respond to bladder stimuli.

Stress Incontinence.

The definition of stress incontinence is loss of urine through a normal urethra as a result of sudden increase in intra-abdominal pressure. As investigations reveal more about the causes of this condition, the definition requires some qualification. The most significant contributing factor is a loss of the normal supports of the bladder base and urethra, which permits these structures to sink to a more dependent position and places them in direct line to receive the impact of increases in intra-abdominal pressure. The loss of support is usually attributable to childbirth injury to the musculofascial layers of the pelvic sling, urogenital diaphragm, and perineum, compounded by atrophy due to age or disease. Additional unfavorable influences are chronic coughing, lifting of heavy objects, obesity, and wearing a tight girdle. The lowering of the bladder neck in the resting state makes it extremely vulnerable to stress from above, which forces it further down and pulls open the internal sphincter before the accessory muscles can compensate voluntarily. Since the increased downward funneling of the lower bladder segment is evident with the individual in the erect but not in the supine position, it seems that gravity plays a role in the appearance of stress incontinence. Probably indirectly as a result of the decreased pelvic supports, the proximal urethra tends to dilate slightly, and its pressure drops below the intravesical pressure, the reverse of the situation in the unafflicted individual. At cinefluoroscopy small wedges of urine can be seen entering the relatively hypotonic proximal urethra following a cough or sneeze. If this urine passes into the distal two-thirds of the urethra, it is lost; otherwise, it returns to the bladder.

Loss of support may not be manifest on physical examination, nor is it limited to parous women. Virginal women may have severe stress incontinence and those with marked anterior vaginal wall bulging may be asymptomatic. In the former group, urgency often overlaps the stress factor, making them virtually indistinguishable; in the latter group, a relatively well-supported urethra and vesical neck or well-developed levator muscles can continue to provide continence. The symptom is more common among postmenopausal women, possibly due to levator atrophy and to tissue changes resulting from estrogen withdrawal. In this connection, women who lead an active sex life seem to be less afflicted. The many inconsistencies in the explanations for stress incontinence in various anatomic situations include its not infrequent appearance in individuals who are normal by both examination and objective testing.

Contributing factors in stress incontinence are obesity, intrapelvic neoplasms pressing on the bladder, and a uterus fixed in acute anteversion by previous surgery. Cure of these disorders by diet or surgery may alone permit compensatory mechanisms to resume a favorable balance.

The term "stress incontinence" is often used inap-

propriately to cover any type of urinary leakage in the female. The diagnosis should properly be made only when all other primary and contributing causes of incontinence have been excluded by comprehensive evaluation.

Effective treatment of mild stress incontinence may be accomplished by prescribing regular exercise of levator and vaginal muscles. The principles of surgery for more severe cases are (1) restoration of urethrovesical supports, usually by plication of submucosal smooth muscle, (2) rebuilding of perineal musculature if defective, (3) establishment of mobility of the urethra and bladder neck, and (4) relocation of the bladder neck from a dependent position forward out of the axis of greatest pressure. More than 50 operations have been devised to meet this contingency. Their success depends not only upon the selection of cases by careful exclusion of other causes of incontinence but also on the technical efficiency of the surgeon in carrying out his chosen plan. The surgical aspects of this problem are considered in Chapter 61.

Detrusor dyssynergia, a common form of urinary incontinence caused by involuntary detrusor contractions, is often confused with stress incontinence. The inappropriate and often violent contractions may be caused by incomplete inhibition at the cortical level or by local inflammation in the trigone and urethra which prematurely triggers the response. Parasympatholytic drugs such as propantheline bromide are helpful in reducing the involuntary spasms but usually are not completely curative.

REFERENCES AND RECOMMENDED READING

Buchsbaum HJ, Schmidt JD: Gynecological and Obstetrical Urology. Philadelphia, WB Saunders, 1978

Cardozo L, Stanton SL, Bennett AE: Design of a urodynamic questionnaire. Br J Urol 50:269, 1978

Cardozo L, Stanton SL, Hafner J et al: Biofeedback in the treatment of detrusor instability. Br J Urol 50:250, 1978

Drutz HP et al: Urodynamic analysis of urinary incontinence symptoms in women. Am J Obstet Gynecol. 134(7):789, 1979

Everett HS, Ridley JE: Female Urology. New York, Harper & Row, 1968

Farber M, Mitchell GW: Anomalies of the kidneys and ureters. Clin Obstet & Gynecol 21:831, 1978

Goss CM: The urogenital system. *In* Goss CM: Gray's Anatomy, 28th ed, pp 1265–1298. Philadelphia, Lea & Febiger, 1966

Graber EA: Stress incontinence in women: A review, Obstet Gynecol Surv 32(7):565, 1977

Harding GKM, Marrie TJ, Ronald AR et al: Urinary tract infection localization in women. JAMA 240:1147, 1978

Hodgkinson CP: Recurrent stress urinary incontinence. Am J Obstet Gynecol 132(8):844, 1978

Hodgkinson CP: Recurrent stress urinary incontinence. Clin Obstet Gynecol 21(3):787, 1978

Hodgkinson CP, Doub HP: Roentgen study of urethrovesical relationships in female urinary stress incontinence. Radiology 61(3):335, 1953

Jones SR et al: Localization of urinary tract infections by detection of antibody-coated bacteria in urinary sediment. N Engl J Med 290(11):591, 1974

Kunin CM: Detection, Prevention and Management of Urinary Tract Infections. Philadelphia, Lea & Febiger, 1972

Lapides J: Symposium on neurogenic bladder. Urol Clin N Am 1:1, 1974

Lee RA et al: Surgical complications and results of modified Marshall–Marchetti–Krantz procedure for urinary incontinence. Obstet Gynecol 53(4):447, 1979

Marshall JR, Judd GE: Guide for the management of women with symptoms arising in the lower urinary tract. Clin Obstet Gynecol 19:247, 1976

Robertson JR: Genitourinary Problems in Women. Springfield, Illinois, Charles C Thomas, 1978

Smith JC, Ardran GM: Prolonged bladder distension as a treatment of urgency and urge incontinence of urine. Br J Urol 46:645, 1974

Stewart BH, Banowsky LH, Montague DK: Stress incontinence: Conservative therapy with sympathomimetic drugs. J Urol 115:558, 1976

Svigos JM, Matthews CD: Assessment and treatment of female urinary incontinence by cystometrogram and bladder retraining programs. Obstet Gynecol 50:9, 1976

Wear JB: Cystometry. Urol Clin N Am 1:45, 1974

Zufall R: Ineffectiveness of treatment of urethral syndrome in women. Urology 12:337, 1978

The various types of pelvic infections are assuming increasing importance because they represent the most common condition that the gynecologist treats. There has been a dramatic increase in the recognition of pelvic infections because of new microbiologic and serologic techniques, because of educational efforts that have increased physician awareness, and because of a rapid increase in the prevalence of sexually transmitted infections (Table 50–1).

The impact of pelvic infections on the physical condition of women ranges from minor annoyance to major morbidity and, in some instances, even death. Additionally, the cost of treating pelvic infections is enormous if direct medical costs and indirect costs, including time lost from work, are calculated. It has been estimated that by the year 2000, one of every two women who reached the reproductive age in the 1970s will have had an episode of pelvic inflammatory disease (PID). Of women with PID, 25% will have been hospitalized, 25% will have had major surgery, and 20% will be sterile.

All genital sites—the vulva, vagina, urethra, cervix, endometrium, fallopian tubes, and ovaries—are susceptible to infectious organisms. Certain agents preferentially infect certain sites and give rise to characteristic symptoms; other agents cause little symptomatology until major pathologic changes occur. Still other organisms are not recognized until congenital neonatal infection occurs or a male partner becomes infected. The gynecologist should have special knowledge of the infections caused by *Neisseria gonorrhoeae, Chlamydia trachomatis, Treponema pallidum,* genital mycoplasma, *Mycobacterium tuberculosis,* and anaerobic bacteria, which may act alone or in concert to produce pelvic infections ranging from acute PID to nonspecific vaginitis.

CHAPTER

50

PELVIC INFECTIONS

David A. Eschenbach

GONORRHEA

Gonorrhea is caused by *Neisseria gonorrhoeae,* a gram-negative diplococcus. The bacteria that attach themselves by pili to columnar or transitional cells are rapidly engulfed by pinocytosis. The organism attracts leukocytes, giving rise to the commonly associated purulent discharge. The disease is usually sexually transmitted, although it can be acquired by the newborn after passing through an infected cervix, thereby causing gonorrheal ophthalmia.

COURSE OF THE DISEASE

N. gonorrhoeae first attaches to tissues of the lower genital tract which are not covered by stratified squamous epithelium: the urethra, the Bartholin glands, and the endocervix. The anus and rectum can also be infected either by colonization from cervical infection or during anal coitus. Urinary frequency, dysuria, and a purulent vaginal discharge are the first symptoms, usually appearing 2 to 5 days after exposure. Many women do not seek medical attention if these symptoms are mild. Occasionally the discharge is locally irritating and causes edema, erythema, and soreness of the vulva. Pharyngitis may occur from *N. gonorrhoeae* pharyngeal infection. In 2% of infected women, disseminated gonococcal infection occurs, causing fever, septicemia, dermatitis, arthritis, endocarditis, or meningitis, in various combinations.

In about 20% of women with untreated gonorrhea, the infection may spread to involve the upper genital tract, resulting in acute PID (Fig. 50–1). Acute PID is the most common and serious sequel of gonorrhea. The mechanical and antibacterial properties of cervical mucus probably provide a barrier against upward extension; during menstruation the mucus barrier is lost and *N. gonorrhoeae* can be disseminated in a rich men-

TABLE 50-1. SEXUALLY TRANSMITTED INFECTIONS

Organisms	Diseases
BACTERIA	
Neisseria gonorrhoeae	Gonorrhea
Chlamydia trachomatis	Chlamydial infection
Treponema pallidum	Syphilis
Hemophilus ducreyi	Chancroid
Calymmatobacterium granulomatis	Granuloma inguinalae
Gardnerella vaginalis	Vaginitis
Group B Beta-hemolytic Streptococcus	Group B infection
MYCOPLASMAS	
Mycoplasma hominis	Mycoplasma infection
Ureaplasma urealyticum	Mycoplasma infection
VIRUSES	
Herpesvirus hominis	Genital herpes
Cytomegalovirus (CMV)	CMV infection
Hepatitis B virus	Hepatitis
Human Papillomavirus	Condyloma accuminata
Molluscum contagiosum virus	Molluscum contagiosum
PROTOZOA	
Trichomonas vaginalis	Vaginitis
FUNGI	
Candida albicans	Vaginitis
PARASITES	
Sarcoptes scabiae	Scabies
Phthirus pubis	Pediculosis pubis

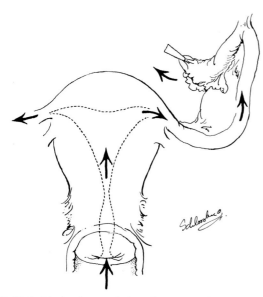

FIG. 50-1. Mode of transmission of gonococcal pelvic infection. Portal of entry is external genitalia. Organism enters cervix, following mucous membrane, passes up through uterine cavity, and attacks fallopian tube. Pelvic peritonitis results from escape of pus from tubal fimbria. (Wharton LR: Gynecology and Female Urology, 1st ed.. Philadelphia, WB Saunders, 1943)

strual blood medium to the uterus and fallopian tubes. A transient endometritis occurs as the organisms pass through the uterine cavity, and reach the fallopian tubes where they produce an acute inflammatory reaction of the tubal mucosa which is invariably bilateral. The tubes characteristically become swollen and reddened as the muscularis and serosa are inflamed. Exudate drips from the fimbriated ends of the tubes, producing a pelvic peritonitis that ultimately gives rise to the filmy peritoneal adhesions typical of healed salpingitis. The swollen and congested fimbriae may adhere to one another.

The process may take any of the following courses:

1. With prompt, appropriate antibacterial therapy the infection may subside with little damage to the reproductive tract.
2. The swollen and congested fimbriae may adhere to one another or to the ovary, trapping the exudate in the tube and giving rise to *pyosalpinx* or to a *tubo-ovarian abscess*.
3. The mucosal folds may adhere to one another, forming glandlike spaces filled, at first, with exudate and later, as the process becomes chronic, by watery secretion, the so-called *follicular salpingitis* (Fig. 50–2).
4. If the infection subsides after agglutination of the

FIG. 50-2. Follicular salpingitis, an end stage of gonorrheal salpingitis. Mucosal folds adherent, giving rise to innumerable round or irregular cystlike cavities lined by cuboidal epithelium. (Kelly HA: Operative Gynecology, Vol 2, plate XI. New York, Appleton, 1898; drawing by Max Brödel)

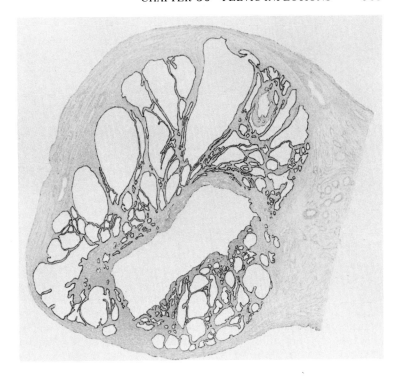

fimbriae and closure of the peripheral end of the tube, watery secretion accumulates and distends the tube forming a *hydrosalpinx,* a retort-shaped structure resembling pyosalpinx (Fig. 50–3).

Hydrosalpinx was formerly regarded as the end stage of pyosalpinx, but the intact, atrophic epithelium and the absence of chronic inflammatory reaction suggest that the primary pathology is closure of the fimbriated end of the tube.

SYMPTOMS AND SIGNS

In the *primary stage* when the disease is first acquired, and when it is most infectious, at least 50% of women have no symptoms. The most common symptoms, when they occur, are dysuria, urinary frequency, and a purulent vaginal discharge. Except for the discharge, which may be milked from the urethra or is present in the vagina, there are few signs of the acute gonococcal infection.

In the *stage of acute salpingitis,* bilateral, severe lower abdominal pain and pyrexia are common. Pelvic, usually not generalized, peritonitis is present, with direct and rebound tenderness, muscle guarding, which prevents abdominal palpation in the lower quadrants,

and tender adnexa on bimanual examination. Movement of the cervix causes pain.

In the *stage of subacute salpingitis,* the infection continues but the signs and symptoms are less overt than are those of the acute stage.

In the *end stage of salpingitis,* the uterus and the adnexa are usually fixed by pelvic peritoneal adhesions. The adnexa are often either adherent to the posterior aspect of the uterus or are prolapsed in the cul de sac, which pulls the corpus uteri into a retroverted position. Notable features are dyspareunia, sterility, and chronic, aching pelvic pain that exacerbates prior to menstruation and subsides to an extent after menstruation.

DIAGNOSIS

The diagnosis of gonorrhea depends upon demonstration of *N. gonorrhoeae.* Among symptomatic women during the initial phase of gonorrhea, the finding of intracellular gram-negative diplococci in the exudate from the cervix or urethra points to gonorrheal infection. If the Gram stain is not conclusive, cultures should be obtained. Gonococcal cultures should be performed on women when symptoms are suggestive of gonorrhea (women with undiagnosed vaginal dis-

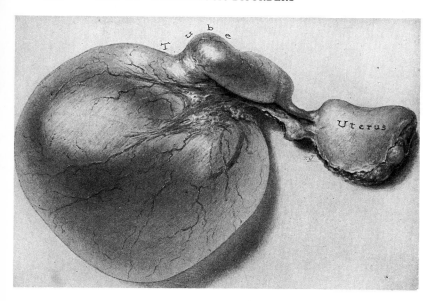

FIG. 50–3. Hydrosalpinx. (Curtis AH, Huffman JW: A Textbook of Gynecology, 6th ed. Philadelphia, WB Saunders, 1950)

charge or dysuria); when other sexually transmitted diseases are present; when Bartholinitis or Skenitis is present; when acute lower abdominal pain is suggestive of acute salpingitis; when suspected disseminated gonococcal infection is suspected; and when women are contacts of males with gonorrhea.

The sites to be cultured are, in order of importance, the cervix, the anal canal, the urethra, and the pharynx. Vaginal discharge should be wiped away from the cervix before obtaining either a culture or Gram stain. Genital samples must be cultured on Thayer–Martin or similar media containing antimicrobial agents that inhibit growth of the normal bacterial and fungal flora.

Serologic tests for active gonococcal infection have such a low predictive value that they are almost without benefit.

Since gonorrhea is a sexually transmitted disease, it follows that gonorrhea is also present in a male partner. The importance of notifying male sexual contacts is emphasized by the fact that more than 40% of the infectious male contacts with gonorrhea are asymptomatic carriers who would otherwise not be treated.

TREATMENT

Drug Therapy

Recent changes have been made in the recommended treatment for both complicated and uncomplicated gonorrhea. The current Center for Disease Control Recommended Treatment Schedules—1979 are as follows:

Uncomplicated Lower Genital Tract Gonorrhea. The drug of choice continues to be aqueous procaine penicillin G (APPG), 4.8 million units injected intramus-cularly at two sites, with 1 g of probenecid by mouth. Alternative treatments are (1) tetracycline hydrochloride 0.5 g by mouth 4 times daily for 5 days (total dosage 10.0 g; tetracycline should not be used in pregnant women), (2) ampicillin 3.5 g with 1 g probenecid by mouth, or (3) amoxicillin 3.0 g with 1 g probenecid by mouth. Patients allergic to penicillin should receive tetracycline, which must be given 1 to 2 hours after meals, since food and milk products interfere with absorption. Women who cannot tolerate tetracycline may be treated with spectinomycin 2.0 g in one intramuscular injection.

Penicillin-resistant Strains of N. gonorrhoeae that elaborate penicillinase are encountered with increasing frequency, making it mandatory that all gonorrhea patients have posttreatment cultures 3 to 7 days following therapy and that any posttreatment isolates be tested for penicillinase production. Patients who fail treatment should receive spectinomycin 2 g intramuscularly.

Patients with gonorrhea who also have incubating syphilis (seronegative, without clinical signs of syphilis) are likely to be cured by all of the above regimens except spectinomycin. In patients treated with spectinomycin, an initial as well as a 6-week follow-up serologic test for syphilis should be performed.

Acute Gonorrheal Salpingitis. *Hospitalization* is appropriate in the following situations: uncertain diagnosis, in which surgical emergencies such as appendicitis and ectopic pregnancy must be excluded; suspicion of pelvic abscess; severe illness; pregnancy; inability of patient to follow or tolerate an outpatient regimen; or failure to respond to outpatient therapy.

The following antimicrobial regimens are appropriate *for outpatients:* either 1) tetracycline 0.5 grams by

mouth 4 times daily for 10 days, or 2) APPG 4.8 million units intramuscularly, ampicillin 3.5 grams, or amoxicillin 3.0 grams, each with 1.0 gram probenecid, each to be followed by ampicillin 0.5 grams, or amoxicillin 0.5 grams orally 4 times daily for 10 days. Tetracycline is to be avoided in pregnant patients, but the other drugs may be used.

For hospitalized patients: Aqueous crystalline penicillin G 20 million units intramuscularly once daily until improvement occurs, followed by ampicillin 0.5 grams 4 times daily to complete 10 days of therapy. An alternative is tetracycline 0.25 grams intravenously 4 times daily until improvement occurs, followed by 0.5 grams orally 4 times daily to complete 10 days of therapy. The tetracycline regimen should not be used in pregnant women.

Surgery

Laporoscopy may be helpful either for diagnosis or to define the extent of the disease. Surgery may be indicated in the case of a ruptured pyosalpinx or ovarian abscess; colpotomy drainage is usually preferable if the lesion is accessible. If laparotomy is performed with a presumptive diagnosis, for example, of appendicitis and acute salpingitis is found instead, the procedure should be limited to the taking of a tubal culture and closure of the abdomen. If laparotomy should be needed for such problems as an unresolved abscess or an adnexal mass that does not subside, surgery should be limited to the most conservative procedures that will be effective. Unilateral abscesses respond to unilateral salpingo-oophorectomy if appropriate antibiotic regimens are used; routine hysterectomy and bilateral salpingo-oophorectomy is rarely needed in young women with limited disease.

Late Sequelae of Gonorrheal Salpingitis. When the outstanding symptom is chronic and recurrent pain, surgery should be deferred as long as possible because of the possibility that removal of the uterus and both tubes and ovaries may be necessary. Mild analgesics (opiates should be avoided if possible) and heat may suffice until the swelling and fixation are reduced. Surgery may be indicated by persistent pain that does not respond to conservative measures, or for recurrent attacks of pelvic pain, or for a pelvic mass that does not resolve. If sterility is the outstanding symptom, surgery may be indicated if the tubal lesion can be shown to be amenable to surgical repair.

CHLAMYDIA

Chlamydia trachomatis is a sexually transmitted organism that is often associated with gonorrhea. Chlamydia infects the same tissues—the urethra, cervix, fallopian tubes, and Bartholin's glands—and produces the same spectrum of symptoms and diseases as gonorrhea. Analogous to gonococcal infection, transmission to males produces both symptomatic and asymptomatic urethritis. Chlamydia causes urethritis, Bartholinitis, cervicitis, endometritis, and salpingitis, including Fitz-Hugh–Curtis perihepatitis. Lymphogranuloma venereum is a chlamydial infection. Neonates born of mothers with genital chlamydia infection have a 40% risk of developing chlamydial conjunctivitis and a 10% to 20% risk of developing chlamydial pneumonia.

C. trachomatis is an obligate intracellular parasite. After attachment to columnar or transitional epithelial cells, it is engulfed by pinocytosis. The intracellular organisms remain within a phagosome membrane that protects them from host defense mechanisms and they replicate until they replace most of the cell and ultimately cause the cell to rupture. The infective particles are released into the extracellular space and the process is repeated. The replication time is relatively slow, explaining the characteristically long latent period between the time of exposure and the onset of symptoms, which ranges from weeks to months.

Chlamydial infections are assuming increasing importance among the sexually transmitted diseases (STD). In many western societies *C. trachomatis* is a more common STD than *N. gonorrhoeae*. The diagnosis is difficult because routine cultures for *C. trachomatis* are not performed among asymptomatic individuals and, hence, it is not often identified until overt infection occurs. The precise attack rate of chlamydial salpingitis is unknown, but it may approximate that of gonorrhea.

For diagnosis, cultures should be taken from both the cervix and urethra, since in many cases organisms will be identified only in one site. Other obvious infected sites should also be cultured. Since the organisms are obligate intracellular parasites, tissue culture methods similar to those used for virus recovery are required. The cultured material should contain tissue cells; exudative material alone is not sufficient. Serologic diagnosis by microimmunofluorescent methods is possible, but it is not widely available. Papanicolaou stains of genital material detect only 40% of infections.

Tetracycline and erythromycin (0.5 g 4 times daily for 7 to 10 days) are the most effective drugs in the treatment of chlamydial infections. Sulfa and sulfatrimethoprin preparations, chloramphenicol, and clindamycin are also effective. Penicillins are much less effective than these antibiotics.

SYPHILIS

Although most women who have syphilis are asymptomatic and have only serologic evidence of infection, physicians must constantly be aware of the possibility

of syphilitic infection. Spirochetes rapidly enter lymphatics after exposure, but a primary lesion, the *chancre*, usually takes about 3 weeks to develop. The classic primary ulcer is painless and firm, with sharply defined, raised edges; however, the majority of syphilitic ulcers are atypical. Therefore, any suspicious genital ulcer should be studied by darkfield examination. Serous material expressed from the ulcer base is mixed with saline, and since *Treponema pallidum* is an anaerobe, this must be immediately placed under a cover slip whose edges are occluded by vaseline. The identification of typical spirochetes by darkfield microscopy establishes the diagnosis of primary syphilis. Serologic tests are usually nonreactive when the chancre first appears but become reactive 1 to 4 weeks later.

Secondary syphilis appears 6 or more weeks later and is characterized chiefly by a symmetric, macular, papular, or papulosquamous rash and generalized, nontender lymphadeopathy. *Condylomata lata* (Fig. 50–4) are highly infectious, hypertrophied, wartlike lesions of secondary syphilis which may occur in moist areas such as the vulva or perineum and must be distinguished from other vulvar lesions. Superficial, painless mucosal erosions of the mouth or vagina, called *mucous patches*, develop in one-third of patients. Systemic symptoms of fever, weight loss, or malaise may occur. Serologic tests are positive.

Untreated patients then enter a *latent phase of syphilis* during which clinical and physical manifestations are absent. Diagnosis is established by serologic tests. Intermittent spirochetal blood stream invasion may occur during the early latent phase of the first 4 years. In pregnancy, the risk of congenital infection of the fetus in the primary and secondary phases of syphilis is 80% to 95%; the risk during the early latent phase is 70%. During the late latent phase, immunity develops, which reduces blood invasion, and the risk of congenital syphilis decreases to 10%. About one-third of patients with untreated late syphilis manifest central nervous system or cardiovascular symptoms of *tertiary syphilis*.

Venereal Disease Research Lab (VDRL) and fluorescent treponemal antibody (FTA) serology should be performed in any patient who has a suspicious lesion; if it is nonreactive or if spirochetes cannot be demonstrated in the discharge, the tests should be repeated in 1 month.

VDRL antibody is a nontreponemal, nonspecific reagin antibody. The antibody can be titrated, and the titer either falls or disappears after therapy of early or secondary syphilis. Accordingly, the VDRL test can be used to judge the activity either of a first episode or of reacquired infection in a patient known to have had syphilis in the past. Treated patients with latent syphilis, however, may retain high, stable VDRL titers. Acute bacterial or viral infections can give rise to acute *false-positive reactions* that last up to 6 months. Several conditions such as aging, addiction to drugs, autoimmune disease, and pregnancy may give rise to chronic, nonspecific, false-positive VDRL reactions. False-positive VDRL titers are usually 1:8 or less. The FTA antibody is a specific antitreponemal antibody and false-positive FTA reactions are rare. A patient with a positive VDRL should have a confirmatory FTA test to exclude a false-positive VDRL reaction. Patients with a false-positive VDRL will have a negative FTA test. In patients with syphilis FTA antibody remains positive indefinitely, and since the test is not titrated, it is unnecessary to repeat FTA testing in a known positive patient.

TREATMENT

The treatment schedules for syphilis which are currently recommended by the USPHS Center for Disease Control are as follows:

Early Syphilis. (Primary, secondary, or latent syphilis of less than 1 year's duration). The drug of choice is benzathrine penicillin G (2.4 million units total, intramuscularly) because it provides effective treatment in a single visit. Alternative choices include

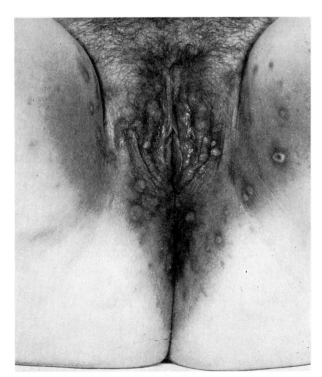

FIG. 50-4. Condylomata lata of vulva and perineum. (Curtis AH, Huffman, JW: A Textbook of Gynecology, 6th ed. Philadelphia, WB Saunders, 1950)

aqueous procaine penicillin G (APPG), 4.8 million units total: 600,000 units by intramuscular injection daily for 8 days or, for patients who are allergic to penicillin, either tetracycline hydrochloride 500 mg 4 times daily by mouth for 15 days, or erythromycin (stearate, ethylsuccinate, or base) 500 mg 4 times daily by mouth for 15 days.

Syphilis of More Than One Year's Duration. Benzathine penicillin G is the drug of choice, 7.2 million units total: 2.4 million units intramuscularly each week for 3 successive weeks. Alternative choices include aqueous procaine penicillin G, 9.0 million units total: 600,000 units intramuscularly daily for 15 days or, for those who are allergic to penicillin, tetracycline hydrochloride 500 mg 4 times daily by mouth for 30 days, or erythromycin 500 mg 4 times daily by mouth for 30 days. As noted elsewhere, tetracycline must not be used in pregnancy.

Patients with syphilis of more than 1 year's duration require a spinal tap to exclude asymptomatic neurosyphilis.

Syphilis in Pregnancy. The treatment of syphilis in pregnancy is discussed in Chapter 27. The treatment is the same as for the corresponding stage of syphilis among nonpregnant women except that tetracycline is not used and special follow-up is required. The *Jarisch–Herxheimer reaction* is common and pregnant women should be hospitalized in anticipation of this possibility. The reaction is ascribed to the sudden massive destruction of spirochetes by antibiotics and it is manifested by fever, myalgia, tachycardia and, occasionally, hypotension. Treatment is stopped if symptoms become severe. The reaction usually begins within 24 hours and subsides spontaneously in the next 24 hours of penicillin treatment.

GENITAL MYCOPLASMAS

Genital mycoplasmas have often been thought of as organisms in search of a disease because they are ubiquitous and not highly virulent. Two genital mycoplasmas are important: *Mycoplasma hominis,* which has been recovered from the vagina in 15% to 70% of women, and *Ureaplasma urealyticum* (formerly called T-strain mycoplasma), which has been recovered from 40% to 95% of women. The phylogenetic position of the organism is between bacteria and viruses.

The most convincing role for mycolasma in human female infections is as a pathogen in salpingitis and postpartum fever. Mycoplasmas can be recovered from the tubes of 2% to 16% of women with salpingitis. In primate model studies, *M. hominis* produces an adnexitis but not salpingitis. Mycoplasmas have been recovered from the blood of 10% to 15% of women with postpartum fever and antibodies to *M. hominis* have been demonstrated in 50% of such women.

The maternal presence of the organism has also been associated with low infant birthweight. Mycoplasmas have been recovered from the fetal tissue of midtrimester spontaneous abortuses, which suggests a relationship between the organism and abortion.

The organism's role in fertility is not settled. In some studies mycoplasmas have been isolated more frequently from infertile than fertile women and in some studies women treated with antibiotics had higher fertility rates than did untreated controls. However, other investigators have failed to confirm these observations.

Both mycoplasmas are sensitive to tetracycline. Erythromycin inhibits *U. urealyticum* but not *M. hominis.* Both are sensitive to aminoglycosides and choramphenicol, but not to sulfa.

GENITAL TUBERCULOSIS

Female genital tuberculosis is relatively uncommon in the United States, and fewer than 1% of salpingitis infections can be attributed to *Mycobacterium tuberculosis.* The reason for this is not entirely clear, since pulmonary tuberculosis remains a problem in many impoverished areas. Although it has been demonstrated that spread of tuberculosis from the primary pulmonary complex to the pelvis usually occurs early during tubercular infection, early detection is rarely feasible. Approximately 10% of patients with pulmonary tuberculosis also develop genital tuberculosis.

PATHOGENESIS

Virtually all genital infections are secondary to a pulmonary infection, which usually spreads by means of the blood stream from the lung focus to the vascular wall of the fallopian tube, generally within 1 year of the primary pulmonary infection (Figs. 50–5, 50–6). Direct extension then occurs from the tube in several directions: to the pelvic peritoneum, to the endometrium, to the cervix, and to the ovary. Less commonly, lymphatic extension to genitalia can occur from abdominal sources or by direct extension from the intestinal tract. Genital tuberculosis rarely is caused by an ascending infection from a sexual partner with tuberculous epididymitis.

The initial tubal lesion may remain localized for a considerable period, in some cases years, or it may extend to the interior tubal mucosal surface. The endosalpingitis results either in (1) an exudative phase with ulcer formation at the site of caseous degeneration, which produces the typical moth-eaten pattern seen on hysterosalpingography, or (2) an adhesive

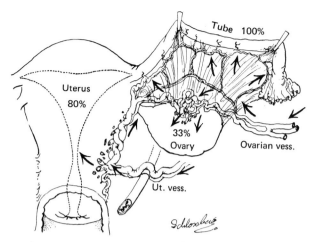

FIG. 50–5. Mode of transmission of tuberculous pelvic infection. Tubercle bacillus invades pelvic organs by way of blood stream from distant focus in lung or other organ. (Wharton LR: Gynecology and Female Urology, 1st ed. Philadelphia, WB Saunders, 1943)

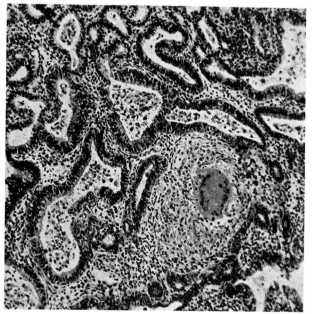

FIG. 50–6. Tuberculosis of fallopian tube (original magnification ×105; Curtis AH, Huffman JW: A Textbook of Gynecology, 6th ed. Philadelphia, WB Saunders, 1950)

phase in which large tubercles are present within the tubes (dense perisalpingeal adhesions are characteristic). In contrast to bacterial salpingitis, tubal occlusion, particularly fimbrial closure, does not occur early in tuberculous disease and the tubes may remain pat-

ent despite relatively marked destruction of the tubal wall.

Tubal infection is present in virtually all women with genital tuberculosis. Endometrial infection is present in 50% to 80% of cases. Because of menstrual sloughing, infected endometrium is shed monthly; after menstruation, the endometrium is again infected by seeding from the tubes. Myometrial infection can occur, but only in the most advanced cases. Cervical infection occurs in only 10% to 25% of patients, resulting in either an ulcerative lesion that can grossly resemble cervical carcinoma, or a papillomatous lesion.

CLINICAL FORMS

Latent Genital Tuberculosis

In this form, tuberculosis appears to be partially or completely arrested following an initial tubal infection and the patient has few or no pelvic complaints. Pelvic physical findings are normal. The diagnosis is made in the course of an investigation of infertility (endometrial biopsy or D & C) or by chance during laparotomy. In these cases a precarious balance exists between the disease and the host defense mechanisms. Active but latent infections have been documented 30 years following an initial infection.

Tuberculous Salpingitis

This is a more advanced infection that may develop immediately after the primary hemotogenous tubal spread, or it may follow a prolonged latent phase. The tubes are grossly enlarged by the inflammatory reaction. Although the symptoms and findings can be identical to those of acute bacterial salpingitis, the clinical manifestations are usually more indolent and prolonged. Additionally, tuberculous salpingitis does not respond to the antibotic therapy used for other forms of salpingitis. Despite these differences, tuberculosis is often recognized only by histologic examination of an excised tube.

Tuberculous Peritonitis

In this form, widespread infection of all peritoneal surfaces produces ascites, adhesions, and innumerable small nodules (tubercles) throughout the abdomen. Usually the serosal surfaces of the pelvic organs are involved and the tubes are often patent. This form results from hematogenous or lymphatic spread.

DIAGNOSIS

A history of pulmonary tuberculosis can often be elicited from patients with genital tuberculosis, but simul-

taneous active pulmonary infection is uncommon. A normal chest film does not exclude genital tuberculosis, since pulmonary lesions are found in only 30% to 50% of cases. The most common complaints are sterility and pelvic pain. Deteriorating health and menstrual abnormalities can also occur. Menorrhagia may be associated with the abdominal pain, but amenorrhea or oligomenorrhea may occur among patients with tuberculous peritonitis. Most women with genital tuberculosis are seen in the second and third decades of life, but because of the frequent tendency for long latency periods, the disease may become active even after the menopause. It must be reemphasized that the clinical picture of tubal tuberculosis can be similar to that of acute bacterial salpingitis. In some cases the clinical picture can be very bizarre and in such cases Kelly's admonition (p. 412) comes to mind: When one is confronted with a pelvic problem that does not conform to expected rules, the first consideration should be ectopic pregnancy and the second should be pelvic tuberculosis. If the signs and symptoms of salpingitis occur in a woman who is considered to be virginal, pelvic tuberculosis should be strongly considered.

A first-strength *tubercular skin test* is of utmost importance, because a negative test virtually rules out the possibility of tuberculosis. Diagnosis can best be established by an endometrial biopsy; this should be performed during the week preceding menstruation, when the endometrium is thickest and is most apt to contain tubercles. A portion of the specimen should be cultured and the remainder should be submitted for histologic examination. Repeated cultures of the menstrual flow have also been utilized with success by some investigators. If cultures of either biopsy specimens or menstrual blood are negative, a curettage may be productive. If *tubercle bacilli* are recovered by culture, antimicrobial susceptibility testing should be performed to predict drug resistance.

Endometrial biopsy, curettage, and culture of menstrual flow or endometrial tissue can provide an exact diagnosis of genital tuberculosis if they are positive but, if negative, the presence of the disease cannot be excluded. If these measures are unrewarding in a patient whose history and pelvic findings suggest genital tuberculosis, diagnostic laparotomy is justified. Diagnostic laparoscopy may be performed if there is minimal likelihood of tuberculous peritonitis, but caution must be used because of the possibility of perforating a loop of adherent bowel. *Hysterosalpingography* may reveal characteristic tubal patterns, but it may also cause severe exacerbation of pelvic tuberculosis and should not be used if there is a likely possibility that this disease is present.

The incidental discovery of reproductive tract tuberculosis, perhaps in the course of an infertility survey, may be the first indication that the patient has tuberculosis. In such patients an effort must be made to determine if other sites (*e.g.,* lungs, urinary tract, bone, and gastrointestinal tract) may also be infected.

TREATMENT

The therapy currently recommended is isoniazid 300 mg daily and ethambutal 1200 mg daily for 18 to 24 months. Patients without adnexal masses should have an endometrial biopsy for culture and microscopic examination 6 and 12 months after the onset of therapy. Persistent organisms should be susceptibility-tested to identify drug-resistant strains. Laparotomy is performed if adnexal masses persist for 4 months; rifampin or streptomycin should be given preoperatively. Bilateral salpingectomy and removal of other tuberculous foci may be performed in young women with minimal disease, but bilateral salpingo-oophorectomy and total hysterectomy are indicated in those who have advanced disease or are of advanced age. Pregnancy following tubal tuberculosis is rare, even among women with minimal disease. If the tubes are damaged by genital tuberculosis, efforts to improve fertility by tubal plastic operations are usually futile.

ANAEROBIC BACTERIA

Anaerobic bacteria are being associated with an increasing number of pelvic infections. The application of modern anaerobic culture techniques has accounted for most of this increased recognition of these infections. Typically, multiple anaerobic species, usually together with one or more aerobic bacteria, combine to form a polymicrobial infection. Intra-abdominal abscess, postoperative pelvic inflammatory disease, and nonspecific vaginitis infections are currently the most important examples of anaerobic bacterial infection.

Anaerobic bacteria are part of the normal cervicovaginal flora. Although many of the mechanisms by which anaerobic bacteria become pathogenic are unknown, two known mechanisms that cause anaerobic infection are tissue trauma that occurs following surgery, which reduces the redox potential, and antibiotic selection that preferentially inhibits aerobic bacteria. The clinician can virtually assume the presence of anaerobes when infection is associated with a foul-smelling odor and abscess formation; only anaerobes produce odorous metabolic products. Anaerobes are virtually always isolated from an abscess if modern anaerobic techniques are used before antibiotic therapy is begun. Anaerobic infections also commonly produce gas formation and thromboembolism.

The most common anaerobic bacteria that are found in genital infections include anaerobic gram-positive cocci (Peptococcus and Peptostreptococcus), gram-negative rods (Bacteroides species—*B. fragilis, B. me-*

laningenicus, B. bivius—and Fusobacterium species), and anaerobic gram-positive rods (Clostridium and Enbacterum species).

The organism should be cultured before the institution of antimicrobial therapy. Since anaerobes are part of the normal flora, deep-tissue cultures are required which are not contaminated by surface bacteria. Unfortunately, 48 or more hours are required for anaerobe recovery, and treatment is usually begun based upon clinical signs. Anaerobic infection should be particularly suspected with abscess formation, a foul odor, gas formation, tissue necrosis, "sterile" cultures from obviously infected sites, and thromboembolism. Antibiotic sensitivity testing is only a rough guide for an organism's susceptibility, but *in vitro* and *in vivo* experience has shown that clindamycin and chloramphenicol are the current antibiotic standards for anaerobes. The newer antibiotics—metronidazole and cefoxitin—are also very effective in treating anaerobic infections.

VULVITIS

Herpes

Today *herpes simplex virus* (HSV) infection is the most common cause of vulvar ulcers and is the most common viral genital infection. Typical HSV genital infection occurs 3 to 7 days after exposure. Primary (first) genital infections consist of multiple vesicles that rapidly ulcerate to produce coalescent ulcerations of the vulva which may be exceedingly painful. The vagina and cervix may also be involved, thereby producing profuse leukorrhea. External dysuria is common and bilateral inguinal lymphadenopathy is usual. Vulvar lesions may last 3 or more weeks, but after this time heal completely. Constitutional symptoms of fever, malaise, headache (aseptic meningitis), and urinary retention (myelitis) may persist for 1 week.

Following the primary infection, latent HSV infection usually occurs in the sacral ganglion and perhaps locally in the dermis. The virus is rarely transmitted during the latency period when there are no symptoms and no physical evidence of infection. However, most patients develop a secondary (recurrent) infection from the latent virus weeks to months after the primary infection. The lesions of the secondary infection are usually less painful, more localized, and last a shorter time (3 to 7 days) than those of the primary infection. Systemic reactions are unusual in secondary HSV.

The infection is caused by *Herpesvirus hominis.* From 75% to 85% of genital infections are caused by type 2 *H. hominis;* the remainder of genital infections are caused by type 1 *H. hominis,* which is the primary cause of lip and perioral infections. The two types of herpes are clinically indistinguishable. The vesicles and ulcers of HSV infection contain many virus parti-

cles that are highly infectious and viral shedding occurs until the lesions reepithelialize. Therefore, genital contact with a person who has either genital or oral lesions leads to a high attack rate. Transmission usually occurs from contact with symptomatic lesions, but asymptomatic lesions may occasionally transmit the disease.

The *diagnosis* of herpes can be made clinically if typical, painful, multiple vulvar ulcers are present. Laboratory confirmation of atypical lesions and lesions that appear during pregnancy is best attained by virus isolation, which usually can be achieved within 48 hours. Papanicolaou or other cytologically examined material can identify intracellular inclusions and multinucleated cells, but unfortunately the cytologic method is only 40% as sensitive as culture in identifying HSV infections. Accordingly, a negative cytologic search in no way excludes HSV infection. Complement fixing and neutralizing antibodies appear within 1 week of the onset of infection; failure of an experienced laboratory to identify antibodies within 3 weeks is evidence against HSV infection. High antibody levels do not protect against recurrent or neonatal HSV infection.

The increased frequency of herpes infection and its serious fetal effects have caused HSV to assume increasing importance in pregnancy. This is discussed in Chapter 27.

HSV infection has been associated with cervical cancer. Women with cervical cancer have a higher prevalence of antibody and usually a higher antibody titer than do controls without cancer. HSV has caused nongenital animal tumors; however, these circumstantial reports suggesting a relationship between herpes and cancer are not sufficient to establish a direct effect of HSV in causing human cancer. Nevertheless, women with HSV infection should receive frequent Papanicolaou smears and colposcopic examinations.

Local therapy of genital herpes is limited to the relief of pain. Most of the local treatment modalities either do not penetrate to virus-containing cells or are administered after the damage has occurred; they neither shorten the duration of symptoms nor prevent recurrent infection. Many local antiviral compounds have been used, but rigorous double-blind and well-controlled studies have shown them to be without effect. The best future hope is the use of systemic antiviral therapy. Local symptomatic therapy is sometimes helpful, *e.g.,* a 10-minute sitz bath 3 to 4 times daily, followed by drying with a bulb light or a hair dryer. Corticosteroids and antibacterial and antifungal ointments are not only without benefit but tend to prevent drying, and so may delay healing.

Condyloma Acuminatum

The genital wart (Fig. 50–7) is caused by a DNA virus of the papova virus group which is distinct from the

papova viruses that cause the common warts. This virus thrives in the moist genital area and is usually sexually transmitted. The incubation period averages 3 months. Warts are most commonly located on the labia and posterior fourchette. They originally appear as individual lesions although, if neglected, large confluent growths up to several centimeters in diameter can occur. Vaginal and cervical warts are common. When white warts are found on the cervix they may be atypical and biopsy or colposcopy may be needed to exclude cervical neoplasia; if so, treatment should be delayed until the nature of the lesion is determined.

Genital warts must be differentiated from the less verrucous, more flat growths of syphilitic *condyloma latum* (see Fig. 50–4) and carcinoma in situ of the vulva; punch biopsies may be required to exclude these lesions. Small- to medium-sized verrucous lesions can usually be treated with 25% podophyllin in tincture of benzoin, which the patient must wash off after 4 hours. Small amounts (0.25 ml) should be used to prevent severe burns; the drug should not be used at all in pregnancy. Large amounts have produced coma in the adult and even fetal death in pregnant women. Atypical lesions should be biopsied before therapy because podophyllin causes bizarre histologic changes that persist for months. Liquid nitrogen or cryocautery should be used if the lesions do not respond to podophyllin or if the woman is pregnant. Recurrence often results from reinfection by an untreated partner or from failure to treat vaginal and cervical lesions.

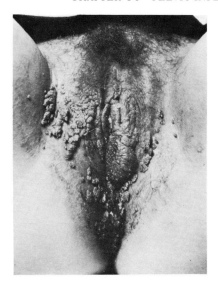

FIG. 50–7. Condylomata acuminata of vulva.

Furunculosis

The hair follicles of the mons and vulva may become infected by staphylococci, giving rise to pustules. This must be distinguished from herpetic and syphilitic lesions. The diagnosis can be made by culture or by the finding of gram-positive cocci in Gram stains of pus taken from the hair follicle. If only a few small lesions are present, they can be treated with hot, wet compresses or hexachlorophene scrubbing. Larger areas require antistaphylococcal antibiotics.

Bartholinitis

Two stages of Bartholin gland infection occur. The first is an acute infection of the duct and lining of the gland, usually by either *N. gonorrhoeae* or *C. trachomatis*. If unchecked, obstruction of the duct results, leading to the second stage, abscess formation. Anaerobic bacteria can be isolated from at least 50% of such abscesses. Rarely, synergistic vulvar gangrene has resulted from Bartholinitis.

Cultures and a Gram stain of material expressed from the duct may identify gonococci. Cervical gonococcal cultures should be obtained and if the patient is

in the initial stage of gonococcal infection, ampicillin or tetracycline should be administered for 7 to 10 days, as discussed previously in this chapter. Patients in the second stage usually require abscess marsupialization or incision with placement of a drain for 3 to 6 weeks. Simple incison and drainage usually lead to recurrent abscess formation. Recurrent infection from vaginal flora and mucus cyst formation are frequent sequelae of Bartholinitis.

Chancroid

The *soft chancre infection* characteristically causes a painful ulcer with a ragged, undermined edge and a raised border. In contrast, the syphilitic chancre is painless and indurated. "Kissing ulcers" on apposing surfaces of the vulva may occur. Tender, unilateral adenopathy is common and suppuration occurs in about 50% of women with lymphadenopathy.

The incubation period of this uncommon, sexually transmitted disease is 2 to 5 days. The infection is caused by *Haemophilus ducreyi*, gram-negative bacteria that form a school-of-fish pattern when seen in the Gram stain preparation. The organism is fastidious and it is best recovered by culturing aspirated lymph nodes on rabbit blood or on the patient's own heat (complement)-inactivated serum.

The differential diagnosis includes syphilis, which is to be excluded by darkfield examinations of the lesion on at least 3 separate days. Chancroid may also resemble genital herpes and lymphogranuloma venereum. Treatment with sulfisoxazole is preferred so that darkfield and serologic studies of syphilis are not obscured; tetracycline therapy is also successful.

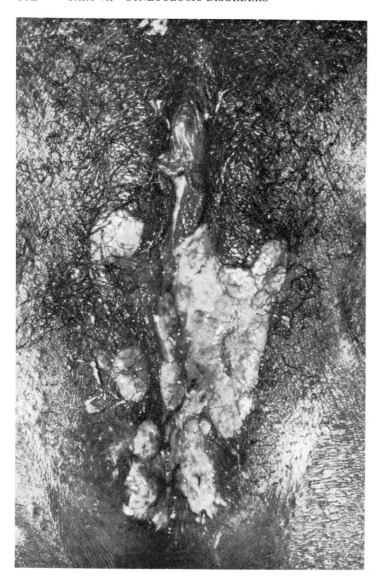

FIG. 50–8. Vulval granuloma inguinale of relatively recent origin, some lesions being separate, other confluent. Margin of lesion is raised and scrolled; base is granular and covered imperfectly by thin, gray slough. (Demis DJ, Crounse RG, Dobson RL, McGuire J (eds): Clinical Dermatology, Vol 3. Hagerstown, Harper & Row, 1972)

Granuloma Inguinale

This chronic granulomatous infection is rare in temperate climates. The organism is usually considered to be sexually transmitted, although gastrointestinal transmission may occur in some cases. The initial papular lesion typically ulcerates and develops into a soft, red, painless granuloma that may be covered by a thin gray membrane. The granuloma may spread over the course of many months to involve the anus and rectum (Fig. 50–8). Lymph nodes are moderately enlarged and painless, but they do not suppurate. Long-standing disease may cause not only genital scarring and depigmentation, but also lymphatic fibrosis with consequent genital edema. Malignancy has been reported in granulomatous areas, but this is unusual.

The infection is caused by a gram-negative bacillus, *Calymmatobacterium granulomatis*, which is difficult to culture because it is an intracellular parasite. The usual identification is made from scraped or biopsied material obtained from the periphery of the lesion. Bipolar staining bacteria are best identified within mononuclear cells (*Donovan bodies*) by Wright or Giemsa staining.

The differential diagnosis includes syphilis, chancroid, and lymphogranuloma venereum. Two to 3 weeks of ampicillin, tetracycline, or erythromycin is the therapy of choice.

Lymphogranuloma Venereum (LGV)

The incubation period for LGV is 2 to 5 days. Thereafter, a transient, primary, painless genital or anorectal ulcer develops. Multiple large, confluent inguinal nodes develop 2 to 3 weeks later and eventually suppurate. Acute infection may cause generalized systemic symptoms. If untreated, the infection enters a tertiary phase which can lead to extensive lymphatic obstruction that, together with continued infection, causes fistulae and ulceration of the anal, urethral, or genital area. Women with LGV are particularly susceptible to rectal stricture. Edema and elephantiasis of the external genitalia and lower extremities are serious sequelae.

The infection is caused by the sexually transmitted organism *Chlamydia trachomatis,* an intracellular bacterium. Usually only L_1, L_2, and L_3 Chlamydia immunotypes, which produce accelerated *in vitro* tissue destruction, cause LGV. The diagnosis can be made by culturing Chlamydia from genital lesions or lymph nodes. Cell culture methods are required to recover the organism. Indirect serologic methods are available. The most specific and sensitive serologic test is the microimmunofluorescent antibody test in which the specific immunotype and titer are identified. Complement fixation (CF) tests are positive in 95% of patients with LGV, but the CF test lacks specificity; it is often falsely positive in patients without LGV due to their exposure to other chlamydial infections. The intradermal *Frei test* is no longer used, since it reacts positively if there should be other prior or concurrent chlamydial infections.

The disease responds to tetracycline, erythromycin, and sulfonamide drugs. Large lymph nodes should be aspirated to prevent chronic drainage. Surgical excision of scarred areas may be necessary.

ACUTE URETHRAL SYNDROME

It is well recognized that no more than one-half of women with symptoms of dysuria and urinary frequency have acute cystitis as defined by pyuria and midstream urine cultures that contain greater than 10^5 organisms per milliliter of coliform or staphylococcal organisms. Until recently, the cause of symptoms in the remaining women was unknown. Some women will have vaginitis. Women with external dysuria consisting of labial pain with urination and a vaginal discharge often are found to have monilial, nonspecific, or trichomonas vaginitis. Women with a recent onset of internal dysuria and urinary frequency who do not have vaginitis are usually considered to have an acute urethral syndrome. The infectious causes of acute urethral syndrome among females has been recently analyzed. About one-half of women with acute urethral syndrome have less than 10^5 coliforms or *Staphylococcus saprophyticus* per milliliter isolated from urine obtained by suprapubic aspirates or urethral catheterization. Virtually all of these women have pyuria, defined as eight or more leukocytes per HPF of urine. An additional one-fourth of patients with this syndrome have "sterile" pyuria; *C. trachomatis* can be isolated from two-thirds of these women with pyuria. Usually no organisms are isolated from the remaining one-fourth of patients without pyuria or bacteriuria. Although women who have recently acquired gonorrheae often develop transient dysuria, gonorrheae is only occasionally isolated from a general group of women with dysuria.

Therapy of acute urethritis consists of therapy for the infectious agent, whether it is coliform, *S. saprophyticus,* or Chlamydia.

A more chronic form of urethritis has been identified by cystoscopy which consists of periurethral gland inflammatory reaction that has responded to some degree to urethral dilatation. However, this entity has not been well studied bacteriologically and it is unknown how many of these patients have a chlamydial or a low-bacterial-count coliform type of urethritis.

VAGINITIS

Vaginal infections are the most common gynecologic complaint. Infectious vaginitis can produce symptoms of increased vaginal discharge, vulvar irritation and pruritis, external dysuria, and a foul odor. Women with infectious vaginitis have either abnormal organisms (Trichomonads), or a quantitative increase in the normal flora (Candida, *G. vaginalis,* anaerobes). At least four entities of infectious vaginitis have been identified: monilial; trichomonal; nonspecific; and, in children, gonococcal. Every effort should be made to establish the diagnosis of one of these specific infections and to avoid the diagnosis of unspecified vaginitis. The establishment of a specific diagnosis is mandatory because the selection of effective therapy is dependent upon a correct diagnosis.

Other conditions that may cause excessive vaginal discharge include cervicitis, a cervical erosion or ectropion, vaginal foreign bodies (most commonly retained tampons), and allergic reactions to douching or vaginal contraceptive agents. The atrophic "vaginitis" among postmenopausal women may produce burning and dyspareunia; an infectious etiology has not been established.

A small amount of vaginal discharge may be normal, particularly at the midcycle when large amounts of cervical mucus production may produce a clear vaginal discharge. A normal vaginal discharge should not have a foul odor, nor should it be pruritic.

EXAMINATION

The external genitalia may be normal, or they may be edematous, erythematous, and excoriated to the point of fissure formation. Occasionally local primary vulvar disease must be excluded from a secondary effect of vaginitis.

On speculum examination the vaginal mucosa may be erythematous or edematous. Discharge characteristics that are important to observe are the viscosity of the discharge, the presence of floccular elements, the color, and the odor. Vaginal discharge should be examined for the pH; in addition, a potassium hydroxide (KOH) odor test and a microscopic exam consisting of a normal saline and 10% KOH wet mount should be done. A drop of each solution is mixed with the discharge. Before placing a cover slip over the two separate drops, the KOH portion is tested for the presence of a fishy amine odor. Microscopic examination of the KOH portion is made for hyphae under the 100× objective and examination of the saline portion is made for trichomonads and clue cells under the 400× objective. Multiple causes of vaginitis are frequent.

Vaginal cultures are not particularly helpful except perhaps in identifying trichomonal infection. Microscopy, the most specific diagnostic method, is only 80% sensitive in identifying various types of vaginitis. Therefore, when infectious vaginitis is suspected among patients who do not have specific diagnoses established, a repeat examination should be performed several days later.

Monilia

The most prominent symptom of monilial vaginitis is intense vulvar and vaginal pruritis. External dysuria is common. A curdlike vaginal discharge and vulvar pain may also occur. Vulvar signs of edema, geographic erythema, and fissures may be present. Classically, the vagina is dry and it has a bright red color mottled by adherent white, curdy placques. However, many women with monilia have little discharge and no erythema.

Candida albicans causes more than 90% of vaginal yeast infections. Other Candida species and Torulopsis can also cause infection. These saprophytic fungi can be isolated from the vagina in 15% to 25% of asymptomatic women. Therefore, the mere presence of vaginal Candida does not identify an infection, but an overgrowth of these organisms can lead to symptomatic vaginitis. An overgrowth is produced by a change in host resistance or in the local bacterial flora, which allows the organisms to proliferate. Several host factors have been associated with monilial infection, the most widely accepted of which are pregnancy, diabetes, and the administration of immunosuppressive drugs and broad-spectrum antibiotics. Because cellular and not humoral immunity is required for resistance to fungal infections, pregnant women and patients receiving immunosuppressive drugs that decrease the cellular immunity are predisposed to excessive fungal growth. Overgrowth is also favored by high blood glucose levels; pregnant women and diabetics with elevated blood glucose levels are susceptible. Women treated with broad-spectrum antibiotics may develop monilial vaginitis as a result of antibiotic suppression of the normal gastrointestinal and vaginal bacterial flora, thereby allowing fungal overgrowth. The role of oral contraceptives in monilial infection remains controversial. These compounds do cause both carbohydrate metabolic alterations and an increased prevalence of monilia in the vagina. However, the rate of symptomatic monilial infection among oral contraceptive users is no higher than among nonusers. A small subset of users, however, may develop repetitive infections. It is not necessary to discontinue oral contraceptives if monilial infection occurs only infrequently unless repetitive infections occur.

The most practical means of diagnosing monilial vaginitis is by microscopic examination of wet mount. Vaginal placques, vaginal discharge, or vulvar scrapings from the edge of the erythematous border is mixed with 10% potassium hydroxide (Fig. 50–9). The mycelial form that usually is found only during an infection can be identified in this preparation in 80% of the cases. The Gram stain, which also identifies the blastospore forms of both noninfectious and infectious states, is slightly more sensitive than wet mounts in identifying fungi. Fungi can be readily recovered on a variety of media. Because they are part of the normal vaginal flora, the recovery of fungi by culture does not necessarily diagnose an infection. Cultures should be limited to patients with suspected monilial vaginitis, including those with unidentified pruritis or suspicious signs that cannot be identified by examination of the wet mount.

In most cases of monilial vaginitis the organisms can also be cultured from the rectum. Since antifungal preparations are not absorbed from the intestinal tract, local vaginal therapy is required. Vaginal nystatin suppositories inserted twice daily for 10 to 14 days are usually effective, and nystatin cream applied to the vulva may relieve the irritation. Two imidazole agents, miconazole and clotrimazole, are more active than nystatin against Candida *in vitro*. These agents should be administered to women with repeated monilial vaginitis because they are more likely than nystatin to completely eradicate fungi from the vagina and also to prevent recurrent infection. Although imidazole drugs are not absorbed to any degree from the vagina, there is some concern over the possibility of fetal teratogenicity; their use in pregnancy should, therefore, be limited to the last 20 weeks. The preparations are inserted vaginally once nightly for 7 days or twice daily for seven doses. More prolonged therapy may be necessary in certain cases. About 15% of male sexual

contacts of women with monilial vaginitis have symptomatic balanitis. It is unclear whether the male infection causes or results from vaginal moniliasis. However, males should be identified and treated to prevent recurrent female infection. Oral antifungal administration to decrease gastrointestinal colonization does not improve therapeutic cure rates or diminish recurrence rates.

The patient who develops frequent recurrences represents the most difficult problem in the treatment of monilial vaginitis. Extended 2- to 3-week vaginal therapy, treatment of the male, and elimination of associated factors are the only ways at present by which to limit these often frustrating infections. A glucose tolerance test should be performed in recurrent or resistant cases to exclude unrecognized diabetes. Also, some women with monilial infection have additional concurrent vaginal infections; a repeated physical and wet mount examination may clarify the problem.

Gentian violet (1% aqueous solution) may still have a place in the treatment of resistant or recurrent infection. It may cause local edema, and leaves an indelible stain on clothing and linens.

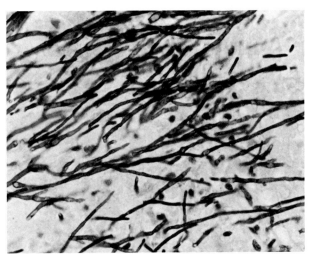

FIG. 50–9. *C. albicans* growing as hyphae and pseudohyphae within infected tissue. (Monif GRG: Infectious Diseases in Obstetrics & Gynecology. Hagerstown, Harper & Row, 1974; PAS, original magnification ×320)

Trichomonas Vaginitis

The characteristic symptoms of Trichomonas infection are a profuse, malodorous, often uncomfortable, sometimes frothy vaginal discharge, internal and external dysuria, and vulvar pruritis. This is probably the most common sexually transmitted organism; it is present in 3% to 15% of asymptomatic women and in 20% to 50% of women who attend clinics for sexually transmitted disease. The organism is most likely to be identified among symptomatic women who have recently acquired the infection. However, many asymptomatic women harbor Trichomonas. Most male contacts of women with trichomoniasis asymptomatically carry the organism in the urethra and prostate.

The classic vaginal discharge is present in only about one-third of women. The vulva may be edematous and moistened by the discharge. Subepithelial hemorrhage of the cervix ("strawberry cervix") is sometimes seen with the naked eye; smaller hemorrhagic areas are usually identified colposcopically. Women with symptomatic trichomoniasis have a discharge that has a pH of greater than 4.5 and forms amines with 10% potassium hydroxide. Motile trichomonads are demonstrated in the saline wet-mount (Fig. 50–10) smear. Trichomonads are larger than white blood cells and they are identified by their rapid, jerking motility. The wet mount usually also contains many polymorphonuclear leukocytes. Nonmotile trichomonads can sometimes be identified by a Pap smear by their characteristic flagellate appearance. Although the wet mount may identify trichomonads with 80% sensitivity among symptomatic women, this method is less than 50% sensitive when used for

asymptomatic women. The organism, *Trichomonas vaginalis,* is an anaerobic protozoan. A culture of *T. vaginalis* is easy to perform but, unfortunately, because a freshly prepared medium is needed, culture has limited practicality and its current use is limited to cases in which the diagnosis is suspected, but the organism cannot be identified in the wet mount or in a Pap smear. Screening cultures of asymptomatic women are not presently recommended except for certain high-risk populations. Women with trichomoniasis should also be cultured for *N. gonorrhoeae,* since as many as 60% of women with proved gonorrhea also have been found to have trichomoniasis. Trichomoniasis frequently causes the symptom that led the patient with gonorrhea to present for care.

T. vaginalis resides not only in the vagina, but also in the urethra, bladder, and Skene glands; therefore, systemic rather than local therapy is required. Metronidazole is effective in treating trichomoniasis; the preferred regimen is 2 g in one dose because of complete patient compliance and high effectiveness. Extended 7-day metronidazole therapy of 500 mg 3 times daily does not increase the 95% cure rate of a single dose. Simultaneous treatment of the male sexual partner is recommended. Recurrent trichomoniasis is usually attributable to a lack of drug compliance or reexposure to untreated sexual partners. The organism remains very sensitive to metronidazole *in vitro* and drug resistance is rare.

Metronidazole therapy is not without controversy because of questions of its possible tumor-causing potential in humans. In animals, large doses (equivalent to 350 to 1000 human doses) cause tumors. The drug

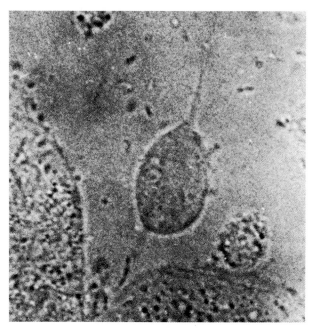

FIG. 50-10. Characteristic configuration of a trichomonad seen in wet smear at high-power magnification. (Monif GRG: Infectious Diseases in Obstetrics & Gynecology. Hagerstown, Harper & Row, 1974)

has also been shown to cause bacterial mutation of the kind associated with a drug's carcinogenic potential. In small series of women evaluated for up to 10 years following metronidazole therapy for trichomoniasis, no increased tumor rates were found. However, these data are only slightly reassuring that the drug does not cause cancer. Because of these concerns, the drug should be avoided in pregnancy, particularly during the first 20 weeks. Unfortunately, other drugs that may be used during pregnancy lack efficacy, and the iodine preparations, which may be somewhat effective, should not be used because the iodine is absorbed in high enough levels to suppress the fetal thyroid. For nonpregnant women, the short-term use of a drug with at most a minimal carcinogenic potential seems justified, especially since this is the only agent that eradicates the disease.

Candida and trichomoniasis often coexist. Persistent discharge after adequate treatment for trichomoniasis should lead to repeated cultures for both Candida and gonorrhea.

Nonspecific Vaginitis

The term *nonspecific vaginitis* is a misnomer, but it is used to identify the vaginitis that results from an overgrowth of both anaerobic bacteria and the organism formerly referred to as *Haemophilis vaginalis*, but now renamed *Gardnerella vaginalis* in recognition of Herman Gardner, who first described the syndrome and identified the organism. Both anaerobes and *G. vaginalis* are normal inhabitants of the vagina, but their overgrowth results in the appearance of a thin, homogeneous, foul-smelling, yellow-gray vaginal discharge that adheres to the vaginal walls and is present at the introitus. In contrast to most other kinds of vaginitis, the vaginal epithelium appears normal. The "fishy," foul odor that is caused by amines produced by the anaerobes is accentuated when 10% potassium hydroxide is added to the discharge.

The diagnosis of nonspecific vaginitis is based upon a pH greater than 4.5, the characteristic homogeneous appearance of the discharge, a fishy amine odor with the addition of 10% KOH, and the presence of clue cells. Clue cells are vaginal epithelial cells to which gram-negative organisms are attached. These cells are epithelial cells that are stippled with adherent bacteria; typically, the cell border is so obscured by adherent bacteria that it cannot be identified. In nonspecific vaginitis, 2% to 50% of the epithelial cells show this distinctive marking, but polymorphonuclear leukocytes and lactobacilli are notably absent. Cultures are not helpful, since anaerobes and *G. vaginalis* can be recovered from normal women. In fact, up to 40% of asymptomatic normal women carry *G. vaginalis*. Although the number of colonies of both organisms is higher among women with nonspecific vaginitis than among normal women, quantitative culture methods are cumbersome and they add only slightly to the specificity of diagnosis.

The factors that lead to an overgrowth of *G. vaginalis* and anaerobes have not been identified. Sexual transmission of the infection has long been considered a risk factor, but this is not proved. *G. vaginalis* can usually be recovered from the urethra of the male sexual contact. Treatment of the male does not prevent recurrence of the infection.

Ampicillin administered orally (500 mg every 6 hours for 7 days) cures 60% of the cases. However, metronidazole (500 mg twice daily for 7 days) is the most effective drug for nonspecific vaginitis. The difference in response between these two drugs is unexplained, since ampicillin inhibits both *G. vaginalis* and the anaerobes that have been isolated from patients with nonspecific vaginitis. Curiously, metronidazole is directly effective only against the anaerobes, although metronidazole metabolites do inhibit *G. vaginalis*. Tetracycline inhibits the growth of both organisms, but it is ineffective in treating nonspecific vaginitis. Local sulfonamide therapy is ineffective because both *G. vaginalis* and the anaerobes are resistant to this drug. At the present time the treatment of the male with ampicillin can only be advocated when nonspecific vaginitis recurs.

CERVICITIS

The majority of hysterectomy specimens contain an area beneath the squamocolumnar junction which is infiltrated by plasma cells and lymphocytes. In the presence of such cells, the pathologist is obliged to make a diagnosis of *chronic cervicitis*. Unless the inflammatory reaction is extensive, there are no symptoms, cultures recover either no organisms, or only organisms that are part of the normal vaginal flora. This condition is not of clinical importance. To qualify as a pelvic infection, the inflammatory reaction must result from the effects of pathogenic organisms or established infection. The common causes of *acute cervicitis* are *N. gonorrhoeae*, *C. trachomatis*, and puerperal infection. The organisms penetrate the columnar epithelium or areas denuded by obstetric or surgical injury. Symptoms are usually limited to a profuse purulent vaginal discharge or intermenstrual bleeding. In more than three-fourths of women who have a purulent or mucoid cervical discharge, *N. gonorrhoeae* or *C. trachomatis* can be isolated separately or in combination from the endocervix.

Infectious ulcers of the cervix caused by herpes virus, syphilis, and chancroid must be distinguished from erosion and the other conditions described in Chapter 53. Depending upon the nature of the lesion, Pap smear, culture, darkfield examination, colposcopy and, in some cases, biopsy may be required.

C. trachomatis may give rise to the friable "papillary erosion" of the cervix in which the columnar epithelium is proliferated above the plane of the squamous epithelium, but many women who do have *C. trachomatis* do not have this lesion. The papillary erosion is also caused by factors other than *C. trachomatis*.

ENDOMETRITIS

Scattered lymphocytes and plasma cells and occasional neutrophils appear normally in the endometrium in the second half of the menstrual cycle, and their presence does not necessarily constitute endometritis. In some cases of abnormal bleeding they may appear in greater number, and in such cases they may represent an abnormal inflammatory reaction. In at least one report, chronic endometritis was related to the isolation of genital mycoplasma from the endometrial cavity.

For the most part, endometritis is an ill-defined entity that produces either uncertain symptoms or none at all, and it should rarely be diagnosed unless a specific etiologic factor is found. *Bona fide* endometritis may occur in the following situations: (1) Puerperal endometritis (see Chap. 40), (2) gonococcal endometritis that occurs among patients with PID, (3) the endometritis that follows instrumentation or surgery, (4) tuberculous endometritis, (5) the purulent endometritis that occurs in pyometra caused by a cervical stricture or following radium insertion, and (6) the endometritis that characteristically occurs in the presence of a tailed intrauterine device (IUD).

The chronic endometritis that is associated with the use of IUDs is well documented. It is clear, however, that it is not the foreign body *per se* that leads to chronic inflammation, but rather the tail of the IUD which acts as a wick for organisms to reach the endometrium from the vagina. Transfundal endometrial cultures of hysterectomy specimens from women who had used tailed IUDs for more than a few weeks uniformly recovered bacteria, while the cultures from women who had used tailless IUDs or no IUD were sterile. The organisms that can be recovered are usually of low pathogenicity, but some more virulent intrauterine bacteria undoubtedly cause the malodorous discharge and the salpingitis that occur more frequently among IUD users than among nonIUD users. In addition, an anaerobe, *Actinomyces israelii*, has been found in Papanicolaou smears from about 5% of women using IUDs, but not among nonIUD users. This organism may colonize the endometrium of IUD users and when it is found in the Pap smear, the IUD should be removed and penicillin should be prescribed for 20 days.

SALPINGITIS

Acute primary salpingitis is a bacterial infection that begins as an endosalpingitis when pathogenic organisms invade the fallopian tube. *Neisseria gonorrhoeae*, *Chlamydia trachomatis*, genital mycoplasma, and normal flora aerobic and anaerobic bacteria cause the overwhelming majority of tubal infections. Virtually all primary salpingitis occurs among sexually active, menstruating, nonpregnant women. Tuberculous, parasitic, or fungal salpingitis is rare in industrialized countries. Most salpingitis occurs spontaneously without instrumentation or trauma to the genital tract; however, approximately 15% follows instrumentation (*e.g.*, IUD insertion, dilatation and curretage, abortion, hysterosalpingography, or tubal insufflation). Salpingitis can also begin as a perisalpingitis secondary to acute appendicitis or other interabdominal bacterial infection, but this kind of infection accounts for less than 1% of the cases of salpingitis.

Acute salpingitis is a common event. Approximately 1% of women between the ages of 15 and 39 years develop salpingitis annually. Young, sexually active women between the ages of 15 and 24 years have the highest rate of infection. As noted at the opening of this chapter, this rate of infection has tremendous national consequences. It is estimated that at least 1 billion dollars is required to treat the 800,000 women

who annually develop acute salpingitis in the United States.

EPIDEMIOLOGY

In most women, but certainly not all, the infection is caused by sexually transmitted organisms. The rate of salpingitis is increased fivefold among women with multiple sexual partners. The rate among younger women may be higher because they are more likely to have multiple partners, or they may be more susceptible to infection because they have less acquired immunity against these organisms than do older women. Previous salpingitis predisposes to the development of subsequent salpingitis, perhaps because a mucosa damaged by a prior infection is more susceptible to infection than normal tissue. In addition, patients with previous uncomplicated gonorrhea have a high rate of subsequent salpingitis, either because women who have once had gonorrhea are likely to have a second gonorrheal infection, or perhaps because in some women infection that may have appeared to be clinically uncomplicated may actually have been a subclinical tubal infection. Subclinical tubal infection would be expected to predispose to the development of clinical salpingitis.

The presence of an IUD is an independent factor in the development of salpingitis. Women using an IUD have a rate of salpingitis which is increased two- to fourfold as compared to women not using an IUD. The highest rate of salpingitis among IUD users occurs within a few weeks of insertion, at which time cervical bacteria are introduced into the endometrial cavity along with the IUD. However, most infections among IUD users occur long after insertion, probably because bacteria "wick" along the IUD tail leading from the vagina to the uterus. Such a mechanism for IUD-associated salpingitis is supported by the isolation of intrauterine bacteria at the time of hysterectomy only among users of tailed IUDs, but not among users of tailless IUDs or women without an IUD. Other mechanisms of IUD infection are possible, such as the enhancement of anaerobic bacterial growth, the presence of a chronic inflammatory reaction, or the production of microulcers by the IUD.

The IUD seems to be a greater factor in producing salpingitis among nulliparous than multiparous women. Also, IUD-induced salpingitis is more commonly nongonococcal than gonococcal. Women using barrier or oral contraceptive methods have a lower than expected rate of salpingitis. The protective effect of oral contraceptives on ascending infection may be due to changes in the cervical mucus, the periodic scanty withdrawal bleeding from an inactive endometrium, or decreased myometrial activity at the times of periodic uterine bleeding.

Socioeconomic factors also influence the rates of salpingitis, which are estimated to be 4% among women of low socioeconomic status and 1% among women of higher socioeconomic status. Women in the former group tend to have a higher rate of sexually transmitted disease; they are less apt to seek medical care for local symptoms and are more apt to have an untreated infectious partner than women of higher socioeconomic status. Other reasons for this difference must be elucidated.

The role of males with untreated gonococcal or chlamydial urethritis is often ignored by gynecologists. More than 75% of male contacts of women with gonococcal salpingitis have not been treated by the time the female develops symptomatic infection. Of the male contacts with infectious gonococcal urethritis, more than one-half are asymptomatic. Among asymptomatic male contacts of women with gonococcal salpingitis, *N. gonorrhoeae* is isolated from 40%. Males with chlamydial, nongonococcal urethritis would also be expected to be a reservoir for chlamydial salpingitis. To reduce the rate of new and recurrent salpingitis, male contacts of women with either gonococcal or nongonococcal salpingitis should be examined and cultured. If infectious organisms are found, they should be appropriately treated. To prevent subsequent PID it is also important that culture and appropriate therapy be provided to the male contacts of *asymptomatic* women identified as having gonorrhea or chlamydia.

BACTERIOLOGY

N. Gonorrhoeae

Formerly *N. gonorrhoeae* was considered to cause the majority of infectious salpingitis. This is no longer true, and in the United States today gonorrhea has assumed a less important position. In most studies *N. gonorrhoeae* can be recovered from only 40% to 50% of women with acute gonococcal salpingitis. However, gonococcal prevalence varies greatly: *N. gonorrhoeae* is isolated from less than 20% of the cases of salpingitis in Sweden, while it is isolated from 80% of salpingitis cases in certain populations in the United States. Among women with both cervical gonorrhea and salpingitis, *N. gonorrhoeae* is the most frequent intra-abdominal isolate, but it is the sole isolate in only 30% of these cases. In the remainder, either no organisms can be isolated or other organisms are isolated either alone or together with *N. gonorrhoeae*. Positive gonococcal cultures are usualy obtained during the early stages of infection. During the later stages of infection the organisms are either present only within epithelial cells or they are inhibited by leukocytes, two factors that make it difficult to isolate the organisms. If positive cultures are obtained in the later stages of gonorrheal salpingitis, organisms other than the gonococcus *can* be isolated either alone or in combination with gonococci.

(indicative of intra-abdominal bleeding) is obtained. A Gram stain of aspirated fluid may suggest a causative organism. A culture of the fluid will be helpful in predicting antibiotic response.

Ultrasound and Computerized Tomography

Ultrasound can be used to distinguish the presence of an abscess from an inflammatory mass within an adnexal mass. It may also be helpful in defining a mass in the very obese or if bimanual examination is unsatisfactory because of muscle guarding. In some cases it may be valuable for follow-up measurement of a mass that is believed to be resolving. More recently, computerized tomography has been used with satisfaction for the same purposes; it may be especially helpful if ultrasound is difficult to perform, as in the presence of peritonitis or a recent abdominal incision. For the most part these tests are not needed; a skillfully performed vaginal examination usually provides the necessary information.

Laparoscopy

Laparoscopy should be used without hesitation when the diagnosis is not clear. The accuracy of this method of diagnosis should approach 100%. It is estimated that for every 100 times a clinical diagnosis of pelvic inflammatory disease is made without visual confirmation, four patients with ectopic pregnancy and three patients with appendicitis are treated for pelvic inflammatory disease, resulting in a critical delay in the correct diagnosis. As noted earlier, about 20 of 100 women with a clinical diagnosis of pelvic inflammatory disease will be found to have no abnormality. In all cases in which laparoscopy is performed, regardless of the findings, cultures should be taken from the fimbriated ends of the tubes.

The pain and tenderness resulting from acute pelvic inflammatory disease should be expected to abate 3 or 4 days after antibiotics are started. If it does not begin to resolve or if it should be worse, laparoscopy is indicated both for confirmation of the diagnosis and direct culture for both aerobic and anaerobic organisms.

Examination of the Male Partner

Examination of the male sexual partner may be helpful in establishing the diagnosis in a woman suspected of having pelvic inflammatory disease. At least 80% of male contacts of women with PID will not have been identified as infectious by the time pelvic inflammatory disease occurs in the female partner. If there is no urethral discharge, urethral material for culture and Gram stain can be obtained using a calcium alginate swab.

TREATMENT

Adequate treatment of salpingitis includes (1) an assessment of severity, (2) antibiotic therapy, (3) additional general health measures, (4) close patient follow-up, and (5) treatment of the male sex partner. Most patients, except for those with the mildest manifestations, should be hospitalized. Specific indications for hospitalization exist for those who have severe manifestations of salpingitis (severe peritonitis, severe nausea, or temperature higher than 38° C), a suspected abscess, outpatient antibiotic failure, or an unclear diagnosis of salpingitis.

After treatment is started, all patients should be examined within 2 to 3 days and again at 7 and 21 days to make sure of a satisfactory response. Ideally, the antibiotic should be selected according to the organism that is recovered from the fallopian tube, but in many cases empiric therapy must be used. If the infection is presumed or is shown to be caused by *N. gonorrhoeae*, the treatment previously outlined should be used. Nongonococcal salpingitis responds to these regimens more slowly than do these caused by *N. gonorrhoeae*. For chlamydia, tetracycline is more effective than penicillins. Doxycycline 100 mg twice daily for 10 days may also be used. The recommended agents must be used in full doses, since subacute salpingitis frequently follows the use of lower doses.

Hospitalized patients with peritonitis but without adnexal abscess usually respond to the regimens of penicillin or ampicillin, or to doxycycline 200 mg intravenously. The combination of penicillin and aminoglycosides or penicillin and doxycycline can also be used. In contrast, if an adnexal abscess is present, even if the systemic manifestations are mild, antibiotics should be selected which inhibit *Bacteroides fragilis*, since 80% of pelvic abscesses contain this organism. A combination of aminoglycoside and clindamycin, or penicillin and chloramphenicol should be used to treat a known or suspected pelvic abscess. Metronidazole and cefoxitin also have been shown to be highly effective against this and other anaerobes associated with pelvic inflammatory disease.

If an IUD is in place, it should be removed 24 to 48 hours after therapy is started.

The position of surgery in dealing with PID is generally as considered earlier in the discussion of gonorrhea.

Other aspects of this problem are considered in Chapter 13.

OOPHORITIS

Oophoritis may occur without accompanying salpingitis in infections such as mumps, septicemia, or other generalized systemic illness. Oophoritis of this type is

bleeding occurs in 35% of women with salpingitis. Such problems as appendicitis and ectopic pregnancy are more likely if there is no recent history of vaginal discharge and dysuria. The risk of sexually transmitted disease can also be helpful in forming a tentative opinion: women who have had multiple sexual partners, gonorrhea, PID, or some other sexually transmitted disease, or a male partner having symptoms of such a disease have an increased risk of PID.

Physical Examination

Patients with salpingitis usually have lower abdominal, cervical, and bilateral adnexal tenderness. However, none of these findings is specific; patients with other disease or with no apparent disease may have similar physical findings, and other associated findings may lack the sensitivity to be useful. For example, although a temperature of 38° C or higher is present more often in patients with than without salpingitis, only 65% of patients with laparoscopically confirmed salpingitis have a temperature of more than 38° C. The clinical findings in 204 patients with a final diagnosis of pelvic inflammatory disease are shown in Table 50–4.

Laboratory Tests

Such nonspecific tests as the white blood count and the sedimentation rate can be helpful only if the results are abnormal; unfortunately, they are often normal. Of the patients with laparoscopically confirmed salpingitis, 50% have a normal white blood count and 25% have a normal sedimentation rate.

Specific laboratory tests such as a cervical Gram stain can be helpful. Properly obtained specimens free of vaginal discharge are 67% sensitive in the diagnosis of women with gonococcal salpingitis. Thus, if one-half of the tested patients have gonococcal salpingitis, one-third of all patients could have the diagnosis established by cervical Gram stain alone.

Cervical culture is mandatory for gonorrhea, and a cervical culture for chlamydia is recommended. However, cervical culture for other organisms is without benefit, since there is no correlation between the presence of other bacteria isolated from the cervix and bacteria isolated from the abdomen.

Culdocentesis

Culdocentesis is helpful if fluid that contains white blood cells (indicative of PID) or nonclotting blood

TABLE 50-3. HISTORIC DATA USEFUL IN PATIENTS WITH PELVIC INFLAMMATORY DISEASE

Age	Contraceptive used
Marital status	Gravidity, parity
Date last menstrual period	Last sexual exposure
Date onset of pain	No. of partners last month, 6 months
Characteristics of pain	History of previous gonorrhea, PID
Fever, chills	History of previous STD
Vaginal discharge	Symptoms in sexual partner
Nausea, vomiting	

PID = pelvic inflammatory disease; STD = sexually transmitted disease (Eschenbach DA: Obstet Gynecol 55:142S, 1980)

TABLE 50-4. CLINICAL FINDINGS IN 204 WOMEN WITH A DIAGNOSIS OF ACUTE PID

Finding	Percent with cervical *N. gonorrhoeae* gonococcal PID (N = 91)	Percent with no cervical *N. gonorrhoeae* nongonococcal PID (N = 113)	P
Abdominal tenderness	99	99	
Severe abdominal tenderness	37	29	
Abdominal rebound tenderness	76	66	
Liver tenderness	33	19	<.05
Purulent vaginal discharge	42	32	
Purulent cervical exudate	47	19	<.0005
Cervical tenderness	98	96	
Adnexal tenderness	100	100	
Unilateral adnexal tenderness	8	6	
Adnexal mass > 6 cm diameter	26	23	

Patient population has been previously reported, PID = pelvic inflammatory disease (Eschenbach DA: Obstet Gynecol 55:142S, 1980)

wall, undoubtedly representing a late end-stage manifestation of the earlier acute capsular inflammation.

Perihepatitis of this kind was formerly believed to be caused solely by *N. gonorrhoeae*, which travel transperitoneally from the fallopian tubes. Recently, culture, serologic, and experimental data have been reported which also link *C. trachomatis* with this syndrome. It has also become apparent that organisms may reach the liver by lymphatic and hematogenous routes, as well as by the more widely accepted transperitoneal migration. The syndrome occurs virtually exclusively among women, although two men with this syndrome have been reported. Salpingitis is almost invariably the source, but the syndrome has also followed appendicitis and other causes of peritonitis.

The Fitz-Hugh–Curtis syndrome is frequently misinterpreted as cholecystitis, viral pneumonia, or pyelonephritis. Liver enzyme levels may be mildly elevated and the gallbladder may not visualize on oral cholecystogram. The syndrome may cause symptoms in 5% to 10% of women with salpingitis, but in another 5% of women the perihepatitis is asymptomatic and the violin-string adhesions may only be recognized as an incidental finding when the surgeon makes his routine exploration of the upper abdomen in the course of laparotomy. Although many women with the Fitz-Hugh–Curtis syndrome note the onset of lower abdominal pain before or at the same time as the upper abdominal pain, in some the upper abdominal pain may be so severe that patients fail to complain of lower abdominal pain. Given the frequency of salpingitis and the infrequency of acute cholecystitis among young women 15 to 30 years of age, the Fitz-Hugh–Curtis syndrome is a more likely cause of upper quadrant pain than cholecystitis and should be suspected in any woman with pleuritic upper quadrant pain who also has physical signs of salpingitis. Laparoscopy is a specific diagnostic tool for unclear cases.

DIAGNOSIS

A tremendously broad spectrum of clinical severity results from salpingitis. Patients without abdominal pain and those with mild manifestations are often not identified. Although severe manifestations are usually recognized, they occur in only 30% of patients. The insistence upon rigid criteria such as fever, severe tenderness, leukocytosis, and an elevated sedimentation rate leads to a failure of diagnosis in nonovert cases. In fact, a clinical diagnosis of salpingitis which relies upon the history, physical examination, and nonspecific laboratory tests is plagued by large false-negative and false-positive errors. Several studies have demonstrated that a clinical diagnosis of salpingitis is confirmed by laparoscopy in only two-thirds of patients (Table 50-2); about 20% of patients had no disease and another 10% had other pelvic conditions, most commonly an ovarian cyst, ectopic pregnancy, appendicitis, or endometriosis. An additional 10% of patients who had a clinical diagnosis of other conditions had salpingitis demonstrated by laparoscopy.

History

The important points in the history of patients with presumed pelvic inflammatory disease are listed in Table 50–3. Lower abdominal pain is the most consistent symptom among women with salpingitis, although in 6% of patients it may be mild or even absent. The pain of an acute attack is present for less than 15 days in 85% of patients who present with PID. Women with gonococcal salpingitis usually have acute onset of pain during menses; in chlamydial salpingitis the onset of pain is usually insidious and is not associated with menses. The abdominal pain is usually continuous, being most severe in the lower quadrants, and equal bilaterally. It is increased by movement, the Valsalva maneuver, and intercourse. Abnormal vaginal

TABLE 50-2. LAPAROSCOPIC OBSERVATION IN PATIENTS WITH A CLINICAL DIAGNOSIS OF PID

Diagnosis	Jacobson and Weström	Chaparro et al	Sweet et al	Total (%)
Salpingitis	532	103	25	661 (62)
Normal findings	184	51	0	235 (22)
Ovarian cysts	12	39	0	51 (5)
Ectopic pregnancy	11	27	1	39 (4)
Appendicitis	24	2	1	27 (3)
Endometriosis	16	0	0	16 (1)
Other	35	1	1	37 (3)
Total				1066 (100)

PID = pelvic inflammatory disease (Eschenbach DA: Obstet Gynecol 55:142S, 1980)

Chlamydia

It is now evident that sexualy transmitted *Chlamydia trachomatis* is as important an organism as the gonococcus in the etiology of acute salpingitis. From 20% to 36% of women with acute salpingitis have cervical *C. trachomatis* and in most of these women the organism can be isolated from the fallopian tube. Up to 30% of women with salpingitis have tubal chlamydial infections. An additional 20% to 30% of patients have antibody changes, suggesting acute chlamydial infection.

Mycoplasmas

Genital mycoplasmas have been recovered from the abdomen in 2% to 16% of patients with salpingitis. In addition, more than 20% of patients with salpingitis have mycoplasmal antibody changes suggestive of invasive infection. These organisms lack the virulence of the gonococcus and chlamydia, and they probably play a lesser role in salpingitis.

Nonsexually Transmitted Aerobic and Anaerobic Bacteria

The fourth group of causative organisms of salpingitis are the nonsexually transmitted aerobic and anaerobic bacteria that are normally present in the cervical and vaginal flora. These organisms can be a direct cause of salpingitis, but more commonly they cause secondary infection in combination with sexually transmitted organisms, IUD use, or instrumentation. In salpingitis caused by these organisms, polymicrobial infection is the rule; infection caused by a single organism is unusual. In such cases, many different gram-positive and gram-negative aerobic organisms have been isolated as well as anaerobic organisms, particularly peptostreptococci and bacteroides species, including *Bacteroides fragilis*. Anaerobic organisms are particluarly common in serious infections and they are almost always found in the presence of abscess formation. The complex relationships that exist between gonococci, chlamydia, and these organisms have not been solved, but it is evident that they commonly invade tissues that have previously been infected by sexually transmitted organisms.

PATHOGENESIS

Salpingitis occurs when the uterus and fallopian tubes are infected by bacteria that are usually confined to the cervix and vagina. The ascent of bacteria from the cervical location to the fallopian tubes probably occurs most commonly during menses. The association between infection and menses is most striking among women who develop gonococcal salpingitis in whom abdominal pain occurs within 7 days of the onset of menses in one-half to two-thirds of patients, suggesting that gonococci are disseminated from their cervical location at the time of menses. As noted earlier, the cervical mucus possesses properties that cause it to act as a barrier to prevent the ascent of organisms into the uterus between menses, but the barrier is lost at menstruation. The movement of organisms from cervix to tubes occurs most commonly during the first menses after the cervical infection is acquired, although it may also occur with subsequent menses. In addition to menses, other risk factors must be operative. Virulent bacteria in the cervix are more likely to cause salpingitis than are nonvirulent bacteria. Endotoxin-producing *gonorrhoeae* and *trachomatis* are two virulent organisms that are capable of causing salpingitis, but virulence occasionally is also manifested by mycoplasma and organisms of the normal flora.

The bacterial virulence can be lessened if the patient develops specific antibodies to the organism. From 10% to 17% of women identified to have cervical gonorrhea develop clinically recognized salpingitis, and probably most of these women develop the tubal infection during the first one or two menstrual periods after the cervical infection is acquired, before specific bactericidal antibodies have developed. A failure to develop antibodies may be associated with an increased risk of salpingitis. Chlamydial salpingitis may be similarly inhibited by specific humoral or local immune systems.

The usual route of infection is the contiguous spread of organisms ascending from the cervix to the endometrial cavity and fallopian tubes. Lymphatic or hematogenous dissemination of organisms from the uterus to the adnexa is uncommon among nonpregnant women except, perhaps, in those with mycoplasma or IUD infections. When the bacteria reach the uterus, they commonly invade the fallopian tubes by contiguous spread along the mucosa (see Fig. 50–1), although it is possible that organisms may be transported to the fallopian tubes by cilia or even carried by their attachment to spermatazoa. Infectious organisms attach to the fallopian tube mucosa and first initiate an endosalpingitis.

The Fitz-Hugh–Curtis Syndrome

Perihepatitis, consisting of capsular inflammation without involvement of the liver parenchyma that has been associated with gonococcal salpingitis is referred to as the Fitz-Hugh–Curtis syndrome. The swelling of the liver capsule gives rise to inspiratory pain, usually in the right upper quadrant. Early in the inflammatory process a purulent or a fibrinous collection appears on the capsular surface. "Violin-string" adhesions form between the liver capsule and the anterior abdominal

who annually develop acute salpingitis in the United States.

EPIDEMIOLOGY

In most women, but certainly not all, the infection is caused by sexually transmitted organisms. The rate of salpingitis is increased fivefold among women with multiple sexual partners. The rate among younger women may be higher because they are more likely to have multiple partners, or they may be more susceptible to infection because they have less acquired immunity against these organisms than do older women. Previous salpingitis predisposes to the development of subsequent salpingitis, perhaps because a mucosa damaged by a prior infection is more susceptible to infection than normal tissue. In addition, patients with previous uncomplicated gonorrhea have a high rate of subsequent salpingitis, either because women who have once had gonorrhea are likely to have a second gonorrheal infection, or perhaps because in some women infection that may have appeared to be clinically uncomplicated may actually have been a subclinical tubal infection. Subclinical tubal infection would be expected to predispose to the development of clinical salpingitis.

The presence of an IUD is an independent factor in the development of salpingitis. Women using an IUD have a rate of salpingitis which is increased two- to fourfold as compared to women not using an IUD. The highest rate of salpingitis among IUD users occurs within a few weeks of insertion, at which time cervical bacteria are introduced into the endometrial cavity along with the IUD. However, most infections among IUD users occur long after insertion, probably because bacteria "wick" along the IUD tail leading from the vagina to the uterus. Such a mechanism for IUD-associated salpingitis is supported by the isolation of intrauterine bacteria at the time of hysterectomy only among users of tailed IUDs, but not among users of tailless IUDs or women without an IUD. Other mechanisms of IUD infection are possible, such as the enhancement of anaerobic bacterial growth, the presence of a chronic inflammatory reaction, or the production of microulcers by the IUD.

The IUD seems to be a greater factor in producing salpingitis among nulliparous than multiparous women. Also, IUD-induced salpingitis is more commonly nongonococcal than gonococcal. Women using barrier or oral contraceptive methods have a lower than expected rate of salpingitis. The protective effect of oral contraceptives on ascending infection may be due to changes in the cervical mucus, the periodic scanty withdrawal bleeding from an inactive endometrium, or decreased myometrial activity at the times of periodic uterine bleeding.

Socioeconomic factors also influence the rates of salpingitis, which are estimated to be 4% among women of low socioeconomic status and 1% among women of higher socioeconomic status. Women in the former group tend to have a higher rate of sexually transmitted disease; they are less apt to seek medical care for local symptoms and are more apt to have an untreated infectious partner than women of higher socioeconomic status. Other reasons for this difference must be elucidated.

The role of males with untreated gonococcal or chlamydial urethritis is often ignored by gynecologists. More than 75% of male contacts of women with gonococcal salpingitis have not been treated by the time the female develops symptomatic infection. Of the male contacts with infectious gonococcal urethritis, more than one-half are asymptomatic. Among asymptomatic male contacts of women with gonococcal salpingitis, N. gonorrhoeae is isolated from 40%. Males with chlamydial, nongonococcal urethritis would also be expected to be a reservoir for chlamydial salpingitis. To reduce the rate of new and recurrent salpingitis, male contacts of women with either gonococcal or nongonococcal salpingitis should be examined and cultured. If infectious organisms are found, they should be appropriately treated. To prevent subsequent PID it is also important that culture and appropriate therapy be provided to the male contacts of *asymptomatic* women identified as having gonorrhea or chlamydia.

BACTERIOLOGY

N. Gonorrhoeae

Formerly N. gonorrhoeae was considered to cause the majority of infectious salpingitis. This is no longer true, and in the United States today gonorrhea has assumed a less important position. In most studies N. gonorrhoeae can be recovered from only 40% to 50% of women with acute gonococcal salpingitis. However, gonococcal prevalence varies greatly: N. gonorrhoeae is isolated from less than 20% of the cases of salpingitis in Sweden, while it is isolated from 80% of salpingitis cases in certain populations in the United States. Among women with both cervical gonorrhea and salpingitis, N. gonorrhoeae is the most frequent intra-abdominal isolate, but it is the sole isolate in only 30% of these cases. In the remainder, either no organisms can be isolated or other organisms are isolated either alone or together with N. gonorrhoeae. Positive gonococcal cultures are usualy obtained during the early stages of infection. During the later stages of infection the organisms are either present only within epithelial cells or they are inhibited by leukocytes, two factors that make it difficult to isolate the organisms. If positive cultures are obtained in the later stages of gonorrheal salpingitis, organisms other than the gonococcus *can* be isolated either alone or in combination with gonococci.

CERVICITIS

The majority of hysterectomy specimens contain an area beneath the squamocolumnar junction which is infiltrated by plasma cells and lymphocytes. In the presence of such cells, the pathologist is obliged to make a diagnosis of *chronic cervicitis.* Unless the inflammatory reaction is extensive, there are no symptoms, cultures recover either no organisms, or only organisms that are part of the normal vaginal flora. This condition is not of clinical importance. To qualify as a pelvic infection, the inflammatory reaction must result from the effects of pathogenic organisms or established infection. The common causes of *acute cervicitis* are *N. gonorrhoeae, C. trachomatis,* and puerperal infection. The organisms penetrate the columnar epithelium or areas denuded by obstetric or surgical injury. Symptoms are usually limited to a profuse purulent vaginal discharge or intermenstrual bleeding. In more than three-fourths of women who have a purulent or mucoid cervical discharge, *N. gonorrhoeae* or *C. trachomatis* can be isolated separately or in combination from the endocervix.

Infectious ulcers of the cervix caused by herpes virus, syphilis, and chancroid must be distinguished from erosion and the other conditions described in Chapter 53. Depending upon the nature of the lesion, Pap smear, culture, darkfield examination, colposcopy and, in some cases, biopsy may be required.

C. trachomatis may give rise to the friable "papillary erosion" of the cervix in which the columnar epithelium is proliferated above the plane of the squamous epithelium, but many women who do have *C. trachomatis* do not have this lesion. The papillary erosion is also caused by factors other than *C. trachomatis.*

ENDOMETRITIS

Scattered lymphocytes and plasma cells and occasional neutrophils appear normally in the endometrium in the second half of the menstrual cycle, and their presence does not necessarily constitute endometritis. In some cases of abnormal bleeding they may appear in greater number, and in such cases they may represent an abnormal inflammatory reaction. In at least one report, chronic endometritis was related to the isolation of genital mycoplasma from the endometrial cavity.

For the most part, endometritis is an ill-defined entity that produces either uncertain symptoms or none at all, and it should rarely be diagnosed unless a specific etiologic factor is found. *Bona fide* endometritis may occur in the following situations: (1) Puerperal endometritis (see Chap. 40), (2) gonococcal endometritis that occurs among patients with PID, (3) the endometritis that follows instrumentation or surgery, (4) tuberculous endometritis, (5) the purulent endometritis that occurs in pyometra caused by a cervical stricture or following radium insertion, and (6) the endometritis that characteristically occurs in the presence of a tailed intrauterine device (IUD).

The chronic endometritis that is associated with the use of IUDs is well documented. It is clear, however, that it is not the foreign body *per se* that leads to chronic inflammation, but rather the tail of the IUD which acts as a wick for organisms to reach the endometrium from the vagina. Transfundal endometrial cultures of hysterectomy specimens from women who had used tailed IUDs for more than a few weeks uniformly recovered bacteria, while the cultures from women who had used tailless IUDs or no IUD were sterile. The organisms that can be recovered are usually of low pathogenicity, but some more virulent intrauterine bacteria undoubtedly cause the malodorous discharge and the salpingitis that occur more frequently among IUD users than among nonIUD users. In addition, an anaerobe, *Actinomyces israelii,* has been found in Papanicolaou smears from about 5% of women using IUDs, but not among nonIUD users. This organism may colonize the endometrium of IUD users and when it is found in the Pap smear, the IUD should be removed and penicillin should be prescribed for 20 days.

SALPINGITIS

Acute primary salpingitis is a bacterial infection that begins as an endosalpingitis when pathogenic organisms invade the fallopian tube. *Neisseria gonorrhoeae, Chlamydia trachomatis,* genital mycoplasma, and normal flora aerobic and anaerobic bacteria cause the overwhelming majority of tubal infections. Virtually all primary salpingitis occurs among sexually active, menstruating, nonpregnant women. Tuberculous, parasitic, or fungal salpingitis is rare in industrialized countries. Most salpingitis occurs spontaneously without instrumentation or trauma to the genital tract; however, approximately 15% follows instrumentation (*e.g.,* IUD insertion, dilatation and curretage, abortion, hysterosalpingography, or tubal insufflation). Salpingitis can also begin as a perisalpingitis secondary to acute appendicitis or other interabdominal bacterial infection, but this kind of infection accounts for less than 1% of the cases of salpingitis.

Acute salpingitis is a common event. Approximately 1% of women between the ages of 15 and 39 years develop salpingitis annually. Young, sexually active women between the ages of 15 and 24 years have the highest rate of infection. As noted at the opening of this chapter, this rate of infection has tremendous national consequences. It is estimated that at least 1 billion dollars is required to treat the 800,000 women

not common, and usually results only in lower abdominal pain that lasts for a few days during the course of an acute infectious illness. The ovarian infection usually subsides without incident, although abscesses can occur. If bimanual examination is not satisfactory, ultrasound scans or polytomography may be used to determine its presence.

Most cases of oophoritis are secondary to salpingitis. The ovary becomes infected by the purulent material that escapes from the fallopian tube. If the tubal fimbriae are adherent to the ovary, the tube and ovary together may form a large retort-shaped, tubo-ovarian abscess. Antibacterial therapy, as previously outlined and also discussed in Chapter 13, is immediately indicated, and surgery is mandatory if the mass should be considered to be leaking or ruptured, or if it fails to resolve.

REFERENCES AND RECOMMENDED READING

Angerman NS, Evans MI, Moravec WD et al: C-reactive protein in the evaluation of antibiotic therapy for pelvic infection. J Reprod Med 25:63, 1980

Bartlett JG, Moon NE, Goldstein PR et al: Cervical and vaginal bacterial flora: Ecolgic niches in the female lower genital tract. Am J Obstet Gynecol 130:658, 1978

Curran JW: Economic consequences of pelvic inflammatory disease in the United States. Am J Obstet Gynecol 138:848, 1980

Eschenbach DA: Acute pelvic inflammatory disease: Etiology, risk factors and pathogenesis. Clin Obstet Gynecol 19:147, 1976

Eschenbach DA, Buchanan TH, Pollock HM et al: Polymicrobial etiology of acute pelvic inflammatory disease. N. Engl J Med 293:166, 1975

Eschenbach DA, Harnish JP, Holmes KK: Pathogenesis of acute pelvic inflammatory disease: Role of contraception and other risk factors. Am J Obstet Gynecol 128:838, 1977

Eschenbach DA, Holmes KK: Acute pelvic inflammatory disease: Current concepts of pathogenesis, etiology, and management. Clin Obstet Gynecol 18:35, 1975

Gall SA, Kohan AP, Ayers OM et al: Intravenous metronidazole or clindamycin with tobramycin for therapy of pelvic infections. Obstet Gynecol 57:51, 1975

Gardner HL: Hemophilus vaginalis after twenty-five years. Am J Obstet Gynecol 137:385, 1980

Goldman P: Drug therapy. Metronidazole. N Engl J Med 303:1212, 1980

Gorbach SL, Bartlett JG: Anaerobic infectioin. N Engl J Med 290:1177, 1237, 1289, 1974

Hager WD, Brown ST, Kraus SJ et al: Metronidazole for vaginal trichomoniasis. Seven-day vs single-dose regimens. JAMA 244:1219, 1980

Holmes KK: The Chlamydia epidemic. JAMA 245:1718, 1981

Holmes KK, Counts LW, Beaty HN: Disseminated gonococcal infection. Ann Intern Med 74:979, 1971

Holmes KK, Eschenbach DA, Knapp JS: Salpingitis: Overview of etiology and epidemiology. Am J Obstet Gynecol 138:893, 1980

Insler V, Bettend FG (eds): The Uterine Cervix in Reproduction, p 71. Stuttgart, Thieme, 1977

Jacobson I, Weström L: Objectivized diagnosis of acute pelvic inflammatory disease. Am J Obstet Gynecol 105:1088, 1969

Johannisson G, Löwhagen G-B, Lycke E: Genital Chlamydia trachomatis infection in women. Obstet Gynecol 56:671, 1980

Josey WE: The sexually transmitted infections. Obstet Gynecol 43:467, 1974

Koehler PR, Moss AA: Diagnosis of intra-abdominal and pelvic abscesses by computerized tomography. JAMA 244:49, 1980

Lal S, Nicholas C: Epidemiological and clinical feature of granuloma inguinalae. Br J Vener Dis 46:461, 1970

Mardh PA, Ripa I, Svensson I et al: Role of Chlamydia trachomatis infection in acute salpingitis. N Engl J Med 296:1377, 1977

McCormack WM, Stumacher RJ, Johnson K et al: Clinical spectrum of gonococcal infection in women. Lancet 1:1182, 1977

McIntosh K: Recent advances in viral diagnosis. Arch Pathol Lab Med 104:3, 1980

Nahmias AJ, Roizman B: Infection with herpes simplex viruses 1 and 2. N Engl J Med 289:667, 719, 781, 1973

Ohm MJ, Galask RP: Bacterial flora of the cervix from 100 prehysterectomy patients. Am J Obstet Gynecol 122:683, 1975

Paavonen J: Chlamydial infections. Microbiological, clinical, and diagnostic aspects. Med Biol 57:135, 1979

Pheifer TA, Forsyth PA, Durfee MA et al: Nonspecific vaginitis: Role of Haemophilus vaginalis and treatment with metronidazole. N Engl J Med 298:1429, 1978

Potterat JJ, King RD: A new approach to gonorrhea control. The asymptomatic man and incidence reduction. JAMA 245:578, 1981

Richart RM (ed): Ovarian abscesses in IUD wearers. Contemp OB/GYN 17:141, 1981

Schacter J: Chlamydial infections. N Engl J Med 298:428, 490, 540, 1978

Schaefer G: Female genital tuberculosis. Clin Obstet Gynecol 19:223, 1976

Spence MR, Gupta PK, Frost JK et al: Cytologic detection and clinical significance of Actinomyces israelii in women using intrauterine contraceptive devices. Am J Obstet Gynecol 131:295, 1978

Spiegel CA, Amsel R, Eschenbach D et al: Anaerobic bacteria in nonspecific vaginitis. N Engl J Med 303:601, 1980

St John RK, Brown ST, Tyler CW: Pelvic inflammatory disease, 1980. Am J Obstet Gynecol 138:845, 1980

Stamm WE, Running K, McKevitt M et al: Treatment of the acute urethral syndrome. N Engl J Med 304:956, 1981

Taylor-Robinson D, McCormack WM: The genital mycoplasmas. N Engl J Med 302:1063, 1980

Thompson SE III, Hager WD, Wong K-H et al: The microbiology and therapy of pelvic inflammatory disease in hospitalized patients. Am J Obstet Gynecol 136:179, 1980

USPHS Center for Disease Control: An outbreak of penicillinase-producing Neisseria gonorrhoeae—Shreveport, Louisiana. Morbid Mortal Week Rep 29:241, 1980

USPHS Center for Disease Control: Gonorrhea. CDC recommended treatment schedules, 1979.

USPHS Center for Disease Control: Recommended treatment schedules for syphilis, 1976.

Wang S-P, Eschenbach DA, Holmes KK et al: Chlamydia trachomatis infection in Fitz-Hugh–Curtis syndrome. Am J Obstet Gynecol 138:1034, 1980

Weström L: Incidence, prevalence, and trends of acute pelvic inflammatory disease and its consequences in industrialized countries. Am J Obstet Gynecol 138:880, 1980

ENDOMETRIOSIS

James A. Merrill

Endometriosis is a protean disease characterized by the presence and proliferation of endometrial tissue outside the uterus. This unique lesion has certain characteristics of malignancy, but is not a true neoplasm. The ectopic tissue shows the ability to grow, infiltrate, spread, and even disseminate in a manner similar to malignant tissue. Histologic changes of malignancy are rare; only when they occur is endometriosis truly malignant in the sense of interfering with vital functions or causing death. Indeed, endometriosis is reversible and often regresses following removal of ovarian activity and possibly under the influence of pregnancy. The ectopic endometrial tissue is usually responsive to the hormonal variations of the menstrual cycle, and the subsequent menstrual-type bleeding is important in pathology and symptomatology of the disease. In this discussion the term *endometriosis* desig-

nates only lesions that exist in sites other than the endometrial surface or myometrium. These include the subperitoneal lesions on the serosal surface of the uterus which react in all respects similarly to lesions elsewhere, but not adenomyosis.

INCIDENCE AND IMPORTANCE

The exact incidence of endometriosis is difficult to determine because the disease exists in many patients without causing significant symptoms. It is found at about 20% of all gynecologic operations, but there is disagreement between the operative and pathologic diagnosis in about 8% of cases. Some place the disagreement rate much higher; at least one investigator has stated that the operative diagnosis is not confirmed pathologically in more than 50% of cases. Endometriosis is a *significant* finding in only about one-third of the patients in whom it is found at surgery. Active endometriosis is found most commonly between the ages of 30 and 40 years. Rarely it is found in patients under 20 years of age, and it is unusual in postmenopausal patients.

Many gynecologists agree that endometriosis is more prevalent among private white patients than among indigent nonwhite patients, and it has been suggested that this is accounted for by late marriage and late childbearing in the high-income groups. Others have questioned the reliability of these impressions. It is possible that the pressure for attention among the people in higher socioeconomic classes is responsible for earlier and more frequent diagnosis.

It is possible that selectivity accounts for both the apparent differences in incidence of this disease and the apparent relation between endometriosis and infertility. The fertility rate of patients with endometriosis is stated to be 66%, as opposed to 88% for the general population. However, infertile patients receive the careful evaluation, including surgical exploration, leading to a diagnosis of endometriosis, more often than do fertile patients with the disease.

It has often been stated that endometriosis improves during and following pregnancy; however, this is difficult to document, and there have been cases in which there was active growth during pregnancy, even requiring surgery. Since endometriosis is usually responsive to cyclic ovarian hormones, the lesions commonly regress following suppression of ovarian activity, artificially or naturally. However, there are well-documented cases of endometriosis becoming active and even symptomatic many years following the menopause. In fact, the author has seen a 74-year-old patient with symptomatic endometriosis of the sigmoid colon.

PATHOLOGY

LOCATION OF LESIONS

Endometriosis has been described in unusual and remote sites in the body, but the majority of lesions are limited to the pelvis (Fig. 51–1). The ovary is the most common site, and involvement is usually bilateral. The next most common site is the peritoneum of the cul-de-sac or pouch of Douglas. Such lesions may extend to involve the rectovaginal septum. The uterosacral ligaments may be involved with or without involvement of the peritoneum of the pouch of Douglas. The round ligament, oviduct, and peritoneal surface of the uterus are next in frequency of occurrence. The rectosigmoid can be involved either as an isolated lesion or as extension from ovarian or uterosacral lesions. Far less common are isolated lesions of the ileum, cecum, appendix, bladder, ureter, cervix, and vagina. Endometriosis is not uncommon in pelvic lymph nodes of patients with pelvic lesions. Unusual sites of endometriotic involvement include the umbilicus, laparotomy scars, episiotomy scars, arms, legs, pleura, lungs, diaphragm, and kidneys.

GROSS APPEARANCE

Endometriosis takes the form of multiple tiny, puckered, hemorrhagic foci referred to as "mulberry spots" or "powder-burn spots." They are usually surrounded by stellate scars and are frequently associated with dense adhesions. The degree of fibrotic reaction is variable. In the ovary, involvement may also exist as typical cysts or endometriomas, rarely larger than 10 cm and filled with thick chocolate-syrup-like material composed of blood and blood pigment, the so-called "chocolate cysts" of the ovary. Not all blood-filled cysts of the ovary are due to endometriosis, however. The adhesions associated with endometriosis of the ovary are far denser than those found with salpingitis or other pelvic inflammatory processes. For this reason endometrial cysts are often ruptured during surgical removal.

Involvement of the peritoneum of the cul-de-sac or pouch of Douglas consists of the puckered bluish-red nodules. Surrounding scar tissue often makes them large enough to be palpated rectovaginally. Lesions in this location occlude the posterior cul-de-sac, fixing the uterus in retroversion. At times the lesions are completely scarred and lose their blue, hemorrhagic appearance. Even in the absence of blood-filled cysts or puckered spots, dense adhesions involving the posterior surface of the uterus and broad ligament should alert the physician to the probabilty of endometriosis.

Lesions in the large bowel rarely penetrate the mucosa. The main pathologic change is fibrotic thickening of the outer coats of the bowel sometimes associated with stricture formation. In this location endometriosis is easily mistaken for carcinoma or diverticulitis of the rectosigmoid. In addition to small lesions in the bladder-flap peritoneum, endometriosis may produce fibrotic nodules in the wall of the bladder which rarely protrude into the lumen.

MICROSCOPIC APPEARANCE

Microscopically, the lesions consist of endometrial glands and stroma, frequently with hemorrhage into the stroma and adjacent tissue. This hemorrhage may result in the accumulation of large numbers of hemosiderin-laden macrophages or pseudoxanthoma cells (Fig. 51–2). The endometrial glands and stroma usually show a response to the phases of the menstrual cycle comparable to that of the uterine endometrium. Occasionally the ectopic endometrium shows a poor secretory response to progesterone. Pregnancy may be accompanied by a typical decidual response of pelvic endometriosis, although the finding of extrauterine decidua alone is not pathognomonic of endometriosis. Decidua without glands occurs in nonpregnant women and during pregnancy may be a mesenchymal response to the pregnancy hormones.

Hemorrhage into the lumen of the endometrial cyst frequently results in pressure atrophy and obliteration of recognizable endometrial tissue in the wall. Such cysts are lined only by granulation tissue, hemosiderin-laden macrophages, and occasionally cholesterol crystal clefts with appropriate foreign body reaction.

There may be a remarkable degree of fibrous proliferation surrounding endometriotic lesions. This is particularly true in the bowel (Fig. 51–3). Because of the reactive phenomena, there are many cases of unquestioned gross endometriosis seen at the operating table in which the removed tissues show no evidence of microscopic endometriosis. Microscopic confirmation of gross endometriosis may be increased if the lesions are marked with a suture by the surgeon before removal.

MALIGNANT CHANGE

Malignant change in endometriosis is extremely rare, but it is now acknowledged that it does occur. Meticulous search of the lesions has revealed, in a few cases, evidences of atypical or adenomatous hyperplasia that might be considered precancerous. Of the endometrioid carcinomas demonstrated to have originated in endometriosis, adenoacanthomas and well-differentiated adenocarcinomas occurred with relatively high frequency, rather more so than among endometrioid

(*Text continues on p. 1008.*)

Diffuse pelvic endometriosis
Ruptured endometrial (chocolate) cyst

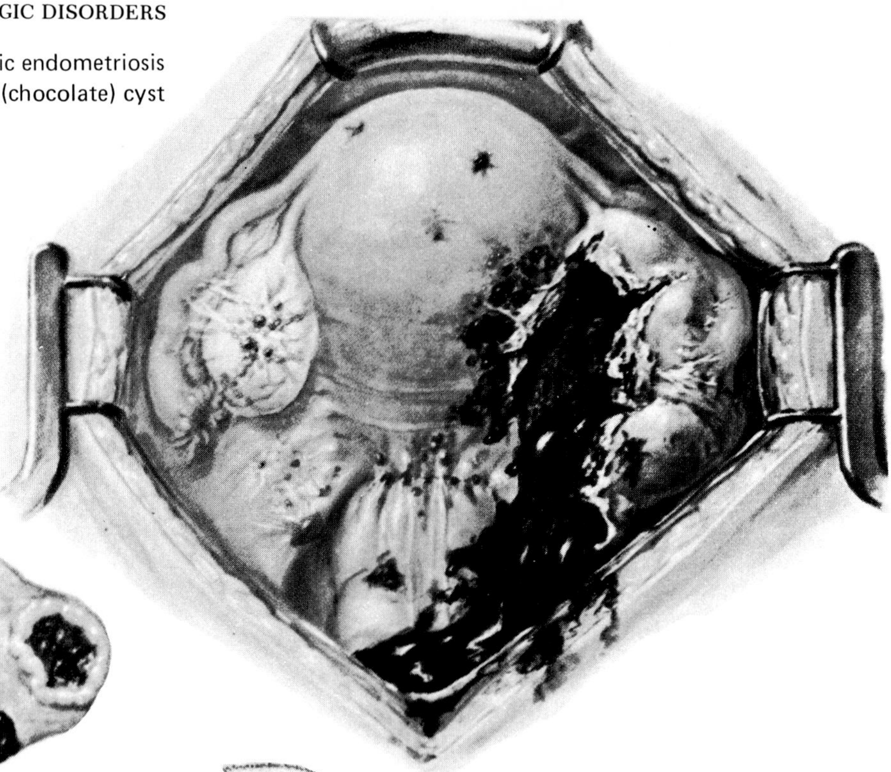

FIG. 51–1. Appearance and various locations of endometriosis. (Drawing by FH Netter. In Ciba Collection of Medical Illustrations, Vol 2. Reproductive System. Summit NJ, © CIBA, 1954)

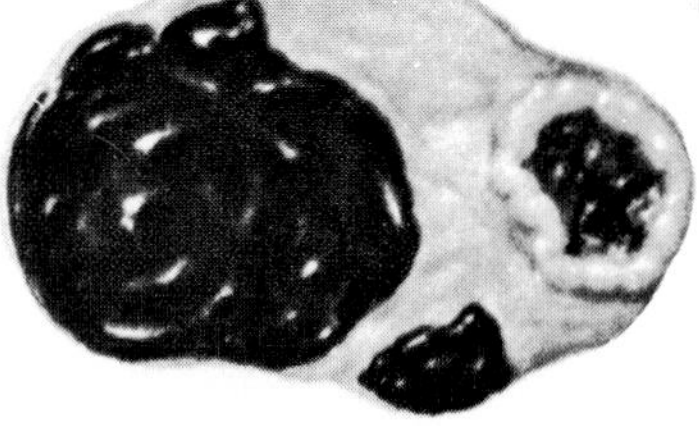

Hemisection of ovary with endometrial cysts and corpus luteum

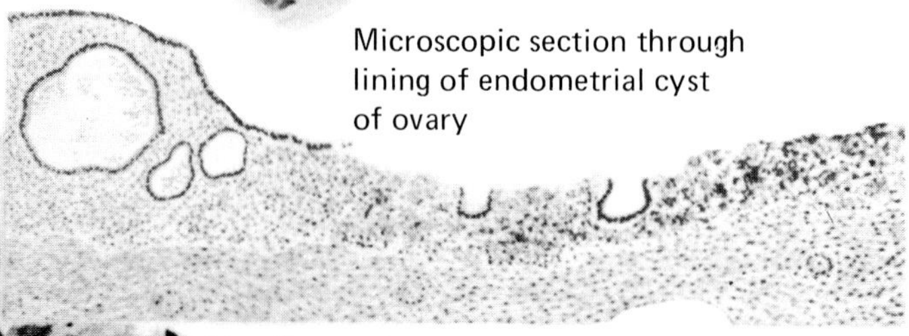

Microscopic section through lining of endometrial cyst of ovary

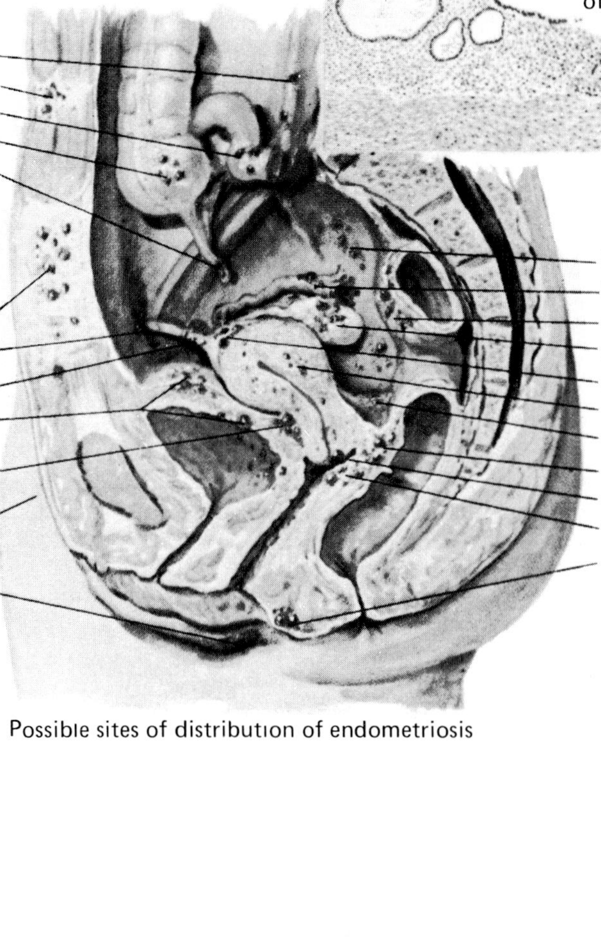

Ureter
Umbilicus
Small bowel
Cecum
Appendix

Laparotomy scar
Inguinal ring
Round ligament
Bladder
Uterovesical fold
Groin
Vulva and Bartholin's gland

Pelvic peritoneum
Fallopian tube
Sigmoid colon
Ovary
Surface of uterus
Myometrium (adenomyosis)
Uterosacral ligament
Rectovaginal septum
Cervix
Vagina
Perineum

Possible sites of distribution of endometriosis

FIG. 51–2. Microscopic appearance of lining of endometrial cyst composed of endometrial epithelium, stroma, and hemosiderin-filled macrophages. Dilated capillaries are characteristic of active lesions of endometriosis.

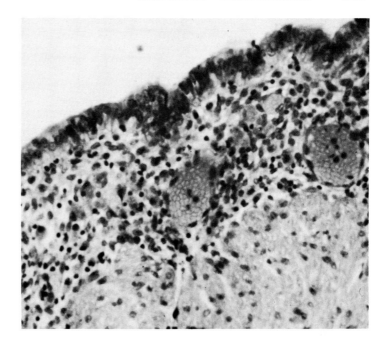

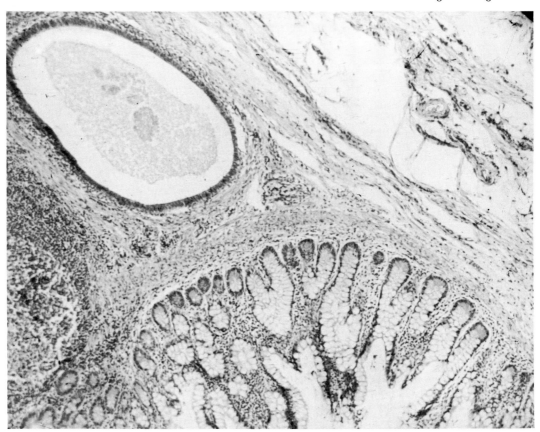

FIG. 51–3. Endometriosis in submucosal region of large bowel.

carcinomas in general; also, the prognosis appears to be somewhat better. A few other epithelial carcinomas (*e.g.,* clear-cell carcinoma) may also have the same source.

The relationship of endometriosis to the later development of cancer has been reviewed by Mostoufizadeh and Scully. An important consideration to which they call attention is the possible risk of estrogen replacement in women with proved endometriosis, since there is no means of monitoring the changes that may occur in retained endometrial tissue.

HISTOGENESIS

There are three major theories of histogenesis of endometriosis: transportation, formation *in situ,* and a combination of these.

TRANSPORTATION

The implantation theory suggests that endometriosis is caused by retrograde tubal flow of menstrual fragments, implantation and growth on the ovary and peritoneal surfaces, followed by secondary seedings from the new foci. Vascular metastasis has also been suggested. The fact that endometrial tissue is found in lymphatics and pelvic lymph nodes is now widely accepted. Moreover, hematogenous spread of endometrial fragments has been observed by many. This offers the best explanation for the rare distant sites of endometriosis. Direct transplantation of endometrium has been suggested by the observation of endometriotic lesions in incisional scars following surgery involving the uterus and in vaginal incisions such as episiotomies. A composite theory of the histogenesis of endometriosis includes (1) direct extension into the myometrium or endosalpinx, (2) exfoliation and implantation of endometrial cells at menstruation or during curettage, (3) lymphatic spread, (4) venous spread and hematogenous metastases to distant organs, and (5) secondary lesions from foci already established.

FORMATION IN SITU

Metaplasia or differentiation of celomic epithelium, possibly triggered by inflammatory or hormonal alterations, has been suggested. This theory gains support from embryologic studies, observations of differentiation of surface epithelium of the ovary into the various cell types of the müllerian duct, and the decidual reaction seen frequently in tissues beneath the pelvic peritoneum during pregnancy. Lesions of endometriosis have been reported to contain tubal and endocervical epithelium. Growth of celomic epithelium, including downward extension into the ovarian cortex and other subsurface connective tissue areas of the pelvis, are observed at sites of irritation and inflammation. A variety of irritants cause metaplasia and growth of celomic epithelium. The theory of embryonic cell rests in the production of endometriosis has largely been discarded.

COMBINATION (INDUCTION)

Hertig and Gore proposed that endometriosis could develop following the formation of a fibrinopurulent exudate, organization of such exudate, and eventual development of metaplastic celomic epithelium with a glandular pattern. A theory of induction has been proposed in which chemical-inducing substances may be liberated from transported endometrium and activate undifferentiated mesenchyme to form endometrial epithelium and stroma. This theory is supported by observations of autologous endometrial implants which reveal that the implant underwent degeneration and that endometrial cysts formed around the degenerating implant. The theory is further supported by Merrill's experimental observations of endometrial tissue that develops in connective tissue adjacent to cell-free extracts of endometrium and adjacent to diffusion chambers containing autologous or heterologous endometrium; such chambers prevent escape of cellular material but allow dispersion of noncellular material from the endometrium. Such an induction theory combines both the transportation and metaplasia theories and appears to be the most likely.

COMMENT

Many observations strongly support the idea that transportation of endometrial fragments by one means or another is important in the development of endometriosis. It has been observed that endometriosis is more common in patients with congenital and acquired deformities of the uterus which favor menstrual regurgitation and that endometriosis is rare or nonexistent in the absence of menstruation. Menstrual fragments have been observed in the lumen of the oviduct as well as in the peritoneal cavity, and endometrial fragments appear in lymphatic and venous channels of the uterus. Menstrual endometrium is viable in tissue culture, but menstrual fragments shed from intraocular transplants in the monkey do not survive or form endometriosis. Transplantation of fragments of endometrium is followed by endometriosis and diversion of menstrual flow into the peritoneal cavity or anterior abdominal wall is followed by endometriosis. Even human endometriosis has been found following experimental subcutaneous injection of menstrual discharge.

None of these experiments conclusively proves that the transported endometrial fragments have grown. It

is equally possible that they degenerate and in the process induce differentiation in the adjacent mesenchyme. Pathologic and experimental investigations demonstrate the metaplastic ability of celomic epithelium lining the peritoneal mesenchyme. Moreover, the influence of irritation, inflammation, and hormonal alteration upon such metaplasia and inclusion cyst formation is noteworthy.

At present it seems likely that no one theory satisfactorily explains all of the lesions of endometriosis, that each may play a role, and that this interesting entity may arise from combinations of influences.

SYMPTOMS

Endometriosis may be extensive without producing any symptoms whatsoever, and the frequency and degree of symptoms are poorly related to extent of the disease. Indeed, many patients with very few small lesions are severely disabled.

Pelvic pain is the most significant symptom of endometriosis. In many, this takes the form of *acquired dysmenorrhea* beginning in the late 20s or early 30s and gradually progressing in severity. The pain is described as dull aching or cramping lower abdominal and back pain, occurring with menstruation and diminishing gradually after the onset of flow. Not all patients have pain that is characteristically related to menstruation. Many complain of vague aching, cramping, or bearing-down sensation in the pelvis or low back, which may or may not become worse during the menstrual period and be somewhat relieved following menstruation. Less often, patients complain of *dyspareunia*, particularly when the uterus is fixed in retroversion and when endometriotic lesions are found in the region of the uterosacral ligaments or the posterior fornix of the vagina. Upon direct questioning, one may obtain a history of *pain with defecation* during menstruation, particularly if the lesions involve the area of the rectovaginal septum.

The mechanism of pain is not altogether clear. Dyspareunia and pain with defecation are related to pressure upon distended lesions or to stretching of adhesions. Pelvic pain and dysmenorrhea may be related to hemorrhagic distention of an endometrial cyst that is restricted by fibrosis or to escape of bloody discharge into the peritoneal cavity. Dysmenorrhea may also be related to increased local concentration of prostaglandins. Rupture of an endometrioma may cause acute peritoneal irritation.

Abnormal uterine bleeding is the presenting symptom almost as often as pain. It has no specific pattern and may be excessive, prolonged, or frequent. This is probably due to involvement of ovaries by the endometriotic lesions and possibly to the frequent association of other pelvic pathology, such as myomas.

Infertility may bring a patient with endometriosis to the physician. It is impossible to determine the true incidence of infertility in patients with endometriosis or the incidence of endometriosis in patients with infertility. Endometriosis has been reported in 8% to 30% of infertile patients studied by endoscopy. Also, it is difficult to explain exactly how endometriosis may interfere with fertility. The oviducts are usually patent and ovulation is not interrupted in most patients. However, it is probable that endometriosis is associated with at least a relative infertility. Certainly, distortion and fixation of the oviducts, fixation of the uterus, and pain during intercourse may be significant factors. Dramatically elevated levels of prostaglandin F have been reported in the peritoneal fluid of patients with endometriosis. PGF stimulates muscular activity of the oviduct in humans.

Unusual symptoms related to involvement of the gastrointestinal tract or urinary tract result from obstruction or interference with function of these organs. Rectal bleeding occurs in approximately 20% of patients with endometriosis of the bowel. Pain and tenderness in the umbilicus, scars, or inguinal region accompany lesions in these locations. Hemoptysis occurring at the time of menstruation has been described in the rare cases of endometriosis involving the lung or bronchus. Exotic symptoms are reported in patients with lesions in unusual sites.

PHYSICAL FINDINGS

The most important clinical finding is multiple tender nodules palpable along the uterosacral ligaments or above the posterior fornix of the vagina. Such nodules are noted to enlarge and become much more tender during menstruation. Often the uterus is fixed in retroposition. Attempts to move it are accompanied by severe pain. Thickening and nodularity of the adnexa may be similar to, and suggestive of, pelvic inflammatory disease. Endometrial cysts of the ovary are rarely movable and usually closely adherent to the uterus, with adjacent induration and tenderness. In rare cases, blue cystic areas may be seen at the umbilicus, in abdominal wound scars, on the cervix or vagina, or elsewhere. These appear or enlarge during menstruation. The lesions of endometriosis have been seen during cystoscopy but are rarely observed during proctosigmoidoscopy.

DIAGNOSIS

Endometriosis should be considered in the young woman with acquired dysmenorrhea, intermittent or constant pelvic pain, dyspareunia, and menstrual abnormality, who has a tender, fixed, retroverted uterus and palpable nodules in the region of the uterosacral ligaments. Endometriosis should be considered in patients with similar symptoms who have unilateral or bilateral adnexal thickening or adnexal masses.

Laparoscopy with visualization of the typical foci may be of great value in confirming the diagnosis. Such an attempt at positive diagnosis is important if expensive hormone therapy is to be considered. Biopsy of externally visible lesions, lesions on the cervix or vagina, or those seen at cystoscopy confirms the diagnosis.

Endometriosis should be a part of the differential diagnosis of malignant disease of the ovary, chronic salpingo-oophoritis, carcinoma of the rectum and colon, diverticulitis, causes of intestinal obstruction, tumors of the umbilicus, inguinal swellings, and causes of hematuria. It is impossible to palpate all small endometriotic lesions, but remembering the protean manifestations of endometriosis may increase the frequency (approximately 20%) of accurate diagnosis.

TREATMENT

The treatment of endometriosis must be influenced by the facts that it is predominantly a disease of women in the childbearing age, that infertility is often a presenting complaint, and that accurate diagnosis is difficult without surgical exploration. Since endometriosis is to some extent responsive to cyclic ovarian hormones, removal of the ovaries and uterus relieves symptoms in the majority of patients. However, such treatment is not compatible with desire for future childbearing and can be recommended only for those patients who have completed childbearing. For the most part, treatment should be designed to produce maximal symptom relief with minimal interference with childbearing function, or it should actually increase fertility potential.

Evaluation of different methods of treatment is complicated by the difficulty in accurate diagnosis and the inherent selection of patients. It is, for example, difficult to compare the results of surgical therapy and hormone therapy if the diagnosis of patients treated surgically is established by pathologic examination and the diagnosis of patients treated with hormones is based only upon clinical findings and has an 80% chance of being inaccurate. Similarly, it is difficult to assign a fertility-promoting effect to therapy when the only patients under study are women under 35 years of age who seriously desire pregnancy, who have limited endometriosis allowing conservative therapy, and who have no other cause of sterility. Such selection, which is common in the management of endometriosis, must be considered when evaluating therapy.

A difficult problem in comparing the results of treatment with different modalities is created by the fact that different series contain patients with different degrees of severity of the disease. For this reason, a number of investigators have proposed classification systems for endometriosis. The factors used to indicate *increase* in the severity of the disease are (1) adhesions, (2) ovarian cysts, (3) scarring and retraction, (4) fixation of pelvic structures, and (5) obliteration of cul-de-sac. The classification proposed by the American Fertility Society is shown in Figure 51–4. Staging is accomplished by systematic clockwise or counterclockwise inspection of the pelvis and assignment of points according to the findings. It is hoped that general use of this classification will permit a more orderly approach to therapy in the different stages and a more accurate appraisal of the effectiveness of different modalities.

Most investigators have shown a direct relationship between the extent of the endometriosis and success of pregnancy following treatment. However, Buttram found no relationship between extent and duration of infertility or between extent and symptoms of dysmenorrhea and dyspareunia.

In general, treatment consists of observation and symptom palliation, surgery, and hormone therapy.

OBSERVATION

Observation, reassurance, and mild analgesia are effective in many patients and should be the initial management of young patients whose symptoms are not severe or incapacitating. If the lesions are small and multiple and are producing few symptoms, it may be best to leave them alone. Indeed, they sometimes become inactive after a while. Time is often helpful, and some procrastination is justified. It is also important to defer active measures in young women attempting pregnancy, since some are of the opinion that pregnancy may result in relief of symptoms or permanent cure. An expectant course should not be followed if large masses are palpated or if the differential diagnosis includes more significant disease. The clinical diagnosis of endometriosis is often inaccurate.

SURGERY

When symptoms are severe, incapacitating, or acute, surgery is indicated. Surgery is indicated if symptoms become worse under medical management or if infertility persists for more than 1 year and no cause other than endometriosis is found. Endometrial cysts of the ovary are indications for surgery if they are larger than 6 to 8 cm in diameter. When surgery is undertaken, every effort should be made to accomplish a conservative procedure that will preserve childbearing function, if this is desired. The extent of surgery also depends upon the extent and location of the lesions and the surgeon's judgment.

Severe symptoms of endometriosis may be dealt with *radically* if the woman is approaching the menopause or has completed childbearing. Bilateral salpingo-oophorectomy and hysterectomy relieve symptoms without risking injury to bowel or other

AMERICAN FERTILITY SOCIETY CLASSIFICATION OF ENDOMETRIOSIS

Patient's name _____

Stage I   (Mild)   1–5
Stage II   (Moderate)   6–15
Stage III (Severe)   16–30
Stage IV   (Extensive)   31–54
Total _____

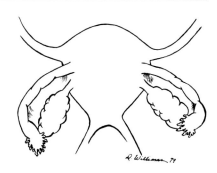

	ENDOMETRIOSIS	<1 cm	1–3 cm	> 3 cm
PERITONEUM		1	2	3
	ADHESIONS	filmy	dense w/ partial cul-de-sac obliteration	dense w/ complete cul-de-sac obliteration
		1	2	3
OVARY	ENDOMETRIOSIS	<1 cm	1–3 cm	> 3 cm or ruptured endometrioma
	R	2	4	6
	L	2	4	6
	ADHESIONS	filmy	dense w/ partial ovarian enclosure	dense w/ complete ovarian enclosure
	R	2	4	6
	L	2	4	6
TUBE	ENDOMETRIOSIS	<1 cm	> 1 cm	tubal occlusion
	R	2	4	6
	L	2	4	6
	ADHESIONS	filmy	dense w/ tubal distortion	dense w/ tubal enclosure
	R	2	4	6
	L	2	4	6

Associated Pathology:

FIG. 51–4. Classification and record of extent of endometriosis as suggested by American Fertility Society. In recording size of lesions, if more than one is present, aggregate size is estimated to arrive at score. Scoring is done at conclusion of laparoscopy or laparotomy and locations entered in sketch. (American Fertility Society: Fertil Steril 32:633, 1979)

structures by attempting to excise every fragment of endometriosis. Even constricting lesions of the bowel or urinary tract may regress following this therapy.

Hysterectomy alone may afford relief of symptoms while maintaining the advantages of ovarian function, even in the presence of some residual areas of endometriosis. Apparently ablation of cyclic menstruation and possible repeated regurgitation of menstrual fragments results in quiescence of remaining areas of endometriosis. Thus, hysterectomy with removal of as many foci of endometriosis as is easily possible, but conservation of all or part of the ovarian tissue, is recommended for the young woman with sufficiently severe symptoms to warrant surgery, who has her family and is not desirous of future childbearing. Estrogen replacement has been given safely to patients following hysterectomy and oophorectomy.

Less radical procedures ("conservative surgery") are indicated in the majority of patients. This generally means excision of all gross endometriosis with preservation of the uterus, tubes, and as much ovarian tissue as possible. This may mean unilateral oophorectomy, resection of endometrial cysts from one or both ovaries, excision of peritoneal lesions, release of adhesions, and resection of portions of rectal or bladder wall. It is possible to excise even fairly large endometrial cysts and conserve functioning ovarian tissue. Some gynecologists recommend suspension of the uterus and presacral neurectomy. A segmental resection and reanastomosis of bowel may be required if castration is not indicated. The results of conservative surgery with regard to relief of symptoms are good. With remaining ovarian function and residual endometriosis, progression is possible, however. The recurrence rate varies from 9% to 29%. The reoperation rate varies from 2% to 46% and is proportional to the frequency with which conservative surgery is the first-chosen treatment. The difficulty in evaluating the effect upon fertility is discussed above; the frequency of subsequent pregnancy may be as high as 60%; however, the average is about 35%.

HORMONE ADMINISTRATION

The use of steroid hormones has been recommended for the patient with symptoms not relieved by reassurance and mild analgesics, who desires subsequent pregnancy, and in whom surgery is either contraindicated or not acceptable, and in the patient with recurrence of symptoms following conservative surgery. The variety of hormones used includes estrogens, androgens, and progestins, in various dose schedules. Antigonadotropins (Danazol) have been used recently in preference to these steroids. It is of interest that almost all doses and combinations of hormones have been successful in the hands of their advocates, almost all of whom report relief of symptoms in approximately

80% of cases. This is about the same percentage of success obtained in selected patients who were not treated. In the majority of cases the relief appears to be temporary and the medication is often associated with annoying side effects. The long-term use of expensive medication should not be undertaken without accurate diagnosis.

Estrogen, in the form of stilbestrol, has been recommended in small doses for the purpose of ovulation suppression and in large doses for the purpose of producing pseudopregnancy and the beneficial effects considered equivalent to those of pregnancy. At present it is generally agreed that this therapy is ineffective because the symptoms and objective findings soon return and intermenstrual bleeding, edema, and nausea may be annoying side effects.

Testosterone and methyltestosterone have been used and reported to be effective in relieving the symptoms of endometriosis. Methyltestosterone linguets, 10 mg daily, have been recommended. This may be reduced to 5 mg daily. The medication is continued for 6 to 12 weeks and, if effective, repeated after 1 to 2 months' rest. The 5-mg dose may be given continuously. Relief of symptoms is reported in 80% of patients, with subsequent pregnancy in 11% to 60% of those complaining of infertility. Side effects of hirsutism, acne, and increased libido are reported but are rare with this dose schedule. The effect of androgens is thought to be suppression of ovulation through the hypothalamus, but there must be a direct effect upon the lesions as well, since ovulation is not always suppressed in patients receiving benefit from the therapy.

Progestin–estrogen treatment is based upon ovulation suppression and the production of pseudopregnancy, with decidual reaction in the endometriotic lesions, atrophy of the glands, eventual fibrosis, and obliteration of the endometriotic lesion (Fig. 51–5). All of the synthetic progestins, in combination with estrogens, have been used in doses that cause months of amenorrhea. The estrogen–progestin oral contraceptives are recommended. If bleeding occurs, the dose is increased and the new dose maintained. An early and an extensively used medication is norethynodrel with mestranol (Enovid®). Largely this has been replaced by low-dose progestin–estrogen contraceptives, used in a continuous fashion, starting with a dose of one tablet daily. This dosage is increased to two tablets after 2 to 3 weeks. If breakthrough bleeding occurs, the dose is increased by one tablet daily and maintained. Medroxyprogesterone acetate (Depo-provera®), 100 mg intramuscularly every 2 weeks for 4 doses and then 200 mg each month for an additional 4- to 6-months period, has been used. Estrogen is given for breakthrough bleeding. Treatment is continued up to 9 months and symptomatic improvement in 85% to 89% of patients has been reported. Subsequent pregnancy has been reported in 30% to 47% of infertile patients. Complaints of nausea, restlessness, edema,

FIG. 51-5. Microscopic section of endometriosis of ovary following 6 months' treatment with synthetic progestins. Stroma demonstrates marked decidual reaction with beginning fibrosis; remaining glands show moderate atrophy. ×100. (Kistner RW: Chap VII-1, In Meigs JV, Sturgis SH (eds): Progress in Gynecology IV, New York, Grune & Stratton, 1963)

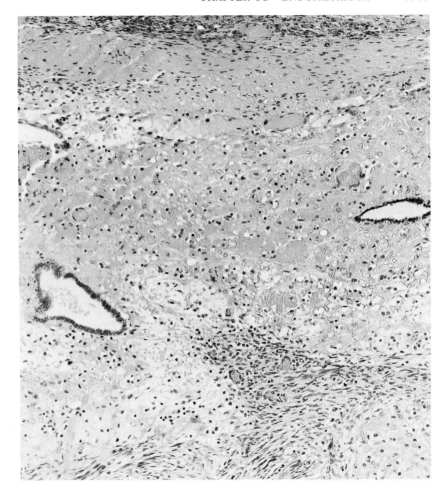

irregular utering bleeding, and excess weight are made by a significant number of patients. The need for surgery after pesudopregnancy is reported in 11% to 51% of patients. Improvement in the endometriosis following therapy persists for varying intervals, but in many cases the findings and symptoms return. Improvement is overestimated when compared to surgical findings. There is little change in the epithelium, mostly evidenced by a decrease in inflammation and adhesions. Some gynecologists feel that there is no evidence that synthetic progestin–estrogen actually cures endometriosis, and that the use of such agents should be considered a temporizing measure for specially selected cases. The use of progestin–estrogen for 5 to 8 weeks prior to contemplated surgery may make the lesions more easily identifiable and may soften the usually dense adhesions.

The therapeutic effect of a synthetic derivative of 17-alpha-ethinyl testosterone (Danazol) is being studied extensively. This drug is an antigonadatropic agent with no significant estrogenic or progestational activity and only minimal androgenic activity. Such treatment induces a state of "pseudomenopause," with anovulation and atrophy of endometrial tissue. Recommended treatment is 800 mg (divided) per day, although 400 to 600 mg daily may be adequate; in some patients 200 mg daily is sufficient. It is recommended that patients with mild disease be treated for 3 to 4 months, moderate disease 6 to 8 months, and severe disease for greater than 8 months or until palpable lesions disappear. The medication is expensive, and is not used if the diagnosis of endometriosis is only presumptive.

Results of treatment are difficult to analyze because of a limited number of patients treated. There are reports of 70% to 100% relief of symptoms during treatment and overall pregnancy rates of approximately 50%, which compare favorably with pregnancy rates following conservative surgery. The relief of symptoms occurs early in the course of therapy, in contrast to pseudopregnancy. Controlled laparoscopic studies re-

veal regression of lesions in 3 to 18 months. In successfully treated patients, most pregnancies occurred in the first year following treatment. Side effects of acne, hot flashes, edema, weight gain, hirsutism, and muscle cramps are uncommonly reported. Danazol therapy largely has superseded the use of pseudopregnancy as the preferred medical therapy; however, additional experience is necessary to establish the ultimate benefit of this drug.

X-RAY TREATMENT

In recurrent cases after failure of conservative surgery, roentgenographic suppression of the ovaries may be effective. The x-ray dose required is not large, but care must be taken to avoid damage to normal structures that are fixed by the dense adhesions.

CONCLUSION

There is no final agreement regarding the most successful therapeutic modality in endometriosis. Each case must be treated individually, based upon the physician's experience and the desires of the patient. Hysterectomy, removal of the adnexa and other tissue containing endometriosis is the optimal treatment for patients who have no desire for fertility and who have significant symptoms. Conservative surgery most often is the recommended treatment for young patients complaining of infertility. Young patients not currently desiring pregnancy may be satisfactorily managed with observation, reassurance, and mild analgesia. Danazol may be used for this group and also for those with recurrence following conservative surgery.

The treatment of the asymptomatic patient is probably not indicated.

REFERENCES AND RECOMMENDED READING

Acosta AA et al: A proposed classification of pelvic endometriosis. Obstet Gynecol 42:19, 1973

Bergman H, Friedenberg RM: Endometriosis: Urologic manifestation. NY State J Med 72:1152, 1972

Brewer JI, Maher FM: Conservatism in endometriosis. Am J Obstet Gynecol 68:549, 1954

Brosset A: Value of irradiation therapy in the treatment of endometriosis. Acta Obstet Gynecol Scand 36:209, 1957

Buttram VC: Conservative surgery for endometriosis in the infertile female. Fert Steril 31:117, 1979

Czernobilsky B, Morris WJ: A histologic study of ovarian endometriosis with emphasis on hyperplastic and atypical changes. Obstet Gynecol 53:318, 1979

Dmowski WP: Endocrine properties and clinical application of danazol. Fertil Steril 31:273, 1979

Garcia C, Sami SD: Pelvic endometriosis: Infertility and pelvic pain. Am J Obstet Gynecol 129:740, 1977

Greenblatt RB, Tzingounis V: Danazol treatment of endometriosis: Long-term follow-up. Fertil Steril 32:518, 1979

Hammond CB, Haney AF: Conservative treatment of endometriosis. Fertil Steril 30:497, 1978

Hertig AH, Gore H: Endometrial cystoma, benign and malignant. In Tumors of the Female Sex Organs, Part 3, p 105. Washington, D.C., Armed Forces Institute of Pathology, 1961

Kempers RD, Dockerty MB, Hunt AB et al: Postmenopausal endometriosis. Surg Gynecol Obstet 111:348, 1960

Kistner RW, Siegler AM, Behrman SJ: Suggested classification of endometriosis. Fertil Steril 30:240, 1978

Levander G, Normann P: Pathogenesis of endometriosis. Acta Obstet Gynecol Scand 34:366, 1955

McArthur JW, Ulfelder H: The effect of pregnancy upon endometriosis. Obstet Gynecol Surv 20:709, 1965

Meigs JV: Endometriosis: Etiologic role of marriage age and parity: Conservative treatment. Obstet Gynecol 2:46, 1953

Merrill JA: Endometrial induction of endometriosis across millipore filters. Am J Obstet Gynecol 94:780, 1966

Mostoufizadeh M, Scully RE: Malignant tumors arising in endometriosis. Clin Obstet Gynecol 23:951, 1980

Panganiban W, Corwog JL: Endometriosis of the intestine and vermiform appendix. Dis Colon Rectum 15:253, 1972

Ridley JH: The histogenesis of endometriosis. Obstet Gynecol Surv 23:1, 1968

Rodman MH, Jones CW: Catamenial hemoptysis due to bronchial endometriosis. N Engl J Med 266:805, 1962

Scott RB, Wharton LR Jr: Effects of progesterone and norethindrone on experimental endometriosis in monkeys. Am J Obstet Gynecol 84:867, 1962

Spangler DB, Jones GS, Jones HW: Infertility due to endometriosis. Am J Obstet Gynecol 109:850, 1971

Yeh TJ: Endometriosis within the thorax: Metaplasia, implantation or metastasis? J Thorac Cardiovasc Surg 53:201, 1967

Regardless of their field of specialization, all physicians who have female patients should have some basic knowledge of gynecologic cancer. These cancers occur frequently, are easily detectable by physical examination, and have symptoms that are usually specific; therefore, an alert consultant and a thorough examination can contribute toward early detection of gynecologic cancer. The physician need not necessarily be a gynecologist or a gynecologic oncologist.

Good management of treatment is next to early detection in importance for survival. Patients must have the best possible care when initially treated because the primary treatment offers the best chance for cure. The difference between the best possible and the most convenient treatment can literally be the difference between life and death if the latter is not adequate. Unless the physician who undertakes the treatment is knowledgeable about modern treatment methods, prepared to deal with failures or complications of treatment, and able to provide posttreatment surveillance, the physician should refer the patient with gynecologic cancer to an institution at which such services are available.

Counseling patients about the treatment of cancer is an important part of the practice of obstetrics and gynecology. Therefore, basic knowledge of therapy updated as new methods are developed is essential preparation for this type of medical practice. The recommended basic knowledge of gynecologic cancers includes an understanding of the predisposing factors, symptomatology, diagnostic methods, the growth and spread patterns of each cancer, treatment modalities, and prognosis.

GYNECOLOGIC MALIGNANCY: GENERAL CONSIDERATIONS

Felix Rutledge

FREQUENCY, AGE RELATIONSHIPS, AND PREDISPOSING FACTORS

Endometrial cancer has displaced cervical cancer as the most common gynecologic malignancy. There are 13,000 new cases and 3,300 deaths annually attributed to adenocarcinoma of the endometrium. In the United States endometrial cancer accounts for 8% of all cancers, cancer of the cervix 5.9%, cancer of the ovary 5%, and cancer of the vulva 1%. Cancer of the vagina has not been well documented but occurs infrequently. A combination of all gynecologic cancers would still reflect occurrence less frequent than cancer of the breast or colon.

Seventy-five percent of endometrial cancer patients are at least 50 years old and 75% have the disease localized when diagnosed. The National Survey in 1970 reported an incidence rate of 20.4 cases per 100,000 white women as compared to 12 cases per 100,000 black women in the United States. The frequency is low in South Africa and Japan, but higher in the United States, the Scandinavian countries, and Germany. These differences exist for unknown reasons. In the United States the single most significant factor increasing the incidence seems to be hormonal, whether due to medication or endogenous production in metabolism of estrogen. The annual risk of endometrial cancer developing in a patient who is postmenopausal is 1 per 1,000.

Though it occurs less frequently than endometrial cancer, carcinoma of the cervix causes more deaths. Cancer of the cervix is more common than cancer of the endometrium if cases of both intraepithelial carcinoma of the cervix and invasive lesions are jointly categorized. Unlike endometrial cancer, however, from one-half to two-thirds of the patients with cancer of the cervix have intraepithelial lesions. Some 30,000 to 40,000 cases of intraepithelial and invasive cervical cancer are discovered annually in the United States, resulting in 8,000 deaths per year. The age distribu-

tion for cancer of the cervix reflects patients much younger than those with cancer of the endometrium. Approximately 10% of the invasive cancer patients are below 35 years of age, whereas over 50% of the intra-epithelial cancer patients are below 35 years of age. The age range for developing carcinoma of the cervix spans a major part of a woman's life.

Carcinoma of the ovary is the leading cause of death in gynecologic cancer. The approximately 17,000 new cases of ovarian cancer per year reflect an incidence rate of 6 per 100,000 of the population. Ovarian carcinoma ranks fourth among causes of death due to cancer among women in the United States. Only cancer of the breast, large intestine, and lung are more lethal. While ovarian cancer has a lower incidence than cancer of the cervix and endometrium, the number of deaths from this disease equals those of cervix and endometrium combined (14 per 100,000). For epithelial cancers of the ovary (which constitute 85% of the total occurrences), the age for development is predominantly in the fourth, fifth, and sixth decades of life. Some special types of ovarian cancer occur in children.

Among gynecologic cancers, cancer of the vulva is the least frequent, accounting for 3% to 5% of all cases. As the average patient's age is in the sixth decade, it is primarily a disease of older women.

Cancer of the cervix occurs in sexually active persons, especially those beginning coitus at an early age. Multiparity increases the occurrence, and the involvement of multiple sex partners seems to be an important factor. At present a venereal viral transmission is suspected, but evidence is still needed to prove an etiologic role. Because in some families a mother–daughter sequence for cancer of the cervix has been observed, heredity is deemed a contributing factor. Epidemiology shows geographic and ethnic variability; for example, blacks and Mexican Americans have a higher incidence than Jews, and in the Middle East there is a relatively low incidence.

Least well understood is the etiology of cancer of the ovary. The epidemiology of this type cancer fails to point out significant roles for environmental, social, fertility, or hereditary factors. No group appears to be protected. Occasionally a family history is notable for the development of ovarian cancer among its females, but a high-risk population cannot be defined at present.

The etiology of cancer of the vulva, like cancer of the cervix, seems venereal-related, especially if there is an association with other vulvar diseases. Herpetic infections are suspected, but at present it is uncertain whether the infection is causative or merely associated. Cancer of the vulva occurs more frequently among patients with condyloma acuminata, granulomatous disease of the vulva, syphilis, and epithelial hyperplastic diseases.

DIAGNOSTIC METHODS

Cancer of the endometrium can be detected by vaginal cytology, but there is a high incidence of false-negative tests. Cells collected from the external os of the cervix can be tested with only a 50% accuracy when there is endometrial cancer in the fundus. The accuracy of tests on cells collected from the uterine cavity or high endocervical canal improves to 70%. Cytologic tests from the uterine cavity have fewer false-negative interpretations. The best diagnostic test for endometrial cancer involves cells or endometrium from the uterine cavity. Many new instruments have been recently perfected for collecting these specimens. These tests can be performed on an outpatient basis or by means of an office procedure more cheaply than by hospitalization. This should be the first step in investigating a patient with or without symptoms, though hospitalization may still be necessary for some.

For cancer of the cervix, vaginal cytology (Pap smear) has proved to be highly accurate for detecting afflicted patients even without symptoms. The Pap smear has discovered cervical cancer and its precursors in very early developmental stages, making early treatment possible and causing a decline in the incidence of invasive cervical cancer. Nevertheless, patients with advanced cancer of the cervix are still encountered, perhaps due to patient neglect or insufficient time for early detection. In a few cases the test may have been at fault, since a Pap smear can fail to detect a lesion. Vaginal cytology is more likely to fail when the cancer is advanced. Approximately one-half of these advanced cancer patients will have a negative Pap smear because large cervical cancers with associated infection produce necrotic debris by serous exudate and hemorrhage, diluting the number of neoplastic cells on the smear. A suitable smear is more difficult to obtain if a cancerous lesion is clinically evident on the cervix.

Cancer of the ovary can be detected only by obtaining an intra-abdominal specimen. Benign masses may feel similar and may even cause ascites. Cells from the peritoneal cavity obtained by needle puncture through the vagina or through the anterior abdominal wall can establish the presence of an intra-abdominal carcinoma, but it cannot diagnose the organ of origin. This approach to diagnosis is not recommended because cancer cells may be liberated. Only by a complete abdominal search and histologic study of tissue samples can ovarian cancer be diagnosed and staged. Laparoscopic examination may provide enough information for a working diagnosis but the abdominal search is limited and staging is inaccurate if metastases are too small. Regrettably, early detection of asymptomatic carcinoma of the ovary is not possible today. Occasionally an early-stage lesion is discovered by routine examination; however, this type of cancer usually grows

and metastasizes rapidly. Disappointingly, immunologic diagnostic methods have proved to be unexpectedly elusive.

Cancer of the vulva should be simple to find and diagnose. Unfortunately, patients often conceal the lesion and physicians sometimes mistake them for benign ones. Symptoms are sometimes treated without examination. There are multiple causes for needless delays in diagnosis of cancer of the vulva. In recent years physicians have become more aware of intraepithelial lesions. These are discovered by biopsy of vulvar lesions that are not typically cancerous. Small early lesions confused with and concealed by condylomatous lesions, leukoplakic and chronic vulvar dystrophies, and minor and subtle surface changes in the vulvar skin may point to intraepithelial carcinoma. There is no typical appearance of intraepithelial cancer of the vulva, though often localized areas of color difference due to increased pigmentation, hyperkeratosis, papillation, and shallow ulceration are indicative. Physicians who have good illumination for inspection of the vulva, who search the region carefully, and who biopsy liberally will more often find early vulvar cancer among their patients.

GROWTH AND SPREAD PATTERNS

Gynecologic cancers generally advance into surrounding tissues and to regional lymph nodes before spreading to establish distant metastases. An exception to this is intraperitoneal spread, notably in cancer of the ovary and occasionally in cancer of the endometrium. Predictably, cancer of the cervix and cancer of the vulva enlarge locally and then progress in a stepwise fashion along the lymphatic pathway as nodes become involved. Cancer of the endometrium may bypass the nearby pelvic nodes, going directly to the para-aortic nodes. Cancer of the ovary freely spreads intraperitoneally once the ovarian surface is penetrated. Metastasis to the pelvic nodes and aortic nodes by ovarian cancer also occurs frequently.

Treatment of metastasis to the inguinal, femoral, external iliac, the obturator, the hypogastric, and to some of the other lower common iliacs is successful. When only a few nodes are involved by small deposits from cancer of the cervix, about one-half of patients can be cured. Excision and irradiation therapy are usually equally effective as treatments. There is little success for treating para-aortic lymph node metastasis. Lymph node metastasis from cancer of the ovary usually has a simultaneous intra-abdominal-spread metastasis; thus, the scope of the treatment must be broader and multidirectional. Knowledge of the growth and spread pattern is essential for proper staging of gynecologic cancer and proper staging is essential for treatment.

TREATMENT MODALITIES

Treatment by surgical excision is the most useful method for gynecologic cancers that develop at either end of the genital tract. These are cancers of the ovary, uterus, and vulva. Most advanced cancers of the cervix and vagina are less suitable for surgery because an adequate margin of cancer-free tissue cannot be excised without invading the nearby bladder or rectum.

Cancer of the endometrium tends to remain confined to the corpus and is thus eminently suitable for resection because the spread is slowed by the thick uterine wall. Seventy-five percent of endometrial cancer patients are in stage I and a large proportion of these patients can, therefore, be cured by hysterectomy alone. However, 75% of patients with endometrial cancer are of postmenopausal age and older, and for this age group the incidence of medical and physical impediments to surgery is high. The treatment for some of these patients must be solely irradiation therapy. For those lesions that have spread beyond the uterus, hysterectomy is still done to remove the primary lesion, and metastases are dealt with by irradiation therapy or chemotherapy. Hysterectomy is the most effective single-treatment method; however, irradiation also plays an important role. Irradiation may be used without hysterectomy, preoperatively, or postoperatively.

Operations for cancer of the ovary range from conservative hysterectomy with bilateral salpingo-oophorectomy for small, localized lesions confined to the ovary, to extensive pelvic and abdominal dissection for advanced cancers of the ovary. Resection of segments of intestine and omentectomy are often necessary. Because most cures are accomplished by resection, an aggressive surgical attack upon advanced cancer of the ovary is warranted. While resection may not remove all of the cancer, if the total tumor burden can be significantly lowered and especially if the size of the remaining tumor masses is less than 2 cm, the effect of either chemotherapy or x-ray therapy is improved. In summary, surgery plays an important role in the management of patients with cancer of the ovary because (1) laparotomy is necessary for diagnosis and staging, (2) most cures are accomplished by total excision, (3) many patients require surgery to relieve intestinal obstruction caused by metastasis, and (4) tumor-reductive surgery is believed to be helpful.

Surgical resection excels over other methods of treatment for carcinoma of the vulva because these cancers are conveniently positioned for surgical removal, and the range needed for resection is minimally restricted. The bladder and rectum are neighboring organs but create a limitation only when the cancer is extensive. When the cancer has spread near the urethra and anus, resection may be incomplete. These pa-

tients receive x-ray therapy either prior to or following vulvectomy. The role of irradiation for advanced cancer of the vulva has been slow to emerge because of a long-standing belief that the normal skin of the perineum tolerates irradiation poorly. With the development of new x-ray machines that spare the skin severe irradiation dermatitis, external irradiation treatment is being reinvestigated as an adjunct to vulvectomy.

For early cancer of the cervix there are two very effective treatment methods: extended hysterectomy and full-dose irradiation therapy. The selection should be based upon which method has less harmful side effects and which is more curative for each cancer. Extended hysterectomy may be preferred because the surgical exploration provides a more accurate prognosis. The possibility of treatment failure because of radioresistance is eliminated. The side effects of irradiation on the bladder and rectum are avoided and the pliability of the mucosa of the vaginal wall is maintained. Extended hysterectomy may also be selected as the initial treatment for the young patient with an early cancer when preservation of the ovaries is desirable. Surgical resection is combined with irradiation therapy for special problem cases: (1) unusual growth pattern of the disease, (2) abnormal anatomic variation, (3) histologic types that are considered to be radioresistive, and (4) for patients whose physical condition is such that surgery poses a lesser risk than irradiation.

Irradiation (radium and x-ray) is applicable for treatment of more patients in early as well as advanced stages. Both intracavitary radium and external therapy are used in the treatment of cervical cancer. The cancerocidal action is the same for both methods. Intracavitary radium provides intense irradiation to a very restricted volume while external x-ray therapy is less restricted and can be directed to areas in which radium treatment is not feasible.

INTRACAVITARY RADIUM

Radium was the first source of radiation used in the treatment of cervical cancer and is still the basic treatment for this disease. Newer sources include isotopes of cobalt, iridium, and gold, each having special merits. Radium is a source of powerful irradiation but has limited depth of penetration. These two qualities make it particularly suitable for the treatment of cervical cancer. Application of radium within the uterus and upper vagina so that the radioactive source is in direct contact with the carcinomatous mass allows a cancerocidal dose to be delivered to the tumor. At the same time, the rectum and bladder receive much less radiation because of the short range of the radium.

EXTERNAL RADIATION

Because intracavitary radium dosage is not adequate for metastasis to regional pelvic wall nodes, x-ray is added in these cases. X-ray has a wider range of effective application, but since the rays must pass through normal tissue before they reach the tumor, they cannot deliver as high a dose as can radium. The development of megavoltage radiotherapy has increased the usefulness of x-ray and is less damaging to abdominal wall tissues; therefore a higher dose can be delivered to the cancerous tissues deep within the pelvis.

COMBINED TREATMENT

Surgery and irradiation may be combined for any of the gynecologic cancers, although the combination is more often used for cancer of the ovary and endometrium than for cancer of the cervix. When the two modalities are combined, less radical surgery or modification of irradiation is necessary to avoid excessive complications.

CHEMOTHERAPY—PRIMARY TREATMENT

Chemotherapy has found its greatest use in carcinoma of the ovary. The epithelial cancers of the ovary are especially responsive to alkylating agents and more recently other agents such as adriamycin and cis-platinum and hexamethylmelamine have been proved beneficial. The discovery of additional effective drugs has led to a combination and simultaneous administration of several agents, especially if the cancer is advanced or the histologic pattern suggests greater aggressiveness. Chemotherapy has partly displaced x-ray therapy as the primary postoperative treatment. Chemotherapy is not employed often as the primary adjunctive treatment for the other gynecologic cancers, since they are much less responsive.

TREATMENT FAILURES

Retreatment for recurrence of gynecologic cancers is practical and successful for some patients. Because this is true, surveillance for persistent or recurrent cancer is a necessary part of good treatment. Follow-up routines for asymptomatic patients include pelvic examination, CT scan,* vaginal cytology, and chest radiography. Some treatment centers include excretory urogram, sonography, and lower colon roentgenogram. Computerized axial tomography is being used increasingly for posttreatment monitoring of the ab-

---

* Computerized tomography scan

dominal cavity. Routine follow-up examinations are advised more frequently during the first 3 years after treatment because 90% of the recurrences and complications occur during that period. After the 3-year period, an annual examination is adequate.

Recurrent cancer of the ovary is very common because more than 80% have already metastasized when they are first discovered. Management of patients with cancer of the ovary usually involves a continual treatment over 1 to 2 years. Of all the gynecologic cancers, cancer of the ovary is most demanding of the physician and necessitates the greatest tolerance by the patient. These patients need close attention from the doctor because the side effects of treatment and discomfort caused by cancer are often severe.

Recurrent endometrial cancer has been successfully treated by progestins and some other drug combinations. Approximately one-third of these patients have some remission with progesterone-type hormones. Alkylating agents, adriamycin, and *cis*-platinum have been demonstrated to be useful, but the response incidence is less than that for cancer of the ovary. Cancer of the cervix and vulva benefit the least from chemotherapy.

RESULTS OF TREATMENT

The results achieved in the treatment of gynecologic cancer at the M. D. Anderson Hospital and Tumor Institute are outlined in Tables 52–1, 52–2, and 52–3. It is emphasized that these are overall results and do not reflect the major or minor deviations from standard therapy occasioned by differences from one patient to another within the several groups. These differences include variations in virulence of the tumor, sensitivity of the tumor to radiation or chemotherapy, host resistance to the tumor, and the patient's ability to withstand the therapy indicated.

The overall 5-year survival of 204 patients with cancer of the vulva is 58%. If those patients not treated because they were preterminal and those treated expecting only palliation are excluded from these calculations, the 5-year survival for 175 such patients is 77.3%. These data are not presented according to stage of disease because the number of cases for each stage would be too small for study.

In Tables 52–1 through 52–3 concerning cervical, endometrial, and ovarian cancer, international staging is used. The stages are defined in the chapters dealing with the individual lesions.

THE TERMINAL CANCER PATIENT

Although the survival rates for most kinds of gynecologic cancer improve each year, many patients are

TABLE 52-1. FIVE-YEAR SURVIVAL AND RATES FOR 916 PATIENTS WITH SQUAMOUS-CELL CARCINOMA OF CERVIX TREATED BY IRRADIATION ONLY (JANUARY 1964 THROUGH DECEMBER 1969)

Stage	No. of patients	Five-year survival rate (%)
Ib	316	91
IIa	178	82
IIb	204	65
IIIa	160	54
IIIb	58	40

(Jampolis S, Andras EJ, Fletcher GH: Radiology 115:681, 1975)

TABLE 52-2. FIVE-YEAR SURVIVAL RATES FOR 737 PATIENTS WITH ADENOCARCINOMA OF ENDOMETRIUM (JANUARY 1948 THROUGH AUGUST 1969)

Stage	No. of patients	Five-year survival rate (%)*
I	516	77.7
II	118	53.9
III	70	18.9
IV	33	3

* All deaths during follow-up observation counted as treatment failure

TABLE 52-3. FIVE-YEAR SURVIVAL RATES FOR 393 PATIENTS WITH SEROUS, MUCINOUS, OR SOLID ADENOCARCINOMA OF OVARY TREATED BY OPERATION AND IRRADIATION

Stage	Five-year survival rate (%)
I	71.7
II	25.8
III	12.0
IV	0

among the less fortunate whose disease cannot be controlled. The care of these patients is just as much the physician's responsibility as is the institution of proper therapy when the disease is at a much earlier stage. Too frequently the physician turns his back when it is clear that the outlook is hopeless, and proceeds to "more interesting" problems when he has exhausted the scientific measures available to him. Support for both the patient and her family is an essential part of the care of all patients, but it is needed especially by those with chronic, advancing disease that cannot be arrested, for whom the resultant physical, social, economic, and emotional problems may be

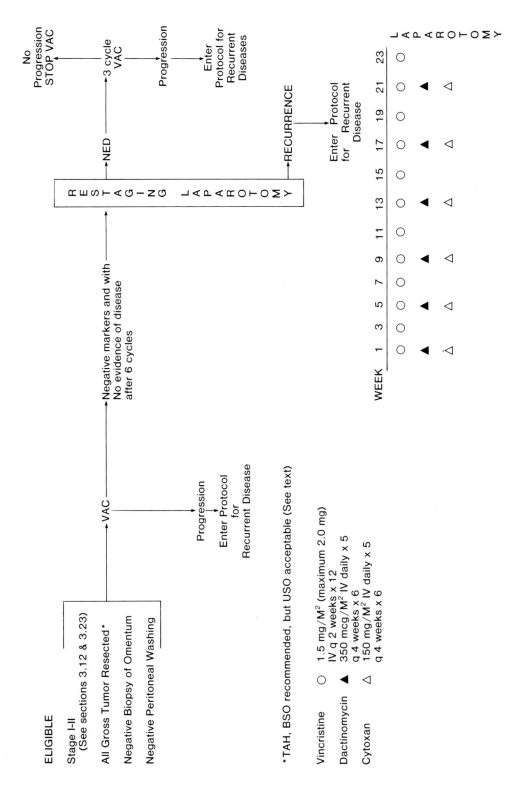

FIG. 52-1. Evaluation of adjuvant vincristine, dactinomycin, and cyclophosphamide therapy in malignant germ-cell tumors of the ovary after resection of all gross tumor. (Gynecologic Oncology Group Protocol).

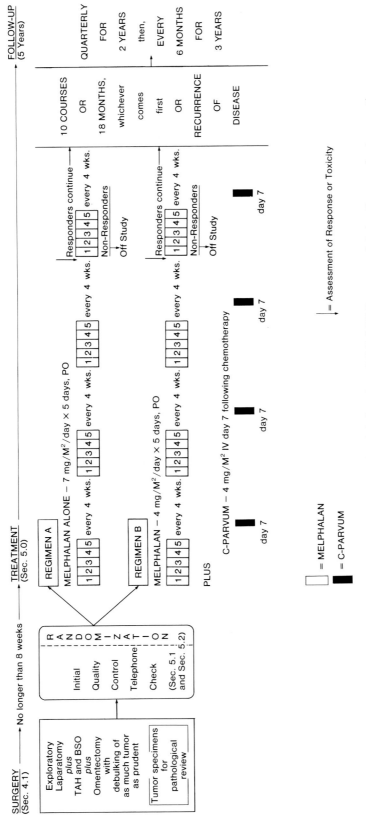

FIG. 52–2. Study Design Protocol Go #25. A randomized comparison of melphalan alone (NSC #8806) versus melphalan therapy plus immunotherapy (*Corynebacterium parvum*—NSC #220537) in the treatment of women with stage III (optimal) epithelial carcinoma of the ovary (phase II). (GOG).

overwhelming. Each patient is unique—there are no absolute measures by which to deal with any of these problems and there is no circumscribed body of knowledge that focuses on the care of the terminal patient. The physician's compassionate understanding and consideration are keystones, and regular visits can provide a degree of reassurance and comfort that is not available from any other source. The physician's role in such cases and his responsibility to the patient and her family are discussed in Norman Miller's sensitive article, written more than 25 years ago, which should be read by all who are concerned not only with those who are numbered among the survivors, but also with those who do not survive.

It is estimated that 60% to 80% of cancer patients suffer pain in the final stages of the disease. Almost all of these patients can be maintained in relative comfort and relatively free of pain if due thought is given to the selection of the drugs that are used. For those who are agitated or depressed, a mild tranquilizer during the day (*e.g.*, diazepam 2 mg t.i.d.) or at bedtime (*e.g.*, haloperidol 10 mg) may reduce the need for analgesia. If nausea should be a problem, such drugs as promethazine, prochlorperazine, or trimethobenzamide may be helpful. For analgesia, aspirin, acetaminophen, and propoxyphene are sometimes completely effective and should be used first in a dose of 650 mg every 3 to 4 hours. Codeine, 30 to 60 mg, may be added if necessary, but a mild laxative may also be needed to counteract the constipating effect. If this is inadequate or unsatisfactory one may advance to oxycodone/APC, which may be more effective and better tolerated. For severe pain, one of the variants of "Brompton's Mixture" is usually suitable. It has the advantage of an oral medication that can be readily used at home and can be adjusted to the needs of the patient. A 20-ml dose (which may be needed every 3 to 4 hours) contains the following: cocaine 10 mg, morphine 10 mg, grain alcohol 2.5 to 5 ml, flavoring syrup, and chloroform water to make 20 ml. The alcohol may be omitted if there should be stomatitis, the morphine content may be increased, if needed, up to 120 mg, or chlorpromazine can be added to potentiate the narcotic effect. Recently a commercial preparation of oral morphine sulfate (10 mg/5 ml) has been made available and appears to be just as effective as Brompton's Mixture. After the first several doses the patient may sleep for prolonged periods; this may be interpreted as due to excessive dosage, but more probably it results from the first real relief for a pain-exhausted patient. A customary dose is 20 mg of the morphine solution every 4 hours; some require doses of up to 75 mg.

Addiction may of course result from the use of narcotics over long periods, with the result that increasing amounts may be needed. However, experience suggests that the opposite may be true, and that over the course of many months the analgesic needs tend to remain stable or to decrease. Addiction *per se* should be of no concern, since the primary objective is to achieve the degree of comfort and freedom from pain that are so important in any terminal illness.

For pain that is entirely intractable the possible need for cordotomy or intrathecal alcohol injection comes to mind. More recently it has been suggested that percutaneous retrograde arterial infusion of nitrogen mustard may be highly effective in dealing with intractable pain due to gynecologic malignancy, producing in most cases marked relief of pain for an average of 6 to 8 weeks.

THE GYNECOLOGIC ONCOLOGY GROUP

The Gynecologic Oncology Group (GOG) * was formed for the purpose of evaluating the efficacy of different modalities or combinations of modalities in the treatment of gynecologic cancer. For the most part there is agreement on the general principles of primary treatment of the various lesions. However, many questions are still unanswered in the area of optimal adjunctive therapy, with reference to the use of radiation, chemotherapy, and immunotherapy either alone or in combination, and it is toward the solution of these questions that the efforts of the GOG are largely directed. The GOG is comprised of members of different institutions that treat large numbers of cases of gynecologic cancer. Protocols have been designed for virtually all kinds, grades, and stages of gynecologic malignancy, and randomized studies of matched cases are in progress to compare the efficacy of one regimen with another. As a result of this large collaborative effort, information will emerge to show which single agents or modalities, or combinations of agents and modalities, are most effective for specific situations, at what intervals they should be used, and how long they should be continued in apparently successful cases. Examples of two of the GOG protocols are shown in the figures on pages 1020–1021.

REFERENCES AND RECOMMENDED READING

Lathrop JC, Frates RE: Arterial infusion of nitrogen mustard in the treatment of intractable pelvic pain of malignant origin. Cancer 45:432, 1980

Miller N: Terminal care of the gynecologic cancer patient. Obstet Gynecol 4:470, 1954

Rutledge F, Boronow RC, Wharton JT: Gynecologic Oncology. New York, John Wiley & Sons, 1976

* The GOG grants are coordinated by the American College of Obstetricians and Gynecologists. Queries about the GOG may be directed to the Chairman, George C. Lewis, Jr., M.D., 1234 Market Street, Philadelphia PA 19107.

BENIGN LESIONS OF THE VULVA

The vulvar skin is of ectodermal origin, and consequently it is subject to diseases that are common to the skin elsewhere as well as to infectious processes that are more or less specific to the genital area.

Benign lesions of the vulva may be classified as follows:

I. Inflammatory lesions
  A. The common dermatitides
    1. Reactive (not allergic)
    2. Intertrigo (seborrheic dermatitis)
    3. Psoriasis
    4. Candidiasis
    5. Tinea (various types)
  B. Viral diseases
    1. Herpes simplex
    2. Condyloma accuminatum
    3. Molluscum contagiosum
  C. Ulcerative lesions
    1. Venereal (syphilis, lymphogranuloma [chlamydia], and granuloma inguinale [*B. Donovanii*])
    2. Autoimmune disease (Behçet's, Crohn's)
    3. Nonspecific (hidradenitis, ecthyma, folliculitis)
II. Traumatic lesions
  A. Hematomas
  B. Lacerations
III. White lesions (excluding neoplasms)
  A. Absence of pigment
    1. Leukoderma (congenital)
    2. Vitiligo (acquired)
  B. Hyperkeratotic lesions
    1. Inflammatory lesions
    2. Benign neoplasms
IV. Dystrophy
  A. Hyperplastic
    1. Typical
    2. Atypical (mild; moderate; marked)
  B. Lichen sclerosus
    1. Typical
    2. Atypical
  C. Mixed dystrophy
    1. Typical
    2. Atypical (mild; moderate; marked)
V. Benign neoplasms
  A. Solid tumors: granular cell myoblastoma; aberrant breast; lipoma; fibroma; hemangioma; hidradenoma; nevus; condyloma; acrochordon (fibroepithelial polyp); endometrioma; pyogenic granuloma
  B. Cystic lesions; inclusion; Bartholin duct; mucinous; canal of Nuck (hydrocele)

CHAPTER 53

LESIONS OF THE VULVA AND VAGINA

J. Donald Woodruff

Since cancer of the vulva may be associated with ulcerative, erythematous, proliferative, or hyperkeratotic lesions, biopsy must be used freely if malignancy is to be diagnosed in its early or even preinvasive stages. The instruments shown in Figure 53–1 are used for single or multiple biopsy of lesions in all cases. It has been suggested previously that simple biopsy of a neoplastic lesion, *e.g.*, melanoma, may be associated with the subsequent rapid spread of the malignancy. Follow-up of these lesions has not documented the validity of this thesis. Thus, it is even more imperative to biopsy all suspicious or controversial lesions in order to prove the true histologic nature of the disease with the knowledge that one can expect no concomitant spread of malignancy from the procedure and the patient can be afforded an accurate evaluation.

The use of 1% toluidine blue as a local nuclear stain may assist in selecting sites for biopsy. The vulva is

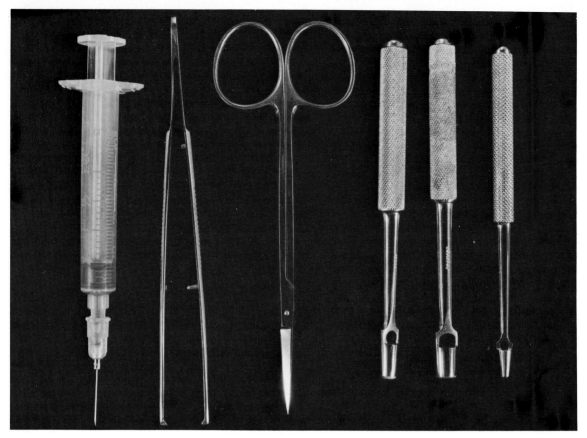

FIG. 53-1. Instruments used for biopsy of vulva. Instruments at *right* are Keys dermatologic punches.

painted with this agent and then washed for 2 to 3 minutes with 1% acetic acid. The stain is removed from normal tissues by the latter agent, but remains as a mark of cellular atypia or ulceration in those areas with retention of the dye. It must be appreciated that there are many false-negative and false-positive results from the use of this diagnostic technique. Acute excoriative processes (*e.g.,* reactive dermatitis) produce superficial ulcerations and the underlying exposed nuclei will absorb the stain; consequently, such processes should be treated and, if nonhealing, erythematous, or ulcerative foci remain, the stain should be applied and suspicious areas biopsied. Conversely, white, hyperkeratotic lesions may *not* absorb the dye and must be biopsied regardless of the results of the toluidine blue study.

The ability of abnormally proliferating lesions to concentrate tetracyclines has been the basis for the use of this agent in identifying the vulvar atypias; however, this "TIFT" test has not been reliable in most investigators' opinions.

INFLAMMATORY LESIONS OF THE VULVA

Vulvitis due to infectious agents is discussed in Chapter 50. The following lesions, in which there is an inflammatory reaction, also should be noted.

The most common benign affliction of the female external genitalia is *reactive dermatitis*. This was formerly called eczema or eczematoid dermatitis; however, the great majority of such dermatoses are due to local irritants, such as tight synthetic underclothing that retains perspiration, aerosol sprays, bubble bath and bath oils, colored toilet paper, detergents used in washing underclothing, perfumed soaps and powders, and a variety of other agents to which the vulva is commonly exposed. Obviously, the treatment is to eliminate the irritant and to use local fluorinated hydrocortisones. The latter agents are extremely powerful and should be used sparingly in strengths of 0.025% to 0.1%. Furthermore, they should be used only for symptomatic relief. Prolonged usage may produce systemic reaction or local fibrosis.

Intertrigo and seborrheic dermatitis are commonly seen in the diabetic. The elimination of moisture and the topical use of fluorinated hydrocortisone creams or lotions for the pruritus are the appropriate approaches to the acute problem. The classic agents used for "dandruff" elsewhere may be applied to the vulva; however, elimination of moisture and local irritants and the use of antipruritic agents are usually sufficient. The chronic hyperkeratotic alterations are "white lesions," as discussed later.

Psoriasis is usually multifocal. The classic picture on extragenital skin is characterized by "silver scales" and associated redness with linear excoriation. On the moist vulva, however, psoriasis appears as an erythematous patch without scales. Consequently, it is most important that the entire patient be examined, not just the vulvar area, if the appropriate diagnosis is to be made.

Candidiasis of the vulva is commonly associated with a vaginal infection, as noted in Chapter 50. Diabetes often accompanies such lesions.

Tinea cruris is usually sharply marginated, affects the adjacent skin surfaces, and is often found elsewhere on the body. Accentuation of the skin markings occurs in the more chronic situations. Lotrimin is most commonly used in the treatment of such lesions. Tinactin is also effective.

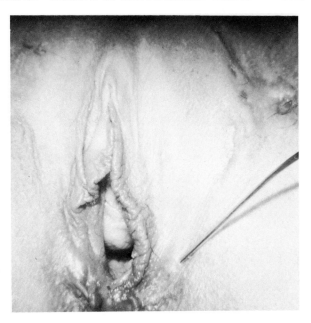

FIG. 53-2. Patient with Crohn's disease (regional enteritis) and concomitant draining sinus. Probe in fistulous tract.

ULCERATIVE LESIONS

Among the ulcerative lesions, special note should be made of *Crohn's disease* (Fig. 53-2). It is not well appreciated that approximately 25% of patients with classic enteritis also have draining sinuses or fistulous tracts in the perineum. Unless this relationship is appreciated, inappropriate therapy may be instituted. Simple incision and drainage of the sinuses may lead to rectovaginal fistula or even breakdown of the perineum. Prednisone is the classic treatment, usually in doses of approximately 40 mg/day. Recently the addition of metronidazole to the therapeutic regimen has made it possible to reduce the dosage of cortisone. Treatment with corticosteroid should be continued indefinitely; however, the author feels that 1 month of metronidazole therapy, 1000 to 1500 mg daily, is adequate.

Behçet's disease, probably an autoimmune disease, is characterized by ulcerations on the vulva and adjacent perineum, associated with similar lesions on the buccal mucous membrane. The third member of this "triple symptom syndrome," iritis, is commonly seen, in the author's opinion. Nevertheless, it should be appreciated that iritis is the most serious manifestation of all, since it may progress to fatal neurologic disease. The fundamental treatment is prednisone 40 mg/day, reduced if possible at the end of 1 month. There are many theories as to the origin of this disease, and thus many therapies have been instituted. Spontaneous regressions and recurrences are common and constitute a major difficulty in management of this disease.

WHITE LESIONS

Leukoderma, cogenital lack of pigment, is common on the vulva, often appears at the time of puberty, and is seldom symptomatic (Fig. 53-3). Associated depigmented areas are often found elsewhere on the body. When symptoms arise in this context, they generally are related to a superimposed dermatitis.

Vitiligo, acquired loss of pigment, is also extremely common and is usually associated with local inflammatory disease (Fig. 53-4). Such alterations are often transitory and migratory. The café-au-lait spots associated with neurofibromatosis (von Recklinghausen's disease) are rare on the vulva.

Hyperkeratotic lesions may be recognized in a variety of circumstances. Increased deposition of keratin (hyperkeratosis) is a protective phenomenon noted particularly on traumatized skin and, therefore, may be associated with any irritation, varying from chronic inflammatory disease to carcinoma. *Intertrigo*, probably the most frequent dermatitis in which hyperkeratosis develops on the vulva, is found most commonly in the interlabial and crural folds and is extremely difficult to combat, particularly in the obese diabetic woman, in whom it is commonly found. Seborrhea

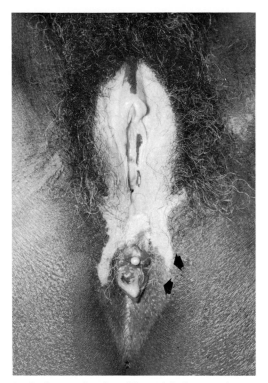

FIG. 53-3. Leukoderma, showing differential pigmentation on labia minora and prepuce. Patient had pruritus at perianal area and small areas of depigmentation due to chronic dermatitis (vitiligo) are apparent, particularly at *arrows*.

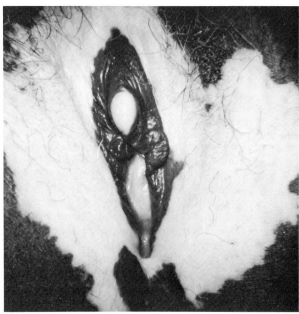

FIG. 53-4. Vitiligo.

(seborrheic dermatitis) is a corollary of intertrigo and is also extremely common in the moist atmosphere of the vulva. Chronic dermatitis results from a variety of locally irritative conditions and similarly produces a thick, protective layer of keratin. The acuminate wart in its initial state is brown or reddish-brown in color and microscopically shows superficial parakeratosis; however, in its later stages it is characterized by the development of hyperkeratosis. Thus, the chronic irritative lesion, regardless of etiology, may eventually produce the superficially protective keratin coat.

Dystrophy means simply a disorder resulting from "abnormal nutrition" and thus has been applied to describe those lesions that are characterized by a keratin layer of varying thickness (accounting for the white or grayish-white color), an abnormal thinning or thickening of the epithelial layer, an underlying chronic inflammatory infiltrate, and varying degrees of change in the subepithelial connective tissue. The latter may, in truth, relate to nutritional deficiencies, as noted by the vascular patterns. These dystrophies are probably the most common lesions, previously diagnosed as leukoplakia.

The term *leukoplakia* means a "white patch," and has been applied to almost every "white" lesion on the vulva. It is therefore highly nonspecific and should be eliminated from the terminology of vulvar disease.

In addition to leukoplakia, a variety of other terms demand careful evaluation and modifications. *Kraurosis* is a clinical designation meaning "shrinkage." The microscopic correlate is lichen sclerosus. Thus, as a specific lesion, the term "kraurosis valvae" should be eliminated in favor of more specific clinical and histopathologic interpretations.

Lichen sclerosus (et atrophicus) has been recognized on the vulva in all age groups (Fig. 53–5). Girls in the first decade of life have been afflicted with this nonspecific, patchy, white alteration of the labial skin. Most of these patients improve at the time of the menarche; however, the lesion may occur throughout the menstrual years, usually beginning as small, bluish-white papules with eventual coalescence into white plaques. In its initial phases, lichen sclerosus is asymptomatic and demands no therapy. It assumes major significance in the postmenopausal patient, in whom it is commonly associated with severe and recalcitrant pruritus. Malignancy may develop in 2% to 3% of these patients if prolonged relief of symptoms is not accomplished.

In the prepubertal patient, relief of symptoms is of major importance. Local hydrocortisone is usually effective. Testosterone is not recommended in such patients; however, 2% progesterone cream may be used if needed for symptomatic relief. It is in the postmenopausal patient that long-term treatment with topical testosterone is most effective. Since persistent therapy with topical fluorinated hydrocortisone may produce fibrosis and scarring of the subepithelial tissues,

steroids should be used primarily for symptomatic relief in the acute case but not as constant therapy over a long time. Progesterone cream has been proposed as an alternative to testosterone preparations, but more trials of this agent are needed. If shown to be effective, they would have the advantage of eliminating the occasional side effects of clitoral enlargement and increased libido associated with testosterone agents.

"*Primary senile atrophy*" and "*atrophic vulvitis*" are nondiagnoses, since there are no such diseases. Most lesions so diagnosed are variations of lichen sclerosus.

The microscopic picture of lichen sclerosus is characterized by moderate hyperkeratosis, a thinning of the epithelium with a loss of the normally arranged cellular layers, underlying collagenization, and inflammatory infiltrate (Fig. 53–6). Similar changes may be seen in the so-called kraurosis; however, the latter term fundamentally means "shrinkage" and is thus a gross clinical, rather than a microscopic, diagnosis. The later stages of lichen sclerosus are commonly associated with dyspareunia due to constriction of the outlet and fissure formation at the fourchette.

Hyperplastic dystrophy is featured by gross lesions that are white or grayish-white and may be either diffuse or focal. The patches are firm and often cartilaginous on palpation (Fig. 53–7). They simulate the general appearance of the lesions previously diagnosed as leukoplakia. Histologically, the keratin layer is usually thicker than that seen with lichen sclerosus and the epithelium is more proliferate, with elongated and often blunted rete pegs. In typical hyperplasia there is an increase in the cellular elements of the epithelium, but no abnormality of maturation. Underlying chronic inflammatory infiltrates vary in degree. Many such alterations are simply due to chronic dermatitis and thus treatment should be symptomatic. Biopsy must be used freely to eliminate the possible coexistence of cellular atypia. As noted above, local fluorinated hydrocortisone is the best of the antipruritic agents. Occasionally, very hypertrophic and often atypically pigmented areas may not respond to either local or systemic hydrocortisones, but the subcutaneous injection of such preparations may be dramatically effective. Small areas of 2 to 3 cm may be injected with 2 to 3 ml of fluorinated hydrocortisone, *e.g.*, Triamcinolone or Kenalog, producing dramatic results not only in elimination of the symptoms but in restoration of the normal coloration. Local measures to eliminate irritation are similar to those described previously and, regardless of the pathology, all patients should be instructed to observe these rules. On occasion these conditions are solitary and can be locally excised. However, multicentric foci must be eliminated by thorough investigation of the adjacent tissue. Diagnosis must be confirmed in all cases by biopsy. Multiple specimens are necessary in most instances, since various patterns often coexist.

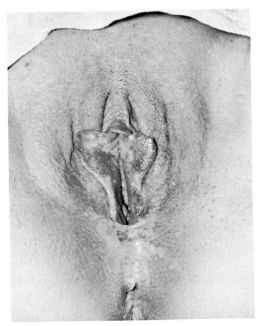

FIG. 53–5. Lichen sclerosus with foci of whitish alterations on labia minora and at fourchette.

Atypical hyperplastic dystrophy is usually a white lesion, but red or pigmented lesions may show similar alterations. These alterations simulate the epithelial changes described for cervical neoplasia, including atypical maturation patterns and intraepithelial "pearl" formation, often occurring adjacent to invasive vulvar cancer (Fig. 53–8) Thus, it is imperative to recognize the differences between cervical and vulvar neoplasia in both the in situ and invasive stages. Finally, it must be noted that histologic abnormalities may be associated with severe viral disease (condylomatous and herpetic). These undoubtedly account for the so-called reversible atypias that have been described recently.

Mixed dystrophy is a combination of "lichen sclerotic changes" with those of hyperplasia. Biopsy is important in identifying the malignant potential of such lesions, and must be used liberally. Colposcopy and cytology have not been helpful in differentiating the degrees of cellular atypia. Biopsy is simple and essentially painless if the area is infiltrated with local anesthetic agent, and the Keyes dermatologic punch is used to remove the tissue (see Fig. 53–1).

In view of these variables and the youth of the patients with in situ neoplasia, now reported to average below the age of 30 years in some clinics, it behooves the clinician to take a very conservative approach to these "neoplasias," always being aware that cancer may develop over a span of many years. Nevertheless, in the study of 106 cases of "in situ vulvar cancer,"

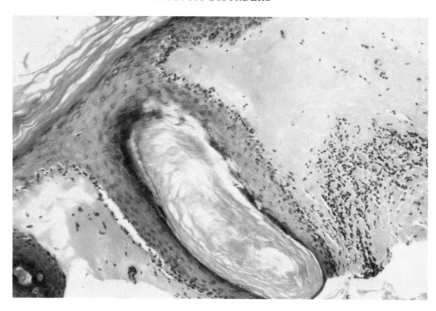

FIG. 53–6. Classic microscopic appearance of lichen sclerosus—Thin epithelieum with underlying collagenation, inflammatory infiltrate, and follicular plugging.

only four cases of invasive malignancy developed in the follow-up period of 2 to 15 years and these were either immunosuppressed or in the older age groups (75 and 83 years).

The basic treatment of all irritative lesions of the vulva must begin with a positive diagnosis; consequently, biopsy is imperative. Assuming that no major atypia is discovered, the next step is to eliminate the irritation. It seems quite possible that the chronic alterations associated with scratching may be of major import in the genesis of neoplasia. The treatment includes the use of topical fluorinated hydrocortisones to control the symptoms and reduce the local inflammatory reaction, the use of estrogen intravaginally in the postmenopausal patient, the treatment of any associated intravaginal infection, and the elimination of local irritants. The latter include colored and perfumed toilet paper, detergents in the wash water, hygiene sprays and local anesthetic ointments, and the use of tight-fitting underclothing composed of "moisture-retaining" synthetics. In the more persistent case, after the above treatments have failed to control the symptoms, alcohol injection of the external genitalia will eliminate the symptoms and not only afford relief to the patient, but allow the skin a chance to recover from the persistent scratching.

SOLID TUMORS

The majority of benign solid tumors, *e.g.*, *lipoma* and *fibroma*, occur only rarely on the vulva and are similar to such lesions elsewhere; thus, they need no special

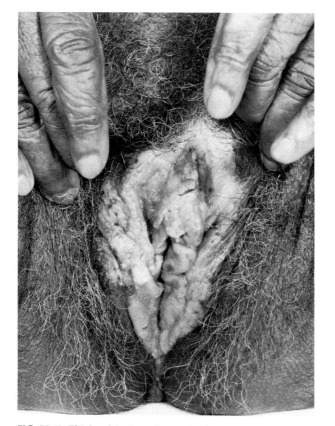

FIG. 53–7. Thick, white hyperkeratotic changes may or may not be associated with hyperplastic dystrophy. Biopsy must be used freely in such cases to rule out malignancy.

FIG. 53–8. Atypical hyperplastic dystrophy.

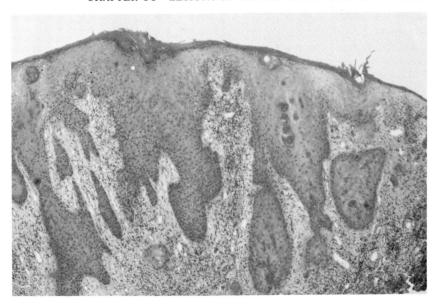

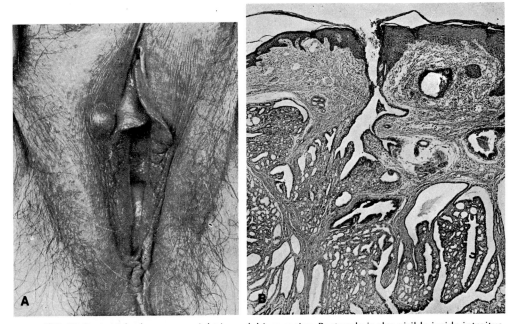

FIG. 53–9. *A.* Hidradenoma on right inner labium majus. Rectocele is also visible inside introitus. *B.* Photomicrograph of hidradenoma of vulva. (Novak ER, Woodruff JD: Gynecologic and Obstetric Pathology. Philadelphia, WB Saunders, 1962)

discussion here. All varieties of *vascular tumors* have been described on the external genitalia; however, the congenital variety deserves special note. Appearing at 2 to 3 months of age, it produces remarkable distortion of the vulva but generally needs and should receive no therapy unless excessive bleeding occurs, since such lesions disappear spontaneously. Small, elevated, hemorrhagic nodes are sometimes mistaken for hemangiomas but are, in truth, tiny varicosities that may produce an occasional episode of irregular bleeding. Varicosities may attain great size and a varicocele, similar to that of the male, develops in the vulva. Such le-

sions are almost always unilateral and are much less common than those that develop as the result of obstruction in the vessels of the spermatic cord. The *hidradenoma* is a rare lesion that, because of the intricate adenomatous pattern, has been confused with malignancy. Malignant alterations are extremely uncommon and the lesion, rarely more than 1 cm in its greatest dimension, can be treated by local excision (Fig. 53–9).

A variety of *pigmented lesions* are seen on the vulva. An irritative focus of chronic dermatitis may be pigmented as may carcinoma *in situ* and the "spreading melanoma." Again, as noted previously, biopsy is imperative to evaluate accurately the histopathology of such lesions.

The *true nevus* should be given special attention, since approximately 3% to 5% of malignant melanomas in the female arise in the vulva. This relatively high percentage of malignant change in the nevus arising in the vulva may be due to the many local irritants to which the vulva is subjected as well as the frequency of junction activity, an alteration of major importance in the development of neoplasia. It has been suggested that the malignant melanoma pursues a more aggressive course during pregnancy. Recent statistics do not substantiate this thesis.

A variety of *papillary lesions* have been recognized on the vulva. The common *acuminate wart*, of viral origin, constitutes a recurring therapeutic problem

and may be a precursor of malignancy. The *fibroepithelial polyp* or *acrochordon* is common in all areas subjected to irritation and needs no treatment other than accurate diagnosis.

Of special interest to both pathologists and clinicians is the *granular–cell myoblastoma*. This benign lesion arising from the nerve sheath is associated with extensive, overlying pseudoepitheliomatous hyperplasia, often misdiagnosed as carcinoma in situ or even early invasive cancer. Careful investigation of the underlying tissue is thus of major importance in order to make an accurate evaluation and institute the appropriate therapy. The finding of large cells with prominent eosinophilic granules makes the accurate diagnosis. Finally, the myoblastoma is not a well-localized tumor and, therefore, is subject to local recurrences. Nevertheless, malignant myoblastomas are uncommon, although multicentric foci arising in diverse areas in the body are not infrequent but should not be interpreted as metastases.

Vulvar endometriosis is uncommon and occurs most commonly in areas subjected to trauma. The incision or excision of the chronically infected Bartholin gland seems to be an ideal precursory event for the development of such lesions. As usual, the characteristic feature is cyclic swelling and pain. Such lesions also develop in the inguinal canal and adjacent mons.

CYSTIC LESIONS

The *sebaceous cyst* is the most common cystic lesion of the vulva (Fig. 53-10). Although a majority of these lesions arise as a result of occlusion of the sebaceous gland on either labia minora or labia majora, microscopically they are epidermal inclusion cysts and in the chronic, quiescent state are lined by stratified epithelium. Prior to the actual development of such lesions, the swelling contains only sebaceous material and thus is not a true cyst. These lesions need no treatment unless they become infected, at which time simple incision and drainage are usually sufficient. If they are recurrently infected, excision may be carried out; however, recurrences are common.

Cystic dilatation of the main Bartholin duct (Fig. 53-11A, B) may be due to chronic inflammatory reactions with scarring and occlusion or to trauma from lacerations or incisions in the area. For the most part, these cysts are asymptomatic and therapy is unnecessary. On occasion they become infected and incision and drainage are indicated. If the infections are recurrent, an attempt should be made to establish a permanent opening by marsupialization of the dilated duct during a quiescent state. Use of the indwelling "WORD" catheter requires only local anesthesia, and can be carried out as an office procedure. Excision is necessary only if marsupialization is unsuccessful in controlling the infection or if the diagnosis of malig-

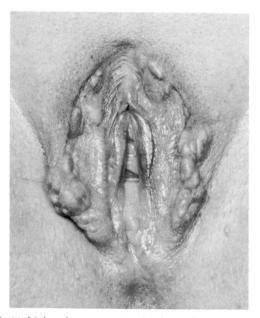

FIG. 53–10. Multiple sebaceous cysts of vulva. (Woodruff JD: Tumors of the Female Genitalia. In Pack GT, Ariel IM (eds): Treatment of Cancer and Allied Diseases, Vol 6. New York, Hoeber, 1962)

FIG. 53-11. *A.* Bartholin duct cyst projecting into introitus. *B.* Various epithelia present in Bartholin gland, primarily transitional in center with mucous secreting acini.

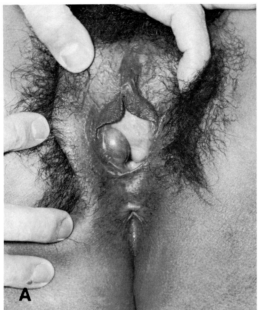

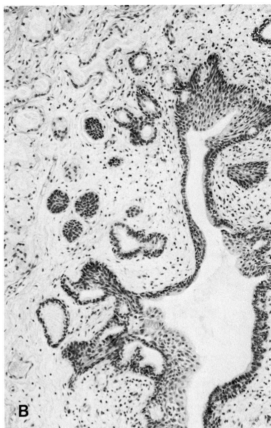

nancy is entertained. It should be noted that the introitus is "ringed" with minor vestibular glands and infection in such structures produces focal areas of erythema and irritation at the introitus. Rarely, cystic dilatations of these glands produce small, superficial, mucinous cysts.

Dysontogenetic cysts, not dissimilar to the above-mentioned mucinous lesions of vestibular gland origin, are found at the introitus and adjacent labia minora. The most frequent site is the area of the urethra. These cysts contain mucoid material and possibly represent the residua of incomplete separation of the cloaca by the urorectal folds; thus, they represent dilatations in rectallike tissue. They may, as noted above, originate by occlusion of the minor vestibular glands that ring the outlet at the introitus. Regardless of origin, these lesions are benign.

Cysts that appear high in the labium majus (*hydrocele of the canal of Nuck*) may simulate the hydrocele in the male. Since the round ligament has an investment of peritoneum, the latter may be occluded in the inguinal canal and allow the accumulation of fluid along the round ligament as it inserts into the labium

majus. It is of major importance to appreciate the origin of such lesions, since simple incision and drainage leads to prompt recurrence.

BENIGN LESIONS OF THE VAGINA

Benign lesions of the vagina include inflammatory reactions (Chap. 50), "leukoplakia" (hyperkeratosis resulting from chronic irritation such as that associated with total prolapse of the uterus), cystic lesions, and solid tumors.

CYSTIC LESIONS

Benign cystic lesions of the vagina are inclusion cysts, Gartner's duct cysts, endometriosis, adenosis, and vaginitis emphysematosa.

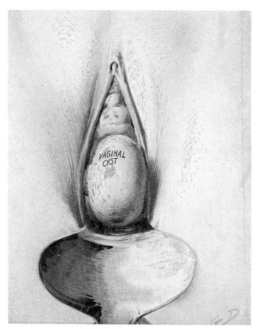

FIG. 53–12. Cyst of anterior vaginal wall. Cyst protrudes through vulva when exposed with speculum. (MacLeod D, Read CD: Gynaecology, 5th ed. London, Churchill, 1955)

The *inclusion cyst* is extremely common, occurring most frequently near the outlet at the site of previous lacerations or episiotomy scar. It seldom attains sufficient size to become symptomatic and associated inflammatory reaction is uncommon. Thus, excision or incision and drainage are rarely necessary. The cyst is filled with desquamated cellular material from the stratified squamous epithelial lining.

Gartner's (mesonephric) duct may be the origin of multiple tiny cystic dilatations or, on rare occasions, a large solitary cyst. The former are palpable only as fine elevations on the mucosal surface of the vaginal fornices or course of the mesonephric duct. They are common and rarely symptomatic. The latter often develops in the midline of the anterior vault and simulates a cystocele (Fig. 53–12). Recognition of the nature of the lesion is important in determining therapy. Removal is usually not needed unless they present symptoms. Although no harm is done if the cyst is inadvertently opened during removal, the surgeon may be dismayed if he erroneously believes he has incised the bladder. Rarely may malignancy develop in these mesonephric remnants.

Endometriosis usually develops as a penetration of cul-de-sac disease. It usually appears in the posterior fornix of the vagina and is characterized grossly by a bluish discoloration produced by the old blood entrapped in the fine fibrous nodules. If penetration is incomplete, the associated nodular induration extending from the uterosacral ligaments into the vagina may simulate cancer. To rule out the latter, the vaginal le-

sion should be biopsied to establish the diagnosis. If the lesion is asymptomatic and is the only abnormality present, no therapy other than accurate evaluation is indicated. Otherwise, appropriate treatment for endometriosis, either medicinal or surgical, should be instituted.

Adenosis varies in gross appearance from diffuse granular thickenings to an irregular, rugose, mucoid lesion. The frequency of adenosis is difficult to access; however, Sandberg suggests that more than 40% of all women demonstrate such subepithelial adenomatous structures. Any area of the vagina may be involved, but most commonly it is the anterior or posterior wall of the upper half of the vault. Probably arising from aberrant ectopic cervical-type "glands" (Fig. 53–13), the lesion is rarely symptomatic and thus therapy is unnecessary. Recently, interest in adenosis vaginae has increased with the appearance of these adenomatous elements in the vaginas of young women whose mothers had received diethylstilbestrol (DES) during pregnancy. The physician may be alerted to this group of lesions by the occasional presence of a transverse septum in the upper third of the vagina or the more frequent occurrence of a collarlike structure around the cervix (Fig. 53–14). Approximately 400 adenocarcinomas have been reported from the population at risk. Such neoplasms develop most commonly in the menarcheal years. Nevertheless, the lesions have been reported in a 7-year-old child, although admittedly the number of occurrences in those younger than 14 years of age is extremely small. Conversely, such malignancies have been discovered in midthird decade of life, the oldest patient at present being 29 years of age. Of importance is the magnitude of this population, which now must approximate more than 1 million young women. Methods of investigation of this special group have challenged the profession. At present, the basic question concerns the chance that the young woman at risk will develop mesonephroid carcinoma of the vagina and the answer currently must be *"rarely,"* or less than 0.1%. The follow-up of the patient at risk should consist of careful palpation of the tissue with inspection and cytopathologic evaluation. Colposcopy has not been of help in identifying the early adenocarcinoma. Most cases of clear cell or mesonephroid carcinoma are brought to light during the first study. However, at least four cases have been discovered in the follow-up study of initially benign adenosis; one of these was a multifocal lesion.

Possibly of more future concern will be the development of epidermoid neoplasia at the many squamocolumnar junctions produced by the change in the embryology of the area. Stafl, in his colposcopic studies, has commented on this variety of histologic alteration. The author notes that benign adenosis can be demonstrated colposcopically in over 90% of the young women at risk. Nevertheless, the incidence of such alterations depends largely upon the stage of the pregnancy at which therapy was instituted, *e.g.*, if treat-

FIG. 53-13. Vaginal adenosis, showing surface-stratified epithelium with underlying glands, one of which contains metaplastic epithelium.

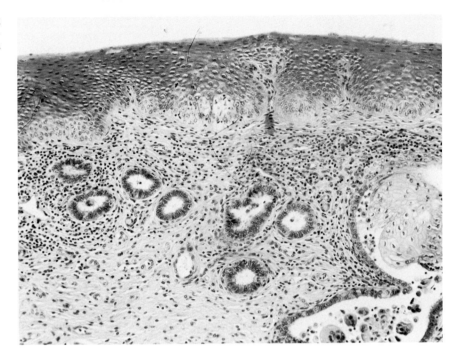

ment was begun prior to the tenth week of gestation, adenosis occurs in approximately 90% of the female progeny. Conversely, if medication was instituted after the 16th week of gestation, the *risk factor* is no greater than that for the female population at large. Microscopic examination of the adenomatous lesion reveals that the epithelia characteristic of the paramesonephric system (*i.e.,* mucinous, endometroid, and endosalpingeal) may be found in many cases; however, the mucinous or endocervical variety is the most common.

Of interest is the rarely diagnosed *vaginitis emphysematosa.* Characterized by widespread submucosal cyst formation, this uncommon lesion is found in the pregnant woman or in the severely decompensated cardiac patient. The blebs are filled with carbon dioxide and definitive infecting agents have not been recovered from the contents. Therapy should be directed at the associated vaginitis, commonly found to be trichomonal in the pregnant woman. Complications have not been reported. Microscopically, the lining of the cavities is characterized by the presence of irregular, "reactive" giant cells (Fig. 53–15).

SOLID TUMORS

Benign solid tumors of the vagina include fibromyoma, papilloma, and condyloma.

Fibroma (fibromyoma), a rare solid tumor, may arise *de novo* from the connective tissue and smooth muscle elements of the vaginal wall. However, many

such lesions are intraligamentary uterine fibromyomas that have become divorced from the fundus and have dissected into the paravaginal area. These lesions, whether primary or secondary, are rarely symptomatic and the incidence of sarcomatous change is negligible. Excision usually is a minor procedure; however, the uterine vessels and/or the ureter may be encountered if dissection is extensive. If any question exists about the nature of the tumor, excision must be carried out, since the treatment of vaginal malignancy is complicated by the necessity for radical surgery or technically difficult radiation. Local excision is often followed by recurrence despite "benign histology."

True *papillary tumors* other than condylomata acuminata are rare. Most lesions so termed are, in truth, fibroepithelial tags (acrochordon). Although vaginal polyps are uncommon, they nevertheless have been classically misinterpreted because of the edematous nature of the lesion. A diagnosis of sarcoma botryoides is often made on the basis of these histologic features. Moreover, in the follow-up of such cases, it has been appreciated that although the polyp may recur, malignancy has not been reported.

Condylomata acuminata are common in the vagina and are associated classically with extensive condylomatosis of the vulva (Figs. 50–4, 53–16). The urethra, cervix, and perianal areas are frequently involved. These lesions may become exuberant, particularly during pregnancy. In the latter situation, they present major complications due to the associated vascularity, edema, and inflammatory reaction. The customary treatment, podophyllin, should not be used during

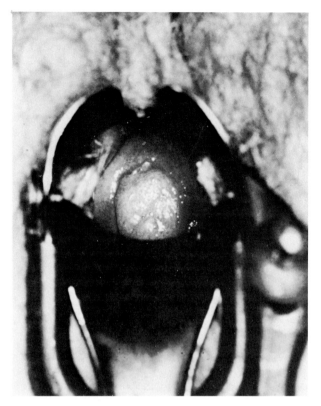

FIG. 53-14. Photograph of cervix of 22-year-old DES-exposed offspring demonstrating complete cervical collar and polypoid structure of central portion of cervix. Note that anterior portion of collar is slightly peaked, giving rise to a deformity referred to as a "cockscomb." (Townsend DE: In Herbst AL (ed): Intrauterine Exposure to Diethylstilbestrol in the Human, p 26. Chicago, American College of Obstetricians and Gynecologists, 1978)

pregnancy. The trauma of delivery may result in vaginal laceration and extensive bleeding. Nevertheless, since the acuminate wart is of viral origin, the lesion may spontaneously regress postpartum with the institution of good local hygiene and the elimination of associated infection. It should be appreciated, however, that laryngeal papillomas in the newborn have been associated with vaginal condylomatosis in the mother. Although these lesions are benign, they do present problems in the care of the neonate.

In the nonpuerperal state, long-term sulfonamide therapy and general cleanliness often result in reduction in the size of the lesion. Podophyllin should be used sparingly in the vagina, since local reactions may be severe. Anaphylactic shock has been reported as a complication of the injudicious use of this cauterizing solution. Local application by the physician to the individual lesion followed by vaginal douche within 2 hours of the application has rarely resulted in any untoward reaction. Although the small individual warts may be so treated, extensive involvement of the vagina may require excision under general anesthesia. In resistant cases 5-flurouracil (Efudex) is often effective.

MALIGNANT TUMORS OF THE VULVA

Vulvar anaplasia comprises 3% to 4% of all primary malignancies of the genital canal. Despite the availability of these lesions for early investigation, there is a longer interval between the appearance of symptoms

FIG. 53-15. Microscopic appearance of vaginitis emphysematosa, showing cystic spaces lined by giant cells.

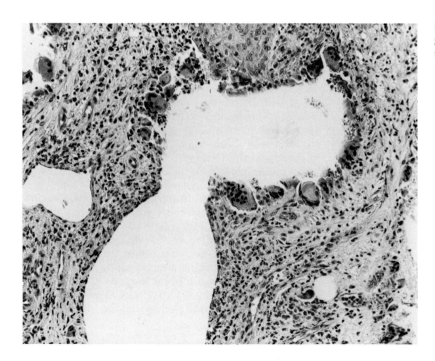

and the establishment of diagnosis of carcinoma of the vulva than for any other primary malignancy of the female genitalia. Much of this delay may result from the reluctance of the elderly patient to seek medical advice; however, the 30% to 35% of cases in which the physician is at fault may be related to the commonplace nature of the initial symptom—pruritus. Too often, treatment is suggested over the telephone before thorough study has been carried out.

As noted previously, the dystrophies may show a variety of histologic alterations, described as typical or atypical hyperplasias. The terms atypia and dysplasia are also used to describe atypical hyperplasia.

Vulvar malignancies may be classified as follows:

I. Primary malignancy
  A. Carcinoma in situ
    1. Bowen's disease
    2. Erythroplasia of Queyrat
    3. Carcinoma simplex
  B. Paget's disease
  C. Invasive cancer
    1. Squamous-cell lesions—Well differentiated, others
    2. Basal-cell carcinoma (histologic variations)
    3. Bartholin gland lesions
      a. Squamous-cell lesions
      b. Transitional lesions
      c. Cribriform (adenocystic) lesions
    4. Verrucous carcinoma—This tumor is locally invasive but not metastasizing. The histology is identifiable and the treatment is wide excision. Recurrences are common and often locally destructive.
  D. Other malignancies—Including melanoma (melanotic and amelanotic), sarcoma, lymphoma, embryonal rhabdomyosarcoma
II. Secondary malignancy

CARCINOMA IN SITU

Carcinoma in situ occurs at any age but is not infrequent during the third and fourth decades of life. Although a common complaint is pruritus, the lesion may present as a lump or may be relatively asymptomatic. The gross appearance varies greatly. The Bowenoid lesion is scaly and characterized by a red background dotted with white, hyperkeratotic islands (Fig. 53–17). Other lesions are almost entirely white, red (erythroplasia of Queyrat), or a combination of these patterns (Fig. 53–18).

A rarely described variety of carcinoma in situ is irregularly pigmented, with a diffuse but hazy background of hyperkeratosis (Fig. 53–19). These variable and bizarre patterns demand that many lesions be biopsied to determine their true nature. Of interest is the increased frequency with which multiple areas of

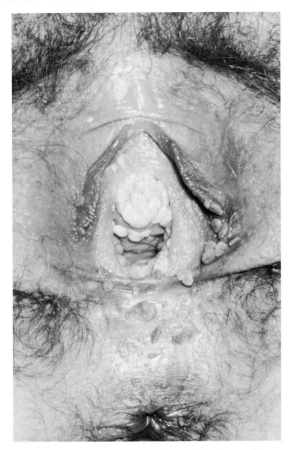

FIG. 53–16. Condylomata acuminata affecting urethea, vagina, and external genitalia.

anaplastic change are noted in the lower genital canal and perianal areas (the anogenital area). Such alterations demand thorough study of the entire region, both initially and at follow-up examinations. Micrographs demonstrate variations in atypical cellular maturation (Figs. 53–20, 53–21).

Of major interest are the variations in the histologic patterns adjacent to invasive cancer and those described as marked atypical hyperplasia or carcinoma in situ. It seems quite possible that viral disease may produce histologic patterns indistinguishable from carcinoma in situ, representing the cases of so-called "reversible atypia."

If multiple foci of malignancy are carefully excluded by use of toluidine blue and random biopsies, wide local excision of the lesion is the acceptable treatment. Thus, although vulvectomy has been the proposed therapy, it is obvious that more conservative approaches are acceptable in most young patients. Conversely, it seems apparent at the present time that carcinoma in situ occurring in the patient over the age

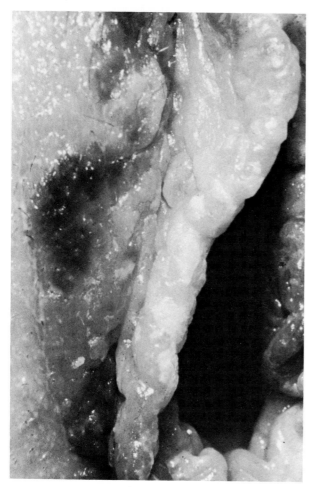

FIG. 53–17. Bowen's disease of vulva. Multiple whitish foci are noted on the *right*. The intervening areas are reddish.

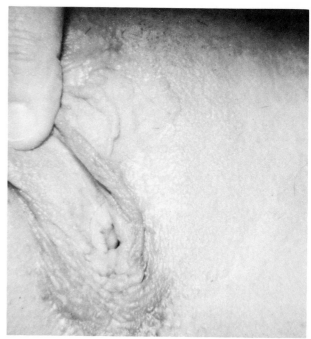

FIG. 53–18. Carcinoma in situ of vulva. Reddish lesion at fourchette, white lesion, left vulva.

of 60 years may be an entirely different disease and thus vulvectomy is more appropriate in such instances unless an isolated focus can be identified. Careful follow-up is essential in either case, since simple excision does not remove the precipitating agent and the potentiality of recurrence always exists, regardless of the surgery, radical or simple. The use of topical chemotherapeutic agents (*e.g.,* 5% fluorouracil cream) have been used with success rates approximating 60% to 75%. Certainly such approaches are worthwhile in the young patient, particularly one whose neoplasia apparently has begun in the background of a condylomatous lesion. More recently an immunologic approach has been used successfully in recurrent, especially pigmented, lesions. The patient is sensitized to dinitrochlorobenzene (DNCB), and the agent is applied locally to the lesions. A severe reaction may occur, and accordingly it is essential to evaluate carefully the strength of the agent needed for each individual patient.

PAGET'S DISEASE

Like its counterpart on the breast, vulvar Paget's disease (Fig. 53–22) is characterized grossly by a fiery red background mottled with white, hyperkeratotic islands and, in this respect, simulates Bowen's disease. Unlike the mammary lesion usually associated with an underlying malignancy, the vulvar disease is intraepithelial in 75% of cases. Nevertheless, the tendency to local recurrence makes the neoplasm a constant threat. Microscopically, the characteristic large, pale cells of apocrine origin are found initially in the basal layer but eventually involve the entire surface epithelium as well as that of the underlying appendages (Fig. 53–23). The positive reaction of the cells to mucicarmine stain serves to differentiate the lesion from Bowen's disease and melanoma.

Therapy primarily demands simple vulvectomy to determine the extent of involvement of the underlying tissues. If invasive disease is recognized in the removed specimen, inguinal and femoral lymph node dissection is indicated. In view of the frequency of recurrence, careful follow-up is mandatory. Radiation has been of little value for the local or metastatic disease. The association with Paget's disease of the breast has been recorded in several studies and, although uncommon in the author's opinion, a thorough study of every patient should be made to rule out a mammary lesion.

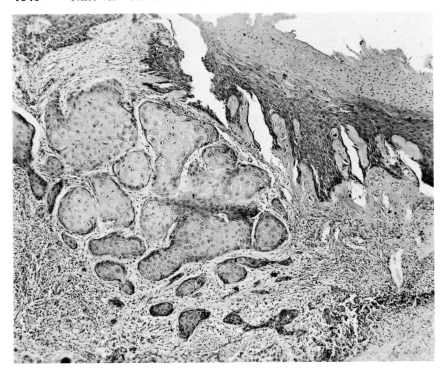

FIG. 53–25. Invasive carcinoma with atypical maturation of invasive epithelium on *left*. At *right*, abnormal changes are characterized by parakeratosis and irregular rete pegs with collagenation (leukoplakia).

the similar lesions on the cervix. Among 58 cases with invasion to a depth of less than 5 mm treated by partial vulvectomy, 5 patients (9%) later died as the result of recurrent or metastatic disease.

Local recurrence, demonstrating either in situ or invasive disease, is a major threat. Approximately 50% of all patients with vulvar malignancy die from direct invasion of local organs. These lesions may be "reoccurrences" rather than recurrences and suggest the possible presence of a persistent carcinogen or the lack of host resistance.

Basal cell carcinoma comprises 5% of all vulvar cancers. Like its counterpart on the skin elsewhere, it is a locally invasive but rarely metastasizing lesion. Wide local excision is the treatment of choice for these tumors.

Although *Bartholin's gland* is an uncommon site for the origin of malignancy, tumors arising in the gland present a wide variety of patterns. The common squamous-cell cancer develops at the orifice of the duct and represents a variant of primary vulvar carcinoma; however, it should not be classified as a Bartholin's gland tumor. The transitional type arises from the characteristic urogenital epithelium of the duct. The true Bartholin gland cancer is a mucoid, cribriform adenocarcinoma developing from the acini of the gland (adenoid cystic tumor). This variety deserves special mention, since it is classically slow-growing, indolent, and locally invasive; however, late metastases occasionally appear in the lungs. The last type usually presents as

an indurated mass in the deep recesses of the perineum, while the former types grossly simulate the common vulvar malignancies. Wide local excision is the treatment for the adenoid cystic lesion, but local recurrences are not uncommon.

OTHER PRIMARY MALIGNANCIES

As noted earlier, the vulva is the site of origin of approximately 2% to 3% of *malignant melanomas* in the female. Since both the spreading and nodular varieties are difficult to differentiate from many of the benign pigmented lesions, biopsy should be used freely. Early diagnosis is of obvious importance. The survival is related directly to the depth of invasion, which is differentiated into five levels: Levels 1 and 2 (involvement of the intrapapillary ridges) are associated with essentially 100% 5-year survival; conversely, the salvage in level 5 tumors (involvement of the reticular dermis) is a miserable 0% to 20%. Surgery is the treatment of choice and at the present time radiation and chemotherapy have added little to the salvage. Current thought suggests there is no need for radical surgery in patients with involvement of only the epithelium and the rete ridge. Breslow has suggested depth measurement as a more accurate determinant of prognosis. For lesions less than 0.75 mm (Clark's level 1) 5-year survival is 100%. However, occasional patients

FIG. 53-24. Invasive cancer characterized by pearl formation without overlying, full-thickness, epithelial changes.

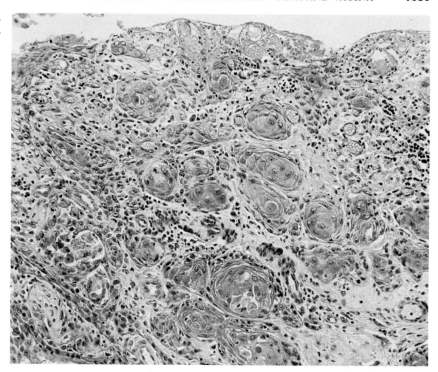

Clinical staging of invasive carcinoma of the vulva

1. Stage I: (TI NO; TI NI)
   a. Tumor confined to vulva, 2 cm or less in largest diameter; no nodes palpable or, if groin nodes palpable, they are mobile, not enlarged, and not clinically suspicious of neoplasm
2. Stage II: (T2 NO; T2 NI)
   a. Tumor confined to vulva and more than 2 cm in largest diameter; status of nodes as in stage I
3. Stage III: (T3 NO; T3 NI; T3 N2; TI N2; T2 N2)
   a. Tumor of any size confined to vulva, with palpable nodes in groin which are enlarged, firm, mobile, and clinically suspicious of neoplasm
   b. Tumor of any size with adjacent spread to urethra, vagina, perineum, or anus with or without suspicious, mobile nodes in groin
4. Stage IV: (TI N3; T2 N3; T3 N3; T4 N3; T4 NO; T4 NI; T4 N2; all other conditions containing M1a or M1b)
   a. Tumor of any size or extent with fixed or ulcerated nodes
   b. Tumor of any size infiltrating mucosa of bladder, rectum, or urethra, or fixed to bone
   c. Tumor of any size with palpable deep pelvic lymph nodes or other distant metastases

TREATMENT

Treatment is fundamentally surgical, with removal of the vulva and the superficial and deep inguinal and femoral nodes. The lymphatic drainage of the vulva is shown in Figure 53–26. Since there is cross-lymphatic circulation, a bilateral procedure should be carried out in most cases (Fig. 53–27). Nevertheless, current studies suggest that unilateral lesions do not have contralateral nodal metastases if the ipsilateral nodes are not involved. Thus, in specific cases unilateral node sampling may eliminate the need for the more extensive operation, which carries a predictably high postoperative morbidity. Lesions larger than 2 cm show increased lymph node involvement, but even with smaller tumors there is dissemination beyond the local area in 15% to 25% of cases. The ulcerative lesion tends to metastasize early in comparison with the exophytic type. An 85% to 90% salvage may be expected if nodes are uninvolved; however, even with metastasis to these regional sentinels, 5-year survival rates approximate 30% to 35%. Various classifications have been proposed, but the above-noted features are of fundamental importance in determining prognosis. The interested student may refer to the works listed under References and Recommended Reading.*

The term *microinvasive cancer of the vulva* demands careful evaluation, since it is not the same as

---

* More recently there has been a resurgence of interest in the use of radiation therapy, particularly for the massive lesion in the elderly patient with medical contraindications to extensive surgery. Results suggest that excision of the tumor mass with follow-up external-beam therapy to the nodes may be an alternative to surgery, particularly in the patient who has positive inguinal nodes, specifically Cloquet's.

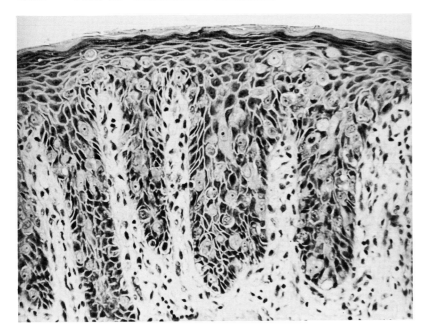

FIG. 53–23. Paget's disease of vulva. Epidermis shows maturation, enlarged rete pegs, and Paget's cells with pale cytoplasm. (×185; Haines M, Taylor CW: Gynaecological Pathology. London, Churchill, 1962)

INVASIVE CARCINOMA

The common vulvar malignancy is a "skin cancer" and thus should be classified as squamous-cell, not epidermoid, carcinoma (Figs. 53–24, 53–25). Approximately 65% to 70% are mature "pearl-forming" tumors and the remainder are poorly differentiated. At present there is no difference in survival between these histologic variants. The average age of all patients with vulvar cancer is 60 to 65 years. Conversely, when the malignancy is preceded by granulomatous disease, a much younger population, aged 35 to 45 years, is affected.

The primary symptom is pruritus, especially if the preceding disease is of the dystrophic type; however, many patients have noted a lump or local irritation for many years. Patients with chronic granulomatous disease or a long-standing benign tumor that has undergone malignant alteration usually complain of mass, local discomfort, and bleeding. Diagnosis is made on examination of the biopsy material. Diagnostic problems lie in differentiating benign proliferating tumors and chronic granulomatous disease from their malignant counterparts.

CLASSIFICATION AND STAGING

The International Federation of Obstetricians and Gynecologists (FIGO) has accepted the following classification of vulvar cancer. To this author the TNM portion of the classification (tumor, nodes, metastases) is cumbersome and would be wisely eliminated.

The final grouping of the FIGO classification, clinical staging, seems sufficient.

TNM Classification

1. *T* *Primary tumor*
   T1 Tumor confined to vulva, 2 cm or less in largest diameter
   T2 Tumor confined to vulva, more than 2 cm in diameter
   T3 Tumor of any size with adjacent spread to urethra and/or vagina and/or perineum and/or anus
   T4 Tumor of any size infiltrating bladder mucosa and/or rectal mucosa, or both, including upper part of urethral mucosa, and/or fixed to bone
2. *N* *Regional lymph nodes*
   NO No nodes palpable
   N1 Nodes palpable in either groin, not enlarged, mobile (not clinically suspicious of neoplasm)
   N2 Nodes palpable in either one or both groins, enlarged, firm, and mobile (clinically suspicious of neoplasm)
   N3 Fixed or ulcerated nodes
3. *M* *Distant metastases*
   MO No clinical metastases
   M1a Palpable deep pelvic lymph nodes
   M1b Other distant metastases
4. If cytology or histology of lymph nodes reveals malignant cells, the symbol + (plus) should be added to N; if such examinations do not reveal malignant cells, the symbol − (minus) should be added to N.

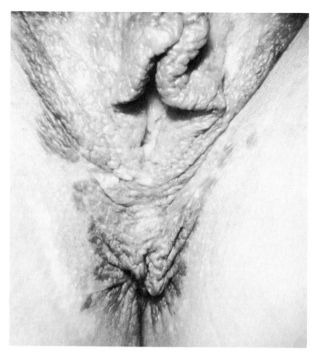

FIG. 53-19. Pigmented carcinoma in situ of vulva.

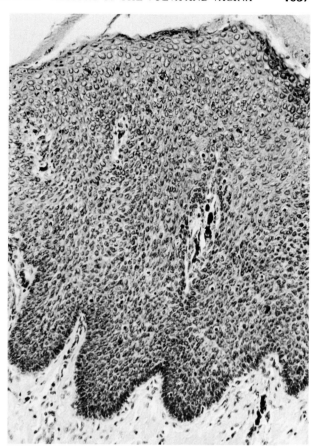

FIG. 53-21. Another pattern of intraepithelial vulvar carcinoma characterized by increase in basal and parabasal cells.

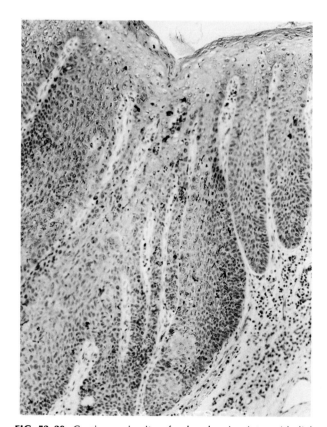

FIG. 53-20. Carcinoma in situ of vulva showing intraepithelial pearl formation and individual cell anaplasia.

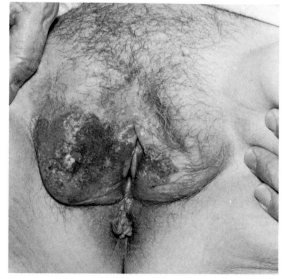

FIG. 53-22. Paget's disease of vulva. Darker areas are grossly red; white patches are evident.

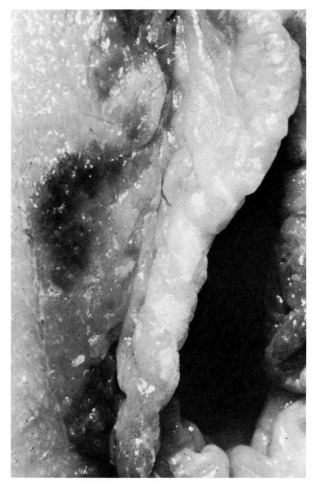

FIG. 53-17. Bowen's disease of vulva. Multiple whitish foci are noted on the *right*. The intervening areas are reddish.

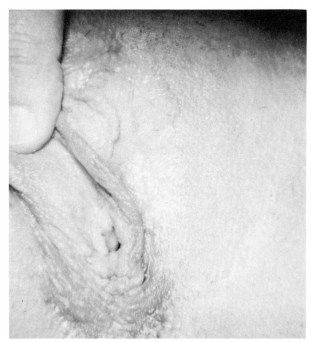

FIG. 53-18. Carcinoma in situ of vulva. Reddish lesion at fourchette, white lesion, left vulva.

of 60 years may be an entirely different disease and thus vulvectomy is more appropriate in such instances unless an isolated focus can be identified. Careful follow-up is essential in either case, since simple excision does not remove the precipitating agent and the potentiality of recurrence always exists, regardless of the surgery, radical or simple. The use of topical chemotherapeutic agents (*e.g.,* 5% fluorouracil cream) have been used with success rates approximating 60% to 75%. Certainly such approaches are worthwhile in the young patient, particularly one whose neoplasia apparently has begun in the background of a condylomatous lesion. More recently an immunologic approach has been used successfully in recurrent, especially pigmented, lesions. The patient is sensitized to dinitrochlorobenzene (DNCB), and the agent is applied locally to the lesions. A severe reaction may occur, and accordingly it is essential to evaluate carefully the strength of the agent needed for each individual patient.

PAGET'S DISEASE

Like its counterpart on the breast, vulvar Paget's disease (Fig. 53–22) is characterized grossly by a fiery red background mottled with white, hyperkeratotic islands and, in this respect, simulates Bowen's disease. Unlike the mammary lesion usually associated with an underlying malignancy, the vulvar disease is intraepithelial in 75% of cases. Nevertheless, the tendency to local recurrence makes the neoplasm a constant threat. Microscopically, the characteristic large, pale cells of apocrine origin are found initially in the basal layer but eventually involve the entire surface epithelium as well as that of the underlying appendages (Fig. 53–23). The positive reaction of the cells to mucicarmine stain serves to differentiate the lesion from Bowen's disease and melanoma.

Therapy primarily demands simple vulvectomy to determine the extent of involvement of the underlying tissues. If invasive disease is recognized in the removed specimen, inguinal and femoral lymph node dissection is indicated. In view of the frequency of recurrence, careful follow-up is mandatory. Radiation has been of little value for the local or metastatic disease. The association with Paget's disease of the breast has been recorded in several studies and, although uncommon in the author's opinion, a thorough study of every patient should be made to rule out a mammary lesion.

and the establishment of diagnosis of carcinoma of the vulva than for any other primary malignancy of the female genitalia. Much of this delay may result from the reluctance of the elderly patient to seek medical advice; however, the 30% to 35% of cases in which the physician is at fault may be related to the commonplace nature of the initial symptom—pruritus. Too often, treatment is suggested over the telephone before thorough study has been carried out.

As noted previously, the dystrophies may show a variety of histologic alterations, described as typical or atypical hyperplasias. The terms atypia and dysplasia are also used to describe atypical hyperplasia.

Vulvar malignancies may be classified as follows:

I. Primary malignancy
  A. Carcinoma in situ
    1. Bowen's disease
    2. Erythroplasia of Queyrat
    3. Carcinoma simplex
  B. Paget's disease
  C. Invasive cancer
    1. Squamous-cell lesions—Well differentiated, others
    2. Basal-cell carcinoma (histologic variations)
    3. Bartholin gland lesions
      a. Squamous-cell lesions
      b. Transitional lesions
      c. Cribriform (adenocystic) lesions
    4. Verrucous carcinoma—This tumor is locally invasive but not metastasizing. The histology is identifiable and the treatment is wide excision. Recurrences are common and often locally destructive.
  D. Other malignancies—Including melanoma (melanotic and amelanotic), sarcoma, lymphoma, embryonal rhabdomyosarcoma
II. Secondary malignancy

CARCINOMA IN SITU

Carcinoma in situ occurs at any age but is not infrequent during the third and fourth decades of life. Although a common complaint is pruritus, the lesion may present as a lump or may be relatively asymptomatic. The gross appearance varies greatly. The Bowenoid lesion is scaly and characterized by a red background dotted with white, hyperkeratotic islands (Fig. 53–17). Other lesions are almost entirely white, red (erythroplasia of Queyrat), or a combination of these patterns (Fig. 53–18).

A rarely described variety of carcinoma in situ is irregularly pigmented, with a diffuse but hazy background of hyperkeratosis (Fig. 53–19). These variable and bizarre patterns demand that many lesions be biopsied to determine their true nature. Of interest is the increased frequency with which multiple areas of

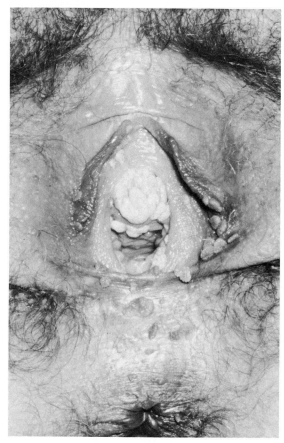

FIG. 53–16. Condylomata acuminata affecting urethea, vagina, and external genitalia.

anaplastic change are noted in the lower genital canal and perianal areas (the anogenital area). Such alterations demand thorough study of the entire region, both initially and at follow-up examinations. Micrographs demonstrate variations in atypical cellular maturation (Figs. 53–20, 53–21).

Of major interest are the variations in the histologic patterns adjacent to invasive cancer and those described as marked atypical hyperplasia or carcinoma in situ. It seems quite possible that viral disease may produce histologic patterns indistinguishable from carcinoma in situ, representing the cases of so-called "reversible atypia."

If multiple foci of malignancy are carefully excluded by use of toluidine blue and random biopsies, wide local excision of the lesion is the acceptable treatment. Thus, although vulvectomy has been the proposed therapy, it is obvious that more conservative approaches are acceptable in most young patients. Conversely, it seems apparent at the present time that carcinoma in situ occurring in the patient over the age

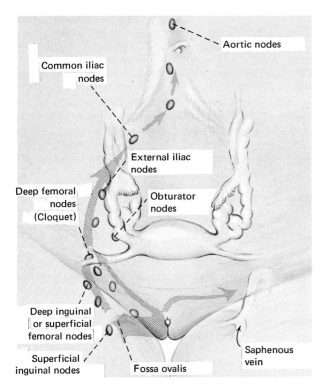

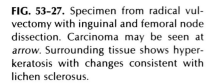

Aortic nodes

Common iliac nodes

External iliac nodes

Deep femoral nodes (Cloquet)

Obturator nodes

Deep inguinal or superficial femoral nodes

Superficial inguinal nodes

Fossa ovalis

Saphenous vein

FIG. 53-26. Lymphatic spread of carcinoma of vulva. Note possible contralateral spread of cancer, especially from anterior vulva and clitoris with possible direct metastasis to Cloquet's node rather than initial involvement of inguinal node. (Modified from Traut HF, Benson RC: Cancer of the Female Genital Tract, 2nd ed. New York, American Cancer Society, 1957)

with lesions extending from 0.75 to 1.5 mm (Clark's levels 1 and 2) are found to have nodal involvement.

Procrastination in treatment is often due to misdiagnosis. Among the last ten cases of malignant melanoma seen by the author, the neoplasm was first diagnosed as a hematoma in two cases and as a hemangioma in one instance. Biopsy is the method of diagnosis, and there is no validity in the opinion that every such lesion must be excised because of the danger of spread induced by biopsy. Furthermore, there is no evidence that the prognosis is worse for lesions that are diagnosed during pregnancy.

Rare cases of *fibrosarcoma* have been reported arising primarily in the external genitalia. Surgery is the treatment of choice, although triple chemotherapy has been suggested by certain authors.

Lymphoma and *embryonal rhabdomyosarcomas* have been reported on the external genitalia. These cases classically arise in young people and the former often represents the superficial demonstration of an underlying lesion.

SECONDARY MALIGNANCIES

Most of these lesions arise in the adjacent area and affect the vulva by direct extension; malignancies of the cervix and rectum are common offenders. Adenocarcinoma of the endometrium and choriocarcinoma show a predilection for metastasizing to the external genitalia and on occasion the diagnosis of trophoblastic malignancy is first made on examination of biopsy material from the vulvar metastasis.

FIG. 53-27. Specimen from radical vulvectomy with inguinal and femoral node dissection. Carcinoma may be seen at *arrow*. Surrounding tissue shows hyperkeratosis with changes consistent with lichen sclerosus.

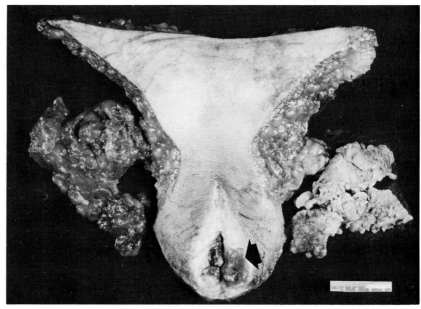

MALIGNANT TUMORS OF THE VAGINA

Primary malignancy arising in the vagina makes up less than 1% of all anaplastic disease arising *de novo* in the genital canal.

Vaginal malignancies may be classified as follows:

I. Primary Malignancy
  A. Carcinoma
    1. Epidermoid carcinoma
      a. In situ
      b. Invasive
    2. Adenocarcinoma
      a. Clear cell (mesonephroid carcinoma arising in adenosis)
      b. Others—Adenocarcinoma in endometrium, *etc.*
  B. Sarcoma
    1. Sarcoma botryoides
    2. Others
      a. Fibro- and leiomyosarcoma
      b. Rhabdomyosarcoma, lymphoma, *etc.*
  C. Melanoma
II. Secondary malignancy, arising from primary lesion in cervix, endometrium, ovary, bowel, vulva, or urinary tract.

The currently accepted FIGO staging for primary carcinoma of the vagina is as follows:

Stage 0:   Carcinoma in situ
Stage I: Carcinoma limited to vaginal wall
Stage II: Carcinoma involving subvaginal tissues but not extending to pelvic sidewall
Stage III: Carcinoma extending to pelvic sidewall
Stage IV: Carcinoma extending beyond true pelvis or involving mucosa of bladder or rectum (extension by bullous edema *per se* does not permit stage IV classification)

IN SITU EPIDERMOID CARCINOMA

In situ carcinoma of the vagina has been described as occurring in three different situations: (1) with other similar lesions in the lower genital canal (regional response to a carcinogen), (2) as residua after incomplete surgery for carcinoma in situ of the cervix, and (3) following radiation for invasive carcinoma of the cervix. Preinvasive changes may be grossly evident prior to the development of invasive disease, but such cases are obviously in a minority. Although asymptomatic, these lesions can be recognized early if routine cytology is performed on all patients and if the possibility of multicentric foci of origin and postirradiation neoplasia is kept in mind.

Similar to invasive disease, in situ malignancy can be treated by surgery and radiation. Since the lesion is superficial, removal is the treatment of choice; however, if the patient is in the third or fourth decade of life, such ablative surgery should be avoided unless the vagina is reconstituted. The latter can be accomplished by immediate covering of the denuded vaginal cavity by skin graft (McIndoe procedure). This procedure has been performed successfully in six consecutive cases in our clinic. More recently the use of local chemotherapeutic agents (topical 5-fluorouracil) has provided a successful and more conservative approach to such lesions. The keratinized tumor and those previously treated with irradiation or other scarifying procedures do not seem to respond as well to the local chemotherapeutic agents as the more classic epidermoid variety.

INVASIVE EPIDERMOID CARCINOMA

This type of cancer is the most common invasive neoplasm of the vagina. Approximately two-thirds of all patients are over the age of 50 years. The common symptom is a bloody vaginal discharge and in many series total vaginal prolapse has been an associated finding (Fig. 53–28). In the more extensive cases, urgency and pain on urination and defecation occur. Diagnosis is confirmed by biopsy. Differential diagnosis lies between primary and secondary malignancy, adenosis, endometriosis, and chronic proliferative inflammatory processes.

Radiotherapy is the most widely accepted treatment for invasive cancer. Intravaginal application of radium or a similar agent plus external radiation are combined as for cervical malignancy, but complications, particularly rectal and vesical, are more common. The use of radium needles has been reported to be effective but should be the option of the radiotherapist in consultation with the clinician.

When invasive carcinoma involves the lower third of the vagina, metastases may appear in the obturator and iliac nodes but not in the inguinal nodes, or the extension may be similar to that of cancer of the vulva (Fig. 53–29). Hence lesions in this area may constitute special problems, depending upon extension. If inguinal nodes are involved, management is usually as that for cancer of the vulva, *i.e.*, radical surgery. Exenterative procedures may be necessary because of frequent involvement of the rectum, bladder, or urethra, or of all three structures.

ADENOCARCINOMA

Primary adenocarcinoma is rare. As noted earlier, interest in recent years has been concentrated on that variety of adenocarcinoma arising in adenosis and de-

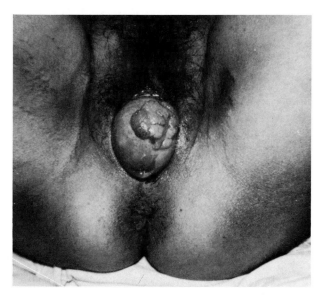

FIG. 53-28. Invasive carcinoma of vagina with total prolapse.

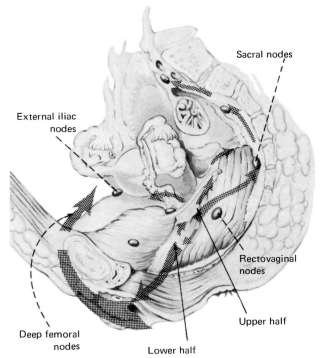

FIG. 53-29. Lymphatic spread of carcinoma of vagina. Extension of cancer of upper half of vagina is similar to that of carcinoma of cervix, while cancer in lower half spreads like vulvar cancer. (Modified from Traut HF, Benson RC: Cancer of the Female Genital Tract, 2nd ed. New York, American Cancer Society, 1957)

veloping most commonly in the young woman (aged 7 to 27 years) whose mother received estrogen therapy during pregnancy. These malignancies are difficult to diagnose in the early stages owing to the infrequency with which the cells are shed from the deeper glandular elements. Colposcopy has offered a means by which the adenosis may be diagnosed but has not been able to determine the early malignant alterations. In view of the rarity of malignant change in such cases (400 cases from a countrywide survey now reside in the registry), it seems that the wisest approach to the patient at risk is careful observance with routine examinations and multiple cytologic and colposcopic studies (Figs. 53–13, 53–30).

If malignancy does arise in the context of adenosis, the treatment most commonly advocated has been surgical. Unfortunately, the latter involves removal of much of the vagina, the uterus, and pelvic lymph nodes. If extension to bladder or rectum is present, even more extensive surgery is necessary. Radiation has been used in a few cases, with reportedly good results. Nevertheless, with only relatively few cases upon which to base judgment, it is difficult, at present, to establish the ideal form of treatment. Preventive measures have been instituted, consisting mainly of the elimination of estrogenic therapy to the pregnant woman.

SARCOMA BOTRYOIDES

Although rare, this grapelike polypoid lesion arising from the lower end at the müllerian tubercle is very aggressive and survivals are few. Occurring in the first

decade of life (two cases have been reported in the newborn), the initial symptom is a bloody vaginal discharge. The gross appearance is almost unmistakable, although foreign bodies and acuminate warts may simulate the botryoid sarcoma. The microscopic picture is characterized by edematous blebs lined by a thin, stratified epithelium. The loose stroma gives the false impression of benignity; however, the elongated, malignant mesodermal elements featuring the rhabdomyoblast can be discerned by careful study.

Therapy has not been satisfactory; however, recently salvage has improved with the use of exenterative surgery (Fig. 53–31), a loathsome procedure in these young children.

OTHER PRIMARY MALIGNANCIES

Fibro- and *leiomyosarcoma* are rare primary malignancies of the vagina, as is the malignant melanoma, although all such lesions have been reported. Prognosis depends upon the extent of the lesion at the time of initial therapy. It should be noted that most of the fibro–leiomyosarcomas in young people are locally aggressive and recurring, but rarely metastasize. The converse is true for the older patient.

Primary endodermal sinus tumors have been re-

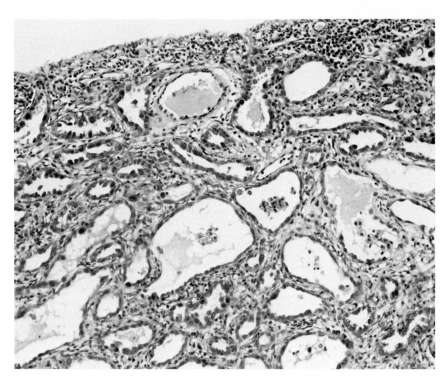

FIG. 53–30. Classic mesonephroid carcinoma arising in vaginal adenosis of 17-year-old girl. Note hobnail pattern.

FIG. 53–31. Sarcoma botryoides, juvenile form. *A.* Gross surgical specimen of lesion from 16-month infant. Tumor arose in vagina and invaded pelvic tissues. Vagina has been split posteriorly to show uterus and tumor. Patient was not given roentgenotherapy, but was treated with Aminopterin, a folic acid antagonist. She was alive and well 8 years later. *B.* Midsagittal section of specimen in *A.* Note lack of involvement of uterus. AFIP Acc. Nos. 218754–693 and 218754–694. (Specimen courtesy of Dr. Sidney Farber. Hertig AT, Gore H: In Anderson WAD (ed): Pathology, 6th ed. St. Louis, CV Mosby, 1971)

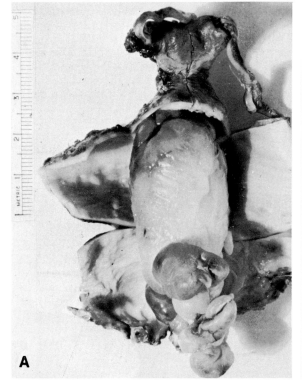

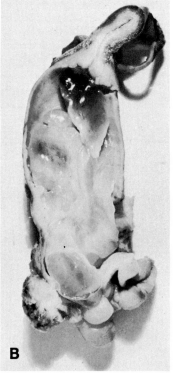

ported as primary lesions in the vagina. Less than 20 cases have now been reported. The vagina actually represents an area close to the terminal portion of the line in the embryo and thus it should not be surprising to see germ-cell tumors in this area. It is important to appreciate their presence, since triple chemotherapy has been effective in controlling these tumors in the ovary and should be instituted for similar lesions in the vagina. Conversely, surgery, as performed for sarcoma botryoides, is certainly not the treatment of choice and irradiation has been classically unsatisfactory for the similar lesion in the ovary.

REFERENCES AND RECOMMENDED READING

Buscema J, Woodruff JD: The significance of the histologic alterations adjacent to invasive vulvar carcinoma. Am J Obstet Gynecol 137:902, 1980

Buscema J, Woodruff JD, Parmley TH, et al: Carcinoma in situ of the vulva. Obstet Gynecol 55:225, 1980

Friedrich EG: Reversible vulvar atypia. Obstet Gynecol 39:173, 1972

Friedrich EG: Vulvar Disease. Philadelphia, WB Saunders, 1976

Friedrich E, Kaufman R, Gardner H, Woodruff JD: The vulvar dystrophies, atypias, and carcinomata in situ: An invitational symposium. J Reprod Med Vol. 17, No. 3, September, 1976

International Society for the Study of Vulvar Disease: New nomenclature for vulvar disease. Obstet Gynecol 47:122, 1976

Japaze, H, Garcia-Bunuel R, Woodruff JD: Primary vulvar neoplasia: A review of in situ and invasive carcinoma, 1935–1972. Obstet Gynecol 49:404, 1977

Kaufman RH, Gardner HL, Brown DJ, et al: Vulvar dystrophies: An evaluation. Am J Obstet Gynecol 120:363, 1974

Woodruff JD, Julian CG, Puray T, et al: The contemporary challenge of carcinoma in situ of the vulva. Am J Obstet Gynecol 115:677, 1973

CHAPTER 54

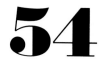

LESIONS OF THE CERVIX UTERI

James A. Merrill
Saul B. Gusberg
Gunter Deppe
Adolf Stafl

BENIGN LESIONS OF THE CERVIX UTERI

James A. Merrill

NONSPECIFIC CHRONIC CERVICAL DISEASE

Chronic cervicitis is characterized by inflammation of the cervical stroma, endocervical glands, and squamous epithelium. The condition is associated with changes in size, shape, and appearance of the cervix and cervical os. Improved obstetric care, the effectiveness of antibiotics in combating acute infections, and the growing trend toward periodic health examinations have done much to reduce the frequency with which the unhealthy or chronically infected cervix is seen.

CLINICAL PICTURE

Chronic cervicitis is a common disorder. Indeed, if one bases the diagnosis on microscopic evidence of inflammation, chronic cervicitis is present in almost every multiparous woman. Few symptoms can be considered specific. The most common symptom is a mucopurulent vaginal discharge; pelvic pain, backache, and dyspareunia are uncommon. Genital spotting or bleeding after douching or intercourse suggests cervical disease. While this may be a symptom of cervicitis, it is more common with malignant than benign disease. Infertility is sometimes attributed to cervical factors, but it is difficult to prove such a causal relation.

Visible and palpatory findings are more reliable than symptoms and serve as the primary basis for diagnosis. The cervix may be hypertrophied and there may be single, bilateral, or multiple lacerations. A tenacious mucopurulent discharge is often seen exuding from the endocervical canal. There may be red areas about the os, occasionally denuded of squamous epithelium. This so-called *erosion* assumes various sizes and shapes, but tends to be irregular. *Nabothian cysts* appear as blue, slightly raised 1-mm to 3-mm nodules on the surface of the cervix and result from mucous distention of endocervical glands or clefts. Healed cervical lacerations often expose portions of the endocervical canal, producing a granular red area termed *eversion*. Erosion, eversion, and ectropion commonly refer to lesions of the exocervix covered by columnar epithelium. Chronic cervical disease may cause tenderness of the cervix or adjacent parametrium. Microscopic examination of the endocervical mucus aids diagnosis. Normal mucus is essentially free of leukocytes; in the presence of chronic inflammation, leukocytes are abundant. It is important to emphasize that all of these findings often are present without producing symptoms.

RELATION TO CANCER

As a cause of significant symptoms, chronic cervicitis is not a great problem. However, there is evidence suggesting some possible relation between benign cervical disease and subsequent malignancy. Carcinoma of the cervix is uncommon in patients who have not been long exposed to chronic inflammation or irritation or who have received adequate treatment for nonmalignant lesions.

CAUSE

Chronic cervicitis may follow the acute infections described in Chapter 50. The most common causes are the trauma and minute lacerations associated with parturition, although cervical inflammation may also

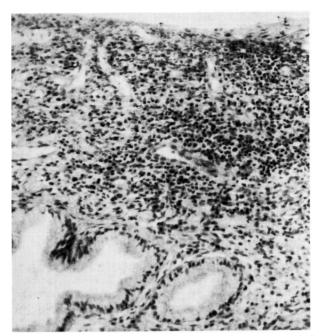

FIG. 54–1. Cervical erosion. Surface squamous epithelium is absent and stroma is densely infiltrated with inflammatory cells.

follow other trauma or instrumentation. Chronic cervicitis is seen commonly in the late postpartum period and becomes worse during pregnancy. Steroid hormones influence the development and appearance of erosions and eversions; thus, cervicitis is commonly observed in women using oral steroid contraception.

PATHOLOGY

Mononuclear leukocytes are collected in the cervical stroma beneath the squamous epithelium and adjacent to endocervical glands. The endocervix may be thrown up into papillary folds, the tips of which are densely infiltrated with leukocytes. There is a proliferation of young capillaries, and the surface epithelium is absent in erosion (Fig. 54–1). With eversion, the endocervical columnar epithelium extends onto the portio.

As a result of inflammation or hormonal variation, the columnar epithelium of the endocervix may be replaced by stratified squamous epithelium, and endocervical glands may become filled with squamous cells. This process is called epidermidalization, squamous metaplasia, prosoplasia, and reserve-cell hyperplasia. *Epidermidalization* refers to the upward growth of squamous epithelium replacing the columnar epithelium. *Squamous metaplasia* implies an *in situ* differentiation of columnar cells into squamous cells (Fig. 54–2), resulting in stratified epithelium with su-

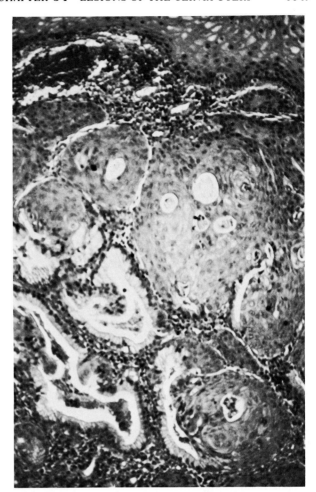

FIG. 54–2. Squamous metaplasia of endocervical glands. Some glands are completely filled with squamous cells; in others, transition from columnar to squamous cells is apparent.

perficial columnar cells and basal cells of squamous appearance. *Reserve-cell hyperplasia* or *prosoplasia* implies growth of cuboidal subcolumnar cells at the squamocolumnar junction which retain the bipotential of differentiation into either columnar or squamous cells. The so-called reserve cells can be identified in the infant cervix and remain throughout adult life. Some authors have suggested that these cells are important in the histogenesis of cancer of the cervix.

A less common pathologic finding is *adenomatous hyperplasia,* an accumulation of closely packed endocervical glands lined by cuboidal epithelium rather than by the typical columnar cells. This lesion, also involving the subcolumnar reserve cells, has been observed in patients taking oral steroid contraceptives. Because of the apparent immaturity of the glands in this situation, the lesion may be mistaken for adenocarcinoma.

TREATMENT

What and how to treat is, in some measure, a matter of philosophy. It is agreed that a patient with symptoms thought to be caused by an unhealthy cervix should be treated. Because evidence suggests a relationship between benign cervical disease and subsequent malignancy, many physicians extend the policy of treatment to include the patient with an unhealthy cervix not causing symptoms and continue treatment until the portio is entirely covered with intact squamous epithelium.

Logically, the treatment of chronic cervical disease should begin with attempts at prevention. Careful management of the obstetric patient, prompt attention to cervical injuries at the time of delivery, and careful treatment of the cervix postpartum reduce the incidence of chronic cervicitis. The best opportunity for treating the cervix is at the postpartum follow-up examination. Before any but the simplest treatment is instituted, adequate measures should be taken to exclude malignant disease. Examination of cervical cells, application of iodine to the cervix (the Schiller test), and biopsy of ulcerated or Schiller-positive areas should be done at the first examination.

We prefer to begin with simple treatment and progress, as needed, to more vigorous forms of therapy. Frequently the diagnostic measures (cervical biopsy) stimulate adequate healing. During pregnancy and in the puerperium, the use of acid douches or jellies may be all that is necessary, since such lesions often heal by physiologic repair mechanisms. Antibiotics have limited value, and systemic administration of antibiotics is indicated only when there is associated infection of the endometrium or parametrial tissues. Sulfonamide-containing vaginal creams may be used if the cervical discharge contains numerous leukocytes and readily apparent bacteria. If the chronic cervical disease is coincident with postmenopausal atrophic vaginal changes, topical application of estrogen is important. Estrogen-containing suppositories or creams are effective.

Chemical cauterization of the cervix may be beneficial in relatively minor chronic cervicitis. Negatol or silver nitrate solution may be applied directly with a cotton-tipped applicator once or twice weekly; a single application is usually without value. Electrocauterization, once the traditional treatment, is accomplished by radial cauterization of the entire surface of the cervix to remove all diseased tissue. Following cauterization, the patient should be instructed to use an antiseptic suppository daily for about 2 weeks.

In recent years, cryosurgery has largely replaced electrocauterization for the treatment of chronic cervicitis. Following cryosurgery, an abnormal-appearing granular cervix may be converted into one that more nearly resembles that of a nulliparous woman. Cryosurgery is performed as an outpatient procedure without anesthesia or analgesia. Liquid freon, carbon dioxide gas, or nitrous oxide may be used as the refrigerant. A probe is chosen that approximates the anatomic configuration of the cervix. Lateral spread of the ice ball usually begins within 10 to 15 seconds after the refrigerant has been circulated. It is important to make certain that the ice extends at least 4 to 5 mm onto the normal-appearing epithelium. Some recommend only a freeze–thaw cycle; others, a freeze, partial thaw, and refreeze cycle. A profuse watery discharge is common for 4 to 6 weeks following cryosurgery.

SPECIFIC CERVICAL DISEASE

ALTERED EPITHELIUM

Congenital erosion is a misnomer for a physiologic process that appears as a symmetric red velvety area surrounding the os. The surface may be slightly elevated in contrast to the shallow depression of the acquired erosion. This condition, common in babies and children, consists of areas of columnar epithelium extending from the cervical canal, over the external os, and onto the portio. Most of these lesions resolve spontaneously. However, a few remain into adult life and result in a clear mucous discharge or become secondarily infected and produce a mucopurulent discharge. The lesion may be encountered at the time of premarital examination. Treatment is seldom necessary but could include cryosurgery.

Leukoplakia describes one or more white, tenacious patches on the portio vaginalis. These cannot be wiped away. Microscopic examination shows surface keratinization of the squamous epithelium with varying degrees of epithelial hyperplasia. In the cervix, leukoplakia is not considered premalignant; however, there may be associated dysplasia. All white plaques should be adequately biopsied and studied microscopically. Specific treatment is not needed, but the lesion should be followed and biopsied again if progression is evident.

CYSTS

A *nabothian cyst* forms as a result of obstruction of the mouth of an endocervical gland and subsequent distention of the gland with mucus. Such cysts rarely produce symptoms or require treatment. They may be evacuated with the electrocautery at the time of surface cauterization or by cryosurgery.

Endometriosis rarely occurs in the cervix. It produces small red or blue, slightly raised cysts 1 to 2 mm in diameter. They may result from seeding at the time of prior curettage. They are pathologic curiosities and require no treatment unless they produce symptoms.

Cysts arising from *remnants of the mesonephric duct* occur in the lateral aspects of the cervix. They are rare and usually measure less than 2.5 mm in diameter. The diagnosis is based upon microscopic examination. The cysts are lined by a low columnar or cuboidal epithelium without intrinsic stroma. Treatment, if necessary, consists of simple excision.

Adenosis describes adenomatous proliferation of endocervical glandular epithelium in the vagina. These lesions, probably of müllerian duct origin, appear as small, slightly raised red foci. Islands of columnar epithelium of endocervical or tubular type are commonly found beneath the lining squamous epithelium of the vagina. Similar lesions may be seen on the portio vaginalis of the cervix. More often, the lesions are seen as extensions of the endocervical mucosa onto all or most of the portio vaginalis. A substantial amount of evidence links the occurrence of adenosis in young women with prenatal exposure to a synthetic estrogen (diethylstilbestrol) or similar nonsteroidal estrogens. Adenosis of the vagina or cervix has been found in as many as 80% of young women so exposed. Clear-cell adenocarcinoma may arise in such areas of adenosis, but this is extremely uncommon. There is no agreement concerning the appropriate method of treating adenosis or whether it need be treated at all. Certainly young women with adenosis should be carefully examined at frequent intervals to be certain that clear-cell carcinoma is not present. Adenosis of the vagina is discussed in Chapter 53.

TUMORS

Aside from chronic inflammation, *polyps* are the most common lesions of the cervix, found at all ages, most often during the reproductive years. They are soft, velvety red lesions, usually pedunculated, protruding from the cervical os. Commonly arising from the lower end of the endocervix, they may arise from the portio vaginalis. They vary in size from a few millimeters to 2 cm in diameter and are rarely larger. The base is usually narrow, but on occasion is broad. They probably develop as the result of inflammatory hyperplasia of endocervical mucosa.

Symptoms are similar to those of chronic cervicitis; the most common is genital bleeding, usually following trauma such as coitus or douching. The diagnosis is made easily by inspection of the cervix. Since many polyps are asymptomatic, genital bleeding should stimulate investigation beyond the polyp for a more significant cause.

Microscopically, the surface is lined by columnar epithelium with areas of ulceration or squamous metaplasia. The stroma frequently is congested and infiltrated by inflammatory cells.

Unless the stalk is large, treatment consists of avulsion of the polyp as an office procedure; however, if

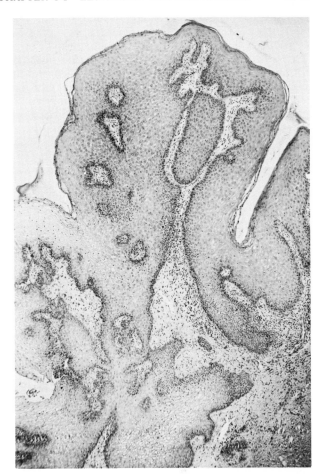

FIG. 54–3. Papilloma of cervix. (Kistner RW, Hertig AT; Obstet Gynecol 6:147, 1955)

there is a history of recent abnormal bleeding, the patient should be admitted to the hospital for curettage. Polyps should be submitted to the laboratory for pathologic examination to exclude coexisting malignancy, although this is uncommon.

Condylomata acuminata rarely involve the cervix and are usually associated with similar lesions of the vulva and vagina.

The cervical *papilloma* (Fig. 54–3) is a soft, gray or red, friable papillary lesion with a broad base, arising from the portio vaginalis. The surface is sometimes hyperkeratotic. It may be indistinguishable from condyloma acuminatum. These lesions, which are rare, are seen more commonly during pregnancy, when they may grow rapidly. They usually regress spontaneously postpartum. There is no evidence that papillomas occurring during pregnancy are related to cervical carcinoma. However, in the nonpregnant state papillomas may show epithelial dysplasia. The symptoms are not

specific, and diagnosis is usually suspected at the time of vaginal examination.

Microscopically, papillomas are composed of stratified squamous epithelium covering fingerlike stalks of fibrous stroma. The stroma may be congested and infiltrated with inflammatory cells. Biopsy may remove a single papilloma. Lesions found in the nonpregnant patient should be excised because of dysplasia. Conservatism and observation are indicated during pregnancy.

Cervical *myomas* and *fibromas* are rare. They appear as smooth, firm masses of varying sizes, replacing a portion or all of the cervix. Large myomas may distort the bladder and produce pressure symptoms. Such tumors are of most concern during pregnancy, when they may interfere with normal vaginal delivery. If the tumor is pedunculated, it may be removed through the vagina; more commonly the tumor must be managed the same as a uterine myoma.

STENOSIS

Stenosis of the cervix may follow chronic cervical infection, treatment for endocervicitis, cauterization or conization of the cervix, cryosurgery, radium therapy, and senile atrophy. Stenosis is usually asymptomatic but may cause abnormal genital bleeding, dysmenorrhea, and infertility. Since stenosis may follow diagnostic conization of the cervix, cervical patency should be ensured by sounding the cervical canal at postoperative examinations. When the stenosis is complete or almost complete, accumulation of cervical or uterine secretions may cause distention of the uterine cavity and secondary infection. Such distention of the uterus with blood (*hematometra*), fluid (*hydrometra*), or exudate (*pyometra*) may be asymptomatic for long periods or may produce cramping abdominal pain. Differential diagnosis includes the soft or cystic tumors occurring in the pelvis. Diagnosis is established by initial inability to pass a uterine sound or small probe and subsequent release of fluid when the canal is opened. It may be necessary to sound the cervical canal under anesthesia. Many gynecologists believe that a gentle attempt to sound the uterine cavity should be a routine part of each pelvic examination. Treatment consists of cervical dilatation and maintenance of patency with a drain.

REFERENCES AND RECOMMENDED READING

Farrar HK Jr, Nedoss BR: Benign tumors of the uterine cervix. Am J Obstet Gynecol 81:124, 1961

Fluhmann CF: The Cervix Uteri and Its Diseases. Philadelphia, WB Saunders, 1961

Fluhmann CF: Histogenesis of acquired erosions of the cervix uteri. Am J Obstet Gynecol 82:970, 1961

Gardner HL: Cervical endometriosis, a lesion of increasing importance. Am J Obstet Gynecol 84:170, 1962

Hellman LM: Changes in cervical epithelium during pregnancy. Prog Gynecol 3:433, 1957

Henderson PH, Buck CE: Cervical leukoplakia. Am J Obstet Gynecol 82:887, 1961

Huffman JW: Mesonephric remnants in the cervix. Am J Obstet Gynecol 56:23, 1948

Kistner RW, Hertig AT: Papillomas of the uterine cervix: Their malignant potentiality. Obstet Gynecol 6:147, 1955

Kolstad P: Diagnosis and management of precancerous lesions of the cervix uteri. Int J Gynaecol Obstet 8:551, 1970

Kyriakos M, Kempson RL, Konikov NF: A clinical and pathologic study of endocervical lesions associated with oral contraceptives. Cancer 22:99, 1968

Marchant PJ: Hemangioma of the cervix. Obstet Gynecol 17:191, 1961

Melody GF: Obstructed cervix: A study of 100 patients. Obstet Gynecol 10:190, 1957

Merrill JA: Treatment of non-malignant unhealthy cervix: Cervicitis. GP 23:94, 1961

MALIGNANT LESIONS OF THE CERVIX UTERI

Saul B. Gusberg, Gunter Deppe

The unique accessibility of the cervix uteri to cell and tissue study and to direct physical examination has permitted the intensive investigation of incipient uterine cancer and has enabled us to learn a great deal about the histogenesis of cervical and endometrial cancer. While this knowledge is as yet incomplete, it has taught us that most of these tumors have a gradual, rather than explosive, onset and that their precursors may exist in a reversible form that is followed by a stage of surface, or in situ, development for some years. While these phases may be asymptomatic, they are detectable by methods now available. This developmental concept of uterine cancer has convinced many gynecologists that complete control of these diseases will be possible in the foreseeable future; we can expect to eradicate death from uterine cancer by the diagnostic and therapeutic techniques now at our command.

PRECURSORS OF SQUAMOUS CELL CARCINOMA

Those lesions in which the full thickness of the epithelium is composed of undifferentiated neoplastic cells are referred to as *carcinoma in situ* (Fig. 54–4), and the term *dysplasia* is used for all other precancerous disorders of the epithelium which are subdivided into mild, moderate, and severe grades (Fig. 54–5). Be-

FIG. 54-4. Carcinoma in situ of cervix. Spindle-shaped, dark-staining epithelial cells rise to surface layers. (McKay DG, Terjan B, Poschyachinda D, Younge PA, Hertig AT: Obstet Gynecol 13:2, 1959)

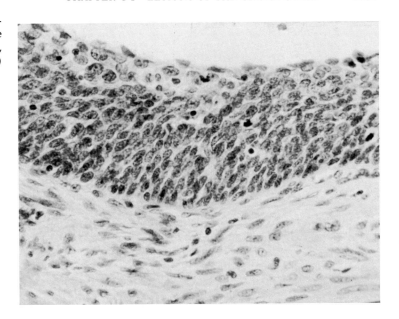

FIG. 54-5. Dysplasia of cervix. This microscopic view shows hyperchromatism and pleomorphism of nuclei of upper half of epithelial layer and evidence of increased growth rate in basal half. This lesion corresponds to CIN 2. (McKay DG, Terjan B, Poschyachinda D, Younge PA, Hertig AT: Obstet Gynecol 13:2, 1959)

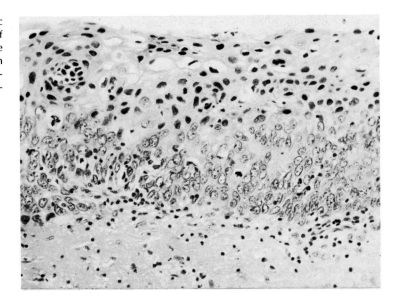

cause of the lack of sharp divisions, these early forms have been called CIN—*cervical intraepithelial neoplasia*—and are divided into three grades: CIN 1 (mild dysplasia), CIN 2 (moderate dysplasia), and CIN 3 (severe dysplasia and carcinoma in situ).

GROSS APPEARANCE

In this early period the squamous epithelium that harbors the incipient tumor has no features discernible by the naked eye which distinguish it from normal squamous epithelium. However, the application of Schiller's iodine solution to the portio of the cervix reveals the area involved by cervical intraepithelial neoplasia in 80% of cases (Fig. 54–6). Schiller's iodine stains normal mucosa dark brown by virtue of its reaction with the glycogen in the cytoplasm of the normal, mature squamous cells. In contrast, the cells in CIN contain less glycogen and fail to stain with the iodine, leaving an unstained region, usually sharply demarcated from the surrounding normal epithelium. The

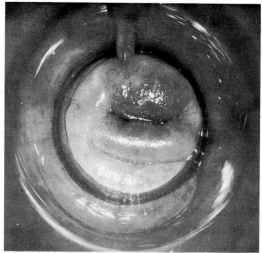

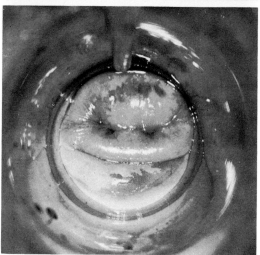

FIG. 54–6. Cervix with CIN. *Top.* Natural appearance. *Bottom.* Stained with Schiller's iodine. Neoplastic focus is outlined as geographic, irregular Schiller-positive area.

of great importance practically. This implies that squamous carcinoma of the cervix *usually arises* in the squamous epithelium at this junction between the two different epithelial types. It is noteworthy that the histologic squamocolumnar junction is not always located at the external os of the cervix. In patients with CIN the squamocolumnar junction is often located out on the portio, owing to eversion of the endocervix or erosion near the os. This spilling out of columnar mucous epithelium onto the portio places most dysplasia within the direct vision and reach of the gynecologist during vaginal examination. However, occasionally the squamocolumnar junction is above the external os, within the endocervical canal, and cannot be directly visualized. Care must be taken in any biopsy method to sample the squamocolumnar junction regardless of its gross anatomic location.

HISTOLOGIC CHARACTERISTICS

Since the unaided eye and the Schiller test are inadequate to establish the diagnosis, the identification of CIN depends entirely upon microscopic examination. Three microscopic methods are available for establishing the diagnosis: (1) biopsy with histologic examination, (2) cervical smear with cytologic examination, and (3) colposcopic examination.

Histologic examination is the definitive diagnostic tool. CIN is, in essence, a disturbance of growth, and the cellular changes are predominantly in the nuclei. Nuclear changes are the hallmarks of neoplasia in most tissues of the body.

Nuclear Pleomorphism. The nuclei of all layers of the squamous epithelium are variable in size and shape. Many nuclei are enlarged and vesicular, some are small, and the nuclear membrane is irregular and wrinkled rather than rounded and smooth. The enlargement of the nucleus results in an increase in the nucleocytoplasmic ratio.

Hyperchromatism. The nuclear material is usually clumped into coarse granules, giving the cell a darker staining quality. Often the nucleus is pyknotic, consisting of one dense ball of DNA in which no nuclear details can be discerned. These pyknotic cells are found in greatest number in the surface layers.

Multinucleation. Cells containing two nuclei are abundant in dysplasia. Cells with as many as ten nuclei in a syncytium are common and are essentially tumor giant cells.

Mitoses. Not only is there an increased number of normal mitoses, but abnormal mitoses are frequent. The latter may have three or four spindles but often

unstained area is referred to as *Schiller-positive.* It is important to emphasize that not all Schiller-positive areas on the portio of the cervix are neoplastic tissue. The majority are benign lesions such as leukoplakia, leukoparakeratosis, erosions, or ectropion. Thus, the usefulness of the Schiller test lies not in its diagnostic ability but in its ability to outline the area that must be biopsied. With the increased practice of colposcopy the nonspecific Schiller's test is being used less frequently in the diagnosis of cervical neoplasia.

CIN is usually found at the junction of the portio squamous epithelium and the columnar mucous epithelium of the endocervix. The fact that the earliest stage of cancer of the cervix is located at the squamocolumnar junction is of great interest theoretically and

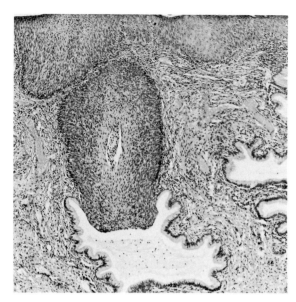

FIG. 54–7. Carcinoma in situ of cervix with involvement of endocervical gland.

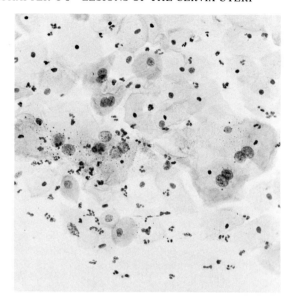

FIG. 54–8. Exfoliated cells from CIN. Neoplastic cells are binucleate and nuclei are considerably larger than those of surrounding normal squamous cells. (Takeuchi A, McKay DG: Obstet Gynecol 15:134, 1960)

take the form of multiple giant chromosomes scattered irregularly throughout the cytoplasm of the cell. These polyploid mitoses are responsible for the appearance of the multinucleated giant cells. From its point of origin at the squamocolumnar juntion CIN spreads out onto the epithelial surfaces. It appears to spread more readily into the endocervix, destroying and replacing the columnar mucous epithelium as it advances. It spreads along the actual lining of the canal, but also grows downward into endocervical glands and may ultimately completely replace the mucous epithelium of the gland (Fig. 54–7). The tumor may spread over a large area and involve many endocervical glands before it invades connective tissue, although the extent varies from patient to patient and some small tumors may invade early. Only the inability to penetrate the basement membrane and to invade the stroma differentiates CIN grade 3 carcinoma in situ from an invasive cancer.

Other Changes. In addition to the changes in individual cells there are changes in the relations of cells to each other. This is best seen in the basal layer that shows a disturbance in polarity, with cells growing haphazardly in every direction instead of having the normal palisaded arrangement. Also, the basal layer, instead of being one cell thick, is usually several cells thick; this change is referred to as *basal cell hyperplasia*. Another abnormality in CIN is the appearance of cornification at the epithelial surface. There may be a thick layer of anuclear cells or a persistence of pyknotic nuclei in cornified cells. This hyperkeratosis and

parakeratosis led to the term *dyskeratosis* as a synonym for this condition.

CYTOLOGIC CHARACTERISTICS

The Papanicolaou stain of cervical smears is primarily used as a screening test for the detection of neoplasia. It has a false-negative rate of 10% to 30%. CIN can be identified by alterations in the nuclei, such as enlargement and irregularity, hyperchromatism and pyknosis, and multinucleated cells (Fig. 54–8). The subclassification of cervical neoplasia into grades can be accomplished by using a cell-counting technique that is based upon the histologic definition of the stages of cervical intraepithelial neoplasia. It relies upon the fact that the greater the degree to which the epithelium is replaced by undifferentiated cells, the more likely such cells are to exfoliate and to be found in the smear. In CIN grade 2, 10% to 20% of the atypical cells are of basal type and in CIN grade 3, 30% or more of the atypical cells are of basal type.

COLPOSCOPIC CHARACTERISTICS

By using a microscope with epiillumination which is capable of magnifying from 6 to 40 times one can observe the histologic appearance of the surface layers of the epithelium of the cervix in the living patient. The

use of the colposcope and interpretation of the findings are discussed later in this chapter.

DEVELOPMENT OF INVASIVE CARCINOMA FROM CERVICAL INTRAEPITHELIAL NEOPLASIA

The cervical cancer precursors form a continuum without clearly identifiable subsets. Different grades are often found adjacent to each other, and one stage of the disease seems to merge into the next. Spontaneous regressions in the absence of biopsy or other types of therapy are unusual. The course of cervical intraepithelial neoplasia in individual patients is unpredictable.

Richart followed 557 women ascertained as having dysplasia by three abnormal pap smears using only cytology and colpomicroscopy as diagnostic procedures. He found that the progression rate increases with increasing grade of CIN and that the transit time to carcinoma in situ was approximately 85 months for very mild dysplasia, 38 months for moderate dysplasia, 12 months for severe dysplasia, and 44 months for all of the dysplasias combined.

Progression rates to invasive cancer are higher in CIN grade 3 (carcinoma in situ) than in earlier states.

The great practical importance of cervical intraepithelial neoplasia is obvious, since recognition at this stage of development permits complete cure of the disease by appropriate treatment.

Invasive carcinoma of the cervix is associated with a high degree of aneuploidy. All grades of CIN may have an aneuploid chromosome distribution pattern and an abnormal nuclear DNA content. These findings support the view that CIN is a preinvasive neoplasm.

EPIDEMIOLOGY

The epidemiology of cervical neoplasia has been studied in great detail and several studies have shown that the disease is found more often in women of low socioeconomic status, women with early age of first coitus, female prostitutes, women having coitus with uncircumcised or multiple partners, and women who are infected with herpesvirus type 2. The occurrence rate of squamous carcinoma of the cervix is very low among Jewish women when compared with non-Jewish women—a ratio of about 1:5. Similarly, carcinoma in situ is one-sixth as common in Jewish as in non-Jewish women. In the opposite direction, black women have twice the occurrence rate of invasive carcinoma of the cervix and twice the rate of in situ cancer when compared with white women. Possibly both genetic and socioeconomic factors are operative. Since squamous cell carcinoma is virtually absent in virgins, it would appear that the carcinogen, whatever its nature, is trans-

mitted by coitus and that cervical neoplasia may be a venereal disease.

INVASIVE CARCINOMA

The neoplastic process becomes potentially dangerous to the patient only when the tumor breaks from its intraepithelial confines and invades the stroma of the cervix. Early invasion occurs predominantly from in situ carcinoma in endocervical glands. Early invasion may occur from multiple sites simultaneously. Long strands or cords of tumor cells may extend for relatively long distances in the cervical connective tissue and, here and there, break their way into lymph vessels and venules. It is curious to note that at the point of invasion the cells tend to become well differentiated. In the in situ stage growth is rapid and little or no differentiation occurs, but invasion of stroma is associated with the development of abundant acidophilic cytoplasm, a forerunner of the "epidermoid pearl" so common in well-developed carcinomas. It may be necessary to take many, even serial, sections of a cervix to find one or two foci of early invasion. Patients with early stromal invasion have survived for a long time with no evidence of recurrence after simple total hysterectomy.

HISTOLOGIC CHARACTERISTICS

Squamous cell carcinoma of the cervix makes up 95% of cervical cancers and can be arbitrarily classified into three basic histologic grades:

Grade I. Well-differentiated squamous-cell carcinoma is composed of sheets and cords of cells with abundant acidophilic cytoplasm, clearly visible intercellular bridges, and often the production of variable amounts of keratin. The formation of the epidermoid pearl is characteristic of these well-differentiated tumors, and relatively few mitoses are found. Grade I tumors constitute about 5% of squamous-cell cancers of the cervix.

Grade II. This is the most common variety and is characterized by masses and cords of spindle-shaped squamous cells with elongated nuclei and scant cytoplasm. There may be a few areas in which the cells have become enlarged and well differentiated to form pearls, but in general there are no intercellular bridges and little keratin formation. Mitoses are frequent (Fig. 54–9); 85% of squamous-cell carcinomas are in this category.

Grade III. Undifferentiated tumors have a rapid growth rate, with numerous mitoses and cells with closely crowded nuclei and scant cytoplasm. These tumors are

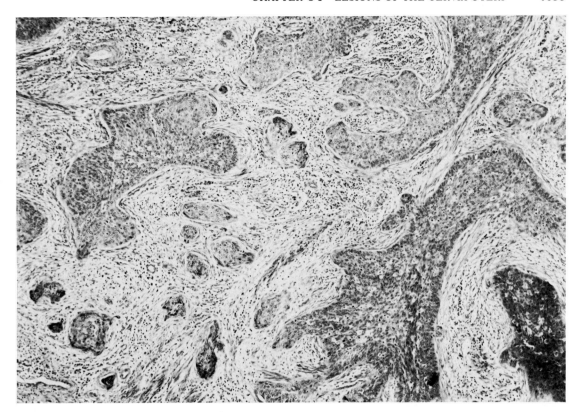

FIG. 54-9. Grade II invasive squamous cell carcinoma of cervix.

difficult to recognize as having originated in squamous cells and constitute approximately 10% of cervical squamous cell tumors.

In general, a tumor is diagnosed according to its best-differentiated portion and graded according to the least-differentiated part. Histologic grading has been used for prognosis and prediction of radiation sensitivity of a given tumor. In practice, histologic grading is useful in describing the variants of cervical cancer for purposes of pathologic diagnosis but is less useful than clinical staging in prognosis or in selection of therapy. Lymphatic penetration and attraction of a collar of lymphocytes can serve as indices of tumor virulence.

GROSS APPEARANCE

As the neoplasm invades, it expands locally and grows out onto the portio and into the stroma of the endocervix. Growth may be predominantly in one of these two directions. Exophytic tumors are more common (64%) than endophytic ones (36%). A friable, granular, red and yellow fungating mass centering around the external os or causing destruction of the entire portio is characteristic. The lesion may be ulcerated

and covered with a patchy necrotic surface, or it may have a purulent, sanguineous, or serous exudate. It usually bleeds readily following slight trauma (Fig. 54–10).

Endophytic tumors may be very deceptive on vaginal examination and present only an enlargement of the cervix with no ulceration or apparent damage to the portio epithelium. A tumor that has remained confined to the cervix up to the time of treatment is comparable to Stage I of the clinical international classification (see section on Clinical Staging).

SPREAD OF TUMOR BEYOND THE CERVIX

Vaginal Extension. The friable fungating tumor may spread outward onto the fornices and down the vaginal wall. If this is the only location in which the tumor has grown beyond the cervix and it does not involve the lower third of the vagina, it corresponds to Stage IIA of the international classification.

Lateral Extension. Extension into one or both broad ligaments is frequent. If one or both broad ligaments are involved and yet the tumor does not extend to the

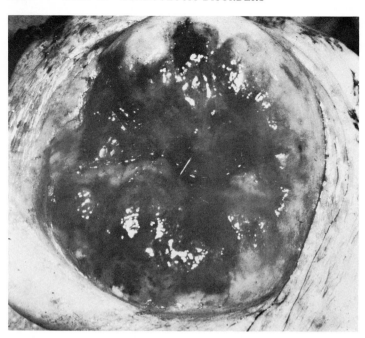

FIG. 54–10. Gross appearance of squamous cell carcinoma of cervix.

lateral wall of the pelvis, the tumor corresponds to Stage IIB.

Endometrial Extension. Direct growth upward into the endometrial cavity occurs, but is not common.

Lymphatic Spread. Lymphatic vessels are invaded even by early tumors. The tumor tends to accommodate itself to the lumen of the lymph channel and propagate along it by direct extension. Tiny fragments of the tumor break off and lodge in the next lymph node, where they die or continue to grow and destroy the lymph node. Tumor emboli are then cast off to the lymph node lying next in the lymphatic chain or, in the case of obstruction to the flow of lymph in the first node, retrograde metastases occur. Although there is considerable variation from one case to the next, the most frequently involved nodes are the paracervical, hypogastric, obturator, and external iliac, which are called the primary lymph nodes. The secondary nodes—the sacral, common iliac, aortic, and inguinal—are less frequently involved. Lymph node metastases are found in approximately the following incidence: Stage I, 15%; Stage II, 30%; Stage III, 50%; and Stage IV, over 60%.

If, at the time of discovery, a tumor extends to the lateral pelvic wall either by continuous involvement of the broad ligaments or by nodular implants on the wall, it corresponds to Stage IIIB of the clinical international classification. A less common variant, corresponding to Stage IIIA, is a tumor involving the lower third of the vagina.

Blood Vessel Invasion. Blood vessel invasion occurs with lymphatic invasion and may be seen even in early tumors, although it is more extensive in the later stages. Arteries are seldom involved; most blood vessel invasion is into venules or veins. Invasion of blood vessels and lymphatics allows spread to distant parts of the body. Approximately 30% of patients dying of cervical cancer have metastases in the liver, lungs, spleen and, rarely, other viscera.

When a cervical cancer has spread to distant lymph nodes and to other viscera, it corresponds to Stage IVB of the clinical international classification. A tumor is classified as Stage IVA when it invades the bladder or rectum, in which case vesicovaginal or rectovaginal fistula may result.

It should be emphasized that the international classification is a clinical preoperative or pretreatment evaluation of the extent of the tumor and may not delineate the actual pathologic or anatomic extent found at the time of surgery or autopsy.

ADENOCARCINOMA

Approximately 5% of cervical cancers arise from the columnar mucous epithelium lining the endocervical canal and endocervical glands and have the histologic pattern of adenocarcinoma. Grossly, the tumors usually arise within the endocervix and grow in a papillary or ulcerative fashion. Occasionally, they develop into polyps. They tend to grow deep into the cervical stroma before they erode onto the portio and may remain clinically silent until late in the life of the tumor.

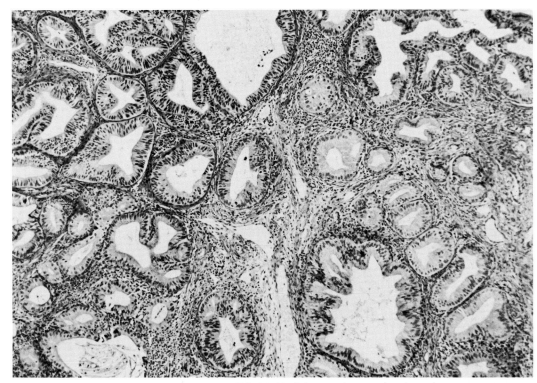

FIG. 54–11. Adenocarcinoma of endocervix.

Growth into the endocervical stroma produces enlargement and often fragility of the cervix. Microscopically, the tumor is usually a mucinous adenocarcinoma associated with papillae and neoplastic glands (Fig. 54–11). As the tumor grows, it becomes less well differentiated and grows in solid sheets of mucin-containing cells with few remnants of its previous glandular architecture. Adenocarcinoma of the cervix has approximately the same prognosis and general clinical behavior as squamous cell carcinoma.

CAUSES OF DEATH FROM CERVICAL CANCER

Cervical cancer causes death by uremia, infection, or hemorrhage. Uremia is caused by compression of the ureter by cancer and fibrous tissue, which produces hydronephrosis and pyelonephritis (see Fig. 49–4). This is the most common cause of death, not only in untreated patients with cervical cancer (60%) but in treated patients as well (50%). Infection, the second most common cause of death, may be a local pelvic abscess or may spread to the peritoneum or bloodstream, causing death from bacterial endotoxin shock. Infection is responsible for approximately 40% of deaths. Uncontrollable hemorrhage causes death in approximately 2% to 7% of patients.

DIAGNOSIS OF CERVICAL CANCER

It is important for us to remember and also to educate our patients about the importance of lawless or noncyclic uterine bleeding, including postcoital spotting, intermenstrual bleeding, and postmenopausal bleeding, since these phenomena may indicate uterine ulceration. The direct transmission of the blood through the vaginal canal to the body surface makes these symptoms apparent to the patient promptly, but we must teach her to consult her physician for diagnostic evaluation. These considerations are of crucial importance in the management of this disease, since the conventional constitutional symptoms of pain and weight loss can make no contribution to the salvation of patients with uterine cancer; these latter symptoms are present in advanced, usually inoperable, disease only.

PREINVASIVE PHASE (CERVICAL INTRAEPITHELIAL NEOPLASIA)

All patients with cervical intraepithelial neoplasia are asymptomatic with respect to these lesions. The median age for CIN is about 10 years younger than the age for invasive cancer of the cervix. Since these cell disturbances do not cause ulceration of the cervix, the patient does not exhibit abnormal uterine bleeding. In

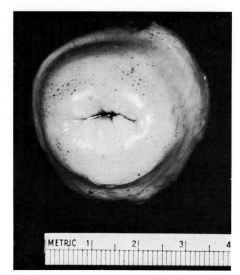

FIG. 54–12. Carcinoma in situ in healthy-appearing cervix. Congestion is operative distortion.

some, the lesion causes enough fragility of the epithelium to result in bleeding on contact, so that an alert patient may note staining after douching, examination, or coitus. In our series, 61% of patients with carcinoma in situ were completely asymptomatic, and more than one-half of the remainder harbored other pelvic abnormalities probably responsible for the symptoms.

The physical examination is not usually helpful in the diagnosis of carcinoma in situ, since there is no characteristic feature of palpation or inspection of the cervix. Intraepithelial carcinoma may be present in a cervix that appears perfectly healthy and epithelialized on speculum examination (Fig. 54–12), or it may be present in an innocent-appearing, so-called erosion or ectropion. In unusual instances one may detect some minimal changes such as exuberance or florid convexity in an erosion, or a whitish leukoplakic cast to the epithelium, but these are uncommon.

Cell Smear

Faced with the problem of detecting these important lesions in patients who are asymptomatic and in whom no significant changes are detectable on examination, one can understand readily the enormous benefit that accrues from the cytologic study method of Papanicolaou. This method may indeed be responsible for the ultimate control of cervical cancer. Certainly, it outstrips by far any therapeutic advance made in the past decade. The reasons for its unique significance are:

1. It is a simple clinical test; obtaining the sample is easy for the physician and free of discomfort to the patient.

2. It is applicable to asymptomatic women as a screening measure, since no lesion need be present to sample. It is a general uterine epithelial sample, in a sense.
3. As a stimulus to biopsy it has enabled tissue documentation of the earliest development of cervical cancer.
4. Its detection efficiency of 90% or more permits treatment at a stage when cure is almost certain. Many women already owe their lives to this method.

Taking the sample of uterine secretion is direct and easy but requires several precautions. The smears must be obtained before bimanual vaginal examination or introduction of lubricating jelly, which distorts the morphologic picture. A clean, dry speculum should be introduced into the vagina and samples taken of secretion from the portio of the cervix at the squamocolumnar junction or transformation zone and from the endocervical canal; we prefer to take the first with an Ayre spatula and the second with a pipet or cotton-tipped swab. Since the cervical cancer precursors have been shown to be a continuum, the designation cervical intraepithelial neoplasia (CIN) grades 1, 2, and 3 has increasingly been utilized in cytologic and histologic classifications of cervical cancer precursors.

A classification introduced by Richart is as follows:

Normal or atypical benign
CIN grade 1 (mild dysplasia)
CIN grade 2 (moderate-severe)
CIN grade 3 (severe dysplasia and carcinoma in situ)
Invasive squamous cell carcinoma
Adenocarcinoma
Atypical cells present; repeat to rule out
Specimen insufficient for diagnosis

The cytologic screening method has been implemented by mass surveys of adult asymptomatic women in various parts of the country. These surveys show a prevalence rate of 0.3% to 1.6% for cervical cancer, the disparity depending upon the type of population sampled. Since increasing age and lower socioeconomic status, together with some ethnic considerations, are associated with a higher incidence of cervical cancer, these differences in case finding are readily understandable.

Biopsy

Since treatment cannot be instituted on the basis of a cell smear without tissue documentation, the abnormal smear must be followed by a cervical biopsy. In the patient whose cervix is normal in appearance or harbors a symmetric, innocent-looking erosion, a general sample must be obtained of the squamocolumnar junction or transformation zone, since this is the site of origin of almost all cervical cancer. This can be done by taking a punch biopsy as an outpatient procedure (no

anesthetic is required), utilizing the Schiller iodine staining method or colposcopy to define areas of abnormality. Unfortunately, the columnar epithelium of the erosion so commonly present in the multiparous cervix also fails to take the Schiller stain, so that the physician's knowledge of the precise area of malignant transformation is not advanced significantly in some cases. More efficient and definitive tissue sampling is achieved by the circumferential (coning) biopsy that encompasses the entire squamocolumnar junction and the lower portion of the cervical canal. For suspicious smears, this may be done as an outpatient procedure using the endocervical punch (Fig. 54–13) or by directed biopsy under colposcopy, but clearly positive smears are best confirmed by a coning biopsy taken under anesthesia with the scalpel. Diagnostic curettage should accompany this to rule out invasive cancer in the canal, since it is clear that the invasive phase of this tumor commonly starts in this region.

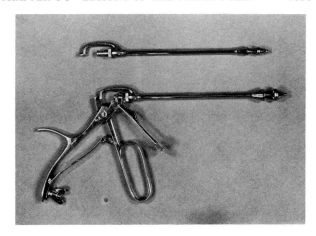

FIG. 54–13. Endocervical punch (SB Gusberg).

Colposcopy

Colposcopy (described later in this chapter) has gained a firm position as the step between an abnormal result of cell study and final diagnosis. It enables localization of the lesion so that a "directed" biopsy can be obtained. Its use may save the patient the expense of hospitalization and anesthesia if dysplasia only is disclosed, but cone biopsy under anesthesia is generally preferred as the definitive diagnostic procedure if the local biopsy discloses later forms of CIN; in this way invasive carcinoma can be ruled out.

Summary

The diagnosis of preinvasive carcinoma of the cervix can be summarized as follows:

Smear suspicious ──────▶ Repeat smear
Repeat smear suspicious ─▶ Colposcopic examination and biopsy (outpatient procedure)
Smear positive ──────▶ Colposcopic biopsy (outpatient procedure) or cone biopsy (hospital procedure)
Colposcopic biopsy shows cancer in situ ──────▶ Cone biopsy
Cone biopsy shows cancer in situ ──────▶ Plan treatment

INVASIVE PHASE

Since the patient usually arrives for diagnostic appraisal with a history of abnormal bleeding, one may expect to find an ulcerated or friable lesion on the cervix. Certainly, the presence of a red, raised, friable

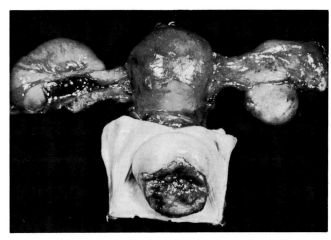

FIG. 54–14. Typical invasive carcinoma of cervix in radical hysterectomy specimen.

lesion such as depicted in Figure 54–14 demands immediate biopsy. No reassurance can be offered such a patient without the completion of diagnostic tests.

Bimanual examination permits an appraisal of cervical infiltration, tumor protrusion, or vaginal extension. Speculum examination allows visual confirmation of this palpation, and rectovaginal examination offers the best appraisal of parametrial infiltration.

Results of cytologic examination are positive except in the unusual massively necrotic lesion whose cell exfoliation is so morphologically disturbed that smear clarity cannot be attained.

Biopsy can be accomplished with a variety of sharp instruments because the friable, raised lesion is easy to sample. Among the most efficient is the Gaylord punch (Fig. 54–15), although scissors, scalpel, curet, or

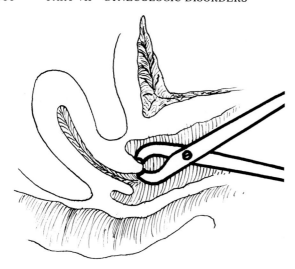

FIG. 54–15. Punch biopsy technique.

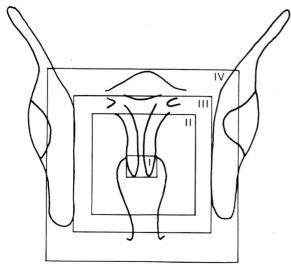

FIG. 54–16. Clinical stages of carcinoma of cervix *I*. Cervix only. *II*. Involvement of parametrium or upper two-thirds of vagina. *III*. Extension to pelvic sidewalls or involvement of lower third of vagina. *IV*. Extension outside reproductive tract. (After DC Morton)

other cutting instrument is frequently equally useful. No anesthetic or other preparation is necessary for such a biopsy and significant bleeding is unusual. Furthermore, there need be no fear of disseminating the cancer, for it is the extruded surface of the tumor that is approached. This diagnostic plan is completed by examination and curettage under anesthesia, for extension in the cervical canal is an important aspect of the growth of this tumor. Precise appraisal of the extent of

the lesion is mandatory before staging can be meaningful and therapy efficient.

CLINICAL STAGING

An international convention of staging permits comparison of results of treatment between institutions and definition of codes of treatment within an institution. *Stage* refers to the clinical extension of disease, *class* to the cytologic smear reading, and *grade* to the differentiation of the tumor by histologic examination.

The staging of cancer of the cervix is a clinical appraisal, preferably confirmed under anesthesia; it is not changed if later findings at surgery or subsequent treatment reveal further advancement of the disease. It is appropriate to consider that Stage I lesions may already have microscopic metastases to the pelvic lymph nodes in some instances, but the gross clinical findings alone are used for the stage designation, in accordance with the international classification. The stage designations for cancer of the cervix are diagramed in Figure 54–16.

The revised FIGO classification is as follows:

Stage 0	Carcinoma in situ, intraepithelial carcinoma
Stage I	The carcinoma strictly confined to the cervix (extension to the corpus should be disregarded)
Stage IA	Microinvasive carcinoma (early stromal invasion)
Stage IB	All other cases of Stage I; occult cancer should be marked "occ"
Stage II	The carcinoma extends beyond the cervix, but has not extended to the pelvic wall; it involves the vagina, but not as far as the lower third
Stage IIA	No obvious parametrial involvement
Stage IIB	Obvious parametrial involvement
Stage III	The carcinoma has extended to the pelvic wall. On rectal examination, there is no cancer-free space between the tumor and the pelvic wall. The tumor involves the lower third of the vagina. All cases with hydronephrosis or nonfunctioning kidney are included.
Stage IIIA	No extension to the pelvic wall
Stage IIIB	Extension to the pelvic wall and/or hydronephrosis or nonfunctioning kidney
Stage IV	The carcinoma has extended beyond the true pelvis or has clinically involved the mucosa of the bladder or rectum. A bullous edema as such does not permit a case to be allotted to Stage IV.
Stage IVA	Spread of the growth to adjacent organs
Stage IVB	Spread to distant organs

Qualifications in Staging Cervical Cancer. Stage IA (microinvasive carcinoma) represents those cases of epithelial abnormalities in which histologic evidence of early stromal invasion is definite. The diagnosis is based upon microscopic examination of tissue removed by biopsy, conization, portio amputation, or removal of the uterus. Cases of early stromal invasion should thus be allotted to Stage IA.

The remainder of Stage I cases should be allotted to Stage IB. As a rule, these cases can be diagnosed by routine clinical examination.

Occult cancer is a histologically invasive cancer that cannot be diagnosed by routine clinical examination. As a rule, it is diagnosed on a cone specimen, the amputated portio, or on the removed uterus. Such cancers should be included in Stage IB and should be marked "Stage IB, occ." Stage I cases can thus be indicated in the following ways:

Stage IA   Carcinoma in situ with early stromal invasion diagnosed on tissue removed by biopsy, conization or portio amputation, or on the removed uterus.

Stage IB   Clinically invasive carcinoma confined to the cervix.

Stage IB   Histologically invasive carcinoma of the cer-
OCC   vix which could not be detected at routine clinical examination but which was diagnosed on a large biopsy, a cone, the amputated portio, or the removed uterus

As a rule, it is impossible to estimate clinically whether a cancer of the cervix has extended to the corpus or not. Extension to the corpus should, therefore, be disregarded.

A patient with a growth fixed to the pelvic wall by a short and indurated but not nodular parametrium should be allotted to Stage IIB. It is impossible at clinical examination to decide whether a smooth and indurated parametrium is truly cancerous or only inflammatory. Therefore, the case should be placed in Stage III only if the parametrium is nodular on the pelvic wall or if the growth itself extends to the pelvic wall.

The presence of hydronephrosis or nonfunctioning kidney due to stenosis of the ureter by cancer permits a case to be allotted to Stage III even if, according to the other findings, the case should be allotted to Stage I or Stage II.

The presence of bullous edema, as such, should not permit a case to be allotted to Stage IV. Ridges and furrows into the bladder wall should be interpreted as signs of submucous involvement of the bladder if they remained fixed to the growth at "palposcopy" (*i.e.*, examination from the vagina or the rectum during cystoscopy). Finding malignant cells in cytologic washings from the urinary bladder requires further examination and a biopsy from the wall of the bladder.

TREATMENT OF CERVICAL CANCER

PREINVASIVE PHASE

The early forms of CIN may be completely removed by biopsy or may be destroyed by cautery or cryosurgery.

The treatment of cancer in situ of the cervix is based upon the reproductive requirements of the patient. Surgery is, in general, preferred to radiotherapy, since morbidity is lower, preservation of normal tissues greater, preservation of ovarian function common, and the problem of radiation resistance nonexistent. If the patient is still in her childbearing years, with her family incomplete, and if her equanimity and responsibility permit her to remain under observation, conization of the cervix is recommended. This coning excision of the transformation zone about the histologic external os and lower canal usually causes the cytologic smear to become negative and preserves the competence of the cervix for childbearing.

Cryosurgery has been recommended for the treatment of some cases of cervical carcinoma in situ. The main disadvantage of this kind of treatment is the absence of a complete tissue sample for histologic study, as can be obtained in the cone specimen. Cryosurgery should be used only after expert colposcopic evaluation and sampling of the most abnormal lesion by colposcopically directed biopsy. The squamocolumnar junction must be fully visualized, the endocervical curettage must be negative, and there must be no colposcopic, histologic, or cytologic suspicion of invasive cervical cancer. Also, cryosurgery for CIN 3 should be used only in patients who are reliable and agreeable to long-term follow-up. Even with these precautions the physician using cryosurgery to deal with cervical carcinoma in situ always takes a calculated risk that the lesion will recur or that an invasive lesion was missed in the preliminary evaluation.

More recently the *carbon dioxide laser beam* has been utilized for the treatment of early cervical neoplasia. This has the advantage of precise destruction of small lesions without destruction of normal tissue. Preliminary results are encouraging, but further study is needed.

The constant surveillance required when such conservative treatment is offered makes it unjustifiable for a patient whose family is complete. In such a patient preferred treatment is total abdominal hysterectomy by the extrafascial technique, with a vaginal cuff and preservation of the ovaries as indicated. While such an individual is also best subjected to regular periodic examination, the cure rate is virtually 100% and vaginal vault recurrences are uncommon.

Carcinoma in Situ in Pregnancy. Routine cytologic smear examinations in pregnant women permit detection of asymptomatic lesions and, occasionally, carcinoma in situ in this younger group. When a positive

smear is encountered, colposcopy and directed biopsy are indicated, though cone biopsy is safe in experienced hands. If cancer in situ only is diagnosed histologically, pregnancy can safely be allowed to continue and vaginal delivery accomplished. Treatment may be postponed for several months, if desirable, so that a choice of methods can be offered. Unless the lesion has been totally removed by the biopsy, however, which would be reflected in the follow-up smears taken during pregnancy, cancer in situ does not regress after pregnancy, since it is not a pregnancy change.

INVASIVE PHASE

In considering the principles of treatment of cancer of the cervix one must remember that clinical staging does not strictly define the limits of the disease. For example, Stage I cancer of the cervix is associated with microscopic metastases to lymph nodes in 15% of cases, and that incidence is higher in more advanced stages. This does not vitiate the importance of staging in the management of this disease, however.

There are now two excellent modes of treatment for invasive cancer of the cervix, and a brief historical review is necessary to place in context the choice of one modality or the other for the individual patient. Simple total hysterectomy, performed first by Freund in 1878, was found quickly to be ineffectual in the treatment of cervical cancer. In 1895 Ries and Clark, in this country, and Wertheim in Vienna, began to perform the radical operation that was intensively studied by Wertheim and came to bear his name.

X-rays also were discovered in 1895 and were applied shortly to all types of external cancer, but it remained for the introduction of the Coolidge tube in 1913 to make radiotherapy constant and reliable. Radium, discovered in 1898, was employed by 1903 for the treatment of cancer of the cervix and by 1920 radiotherapy was well defined by the group headed by Regaud and working at the Curie Institute in Paris. Thereafter, radiotherapy gained widespread popularity, because it appeared to be more efficient than surgery in the cure of cancer of the cervix and had a much lower morbidity and negligible mortality. In the next 25 years this method was considered to be the standard one for the treatment of this disease in most large clinics throughout the world. In only a few centers did radical hysterectomy retain its popularity.

The renaissance of radical hysterectomy in this country was initiated by Meigs of Harvard University in 1944, and very shortly this procedure was adopted by many clinics in this country. Dissatisfaction had been expressed with the limitations of radiotherapy because 1) some lesions were not radiosensitive, 2) some patients with limited clinical disease already had microscopically disseminated disease in the lymph nodes which was alleged to be radioresistant, 3) radiation injuries were apparent, and 4) gynecologists were, by definition, surgeons rather than radiotherapists and felt more comfortable with surgery. With the introduction of modern techniques of surgery, modern anesthesiology, antibiotics, and greater understanding of electrolyte balance, it appeared that the enormous morbidity once attendant upon radical hysterectomy could be strikingly reduced.

In the succeeding decade it became apparent that radical hysterectomy in skilled hands was a relatively safe operation. Several other factors, however, introduced a new balance in the consideration of radiotherapy versus surgery: it was demonstrated that the number of radiation-resistant lesions was relatively small, that radiation injury in skilled hands was limited, and that while the mortality from radical surgery was reducible, there seemed to be an irreducible number of injuries attendant upon this operation, especially with respect to ureterovaginal fistula. With increasing confidence that radiotherapy could deal with disease in lymph nodes as well as the primary lesion, even harder decisions were required. During this decade it was apparent that if radical hysterectomy was confined to patients who were relatively young, lean, and in otherwise good health, and was done in a good hospital by a skilled surgical team, an excellent cure rate could be obtained; the place of this operation in the therapeutic armamentarium was clearly established. If radiation therapy was reserved for the remaining patients who were not suitable for operation, it was obvious that these poorer quality patients would have a poorer rate of cure even for same-stage disease. However, when attempts were made to select patients impartially for surgery or radiotherapy, it became evident that without rigid selection in favor of surgery, radiotherapy would attain an equal rate of cure. It was then clear that a choice for the individual patient could be based upon the therapist's experience or training or on the biologic nature of the tumor.

It was logical at this point for investigators to turn their attention to radiosensitivity testing of cervical cancer. For many years investigators of this disease had studied serial biopsies stained by conventional hematoxylin and eosin methods to assay such tumors' sensitivity to and curability by standard radiation. This technique was finally codified by Glucksmann, who studied the growing edge of the lesion, counted active and inactive cells after therapeutic radiation, and showed the accuracy of his predictions of radiocurability to be high. The size of the biopsy required by his technique, penetrating the normal surrounding tissues, and the need for giving full radiation while the testing was going on reduced the value of this method in the eyes of some observers. During this same period

FIG. 54–17. Plan of treatment for carcinoma of cervix with radiosensitivity testing (RST). *Ib,* tumor > 2.5 cm in our classification; *Ic,* tumor < 2.5 cm in our classification.

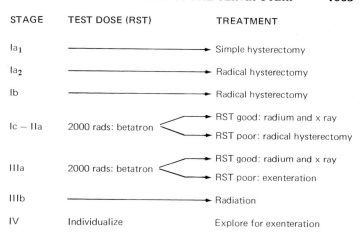

STAGE	TEST DOSE (RST)	TREATMENT
Ia₁		Simple hysterectomy
Ia₂		Radical hysterectomy
Ib		Radical hysterectomy
Ic – IIa	2000 rads: betatron	RST good: radium and x ray / RST poor: radical hysterectomy
IIIa	2000 rads: betatron	RST good: radium and x ray / RST poor: exenteration
IIIb		Radiation
IV	Individualize	Explore for exenteration

the studies of Graham in Boston demonstrated the value of host response as measured by the qualities of the normal vaginal cells surrounding a cancer both before and during radiation; this has been widely investigated since that time. The third technique, introduced in this field by our own group, involved cytomorphologic and cytochemical testing following a test dose of radiation. It has been found to offer a basis for selecting treatment in terms of the patient's biologic requirements. This technique utilizes a test dose of radiation which is small enough to be unimportant if a final radiotherapeutic plan is made and causes no complication if surgical treatment is to be undertaken. Small biopsies, which can also be used for imprint smears, are taken from the healthy sectors of the tumor and sectioned; these are stained cytochemically for evaluation of the nuclear components, especially the chromatin material and nucleoli. There are three types of reactions indicating sensitivity to radiation: 1) death and dissolution of cells; 2) maturation of cells, or differentiation; and 3) radiocytologic reactions indicating the probability of irreversible cell damage, such as increased size of nucleus, increased size of nucleolus, and initial chromatin increase followed by relative decline. This latter reaction occurs because the reproductive apparatus of the cell is more sensitive to damage than is the protein-forming apparatus found in the nucleolus, *i.e.,* the nuclear RNA.

These techniques of radiosensitivity testing have afforded valuable information about cervical cancer responses to treatment, but they are still incomplete. With the knowledge that the virulence of the tumor and the excellence of treatment, as well as radiosensitivity, affect the outcome, a complex judgment is required. In an effort to offer each patient the method of treatment best suited to her needs, we have adopted the treatment scheme depicted in Figures 54–17 and 54–18.

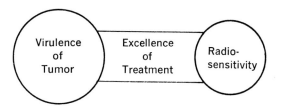

FIG. 54–18. Factors in cure of cancer of cervix.

While the majority of cervical cancers are radiosensitive and radiotherapy is more or less standard today in most clinics, surgery is preferable in an early lesion in a young, otherwise healthy woman, since this form of treatment will leave her tissues in a better state of preservation over the years. Surgery should, of course, be used in patients with radiation-resistant lesions, since these, though possibly curable by higher intensity radiation, may exact a penalty in complications which is unacceptable when surgical treatment is available.

Radical hysterectomy is a difficult operation requiring seasoned surgical judgment in addition to conventional technical skill because it involves removal of the uterus, tubes, ovaries, upper third of the vagina, and all of the parametrium on each side, as well as pelvic lymph node dissection encompassing the four major pelvic lymph node stations: ureteral, obturator, hypogastric, and iliac. The magnitude and complexity of this procedure may be judged by the knowledge that these tissues are bordered and constrained by vital structures such as the bowel, the bladder, the ureters, and the great vessels traversing the pelvis. Late-stage disease presents the problem of a high percentage of aortic lymph node involvement. The treatment of positive aortic nodes by radiotherapy has been associated with an increase in complications, without a propor-

tionate increase in cure. Ultimate management of this group of patients might necessitate the addition of a systemic treatment such as chemotherapy or immunotherapy. Despite the availability of chemotherapeutic agents for many years, chemotherapy has been minimally tested in the treatment of carcinoma of the cervix. The use of chemotherapeutic agents for patients with cervical cancer initially being treated with extensive surgery with or without radiotherapy is difficult because of decreased pelvic tissue vascularity, decreased renal function due to ureteral involvement, and compromised bone marrow secondary to previous therapy. A further problem is pelvic scarring, which does not allow adequate measurement of disease and evaluation of response. Recent clinical trials with cisplatinum (II) diamminedichloride show that DDP is an active drug against squamous cell carcinoma of the cervix and may be beneficial to patients with advanced disease.

In the case of advanced disease that has failed to respond to radiation, pelvic exenteration may offer the possibility of cure to a patient whose local disease is so massive that it threatens disaster by ureteral compression and uremia, and yet is confined to the pelvis without distant metastases. This massive surgical approach is more applicable to those with so-called *geographic spread, i.e.,* a more or less local tumor with accidental, so to speak, involvement of bladder and rectum, than to those with the unfortunately more conventional biologic spread by way of lateral parametrial lymphatic permeation to sidewall fixation.

The management of cervical cancer in pregnancy introduces special problems, considered in Chapter 27.

PROGNOSIS FOR CERVICAL CANCER

The outlook is highly favorable for patients with early cervical cancer. Indeed, a cure rate of 100% can be expected for stage 0 lesions. Prognosis is less hopeful for more advanced lesions, but with appropriate modern treatment the following cure rates can be expected: Stage I, 85%; Stage II, 50% to 60%; Stage III, 30%; and Stage IV, 5% to 10%. Clearly, the earlier the lesion is diagnosed and treated, the better are the prospects for cure.

REFERENCES AND RECOMMENDED READING

Averette HE, Denton RC, Ford JH, Jr: Exploratory celiotomy for surgical staging of cervical cancer. Am J Obstet Gynecol 113:1090, 1972

Baggish MS: High-power density carbon dioxide laser therapy for early cervical neoplasia. Am J Obstet Gynecol 136:117, 1980

Barron BA, Richart, RM: A statistical model of the natural history of cervical carcinoma based on a prospective study of 557 cases. J Nat'l Cancer Inst 41:1343, 1968

Bruckner HW, Cohen CJ, Deppe G, et al: Chemotherapy of gynecological tumors with platinum II. J Clin Hematol Oncol 7:619, 1977

Cohen CJ, Castro-Marin A, Deppe G, et al: Chemotherapy of advanced recurrent cervical cancer with Platinum II—preliminary report. Abstr, Am Soc Clin Oncol 19:401, 1978

Cohen CJ, Deppe G, Castro-Marin CA, et al: Treatment of advanced squamous cell carcinoma of the cervix with cis-platinum (II) diamminedichloride (NSC 119875). Am J Obstet Gynecol 130:853, 1978

Gusberg SB, Herman GG: Radiosensitivity testing of cervix cancer by the test dose technique. Am J Roentgenol 88:60, 1962

Gusberg SB, Yannopoulos K, Cohen CJ: Virulence indices and lymph nodes in cancer of the cervix. Am J Roentgenol Radium Ther Nucl Med 3:273, 1971

Gusberg SB: Cancer of the cervix: Cancer in situ and pathogenesis. In Gusberg SB, Frick HC, II (eds): Corscaden's Gynecologic Cancer. Baltimore, Williams & Wilkins, 1978

Gusberg SB: Cancer of the cervix: Diagnosis and principles of treatment. In Gusberg SB, Frick HC, II (eds): Corscaden's Gynecologic Cancer. Baltimore, Williams & Wilkins, 1978

Hinselmann H: Verbesserung der Inspektionsmöglichkeit von Vulva, Vagina und Portio. Munch Med Wochenschr 77:1733, 1925

Kolstad P, Stafl A: Atlas of Colposcopy. Baltimore, University Park Press, 1972

Nelson JH, Jr, Macasaet MA, Lu T, et al: The incidence and significance of para-aortic lymph node metastases in late invasive carcinoma of the cervix. Am J Obstet Gynecol 118:749, 1974

Richart RM, Barron, BA: A follow-up study of patients with cervical dysplasia. Am J Obstet Gynecol 105:386, 1969

Richart RM: Cervical intraepithelial neoplasia: A review. In Sommers SC (ed): Pathology Annual. New York, Appleton-Century Crofts, 1973

Symmonds RE, Pratt JH, Webb MJ: Exenterative operations: Experience with 198 patients. Am J Obstet Gynecol 121:907, 1975

Thigpen T, Shingleton H: Phase II trial of cis-Platinum (II) diamminedichloride in treatment of advanced squamous cell carcinoma of the cervix. Abstr, Am Soc Clin Oncol 19:332, 1978

Townsend DE, Ostergard DR, Mishell DR, Jr, et al: Abnormal Papanicolaou smears: Evaluation by colposcopy, biopsies and endocervical curettage. Am J Obstet Gynecol 108:429, 1970

UICC/American Joint Committee for Cancer Staging: Classification and staging of malignant tumors in the female pelvis. ACOG Technical Bulletin, No. 47, June 1977

Wasserman TH, Carter SK: The integration of chemotherapy into combined modality treatment of solid tumors. VIII. Cervical Cancer. Cancer Treat Rev 4:25, 1977

Wertheim E: Radical abdominal operation in carcinoma of the cervix uteri. Surg Gynecol Obstet 4:1, 1907

Wharton JT, Jones HW, Day TG, et al: Preirradiation celiotomy and extended field irradiation for invasive carcinoma of the cervix. Obstet Gynecol 49:333, 1977

Yannopoulos K, Gusberg SB: Radiosensitivity testing, virulence indices and stromal reaction in carcinoma of the cervix uteri. Pathol Annu 12:131, 1977

COLPOSCOPY

Adolf Stafl

Colposcopy was developed by Hinselmann in 1925, and although it was used extensively in German-speaking countries and in South America, it made relatively little impression in the English-speaking world, except in Australia. The delay in adoption of colposcopy in Great Britain and the United States was due mainly to Hinselmann's highly technical and difficult terminology, most of which originated from visual impressions not necessarily related to the underlying histopathologic processes. The development of diagnostic exfoliative cytology also delayed the introduction of colposcopy in English-speaking countries. Learning how to take an adequate cervical smear is certainly much easier than learning how to use the colposcope. Training in colposcopy is time-consuming, but without adequate training adequate results are impossible.

Colposcopy and cytology were long considered competitive methods of early cancer detection. The fact is, however, that each method has its particular limitations and strengths in cancer detection and the two methods complement one another. Cytology is a laboratory method of detection; colposcopy is a clinical method. Each deals with a different aspect of neoplasia. Cytology evaluates the morphologic changes in the exfoliated cells; colposcopy evaluates the changes in the terminal vascular network of the cervix which reflect the biochemical and metabolic changes in the tissue.

In recent years colposcopy has attracted a wide interest in the United States and is used by an increasing number of physicians. Its acceptance has been stimulated by new colposcopic terminology, new concepts in the natural history of cervical neoplasia, the change in priorities in the clinical application of colposcopy, and the improvement of training in the method's use.

TECHNIQUE

The colposcope (Fig. 54–19) is basically a stereoscopic microscope by which the cervix can be visualized in bright light at a magnification of 6 to 40 times. The examination technique is rapid, requiring little more time than inspection of the cervix with an unaided eye. After a specimen for cell study has been obtained, the mucus is carefully removed from the cervix by means of a swab of dry gauze. Cottonwool swabs should be avoided because fibers are left behind. The colposcope

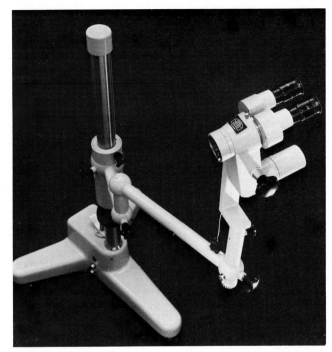

FIG. 54–19. Zeiss colposcope.

is then focused on the cervix. During inspection the surface of the cervix should be moistened with normal saline. A dry epithelial surface is insufficiently transparent and allows only a poor view of the vascular pattern. In routine colposcopic examination, a magnification of 16 is used. Optimal contrast of the vessels is achieved by the insertion of the green filter. After inspection of the saline-moistened cervix, a generous amount of 3% acetic acid is applied to the cervix. The acetic acid helps to coagulate the mucus, which can then be easily removed from the clefts and folds of columnar epithelium. After the application of acetic acid, areas of columnar epithelium stand out as typical grapelike structures. At the same time the acetic acid causes the tissue to swell and the transparency of the tissue is greatly reduced. Metaplastic, dysplastic, and carcinoma in situ epithelium assumes a whitish appearance over a fairly well-demarcated area. The effect of the acetic acid lasts only a few minutes, but the cervix may again be soaked with acetic acid if further examination is desirable.

TERMINOLOGY

In 1978 during the III World Congress for Cervical Pathology and Colposcopy in Orlando, Florida, a new colposcopic terminology was adopted. Colposcopic find-

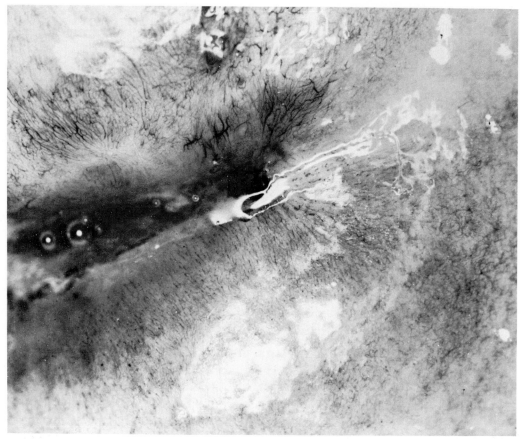

FIG. 54–20. Original squamous epithelium. Superficial spiderlike network of capillaries is barely visible. (× 16; Kolstad P, Stafl A: Atlas of Colposcopy. Oslo, Universitetsforlaget, 1972)

ings are divided into four groups: normal, abnormal, unsatisfactory, and other. These are described below.

NORMAL COLPOSCOPIC FINDINGS

Original Squamous Epithelium. This is the smooth, pink, featureless epithelium originally established on the cervix and vagina. No remnants of columnar epithelium are identified, such as mucus-secreting epithelium, cleft openings, or nabothian cysts (Fig. 54–20).

Columnar Epithelium. This is a single layer of tall, mucus-producing epithelium that extends into the endocervix from the original squamous epithelium or the metaplastic epithelium. The area covered with columnar epithelium has an irregular surface with long stromal papillae and deep clefts. After application of acetic acid, this epithelium has a typical grapelike structure.

Columnar epithelium may be present on the portio or may extend into the vagina (Fig. 54–21).

Transformation Zone. This is the area between the original squamous epithelium and the columnar epithelium in which metaplastic epithelium in varying degrees of maturity is identified. Components of a normal transformation zone include islands of columnar epithelium surrounded by metaplastic epithelium, gland openings, and nabothian cysts. In a normal transformation zone there are no colposcopic findings suggestive of cervical neoplasia (Fig. 54–22).

ABNORMAL COLPOSCOPIC FINDINGS

Atypical Transformation Zone. An atypical transformation zone contains one or more of the following findings that are suggestive of cervical neoplasia:

1. *White epithelium.* A focal, abnormal colposcopic lesion seen after application of acetic acid. The white

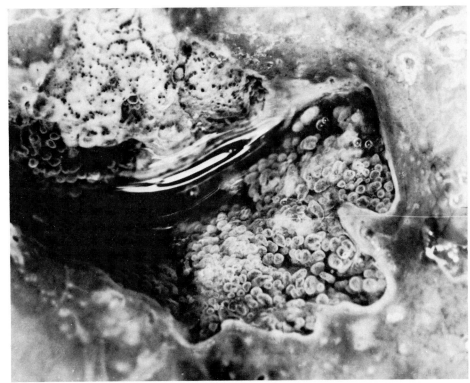

FIG. 54–21. Normal columnar epithelium. On posterior lip there is an area covered with columnar epithelium, with typical grapelike structure visible after application of acetic acid. (× 16; Kolstad P, Stafl A; Atlas of Colposcopy. Oslo, Universitetsforlaget, 1972)

FIG. 54–22. Normal transformation zone. Islands of columnar epithelium, tongues of squamous metaplasia, and gland openings are visible. (× 25)

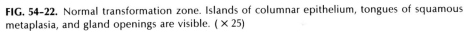

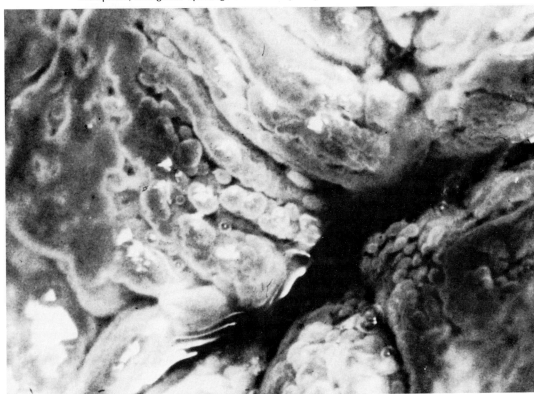

epithelium is a transient phenomenon seen in the area of increased nuclear density (Fig. 54–23, Color Plate).

2. *Punctation.* A focal abnormal colposcopic lesion with a stippled vascular pattern caused by capillary loops in stromal papillae. The vascular changes are sharply demarcated against normal epithelium (Fig. 54–24.

3. *Mosaic.* A focal abnormal colposcopic lesion in which the tissue has a mosaic pattern. The fields of mosaic are separated by reddish borders (Fig. 54–25).

4. *Hyperkeratosis.* A focal colposcopic pattern in which hyperkeratosis or parakeratosis appears as an elevated whitened plaque. This whitened plaque is identified before the application of acetic acid. At times, hyperkeratosis may be identified outside the transformation zone.

5. *Abnormal blood vessels.* A focal abnormal colposcopic pattern in which the blood vessel pattern appears not as punctation, mosaic, or delicately branching vessels, but rather as irregular vessels with abrupt courses appearing as commas, corkscrew capillaries, or spaghettilike forms running parallel to the surface (Fig. 54–26).

Suspect Frank Invasive Cancer. This is colposcopically obvious invasive cancer that is not evident on clinical examination (Fig. 54–27).

UNSATISFACTORY COLPOSCOPIC FINDINGS

This designation is applied when the squamocolumnar junction cannot be visualized.

OTHER COLPOSCOPIC FINDINGS

These include the following conditions:

1. Vaginocervicitis, a diffuse colposcopic pattern of hyperemia in which the blood vessels appear in a stip-

FIG. 54–24. Punctation. Sharply demarcated lesion on posterior lip of cervix with punctation vessels. Biopsy from this area showed carcinoma *in situ* (× 16; Kolstad P, Stafl A: Atlas of Colposcopy. Oslo, Universitetsforlaget, 1972)

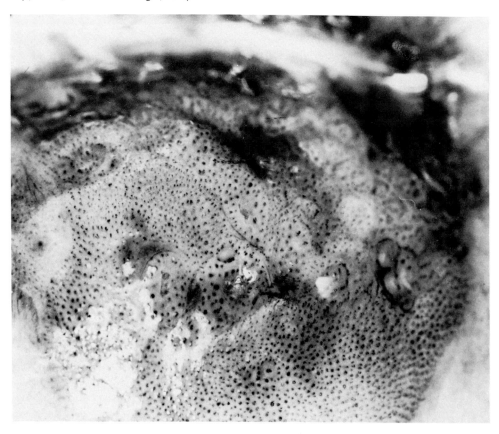

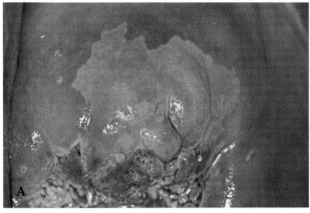
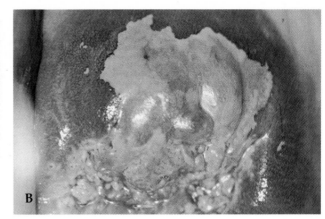

FIG. 54–23. White epithelium. *A.* Sharply demarcated area of white epithelium visualized after application of acetic acid. Borders are irregular. Biopsy from this area showed mild dysplasia. In lower portion of picture, normal columnar epithelium is present. *B.* Same cervix after Schiller test. Neither area covered with white epithelium nor area covered with columnar epithelium takes iodine stain. Thus, the Schiller test cannot distinguish between dysplasia and normal columnar epithelium.

FIG. 54–29. White epithelium with punctation. *A.* Cervix before application of acetic acid. Lesion is darker than surrounding normal epithelium and punctation vessels are visible. *B.* Cervix after application of acetic acid. Note remarkable change in color. Lesion is much whiter than surrounding normal epithelium. Biopsy from this area showed severe dysplasia.

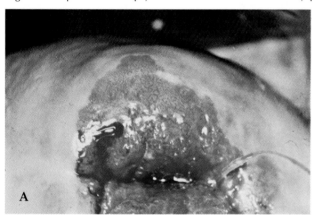
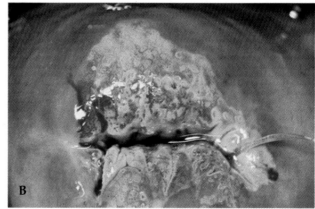

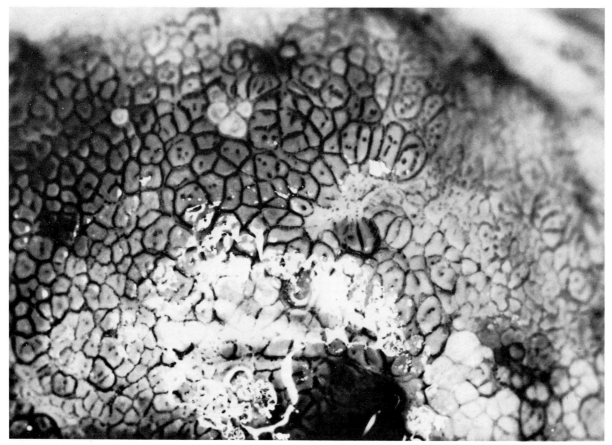

FIG. 54–25. Mosaic pattern. Coarse mosaic with significantly increased intercapillary distance. Biopsy from this area showed carcinoma *in situ*. (× 16; Kolstad P, Stafl A: Atlas of Colposcopy. Oslo, Universitetsforlaget, 1972)

pled pattern, similar to the vascular pattern in punctation (Fig. 54–28).

2. True erosion, an area denuded of epithelium usually caused by trauma
3. Atrophic epithelium, an estrogen-deprived squamous epithelium in which the vascular pattern is more readily identified owing to the relative thinness of the overlying squamous epithelium
4. Condyloma and papilloma, exophytic lesions that may be inside or outside the transformation zone

CORRELATION OF COLPOSCOPIC AND HISTOLOGIC FINDINGS

Table 54–1 correlates the colposcopic terminology with the colposcopic appearance and the expected histologic changes. Normal colposcopic findings show, histologically, original cervical epithelium (either squamous or columnar) or metaplastic squamous epithelium. In patients with normal colposcopic findings when the squamocolumnar junction is fully visible, cervical neoplasia should not be present in the tissue.

The most common abnormal colposcopic findings are white epithelium, punctation, and mosaic. Since pathogenesis of these patterns is similar, combinations of these findings are common. The histologic counterparts of these patterns range from minimal dysplastic changes to carcinoma in situ. For prediction of histopathologic changes in directed biopsy, it is not important whether the lesion viewed colposcopically appears as white epithelium, punctation, or mosaic; however, the histopathologic changes can be predicted by reference to the following easily observable colposcopic features: 1) vascular pattern, 2) intercapillary distance, 3) surface pattern, 4) color tone, and 5) clarity of demarcation.

The *vascular pattern* is one of the most important diagnostic features. Changes in the vascular pattern

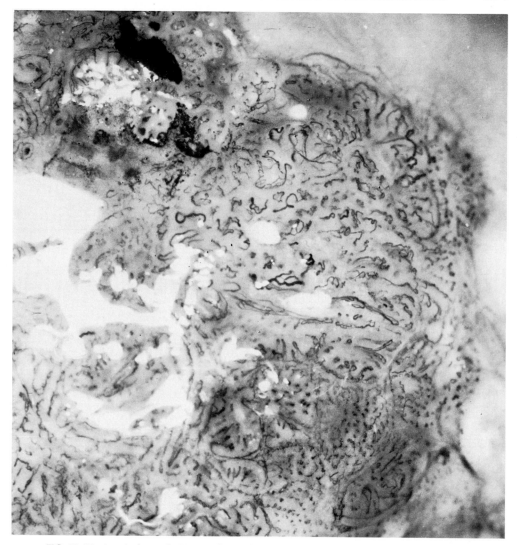

FIG. 54–26. Atypical vessels. Terminal vessels are irregular in size, shape, and arrangement. Biopsy showed microinvasive carcinoma. (× 16; Kolstad P, Stafl A: Atlas of Colposcopy. Oslo, Universitetsforlaget, 1972)

correspond closely to the degree of histologic changes. It is generally accepted that the first change in carcinogenesis is at the cellular biochemical level and can be detected only by very sophisticated laboratory methods that are not clinically applicable. During the first stage of carcinogenesis, the morphology of the tissue is unaltered. The blood vessels, however, react to these changes in tissue metabolism and cell biochemistry, and such vascular alterations constitute the first morphologic abnormality in the development of cervical neoplasia. These changes are clearly visible through the colposcope, but are not detectable in routine histologic sections. For a detailed description of the differ-

ent patterns of vessels and their diagnostic significance, the reader is referred to the colposcopic literature.

Intercapillary distance refers to the amount of cervical tissue that separates blood vessels. During a colposcopic examination the intercapillary distance in a colposcopically abnormal lesion can be estimated by comparing it with that of the capillaries in the adjacent normal epithelium. In cervical neoplasia, the intercapillary distance increases as the stage of the disease advances.

The colposcope provides a stereoscopic magnification that greatly facilitates the study of the *surface*

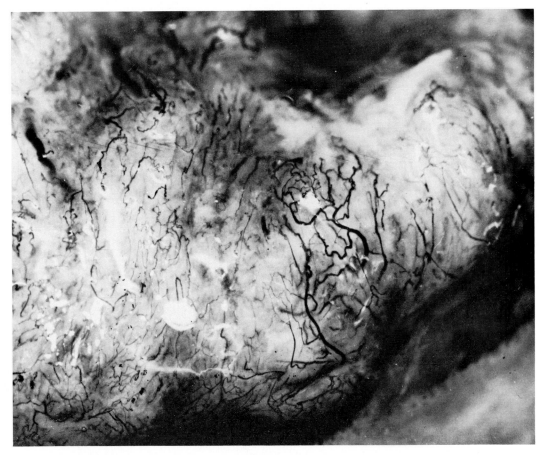

FIG. 54–27. Suspect frank invasive cancer. Atypical branching and network vessels are compatible with frank invasive cancer. Biopsy confirmed diagnosis. (× 16; Kolstad P, Stafl A: Atlas of Colposcopy. Oslo, Universitetsforlaget, 1972)

contour. This can be described as smooth, uneven, granulated, papillomatous, or nodular. Normal squamous epithelium or minimal dysplasia has a smooth surface; carcinoma *in situ* and particularly early invasive cancer have an uneven, slightly elevated surface.

Colposcopic lesions show different *color tones,* varying from white to deep red. The difference between the surface color of the cervix before and after the application of acetic acid is diagnostically significant. When there is a marked change from deep red to white after application of acetic acid, a more severe histologic lesion may be expected (Fig. 54–29, Color Plate). It is, therefore, very important to examine the cervix colposcopically both before and after application of acetic acid.

An important feature of a colposcopically abnormal lesion is the *border between the lesion and the adjacent normal tissue.* The borderline between normal squamous epithelium and inflammatory changes or minimal dysplasia is quite diffuse and irregular. Severe

dysplasia or carcinoma in situ usually produces a lesion with sharp borders that distinctly demarcate it from the adjacent normal epithelium.

CLINICAL APPLICATIONS OF COLPOSCOPY

In recent years clinical use of colposcopy as a screening procedure for cervical cancer has declined, and the method has assumed a more important role in the evaluation of patients with abnormal cell studies. In Europe, colposcopy has been promoted primarily as a cancer-detection technique, placing it in competition with cytologic examination. Each method has its particular limitations and strengths in cervical cancer detection; these are summarized in Table 54-2. Without doubt cell study is the better method for cervical cancer screening. Cervical smears can be obtained by any trained medical personnel and their examination can detect lesions in the endocervical canal; moreover,

TABLE 54–1. CORRELATION OF COLPOSCOPIC AND HISTOLOGIC FINDINGS

Colposcopic Term	Colposcopic Appearance	Histologic Correlate
Original squamous epithelium	Smooth, pink Indefinitely outlined vessels No change after application of acetic acid	Squamous epithelium
Columnar epithelium	Grapelike structures after application of acetic acid	Columnar epithelium
Transformation zone	Tongues of squamous metaplasia "Gland openings" Nabothian cysts	Metaplastic squamous epithelium
White epithelium	White, sharp-bordered lesion visible only after application of acetic acid No vessels visible	From minimal dysplasia to carcinoma *in situ*
Punctation	Sharp-bordered lesion Red stippling Epithelium whiter after application of acetic acid	From minimal dysplasia to carcinoma *in situ*
Mosaic	Sharp-bordered lesion Mosaic pattern Epithelium whiter after application of acetic acid	From minimal dysplasia to carcinoma *in situ*
Hyperkeratosis	White patch Rough surface Already visible before application of acetic acid	Usually hyperkeratosis or parakeratosis; seldom carcinoma *in situ* or invasive carcinoma
Atypical vessels	Horizontal vessels running parallel to surface Constrictions and dilatations of vessels Atypical branching, winding course	From carcinoma *in situ* to invasive carcinoma

the method is economical. the limitations of cell study include the fact that inflammation, atrophy, and folic acid deficiency may produce suspicious changes in the cell morphology that are not related to cervical neoplasia. Also, there are many procedural steps between the patient and the cytopathologist, and diagnostic errors can and do occur. The diagnostic accuracy of cell study has been exaggerated. Reports from the literature show a false-negative rate of 2% to 5%. However, these rates are obtained by the best cytologists under specially controlled research conditions that cannot be reproduced in routine practice. The practical false-negative rate for a study of a single Papanicolaou smear is estimated at 15% to 20%. The true false-negative rate of cell study is difficult to determine because a cervix that appears normal and has normal cells is not examined further. Theoretically, the only accurate way of evaluating the false-negative rate of cell study is to perform a cervical conization biopsy in all patients, including those whose cells are normal, and to study the cone in serial sections. For obvious reasons, such an evaluation cannot be done. Any other method is a compromise and is associated with varying degrees of inaccuracy. Many studies have compared the accuracy of colposcopy and cell study, and there is general agreement that the combination of both methods increases the diagnostic accuracy over that of either method separately. Navratil, who simultaneously applied both methods to a series of 55,000 patients, of whom 838 had cervical carcinomas, found that 87% of the neoplastic lesions were diagnosed by cell study and 79% by colposcopy. With the simultaneous use of both methods, 98.8% of lesions were recognized on initial examination.

Although routine colposcopy might detect cervical neoplasia missed through cytologic screening, it is doubtful if the time and effort involved would justify its use. Even in populations with a relatively high prevalence of cervical neoplasia, it would be necessary to examine 2000 patients by colposcopy to detect a single case of cervical neoplasia missed by cell study. This application of colposcopy is, therefore, still questionable because it is not economical and because too few physicians are trained in the technique. In the future, however, this situation may change. By including colposcopic training in most residency programs or by training paramedical personnel in basic colposcopy, it may be possible to achieve the ideal goal of examining all patients both cytologically and colposcopically. Routine colposcopy requires almost the same time as

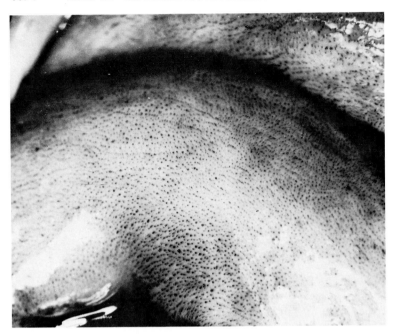

FIG. 54–28. Original squamous epithelium with inflammatory changes. Terminal vessels in *Trichomonas* infection may give colposcopic picture resembling punctation; however, capillaries are diffusely distributed over both ectocervix and vaginal wall. (× 16; Kolstad P, Stafl A: Atlas of Colposcopy. Oslo, Universitetsforlaget, 1972)

the visual examination of the cervix and does not significantly prolong the gynecologic examination.

At present the main value of colposcopy is in the evaluation of patients whose cell studies are abnormal and who are at high risk (due to intrauterine exposure to diethylstilbestrol or clinical evidence of adenosis). Colposcopy makes it possible to localize the lesion, evaluate its extent, and obtain a directed biopsy from which the histopathologic diagnosis can be established. Colposcopy is very accurate in differentiating invasive from noninvasive lesions and inflammatory atypia from neoplasia. In patients with abnormal cells, colposcopy can immediately differentiate between inflammatory and neoplastic changes. The limitation of colposcopy is its inability to detect a lesion deep in the endocervical canal. However, in this latter situation results of the colposcopic evaluation are not negative but rather unsatisfactory because the squamocolumnar junction is not visible. Further diagnostic steps are required. The frequency of unsatisfactory colposcopy findings in premenopausal women is 12% to 15%. After menopause the frequency of unsatisfactory colposcopy rises significantly and, therefore, the value of colposcopy in the evaluation of the cervix of postmenopausal women is somewhat more limited. However, in patients whose squamocolumnar junction is fully visible, the false-negative rate of colposcopy is very low. This was demonstrated by Stafl and Mattingly from the results of the Wisconsin Colposcopy Program, in which the false-negative rate of directed biopsy was 0.3%.

Clinical diagnosis of lesions demonstrated to contain abnormal cells should be done only by an experienced colposcopist. Not every gynecologist should attempt to master the technique. Such an effort is uneconomical and time-consuming, and an individual physician is unlikely to see enough candidates for colposcopy to maintain his expertise at a high level. It is more reasonable to train a few physicians in a community or re-

TABLE 54–2. ADVANTAGES AND DISADVANTAGES OF COLPOSCOPY AND CELL STUDY

Advantages	Disadvantages
CELL STUDY	
Ideal for mass screening Economical	Cannot localize lesion
Specimen can be obtained by any medical personnel	Inflammation, atrophic changes, folic acid deficiency may produce suspicious changes
Detects lesions in endocervical canal	Many steps between patient and cytopathologist allow misdiagnosis
Detects adenocarcinoma	Value of single smear is limited
COLPOSCOPY	
Localizes lesion	Inadequate for detection of endocervical lesions
Evaluates extent of lesion	Difficult training
Differentiates between inflammatory atypia and neoplasia	
Differentiates between invasive and noninvasive cervical lesions	
Enables follow-up	

gion to whom patients with abnormal cytologic results can be referred for colposcopic consultation.

The increased interest in colposcopy carries the potential danger of unrestricted use and abuse of the technique. Like every diagnostic method, colposcopy has limitations that must be fully recognized. The importance of adequate training and experience cannot be overemphasized. Inexperience can lead to serious mistakes in the diagnosis and management of cervical cancer which might significantly discredit colposcopy. The limitation of colposcopy in the diagnosis of lesions in the endocervical canal should be fully appreciated, and when the squamocolumnar junction is not fully visible, other methods of evaluation (endocervical curetting, conization) must be utilized. It should also be recognized that while the diagnosis of carcinoma in situ is often relatively easy, the proper evaluation of vascular changes suggesting invasion requires much longer experience. When used intelligently with thorough understanding of all the morphologic details, colposcopy is an important diagnostic tool, both for clinical practice and research.

REFERENCES AND RECOMMENDED READING

Bolten KA: Practical colposcopy in early cervical and vaginal cancer. Clin Obstet Gynecol 10:808, 1967

Bolten KA, Jacques WE: Introduction to Colposcopy. New York, Grune & Stratton, 1960

Coppleson M, Pixley F, Reid BL: Colposcopy: A Scientific and Practical Approach to the Cervix in Health and Disease. Springfield IL, Charles C Thomas, 1971

Hinselmann H: Verbesserung der Inspektionsmoglichkeit von Vulva, Vagina und Portio. Munch Med Wochenschr 77:1733, 1925

Kolstad P, Stafl A: Atlas of Colposcopy. Baltimore, University Park Press, 1972

Mestwerdt G, Wespi HJ: Atlas der Kolposkopie, 3rd ed. Stuttgart, Fischer, 1961

Stafl A: Use of the azocoupling method for identification of alkaline phosphatase in study of the capillary network of the cervix uteri. Cesk Morfol 10:336, 1962

Stafl A: The clinical diagnosis of early cervical cancer. Obstet Gynecol Surv 24:976, 1969

Stafl A, Dohnal V, Linhartova A: Uber kolposkopische, histologische und Gefassbefunde an der Krankhaft veranderten Portio. Geburtshilfe Frauenheilkd 23:437, 1963

Stafl A, Friedrich EG Jr, Mattingly RF: Detection of cervical neoplasia: Reducing the risk of error. Clin Obstet Gynecol 16:238, 1973

Stafl A, Linhartova A: Die Umwandlungszone und ihre Genese. Arch Gynaekol 204:228, 1967

Stafl A, Linhartova A, Dohnal V: Das kolposkopische Bild der Felderung und seine Pathogenese. Arch Gynaekol 199:223, 1963

Stafl A, Linhartova A, Dohnal V: Das kolposkopische Bild des Grundes, des papillaren Grundes, der atypischen Umwandlungszone und deren Pathogenese. Arch Gynaekol 204:212, 1967

Stafl A, Mattingly RF; Isoantigens ABO in cervical neoplasia. Gynecol Oncol 1:26, 1972

Stafl A, Mattingly RF: Colposcopic diagnosis of cervical neoplasia. Obstet Gynecol 41:169, 1973

Stafl A, Mattingly RF: Vaginal adenosis: A precancerous lesion? Am J Obstet Gynecol 120:666, 1974

Stafl A, Mattingly RF: Angiogenesis of cervical neoplasia. Am J Obstet Gynecol 121:845, 1975

Stafl A, Mattingly RF, Foley DV, Fetherston WC: Clinical diagnosis of vaginal adenosis. Obstet Gynecol 43:118, 1974

Tredway DR, et al: Colposcopy and cryosurgery in cervical intraepithelial neoplasia. Am J Obstet Gynecol 114:1020, 1972

LESIONS OF THE CORPUS UTERI

James A. Merrill
Saul B. Gusberg
Gunter Deppe

BENIGN LESIONS OF THE CORPUS UTERI

James A. Merrill

BENIGN LESIONS OF THE ENDOMETRIUM

The growth and development of the endometrium reflect accurately the aging process and hormonal changes in women. This is observed best during the phases of the menstrual cycle and in the changes occurring during intrauterine or extrauterine pregnancy. Likewise, the endometrium may reflect abnormal endocrine states and is responsive to the exogenous administration of hormones, occasionally with the production of pathologic conditions.

IRREGULAR SHEDDING AND RIPENING

Irregular shedding of the endometrium indicates a specific clinicopathologic syndrome characterized by prolongation of regular cyclic menstrual bleeding, which is often increased in amount. Irregular shedding is found in approximately 3% of patients with abnormal uterine bleeding. The diagnosis is based upon the history and is substantiated by curettage of the uterus done toward the end of a period of prolonged bleeding, beyond the time when endometrial regeneration normally would have occurred. Thus, curettage must be done beyond the fifth or sixth day of menstrual flow. Microscopic examination of endometrial curettings shows areas of typical postovulatory menstrual endometrium as well as areas of early proliferative endometrium.

This abnormality of endometrial growth is apparently produced by prolonged or excessive output of progesterone by the corpus luteum. A cystic corpus luteum or a corpus luteum cyst occasionally is associated. Both the clinical symptoms and the endometrial pathology have been produced by administration of progesterone during the premenstrual phase of the cycle. The curettage of the uterus required for diagnosis is usually therapeutic.

A somewhat related condition is referred to as *irregular ripening* of the endometrium. Microscopic examination of endometrium removed during the postovulatory phase of the menstrual cycle reveals a patchy mixture of proliferative and secretory endometrium. Such a diagnosis requires that the histologic changes be observed in the superficial layer of the endometrium. The symptoms and treatment are similar to those of irregular shedding and it is possible that the two conditions are the same.

ENDOMETRIAL HYPERPLASIA

Endometrial hyperplasia is a common pathologic finding in patients with excessive, irregular, or prolonged menstruation. It also occurs in patients without symptoms or signs and may cause or accompany postmenopausal bleeding. Progressive changes of endometrial hyperplasia may lead to malignancy. The pathologic physiology is thought to be excessive or continued and unopposed estrogen activity. Estrogen production need not be excessive if it is prolonged and unopposed by progesterone from a corpus luteum. Anovulation is the most common cause of such altered hormone production, although anovulatory cycles are not always associated with endometrial hyperplasia or with abnormal bleeding. Thus, hyperplasia is encountered most commonly at the two extremes of menstrual life, postpuberty and the menopause, since both of these epochs are associated with failure of ovulation. Hyper-

plasia of the endometrium may also result from excess estrogen production from such sources as functioning ovarian tumors, polycystic ovarian disease, and abnormalities of the adrenal cortex and possibly other endocrine glands. Administration of hormones or medications with a hormonally active metabolite may cause hyperplasia; digitalis, for example, is known to result in estrogen activity. A careful history should be taken to exclude all sources of exogenous hormone, especially in menopausal or postmenopausal women.

The actual mechanism of uterine bleeding is not clear. In addition to increased volume of tissue, there may be altered vasculature including fibrosis and elastosis of spiral arterioles that may interfere with their contraction. It is apparent, however, that the frequency and extent of the bleeding are not dependent upon the degree of hyperplastic change. Profuse bleeding may occur with minimal hyperplasia.

Pathology

The uterus may be enlarged, but commonly is of normal size. The endometrium may be enormously thickened and polypoid (Fig. 55–1), even to the point of being confused with carcinoma. Endometrial curettings are abundant, soft, and succulent. Friability suggests malignancy, but may occur with hyperplasia. Occasionally the curettings are not abnormal grossly. Endometrial hyperplasia is often associated with endometrial polyps, myomas, and adenomyosis.

The most common type of endometrial hyperplasia is *cystic* or Swiss-cheese *hyperplasia* (Fig. 55–2). Microscopically, the endometrial glands are dilated, increased in number, and lined by pseudostratified, regular columnar epithelium, without evidence of secretory activity. The cells are tall, but not atypical.

The degree of cystic dilatation is quite variable. The stroma, consisting of cells with little cytoplasm, is dense and contains focal collections of lymphocytes and thin-walled vascular channels. Mitoses are numerous in the epithelium and stroma. During the bleeding phase, areas of necrosis and thrombi are seen.

Adenomatous hyperplasia, which represents a more active or advanced phase of hyperplasia, is characterized by an abundance of closely packed glands, some of which are cystically dilated, with small outpouchings. An aggregation of "daughter" glands may surround a larger gland, or there may be a cluster of varying-sized glands with little or no intervening stroma (Fig. 55–3). The stromal proliferation is similar to that described for cystic hyperplasia. However, unlike cystic hyperplasia, the epithelium may show cellular irregularities or be stratified, producing papillary projections into the lumina of the glands. (See also Developmental Stages of Endometrial Cancer, p. 1092.)

Cystic endometrial changes occur in postmenopausal women, probably as the result not of estrogen stimulation but of atrophy, with occlusion of gland mouths

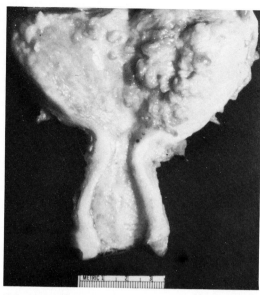

FIG. 55–1. Gross appearance of marked polypoid hyperplasia of endometrium.

and accumulation of secretion within the glands. The endometrium is thin, consisting of many thin-walled, dilated glands and scant stroma. Indeed, the stromal cells and epithelial cells show more atrophy than proliferation. We refer to this lesion as *cystic atrophy* instead of including it as one of the hyperplastic lesions of the endometrium.

Progestational hyperplasia refers to the glandular changes that occur in the endometrium in early pregnancy due to increased and increasing levels of ovarian steroid hormones. In the usual nonpregnant menstrual cycle, endometrial glands and stroma show regressive changes commencing about Days 21 to 23 of the cycle. If pregnancy occurs during that cycle, regression does not occur and there is continued growth and proliferation, particularly of the secretory glands. This growth may be so exuberant as to be misinterpreted as a pathologic hyperplasia. Furthermore, occasionally in early pregnancy, atypical glandular cellular changes are observed. These pregnancy changes have been misinterpreted as malignancy, particularly clear-cell carcinoma. Such findings are likely to be observed in endometrial curettings obtained from women with abnormal uterine bleeding in whom pregnancy is not suspected. This has been described specifically in patients with ectopic tubal gestation (the Arias–Stella reaction). The atypical changes are entirely physiologic and represent no evidence of neoplastic growth. In a small number of patients receiving high doses of synthetic progestins, atypical stromal changes may be seen. In these endometria, atypical glandular components are not present.

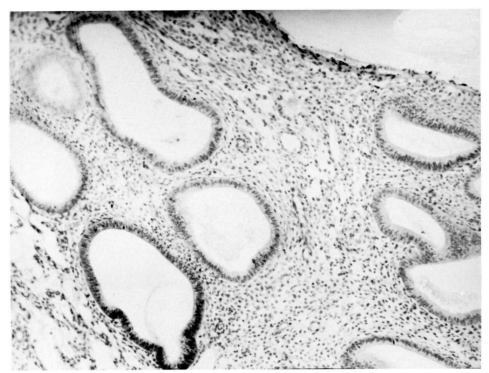

FIG. 55–2. Cystic hyperplasia of endometrium. In addition to glandular changes, stroma contains numerous thin-walled vascular channels, which may partially explain excessive menstrual bleeding in this condition.

Relation to Cancer

In the majority of cases, the microscopic pattern of hyperplasia is clearly benign. In a few, there is marked proliferative activity and even atypia of cellular detail and growth pattern. In these cases, the interpretation of curettings is not easy and the criteria of malignancy vary considerably among pathologists. Indeed, the author is certain that the changing histologic criteria of cancer and hyperplasia account for some of the recent reported increase in incidence of endometrial cancer. The atypical, probably premalignant, varieties of endometrial hyperplasia, especially adenomatous hyperplasia, and their relation to cancer are discussed later in this chapter. The physician should become familiar with the meaning of the diagnostic terms used by *his* pathologist. The hyperplastic abnormalities, some of which may be premalignant, go by various terms, and intelligent management of the patient necessitates an awareness of each. As we use the terms, cystic hyperplasia and usually adenomatous hyperplasia are considered benign. Adenomatous hyperplasia with areas of *anaplasia* or *atypia* is viewed with suspicion. However, such lesions may be reversible and should not be considered categorically as premalignant. *Carcinoma in situ* of the endometrium is used by us to indicate the lesion that is probably not reversible. The same lesions may be referred to by other names in other clinics. *The terminology is not important, as long as you know what your pathologist means by it.* Occasional difficulties in the pathologic evaluation of hyperplastic lesions make the gynecologist's decision regarding treatment a difficult one.

Treatment

Certainly initial therapy in *all* cases should be dilatation and curettage of the uterus. In benign hyperplasia this can be expected to produce immediate cure in about 50% to 70% of patients. In others, there may be recurrence in 4 to 8 months. For recurrent bleeding, hormone therapy as outlined in Chapter 46 may be appropriate and effective. Initiation of ovulation or the use of cyclic progesterone or progestins corrects the pathophysiology most effectively. The presence of *atypical* adenomatous hyperplasia in curettings is an indication for strict surveillance of the patient, with repeat curettage within 2 to 4 months. If the process is less active at that time, the patient may be safely followed. If the process shows a greater degree of activity or atypia, hysterectomy should be considered. The potential of malignancy is related to progression of hy-

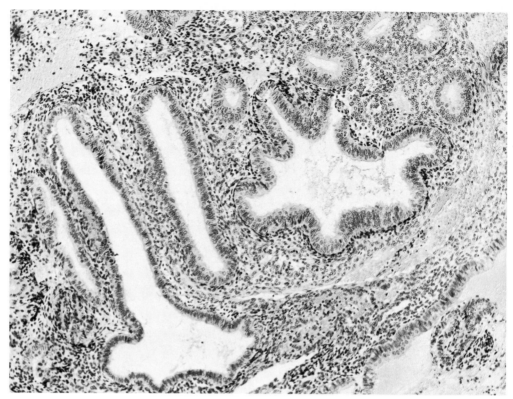

FIG. 55-3. Adenomatous hyperplasia of endometrium. Note intraluminal papillary projections and "daughter" glands. (Kistner RW: Clin Obstet Gynecol 5:1166, 1962)

perplastic activity. More radical therapy is indicated in the postmenopausal woman.

ENDOMETRIAL POLYPS

Endometrial polyps are sessile or pedunculated projections of the endometrium (Fig. 55–4). They develop as solitary or multiple soft tumors, frequently composed of hyperplastic endometrium. Diffuse endometrial hyperplasia may consist of multiple polypoid projections. The cause of most endometrial polyps is best explained as similar to that of endometrial hyperplasia.

Most polyps are asymptomatic, and it is difficult to determine which symptoms actually are due to endometrial polyps, since they are frequently associated with leiomyomas of the uterus and endometrial hyperplasia. Polyps are often an incidental discovery at the time of curettage or hysterectomy. When symptoms do exist, the clinical picture is one of nonspecific abnormal uterine bleeding. Endometrial polyps occasionally cause postmenopausal bleeding. It is not clear that polyps bear any relation to endometrial cancer, except possibly those found in postmenopausal women.

Incidence

These lesions are common, but their exact incidence is not known. The age range is from 12 to 81 years, although they are most frequently found in women between 30 and 59 years of age.

Pathology

Polyps vary in size from a local elevation of the endometrium to a growth filling the endometrial cavity. They may be sessile or pedunculated. Most arise in the fundus or cornua of the uterus, but may protrude through the cervix. These are usually firmer and less red than cervical polyps. In the majority of cases the polyp is made up of endometrium similar to that seen in the basalis and does not show secretory changes. Less than one-third of the polyps contain functional endometrium, similar histologically to the endometrium from which they arise. Polyps frequently show a microscopic picture of cystic hyperplasia and, less commonly, one of adenomatous hyperplasia. The tip of the polyp may be necrotic and inflamed, particularly if it is long and protrudes into the cervix (Fig. 55–5). Squamous metaplasia of the lining surface has been observed.

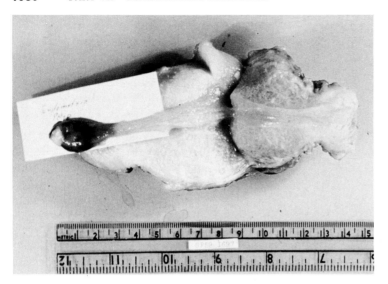

FIG. 55–4. Endometrial polyp. This polyp has long pedicle and protruded through cervical os; because of this, tip of polyp was hemorrhagic and necrotic.

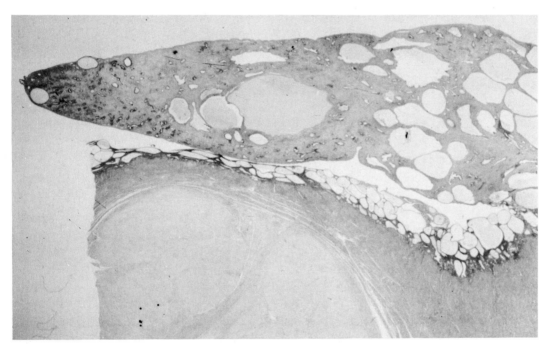

FIG. 55–5. Submucous myoma, cystic atrophy of endometrium, and endometrial polyp with cystic hyperplasia and slight congestion of tip. These were unexpected findings in uterus removed from postmenopausal patient.

Diagnosis and Treatment

The diagnosis is usually established at the time of curettage or hysterectomy. Occasionally a polyp may protrude through the cervical os and be mistaken for a cervical polyp. Polyps may be diagnosed from hysterosalpingograms, in which they produce a depression in the outline of the uterine cavity. Polyps are often missed at curettage unless the curettage is accompanied by the insertion of a grasping instrument in the uterine cavity. For this reason, no curettage should be considered complete unless a polyp forceps is introduced prior to and following the actual curetting.

Endometrial polyps should be considered benign, al-

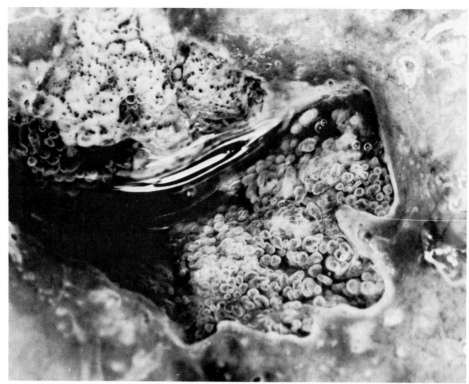

FIG. 54-21. Normal columnar epithelium. On posterior lip there is an area covered with columnar epithelium, with typical grapelike structure visible after application of acetic acid. (× 16; Kolstad P, Stafl A; Atlas of Colposcopy. Oslo, Universitetsforlaget, 1972)

FIG. 54-22. Normal transformation zone. Islands of columnar epithelium, tongues of squamous metaplasia, and gland openings are visible. (× 25)

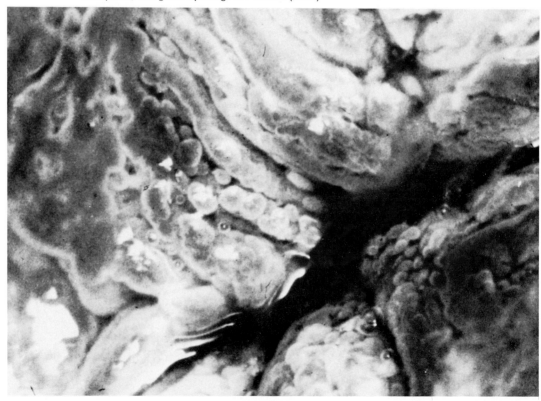

though carcinoma of the endometrium coexists with them in about 10% of postmenopausal women. However, the carcinoma is usually not in the polyp. Thus, polyps require no special treatment other than removal, although in postmenopausal women they must be regarded with suspicion of malignancy.

BENIGN LESIONS OF THE MYOMETRIUM

LEIOMYOMAS

A leiomyoma is a well-circumscribed, but nonencapsulated, benign uterine tumor, composed mainly of smooth muscle but with some fibrous connective tissue elements. The tumor is also called myoma, fibromyoma, fibroma, and fibroid. The term "fibroid" has been firmly established in medical parlance by usage, although "myoma" is more accurate.

Incidence

The exact incidence of leiomyomas is uncertain; however, they constitute the most common pelvic tumor, and it has been estimated that one out of every four or five women over the age of 35 years has a uterine myoma. Although most myomas produce no symptoms, it has been estimated that 60% of all pelvic laparotomies in women are done for the reason (or excuse) of myomas. The lesion is most frequently found in the fourth and fifth decades of life and more commonly in the black than in the white patient. Interestingly enough, however, the incidence of myomas in the African Negro is reported to be very low, suggesting causative factors other than heredity.

Location

Myomas are classified according to their location in the uterus. *Intramural* tumors, which are most common, are situated in the muscle wall without close proximity to either the mucosa or the serosa. With growth, these tumors distort the cavity as well as the external surface of the uterus. Single large intramural tumors may produce symmetric enlargement of the uterus. *Subserous* tumors (Fig. 55–6) are located directly beneath the serosa and project from the external surface of the uterus, producing the typical knobby configuration of the fibroid uterus. With growth, the subserous tumor may become pedunculated, attached to the uterus by a broad or long thin pedicle. On occasion such a pedunculated tumor may become attached to adjacent viscera, peritoneum, or omentum, lose its primary blood supply, and develop a secondary blood supply from the adherent structure. These tumors are referred to as *parasitic;* fortunately, they are rather rare. *Intraligamentous* tumors result from growth of a subserous tumor into the broad ligament. These may impinge on the ureter or even the pelvic blood vessels. They have special significance with respect to difficulty of surgical removal. *Submucous* tumors are present just beneath the endometrium (Fig. 55–7). With growth, they displace and thin the endometrium over their surface, which may become the site of necrosis and infection. Submucous tumors may also become pedunculated and eventually protrude into the cervical canal or the vagina. In this situation, infection is common.

Pathology

The corpus is the most common site of origin of myomas. They are usually multiple, of various sizes,

FIG. 55–6. Uterus containing numerous pedunculated subserous myomas. Tumors of this sort may be mistaken for ovarian neoplasms.

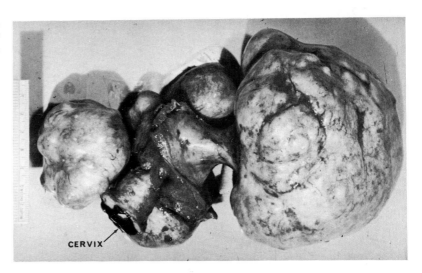

CERVIX

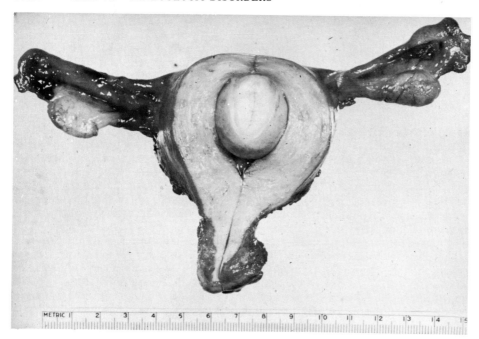

FIG. 55–7. Uterus containing submucous myoma that completely fills uterine cavity.

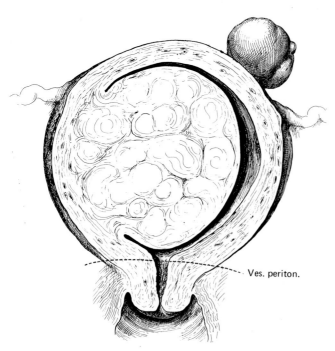

Ves. periton.

FIG. 55–8. Large submucous myoma. Great distortion of uterine cavity shows futility of attempted curettage in such circumstance. (Drawing by M Brödel In Kelly HA: Operative Gynecology, Vol 2. New York, Appleton, 1903

and distort the contour of the uterus (Fig. 55–8). A single myoma may produce a rather uniform enlargement of the uterus simulating pregnancy.

Tumor size varies from the small 1-cm seedling myomas to those weighing as much as 147 lb. They are firm and well demarcated from the surrounding myo-metrium. On sectioning, the tumor bulges from the surface and the pseudocapsule, produced by compression of adjacent myometrial tissue, becomes readily apparent. The surface is smooth, glistening white with a whorled and fasciculated pattern.

Microscopic examination discloses bundles of

FIG. 55-9. Microscopic section of be-nign myoma. Smooth muscle cells are seen in cross section and longitudinal section.

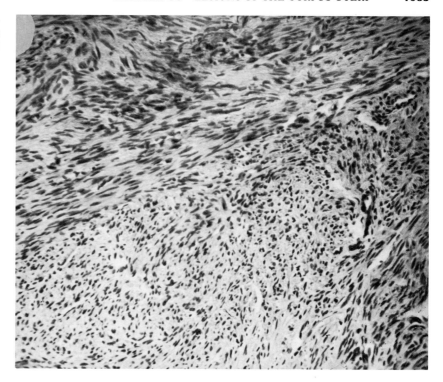

smooth muscle arranged in interlacing patterns, sepa-rated by fibrous connective tissue. There are relatively few blood vessels. The arrangement in bundles allows groups of smooth muscle cells to be seen variously in cross section or longitudinal section, giving a typical microscopic appearance (Fig. 55-9). The tumors have no true capsule. At the margin there is usually an area of compressed myometrium forming a pseudocapsule. The artifact of fixation results in a space between the myoma and the adjacent compressed myometrium. Mitoses are rarely seen.

Histogenesis

Although myomas are common, their origin and devel-opment are not well understood. The tumors undoubt-edly arise from smooth muscle within the myome-trium. It has been suggested that they arise from persistent small, embryonic cell rests. Evidence has been offered that the tumors arise from the smooth muscle of blood vessel walls within the myometrium. It has further been suggested that myomas develop in response to estrogen stimulation; the evidence for this theory is far from convincing. The most impressive ob-servation is that the tumors occur most commonly during the reproductive years and usually undergo re-gression, often complete, following the menopause. Oral contraceptives may cause myomas to enlarge. Also, it is generally held that leiomyomas increase in

size during pregnancy, when estrogen production is high. However, Randall and Odell found little evidence that these tumors actually proliferate during preg-nancy.

Degeneration and Complications

Myomas are subject to a variety of degenerative phe-nomena (Figs. 55-10, 55-11). Some have clinical sig-nificance, but the majority are pathologic findings unrelated to the clinical picture. The majority of these degenerative changes result from alteration in the blood supply of the tumor occurring with rapid growth, pregnancy, mechanical accident, or postmenopausal atrophy. The most common type of degeneration is *hyalinization*. A great many myomas, even small ones, reveal some degree of hyaline change. On cut section, the surface appears homogeneous and has lost some of the whorled, fascicular pattern. Microscopically, broad zones of hyaline connective tissue replace the smooth muscle cells. Somewhat less common is *cystic degen-eration*. Small or large areas undergo liquefaction and myxomatous change resulting in cystic foci. When these are present to a substantial degree, the consis-tency of the tumor is soft, and on section, the cystic areas are obvious grossly. *Calcification* of myomas is an interesting degenerative change occurring more commonly in the postmenopausal woman (Fig. 55-12). The areas of calcification may be scant or dif-

(*Text continues on p. 1086.*)

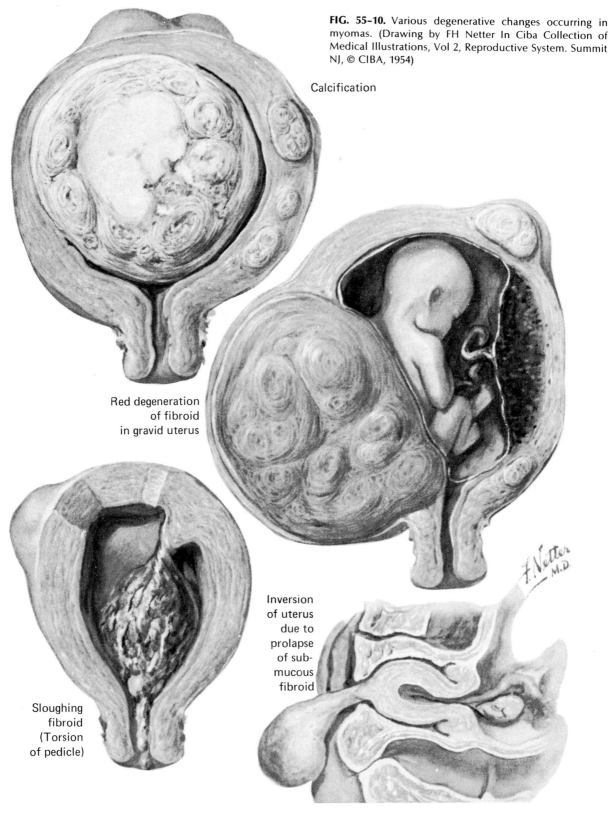

FIG. 55-10. Various degenerative changes occurring in myomas. (Drawing by FH Netter In Ciba Collection of Medical Illustrations, Vol 2, Reproductive System. Summit NJ, © CIBA, 1954)

Calcification

Red degeneration
of fibroid
in gravid uterus

Sloughing
fibroid
(Torsion
of pedicle)

Inversion
of uterus
due to
prolapse
of sub-
mucous
fibroid

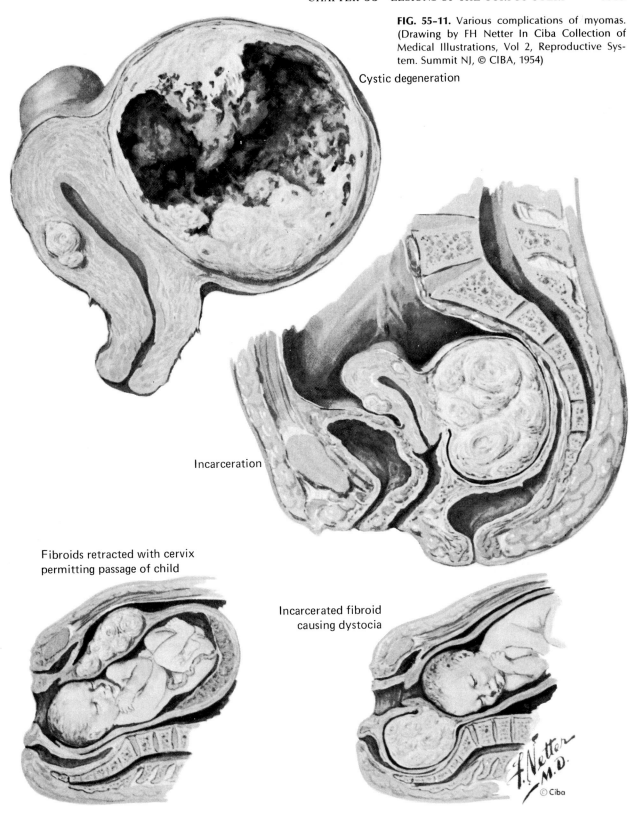

FIG. 55-11. Various complications of myomas. (Drawing by FH Netter In Ciba Collection of Medical Illustrations, Vol 2, Reproductive System. Summit NJ, © CIBA, 1954)

Cystic degeneration

Incarceration

Fibroids retracted with cervix permitting passage of child

Incarcerated fibroid causing dystocia

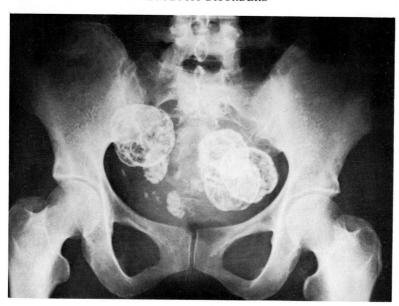

FIG. 55–12. Radiograph of abdomen showing many calcified uterine myomas.

fuse. When diffuse, the tumor may be visualized roent-genographically. Occasionally such a myoma is an incidental finding during radiographic examination of the abdomen. Rarely, there is heterotopic bone formation. *Fatty degeneration* of myomas is observed usually as an incidental microscopic finding. *Necrosis* may result from torsion or twisting of a pedunculated myoma and may be associated with abdominal pain, tenderness, fever, and leukocytosis. This may occur as an acute accident. A special variety of necrosis is *carneous* or *red degeneration*. This is said to occur in 8% of tumors complicating pregnancy. The change is due to aseptic necrosis associated with hemorrhage into the substance of the tumor and subsequent hemolysis. Grossly these tumors become beefy red and soft and clinically produce pain and tenderness.

Infection of a myoma may occur in association with adjacent pelvic inflammatory disease but is most common in the submucous pedunculated myoma, which becomes necrotic first and inflamed secondarily.

Degeneration is important in two respects: 1) it may produce symptoms and signs that require treatment, including surgery, and 2) on the basis of gross appearance, a benign, degenerated leiomyoma may be confused with a sarcoma. Sarcomatous transformation of a myoma does occur, but the incidence is less than 1% and, in general, should not influence the clinical management of patients with leiomyomas.

Physical Signs

A presumptive diagnosis of leiomyoma of the uterus may be made by abdominal palpation if the uterus is displaced out of the pelvis or if the tumors are large. They are palpated as firm, irregular nodules arising from the pelvis and extending into the lower abdomen.

Generally, the nodular mass is movable. If tumors are pedunculated they may be moved separately. If the tumor mass fills the pelvis, mobility is restricted, and similar restriction may result from associated inflammatory involvement of the supporting tissues.

Bimanual pelvic examination is more revealing. Diagnosis is relatively simple if the uterus can be outlined easily and its contour is distorted by multiple smooth, round nodules. These masses may be small irregularities on the surface of the uterus, no larger than 1 cm, or masses that fill the pelvis and lower abdomen. The examination should be done carefully to make certain that the masses are part of the uterus. A normal uterus may be displaced posteriorly by a solid ovarian tumor. Sounding the uterus gives the direction of the uterine cavity and its depth. Frequently the uterine cavity is enlarged by myomas and directed toward the myomas. If the cavity is of normal size and deviated away from the masses, an extrauterine tumor must be considered. It is possible, of course, for a solitary myoma to displace the major portion of a normal-sized uterus. A pedunculated, submucous myoma may be seen protruding from the cervical os as a grayish-pink smooth mass. If there is infection or necrosis, the surface may be red and friable. It is possible to diagnose a submucous myoma at the time of uterine curettage. An irregularity of the cavity is felt by the uterine sound or by the curet when it is brought down the anterior or posterior wall. One should not mistake the cornual areas for myomas, however.

Symptoms

Most myomas, even large ones, produce no symptoms. Indeed, many more are discovered as an incidental finding than are associated with symptoms, despite the

great frequency with which such tumors are removed in the operating room. The mere presence of uterine myomas does not mandate active treatment.

The asymptomatic tumor may present a problem in differential diagnosis. Symmetric enlargement of the uterus may be confused with pregnancy. Usually the menstrual history and typical changes in the cervix and vagina make the pregnancy apparent. The myomatous uterus has a firm consistency as opposed to the soft, pregnant uterus. An hCG test for pregnancy should be done if any doubt exists. If the tumor is pedunculated, it may be difficult to distinguish from an ovarian tumor; indeed, the distinction may be impossible and exploratory surgery may be required to exclude ovarian neoplasm, particularly in postmenopausal patients. Adnexal inflammatory masses and endometriosis can usually be distinguished from a solitary subserous or pedunculated myoma on the basis of symptoms and associated findings of pelvic scarring or fixation. Ultrasound may help to make the distinction.

Bleeding. Any pattern of abnormal uterine bleeding may occur, but the most common is excessive or prolonged menses. This may produce a rather profound anemia. It is important to remember that the patient with myomas may have abnormal uterine bleeding from causes other than the myomas. The patient's endocrine status and endometrium must be carefully evaluated.

The exact mechanisms by which myomas of the uterus cause bleeding abnormalities are not altogether clear. In many cases bleeding is probably due to associated endocrine disorders such as anovulation. Indeed, such underlying abnormalities in endocrine function may have a causal relation to the tumors themselves. In one study, 36% of myomatous uteri were found to have endometrial hyperplasia. Submucous myomas may produce bleeding because of congestion, necrosis, and ulceration of the surface. Excess bleeding may result from the increased surface area of the endometrium when tumors enlarge and distort the endometrial cavity. The surface area of the normal uterine cavity is about 15 cm^2. In the presence of the multiple myomas it may be as great as 225 cm^2. Large tumors also may produce mechanical interference with the blood supply to the endometrium, and the presence of intramural tumors may interfere with the ability of the uterus to contract and effectively occlude blood vessels at the time of menstruation. Large vascular channels are frequently seen in the endometrium adjacent to myomas.

Pressure. Pressure on the bladder produces urinary frequency, urgency and, rarely, inability to void. Constipation results from pressure on the rectum. With extremely large tumors, pressure on the pelvic vessels may result in edema or varicosities of the legs. Rarely, ureteral pressure produces hydroureter and/or hydronephrosis.

Pain. Pain and tenderness may result from degeneration of the myoma. The onset is gradual and the pain intermittent. A dull aching soreness is usual, but the pain may be colicky. Fever and leukocytosis accompany severe degeneration. A tumor with a long pedicle may twist and produce acute pain, tenderness, nausea, and signs of peritoneal irritation. The pressure of large tumors on adjacent viscera may result in pain. With growth, stretching of old inflammatory adhesions may result in bilateral pelvic discomfort. Cramping pain may be associated with attempts at passage of a submucous tumor from within the uterine cavity. Intramural tumors may aggravate or produce dysmenorrhea, although other sources of dysmenorrhea should be considered first. The most common type of discomfort, particularly with large tumors, is a sensation of pelvic heaviness or "bearing down."

Distortion of the Abdomen. The patient herself may notice the presence of a tumor by self-examination or noticeable alterations in girth and abdominal contour.

Infertility. Myomas are sometimes found in the process of evaluating infertile patients. Their presence should not be interpreted immediately as having a causal relation to the infertility. Myomas *may* impair fertility, particularly if they occlude the endocervical canal, sufficiently distort the isthmic portions of the oviducts, or cause sufficient thinning and change in the endometrium to impair proper implantation. However, many patients, even those with sizable uterine tumors, are normally fertile and maintain pregnancy to term. Other causes of infertility should always be sought.

Pregnancy Complications. Uterine myomas may present symptoms only during pregnancy. The management of this special situation is considered below.

Treatment

Observation and Reassurance. In many, if not most, cases treatment is not necessary when a diagnosis of uterine myoma is made, particularly if the patient is asymptomatic, has small tumors, or is postmenopausal. These patients should be carefully examined every 3 to 6 months to check for unusual growth or complications. Abnormal uterine bleeding due to fibroids requires diagnostic curettage, but if no malignancy is found, it often can be controlled by appropriate supportive therapy and endocrine management. This is recommended for the patient who is approaching the menopause. If the bleeding can be controlled for a short time, it will cease spontaneously at the menopause and the myomas will regress.

Treatment may be indicated for patients with asymptomatic tumors if the differential diagnosis includes another lesion of greater significance (such as an ovarian tumor), if the tumor is unusually large

(particularly if it produces abdominal distortion), and possibly if infertility is present with no other apparent cause. How large is a "large" tumor? Many consider a myomatous uterus larger than a 3-month pregnancy an indication for treatment. Sudden growth of a tumor, particularly in a postmenopausal woman, is indication for treatment.

Surgery. For patients with significant symptoms, surgery is the preferred method of treatment. Myomectomy (the removal of tumors) can be done to preserve the uterus for future childbearing. This is accomplished through the vagina in cases of pedunculated submucous myomas, employing a wire loop and electrocautery. Myomectomy is more commonly done by the abdominal approach. A single pedunculated subserous tumor can be removed easily, but it is also possible at one time to remove a great many intramural and even submucous tumors from the uterus. Myomectomy is the operation of choice when the indication is infertility or when a tumor is to be removed because its location is likely to interfere with normal delivery. Occasionally myomectomy is indicated because the patient has a strong desire to retain menstrual function, although future childbearing is not a special consideration. Multiple myomectomy has a high frequency of postoperative complications in terms of adhesions and bowel obstruction, and there is a relatively high incidence of recurrence. Thus, removal of a single pedunculated tumor may be of value, but multiple myomectomy should be done only in selected young, otherwise fertile patients who are desirous of having more children.

For the majority of patients with symptoms thought to be related to myomas, the treatment should be total hysterectomy. If the tumors are small, the hysterectomy may be done vaginally, particularly if there is associated pelvic relaxation. Most often we prefer the abdominal approach for ease of operating and ability of inspecting the remainder of the pelvis carefully. Since large tumors and intraligamentous tumors may distort the ureters from their usual course and make them more liable to surgical trauma, catheters should be placed in the ureters prior to surgery to enable the surgeon to locate the ureters and avoid accidental injury. There is no reason to remove the ovaries when doing a hysterectomy for uterine myomas. *Hysterectomy should not be done without prior curettage of the uterus to rule out intercurrent endometrial or cervical disease.*

Radiation. In the past, radiation has been used for the treatment of myomas. In some clinics it is occasionally used today. It is mentioned here only to be condemned, since radiation has no place in the treatment of uterine myomas.

Myomas in Pregnancy

Reports indicate that the incidence of uterine myomas during pregnancy varies from 0.3% to 7.2%. The tumors almost always precede the pregnancy, although they may not become apparent until pregnancy occurs. During the course of pregnancy myomas usually increase in size. However, this is largely due to edema and degeneration and probably does not represent true proliferation of the tumor. The frequency of spontaneous abortion is increased in patients with uterine myomas. No treatment is indicated during the pregnancy; moreover, it is difficult to predict which cases will proceed without mishap. Fortunately this is not a common cause of abortion.

During the second and third trimesters, increase in the size of tumors may produce or increase pressure symptoms. Degeneration of intramural tumors due to alterations in blood supply or twisting of pedunculated tumors produces symptoms of gradual or acute pain, usually associated with localized tenderness. This may be difficult to distinguish from other acute intra-abdominal accidents or inflammation, and surgery may be necessary for this reason. However, in the majority of patients, degeneration rarely constitutes an indication for surgical intervention. The patient is best treated by bedrest, symptom relief, and careful observation. Myomectomy, which is indicated rarely, is followed by an increased incidence of abortion and premature labor.

During late pregnancy and delivery, myomas may produce fetal malpresentation, uterine inertia, or mechanical dystocia, depending upon the number, size, and location of tumors. A large tumor in the lower uterine segment or cervix may actually block descent of the head into the pelvis. Fortunately, most such tumors rise out of the pelvis as pregnancy progresses. Dystocia is more likely to occur with true cervical myomas. Such situations require expert obstetric judgment and, on occasion, cesarean section. If cesarean section is accomplished, myomectomy is not advisable at the same operation.

Postpartum hemorrhage is more likely to occur when the uterus contains myomas. This complication should be anticipated and appropriate precautions taken to avoid unnecessary blood loss or to combat it if it occurs. Because of the sudden change in the shape and position of the uterus, twisting or vascular accidents of pedunculated tumors may complicate the puerperium.

The management of a pregnant patient with myomas is essentially no different from the management of a normal pregnant woman. Close observation is necessary; hospitalization, analysis and, rarely, surgery may be needed, but in the majority of cases a safe vaginal delivery can be anticipated.

ADENOMYOSIS

Adenomyosis is a benign disease of the uterus characterized by areas of endometrial glands and stroma within the myometrium. There is usually no direct connection between these heterotopic foci and the endometrium lining the uterine cavity. The lesion is not a tumor, but a hyperplastic growth, and may be localized or diffuse. *Adenomyoma* refers to a localized tumorlike mass composed of hyperplastic smooth muscle admixed with foci of endometrium. While adenomyosis has certain morphologic similarities to endometriosis, it is not, in the author's opinion, truly related to endometriosis, nor should it be considered to be part of the endometriosis complex. The term "endometriosis interna" should not be used to refer to adenomyosis. Endometriosis is not commonly found in association with adenomyosis.

Clinical Picture

Adenomyosis is usually diagnosed by the pathologist as an incidental finding in a uterus removed because of functional symptoms, intractable abnormal bleeding, or suspicion of myomas. Adenomyosis is found in approximately 20% of removed uteri and probably is of more clinical significance than is generally recognized. In one study, adenomyosis was found to be diagnosed correctly before surgery in only 10% of cases. This disease is observed most commonly in women during the fifth and sixth decades; classic manifestations are progressively heavy menstrual bleeding, increasingly painful dysmenorrhea, and a gradually enlarging, tender uterus. Adenomyosis does not produce symptoms following the menopause. All or part of this classic symptom complex occurs with other more common or more readily diagnosed conditions. Moreover, adenomyosis and uterine myomas frequently coexist, and some believe that endometrial hyperplasia commonly occurs in the same uterus. Myomas are a much more common cause of uterine enlargement than is adenomyosis, and endometrial hyperplasia is a more common cause of abnormal bleeding. Even endometrial hyperplasia, if marked, may cause a diffuse enlargement of the uterus. Secondary dysmenorrhea, a common complaint of women with adenomyosis, is more common in patients without definite pelvic disease and in those with endometriosis.

Thus, adenomyosis should be considered when a patient in her 40s complains of prolongation and increase of menstrual flow and dysmenorrhea, and is found to have a globular, firm, tender uterus that is one or two times enlarged. It should be apparent, however, that only a few such patients will be proved to have adenomyosis. Increased awareness may increase the frequency with which an accurate diagnosis is made, but it should not constitute a reason for increasing the frequency of hysterectomy or neglecting a careful search for other important disease.

Pathology

The uterus is firm, enlarged, and somewhat globular. On section, the myometrium is greatly thickened and the cut surface irregular, with a somewhat knobby appearance. There may be tiny foci of translucent tissue protruding from the cut surface. Miscroscopic examination shows areas of endometrial glands and stroma scattered throughout the myometrium (Fig. 55–13). By tradition, the diagnosis is made when such foci are separated from the basal layer of lining endometrium by more than one low-power microscopic field. The ectopic endometrium is rarely responsive to cyclic ovarian hormones and usually resembles nonsecretory basal endometrium. In this regard the appearance is like the endometrium found in endometrial polyps. There are occasional examples of cystic hyperplasia in adenomyotic foci. Occasionally during pregnancy the areas undergo a decidual change, and rarely a typical response to the progestational phase of the menstrual cycle is seen.

An adenomyoma may be difficult to distinguish grossly from a myoma. The cut surfaces reveal the nodule to be poorly demarcated from the surrounding myometrium, and it does not bulge above the myometrium as the typical myoma does. There is no cleavage plane or pseudocapsule. Microscopically, the adenomyoma resembles a myoma with foci of endometrium.

Histogenesis

There are numerous theories of histogenesis, none of which is proved. It is commonly accepted that adenomyosis arises by downward extension of the basal portion of endometrium into the underlying myometrium. This explains the infrequency with which adenomyosis shows cyclic response to ovarian hormones. The mechanism of symptom production is similarly difficult to explain and is often related to coexisting pathologic conditions of the uterus or ovary. Prolonged or excessive menstrual flow has been explained by interference with adequate myometrial contraction. Conversely, the adenomyotic foci have been credited with irritation of uterine muscular contractility and resultant dysmenorrhea. Areas of adenomyosis are rarely the sites of malignant change, although this has been described. In cases of well-differentiated adenocarcinoma of the endometrium, it may be difficult to differentiate areas of adenomyosis from areas of myometrial invasion.

Treatment

Hysterectomy is the treatment of choice for the patient with symptomatic adenomyosis, even though it is fre-

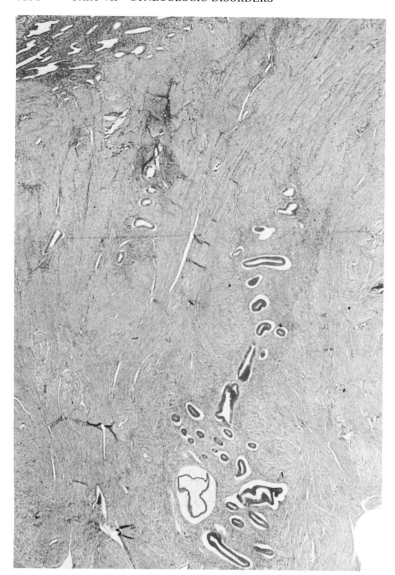

FIG. 55-13. Microscopic section of uterus with adenomyosis. Foci of endometrium are present deep to endometrium within myometrium.

quently undertaken on the basis of an incorrect preoperative diagnosis.

STROMAL ADENOMYOSIS

This lesion is variously referred to as *endolymphatic stromal myosis, stromatosis, stromal endometriosis,* or stromal adenomyosis. Some examples are actually endometrial sarcoma or mixed müllerian tumors. The truly benign variety is morphologically similar to adenomyosis, except that the ectopic areas consist only of endometrial stroma without glands. The gross appearance of the benign condition is no different from that of adenomyosis. Microscopic examination demonstrates multiple foci of compact endometrial stromal cells, similar to those seen in the proliferative phase of the menstrual cycle, throughout the myometrium. Sometimes these foci extend into lymphatic or venous channels. No specific clinical picture is associated with stromal adenomyosis. The exact diagnosis rests upon the pathologist's interpretation of microscopic findings. In the truly benign variety—without vascular involvement—hysterectomy is adequate treatment.

UNUSUAL TUMORS

Other benign tumors of the uterus are hemangioma, lymphangioma, lipoma, and cysts of mesonephric origin. Few cases of each have been reported. There are no specific clinical syndromes and the precise histo-

genesis of these tumors is not known. They are usually noted as incidental findings or mistaken for myomas. Hysterectomy is the usual treatment.

Lymphangiomas may resemble soft myomas. They are usually small, circumscribed nodules composed of a maze of lymphatic channels with a background of fibrous connective tissue. Lymphangiomas must be distinguished from lymphangiectatic changes in a myoma. They are very rare indeed. *Hemangiopericytoma* is a rare tumor composed of nonneoplastic capillaries surrounded by collars of neoplastic capillary pericytes. It is usually found incidentally, sometimes confused with stromal adenomyosis, and the prognosis is good. *Lipomas* are lobulated, encapsulated yellow growths consisting of adult adipose tissue. It is usually possible to distinguish a myoma with fatty degeneration from a lipoma by the remaining areas of smooth muscle in the former. Cysts or small adenomatous growths in the lateral wall of the uterus are rare. These lesions presumably arise from remnants of the mesonephric duct or tubules. Even more rarely such lesions give rise to malignant neoplasms.

SUBINVOLUTION OF THE UTERUS: FIBROSIS UTERI

Subinvolution of the uterus, or fibrosis uteri, is a diffuse, symmetric enlargement of the uterus occasionally found in multiparous women and credited with various symptoms, notably abnormal uterine bleeding. Some believe this to be a significant abnormality of the uterus resulting from incomplete puerperal involution, with retention or deposition of excess elastic connective tissue. For whatever reason, parous women have larger uteri than nonparous women. This condition *per se* has no clinical importance, is never an indication for surgery, and should be disregarded in a consideration of diseases of the uterus.

REFERENCES AND RECOMMENDED READING

BENIGN LESIONS OF THE ENDOMETRIUM

Benson RC, Miller JN: Surgical curettage. Obstet Gynecol 8:523, 1956

Bergman P: Traumatic intra-uterine lesions. Acta Obstet Gynecol Scand 40 (Suppl 4):1 1961

Cohen CJ, Gusberg SB: Screening for endometrial cancer. Clin Obstet Gynecol 18:27, 1975

Gusberg SB, Kaplin AL: Precursors of corpus cancer. Am J Obstet Gynecol 87:662, 1963

Hertig AT, Sommers SC: Genesis of endometrial cancer. One study of prior biopsies. Cancer 2:946, 1949

Holstrom EG, McLennan CE: Menorrhagia associated with irregular shedding of the endometrium. Am J Obstet Gynecol 53:727, 1947

Katayama KP, Jones HW: Chromosomes of atypical hyperplasia and carcinoma of the endometrium. Am J Obstet Gynecol 97:978, 1967

Kistner RW, Gore H, Hertig AT: Carcinoma of the endometrium: A preventable disease? Am J Obstet Gynecol 95:1011, 1966

Overstreet EW: Clinical aspects of endometrial polyps. Surg Clin North Am 42:1013, 1962

Sutherland AM: Tuberculosis of the endometrium. J Obstet Gynaecol Br Commonw 63:161, 1956

Traut HF, Kuder A: Irregular shedding and irregular ripening of the endometrium. Surg Gynecol Obstet 61:145, 1935

Wentz WB: Treatment of persistent endometrial hyperplasia with progestins. Am J Obstet Gynecol 96:999, 1966

BENIGN LESIONS OF THE MYOMETRIUM

Baruah BD, Barkakati D: Endometrial changes in uterine myoma. J Obstet Gynecol India 12:246, 1961

Benson RC, Sneeden VD: Adenomyosis: A reappraisal of symptomatology. Am J Obstet Gynecol 76:1044, 1958

Buttram VC Jr, Reiter RC: Uterine leiomyomata: Etiology, symptomatology and management. Fertil steril 36:433, 1981

Emge LA: Problems in the diagnosis of adenomyosis uteri. West J Surg 64:291, 1956

Marcus CC: Relationship of adenomyosis uteri to endometrial hyperplasia and endometrial carcinoma. Am J Obstet Gynecol 82:408, 1961

Miller NF, Ludovici PP: On the origin and development of uterine fibroids. Am J Obstet Gynecol 70:720, 1955

Parks J, Barter RH: The myomatous uterus complicated by pregnancy. Am J Obstet Gynecol 63:260, 1952

Randall JH, Odell LD: Fibroids in pregnancy. Am J Obstet Gynecol 46:349, 1943

Schwarz O: Benign diffuse enlargement of the uterus. Am J Obstet Gynecol 61:902, 1951

Stearns HC: A study of stromal endometriosis. Am J Obstet Gynecol 75:663, 1958

Strassman EO: Plastic unification of double uterus. Am J Obstet Gynecol 64:25, 1952

MALIGNANT LESIONS OF THE CORPUS UTERI

Saul B. Gusberg, Gunter Deppe

CARCINOMA OF THE ENDOMETRIUM

In the reproductive period the endometrium is a constantly changing tissue. It is the only tissue of the body that normally undergoes necrosis and is rebuilt again on a virtually monthly basis. Histologic examination of the endometrium during the menstrual cycle reveals that the cyclic changes (proliferation, secretion, and necrosis) occur in the superficial three-fourths of the endometrial lining and that the basal region does not undergo these changes; it has a rather constant and inactive histologic appearance and remains behind while the larger surface layer is sloughing. It is from this basal layer that the new endometrium arises each month. It is also from the basal layer that carcinoma of the endometrium arises when the appropriate biologic

background exists. One might consider this basal layer as the "growth" layer of endometrium.

The basic condition associated with the development of adenocarcinoma of the endometrium is failure of ovulation over a long time. Evidence that this is the case is readily obtained from an analysis of the clinical conditions associated with carcinoma of the endometrium.

1. *The menopause.* About 75% of all endometrial cancers occur in postmenopausal women. The peak incidence for this tumor is between the ages of 50 and 60 years, an average of some 10 years after the cessation of ovulation.

2. *Failure of ovulation in young women.* When cancer of the endometrium develops in a premenopausal woman, there is frequently a history of long periods of amenorrhea and menorrhagia. These patients usually do not have regular menses but have either irregular bleeding at widely spaced intervals or excessive bleeding at irregular intervals. Examination of the endometrium during these bleeding episodes usually does not reveal the pattern of menstruation. These patients are anovulatory and are bleeding for an entirely different reason.

3. *Endogenous estrogen excess.* Women with ovarian tumors that secrete estrogen (thecomas and granulosa cell tumors) appear to have a higher incidence of endometrial cancer than other women. In patients with these tumors the amount of estrogen excreted in the urine daily may fall considerably below that of normal women, yet it is enough to suppress pituitary secretion of follicle-stimulating hormone and to prevent ovulation. The duration of anovulation depends upon the continued secretion of hormone by the tumor, but often extends for long periods.

4. *Exogenous estrogen administration.* A greater than expected number of patients who have been given estrogenic substances for many years on a therapeutic basis, have ultimately developed endometrial carcinoma.

5. *Endometrial polyps.* The origin of adenocarcinoma of the endometrium within endometrial polyps is a special case of the general rule. The benign endometrial polyp arises from the basal layer of the endometrium. The core of all benign polyps is composed of this tissue, even though the surface layers of some polyps respond to the cyclic changes in the ovaries. The core, and in many instances the entire polyp, usually does not undergo cyclic changes and remains static for long periods. As far as this small focus of tissue is concerned, the patient might as well be anovulatory, since it ignores the hormone fluctuations anyway. Thus, some patients with endometrial cancer have normal regular menses; however, these are exceptions to the general rule. The origin of the endometrial cancer, however, is the same unstimulated growth layer of the endometrium, which in this instance has isolated itself from its hormone environment and is focal.

Thus, adenocarcinoma is always preceded by long-term inactivity of basal endometrium, most frequently as a result of the cessation of ovulation. However, it should be emphasized that this is a predisposing, not a causative, factor. Some more fundamental change, at present unknown, must be added to the predisposing factor for cancer to appear. This is obvious because all patients who are postmenopausal are anovulatory, but not all those who have estrogen-secreting tumors, or are given exogenous estrogens, or have endometrial polyps develop endometrial cancer. In fact, the overwhelming majority do not.

Of great interest, clinically, is the fact that patients with endometrial cancer are likely to represent a phenotype consisting of obesity, diabetes or a diabetic glucose-tolerance curve, and hypertension. Almost 50% of patients with endometrial cancer are obese, 10% have clinical diabetes, over 50% have a diabetic glucose-tolerance curve, and over 50% are hypertensive. The presence of this phenotype should alert the clinician to the possibility of endometrial cancer. Whether the metabolic changes are in any way directly connected with the development of cancer remains to be determined. There is evidence that obesity and altered steroid metabolism coincide frequently.

DEVELOPMENTAL STAGES OF ENDOMETRIAL CANCER

Cystic Hyperplasis

When endometrium remains static for a long time, many of its glands become cystic (Fig. 55–14). This cystic hyperplasia of the endometrium is common in postmenopausal women, in anovulatory young women, in patients with thecomas or granulosa cell tumors, in women given exogenous estrogens, and in women with endometrial polyps. Cystic hyperplasia is one of the early stages in the development of carcinoma. This is best demonstrated by studies of biopsies or curettings taken from patients years prior to the appearance of cancer. However, *this is a reversible stage* in the development of cancer, since only 1.5% of patients with cystic hyperplasia actually develop cancer.

Adenomatous Hyperplasia

If cystic hyperplasia persists for years, it undergoes a gradual transformation. The cysts tend to collapse and leave radially symmetric projections of smaller glands at their periphery. Small satellite glands appear around the cysts. These smaller glands crowd closely together, become irregular in size and shape, and may form a rather complex glandular tissue. The epithelium lining

FIG. 55-14. Cystic hyperplasia of endometrium.

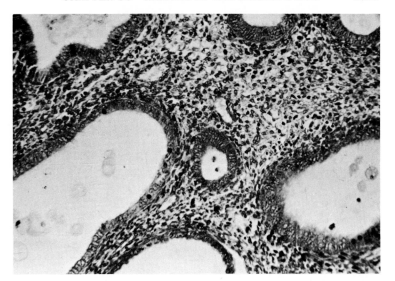

these glands is dark-staining, due to the basophilic cytoplasm and dense nuclei (Fig. 55–15). This adenomatous transformation is the early phase of adenomatous hyperplasia (Types I and II) and may be found side by side with cystic hyperplasia.

Dysplasia and Carcinoma In Situ (Stage 0 Cancer of Endometrium or Severe Adenomatous Hyperplasia, Type III)

As time passes, the cells lining the glands of adenomatous hyperplasia undergo a transformation. The cells become larger and paler-staining, owing to the acquisition of abundant acidophilic cytoplasm and to the enlargement of the nuclei, which are now vesicular and light-staining. The cells are not only enlarged but lose their polarity, and instead of lining up in an orderly fashion, grow in a haphazard manner in all directions. They frequently bud into the lumen. This change has been called "anaplasia" or "dysplasia" because it gives these glands the same cytologic appearance as those in obvious endometrial carcinoma. This similarity allows us to recognize these initial stages of the neoplastic process. The cellular alteration is best recognized by comparing the anaplastic gland with its neighbors, whose cells often retain the dark-staining reaction of benign endometrial growth.

When anaplastic (pale-staining) epithelium lines many glands (10 to 30) in a low-power microscopic field, the neoplasm has reached the stage of carcinoma in situ, designated as severe adenomatous hyperplasia (dysplasia) or Stage 0 cancer of the endometrium by some investigators. Not only do the epithelial cells resemble cancer cells, but the glands have enlarged and expanded against the surrounding stroma and have come to lie back to back (Fig. 55–16). This tiny focus

of neoplastic glands has not yet grown to the point of invading lymphatics or blood vessels and hence fulfills the requirements of the definition of carcinoma in situ. Great care must be taken to distinguish neoplastic changes from benign inflammatory or secretory changes in endometrial glands. As is true for the cervix, carcinoma in situ of the endometrium may be found alongside an invasive cancer, and the peak age incidence occurs several years prior to the peak age incidence of invasive carcinoma.

In summary, the stages in the development of endometrial carcinoma are cystic hyperplasia, adenomatous hyperplasia, anaplasia (dysplasia), and carcinoma in situ. A few patients on whom multiple biopsies were taken over long periods have been observed to go through all of these stages. This same progression has been noted in animals developing carcinoma upon exposure of the endometrium to methylcholanthrene.

Invasive Carcinoma

Prior to invasion, the tumor cannot be recognized grossly. The next stage in the development of endometrial cancer is that in which the neoplastic glands have grown and produced a grossly visible tumor, usually a sessile polypoid mass. The tumor has encroached on the surrounding connective tissue and projects into the lumen of the uterine cavity, but has not yet invaded the myometrium or the blood vessels. Between 20% and 40% of endometrial cancers are confined to the endometrium.

Histologic Characteristics. Well-differentiated adenocarcinoma of the endometrium is composed of closely packed neoplastic glands lined by pale acidophilic cells with large vesicular nuclei. Papillary processes into the

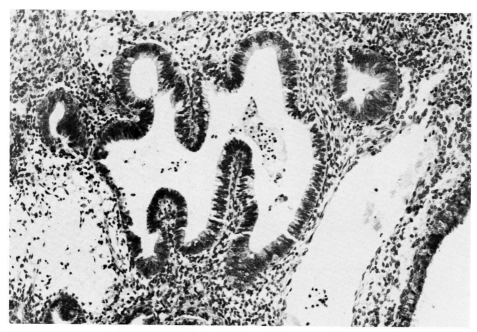

FIG. 55–15. Adenomatous hyperplasia of endometrium. Glands are distorted, but lining epithelium is still dark-staining and resembles proliferative phase.

gland lumina are common and multiple secondary glands are often formed within the epithelium itself. The stroma is almost completely crowded out by the glandular growth. In about 20% of these tumors the gland epithelium is converted focally into squamous-cell nests (Fig. 55–17). These nests seldom have the appearance of malignant squamous epithelium but do develop in distant metastatic sites and are apparently an integral part of the tumor. Masses of squamous cells in an adenocarcinoma give it the name *adenoacanthoma*. The clinical behavior of adenoacanthoma is essentially the same as that of adenocarcinoma. This lesion must be differentiated from *adenosquamous tumors,* which are more virulent.

As endometrial cancers continue to grow, they tend to become less differentiated. The neoplastic glands become smaller, the papillary projections become increasingly complex, and ultimately a solid, rapidly growing, undifferentiated carcinoma appears. These variations in differentiation can be graded histologically, and when the *histologic grade* is compared with the 5-year survival rate, an inverse relation exists. Thus, histologic grading is of prognostic value (Table 55–1).

Gross Appearance. Carcinoma of the endometrium develops as a polypoid, soft, friable mass, either focally or diffusely, throughout the uterine cavity (Fig. 55–18). The surface of the tumor may be necrotic, ulcerated, or hemorrhagic, but often has a glistening mucoid ap-

pearance. This tumor has a great tendency to produce mucus that, when mixed with blood from the necrotic parts, gives rise to the mucoid, bloody vaginal discharge that is clinically characteristic of endometrial cancer.

Spread of the Tumor. After extending locally into the surrounding endometrium, the tumor invades the myometrium. It may involve only the inner portion of the myometrium or may extend through it and burst out on the serosal surface. Rarely it spreads in the pelvic peritoneum and implants on the serosal surface of other pelvic and abdominal viscera. While growing in the myometrium, it may invade lymph vessels and gain access to the pelvic lymph nodes. The nodes of the upper portion of the broad ligaments are primarily involved, but from this region the tumor may spread to the para-aortic and vena caval nodes (Fig. 55–19). Recent experience with pretreatment surgical staging suggests that poorly differentiated cancers of the endometrium, even in very early stages, frequently metastasize to the periaortic lymph nodes.

Deep pelvic lymph nodes in the ureteral, iliac, obturator, and hypogastric areas may be affected with cervical involvement or deep myometrial extension. Lymphatic spread accounts for metastases in the vault of the vagina, around the rectum, and in the ovary. Invasion of blood vessels accounts for the involvement of liver, lungs, and bone marrow.

FIG. 55–16. Carcinoma in situ of endometrium—Type III adenomatous hyperplasia (dysplasia). Neoplastic gland is lined by large, pale acidophilic cells; papillary projection enters lumen from *right*. Cellular alteration is more obvious by comparison with two nonneoplastic glands on *left*.

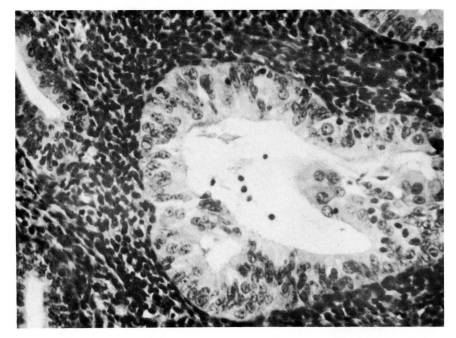

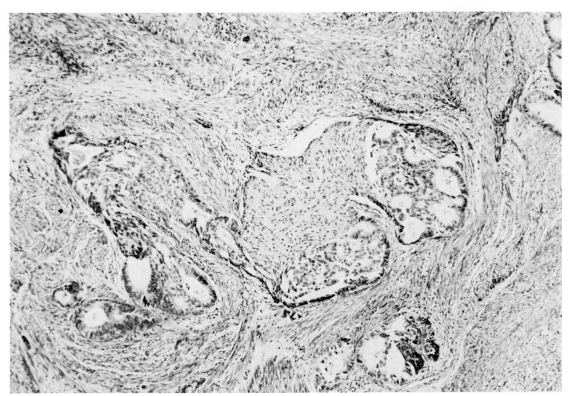

FIG. 55–17. Adenoacanthoma of endometrium. Squamous element forms in center of adenocarcinomatous tissue. This tumor is invading myometrium.

TABLE 55–1. RELATION OF HISTOLOGIC GRADE OF CANCER AND 5-YEAR SURVIVAL

Grade	% patients	% survival
I	14	76
II	50	57
III	32	39
IV	3	25

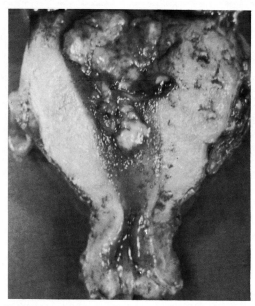

FIG. 55–18. Adenocarcinoma of endometrium with invasion of uterine wall.

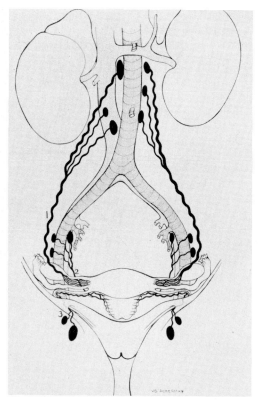

FIG. 55–19. Schematic representation of lymphatics of uterine corpus, showing (*1*) uteroovarian pedicle, (*2*) external iliac pedicle, and (*3*) round ligament pedicle leading to inguinal lymph nodes. (del Regato JA, Spjut HJ: Ackerman and del Regato's Cancer. Diagnosis, Treatment and Prognosis, 5th ed. St. Louis, CV Mosby, 1977)

OTHER MALIGNANT TUMORS OF THE CORPUS

MIXED MESODERMAL TUMORS

The hallmark of mixed mesodermal tumors is their composition of malignant epithelial and malignant connective tissues. They are highly malignant and often kill the patient within 2 years of the time of their discovery. Such a tumor can often be recognized grossly because, characteristically, it forms a large, friable, bulky polypoid mass that often originates at or near the fundus of the uterus and distends and dilates the uterine cavity. It sometimes reaches a relatively large size and may first be detected as a polypoid mass at the external os of the cervix. The tip of the tumor is often necrotic and hemorrhagic.

Histologically these tumors are quite variable. Some are composed of poorly differentiated adenocarcinoma with a sarcomatous stroma that has the appearance of fibrosarcoma. In others the malignant connective tis-

sue contains striated muscle and is essentially a rhabdomyosarcoma (Fig. 55–20). In many, cartilage appears, but rarely is bone found. Sometimes the epithelial component is essentially squamous-cell nests. Mixed mesodermal tumors of the adult woman are thought to be related to sarcoma botryoides, which is predominantly a tumor of the cervix and vagina in children. These tumors spread rapidly to the lymphatics and bloodstream, and metastases are found in pelvic, inguinal, retroperitoneal, and mediastinal lymph nodes as well as in the pleura, lungs, pericardium, liver, kidneys, and bones.

SARCOMAS

Endometrial Stromal Sarcoma

Sarcoma of the endometrial stroma presents the paradox of a well-differentiated but highly malignant connective tissue tumor. Only 20% of patients survive 5 years or longer after discovery of the tumor.

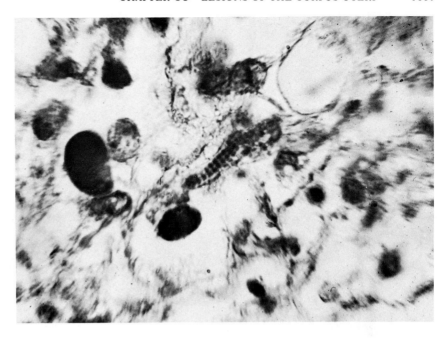

FIG. 55–20. Mixed mesodermal tumor of uterus. Basic constituents are multiple types of sarcoma. In center is striated muscle indicating that this portion is essentially rhabdomyosarcoma.

Grossly, this tumor is polypoid, with its attachment usually at the fundus of the uterus. It has a smooth, homogeneous, soft texture, although there may be foci of hemorrhage or necrosis, especially at its tip. It may occasionally occur as a sessile mass spreading into the endometrium on either side.

Microscopically, it is composed of typical endometrial stromal cells that have oval or elongated dark nuclei and very little cytoplasm. The cells are very regular and monotonously similar, with little pleomorphism. Few mitoses are found in this relatively homogeneous mass of cells (Fig. 55–21).

The tumor extends locally into the endometrium and myometrium and metastasizes by way of the bloodstream to distant organs such as the lungs and liver.

Endolymphatic Stromal Myosis

Endolymphatic stromal myosis is a rare condition that has a curious growth pattern and seems to represent a relatively low-grade variant of endometrial stromal sarcoma. The name is derived from the fact that this tumor is composed of endometrial stromal tissue that grows around and within lymph vessels of the myometrium. Extrauterine extension may occur via these channels.

Often this tumor is found only upon microscopic examination; however, it may reach a size that is grossly visible. When it does, it causes a focal or diffuse enlargement of the uterine muscle. Its cut surface resembles white or yellowish nodules interspersed between coarse strands of smooth muscle. It bears some resemblance grossly to adenomyosis.

Microscopically, this tumor is composed of oval or elongated endometrial stromal cells with very little cytoplasm and the same monotonous regularity seen in endometrial stromal sarcoma. There are few mitoses and no pleomorphism. These cells grow in large, irregular sheets in the region of the adventitia of blood vessels and lymph vessels. They have a curious propensity to expand into the lumina of lymph vessels and to cause enormous dilatation of these vessels without actually obstructing the flow of lymph. A sickle-shaped lymph channel usually lies alongside the invading tumor mass (Fig. 55–22).

With surgical removal of the uterus most patients are cured, but in about 20% the tumor recurs in the pelvic lymphatics and causes death by local growth in the pelvis and compression of ureters and bowel. It should be treated with radical surgery because of its invasive property.

Leiomyosarcoma

Malignant tumors of the uterine smooth muscle may arise directly from the myometrium, but in all likelihood the majority arise from preexisting leiomyomas. Approximately 0.40% of uterine myomas are sarcomatous.

Leiomyosarcomas have the same general gross features as their benign counterpart. They may be subserous, intramural, or submucous in location and tend to be circumscribed, although a few spread diffusely

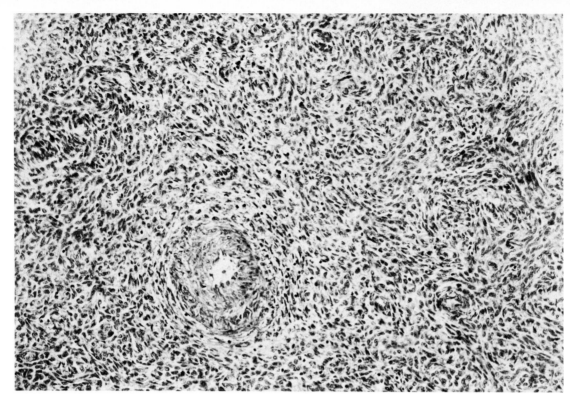

FIG. 55–21. Endometrial stromal sarcoma. Cells are typical stromal cells and have uniform, regular appearance that belies highly malignant character of this tumor.

FIG. 55–22. Endolymphatic stromal myosis. Masses of endometrial stroma grow alongside and extend within lymph channels of myometrium.

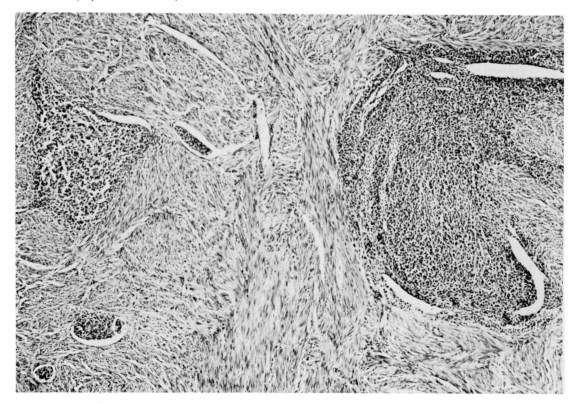

FIG. 55–23. Leiomyosarcoma of myometrium.

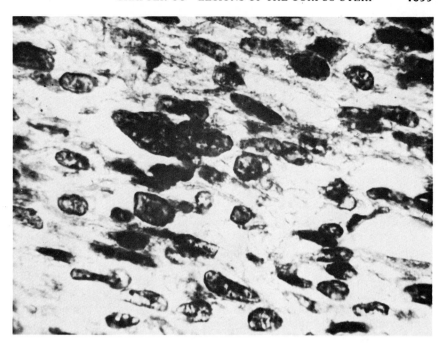

throughout the uterus. They tend to be yellowish-white or pink and, in general, are softer than the usual myoma, although identification of leiomyosarcoma depends upon microscopic examination.

Histologically these tumors resemble benign myomas inasmuch as both are composed of spindle-shaped cells that contain typical thick myofibrils when stained with phosphotungstic acid and hematoxylin. The sarcomas differ in having more numerous mitoses, larger cells with more rounded nuclei, nuclei of varying size and shape, and often multinucleated tumor giant cells (Fig. 55–23). When the sarcoma can be demonstrated to have arisen from a benign leiomyoma, the sarcomatous transformation is usually found in the center of the tumor and only rarely at the periphery.

These tumors extend locally but have a tendency to invade blood vessels and metastasize by way of the bloodstream. It is difficult to predict the clinical behavior of these tumors. Most are discovered after hysterectomy or myomectomy. Hysterectomy usually eradicates the tumor that is confined to the center of a myoma and, in most cases, the entire primary tumor can be readily removed. In a few cases, however, metastases appear, sometimes in bizarre locations such as striated muscle, perhaps several years after removal of the primary tumor.

Enlargement of the uterus after menopause may indicate a sarcomatous change or an adnexal mass that has been misinterpreted as uterine. In these instances abdominal exploration should be undertaken, for the treatment of uterine sarcoma is primarily surgical and

hysterectomy should be attempted. If the enlargement is accompanied by bleeding, local infection, or fever, curettage may secure the tissue necessary for diagnosis; endometrial sarcoma and mixed mesodermal tumors may produce these symptoms.

Adjuvent radiotherapy may help in the case of endometrial sarcoma but it is fruitless in leiomyosarcoma. Uterine sarcomas respond to chemotherapy with Adriamycin in about one-third of cases.

The incidence of leiomyosarcoma in fibroids is so low that prophylactic removal of the fibroids is clearly contraindicated.

Prognosis on the basis of histologic appearance may be misleading. Some tumors that are histologically entirely benign may metastasize. The best example of this is the *benign metastasizing leiomyoma.* Other tumors that present a very malignant appearance with numerous mitoses and multinucleated cells are eradicated by simple, total hysterectomy.

DIAGNOSIS OF ENDOMETRIAL CANCER

PREINVASIVE CANCER

Clinical Diagnosis

Adenomatous hyperplasia of the endometrium (also called Stage 0 cancer of the endometrium or, in its more intense form, cancer in situ), like cancer in situ of the cervix, is a preinvasive lesion. Some investigators prefer the term adenomatous hyperplasia or Stage 0 to cancer in situ because of the difficulty of defining

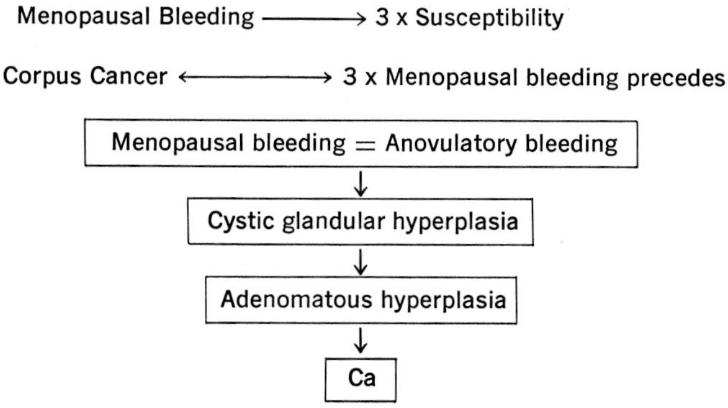

Menopausal Bleeding ────────→ 3 x Susceptibility

Corpus Cancer ←────────→ 3 x Menopausal bleeding precedes

```
┌─────────────────────────────────────────┐
│ Menopausal bleeding = Anovulatory bleeding │
└─────────────────────────────────────────┘
                    ↓
        ┌──────────────────────────┐
        │ Cystic glandular hyperplasia │
        └──────────────────────────┘
                    ↓
        ┌──────────────────────────┐
        │  Adenomatous hyperplasia  │
        └──────────────────────────┘
                    ↓
                ┌──────┐
                │  Ca  │
                └──────┘
```

FIG. 55–24. Precursors of carcinoma of endometrium.

morphologically a noninvasive endometrial cancer in an area in which stromal replacement is such an impure criterion of malignancy. Whatever the term, the lesion's biologic implication as a cancer precursor is clear and developmental phases can be defined. A recent prospective study disclosed development of invasive endometrial cancer from adenomatous hyperplasia in 12% of patients in a relatively short (5- to 10-year) follow-up (Fig. 55–24). Other studies revealed later cancer in 15% to 25% of patients.

The problem of dysfunctional uterine bleeding is intertwined with that of endometrial cancer, since abnormal bleeding, especially in women in the climacteric years, cannot be considered benign or dysfunctional until tissue sampling has excluded malignant disease. The highest incidence of adenomatous hyperplasia occurs in patients between the ages of 45 and 50 years, about 10 years younger than the median age of frank cancer of the endometrium. In addition, these problems are considered together because 1) patients who have dysfunctional bleeding at the menopause have a higher prospective incidence of later endometrial cancer; 2) patients who develop endometrial cancer postmenopausally have a higher incidence of prior menopausal bleeding than do controls; 3) patients who develop endometrial cancer premenopausally have a significantly high incidence of prior dysfunctional bleeding; and 4) patients who have bled postmenopausally because of long-term administration of estrogens or the presence of a functioning ovarian tumor have a high rate of coincident cystic glandular hyperplasia, adenomatous hyperplasia, and adenocarcinoma.

Thus it is not logical to dismiss a patient with abnormal bleeding in the climacteric years with reassurance of its simple endocrine cause without completion of the diagnostic convention that enables one to document this. Of course, an individual with postmenopausal bleeding, having no ordinary endocrine excuse, is usually promptly subjected to diagnostic curettage. It is also important to practice cancer prophylaxis and

careful preventive medicine by attempting restoration of ovulation, or at least restoration of progestational activity, in younger women who bleed abnormally in a dysfunctional pattern.

Physical Examination

Most patients with incipient or early endometrial cancer have no abnormality detectable by pelvic examination. The corpus is usually normal in size and configuration. The absence of abnormal findings on pelvic examination, therefore, does not enable the physician to rule out such a malignant transformation, and when his patient presents a bleeding aberration, he must pursue the diagnosis by examining tissue or cell samples to obtain documentary evidence of the cause of this bleeding.

Histologic Study

Accurate histologic samples of the endometrial cavity can be obtained with ease by means of an aspiration curette. This device consists of a cannula curette only 3 mm in its outside diameter, which is connected to a negative-pressure source. It is an outpatient method, requires no anesthesia, and has a high degree of patient acceptance. With the aspiration curettage one can obtain an excellent general sample of endometrium, and the procedure should be used without hesitancy whenever the information it supplies can be useful in diagnosis. Its particular value in endometrial cancer is the diagnosis of precursor lesions that can be acted upon, thus preventing the development of invasive cancer.

Diagnostic Curettage

This simple, painless surgical procedure, which does not require a significant convalescent period, is the definitive technique for obtaining endometrial tissue to establish or rule out the presence of endometrial cancer or its precursors. It requires a very brief hospital stay, provides a suitable tissue sample, gives the operator a clue to the gross extent of the lesion, and is virtually free of complication. We have seen no danger of spreading cancer by this method, and in the hands of most gynecologists it has proved most accurate in disclosing the presence of endometrial malignancy. In our experience, analysis of endometrial tissue obtained by curettage rarely fails to detect existing cancer, even in the presence of fibroids distorting the endometrial cavity.

Hysterography

The use of radiopaque media for diagnostic uterine radiography has increased in popularity in recent years, and some advocate its use for endometrial cancer de-

tection. We consider that its use for this purpose is theoretically more favorable to cancer dissemination and practically less accurate for diagnosis than curettage. We have, therefore, reserved its use to those patients who have resumed abnormal bleeding after curettage failed to disclose disease on the chance that an endometrial polyp or small submucous fibroid has been missed.

INVASIVE CANCER

Bleeding or blood-streaked watery discharge in postmenopausal women is a serious symptom. It is notable that pain or constitutional reaction is usually absent.

It is interesting to compare the phenotypes of individuals with endometrial cancer and with cancer of the cervix. The former patients are frequently obese, infertile, and of higher socioeconomic status than the latter.

Physical examination may be uninformative, since the cervix and corpus may be normal to inspection and palpation. The value of the cytologic smear and endometrial biopsy is outlined above, and it is clear that the final judgment rests with the diagnostic curettage, especially when performed in fractional or regional fashion. This enables the operator to evaluate first penetration into the cervical canal and its substance, then to obtain tissue selectively from the walls of the endometrial cavity and its roof or fundus, to assay the size of the tumor and the size of the cavity, and finally to obtain tissue for microscopic examination; lack of differentiation in these tumors is related directly to the expected penetration of the myometrium and ultimate virulence. Thus, these three critical parameters—size of uterine cavity, involvement of cervix, and differentiation—can be used to set up a meaningful classification (Fig. 55–25). This classification is most helpful in selecting treatment and offering a prognosis. The international staging has incorporated these parameters (Table 55–2).

TABLE 55–2. INTERNATIONAL STAGE DESIGNATIONS FOR CANCER OF THE ENDOMETRIUM (FIGO)

Stage	Description
0	Adenomatous hyperplasia or cancer *in situ*
I	Cancer confined to corpus
Ia	Cavity 8 cm or less
	G_1 Highly differentiated
	G_2 Partly differentiated
	G_3 Undifferentiated
Ib	Cavity more than 8 cm
	G_1 Highly differentiated
	G_2 Partly differentiated
	G_3 Undifferentiated
II	Cancer involves corpus and cervix
III	Cancer extends outside uterus but not outside true pelvis.
IV	Cancer extends outside true pelvis or involves mucosa of bladder or rectum.

G, histologic grade of tumor

TREATMENT OF ENDOMETRIAL CANCER

PREINVASIVE CANCER

Treatment of adenomatous hyperplasia or Stage 0 lesions depends upon the age and reproductive needs of the patient. In young women for whom preservation of the uterus is important it has been demonstrated in recent years that restoration of ovulation and of progestational endometrium by endogenous or exogenous means can reverse the pattern.

In women who have developed dysfunctional bleeding of the menopause a scheme of treatment may be developed, based upon the histologic characteristics of the endometrial sample obtained at diagnostic curettage, that relieves the presenting symptoms and, in addition, effects prophylaxis (Fig. 55–26).

Observation or endocrine manipulation of patients with adenomatous hyperplasia who are beyond their reproductive years is both illogical and radical and should be carried out only under special circumstances. Hysterectomy is the treatment of choice.

Stage I	Uterus normal size	
Stage II	Uterus mildly enlarged up to 10 cm depth	Downstage for anaplastic tumor or cervix involvement
Stage III	Uterus markedly enlarged over 10 cm depth	
Stage IV	Contiguous organs involved or distant metastases	

FIG. 55–25. Gusberg–Mount Sinai Hospital clinical classification of carcinoma of endometrium.

INVASIVE CANCER

The contribution of clinical staging to the selection of treatment for the individual patient with uterine cancer is suggested above. A clinical classification of the disease based upon three important parameters further contributes to choice of treatment:

1. *Size of the uterus.* This is a fairly good index of tumor growth, since the tumor tends to grow locally for long periods and expand the uterus by local extension. The size may be estimated by the depth of uterine sounding.

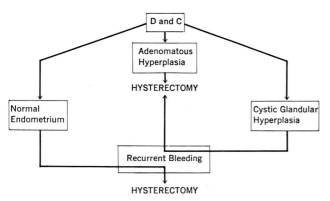

FIG. 55–26. Treatment of dysfunctional bleeding at menopause.

2. *Involvement of isthmus and cervix.* This indicates the need for treatment of lower parametrial lymphatic channels and primary pelvic lymph nodes. It can usually be diagnosed on fractional curettage, though some have suggested the use of hysterography. Aggressive radiotherapy and surgery to eradicate carcinoma in the cervix may improve the poor prognosis in this group.

3. *Lack of tumor differentiation.* This indication of deep myometrial penetration and possible node involvement warns that aggressive treatment is required. Examination of a frozen section at curettage can supply this information in spite of its deficiency for more subtle histologic description.

The traditional treatment for endometrial cancer is simple total hysterectomy and bilateral salpingo-oophorectomy. Routine radical pelvic dissection seems unjustified in patients who are frequently elderly, usually obese, and often hypertensive, with lesions most frequently confined to the corpus and, if spread beyond this, more often out of the pelvis than in it.

In recent years the combination of preoperative radium application followed by abdominal hysterectomy has gained favor in American clinics as the treatment of choice in this disease. The advantages claimed for this preparation for operation by radium include 1) devitalization of the tumor surface to increase the efficiency of later surgery by preventing spill and implantation metastases, 2) diminution in uterine size to facilitate operation and increase surgical clearance, 3) fibrosis of the uterus to seal lymphatics and prevent operative rupture, 4) improvement in the cure rate. Postoperative x-ray therapy is usually reserved for those patients in whom surgery revealed cancer spread beyond the uterus or deep in myometrial lymphatics. The position and technique of radiation in the treatment of cancer of the endometrium are discussed in Chapter 60.

Total abdominal hysterectomy has been found to be efficient and safe for the treatment of endometrial

FIGO Stage I_{AG1}--------TAH + BSO • optional postop vault radium

STAGE I_{AG2+G3}
STAGE I_{BG1} }----Combined treatment preop radiation

STAGE I_{BG2+G3} ⟩Preop rad • TAH + BSO + lymphadenectomy
STAGE II ⟩Preop rad • radical hysterectomy
STAGE III ⟩Preop rad • TAH + BSO + ext radiation

STAGE IV---------Individualize

Postop irradiation for deep myometrial infiltration

FIG. 55–27. Treatment of corpus cancer. (From Gusberg SB: Cancer 38:603, 1976)

cancer. When combined with radium implantation, it is usually performed 4 to 6 weeks following the radium placement, though some studies suggest that earlier operation offers no increased technical hazard. Whether this earlier timing of operation confers as much radiotherapeutic benefit has not been established. A commonly used procedure, and the one favored by our group, is total abdominal hysterectomy and bilateral salpingo-oophorectomy, by the extrafascial technique. This may be followed by external irradiation for tumors with high virulence factors. Radical hysterectomy should be reserved for patients of favorable operability in whom deep myometrial invasion or involvement of isthmus and cervix is highly likely. For such patients the risk of more radical operation may be justified in order to gain surgical removal of nodes and parametrium. Patients with poorly differentiated endometrial carcinoma have a high incidence of positive aortic lymph nodes. Hormonal or cytotoxic chemotherapy, or both, may be helpful for such patients.

Treatment with progestational agents in women with advanced or recurrent endometrial carcinoma has shown a response in about one-third of patients. The mode of action of progestins is not known. Measurement of cytoplasmic progesterone and estrogen receptors or estradiol 17-beta dehydrogenase in the tumors may help to identify the hormone-dependent endometrial cancers. By predicting which cancers will respond, one can improve the usefulness of progestins and administer cytotoxic chemotherapy earlier to those tumors found to be hormone-independent. At present there is no evidence of benefit from use of prophylactic progestational agents in Stage I disease.

Adriamycin alone, combinations of Adriamycin, cyclophosphamide and 5-fluorouracil or Alkeran and 5-fluorouracil administered with medroxyprogesterone acetate have produced objective tumor regressions in patients with metastatic endometrial carcinoma. Pro-

FIG. 55-28. Treatment of corpus cancer. (From Gusberg SB: Cancer 38:603, 1976)

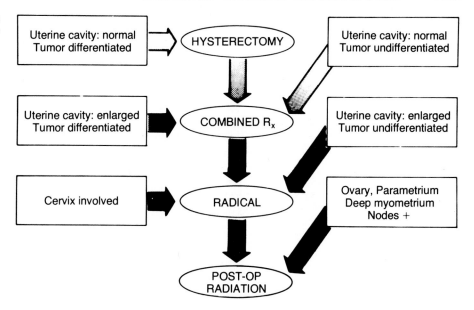

spective controlled trials are required before any definite assessment of cytotoxic chemotherapy can be made. These principles of treatment for endometrial adenocarcinoma are summarized in Figures 55–27 and 55–28.

PROGNOSIS FOR ENDOMETRIAL CANCER

The prognosis for adenocarcinoma of the endometrium is generally good with most forms of treatment, due especially to the fact that it tends to remain localized for a considerable period of time and that it is usually susceptible to local treatment. For operable lesions, irradiation alone can provide good results (50% or better), for surgery alone, good results are obtained in 60% of cases, and for combinations of irradiation and surgery, 75%. The survival rate for patients with inoperable lesions treated by irradiation alone is somewhat better than 20%. As is true of most cancers, the prognosis in endometrial cancer is clearly correlated with many factors, including clinical extent of disease, histologic grade of the tumor, extension to the cervix, and degree of involvement of the myometrium.

REFERENCES AND RECOMMENDED READING

MALIGNANT LESIONS OF THE CORPUS UTERI

Bruckner HW, Deppe G: Intensive combination chemotherapy of advanced endometrial carcinoma with Adriamycin, cyclophosphamide, 5-fluorouracil, and medroxyprogesterone acetate. Obstet Gynecol 50:105, 1977

Christopherson WM, Williamson EO, Gray LA: Leiomyosarcoma of the uterus. Cancer 29:1512, 1972

Cohen CJ, Gusberg SB: Screening for endometrial cancer. Clin Obstet Gynecol 18:27, 1975

Cohen CJ, Deppe G, Bruckner HW: Treatment of advanced adenocarcinoma of the endometrium with Melphalan, 5-fluorouracil, and medroxyprogesterone acetate—A preliminary study. Obstet Gynecol 50:415, 1977

Cohen CJ, Deppe G: Sarcoma and Lymphoma. In Gusberg SB, Frick HC (eds): Corscaden's Gynecologic Cancer, 5th ed. Baltimore, Williams & Wilkins, 1978

Cramer DW, Cutler SJ, Christine B: Trends in the incidence of endometrial cancer in the USA. Gynecol Oncol 2:130, 1974

Creasman WT, Boronow RC, Morrow CP, DiSaia PJ, Blessing J: Adenocarcinoma of the endometrium: Its metastatic lymph node potential. Gynecol Oncol 4:239, 1976

Creasman WT, Weed JC: Screening techniques in endometrial cancer. Cancer 38:436, 1976

DiSaia PJ, Castro JR, Rutledge FN: Mixed mesodermal sarcoma of the uterus. Am J Roentgenol Radium Ther Nucl Med 117:632, 1973

Donovan JF: Nonhormonal chemotherapy of endometrial adenocarcinoma: A review. Cancer 34;1587, 1974

Gray LA, Christopherson WM, Hoover RN: Estrogens and endometrial carcinoma. Obstet Gynecol 49:385, 1977

Gurpide E: Endocrinologic aspects of gynecologic cancer. In Gusberg SB, Frick HC (eds): Corscaden's Gynecologic Cancer, 5th ed. Baltimore, Williams & Wilkins, 1978

Gusberg SB: Precursors of corpus carcinoma. I. Estrogens and adenomatous hyperplasia. Am J Obstet Gynecol 54;905, 1947

Gusberg SB, Kaplan AL: Precursors of corpus cancer. IV. Adenomatous hyperplasia as stage 0 carcinoma of the endometrium. Am J Obstet Gynecol 87:662, 1963

Gusberg SB: Dysfunctional and the neoplastic: Clinical investigation in the service of patient care in endometrial cancer. Am J Obstet Gynecol 116:175, 1973

Gusberg SB, Chen SY, Cohen CJ: Endometrial cancer: Factors influencing the choice of treatment. Gynecol Oncol 2:308, 1974

Gusberg SB: Evolution of modern treatment of corpus cancer. Cancer, 38:603, 1976

Gusberg SB: The individual at high risk for endometrial carcinoma. Am J Obstet Gynecol 126:535, 1976

Gusberg SB: Cancer of the endometrium: Diagnosis and histogenesis. In Gusberg SB, Frick HC (eds): Corscaden's Gynecologic Cancer, 5th ed. Baltimore, Williams & Wilkins, 1978

Gusberg SB: Cancer of the endometrium: Classification and treatment. In Gusberg SB, Frick HC (eds): Corscaden's Gynecologic Cancer, 5th ed. Baltimore, Williams & Wilkins, 1978

Kohorn, EI: Gestagens and endometrial carcinoma. Gynecol Oncol 4:398, 1976

Krieger PD, Gusberg SB: Endolymphatic stromal myosis— A grade I endometrial sarcoma. Gynecol Oncol 1:299, 1973

MacMahon B: Risk factors for endometrial cancer. Gynecol Oncol 2:122, 1974

Morrow CP, DiSaia PJ, Townsend DE: Current management of endometrial cancer. Obstet Gynecol 42:399, 1973

Martel R, Koss LG, Lewis JL, D'Urso JR; Mesodermal mixed tumors of the uterine corpus. Obstet Gynecol 43:248, 1974

Ober, WB; Uterine sarcomas: Histogenesis and taxonomy. Annu NY Acad Sci 75:568, 1959

Reagan JW: The changing nature of endometrial cancer. Gynecol Oncol 2:144, 1974

Thigpen JT, Buchsbaum HJ, Mangan C, et al: Phase II trial of adriamycin in the treatment of advanced or recurrent endometrial carcinoma: A gynecologic oncology group study. Cancer Treat Rep 63:21, 1979

Vellios F: Endometrial hyperplasia and carcinoma in situ. Gynecol Oncol 2:152, 1974

Watring WG, Byfield JE, Lagasse LD, et al: Combination Adriamycin and radiation therapy in gynecologic cancer. Gynecol Oncol 2:518, 1974

BENIGN LESIONS

A variety of cysts and tumors arise in the pelvic supporting structures and fallopian tubes (oviducts). Such lesions are usually benign and originate from peritoneal inclusions or embryonic remnants. The embryologic development of the oviducts and broad ligament accounts for mesonephric and paramesonephric derivatives capable of giving rise to cystic structures. The majority are small, multiple, not associated with any clinical syndrome, and without clinical significance. An awareness of them is important, however, since they are often encountered at the time of pelvic surgery, and intelligent management requires an appreciation of their nature. Occasionally a cystic structure in the broad ligament reaches sufficient size to be palpated or to produce symptoms from pressure on adjacent structures, twisting of a pedicle, rupture, or hemorrhage. Under these circumstances, the lesion is often mistakenly thought to be of ovarian origin. Surgical removal is required.

Cysts of the broad ligament are of mesonephric or paramesonephric origin. They may be intraligamentous or pedunculated, but the location is not diagnostic of origin. Most broad ligament cysts can be classified by the character of their lining epithelium. *Pedunculated cysts* of the broad ligament are common and are referred to as *hydatids of Morgagni* (Fig. 56–1). The cyst is small and translucent, with a long, slender pedicle attached near the fimbria of the oviduct, frequently bilaterally. It rarely exceeds 1 cm in diameter. *Intraligamentous cysts* may be small or may reach 10 to 15 cm in diameter or greater. They are thin-walled and unilocular. These cysts are commonly referred to as *parovarian cysts* because of their location. The ovary is intact and separate from the cyst, and the oviduct is stretched across the circumference. If large, such intraligamentous cysts should be removed. Malignant change is rare and can be ignored. The student is referred to the excellent review by Gardner *et al.* for further discussion of the microscopic pathology.

The most common tumorlike lesions of the oviduct are *Walthard's cell rests* (Figs. 56–2, 56–3). They are seen on the peritoneal surface of the oviduct and adjacent broad ligament as multiple, small (1 to 2 mm), glistening, soft, waxlike cysts. They are benign and probably arise from inclusions of surface celomic epithelium. At times, they must be differentiated from tubercles. This is usually possible because of their typical glistening, noninflamed appearance. Microscopic examination reveals subperitoneal nests of squamous-like epithelial cells, some of which show central cystic change.

Salpingitis isthmica nodosa is an uncommon lesion of the oviduct characterized by one or more nodular thickenings of the isthmus (Fig. 56–4). Microscopically, there is a thickening of the smooth muscle surrounding the isthmic lumen of the oviduct. Within the

CHAPTER 56

LESIONS OF THE FALLOPIAN TUBE

James A. Merrill

smooth muscle are discrete acini, or glandlike spaces, lined by immature tubal-type epithelium. Unlike the epithelium of the major portion of the oviduct, this epithelium tends to be cuboidal rather than columnar. The lesion can be distinguished easily from endometriosis of the oviduct. Opinions differ as to its genesis. Many consider it to be an aftermath of inflammation of the oviduct; others favor a congenital origin from embryonic rests. The author believes the lesion arises from downgrowth of the epithelium of the oviduct in a manner similar to that which occurs in adenomyosis. Salpingitis isthmica nodosa rarely requires specific treatment.

Accessory oviducts or *diverticula* of the oviducts are developmental anomalies that may be confused with broad ligament cysts or salpingitis isthmica nodosa. The microscopic pattern of typical tubal plicae and epithelium is diagnostic.

Several rare *benign tumors of the oviduct* have been
(*Text continues on p. 1108.*)

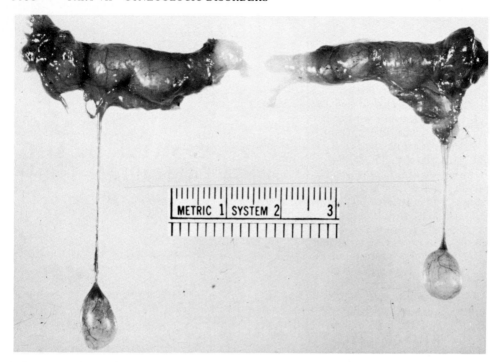

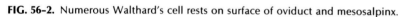

FIG. 56–1. Hydatids of Morgagni attached to mesosalpinx of each oviduct.

FIG. 56–2. Numerous Walthard's cell rests on surface of oviduct and mesosalpinx.

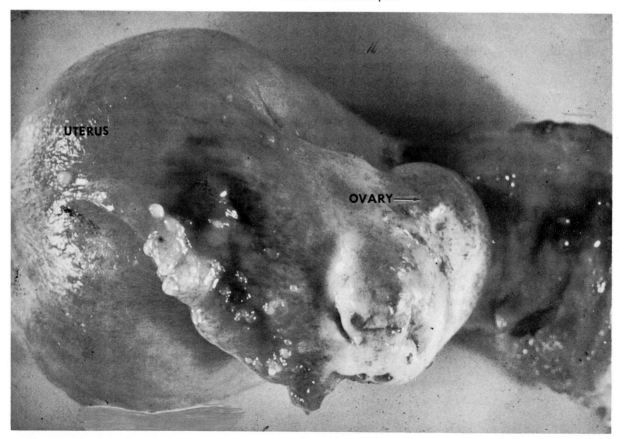

FIG. 56–3. Microscopic section of mesosalpinx showing Walthard's cell rests. One on surface is solid mass of cells, other shows cystic change.

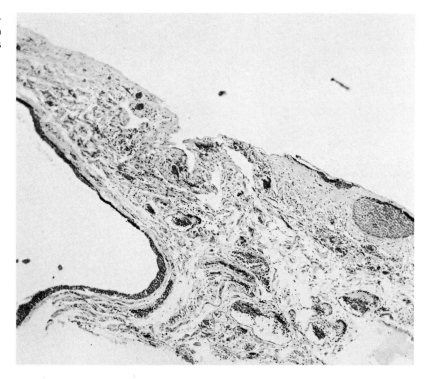

FIG. 56–4. Microscopic section of oviduct with salpingitis isthmica nodosa. Central lumen is intact; smooth muscle of wall of oviduct contains numerous glandlike spaces.

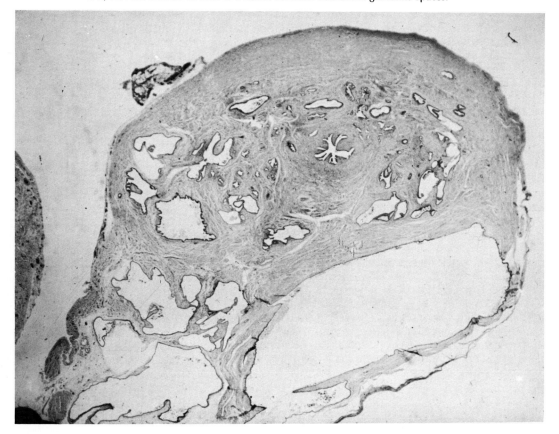

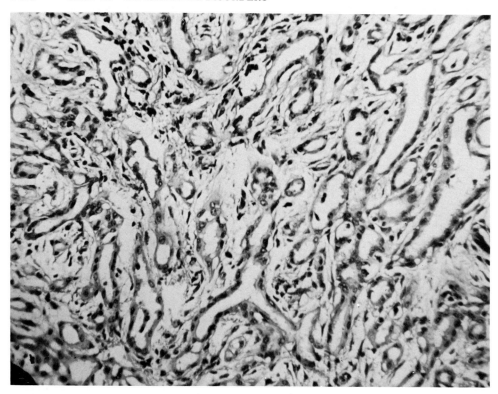

FIG. 56–5. Microscopic section of adenomatoid tumor of oviduct.

described: dermoid cysts, hemangiomas, lymphangiomas, leiomyomas, and adenomatoid tumors. The adenomatoid tumors are the most common and are usually small and circumscribed, confined to the muscular wall. (Fig. 56–5). They are composed of small, glandlike spaces lined by cells of mesothelial, endothelial, or epithelial appearance. There is no agreement as to their origin. They are usually incidental findings, and all such tubal lesions reported to date have been benign.

Myomas arise in the round ligament (Fig. 56–6). They commonly become pedunculated and pose the problems of treatment and differential diagnosis described in Chapter 55. In gross and microscopic appearance they resemble myomas of the uterus.

Adrenal rests are found in the broad ligament (Fig. 56–7). In a review of autopsy material from 98 infants and children, broad ligament or mesovarian adrenal rests were present in three. This is explained by the proximity of the anlage of the adrenals to the genital ducts. Adrenal rests may be grossly visible but are more often microscopic. They are small nodules, firm, smooth, and yellow. Microscopic appearance is typical of adrenal cortical tissue. It is extremely rare that adrenal rests produce endocrine symptoms.

Endometriosis frequently involves the broad ligament, oviducts, and uterosacral ligaments. It is discussed in Chapter 51.

MALIGNANT LESIONS

Cancer of the fallopian tube is uncommon, constituting less than 1% of all cancer of the female genital tract. The recorded cases of cancer of the oviduct—less than 1000—suggest the probability of three cases per million women per year. Furthermore, this malignancy is difficult to diagnose. In at least two cases (Mitchell; Starr) very early tubal cancers were found accidentally on microscopic examination of tubal fragments resected for postpartum sterilization.

Suspected tumor of the ovary or uterus is the usual reason for surgery in the patient with cancer of the oviduct; in many cases both tube and ovary are involved, and less often tube and endometrium. Thus, it may be difficult to decide which site is primary. It has been suggested that some of these multiple lesions represent multicentric foci of origin. As is true of other cancers, the success of treatment is directly correlated with the extent of the disease at the time of treatment. Unfortunately, owing to the difficulty of diagnosis, many tubal neoplasms are diagnosed late.

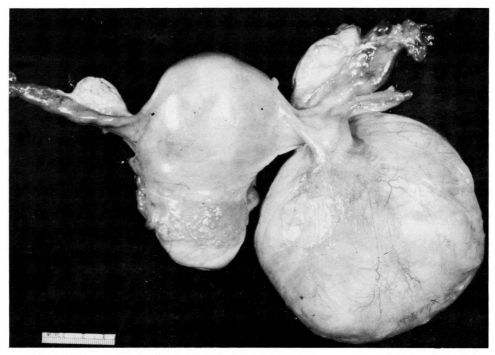

FIG. 56–6. Myoma of round ligament. Uterus, oviducts, and ovaries are normal.

FIG. 56–7. Section of ovary, mesosalpinx, and oviduct from newborn infant. Mesosalpinx contains well-defined adrenal rest surrounded by remnants of wolffian duct. (Merrill JA: Am J Obstet Gynecol 78:1258, 1959)

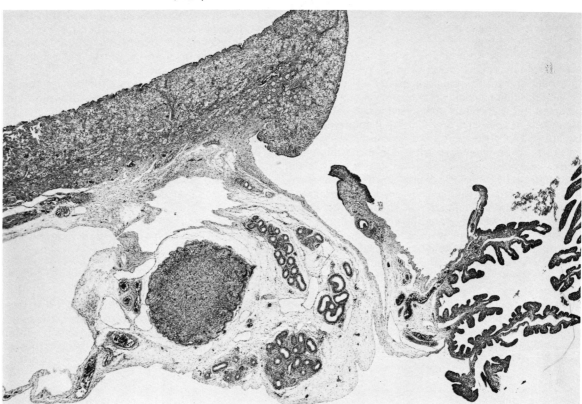

More than 90% of the primary cancers of the oviduct are carcinoma. Leiomyosarcomas, mixed tumors, and trophoblastic tumors rarely arise in the oviduct.

PRIMARY CARCINOMA

Most primary tubal carcinomas are papillary adenocarcinoma, although squamous cell carcinoma and carcinoma in situ can arise from the tubal epithelium.

Age

The age reported for patients with primary tubal carcinoma ranges from 17 to 80 years. The highest incidence of this disease occurs during the fifth decade of life. Women with carcinoma of the oviduct are frequently infertile.

Symptoms

Symptoms are rare in patients with early tubal carcinoma. About 20% of all patients have no symptoms. In those who do have symptoms, the most common are vaginal discharge, abnormal vaginal bleeding, irregularities of menstruation, and pain. The discharge is often yellow or slightly blood-tinged (honey-colored). A classic, but rare, symptom of episodic vaginal discharge known as *hydrops tubae profluens* has been described with both carcinoma of the oviduct and hydrosalpinx. In this circumstance, cramping pelvic pain and an adnexal mass disappear with a sudden serous or serosanguineous discharge.

Diagnosis

An adnexal mass is the most common physical finding in a patient with tubal carcinoma. However, 50% of women have no palpable pelvic mass. Carcinoma of the fallopian tube is rarely diagnosed prior to surgery. Most tubal carcinomas are found in patients undergoing surgery for a preoperative diagnosis of ovarian neoplasm, uterine myoma, or tubo-ovarian inflammatory disease. Laparotomy may disclose a rare early lesion not suspected on the basis of preoperative pelvic examination. The triad of pain, discharge, and adnexal mass occurs in about 50% of patients. The possibility of carcinoma of the oviduct should be considered in a postmenopausal nulliparous woman with a serous or serosanguineous discharge and an adnexal mass. Some cases have been suspected when cytologic examination of vaginal smears repeatedly showed abnormal cells even though material obtained from cervical biopsies and endometrial curettings was normal. However, the reported accuracy of cytologic examination of vaginal smears as a diagnostic procedure for carcinoma of the oviduct is disappointingly low, varying from 0% to 60%.

Laparoscopy and hysterosalpingography have been suggested as aids in the diagnosis of carcinoma of the oviduct.

Pathology

At surgery, an oviduct harboring a carcinoma frequently resembles a subacutely or chronically infected tube with pyosalpinx or hydrosalpinx. The tumors are bilateral in 15% to 30% of cases. Ascites is a rare associated finding. Adhesions to adjacent peritoneal surfaces are often less tenacious than the adhesions usually associated with pelvic inflammation disease. The appearance of the opened tube, packed with friable papillary excrescences, is characteristic. Less often there is a localized, soft, friable tumor mass. There may be soft, yellow areas of necrosis or soft, red-brown areas of hemorrhage. In some situations, the entire lumen is filled with tumor, some of which may protrude from the fimbriated end. The carcinoma in the oviduct may be continuous with an ovarian neoplasm. In these circumstances, it is impossible to say whether the tumor first appeared in the tube or the ovary.

The microscopic pattern is that of a papillary adenocarcinoma (Fig. 56–8). Well-differentiated tumors are composed of delicately branched processes covered by a thin layer of columnar epithelial cells. The pattern may resemble that of a papillary serous cystadenocarcinoma of the ovary. Less well-differentiated tumors have a trabecular or aveolar pattern. The muscular wall of the tube is usually invaded and the tumor may completely fill the lumen of the tube and replace all normal tubal epithelium. For certain diagnosis of primary carcinoma of the oviduct, the lesion should be confined to the endosalpinx and there should be a microscopically identifiable transition between the anaplastic epithelium of the malignant neoplasm and the adjacent benign tubal epithelium (Fig. 56–9).

The adenomatous salpingitis that characterizes tuberculosis of the oviduct may, on occasion, be confused with tubal carcinoma. However, in the case of inflammation, the cellular characteristics of neoplasia are absent. The presence of typical granulomatous inflammation makes the diagnosis of malignancy doubtful.

Squamous carcinoma, adenocanthoma, and transitional-cell carcinoma have been reported to occur in the tube.

Associated Disease

Because carcinoma of the oviduct grossly resembles hydrosalpinx and pyosalpinx, and because carcinoma of the tube is often found in association with healed or subacute salpingitis, it has been suggested that chronic inflammation may be a predisposing factor.

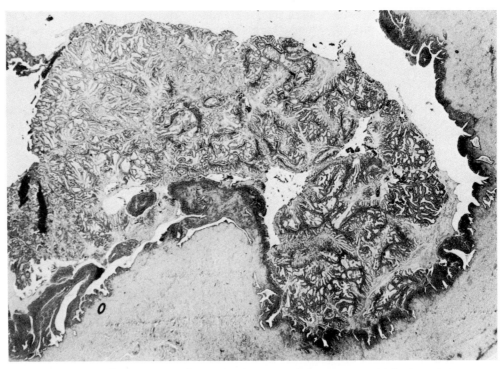

FIG. 56–8. Papillomatous growth pattern of primary adenocarcinoma of fallopian tube. (× 50)

FIG. 56–9. Early primary adenopapillary carcinoma of fallopian tube. (× 10)

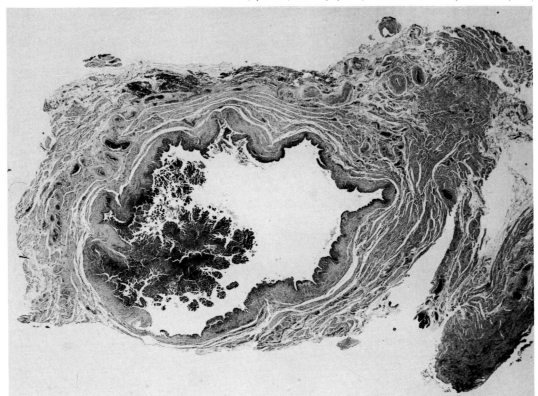

The observation of a relatively high incidence of infertility among patients with carcinoma of the fallopian tube further suggests preexisting tubal disease in these patients. It is possible, of course, that the tubal inflammation seen at the time carcinoma of the oviduct is diagnosed is secondary to necrosis and infection within the tumor itself.

Spread

Carcinoma of the oviduct usually spreads by direct extension rather than by way of the lymphatics until late in the history of the disease. Peritoneal implants are likely if the tubal lumen is patent through the fimbriated end. Usually, however, inflammatory adhesions obliterate the fimbriae. The regional pelvic nodes, local peritoneum, ovary, bladder, rectum, and vagina are usually involved prior to the development of extrapelvic spread. Peritoneal spread has not been reported to be as extensive as that observed with ovarian cancer.

Staging

As in all malignant tumors, staging is essential for comparison of cases and evaluation of therapy. Since the *Fédération Internationale de Gynécologie et Obstetrique* (FIGO) has not yet addressed this question for tubal carcinoma, no uniform staging has been adopted. Several have suggested, and used, a staging system similar to that for carcinoma of the ovary. A simpler staging system, also used by several authors, is as follows:

Stage I: Carcinoma limited to the tube; no extension to the serosa

Stage II: Carcinoma extending to the tubal serosa or adjacent pelvic viscera

Stage III: Carcinoma extending beyond the pelvis, but still confined to the abdominal cavity

Stage IV: Extra-abdominal metastases

Treatment

The preferred treatment for carcinoma of the oviduct is total abdominal hysterectomy and bilateral salpingo-oophorectomy. The place of omentectomy has not been determined. Peritoneal washings should be taken unless it is obvious that the disease has spread beyond the tube. More extensive procedures may be indicated if the lesion has spread to adjacent organs or structures. The value of extensive procedures, such as exenteration and lymph node dissection, cannot be stated because they have not been performed often enough to permit valid assessment of the results. Postoperative external beam irradiation is commonly given, although the effectiveness has not been satisfactorily evaluated.

Intraperitoneal insertion of colloidal isotopes and systemic chemotherapy have been used, but the experience is inadequate to allow conclusions regarding efficacy.

Prognosis

The prognosis for survival depends upon the extent of the malignancy. If spread beyond the tube is grossly apparent, the prognosis is extremely poor. The 5-year survival rates vary from 0% to 44%. Bilateral tubal carcinoma is associated with a poorer prognosis than is unilateral disease. There appears to be little correlation between prognosis and the microscopic differentiation of the tumor, although solid tumors seem to have a worse prognosis than papillary ones.

METASTATIC CANCER

Cancer metastatic to the oviducts occurs much more commonly than primary carcinoma. Indeed, metastasis or direct extension from lesions arising in the adjacent organs accounts for 80% to 90% of malignancies found in the oviduct. Most of these tumors originate in the ovary or uterus. Metastases from the breast or gastrointestinal tract also have been reported. Metastases may extend along the serosa, through subepithelial or subserosal lymphatics, or directly along the lumen of the endosalpinx. The histologic pattern, which shows conspicuous lymphatic involvement and intact tubal epithelium (Fig. 56–10), is easily distinguished from primary tubal carcinoma.

When both tube and ovary are involved, the salvage is poor, regardless of which was the primary site of the neoplasm.

RARE MALIGNANT TUMORS

Sarcoma

A few cases of primary sarcoma (usually leiomyosarcoma) of the oviduct have been reported. The prognosis is poor, similar to that for sarcomas elsewhere. Treatment primarily is surgical.

Mixed Müllerian Tumor

A primary, malignant, mixed müllerian tumor has occasionally been seen in the oviduct. The clinical findings and gross pathology are similar to those of primary adenocarcinoma of the oviduct. Microscopically, the lesions, which have been bilateral in one-third of cases, are similar to tumors in the myometrium with various types of neoplastic immature connective tissue and epithelium. Treatment is similar to that for primary tubal carcinoma.

FIG. 56–10. Secondary tubal carcinoma showing intact tubal epithelium and carcinoma areas in lymphatics. Primary cancer was located in endometrium. (× 20)

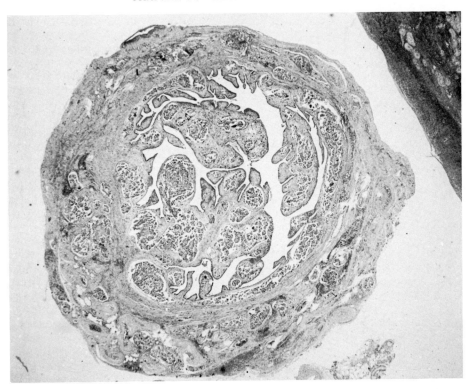

Trophoblastic Tumors

Rare primary tubal choriocarcinoma has been reported. The tumor presumably has followed ectopic tubal pregnancy. Success with chemotherapy is similar to that for gestational choriocarcinomas arising in the uterus.

REFERENCES AND RECOMMENDED READING

Anbrokh YM: Histological characteristics and questions concerning histogenesis of cancer of the fallopian tubes. Neoplasms 17:631, 1970

Benedet JL, White GW, Fairley RN, et al: Adenocarcinoma of the fallopian tube. Experience with 41 patients. Obstet Gynecol 50:654, 1977

Boutselis JG, Thompson JN: Clinical aspects of primary carcinoma of the fallopian tube: A clinical study of 14 cases. Am J Obstet Gynecol 111:98, 1971

DeQueiroz AC, Roth LM: Malignant mixed Müllerian tumor of the fallopian tube. Report of a case. Obstet Gynecol 36:554, 1970

Dodson MG, et al: Clinical aspects of fallopian tube carcinoma. Obstet Gynecol 36:935, 1970

Dowdeswell RH, Pratt THR: Benign teratoma of fallopian tube. A case report. Obstet Gynecol 36:554, 1970

Dowdeswell RH, Pratt THR: Benign teratoma of fallopian tube. A case report. Obstet Gynecol 39:52, 1972

Ebrahimi T, Okagaki T: Hemangioma of the fallopian tube. Am J Obstet Gynecol 115:864, 1973

Federman Q, Toker C: Primary transitional cell tumor of the uterine adnexa. Am J Obstet Gynecol 115:863, 1973

Gardner GH, Greene RR, Peckham B: Normal and cystic structures of the broad ligament. Am J Obstet Gynecol 55;917, 1948

Hertig AT, Gore H: Tumors of the Female Sex Organs, Part 4. Washington DC, Armed Forces Institute of Pathology, 1961

Mazzarella P, et al: Teratoma of the uterine tube. A case report and review of the literature. Obstet Gynecol 39:381, 1972

Mitchell RM, Mohler RW: Primary carcinoma of the fallopian tube. Am J Obstet Gynecol 50:283, 1945

Momtazee S, Kempson RL: Primary adenocarcinoma of the fallopian tube. Obstet Gynecol 32:649, 1968

Okagaki T, Richard RM: Neurilemoma of the fallopian tube. Am J Obstet Gynecol 106:929, 1970

Palomaki JF, Blair OM: Hilus cell rest of the fallopian tube. A case report. Obstet Gynecol 37:60, 1971

Salazar H, et al: Ultrastructure and observations on the histogenesis of mesotheliomas, "adenomatoid tumors," of the female genital tract. Cancer 29:141, 1972

Sedlis A: Carcinoma of the fallopian tube. Surg Clin N Am 58:121, 1978

Starr AJ, Ruffalo EH, Shenoy BV, et al: Primary carcinoma of the fallopian tube: A surprise finding in a postpartum tubal ligation. Am J Obstet Gynecol 132:344, 1978

Woodruff JD, Pauerstein CJ: The Fallopian Tube. Baltimore, Williams & Wilkins, 1969

CHAPTER

LESIONS OF THE OVARY

James A. Merrill
James H. Nelson, Jr.
Thomas E. Dolan

BENIGN LESIONS OF THE OVARY

James A. Merrill

The consideration of ovarian neoplasms has always stirred great interest among gynecologists. The very history of modern gynecology begins with Ephraim McDowell's successful removal of a large ovarian tumor in 1809, which is described on page 20. This, the first successful removal of an abdominal tumor, was a landmark in abdominal surgery. Equally fascinating has been the wide variety of histologic patterns found in ovarian neoplasms and the corresponding array of clinical findings.

More than any other gland or organ in the body, the ovary has the potential of producing an unusual num-

ber of neoplasms of both epithelial and connective tissue origin. Knowledge of the physiology and anatomy of the ovarian cycle is required for correct evaluation of the pathologic nature of an ovarian enlargement, and the immediate treatment and ultimate prognosis depend upon the pathologic interpretation. The mature ovary is a complex gland consisting of different types of connective tissue as well as cells with specific differentiation and function. Moreover, the adult ovary contains embryonic remnants, in addition to cells, capable of differentiation into various morphologic and functional types. The cyclic growth, enlargement, and subsequent atresia of follicles form the basis for most nonneoplastic enlargements of the ovaries.

The embryonic gonads develop in the genital ridge, ventral to the mesonephros and adjacent to the primordial adrenal. In the ovary, these intimate relations result in embryonic rests that persist past fetal life. We should expect to find neoplasms in the ovary arising from these structures and, indeed, such tumors are present. The gonad develops from a mass of specialized mesenchyme. Differentiation of this mesenchyme results in the follicular apparatus of the ovary (granulosa and theca cells) and components of the tubular apparatus of the testis. This bipotential capacity of the embryonic gonad is best demonstrated in the ambiguous gonads of intersex patients. In the mature ovary this specialized mesenchyme persists as the ovarian cortical stroma and probably retains some of its original potential for differentiation, accounting for the hormone-producing, mesenchymomas composed of "female-directed" or "male-directed" cells. The surface epithelium of the ovary, so-called *germinal epithelium,* is derived from celomic epithelium and has the same potential for development as the primitive müllerian duct. Cystic neoplasms arising from these cells result in the most common of ovarian tumors, composed of various epithelia. The oocytes migrate to the embryonic gonad and exert an organizing effect upon the stroma. These primordial germ cells retain a vast potential for differentiation, and an almost limitless variety of tissues arises from neoplastic growth of these cells.

These observations form the basis for the many theories of histogenesis of ovarian neoplasms.

Many ovarian neoplasms are asymptomatic and many functional cystic enlargements of the ovary are found, and unfortunately removed, incident to abdominal surgery for other indications. It is not uncommon for a surgeon operating for appendicitis to find an ovary that appears "cystic" or contains a "cyst." Failure to understand the significance of such findings results in sacrifice of the ovary or a portion thereof. Efforts should be made to diagnose true ovarian neoplasms early and at the same time recognize the functional nature of nonneoplastic ovarian enlargements.

Ovarian tumors have been described in patients of

all ages, including intrauterine fetuses, newborn infants, children, and nonagenarians. However, they are most prevalent during the reproductive years, and benign tumors occur most often in women in their 40s. Ovarian tumors are likely to be malignant when they occur in youngsters and women past 50 years of age.

SYMPTOMS OF OVARIAN ENLARGEMENT

Not only are many ovarian tumors asymptomatic, but the symptoms are notoriously late in appearing. This is true of benign and malignant tumors alike. Ovarian enlargement or neoplasia may be discovered first during a premarital or prenatal examination, a school or employment physical examination, or a periodic health examination. With a few notable exceptions, what symptoms are present are not characteristic of any specific tumor.

Pressure. An enlarging tumor may press upon the bladder, producing overflow incontinence or urinary frequency. Occasionally a tumor becomes impacted in the pelvis and obstructs either the urethra or the ureters. Similarly, a tumor, particularly a solid tumor, may press upon the rectum and produce constipation. More commonly, a sizable tumor or cyst produces an ill-defined pressure sensation or "heaviness" in the pelvis. When tumors reach great size they interfere with venous and lympahtic drainage from the lower extremities, resulting in edema of the legs or varicosities. They may also produce venous distention over the abdomen and elevate the diaphragm sufficiently to cause shortness of breath.

Size. Occasionally a very large tumor produces as its only symptom—an increase in girth (Fig. 57–1). The patient describes a progressive increase in the size of her abdomen and the frequent need to buy new clothes or to let out the waist of old ones. Often this is erroneously accredited to middle-age spread.

In infants and children, ovarian tumors are often noticed by parents at the time of bathing or changing clothes. In the rare instances of tumors diagnosed in the newborn, suspicion is aroused solely by the obvious appearance of an abdominal mass.

Pain. Pain is a rare symptom of an uncomplicated ovarian tumor, even one of considerable size. Pain may result from rupture, torsion of the pedicle, or distention of a cyst through rapid enlargement or hemorrhage. Ovarian pain is a constant aching referred to the ipsilateral iliac or inguinal region and into the inner aspect of the upper thigh. Pain occasionally radiates into the vulva. An ovarian tumor may produce dyspareunia, particularly if it is situated deep in the cul-de-sac. Pain may result from adhesions to adjacent

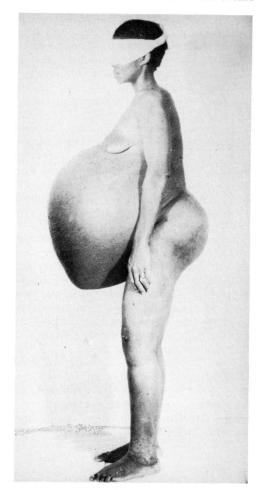

FIG. 57–1. Patient with huge benign cystadenoma of ovary. Cyst weighed 128 lb; following removal, patient weight 126 lb. There was marked edema of lower extremities. (JW Kelso)

structures or pressure upon them. However, most pain is the result of some acute accident or complication.

Menstrual Abnormalities. Tumors with endocrine function are often the cause of menstrual abnormalities. Estrogen-producing tumors may cause oligomenorrhea or amenorrhea, followed by irregular, excessive, or prolonged menses. The masculinizing tumors are often associated with amenorrhea or oligomenorrhea, without prolonged or excessive menses. Certain tumors, not ordinarily regarded as having functional potential, may be accompanied by endocrine activity, menstrual aberrations, and endometrial hyperplasia; this is related to functional activity of the stroma of such tumors as cystadenomas, Brenner tumors, and adenofibromas. However, abnormal bleeding is more often unrelated to the ovarian neoplasm.

Hormone Changes. In addition to menstrual abnormalities, some tumors with endocrine function are associated with other clinical manifestations of hormone production. Ovarian mesenchymomas, which include granulosa–theca-cell tumors, Sertoli–Leydig tumors (arrhenoblastomas), and lipoid tumors, may be associated with feminization or masculinization. In the prepubertal girl, feminization is manifested as sexual precocity, with menstrual flow and breast development. In the postmenopausal woman, the only significant finding is often return of uterine bleeding. Feminizing tumors in women of childbearing age may cause alterations in secondary sex characteristics, but commonly the symptoms are related to overstimulation of the endometrium and lower genital tract. The same tumors may produce masculinization, characterized by hirsutism, enlargement of the clitoris, anovulation, amenorrhea, breast atrophy, and deepening of the voice. Tumors derived from adrenal rests may produce some of the symptoms of Cushing's disease, and an interesting but rare tumor, struma ovarii, may produce symptoms of hyperthyroidism.

These symptoms are usually dramatic, but the tumors that produce them consitute a small portion of the total number of ovarian neoplasms.

Infertility. Ovarian tumors can be associated with infertility. Except in the Stein–Leventhal syndrome and in conditions related to polycystic ovarian disease, there is seldom a direct relation between the ovarian enlargement and the infertility.

COMPLICATIONS

The most dramatic symptoms occurring with ovarian neoplasms are the result of secondary changes or complications. This is particularly true of benign tumors.

Vascular Accident. Hemorrhage into a cyst is usually a slow process producing gradual distention and minimal symptoms. If the hemorrhage is sudden and large in amount, it produces acute abdominal pain with typical ovarian radiation and signs of peritoneal irritation. The tumor is tender, and motion of the cervix or uterus produces pain. Hemorrhage from a cyst may escape into the peritoneal cavity, resulting in abdominal distention, tenderness, and rebound tenderness. If the cyst has collapsed, the diagnosis is difficult unless its presence was suspected earlier. Rarely, necrosis occurs, more commonly in malignant than in benign ovarian enlargements.

Torsion. Many of the benign tumors, both cystic and solid, develop a tenuous pedicle which is triradiate—the infundibulopelvic ligament, the utero-ovarian (suspensory) ligament and oviduct, and the mesosalpinx (Fig. 57–2). Neoplasms that rise out of the pelvis and are not large enough to be fixed in position may undergo complete or partial torsion of the pedicle. In one study, torsion was found to be present in 12% to 14% of patients operated on for tumors. If the torsion is incomplete, the result is congestion and enlargement of the neoplasm with thrombosis of vessels. If the torsion is complete and obstructs the arterial blood supply, gangrenous necrosis results. Thus, the symptoms may be gradual pain and tenderness in the region of the tumor or the abrupt onset of pain typical of an acute abdominal condition. Torsion occurs somewhat more commonly in pregnant women and in children. In the latter it is frequently confused with acute appendicitis.

Rupture. As a result of hemorrhage or torsion, an ovarian cyst may rupture and spill its contents into the peritoneal cavity. This results in intensification of the symptoms or occasionally a temporary reduction if the symptoms have been the result of distention of the cyst. Rupture may also occur as a result of trauma, such as a fall, a blow to the abdomen, and intercourse. Rupture of small, thin-walled ovarian cysts is not rare following vigorous bimanual examination, particularly when this is done under anesthesia. When the cyst contains serous fluid there may be few or no symptoms. If a benign cystic teratoma (dermoid) ruptures, the irritating sebaceous material produces an intense chemical peritonitis. Pseudomyxoma peritonei produces a specific diffuse accumulation of tenacious mucinous material throughout the abdomen. This is discussed more specifically in connection with mucinous cysts.

Infection. Ovarian neoplasms rarely become infected. If they do, it is usually secondary to necrosis, hemorrhage, or salpingitis. It is often impossible to distinguish an infected ovarian tumor from a tubo-ovarian abscess.

PHYSICAL FINDINGS

The physical findings in patients with ovarian neoplasms vary with the nature of the tumor: its consistency, surface contour, position, mobility, and benign or malignant nature. Most benign tumors are unilateral, separate from the uterus, and freely movable. Bilaterality or fixation should arouse suspicion of malignancy. The majority of benign tumors are cystic and pedunculated. They are palpated as smooth, tense masses, readily movable, frequently from one side of the pelvis to the other. Since the pedicles are sometimes long, the neoplasm may be palpated on the side of the pelvis opposite its origin and is often found in different locations at different examinations. The external surface of cystic tumors is usually smooth and regular, but there may be nodular areas, irregularities,

FIG. 57-2 *A.* Left ovarian cyst with twisted pedicle, including uterine tube, ovarian ligament, and round ligament. *B.* pedicle untwisted to show its anatomic elements, extent to which round ligament is involved, and hemorrhagic infarct. (Drawing by Max Brödel. In Kelly HA: Operative Gynecology, Vol 2. New York, Appleton, 1903)

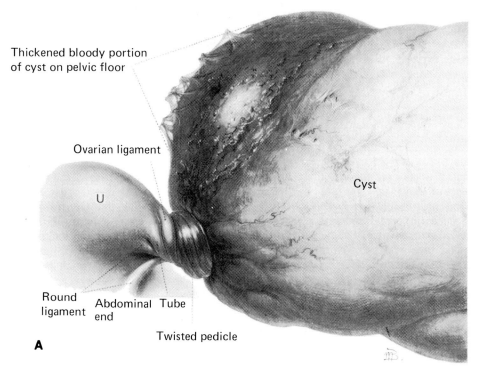

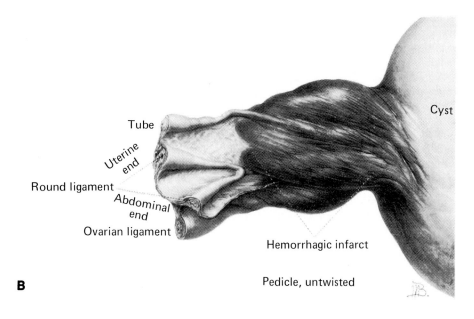

or even solid portions. Benign solid tumors are similarly smooth, also with occasional bosses, but of firm consistency. Some cystic tumors, the benign cystic teratoma (dermoid) in particular, often rise out of the pelvis and are palpated in the abdomen. Most benign tumors are movable, but a tumor may be fixed because it fills the available space in the pelvis or because the pedicle is very short. Small tumors, either cystic or solid, may be palpated best by rectal examination, noting the mass within the cul-de-sac. Presence of definite nodules on the surface of an ovarian tumor is uncommon if the tumor is benign.

It may be difficult to distinguish a huge cyst from ascites. If the abdominal distention is due to an ovarian cyst, there may be distention of veins over the lower abdomen and an absence of the shifting dullness characteristic of ascites. Percussion is dull over all of the abdomen except the flanks, where the displaced intestines lie. The percussion note does not change with changes in position. Distortion of the uterus with displacement of the cervix behind the symphysis pubis and elongation of the vagina is suggestive of a large ovarian cyst. Ascites may be present with small, benign ovarian tumors. *Meigs's syndrome* consists of ascites and hydrothorax in association with fibroma or thecoma of the ovary. In fact, the ascites may make it difficult to accurately palpate a small tumor. Nonneoplastic cystic enlargement of the ovaries may make the ovaries readily palpate but not otherwise abnormal.

DIAGNOSIS

Although the presence of an ovarian neoplasm is sometimes suggested by one or more symptoms, particularly those of acute or sudden onset, the most important factor in diagnosis is the interpretation of an enlargement or mass in the region of the ovary. The diagnosis may be made with reasonable certainty in many cases. However, the differential diagnosis of an adnexal mass must include distended bladder, redundant sigmoid or low-lying cecum, pelvic abscess, ectopic pregnancy or hydrosalpinx, uterine myoma, desmoid tumor or urachal cyst, impacted feces, carcinoma of the sigmoid, diverticulitis of the sigmoid, adherent bowel or omentum secondary to surgery or infection, pelvic kidney, retroperitoneal neoplasm or abscess, hematoma of the rectus muscle, ascites, and bicornuate uterus with pregnancy in one horn.

The examination must be done with care. The bladder always should be empty. Many gynecologists have observed the rapid disappearance of an apparent ovarian cyst following catheterization of the bladder. Likewise, the rectum should be empty, and on occasion it may be advisable to repeat the examination following an enema. It is sometimes helpful to examine the patient in the knee–chest position. In this position an ovarian tumor on a pedicle may be easily displaced out of the pelvis, whereas a uterine myoma or a fixed inflammatory mass of either adnexal or bowel origin will not be displaced. If the mass is high on either side, not adjacent to the uterus, particularly if mobility is limited, a lesion of the sigmoid or cecum should be suspected. Ascites should be suspected if it is difficult to outline the contour of the supposed ovarian cyst and especially if there is a demonstrable fluid wave or shifting dullness. A history of systemic disease that might result in ascites is helpful.

X-Ray Examination. X-ray studies are sometimes of value. Injection of air or carbon dioxide into the peritoneal cavity with the patient in Trendelenburg's position has been used to outline the structures of the pelvis on the x-ray film. This technique, referred to as *gynecography* (see Fig. 57–8), may demonstrate small cystic enlargements of the ovaries such as are seen in polycystic ovarian disease. For the majority of ovarian neoplasms such a study is not necessary and has been replaced largely by ultrasonography or, in some cases, tomography. Roentgenography may demonstrate calcification or formed teeth within a benign, cystic teratoma. Diffuse calcification in an ovarian neoplasm should arouse suspicion of a malignant, serous cystadenocarcinoma (containing psammoma bodies). Intravenous urography and roentgenography following barium enema are helpful in detecting displacement of ureter or bowel, which might complicate the surgical approach to a tumor.

Ultrasound. Ultrasound may be useful in the diagnosis of ovarian neoplasms. It can localize pelvic and intra-abdominal masses, distinguish cystic from solid tumors, and discriminate between uterine and adnexal masses (see Chap. 58).

Endocrine Studies. Endocrine assays that may be of value in the diagnosis of hormone-producing ovarian leisons are pituitary gonadotrophin determination, serum estrogens and testosterone determinations, 17-ketosteroid determination and fractionation, and thyroid function studies. The interpretation of such assays is mentioned below in connection with the specific neoplasms.

If there is any doubt at the first examination, the patient should be reexamined, possibly under anethesia. Gynecography, laparoscopy, and ultrasonography are usually of limited value except in those cases in which a question exists concerning actual ovarian enlargement.

TREATMENT

The management of actual or suspected ovarian neoplasms is basically surgical. Operation is indicated for the relief of symptoms, and when there are no symptoms, surgery is performed to exclude malignancy. Indeed, it is not unrealistic to consider every ovarian neoplasm to be potentially malignant. The likelihood of malignancy of all ovarian neoplasms is between 15% and 25% and is even greater among children and postmenopausal women. Therefore, the need for accurate diagnosis is clear. Occasionally it is possible to differentiate benign from malignant tumors on the basis of history and physical examination, but usually an accurate diagnosis can be made only following gross and microscopic examination of the tumor.

SURGERY

Exploratory operation is essential for all patients in whom an ovarian neoplasm is suspected. This concept should *not* be extended to include all patients with an enlargement of the ovary, since many ovarian enlargements simply represent extensions of the normal cystic response of the ovary to changing physiology. Which patients need surgery has to be decided rather arbitrarily. Many gynecologists rely upon the size of the ovarian enlargement. We consider ovarian enlargements greater than 7 cm in diameter as probably neoplastic and those under this size as probably nonneoplastic; 7 cm is an easy size to remember because it is exactly the diameter of a new tennis ball. Other gynecologists draw the line at 6 or 5 cm. According to one study, 93.6% of ovarian cysts less than 5 cm in diameter were nonneoplastic. Since the probability of malignancy is greater in solid than in cystic tumors, we prefer to operate on most patients with solid tumors, even those smaller than 7 cm. It is often of value to reexamine the patient and note changes in the size of an ovarian enlargement. A patient found to have a mass about 7 cm in diameter should be reexamined in several weeks. Attention should be given to the phase of the ovarian cycle, for the enlargement of a corpus luteum prior to menstruation may not be apparent in the postmenstrual phase. If follow-up examination reveals gradual enlargement of a cystic mass, even though it is smaller than 7 cm, this suggests neoplastic growth. If the tumor regresses in size or disappears, it is safe to assume the enlargement was functional.

Oral contraceptives have been recommended to accelerate involution of nonneoplastic ovarian enlargement. Since most of these cysts are gonadotropin-dependent, the inhibitory effect of ovarian steroids upon release of pituitary gonadotropins diminishes the stimulus to cyst formation and persistence. Spanos studied patients with unilateral cystic adnexal masses. Oral contraceptives were prescribed and the mass disappeared in 72% of patients reexamined in 6 weeks. All patients with a persistent mass were found to have a neoplasm at laparotomy.

A plan of observation and follow-up is not applicable to the infant or young girl. In these patients, any enlargement mandates surgical exploration. The same is true for the postmenopausal woman. The probability of malignancy increases sharply after the age of 50 years, and all ovarian enlargements in postmenopausal women should be investigated surgically. In the young woman, however, careful repeat examination may show surgery to be unnecessary.

When surgery is the treatment of choice, the type and extent needed can only be determined at the operating table on the basis of the pathologic findings considered in the light of the patient's age, general health, and desire for future childbearing. Treatment may consist of 1) nothing, 2) excision of the lesion preserving the remainder of the ovary, 3) unilateral removal of the adnexa, 4) bilateral removal of the adnexa with hysterectomy, or 5) occasionally more radical procedures. We are opposed to tapping large ovarian cysts to reduce their size to make removal less difficult. Even when the greatest caution is exercised, cells may be spilled into the peritoneal cavity and cause irritation and metastatic implantation.

Differentiation of Benign and Malignant Tumors

Much depends upon gross diagnosis. For practical purposes ovarian enlargements may be classified as 1) functional or nonneoplastic, 2) obviously malignant, 3) probably benign, and 4) questionable.

Functional Cystic Enlargements. At the outset it is essential to distinguish functional enlargements from neoplasms. Functional enlargements tend to be multiple, small, smooth, thin-walled, filled with clear fluid, and bilateral (Fig. 57–3). The corpus luteum is recognized by its characteristic shape and yellow color. Functional cysts rarely require surgical treatment, unless there is associated bleeding, as may occur from a corpus luteum or corpus luteum cyst. These may be managed by suture of the rupture site or excision of the cyst.

Obviously Malignant Tumors. Many malignant neoplasms of the ovary can be diagnosed accurately by inspection of the tumor, the peritoneal cavity, and the relation of the tumor to adjacent structures. The characteristics of malignant tumors and their management are discussed later.

Probably Benign Tumors. Some benign ovarian neoplasms can be diagnosed accurately at the time of surgery by gross inspection, section of the tumor and, occasionally, microscopic examination of frozen sections. This is so for the unilocular, thin-walled, simple serous cystoma and some of the nonpapillary cystadenomas. The benign cystic teratoma (dermoid) is easily diagnosed on the basis of its smooth, gray exterior and an interior filled with sebaceous material, hair, and sometimes calcified matter or teeth. Benign fibroma may be suspected if the tumor is unilateral, very firm, and has a glistening gray external surface and a compact, smooth, cut surface. Microscopic examination of a frozen section confirms the suspicion. A conservative operative approach is indicated if the woman is in the reproductive years and especially if she is young and desirous of further childbearing. If significant normal ovarian tissue is present, the lesion may be excised alone. In the majority of cases it is preferable to remove the entire ovary containing the cyst or tumor.

Neoplasms of Questionable Nature. Unfortunately, it is often difficult to determine the malignant or benign

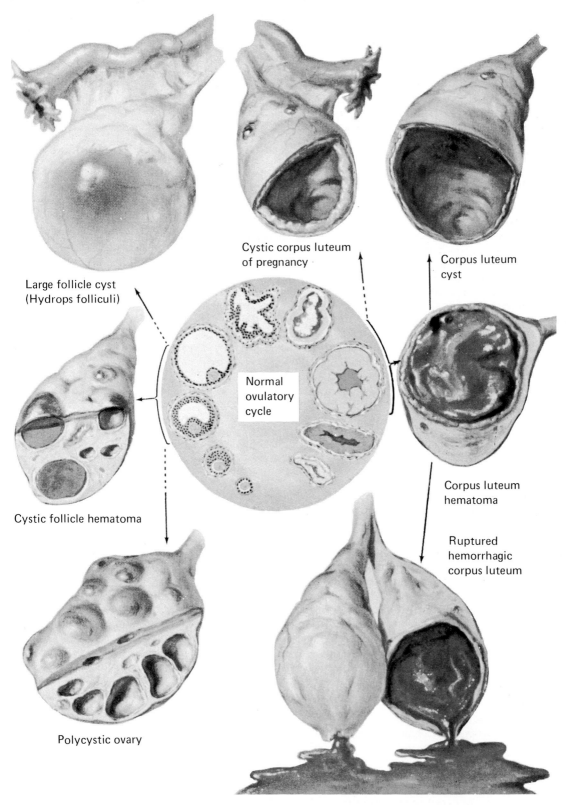

FIG. 57-3 Physiologic, nonneoplastic cystic enlargements of ovaries. (Drawing by FH Netter In Ciba Collection of Medical Illustrations, Vol 2, Reproductive System. Summit NJ, © CIBA, 1954)

nature of an ovarian neoplasm without histologic examination. Leads can be gained from examination of the external surface and interior of a tumor. Solid tumors, particularly of a soft or semisolid consistency, are more likely to be malignant than are completely cystic tumors. Bilateral tumors should arouse suspicion of malignancy. The presence of papillary excrescences on the surface of a cystic tumor commonly indicates malignancy. However, if the papillary processes are firm, broad-based, and not friable, they may be part of a benign process; thus, they cannot be considered absolute indications of malignancy. Fixation of the neoplasm to adjacent tissues should be taken as evidence of probable malignancy.

All ovarian neoplasms should be opened in the operating room and examined by the surgeon or the findings reported to him by a pathologist. The external surface of a neoplasm may appear benign, whereas the interior reveals obvious evidences of malignancy. Hemorrhage, areas of necrosis, or small, friable papillary excrescences within the interior of a cyst suggest malignancy, as does a coarsely granular, fleshy, or semisolid cut surface. The finding of sebaceous material suggests a benign cystic teratoma (dermoid). The presence of tenacious mucinous fluid indicates a mucinous neoplasm, which has a relatively low incidence of malignancy. Solid areas within an otherwise cystic tumor should arouse suspicion of its malignant nature. A biopsy for frozen-section examination should be taken from any solid or otherwise suspicious area. However, frozen-section examination is often of limited value. The microscopic distinction between a malignant and benign process is difficult under the best circumstances and is sometimes impossible with a frozen-section preparation.

Conservative Approach

If the lesion is thought to be benign, the opposite ovary and the uterus may be conserved if they are normal. Most physicians prefer to remove the opposite ovary and uterus in postmenopausal patients. A conservative approach is justified in the management of the questionable lesion if the patient is young and wants additional children. Simple oophorectomy is done, and further decisions regarding therapy are reached following the final pathologic interpretation of the specimen. If the patient is premenopausal or postmenopausal, questionable lesions should be treated by bilateral salpingo-oophorectomy and hysterectomy.

Decision to conserve the opposite ovary is dependent upon its being normal and not the site of a second neoplasm. This is particularly true when the gross diagnosis of the primary tumor is in question. The external surface should be carefully examined. If the primary neoplasm is thought to be a benign cystic teratoma (dermoid), a serous cystadenoma, or a predominantly solid tumor, it is advisable also to split the opposite ovary and inspect the interior. The frequency of bilateral occurrence of these tumors warrants this approach. If evidence of another neoplasm is found, the tumor should be excised or the ovary removed.

Sectioning an ovary for inspection is a simple procedure and apparently does no harm. The incision should be made in the sagittal plane, which allows for examination of the ovary down to the hilus, where certain tumors originate. Failure to inspect the opposite ovary adequately may result in leaving behind another tumor which subsequently will require surgery.

HISTOGENESIS

The most common enlargements of the ovary are those arising from physiologic cystic proliferation of the normal follicular apparatus of the ovary; these are not true neoplasms. Sometimes they represent a failure of normal regression or involution.

In general, the benign true neoplasms of the ovary arise either from normal constituents of the ovary or from congenital rests or heterotopic implants. The tumors developing from structures of the ovary are 1) the majority of the cystic tumors, which arise from the surface (germinal) epithelium, 2) the hormone-producing tumors, which arise from the specialized stroma of the ovarian cortex, 3) the rare tumors also found in sites other than the ovary, which arise from the nonspecialized connective tissue of the ovary, and 4) the benign and malignant teratomas, which arise from the germ cells. Tumors arising from congenital rests or heterotopic implants include adrenal tumors, hilus-cell tumors, and mesonephric and metanephric rest tumors.

CLASSIFICATION

Classifications of tumors or enlargements of the ovary have evolved through a need to understand the origin and function of these lesions and their clinical significance. As more is learned about the physiology and metabolism of the ovary, it becomes apparent that all of the classifications have serious shortcomings. Nonetheless, some form of organization is necessary to permit an orderly discussion of the varieties of ovarian enlargements. The following outline serves this purpose:

A. Functional cysts
    1. Follicle cyst
    2. Corpus luteum cyst
    3. Theca lutein cyst
    4. Polycystic ovary
B. Hyperplasias
C. Endometrial cysts
D. True neoplasms
    1. Common surface epithelial neoplasms
        a. Germinal inclusion cyst

    b. Serous cystadenoma
    c. Mucinous cystadenoma
    d. Cystadenofibroma
    e. Endometrioid tumor
2. Sex chord–mesenchymal tumors (gonadal stromal tumors)
    a. Granulosa cell tumor
    b. Theca cell tumor
    c. Sertoli–Leydig cell tumor (arrhenoblastoma)
    d. Gynandroblastoma
    e. Hilus cell tumor
    f. Lipoid cell tumor
3. Nonintrinsic connective tissue tumors
    a. Fibroma
    b. Rare tumors
4. Germ cell tumors
    a. Mature teratoma
        1) Cystic teratoma (dermoid)
        2) Struma ovarii
    b. Immature teratoma
    c. Embryonal teratoma
    d. Extraembryonal teratoma (endodermal sinus tumor)
    e. Germinoma
    f. Gonadoblastoma
    g. Choriocarcinoma
5. Tumors of uncertain origin
    a. Brenner tumor
    b. Adrenal tumor
    c. Mesonephroma (clear cell)
    d. Lipoid cell tumor
6. Metastatic tumors
    a. Krukenberg
    b. Breast
    c. Other

FUNCTIONAL OVARIAN CYSTS

Follicle Cyst

Mature or atretic follicles that become distended with pale, straw-colored fluid are frequently found in the ovary. Enlargement of atretic follicles to the point of producing grossly visible cystic changes is common during infancy and childhood and may, rarely, enlarge one or both ovaries. Following puberty, grossly cystic follicles are less common but still constitute the most frequently seen cystic enlargement of the ovary.

Follicle cysts are the result of failure of ovulation, with continued growth of the follicle. They are usually multiple and occur in both ovaries (Fig. 57–4). Rarely larger than 3 cm in diameter, follicle cysts occasionally attain a larger size. They do not always alter the external surface of the ovary but may produce yellow blebs on the surface. When cut, they are seen to be thin-walled and filled with a clear serous fluid. Microscopically, the cystic space is lined by a layer of granulosa and underlying theca cells, occasionally flattened or obliterated by the intracystic pressure (Fig. 57–5).

Follicle cysts rarely produce symptoms unless they are large or complicated by rupture or hemorrhage. However, they are often associated with endometrial hyperplasia and uterine myomas. Although earlier writers ascribed a hyperestrogen function to this ovarian change, this concept is less generally accepted at present. The cysts vary in size from time to time and may disappear between examinations. A diagnosis is usually made at the operating table and treatment consists of nothing, puncture of the cyst, or excision of the cyst if it is large or hemorrhagic.

Corpus Luteum Cyst

The corpus luteum which develops following ovulation is normally a cystic structure, albeit small and often only potentially cystic. During pregnancy, with growth and continued function, the corpus luteum becomes truly cystic and at times sufficiently large to be palpated on bimanual pelvic examination. This cystic corpus luteum is not difficult to diagnose or explain. In the absence of pregnancy, the corpus luteum normally collapses and in due time is replaced by hyaline connective tissue to form the corpus albicans. Occasionally, in the nonpregnant state, the corpus luteum becomes cystic, either as a result of unusual continued growth or of hemorrhage into the lumen.

Such cystic enlargement rarely exceeds 4 cm in diameter but has been observed as large as 11 cm. Grossly, the cyst protrudes from the contour of the ovary and the wall appears convoluted, with yellow-orange areas alternating with the usual gray surface. If the cyst is filled with blood, a dark red or purple discoloration is seen. Microscopically, all elements of the corpus luteum are present in the cyst wall. Depending upon the age of the cyst and the degree of intracystic pressure, luteinized granulosa and theca cells may be easily recognizable or may be distorted. The center of the cyst contains blood, serous coagulum, and some connective tissue organization.

Symptoms are related to large size or complications of torsion, rupture, or hemorrhage. The greatest clinical significance of a corpus luteum cyst is that it can simulate ectopic pregnancy. Continued hormone production may cause amenorrhea and subsequent irregular uterine bleeding. In such cases, the ovarian enlargement must be distinguished from swelling of the oviduct. Sudden hemorrhage into the cyst can produce pelvic pain of an aching or colicky type. If the cyst ruptures, the associated findings of intra-abdominal hemorrhage complete the picture of ectopic gestation. More commonly, cystic corpora lutea and corpus luteum cysts produce no symptoms and undergo absorption or regression.

If the symptoms warrant operation, treatment

FIG. 57-4. Uterus and ovaries. Note numerous small follicle cysts on surface of ovaries.

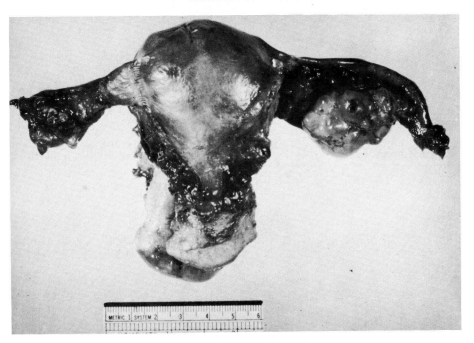

usually consists of excision of the cyst and conservation of the remaining ovary.

Theca Lutein Cyst

During pregnancy atretic follicles are numerous in the ovaries. Occasionally they undergo cystic enlargement. Bilateral ovarian enlargement due to multiple theca lutein cysts occurs in 50% to 60% of women with hydatidiform mole, 5% to 10% of women with choriocarcinoma, and a few women who have multiple gestation. Cyst formation is best explained as a response to the increased production of chorionic gonadotropin.

The cysts are almost always bilateral, and the enlargement may exceed 15 cm. The external surface of the ovary is slightly lobulated, smooth, and blue or gray. The cut surface discloses many thin-walled, clear-fluid-filled cystic spaces with a gray lining. Microscopically, the cysts are lined by theca cells showing varying degrees of luteinization and a central layer of fibrous connective tissue (Fig. 57-6). Granulosa cells may be present but usually are not. Central to the zone of fibrous connective tissue there may be organized blood.

Theca lutein cysts rarely produce symptoms of their own and are usually found incidentally in a patient with hydatidiform mole (Fig. 57-7). Indeed, the finding of bilaterally enlarged ovaries offers strong support to the diagnosis of hydatidiform mole. These cysts may undergo the same complications as other ovarian enlargements. Despite the occasional enormous size of

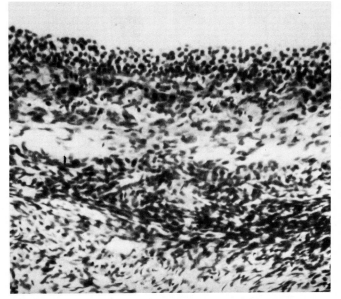

FIG. 57-5. Microscopic section of wall of follicle cyst showing lining granulosa cells.

theca lutein cysts, they are physiologic and should be removed only when this is dictated by the nature of the intrauterine pathology. Following evacuation of a hydatidiform mole or termination of a pregnancy, complete regression of the cysts and return of the ovary to normal size may be anticipated.

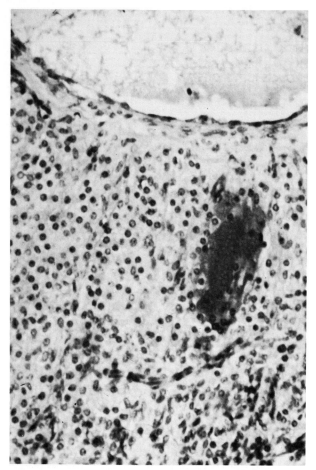

FIG. 57-6. Microscopic section of wall of theca lutein cyst showing vertically arranged luteinized theca cells. There is slight fibrosis of central lining.

HYPERPLASIAS

Polycystic Ovary

Bilateral polycystic enlargement of the ovaries is found in adolescent girls and young women with a complex of symptoms and endocrine abnormalities related to anovulation (Fig. 57–8). These ovaries are enlarged, tense, and oval (Fig. 57–9). The external surface is smooth and white, sometimes revealing subcapsular cysts. The tunica is thick, tough, and white. The ovarian cortex is represented by a thick fibrous capsule surrounding ovarian stroma containing multiple follicle cysts. Microscopically, the follicle cysts demonstrate prominent hyperplasia of the theca interna cells, which are frequently luteinized (Fig. 57–10). Atretic follicles are numerous, with similar hyperplasia and luteinization of theca cells surrounding the lumen. Primordial follicles are not present in the thickened tunica but are commonly aligned immediately beneath this zone in the ovarian stroma. Evidence of present or prior ovulation is usually not seen.

These ovarian changes may result from a specific type of ovarian insufficiency without clearly demonstrable causes outside of the ovary. Indeed, in 1935 Stein and Leventhal reported seven cases of a possible syndrome consisting of bilateral polycystic ovarian enlargement, amenorrhea or irregular menses, infertility, and often masculinization. Similar cystic ovarian enlargement is not uncommon in patients with various types of adrenal hyperplasia and has been observed with pituitary and hypothalamic tumors, increased intracranial pressure, adrenal tumors, and chronic inflammatory disease of the pelvis. Moreover, similar changes have been observed in ovaries containing

FIG. 57-7. Bilateral theca cysts associated with hydatidiform mole.

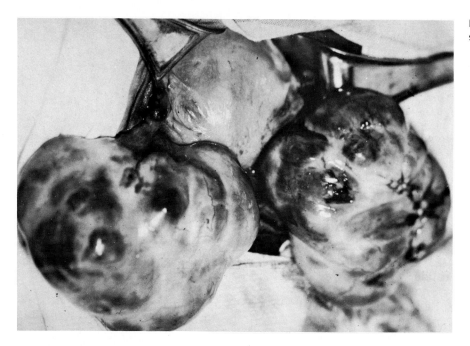

small, masculinizing mesenchymomas. The ovaries of prepubertal girls from 10 to 15 years old are morphologically similar to the polycystic ovaries just described. All of these observations suggest that the microscopic morphology of the polycystic ovary is specific only in *anovulation*. Furthermore, the similarity between the morphology of the polycystic ovary in the abnormal postpubertal woman and the normal prepubertal girl, as well as certain features of the clinical findings in the former patients, suggest that the clinical syndrome of the polycystic ovary is related to acyclic hypothalamic activity and failure to initiate regular ovulation at puberty.

For many years there has been interest in *polycystic ovarian disease* and its variations, and there have been efforts to explain the altered ovarian physiology. As a result of this enthusiasm, the polycystic ovary syndrome has, in general, become more elusive and hard to define. If we eliminate the nonovarian causes of anovulation and related symptoms of amenorrhea, infertility, and possibly hirsutism, we may describe a complex that warrants the designation syndrome (Stein–Leventhal or polycystic ovary syndrome). Characteristically, these young patients, who may still be in adolescence or slightly beyond, have never developed regular ovulatory cycles. A few have never menstruated, but most have had irregular menstrual periods that have gradually become more abnormal. In some cases this menstrual abnormality is first manifested by excessive or prolonged bleeding due to endometrial hyperplasia. Eventually, the periods may become infrequent, scanty, or absent. Infertility exists and is commonly the most serious problem among the patients who are married. There may be hirsutism but rarely, if ever, true masculinization. Obesity is sometimes noted. Ovarian enlargement, while common, may be absent or unilateral. This may be demonstrated by pelvic examination, ultrasonography, laparoscopy, or exploratory laparotomy. The uterus and breasts are said to be frequently hypoplastic, although this has not been common in our experience. The endocrinologic aspects of this syndrome and its diagnosis and treatment are considered in Chapter 46.

A somewhat related ovarian abnormality is *hyperthecosis*. The clinical manifestations may resemble those of the polycystic ovary syndrome, usually with more marked hirsutism and even true masculinization. The ovaries show varying degrees of enlargement The characteristic histologic finding is extreme hyperplasia of theca cells throughout the ovarian stroma; some of the cells are luteinized. These morphologic findings may be present with or without the other histologic changes characteristic of the polycys-

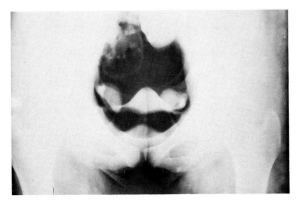

FIG. 57–8. X-ray gynegram of adolescent patient demonstrating bilateral polycystic enlargement of ovaries.

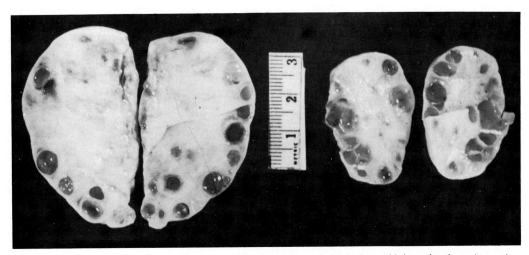

FIG. 57–9. Gross appearance of cut surface of bilateral polycystic ovaries.

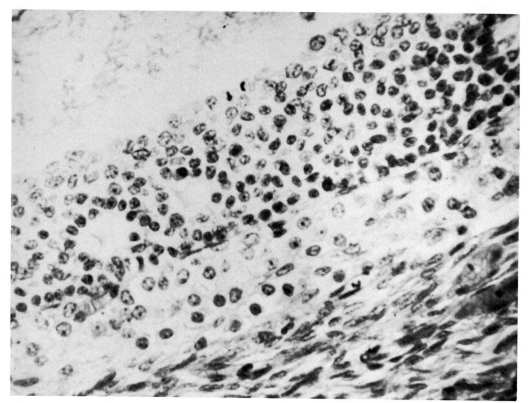

FIG. 57–10. Polycystic ovary. Microscopic section of follicle cyst with inner lining of granulosa cells and outer zone of hyperplastic luteinized theca cells. Theca cells are large with abundant pale cytoplasm. Note Call–Exner body in granulosa layer.

tic ovary. The cause of this lesion is unknown, but in all probability it is related to either polycystic ovary disease or adrenal hyperplasia.

ENDOMETRIAL CYSTS

Endometriosis (detailed in Chap. 51) is mentioned here because it may produce single or multiple cysts (*endometrioma*) in the ovary which may reach significant proportions. Endometriosis has a specific symptom complex, but the large endometrial cysts alone may produce symptoms similar to those of other ovarian cysts and tumors.

TRUE OVARIAN NEOPLASMS

COMMON SURFACE EPITHELIAL NEOPLASMS

Germinal Inclusion Cyst

Germinal inclusion cysts are common microscopic findings in the ovaries of menopausal or postmenopausal women. They are superficial, beneath the surface

epithelium, and unilocular. The lining epithelium is usually columnar with elongated basophilic nuclei. Cilia are occasionally present. Since this is the characteristic epithelium of serous cystomas, cystadenomas, and cystadenocarcinomas, it is probable that inclusion cysts are the forerunners of more significant cystic tumors of the ovary. Somewhat similar lesions are seen in ovaries with surface inflammation or adhesions, in which an actual infolding of the surface epithelium is observed. A similar process of epithelial inclusion is probably the mechanism by which all cystic epithelial ovarian tumors are formed.

Serous Cystadenoma

The serous cystadenoma and the mucinous cystadenoma are the most common benign ovarian neoplasms, constituting 15% to 23.5% of all benign ovarian tumors. Serous cystadenomas occur most commonly between the ages of 20 and 50 years and reach their peak incidence in the third and fourth decades of life. The reported frequency of bilaterality varies from 18% to 50%. Those with papillary projections are more often bilateral. Most serous cystic

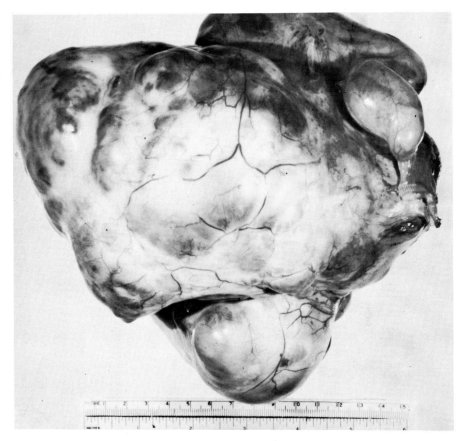

FIG. 57–11. Serous cystadenoma. Surface is lobulated and glistening. Tumor has assumed shape of bony pelvis with growth. Hydrosalpinx is attached to superior surface of cyst.

tumors are benign; however, an indefinite number (32% to 45%, according to various studies) become malignant. This does not indicate the frequency with which a histologically benign serous cystadenoma becomes malignant, but does indicate a significant potential for malignancy. The frequency of malignant change, like bilaterality, is greater in those tumors with papillary processes.

The serous cystadenoma (Fig. 57–11) is a unilocular, parvilocular, or multilocular cystic neoplasm derived from the surface epithelium of the ovary and lined by epithelium that resembles the mucosa of the oviduct. The external surface is smooth or lobulated, gray or bluish-gray, and darker if there has been hemorrhage into the cyst. External papillary projections occur in 10% to 30% of tumors. They are firm, white, and broad-based. Softness and friability suggest malignancy. The benign serous cystadenoma is usually of moderate size and varies from 5 to 10 cm in diameter; occasionally it fills the entire abdomen. The cut surface reveals a single or multiple locule(s) with a smooth gray lining and containing clear, yellow fluid. The majority are unilocular and thin-walled. Less common are those with multiple locules and numerous thin septa. Papillary processes similar to those described on the external surface may be present. It is

not rare to find solid portions, but this should suggest malignancy. Occasionally one or more of the locules contains blood.

Microscopically, the epithelial lining of a serous cystadenoma varies from simple cuboidal to tall columnar with elongated nuclei, resembling the epithelium of the oviduct (Fig. 57–12). Cilia are observed in some cases. The stroma varies from an edematous to a densely fibrous type and is variable in amount. The papillary processes are broad, fibrous, and covered by a single layer of epithelium (Fig. 57–13). Occasionally small calcific concretions, known as *psammoma bodies* (see Fig. 57–34), are found in the stroma adjacent to the epithelium. These deposits, if present in large numbers, may be visible on x-ray examination of the abdomen.

The microscopic evaluation of malignancy in this group of tumors may pose considerable difficulty. Indeed, in some tumors of a borderline nature a piling up of epithelial cells and slight degrees of dedifferentiation make it impossible to distinguish between a benign and a malignant process. In these cases only the clinical course indicates the biologic nature of the tumor. The problem of borderline malignancy is discussed on page 1162.

No symptoms are specific for this tumor. The diag-

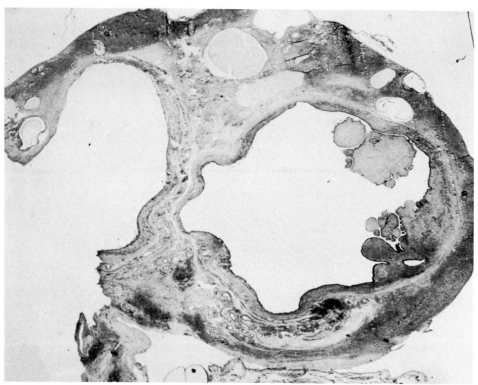

FIG. 57-12. Microscopic view of papillary serous cystadenoma. Tumor did not enlarge ovary and was not visible externally. Papillary processes are blunt and broad-based, lined by single layer of epithelium. This lesion represents early phase in histogenesis of serous tumor of ovary.

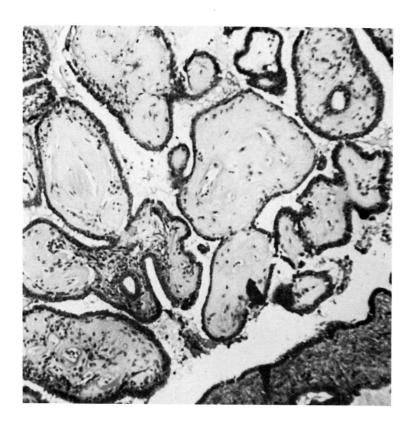

FIG. 57-13. Microscopic section of papillary serous cystadenoma. Papillae are small and delicate but lined by single layer of epithelium.

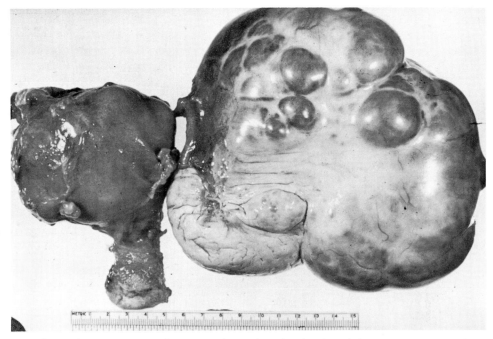

FIG. 57-14. Mucinous cystadenoma. Surface is bosselated and a solid portion is present in lower pole.

nosis is commonly made after pelvic examination in a patient who is asymptomatic or has noticed gradual abdominal enlargement.

Treatment must be planned with knowledge of the frequency of bilateral involvement, the potential for malignancy, and the fact that papillary processes and hemorrhage suggest malignancy. In patients past the childbearing age, treatment should consist of bilateral salpingo-oophorectomy and hysterectomy. Conservatism is recommended for most others.

Mucinous Cystadenoma

Mucinous cystadenomas are unilocular or multilocular cystic ovarian tumors occurring as often as, or more often than, the serous cystadenoma. According to various studies, they constitute 16% to 30% of all benign ovarian neoplasms. Unlike the serous tumors, they are bilateral in only 5% to 7% of cases. Moreover, the incidence of similar tumors appearing later in the conserved opposite ovary is extremely low. These tumors rarely become malignant. Mucinous cystadenomas occur most frequently during the third and fifth decades of life, and only occasionally (10%) after the menopause. They may complicate pregnancy.

There are two theories of histogenesis. The most commonly accepted is an origin from the surface epithelium of the ovary with differentiation to the endocervical type of müllerian duct epithelium. The other theory holds that the epithelium is intestinal in type and arises from a monophyletic teratoma in which only one type of tissue persists. It is possible that the cysts arise in both fashions.

Mucinous tumors are often much larger than the serous cystadenoma and usually account for the legendary huge cysts that are reported. They range from 1 to 50 cm in diameter, with the majority being 15 to 30 cm. Ordinarily they are completely cystic and multilocular. The external surface is smooth, occasionally lobulated, pinkish-gray, and without extracystic papillar growths (Figs. 57–14, 57–15). The cut surface shows individual cysts or locules, varying in size and containing a sticky, slimy, or viscid material. The interlocular septa are very thin. Intracystic papillary processes are present in 10% to 25% of cases, and as is true for the serous tumor, are even more common in the malignant variety.

Microscopically, the locules and cysts are lined by a typical tall columnar "picket-fence" type of cell, with a basally situated nucleus and superficial accumulation of mucin within the cytoplasm (Fig. 57–16). The cell resembles the secretory cell of the endocervix and intestine. Argentaffin cells also may be present. Dense connective tissue stroma is scant and forms a capsule.

The usual treatment for the obviously benign mucinous cystadenoma is unilateral oophorectomy. In older women bilateral oophorectomy and hysterectomy is preferable.

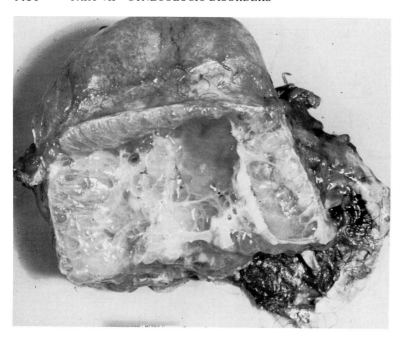

FIG. 57–15. Mucinous cystadenoma coexisting with cystic teratoma (dermoid). Coexistence of these two tumors supports theory of origin of mucinous tumors from benign teratomas.

Pseudomyxoma peritonei is a complication that may result if the contents of a mucinous cyst are spilled into the peritoneal cavity by rupture, extension, or at surgery. This is a good reason not to tap or aspirate ovarian cysts at operation. Fortunately, pseudomyxoma does not always develop with spillage. The process is biologically malignant, although it is histologically benign. Diffuse implants develop on all the peritoneal surfaces, with tremendous accumulation of mucinous material within the peritoneal cavity. Rarely is there spread beyond the peritoneum of invasion of vital structures. Microscopic examination of the implants reveals the morphology of a benign mucinous tumor. In fact, areas of epithelium are scant and hard to find. The clinical course is usually progressive malnutrition and emaciation. The fluid is difficult to remove because of its viscosity, and repeated laparotomies may be required. The interesting association of mucinous cysts of the ovary and *mucocele of the appendix* has been reported.

Cystadenofibroma

The cystadenofibroma is a variant of the serous cystadenoma and much less common. This tumor is partially cystic and partially solid. The age distribution is similar to that of the serous tumors. It is usually benign and unilateral.

The external surface is gray or white, composed of multiloculated cystic areas and lobulated solid portions with large broad papillae or deep sulci. The papillae are firm and nonfriable. The cut surface reveals numerous amber fluid-filled cysts within firm, glistening grayish-white lobules. Microscopically, the solid areas are composed of whorls of fibrous connective tissue containing various amounts of ovarian stroma and are lined by typical surface or germinal epithelium. The cystic spaces are similar to those of serous cystadenoma. The cystadenofibroma can be distinguished from a fibroma with cystic degeneration by the papillary or gyrated character of the surface. Similar gross and microscopic findings are not uncommon in normal-sized postmenopausal ovaries.

Treatment varies with age and associated findings.

Endometrioid Tumor

Ovarian tumors with a pattern resembling endometrial tumors have been reported to occur with significant frequency. In the past, these tumors have been considered to arise from areas of endometriosis. It seems probable that they may arise *de novo* just as the serous and mucinous tumors do. The majority are malignant.

SEX CHORD–MESENCHYMAL TUMORS (GONADAL STROMAL TUMORS)

The *mesenchymomas* constitute a group of tumors frequently demonstrating endocrine function. They all have certain morphologic similarities, and each probably arises from ovarian cortical stroma (or embryonic

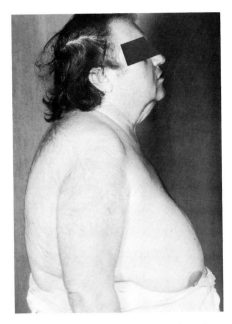

FIG. 57-20. Patient with marked masculinization resulting from hilus cell tumor. Same appearance may be associated with other masculinizing tumors of ovary.

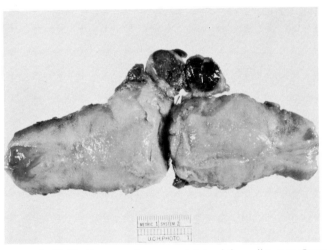

FIG. 57-21. Uterus and ovary containing hilus cell tumor. Ovary was not enlarged. (Merrill JA: Am J Obstet Gynecol 78:1258, 1959)

comas (often luteinized) show evidence of excess androgen production. An unusual associated finding is ascites and hydrothorax (Meigs' syndrome) without metastasis or implants.

Treatment usually consists of removal of the involved ovary in young patients, and bilateral salpingo-oophorectomy and hysterectomy in older patients.

Sertoli–Leydig Cell Tumor

Sertoli–Leydig cell tumor is a rare tumor of the ovarian stroma occasionally associated with virilizing symptoms. It has a malignant potential of about 25%.

Gynandroblastoma

This is an extremely rare tumor described by Meyer in 1930. Its ability to produce both masculinizing (hirsutism, hypertrophy of the clitoris, voice change) and feminizing (vaginal bleeding due to endometrial hyperplasia) effects is attributed to the mixed and varied histologic pattern in which elements of both Sertoli–Leydig and granulosa cell tumor may be present side by side or intermixed.

Hilus Cell Tumor

Hilus cell tumors are extremely rare; approximately 30 have been described in the literature. The tumors are small and produce relatively little enlargement of the ovary. They have been discovered most often in postmenopausal women with hirsutism who have had menstrual abnormalities (oligomenorrhea and amenorrhea), infertility, enlargement of the clitoris, and related features of masculinization (Fig. 57–20). Metabolites of the tumors are excreted as 17-ketosteroids. Only one malignant tumor has been described.

Grossly, they are circumscribed, solid, soft, and yellow or brown (Fig. 57–21). Microscopically, they consist of nonencapsulated sheets or cords of polyhedral cells similar to the normally occurring hilus cells of the adult ovary (Fig. 57–22). The cytoplasm contains lipochrome pigment and eosinophilic crystalloids.

Unilateral oophorectomy is recommended. It may be necessary to bisect the ovary to discover the tumor.

Lipoid Cell Tumor

Because it is often difficult to distinguish between hilus cell tumors, luteinized thecomas, adrenallike tumors, and pure Sertoli cell tumors, pathologists increasingly favor the use of lipoid cell tumor for this group of masculinizing tumors. The pregnancy luteoma is sometimes included, although this is probably a nonneoplastic hyperplasia of luteinized theca cells.

NONINTRINSIC CONNECTIVE TISSUE TUMORS

Fibroma

The ovarian fibroma is a connective tissue tumor composed of fibrocytes and variable amounts of collagen. The fibroma occurs most frequently in middle age, with an average age incidence of 48 years. These tumors probably arise from the nonintrinsic connective tissue of the ovarian cortical stroma, although they

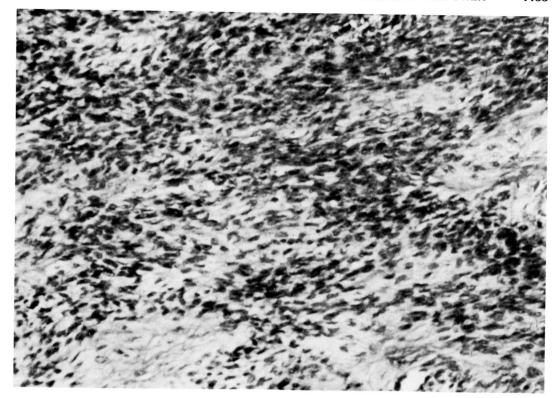

FIG. 57-19. Microscopic view of thecoma. Fat stain reveals fat within cystoplasm of plump, spindle-shaped cells.

proved to be biologically malignant (see Malignant Lesions of the Ovary).

Thecoma

Most granulosa cell tumors contain varying amounts of theca, and it has been stated that the endocrine function of granulosa cell tumors is related to the thecal component. There are tumors, however, composed principally or entirely of theca cells (12% of the feminizing mesenchymomas). Thecomas are much rarer than granulosa cell tumors and constitute about 2% of all ovarian tumors. They occur at all ages from 1 to 92 but are uncommon in women under the age of 35. They are most often found in postmenopausal women.

The evidence is good that thecomas arise from the ovarian cortical stroma. Indeed, transition from cortical stromal hyperplasia to thecoma has been observed, and it is not uncommon to find cortical stromal hyperplasia in the opposite ovary.

Theca cell tumors are unilateral and practically never malignant; fewer than 20 cases of malignant thecoma have been reported. The encapsulated tumor may be so small that the external contour of the ovary is unaltered, or it may become as large as 15 to 20 cm in diameter. The external surface is firm, ovoid or round, smooth, and gray, occasionally streaked with yellow. The cut surface is firm, uniform, and gray, frequently showing yellow foci which represent luteinization with fat deposition (Figs. 57–17, 57–18). Microscopic examination reveals interlacing bands of plump, spindle-shaped theca cells with intervening zones of hyalinization (Fig. 57–19). Fat stains frequently reveal the presence of fat within the cells. Occasional tumors show marked luteinization. Thecomas have been found within polycystic ovaries. The similarity between the two suggests a common endocrine pathogenesis.

Symptoms are related to estrogen production. However, it has been stated that in 25% of cases there is no evidence of hormonal activity. Since the tumors are most common in the postmenopausal period, the most frequent symptom is postmenopausal uterine bleeding. Menopausal bleeding or hypermenorrhea with endometrial hyperplasia are less common symptoms. A small but significant number of patients with the-

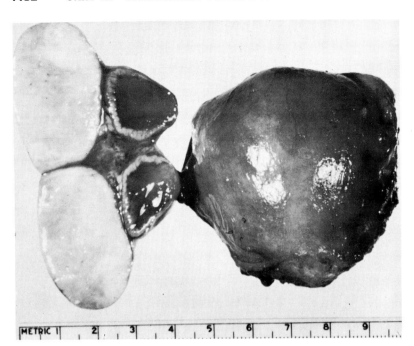

FIG. 57–17. Thecoma of ovary. Cut surface is white streaked with yellow. Note also hemorrhagic corpus luteum.

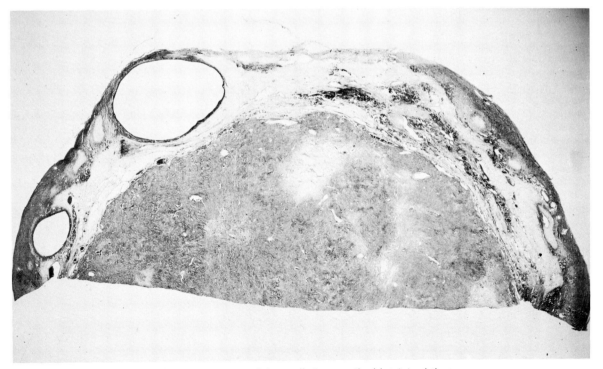

FIG. 57–18. Section through polycystic ovary containing well-circumscribed luteinized thecoma. Note follicle cysts in cortex of ovary. Patient's symptoms included hirsutism, oligomenorrhea, and infertility.

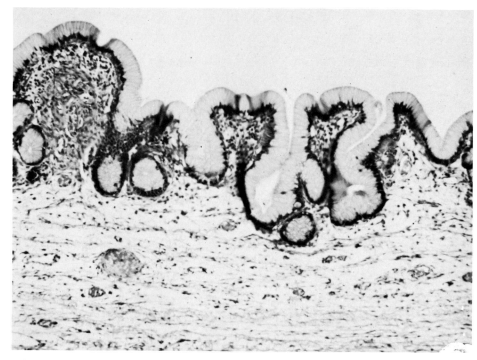

FIG. 57-16. Microscopic appearance of lining of mucinous cystadenoma. Picket-fence epithelium is characteristic of this tumor.

gonadal stroma) or its follicular wall derivatives. Recently there has been a trend to refer to these tumors simply as *feminizing mesenchymomas* (granulosa and theca cell tumors) and *masculinizing mesenchymomas* (arrhenoblastoma, hilus cell tumor, lipoid tumors), depending upon histology. It is apparent that the morphology is often amazingly similar and that tumors of each morphologic type may demonstrate clinical features of estrogen or androgen production and, on occasion, both. The granulosa-cell tumor, which is generally feminizing, has been reported to produce masculinization. The theca cell tumor, which also is usually femininizing, may produce virilization; hyperplasia of the theca cell in the polycystic ovary syndrome is often associated with features of androgen activity. The masculinizing tumors (arrhenoblastoma, androblastoma, or Sertoli–Leydig cell tumors) have rarely been associated with estrogen activity. Thus, any attempt to limit the production of specific hormones to a specific cell or a specific tumor of the ovary is not realistic in the light of clinical findings or present knowledge of steroid biosynthesis in the ovary. *Any cell or tissue that is capable of steroid biosynthesis is capable of producing progestrone, estrogens, and androgens.* The predominance depends upon the rates of biosynthesis and the enzymes required for the various

steps thereof. It is postulated that all of these tumors arise from the mesenchymal ovarian stroma, which retains most of its embryonic multidifferentiating potential. This potential may be exploited both in degree and direction by tumorigenic stimuli. Abnormal hormone production probably occurs as a result of subsequent imbalance of normal enzyme activity and disruption of the usual steroid metabolic pathways.

In considering the clinical importance of this group of hormonally active tumors, it is impossible to stress too strongly the fallacy of emphasizing the histology rather than the metabolic activity of the tumor. However, histologic classification remains a handy means of considering the pathology of these tumors and is a necessity in deciding the malignant potential.

Granulosa Cell Tumor

These tumors, composed predominantly of granulosa cells, commonly produce menometrorrhagia, menopausal bleeding, postmenopausal bleeding, and enlargement of the external genitalia and breasts. Occurring at any age, about 50% are found in postmenopausal patients. They may occur in youngsters and must be distinguished from constitutional precocity. Possibly one-third of these tumors have

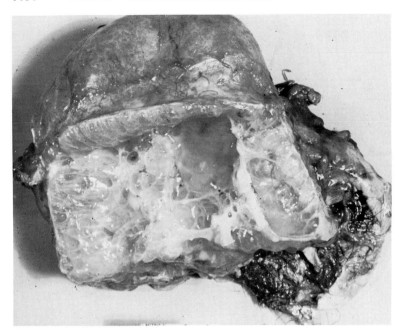

FIG. 57-15. Mucinous cystadenoma coexisting with cystic teratoma (dermoid). Coexistence of these two tumors supports theory of origin of mucinous tumors from benign teratomas.

Pseudomyxoma peritonei is a complication that may result if the contents of a mucinous cyst are spilled into the peritoneal cavity by rupture, extension, or at surgery. This is a good reason not to tap or aspirate ovarian cysts at operation. Fortunately, pseudomyxoma does not always develop with spillage. The process is biologically malignant, although it is histologically benign. Diffuse implants develop on all the peritoneal surfaces, with tremendous accumulation of mucinous material within the peritoneal cavity. Rarely is there spread beyond the peritoneum of invasion of vital structures. Microscopic examination of the implants reveals the morphology of a benign mucinous tumor. In fact, areas of epithelium are scant and hard to find. The clinical course is usually progressive malnutrition and emaciation. The fluid is difficult to remove because of its viscosity, and repeated laparotomies may be required. The interesting association of mucinous cysts of the ovary and *mucocele of the appendix* has been reported.

Cystadenofibroma

The cystadenofibroma is a variant of the serous cystadenoma and much less common. This tumor is partially cystic and partially solid. The age distribution is similar to that of the serous tumors. It is usually benign and unilateral.

The external surface is gray or white, composed of multiloculated cystic areas and lobulated solid portions with large broad papillae or deep sulci. The papillae are firm and nonfriable. The cut surface reveals numerous amber fluid-filled cysts within firm, glistening grayish-white lobules. Microscopically, the solid areas are composed of whorls of fibrous connective tissue containing various amounts of ovarian stroma and are lined by typical surface or germinal epithelium. The cystic spaces are similar to those of serous cystadenoma. The cystadenofibroma can be distinguished from a fibroma with cystic degeneration by the papillary or gyrated character of the surface. Similar gross and microscopic findings are not uncommon in normal-sized postmenopausal ovaries.

Treatment varies with age and associated findings.

Endometrioid Tumor

Ovarian tumors with a pattern resembling endometrial tumors have been reported to occur with significant frequency. In the past, these tumors have been considered to arise from areas of endometriosis. It seems probable that they may arise *de novo* just as the serous and mucinous tumors do. The majority are malignant.

SEX CHORD-MESENCHYMAL TUMORS (GONADAL STROMAL TUMORS)

The *mesenchymomas* constitute a group of tumors frequently demonstrating endocrine function. They all have certain morphologic similarities, and each probably arises from ovarian cortical stroma (or embryonic

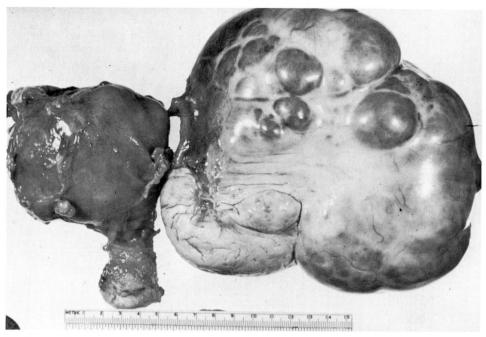

FIG. 57–14. Mucinous cystadenoma. Surface is bosselated and a solid portion is present in lower pole.

nosis is commonly made after pelvic examination in a patient who is asymptomatic or has noticed gradual abdominal enlargement.

Treatment must be planned with knowledge of the frequency of bilateral involvement, the potential for malignancy, and the fact that papillary processes and hemorrhage suggest malignancy. In patients past the childbearing age, treatment should consist of bilateral salpingo-oophorectomy and hysterectomy. Conservatism is recommended for most others.

Mucinous Cystadenoma

Mucinous cystadenomas are unilocular or multilocular cystic ovarian tumors occurring as often as, or more often than, the serous cystadenoma. According to various studies, they constitute 16% to 30% of all benign ovarian neoplasms. Unlike the serous tumors, they are bilateral in only 5% to 7% of cases. Moreover, the incidence of similar tumors appearing later in the conserved opposite ovary is extremely low. These tumors rarely become malignant. Mucinous cystadenomas occur most frequently during the third and fifth decades of life, and only occasionally (10%) after the menopause. They may complicate pregnancy.

There are two theories of histogenesis. The most commonly accepted is an origin from the surface epithelium of the ovary with differentiation to the endocervical type of müllerian duct epithelium. The other theory holds that the epithelium is intestinal in type and arises from a monophyletic teratoma in which only one type of tissue persists. It is possible that the cysts arise in both fashions.

Mucinous tumors are often much larger than the serous cystadenoma and usually account for the legendary huge cysts that are reported. They range from 1 to 50 cm in diameter, with the majority being 15 to 30 cm. Ordinarily they are completely cystic and multilocular. The external surface is smooth, occasionally lobulated, pinkish-gray, and without extracystic papillar growths (Figs. 57–14, 57–15). The cut surface shows individual cysts or locules, varying in size and containing a sticky, slimy, or viscid material. The interlocular septa are very thin. Intracystic papillary processes are present in 10% to 25% of cases, and as is true for the serous tumor, are even more common in the malignant variety.

Microscopically, the locules and cysts are lined by a typical tall columnar "picket-fence" type of cell, with a basally situated nucleus and superficial accumulation of mucin within the cytoplasm (Fig. 57–16). The cell resembles the secretory cell of the endocervix and intestine. Argentaffin cells also may be present. Dense connective tissue stroma is scant and forms a capsule.

The usual treatment for the obviously benign mucinous cystadenoma is unilateral oophorectomy. In older women bilateral oophorectomy and hysterectomy is preferable.

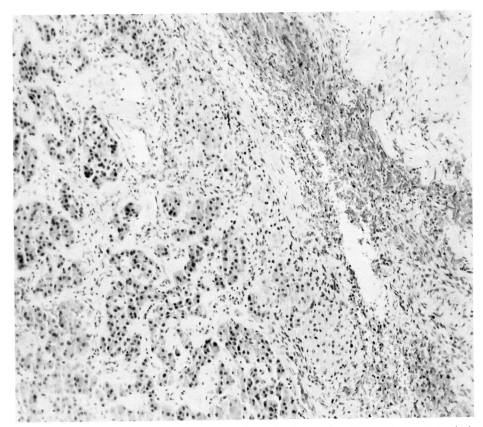

FIG. 57-22. Ovarian hilus cell tumor. Microscopic section from edge of tumor demonstrates lack of encapsulation and nests of cells comprising growth. (Merrill JA: Am J Obstet Gynecol 78:1258, 1959)

may represent the inactive end stage of theca cell tumors. The frequency of bilaterality is between 2.9% and 10%.

The average size of ovarian fibromas is 6 cm, with 4.5% of the tumors larger than 20 cm. At operation the tumor is firm or hard and smooth; the external and internal surfaces are grayish-white and glistening (Fig. 57–23). The cut surface is composed of homogeneous fibrous tissue, but may contain cysts. Microscopically, the tumor consists of small, thin spindle-shaped cells arranged in bundles, giving an overall fasciculated appearance. Small tumors are usually cellular; large tumors more fibrous. As mentioned, differentiation from thecoma may be difficult.

There are no specific symptoms other than the occasional finding of ascites and less often hydrothorax. The explanation of this occurrence with benign solid tumors is not clear and of no special relevance. The effusion disappears following removal of the tumor. Simple removal of the tumor is adequate therapy for this group of findings, which is known as *Meigs syndrome.*

GERM CELL TUMORS

Benign Cystic Teratoma (Dermoid Cyst)

Dermoid cysts are relatively common, probably derived from primordial germ cells, and composed of any combination of well-differentiated ectodermal, mesodermal, and entodermal elements. They are slightly less common than the serous and mucinous cystadenomas, probably making up 18% to 25% of all ovarian neoplasms. The tumors may occur at any age, but the peak incidence is reported between 20 and 40 years. The tumors are almost always benign, although there is a malignant counterpart in the solid teratoma. In the unusual cases of malignancy, the malignant element is usually squamous epithelium.

Dermoids are bilateral in approximately 12% of patients, and the majority measure 5 to 10 cm in diameter. At operation the tumors are round, with a smooth, glistening gray surface. At body temperature they have the consistency of other tensely cystic tumors. Outside the body they have a soft pultaceous consistency. On

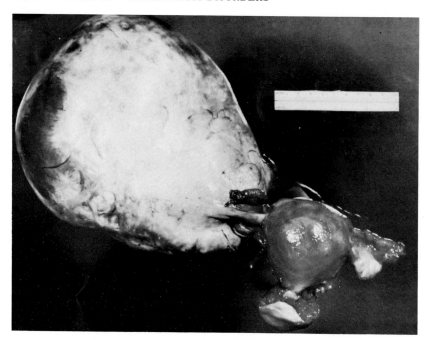

FIG. 57–23. Fibroma of ovary. External surface is firm, smooth, and white.

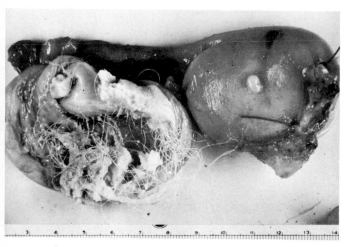

FIG. 57–24. Benign cystic teratoma of ovary. Tumor has been sectioned; sebaceous material and hair are apparent.

sectioning, they are usually unilocular and filled with thick sebaceous material and tangled masses of hair (Fig. 57–24). There is often a solid portion at one pole of the cyst which contains the bulk of the cellular elements and the various dermal structures. In possibly 30% to 50% of cases the cyst contains formed teeth. Microscopically, a wide variety of tissues are found (Fig. 57–25). Most common are tissues normally found above the diaphragm: skin, sweat glands, respi-

ratory epithelium, cartilage, salivary glands, and nervous tissue. Ectodermal structures are almost always present, with mesodermal and entodermal structures only slightly less frequent.

Because teeth are commonly present, x-ray of the abdomen may aid in diagnosis. Moreover, a dermoid cyst often has a long pedicle, allowing it to be palpated in the abdomen or anterior to the uterus. The frequency of torsion is relatively great. Since these tumors occur in young patients, treatment usually consists of excision of the cyst, conserving the remaining portion of the ovary. Many recommend that the opposite ovary be incised and inspected for a second tumor.

Struma Ovarii

Struma ovarii is a unique benign cystic teratoma, in which thyroid tissue constitutes the entire, or nearly entire, cellular portion of the neoplasm. In external appearance this tumor is not distinguishable from a dermoid cyst. On sectioning, locules of typical colloid may be seen (Fig. 57–26). The locules are of various sizes and have a yellowish-brown color. Microscopically, well-differentiated thyroid tissue is seen.

About 5% of strumas produce symptoms or signs of thyrotoxicosis, and possibly 10 patients have been reported with evidence of hyperthyroidism that was relieved by removal of the ovarian tumor. Rarely

FIG. 57-25. Microscopic section of benign cystic teratoma showing thyroid tissue, respiratory epithelium, salivary glands, and cartilage. This section duplicates structures of anterior part of neck.

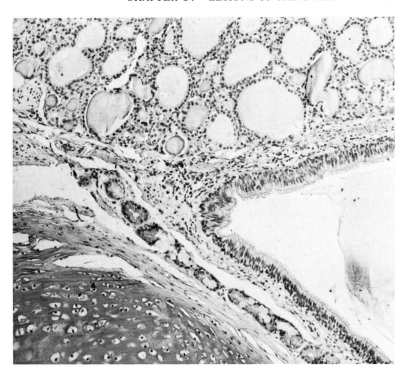

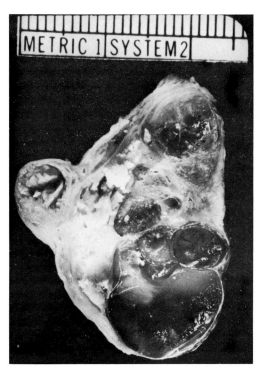

FIG. 57-26. Gross section of struma ovarii. Locules of colloid are easily identified.

thyrotoxicosis is unrelieved by thyroidectomy but finally is relieved when a struma ovarii is detected and removed.

Gonadoblastoma

Gonadoblastoma, described by Scully, is an unusual tumor that recapitulates the embryonic development of the gonad. It is usually a unilateral, soft, solid tumor 5 to 15 cm in size, composed of large germ cells, sex chord elements, calcific concretions, and cellular stroma resembling Leydig or theca cells. Gonadoblastomas are found principally, but not always, in streak gonads of phenotypic females with gonadal dysgenesis and a Y chromosome in the karyotype. The tumors themselves are almost invariably benign, but the germ cell component may give rise to highly malignant germ cell tumors including dysgerminoma, endodermal sinus tumor, and embryonal carcinoma. Consequently, even in the absence of a palpable tumor it is advisable to remove the gonads of phenotypic females with gonadal dysgenesis and a Y chromosome in the karyotype. If a Y chromosome is absent, the risk of gonadoblastoma is extremely small; however, among approximately 80 cases of this tumor which have been reported, one occurred in a patient with a 45,XO karyotype, and three in patients with 46,XX pattern.

TUMORS OF UNCERTAIN ORIGIN

Brenner Tumor

The Brenner tumor is a fibroepithelial tumor with gross characteristics similar to the fibroma. It constitutes approximately 1% to 2% of all ovarian tumors and is practically never malignant. Brenner tumors have been reported in patients 6 to 81 years of age; however, approximately one-half the patients are over the age of 50 years. One study indicates that approximately 13% of the tumors are bilateral; figures as low as 5.9% have been given by others.

According to the most widely accepted theory of histogenesis, Brenner tumors arise from Walthard's cell rests, which themselves are a modification and inclusion of the surface epithelium (germinal epithelium) of the ovary. Careful examination of tumors has revealed continuity between the epithelial nests of the tumor, superficial Walthard's cell rests, and the surface epithelium. Brenner tumors and mucinous cystadenomas occasionally coexist. This is explained as metaplasia either of the mucinous epithelium to the squamoid type or of the epithelial nests of the Brenner tumor to a mucinous type. The association of these two tumors is compatible with a theory of origin from the surface epithelium of the ovary. Coexistence of other genital tumors has been reported.

The tumors vary from microscopic size to 30 cm in diameter. The average tumor is between 10 and 15 cm in diameter. They are usually solid but may be partially cystic. The surface is smooth and grayish-white, with irregular lobulation. The cut surface is grayish-white and whorled. The cystic areas vary in size and contain clear serous fluid. Microscopically, the solid portion of the tumor consists of abundant fibrous connective tissue and typical nests of squamouslike epithelial cells with characteristic longitudinal grooving of the nucleus (Fig. 57–27). Frequently the centers of these nests become cystic. The cells lining the central cavity are cuboidal, low columnar, or occasionally typical of mucinous epithelium.

A few Brenner tumors have been associated with postmenopausal bleeding, and it has been suggested that they occasionally contain hormonally active stroma. In common with the fibroma and thecoma, Meigs's syndrome of ascites and hydrothorax occurs with Brenner tumors.

Treatment usually consists of simple excision or oophorectomy.

Adrenal Rest Tumor

The adrenal rest tumor, often referred to by other terms, is one of the group of lipoid masculinizing tumors of the ovary related in morphology and symptomatology to the hilus cell tumor, the luteinized thecoma, and Sertoli–Leydig tumors. It resembles the cortical tissue of the adrenal, grossly and microscopically. According to a survey of 56 adrenal rest tumors reported in the literature, the tumors were usually unilateral and varied in size from 1 to 30 cm (42% were 5 cm or less in diameter, and 81% were 11 cm or less). They occurred in patients aged 6 to 71 years, the aver-

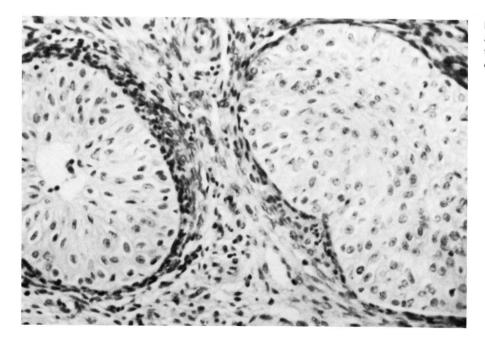

FIG. 57–27. Microscopic appearance of cell nest in Brenner tumor. Note beginning cystic change in one of the cell nests.

age age being 32 years. About 21% were considered malignant.

The most likely theory of histogenesis supposes an origin from embryonic rests of adrenal cortex in the ovary. Adrenal rests are relatively common in the ovaries and mesovarium of newborns.

Grossly, the tumors are usually encapsulated and lobulated. They are solid, rubbery, and usually yellow. Microscopically, the cells are typically those of the adrenal cortex and are arranged centripetally in strands separated by capillary networks. The cytoplasm contains lipid and brown pigment granules.

Essentially all patients have some features of masculinization including voice change, hypertrophied clitoris, atrophy of the breasts, and amenorrhea. Of the 56 patients reported in the literature, 30 had one or more features of Cushing's syndrome and most had elevated levels of urinary 17-ketosteroids, which rapidly fell to normal following removal of the tumor.

Treatment is oophorectomy.

REFERENCES AND RECOMMENDED READING

Abel MR: The nature and classification of ovarian neoplasms. Can Med Assoc J94:1102, 1966

Aiman J, Edman C, Worley RJ, et al: Androgen and estrogen formation in women with ovarian hyperthecosis. Obstet Gynecol 51:1 1978

Anderson WR, et al: Granulosa–theca cell tumors: Clinical and pathologic study. Am J Obstet Gynecol 110:32, 1971

Arey LB: Origin and form of the Brenner tumor. Am J Obstet Gynecol 81:743, 1961

Azoury RS, et al: Coexistence of Brenner tumors with epithelial neoplasia. Gynecol Oncol 6:54, 1978

Babaknia A, Calsopoulos P, Jones HW Jr: The Stein–Leventhal syndrome and coincidental ovarian tumors. Obstet Gynecol 47:223, 1976

Barbor HRK: Gyneological tumors in childhood and adolescence. Obstet Gynecol Surv 28:357, 1973

Barclay DL, Forney JP, Yellios F, et al: Hyperreactio luteinalis: Postpartum persistence. Am J Obstet Gynecol 105:642, 1969

Beck RP, Latour JPA: Review of 1019 benign ovarian neoplasms. Obstet Gynecol 16:478, 1960

Beck RP, Latour JPA: Atypical fibromas and thecomas of the ovary. Obstet Gynecol 19:228, 1962

Busby T, Anderson GW: Feminizing mesenchymomas of the ovary. Am J Obstet Gynecol 68:1391, 1954

Caspi E, et al: Ovarian lutein cysts in pregnancy. Obstet Gynecol 42:388, 1973

Chalvardjian A, Scully RE: Sclerosing stromal tumors of the ovary. Cancer 31:664, 1973

Danforth DN: The cytological relationship of the Walthard cell rest to the Brenner tumor of the ovary and to the pseudomucinous cystadenoma. Am J Obstet Gynecol 43:948, 1942

De Alvarez RR, et al: Virilizing lipoid tumors of the ovary. Obstet Gynecol 35:956, 1970

De Bacalao EB, Dominquezl: Unilateral gonadoblastoma in a pregnant woman. Am J Obstet Gynecol 105:1279, 1969

Doss N, Leverich EB, Kemmerly JR; Covert bilaterality of mature ovarian teratomas. Obstet Gynecol 50:651, 1977

Dunnihoo DR, et al: Hilar cell tumors of the ovary: Report of two new cases and review of the world literature. Obstet Gynecol 27:703, 1966

Emig OR, Hertig, AT, Rowe FJ: Gynandroblastoma of the ovary: Review and report of a case. Obstet Gynecol 13:135, 1959

Fox H, Agrawal K, Langley FA: A clinicopathologic study of 92 cases of granulosa cell tumor of the ovary with special reference to the factors influencing prognosis. Cancer 35:231, 1975

Graber GA, O'Rourke JJ, Sturman M: Arrhenoblastoma of the ovary. Am J Obstet Gynecol 81:773, 1964

Gusberg SB, Danforth DN: Clinical significance of struma ovarii. Am J Obstet Gynecol 48:537, 1944

Hutchinson JR, Taylor HB, Zimmermann EA: Stein–Leventhal syndrome and coincident ovarian neoplasms. Obstet Gynecol 28:700, 1966

Marcus CC, Marcus SL: Struma ovarii. Am J Obstet Gynecol 81:752, 1961

Meigs JV: Pelvic tumors other than fibromas of the ovary with ascites and hydrothorax. Obstet Gynecol 3:471, 1954

Merrill JA: Morphology of the prepubertal ovary: Relationship to the polycystic ovary syndrome. South Med J 56:225, 1963

Norris HJ, Taylor HB: Virilization associated with cystic granulosa tumors. Obstet Gynecol 34:629, 1969

Novak ER, Long JH: Arrhenoblastoma of the ovary: A review of the ovarian tumor registry. Am J Obstet Gynecol 92:1082, 1965

Pedowtiz P, Pomerance W: Adrenal-like tumors of the ovary. Obstet Gynecol 19:183, 1962

Randall CL, Hall DW: Clinical considerations of benign ovarian cystomas. Am J Obstet Gynecol 62:806, 1951

Scully RE: Tumors of the Ovary and Maldeveloped Gonads. Washington DC, Armed Forces Institute of Pathology, 1979

Spanos WJ: Preoperative hormonal therapy of cystic adrenal masses. Am J Obstet Gynecol 116:551, 1973

MALIGNANT LESIONS OF THE OVARY

James H. Nelson, Jr.
Thomas E. Dolan

Malignant neoplasms of the ovary are the fourth leading cause of death from cancer among American women, following cancer of the breast, colon, and lung. Their diagnosis and management present a major challenge. Because of the tumors' silent growth and relative inaccessibility to diagnostic methods, most patients are first seen with far advanced lesions. For this reason, 5-year survival rates remain relatively poor. However, mean survival time and the quality of life during the period of extended survival have improved, owing to a more aggressive surgical approach and advancements in radiotherapy and chemotherapy.

In the past, elaborate classifications and contradictory approaches to management were sources of much confusion. In recent years these problems have been

largely resolved, permitting a much more rational approach to this disease.

EPIDEMIOLOGY

Statistics compiled by the American Cancer Society predicted 18 cases of ovarian cancer per 100,000 women in the United States in 1979, a total of 18,000 cases; for the same year 11,000 deaths from ovarian carcinoma were predicted. Although the incidence decreased 10% from 1947 (14.7/100,000) through 1969 (13.3/100,000), it is again on the rise and mortality has actually increased from 7.6/100,000 in 1950 to 11/100,000 in 1979. The overall 5-year survival rate was 25% in 1950 and 32% in the '70s. Despite the low overall survival rate, mean survival time has improved.

The therapeutic approach changed radically from 1965 through 1969. From 1940 to 1949, 38% of patients were treated by surgery alone, 21% by surgery and radiation, and 13% by radiation alone; 27% received no therapy. From 1965 to 1969, 13% of patients were treated by surgery alone, 15% by surgery and radiation, 18% by surgery and chemotherapy, 23% surgery, radiation, and chemotherapy, 18% by radiation and chemotherapy, and 7% by radiation alone; 8% received no treatment. In these two periods the use of surgery increased from 54% to 71%; the use of chemotherapy, from 0 to 55%; and the use of radiotherapy, from 34% to 50%. The proportion of untreated patients declined from 27% to 8%.

Of the 9978 deaths from ovarian cancer reported by the U.S. Bureau of Vital Statistics for 1971, 2477 (25%) occurred in women between the ages of 35 and 54, 5333 (53%) in women 55 to 74, and the remaining 2168 (22%) in girls 1 to 15 years of age or women older than 75. Some 60% of malignant ovarian tumors are said to occur in women 40 to 60 years old; 20% occur in women under 40, and the remaining 20% in women over 60. Way reports that 90% of ovarian neoplasms in women aged 20 to 40 are benign, and nearly 50% in women over 50 are malignant. About 15% of all ovarian tumors are malignant.

Although exact causes cannot be established, it is agreed that several *factors predispose*. Women of lower parity, especially those with history of infertility, repeated spontaneous abortion, and delayed onset of childbearing appear more apt to develop ovarian carcinoma. There is a family history of malignancy in 20% to 25% of patients who have ovarian carcinoma, but this is generally true of most malignancies. The M.D. Anderson Hospital and Tumor Institute is investigating pedigrees of ovarian cancer patients. Preliminary results suggest a definite family tendency.

Some 50% of all women with ovarian carcinoma are postmenopausal, 25% have normal menses, and 25% have abnormal menses. Ovarian carcinoma occurs more frequently in Caucasian women of European and North American origin than in women of African or Asian origin (Table 57–1). The racial distribution of ovarian carcinoma appears to parallel that of carcinoma of the breast and carcinoma of the endometrium.

Environmental factors are implicated as causative factors for ovarian carcinoma but there is no solid proof. The highest rates are found in industrial countries, suggesting that physical or chemical factors may be a cause. One exception to this hypothesis is Japan, which is highly industrialized but has a low overall incidence of the disease.

Mumps virus has been considered, but the relationship is only speculative and is not yet supported by valid data.

EMBRYOLOGY AND HISTOGENESIS

A knowledge of the development of the ovary is important to an understanding of the natural history of ovarian carcinoma, because the tumors differ histologically and most are probably embryonic in origin. The embryology of the ovary is detailed in Chapter 5.

In brief, the development of the ovary may be divided into four stages. The ovary arises as a mass of mesenchyme on the dorsal wall of the abdominal cavity of the embryo in the first stage. In the second stage, epithelium from the pelvic celiac cavity surrounds this mass. Ova are believed to come from this epithelium according to one theory; in another, they are considered to arise from the hindgut and to migrate into the mass. During the third stage, a peripheral cortex and central medulla form. The connective tissue surrounding the ova becomes highly specialized and gives rise to the granulosa and theca cells of the follicles. In the depth of the embryonal ovary and arising from connective tissue are structures resembling epithelial tissue; thus, the lining of the follicle cysts that arise from granulosa cells is epithelial in appearance, yet its origin is not epithelial. The last stage is characterized by the development of the cortex and a central me-

TABLE 57–1. RACIAL DISTRIBUTION OF CARCINOMA OF THE OVARY

Country and race	Incidence per 100,000 women
United States	
Whites	15
Blacks	8
Latins	6
Sweden	21
Israel	11
Japan	3

(Data from Kolstad P: American-European Conference on the Ovary, 1974)

TABLE 57-2. INTERNATIONAL STAGING DESIGNATIONS FOR CANCER OF THE OVARY (FIGO)

STAGE I	Growth limited to the ovaries
Stage IA	Growth limited to *one* ovary; no ascites
	(1) No tumor on the external surface; capsule intact
	(2) Tumor present on the external surface and/or capsule ruptured
Stage IB	Growth limited to *both* ovaries; no ascites
	(1) No tumor on the external surface; capsules intact
	(2) Tumor present on the external surface and/or capsules ruptured
Stage IC	Tumor either Stage IA or Stage IB, but with ascites* present or positive peritoneal washings
STAGE II	Growth involving one or both ovaries with pelvic extension
Stage IIA	Extension and/or metastases to the uterus and/or tubes
Stage IIB	Extension to other pelvic tissues including the peritoneum and the uterus
Stage IIC	Tumor either Stage IIA or Stage IIB, but with ascites* present or positive peritoneal washings
STAGE III	Growth involving one or both ovaries with intraperitoneal metastases outside the pelvis and/or positive retroperitoneal nodes
	Tumor limited to the true pelvis but with histologically proven malignant extension to small bowel or omentum
STAGE IV	Growth involving one or both ovaries with distant metastases
	If pleural effusion is present there must be positive cytology to allot a case to Stage IV
	Parenchymal liver metastases equals Stage IV

Special Category: Cases that are thought to be ovarian carcinoma, but whose origin has been impossible to discern.
* *Ascites* is a peritoneal effusion that, in the opinion of the surgeon, is pathologic or clearly exceeds normal amounts.

dulla. It is interesting to note, however, that although nearly 85% of ovarian carcinomas are epithelial in origin, they do not necessarily arise from tissues peculiar to the ovary. For example, a mesothelioma may originate anywhere in the celiac cavity.

Some consider the very early gonad neither ovarian nor testicular, and believe that its development depends upon whether its germ cells are spermatozoa or ova. It is conceivable, therefore, that certain testicular cells are present in the ovary even without spermatozoa and are the origin of masculinizing endocrine tumors.

The adrenal glands and the kidneys develop in close proximity to the ovary, and both hypernephromas and mesonephromas of the ovary have been described.

STAGING

The staging of ovarian cancer has been of immense value not only for comparing the results of treatment within a single institution and among many institutions, but also for establishing protocols of therapy for different stages of tumors. The staging of ovarian cancer is less straightforward than that for other pelvic cancers, whose extent can usually be determined by clinical examination prior to surgery. Visualization of the ovaries and exploration of the abdomen at laparotomy are necessary before a stage can be ascribed to a particular ovarian cancer. Accordingly, *ovarian cancer is staged on the basis of all of the information regarding the lesion,* including the results of curettage, ex-

amination of the tumor at laparotomy, data from radionuclide or other scanning, ascites or spill (either spontaneous or from rupture at the time of surgery), and the results of peritoneal washings. When the patient's condition does not permit abdominal exploration, a tumor presumed to be ovarian is assigned to a special category.

The international system for staging ovarian cancer that is now generally used and that should be applied to all such tumors, is shown in Table 57–2.

The importance of careful staging, especially in stage II lesions, needs repeated emphasis. A report from the National Cancer Institute indicated the need for upstaging in 40% of the patients referred to that institution with a diagnosis of Stage IIB carcinoma of the ovary.

CLASSIFICATION AND BIOLOGIC BEHAVIOR

The classification of ovarian tumors is complex because various elements in the ovary can give rise to many different kinds of tumors. Over the years innumerable classifications have been suggested, none of which is universally accepted. In 1961, the following histologic classification was proposed for epithelial tumors, which constitute 85% of ovarian tumors:

A. Serous cystomas
  1. Serous benign cystadenomas
  2. Serous cystadenomas with proliferating activity

of epithelial cells and nuclear abnormalities, but with no infiltrative destructive growth (low potential malignancy)
   3. Serous cystadenocarcinomas
B. Mucinous cystomas
   1. Mucinous benign cystadenomas
   2. Mucinous cystadenomas with proliferating activity of epithelial cells and nuclear abnormalities, but with no infiltrative destructive growth (low potential malignancy)
   3. Mucinous cystadenocarcinomas
C. Endometrioid tumors
   1. Endometrioid benign cysts
   2. Endometrioid tumors with proliferating activity of epithelial cells and nuclear abnormalities, but with no infiltrative destructive growth (low potential malignancy)
   3. Endometrioid adenocarcinomas
D. Clear-cell tumors (mesonephric tumors)
   1. Benign mesonephric tumors
   2. Mesonephric tumors with proliferating activity of epithelial cells and nuclear abnormalities, but with no infiltrative destructive growth (low potential malignancy)
   3. Mesonephric cystadenocarcinomas
E. Concomitant carcinomas, unclassified carcinomas (tumors that cannot be assigned to Group A, B, C, or D.)

In 1973 a classification was suggested for the remaining 15%, the so-called *special tumors* (including the nonepithelial, germ cell, sex chord–mesenchymal, and mixed tumors):

A. Stromal epithelial tumors (primarily stromal)
   1. Brenner tumors
   2. Tumors with functioning matrix
B. Stromal tumors
   1. Fibroma
   2. Fibrothecoma
   3. Sarcoma
C. Sex chord–mesenchymal tumors
   1. Tumors of the female cell type
      a. Granulosa cell tumors
      b. Theca cell tumors
      c. Granulosa–theca cell tumors
   2. Tumors of the male cell type
      a. Sertoli cell (testicular tubular adenoma) tumors
      b. Leydig cell (hilus cell) tumors
      c. Sertoli–Leydig cell tumors (arrhenoblastoma, androblastoma)
   3. Lipoid cell tumors
D. Germ cell tumors
   1. Dysgerminoma
   2. Endodermal sinus tumor
   3. Choriocarcinoma
   4. Embryonal carcinoma
   5. Polyembryoma
   6. Polyvesicular vitelline tumor
   7. Solid teratoma
   8. Cystic teratoma (dermoid cyst)
E. Gonadoblastoma
   Mixed germ cell–sex chord mensenchymal tumors
F. Metastatic tumors of the ovary

Epithelial tumors are disseminated by transperitoneal implantations (or stimulation of totipotential cells) on serosal surfaces. This produces an overall bulk effect which can interfere with gastrointestinal function, produce serous effusions, and institute metabolic competition, resulting in acute and chronic inanition. Mechanical intestinal obstruction occurs when the tumor produces compression, angulation, or fixation of the bowel. Lymphatic spread has not been regarded as an important means of dissemination, but this concept is changing. The paraaortic lymph nodes are often involved. Lymphatic spread to the diaphragm is also common. Invasion of blood vessels with hematogenous spread is a late manifestation.

Aure, Hoeg, and Kolstad reported on long-term follow-up of patients with epithelial tumors. Their objective was to study the prognostic significance of the histologic classification system. Figure 57–28 shows survival in relation to anatomic extent and operability of the tumor. It seems clear that prognosis is greatly improved when the tumor can be completely removed. Figure 57–29 shows the survival rates associated with the various epithelial tumors of all stages and Figure 57–30 illustrates survival rates for patients with Stage I tumors. In this series the different types of treatment were equally distributed among the various histologic tumor groups; however, many of the tumors were discovered and treated before the modern aggressive approach was developed and before the advent of modern radiotherapy and chemotherapy.

PATHOLOGY

The clinician should have a thorough appreciation of the clinical and histologic characteristics of the different ovarian tumors. Many cancers of the ovary bear a direct relation to their benign counterparts discussed earlier in this chapter. Some of the benign lesions are mentioned here because of their propensity for malignant change.

EPITHELIAL TUMORS

Most ovarian neoplasms are epithelial tumors; approximately 52% are of the serous and mucinous types. Varying degrees of malignancy exist and are related to

FIG. 57-28. Survival rates (life-table technique) for patients with ovarian carcinoma in relation to stage and operability of tumor. Numbers of patients in parentheses. (Aure JC, Hoeg K, Kolstad P: Obstet Gynecol 37:1, 1971)

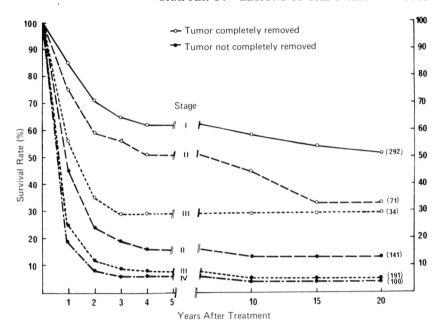

FIG. 57-29. Survival rates for patients with different histologic types of ovarian carcinoma, all stages. Numbers of patients in parentheses. *A2,* serous tumors with low potential malignancy; *B2,* mucinous tumors with low potential malignancy; *A3,* serous carcinomas; *B3,* mucinous carcinomas; *C3,* endometrioid carcinomas; *D3,* mesonephroid carcinomas of clear-cell type; *4T,* mesonephroid carcinomas with tubular pattern; *E,* undifferentiated carcinomas. (Aure JC, Hoeg K, Kolstad P: Obstet Gynecol 37:1, 1971)

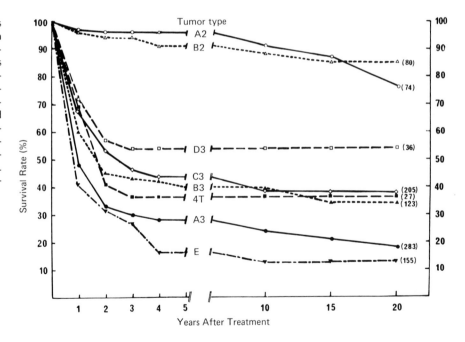

such histologic factors as nuclear atypia, mitotic activity, and presence or absence of stromal invasion. In the classification outlined above, the degree of malignancy is based upon presence or absence of stromal invasion. The diagnosis of a lesion as borderline is based upon the amount of stromal involvement in the primary lesion only, regardless of whether the disease has already spread beyond the ovary.

Serous Tumors

Serous tumors of the ovary, whether benign or malignant have similar gross and histologic features (Figs. 57-31, 57-32, 57-33). Therefore, it is essential that many microscopic fields be examined before the lesion is diagnosed as benign. For gross evaluation each cyst must be carefully opened and examined for solid areas or papillary projections. A malignant ovarian tumor is

(*Text continues on p. 1147.*)

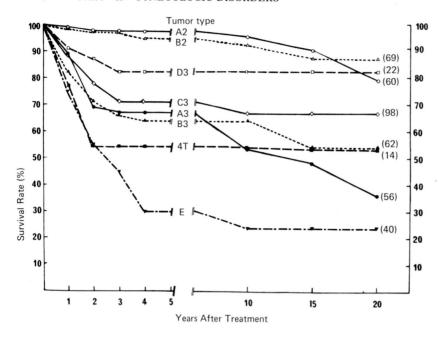

FIG. 57–30. Survival rates for patients with stage I ovarian carcinoma in relation to histologic type of tumor. Numbers of patients in parentheses. *A2,* serous tumors with low potential malignancy; *B2,* mucinous tumors with low potential malignancy; *A3,* serous carcinomas; *B3,* mucinous carcinomas; *C3,* endometrioid carcinomas; *D3,* mesonephroid carcinomas of clear-cell type; *4T,* mesonephroid carcinomas with tubular pattern; *E,* undifferentiated carcinomas. (Aure JC, Hoeg K, Kolstad P: Obstet Gynecol 37:1, 1971)

FIG. 57–31. Proliferating serous papillary cystadenoma without stromal invasion (possibly malignant). (×50)

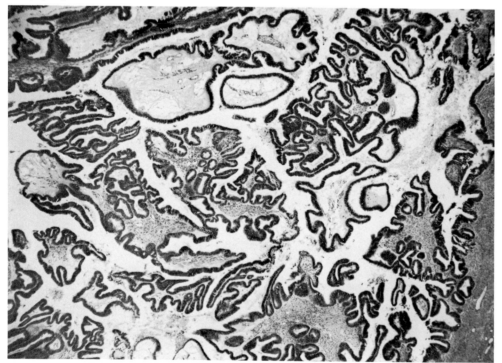

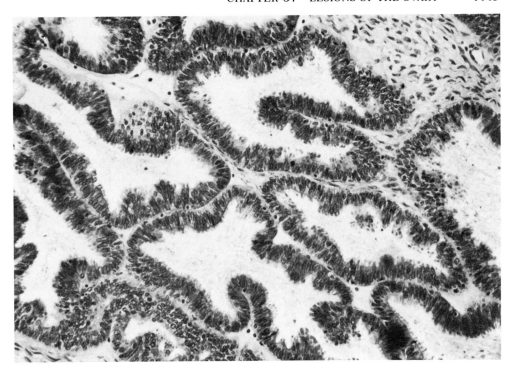

FIG. 57–32. High-power view of tumor shown in figure 57–31. Note marked proliferative activity in epithelium, with disparity of cells and nuclei. This tumor type must be regarded as potentially malignant. (×200)

FIG. 57–33. Papillary serous cystadenocarcinoma (×50)

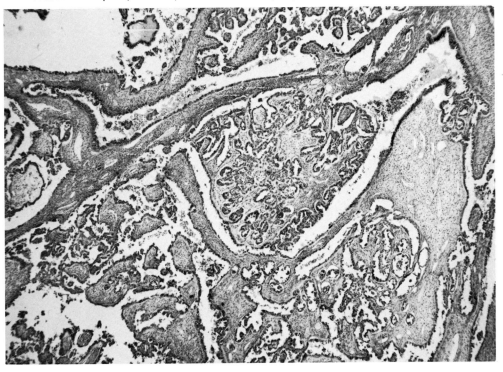

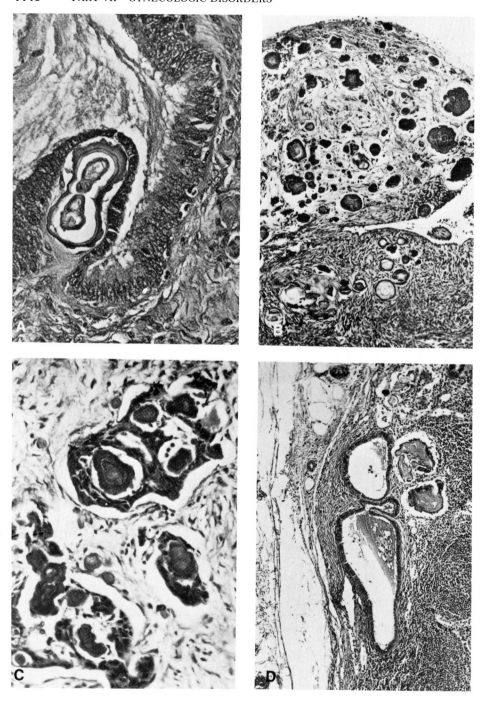

FIG. 57-34. Serous cystadenocarcinoma. *A.* Psammoma body within stroma adjacent to epithelium of serous cystadenoma of ovary. (original magnification ×400) *B.* Fibrous adhesions and cortex of a senescent ovary containing numerous psammoma bodies. (×125) *C.* Psammoma body formation in stroma associated with serous cystadenocarcinoma. (×220). *D.* Pelvic lymph node showing mullerian-type epithelium and associated psammoma body in a peripheral sinus. (×75) (Hertig AT, Gore H: Tumors of the Female Sex Organs, Part 3, Tumors of the Ovary and Fallopian Tube. Atlas of Tumor Pathology, Sect 9, Fasc 33. Washington DC, Armed Forces Institute of Pathology, 1961)

more often bilateral than is a benign tumor. This is especially true of the serous tumors. In Tweeddale and Pederson's series, 19.2% of malignant serous tumors were bilateral, a finding that is in agreement with many single case reports. More than 50% of serous tumors are larger than 15 cm in diameter at the time of surgery.

The fluid contained in 72% of serous carcinomas is watery in consistency, rich in the serum proteins albumin and globulin, and, of course, cancer cells. In 28% the fluid has mucinous characteristics. The fluid is usually clear to very light yellow, but can be hemorrhagic, especially in malignant tumors, perhaps owing to invasion, rapid growth, or an association with endometriosis. Estrogen may be present in the fluid, but this is not constant or well understood. Serous tumors are also characterized by an admixture of solid and cystic areas. The solid component is more common in malignancy. Examination of papillary serous cystadenocarcinomas, using both light and electron microscopy has disclosed five cell types: Types A and B are similar to those seen in the fallopian tube; Type C is similar to the corresponding cell of the endometrium; Type D is composed of secretory cells that resemble endocervical epithelial; and Type E is a cell unlike any previously described in the female reproductive tract. Identification of these different cell types lends credence to the hypothesis that serous tumors originate from germinal epithelium. Differentiation of benign, borderline, and malignant tumors can be difficult, and since different areas of a single tumor may vary in histologic appearance, diagnosis cannot reliably be based upon a single sample.

As a general rule, when the constituent cells closely mimic the normal fallopian tube lining, the tumor is benign. Early malignant change includes loss of cell polarity and cell differentiation, frequent mitoses (in benign tumors the number of mitoses rarely exceeds one per high-power field), and hyperchromatism. Desmoplastic tumor stroma is present in 75% of malignant serous tumors. Even with careful study a definitive diagnosis cannot always be made; approximately 20% of serous tumors are designated as borderline.

Calcospherites (*psammoma bodies*) are present in about 20% of serous cystadenocarcinomas (Fig. 57–34) and are thought to occur as a result of degeneration and calcification of small papillae. They may be found in the primary tumor, in metastatic sites, and even many years after removal of the primary tumor. They can occasionally be seen on x-ray films.

Grading of Serous Tumors. The most generally used grading system for serous tumors is based upon a histologic scheme in which Grade I is the most highly differentiated and Grade IV the most anaplastic lesion. The frequency distribution characteristic of serous carcinomas is presented in Table 57–3. These data suggest that many serous carcinomas are anaplastic.

TABLE 57–3. FREQUENCY DISTRIBUTION OF VARIOUS GRADES OF SEROUS OVARIAN TUMORS

Grade	No. of Patients	Percent of Patients
I	59	17.8
II	84	25.4
III	110	33.2
IV	78	23.6
Total	331	100.0

(This is in sharp contrast to mucinous carcinomas of which more than 95% are Grade I and II lesions and Grade IV is uncommon.)

Metastasis of Serous Tumors. By the time serous tumors are detected clinically, about two-thirds have already metastasized by transperitoneal implantation or transport through the lymphatics, the tubes and uterine cavity, or the blood stream. Peritoneal implantation is the most common form of spread and occurs more often in serous than in mucinous tumors. Common abdominal sites for metastases include the omentum, small and large intestines, and the parietal portion of the peritoneum. It has been generally considered that metastases resulting from lymphatic spread occur later than those that result from seeding, but recent studies suggest this may be in error. Lymphatic spread is through the iliac, lumbar, mesenteric, and para-aortic nodes (see Figs. 57–35 and 57–36).

Mucinous Tumors

Mucinous tumors may reach enormous size, filling the entire abdominal cavity (see Fig. 57–1). The largest reported weighed 328 lb, including the fluid removed at preoperative paracentesis; most are found and removed before they attain this huge size. Mucinous tumors tend to be larger as a group than serous tumors, but occasionally serous tumors are also very large. Mucinous tumors, once thought to carry a better prognosis, are now known to be about equally virulent, stage for stage and grade for grade, as serous tumors.

Mucinous tumors occur about one-third as often as serous tumors. Grossly, they are usually lobulated and have a smooth outer surface that may or may not be adherent to neighboring organs. The cyst wall is generally thin, translucent, and white or blue-white. Ovarian tissue is frequently totally replaced. The contained fluid is usually thick and viscid, but may be watery. It is usually straw-colored but may be light brown or chocolate-colored from intraluminal bleeding. Papillary growths in the wall occur in only 5% to 10%. Each cyst should be opened and examined for solid areas, since these are most likely to be malignant.

Characteristically, these tumors are composed of locules or compartments separated by septa of fibrous

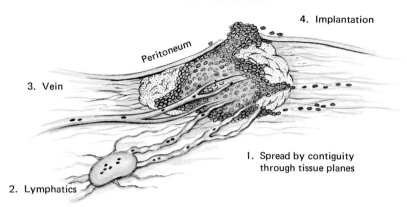

FIG. 57–35. Four mechanisms of dissemination of cancer cells. (Cole WH, McDonald GO, Roberts SS, Southwick HW: Dissemination of Cancer. New York, Appleton, 1961)

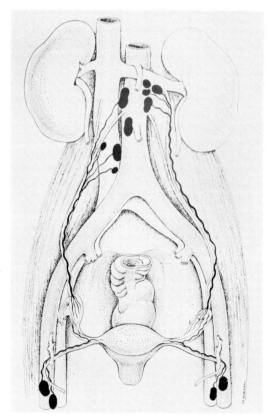

FIG. 57–36. Anatomic sketch of lymphatics of ovary, showing drainage by paraaortic lymph nodes. There is inconstant drainage toward external iliac nodes. (Ackerman LV, del Regato JA: Cancer: Diagnosis, Treatment, and Prognosis, 4th ed. St. Louis, CV Mosby, 1970)

tissue, but unilocular cysts do occur. Mucinous tumors are less often bilateral than serous tumors. Microscopically (Fig. 57–37), the most characteristic finding is the typical picket-fence epithelium, which resembles that of the endocervix. Mucinous epithelium is found routinely in no other ovarian tumor ex-

cept the teratoma. Malignant degeneration occurs in 5% to 10% of benign mucinous cysts, an incidence much lower than that of serous tumors. If a mucinous cyst ruptures spontaneously or during surgery, mucinous epithelium may become implanted. Such seeded cells may continue their secretory activity, with gradual accumulation in the peritoneal cavity of huge amounts of gelatinous material, usually lemon yellow in color, the so-called *pseudomyxoma peritonei* (Fig. 57–37). This may cause bowel obstruction or other gastrointestinal complications. The same clinical entity can result from rupture of a mucocele of the appendix.

Endometrioid Adenocarcinoma

The term "endometrioid carcinoma" reflects the tumor's histologic resemblance to adenocarcinoma of the endometrium. Although the term was not intended to imply that the tumor necessarily arises in areas of endometriosis, it has become apparent that most do have this source (Fig. 57–38). The tumors may be solid or cystic and range up to 20 cm in diameter. About 25% to 30% are bilateral. Microscopic examination shows the same variability as in endometrial carcinoma, including acanthomatous change. The prognosis is better than for most other solid cancers of the ovary.

Mesonephroid (Clear-cell) Tumors

The mesophroma was first described by Schiller in 1939. The tumor is of epithelial origin, but there is no agreement about whether it indeed arises from mesonephric epithelial rests. It is generally agreed that the lesions constitute a definite pathologic group, and the term *clear-cell carcinoma* is now accepted. The name reflects the presence of these tumors of the classic glomeruluslike structure with the clear cell which characterizes the hypernephroid lesion of the kidney (Figs. 57–39, 57–40).

Grossly, clear-cell tumors may be cystic or solid and contain chocolate-colored fluid and yellowish, pale-

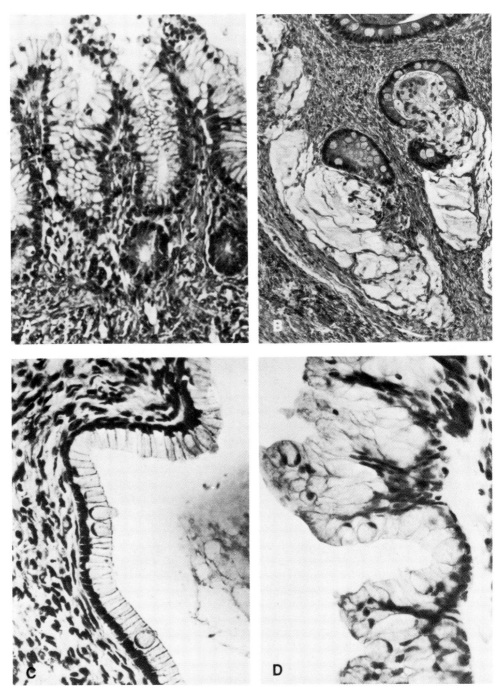

FIG. 57–37. Mucinous tumor *A*. Intestinal type of epithelium occurring as a single focus within otherwise typical mucinous cystadenoma. Most mucinous cystadenomas derive from germinal epithelial inclusion cysts of müllerian potential and resemble mucus-secreting glands of endocervix (×250) *B*. Small area of myxoma ovarii related to myxoma peritonei, incidental finding in large mucinous cystoma that also contained a Brenner tumor. This illustrates that mucinous material originates from intestinal type epithelium and gains access to stroma by rupture of previously intact gland or cyst. (×160) *C*. High-power detail of epithelium from mucinous cystadenoma. A few goblet cells are seen within tall picket-fence mucinous epithelium. (×275) *D*. Mucinous cystadenoma or low-grade cystadenocarcinoma showing a papillary pattern of underlying stroma indicating low potential malignancy. (Hertig AT, Gore H: Tumors of the Female Sex Organs, Part 3, Tumors of the Ovary and Fallopian Tube. Atlas of Tumor Pathology, Sect 9, Fasc 33. Washington DC, Armed Forces Institute of Pathology, 61)

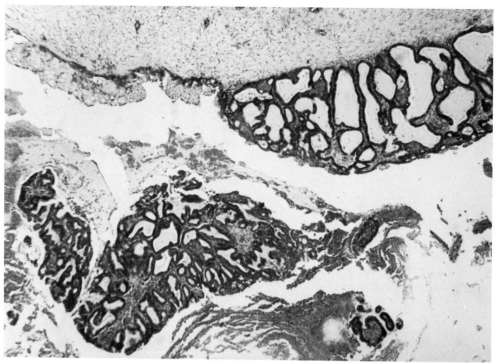

FIG. 57–38. Endometrioid adenocarcinoma of ovary. Junction of carcinoma with lining of benign endometrial cyst of ovary can be seen at *upper left.* (×50)

brown polypoid masses. They may be related to endometrioid tumors and are often associated with endometriosis elsewhere in the pelvis. About 90% are unilateral. The 5-year survival rate approaches 50%.

CONCOMITANT CARCINOMA, UNCLASSIFIED CARCINOMA

The group includes undifferentiated (primary solid), papillary, medullary, scirrhous simplex, areolar, and plexiform carcinomas. These tumors often contain a mixture of two or more of the previously described cell types, which are so undifferentiated that they cannot be recognized as a definite subgroup. The tumors are often bilateral and the survival rate is poor.

THE SPECIAL TUMORS

Stromal Epithelial Tumors (Predominantly Stromal)

This group includes 1) tumors with predominantly gonadal mesenchyme plus an epithelial component that varies from the simple mesothelium of the surface fibromatous papillomas to the stratified squamoid epithelium of the Brenner tumor, 2) fibrocystadenomas, and 3) tumors with functioning matrix. Some of these

lesions are quite large, but some are so small the ovary may appear grossly normal. They are rarely functional, with the possible exception of the Brenner tumor, which is reported to have a very limited association with hyperplasia and adenocarcinoma of the endometrium. These tumors are most frequently seen in postmenopausal patients but also occur in women of childbearing age. Tumor growth is usually slow, and few if any clinical symptoms are present.

Grossly, stromal epithelial tumors are similar to fibromas; they are sometimes, but rarely, malignant and usually unilateral. Numerous sections should be examined, however, to rule out malignancy. Microscopically, there are two essential findings: the characteristic nests of epithelial cells and the concentration of mesenchymal tissue surrounding the epithelial islands (see Fig. 57–27). Both findings must be present for a diagnosis of Brenner tumor. The grooved nucleus is also a characteristic finding in all benign and in most malignant Brenner tumors.

Stromal Tumors

Solid stromal tumors are usually unilateral and benign. However, some solid stromal ovarian tumors, especially if bilateral, may be metastatic from other areas, and careful search should be made for a primary lesion in another site. The benign solid tumors include

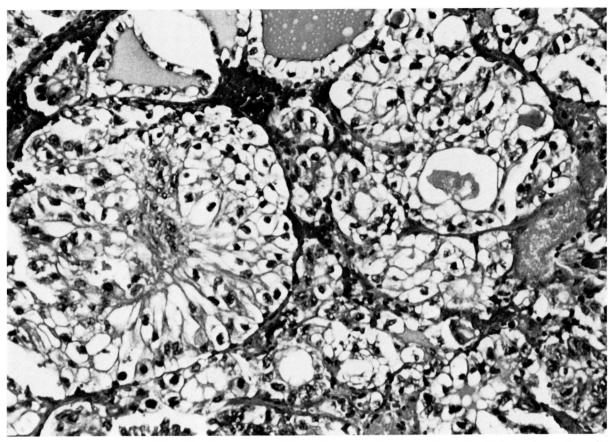

FIG. 57–39. Mesonephroma (clear-cell carcinoma) showing clear cells with hyperchromatic nuclei (×100) (E dePapp)

fibromas, fibrothecomas, angiomas, lymphangiomas, and neuromas; although malignant change is uncommon, it can occur. Microscopic examination shows spindle-shaped fibroblasts, fibrocytes, and an abundant collagenous stroma. Sarcomas are rare, occurring 40 times less often than carcinoma, but they are highly malignant. Included are teratoid sarcomas, mesenchymal or stromal sarcomas, and müllerian or paramesonephric sarcomas. Lymphomas also are rare and are associated with primary lesion elsewhere, usually in the gastrointestinal tract.

Germ Cell Tumors

Except for the malignancies that can arise in benign cystic teratomas, the malignant germ cell tumors occur in children and young adults. Understanding the various elements that can arise in these tumors requires understanding the origin of tissues from the fertilized ovum. The blastocyst differentiates into extraembryonal elements (classically the trophoblast), and the tissues derive from the three germ layers—ectoderm, mesoderm, and endoderm. In tumors, these elements may exist in either mature or immature forms, and the ability of the tumor tissue to mature determines the overall prognosis. Tumors composed of mature elements (*i.e.,* benign cystic teratomas) have an excellent prognosis; those composed of immature elements (*e.g.,* endodermal sinus tumor), grow in an undisciplined manner and cause the eventual, often prompt, death of the patient. Figure 57–41 diagrams the origin of germ-cell tumors.

The *dysgerminoma** is reputedly one-third as com-

* This tumor, like so many others, was first described by the preeminent gynecologic pathologist, Robert Meyer. He designated it a "disgerminoma," selecting the prefix because "such tumors arise from a type of cell which should become sex cells, but for some unknown reason lose that quality." In his autobiography, Dr. Meyer comments on the dissension over the spelling: "The genesis of this tumor should be in the foreground of further discussion instead of arguments about the spelling of the word. Webster says 'dis' is in English a prefix denoting: (i) reversal, undoing, depriving, or negation; (ii) undoing or depriving of a character or quality. This was what my theory was meant to express—the losing of a quality. But, for myself, it is absolutely unimportant whether one spells disgerminoma with a 'y.' " (Editor)

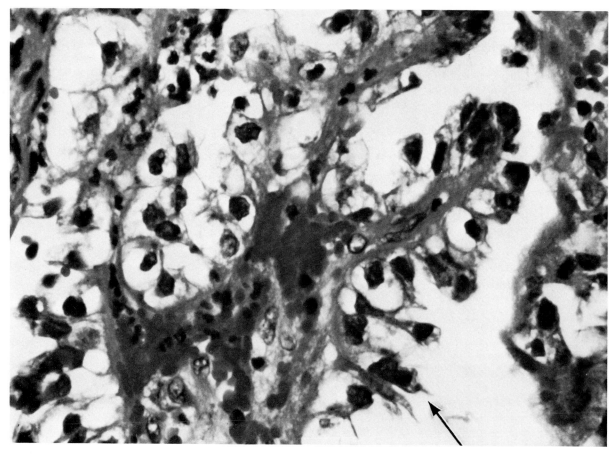

FIG. 57–40. Mesonephroma (clear-cell carcinoma) showing hobnail cells (*arrow*). (×160) (E de-Papp)

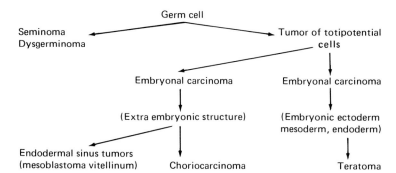

FIG. 57–41. Diagrammatic representation of origin of germ cell tumors.

mon as the granulosa cell tumor, although some feel that it is equally common. There is considerable controversy over the malignant potential of this tumor: the 5-year survival varies in different series from 27% to 95%. It appears less malignant than the common forms of primary ovarian carcinoma. Dysgerminomas vary in size from a few centimeters to a size that fills the abdominal cavity. Characteristically, the lesion has a smooth, dense capsule, a rubbery consistency, and a cut surface that is pink mottled with areas of yellow. Microscopically, the dysgerminoma is characterized by large round, ovoid, or polygonal cells (Fig. 57–42). Cytoplasm is abundant and the nucleus large and round. The cells are arranged in alveoli or nests separated by septa of hyalinized fibrous tissue.

The *choriocarcinoma* of the ovary, an embryonal

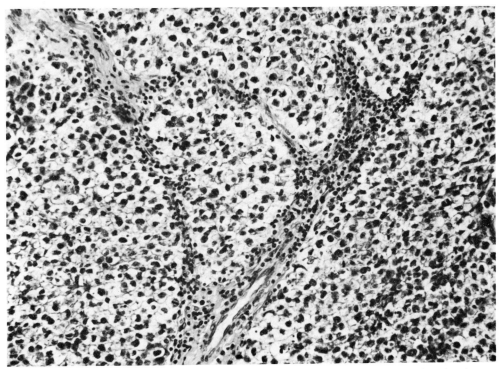

FIG. 57-42. Dysgerminoma. Large round, ovoid, or polygonal cells are arranged in alveolar nests separated by septa of hyalinized fibrin tissue. Note abundant clear cystoplasm with large nucleus. Lymphocytes are in background. (×200)

carcinoma of extraembryonic origin, is extremely rare and highly malignant. It can arise from a teratoma or an ovarian pregnancy, or may be metastatic from choriocarcinoma originating elsewhere. This disease is discussed in Chapter 21.

Teratomas containing immature elements are rare, constituting only 0.2% of all ovarian tumors. They are usually solid, but commonly have areas of degeneration. The microscopic patterns vary from those containing extraembryonal elements, the endodermal sinus, or trophoblast, to those containing embryonal components showing varying degrees of differentiation (Figs. 57–43, 57–44). The prognosis is poor for the tumors with immature elements and better for those with mature elements. About 10% to 15% of teratomas are bilateral. A very unusual and poorly differentiated form of the embryonal teratomas is the *polyembryonic embryoma,* a tumor containing multiple, perhaps hundred of, early embryonic formations.

In adults, 1% to 3% of cystic teratomas (benign cystic teratoma or dermoid cyst) are malignant. Usually malignancy develops in the ectodermal element, forming squamous cell carcinoma. This lesion is quite different from the embryonic forms of solid teratoma. Any of the elements may be malignant and occasionally sarcomas, adenocarcinomas, and carcinoid tumors are present. Malignant dysgerminoma may be superimposed.

In recent years much has been written of the *endodermal sinus tumor,* a rare, highly lethal germ cell tumor occurring principally in young women. Like many other tumors, survival rates have improved as the result of new techniques of adjunctive therapy.

Gonadoblastoma

The gonadoblastoma, arising in an abnormal testis or in a dysgenetic ovary, is encountered most often in phenotypic females showing virilization. This neoplasm is classified between the dysgerminoma and the sex chord–mesenchymal tumors, containing not only germ cells but also elements derived from the gonadal sex chords and mesenchyme. The sex chord components resemble immature Sertoli or granulosa cells, but are not specifically identifiable as either. The tumors are almost invariably benign, but their frequent association with such tumors as dysgerminoma causes them to be considered among malignant tumors (see page 1137).

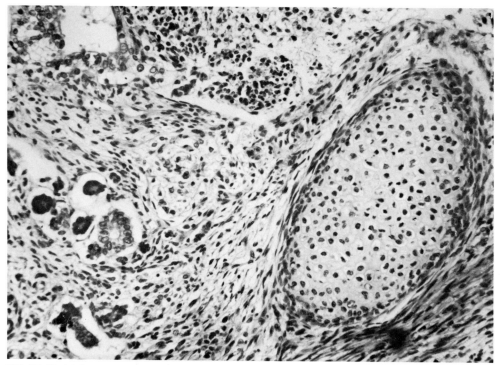

FIG. 57–43. Malignant teratoma of ovary. Note area of immature cartilage and glandlike structures in undifferentiated stroma. (×200)

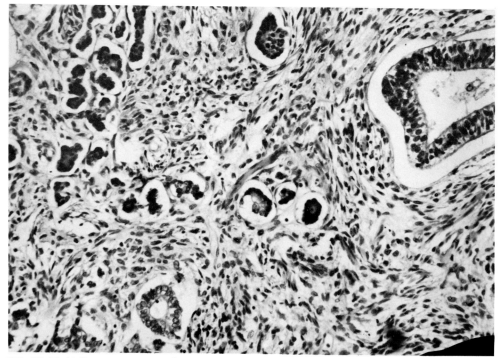

FIG. 57–44. Malignant teratoma of ovary (same tumor as shown in Fig. 57–43). Note irregular glands embedded within pleomorphic stroma. (×200)

Sex Chord-Mesenchymal Tumors

All tumors in this group have malignant potential. They appear to arise from the mesenchyme of the embryonic gonad and include the feminizing tumors (granulosa and theca cell), virilizing tumors (arrhenoblastoma, adrenal, and hilus cell tumors), and lipoid tumors. They may contain granulosa cells, theca cells, lutein cells, Sertoli cells, and Leydig cells—alone or in combination.

The most important feminizing tumor in this group, which may be malignant, is the *granulosa cell tumor* (Fig. 57–45). Granulosa cell tumors of the ovary represent about 10% of all solid ovarian tumors. They are bilateral in about 5% of patients. Malignant change occurs in about 30%. The tumors secrete estrogen, which frequently causes endometrial proliferation and, consequently, abnormal uterine bleeding. Endometrial carcinoma is reported to be associated with about 20% of granulosa cell tumors. They may occur at any age and the clinical manifestations depend upon age. For example, precocious puberty occurs when this tumor develops prior to menarche.

The lesions vary in size from a few millimeters to large masses that fill the abdomen. Microscopically, the pattern is highly variable (Fig. 57–46), and this has led to confusion regarding nomenclature and classification. Microfollicular, macrofollicular, trabecular, cylindromatous, insular gyriform, solid tubular, and sarcomatoid or diffuse patterns may be found. Diagnosis must be based upon examination of many sections. In the most common variety, the granulosa cells tend to be clustered at intervals in small groups or rosettes around a central lumen, producing a resemblance to primordial follicles. These tiny structures are known as *Call–Exner bodies*. Survival rates for patients with granulosa-cell carcinoma are generally good, perhaps because the endocrine effects signal the tumor's presence at a fairly early stage. Kottmeier states that these tumors occur in two distinct forms: a well-differentiated form associated with an excellent survival rate of 87%, and a less well-differentiated or sarcomatoid tumor with a 5-year survival rate of 64%. The malignant properties of the granulosa cell appear to be low grade, and recurrences are sometimes detected 15 to 20 years after removal, with apparent cure, of the primary tumor. Novak and Woodruff state that it is difficult, if not impossible to evaluate the malignant trends of the special tumors by mitosis count or any close scrutiny of the individual tumor cells. Distant metastases are rare, and recurrences are often responsive to therapy. These patients must be followed very carefully for a long time after primary treatment.

The virilizing tumors represented chiefly by the *arrhenoblastomas* (Fig. 57–47), are rare. The group includes tumors with Sertoli cells (testicular tubular adenoma), Leydig cells (hilar cells tumors), and combinations that may be either masculinizing or

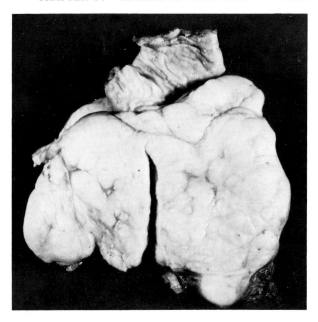

FIG. 57–45. Granulosa-cell carcinoma. Preparation artifact is caused by midline split. Note solid fat appearance. (N Peralta)

inert. It has been suggested that this group of tumors be termed "mesenchymal" or "gonadal stromal" tumors with a qualifying prefix: inert, masculinizing, or feminizing. The proposal is based upon the endocrine effect of these tumors and the evidence that they all arise from mesenchyme. Malignant change is less frequent than in other more common types of ovarian cancers, but may be greater than some believe. Reported mortality rates range from about 10% to more than 30%. Mathet and Novak and Long consider it almost impossible to formulate any prognosis in the case of these neoplasms, at least partly because the higher reported figures for malignancy may be due to the erroneous inclusion of carcinomas having an androgen-secreting stroma.

The *lipoid cell tumor*, which appears to have a common origin with the adrenal and hilus cell tumors, produces varying hormone effects. These tumors are rare, but approximately 20% are malignant.

METASTATIC CARCINOMA

Metastatic ovarian carcinomas are usually bilateral, firm, and solid. About 6% of ovarian cancers encountered during exploration for a pelvic or abdominal mass are metastatic, usually from primary cancers of the intestine, breast, thyroid, or lymphatic tissue. The term *Krukenberg tumor* (Figs. 57–48, 57–49, 57–50) should be reserved for ovarian metastases that contain significant numbers of signet ring cells and a cellular

(*Text continues on p. 1158.*)

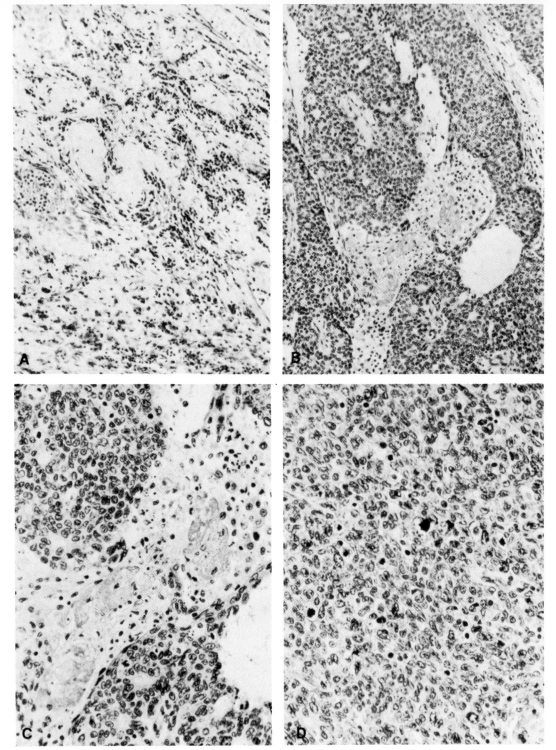

FIG. 57–46. Granulosa cell tumors. *A.* Granulosa-cell tumor with prominent hyalinization of the theca externa stromal elements. Small, irregular strands of epithelial cells are granulosa cells; broad pale bands are hyalinized theca. (×120) *B.* Granulosa cell carcinoma. Note general resemblance of microscopic pattern to that of granulosa cell tumor. Large trabeculae of relatively small cells with occasional Call-Exner bodies are characteristic. Broad pale stromal zones represent theca externa and interna. (×105) *C.* High-power view of *B.* Note thrombosed vessels in stroma and Call–Exner bodies in lower part of photomicrograph. (×120) *D.* High-power view of *B.* Note pleomorphism and numerous mitoses. (×210) Hertig AT, Gore H: Tumors of the Female Sex Organs, Part 3, Tumors of the Ovary and Fallopian Tube. Atlas of Tumor Pathology, Sect 9, Fasc 33. Washington DC, Armed Forces Institute of Pathology, 1961)

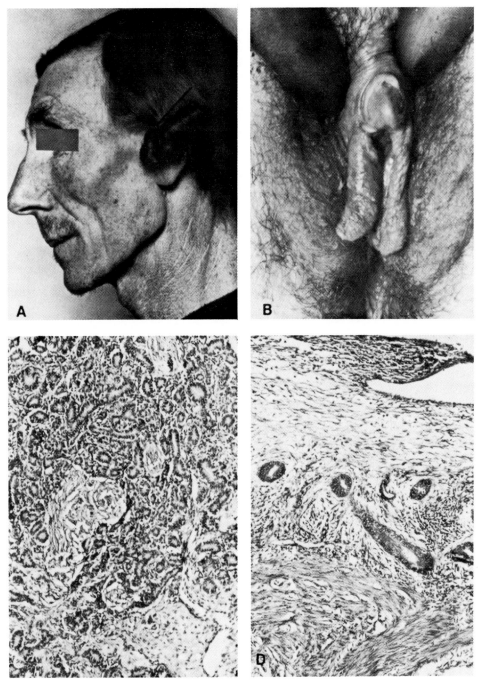

FIG. 57–47. Arrhenoblastoma. *A.* Laryngeal hypertrophy, hirsutism (regular shaving was required), and general masculine facies in 50-year-old woman. *B.* Enlarged clitoris prior to removal of well-differentiated tubular arrhenoblastoma. *C.* General architecture of tubular arrhenoblastoma. Note tubular pattern and broad sheets of stroma; cells have a swollen, pleomorphic appearance. (×100) *D.* Endometrium from same patient. Note inactive straight or tubular, sparsely distributed glands and relatively prominent endometrial stroma. (×100) (Hertig AT; Gore H: Tumors of the Female Sex Organs, Part 3, Tumors of the Ovary and Fallopian Tube. Atlas of Tumor Pathology, Sect 9, Fasc 33. Washington DC, Armed Forces Institute of Pathology, 1961)

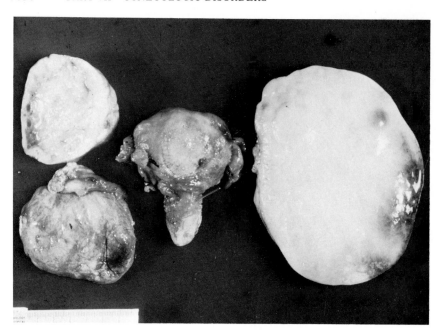

FIG. 57–48. Gross appearance of bilateral Krukenberg tumor of ovary. Uterus also shown. Note that right ovary is bivalved. (N Peralta)

stroma derived from the ovarian stroma. This restriction is important because tumors with these microscopic characteristics have distinctive pathologic and clinical features. Almost all have metastasized from the stomach, but some have arisen in the breast, intestine, or another mucus-gland-containing organ. Microscopic evaluation usually, but not always, delineates the primary site.

The frequency with which the various ovarian cancers are encountered at surgery is shown in Table 57–4.

SYMPTOMS AND SIGNS

One of the perplexing problems of ovarian neoplasia is the silent nature of the lesions until they are well advanced in their malignant growth pattern. This *lack of symptoms,* especially in the early stages of the disease, has led to the designation of ovarian cancer as the "silent killer." In four large series reported from the 1940s through the 1970s (Table 57–5) there is a consistent pattern of increase in abdominal girth, vague lower abdominal discomfort, dyspepsia, weight gain or loss, and other GI abnormalities that usually occur late in the disease. The problem is further compounded by patient delay and physician delay from the time of onset of earliest symptoms to the diagnosis and definitive therapy. All postmenopausal women who present with vague GI complaints or changes in weight should be evaluated with a high index of suspicion for ovarian cancer. Unfortunately, many women have no symptoms sufficient to initiate a report to the doctor. Most

malignant tumors are largely cystic and do not compromise physiologic, biochemical, or biologic function until late in the course of the disease. Most produce few, if any, symptoms until discomfort arises because of their size or as a result of metastases. Because ovarian neoplasms grow quietly and painlessly, any abdominal enlargement requires that the physician rule out an ovarian neoplasm.

Physical findings can also be absent until the later stages of tumor growth. Any palpable ovarian mass in a premenarchal or postmenopausal woman should be considered abnormal. In a menstruating woman an enlarged ovary should be suspect, but caution is mandatory, since a functional or benign cyst also produces ovarian enlargement. Any mass greater than 5 cm in any woman should be considered suspect. If there is any doubt, an ultrasound scan or laparoscopy may be helpful.

Ascites with shifting dullness, a fluid wave, and palpable abdominal masses are common findings when the tumor has metastasized to the omentum. Although ascites usually suggests a malignancy, it can also occur with a benign tumor (Meigs' syndrome).

A mass in the anterior cul-de-sac is most commonly associated with a benign cystic teratoma or an endometrioma, whereas masses in the posterior cul-de-sac are more commonly associated with malignant tumors. A solid, bilateral, fixed mass greater than 10 cm in diameter is more often malignant. A common mistake is to confuse an ovarian neoplasm with a leiomyoma. On the other hand, a unilateral, cystic, mobile, smaller mass is most often benign.

Metastases often lead to pleural effusions, and

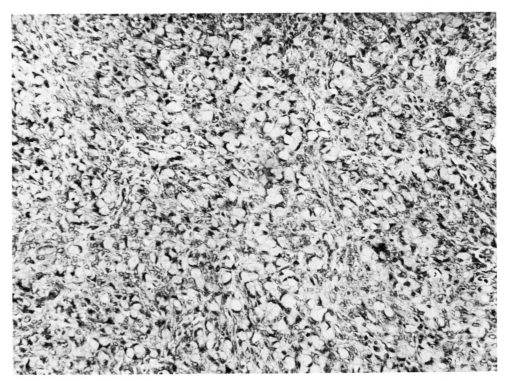

FIG. 57–49. Krukenberg tumor of ovary. Polyhedral epithelial cells intermingle with fibrous tissue stroma. Primary tumor was located in stomach. (×200)

FIG. 57–50. High-power view of tumor shown in Figure 57–49. Note spongy cytoplasm of tumor cells and location of nucleus at periphery of cell, imparting typical signet-ring form. (×600)

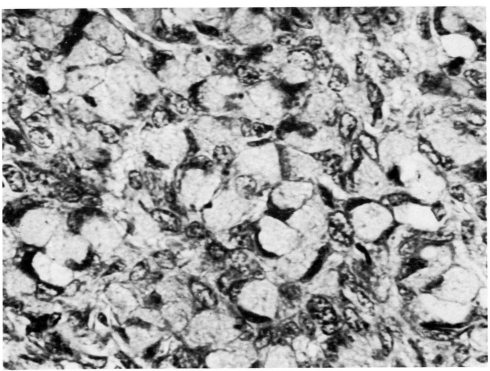

malignant cells can be found in other lymph-bearing areas of the body, especially the supraclavicular, axillary, and inguinal nodes. The most common sites of metastases in ovarian cancer are listed in Table 57-6.

DIAGNOSIS

The low survival rate of patients with carcinoma of the ovary is due not only to the virulence of the disease but also, and of preeminent importance, to the difficulty and at times the impossibility of early diagnosis. Despite the low yield, pelvic examination remains the most reliable method of detecting early disease. The following should be axiomatic: 1) unless there are specifically extenuating circumstances, all ovarian tumors 7 cm in diameter should be removed at once, regardless of the patient's age (a tennis ball is 7 cm in diameter); 2) in women of childbearing age ovarian tumors 5 cm in diameter that persist at a second examination

6 weeks later should be removed; and 3) in postmenopausal women, palpable enlarged ovaries, regardless of size, should be removed. Barber and Graber have coined the phrase "postmenopausal palpable ovary syndrome," which directs attention to the important fact that the ovaries of postmenopausal women are not normally palpable. If they can be felt, they are enlarged, and exploration is recommended. If this dictum is followed some unnecessary laparotomies will be performed; but some very early ovarian cancers will also be found.

The ultimate diagnosis of ovarian neoplasia depends upon surgical exploration.

Although preoperative evaluations are helpful and important, preoccupation with a stipulated group of diagnostic procedures that must be done before surgery is unwise. The major evaluation is as follows:

1. Careful history, with attention to all systems
2. Physical examination
3. Pelvic examination and cervical and vaginal smears
4. CBC and urinalysis
5. Blood chemistries and coagulation studies
6. Chest x-ray
7. IVP
8. Barium enema
9. GI series, proctosigmoidoscopy, liver scan, bone scan when indicated.

These tests done in rapid sequence can be very debilitating; the preoperative survey should be designed to provide the information needed for an intelligent approach to the abdominal surgery, and the remaining tests should be carried out after surgery.

Ultrasound or CT scan of the pelvis and abdomen can usually delineate a mass but cannot distinguish whether the mass is benign or malignant. They can also be helpful in directing paracentesis so as to avoid rupture of a cyst and spread with possible implantation of tumor to uninvolved areas. These tests are also useful in following the response of residual masses to chemotherapy or other adjunctive therapy.

Routine paracentesis or cul-de-sac aspiration to obtain samples for cell study is not recommended even in

TABLE 57-4. INCIDENCE OF VARIOUS TYPES OF OVARIAN CANCER DISCOVERED AT OPERATION

Tumor type	Incidence (%)
Serous borderline tumor	10–15
Serous carcinoma	25–35
Mucinous borderline tumor	5–10
Mucinous carcinoma	5–10
Endometrioid borderline tumor	1–2
Endometrioid carcinoma	15–20
Clear-cell carcinoma	4–6
Undifferentiated carcinoma and adenocarcinoma, otherwise unclassified	5–10
Dysgerminoma	1–2
Embryonal teratoma	1–2
Malignant tumor in dermoid cyst	1–2
Granulosa cell tumor	5–10
Metastatic cell tumor	4–8
Other	1–2

(From Scully RE: Hum Pathol 1:73, 1970)

TABLE 57-5. INITIAL SYMPTOMS OF PATIENTS WITH OVARIAN CARCINOMA

Symptom	Percent of Patients Reported by			
	Meigs	Kistner	Parker	DiSaia
Abdominal swelling	50	50.7	46	70
Abdominal discomfort	68	56.7	56	50
Gastrointestinal abnormality	—	16.3	—	20
Urinary abnormality	25–41	16.9	18	15
Abnormal bleeding	25–30	34.4	22	15
Weight loss	33–40		31	15
No symptoms			32	

TABLE 57–6. LOCATION OF METATASES NOTED AT OPERATION AND AUTOPSY IN 86 PATIENTS WITH OVARIAN CARCINOMA

Location	No. of patients	Percent
Peritoneum	75	87
Omentum	61	71
Opposite ovary	61	71
Uterus	16	19
Vagina	11	13
Lymph nodes		
Pelvic	69	80
Aortic	67	78
Mediastinal	43	50
Supraclavicular*		
Left	23	50
Right	21	46
Inguinal		
Left	37	43
Right	31	36
Axillary		
Left	25	29
Right	21	24
Pleura		
Left	25	29
Right	32	37
Lung	32	27
Liver	29	34
Bone	12	14
Spleen, kidney, adrenal, skin	5–7	6–8
Vulva, brain	1	1

* Examined in 46 cases only. (Bergman F: Acta Obstet Gynecol Scand 46:211, 1966)

patients with ascites. However, in patients with advanced or inoperable disease it may be helpful in establishing a tentative diagnosis.

Immunodiagnosis of ovarian malignancy is a field of intense investigation, but the techniques are not yet applicable for general clinical use. Much work is being done to improve the purity of the necessary antigens to the point where they can be used to detect subclinical disease and to evaluate the response to therapy. Sufficient progress is being made to suggest that these objectives will ultimately be met. An immediate objective would be the finding of a tumor marker in the serum or excreted in the urine; *carcinoembryonic antigen* (CEA) and *alpha fetoprotein* (AFP) may turn out to be of clinical value in this respect and to monitor progress after therapy. CEA is present in the serum of 35% of patients with ovarian cancer but not in the presence of benign tumors. AFP is present in amounts above 10 ng/ml of serum and ascitic fluid of patients with teratomas containing significant vitelline components (*e.g.*, endodermal sinus tumor), and in lesser amounts in some patients with epithelial ovarian cancer.

MANAGEMENT

In addition to the virulence of most ovarian cancers, two additional factors must be considered in planning therapy: 1) because the commonest method of spread of ovarian cancer is by the seeding of peritoneal surfaces from excrescences on the external aspect of the tumor, serosal implants widely distributed through the abdomen may be an early feature of even relatively small ovarian cancers: and 2) because the major lymphatic drainage from the ovaries is via the collecting trunks that extend upward with the utero-ovarian vessels and terminate in the para-aortic nodes at the level of the lower pole of the kidney, when the disease is diagnosed it may already have spread to a level above the pelvis. For these reasons, regardless of the apparent localization of a malignant ovarian tumor, one must consider the possibility that the disease has spread outside the pelvis and that peritoneal surfaces are involved.

The three accepted modalities for the treatment of ovarian cancer are surgery, radiation, and chemotherapy. Immunotherapy is also under investigation, but at present little is known of its efficacy. Of these, surgery must be regarded as the primary therapy. The others are used as supplementary or adjunctive therapies.

SURGERY

Surgery is always the first step in the treatment of ovarian cancer. It is essential for diagnosis of the disease and for determining the type and stage of the tumor; it is needed for histologic grading; if it is done early enough it may be curative; if it is done late in the disease it is essential for the removal of as much of the tumor as possible, since the outlook is related directly to the amount of tumor remaining in the abdomen after surgery. In addition, it is essential for the thorough and systematic exploration of the abdomen that is needed for formulating the subsequent treatment plan.

The *abdominal incision* should be of the midline type (not transverse) and should be large enough to permit both thorough exploration and intact removal of the entire tumor, if it is feasible.

Any *peritoneal fluid* encountered upon opening the peritoneal cavity should be aspirated and submitted for cytologic study. In the absence of peritoneal fluid, "4 washings" should be taken by lavaging the peritoneal surfaces with 100 ml of saline as follows: washings from the undersurface of the diaphragm are taken as one specimen; lateral to the ascending and descending colon as the second and third specimens; and the pelvic peritoneal surfaces as the fourth specimen. Peritoneal washings are of no interest if there is clear extension of the disease to peritoneal surfaces or to the omentum or if the entire tumor cannot be removed.

They are immensely valuable if the disease appears to be limited to the ovary, since knowledge of the presence or absence of cancer cells in the washings is of vital importance in the decisions regarding the desirablility and kind of postoperative therapy.

Whenever feasible, frozen-section diagnosis should be utilized early in the operation, since the extent of the procedure may depend upon it.

The *abdominal exploration* is extremely important, and to be thorough it usually requires use of a fiberoptic endoscope for visualization of the upper abdomen. One should visualize and palpate all peritoneal surfaces, including the underside of the diaphragm, the liver, the omentum, and the large and small bowel mesentery. Fatty streaks in the diaphragm should be noted especially, since this is the site of lymphatics that can harbor malignant cells. If the ovarian tumor is small, the exploration should be carried out before undertaking the pelvic operation; if the tumor is large the exploration may have to be deferred until it has been removed.

The *basic operation for ovarian carcinoma* is total abdominal hysterectomy, bilateral salpingo-oophorectomy, and omentectomy. With a few exceptions (see below) this therapy should be applied to all ovarian cancers. Two reports (Munnell and Parker *et al.*) have shown that the 5-year survival of patients with Stage I ovarian carcinoma is improved in those who had undergone omentectomy. Detection of microscopic metastases to the omentum even when obvious tumor involvement is absent also argues for removal of the omentum. When the omentum is grossly involved by disease, omentectomy is clearly indicated. If the omentum is not grossly involved, a biopsy should be done and the specimen examined. Hysterectomy is an integral part of the treatment, since the tumor may affect the uterus by direct extension, retograde lymphatic flow, serosal implants, or transtubal spread. The endometrium should be inspected for a second primary lesion. Bilateral salpingo-oophorectomy is almost always indicated to avoid missing an occult tumor and to prevent later development of a new tumor in the opposite ovary.

As much of the tumor as possible should be removed. Roughened or suspicious peritoneal surfaces should be removed for biopsy as needed. Adhesions should be excised, not incised, since they often contain microscopic disease.

Judgment is needed to determine how radical the surgery should be. Complete removal may require resection of portions of the bladder, colon, or loops of small intestine, and the wisdom of this must be weighed so as not to endanger the patient's life. There appears to be no place for pelvic exenteration in this disease and there is no evidence that radical hysterectomy or lymphadenectomy improves survival. However, a maximal surgical effort should be made to remove the entire tumor as well as obvious implants that may be accessible.

Surgical Options

As noted above, the first and basic therapy for ovarian cancer is removal of the adnexa, the uterus, and at least part of the omentum. However, exception to this rule can be made in three major circumstances:

Borderline Malignant Epithelial Neoplasms. Time has supported the concept of a group of ovarian neoplasms in which the histologic and biologic features are neither clearly benign nor obviously malignant. In 1973 FIGO classified these neoplasms as "borderline" or of low malignant potential. They comprise 15% of all epithelial ovarian neoplasms and formerly were designated as "proliferative cystomas." Although the 10-year survival rate is 95%, it is now recognized that they may have a very long latency period (up to 20 years) after which both recurrence and death have been reported. Accordingly, the preferable treatment for such tumors is to remove the uterus, both adnexa, and part of the omentum. However, if it is essential to preserve childbearing potential it is permissable in borderline epithelial tumors to perform a conservative procedure; but the patient must understand the possiblity of late recurrence and the need for long-term follow-up.

Malignant Germ Cell Tumors. Malignant germ cell tumors ordinarily occur in young women in whom conservatism is desirable unless there is compelling evidence that this is not appropriate (*e.g.*, bilateral disease, age over 35, no need to preserve childbearing potential). In some of the germ cell tumors unilateral salpingo-oophorectomy may suffice if the disease is limited to one ovary and if abdominal exploration and peritoneal washings are wholly negative. The dysgerminoma is the prototype for this kind of therapy, and there is ample precedent for its use. More recently this conservative therapy has also been used as primary treatment for such tumors as embryonal carcinoma, endodermal sinus tumor, immature teratoma, choriocarcinoma, and "anaplastic dysgerminoma" (a dysgerminoma showing marked anaplasia and pleomorphism and in excess of three mitotic figures per high-power field). Preliminary reports are enthusiastic, but more information is needed before accepting the propriety of conservativism in malignant germ-cell tumors other than the "pure" dysgerminoma.

In the dysgerminoma, adjunctive therapy (see below) is used only for recurrence; in the other malignant germ cell tumors chemotherapy is an essential part of treatment. In the latter group, removal of all gross tumor is desirable, but evidence is accumulating to the effects that 1) hysterectomy and removal of a normal-appearing contralateral ovary adds nothing to the survival rate, and 2) chemotherapy is essential regardless of whether the disease is limited to one ovary, and it may be curative even if peritoneal washings are

Hasleton PS, Kelehan P, Whittaker JS, et al: Benign and malignant struma ovarii. Arch Pathol Lab Med 102:180, 1978

Hertig AT, Gore H: Tumors of the Female Sex Organs, Part 3, Tumors of the Ovary and Fallopian Tube. Atlas of Tumor Pathology, Sect 9, Fasc 33. Washington DC, Armed Forces Institute of Pathology, 1961

`Hreshchyshyn MM, Park RC, Blessing JA, et al:** The role of adjuvant therapy in Stage I ovarian cancer. Am J Obstet Gynecol 138:139, 1980

Humphrey L, Panoussopoulos D, Volenec J, et al: Role of tumor immunity in ovarian cancer. S Med J 70:10, 1977

Izbicki RM, Baker LH, Samson MK, et al: 5-FU infusion and cyclophosphamide in the treatment of advanced ovarian cancer. Cancer Treat Rep 61:8, 1977

Jackson SM: Ovarian dysgerminoma. Br J Radiol 40:459, 1967

Jensen RD, Norris HJ: Epithelial tumors of the ovary. Arch Pathol 94:29, 1972

Joly DJ, Lilienfield AM, Diamond EL, et al: An epidemiologic study of the relationship of reproductive experience to cancer of the ovary. Am J Epidemiol 99:190, 1974

Julian CG, Goss J, Blanchard K, et al: Biologic behavior of primary ovarian malignancy. Obstet Gynecol 44:6, 1974

Julian CG, Inalsingh CHA, Burnett LS: Radioactive phosphorus and external radiation as an adjuvant to surgery for ovarian carcinoma. Obstet Gynecol 52:2, 1978

Julian CG, Woodruff JD: The biologic behavior of low-grade papillary serous carcinoma of the ovary. Obstet Gynecol 40:860, 1973

Kalpaktsoglou PK, Ioannidou GB, Kondyli AP, et al: Immunochemotherapy in adenocarcinoma of the ovary. Acta Obstet Gynecol Scand 57:85, 1978

Kardinal CG, Luce JK: Evaluation of a hexamethylmelamine and 5-fluorouracil combination in the treatment of the advanced ovarian carcinoma. Cancer Treat Rep 61:9,1977

Karlen JR, Akbari S, Cook WA: Dysgerminoma associated with pregnancy. Obstet Gynecol 53:330, 1979

Kjorstad KE, Welander C, Kolstad P: Preoperative irradiation in stage III carcinoma of the ovary. Acta Obstet Gynecol Scand 56:449, 1977

Klemi PJ, Gronroos M: Endometrioid carcinoma of the ovary. A clinicopathologic, histochemical, and electron microscopic study. Obstet Gynecol 53:572, 1979

Knauf S, Urbach GI: A study of ovarian cancer patients using a radioimmunoassay for human ovarian tumor-associated antigen OCA. Am J Obstet Gynecol 138:1222, 1980

Koller O, Gjonnaess H: Dysgerminoma of the ovary: A clinical report of 20 cases. Acta Obstet Gynecol Scand 43:268, 1964

Kolstad P, Davy M, Hoeg K: Individualized treatment of ovarian cancer. Am J Obstet Gynecol 128:617, 1977

Kolstad P, Davy M, Scheinert H: Individualized treatment of ovarian neoplasia. Carcinoma Ovary 73:1137, 1968

Kottmeier HL: Ovarian cancer with special regard to radiotherapy. Am J Roentgenol Radium Ther Nucl Med 111:417, 1971

Kottmeier HL (ed): Annual report on the Results of Treatment of Carcinoma of the Uterus, Vagina, and Ovary, Vol 15, International Federation of Gynaecology and Obstetrics, 1973

Kulpers, T: Report on treatment of cancer of the ovary. Br J Radiol 49:526, 1976

Laverty CRA, Brown JB, Fortune DW: Hormonal function of ovarian tumors. Contemp Ob/Gyn 5:77, 1975

Lele SB, Piver S, Barlow JJ: Chemotherapy in ovarian carcinoma recurrent after radiation therapy. Obstet Gynecol 51:1, 1978

Levi MM, Parshley MS, Mandl I: Antigenicity of papillary serous cystadenocarcinoma tissue culture cells. Am J Obstet Gynecol 102:433, 1968

Levin L, McHardy JE, Poulton TA, et al: Tumour-associated immunity and immunocompetence in ovarian cancer. Br J Obstet Gynaecol 83:393, 1976

Levin L, McHardy E, Poulton TA, et al: Tumour-associated immune responses and isolated carcinoembryonic antigen and alpha feto-protein levels related to survival in ovarian cancer patients. Br J Cancer 33:363, 1976

Lewis ACW, Davison BCC: Familial ovarian cancer. Lancet 2:235, 1969

Lewis GC, Blessing J: Ovarian cancer. Cancer 40:588, 1977

Li FP, Rapoport AH, Fraumeni JF, et al: Familial ovarian carcinoma. JAMA 214:1559, 1970

Li MC, Hsu KP: Combined therapy for ovarian carcinoma. Clin Obstet Gynecol 13:928, 1971

Lifshitz S, Newland WH, Dolan T, et al: Ovarian carcinoma presenting as a vaginal lesion. JAMA 239:17, 1978

Lokey JL, Baker JJ, Price NA, et al: Cisplatin, vinblastine, and bleomycin for endodermal sinus tumor of the ovary. Ann Intern Med 94, 56, 1981

Long ME, Taylor HC Jr: Endometrioid carcinoma of the ovary. Am J Obstet Gynecol 90:936, 1964

Lucraft HH: A review of thirty-three cases of ovarian dysgerminoma emphasizing the role of radiotherapy. Clin Radiol 30:585, 1979

Lynch HT, Albano W, Black L, et al: Familial excess of cancer of the ovary and other anatomic sites. JAMA 245:261, 1981

Lynch HT, Organ CH, Harris RE, et al: Familial cancer: Implications for surgical management of high-risk patients. Surgery 83:1, 1978

Malkasian GD, Symmonds RE: Solid malignant ovarian teratoma: Case of an 8-year survival. Am J Obstet Gynecol 110:1020, 1971

Markovits P, Bergiron C, Chauvel C: Lymphography in the staging, treatment planning, and surveillance of ovarian dysgerminomas. Am J Roentgen 128:835, 1977

McGowan L, Bunnag, B: The evaluation of therapy for ovarian cancer. Gynecol Oncol 4:375, 1976

McGowan L, Davis RH, Bunnag B: The biochemical diagnosis of ovarian cancer. Am J Obstet Gynecol 116:760, 1973

McGowan L, Stein DB, Miller W: Cul-de-sac aspiration for diagnostic cytologic study. Am J Obstet Gynecol 96:413, 1966

McKay DG: Origins of ovarian tumors. Clin Obstet Gynecol 5:1181, 1962

Meigs JV: Cancer of the ovary. Surg Gynecol Obstet 71:44, 1940

Meyer R: The pathology of some special ovarian tumors and their relation to sex characteristics. Am J Obstet Gynecol 22:697, 1931

Moore JG, Schifrin BS, Erez S: Ovarian tumors in infancy, childhood, and adolescence. Am J Obstet Gynecol 99:913, 1967

Morton DG: Ovarian carcinoma. Am J Obstet Gynecol 95:359, 1966

Munnell EW: The changing prognosis and treatment in cancer of the ovary. Am J Obstet Gynecol 100:790, 1968

Munnell EW: Is conservative therapy ever justified in stage I (IA) cancer of the ovary? Am J Obstet Gynecol 103:641, 1969

Munnell EW, Taylor HC Jr: Ovarian carcinoma: A review of 200 primary and 51 secondary cases. Am J Obstet Gynecol 58:943, 1949

Nelson JH, Urcuyo R: Pretreatment staging. Cancer 38:458, 1976

Barber HRK, Graber EA: The PMPO syndrome (post-menopausal palpable ovary syndrome). Obstet Gynecol 38:921, 1971

Barber HRK, Kwon T, Buterman I, et al: Current concepts in the management of ovarian cancer. J Repro Med 20:1, 1978

Barlow JJ, Piver MS: Methotrexate (NSC-740) with citrovorum factor (NSC-3590) rescue, alone and in combination with cyclophosphamide (NSC-26271), in ovarian cancer. Cancer Treat Rep 60:5, 1976

Barlow JJ, Piver MS: Single agent vs combination chemotherapy in the treatment of ovarian cancer. Obstet Gynecol 49:5, 1977

Bauermeister D: Diagnostic laparoscopy from the pathologist's viewpoint. J Reprod Med 18:5, 1977

Bergman F: Carcinoma of the ovary. Acta Obstet Gynecol Scand 45:211, 1966

Bolandgray A, Mehellati KA, Ardekang MS: Early detection of ovarian malignancy by culdocentesis. J Reprod Med 9:32, 1972

Boronow RC, Barber HRK, Cohen JC, et al: Immunologic diagnosis of ovarian cancers. Contemp Obstet Gynecol 4:53, 1974

Buchler DA, Kline JC, Davis HL, et al: Stage III ovarian carcinoma: Treatment and results. Therap Radiol 122:469, 1977

Buka NJ, MacFarlane KT: Malignant tumors of the ovary. Am J Obstet Gynecol 90:383, 1964

Burns BC, Rutledge FN, Smith JP, et al: Management of ovarian carcinoma: Surgery, irradiation, and chemotherapy. Am J Obstet Gynecol 98:374, 1967

Bush RS, Allt WEC, Beale FA, et al: Treatment of epithelial carcinoma of the ovary: Operation, irradiation, and chemotherapy. Am J Obstet Gynecol 127:692, 1977

Clark DGC, Hilaris BS, Ochoa M Jr, et al: Interdisciplinary approach to advanced ovarian cancer. Surg Clin North Am 54:897, 1974

Copenhaven EH, Abre-Rustun S: Management of primary carcinoma of the ovary. Surg Clin North Am 47:715, 1967

Curling OM, Potsides PN, Hudson CN: Malignant change in benign cystic teratoma of the ovary. Br J Obstet Gynaecol 86:399, 1979

Curry SL, Smith JP, Gallagher HS: Malignant teratoma of the ovary: Prognostic factors and treatment. Am J Obstet Gynecol 131:845, 1979

Creasman WT, Fetter, BF, Hammond CB, et al: Germ cell malignancies of the ovary. Obstet Gynecol 53:226, 1979

Danforth DN, Bird CC, Victor TA: Endodermal sinus tumor of the ovary. Obstet Gynecol 51:2, 1978

Daniels RJ: Granulosa-cell carcinoma of ovary. Proc R Soc Med 59:835, 1966

DePalo GM, De Lena M, Bonadonna G: Adriamycin versus adriamycin plus malphalan in advanced ovarian carcinoma. Cancer Treat Rep 61:3, 1977

DiSaia PJ, Morrow CP, Townsend DEL: Synopsis of Gynecologic Oncology. New York, Wiley, 1975

DiSaia PJ, Morrow CP, Haverback BJ, et al: Carcinoembryonic antigen in cancer of the female reproductive system. Cancer 39:2365, 1977

DiSaia PJ, Townsend D, Morrow CP: The rationale for less than radical treatment for gynecologic malignancy in early reproductive years. Obstet Gynecol Surv 29:9, 1974

Dockerty MB: Ovarian neoplasms: A collective review of the recent literature. Int Abstr Surg 81:179, 1945

Dockerty MB: Primary and secondary ovarian adenoacanthoma. Surg Gynecol Obstet 99:392, 1954

Doshi N, Tobon H: Primary clear-cell carcinoma of the ovary. Cancer 39:2658, 1977

Eastwood J: Mesonephroid (clear-cell) carcinoma of the ovary and endometrium. Cancer 41:1911, 1978

Edgehill AR, Gardiner J, Hayes JA: Mixed mesodermal tumor of the ovary. Am J Obstet Gynecol 97:578, 1967

Ein SH: Malignant ovarian tumors in children. J Pediatr Surg 8:539, 1973

Einhorn LH, Williams SD: The role of cis-platinum in solid-tumor therapy. N Engl J Med 300:298, 1979

Ellis H, Stoker TA: Second-look operation for ovarian dysgerminoma. Postgrad Med J 48:59, 1972

Felmus LB, Pedowitz P: Clinical malignancy of endocrine tumors of the ovary and dysgerminoma. Obstet Gynecol 29:344, 1967

Fenoglio CM, Richart RM: Tumor antigens: How can they be used? Contemp Ob/Gyn 16:141, 1980

Fisher RI, Young RC: Chemotherapy of ovarian cancer. Surg Clin N. Am 58:1, 1978

Frei E III: Effects of dose and response. In Holland, JF, Frei, E III, (eds): Cancer Medicine, pp 717–730. Philadelphia, Lea & Febiger, 1973

Frei E III, Lazarus H: Predictive tests for cancer chemotherapy. N Engl J Med 298: 1358, 1978

Friberg LG, Kullander S, Persijn JP, et al: On receptors for estrogens (E_2) and androgens (DHT) in human endometrial carcinoma and ovarian tumours. Acta Obstet Gynecol Scand 57:261, 1978

Frick G, Johnsson, JE, Landberg T, et al: Relaparotomy in advanced ovarian carcinoma. Acta Obstet Gynecol Scand 57:165, 1978

Fuller ME: Oral contraceptive therapy for differentiating ovarian cysts. Postgrad Med 50:143, 1971

Gallion H, Van Nagell JR, Powell DF, et al: Therapy of endodermal sinus tumor of the ovary. Am J Obstet Gynecol 135:447,1979

Gentil F, Junqueira AC (eds): Ovarian cancer. UICC Monograph Series, Vol 11 New York, Springer Verlag, 1968

Gibbs EK: Suggested prophylaxis for ovarian cancer. Am J Obstet Gynecol 111:756, 1971

Glatstein E, Fuks Z, Bagshaw M: Diaphragmatic treatment in ovarian carcinoma: A new radiotherapeutic technique. Int J Rad Oncol Biol Phys 2:357, 1977

Goldston WR, Johnston WW, Fetter BF, et al: Clincopathologic studies in feminizing tumors of the ovary. Am J Obstet Gynecol 112:422, 1972

Graham JB, Graham RM, Schueller DF: Preclinical detection of ovarian cancer. Cancer 17:1414, 1964

Graham RM, van Niekerk WA: Vaginal cytology in cancer of the ovary. Acta Cytol 6:496, 1962

Greene RR: Feminizing tumors of the ovary and carcinoma of the endometrium. Obstet Gynecol Ann p 393, 1973

Griffiths CT: Ovary and fallopian tube. In JF Holland, Frei E III (eds): Cancer Medicine, pp 1710–1720, Philadelphia, Lea & Febiger, 1973

Griffiths CT, Grogan RH, Hall TC: Advanced ovarian cancer: Primary treatment with surgery, radiotherapy, and chemotherapy. Cancer 29:1, 1972

Hadfield GJ: Urologic problems following treatment of ovarian carcinoma. Br J Urol 41:676, 1969

Hannemann JH: Radiation therapy in selected ovarian cancers. Rocky Mt Med J 69:57, 1972

Hart WR, Norris H Jr: Borderline and malignant mucinous tumors of the ovary: Histologic criteria and clinical behavior. Cancer 31:1037,1973

Hart WR: Ovarian epithelial tumors of borderline malignancy (carcinomas of low malignant potential). Human Pathol 8:5, 1977

Acute leukemia appears to be a rare but possible side-effect among long-term survivors who have been treated with either chemotherapy or radiation.

Immunotherapy

Studies are now in progress to determine whether immunologic intervention may have a place in the adjunctive treatment of ovarian cancer. The details of this relationship are discussed in Chapter 12. The immunotherapeutic agents that are now under clinical investigation include *Corynebacterium parvulum,* BCG, irradiated tumor cells, and neuramidase-treated tumor cells.

THE "SECOND-LOOK" OPERATION

The second-look operation is designed to evaluate the effect of radiation or chemotherapy when ovarian cancer has been diagnosed by prior laparotomy. It is applicable in two situations: 1) when a tumor found to be inoperable initially has, as a result of therapy, regressed sufficiently to suggest that operation may now be feasible; and 2) when, after 10 to 12 courses of chemotherapy, it seems useful to evaluate the effects of therapy so the treatment can be modified, if necessary, or discontinued if no cancer is found. When a second-look is decided upon, laparoscopy may be extremely helpful as a preliminary step. If tumor is found to be present and can be evaluated laparoscopically, laparotomy may not be needed. If no tumor can be seen by laparoscopy, then laparotomy is needed for the abdominal exploration that is required for the determination of cure.

MANAGEMENT OF THE PATIENT WITH ADVANCED OVARIAN CARCINOMA

The most difficult problem in the treatment of ovarian carcinoma is the management of the patient with advanced disease. Such a patient requires tremendous emotional support from the physician. The patient will tax to the utmost his ability to utilize the interdisciplinary approach of surgery, chemotherapy, and radiotherapy. The ultimate goal in the management of such a patient is to eradicate her disease. Though this goal may not be attainable, the prolongation of life for 1 or 2 years is worthwhile, if the quality of life is acceptable.

Probably the most common clinical problems in advanced disease are ascites and pleural effusion. When intractable and symptomatic, they should be treated aggressively by paracentesis or thoracocentesis, followed by chemotherapy or radiotherapy. For intractable pleural effusions, placement of chest tubes with sclerosing agents is helpful.

In recurrent ovarian carcinoma, intestinal obstruction is frequent and can be a major problem when complicated by the effects of radiation or chemotherapy. Usually it is best dealt with by conservative management in the form of intravenous administration of fluids, hyperalimentation, and nasogastric decompression. Surgery for recurrent disease should be limited to the simplest and quickest procedure that will contribute to palliation. Bowel is often involved by tumor to the extent that a clean resection cannot be accomplished, and after extensive resection the incidence of fistula formation is very high (34% has been reported). Therefore, a bypass procedure without any resection (*e.g.,* an ileotransverse colon side-to-side anastomosis or similar procedure) is preferred. A diverting colostomy or ileostomy is rarely helpful, but may be the treatment of choice if the involved intestines cannot easily be mobilized.

The point at which the physician must admit defeat and discontinue therapeutic attempts is difficult to determine. If a reasonable quality of life can be sustained, one must continue to combat the disease aggressively. The clinician may ultimately be faced with the question of whether he is prolonging life or prolonging agony. If indeed the latter is true, only conservative measures should be taken to make the patient as comfortable as possible. Finally, the physician must recognize that his most important responsibility is to relieve the pain that is so pronounced in the terminal phases of this disease. Measures for dealing with this problem are outlined in Chapter 52.

REFERENCES AND RECOMMENDED READING

MALIGNANT LESIONS OF THE OVARY

Abell MR, Halz F: Ovarian neoplasms in childhood and adolescence. II. Tumors of non-germ-cell origin. Am J Obstet Gynecol 93:850, 1965

Abell AR, Johnson VJ, Holz F: Ovarian neoplasms in childhood and adolescence. I. Tumors of germ cell origin. Am J Obstet Gynecol 92:1059, 1965

Acosta A, Kaplan AL, Kaufman RH: Gynecologic cancer in children. Am J Obstet Gynecol 112: 944, 1972

Allen MS, Hertig AT: Carcinoma of the ovary. Am J Obstet Gynecol 58:640, 1949

Anstey JT, Blythe JG: Fibrin degradation products and the diagnosis of ovarian carcinoma. Obstet Gynecol 52:605, 1978

Ashley DJB: Origin of teratomas. Cancer 32:390, 1973

Aure JC, Hoeg K, Kolstad P: Clinical and histologic studies of ovarian carcinoma. Obstet Gynecol 37:1, 1971

Averette HE, Hoskins WJ, Dudan RC, et al: Carcinoma of the ovary. In Nealon, TF Jr., Management of the Patient with Cancer. 2nd ed. (ed): Philadelphia, WB Saunders, 1976

Bagley CM, Robert CY, Canellos GP, et al: Treatment of ovarian carcinoma: Possibilities for progress. N Engl J Med 287:856, 1972

Barber HRK: Manual of Gynecologic Oncology. Philadelphia, JB Lippincott, 1980

Barber HRK, Graber EA: Managing ovarian tumors of childhood and adolescence. Contemp Obstet Gynecol 3:123, 1974

positive and there is evidence the disease has spread beyond the involved ovary.

Extensive Disease. In the presence of extensive disease, it may be technically impossible to cleanly remove the uterus, the adnexa, and the omentum. In such cases it is of first importance to obtain tissue for histologic diagnosis and to remove as much of the tumor as possible. This is termed *"debulking"* and is extemely important, since the effectiveness of adjuvant therapy varies inversely with the bulk of tumor remaining after surgery. The elegant term for this procedure is *"cytoreductive surgery."* In theory, the procedure removes large numbers of cells in the resting stage (G-0), causing the residual cells to be propelled into the more vulnerable pool of proliferating cells. Regardless of the exact explanation, the response to adjuvant therapy, and survival, correlate inversely with residual tumor volume. One's objective should be to leave no tumor masses larger than 1 to 2 cm in diameter. Among Stage III patients in whom residual tumor masses were 1 cm in diameter or less the M. D. Anderson Hospital and Tumor Institute reports 2-year survival of 70% and 5-year survival of 50%, results that cannot be matched if larger fragments of tumor are left behind.

ADJUNCTIVE (SUPPLEMENTARY) THERAPY

The accepted modalities for adjunctive therapy of malignant ovarian neoplasms are radiation and chemotherapy. There is much current interest in the possibility that immunotherapy may be beneficial as supplemental treatment for some forms of ovarian cancer, but the question is still unsettled.

The value of both radiation and chemotherapy is well established, but much remains to be learned about their limitations and the techniques that offer greatest benefit in given situations. As noted on page 1022, the massive study now being conducted by the Gynecologic Oncology Group (GOG) will ultimately provide answers to the questions of which adjunctive modality or combination of modalities or agents is most effective in what situations, in what dosages, and over what periods of time. In the meantime certain principles of adjunctive therapy have emerged, but the nuances and important variations of such therapy must await the results of these studies.

Radiation Therapy

The subject of radiation therapy in gynecologic cancer is discussed in Chapter 60. There are at least two kinds of ovarian cancer in which this therapy is recommended in preference to chemotherapy:

1. In Stage I disease the survival appears to be improved by the postoperative intraperitioneal instilla-

tion of radioactive phosphorus, P^{32}. This is a beta-emitter whose rays penetrate to a depth of not more than 1 to 2 mm. Its particular usefulness is the destruction of isolated malignant cells or cell aggregates that may be free in the abdominal cavity. Use of this device is facilitated by placing the end of a polyethylene tube in the cul de sac and bringing it through a stab wound in the flank at the time of the original surgery. P^{32} may also be used in Stage IIa, but it is not applicable if any gross disease remains in place after surgery.
2. Recurrent dysgerminoma is usually sensitive to external irradiation, and this is the treatment of choice for such lesions. The other germ cell tumors appear to be refractory to radiation.

Opinion is divided as to the effectiveness of radiation therapy as primary adjunctive treatment of ovarian cancer, and this is one of the questions that will be clarified as the GOG study unfolds. At present it does seem clear that some ovarian malignancies are more radiation-sensitive than other. Some have reported favorable results with surgery plus radiation in patients with Stage II disease confined to the pelvis but not surgically resectable, and in recurrence confined to the pelvis. One of the difficulties, of course, is determining if the disease is, in fact, confined to the pelvis; if there is extension outside the true pelvis, the results of radiotherapy are poor.

Chemotherapy

Chemotherapy has now become established as an important modality in the management of ovarian cancer. The optimal regimens for the different tumors have not been established, and this is one of the questions to which the GOG study is directed. One of the early answers to emerge from this study has to do with the rare and highly lethal germ cell tumors, in which experience with 39 patients is reported: radiation was found to have no virtue, and in unilateral disease the dismal outlook was not improved by removing more than the affected ovary. Of most interest, the VAC combination of vincristine, actimomycin D, and cyclophosphamide clearly improved the chance of survival.

It will not be possible to make specific recommendations of optimal chemotherapeutic regimens until the results of the study of large numbers of randomized patients are known. At present, the following general practices appear to be in use: 1) for patients with ovarian cancer Stages IA (ii), IB, IC, and II—an alkylating agent may be used after complete removal of the tumor, with or without the addition of radiotherapy; 2) for Stage III lesions: following surgical removal of as much of the tumor as possible chemotherapy in the form of either a single alkylator or combination chemotherapy; 3) for Stage IV lesions chemotherapy may be used as initial treatment with either a single alkylator or combination chemotherapy.

They are immensely valuable if the disease appears to be limited to the ovary, since knowledge of the presence or absence of cancer cells in the washings is of vital importance in the decisions regarding the desirablility and kind of postoperative therapy.

Whenever feasible, frozen-section diagnosis should be utilized early in the operation, since the extent of the procedure may depend upon it.

The *abdominal exploration* is extremely important, and to be thorough it usually requires use of a fiberoptic endoscope for visualization of the upper abdomen. One should visualize and palpate all peritoneal surfaces, including the underside of the diaphragm, the liver, the omentum, and the large and small bowel mesentery. Fatty streaks in the diaphragm should be noted especially, since this is the site of lymphatics that can harbor malignant cells. If the ovarian tumor is small, the exploration should be carried out before undertaking the pelvic operation; if the tumor is large the exploration may have to be deferred until it has been removed.

The *basic operation for ovarian carcinoma* is total abdominal hysterectomy, bilateral salpingo-oophorectomy, and omentectomy. With a few exceptions (see below) this therapy should be applied to all ovarian cancers. Two reports (Munnell and Parker *et al.*) have shown that the 5-year survival of patients with Stage I ovarian carcinoma is improved in those who had undergone omentectomy. Detection of microscopic metastases to the omentum even when obvious tumor involvement is absent also argues for removal of the omentum. When the omentum is grossly involved by disease, omentectomy is clearly indicated. If the omentum is not grossly involved, a biopsy should be done and the specimen examined. Hysterectomy is an integral part of the treatment, since the tumor may affect the uterus by direct extension, retograde lymphatic flow, serosal implants, or transtubal spread. The endometrium should be inspected for a second primary lesion. Bilateral salpingo-oophorectomy is almost always indicated to avoid missing an occult tumor and to prevent later development of a new tumor in the opposite ovary.

As much of the tumor as possible should be removed. Roughened or suspicious peritoneal surfaces should be removed for biopsy as needed. Adhesions should be excised, not incised, since they often contain microscopic disease.

Judgment is needed to determine how radical the surgery should be. Complete removal may require resection of portions of the bladder, colon, or loops of small intestine, and the wisdom of this must be weighed so as not to endanger the patient's life. There appears to be no place for pelvic exenteration in this disease and there is no evidence that radical hysterectomy or lymphadenectomy improves survival. However, a maximal surgical effort should be made to remove the entire tumor as well as obvious implants that may be accessible.

Surgical Options

As noted above, the first and basic therapy for ovarian cancer is removal of the adnexa, the uterus, and at least part of the omentum. However, exception to this rule can be made in three major circumstances:

Borderline Malignant Epithelial Neoplasms. Time has supported the concept of a group of ovarian neoplasms in which the histologic and biologic features are neither clearly benign nor obviously malignant. In 1973 FIGO classified these neoplasms as "borderline" or of low malignant potential. They comprise 15% of all epithelial ovarian neoplasms and formerly were designated as "proliferative cystomas." Although the 10-year survival rate is 95%, it is now recognized that they may have a very long latency period (up to 20 years) after which both recurrence and death have been reported. Accordingly, the preferable treatment for such tumors is to remove the uterus, both adnexa, and part of the omentum. However, if it is essential to preserve childbearing potential it is permissable in borderline epithelial tumors to perform a conservative procedure; but the patient must understand the possiblity of late recurrence and the need for long-term follow-up.

Malignant Germ Cell Tumors. Malignant germ cell tumors ordinarily occur in young women in whom conservatism is desirable unless there is compelling evidence that this is not appropriate (*e.g.*, bilateral disease, age over 35, no need to preserve childbearing potential). In some of the germ cell tumors unilateral salpingo-oophorectomy may suffice if the disease is limited to one ovary and if abdominal exploration and peritoneal washings are wholly negative. The dysgerminoma is the prototype for this kind of therapy, and there is ample precedent for its use. More recently this conservative therapy has also been used as primary treatment for such tumors as embryonal carcinoma, endodermal sinus tumor, immature teratoma, choriocarcinoma, and "anaplastic dysgerminoma" (a dysgerminoma showing marked anaplasia and pleomorphism and in excess of three mitotic figures per high-power field). Preliminary reports are enthusiastic, but more information is needed before accepting the propriety of conservativism in malignant germ-cell tumors other than the "pure" dysgerminoma.

In the dysgerminoma, adjunctive therapy (see below) is used only for recurrence; in the other malignant germ cell tumors chemotherapy is an essential part of treatment. In the latter group, removal of all gross tumor is desirable, but evidence is accumulating to the effects that 1) hysterectomy and removal of a normal-appearing contralateral ovary adds nothing to the survival rate, and 2) chemotherapy is essential regardless of whether the disease is limited to one ovary, and it may be curative even if peritoneal washings are

TABLE 57-6. LOCATION OF METATASES NOTED AT OPERA-TION AND AUTOPSY IN 86 PATIENTS WITH OVARIAN CARCINOMA

Location	No. of patients	Percent
Peritoneum	75	87
Omentum	61	71
Opposite ovary	61	71
Uterus	16	19
Vagina	11	13
Lymph nodes		
Pelvic	69	80
Aortic	67	78
Mediastinal	43	50
Supraclavicular*		
Left	23	50
Right	21	46
Inguinal		
Left	37	43
Right	31	36
Axillary		
Left	25	29
Right	21	24
Pleura		
Left	25	29
Right	32	37
Lung	32	27
Liver	29	34
Bone	12	14
Spleen, kidney, adrenal, skin	5–7	6–8
Vulva, brain	1	1

* Examined in 46 cases only. (Bergman F: Acta Obstet Gynecol Scand 46:211, 1966)

patients with ascites. However, in patients with advanced or inoperable disease it may be helpful in establishing a tentative diagnosis.

Immunodiagnosis of ovarian malignancy is a field of intense investigation, but the techniques are not yet applicable for general clinical use. Much work is being done to improve the purity of the necessary antigens to the point where they can be used to detect subclinical disease and to evaluate the response to therapy. Sufficient progress is being made to suggest that these objectives will ultimately be met. An immediate objective would be the finding of a tumor marker in the serum or excreted in the urine; *carcinoembryonic antigen* (CEA) and *alpha fetoprotein* (AFP) may turn out to be of clinical value in this respect and to monitor progress after therapy. CEA is present in the serum of 35% of patients with ovarian cancer but not in the presence of benign tumors. AFP is present in amounts above 10 ng/ml of serum and ascitic fluid of patients with teratomas containing significant vitelline components (*e.g.*, endodermal sinus tumor), and in lesser amounts in some patients with epithelial ovarian cancer.

MANAGEMENT

In addition to the virulence of most ovarian cancers, two additional factors must be considered in planning therapy: 1) because the commonest method of spread of ovarian cancer is by the seeding of peritoneal surfaces from excrescences on the external aspect of the tumor, serosal implants widely distributed through the abdomen may be an early feature of even relatively small ovarian cancers: and 2) because the major lymphatic drainage from the ovaries is via the collecting trunks that extend upward with the utero-ovarian vessels and terminate in the para-aortic nodes at the level of the lower pole of the kidney, when the disease is diagnosed it may already have spread to a level above the pelvis. For these reasons, regardless of the apparent localization of a malignant ovarian tumor, one must consider the possibility that the disease has spread outside the pelvis and that peritoneal surfaces are involved.

The three accepted modalities for the treatment of ovarian cancer are surgery, radiation, and chemotherapy. Immunotherapy is also under investigation, but at present little is known of its efficacy. Of these, surgery must be regarded as the primary therapy. The others are used as supplementary or adjunctive therapies.

SURGERY

Surgery is always the first step in the treatment of ovarian cancer. It is essential for diagnosis of the disease and for determining the type and stage of the tumor; it is needed for histologic grading; if it is done early enough it may be curative; if it is done late in the disease it is essential for the removal of as much of the tumor as possible, since the outlook is related directly to the amount of tumor remaining in the abdomen after surgery. In addition, it is essential for the thorough and systematic exploration of the abdomen that is needed for formulating the subsequent treatment plan.

The *abdominal incision* should be of the midline type (not transverse) and should be large enough to permit both thorough exploration and intact removal of the entire tumor, if it is feasible.

Any *peritoneal fluid* encountered upon opening the peritoneal cavity should be aspirated and submitted for cytologic study. In the absence of peritoneal fluid, "*4 washings*" should be taken by lavaging the peritoneal surfaces with 100 ml of saline as follows: washings from the undersurface of the diaphragm are taken as one specimen; lateral to the ascending and descending colon as the second and third specimens; and the pelvic peritoneal surfaces as the fourth specimen. Peritoneal washings are of no interest if there is clear extension of the disease to peritoneal surfaces or to the omentum or if the entire tumor cannot be removed.

Norris HJ, Chorlton IC: Functioning tumors of the ovary. Clin Obstet Gynecol 17:189, 1974

Norris HJ, Jensen RD: Relative frequency of ovarian neoplasms in children and adolescents. Cancer 30:713, 1972

Norris HJ, Taylor HB: Prognosis of granulosa theca tumors of the ovary. Cancer 21:255, 1968

Novak ER, Kutchmeshgi J, Mupas RS, et al: Feminizing gonadal stromal tumors: Analysis of the granulosa-theca cell tumors of the ovarian tumor registry. Obstet Gynecol 38:701, 1971

Novak ER, Woodruff JD: Novak's Gynecologic and Obstetric Pathology, 7th ed. Philadelphia, WB Saunders, 1974

Obel EB: A comparative study of patients with cancer of the ovary who have survived more or less than 10 years. Acta Obstet Gynecol Scand 55:429, 1976

Omura G, DiSaia P, Blessing J, et al: Chemotherapy for mustard-resistant ovarian adenocarcinoma: A randomized trial of CCNU and Methyl-CCNU. Cancer Treat Rep 61 (8), 1977

Ozols RF, Fisher RI, Anderson T, et al: Peritoneoscopy in the management of ovarian cancer. Am J Obstet Gynecol 140:611, 1981

Parker BR, Castellino RA, Fuks ZY, et al: The role of lymphangiography in patients with ovarian cancer. Cancer 34:100, 1974

Parker RT, Parker CH, Wilbanks GD: Cancer of the ovary: Survival studies based upon operative therapy, chemotherapy, and radiotherapy. Am J Obstet Gynecol 108:878, 1970

Parmley TH, Woodruff JD: The ovarian mesothelioma. Am J Obstet Gynecol 120:234, 1974

Pattillo RA: Immunotherapy and chemotherapy of gynecologic cancers. Am J Obstet Gynecol 124: (8), 808, 1975

Pezner RD, Stevens KR, Tong D, et al: Limited epithelial carcinoma of the ovary treated with curative intent by intraperitoneal instillation of radiocolloids. Cancer 42:2563, 1978

Piver MS: Reviews: Guidelines for the management of patients with ovarian adenocarcinoma. Obstet Gynecol 40:411, 1972

Piver MS, Barlow JJ, Bhattacharya M: Diagnosing, staging, and treating early ovarian carcinoma. Contemp Ob/Gyn, 14:33, 1979

Piver MS, Barlow JJ, Lele SB: Incidence of subclinical metastasis in stage I and II ovarian carcinoma. Obstet Gynecol 52: (1), 100, 1978

Piver MS, Lele FS, Barlow JJ: Preoperative and intraoperative evaluation in ovarian malignancy. Obstet Gynecol 48:312, 1976

Piver MS, Lele SB, Barlow JJ, et al: Second-look laparoscopy prior to proposed second-look laparotomy. Obstet Gynecol 55:571, 1980

Piver MS, Lopez RG, Zynos F, et al: The value of pre-therapy peritoneoscopy in localized ovarian cancer. Am J Obstet Gynecol 127 (3), 1977

Plentyl AA, Friedman EA: Lymphatics of the Female Genitalia: the Morphologic Basis of Oncologic Diagnosis and Therapy. Philadelphia, WB Saunders, 1971

Pollock, AV: The treatment of resistant malignant ascites by insertion of a peritoneao-atrial Holter valve. Br J Surg 62:104, 1975

Randall CL, Hall DW, Armenia CJ: Pathology in the preserved ovary after unilateral oophorectomy. Am J Obstet Gynecol 84:1233, 1962

Raventos A, Lewis GC, Chidiac J: Primary ovarian cancer: A twenty-five-year report. Am J Roentgenol Radium Ther Nucl Med 89:524, 1963

Roberts DK, Marshall RB, Wharton RB, et al: Ultrastructure of ovarian tumors. I. Papillary serous cystadenocarcinoma. Cancer 25:947, 1970

Rosenshein NB, Leichner PK, Vogelsang G: Radiocolloids in the treatment of ovarian cancer. Obstet Gynecol Surv 34:708, 1979

Schwartz PE, Smith JP: Second-look operations in ovarian cancer. Am J Obstet Gynecol 138:1124, 1980

Santesson L, Kottmeire HL: General classification of ovarian tumors in ovarian cancer. In Gentil F, Junqueira (eds): UICC Monograph Series, Vol 11. New York, Springer Verlag, 1968

Santesson L, Marrubini G: Clinical and pathological survy of ovarian embryonal carcinomas, including so-called "mesonephromas" (Schiller) or "mesoblastomas" (Teilum) treated at the Radiumhemmet. Acta Obstet Gynecol Scand 36:399, 1957

Schiller W: Mesonephroma ovarii. Am J Cancer 35:1, 1939

Scully, RE: Gonadoblastoma: A gonadal tumor related to the dysgerminoma (seminoma) and capable of sex hormone production. Cancer 6:455, 1953

Scully RE: Gonadoblastoma. Cancer 25:1340, 1970

Scully RE: Ovarian tumors. Am J Pathol 87:685, 1977

Scully RE: Ovarian tumors of germ cell origin. In Sturgis SH, Taymor ML (eds): Progress in Gynecology, Vol 5. New York, Grune & Stratton, 1970

Scully RE: Recent progress in ovarian cancer. Human Pathol 1:73, 1970

Scully RE: Tumors of the Ovary and Maldeveloped Gonads. Atlas of Tumor Pathology, Second Series, Fascicle 16. Washington, D.C., Armed Forces Institute of Pathology, 1979

Scully RE, Barlow JF: "Mesonephroma" of ovary: Tumor of müllerian nature related to the endometrioid carcinoma. Cancer 20:1405, 1967

Scully RE, Richardson GS, Barlow JF: The development of malignancy in endometriosis. Clin Obstet Gynecol 9:384, 1966

Silverberg E, Holleb AI: Cancer statistics 1974: World-wide epidemiology. CA 24:2, 1974

Silverberg E, Holleb AI: Major trends in cancer: 25-year survey. CA 24:2, 1974

Simmons RL, Sciarra JJ: Treatment of late recurrent granulosa cell tumors of the ovary. Surg Gynecol Obstet 124:65, 1967

Slayton RE, Hreshchyshyn MM, Silverberg SG, et al: Treatment of malignant ovarian germ cell tumors. Response to vincristine, dactinomycin, and cyclophosphamide. Cancer 48:390, 1978

Smith JP, Rutledge FN, Satow WW: Malignant gynecologic tumors in children: Current approaches to treatment. Am J Obstet Gynecol 116:261, 1973

Smith WG, Day TG, Smith JP: The use of laparoscopy to determine the results of chemotherapy for ovarian cancer. J Reprod Med 18 (5), 1977

Soloway I, Latour JPA, Young MHV: Krukenberg tumors of the ovary. Obstet Gynecol 8:636, 1956

Stewart RS, Woodard DE: Malignant ovarian hilus cell tumor. Arch Pathol 73:91, 1962

Stone M, Bagshawe KD, Kardana A, et al: Human chorionic gonadotrophin and carcino-embryonic antigen in the management of ovarian carcinoma. Br J Obstet Gynaecol 84:375, 1977

Symmonds RE, Tauxe WN: Gallium-67 scintigraphy of gynecologic tumors. Am J Obstet Gynecol 42:137, 1973

Talerman A, Van der Pompe WB, Haije WG, et al: Alpha-foetoprotein and carcinoembryonic antigen in germ cell neoplasms. Br J Cancer 35:288, 1977

Taylor HB: Functioning ovarian tumors and related conditions. Pathol Annu 1:127, 1966

Taylor HC Jr: Changing conceptions of ovarian tumors. Am J Obstet Gynecol 40:566, 1940

Teilum G: Special tumors of the ovary and testis and related extragonadal lesions: Comparative pathology and histological identification. Philadelphia, JB Lippincott, 1971

Tepper E, Sanfilippo LJ, Gray J, et al: Second-look surgery after radiation therapy for advanced stages of cancer of the ovary. Am J Roentgenol Radium Ther Nucl Med 112:755, 1971

Terz JJ, Barber HRK, Brunschwig A: Incidence of carcinoma in the retained ovary. Am J Surg 113:511, 1967

Thompson JP, Dockerty MB, Symmonds RE, Hayles AB: Ovarian and paraovarian tumors in infants and children. Am J Obstet Gynecol 97:1059, 1967

Tobias JS, Griffiths CT: Management of ovarian carcinoma: Current concept and future prospects (Part Two). N Engl J Med 294:877, 1976

Tweeddale DN, Pederson BL: Serous neoplasms of the ovary (with observations on related neoplasms) Am J Med Sci 701:113, 1965

Underwood PB: Ovarian Conservatism. S Med J 69 (4), 1976

Van Nagell JR, Donaldson ES, Gay EC, et al: Carcinoembryonic antigen in ovarian epithelial cystadenocarcinomas: The prognostic value of tumor and serial plasma determinations. Cancer 41:2335, 1978

Vogl SE, Greenwald E, Kaplan BH, et al: Ovarian cancer. Effective treatment after alkylating-agent failure. JAMA 241:1908, 1979

Wallach RC, Blinick G: The second-look operation for carcinoma of the ovary. Surg Gynecol Obstet 131:1085, 1970

Wangensteen OH, Lewis FJ, Tangen LA: The "second look" in cancer surgery. Lancet 71:303, 1951

Way S: Treatment of ovarian carcinoma. Proc Roy Soc Med 62:9, 1969

Way S: Malignant Disease of the Female Genital Tract, Philadelphia, Blakiston, 1951

Webb MJ, Decker DG, Mussey E, et al: Factors influencing survival in stage I ovarian cancer. Am J Obstet Gynecol 116:222, 1973

Weiss NS, Silverman DT: Laterality and prognosis in ovarian cancer. Obstet Gynecol 49 (4), 421, 1977

Weiss NS, Peterson AS: Racial variation in the incidence of ovarian cancer in the US. Am J of Epidemiol 107 (2), 1978

Welander C, Kjorstad KE, Kolstad P: Postoperative irradiation and chemotherapy in patients with advanced ovarian cancer. Acta Obstet Gynecol Scand 57, 1978

Wharton JT, Rutledge F, Smith JP, et al: Hexamethylmelamine: An evaluation of its role in the treatment of ovarian cancer. Am J Obstet Gynecol 133:833, 1979

White KC: Ovarian tumors in pregnancy: A private hospital ten-year survey. Am J Obstet Gynecol 116:544, 1973

Wider JA, O'Leary JA: Dysgerminoma: A clinical review. Obstet Gynecol 31:560, 1968

Williams TJ: Management of ovarian carcinoma in young women. Clin Obstet Gynecol 19:673, 1976

Williams TJ, Dockerty MB: Status of the contralateral ovary in encapsulated low-grade malignant tumors of the ovary. Surg Gynecol Obstet 143, 1976

Williams TJ, Symmonds RE, Litwak O: Management of unilateral and encapsulated ovarian cancer in young women. Gynecol Oncol 1:143, 1973

Williams TJ, Whitehouse JMA: Cis-platinum: a new anticancer agent. Br Med J 1:1689, 1979

Willis RA: A review of 500 consecutive cancer autopsies. Med J Aust 2:258, 1941

Winkelstein W, Sacks ST, Ernster VL, et al: Correlations of incidence rates for selected cancers in the nine areas of the third national cancer survey. Am J Epidemiol 105 (5), 1977

Wisniewski M, Deppisch LM: Solid teratomas of ovary. Cancer 32:440, 1973

Woodruff JD, Bie LS, Sherman RJ: Mucinous tumors of the ovary. Obstet Gynecol 16:699, 1960

Woodruff JD, Julian CG: Histologic grading and morphologic changes of significance in the treatment of semi-malignant and malignant ovarian tumors. Proc Nat'l Cancer Conf 6:346, 1970

Woodruff JD, Murphy YS, Bhaskar TN, et al: Metastatic ovarian tumors. Am J Obstet Gynecol 107:202, 1970

Woodruff JD, Noli Castillo RD, Novak ER: Lymphoma of the ovary: A study of 35 cases from the ovarian tumor registry of the American Gynecological Society. Am J Obstet Gynecol 85:912, 1963

Woodruff JD, Novak ER: Papillary serous tumors of the ovary. Am J Obstet Gynecol 67: 1112, 1954

Woodruff JD, Novak ER: The Krukenberg tumor: Study of 48 cases from the ovarian tumor registry. Obstet Gynecol 15:351, 1960

Woodruff JD, Protos P, Peterson WF: Ovarian teratomas: Relationship of histologic and oncogenic factors to prognosis. Am J Obstet Gynecol 102:702, 1968

Woodruff JD, Perry H, Genadry R, et al: Mucinous cystadenocarcinoma of the ovary. Obstet Gynecol 51:483, 1978

Young RD, Fisher R: The staging and treatment of epithelial ovarian cancer. Can Med Assoc J 119:249, 1978

ULTRASOUND

The principles and technology of ultrasonic imaging are outlined in Chapter 28. At present the principal uses of ultrasound in gynecology are 1) localization of palpable pelvic masses and 2) distinction between solid and cystic pelvic masses. Many ovarian masses are cystic or have cystic components, so that ultrasound is especially well adapted to displaying them. Exposure to ionizing radiation entails less risk for the average gynecologic patient, usually beyond the childbearing age, than for the pregnant patient; therefore, roentgenographic imaging techniques are employed more freely in gynecology than in obstetrics.

Ultrasonic diagnosis of pelvic masses can be difficult, but certain details of technique can reduce the difficulty considerably. It is important that the bladder be full. The examination should include both transverse and longitudinal scans. A special effort should be made to identify the relationship between an abnormal mass and the uterus. If the uterus is separate from an abnormal mass, the differential diagnosis is narrowed considerably. When a pelvic mass is detected, it is useful to review the intravenous urogram for evidence of hydronephrosis. If no urogram is available, it is a simple matter to examine the kidneys ultrasonically. Hydronephrosis in the presence of a pelvic mass suggests that the mass is malignant.

It is best if the person responsible for interpreting the study personally conducts part of the examination. An ultrasonic examination is like a fluoroscopic examination. Interpretation of the films without detailed knowledge of how they were obtained is possible but can be hazardous.

Overall, the purpose of an ultrasonic examination of the pelvis is to elucidate equivocal physical findings, to determine the size and location of mass lesions, to narrow the diagnostic possibilities, and occasionally to suggest that a mass is malignant.

ULTRASOUND, ROENTGENOGRAPHY, AND RADIONUCLIDE IMAGING IN GYNECOLOGIC DIAGNOSIS

Bruce D. Doust
Vivienne L. Doust

ULTRASONIC PROPERTIES OF PELVIC MASSES

Some pelvic masses have ultrasonic properties that are relatively specific, so that it is sometimes possible to predict the nature of a mass on the basis of its ultrasonic appearance. For instance, many dermoids have a powerfully echoing nodule within them (Fig. 58–1). However, there is considerable overlap in the appearances of pelvic masses, and it is often not possible to do more than offer a range of diagnostic possibilities.

Ultrasonic Diagnosis of Fibroids

Generally, a fibroid uterus is enlarged, has an irregular outline, and transmits sound poorly. Fibroids are commonly multiple. It is usually possible to demonstrate the continuity of a fibroid with the uterus, an observation that eliminates the ovary as the origin of the mass and so narrows the differential diagnosis considerably. However, a subserosal fibroid may be ultrasonically indistinguishable from a solid ovarian tumor.

Typically, there are generalized echoes within a fibroid. The characteristic swirl pattern of the smooth muscle fibers can sometimes be demonstrated ultrasonically. Between adjacent myomata echoing bands of tissue can sometimes be demonstrated (Fig. 58–2). There is a wide variation in the ultrasonic properties of fibroids, even in the same individual. Calcified or degenerated fibroids echo strongly, while some fibroids are almost echo-free. In pregnancy, fibroids often become more homogeneous than usual and may even be confused with a cystic lesion. After delivery, they revert to their usual appearance.

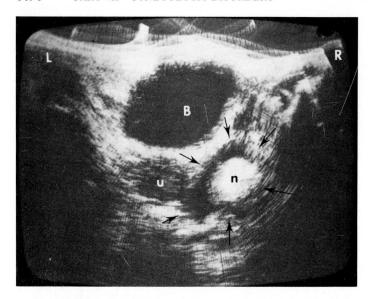

FIG. 58–1. Ovarian tumor (dermoid); gray-scale image. Transverse scan 1 cm above pubic symphysis shows large rounded lesion (*arrows*) containing strongly echoing mural nodule (*n*) surrounded by echo-free annulus representing fluid. Strength of echoes from mural nodule suggests calcification, which in turn suggests that lesion is a dermoid. (*u*, uterus; *B*, bladder)

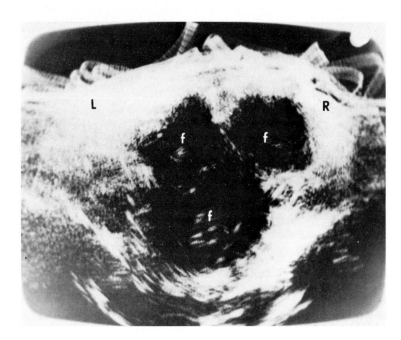

FIG. 58–2. Fibroid uterus; gray-scale image. Transverse scan is horizontal section taken cranial to bladder, about 6 cm above pubic symphysis. Anterior abdominal skin is at *top* of picture. Patient's right is at *right* of picture. There is a trilobed mass containing few echoes in central part of picture. This mass is composed of at least 3 fibroids (*f*), separated by bands of echoing material, probably representing compressed tissue.

Ultrasonic Diagnosis of Carcinoma of the Corpus Uteri

Uterine carcinoma may cause diffuse or localized uterine enlargement with poorly defined areas of diminished echogenicity. Extension of the tumor to the pelvic wall or floor can sometimes be detected; however, the changes are not specific, and ultrasound is not usually employed in the diagnosis or staging of uterine carcinoma.

Ultrasonic Diagnosis of Salpingitis and Tubo-ovarian Abscess

A tubo-ovarian abscess typically appears as a rounded mass with an echo-free center and well-defined wall, usually situated lateral to the uterus and posterolateral to the urinary bladder. Tubo-ovarian abscesses may also be seen in the midline, either cranial to the bladder or in the Pouch of Douglas. There is often some weakly echoing debris within a tubo-ovarian abscess.

FIG. 58-3. Bilateral pyosalpinx; gray-scale image. Transverse scan 1 cm above pubic symphysis. Patient's right at *right* side of picture. Bladder (*B*) is moderately distended. Behind and to left of uterus (*u*) is a sausage-shaped echo-free structure—the dilated, fluid-filled (*black*) left fallopian tube (*ft*). Right fallopian tube is also abnormally large, and is fluid filled. Shape of left tube distinguishes it from an ovarian cyst. Strong echo within uterus is due to menstrual blood in uterine cavity, suggesting that patient is not pregnant, thus eliminating diagnosis of ectopic pregnancy.

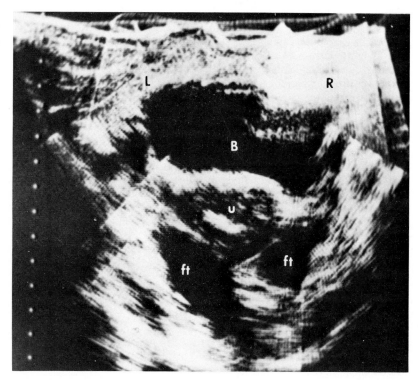

Not uncommonly, the masses are bilateral, and they can usually be demonstrated as separate from the uterus.

In patients with acute symptoms, the important differential diagnosis of salpingitis is tubal pregnancy (Fig. 58–3). In tubal pregnancy, the uterus is usually larger (although variations in the size of a normal uterus make this sign difficult to evaluate), and there are diffuse echoes arising from the decidual reaction. In salpingitis these internal echoes are less prominent. Occasionally, a clearly defined amniotic sac or even a fetus can be seen within a tubal pregnancy and, when this is the case, the diagnosis is obvious; however, the differential diagnosis is often difficult.

In patients without acute symptoms, the hydrosalpinx must be differentiated from an ovarian cyst, particularly a corpus luteum cyst, which may contain blood. Again, equivocal appearances are not rare.

Ultrasonic Diagnosis of Ovarian Cysts and Tumors

Small follicular cysts between 1 and 2 cm in diameter are often seen in asymptomatic patients (Fig. 58–4). They usually have a sharply defined, smooth wall and are unilocular and echo-free. They may be bilateral. In Stein–Leventhal syndrome, the cysts are generally numerous and may be too small to be resolved as separate cysts on ultrasonic examination.

Corpus luteum cysts with bleeding into the cavity may be considerably larger and sometimes show strongly echoing clot or solid material in the dependent portion of the cyst.

Pseudomucinous cystadenomas are typically septated cystic masses that may become very large.

Dermoids characteristically contain an area of very strongly echoing material. (see Fig. 58–1) Typically, an echo-free crescent of fat surrounds a strongly echoing mural nodule composed of hair and other solid elements.

Small ovarian cysts or tumors lie posterolateral to the uterus. Larger masses usually move medially and forward to lie on the urinary bladder; less commonly, they lie in the pouch of Douglas. If a mural nodule can be seen, the mass is more likely to be malignant (or a dermoid). Occasionally, cystic ovarian tumors become so large that they almost fill the abdomen and may be difficult to distinguish clinically from ascites. The ovarian tumor occupies the central part of the abdomen, which is, therefore, echo-free; the liver and bowel are displaced cranially and laterally. In the patient with ascites, on the other hand, the central portion of the abdomen contains loops of bowel and the echo-free ascites is situated in the flanks. If internal septa are seen, the diagnosis is even more certainly ovarian tumor.

The ultrasonic features that suggest malignancy are as follows:

1. Thickening or irregularity of the wall of a cystic lesion
2. Nodules or papillary masses arising from the wall or from septa within a cystic lesion
3. A complex or solid mass of ovarian origin, particularly in an older patient
4. Ascites
5. Hydronephrosis

Ultrasonic Diagnosis of Endometriosis

The ultrasonic appearances of endometriosis is quite variable. A chocolate cyst is usually regular, rounded, unilocular, and largely echo-free. It may contain varying amounts of debris due to the presence of altered blood. However, some endometriomata may appear as solid or complex adnexal masses with no distinctive ultrasonic properties. The clinical history may assist in diagnosis.

LOCALIZATION OF INTRAUTERINE CONTRACEPTIVE DEVICE BY ULTRASOUND

When the strings attached to an intrauterine contraceptive device cannot be seen protruding from the cervical os, suspicion arises that the device is no longer in the uterine cavity. It may be that the IUD is in place and the strings are within the uterus, or that the strings have separated from the device. Alternatively,

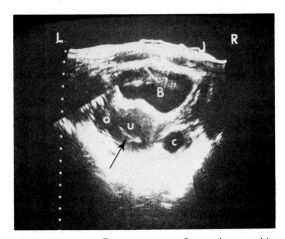

FIG. 58–4. Ovarian cyst. Transverse scan 5 cm above pubic symphysis. Patient's right is to left of picture. Uterus (*u*) is displaced a little to right and contains a strong linear echo (*arrow*) representing an intrauterine contraceptive device. To left of uterus is a small, sharply defined, echo-free area representing an ovarian cyst (*c*). Right ovary (*o*) is better seen than usual, but is normal. White area in superficial third of bladder (*B*) is an artefact caused by reverberation of sound to and fro between the anterior bladder wall and transducer face.

the device may have fallen out, may be outside the uterus, or maybe within the pelvic or abdominal cavity. IUDs are made of metal or plastic and can be readily identified both ultrasonically and roentgenographically.

Ultrasonic scanning allows identification of both the device and the uterus, so that the relation between the uterus and the device can be determined. A real-time scanner facilitates this task and can usually detect an IUD that has perforated the uterus and lies free. Plain radiographs do not show the outline of the uterus, so that the relationship of the device to the uterus may be difficult to determine.

Radiographic techniques for identifying the position of the uterus are more traumatic than ultrasonic procedures because they involve insertion of a second IUD, a sound, or hysterosalpinography. The possibility of physical or radiation damage to an unsuspected early pregnancy is a good reason for avoiding roentgenographic methods if an ultrasonic service is available.

Each type of IUD has a characteristic appearance on an ultrasonic scan. The ultrasonic display is laminagraphic, so that the images are actually cross sections of the device. For instance, a Lippes' loop appears as a series of short linear echoes arranged at regular intervals in a straight line. Each line or dot represents a cross section through one of the transverse bars of the device.

If ultrasonic examination fails to show an intrauterine device or a pregnancy, the most reasonable next step is a plain radiograph of the abdomen. This is more convenient and reliable than further searching for the IUD with ultrasound.

ULTRASONIC TIMING OF OVULATION

Artificial insemination with donor sperm is an increasingly popular means of achieving pregnancy in women whose husbands are infertile. To ensure that the procedure has the best possible chance of success, the semen must be introduced at or near the time of ovulation. Careful daily ultrasonic examinations around the time of ovulation can detect the ovarian follicle. The follicle appears as a small, well-defined, echo-free adnexal mass. Ovulation is accompanied by rupture of the follicle, which then disappears or alternatively develops strong echoes (due to clotted blood) within it. Use of this technique in conjunction with serial estimates of circulating hormone levels has been reported to increase the frequency of successful insemination.

ULTRASOUND AS AN ADJUNCT TO RADIATION THERAPY

An ultrasonic B-mode scan provides an undistorted outline of the abdominal wall, the kidneys, and some tumor masses and shows the depth of the tumor below

the skin surface. Serial ultrasound examinations can also be used to follow a tumor's response to therapy. These techniques have, for the most part, been superseded by computerized axial tomography (discussed later) which provides this information more simply, but ultrasound is still useful if computerized axial tomography is not available.

COMPARISON OF ULTRASONOGRAPHY WITH RADIOGRAPHIC MEANS OF IMAGING THE PELVIC CONTENTS

Ultrasonography is less traumatic, is free of radiation hazard, and provides more information than pelvic pneumography, a technique that has been largely superseded.

The relative value of ultrasonography and computed tomography (CT) in the evaluation of pelvic pathology is not yet settled; however, some generalizations are possible. Demonstration of the ovaries is easier and more often satisfactory by means of ultrasonography than by CT unless the patient is obese and there is much pelvic fat. Ultrasound does not expose the ovaries to radiation, a consideration that may be important in younger patients. CT allows estimation of the vascularity of a tumor and assessment of the extent of pelvic wall and lymph node involvement. Thus, it appears that ultrasound is more satisfactory as the initial means of diagnosing pelvic masses, but that CT is superior in assessing the extent of pelvic malignancy.

ULTRASONIC MAMMOGRAPHY

A palpable breast mass can be examined ultrasonically with a conventional contact scanner to determine whether the mass is solid or cystic. Cystic lesions can be evaluated by needle aspiration, so that patients who have cysts may be spared open biopsy. This form of ultrasonic examination has gained only limited acceptance due to the difficulty of performing contact scans of the breast. Breast tissue is mobile and it is almost impossible to keep the breast still during a contact scan.

Water-bath scanners have made ultrasonic survey examinations of the breast practical. A technique of scanning through a water-bath suspended over the breast, with the patient lying supine, has been used with some success in Japan, and appears satisfactory when the breasts are small. Another approach uses an automated water-bath scanner on which the patient lies prone with the breasts suspended in the water. Eight transducers are mounted on a motor-drive gantry at the bottom of the bath. The advantage of this technique is that the breast configuration remains constant throughout the examination, and compression of the breast tissue is avoided. Numerous scans in both longitudinal and transverse planes are performed. The technique requires more time and more specialized equipment than does x-ray mammography, but is free of any radiation hazard.

Indications

Ultrasonic mammography is useful in determining the nature of a palpable breast mass and possibly as a means of screening selected asymptomatic populations for breast cancer.

Concern for the potentially carcinogenic effects of exposure to x-rays during repeated routine x-ray mammography has prompted the search for other methods of examining the breasts, particularly for use in women under 40 years of age. Ultrasonic imaging is particularly suitable for use in younger women because the plentiful glandular tissue in the young breast (which can interfere with x-ray mammography) has little effect on the ultrasonic mammogram. Moreover, young women are likely to receive considerable radiation in the course of their lifetimes from repeated screening x-ray mammography, a hazard that is considerably reduced in older women. Accordingly, the major role of ultrasonic mammography will probably be for screening younger women and women with radiographically dense breasts. Its accuracy appears now to be comparable to that of conventional x-ray mammography.

Interpretation

The ductal and glandular pattern of the normal breast can be seen converging on a point immediately behind the nipple. Prominent ducts are tubular and conduct sound well. Glandular tissue is distributed fairly evenly throughout the breast in a lobular pattern and does not cause a sonic shadow.

Cysts, as seen in fibrocystic disease, are echo-free, have sharp walls, and conduct the sound extremely well, so that echoes from structures deep to the cyst are stronger than the echoes from similar structures underlying solid tissue.

Solid masses have internal echoes. Fibroadenomas usually have diffuse, moderately strong internal echoes, sharp, fairly well-defined borders, and conduct sound well. Benign solid lesions contain echoing material but may not be readily distinguishable from carcinomas.

Carcinomas vary in the strength of their internal echoes, have ragged margins, and conduct sound poorly. Typically, a carcinoma attenuates sound most markedly at its edges, so that the sonic shadow deep to a carcinoma is less dense beneath the middle of the lesion than at the edges. This phenomenon has been called the "tadpole" sign.

Unfortunately, there is no ultrasonic property that

specifically indicates malignancy, and ultrasonic examination must be used in conjunction with clinical evaluation. At the present state of our knowledge it is probably advisable that masses that cannot be positively categorized as cysts on ultrasonic examination be examined by x-ray mammography or biopsied, or at least pursued clinically.

ROENTGENOGRAPHY

PLAIN ROENTGENOGRAPHY

The most important contribution of plain roentgenography in the evaluation of gynecologic disease is the incidental identification of pelvic masses in the course of investigating other abnormalities. For instance, uterine myomas are often detected for the first time on intravenous urograms done in the course of evaluating a patient with hypertension (Fig. 58–5). A plain x-ray film of the abdomen in a patient with salpingitis may show dilated small bowel loops in the right or left lower quadrant—a manifestation of ileus due to localized peritonitis. When seen on the right, these roentgenographic appearances may suggest appendicitis.

There are a few conditions that have specific plain-film manifestations. Uterine myomas usually lie in the midline immediately cranial to the bladder and may be extensively calcified. Dermoids (ovarian teratomas) often contain teeth or tooth remnants that are densely calcified (Fig. 58–6). Many teratomas also contain large amounts of fat, which has a lower radiographic density than the remainder of the pelvic contents. Ascites causes bulging of the flanks and gives an overall hazy appearance to the abdominal x-ray film. The outlines of the liver, kidneys, and psoas muscles are lost because the fat that outlines them is obscured by fluid.

Fat planes may also be obscured by conditions other than ascites, *e.g.*, cachexia and retroperitoneal inflammation. On the other hand, anterior intraperitoneal masses such as large ovarian tumors do not obscure the outlines of the kidneys and the psoas muscles. This finding is occasionally useful when an ovarian mass is so large that it is difficult to distinguish it clinically from ascites.

Cystadenocarcinomas of the ovary may contain fine granular calcifications that may also be present in their peritoneal metastases. Widespread, fine intra-abdominal calcification is occasionally visible on a plain abdominal radiograph. Rarely, pseudomyxoma peritonei produces ringlike intra-abdominal calcification.

Plain x-ray films of the abdomen may also demonstrate spread of malignancy to the pelvis and vertebral column. Bony metastases characteristically appear as osteolytic lesions that are multiple and of several different sizes, with poorly defined margins. Most bony metastases are osteolytic; however, sclerotic metastases occur occasionally. The list of neoplasms that can cause osteosclerotic metastases varies from authority to authority, and one is left with the impression that almost any tumor can rarely produce a sclerotic metastasis. Carcinomas of the breast and bladder are probably the commonest sources of sclerotic metastases in the female, but it should be emphasized that in females osteolytic metastases are far more common than osteosclerotic metastases.

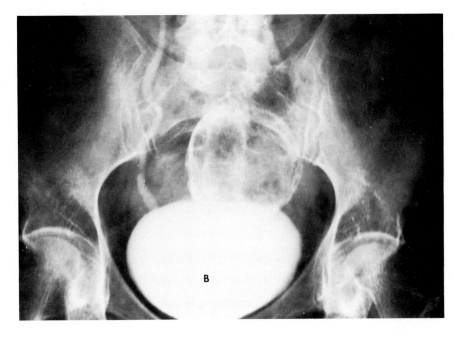

FIG. 58–5. AP film of pelvis taken as part of intravenous pyelography and showing uterine myoma. Bladder (*B*) and right ureter are opacified. A large, rounded, calcified myoma is immediately cranial to bladder.

Between 25% and 50% of the bone mineral must be lost before bone loss is recognizable on plain radiographs. Therefore, there can be extensive bony metastases that are not radiographically recognizable. Radionuclide bone scanning (p. 1188), particularly with methylene diphosphonate Tc 99m, is a much more sensitive index of metastatic bone involvement than plain roentgenography. Radiographic skeletal surveys performed in search of asymptomatic metastases are a waste of time if radionuclide bone scanning is available.

HYSTEROSALPINGOGRAPHY

In hysterosalpingography a radiopaque contrast agent is instilled through the cervix so that it fills the cervical canal and the body of the uterus; it then flows on through the fallopian tubes to spill into the peritoneal cavity.

Indications

Hysterosalpingography is used most commonly in the investigation of infertility in order to determine whether the infertility is caused by an anatomic, surgically remediable defect such as tubal occlusion. It is also used to determine the extent of the irregularity produced in the anterior uterine wall by previous cesarean section, to confirm that interruption of the fallopian tubes for elective sterilization has been successful, and to investigate the cause of dysmenorrhea, postmenopausal bleeding, or repeated abortion. The procedure itself may have a therapeutic effect on some hitherto infertile patients.

Contraindications

Hysterosalpingography should not be performed until at least 6 weeks after the end of a normal pregnancy, an abortion, or a dilatation and curettage procedure. It should also be avoided in patients with active pelvic inflammatory disease, vaginitis or cervicitis, or severe systemic illness that would make patient cooperation difficult or extravasation of contrast agent into the circulatory system particularly hazardous.

Technique

Preferably, the examination should be done around the time of ovulation when normally the sphincters are relaxed and it is easiest to fill the fallopian tubes. A mild sedative or an antispasmodic may be useful. The contrast agent may be either aqueous or oily. An oily contrast agent may leave a long-term residue if it spills into the peritoneal cavity. Because it is rapidly absorbed, an aqueous contrast agent leaves no residue if it spills into the peritoneal cavity. However, peritoneal

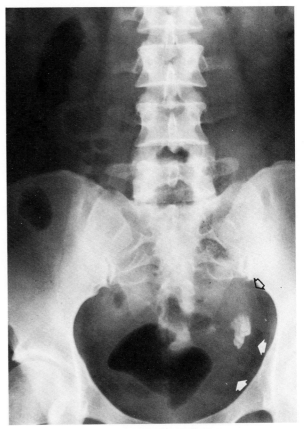

FIG. 58–6. AP film of pelvis showing soft-tissue mass in left side of pelvis, partly outlined by *arrows.* Within this mass are two well-formed teeth, making the diagnosis of ovarian dermoid virtually certain.

spillage of aqueous contrast agent may be painful. Theoretically, aqueous material is a little safer than oil if it extravasates into the uterine vasculature. Oily contrast medium allows follow-up examination 24 or 48 hours later to check for late spillage. This extra test for tubal patency cannot be done with aqueous medium because it is absorbed within the first 24 hours.

A preliminary plain film of the pelvic area should be taken to ensure that no contrast agent remains from a previous examination. The syringe and the cannula should be checked for patency and proper functioning. The cannula should have a soft rubber tip. All gas bubbles should be removed from the contrast agent, and the cannula and syringe should be entirely filled before the examination begins.

The examination should be done on a fluoroscopy table equipped with a spot-film device. A plastic rather than metallic speculum should be used, since metallic specula block the x-ray beam and may obscure important detail, particularly in the cervix. Contrast agent

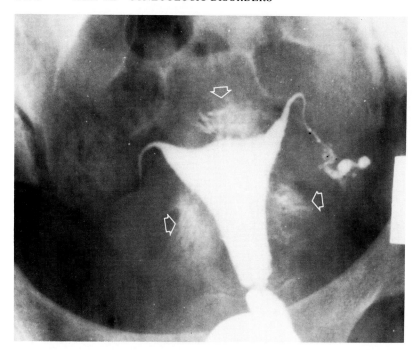

FIG. 58–7. Hysterosalpingogram showing tubal obstruction and extravasation of contrast agent into myometrium. Intramural contrast is present bilaterally and in fundus (*arrows*). Left fallopian tube is almost completely filled. Right tube is filled only in its juxtauterine part. Subsequent films showed no further filling of tubes and no evidence of spillage of contrast into peritoneal cavity.

should be injected slowly with gentle pressure, under fluoroscopic control. During injection, gentle caudal traction should be exerted on the tenaculum to maintain a seal between the cervical os and the cannula and to bring the body of the uterus into a position more nearly at a right angle to the x-ray beam. Failure to pull down on the uterus can give rise to unfamiliar, foreshortened images of the uterine cavity.

Spot films should be taken during the filling phase, lest intrauterine and cervical pathology be missed. Fluoroscopy during filling helps to detect extravasation of contrast agent (Fig. 58–7). Failure of the contrast agent to enter the fallopian tubes may be due to spasm of the intramural portion of the tube and calls for continuous gentle pressure on the syringe plunger, together with variation in the traction on the tenaculum. Once the uterus and fallopian tubes have been filled, anteroposterior and both oblique films should be taken. If the purpose of the examination is to evaluate the scar from the previous cesarean section or if the AP and oblique views are confusing, a lateral view of the uterus should be taken. After the examination, the patient should walk about for approximately 30 minutes; then, another AP film should be taken to distinguish between intraperitoneal (spilled) contrast and contrast in the distal portion of an obstructed fallopian tube. These conditions may appear similar early in the examination. If oily medium has been used and no spillage is seen, further films taken after 24 hours may be useful.

Interpretation

In cases of incompetent cervix the cervical canal may appear widened. Widening may not be obvious in the early films but becomes apparent only after injection of sufficient contrast agent to distend the cervical canal. Abnormalities of uterine position (*e.g.,* retroversion and lateral deviation) can readily be diagnosed. It is important to distinguish between a laterally deviated uterus and the single horn of a bicornuate uterus. The latter is, in general, smaller and more markedly deviated from the midline. Filling of a second horn or observation of a second cervical canal on direct examination through the speculum may also clarify the matter.

Arcuate and bicornuate uteri are gradations in the failure of the two müllerian systems to fuse. The fundus of the normal uterine cavity is convex, or only slightly concave (Fig. 58–8). In an arcuate uterus the fundus is indented caudally more than 1 cm. A bicornuate uterus represents a more severe failure of fusion. In a bicornuate uterus, indentation is deep, the angulation between the cornua is wide, and each horn is fusiform and convex on its lateral aspect. Since associated renal tract abnormalities are more common in a patient with a bicornuate uterus or other genital anomaly, intravenous urography should be considered as a follow-up investigation.

Hysterosalpingography also allows the identification of filling defects within the uterine cavity such as

polyps and subserous myomas. These filling defects may be difficult to differentiate from air bubbles in the contrast agent. Roentgenographic determination of the pathologic nature of the filling defect is less important than accurate identification of its site, so that subsequent curettage will be more likely to obtain tissue from the lesion.

Adenomyosis (endometrial tissue invading the uterine wall) may produce diverticular outpouchings along the borders of the uterine cavity and the fallopian tubes, occlusion or narrowing of the fallopian tubes, or generalized thickening of the uterine wall. The outpouchings resemble colonic diverticula, but are smaller and may be more spiculated. Aqueous contrast agent is said to demonstrate this condition better than oily medium.

The presence of intrauterine synechiae (adhesions) is known as the Asherman syndrome. These adhesions are caused by trauma such as repeated curettage, manual removal of the placenta, or intraluminal therapeutic radiation. The syndrome is characterized roentgenographically by irregular filling defects within the uterus which are not obliterated by increased amounts of contrast agent.

Abnormalities of the fallopian tubes are probably better examined by hysterosalpingography than by any other methods (Figs. 58–7, 58–9). Tubal patency is proven if contrast agent spills into the peritoneal cavity. Absence of spill can be due to incomplete filling of the tubes, as well as to tubal occlusion, so that a special effort should be made to fill the tubes during injection and to document on film the extent of filling achieved during the injection.

Delayed films are particularly important when tubal obstruction is suspected. If the tubes appear occluded, a repeat examination may be necessary after an antispasmodic has been given (to eliminate tubal spasm as the cause of occlusion).

Pyosalpinx (Fig. 58–9) is readily diagnosed by hysterosalpingography and is commonly associated with tubal obstruction. The tube enlarges and becomes irregular in caliber. Dilatation may be generalized or principally localized to one section of the tube.

Occasionally, hysterosalpingography is used to determine the position of an IUD. Usually, however, ultrasound investigation is more satisfactory for IUD localization.

INTRAVENOUS UROGRAPHY

In intravenous urography, the kidneys, pelvicalyceal systems, ureters, and bladder are opacified by the excretion of an intravenously administered, iodine-containing, water-soluble radiopaque material. This widely used examination depends for its success upon adequate renal function, *i.e.,* on the kidney's ability

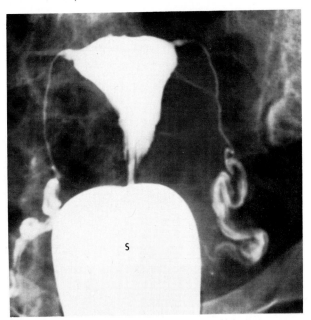

FIG. 58-8. Hysterosalpingogram showing normal uterus and tubes. Uterine cavity is of normal shape. Fundus extends slightly cranial to a line joining fallopian tubes. Fallopian tubes are patent and spillage of contrast agent into peritoneal cavity can be seen bilaterally. A metal speculum (S) has been used. A plastic speculum is more satisfactory because it does not block x-ray beam.

to concentrate the contrast agent. In general, it is not worth attempting intravenous urography if the patient's blood urea nigrogen is in excess of 100mg/100ml.

Before the examination, the bowel must be emptied; thus, purgatives and at least one cleansing enema must be given during the 24-hour period prior to the study. The patient should be mildly underhydrated by withholding fluids overnight in order to ensure a high concentration of contrast agent in the renal tract. The patient should void immediately before the examination to avoid diluting the contrast with residual bladder urine. The examination itself usually takes from 30 minutes to 1 hour.

Intravenous urography is associated with a small mortality (about one in every 20,000 examinations) and a significant morbidity. About one patient in 500 suffers a serious, nonfatal reaction to the injected contrast agent. Pretesting with a small dose of contrast agent is not helpful in preventing fatal reactions.

In gynecology, intravenous urography is particularly useful in assessing the patient with a pelvic mass or pelvic malignancy, or, occasionally, cystocele. Among other things, it allows for evaluation of the structure and function of each kidney, the patency of each ure-

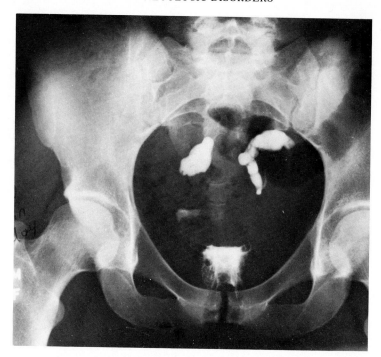

FIG. 58–9. Hysterosalpingogram showing bilateral pyosalpinx with no spillage of contrast agent. Film was taken 30 minutes after instillation of water-soluble contrast agent through cervix. In interval patient was ambulatory. Both fallopian tubes are dilated. There is no evidence of spillage of contrast into peritoneal cavity. Contrast in fallopian tubes may be mistaken at fluoroscopy for peritoneal spillage. A film taken at 30 minutes is of great assistance in avoiding this error.

ter, the degree of displacement of the ureters, and displacement and distortion of the bladder. The procedure is also helpful in the postoperative assessment of some of the complications of pelvic surgery. The ureters pass close to the uterine cervix and below the uterine artery. During hysterectomy, the ureter may be divided or obstructed by kinking or by a suture. A divided ureter is manifested on the urogram by contrast agent spilling from the cut end of the ureter into the retroperitoneum or peritoneal cavity. When postoperative urography shows evidence of ureteral obstruction (a dense nephrogram, poor, delayed excretion of contrast, hydronephrosis, and/or hydroureter), the study must be compared with the preoperative study to distinguish changes caused by the surgical procedure from those due to preexisting urinary tract disease. Thus, lack of a preoperative study may result in confusion. The urethra and the bladder can be demonstrated during intravenous urography if AP and lateral or oblique films are taken during voiding and the concentration of the contrast agent is high.

RETROGRADE PYELOGRAPHY

In retrograde pyelography a cystoscope is passed through the urethra into the bladder. Catheters are then passed through the cystoscope and into the ureteral orifices, a procedure that requires some experience and skill and which, in some cases, is impossible.

Each catheter is cautiously advanced up the ureter until the tip encounters obstruction or until it is in the renal pelvis. Small amounts of water-soluble contrast agent are then injected gently, preferably under fluoroscopic control, until the pelvicalyceal system and ureter are filled. AP films of the abdomen are then taken. After the ureteral catheter has been removed, it is sometimes useful to take films to assess the drainage of the contrast agent from the pelvicalyceal system. Retrograde pyelography is more traumatic than intravenous urography and usually provides less information. It is rarely needed for gynecologic diagnosis and is used most commonly when renal function is considerably reduced or when an intravenous urogram has failed to provide needed information.

BARIUM ENEMA

A barium enema is performed by introducing a tube into the rectum and allowing an aqueous suspension of barium sulfate to flow around the large bowel until it fills the appendix or refluxes into the terminal ileum. The barium enema is one of the safest and most useful radiologic examinations. It is the best initial examination for the detection of colonic lesions proximal to the rectum. Virtually all of the fecal material must be removed from the bowel prior to the study; purgatives and enemas must be administered prior to the examination and, therefore, preparation for a barium enema

is usually unpleasant, particularly for elderly, fragile patients.

In gynecologic diagnosis, barium enema examinations are valuable in demonstrating displacement of the rectosigmoid colon by an extrinsic mass, involvement of the colon by endometriosis or gynecologic cancer, and in demonstrating that a pelvic mass is colonic rather than gynecologic in origin.

Significant rectal lesions may not be demonstrable by barium enema. Digital examination and proctoscopy should be used to examine the rectum.

Since barium sulfate interferes with the transmission of ultrasound, it is preferable to schedule ultrasonic examinations prior to a barium examination.

RADIOGRAPHIC LOCALIZATION OF INTRACAVITY RADIATION SOURCES

Carcinoma of the cervix and uterine body is sometimes treated by placing radiation sources into the uterine cavity and the fornices of the vagina, as discussed in Chapter 60. The precise relation of these sources to each other and to the uterus must be known, so that the radiation dose to the tumor can be maximized without causing necrosis of the adjacent bladder and bowel. These relations can be determined by placing the radioactive sources in the uterine cavity and the lateral vaginal fornices, taking AP and lateral films, and calculating the geometry. Another method of ensuring correct placement is by positioning nonradioactive applicators in the uterine cavity and fornices and checking their positions before the radioactive material is inserted. AP and true lateral films of the pelvis are taken, and the tube–film distance is measured. After correction for magnification, the relationship of the containers to each other and to the pelvis can be measured from the films and adjusted if necessary. The radiation dose to all of the structures in the area (isodose curves) can then be predicted mathematically. When all of the dose calculations are complete and deemed satisfactory, the applicator is loaded and left in place until the required dose of radiation has been administered.

One would expect that intracavitary sources could be localized by computerized tomography. There are reports that a few centers use this technique, but as yet its use is not widespread. Metallic containers cause troublesome artefacts in computed tomographic images.

LYMPHANGIOGRAPHY

The treatment of carcinoma depends, among other things, upon how and to what extent the malignancy has spread. Involvement of the iliac and para-aortic lymphatics by carcinoma of the cervix or, less commonly, of the uterine body, and of inguinal nodes by carcinoma of the vulva, can be assessed by lymphangiography.

Technique

The skin on the dorsum of the feet and between the toes is cleaned and a small amount of a strongly colored dye, such as Evans blue, is injected subcutaneously into one or more web spaces of each foot. The dye is taken up by the lymphatics so that after about 30 minutes they can be seen through the skin. A large lymphatic on the dorsum of each foot is then selected and exposed through a small skin incision. A fine 27- or 30-gauge, specially designed lymphography needle is then introduced into the lymphatic and tied in place. Oily contrast agent is injected slowly over a period of about 1 hour.

The contrast agent passes up the lymphatic channels and fills successively the inguinal, external iliac, common iliac, and para-aortic nodes; the internal iliac nodes do not fill. Excess contrast passes into the cisterna chyli and, by way of the thoracic duct, to the left subclavian vein. It then passes into the lungs to produce innumerable minute oil emboli.

Plain radiographs of the abdomen are taken during the injection, and injection is continued until opacification has progressed well up the para-aortic lymph node chains or until a maximum of 8 ml of contrast agent has been injected into each foot. Films are then taken in the AP and both oblique projections. Occasionally, fluoroscopic spot films, tomography, and magnification views are helpful. Further films are taken 24 hours after injection.

Precautions

Occasionally, an inexperienced operator mistakes a vein for a lymphatic; a film of the leg can be used to confirm lymphatic filling. In a patient with a strong allergic history of asthma or eczema, or a previous adverse reaction to intravenous contrast agent, the necessity for and advisability of the study should be carefully considered before administering the contrast agent. In a patient with serious pulmonary disease, the volume of contrast agent should be kept to the minimum consistent with an adequate study. The abdominal lymphatics should be monitored by abdominal radiographs and the injection should be suspended before excess contrast agent passes into the thoracic duct. In general, oil embolus due to excess oily contrast agent has no clinically recognizable adverse effects. However, in a patient with serious lung disease, cardiorespiratory difficulty may develop, probably due to embolic blockade of the pulmonary capillary bed. The possibility of oil embolus to the systemic circula-

tion in patients with right-to-left shunts makes lymphangiography more than usually hazardous for them. Occasional deaths have been attributed to the procedure.

Interpretation

In the normal person, during the filling phase, contrast agent can be seen in several lymphatic channels, which usually have a beaded appearance. The inguinal lymph nodes are commonly enlarged, have irregular outlines, and often show some filling defects. These findings do not suggest malignancy when seen in the inguinal nodes, but are probably the result of repeated inflammation from minor infections of the feet and toes. This irregularity is particularly troublesome in assessing the spread of carcinoma of the vulva. The external and common iliac and the para-aortic nodes are much more regular. They have smooth, oval outlines and generally are free from defects. In older patients, there may be small defects caused by fatty deposits within the nodes. These defects do not represent ma-

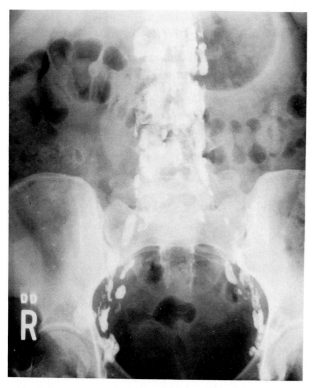

FIG. 58–10. Lymphangiogram showing normal node chains— AP film taken 24 hours after injection of contrast into lymphatics of both feet. Lymph node chains are symmetric. Para-aortic node chains have filled up to the level of L1. Minor irregularities of nodes of both external iliac chains are within normal limits.

lignancy. Provided the injections in both feet have been technically satisfactory, the lymph node chains on either side of the midline should be nearly symmetric. Filling of lymph nodes should proceed through the level of the upper lumbar spine on both sides (Fig. 58–10). The internal iliac nodes do not fill.

A metastatic deposit within a lymph node characteristically appears as a sharply demarcated, peripherally located filling defect within the node (Fig. 58–11). The lymph node looks as if a bite has been taken out of its edge. Extensive metastatic involvement may result in total obstruction of lymph flow through the node. Then, comparison with the contralateral node chain shows asymmetry, and unusual collateral lymph channels fill with contrast. Also, contrast material in the lymph vessels in the 24-hour film (Fig. 58–11) suggests obstruction and, therefore, metastatic involvement. Lymph nodes that do not fill must be assumed to be involved by malignancy.

Lymphangiography may be used to follow the effects of drug or radiation therapy. Normally the pelvic lymph nodes are bigger than the para-aortic nodes. After radiation therapy to the pelvis, this relation is reversed. Follow-up studies may not require further injection of contrast agent, since contrast clears from the lymph nodes slowly (over several months).

Probably the most common reason for performing lymphangiography is to assess the extent of lymphoma. Lymphomatous nodes are diffusely enlarged, have a foamy appearance, are not obstructed, and do not have peripheral filling defects.

Limitations

The principal limitation of lymphangiography in assessing metastatic spread of carcinoma is that the injection technique cannot fill all nodes draining the primary tumor. Most notable is the failure to fill the internal iliac chain, a group of nodes likely to be involved early by metastatic pelvic malignancy. The nodes in the upper abdomen are usually not completely filled and mesenteric nodes do not fill. Also, microscopic involvement of lymph nodes may be clinically significant but undetectable by lymphangiography. Therefore, lymphangiography generally underestimates the degree of metastatic involvement of the lymphatic system.

Computed tomography can also be used to assess the abdominal and pelvic lymph nodes. It is generally complementary to lymphangiography, being especially useful in showing pelvic, mesenteric, and upper abdominal nodes. Computed tomography does not demonstrate lymph node involvement unless the nodes are enlarged and does not differentiate between benign and malignant causes of enlargement, so that in some respects it is inferior to lymphangiography.

COMPUTED TOMOGRAPHY

Computed tomography (CT) is a radiographic technique for obtaining cross-sectional images of the body. It has caused much interest, concern, and dispute in recent years because it is a powerful and atraumatic diagnostic tool, but requires equipment that is at present very expensive. A detailed description of the technology of CT is beyond the scope of this account. However, a brief outline of principles is appropriate.

If an x-ray tube is covered with a lead shield in which a narrow slit has been cut, one obtains a thin, fan-shaped beam of x-rays. If this tube is used to take a conventional radiograph, a slitlike picture of a slice of tissue is obtained. The amount of blackening at each point on the x-ray film depends upon the amount of tissue through which the x-ray beam passed on its way from the x-ray tube to the film and the degree to which the x-ray beam is attenuated by each piece of tissue.

If the strip of film is replaced by a row of electronic x-ray detectors and each detector responds to the x-rays that strike it by producing an electrical signal, then the electrical signals from each detector represent the sum of the densities of all of the structures through which the x-ray beam passed on its way to that detector. If an x-ray tube and the detectors are mounted on opposite sides of a circular gantry so that they both travel in a circle around the patient, then numerous, very short x-ray exposures can be made as the x-ray tube and detectors rotate. All of the electronic signals generated by these multiple x-ray exposures, together with signals representing the position of the gantry at the time of each exposure, are stored in a computer memory.

This colossal mass of raw electronic data is then processed mathematically. The object of the processing is to determine the attenuation coefficient of each tissue element in the body section under examination. It is possible to do this because every structure in the slice of tissue is inspected from many angles as the gantry rotates, so that each tissue element makes a contribution to several hundred detector readings.

The problem is further complicated because calculations are also required to allow for overlapping and incomplete sampling of tissue elements, to locate each element in its proper position in the image, to compensate for unevenness of x-ray output and instability in the x-ray detectors, to improve resolution, to eliminate artefacts, and so forth. The algorithms (programs of mathematic manipulation) that are used to accomplish all of these operations have been the subject of intense research by the manufacturers of CT equipment, and striking improvements in image quality and speed of reconstruction have been achieved by refinement of the algorithms. The latest CT scanners complete the radiographic exposure in less than 5 seconds

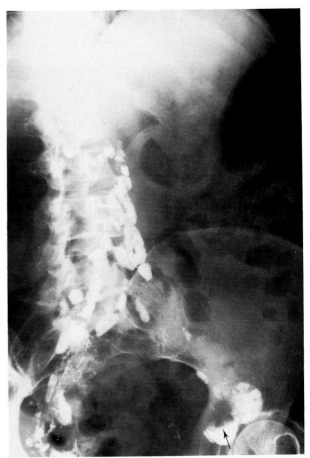

FIG. 58–11. Lymphangiogram showing lymphatic spread of carcinoma of uterus—Oblique film taken 24 hours after injection. Note large, sharply marginated filling defect in left external iliac node (*thin black arrow*). Almost no filling of left common iliac chain has occurred, suggesting extensive involvement by metastatic malignancy. Contrast agent can be seen in the right common iliac lymphatic vessels (*open arrow*). This is abnormal in a 24-hour film and suggests obstruction by metastatic involvement.

and perform all of the required calculations in about 45 seconds.

The principal advantages of CT over other forms of radiographic examination are as follows:

1. The procedure is noninvasive.
2. Much anatomic detail can be demonstrated even without the use of contrast agents. The intrinsic differences in radiographic density between fat and other body tissues are enough to allow clear demonstration of most structures. (In patients who have little fat, CT images are less satisfactory.) Intrave-

nous administration of contrast agent allows vessels to be positively identified and tumor vascularity to be assessed. Rectal and oral contrast aid in distinguishing bowel from other pelvic organs. In many examinations, the patient receives contrast by all three of the above routes.

3. The display is in the form of a cross section through the body, a format that shows anatomic relationships that might otherwise be obscure.

4. The contrast and the density of the image can be manipulated after the examination has been completed, without further radiation to the patient.

5. The radiographic density of organs or masses can be estimated. These density values are sometimes helpful in determining the nature of the structure being examined.

6. The examination is unaffected by bowel gas, colostomies, and surgical dressings; however, metallic clips do cause troublesome artefacts.

Comparison of Computed with Conventional Tomography

In a conventional tomogram the shadows of all of the tissues through which the x-rays pass are recorded on the film. The shadows of structures above and below the plane of interest are blurred and spread evenly over the film so that they are less obtrusive, but they are not eliminated. Thus, a conventional tomogram appears gray, and the contrast between the structures of interest and the background is low; very little can be done to change this. On the other hand, in a computed tomogram there are no background shadows, and contrast and overall density can be manipulated at will.

Computed Radiographs

In addition to producing cross-sectional images, modern CT scanners can produce pictures that resemble conventional radiographs. To do this, the x-ray tube and the detectors remain stationary while the patient is moved through the x-ray beam on a motor-driven table, while numerous exposures are made. If the x-ray tube is in front and the detectors behind the patient, an AP view results. If the x-ray tube and the detectors are positioned on either side of the patient, a lateral view is produced. At present, computed radiographs are generally inferior to those produced conventionally. They are valuable for determining the levels at which CT sections should be performed to ensure a complete examination of an organ or region, so that extremely accurate planning and rapid performance of each computed tomographic study is possible. The technique promises to provide additional diagnostic information in its own right because computer techniques can be used to manipulate the image and so render subtle abnormalities more readily visible. However, these applications are still experimental.

Applications of Computed Tomography in Gynecologic Diagnosis

CT is primarily useful to the gynecologist for 1) demonstrating the nature and extent of pelvic masses, 2) examining the pelvic and para-aortic lymph node chains as part of the examination for metastatic deposits from gynecologic cancer, and 3) examining liver, lungs, and brain for metastases.

Pelvic Masses. CT allows demonstration of the mass itself, the relationship of the mass to loops of bowel and to the bladder and ureters, and the extent of tumor invasion of the pelvic wall (Fig. 58–12). It does not demonstrate mucosal involvement of the bowel as well or as inexpensively as the barium enema examination and appears inferior to ultrasound in the delineation of normal ovaries and small ovarian cysts. It is the best method available for demonstrating soft-tissue infiltration. It is probably less sensitive than the radionuclide bone scan (p. 1188) in the detection of early bone involvement. It seems to be particularly valuable in demonstrating invasion of the tissue planes around the urinary bladder by bladder or uterine cancer, and for evaluating the tumor response to therapy (Fig. 58–13).

Detection of Lymph Node Metastases. CT has proved useful in demonstrating the internal iliac lymph node chain, the para-aortic nodes of the upper abdomen, particularly those above the cisterna chyli, and the mesenteric nodes, areas that are not usually opacified by lymphangiography, and also demonstrates lymph node enlargement without the need for added contrast. It is common for abnormal nodes that are not opacified during lymphangiography to be demonstrated by CT. Unfortunately, CT also has its limitations, since metastases that do not enlarge the lymph node are undetectable by this technique. Microscopic metastases, although clinically of great significance, are not detectable by either method.

Detection of Metastases Elsewhere in the Body. The radiographic density of metastases is usually different from that of the normal tissue that surrounds them. This difference in density can often, but not always, be enhanced by intravenous infusion of contrast agent. In the case of liver metastases, intravenous contrast usually increases the radiographic density of the normal parenchyma, so that the normal tissue becomes more dense than the metastases.

Hepatic metastases are probably better sought by CT than by any other method; radionuclide scans and ultrasound are the only other atraumatic methods, but they appear to be less sensitive. There are, of course, isolated instances in which the ultrasound or radionuclide scan is superior. CT is the best means of seeking cerebral metastases. Pulmonary metastases may be resected if it is probable that all of them can be re-

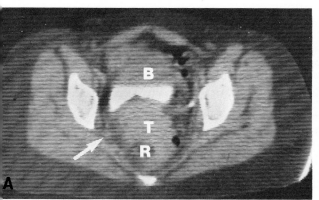
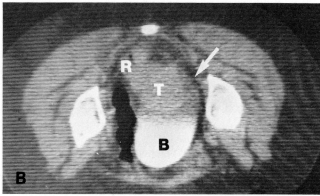

FIG. 58–12. Computed tomogram, recurrent carcinoma of cervix, patient supine. *A.* Recurrent tumor (*T*) indents posterior wall of bladder (*B*) and surrounds anterior and left side of rectum (*R*). Linear strands of tumor are attached to right pelvic sidewall (*arrow*). *B.* Prone scan. Tumor (*T*) protudes into bladder (*B*) and is fixed to rectum (*R*) and pelvic sidewall. Cystoscopy, sigmoidoscopy, and laparotomy confirmed findings. (Walsh JW, Amendola MA, Hall DJ, et al: Am J Roentgenol 136:117, 1981)

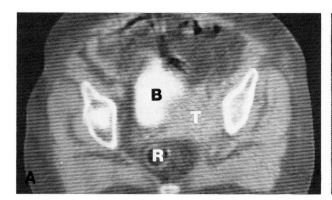
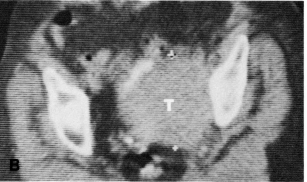

FIG. 58–13. Computed tomogram, recurrent carcinoma of cervix. *A.* Recurrent tumor (*T*) between bladder (*B*) and rectum (*R*) attached to left pelvic sidewall with loss of all fat planes. *B.* Follow-up scan 7 months after *cis*-platinum chemotherapy. Massive enlargement of tumor (*T*). (Walsh JW, Amendola MA, Hall DJ, et al: Am J Roentgenol 136:117, 1981)

moved and there are no other deposits. Customarily the patient is examined initially by means of plain films and conventional laminograms, because these methods of examination are less expensive; if x-ray demonstrates no lesions that would make resection impractical, CT is used as a final check.

Computerized Emission Tomography

The principles of CT can be adapted to make a two-dimensional image showing the distribution of a radionuclide within the body. In this case, the source of radiation is the radionuclide rather than an x-ray tube.

It is hoped that this technique will enhance the quality of images obtainable with radionuclides, but at present the technique is still being developed.

ANGIOGRAPHY

Arteriography is used in gynecology to demonstrate the blood supply to a pelvic mass as an aid in planning the surgical approach to the lesion. It may also be used to assess the spread of malignancy to the pelvic wall

and to demonstrate vascular metastases to the liver. Avascular metastases, even if very large, may produce little change in the hepatic arteriogram.

When a patient is bleeding intractably from a pelvic malignancy, arteriography may be used to determine the site of bleeding. The arteries supplying the bleeding area can then be selectively catherized and small pieces of solid material injected through the catheter so that the artery is obstructed and the bleeding stopped. Autologous clot, gelfoam, and small spiral fragments of stainless steel wire to which wool fibers have been attached (to promote thrombosis) have been described as embolizing agents. This technique can also be used to infarct inoperable vascular tumors or to reduce tumor vascularity prior to surgical resection.

Venography may be used to determine whether malignancy has spread to the iliac veins and inferior vena cava.

GENITOGRAPHY

In genitography, the contrast agent is injected into all of the perineal openings so that the internal genital passages are displayed. This technique is sometimes helpful in assigning sex in cases of ambiguous external genitalia.

BEAD CHAIN CYSTOURETHROGRAPHY

As discussed in Chapter 49, the ability of the bladder to retain urine depends upon a number of factors, including the competence of the urethral sphincters and the angle between the urethra and the base of the bladder (posterior urethrovesical angle). If the information is needed, bead chain cystourethrography can be used to measure the length of the urethra, the angle between the line of the urethra and the vertical plane, and the posterior urethrovesical angle.

THERMOGRAPHY

Thermography has been used extensively in an effort to detect breast lesions. A thermogram is a picture of the infrared radiation (the heat) coming from any part of the body. Thermograms may be obtained with an infrared camera or by bringing a sheet containing liquid crystals into contact with the breast. (The color of a liquid crystal depends upon its temperature.) The infrared camera produces an image in which the hottest parts of the breast appear black and the coldest parts appear white (or vice versa). Cameras producing color displays are also available, each 1° C-interval being displayed as a separate color.

Technique

The patient is placed in a draft-free room in which the temperature is about 20° C. All clothing above the waist is removed. The patient remains thus for about 15 minutes while the skin cools. At the end of the cooling period, infrared photograhs of the breast and chest wall, or of the liquid crystal sheet in contact with the breast, are taken. Two pictures (AP and oblique) are taken of each breast.

Interpretation

The rationale of this technique is that a carcinoma of the breast, even if deep-seated, is associated with a generalized increase in the blood flow to the affected breast, or with a redistribution of blood within the breast. The affected breast may show more prominent veins than does the contralateral normal breast. Since carcinomas have a high metabolic rate, the carcinoma itself may be hotter than the surrounding breast tissue (Fig. 58–14). Unfortunately, abscesses and other inflammatory processes also produce an increase in blood flow and a localized or generalized rise in temperature; on the other hand, some carcinomas do not produce thermographically recognizable changes. Therefore, both false-negative and false-positive results are not rare. An error rate of about 30% has been reported. Other reports have suggested better (and worse) results, but in all published series the error rate is substantial. Thermography is no longer being used in the National Cancer Institute Breast Cancer Detection Demonstration project.

MAMMOGRAPHY

Mammography provides detailed x-ray images of intramammary structures. Two forms of mammography are currently in use: film mammography and Xeromammography. The clinical use of these techniques is discussed in Chapter 59.

Xeromammography. When x-rays strike a charged, selenium-coated plate, they dissipate some of the charge. The amount of charge dissipated is in proportion to the amount of x-rays striking the plate. Thus, a latent image in the form of a pattern of varying electrical charges is created on the surface of the plate.

If the plate is then placed in a chamber into which charged pigment particles are blown, some particles are attracted by the charge on the plate and settle on its surface. The amount of pigment at each point on the plate depends upon the charge at that point. The resultant image is then transferred to a piece of plastic-coated paper by pressing the plate and the paper together and exposing the paper to heat. The entire pro-

cess is performed automatically in a commercially available processor.

At the boundary between two differently charged areas, the electric field is distorted, causing an excessive amount of pigment to be deposited on the denser side of the boundary, while a disproportionately small amount of pigment is deposited on the less dense side. Thus, edges are sharply displayed, even though the difference in radiographic density between adjacent structures may be very slight. Apart from this strong edge-enhancement effect, xeroradiography provides a low-contrast image that satisfactorily demonstrates the entire breast and the retromammary structures, all in one exposure (Fig. 58–15).

Film Mammography. The differences in radiographic density between the components of the breast are slight. Low-energy x-rays and high-contrast film must be used to display these slight differences in density.

To maximize the contrast of the image and to provide the sharp detail necessary for useful interpretation, special high-contrast film that has emulsion on one side only (conventional x-ray film has an emulsion on both sides) is used in combination with special cassettes containing a single, fine-grain intensifying screen.

To enhance the visibility of intramammary detail, the breast is drawn over a plate or film holder and compressed with a plastic cone or a balloon so that the breast tissue is spread out. Mediolateral, craniocaudal, axillary, and often lateromedial views of each breast are taken.

For Xeromammography the dose of radiation to the skin of the breast is less than 1 rad per image. Film mammography using modern film-screen combinations requires a slightly lower dose. These figures are only approximate, since reported values vary. With both Xeromammography and film mammography, the radiation exposure to the gonads and the eyes is negligible, so that the only hazard from the examination is the direct effect of radiation on the breast tissue itself.

Interpretation

Malignancy is suggested by

1. An increase in the vasculature of one breast. (Unfortunately, increased vascularity can occur with inflammatory disease as well as malignancy.)
2. A mass whose borders are not sharp
3. Strands of tissue running from a mass to the skin, the nipple, or the chest wall (Fig. 58–16)
4. Thickening due to edema of the skin of the breast
5. Very fine punctate calcifications within a mass (Fig. 58–17)

Calcification may be so fine that it can be detected on the mammogram only with the aid of a magnifying

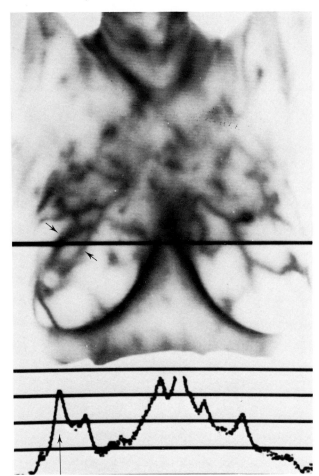

FIG. 58–14. Thermogram showing carcinoma of right breast. Compare hot (*black*) area in upper part of right breast (*arrows*) with corresponding area of left breast. Densitometer scan at bottom of figure shows a tall peak (*arrow*) representing hot area in right breast.

glass. Malignant calcification must be distinguished from vascular calcification, which follows the course of blood vessels. Other benign forms of calcification are, in general, coarser than the calcification of malignancy. Comedocarcinoma (a form of intraductal carcinoma) also calcifies. Its calcification is often widespread and consists of fine, short, linear flecks. Secretory disease may also be associated with calcification that is similar to but, in general, coarser than that of comedocarcinoma.

Benign breast masses (*e.g.*, fibroadenoma) have sharply defined margins and do not show skin thickening or stranding (Fig. 58–18). Increased vasculature is commonly seen with inflammatory disease and benign masses may be calcified. Hyperplastic cystic dis-

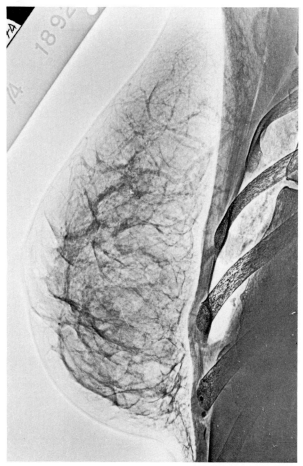

FIG. 58–15. Xeromammogram showing normal breast—Mediolateral view. Nipple, skin, vasculature, ductal structures, and retromammary tissues are all clearly seen. No masses are present.

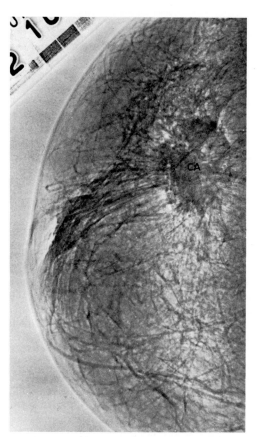

FIG. 58–16. Xeromammogram showing carcinoma of breast—Craniocaudal view. Carcinoma (*CA*) is about 2 cm in diameter and has poorly defined border. Note strands of dense tissue running forward from mass to subareolar region. Increased breast vascularity, skin thickening, and calcification (features often seen in malignancy) are not seen in this example.

ease appears as a series of homogeneous densities (representing retention cysts) together with accentuation of the ductal pattern. Calcification may be present; benign calcification is, in general, coarser than malignant calcification.

In many cases the distinction between a benign and a malignant mass is straightforward; however, difficult and borderline cases are not rare, and carcinoma may be present in a breast that is roentgenographically normal. Therefore, mammographic normalcy does not guarantee absence of breast cancer; when any doubt exists, tissues should be excised for histologic analysis, or a follow-up examination should be done in 3 months. Mammography should not be the sole diagnostic modality. Palpable carcinomas do occur in the presence of normal mammograms, although they are rare. (Fuller accounts of mammography are available in work published by Wolfe.)

GALACTOGRAPHY

Galactography is a radiographic investigation involving injection of contrast agent into a mammary duct (Fig. 58–19). It is used primarily when an intraductal lesion (*e.g.*, a papilloma) is suspected. Occasionally, galactograms are used to aid in the localization of a breast mass and to differentiate a cystic from a solid breast mass.

RADIONUCLIDE IMAGING

Images that are produced with x-rays and ultrasound result from energy that originates outside the patient. Radionuclide imaging is fundamentally different in that the radiation that forms the image originates

inside the body. The radiation is emitted by pharmaceuticals containing elements that are radioactive.

A radioactive atom is one that has an unstable nucleus. As the nucleus undergoes internal rearrangement, radiation is emitted. The only useful form of radiation for medical imaging purposes is the gamma ray, a form of electromagnetic radiation that is closely related to x-ray. Gamma rays with a photon energy in the range of 75 to 200 KeV are the best for imaging. Positron imaging systems that use gamma rays with a photon energy of about 500 KeV are gaining popularity and may well be the wave of the future, but they are not yet in widespread use.

By far the most useful radionuclide is ^{99m}Technetium. This radionuclide has a short half-life (6 hours) and emits only gamma rays, two properties that keep the dose of radiation to the patient low and so allow large doses of the radionuclide to be given without undue radiation risk. (It is desirable to give a large dose of radionuclide because the larger the dose, the easier it is to obtain a high quality image.) ^{99m}Tc is easily obtained from commercially available generators containing ^{99}Molybdenum. The ^{99}Mo decays to ^{99m}Tc, which is periodically eluted from the generator by flushing with saline.

The Technetium is given the desired biologic properties by incorporating it into a suitable molecule or particle. For instance, if one wishes to obtain a radionuclide image of the skeleton, the ^{99m}Tc is incorporated into a molecule that binds to bone.

Radionuclide images are obtained with an instrument known as a gamma camera. On the face of the camera there is a collimator, a lead plate about 1-inch thick through which several hundred holes are drilled. The collimator serves both to limit the field of view of each point on the crystal detector lying behind the collimator, and to cut off stray radiation, thereby improving the resolution of the image.

The crystal detector consists of a large sodium iodide crystal about 12 inches in diameter, which contains a small amount of an impurity such as Thallium (introduced to increase its sensitivity). When gamma rays strike the crystal they cause it to emit a flash of light. As the collimator limits the field of view of each part of the crystal to the tissue that is immediately in front of it, the location of the radionuclide that emitted the gamma ray responsible for the flash is determined from the location of the flash.

Behind the crystal there is an array of photomultiplier tubes. The flashes of light emitted by the crystal are picked up by the photomultiplier tubes, which then each generate an electrical pulse. After electronic processing, the pattern of radioactivity is displayed as a pattern of flashes on a cathode-ray tube, which is then photographed to produce the final image.

Modern gamma cameras can acquire image data very rapidly and can produce images of dynamic processes such as blood flow and left ventricular func-

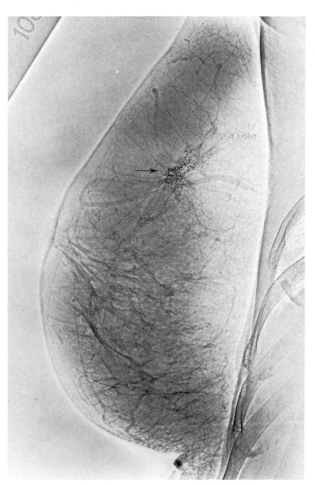

FIG. 58–17. Xeromammogram showing malignant calcification in carcinoma of breast. Calcified carcinoma (*arrow*) can be seen in upper part of breast. Malignant calcification is typically very fine and may be much more difficult to see than in this example.

tion. Dynamic studies do not have much place in gynecology.

Apart from the intravenous injection, radionuclide examinations are painless. There is an unavoidable delay between the injection of the radionuclide and the commencement of imaging due to the time needed for the radionuclide to clear from the blood and to concentrate in the tissue of interest. With modern radiopharmaceuticals (other than Gallium) this delay ranges from a few seconds to 2 hours. Several minutes are usually required to collect the data needed to form a good image, during which time the patient must remain motionless. The dose of radiation received by the patient from most modern radionuclide studies is low, and repeated studies can safely be performed in all but pregnant patients.

Present day radionuclide images have a much lower

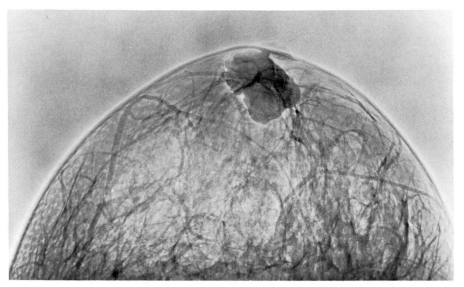

FIG. 58-18. Xeromammogram showing benign breast mass (fibroadenoma); Craniocaudal view. A lobulated, sharply defined, uncalcified mass can be seen immediately subjacent to nipple. Skin thickening, calcification, increased vasculature, and stranding are absent. Nipple is not retracted. This is typical appearance of fibroadenoma. (Courtesy of J. Milbraith)

spatial resolution than x-ray or ultrasonic images. Their value lies in their sensitivity to alterations in physiologic processes (*e.g.*, osteoblastic activity) that are not easily detected by other methods. However, alterations in a physiologic process may be due to many causes, so that radionuclide studies tend to give non-specific results. It is especially important to interpret radionuclide studies in the light of clinical and other data. For instance, areas of increased osteoblastic activity may be due to metastases, healing fractures, osteoporosis with unusual bone stress, osteomyelitis, arthritis, etc. Although each may give some distinctive feature to the radionuclide bone scan, there are many similarities; in such instances, the precise pathologic diagnoses usually must be determined by other means.

RADIONUCLIDE DETECTION OF METASTASES TO BONE

Metastases in bone may be advanced enough to produce symptoms and yet be undetectable on roentgenographic examination of the skeleton. Radionuclide bone scanning is a much more sensitive means of detecting bony metastases than plain x-ray films. A number of radiopharmaceuticals are available for bone scanning. These are taken up by osteoblasts, resulting in an area of increased radioactivity that also represents an area of increased osteoblastic activity. Bone scanning alone gives no firm indication that the increase is caused by metastasis. Currently the most popular agent used for such scans is ^{99m}Tc-labeled methylene diphosphonate.

Technique

Approximately 20 mCi of ^{99m}Tc-labeled methylene diphosphonate is injected intravenously. Part of the in-

jected radionuclide is taken up by areas of osteoblastic activity, while the remainder is rapidly cleared from the circulation by the kidneys. The best images are usually obtained after an interval of 1 to 2 hours. If renal function is reduced, clearing of the excess radionuclide from the blood is slower and less complete, and inferior images are the usual result.

Survey views of the entire skeleton are taken, together with special views of areas of particular concern.

Interpretation

Normal bone takes up more radionuclide around the joints than elsewhere, but these areas of increase are symmetric. Metastases appear as areas of increased radioactivity that are asymmetric or located away from joints.

When areas of abnormality are noted on the radionuclide bone scan, it is essential to obtain radiographs of the affected bones as aids to interpretation. Areas of increased radionuclide uptake that are not adjacent to joints and are not associated with any radiologically demonstrable abnormality are likely to be due to metastases.

RADIONUCLIDE DETECTION OF METASTASES TO OTHER ORGANS

Liver metastases can be detected by scanning after intravenous injection of ^{99m}Tc-labeled colloidal sulfur. The colloidal particles are taken up by the Kupffer cells, reticuloendothelial phagocytic cells within the liver. Imaging may be commenced immediately after the injection. Metastases usually appear as multiple round areas of diminished radioactivity. Hepatic metastases smaller than 2 cm in diameter cannot be rou-

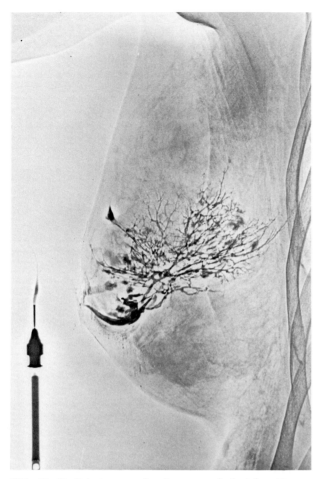

FIG. 58-19. Galactogram showing normal ductal pattern—Xeroradiographic study, mediolateral view. Film was taken immediately after injection of about 0.5 ml water-soluble contrast agent into a mammary duct. Branching pattern is normal. There is some filling of peripheral lobules, but no evidence of intraductal filling defects.

tinely detected by radionuclide scanning, even with the best equipment. The margins of normal liver images are often irregular, and these irregularities are sometimes difficult to distinguish from defects due to subcapsular metastases.

Cerebral metastases, particularly if located high in the cerebral hemisphere, can often be demonstrated by a two-stage radionuclide procedure. Initially, a flow study is performed. A bolus of 20 mCi of ^{99m}Tc-DTPA is administered by rapid intravenous injection and images of the skull are taken every 2 seconds. This study demonstrates the major cerebral arteries and veins and areas of abnormally increased or decreased perfusion. Between 1 and 2 hours after injection, multiple views of the head are taken.

Abnormalities in cerebral radionuclide images are

due to changes in the blood–brain barrier. If the blood–brain barrier is intact, the radiopharmaceutical is excluded from the brain; that is, in a normal brain scan, radioactivity can be seen in the venous sinuses, the facial vasculature, and in the temporal muscles, but not in the brain. Metastases disrupt the blood–brain barrier and so appear as areas of abnormally increased radioactivity. The popularity of radionuclide brain scanning has declined since the introduction of CT.

RADIONUCLIDE LYMPHOGRAPHY

If a radionuclide-labeled colloid of appropriate particle size is injected subcutaneously, it is taken up by the lymphatics and transported to the regional nodes, so that images of the draining lymph nodes can be obtained. This technique is generally inferior to conventional lymphangiography because, when compared to radiographic images, the resolution of a radionuclide image is poor. Radionuclide lymphography is useful when conventional lymphangiography cannot be done. Its principal application is in the delineation of the internal mammary lymph node chain in patients with breast carcinoma.

REFERENCES AND RECOMMENDED READING

Barash IM, Pasternack BS, Venet L, et al: Quantitative thermography as a predictor of breast cancer. Cancer 31:769, 1973

Buice JW, Gould DM: Abdominal and pelvic pneumography. Radiology 69:704, 1957

Dodd GD: Present status of thermography ultrasound and mammography in breast cancer detection. Cancer 39 (Suppl 6):2796, 1977

Ege GN: Internal mammary lymphoscintigraphy. Radiology 118:101, 1976

Gold WM, Youker J, Anderson S, et al: Pulmonary-function abnormalities after lymphangiography. N Engl J Med 273:519, 1965

Goldberg BB: The identification of placenta previa. Radiology 128:255, 1978

Isard HJ, Ostrum BJ: Breast thermography: The mammatherm. Radiol Clin N Am 12:167, 1974

Jellins J, Kossoff G, Reeve TS: Detection and classification of liquid-filled masses in the breast by gray-scale echography. Radiology 125:205, 1977

Kelly MT, Santos-Ramos R, Duenhoelter J: The value of sonography in suspected ectopic pregnancy. Obstet Gynecol 53:703, 1979

Kinsella TJ, Bloomer WD: New therapeutic strategies in radiation therapy. JAMA 245:1169, 1981

Kobayashi T: Gray-scale echography for breast cancer. Radiology 122:207, 1977

Lee JKT, Stanley RJ, Sagel SS, et al: Accuracy of CT in detecting intraabdominal and pelvic lymph node metastases from pelvic cancers. Am J Roentgenol 131:675, 1978

Milbrath JR, Wilkinson EJ, Friedrich EG: Xeroradiography of

radical vulvectomy specimens. Am J Roentgenol Radium Ther Nucl Med 125:486, 1975

Myrden JA, Hiltz JE: Breast cancer following multiple fluoroscopies during artifical pneumothorax treatment of pulmonary tuberculosis. Can Med Assoc J 100:1032, 1969

Photopoulos GJ, McCartney WH, Walton LA, et al: Computerized tomography applied to gynecologic oncology. Am J Obstet Gynecol 135:381, 1979

Sample WF, Lippe BM, Gyepes MT: Gray-scale ultrasonography of the normal female pelvis. Radiology 125:477, 1977

Shopfner CE: Radiology in pediatric gynecology. Radiol Clin N Am 5:151, 1967

Siegler AN: Hysterosalpingography. New York, Medcom Press, 1974

Swartz HM, Reichling BA: The risks of mammograms. JAMA 237:965, 1977

Swartz HM, Reichling BA: The safety of x-ray examination or radioisotope scan. JAMA 239:2031, 1978

Thompson HE, Bernstine RL: Diagnostic Ultrasound in Clinical Obstetrics and Gynecology. New York, Wiley, 1978

Wallace S, Jing B: Lymphangiography in tumors of the female genital system. Radiol Clin N Am 12:79, 1974

Walsh JW, Amendola MA, Hall DJ, et al: Recurrent carcinoma of the cervix: CT diagnosis. Am J Radiol 136:117, 1981

Walsh JW, Taylor KJ, Wasson JF, et al: Gray-scale ultrasound in 204 proven gynecologic masses: Accuracy and specific diagnostic criteria. Radiology 130:391, 1979

Wolfe JN: Xeroradiography. Springfield IL, Charles C Thomas, 1972

Wolfe JN: Analysis of 462 breast carcinomas. Am J Roentgenol Radium Ther Nucl Med 121:846, 1974

Wolfe JN: Mammography. Radiol Clin N Am 12:189, 1974

Among diseases of the female breast, cancer is preeminent. It is more likely to be responsible for the death of women 40 to 55 years of age than any other cause. The total annual mortality from childbearing (320 in 1978) and all gynecologic neoplasms (22,800) falls far short of the 35,000 deaths that now result from cancer of the breast in the United States each year. In 1981 an estimated 108,000 new cases are expected, and the incidence—now 76 per 100,000 female population per year—is gradually rising.

Consistent with national frequencies, 7% or approximately one of every 13 of an obstetrician–gynecologists's patients can be expected to develop cancer of the breast at some time during her adult life. Three percent of these will be coincident with a pregnancy, but most occur in the decade prior to menopause and in the two decades that follow (40 to 70 years of age). Risk climbs with age, so there is no respite for the elderly, and only the declining number of the latter maintains the average age of all patients as low as 59 years.

Presently, 23,376 practicing obstetricians and gynecologists repeatedly examine several million women on a regular basis and have the opportunity to detect cancer of the breast in its earliest clinical stages. This opportunity is emphasized by the American College of Obstetricians and Gynecologists which recommends that 1) examination of the breast be an integral part of the gynecologic examination, 2) patients be instructed in the importance and technique of breast self-examination (BSE), 3) use be made of mammography and needle aspiration as effective techniques for early detection, 4) ambulatory facilities for breast biopsy be encouraged, 5) breast biopsies be performed by properly trained individuals, 6) women at high risk for breast cancer be recognized and innovative detection programs be initiated for them, and 7) training for obstetricians and gynecologists include instruction in early diagnosis and treatment options.

Emphasis upon early detection of breast cancer stems from the striking improvement in the prospects for cure when tumors are small and without signs of spread beyond the breast. Noninvasive or minimally invasive cancers presently can be cured in greater than 95% of cases. While early detection is an opportunity for all physicians, the obstetrician–gynecologist is in a position to play a particularly important role in the diagnosis of breast disease.

WOMEN AT HIGH RISK FOR BREAST CANCER

Development of breast cancer is not a random event; demographic and personal characteristics can be identified which confer greater than average risk. This information serves to focus attention upon individuals at

CHAPTER

DISEASES OF THE BREAST

William L. Donegan

greater risk and to improve the efficiency of screening efforts (Table 59–1).

Most importantly, the disease is sex- and age-related. Ninety-nine percent of breast cancers occur in women. It is infrequent below the age of 30 years (<1.5% of cases) but steadily climbs in frequency after the age of 35 years. Almost 85% of patients are 40 years of age or older. Western women are considerably more likely to develop the disease than are Oriental women, Dutch women have greater risk than any other nationality, and breast cancer is uncommon in Japan. In the United States, Jews and women of high socioeconomic status are notably susceptible.

Mortality from breast cancer in the United States has an uneven geographic distribution, the highest death rates being almost entirely confined to the northeastern part of the country and centered in urban and highly industrialized areas.

TABLE 59–1. RISKS FOR DEVELOPMENT OF BREAST CANCER

WOMEN AT HIGH RISK OF BREAST CANCER

Age > 40 years
Caucasian
Obesity
Urban residence
High socioeconomic group
Jewish
Mother or sister with breast cancer
Previous benign breast disease
Previous cancer of one breast
Previous cancer of the endometrium, ovary, or colon
Excessive irradiation of the breast
Cowden's disease (multiple hamartoma syndrome)
Prolonged exogenous estrogen exposure
Early menarche (< 12 years of age)
Late menopause (> 50 years of age)
Aggregate lifetime menstrual cycles $\geq$ 30 years
Nulliparous
First full-term pregnancy after the age of 30 years

WOMEN AT LOW RISK OF BREAST CANCER

Surgical castration before the age of 37 years
Oriental
First full-term pregnancy before 18 years of age
Age < 30 years

The exceptionally high frequency of breast cancer in men with Klinefelter's syndrome (XXY sex chromosomes), in association with Cowden's disease of women or multiple hamartoma syndrome (Fig. 59–1), and with the allele for wet ear wax, as well as its tendency to occur in some families, all suggest a genetic predisposition. Close relatives of breast cancer patients are three times more likely than expected to have the disease, with the risk highest for daughters, sisters, and mothers in ascending order. If the disease involves both breasts, the risk to relatives increases to fivefold and to nine times the expected if the patient is also premenopausal. Curiously, familial risk is not as obvious if the patient is postmenopausal.

Environmental factors associated with increased risk include high fat consumption, obesity, and carcinogen exposure. Women whose breasts were irradiated with excessive fluoroscopy or for postpartum mastitis, or by atomic explosions are at excess risk. The fact that viruses (MMTV) transmit breast cancer in mice and that certain polycylic hydrocarbons, e.g. dimethybenzanthracine can regularly cause breast cancer in rats after a small single dose make both viruses and chemicals candidates for human carcinogens.

Although excess risk associated with the ingestion of estrogens has not been proved, considerable suspicion is justified. In 1976 Hoover found that women treated with conjugated estrogens for natural or surgical menopause developed an excess frequency of breast cancer after a latent period of 10 years and had twice the expected risk after 15 years. Cyclic use, high doses, and development of fibrocystic disease while on estrogens increased the risk, and the protective effect of nulliparity and of early castration was lost. No overall excess risk has been associated with oral contraceptives, and they may possibly prevent fibrocystic disease, but young women with established fibrocystic disease who use oral contraceptives for extended periods is another matter. Fasal and Paffenbarger observed that after 6 years of oral contraceptive use, these women had 11 times the usual frequency of breast cancer. The importance of these observations should not be lost upon the practicing obstetrician–gynecologist. If estrogens for contraception or postmenopausal replacement are deemed desirable, the potential hazard should be made clear to the patient in advance. It is highly questionable whether premenopausal women with fibrocystic disease or a strong family history of breast cancer should receive oral contraceptives at all.

The increased frequency of breast cancer in Japanese women who relocate in the United States is further evidence for the role of environmental carcinogens in this disease.

A consistent finding in several reports is the predisposition of patients treated for cancer of the endometrium to a subsequent cancer of the breast, both perhaps being related to a particular hormonal milieu or other common stimulus. It is not clear that women with an initial breast cancer are more susceptible than usual to cancer at another site, although ovarian cancer is a possibility.

Among the most potent predispositions for the development of a new breast cancer is the fact of having been treated for cancer of the opposite breast. The frequency varies from two to five times the expected rate and makes the remaining breast of a mastectomized woman worthy of special attention on follow-up examinations. This liability is concentrated in women whose first cancer was noninvasive, multifocal, or of lobular type, and in those less than 50 years of age or with a family history of breast cancer.

Clinically recognizable fibrocystic disease of the breast is widely recognized as placing a woman at risk. Those who have had gross cysts or a biopsy showing fibrocystic disease, particularly epithelial proliferative changes, are from three to five times more likely than others to develop mammary carcinoma. Cellular atypia is particularly ominous. The relationship between mammographic tissue patterns and of abnormal thermograms and risk is controversial at present.

Other personal characteristics associated with increased prospects of breast cancer implicate endocrine function: an early menarche (less than 12 years of age), 30 or more years of active menstrual activity, a late menopause, two or fewer pregnancies, and a late

initial full-term pregnancy. Women who give birth to their first child after the age of 35 years have a twofold higher risk than women less than 20 years of age at first childbirth. Nulliparous women are at less risk than primiparas 35 years of age or older. This is a potentially important consideration in family planning and counseling. The important relationship between ovarian function and breast cancer is further illustrated by the fact that castration before the age of 40 years reduces the incidence of breast cancer by 75% regardless of previous parity. Subsequent to the fourth decade, when ovarian function has begun to decline, oophorectomy or irradiation castration provides no protection. Finally, biochemical features of high risk include a low ratio of urinary estriol to total estrogens and a subnormal excretion of androgen metabolites, both suggesting an overbalance of estrogenic influences.

Contrary to earlier beliefs, epidemiologic studies fail to confirm any protection against breast cancer attributable to breast-feeding; therefore, this can no longer be included among its virtues. As virus particles similar to those of the mouse mammary tumor virus can be found in human milk and human cancers, thereby perpetuating the possibility of viral transmission, one might question the advisability of recommending breast-feeding to women of high-risk groups.

Epitomizing high risk for breast cancer would be an elderly, obese, Caucasian woman on long-term estrogen replacement who had been successfully treated for an endometrial carcinoma and cancer of one breast. Also factors to consider would be 1) if her menarche was early and her menopause late, 2) if she delivered her first and only child at the age of 35 years, 3) if her remaining breast had been irradiated for postpartum mastitis and subsequently biopsied, with a diagnosis of fibrocystic disease featuring ductal epithelial proliferation with atypia, and 4) if urinalysis showed a low estriol ratio and was consistent with subnormal androgen production. Such patients are few.

Factors of risk are additive, but to what ultimate extent is uncertain. In 1977, Farewell and associates considered family history, early age at menarche, and late first childbirth and found that the probability of breast cancer progressively doubled with the addition of each.

SIGNS AND SYMPTOMS OF BREAST CANCER

With few exceptions, breast cancers develop from the epithelial lining of mammary ducts; fewer than 1% are of connective tissue origin. Hyperplasia of ductal cells, either those of the collecting ducts or those within the lobules, increasing cellular atypia, progression to purely intraductal (in situ) carcinoma, and finally to stromal invasion represent the course by which carci-

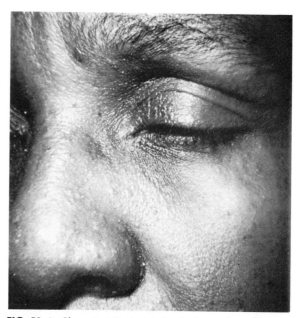

FIG. 59-1. Characteristic facial skin lesions of Cowden's syndrome. Small raised tumors (tricholimomas) are distributed on face and hands, but in other cases occur also in oral cavity. This patient had a mastectomy for carcinoma of breast and also had a thyroidectomy and a hysterectomy for tumors in these organs. An upper GI series showed polypoid lesions of gastric mucosa. Women with Cowden's disease (multiple hamartomas) frequently have symptomatic fibro-cystic disease of the breast and are at high risk for mammary carcinoma. Ten of the 21 cases reported through September of 1977, as well as this patient, have had cancer of the breast (Brownstein, et al: Cancer, 41:2393, 1978).

nomas evolve. These changes frequently occur simultaneously within many ducts; on careful examination, multiple sites of microscopic invasive or noninvasive cancer can be found in 50% of breasts removed for what appears clinically to be a single focus of cancer. The microscopic, asymptomatic growth phase is probably of protracted duration. Based upon observed gross doubling times (the period required for an exponentially growing tumor to double its volume), a cancer that evolves from a single cell may require an average of 7 years to become large enough to feel on palpatory examination (*i.e.*, a mass 1 cm in diameter). At this modest size already 20% of cancers have produced metastases. If cancers can be detected and treated while "minimal" (*i.e.*, less than 5 mm in diameter) or while still noninvasive, metastasis is unlikely and cure is highly probable.

The initial sign of cancer is a mass in almost 80% of cases, and it is usually discovered by the patient. The mass is characteristically nontender but may be associated with discomfort, tenderness, or a drawing sen-

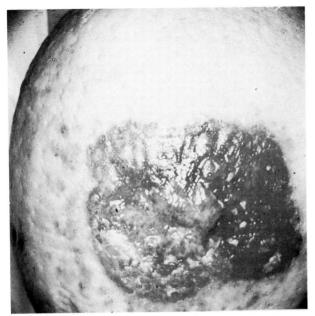

FIG. 59–2. The lesion on this nipple represents Paget's disease, intraepithelial cancer associated with underlying malignancy. Paget's disease can have several appearances but characteristically presents as a moist, nonhealing ulcer. In this instance it has destroyed the nipple and extended beyond it.

sation. Attachment to or dimpling of the overlying skin is highly suggestive of malignancy. Although cancer can arise at any location within the breast, the upper outer quadrant is most often the site, possibly because most tissue is concentrated in this location. The left breast is involved slightly more often than the right.

Nipple discharge from in situ or invasive cancer within ducts is second only to a mass as the first sign of cancer; it can be bloody, nonbloody, clear, or of any color. Some discharge can be expressed from the breasts of most nonlactating women, but it is ordinarily obtainable from both sides, is nonbloody, small in quantity, and issues from more than one ductal orifice. Occasionally blood-tinged discharge can be expressed from the breasts of pregnant women, and persistent milky discharge is not unusual in parous women. Bilateral discharge from otherwise normal breasts is drug-induced, physiologic, or secondary to a diffuse process such as fibrocystic disease. Cytology is rarely helpful in these instances.

Unilateral discharge from a single orifice is highly suggestive of a local lesion. Bloody fluid suggests a duct papilloma or carcinoma. The probability that cancer is the cause increases with age and in the presence of a mass.

Less frequent initial signs of malignancy include nipple retraction, localized edema of the skin, erythema, ulceration of the breast, pain, and ecchymoses.

Persistent erosion or crusting of the nipple may be a

sign of Paget's disease, *i.e.*, intraepithelial carcinoma associated with cancer in the underlying ducts (Fig. 59–2). A lesion of the nipple which does not respond rapidly to topical treatment within 2 weeks should, therefore, be biopsied. Paget's disease of the nipple may or may not be accompanied by a palpable mass.

"Inflammatory" carcinoma mimics, in all respects, an acute infection with erythema, edema of the skin, enlargement of the breast, and discomfort. Too often it is mistaken for an infection and treated for prolonged periods unsuccessfully with antibiotics and local heat (Fig. 59–3).

Upon occasion an enlarged axillary lymph node due to metastases is the only sign of an occult carcinoma within the breast. The latter may be detectable only by mammography.

An increasing number of cancers are detected by routine mammograms in the absence of physical signs or symptoms. The radiographic changes that betray these early lesions include clusters of innumerable fine calcifications, small stellate densities, and focal architectural disturbances of the mammary parenchyma.

As cancer advances, other signs appear: nipple retraction, ulceration of the skin, retraction of the entire breast, pink satellite nodules within the skin, extensive edema and erythema of the skin, fixation to the chest wall, swelling of the arm due to extensive involvement of the axilla, and enlarged supraclavicular lymph nodes (Fig. 59–4). Beyond the breast and its regional lymph nodes, mammary cancer can spread to any site in the body. Favored sites are distant lymph nodes, bones of the axial skeleton, the pleura, and lungs. The liver is often eventually involved and intracranial metastases are betrayed by neurologic disturbances.

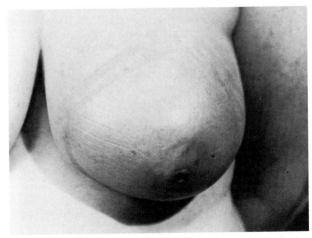

FIG. 59–3. Inflammatory carcinoma of this breast demonstrates characteristic features, *i.e.*, diffuse swelling without a distinct mass, erythema, and cutaneous edema. It can be confused with nonneoplastic inflammatory processes.

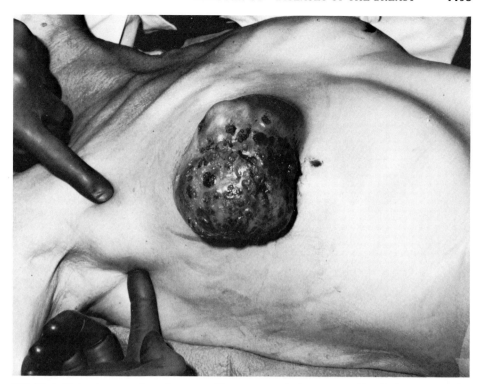

FIG. 59–4. Natural progression of untreated breast cancer is demonstrated by this large tumor that permeates and ulcerates overlying skin, is attached to underlying pectoralis major muscle, and is associated with enlarged tumor-bearing axillary lymph nodes. Cure is unlikely when disease has reached this extent.

Pleural effusions can be troublesome and retroperitoneal involvement can obstruct the ureters. Additional spread within the skin is not unusual, sometimes surrounding the chest like a constrictive breast plate, so-called *carcinoma en curaisse.* Involvement of bones with lytic, sometimes blastic, metastases leads to pain, pathologic fractures, and potentially lethal hypercalcemia.

Cancer may appear in the opposite breast as a component of generalized dissemination, but it should also be appreciated that approximately 5% of patients treated for one cancer develop an independent second cancer in the remaining breast. This may be discovered simultaneously with the first, but more often it is a subsequent development and, in the absence of dissemination, it also may be curable with vigorous treatment.

DIFFERENTIAL DIAGNOSIS

Several diseases of the breast present with signs or symptoms similar to cancer and must be distinguished from it; some are far more common. A biopsy is often necessary for secure diagnosis.

FIBROCYSTIC DISEASE

Symptomatic fibrocystic disease of the breasts is a condition of the reproductive years, probably originating in hormonal imbalance. A relative estrogen excess or a progesterone deficiency in the luteal phase of the menstrual cycle may be responsible. Characteristic symptoms are cyclic pain and tenderness of one or both breasts, more prominent immediately prior to menses. Signs include irregular firmness and granularity of the breast tissue, masses, and expressible nipple discharge. These changes often wax and wane, paralleling symptoms.

A variety of histologic changes are involved, including gross and microscopic cysts, epithelial proliferation within ducts sometimes to the point of diffuse papillomatosis or papilloma formation, proliferation of ducts (adenosis) associated with a varying degree of sclerosis (sclerosing adenosis), focal sclerosis (fibrous disease), and apocrine metaplasia of epithelium. Any or all of these changes can result clinically in masses, dominant nodules, and nipple discharge. Masses and cysts are often transient, and cysts can usually be identified with fine-needle aspiration, but persistent masses raise the possibility of cancer.

Symptomatic measures such as firm support with a well-fitting bra, mild analgesics, and local heat can provide relief. According to a recent theory, the problem is aggravated by ingestion of foods and drinks containing methylxanthines, and improvement can be obtained by eliminating tea, coffee, cola drinks, and chocolate from the diet (Minton, 1979). Methylxanthines stimulate cyclic AMP and increase metabolic activity in the breast. Occasionally, hormonal therapy with progesterone during the second half of the menstrual cycle or administration of anti-estrogens is justified. Difficult cases incapacitated by discomfort and requiring multiple diagnostic biopsies occasionally require subcutaneous mastectomy with prosthetic implants for relief.

As the cause of most complaints related to the breast, fibrocystic disease continues to be prominent in clinical practice. It is important to appreciate that fibrocystic disease is a marker, or possibly a precursor, of malignant change. Women with proved fibrocystic disease have three times the general risk for developing breast cancer. They are a well-defined high-risk group with a difficult problem: any abnormality is most likely to be further fibrocystic changes, but is also more likely than usual to be breast cancer (Fig. 59–5).

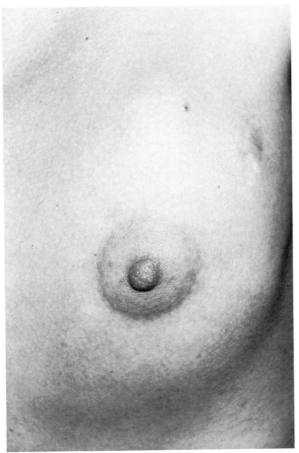

FIG. 59-5. Association between fibrocystic disease and carcinoma as illustrated by this young patient who presented with mass in upper midline of the breast which subsequently proved to be cancerous. Scar in upper outer quadrant marks site of previous biopsy that revealed fibrocystic disease.

BENIGN NEOPLASMS

Fibroadenomas

Fibroadenomas are the most common benign neoplasms of the breast, with a peak incidence in the third and fourth decades of life. Nevertheless, they can still be found in the breasts of elderly women.

The physical findings are characteristic. Fibroadenomas are spherical, firm, well-defined, and convey a palpatory sensation of easy mobility (Fig. 59–6). They occur more frequently in black women and are bilateral and multiple in approximately 15% of cases. Some are soft, demonstrate continued progressive growth, and can reach large size.

While the physical features of fibroadenomas are distinctive, they can be duplicated by the rare and treacherous cystosarcoma phyllodes, a sarcoma possibly having its origin in fibroadenomas. Mammographically, the latter have the same round shape and smooth borders as cysts, but some contain large distinctive calcifications. Fibroadenomas are best removed on an elective basis, both for definitive diagnosis and to avoid progressive growth.

Lipomas

Benign lipomas of the breast are frequent and vary considerably in size. Differential diaganosis is not usually a problem, since large tumors are typically superficial, soft, and lobulated, but small lipomas can be deceptively firm. These tumors are usually in the subcutaneous tissues, but may be located in any quadrant of the breast. The contour of the breast may be distorted, albeit smoothly so, and cutaneous or deep attachment is not usually a feature (Fig. 59–7). The mass transilluminates easily, and a mammogram char-

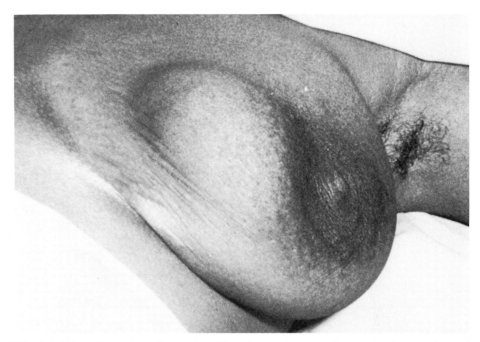

FIG. 59–6. This well-marginated tumor is a fibroadenoma, the most frequent benign neoplasm of the breast. Fibroadenomas predominate in third and fourth decades of life and present as nontender, firm, round, highly mobile masses. Clefts are found on cut surface, and represent distorted mammary ducts. Elective removal is appropriate.

acteristically shows the radiolucency of fat with some compression of adjacent mammary parenchyma.

Adenoma of the Nipple

This unusual benign neoplasm of both men and women produces firmness and soreness of the papilla of the nipple, often with crusting and a bloody discharge. A discrete hard lump may be present. Grossly, it mimics Paget's disease and, microscopically, has occasionally been mistaken for carcinoma. A biopsy is diagnostic, and local excision is curative.

INFLAMMATIONS

Abscesses

Typical bacterial infections and abscesses are found most often in the postpartum period and are attributed to cracked nipples. They respond to appropriate antibiotics and to incision and drainage of pus when it is present. Abscesses in the breast of postmenopausal women are uncommon, are usually in the subareolar area, and result from ductal ectasia.

Squamous metaplasia within major lactiferous ducts of both the young and old can lead to repeated periareolar abscesses that drain at the areolar margin

and chronic sinuses communicating with the ductal system (Fig. 59–8). Patients have a characteristic history of repeated infections and multiple incisions for drainage. Complete removal of the abnormal ducts, ordinarily the entire major duct system, is necessary for relief of the problem.

Carcinoma of the breast should not be missed in the differential diagnosis of inflammations or abscesses. Erythema, edema, tenderness, and swelling are characteristic features of inflammatory carcinoma. Fortunately, this virulent form of the disease comprises only 2% of all cases. Diffuse induration rather than a discrete mass is the rule, and a mammogram provides no clue to set it apart from other sources of inflammation. Diagnosis depends upon suspicion and a specimen of tissue and skin for microscopic examination. The histologic hallmark is cancer in dermal lymphatics. Failure of a postpartum infection to resolve promptly and infections in postpartum breasts are suspicious of cancer and warrant biopsy. An incision and drainage for abscesses should be routinely accompanied by a tissue specimen.

Fat Necrosis and Plasma Cell Mastitis

These two diverse entities can mimic almost all signs of breast cancer; they are able to produce a mass, and

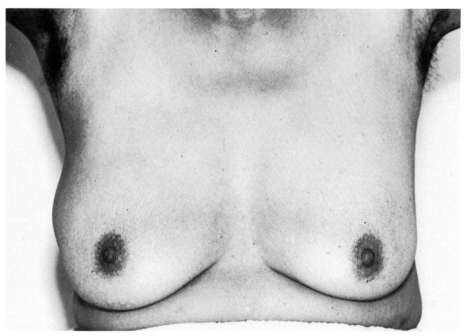

FIG. 59–7. Benign lipoma distorts lateral contour of right breast. These neoplasms are generally identifiable by characteristic physical and mammographic features.

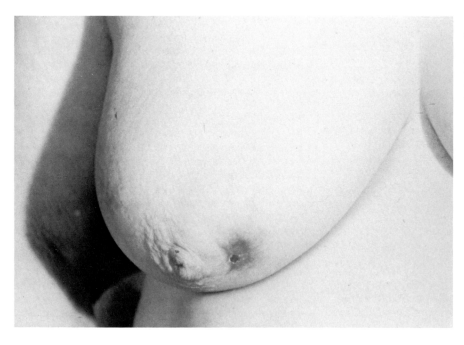

FIG. 59–8. Chronic sinus at margin of areola and a history of multiple abscesses in this area is typical of complications associated with ductal ectasia. Resection of major lactiferous ducts is usually necessary for cure.

cause nipple retraction and skin dimpling. Mammograms are also highly suggestive of cancer with spiculated density and clustered calcification.

Fat necrosis is usually a sequel of direct trauma. The history is suggestive and a bruise may have been noted by the patient. Prominent histologic features are fibrosis intermixed with foamy macrophages, histiocytic giant cells, fat droplets, and necrotic debris. Calcification may be present.

Plasma cell mastitis, an inflammatory mass characterized by prominent infiltration of plasma cells, probably has its origin in ductal ectasia, a process in which squamous metaplasia within lactiferous ducts results in an accumulation of keratinous debris. This inspissated material eventually erodes the ductal wall, thereby inciting the characteristic tissue response.

Excisional biopsy is usually necessary for diagnosis of both of these lesions.

Mondor's Disease

Thrombosis of the thoracoepigastric vein, which courses lateral to or across the breast (Mondor's disease), can present clinically either as an asymptomatic or tender subcutaneous fibrotic cord. The cord may attach to the dermis to produce a cutaneous furrow on the breast with retraction of the skin, most prominent when the arm is abducted. It is often associated with operations upon the breast or thorax and is self-limited, completely resolving with time. The clinical features are usually characteristic but can sometimes be confused with cancer. In situations of uncertainty, a biopsy is necessary. If the cord traverses the axilla (Fig. 59–9), it can cause limitation of shoulder motion and may require transection, but this is unusual.

DETECTION AND DIAGNOSIS

MEDICAL HISTORY

Evaluation of the patient for breast disease begins with a physical examination, and a complete physical examination includes a history relevant to breast disease. After defining the presenting problem, the physician should inquire about previous breast disease, known risk factors, and current medications, particularly oral contraceptives and other hormones. A history of oophorectomy is noteworthy as well as previous treatment for cancers that may increase the risk for breast cancer, *e.g.,* carcinoma of the endometrium and of the colon. The age of menarche, the number of pregnancies and live births, the age at first childbirth, and the date of last menses are important considerations. If previous operations included a hysterectomy, pertinent information includes its cause, whether the ovaries were removed and, if not, whether symptoms suggestive of menopause subsequently have been ex-

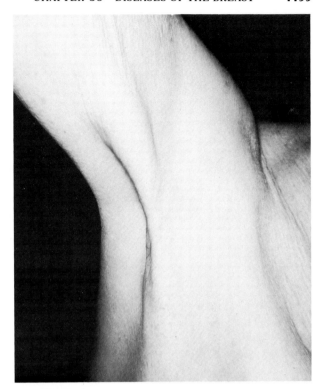

FIG. 59-9. Firm subcutaneous band crossing axilla represents a form of Mondor's disease. Thrombophlebitis, usually of thoraco-epigastric vein, is responsible and sometimes has been confused clinically with infiltrating mammary carcinoma.

perienced. Inquiry should be made about breast cancer in other family members.

VISUAL EXAMINATION

General physical features of pertinence are signs of Cowden's disease, a previous mastectomy, or, in males, features of Klinefelter's syndrome. The breasts are examined visually and with palpation, and attention is given to the regional nodes in the axilla and the supraclavicular and infraclavicular areas.

No special equipment is necessary to perform an adequate examination. The examination is begun with the patient comfortably seated and disrobed to the waist. If the patient has a complaint specifically related to the breast such as a lump or point of tenderness, it is useful at this point for her to indicate the site so that it can receive special attention during the examination, the details of which are shown in Figure 59–10.

Considerable variation exists among patients with respect to the size of breasts and their general configuration, but outlines are normally curvilinear. These constitutional differences are all subject to change

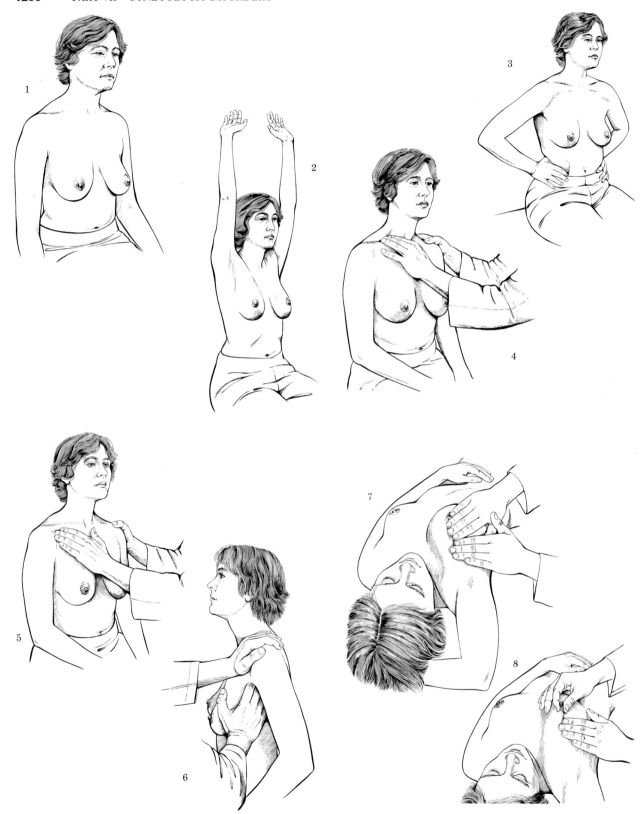

with age, pregnancy, and hormonal stimulation. Perfect symmetry is rarely found, and one must have an appreciation for the range of normal. Attention is given to unusual asymmetry in size or shape, color of the skin and its venous pattern, skin changes, and nipple excoriations, deviation, or inversion. Enlarged nodes may be visible in the supraclavicular areas.

The patient is instructed, in turn, to fully extend both arms above her head and then to place the hands upon her hips and press inward, tightening the pectoralis major muscles. These positions change the relationship between the breasts and both the deep pectoral fascia and the skin; if abnormal attachments are present they will produce signs of retraction or dimpling.

PALPATION

With the patient still seated, the supraclavicular, infraclavicular, and axillary areas are palpated for lymph nodes. Infraclavicular (actually apical axillary) lymph nodes can be felt in the deltopectoral triangle if they are enlarged. The coracoid process of the scapula, which may be prominent at this site, can mimic a hard, fixed lymph node, but betrays its true nature by being present on both sides. The axilla is best examined with the patient's arm relaxed at her side, only slightly abducted, a position that loosens the axillary fascia and facilitates palpation. The left axilla is examined with the right hand while the examiner's left hand is placed upon the patient's shoulder to prevent upward motion. The fingertips are inserted high but gently into the axilla in a slightly cupped position and then withdrawn downward along the chest wall. This maneuver traps axillary lymph nodes so that they can be readily appreciated as they escape from beneath the fingers. If the heel of the hand that is on the shoulder is pressed

gently upon the pectoralis major, the axillary contents are centralized for a better examination. Nevertheless, both the anterior and the posterior portions of the axilla should be explored. The right axilla is examined by reversing the position of the hands. The size, number, consistency, location, tenderness, and mobility of nodes are important to note.

The examination is continued with the patient in the supine position and ideally with a small pad or pillow beneath the back to elevate the side being examined. This flattens and distributes the breast evenly upon the chest wall and thins the parenchyma. The arm should be abducted. All portions of the breast are examined using the volar surfaces of the fingertips. The examiner should appreciate that breast tissue can reach to the costal margin inferiorly, to the clavicle superiorly, to the midline of the chest, and to the posterior axillary line as well as into the lower axilla. A systematic palpation is best, using the fingers of both hands and proceeding progressively around the breast from center to periphery as if examining each spoke of a wheel. Some examiners prefer to begin peripherally and palpate in diminishing concentric circles centered upon the areola. Fine rotating motions of the fingers serve to displace the underlying glandular tissue back and forth beneath the skin and permit a better appreciation of its consistency, which may vary from soft and lobular to finely or coarsely granular. The axillary extension of the breast should not be forgotten.

Masses or dominant nodules are described in detail and measured with a tape or caliper. The breast may be conceptualized as four quadrants—the upper outer, upper inner, lower outer, and lower inner—as well as a central portion beneath the areola. Masses are described in terms of their location in these quadrants, their size, shape, consistency, mobility, sensitivity, and attachment to skin or deep tissues. Fixation of an otherwise mobile mass when the patient presses her hand upon her hip is a sign of attachment to the deep pectoral fascia or to the pectoralis major muscle itself. Dimpling or inability to move the skin independently of the mass connotes skin attachment. Complete immobility of a mass implies fixation to ribs and intercostal muscles, i.e., the chest wall.

Simultaneous palpation of corresponding quadrants of the breasts is sometimes of value in deciding whether an abnormality is present. A significant asymmetry can be made more obvious with this technique.

Finally, the nipple and areola are examined for underlying masses, inversion, or discharge. A persistent excoriation or "dermatitis" may be a sign of Paget's disease of the nipple and an underlying carcinoma. Women not infrequently report a long history of nipple inversion; but if this is a recent change and the nipple cannot be at least temporarily everted, it is a serious omen. Finally, the nipple is gently squeezed to elicit discharge. The characteristics of a discharge and the number of ducts involved are important observations.

◀ **FIG. 59–10.** *1.* Examination of breasts begins with inspection; patient is disrobed to waist and comfortably seated facing examiner. Asymmetry, prominent veins, and skin changes may be signs of disease. *2.* Patient raises arms above head, thereby altering position of breasts. Immobility or abnormal cutaneous attachments may become evident. *3.* Inward pressure on hips tenses pectoralis major muscle. Abnormal attachments to its overlying fascia and skin can produce retraction or dimpling of skin. *4.* Palpatory examination is performed of supraclavicular lymph nodes. *5.* Delto-pectoral triangle is palpated for evidence of infraclavicular nodal enlargement. *6.* Each axilla is examined for nodal enlargement. Proper placement of examiner's hands and of patient's arm is important. *7.* Thorough palpatory examination of entire breast for masses is performed with patient in supine position. A fine rotational movement of hands is useful to appreciate consistency of underlying tissues. *8.* Nipple is compressed to elicit discharge.

FINE-NEEDLE ASPIRATION

Since cysts of the breasts are frequent and breast cancers are rarely cystic, a reliable distinction between a solid mass and a cyst has considerable value. The distinction cannot be made reliably with palpation, transillumination, or mammograms. Fine-needle aspiration provides a rapid and relatively painless method of distinguishing between solid masses and cysts and can be performed at the time of a physical examination with readily available materials and without anesthesia. A 5- or 10-cc syringe, a 1.5-inch sharp 20-gauge needle, and an antiseptic solution such as 70% alcohol or an iodophor are sufficient (Fig. 59–11).

With the patient in the supine position and advised as to the nature of the procedure, the skin over the mass is prepared with the antiseptic solution. The mass is stabilized with the free hand, and with the other the needle is passed into the mass and it is aspirated. Increased resistance to passage of the needle ordinarily indicates a solid mass and reduced resistance a cyst. Simple cysts will produce nonbloody fluid

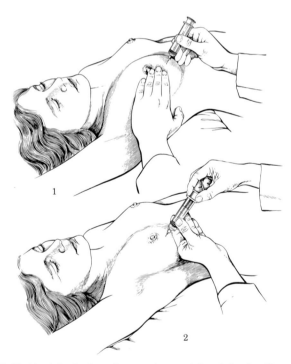

FIG. 59–11. *1.* Aspiration of masses is a useful and simple office procedure. After preparing skin with antiseptic solution, mass is stabilized using index and middle fingers of left hand and a #20 needle fitted to a syringe is introduced into it with one motion. No local anesthesia is necessary because discomfort is minimal. *2.* With needle and syringe stabilized, aspiration is performed. All fluid that can be obtained is withdrawn. After needle is removed, site is reexamined to determine if mass is persistent.

that may be thick or thin and vary from colorless to white, yellow, brown, or green. Milk is obtained from galactoceles. Upon aspiration of all fluid the cyst wall collapses and the mass disappears. If a mammogram is normal and reexamination in 2 to 3 weeks reveals no recurrence of the cyst, no further intervention is necessary.

A biopsy is indicated if 1) no fluid is obtained on aspiration, 2) the mass does not completely disappear after all fluid is removed, 3) the fluid obtained is bloody, 4) the mammogram is suspicious of cancer, or 5) the cyst reappears after two apparently successful aspirations. These signs suggest a solid tumor (which may be cancer) or an intracystic or partially cystic cancer. It is not necessary to routinely examine the cytology of an innocent-appearing cyst aspirate; rarely is this useful.

CYTOLOGY

The cytologic examination of nipple discharges, cyst aspirations, and tissue fluid from solid masses is of limited value. Although morphologically malignant cells from nipple discharge cannot be ignored and serve as an impetus for further diagnostic measures, false-positives are not infrequent, and false-negatives in the presence of cancer are common. Therefore, cytology cannot be considered diagnostic, and the absence of malignant cells should not lead to complacency. A positive cytologic examination of cyst fluid in the absence of other indications for biopsy is sufficiently rare that the examination can hardly be justified as a routine.

Indisputably malignant cells seen in the tiny amount of tissue fluid obtained from aspiration of a solid mass is a reliable indicator of cancer, but failure to identify malignant cells in the aspirate does not rule out cancer. It is not possible to determine from the aspirate whether a cancer is invasive or not, making difficult the selection of a proper surgical procedure. Thus, while the finding of malignant cells may expedite an evaluation and justify staging, it still does not obviate a biopsy.

MAMMOGRAPHY

Mammograms, soft-tissue radiographs of the breast, deserve special attention in early detection of breast cancer because they offer several unique capabilities. Cancers too small to be felt (*e.g.*, 0.2 cm in diameter) can be detected with mammography, making this a logical extension of the physical examination. Furthermore, mammograms can reveal signs of cancer in the absence of symptoms and, therefore, are useful for screening asymptomatic, apparently healthy women. Finally, the probable nature of a palpable mass can be determined by mammography with considerable, but not absolute, accuracy.

Mammograms are most useful for older women whose breasts are largely fatty and less dense than those of young women. Radiographically dense cancers are more easily visualized against this background.

Two views of each breast at right angles to one another, mediolateral and craniocaudal views, are a standard examination. Together they entail a total radiation exposure to each breast of less than 1 roentgen. Either of two techniques may be used: film mammograms, which have the appearance of radiographs, and Xerograms, opaque blue-and-white images produced on paper backing. Both involve equally low radiation exposure. Examples of normal and abnormal Xeromammograms are shown in Figures 58–15 through 58–18. Interpretation of the films is discussed in Chapter 58.

It is important to understand that mammograms do not substitute for a physical examination. Approximately 10% of early cancers are detected by physical examination alone and are not visualized by mammograms; thus, a normal mammogram provides no assurance that cancer is absent. The images depend upon differing radiographic densities within the breasts, and some tumors that are easily palpable can escape detection by mammography, presumably because of insufficient difference in radiographic density from the surrounding breast tissue. In other instances proximity to the chest wall or location at the periphery of the breast may place them outside the standard image of a routine examination. It is also important to appreciate that mammograms are not sufficiently accurate to diagnose the nature of a palpable mass. Radiographic lesions judged radiographically suspicious for cancer by trained radiologists prove benign in 10% to 12% of cases, and about 5% of radiographically benign lesions prove on biopsy to be cancers. Subclinical lesions judged suspicious of cancer prove to be malignant neoplasms in one of six instances. Inaccuracy stems from the fact that slowly growing malignancies can appear well circumscribed and mimic the characteristics of fibroadenomas, cysts, and other innocent lesions, while a number of benign processes, such as fat necrosis, sclerosing adenosis, and biopsy scars, mimic to perfection the radiographic signs of cancer. Since the fibrosis of previous surgery and common skin lesions such as nevi can be misleading on mammograms, the accuracy of the examination is improved if a physical examination is performed by the radiologist or if pertinent information from the patient's history and physical examination is furnished by the clinician.

Indications for mammography are well established. Symptomatic adults should have mammograms in conjunction with a physical examination whenever a complaint is related to the breast, whether or not an abnormality is visible or palpable. Mammograms should be performed prior to biopsy or any other operation upon the breast. They are also indicated even if cancer in one breast may be clinically obvious, in order to check the possibility of subclinical cancer in the opposite breast.

Current recommendations of the National Cancer Institute are that asymptomatic women have mammograms performed annually in conjunction with a physical examination for early detection 1) if they are 50 years of age or older, 2) if they are 40 to 49 years of age with a history of cancer in a mother, sister, or daughter, and 3) at any age if they have had one breast removed for cancer.

Among the indications for mammography must be included the localization of nonpalpable lesions for biopsy, and specimen radiography. The localization technique permits accurate removal of nonpalpable lesions. Using the two mammographic views, two topographic coordinates can be established for any subclinical lesion. A drop of visible and radiographically opaque dye previously mixed is injected at the junction of the coordinates, after which a second mammogram is performed. The relationship of the radiopaque "spot" to the lesion is observed, and the visible blue dye then serves to guide the surgeon. The occult lesion can be removed cosmetically with minimal sacrifice of tissue, an important point considering that most biopsies prove benign and that some women require multiple biopsies. If suspicious calcifications are the target of a biopsy, a specimen radiograph (*e.g.,* a roentgenogram of the tissue removed) can serve to assure that all suspicious calcifications are present in the specimen and have been removed.

Mammography is also useful in conjunction with a physical examination of the breasts in search for the source of metastatic adenocarcinoma when the breasts are among the possible sites of an occult primary.

The following may be considered contraindications to mammography: 1) women less than 18 years of age, 2) pregnancy—radiation exposure is undesirable, and the breasts are dense and unlikely to provide a satisfactory image, and 3) asymptomatic women less than 40 years of age who have no personal history of breast cancer.

The potentially carcinogenic influence of mammograms due to radiation of the breast cannot be ignored but should not be exaggerated. The value of mammography as a detection device is indisputable; the carcinogenic potential is still theoretic. It is estimated that mammograms might result in six cancers per 1,000,000 women per year per roentgen of exposure after a latent period of 10 years (Breslow, *et al.*). This risk, though small, serves to emphasize that the indications for mammography should remain well defined and be observed.

BIOPSY

Physical signs or mammographic lesions suggestive of cancer provide the indications for biopsy. Most frequently these indications are a persistent mass or a

suggestive nipple discharge, but with current efforts for early detection and screening, asymptomatic lesions found with mammography are an increasing indication.

A persistent mass or dominant nodule must be biopsied, despite a normal or "negative" mammogram. In the premenopausal breast an equivocal mass or one of recent origin may be observed through one menstrual cycle to determine if it persists despite hormonal change. A brief trial off oral contraceptives is also worthwhile, and fine-needle aspiration can be employed immediately to identify a benign cyst; otherwise, a histologic diagnosis must be made.

The traditional procedure, *i.e.*, hospital admission with biopsy under general anesthesia, immediate diagnosis with frozen section, and mastectomy if indicated in one stage, is rapidly changing. In response to economic pressures, controversy about treatment, and the evidence that a short delay between biopsy and surgical treatment does not compromise chances for cure, many biopsies are now performed as an outpatient procedure often under local anesthesia. Since only one of five or six biopsies reveals cancer, this is not only expedient but also spares the time and expense of many needless hospitalizations. A two-step procedure in which there is a deliberate interval between biopsy and treatment is gaining acceptance. This permits the diagnosis to be made securely on the basis of thorough histologic examination of permanent sections rather than a frozen section, an advantage when one considers that many cancers are diagnosed so early that a distinction is sometimes difficult between hyperplasia and early cancer. With a diagnosis firmly established, thoughtful consideration can be given to staging and to the options for treatment. If the patient is interested, the possibilities for future reconstruction of the breast can be discussed.

Biopsies should be performed by a surgeon who is well informed about the management of breast diseases and skilled in the technique of biopsy and mastectomy. Biopsies must be performed with proper indications, with due consideration of cosmetics and with accuracy, so that a correct diagnosis is obtained. Complications such as infection or hematoma can delay further treatment inordinately, and misplaced or unnecessarily extensive biopsies can compromise the options for treatment or permit only a suboptimal result.

Only microscopic analysis of a tissue specimen provides a definitive diagnosis of mammary cancer. No other procedure provides sufficient diagnostic assurance to permit treatment for cancer of the breast. A suitable tissue specimen can be obtained with a biopsy needle, an incisional biopsy, or an excisional biopsy. Several types of needles permit a core of tissue to be removed from suspicious masses under local anesthesia in an office or clinic. This is useful for large tumors that are easy targets or for cases in which a mastectomy or tumor removal is not anticipated. A negative result is nondiagnostic.

An incisional biopsy can be performed under local or general anesthesia. Small masses are completely removed (excisional biopsy); a small specimen from a large mass (incisional biopsy) will usually identify it as cancer. In most instances it is possible to use a cosmetic para-areolar incision for biopsies.

ESTROGEN-RECEPTOR PROTEIN

An important consideration at the time of biopsy if the entire tumor is removed, or if no mastectomy is contemplated, is special care of the specimen so that an estrogen-receptor protein (ER) analysis can be performed on the fresh or frozen tumor tissue. An adequate amount of tissue (usually $\geqq 500$ mg) and immediate cooling are necessary. The presence of this special cytoplasmic protein that binds estradiol identifies the tumor as being hormonally dependent (*i.e.*, having a 67% probability of responding to hormone or endocrine therapy), and the probability of hormone responsiveness increases with the concentration of ER. More importantly, its absence signifies that such therapy will almost certainly be of no use (< 8% chance of a response). This information is of considerable importance if adjuvant therapy in conjunction with mastectomy or if palliative therapy for recurrence is being considered. Since recurrent tumors after mastectomy may prove inaccessible, routine assay of primary tumors at the time they are removed is a wise precaution. If tumor tissue contains progesterone receptors as well as estrogen receptors, the likelihood of a response to hormonal or endocrine therapy is raised to almost 90%. Of additional importance is that the presence of ER signifies a relatively good prognosis. Analysis of tumor tissue for hormone-receptor proteins has rapidly become a routine procedure in the management of patients with cancer of the breast (Degenshein, *et al.*, 1979).

INVESTIGATIONAL TECHNIQUES OF DETECTION

Still under investigation for detection of breast disease are computed tomography, thermography, and ultrasound. *Computed tomography* can be performed with acceptable levels of radiation exposure but is a cumbersome and lengthy procedure. Its advantage over mammography is perhaps in the evaluation of very dense breasts. However, in one study 35% of subsequently proved carcinomas were missed by this technique; difficulties included failure to detect microcalcifications.

Thermography (see p. 1184), which produces a visual pattern of heat from the skin of the breast, depends for detection upon the fact that many cancers have a high metabolic rate and are, therefore, hotter than surrounding tissues. It has the advantage of involving no irradiation exposure or direct contact with the pa-

tient, but interpretation is subjective, false-positive rates are high, and many cancers produce no abnormalities.

Ultrasound examination of the breast is superior to x-ray mammography in the visualization of discrete cysts in breasts with dense tissues. Cysts measuring 0.2 to 0.4 cm can be identified using this technique and distinguished from solid lesions. It involves no irradiation, and at present there is no evidence that damage to tissues occurs or that the examination facilitates the spread of cancer (see also p. 1173).

BREAST SELF-EXAMINATION

Most cancers (70% in a survey of tumor registries by the American College of Surgeons) continue to be found by patients themselves as a lump or nipple discharge. Yet too few women do routine self-examinations, a practice that should be encouraged. The objective is to detect tumors at the smallest possible size when they are most likely to be localized and curable. Many neglect this examination for fear of making an unwanted discovery, but most are willing to do so if instructed properly (Fig. 59–12). Women expect their obstetrician–gynecologist to be informed on this subject, and the initial office visit is an opportune time at which to provide instruction. Supplementary literature on breast self-examination is available from the American Cancer Society, the Department of Health and Human Services, and other sources.

Self-examination should begin when a woman reaches adulthood. The examination is performed monthly, an interval generally sanctioned as convenient and not unduly repetitious, the best time for premenopausal women is during the week after menstruation ceases. Most women's breasts are less tender and swollen at this time, permitting a thorough examination without discomfort. Inconsequential changes are also least likely to be present. After menopause, when cyclic changes have ceased, timing is not critical and, since menses no longer serve as a reminder, any regular time such as the first day of the month may be chosen for the examination. The time of bathing provides several conveniences: privacy, freedom from clothing confinements, and the opportunity to examine the breast with the skin wet and soapy, which seems to aid palpation by providing additional sensitivity.

The breasts are both viewed and manually examined. While standing before a mirror, the woman should view her breasts first facing forward with the arms relaxed at the sides and then alternately turning the torso to each side. Notable is asymmetry (some is normally present, since the breasts are seldom of equal size), unusually prominent veins, nipple deviation or inversion, and prominences or skin changes. Dimpling of the skin is particularly noteworthy. The arms are moved in various positions to elicit dimpling that may not be obvious otherwise. These positions include fully extending the arms above the head, placing them on top of the head and, finally, placing the hands upon the hips and pressing inward to tighten the pectoral muscles.

The palpatory examination should be performed thoroughly and systematically, including the entire breast, from clavicle to costal margin and from midline to lateral chest. Ideally, the examination is performed in the supine position; raising the side to be examined by placing a pillow under the back facilitates palpation by flattening and distributing the breasts more evenly on the chest wall. The flats of the fingers, not the tips, are used, pressing firmly with a fine rotating motion. Palpation proceeds from the periphery in a diminishing spiral toward the nipple. Alternatively, the breast may be considered to be a wheel with radiating spokes, and each spoke is examined, in turn, from nipple to periphery.

This portion of the examination can also be done effectively in the shower or in the bathtub, in which case one has the advantage of wet and soapy skin. The axillary extension of the breasts should not be missed and an axillary examination can be added. Attention is also given to the nipple, which is palpated, and a gentle squeeze can elicit discharge if it is present.

As a woman becomes familiar with her breasts through repeated examinations, she is better able to appreciate significant changes. She should be aware that most lumps are not cancers, but that persistent masses, discharge, or skin changes should prompt medical consultation.

STAGING OF BREAST CANCER

The choice of treatment for cancer of the breast is guided by the stage, or apparent extent, of the tumor. The "clinical" stage is determined by physical examination, radiographs, blood tests, and isotopic scans. Examples of current clinical classifications are the Columbia Clinical Classification and the TNM systems of The American Joint Committee for Cancer Staging and End Results Reporting (Fig. 59–13) and of the International Union Against Cancer. Tumors localized to the breast (Stage I) and those with limited spread to axillary lymph nodes (Stage II and many of Stage III) are generally treated by mastectomy. Localized cancers are highly curable by mastectomy and almost uniformly so if the tumor is still noninvasive. The expectation of surgical cure is less in cases with clinically involved axillary nodes, but still can be obtained in a substantial number of cases. Locally unresectable and disseminated cases (Stage IV) are treated for palliation by irradiation to the breast and regional nodes and with hormonal, endocrine, or chemotherapy.

The extent of disease determined from resected tissues constitutes the "pathologic" stage. The pathologic stage of cases treated surgically is based primarily upon the absence (Stage I) or presence (Stage II) of metastases in axillary lymph nodes. This is the single

(*Text continues on p. 1208.*)

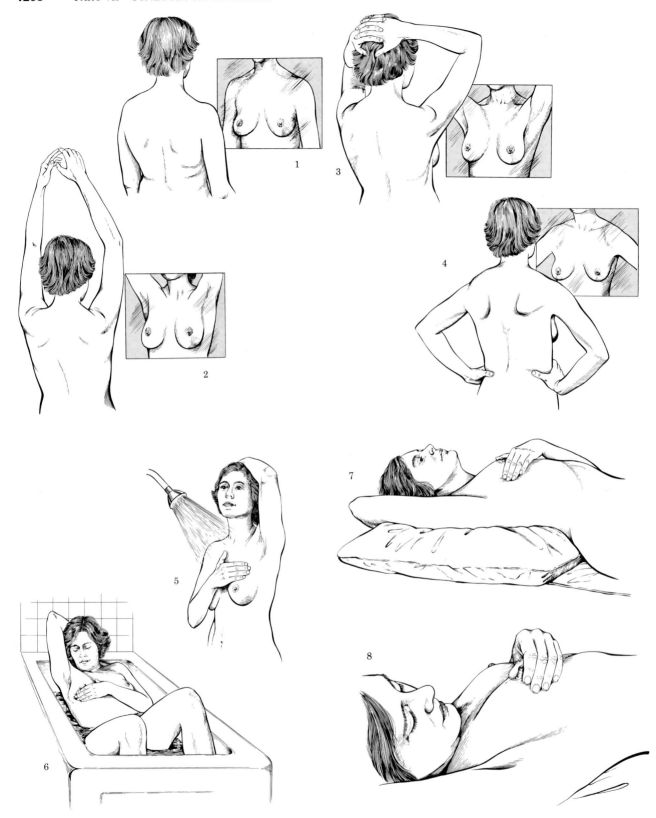

◄**FIG. 59-12.** *1.* Breast self-examination is begun with inspection using a mirror. Attention is given to contours of breast and to skin. *2.* Arms are extended high above head, watching for abnormal motion or skin retraction. *3.* Pressure is placed on back of head to tense the pectoralis major muscles that underlie mammary tissues. *4.* Inward pressure on hips serves to tense pectoralis major muscles. Retraction of skin is a sign of abnormality. *5.* Wet soapy skin facilitates manual examination of breast for lumps. *6.* Tub bathing provides an optimal time for discovering lumps. Wet skin permits easy motion of examining hand, and reclining position flattens breast tissues upon chest wall. *7.* Palpatory examination is best performed in supine position with side to be examined elevated on a pillow or blanket. Lumps are most evident when breast is flattened and evenly distributed upon chest wall. As a woman gains familiarity with appearance and feel of her breasts through repeated examinations, she becomes more capable of appreciating changes. *8.* Self-examination is completed with a squeeze of nipple to detect abnormal discharge.

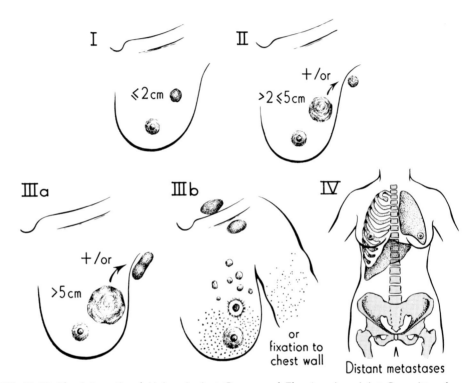

FIG. 59-13. The International Union Against Cancer and The American Joint Committee for Cancer Staging and End Results Reporting recognizes four clinical stages of invasive mammary carcinoma. *Stage I* includes tumors confined to breast and no more than 2 cm in diameter. *Stage II* includes larger tumors localized to breast but not exceeding 5 cm in diameter or cancers with small, mobile, clinically involved axillary lymph nodes. *Stage IIIa* consists of large tumors exceeding 5 cm in diameter or cancers that have produced clinically enlarged axillary lymph nodes fixed to one another or to adjacent tissues. *Stage IIIb* designates more advanced, but still undisseminated cancers with evidence of direct involvement of skin such as edema, ulceration, or satellite nodules and those with fixation to chest wall or with clinically evident supraclavicular or infraclavicular nodal metastases. Cases with edema of ipsilateral arm are also Stage IIIb. All cases with distant metastases are *Stage IV*. Noninvasive cancers are classified separately as *Stage TIS* (tumor-in-situ), not pictured here.

most important prognosticator, and cure becomes progressively less likely with the presence and the extent of nodal involvement. The importance of this information for prognosis, and the reason further treatment is usually considered for patients with metastases, are evident from Table 59–2. When metastases are present in nodes, surgical treatment is often supplemented by systemic chemotherapy or irradiation to the thorax in order to reduce or delay recurrence.

Staging is also useful for estimating the prognosis after treatment and for comparing the results of different treatments. The prognoses of white and black women according to the Cancer Surveillance, Epidemiology, and End Results (SEER) program of the U.S. Department of Health, Education, and Welfare are shown in Table 59–3. This four-stage system, recognized by the American College of Surgeons, is based upon both clinical and histologic information to categorize cases as being 1) in situ, 2) localized to the breast, 3) regionalized (involvement of adjacent tissues or signs of early axillary nodal involvement), and 4) disseminated.

TREATMENT OF BREAST CANCER

Surgical removal of the breast is the preferred treatment for potentially curable cases of breast cancer. Removal of the entire organ is predicated upon the fact that cancer is often multifocal in the breast rather than confined to a single site. The knowledge that regional lymph nodes in the axilla contain metastases in at least 40% of cases whether or not they appear clinically involved has provided the rationale for routinely removing regional lymph nodes and varying amounts of intervening tissues.

RADICAL MASTECTOMY

Until recently en bloc removal of the entire breast, the underlying pectoralis major and pectoralis minor muscles, and the entire axillary contents—the so-called radical mastectomy—was the standard treatment for operable breast cancer. This operation has been supplanted by an increasing turn to the less extensive modified radical mastectomy, a procedure that is equally effective and is less deforming. Approximately 60% of all women treated with radical or modified mastectomy survive for at least 5 years. The results as influenced by axillary nodal status are shown in Table 59–2.

MODIFIED RADICAL MASTECTOMY

Modified radical mastectomy is presently the operation most widely used for carcinoma of the breast. This surgical procedure allows for the removal of the entire breast and a varying amount of axillary tissue but spares the pectoralis major muscle, thereby preventing deformity of the anterior chest wall and facilitating subsequent reconstruction of the breast should the patient desire it. The Patey version of the modified radical mastectomy entails removal of the entire axillary contents including the pectoralis minor muscle; the Auchincloss version spares the pectoralis minor muscle while removing lymph nodes from the low and mid-axilla. The latter is frequently employed when limited involvement of axillary lymph nodes is suspected.

TABLE 59–2. SURVIVAL OF PATIENTS TREATED WITH RADICAL MASTECTOMY ACCORDING TO AXILLARY NODAL STATUS

| Category | No. | Percent Survival | |
		5 years	10 years
All cases	406	63.5	45.9
Negative axillary nodes	207	78.1	64.9
Positive axillary nodes	207	46.5	24.9
1–3 positive nodes	107	62.2	37.5
≧ 4 positive nodes	100	32.0	13.4

(Fisher, et al: Surg Gynecol Obstet 140:528, 1975)

TABLE 59–3. STAGE OF BREAST CANCER VERSUS PROGNOSIS

| Stage | Relative Survival (%)* | | | |
| | 5-year | | 10-year | |
	White	Black	White	Black
All Stages	64	46	52	41
Localized	84	77	74	77
Regional	54	44	39	34
Disseminated	7	6	2	4

* Survival after correcting for deaths unrelated to breast cancer (Cancer Patient Survival, Report No. 5, 1978)

TOTAL MASTECTOMY WITH LOW AXILLARY DISSECTION

In this operation the surgeon removes the entire breast and all lymph nodes lateral to the pectoralis minor muscle (*i.e.,* the low axillary lymph nodes). Its major indication is noninvasive carcinoma of the breast, and it has the primary objective of removing all mammary parenchyma, including the axillary tail of Spence, and providing a limited sampling of axillary lymph nodes.

EXTENDED RADICAL MASTECTOMY

This surgical procedure adds en bloc removal of the internal mammary lymph nodes to the radical mastec-

tomy. Although these lymph nodes contain metastases in approximately 25% of surgical cases, their removal is technically difficult and results are not significantly better. In general, metastases at this site can be controlled equally well with irradiation.

SEGMENTAL MASTECTOMY

Surgical removal of less than the entire breast has obvious cosmetic advantages but relies upon high-dose irradiation to control any cancer in the remaining breast tissue and regional lymph node groups. Whether this approach is equally as curative as more extensive surgery is presently under investigation at a number of medical centers, and early results are promising (Veronesi). It is apparent that gross residual cancer and low doses of irradiation lead to unsatisfactory results (Margolese).

IRRADIATION

Information is becoming available regarding the treatment of operable stages of breast cancer, primarily with high energy irradiation. In these stages surgery is limited to preliminary local excision of the tumor mass (lumpectomy) for estrogen receptor determination and sampling of ipsilateral axillary lymph nodes for the purpose of pathologic staging. There is still not enough experience with this procedure and cases are highly selected, but control of cancer in the breast and in regional lymph nodes appears to be comparable to that achieved with standard forms of mastectomy after limited periods of observation. The cosmetic results are generally good, but complications of irradiation, sometimes necessitating removal of the breast, occur in 10% to 17% of cases. Also, the long-term morbidity, which may include carcinogenesis, is yet to be evaluated.

Irradiation to the breast and regional lymphatics provides the best method for local control of unresectable advanced breast cancers. Limited mastectomy, when it is technically feasible, to eliminate gross tumor seems to improve the chances for effective palliation.

Postoperative irradiation to the mastectomy site and the axillary, supraclavicular, and internal mammary lymph nodes is often employed when metastases are found in the axillary lymph nodes removed with mastectomy, or when cancers are located medially in the breast, suggesting increased likelihood that internal mammary lymph nodes contain metastases. This supplemental treatment undoubtedly reduces the frequency of recurrence in the irradiated areas but does not improve the prospects for cure; its use is declining in favor of systemic adjuvant chemotherapy.

Preoperative irradiation to the breasts and regional lymph nodes is sometimes used for locally advanced tumors prior to mastectomy and has theoretic advantages, but benefits in terms of improved cures are difficult to demonstrate.

Localized irradiation of painful bony metastases can produce dramatic relief of pain and promote osseous repair. It is often employed for this purpose in cases with disseminated cancer in conjunction with other therapy. Whole brain irradiation is also particularly useful for controlling symptomatic intracranial metastases.

CHEMOTHERAPY

A broad spectrum of cytoxic agents provide effective palliation for breast cancer and are often used in three to five drug combinations. Adriamycin, Cytoxan, Methotrexate, and Fluorouracil are the most successful. Systemic chemotherapy has two roles in management: 1) systemic adjuvant therapy designed to improve the results of mastectomy and 2) palliative treatment of advanced disease. Prolonged treatment with chemotherapy after mastectomy is justified when lymph nodes contain metastases, since these patients are at high risk for recurrence. Adjuvant chemotherapy results in definite prolongation of disease-free survival as well as reduction in local recurrence of tumor. The most impressive benefits are achieved with combinations of drugs and are seen in premenopausal women, but postmenopausal women also can benefit.

Systemic chemotherapy has a well-established place in the treatment of patients with disseminated breast cancers. Forty percent to 60% of cancers regress in response to treatment, and regressions are associated with extended survival. Chemotherapy is, in fact, the initial management of patients who are unlikely to respond to hormone or endocrine therapy, e.g., those whose tumors contain no estrogen-receptor protein or those who have predominantly visceral metastases.

ENDOCRINE AND HORMONE THERAPY

Approximately one-third of patients with disseminated breast cancer will derive worthwhile benefit from oophorectomy, adrenalectomy, or hypophysectomy, or from the administration of estrogens, androgens, progesterones, or anti-estrogens. Knowledge of the estrogen-receptor protein (ER) content of the patient's tumor considerably improves selection for therapy. The presence of ER increases the likelihood of a beneficial response to 60% to 70%. If ER is lacking, fewer than 10% will respond. It has, therefore, become routine to perform the assay on primary tumors removed with mastectomy in case inaccessible metastases should appear later; in advanced cases, primaries or metastases may be biopsied or removed simply to obtain tissue for assay.

BREAST CANCER DURING PREGNANCY

Special problems are posed when breast cancer occurs in conjunction with pregnancy. Since only 20% of breast cancers occur in premenopausal women, this concurrence is unusual, and few clinicians face the problem during their professional careers. Breast cancer has the reputation of being a more virulent disease than usual in the pregnant or lactating female, but there is mounting evidence that the disappointing experiences reported in the past have resulted from tardy diagnosis and less than vigorous treatment.

The principles of prompt diagnosis and optimal treatment are the same as those in the absence of pregnancy. Opinion at present is to treat the cancer and not be distracted by the pregnancy. When the extent of disease is comparable, the prognosis for cure of the young is essentially that for the elderly and of the pregnant, essentially that for the nonpregnant.

Only 3% of breast cancers are diagnosed during pregnancy or the puerperium. From another perspective, no more than three of every 10,000 pregnancies are accompanied by cancer of the breast. The rising age-specific incidence of breast cancer after the age of 30 years converges with the declining frequency of pregnancies after this age to place most patients with this convergence of circumstances early in their fourth decade of life.

The relatively poor prognosis of pregnant patients can be directly related to the extent of disease at the time of treatment, particularly the high frequency of axillary node involvement, which continues to range from 50% to 85% in surgical cases.

Both physiologic changes and suboptimal management may be disadvantageous to pregnant patients. Rising levels of plasma corticosteroids and perhaps the rise of prolactin and depressed cellular immunity might be expected to enhance the growth and spread of mammary carcinoma. Enlargement and increased vascularity of the breast not only tends to obscure and delay the detection of masses but to invite dissemination through hematogenous and lymphatic routes as well. Too often, however, physician delay results from failure to appreciate the significance of a breast mass or uncertainty about management in this situation.

The signs and symptoms of breast cancer in pregnant women are identical to those in nonpregnant women, and the frequency with which masses prove to be cancerous is also comparable (*e.g.*, approximately one per five biopsies).

Expeditious management serves the patient best and involves only small risk for the fetus. Mammograms are neither desirable nor useful because the breasts are too dense. Furthermore, biopsies should be performed under local anesthesia whenever possible in order to minimize the risk of spontaneous abortion. The increasing trend to outpatient biopsy under local anesthesia is particularly attractive for the pregnant patient. If a mastectomy is necessary, procrastination because of the pregnancy or other reasons is unwise. With modern anesthesia the fetal loss when biopsies or mastectomies are performed under general anesthesia is small (1.2% in Byrd's series).

From 70% to 90% of cases are diagnosed in operable stages, and their prognosis for 5-year cure with mastectomy approximates 50%, only 10% lower than that for nonpregnant patients. Still, more than half are found to have metastases in axillary lymph nodes, and this continues to be a potent prognostic influence. When nodes are involved, the 5-year survival reported in the last 40 years approximates 25%, rising to 60% when nodes are free.

Other influences upon the results of mastectomy are the clinical stage and the trimester of pregnancy in which the cancer is discovered and treated. Prognosis is appreciably better during the first trimester of pregnancy or during the postpartum period. Poor results are associated with the second and third trimesters of pregnancy. This may be an illusion created by the difficulty of detecting cancers in early stages during late pregnancy and possibly by procrastination in their treatment.

THERAPEUTIC ABORTION

As adjuvants to potentially curative mastectomy, therapeutic abortion and prophylactic castration have not improved the outlook for cure and are not justified as routine measures. Patients at high risk for treatment failure because of axillary metastases may be candidates for systemic adjuvant chemotherapy or postoperative irradiation. Adjuvant chemotherapy has resulted in a substantial improvement in the disease-free survival of premenopausal patients, but during pregnancy entails the risk of abnormal fetal development or spontaneous abortion, particularly in the first trimester. Complete protection of the fetus is also not possible during chest wall irradiation. Therefore, if chemotherapy or postoperative irradiation is to be used, it is best delayed until after delivery or preceded by therapeutic abortion.

Effective palliation of advanced and disseminated breast cancer during pregnancy ordinarily requires therapeutic abortion. Continued placental function negates the value of therapeutic castration or adrenalectomy, and intensive chemotherapy or irradiation is hazardous to normal fetal development. If palliation is not urgent and is consistent with the patient's wishes, treatment might be delayed for a short period to permit a normal delivery or obtain a viable fetus.

PREGNANCIES SUBSEQUENT TO MASTECTOMY

No more than 7% of fertile women become pregnant after mastectomy and 70% of these do so within the

first 5 years. The evidence is clear that despite the theoretic disadvantages of pregnancy after a mastectomy for carcinoma of the breast, it does not promote recurrence. This is true whether the pregnancy occurs early or late; thus it is unlikely to be a selective phenomenon in which only those with a favorable prognosis survive long enough to become pregnant. On these grounds, therefore, recommendations for prophylactic castration or contraception have little support.

Future pregnancies would seem unwise, however, if the probability of recurrence and death is high, eventualities that would prevent the patient from assuming the continuing responsibilities of motherhood. The highest risk of recurrence is during the first 2 years after mastectomy, and this gradually declines, reaching a permanently low level after 8 to 10 years.

The 10-year risk of recurrence observed for nonpregnant women with axillary metastases is high, approximating 67%, with risk concentrated in the first 5 years. Most authorities recommend, therefore, that women with metastases in axillary lymph nodes delay a subsequent pregnancy for 2 to 5 years until some assurance of continued well-being can be established. Failure rates after mastectomy for those with four or more positive nodes is sufficiently high (*i.e.*, 86% within 10 years), that little reassurance can be given. With uninvolved axillary lymph nodes the risk of recurrence is considerably lower (*i.e.*, 24% within 10 years), and pregnancy is unlikely to be complicated by recurrence. Nevertheless, risk is still concentrated in the first 3 postoperative years.

The point must be made that although the risk of recurrence diminishes with time, it is never eliminated. Recurrence can appear after many years, following one or more successful and uncomplicated pregnancies.

REFERENCES AND RECOMMENDED READING

American Joint Committee for Cancer Staging and End-results Reporting: Manual for Staging of Cancer, pp 101–107. Chicago, Whiting Press, 1978

Anderson DE: A genetic study of human breast cancer. J Natl Cancer Inst 48:1029, 1974

Bandeian J, Horton CE, Rosato FE: Evaluation of patients after augmentation mammoplasty. Surg Gynecol Obstet 147:596, 1978

Bassett LW, Gold RH, Cove HC: Mammographic spectrum of traumatic fat necrosis: The fallibility of "pathognomonic" signs of carcinoma. Am J Roentgenol 130:119, 1978

Bedwinek JM, Perez CA, Kramer S, et al: Irradiation as the primary management of stage I and II adenocarcinoma of the breast. Cancer Clinical Trials 3:11, 1980

Best JJK, Asbury DL, George WD, Sellwood RA, Isherwood I: Computed tomography (CT) of the breast. Clin Oncol 3(4):394, 1977

Breslow L, Thomas LB, Upton AC: Final reports of the National Cancer Institute ad hoc working groups on mammography in screening for breast cancer and a summary report of their joint findings and recommendations. J Natl Cancer Inst 59(2):468, 1977

British Breast Group: Steroid-receptor assays in human breast cancer. A statement by the British Breast Group and colleagues. Lancet 1:298, 1980

Brownstein MH, Wolf M, Bikowski JB: Cowden's disease. A cutaneous marker of breast cancer. Cancer 41:2393, 1978

Byrd BF, Jr., Bayer DS, Robertson JC et al: Treatment of breast tumors associated with pregnancy and lactation. Ann Surg 155:940, 1962

Coombs LJ, Lilienfeld AM, Bross IDJ, Burnett WS: A prospective study of the relationship between benign breast diseases and breast carcinoma. Prev Med 8:40, 1979

Degenshein GA, Ceccarelli F, Bloom ND, Tobin EH: Hormone relationships in breast cancer: The role of receptor-binding proteins. In Ravitch MM (ed): Current Problems in Surgery, Vol. 16, No. 6, pp 1–59. Chicago, Year Book Medical Publishers, 1979

Donegan WL: Breast cancer and pregnancy. Obstet Gynecol 59(2):244, 1977

Farewell VT, Math B, Math M: The combined effect of breast cancer risk factors. Cancer 40:931, 1977

Fasal E, Paffenbarger RS: Oral contraceptives as related to cancer and benign lesions of the breast. J Nat Cancer Inst 55(4):767, 1975

Fisher B, Slack N, Katrych D, Wolmark N: Ten-year follow-up results of patients with carcinoma of the breast in a cooperative clinical trial evaluating surgical adjuvant chemotherapy. Surg Gynecol Obstet 140:528, 1975

Gapinski PV, Donegan WL: Estrogen receptors and breast cancer: Prognostic and therapeutic implications. Surgery 88:386, 1980

Golinger RC: Hormones and the pathophysiology of fibrocystic mastopathy. Surg Gynecol Obstet 146:273, 1978

Gray LA, Sr: Breast pain: Causes, workup, and treatment. CONSULTANT, 1976

Harmer MH (ed): TNM Classification of Malignant Tumors, 3rd ed. pp 47–56. Geneva, International Union Against Cancer, 1978

Harris JR, Levene MB, Hellman S: Results of treating stage I and II carcinoma of the breast with primary irradiation therapy. Cancer Treatment Reports 62:985, 1978

Hoover R, Gray LA Sr, Cole P, MacMahon B: Menopausal estrogens and breast cancer. N Engl J Med 295(8):401, 1976

Hubay CA, Barry FM, Marr CC: Pregnancy and breast cancer. Surg Clin N Am 58(4):819, 1978

Leavitt T Jr: The role of the obstetrician–gnecologist in the diagnosis and treatment of breast cancer. BREAST 4(3):19, 1978

Leis HP Jr: The diagnosis of breast cancer. CA 27(4):209, 1977

Lipsett MB: Estrogen use and cancer risk. J Am Med Assoc 237(11):1112, 1977

Lipsett MB: Postoperative radiation for women with cancer of the breast and positive axillary nodes. Should it continue? N Engl J Med 304:112, 1981

Margolese RG: Current concepts in the management of primary breast cancer. Can J Surg 20(3):199, 1977

Minton JP, Foecking MK, Webster DJT, Matthews RH: Caffeine, cyclic nucleotides, and breast disease. Surgery 86(1):105, 1979

Nemoto T: Changing treatment for breast cancer: A survey of surgeons. BREAST 4(1):16, 1978

Perry S: Recommendations of the Consensus Development Panel on Breast Cancer Screening. Cancer Research 38:476, 1978

Peters TG, Donegan WL, Burg EA: Minimal breast cancer: A clinical appraisal. Ann Surg 186(6):704, 1977

Rosemond GP, Maier WP, Brobyn TJ: Needle aspiration of breast cysts. Surg Gynecol Obstet 128:351, 1969

Sitruk-Ware R, Sterkers N, Mauvaris-Jarvis P: Benign breast disease I: Hormonal investigation. Obstet Gynecol 53:457, 1979

Urban JA, Egeli RA: Non-lactational nipple discharge. CA 28(3):130, 1978

Veronesi U, Saccozzi R, Del Vecchio M, et al: Comparing radical mastectomy with quadrantectomy, axillary dissection, and radiotherapy in patients with small cancers of the breast. N Engl J Med 305:6, 1981

Wolfe JN: Breast patterns as an index of risk for developing breast cancer. Am J Roentgenol 126:1130, 1976

PART **VIII**

RADIATION AND SURGERY IN GYNECOLOGY

CHAPTER 60

RADIATION THERAPY IN GYNECOLOGY

Philip J. DiSaia
James F. Nolan
A. N. Arneson

All life on this planet has evolved in a milieu in which the major source of energy essential for most biologic processes is in the form of radiant energy (*radiation*). Various forms of radiation influence living material in a variety of ways: sunlight provides heat, light, and energy for plant photosynthesis; radio waves provide a means of communication. These radiations are not harmful in ordinary quantities, but actually benefit life processes. However, certain types of high-energy (*ionizing*) radiations are not so harmless, but provide useful tools in gynecology, both for diagnostic and therapeutic purposes. These high-energy radiations can be traumatic to biologic material, and their use in oncology depends upon their ability to inflict an injury from which normal tissue recovers more effectively than malignant tissue. They are known to produce deleterious effects on all forms of life from the relatively simple unicellular plants and animals to the complex higher organisms.

The change produced by ionizing radiations is some-times grossly apparent and may be visible soon after exposure of the living organism, but more often the radiation does not appear (on cursory examination) to have affected the organism at all. It may produce small changes that can be detected only by careful chemical or microscopic study and that may not become apparent for many years or, indeed, may manifest themselves only in the offspring of the irradiated organism. The attitude concerning radiation exposure should always be that diagnostic tests, therapeutic radiation, or radiation acquired incidentally from the environment may all be detrimental. Although in many instances the chance of injury is slight, the possibility of damage from a known exposure must always be weighed against the importance of the information to be gained or effect desired. Certainly, incidental exposure must be avoided through control of environmental hazards wherever possible.

NATURE AND EFFECTS OF IONIZING RADIATION

The radiation emitted by radium is used in the treatment of a wide variety of malignancies. In addition, over the past three decades, machines capable of producing radiant energy of high intensity (supervoltage, megavoltage) have become available and are used extensively in the treatment of malignancies. Those machines that emit energies greater than 1 million electron volts (1 mev) are the most commonly used at the present time. Among these pieces of equipment are cobalt generators, betatrons, and linear accelerators (see Table 60–1).

PHYSICAL AND CHEMICAL NATURE

The physical forces of concern here are called *ionizing radiations* because of their characteristic ability to transfer their energy to matter by separating orbital electrons from their atoms and thus forming physical ion pairs. The term is an inclusive one, since the phenomenon may be caused by particulate radiations as well as electromagnetic waves. This discussion is limited to those electromagnetic radiations with wavelengths in the range of 10^{-7} to 10^{-10} cm (10 to 10^{-3}Å). Those radiations that originate from decay of an atomic nucleus are termed γ-*rays* (*gamma rays*); those that originate outside the atomic nucleus are termed *x-rays* and are produced when high-energy charged particles (electrons) bombard a suitable target such as tungsten. When these fast-moving electrons approach the fields around the nuclei of the atoms of the target material, they are deflected from their path and energy is emitted in the form of electromagnetic radiation. These emitted x-rays may have any energy from zero to a maximum as determined by the kinetic energy of the impinging electrons. Machines such as the betatron are capable of generating electrons at high accelera-

TABLE 60-1. MODALITIES OF EXTERNAL RADIATION

Modality	Voltage	Source
Low voltage (superficial)	85–150 kv	X-ray
Medium voltage (orthovoltage)	180–400 kv	X-ray
Supervoltage	500 kv–8 mv	X-ray
		^{60}Co
		^{137}Cs
		^{226}Ra
Megavoltage	Above supervoltage energy	Betatron
		Synchrotron
		Linear accelerator

tions and, therefore, the x-rays generated by these machines are quite high in energy. A continuous spectrum of x-rays of various energies can be produced when a large number of impinging electrons is involved. Other x-rays are produced when a high-speed electron impinging on the target material knocks out an orbital electron (ionization) from a target atom. When this electron is from an inner shell, its place is immediately taken by an electron from an outer shell, and during this latter transition an x-ray is given off. The photon energy of that x-ray represents the difference in energies of the inner and outer orbital electron levels. It should be remembered that γ-rays and x-rays can be collectively termed *photons,* and it is the energy of the photon, not its source, that is important.

The interaction of photons with matter takes place primarily through three mechanisms: the photoelectric effect, Compton scattering, and pair production. All of these processes result in either ionization of molecules within the target or free radical formation. Free hydrogen atoms and free hydroxyl radicals commonly result from the bombardment of water by high-energy photons (Fig. 60–1).

About one-half of the H atoms encounter OH radicals and form H_2O_2. In the irradiation of water by electrons or photons, very few of the H atoms or OH radicals are formed close enough to one another to react quickly before they diffuse. The addition of O_2, however, causes the H atoms to react to form the radical HO_2. This is less reactive than the OH radical and permits the decomposition of water to H_2O_2 to proceed. These excited and ionized molecules are very unstable and react with proteins and other key substances within the cell. Multiple other events may occur with photon bombardment: longchain molecules may be split and regrouped, aggregates may be produced, and ring forms may be disrupted indiscriminately. Certain chemical bonds may be vulnerable to inactivation by oxidation, resulting in loss of functional capacity. All of these chemical changes may ultimately be translated into biologic injury at the cellular level.

BIOLOGIC EFFECTS

The mechanism of cell injury from radiation is varied, and the effects may become manifest at different time intervals after the primary event depending upon the type of intracellular target affected and the time in which certain chemical constituents are called upon to perform. Thus, following some injury by ionization, a mature cell in a state of low metabolic activity may be grossly unaffected while an actively growing cell may be destroyed. Cells in the act of dividing are more vulnerable than those resting between mitoses. Low oxygen tension, dehydration, freezing, and the presence of chemical reducing agents may significantly protect cells from radiation injury. Radiation injury manifests itself as swelling of the cell, vacuolization of the cytoplasm, giant-cell formation, and fragmentation or partial separation of the chromosomes at the time of division. There occurs, after a latent period, evidence of cell death with loss of nuclear and cytoplasmic structure. Response is the typical inflammatory reaction— edema, capillary dilatation and proliferation, infiltration of round cells, and a fibroblastic response. This immediate reaction is followed by gradual fibrosis, avascularity, and a walling off of the injured area (see Fig. 60–2). Very late changes are scarification and contracture, with occasional inelastic dilated blood vessels pinched off by essentially avascular stroma.

The selective destruction of tissues forms the basis of therapeutic radiology. Neoplastic cells are always more easily killed by radiation than are their parent cells of the surrounding normal tissues. The magnitude of the difference in radiovulnerability between normal and cancerous tissues determines, in large part, whether the particular portion of the disease considered for radiation can be eradicated. This relative difference in local radiovulnerability is referred to as a difference in *radiosensitivity.* Radiosensitivity and radiocurability are not identical in meaning. Relatively radioresistant tumors accessible to high-dose local radiotherapy are curable, whereas radiosensitive tumors that are at the start of therapy or shortly thereafter widely metastasized can only be controlled locally. An excellent example of a relatively radioresistant tumor is squamous cell carcinoma of the cervix. Yet this malignancy remains one of the most curable tumors because of its accessibility to high-dose radiation and the relatively radioresistant nature of the hosting normal tissues (cervix and vagina). The ability to place in juxtaposition to the malignancy a dose of radium that is tolerated by the surrounding normal tissue contributes to success.

As a result of the chemical changes described above, very large molecules (common in biologic systems) undergo a variety of structural changes that may lead to altered function. *Degradation,* or breaking into smaller units, has been shown to occur when large molecules are radiated. *Cross-linking* is another common structural change. A long molecule that is some-

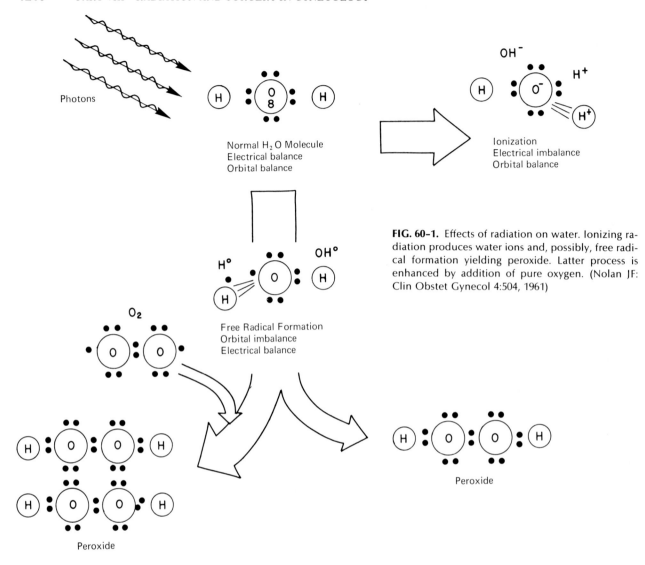

FIG. 60-1. Effects of radiation on water. Ionizing radiation produces water ions and, possibly, free radical formation yielding peroxide. Latter process is enhanced by addition of pure oxygen. (Nolan JF: Clin Obstet Gynecol 4:504, 1961)

what flexible in structure can undergo intramolecular cross-linking when a chemically active locus is produced on it and when this spot can come in contact with another reactive area. If the cross-linking is extensive, not only are the molecules incapable of normal function, but they may no longer be soluble in the system. Many macromolecules are held in a rigid configuration by intramolecular cross-linking bonds, *i.e.,* specific chemical groups are linked together, frequently by hydrogen atoms, to form a three-dimensional structure. The hydrogen bonds are among the weakest in the molecule and, thus, are the first to be broken by radiation. Such structural changes can lead to severe alterations in the biochemical properties of the molecule.

In this manner, radiation effects on molecules such as proteins, enzymes, nucleic acids, and certain lipids can profoundly affect the cell, which in turn can alter the organ and organism. The initial chemical change occurs in but a fraction of a second and is rarely detected directly. Some of these chemical changes are repaired almost immediately; others that occur within less important structures may result in alterations that are rarely recognizable. In the majority, the transition between a chemical change in a system and the biologic manifestation of this change is complicated and often obscure. Absorption and utilization of energy by a cell is a complex chain of events in which multiple proteins are involved; radiation damage to these vital proteins can result in loss of cell membrane integrity and even cell death.

Although a variety of morphologic and functional changes have been described in irradiated cells, the bulk of both direct and inferential evidence suggests

that the cell nucleus is the major site of radiation damage leading to cell death. For example, it has been calculated that 1 million rads is required to damage a cell membrane.* In contrast, chromosomal aberrations and mutations can be produced by low radiation doses. Since only a few hundred rads are needed to kill most proliferating cells in tissue culture, it seems most logical that the nuclear changes produced by the low doses are responsible for cell death.

GENETIC EFFECTS

It is not possible to assign a specific mutation rate to a specific radiation dose. Gene loci differ markedly in their mutability, and the rather random damage exerted by radiation on any particular chromosome makes predictability exceedingly difficult. Certainly mitotic stage, cell type, sex, species, and dose rate all influence the rate of mutation production in lower animals and bacteria. Data accumulated in lower animals are difficult to extrapolate to man and, therefore, predictions about mutation rates cannot be expected on the basis of the evidence accumulated from various types of radiation exposure; direct evidence of radiation-induced mutation in man is lacking. The largest group of humans available for study are descendants of those exposed to radiation in Hiroshima and Nagasaki, and while there has been no detectable effect on the frequency of prenatal or neonatal deaths or on the frequency of malformations in the offspring of these persons, this does not mean that no hereditary effects have been produced by the radiation. The number of exposed parents was small and doses were so low that it would be surprising if an increase in mutation had been detected to date. Several generations are needed to reveal recessive damage.

It is, however, logical to expect that radiation exposure will increase the mutation rate in humans. This expectation is based largely upon experiments on mice. It is estimated that the dose that will double the spontaneous mutation rate for man lies between 10 and 100 rads. For an acute exposure to radiation the probable value is between 15 and 30 rads and for chronic irradiation it is probably around 100 rads. The Committee of Genetics of the Atomic Energy Commission has recommended that no individual from conception to the age of 30 years be subjected to more than 10 rads. With appropriate shielding to prevent scatter, improved x-ray film, image intensifiers, and the like it is possible to attain satisfactory roentgenographic visualization of internal structures with reduced exposure. The average radiation doses to a developing fetus and to the maternal gonads inflicted by some common diagnostic techniques are shown in Table 60–2.

EFFECTS ON THE FETUS

The classic effects of radiation on the mammalian embryo are 1) intrauterine and extrauterine growth retardation, 2) embryonic, fetal, or neonatal death, and 3) gross congenital malformations. The structure most readily and consistently affected by radiation is the central nervous system. If the *in utero* absorbed dose is below 25 rads, these classic effects of radiation are never observed together in experimental animals or, in all likelihood, in the human. Not only are the absorbed dose and the stage of gestation important in determining the effect of radiation on a mammalian embryo, but the dose rate must also be considered. Embryonic damage can be reduced significantly by decreasing the dose rate to allow recovery processes to function. Gross malformations occur most often when the fetus is irradiated during the early organogenic period, although cell, tissue, and organ hypoplasia can be produced by radiation throughout organogenic, fetal, and neonatal periods, if the dose is high enough. There is no stage of gestation during which exposure to 50 rads is not associated with significant probability of observable embryonic defect: death during the preimplantation period, malformations during the early organogenic stage, and cell deletions and tissue hypoplasia during the fetal stages. Animal experiments indicate that all embryos exposed to 100 rads or more after implantation exhibit some degree of growth retardation. Finding and recognizing radiation-induced deleterious effects in offspring irradiated *in utero* become increasingly difficult with decreasing doses (less than 10 rads) because such small doses are unlikely to produce such defects and because the natural incidence of defects is high. From the clinical point of view, an absorbed dose of 10 rads to the fetus at any time during gestation can be considered a practical threshold for the induction of congenital defects, below which the probability of producing adverse effects becomes exceedingly small. Diagnostic x-ray procedures (Table 60–2) should be avoided in the pregnant woman unless there is overwhelming urgency. In women of childbearing age, possible damage to an early conceptus may be prevented by performing such tests immediately after the commencement of a menstrual period (see also page 571).

GENERAL CONCEPTS OF RADIATION THERAPY

The technical modalities used in modern radiation therapy may be classified as external irradiation and local irradiation. *External irradiation* applies to radiant energy from sources at a distance from the body

---

* Quantity of radiation is expressed in roentgens (R) or rads. The roentgen is the unit of exposure, the rad the unit of absorbed dose. In the case of *x*- or γ-rays, exposure to 1 R results in an absorbed dose in soft tissue that is equivalent to 1 rad.

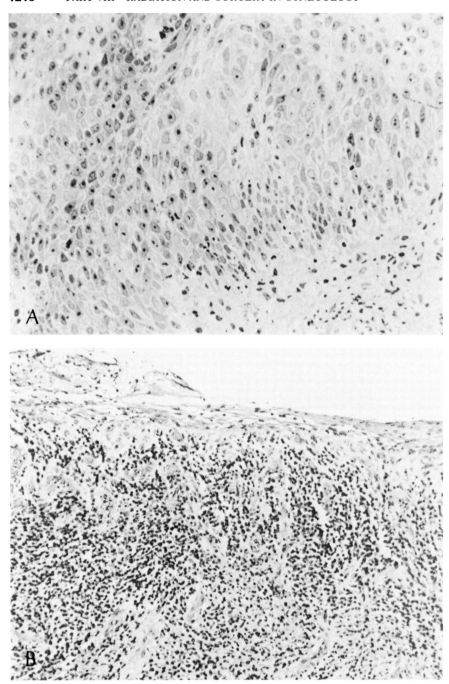

FIG. 60-2. *A.* Photomicrograph of benign cervical squamous epithelium immediately after re-moval of intracavitary radiation applicator. An estimated 15,000 rads had been absorbed in this area at the time of this biopsy. Note the intercellular edema and general acute necrosis. The base-ment membrane area appears smudged. Thick section was embedded in Epon after glutaralde-hyde fixation (× 298). *B.* The cervical squamous epithelium 6 weeks after radiation (intracavitary radioactive source) is thin and still coated with exudate in focal areas (*left*). Epithelial cells are va-cuolated. The underlying stroma is densely infiltrated by plasma cells and lymphocytes. Capillary endothelial cells appear swollen; some capillaries are occluded by fibrin thrombi. Estimated dose to epithelium in this area is approximately 30,000 rads. The patient had endometrial adenocarci-noma that did not involve this area prior to treatment (× 128).

(*Continued on next page*)

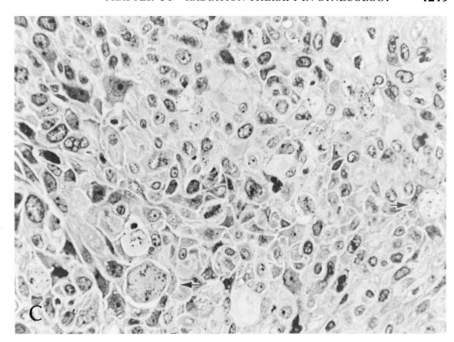

FIG. 60-2 (*Continued*). *C.* Epidermoid carcinoma of cervix immediately after removal of intracavitary radiation source. The most dramatic morphologic change is in cells undergoing mitosis. Note the swelling and disruption of mitotic spindles (*arrow*). Cytoplasm and nuclei of interphase cells are vacuolated; cytoplasm generally appeared swollen when compared to tumor pattern prior to radiation (× 255). (Kraus KT: Irradiation changes in the uterus. In Norris HJ, Hertig AT, Abell MR (eds): The Uterus. Baltimore, Williams & Wilkins, 1973)

TABLE 60-2. AVERAGE RADIATION DOSE TO FETUS AND TO MATERNAL GONADS FROM VARIOUS DIAGNOSTIC EXAMINATIONS

Examination	Dose to fetus and maternal gonads (millirads)
Lower extremity roentgenography	1
Cervical spine roentgenography	2
Skull roentgenography	4
Chest roentgenography	8
Pelvimetry	750
Chest fluoroscopy	70
Cholecystography	300
Lumbar spinal roentgenography	275
Abdominal roentgenography	185/film
Hip roentgenography	100
Intravenous or retrograde pyelography	585
Upper gastrointestinal roentgenography	330
Lower gastrointestinal roentgenography	465

(*e.g.*, therapy with ^{60}Co, linear accelerator, betatron, or standard orthovoltage x-ray machines). *Local irradiation* applies to radiant energy from sources in direct proximity to the tumor. Examples are intracavitary irradiation by means of applicators loaded with radioactive material such as radium or cesium (vaginal ovoids, vaginal cylinder, or Heyman capsules), interstitial irradiation usually delivered in the form of removable needles containing either radium or cesium, and direct therapy (*e.g.*, transvaginal) usually delivered by means of cones from an orthovoltage machine.

EXTERNAL IRRADIATION

The energy and penetrating power of ionizing radiation increase as the photon wavelength decreases. Thus, differences in the physical characteristics of the radiation utilized are of great importance in therapeutic radiology (Table 60–3). The clinically important changes occur with radiation generated in the range of 400 to 800 kv. Above this energy, the advantages are reduced absorption of radiation in bone, less damage to the skin at the portal of entry, better tolerance of the vasculoconnective tissue, greater radiation at the depth relative to the surface dose, and reduced lateral scatter of radiation in the tissues (Table 60–1).

The reduced skin effect of supervoltage radiation as compared with orthovoltage radiation is based upon the physical fact that, with higher energy radiation, forward scattering (in the direction of the primary beam) of radiation in the absorber is greater and lateral scattering less. With supervoltage radiation the

TABLE 60-3. THE ELECTROMAGNETIC SPECTRUM

Type of wave	Wave energy	Wavelength
Radio	10^{-10}–10^{-4} ev	3×10^5–1 cm
Infrared	0.01–1 ev	0.01–10^{-4} cm
Visible	2–3 ev	7000–4000 Å
Ultraviolet	3–124 ev	4000–100 Å
X-ray	124 ev–124 mev	100–0.0001 Å

An electron volt (ev) is the energy of motion acquired by an electron accelerated through a potential difference of 1 volt; 1 kiloelectron volt (kev) = 1000 ev; 1 millielectron volt (mev) = 1 million ev

1 angstrom (Å) = 10^{-8} cm

maximal ionization occurs below the level of the epidermis. For example, with ^{60}Co teletherapy, maximal ionization occurs about 5 mm below the surface, while the surface dose may be only 40% of this maximum (Fig. 60–3). As the energy of radiation increases, it becomes more penetrating; as photons and resultant electrons become more energetic, they travel a greater distance into absorbing material. Therefore, the percentage of radiation at any specific depth, compared with the surface dose, increases as the energy increases. This advantage of supervoltage and megavol-

tage is of clinical importance in the treatment of tumors located deep within the organism (*e.g.*, carcinoma of the bladder and endometrium) where the introduction of a sufficiently high dose with orthovoltage radiation is difficult or impossible.

In the supervoltage range, absorption of radiation in bone approximates that in water or soft tissue per unit density, whereas with orthovoltage absorption of radiation is considerably greater in bone than in soft tissue. The vasculoconnective tissue immediately adjacent to the bone around the haversian canals receives a higher dose because of static irradiation. This higher dose increases the risk of bone necrosis by destruction of the osteoblastic elements and damage to the vascular system. Furthermore, preferential absorption by bone leads to a reduction in the dose at the point of interest when thick bone must be traversed by the radiation. In addition, it has been observed clinically that, as radiation energy increases, similar tumor effects can be produced with less damage to important adjacent normal structures. The incidence of mucosal and skin reactions is reduced and apparently there is less damage to the vasculoconnective tissue. This greater tolerance of vasculoconnective tissue to a higher dose of properly protracted supervoltage radiation therapy is one of the factors that permits the planned combination of preoperative radiation and surgery without appreciably in-

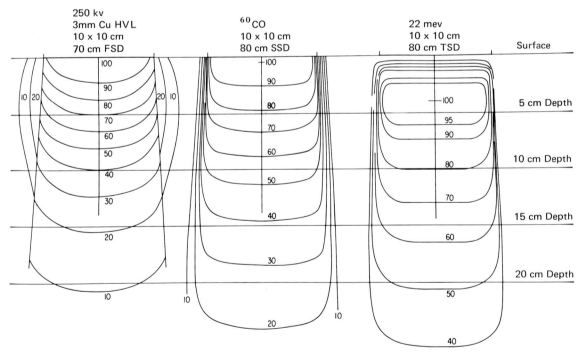

FIG. 60-3. Three isodose curves showing differences in tissue penetration by same radiation dose generated by orthovoltage (250 kv), supervoltage (^{60}Co), and megavoltage (22 mev). CuHVL is copper half value layer; FSD, focal skin distance; SSD, source skin distance; TSD, tumor source distance.

creasing the surgical risks beyond those associated with surgery alone.

LOCAL IRRADIATION

Local application of radiation permits delivery of very high doses to restricted tissue volumes. In this situation the physical principle that the intensity of irradiation rapidly decreases with distance from the radiation source (inverse square law) is used to advantage. Local irradiation is suitable for a small tumor with well-defined limits and a clinical situation in which it is desirable to restrict the volume of tissue irradiated. A larger volume of tissue is best treated with external irradiation. Radium is the element most frequently used for local application, both in tubes and needles. For the other materials (Table 60–4) available for local application, the major disadvantage is an appreciably shorter half-life. Several, however, have an advantage in that they can be incorporated in a solid material such as ceramic and need not be used as a powder or gas, as is the case with radium. Radium tubes and needles contain radium powder, and many of its decay products are in gas form within the same container. ^{198}Au has been used as a permanent tumor implant; disadvantages are difficulty of preparation, the rather rapid radioactive decay, and the difficulty of obtaining homogeneity of dose. Although ^{198}Au was frequently used in the past, it is not currently available.

Dosimetry is the measurement or calculation of the dose the patient receives. If the radiation intensity decreases rapidly with increasing depth in tissue, as is the case with local irradiation, the tissue adjacent to the radiation source may theoretically be treated adequately without damage to the underlying structures. The effectiveness of this distribution of radiation is, of course, dependent upon careful application of the source. Interstitial application of a radioactive source is a great deal more difficult than intracavitary application. A system of multiple discrete sources often results in a less homogeneous isodose pattern than irradiation from an external source or from a well-placed intracavitary source.

Some of the high cure rates possible in gynecologic cancer are due to the accessibility of vaginal and uterine cancer to local irradiation. This accessibility allows relatively high doses of radiation to be delivered to the neoplasm with relatively safe amounts of normal tissue exposure.

Another form of local irradiation that has value in the treatment of some vaginal and cervical malignancies is transvaginal radiation therapy. Utilizing a 140 to 250 kv unit and vaginal cones constructed of metal or Bakelite, an orthovoltage beam can be directed topically to the lesion. With these low-energy photons, there is a fast falloff of the depth dose so that almost all of the energy is absorbed in the central tumor mass, giving an effect quite similar to that achieved with radium therapy.

THE CONCEPT OF NOMINAL STANDARD DOSE

The work of Ellis has introduced a new expression of the biologic effect of radiation—*rad equivalent therapy* (RET). From a consideration of isoeffect relations in clinical radiotherapy, Ellis proposed that the tolerance dose of normal tissue (D) could be related to the overall treatment time (T) and the number of fractions (N) by the expression

$$D = (NSD) \times T^{0.11} \times N^{0.24}$$

This expression, which has come to be known as the Ellis *nominal standard dose* (NSD) equation, is based specifically upon the isoeffect curve for skin, the overall slope of which is 0.33. In the Ellis equation this slope has been allocated partly to overall time, with an index of 0.1, and partly to the number of fractions, with an index of 0.24. The suggested dependence on time is close to that observed experimentally for pigskin by other investigators and appears to be a valid deduction on a theoretic basis. The concept of the NSD has the obvious advantage of providing a simple basis for comparison of techniques in the same Center and among Centers, and a further advantage of allowing the therapist to total the effect of two different types of treatment such as intracavity application of radium and external beam irradiation. Thus, one can calculate the nominal single dose for any radiation treatment plan and express it in standard units. The greatest assistance gained in the day-to-day use of the NSD concept involves the comparison of two treatment regimens that differ in total dose, overall time, and fractionation pattern.

That this equation accurately assesses the normal tissue tolerance is yet to be proved in a wide spectrum of tissues. In addition, one of the principal weaknesses of the NSD system is that it does not include a systematic allowance for field size.

TABLE 60–4. ISOTOPES COMMONLY USED IN RADIATION THERAPY

Isotope	Energy (mev)	Half-life
^{137}Cs	0.662	30 years
^{60}Co	1.173, 1,332	5.3 years
^{192}Ir	0.47	74 days
^{226}Ra	0.8	1620 years
^{222}Rn	0.8	3.83 days
^{182}Ta	1.18	115 days

^{226}Ra, ^{137}Cs, ^{192}Ir, and ^{182}Ta are suitable for temporary implants; and ^{222}Rn are suitable for permanent implants which remain in the patient; ^{60}Co has some uses in intracavitary therapy.

USE OF IONIZING RADIATION IN GYNECOLOGY

For practical purposes modern use of ionizing radiation in gynecology is limited to the treatment of malignant diseases. The student should understand, however, that in the recent past radiation was used for sterilization, in the treatment of dysfunctional or climacteric bleeding, to produce ovulation in cases of infertility, and in the treatment of eczematoid and other benign diseases of the vulva. A single dose of 400 to 500 rads is often sufficient to permanently arrest menses in a premenopausal woman. However, a dose of 1200 to 2000 rads in 10 days to 2 weeks is often required to produce complete arrest of ovarian steroidogenesis in younger patients. This technique for producing cessation of menses still has applicability in some women with severe menorrhagia who are not good surgical candidates, *e.g.,* a premenopausal, acutely leukemic woman with thrombocytopenia and menorrhagia. However, with this possible exception, all of these benign conditions are now managed by other means.

TOLERANCE OF PELVIC ORGANS

Radiation tolerance of organs of the pelvis varies slightly from patient to patient and is, of course, subject to the factors mentioned above such as volume, fractionation, and energy of radiation received. The administration of radium by different techniques may also result in different dose distributions and considerable differences in tolerance. The more advanced the lesion, the greater the dose necessary for eradication and the greater the likelihood of morbidity. With advanced disease, higher risks of injury are not only present but justified. In advanced cervical, vaginal, or corpus cancer the integrity of the bladder and rectum may be already compromised, with the result that serious sequelae may follow radiation of such lesions.

The cervix and corpus of the uterus can tolerate very high doses of radiation. In fact, they withstand higher doses than any other comparable volume of tissues in the body; doses of 20,000 to 30,000 rads in about 2 weeks are routinely tolerated. This remarkable tolerance level permits a large dose and allows a very high percentage of control of cervical cancer. The unusual tolerance of the uterus and the vagina to radiation accounts for the success of radium in the treatment of cervical lesions. In addition to the tissue tolerance, the epithelium of the uterus and vagina appears to have unusual ability to recover from radiation injury.

The sigmoid, rectosigmoid, and rectum are more susceptible to radiation injury than other pelvic organs. The frequency of injury to large bowel often depends upon its relation to the distribution of radium as well as to the total dose administered by both external beam and intracavitary radium sources. With external beam alone the large bowel is the most sensitive of pelvic structures to radiation. An acute early reaction is heralded by diarrhea and tenesmus. A later manifestation of injury (usually occurring 6 to 12 months following treatment) is chronic pelvic pain associated with constriction of the bowel lumen and partial bowel obstruction. The maximal dose that the rectum will tolerate depends upon multiple factors, including the time–dose relation of both external beam and local radium source. Kottmeier calculated that the dose to the bladder and rectum from the Stockholm technique of intracavitary application of radium is about 4000 rads/3 cm^2 of rectum and bladder.

The bladder tolerates slightly more radiation than the rectum according to most calculations. A convenient rule of thumb proposed by Fletcher gives upper limits of radiation and indirectly estimates the tolerance of the bladder and rectum: the sum of the central dose by external beam plus the number of milligram-hours of radium administered by intracavitary techniques should never exceed the number 10,000. (This rule of thumb may not be valid unless the Fletcher–Suit radium system is used.) Thus, if a heavy dose of intracavitary radium is applied centrally for a small lesion, the amount of external beam applied centrally must be kept to a minimum. Conversely, if the lesion is large and the vaginal geometry poor, a minimal intracavitary dose can be given and the dose administered centrally by external beam may be quite high (6000 to 7000 rads).

Since irradiation for carcinoma of the cervix is primarily directed to the pelvic contents, only limited portions of small bowel are included. The small bowel is normally in constant motion, and this tends to prevent any one segment from receiving an excessive dose. If loops of small bowel are immobilized as the result of adhesions from previous pelvic surgery, they may be held directly in the path of the radiation beam and thus be injured. The resultant injury usually becomes symptomatic 1 year or more after the completion of radiation and is manifest as a narrowed lumen with or without associated mucosal ulceration.

It is important for students of this subject to understand the concept of permanent injury to normal tissue. When any area of the body is subjected to tumoricidal doses of radiation, the normal tissues of that area suffer an injury that is only partially repaired, even if the individual survives several decades following treatment. Radiobiologists estimate that in the case of injury to normal tissues, only 5% to 20% of the damage is repaired. Thus, the normal tissues in the irradiated area can retain a very considerable handicap. Should a second malignant neoplasm arise in that same area many years later additional tumoricidal radiation would result in a normal tissue injury level that could be unacceptable. Thus, the same area must not be

subjected to tumoricidal radiation on more than one occasion; the result will inevitably be massive loss of normal tissue.

CANCER OF THE VAGINA AND VULVA

Squamous cell carcinoma of the vagina usually occurs in elderly women who are not good candidates for surgery. Thus, the role of radiation in this disease is quite prominent. Most lesions are treated by whole pelvis irradiation, which effectively treats the pelvic lymph nodes and also markedly reduces the size of the central lesion. The central lesion is then additionally treated by local irradiation delivered by a transvaginal cone or by interstitial implantation of radium within the lesion. Overall cure rates of 40% to 50% with radiation therapy have been reported from some institutions. Indeed, about 80% of Stage I lesions are effectively eradicated.

Although some very large squamous cell cancers of the vulva have responded dramatically to radiation therapy, it is generally considered that ionizing radiation is not the treatment of choice for this lesion. Whereas the normal tissues of the cervix and vagina can tolerate large doses of radiation, the vulva is exquisitely sensitive to ionizing radiation. Some radiobiologists explain this on the basis that this area contains a disproportionately large number of end arteries whose damage by radiation results in vasculitis and radiation necrosis. Radiation to the vulva is inevitably associated with severe vulvitis that almost invariably requires interruption of therapy. Thus, surgical excision of the vulvar lesion by means of a radical vulvectomy remains the treatment of choice. The rationale for a combination of wide local surgery followed by a radiation to the regional nodes has some merit, especially in patients who are unable to undergo surgical removal of these regional nodes (see also Chapter 53).

CANCER OF THE CERVIX

The justification for external pelvic irradiation in cervical cancer can be summarized in the following manner. First, as noted previously, intracavitary radium obeys the inverse square law of all radiation that emanates from radioactive isotopes (Fig. 60–4) and, therefore, it cannot safely deliver a cancericidal dose beyond 3 cm from the external cervical os. Second, structures other than the uterus, upper part of the vagina, and medial portions of the broad ligament (lateral portions of the broad ligament, uterosacral ligaments, uterovesical ligaments, and pelvic lymph nodes) also must be considered within the spread pattern of uterine cancer and, therefore, within the field to be treated. Third, the amount of intracavitary radium that can be safely applied is limited by the sensitivity of neighboring structures such as the bowel and bladder. Although the normal tissue of the uterus and vagina is extremely radioresistant, certain limits to the quantity of intracavitary radium must be set. External

FIG. 60–4. Radiation effects at various distances from 1-mg point source of radium and 1-mg 2-cm-long tubular source of radium.

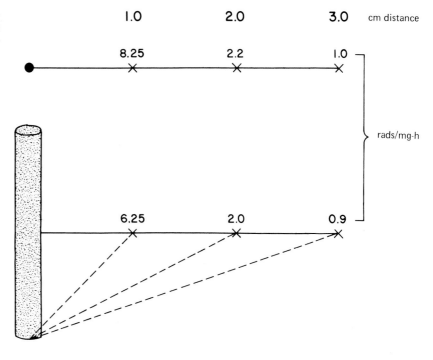

pelvic irradiation remains the only method capable of delivering an effective dose homogeneously throughout the large volume of tissue at risk.

In the treatment of cervical cancer the careful combination of external irradiation and intracavitary application of radium (many institutions now use cesium) is crucial. In early Stage Ib lesions, in which regional metastases are unlikely, intracavitary radium may be used alone, delivering a total of 10,000 mg-hr in two applications by the Fletcher technique. Conversely, for Stage III lesions (especially with poor vaginal geometry for radium) external beam irradiation may be the major component of the treatment plan and whole pelvis irradiation can be 6000 to 7000 rads. The distribution of disease must be carefully assessed by palpation and diagnostic techniques, and intracavitary application of radium and external beam irradiation must be applied judiciously to direct the greatest dose to the tumor that is compatible with acceptable morbidity.

The objective of treatment is twofold: 1) to sterilize the central lesion and 2) to destroy any islands of neoplasm in the paracervical tissues and regional lymph nodes. Almost always, external irradiation is used first to destroy metastases to the lateral lymph nodes and to reduce the size of the central lesion. Reduction in the size of the central lesion is desirable, since the lateral effect of a radium source diminishes according to the square of the distance (the inverse square law); hence, the smaller the cervix the greater the radium effect lateral to the cervix. The use of external irradiation initially prior to local radium therapy also allows

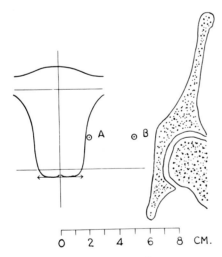

FIG. 60–5. Technique for determining radiation dose to various areas of pelvis. *Point A* is 2 cm lateral to cervical canal and 2 cm superior to lateral vaginal vault. *Point B* is 3 cm lateral to Point A. Calculation of radiation dose to Point A indicates radiation delivered to paracervical structures that may be involved by cervical cancer; calculation of radiation dose at Point B indicates radiation delivered to pelvic lymph glands draining cervix.

resolution of badly infected cervical lesions and shrinkage of fungating exophytic lesions that interfere with the accurate placement of radium.

In order to quantitate the amount of radiation reaching certain areas in the pelvis, concomitant with the development of the Manchester system (see below), British workers suggested specific landmarks designated as Point A and Point B. They defined a point 2 cm above the mucosa at the lateral vaginal fornix and 2 cm lateral to the uterine canal as Point A and another point 5 cm lateral using the same landmarks as Point B (Fig. 60–5). This enables calculation of the dose (of both radium and x-ray) delivered and of the dose absorbed in the paracervical triangle (Point A) and in the region of the pelvic nodes (Point B). It was suggested that to control squamous cell carcinoma of the cervix, a tumor dose of 7000 to 8000 rads was necessary, and most followers of the Manchester system attempted to administer a minimum of 7000 rads to Point A. This precipitated concern for positioning of the radium, since it was desirable to keep the rectal dose at 6000 rads to Point A. Careful placement of radium makes this possible.

Application of Radium

Stockholm Technique. The Stockholm technique (Fig. 60–6A) usually employs two intracavitary applications of radium 3 weeks apart. Each application is of approximately 25 to 28 hours' duration and the intrauterine applicator contains between 50 and 75 mg of radium. In an attempt to reduce the chance of overdose to the cervix and adjacent midline structures, the lower 2 cm of the uterine tandem contains no radium; the uterine applicator is otherwise evenly distributed with sources. The vaginal applicator consists of boxes or cylinders in series. In this manner, two to four rows of sources can be utilized to cover the cervical lesion and a total of 60 to 80 mg radium is commonly used. This technique utilizes a rather "hot loading" of radium over a relatively brief period. In the Stockholm technique the dose at Point A averages slightly less than 6000 rads; the dose at Point B is usually about 1900 rads.

Paris Technique. This technique (Fig. 60–6B) was initiated by the Curie Foundation and also employs a uterine tandem and vaginal sources. The tandem extends the length of the uterine cavity and in a typical case contains 6.6 mg radium in the cervical canal and two sources of 13.3-mg cephalad for a total of three sources within the tandem. A 10- or 15-mg source can be substituted for the 13.3-mg source. In the typical case, two cork cylinders containing 13.3 or 15 mg radium are pushed into the lateral vaginal fornices by a connecting spring. A third cork containing 6.6 mg is placed directly against the external os. With the Paris technique the dose at Point A is similar to that deliv-

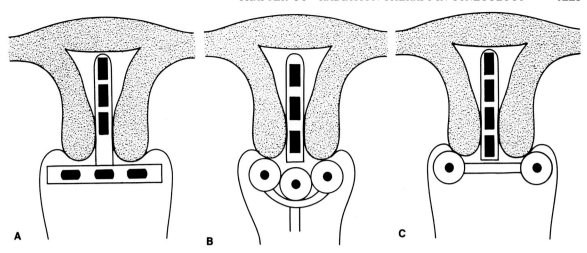

FIG. 60-6. Application of radium in treatment of cervical cancer. *A.* Stockholm technique. *B.* Paris technique. *C.* Manchester technique.

FIG. 60-7. Isodose curves showing dose delivered by Manchester technique to different depths in two cases in which differing amounts of radium could be used. In each, dose is calculated as 100% at Point A, or χ number of rads. Other numbers show percentage of this dose delivered at other depths. *A.* Standard applicators for large vagina. *B.* Standard applicators for small vagina. Note: the dose at Points A and B is considerably improved by utilizing larger vaginal ovoids. Thus, with the larger ovoids the same maximal normal tissue tolerance of the bladder, rectum, and vaginal mucosa is arrived at with more radiation being delivered to the parametria as represented by Point A and Point B. (Paterson R: The Treatment of Malignant Disease by Radiotherapy. London, Arnold, 1963)

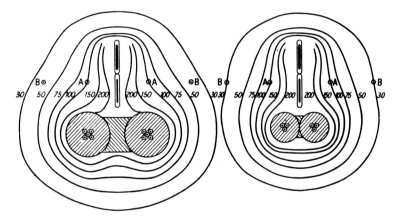

ered by the Manchester technique. When equivalent milligram-hours are used, this dose is in the neighborhood of 5700 rads in 6 days. One treatment period of 96 to 200 hours is the rule for the Paris technique.

Manchester Technique. The Manchester technique (Fig. 60–6C), a convenient and popular modification of the Paris system, differs from the Paris technique in that the source placed in the neighborhood of the cervical canal is considered as unit strength and the remaining sources in the corpus and vagina are applied as multiples of this unit and are selected and arranged to produce the equivalent isodose curves in each case and an optimal dose to preselected points in the pelvis (Points A and B). Thus, the Manchester system is designed to yield constant isodose patterns regardless of the size of the uterus and vagina (Fig. 60–7). A modi-

fication of the Manchester technique is the Nolan applicator (Fig. 60–8). Another modification that has gained wide popularity because of its ability to accommodate to after-loading is the Fletcher–Suit radium system (Fig. 60–9).

External Pelvic Irradiation

Whole pelvis irradiaton is usually administered through an anterior and posterior field approximately 15 to 18 cm^2 (Fig. 60–10). When the lesion is central and small, it may be judicious to conserve the tolerance of the bladder and rectum for radium and use a 4-cm lead block in the midline of the field. This technique, called *parametrial irradiation* (Fig. 60–11), allows the parametrium and pelvic wall to be irradiated homogeneously and conserves the tolerance of

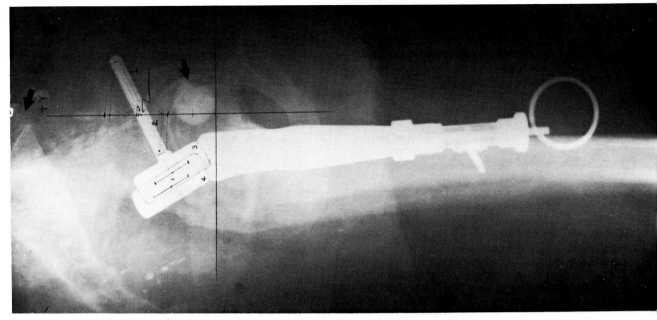

FIG. 60-8. Lateral view of Nolan applicator in place. *Arrows* point to Hypaque-filled Foley balloon (marking trigone of bladder) and sacral promontory (marking point at which posteriorly placed tandem can impinge on rectosigmoid).

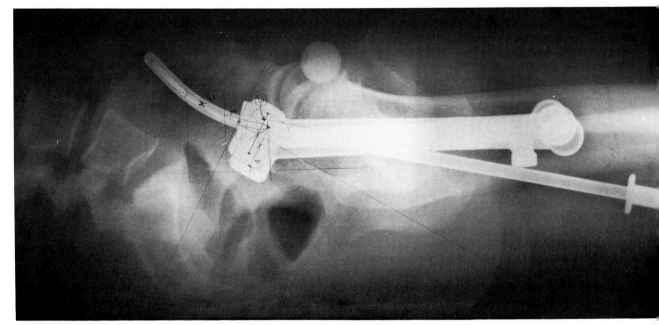

FIG. 60-9. Fletcher–Suit after-loading radium system. All radium is placed into hollow tandem and ovoids after placement films (similar to that seen here) are inspected and approved. Metal seed in posterior lip of cervix can be seen above ovoids, marking cervical tissue on film.

all grossly visible tumor considerably enhances the response to radiation therapy. Although bulky ovarian cancer within the pelvis may respond satisfactorily to standard pelvic irradiation, large residual areas of disease in the upper abdomen present a difficult problem for the radiotherapist. Indeed, the difficulty arises whenever the entire abdomen is at risk, since tolerance for whole abdomen irradiation is quite low and the dose that can be safely delivered is well below a tumoricidal dose. The abdomen tolerates a dose above 2500 rads very poorly. Fletcher has proposed that the peritoneal cavity be irradiated by "moving strip technique" in which small segments of the abdomen are systematically irradiated at high intensity. This technique theoretically keeps the morbidity at an acceptable level and permits radiobiologically greater effective doses to be delivered. Many institutions have been unable to adopt this technique successfully and its value remains uncertain. Several studies have illustrated at least equal effectiveness of chemotherapy as compared with radiotherapy in the postoperative treatment of patients with advanced ovarian cancer (see Chapter 57). Certainly chemotherapy should be seriously considered when bulky residual disease remains in the upper abdomen following radiation therapy. Several current, prospective, randomized studies may settle the issue of whether chemotherapy is also equally valuable in patients with minimal residual disease following surgery. Two studies recently concluded suggest that single-agent (Alkeran) chemotherapy is indeed as effective as full-dose radiation therapy, even for patients with minimal residual.

There is much current interest in a treatment technique for Stage I and Stage II ovarian cancer which requires the postoperative intraperitoneal instillation of P^{32}. This technique has considerable theoretic merit, if all gross disease is removed following hysterectomy and bilateral salpingo-oophorectomy and there remain only microscopic implants or cellular spill for postoperative therapy. P^{32} emits beta rays, which penetrate only to a depth of 1 mm or so. The colloidal substances have been shown to adhere to or be phagocytized by peritoneal surfaces and thus can discharge their ionizing radiation to malignant cells in situ.

NEW THERAPEUTIC STRATEGIES

Radiation therapy is an integral part of curative cancer therapy; however, the tolerance of normal tissues traversed by radiation and the resistance that tumor cell populations can develop have limited the curability of certain tumors, especially those in higher clinical stages. Research in radiobiology and radiation physics may provide methods to increase cure while decreasing morbidity. Computer-controlled dynamic treatment radioprotector drugs, hyperbaric oxygen, carbogen breathing during irradiation, particle irradiation, and hypoxic cell-sensitizing drugs are at this time undergoing clinical evaluation in various studies with some preliminary but encouraging results. The reader is referred to the article by Kinsella and Bluma for reviews of this material.

REFERENCES AND RECOMMENDED READING

Arneson AM, Nolan JF: Radiation therapy. Clin Obstet Gynecol 4:443, 1961

Brown GR, Fletcher GH, Rutledge FN: Irradiation of "in situ" and invasive squamous cell carcinomas of the vagina. Cancer 28:1278, 1971

Deeley TJ: Modern Radiotherapy: Gynecologic Cancer. New York, Appleton, 1971

Delclos L, Quinlan ET: Malignant tumors of the ovary treated with megavoltage postoperative irradiation. Radiology 93:659, 1969

DiSaia PJ, Morrow CP, Townsend DE: Synopsis of Gynecologic Oncology. New York, Wiley & Son, 1975

Ellis F: The relationship of biological to dose-time fractionation factor: Radiotherapy. Curr Top Radiation Res 4: 359, 1968

Fletcher GH: Correlated Seminar, Part II, Radiation Therapy of Cancer of the Cervix. Twelfth Annual Clinical Meeting, American College of Obstetricians and Gynecologists, 1964

Fletcher GH: Cancer of the uterine cervix. Am J Roentgenol Radium Ther Nucl Med 111:225, 1971

Fletcher GH: Textbook of Radiotherapy, 2nd ed. Philadelphia, Lea & Febiger, 1973

Fletcher GH, Rutledge FN, Chau PM: Policies of treatment in cancer of the cervix uteri. Am J Roentgenol Radium Ther Nucl Med 87:6, 1962

Fletcher GH, Rutledge FN, Delclos L: Adenocarcinoma of the uterus. In Vaeth JM (ed): Frontiers of Radiation Therapy and Oncology. White Plains NY, Karger, 1970

Glasser O, Quimby EH, Taylor LS et al: Physical Foundations of Radiology, 3rd ed. New York, Hoeber, 1961

Hall, EJ: Radiobiology for the Radiologist. Hagerstown, Harper & Row, 1973

Kinsella PJ, Bluma WD: New therapeutic strategies in radiation therapy. JAMA 245:169, 1981

Rosenshein NB, Leichner PK, Vogelsang G: Radiocolloids in the treatment of ovarian cancer. Obstet Gynecol Surv 34:708, 1979

Swartz HM: Hazards of radiation exposure for pregnant women. JAMA 239: 1907, 1978

FIG. 60-12. Preoperative application of radium for uterine cancer. Heyman capsule packing can be seen in endometrial cavity and ovoids in vaginal fornices. (Costolow WE, et al: Am J Roentgenol Radium Ther Nucl Med 71:669, 1954)

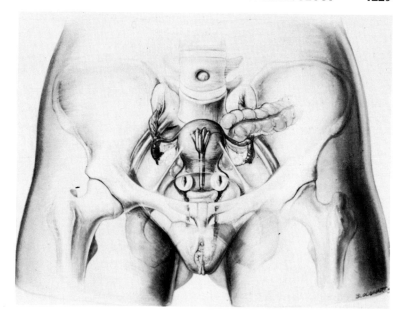

pathologic findings may be obscured. Immediate hysterectomy allows them to be revealed and may influence the decision for further treatment in the form of whole pelvis irradiation that would include the pelvic nodes.

Postoperative Application of Radium to Vaginal Vault

Several recent studies have suggested strongly that postoperative adjunctive radiation therapy for endometrial carcinoma is as effective as preoperative radiation in the prevention of vaginal cuff recurrence. Indeed, some institutions advocate primary hysterectomy with bilateral salpingo-oophorectomy when there is no indication of cervical involvement or anaplastic histology. The specimens are then carefully reviewed by the pathologist and if an occult area of undifferentiated disease, occult involvement of the cervix or isthmus, deep myometrial invasion, or adnexal metastases is found, postoperative whole pelvis irradiation is applied. If none of these indicators of nodal involvement is found, the post-operative radiation therapy may take the form of cuff irradiation delivered by a variety of radium applicators as soon as 1 week following hysterectomy. This cuff irradiation, which may also be delivered by transvaginal cone, is relatively simple and usually can be accomplished without additional anesthetic.

Radiation Treatment of Recurrent Cancer

The development of a pelvic mass in a patient previously treated for endometrial carcinoma may indicate a pelvic sidewall recurrence. Laparotomy should be performed, if possible, to confirm the diagnosis and delineate the extent of the disease. If whole pelvis irradiation has not already been utilized, consideration should be given to outlining the recurrence with metal clips and delivering external irradiation to the affected area after the operation. If the recurrence is at the apex of the vaginal vault, treatment depends upon the size of the lesion. External irradiation should be considered if normal tissue tolerance has not been approached by previous radiation therapy. For vaginal recurrence external irradiation is usually supplemented by direct application of radium or the use of a transvaginal cone. Unfortunately, these pelvic recurrences are often in a field of fibrosis and avascularity secondary to previous radiation therapy, and it is for this reason that the response of pelvic recurrence to systemic progestin therapy is much less favorable than that for distant recurrences.

CARCINOMA OF THE OVARY

Some 80% of primary ovarian carcinomas arise from germinal epithelium, and this histogenesis is associated with limited radiosensitivity. In general, except for dysgerminoma, ovarian carcinomas are not easily treated with radiation. Although the adenocarcinomas have limited radiosensitivity, other ovarian tumors, such as malignant teratoma or embryonal carcinoma, are notoriously poor in their response to radiation. In addition to the limited radiovulnerability of these lesions, radiation therapy is severely handicapped by the fact that the disease is often widely distributed within the peritoneal cavity. Complete surgical extirpation of

TABLE 60-5. SURVIVAL RATES FOR SQUAMOUS CELL CARCI-
NOMA OF CERVIX TREATED BY RADIATION
ONLY, SEPTEMBER 1954 THROUGH DECEMBER
1967, M. D. ANDERSON HOSPITAL AND TUMOR
INSTITUTE

Stage	5-year survival rate* (%)	10-year survival rate* (%)
Cervical carcinoma, intact uterus (1705 patients†)		
Ib	91.5	90.0
IIa	83.5	79.0
IIb	66.5	57.0
IIIa	45.0	39.5
IIIb	36.0	30.0
IV	14.0	14.0
Carcinoma of cervical stump (189 patients)		
Ib	97.0	97.0
IIa	93.0	89.0
IIb	67.0	67.0
IIIa	61.0	61.0
IIIb	32.0	32.0
IV	0	0

* Modified life table method. Patients dying from intercurrent disease are excluded.
† Includes patients treated incompletely or for palliation
(Fletcher GH: Am J Roentgenol Radium Ther Nucl Med
111:225, 1971)

cancer that has extended to involve the endocervical
canal. However, this remains controversial.

Preoperative Application of Radium

The basic treatment for uterine corpus cancer is hysterectomy. However, the pelvic recurrence rate and
incidence of cuff metastases can be lowered and the
overall survival rate improved by the use of adjunctive
radiation therapy, especially in a patient who harbors
an anaplastic lesion in an enlarged uterus. Although
external irradiation is often utilized, radium implantation either with or without external beam irradiation is
effective. The simple tandem or string of radium
sources is rarely adequate to irradiate uniformly the
enlarged and irregular uterus so often associated with
corpus cancer. Instead, a packing technique is used in
which small radium sources in uniformly sized capsules are individually introduced and firmly packed to
fill the uterine cavity (Fig. 60–12). It is important also
to irradiate the endocervical canal and the vaginal fornices, and this is usually accomplished by a placement
of short uterine tandem and the usual vaginal ovoids.
Intrauterine radium is usually delivered in two applications of 2500 mg-hr each separated by a 2- to 3-week
interval, or as a single application of 3500 mg-hr if necessary. The value of radiation preoperatively lies in its
ability to shrink the uterus and partially debilitate the
malignant cells, leaving them less suitable for implantation. It is also thought that preoperative irradiation
minimizes the possibility of dissemination of viable
cancer at the time of the surgical procedure.

Preoperative External Radiation

The contribution of intrauterine radium to the parametrium and pelvic nodes is minimal and where these
are at risk as possible sites of viable malignant cells (as
when the cancer has extended to involve the cervix),
appropriate therapy must be instituted. The parametrium and pelvic nodes must be treated in a manner
similar to that utilized for cervical cancer. Data so far
collected suggest that cervical or isthmic involvement,
deep myometrial invasion, and/or anaplastic histology
significantly increase the possibility of pelvic dissemination and mandate whole pelvis irradiation (preferably with an external beam). The customary dose is
4000 to 5000 rads if pelvic wall disease is suspected.
This is often followed by one radium application delivering approximately 2500 mg hr and then a simple extrafascial hysterectomy in 4 to 6 weeks. External therapy will usually shrink the uterus significantly,
allowing safe use of a simple intrauterine tandem instead of the more difficult packing of capsules.

If the patient with endometrial cancer is elderly and
unable to tolerate several anesthetics, one anesthetic
can be eliminated by substituting external irradiation
for intracavitary radium application. It is hoped, then,
that the patient will be able to tolerate a single anesthetic so that hysterectomy and bilateral salpingo-oophorectomy can be performed.

Timing of Hysterectomy after Radiation

The interval between the completion of radiation and
the performance of hysterectomy is the subject of controversy. Classically, a 6-week interval following completion of radiation therapy is advised prior to hysterectomy, but several studies suggest that it is not
necessary. The 6-week treatment-free interval does,
however, allow maximal shrinkage of the uterus and
resolution of most of the acute inflammatory process
associated with radiation therapy. If whole pelvis irradiation has been utilized, the treatment-free interval
also allows recovery from the side affects of this therapy, such as diarrhea, crampy abdominal pain, and
often a state of negative nitrogen balance. On the other
hand, if radium alone has been used in the preoperative treatment, it may be advisable to do the hysterectomy as quickly as possible thereafter to prevent the
distortion that results from radiation. As stated previously, patients with deep myometrial invasion or occult involvement of the cervix or isthmus often have
pelvic node metastases. During a 6-week waiting period, shrinkage of the uterine tumor occurs and these

FIG. 60-10. Whole pelvis irradiation for cervical cancer extending to involve upper part of vagina. Lower margin of 18 × 18-cm field is well below pubic symphysis. Lead tapes (*white strips*) show technique of excluding corners of a square field and thus reducing volume irradiated by roughly 10%.

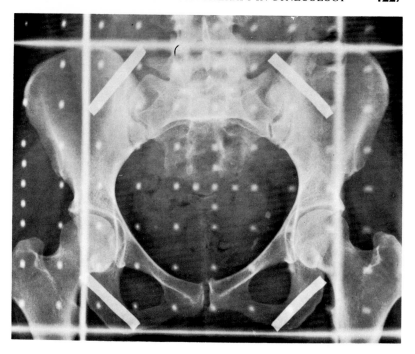

the midline structures for future intracavitary techniques. Supervoltage or megavoltage radiation has the advantages mentioned earlier, and whenever possible should be utilized for whole pelvis or parametrial irradiation.

Individualized therapy with judicious use of both external-beam and intracavitary irradiation can result in gratifying survival rates (Table 60–5).

Other considerations with regard to the treatment of cancer of the cervix are discussed in Chapter 54.

CARCINOMA OF THE ENDOMETRIUM

The most common malignant lesion of the uterine corpus is endometrial carcinoma, and this lesion often invades deeply into the myometrium. Thus, placing radium sources in close proximity to the disease so as to deliver optimal radiation to all the central lesion is usually not possible. As noted in Chapter 55, removal of the uterus along with both adnexa has proved essential for optimal results; when large series of patients are analyzed, it is apparent that the addition of hysterectomy to the treatment plan for endometrial cancer improves survival by at least 20%, even when the data are corrected for death due to intercurrent disease. Thus, unlike cervical cancer, treatment of endometrial cancer by irradiation alone is not advisable. Some institutions believe that radiation alone constitutes adequate treatment of Stage II endometrial

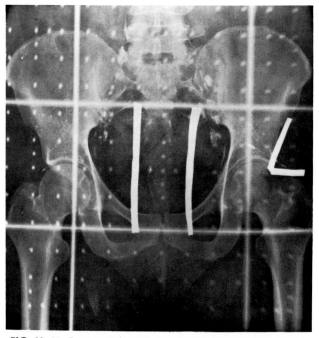

FIG. 60-11. Parametrial irradiation for cervical cancer. A 4-cm lead block is placed between strips of lead tape, sparing midline. Note that height of field is considerably reduced compared with that in Figure 60-10: Only a 10-cm height need be blocked in midline, and in larger field top center portion should not be spared since this represents node-bearing areas.

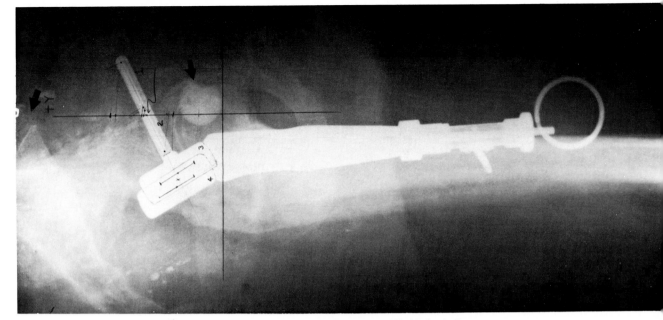

FIG. 60-8. Lateral view of Nolan applicator in place. *Arrows* point to Hypaque-filled Foley balloon (marking trigone of bladder) and sacral promontory (marking point at which posteriorly placed tandem can impinge on rectosigmoid).

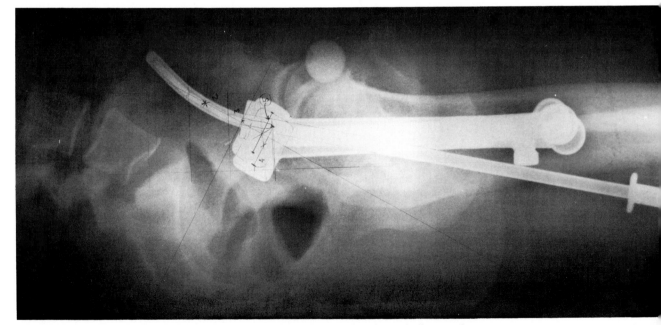

FIG. 60-9. Fletcher–Suit after-loading radium system. All radium is placed into hollow tandem and ovoids after placement films (similar to that seen here) are inspected and approved. Metal seed in posterior lip of cervix can be seen above ovoids, marking cervical tissue on film.

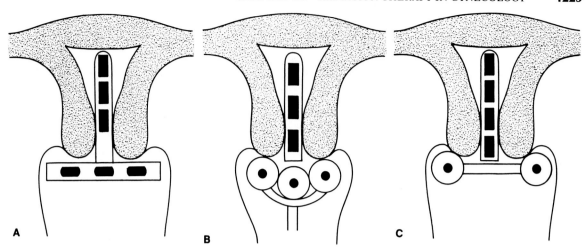

FIG. 60-6. Application of radium in treatment of cervical cancer. *A.* Stockholm technique. *B.* Paris technique. *C.* Manchester technique.

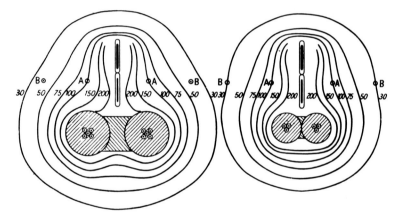

FIG. 60-7. Isodose curves showing dose delivered by Manchester technique to different depths in two cases in which differing amounts of radium could be used. In each, dose is calculated as 100% at Point A, or χ number of rads. Other numbers show percentage of this dose delivered at other depths. *A.* Standard applicators for large vagina. *B.* Standard applicators for small vagina. Note: the dose at Points A and B is considerably improved by utilizing larger vaginal ovoids. Thus, with the larger ovoids the same maximal normal tissue tolerance of the bladder, rectum, and vaginal mucosa is arrived at with more radiation being delivered to the parametria as represented by Point A and Point B. (Paterson R: The Treatment of Malignant Disease by Radiotherapy. London, Arnold, 1963)

ered by the Manchester technique. When equivalent milligram-hours are used, this dose is in the neighborhood of 5700 rads in 6 days. One treatment period of 96 to 200 hours is the rule for the Paris technique.

Manchester Technique. The Manchester technique (Fig. 60–6C), a convenient and popular modification of the Paris system, differs from the Paris technique in that the source placed in the neighborhood of the cervical canal is considered as unit strength and the remaining sources in the corpus and vagina are applied as multiples of this unit and are selected and arranged to produce the equivalent isodose curves in each case and an optimal dose to preselected points in the pelvis (Points A and B). Thus, the Manchester system is designed to yield constant isodose patterns regardless of the size of the uterus and vagina (Fig. 60–7). A modi-

fication of the Manchester technique is the Nolan applicator (Fig. 60–8). Another modification that has gained wide popularity because of its ability to accommodate to after-loading is the Fletcher–Suit radium system (Fig. 60–9).

External Pelvic Irradiation

Whole pelvis irradiaton is usually administered through an anterior and posterior field approximately 15 to 18 cm² (Fig. 60–10). When the lesion is central and small, it may be judicious to conserve the tolerance of the bladder and rectum for radium and use a 4-cm lead block in the midline of the field. This technique, called *parametrial irradiation* (Fig. 60–11), allows the parametrium and pelvic wall to be irradiated homogeneously and conserves the tolerance of

This chapter is intended as an overview of the subject of gynecologic surgery. Its purpose is to provide the student with an immediate reference to the objectives and basic principles of the surgical procedures that are an integral part of the discipline of obstetrics and gynecology, and to indicate what some of them entail. For greater detail the student is urged to consult the standard works and periodicals, some of which are listed at the end of this chapter.

The fascinating story of the development of gynecology as a surgical specialty is outlined in Chapter 1 and will be of much interest as a background for the ingenuity and precision of modern techniques.

PREOPERATIVE INVESTIGATION

HISTORY AND PHYSICAL EXAMINATION

The preoperative appraisal of the patient's physical status should be comprehensive and detailed. Oriented toward detecting unsuspected pathology and impaired physiologic tolerance, the basic history, physical examination, and laboratory studies serve as broad screening procedures to uncover vital functions that need preliminary treatment and more precise evaluation before the patient is subjected to an anesthetic and an operative procedure. Although the conditions listed below are not necessarily absolute contraindications to gynecologic operations, elective procedures should be delayed until special studies are performed to establish accurate diagnosis and functional status when the following are suspected: impaired cardiac function; chronic and acute pulmonary disease; renal disease and urinary tract infection; arterial and venous insufficiency from thrombosis, embolism, vascular occlusion, or vascular ectasia; water, nutrition, and vitamin starvation states; metabolic diseases, particularly diabetes, hypoadrenalism, and hyperthyroidism; actual or incipient psychiatric disorders; infectious dermatitis; hypersensitivity to drugs such as antibiotics, sedatives, and antiseptics; arterial hypertension, particularly if there is a history of previous vascular accident; and hematologic defects such as sicklemia, defective coagulation, and blood cell neoplasia.

In the gynecologic patient it is essential that an unsuspected pregnancy not be jeopardized; the slightest suggestion that pregnancy exists, regardless of the history, is reason to delay the operation. The date of the last menstrual period should be boldly displayed on the front page of the history and on the anesthetic sheet.

EFFECT OF IATROGENIC FACTORS

In preoperative evaluation of the gynecologic patient, attention must be paid to iatrogenic factors that may adversely influence the tolerance of the patient to the

OPERATIVE GYNECOLOGY

C. Paul Hodgkinson
Bruce H. Drukker

operative procedure. Particularly in the patient with hypertension or a degenerative disease, specific inquiry should be made about drugs she has received. Recent experience has shown that certain drugs given for the treatment of hypertension may cause the commonly administered anesthetic agents to have a highly potentiated or unusual pharmacologic action.

The thiazide compounds, for example, cause potassium depletion, which may alter cardiac function or enhance the reaction to digitalis and D-tubocurarine. Hypotension may be accentuated owing to the altered reactivity to norepinephrine. Thiazide compounds should be discontinued for at least 4 days before an elective operation.

If possible, one should avoid the administration of an anesthetic to a patient receiving rauwolfia alkaloids. The catecholamine depletion effects of rauwolfia plus the effects of anesthesia severely depress sympathetic

control of vascular tone, producing a prolonged hypotension that is recalcitrant to therapy. At least 2 weeks should elapse from the time the drug is stopped before surgery is undertaken. Similar but less severe reactions have been observed following the administration of guanethidine. This drug should be stopped 10 days before surgery. Also, it is important to keep in mind the depressant-potentiating effects of the ataractic drugs.

Patients who have received adrenocorticosteroids within 1 year withstand poorly the stress of an operation. As a rule of thumb, for a patient currently under therapy the dose of corticoids should be doubled 24 hours prior to surgery. For a patient not presently under therapy but who has received corticoids within the year previous to the date of the operation, corticoid therapy in a dose equivalent to 200 mg cortisone should be instituted 24 hours before the time of the operation and continued for 4 days postoperatively; then the dose may be gradually reduced preliminary to discontinuation of the drug.

The hazard of surgery is increased for the patient undergoing anticoagulant therapy. A patient receiving heparin should not undergo an operation until the drug has been discontinued for 24 hours. In an emergency, heparin effects can be neutralized immediately by protamine sulfate given intravenously in a dose equal to the last dose of heparin. A patient receiving long-acting anticoagulants of the coumarin series should not have surgery until the prothrombin time reaches 18 seconds or less, which generally requires several days. In an urgent situation, vitamin K_1 can be used to shorten the prothrombin time, but in a patient with myocardial or cerebral damage gradual spontaneous prothrombin-time recovery is preferable. Some patients, notably arthritics, may consume aspirin each day. If it is not stopped 48 hours before surgery, the platelets will be depleted and heavy bleeding may be encountered.

EFFECT OF ADVANCED AGE

Advanced age in itself is not a contraindication to surgery. The elderly patient must be carefully surveyed for critical depression of vital functions, and the urgency of the operation must be weighed against the general physical status. Particular attention must be paid to the efficiency of the peripheral circulation. It is important to remember that the elderly patient has an increased sensitivity to drugs and anesthetics: opiates, barbiturates, and belladonna-like drugs must be given with caution. Generally the older patient tolerates operative procedures as well as any other healthy adult, but her ability to withstand postoperative complications is definitely reduced.

Although the highly sophisticated tests employed to evaluate the function of the various organs are desirable and of great value, sometimes clinical evaluation of overall tolerance according to the patient's day-by-day activities gives more practical knowledge of her ability to withstand an operation. It is advisable to inquire if she does her own housework and her own marketing, how far she walks to the store, whether she carries her own packages, how many times during the day she climbs stairs, and whether she manages her own affairs. The elderly patient who performs such tasks will have little difficulty withstanding the trauma of most any operation. Prompt resumption of ambulatory activity is essential for the elderly patient; she should be ambulatory within 24 hours following operation.

Some of the tests involved in a "standard preoperative survey" can be very rigorous for elderly or debilitated patients. Such tests, of course, should be used if they are needed, but they should not be orderd merely by rote.

EMERGENCY OPERATIONS

Evaluation of the patient prior to an emergency operation performed for a life-threatening condition should be comprehensive, but some diagnostic procedures done before elective operations necessarily are bypassed. The deterioration of the patient's physiologic functions demands prompt institution of supportive therapy in preparation for operation. Hypovolemic shock from vaginal or intra-abdominal hemorrhage, and pain and neurogenic shock from acute torsion of the pedicle of a pelvic viscus, are the conditions that constitute most of the gynecologic emergencies. In elective operations 10 g hemoglobin per 100 ml blood is the borderline value for adequate oxygen transport during anesthesia. In severe shock from massive hemorrhage (*e.g.*, ruptured tubal pregnancy or incomplete abortion), surgery must be performed when the hemoglobin value is far below this level and in some cases when blood pressure is barely obtainable. In such instances decisions concerning the time to induce anesthesia and to operate must depend upon minimal evidence that the patient is responding to therapy. When whole blood and fluids are being administered through large-bore (17-gauge) needles installed in at least two adequate veins, slight elevation of the blood pressure and slowing of the pulse can usually be taken as indications that the patient will tolerate light general anesthesia and a rapidly performed operation. Immediate ligation of the points of hemorrhage is usually promptly followed by elevation of the blood pressure and slowing of the pulse.

An important item easily forgotten in the haste of an emergency is to inquire about the time of, and what was eaten at, the last meal.

BASIC OPERATIVE TECHNIQUES

Although the operative techniques employed by the gynecologist are directed principally toward those structures primarily involved in the process of reproduction in the female, the scope of knowledge and experience must include the principles of surgery as they apply to the abdomen, urinary tract, and breast.

It is the responsibility of each physician who performs abdominal operations, regardless of special interests, to have mastered the principles and techniques of intestinal resection and anastomosis, blood vessel repair, bladder and ureter repair, and reconstruction methods for the abdominal wall and perineum. All who enter an operating room should have thorough knowledge of cardiac resuscitation. The gynecologist must be thoroughly grounded in the basics of blood transfusion, fluid and electrolyte balance, wound healing, infections, shock, hemorrhage, trauma, and the like. As a surgical specialist, the operating gynecologist must have had training and experience sufficient to discriminate between good and bad technique, good and bad judgment, and devotion to patient and mercenary interests.

W. Wayne Babcock epitomized the attributes of one who would presume to operate as follows: "The highest art is the protection of the patient and his tissues . . . by the selection of the best procedure that the patient can endure, by delicacy and skill in manipulation of the tissues, by absence of bruising, crushing, or laceration, by conservation of blood and body heat, by protection of nerves, blood vessels, and other important structures, and by avoidance of strangulating constriction in the closing of wounds." Regardless of the extent or complexity of a surgical procedure, the use of large clamps, big needles, heavy suture material, scissors dissection, large gauze packs, sponging by wiping, mass ligatures, and heavy retraction is reflected in a slightly lessened chance for recovery, increased postoperative pain, prolonged convalescence, greater postoperative morbidity, and an increased likelihood of postoperative complications.

Conversely, good technique can be measured by an operator's skill in incising tissues with the sharp scalpel rather than crushing them with scissors, by willingness to forego the convenience of large clamps and mass ligature for the use of precise crushing with smaller clamps and precise ligating with finer ligatures, by avoidance of large packs and forceful retraction, by ability to select the proper size and type of suture material for the tissue involved, by the precision used in placing needles, and by the careful attention given to the tension of well-seated knots. Finally, effectiveness is enhanced in proportion to the patience and courtesy shown to assistants.

OPERATIONS

Local Excision and Biopsy

Many pedunculated and intradermal lesions are treated by circular, full-thickness skin excision and closure with interrupted nonabsorbable sutures of silk, cotton, or plastic. All excised material should be subjected to pathologic examination. Infected cysts should be drained by incisions and not closed. Prior to biopsy, all suspicious ulcerative lesions should be studied by dark-field microscopy and tests performed for granulomatous lesions of venereal origin.

For office biopsy, toluidine blue is used to designate appropriate sites (see p. 1023), which are removed with a Keys dermatologic punch. If many biopsies are needed, it is usually preferable that they be done in the hospital under general anesthesia.

All white lesions, persistent skin thickenings, and nonvenereal ulcerations—collectively better classified as "chronic dystrophic dermatitis"—may be treated by systematic multiple biopsy according to a vulvar map (Fig. 61–1) constructed for each patient. Because car-

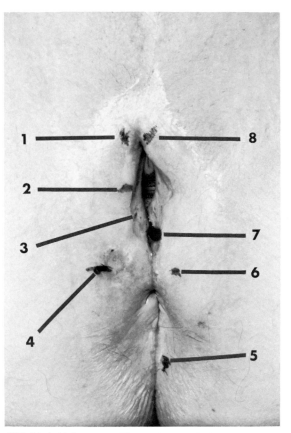

FIG. 61-1. Vulvar map. Biopsy sites marked for excision.

cinoma of the vulva is a field-change phenomenon, every lesion and several areas of noninvolved skin should be marked with a colored dye (1% gentian violet) prior to biopsy. The vulvar map should be drawn in the patient's record and each biopsy site numbered in an anticlockwise position starting at the operator's upper left. Full-thickness skin biopsy specimens should be obtained and placed in bottles appropriately numbered for pathologic examination. Skin closure should be accomplished by interrupted sutures of nonabsorbable material.

Simple Vulvectomy

This procedure is used for biopsy of extensive lesions and as treatment for recalcitrant pruritus and chronic dystrophic dermatitis. It involves the excision of the full thickness of the skin from the level of the hymenal ring outward, leaving a 0.5-cm skin margin around the external urinary meatus and usually including the skin over the labia minora, clitoris, and much of the labia majora, and the skin of the perineum down to the level of the anus. Either the sharp scalpel or cutting-current electrocoagulation may be used.

Basic Technique. 1) A circular incision is made through the skin at the level of the hymen, leaving a 0.5-cm margin around the external urinary meatus. 2) An outer circular incision is made to include the vulvar lesion. 3) Dissection is done from below upward to ex-

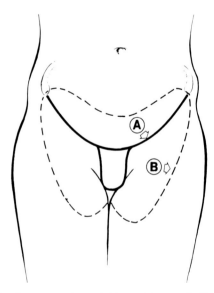

FIG. 61–2. Radical vulvectomy. Lines of skin excision are indicated by *heavy solid lines* (A); *dotted lines* (B) show extent of dissection of skin flaps. If there is clinical suggestion that malignancy involves skin of groin, wide excision of skin must be practiced and wound allowed to close by secondary intention.

cise the full thickness of the skin. 4) Meticulous hemostasis is accomplished by ligature or electrocoagulation. 5) Skin edges are closed with interrupted nonabsorbable sutures with ends cut at least 2-cm long to aid in subsequent identification.

Radical Vulvectomy

This procedure is performed for invasive carcinoma of the vulvar skin, external urinary urethra, outer half of the vagina, anus, and all lesions that drain into the iliofemoral lymph nodes. Adequate, radical vulvectomy is defined as 1) removal of the entire vulva to the level of a curvilinear line over the mons pubis extending between the anterior superior spines of the ilia and 2) bilateral excision of superficial and deep inguinal lymph nodes, of the lymph-node-containing fat, of the segment of the greater saphenous vein in Scarpa's triangle, and of the deep external and internal iliac and obturator lymph nodes. The procedure is best performed in one stage, simultaneously by two teams, starting with the groin dissections. If the patient's condition does not permit a one-stage procedure, vulvectomy should be done first and groin dissections delayed until the skin of the vulva has healed.

Basic Technique. 1) Skin incision is made curving downward from each anterior superior iliac spine to the level of the upper border of the symphysis (Fig. 61–2). 2) The skin flaps are dissected upward and downward to expose oblique muscle and Scarpa's triangle, which is excised en bloc; in Scarpa's triangle this includes the segment of the saphenous vein up to its anastomosis with the superficial femoral. 3) The round ligament and the lymph nodes in the inguinal canal are excised to the level of the peritoneum. 4) The lymphatics and lymph nodes along the femoral vessels and the external and internal iliac and obturator lymph nodes are excised, including Cloquet's node, which is constantly found in the femoral canal (Fig. 61–3). 5) Adequate hemostasis is obtained and the skin of the groin is closed, sweeping all dissected tissue to the center of the incision. 6) The vulvectomy incision extends around the entire vulva to the level of the upper border of the anus. 7) The inner vulvectomy incision is made at the level of the hymenal ring, excluding 0.5 cm of periurethral skin unless the urethra is involved, in which case the incision must be more extensive. The lower half of the urethra may be sacrificed without loss of urinary control. 8) Beginning at the perineal incision (Fig. 61–4), all tissue to the level of the inferior fascia of the urogenital diaphragm is excised, including the bulbocarvernosus and ischiocavernosus muscles, the clitoris and each crus attached to the pubic rami, Bartholin's glands, the bulbs of the vestibule, and the terminal pudendal blood vessels and nerves (Fig. 61–5). 9) Multiperforated No. 20 soft rubber catheters with constant pump suction are used

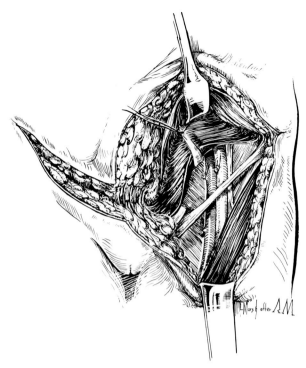

FIG. 61-3. Radical vulvectomy. All fat and lymphatic tissue must be removed from Scarpa's triangle and along external iliac vessels. Round ligament has been cut and proximal end displaced upward; distal end will be excised with vulva. Inguinal ligament may be cut or left intact.

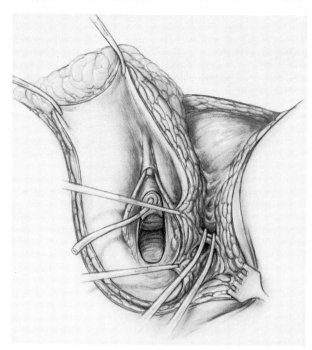

FIG. 61-4. Perineal incision includes wide margin of skin and excision of all tissue to level of inferior surface of pelvic diaphragm. Inner incision is made at level of introitus, leaving, if possible, 0.5-cm margin around external urinary meatus.

to drain the iliac, femoral, and pudendal areas (Fig. 61–6). 10) The perineal skin is closed, when possible, with interrupted nonabsorbable sutures, and the area is dressed with elastic bandages for uniform compression. If the skin edges cannot be approximated, as is often the case, they are left to granulate.

Operations on Bartholin's Glands

Compound racemose glands with a single duct emerging between the midlevel of the labia minora and the hymenal ring, Bartholin's glands are subject to acute suppurative abscess formation and chronic noninfected cystic dilatation. They lie posterior and somewhat inferior to the highly vascular bulbs of the vestibule and are in relatively close proximity to the rectum. Acute hemorrhage, extensive dissecting hematoma, and perforation of the rectum with persistent fistula are major complications of operations on Bartholin's glands. Although acute suppurative bartholinitis is a regular complication of gonorrhea, Bartholin gland suppuration also occurs from staphylococcal, streptococcal, and coliform organisms.

An abscess may be incised and drained or marsupialized (Figs. 61–7, 61–8). A noninfected cyst

can be treated by excision or marsupialization. In acute infections, because Bartholin's glands lie deep to the fat and fascia of the labia, marked swelling and edema of the overlying labia majora give the erroneous impression that the abscess is pointing in this direction. Spontaneous rupture of an abscess occurs into the vestibule near the location of the duct. The best operative approach is through incisions made in the vestibule parallel to the hymenal ring. Because the gland is closest to the surface in this area, less pain, hemorrhage, and postoperative scarring result from incisions made in this area than from incisions made directly through the area of maximal swelling in the labia majora. Frequently, because of pain following operations on Bartholin's glands, inability to void may be bothersome for several days. Intermittent catheterization, sitz baths, and reassurance are sufficient treatment until postoperative edema and pain subside.

Incision and Drainage. Incision and drainage are used primarily for acute suppuration with abscess formation.

Basic Technique. 1) By means of moist gauze, the inflamed labia majora are displaced manually, laterally, until the vestibule is displayed. 2) An area of fluctua-

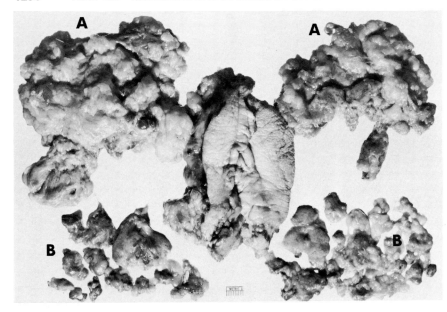

FIG. 61-5. Vulvar skin and excised fat and lymphatic tissue from radical vulvectomy. Masses *A* were removed from above inguinal ligament and include tissue from region of external iliac vessels; masses *B* were removed from Scarpa's triangle.

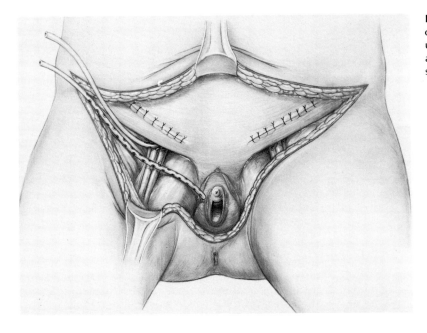

FIG. 61-6. Multiperforated No. 20 soft rubber catheters with constant pump suction are used to drain iliac, femoral, and pudendal areas. They should remain until danger of seroma collection is past.

tion is palpated and an incision is made directly into it with a sharp scalpel, beginning near the posterior margin of the vestibule and directing the incision upward. High incisions should be avoided for fear of opening into the highly vascular bulb of the vestibule; for the same reason it is best *not* to open the abscess in the office. 3) Petroleum jelly or antibiotic-impregnated gauze tape is used for packing for 24 hours to control bleeding. 4) To control profuse hemorrhage, a tightly placed vaginal pack is of value. 5) Hot sitz baths for 20 minutes three times daily and continued drainage reduce pain.

Marsupialization. Marsupialization is used primarily for infected Bartholin gland cysts. Pain is minimal and recurrence is unusual.

Basic Technique. 1) The gland is exposed by lateral retraction of the labia majora. 2) An incision is made into the gland at the inferior level of the vestibule. 3) A cir-

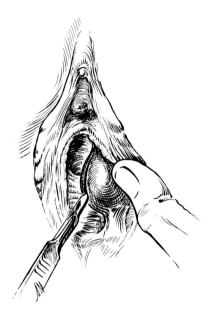

FIG. 61-7. Incision for Bartholin gland cyst or abscess. Incision should be made over medial surface of introitus on line parallel with posterior margin of hymenal ring. At this point Bartholin gland cyst or abscess is most superficial. Incision area is exposed by displacing cyst outward.

cular area of the cyst wall and the overlying skin is excised. 4) The cyst is sutured open by uniting the cyst wall with the skin edge. 5) No packing is used (Fig. 61–8).

Excision. Excision of a Bartholin gland cyst is done in the absence of infection. It prevents recurrence and should always be used if there is suspicion of tumor, for biopsy purposes. Pain and a varying degree of ecchymosis of the skin of the perineum are usual following excision operations; the patient should be advised of this preoperatively.

Basic Technique. 1) The labia are retracted laterally to expose the vestibule. 2) A liberal incision is made extending inferolaterally from a point about 1 cm from the external urinary meatus parallel to the hymenal ring to the posterior margin of the vestibule. 3) With Allis forceps on the skin edges for retraction, dissection of the cyst from surrounding tissues is begun posteroinferiorly to avoid early bothersome bleeding. 4) In the area of the vestibular bulb brisk bleeding is best controlled with suture ligatures. 5) After removal of the cyst, closure of the tissue space is best accomplished with a continuous suture of No. 3-0 absorbable material. 6) Accidental opening of a cyst during excision, even in the presence of chronic infection, does not preclude closure of the tissue defect.

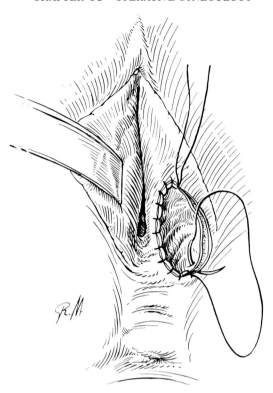

FIG. 61-8. Marsupialization of Bartholin gland cyst. Skin edge is joined to cyst wall using continuous locking suture or with interrupted sutures. No. 3-0 absorbable suture is highly suitable. Exposure is aided if traction is made on a continuous locking suture.

Operation for Urethral Caruncles

Urethral caruncles are benign protrusions of the posterior urethral mucosa resulting from anestrogenic atrophy of menopause; they may be granulomatous, papillomatous, or angiomatous, and asymptomatic, painful, or hemorrhagic. If asymptomatic, sessile, and noninfected, they become less prominent with the use of estrogen-containing vaginal creams. If multiple, painful, infected, and easily traumatized, they should be excised and subjected to microscopic study.

Repair of Prolapse of Urethral Mucosa

Prolapse of urethral mucosa occurs in the anestrogenic states of the very young and the very old from the stress of increased intra-abdominal pressure caused by crying, coughing, straining, and the like. Occasionally it results from an intraurethral polyp. It occurs as a sleevelike prolapse of the mucosal layer of the urethra through the external urinary meatus and is subject to severe congestion and gangrene from constriction. Clinically it appears as a blue-black, but-

tonlike swelling with a central dimple on the distal end of the urethra. It should be excised and the edges of the mucosa united with No. 3-0 absorbable suture.

Operations on the Hymen

The hymen may be imperforate or stenotic. If imperforate, retention of menstrual blood leads to hematocolpos and hematometra following menarche. Treatment is by excision of the hymen and suture of the skin edges with No. 3-0 absorbable material. Simple incision of the hymen is not sufficient.

Stenosis rarely is sufficient to prevent sexual intercourse. If stenosis is suspected during premarital examination, it is best unmentioned. The unwary physician who unwisely predicts difficulty with sexual intercourse may contribute to iatrogenic sexual neurosis. Treatment should be recommended after several weeks of marriage. Excision of the stenotic hymen and manual vaginal dilatation are sufficient.

Operations on the Perineum

The female perineum may be excessively long or excessively short; either condition may be congenital or acquired.

Congenital elongation of the perineum due to excessive fusion of the labioscrotal folds may be idiopathic or the result of administration of androgens to the mother during pregnancy. If idiopathic, other genitourinary tract defects of an intersex nature should be suspected. If iatrogenic, the clitoris may also be enlarged, and care must be taken that the proper sex is assigned at birth. Sex chromosome studies are essential. The development of the internal generative organs in the female is essentially normal if the perineal elongation is iatrogenic. Treatment is by longitudinal incision in the median raphe and suture of the edges with fine gut. Agglutination of the labia occurs in infancy and early childhood and is usually correctable by gentle manual separation without anesthesia and by application of estrogen creams.

Acquired elongation of the perineum ("dashboard perineum") results from overzealous repair of the perineum incidental to delivery or posterior colpoplasty. Correction is by transverse repair of a longitudinal incision made through the mucosa and underlying perineal body.

An excessively short perineum may occur as a developmental defect that may be so extensive as to involve the anal sphincter and anus, giving rise to congenital rectovaginal fistula. Successful plastic reconstruction of the perineum may be limited because of agenesis.

Acquired shortness of the perineum is the result of laceration, which may be complete or incomplete and may be of obstetric, surgical, or traumatic origin. First-degree lacerations involve the mucosa and a short segment of the perineal body; second-degree lac-erations involve the entire perineum down to, but not through, the anal sphincter; third-degree (complete) lacerations extend through the anal sphincter and the rectal mucosa.

Incomplete lacerations may be repaired by denuding a diamond-shaped area of mucosa at the mucocutaneous junction over the lacerated perineum and repairing the defect in the longitudinal direction to restore the triangular shape of the perineum.

Successful repair of lacerations that extend into the rectum depends upon the prevention of infection. Direct repair by excision of the scarred margins of the laceration is associated with unpredictable success, although more consistently good results with this technique have been obtained since antibiotics and bowel sterilization procedures have become available. Two techniques that exclude the bowel lumen from the suture line have been highly successful. In the Warren technique, a flap of posterior vaginal wall is everted anteriorly like a hinge over the rectal wall defect. The anal sphincter and perineal body are approximated over this flap. A somewhat similar method, known as the Noble–Mengert technique, involves pulling the liberated anterior rectal wall outward beyond the level of the perineal body and repairing the anal sphincter and the perineum above (Fig. 61–9). The outer edge of the anterior rectal wall is sutured outside to the skin of the perineum.

OPERATIONS ON THE VAGINA

EXCISION OF A VAGINAL SEPTUM

The typical complete vaginal septum extends between the anterior and posterior vaginal walls and is made up of apposing vaginal wall layers. It extends from the vaginal introitus to the cervix and divides the vagina into symmetric halves. Usually the condition is classified as double vagina because each vaginal tube leads to one or two cervices, which are separated by the septum. All degrees of variation of vaginal septa are observed, and frequently no surgical treatment is necessary. When the vaginal septum is part of genital tract duplication, there is little advantage to the patient from excision unless the septum interferes with intercourse. A partial or incomplete septum may interfere with delivery. For example, one infant delivering by the breech was observed to straddle a firm septum, thereby arresting the progress of labor until the septum was divided. If operation is deemed necessary, total excision is better than simple division. Bleeding may be excessive unless ligation is performed as the septum is excised. It is well to begin at the junction of the septum with the posterior vaginal wall and progress backward to the cervix in short steps. The vaginal mucosa edges should be approximated with a continuous locking stitch of No. 3-0 absorbable suture.

FIG. 61-9. Noble–Mengert technique for repair of complete ▶ perineal tear. After transverse linear incision has been made in rectovaginal septum at rectovaginal border, cleavage plane is dissected to level of cervix. This allows anterior rectal wall to stretch and be easily displaced to level of perineal skin. Anal sphincter is approximated in midline over mobilized anterior rectal wall. Perineum is reconstructed by interrupted No. 2-0 absorbable sutures.

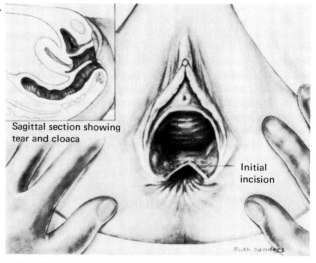

Sagittal section showing tear and cloaca

Initial incision

Stricture of the vagina may be corrected by making longitudinal incisions through the full thickness of the mucosa and suturing the defect transversely.

CONSTRUCTION OF VAGINA

In congenital absence of the vagina, operation is best delayed until marriage is contemplated unless the patient has a functioning uterus producing hematometra. The split-thickness skin graft technique of McIndoe has superseded the other methods that employed small bowel (Mori–Baldwin method), rectum (Shirodkar, Schubert, Pratt), pedicle skin flaps from the thigh (Frank, Geist), vulvar skin flap (Grossman), fetal membrane (Burger, Brindeau, von Mikulicz–Radicki, Caffier), test tube pressure (Frank, Falls), and the blunt dissection and obturator method (Wharton).

Basic Technique, McIndoe Procedure. 1) After perineal incision, blunt dissection is done to adequate depth of the space between the urethra and bladder and the rectum. 2) A suitably sized plastic mold is prepared to fill the cavity and to extend slightly externally. 3) The mold is covered with split-thickness skin graft about 0.012 inches thick; the skin surface is placed adjacent to the mold. 4) The mold is inserted in place by elastic pressure straps.

Because of difficulty in maintaining mold immobility and because infection is the main reason for failure, the author has modified the technique by suturing the skin of the introitus closed over the skin mold. Six weeks later the introitus is opened and the mold is removed. Absolute hemostasis is essential if the introitus is to be closed. The skin take is usually 100%. This procedure simplifies postoperative care and relieves the worry of mold mobility and infection. After removal of the mold, the introitus is kept open by insertion of a plastic mold several times daily.

REPAIR OF OBLITERATED VAGINA

The split-thickness skin technique is less suitable for radiation, operative, and traumatic obliteration of the vagina because of excessive scar tissue. In such cases, the sigmoid colon substitution technique is best.

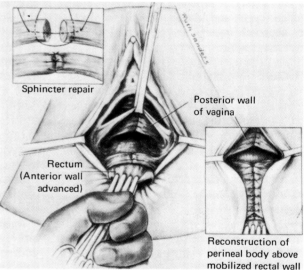

Sphincter repair

Posterior wall of vagina

Rectum (Anterior wall advanced)

Reconstruction of perineal body above mobilized rectal wall

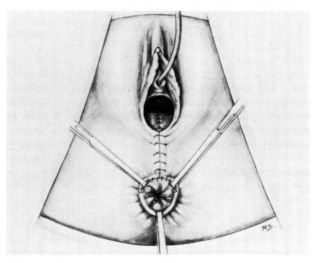

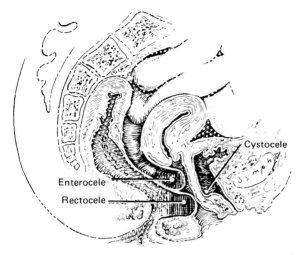

FIG. 61–10. Anatomic relations of cystocele, enterocele, and rectocele.

REPAIR OF ACUTE INJURIES

Acute injuries from accidental trauma occur at all ages. In infants and children every suspected laceration should be investigated in good light with adequate exposure under general anesthesia. Traction on a continuous locking suture aids in repairing the apex of an obscure laceration.

Stenosis and atrophy of the vaginal vault incidental to radiation therapy responds poorly to operative efforts. Adequate correction requires excision of the involved area and replacement with a graft. Stenosis resulting from operations can usually be corrected by dilatation, although occasionally excision of scar tissue is necessary. In postmenopausal patients vaginal application of estrogen creams or suppositories is beneficial.

REPAIR OF DEFECTS CAUSED BY CHILDBIRTH INJURIES

Trauma during parturition is the most common cause of anatomic vaginal defects. The fundamental pathology is attenuation or laceration of the endopelvic vaginal fascia and attenuation or laceration of the paravaginal fibrous supporting ligaments, including the uterosacral ligaments and the cervicosacral fibrous bands. If the cervix is taken as the focal point of obstetric injury, and if the wedge of the presenting part of the baby is considered to be the dilating force of trauma, then it is reasonable to expect fascial damage to be most marked in the area adjacent to the cervix and least marked at points most distant from the cervix. The central dilating force of the cervix produces

concentric rings of diminishing trauma toward the periphery. An attenuated or torn paravaginal fascia lacks contractive capacity and tends to heal to whichever structures it happens to contact. Usually it attaches to an area of the vaginal wall more distant from the cervix than its original attachment. This leaves a zone of deficient support between the cervix and the new point of attachment of the paravaginal fascia. Subsequently, the force of gravity and increased intra-abdominal pressure act directly upon the weakened vaginal wall area to give rise to vaginal wall protrusions that are named according to the contiguous organ involved (Fig. 61–10). *Cystocele* is a vaginal wall protrusion that affects the bladder. *Urethrocele* results from more extensive fascial damage and involves the urethra. *Rectocele* permits protrusion of the rectal wall. In a pathologic sense these conditions represent a diastasis of vaginal wall supports rather than true hernias because no peritoneal sac is present. Rarely is a single defect observed. An *enterocele,* however, is a true hernia with a well-developed peritoneal sac that protrudes through a precise defect in the paravaginal fascia posterior to the cervix and adjacent to the cul-de-sac of Douglas.

Principles of repair of vaginal wall protrusions, except for enterocele, are essentially similar. The vaginal mucosa is dissected laterally from midline incisions until the weak vaginal wall is replaced by a strong vaginal wall. The attenuated vagina wall is excised and the defect repaired by suturing together the vaginal mucosa combined with its supporting fascia. Two types of dissection may be used. If scissors are employed for dissection, the line of fusion between the vagina and the paravaginal fascia is not detached, and the type of repair is designated *full thickness.* If the scalpel is used for dissection, the fused fascia and vagina are separated, and the defect may be closed by approximating corresponding anatomic layers.

Repair of Urethrocele and Cystocele

Urethrocele and cystocele are repaired by one continuous procedure.

Basic Technique. 1) A midline incision is made through the anterior vaginal mucosa from the external urinary meatus to the cervix, where it joins with a short transverse incision through the mucosa over the anterior cervix: the inverted-T incision. 2) Lateral dissection is continued until the margin of the defect is identified. If scissors dissection is used, the margin of the defect is identified by palpation; if scalpel dissection is used, the torn fascial margin is visualized. 3) The bladder is detached from the anterior cervix and elevated to a higher level with several interrupted sutures. 4) Attenuated vaginal mucosa is excised. 5) In full-thickness repair, interrupted stitches of No. 2-0 absorbable suture are used to approximate the cut edges

of the vaginal mucosa. 6) If layers have been developed by sharp scalpel dissection, fascia and mucosa edges are approximated separately.

Repair of Rectocele and Perineum

Rectocele and perineum are usually repaired together.

Basic Technique. 1) An incision is made in the midline or, if lacerated, a diamond-shaped area of mucosa is excised. The incision is carried through the vaginal mucosa in the midline to join with a short transverse incision posterior to the cervix. 2) Lateral dissection of the vaginal mucosa is continued until the margin of the defect is identified. Dissection may be either full thickness or in layers. 3) Repair is begun posteriorly using either continuous or interrupted sutures of No. 2-0 absorbable material by bringing to the midline, posterior to the cervix, the diverging fibers of the paravaginal fascia, either as separate layers or as a single full-thickness layer. 4) When the perineum is reached, sutures are made to include the medial margins of the puborectalis fibers of the levator ani muscles, and the triangular shape of the perineum is restored.

Repair of Enterocele

Enterocele is repaired according to principles that apply to abdominal hernia.

Basic Technique. 1) The posterior vaginal wall is incised with an inverted-T incision. 2) The vaginal wall flaps are dissected laterally to uncover the peritoneal sac. 3) The peritoneal sac is identified and dissected from the adjacent paravaginal fascia to the level of the neck. 4) The sac is opened to ensure high mobilization. 5) The neck of the sac is closed with a purse-string suture at the highest level possible, being certain that no sutures pass through the anterior rectal wall, which may be adherent posteriorly. 6) The redundant peritoneum is excised and the neck fixed to the uterosacral ligaments near their junction with the cervix. 7) The posterior paravaginal fascia and vaginal mucosa are closed as in rectocele repair.

Repair of Cystocele by Uterine Interposition

The uterine interposition operation for cystocele repair (Watkins) is an obsolete procedure. It is mentioned for its historic interest and because a knowledge of this procedure is needed if one should be called upon to remove the uterus of a patient who previously has had such an operation, since the relations are greatly distorted. The technique involves transposing the uterine fundus through an opening in the vesicouterine fold of peritoneum to a position inferior to the bladder by suturing the fundus to the inferior pubic rami.

Basic Technique. 1) An inverted-T incision in the anterior vaginal wall is employed. 2) Lateral vaginal flaps are developed. 3) The pubocervical fascia is detached from the anterior cervix, and the peritoneum is opened anterior to the uterus. 4) The fundus is drawn through the peritoneal opening by traction, and the peritoneal opening is closed with sutures of No. 3-0 absorbable material. 5) The fundus is fixed to the inferior pubic rami with several No. 2-0 absorbable sutures. 6) Usually the cervix is partially amputated to provide easier rotation of the fundus. 7) The vaginal incision is closed with interrupted sutures of No. 2-0 absorbable material.

REPAIR OF UTEROVAGINAL PROLAPSE

The Manchester operation is indicated, in lieu of vaginal hysterectomy, for the correction of first-degree uterovaginal prolapse when it is desirable to retain the normal uterus for menstrual function or when it is felt that the lateral uterine ligaments are sufficiently strong to support the uterus adequately. Pregnancy and successful delivery have followed the Manchester operation, but there is a high incidence of relative infertility and late abortion, since the cervix has been amputated. Technically, the procedure is somewhat simpler than vaginal hysterectomy, but anatomic precision is less gratifying. It is also called the Donald–Fothergill operation. The principles of the procedure are 1) anterior colporrhaphy, 2) amputation of the cervix, 3) establishment of absence of uterine malignancy, 4) plication of the paracervical fascia anterior to the uterus, and 5) posterior colporrhaphy.

COLPOCLEISIS

Colpocleisis, obliteration of the vagina, may be complete or partial. It is used to correct primary or recurrent complete vaginal prolapse in the elderly patient who has no further interest in sexual intercourse and whose physical condition is too debilitated to permit vaginal reconstructive procedures. It is seldom used by the skillful gynecologist.

Complete colpocleisis is performed for recalcitrant vaginal vault prolapse after hysterectomy. It involves excision of all the vaginal mucosa to the level of the introitus. The cavity remaining is obliterated with absorbable sutures, and the introitus is closed by approximating in the midline the edges of the levator ani muscles.

Partial colpocleisis (LeFort's operation) is employed when the uterus remains. The principle is to create a broad transverse vaginal septum leaving laterally an inverted-U-shaped tube lined with vaginal mucous membrane extending from the cervix to permit drainage.

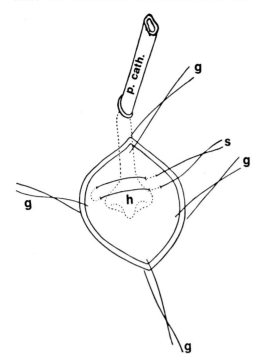

FIG. 61–11. Kelly operation for stress urinary incontinence. Original Kelly diagram of vesical sphincter plication. *h*, head of catheter marking neck of bladder; *g*, guy sutures holding wound open; *s*, suture at neck of bladder reuniting sphincter muscle. (TeLinde RW: Operative Gynecology, 3rd ed. Philadelphia, JB Lippincott, 1962)

Basic Technique. 1) Dilatation of the cervix and curettage of the uterus with biopsy of the cervix are done to eliminate malignancy. 2) From the anterior and posterior walls of the vagina are excised broad rectangular areas of vaginal mucosa extending from the introitus to within 2 cm of the cervix. 3) The cervix is inverted by suturing together the anterior and posterior raw surfaces; simultaneously, the anterior and posterior edges of the vaginal mucosa are approximated to form an inverted-U-shaped tube lined by mucous membrane of the vaginal wall.

RELIEF OF STRESS URINARY INCONTINENCE

This condition, which affects over 50% of adult females, is characterized by the loss of urine in spurts through the intact urethra as the result of a sudden elevation of intra-abdominal pressure such as occurs with coughing, laughing, or sneezing. Radiographic studies of the bladder and the urethra show the essential pathology to be downward displacement of the internal urinary meatus to the lower-most bladder level during the straining effort. If the bladder rotates pos-

teriorly during straining to a level lower than the urethrovesical junction, stress incontinence does not occur. The basic principle of operative repair for stress urinary incontinence is to elevate the urethrovesical junction to a higher level than the base of the bladder. The choice of operative technique depends upon the position of the urethrovesical junction as revealed by the anteroposterior radiograph. If, during straining, the urethrovesical junction descends lower than 4 cm below the inferior edge of the symphysis, vaginal repair should be performed according to the principles of Kelly. If the descent of the urethrovesical junction is less than 4 cm below the inferior edge of the symphysis, retropubic urethropexy performed through a lower abdominal incision is preferable. Operations primarily devised to tighten a "uretheral sphincter," unless combined with urethrovesical elevation, have been notoriously unsuccessful.

Kelly Operation

As first described in 1914, the operation consisted of elevation of the urethrovesical junction by plication of the pubocervical fascia beneath the urethrovesical junction (Fig. 61–11).

Basic Technique. 1) A longitudinal incision is made in the anterior vaginal mucosa at the level of the urethrovesical junction. 2) Lateral dissection of the vaginal flaps is accomplished. 3) The internal urinary meatus is located by palpation of a mushroom catheter placed in bladder. 4) At the highest level possible on each side of the urethrovesical junction are placed two to four mattress sutures of No. 0 absorbable material to effect urethrovesical elevation. 5) The vaginal mucosa is closed with absorbable sutures.

With the technique originally described by Kelly, good elevation of the urethrovesical junction was effected and the percentage of cures of incontinence was high. However, the operation did little to correct the urethrocele anterior to the Kelly stitches or to correct the cystocele posterior. Kennedy advocated plication of the paraurethral fascia in addition to the Kelly stitches to tighten the urethra. The combined procedure is known as the Kelly–Kennedy operation for stress urinary incontinence. Others have recommended simultaneous repair of the cystocele. However, with this there is the danger of negating the beneficial effects of urethrovesical elevation and thereby canceling the salutary effects of the Kelly technique. If the cure of stress urinary incontinence is the prime objective of operation, overcorrection of the cystocele must be avoided.

Retropubic Urethropexy

Retropubic urethropexy has been accomplished by passing slings of fascia, round ligaments, plastic, or

various animal membranes around the urethra from above. The technique is popularly known as the Goebell–Frangenheim–Stoeckel operation. Usually, elevation of the urethrovesical junction is accomplished by upward tension mediated through a strip of fascia obtained from the anterior rectus sheath and passed through a suburethral tunnel dissected beneath the urethra from exposure through the space of Retzius. All techniques that involve making a suburethral tunnel from the suprapubic approach carry the same disadvantage: urinary fistula from perforation of the urethra. Aldridge has combined the vaginal and abdominal operations by supporting the urethrovesical junction from below with fascia passed from above after the urethra first has been dissected free in the course of a vaginal plastic operation. The Aldridge operation avoids the high complication rate of suburethral tunneling from above, but apparently does so with some compromise of urethrovesical elevation.

The Marshall–Marchetti–Krantz technique has been widely adopted for the management of urinary stress incontinence. This technique involves elevating the anterior vaginal wall to a high retropubic level by vaginal finger pressure from below and fixing the paraurethral tissue to the retropubic periosteum. In properly selected patients, the technique accomplishes good urethrovesical elevation and is highly successful. The major complication of the procedure is pubic osteitis, a prolonged and painful disability.

Experience has shown that without compromising the principles of the Marshall–Marchetti–Krantz operation, the complication of pubic osteitis can be avoided by approximating the anterior paravaginal tissues to the iliopectineal line (Cooper's ligament) at the pelvic brim (Burch's modification, Fig. 61–12). The articles by Burch and by Durfee contain helpful technical details.

This operation provides excellent retropubic elevation of the urethrovesical junction and broad vaginal wall support to the inferior urethra (Fig. 56–12B). In properly selected patients the results are excellent and very durable, even after subsequent vaginal delivery.

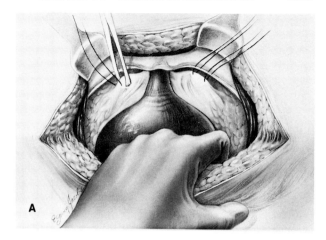

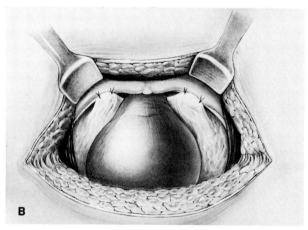

FIG. 61-12. Retropubic urethropexy, vaginal wall technique. *A.* On right, sutures have been passed through white paravaginal fascia, made evident by upward pressure cone, and through iliopectineal line at pelvic brim. Bladder and urethra must be displaced medially. On left, pressure cone has been grasped with Allis clamp. Should sutures pass into vagina, little concern need be given because complications are rare. *B.* After sutures are tied, urethrovesical junction is elevated to high, fixed retropubic position. Urethra is supported by broad vaginal wall sling. Bladder is free to rotate backward and downward during time of increased intraabdominal stress.

REPAIR OF VAGINAL FISTULAS

Vaginal fistulas are named from the viscera involved: they may be *simple* if the tract connects with two structures or *compound* if the tract connects with more than two structures. Rectovaginal and vesicovaginal are simple types, while vesicouretero-vaginal and rectoentero-vaginal are examples of compound types. Many different combinations are possible, as noted in Figure 48–15.

The basic principles of successful repair for all vaginal fistulas are 1) accurate diagnosis, 2) absence of infection, 3) absence of tissue inflammation, 4) adequate exposure, 5) complete excision of the fistula tract, 6) complete liberation of scar tissue and tissue plane adhesions, 7) accurate cut-edge to cut-edge approximation of the mucosa of the viscus, 8) ample reinforcement of the closure line by suture in layers of the investing fibrous tissue and the vaginal wall, 9) avoidance of hematoma and postoperative infection, and 10) elimination of the pressure of distention in the viscus repaired until solid healing has occurred.

Because fistulas vary in type, it is impossible to outline precisely the basic steps of a specific procedure.

The operator must be prepared to handle any situation encountered according to basic principles.

Repairs of Vesicovaginal Fistula

In vesicovaginal fistula, careful preoperative diagnosis must establish the relation of the ureteral openings to the fistula and make certain that multiple fistulas are not present. Many failures have resulted because the ureteral orifice was inadvertently included in the suture line. Lack of success has resulted also from failure to eradicate infection preoperatively; indwelling catheters should be removed at least 5 days before surgery. The time of the operation is most important: as a rule from 4 to 6 months are required for subsidence of local tissue inflammation. Recently, the administration of 300 mg cortisone daily for 2 to 3 weeks has been advocated to shorten the inflammatory phase of acute fistula, thereby permitting earlier surgery for closure. Although many gynecologists use silver-wire sutures, as was advocated first by Marion Sims, others employ fine absorbable sutures. Nonabsorbable sutures must not be buried beneath the bladder mucosa because in time they work their way into the bladder to provoke infection and calculus formation.

Repair of Rectovaginal Fistula

In repair of rectovaginal fistula, infection is the great obstacle to success. Several means of preventing fecal contamination of the suture line are possible. In low rectovaginal fistula the suture line may be protected by turning down a flap of upper vaginal mucosa, as in the Warren method, or by pulling down a liberated segment of the anterior rectal wall, as in the Noble–Mengert technique. In both of these techniques the suture lines used to repair the rectal sphincter and the perineum are isolated from the bowel lumen by an intact tissue layer. Preliminary bowel preparation by thorough mechanical and cathartic cleansing and the use of a diet that does not produce a residue are essential. Intestinal antibiotics and chemotherapeutic agents administered in adequate dosage not only reduce the infection danger by largely eliminating fecal bacteria but offer the mechanical benefits of reducing and liquefying fecal bulk. If the fistula is recurrent, has been caused by radiation, is located high, or is very large, preliminary diversion by colostomy is necessary. Because the objectives of preliminary colostomy are to relieve the fistula of the trauma of fecal bulk and of contamination by fecal bacteria, the ends of the colostomy should be separated by at least 15 cm. If the stoma of the distal loop is continually bathed by feces, the cilia of the mucosa continue to sweep small amounts of fecal material into the bowel lumen of the lower loop to perpetuate the infection hazard. Following diversion colostomy with complete separation of the stomas, the author has observed several very large radiation fistulas to close spontaneously. Partial or complete severing of a bowel loop brought out over a glass rod, without complete separation of the ends, is an inadequate colostomy technique for diversion in rectovaginal fistula.

TREATMENT OF HEMATOCOLPOS

Cystic dilatation of the entire vagina by hematocolpos occurs following the onset of menstruation if the hymen is imperforate. The condition is usually observed in a patient in her early teens, after several menstrual periods have occurred without external bleeding. Rectovaginal examination shows a large, tender, cystic mass filling the pelvis. Usually the hymen bulges as a blue membrane occluding the vaginal orifice. Operative excision of the entire hymen effects a cure. Subsequent vaginal dilatation is advisable to prevent postoperative adherence. Simple incision of the hymen is insufficient because it is usually followed by stenosis.

Occult hematocolpos occurs when there is a functional second uterus connected with a second vagina that ends blindly. Examination discloses a large cystic mass lying anterolateral to the vagina. It produces periodic pain. Treatment consists of excision of the intervening vaginal wall according to the principles of marsupialization.

TREATMENT OF VAGINAL CYSTS

Vaginal wall cysts are of the retention type and generally result from endometriosis or from a small piece of vaginal wall being buried at the time of repair of vaginal wall laceration. Simple excision or electrocoagulation is sufficient treatment.

Paravaginal cysts are usually of Gartner's duct origin and may be simple or complicated. Isolated cysts are easily cured by excision. Multiple cysts may extend far into the broad ligament and lead the unwary into a complicated operation for which the surgeon is not prepared. When paravaginal cysts are suspected, preliminary investigation should be made for other congenital anomalies of the genitourinary system.

EXCISION OF SUBURETHRAL DIVERTICULUM

A suburethral diverticulum is a prolapse of the urethral wall through a defect in the periurethral (endopelvic) fascia. Anatomically it may be divided into a neck and a cystic dilatation, which are generally found initially on the inferior surface of the urethra. It can be palpated on vaginal examination as a cystic, rounded structure in the space between the anterior vaginal wall and the urethra (Fig. 61–13). Occasionally the diverticulum may arise from the lateral or anterior surfaces of the urethra. Using a special balloon-type

catheter to occlude the inner and outer ends of the urethra, the diverticulum can be visualized radiographically following injection of radiopaque contrast medium. Although primarily a urologic condition, suburethral diverticulum is important to the gynecologist because it may be mistaken for a vaginal wall cyst.

As long as the neck remains patulous, permitting free passage of urine between the diverticulum and the urethra, symptoms are minimal. Complete or ball-valve occlusion of the neck may result in acute infection, sudden enlargement, urethral occlusion, suppuration, abscess formation, and sinus tract and fistula formation.

Basic Technique. 1) An 18-Foley catheter is placed into the urethra. 2) The vaginal mucosa is incised longitudinally to the level of the diverticulum. 3) Careful dissection is performed to the neck of the diverticulum. 4) The diverticulum is completely excised at the level of the neck. 5) With excision of the neck of the diverticulum, the catheter in the urethra is visualized. 6) The urethral mucosa is carefully approximated using closely placed interrupted sutures of No. 4–0 absorbable material. 7) The defect in the periurethral endopelvic fascia is reapproximated and reinforced with as many layers as possible. 8) The vaginal mucosa is closed. 9) Bladder drainage is accomplished by suprapubic trochar cystostomy. 10) Culture and antibiotic sensitivity tests are done on material from the urethral surface of the diverticulum, and appropriate antibiotics are given in high dosage for at least 7 days. Note that in a large urethral diverticulum that has caused severe damage to the urethral wall, primary sutures are frequently insecure and blood supply may be somewhat inadequate. Reinforcement of the suture line by transplantation of a labial fat pad to the suburethral area provides support and improves chances for primary healing without fistula formation.

TREATMENT OF VAGINAL TUMORS

Benign tumors of the vagina are relatively rare. Fibromas, lipomas, myomas, and hemangiomas usually can be removed by enucleation.

Malignant tumors of the vagina may be primary or metastatic. If primary, they are epidermoid in type (rarely adenocarcinoma) and generally involve the upper half of the vagina. Initial treatment should be by combined local and external radiation. Radical vaginectomy is reserved for lesions that inadequately respond to radiation. Because of variations in lymphatic drainage, radical vaginectomy varies according to the site of the lesion. If the upper third of the vagina is involved, radical vaginectomy consists of excision of the entire vagina, the uterus, the adnexa, the paravaginal and parauterine tissues, and the pelvic lymphatics. Lesions confined to the middle third of the vagina additionally should be treated by radical vulvectomy. In le-

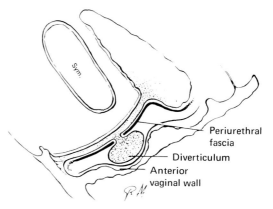

FIG. 61-13. Urethrovaginal relations of a suburethral diverticulum.

sions confined to the lower third of the vagina, treatment should consist of simple vaginectomy plus radical vulvectomy. Amputation of the urethra is generally necessary in anterior vaginectomy; the distal two-thirds of the urethra may be excised without producing urinary incontinence.

Sarcoma of the vagina, including sarcoma botryoides observed in children, is usually recalcitrant to all forms of therapy, although occasional patients apparently cured by radical vaginectomy have been reported.

Vaginal metastasis most frequently occurs from carcinoma of the cervix, carcinoma of the uterine fundus, and choriocarcinoma. Except for biopsy for diagnosis and local excision or simple vaginectomy in recurrent preinvasive carcinoma of the vaginal vault, therapy is generally limited to radiation, and surgery is not indicated.

OPERATIONS ON THE UTERUS

ANATOMIC CONSIDERATIONS

From the viewpoint of operative gynecology, it is important to recall that the uterus is derived by fusion and anteromedial migration of the caudal ends of the müllerian ducts; that, in conjunction with the complex anatomic changes incident to the biped state and the effects of gravity, the intra-abdominal position of the uterus in the infant changes in the adult to an intrapelvic position; that, except indirectly, the uterus has no bony points of fixation; and that it is suspended in the pelvis by musculofibrous modifications of the endopelvic fascia which pass from the pelvic wall to the cervix. Particularly in the adult in the erect position, insufficient emphasis has been given to the importance of the peculiar anatomic characteristics of the uterosacral musculofibrous supports that extend posterolaterally from the cervix to the presacral fascia.

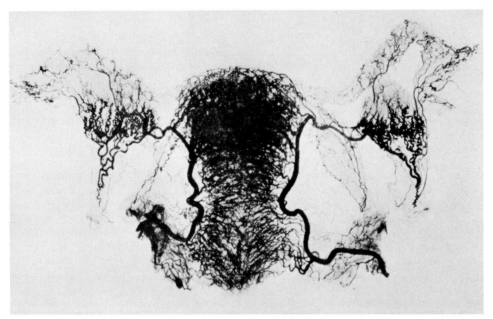

FIG. 61-14. Double blood supply to uterus. Uterus is suspended between a right and a left arterial loop, giving a bilateral, double-access to arterial blood supply. Arterial blood passes to uterus by secondary arteries which spring from each arterial loop.

Congenitally, or due to obstetric trauma, these supporting masses of tissue may be long or short, strong or weak. If they are short, the cervix is maintained in the posterior pelvis, and the fundus falls anteriorly (uterine anteversion and anteflexion). If the ligaments are long, the cervix is located in the anterior position, and the fundus is displaced backward by the distended bladder and the force of gravity (uterine retroversion and retroflexion). If the uterosacral supports are strong, the position of the cervix is relatively fixed; if they are weak, the cervix is mobile and from the force of gravity falls downward and outward (uterine prolapse).

It is important to keep in mind the unique characteristics of the double blood supply to the uterus (Fig. 61-14). The primary uterine and ovarian arteries that supply blood to the uterus never actually enter the uterus. These two arteries inosculate near the uterine cornua to form bilaterally a highly coiled single vessel, which in reality is an arterial loop extending from the midaorta to the anterior division (pudendal artery) of the internal iliac artery. The uterus is suspended between the two arterial loops, which shunt blood to the uterus by secondary arcuate arteries that perforate the myometrium. Thus, nature has provided for generous blood supply under highly mobile conditions. The veins, in general, follow the arteries, although in highly vascular states such as pregnancy and the presence of a large abdominal tumor much blood is returned to the general circulation by means of the vertebral system of veins.

An anatomic consideration of extreme importance to the gynecologist is the lower urinary tract. Although the anatomic relations of the ureters, bladder, and urethra are precisely detailed in Chapters 3 and 49, certain principles of surgical significance should be mentioned here. Except for the distal half of the urethra, the entire urinary tract is invested between layers of the transversalis fascia and its modifications. Until the ureter passes through the broad ligament, it is intimately associated with the peritoneum. It is necessary for the gynecologist constantly to remind himself that the position of the ureter may rather drastically change when the peritoneum of the pelvis is distorted by a tumor or by the blade of a retractor. An intraligamentous cyst or a cervical myoma may force the ureter to a medial position so that it lies deep in a groove between the tumor and the uterus. Because the uterine artery passes over the ureter, extreme uterine prolapse may drag the lower ureter sharply downward and produce sufficient angulation to cause temporary ureteral obstruction.

OPERATIONS BY THE VAGINAL ROUTE

Regardless of the age of the patient or the type of operation to be performed, a smear for cytologic study is an essential preliminary to an elective operation on the cervix or, indeed, to any gynecologic operation.

The first step in any vaginal operation that is performed under anesthesia is bimanual examination to

verify the size and position of the uterus and to note whether adnexal masses are present that could not be felt before.

Cervical Dilatation and Uterine Curettage (D&C)

This procedure is used for diagnosis and in some instances for treatment of intrauterine disorder. It is the most frequently performed gynecologic operation and should be performed in "fractional" manner except in incomplete abortion, when this is not needed.

Basic Technique. 1) The position of the uterus is determined by bimanual examination. 2) The cervical canal is straightened by firm outward traction on the cervix. 3) The external os (only) is dilated sufficiently to admit a small curette into the cervix. (Dilators of the more pointed Pratt type are less traumatic than the blunt-ended Hegar dilators). 4) The cervical canal is systematically curetted. Any returns from the cervix are placed in a separate bottle of fixative. 5) A uterine sound is introduced to the uterine fundus to note the depth and course of the uterine cavity. 6) The internal os is dilated with graduated dilators up to a number 21 or 22 French. 7) A sharp curette of medium size is introduced to the top of the fundus, and with light, retrieving strokes the entire uterine cavity is systematically curetted. 8) The uterine cavity is explored with a ureteral stone forceps by opening, closing, and withdrawing the blades. 9) All tissue is transferred to a second bottle of fixative. 10) Cervical biopsy may be done.

It is important to remember that perforation of the uterus occurs because of a thrusting motion, rather than a retrieving motion (Fig. 61–15). Because the presenting edges of the "sharp" and "dull" curet are equally blunt, perforation with one instrument is just as likely as with the other. In fact, because the dull curet is less efficient, it is likely to be used with a heavier hand and so may be the more dangerous instrument of the two. The accidental perforation of the uterus calls for individualized treatment. If it occurs in a small, firm uterus that contains neither infection nor malignancy, watchful waiting is usually sufficient. If it occurs in a uterus that contains endometrial carcinoma, immediate hysterectomy is best. Abdominal surgery is necessary if injury to the bowel or bladder is suspected or if bleeding is excessive and persistent.

Biopsy of the Cervix

An adequate biopsy of the cervix is one that is sufficient to establish a diagnosis of unquestioned accuracy. The amount of tissue obtained may vary from a sample a few millimeters in diameter, such as a tiny fragment of tissue manually detached from a friable malignant mass, to a specimen consisting of the entire cervix. It is important to remember that for a diagnosis

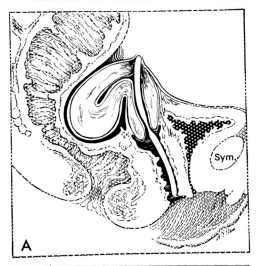

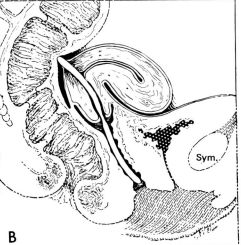

FIG. 61–15. Uterine perforation. *A.* Uterus in retroflexion. *B.* Uterus in anteflexion. (TeLinde RW: Operative Gynecology, 3rd ed. Philadelphia, JB Lippincott, 1962)

of malignant invasion, the pathologist needs no more than the surface epithelium and a shallow layer of the underlying stroma; an excessively extensive biopsy may delay definitive operative treatment. However, in a patient with a positive Papanicolaou smear in whom no gross lesion can be identified and colposcopy is negative, the biopsy should include the lining of the endocervix as well as the entire epithelial surface of the external cervix (Fig. 61–16). Tissue for microscopic study should be obtained with a sharp cutting edge of a cold scalpel, not with cutting–current electrocoagulation. The practical value of tissue obtained as a continuous sheet by conization over that obtained as multiple bites of tissue by punch biopsy remains a moot question.

If a cervical lesion is clearly suspicious, colposcopi-

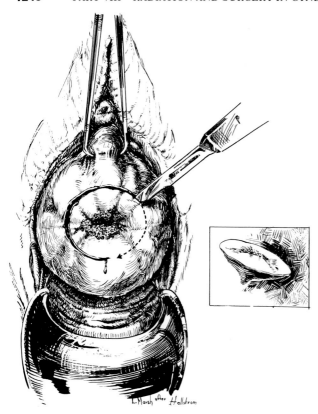

FIG. 61-16. Conization of cervix for biopsy.

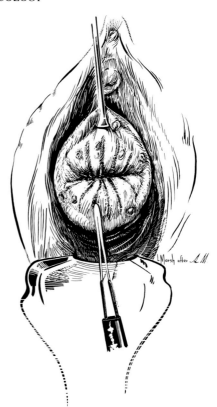

FIG. 61-17. Cauterization of cervix. From six to ten linear applications are made, depending upon size of lesion.

cally directed biopsy may solve the problem. If not, punch biopsy of the cervix should be performed before dilatation and curettage.

Cauterization of the Cervix

Cauterization of the cervix is usually done to relieve chronic cystic cervicitis (nabothian cysts), although it can be used to some advantage in ectropion of the cervix and chronic noncystic cervicitis with discharge. It is of little value in the pseudoerosion of nulliparous women.

The intention of cauterization is to destroy the deep cervical glands leaving in-between islands of untreated cervix for healing (Fig. 61–17). When cystic cervicitis is less extensive, individual cysts may be cauterized separately. The best heat is obtained when the cautery tip is a glowing dull red. No anesthesia is needed.

Cryosurgery of the Cervix

Cryotherapy—treatment by freezing—of the cervix is an alternate technique to hot cauterization for chronic cervicitis, cystic or noncystic, and for ectropion. The objective of cryotherapy is limited-depth destruction of the portion of the cervix involved (Fig. 61–18). Two systems for rapid refrigeration of tips of sophisticated cervical probes have been developed, one using liquid nitrogen and the other using liquid freon. The requirements for therapy are an operating temperature of $-50°$ C to $-60°$ C and an operating time of 120 to 180 seconds. Cryosurgery is an acceptable method of treating benign chronic cervicitis and erosion. There is difference of opinion regarding its use for treatment of carcinoma in situ.

Basic Technique. 1) No anesthesia is needed. 2) The cervix is exposed and vaginal folds held away. 3) The probe is applied to the cervix, usually with the tip within the cervical canal. 4) The temperature is rapidly lowered to $-50°$ C to $-60°$ C and held for 120 to 180 seconds. 5) The tip is rapidly warmed to allow detachment of the probe from the frozen area of the cervix.

Compared with the hot cautery, cryosurgery is characterized by less pain and relative freedom from post-treatment complications such as bleeding, discharge, and infection.

Excision of Cervical Lips

This procedure is seldom indicated but may be helpful for a multipara with everting cervical lips secondary to lacerations of childbirth, evoking ectropion and chronic vaginal discharge.

Basic Technique. 1) Wedge-shaped areas on the inner surface of the everting cervical lips are excised. 2) The approximating edges of the lacerations are freshened. 3) The cervical mucosa is liberated until it is sufficiently free to cover the raw area over the cervical lips. 4) The cervical mucosa is inverted to the level of the external os with a mattress or Sturmdorf-type suture of No. 0 absorbable material. 5) The lacerations are repaired with interrupted sutures of No. 0 absorbable material.

Hysteroscopy

A special endoscope has been designed to visualize the uterine cavity. The cervix is first dilated under paracervical block and the uterus is distended continuously with 5% dextrose. The real value of the instrument has not been determined except for retrieval of a tailless IUD when other methods have failed.

Amputation of the Cervix

This procedure, applicable for patients who fail to respond to cauterization, is infrequently used and is often followed by sterility. High amputation of the cervix may expose endometrium and provoke irregular vaginal bleeding. Subsequent delivery may be precipitous; if enough of the cervix is removed, late abortion should be expected.

Excision of a Cervical Polyp

Although cervical polyps are seldom malignant, they do provoke vaginal discharge and occasionally bleeding. They may be high or low, sessile or pedunculated. The object of excision of the polyp is to remove sufficient base to prevent recurrence. Snipping off or avulsing the polyp in the office at the level of visibility may be insufficient.

Basic Technique. 1) The cervix is adequately dilated. 2) If the polyp is low and sessile, it should be excised by a wedge-shaped incision and the defect closed with interrupted gut sutures. 3) If pedunculated and high, it is best excised with a snare as close to the base as possible. 4) Curettage of the uterus should be performed and the endometrial cavity searched for polyps with the ureteral stone forceps.

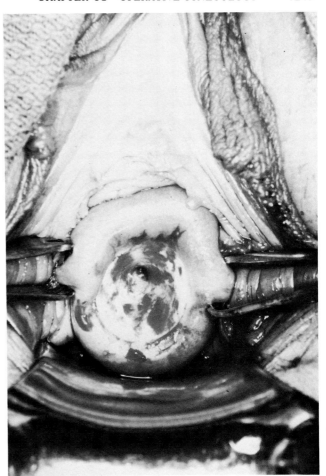

FIG. 61-18. Cervical ice ball after 60 seconds' exposure at −60° C.

Posterior Colpotomy

Posterior colpotomy may be performed for diagnosis of obscure pelvic pathology if laparoscopy is not applicable; for treatment, to drain pus confined to the cul-de-sac; and for execution of certain operative procedures, such as salpingectomy for ectopic pregnancy and tubal ligation.

The objective of posterior colpotomy is to provide access, both visual and manual, to the pelvic organs. Its use should be reserved for the patient whose vagina is sufficiently spacious to permit adequate retraction.

Basic Technique. 1) External cervical traction is obtained by a tenaculum attached to the posterior cervical lip. 2) Adequate retraction of the posterior vaginal wall is necessary. 3) A transverse incision is made through the vaginal mucosa of the posterior vaginal fornix and the peritoneum between the uterosacral lig-

aments. 4) Manual exploration of the pelvis is accomplished. 5) Visual examination is done of mobile structures brought into the incision with sponge-tipped forceps, Babcock clamps, and forceps. 6) The intended surgical procedure is performed. 7) The peritoneum and vaginal mucosa are closed separately with No. 2-0 absorbable sutures.

Drainage of the Pelvis

Gynecologic intraperitoneal pyogenic infections may point in the cul-de-sac, rectum, small or large bowel, or through adhesions into the upper abdomen. Retroperitoneal pyogenic infections may point in the groin at the level of the inguinal ligament. Drainage is indicated for localized abscess formation and occasionally in conjunction with abdominal operations when there has been extensive intraperitoneal spill of purulent material. Drainage of pelvic abscess, regardless of location, should be delayed until pointing is clearly evident on clinical examination. In the presence of hard, brawny induration (characteristic of cellulitis), incision and drainage should be delayed. Complications of inappropriate incision and drainage are hemorrhage, extended infection, opening into an ovarian cyst, laceration of bowel, and fistula formation. "If in doubt about fluctuation, delay incision and drainage," is a good rule to follow.

Posterior Culdostomy. Posterior culdostomy is indicated for an abscess that points into the cul-de-sac of Douglas and that can be detected by manual vaginal examination as a softened, fluctuant area in the posterior fornix.

Basic Technique. 1) External cervical traction is obtained by a tenaculum attached to the posterior cervix. 2) A 15-gauge needle is passed into the area of maximal softening. 3) Aspiration is done, using a glass syringe, to obtain pus, of which both aerobic and anaerobic cultures are made. 4) The abscess cavity is opened into by means of a transverse or vertical incision. 5) The opening is enlarged by opening the blades of a Kelly clamp or scissors, as in Hilton's method. 6) Two or more large gauze-filled rubber drains are inserted into the abscess cavity and maintained in place by sutures passed through the edge of the vaginal incision.

Proctostomy. Proctostomy is indicated for pelvic abscesses that point into the rectum.

Basic Technique. 1) Gradual digital dilatation of the anal sphincter is accomplished. 2) The anterior rectal wall is exposed with narrow-bladed retractors. 3) A 15-gauge needle is inserted into the area of maximal softening, and aspiration is done to obtain pus. 4) A transverse incision is made through the anterior rectal wall into the abscess cavity. 5) The incision is enlarged by

opening the blades of a large Kelly clamp or scissors, as in Hilton's method. 6) No drains are needed; healing without fistula or sinus formation can be expected.

Drainage of Inguinal Abscess. Drainage of inguinal abscesses is indicated for retroperitoneal infections with dissection to the inguinal areas. Clinically such abscesses appear as hot, tender, indurated inguinal swelling that gradually show evidence of pointing, as indicated by dusky-red skin discoloration and a detectable area of central softening.

Basic Technique. 1) A 15-gauge needle is inserted into the area of central softening, and aspiration is done, using a glass syringe, to obtain pus. 2) The skin is incised in the direction of the inguinal ligament over the area of softening. 3) The aponeurosis of the external oblique muscle is incised in the line of the direction of the fibers. 4) The opening is enlarged by blunt-finger dissection of the fibers of the external oblique muscle. 5) The retroperitoneal abscess cavity is explored digitally, using care to avoid the underlying external iliac vessels. 6) Gauze-filled rubber drains are inserted into the abscess cavity.

Drainage Plus Pelvic Laparotomy. Drainage in conjunction with pelvic laparotomy is indicated when there has been extensive spill of purulent material throughout the abdominal cavity and when an opened abscess cavity cannot be completely excised. Pelvic drainage is best accomplished by passing drains through the posterior vaginal fornix and vagina from within the abdominal cavity. Adhesions and obliteration of the cul-de-sac of Douglas make the posterior vaginal fornix difficult to identify from within the abdomen. This identification can be safely accomplished by having an assistant work beneath the drapes to direct the point of a dressing forceps into the posterior vaginal fornix. When firm pressure is made inward and upward, the point of the forceps can be identified by palpation from within the abdomen. After making certain the area is free of bowel, an incision is made over the point of the forceps to permit its entry into the pelvic cavity. The ends of two or more gauze-filled rubber drains are placed between the jaws of the forceps and pulled into the vagina (Fig. 61–19).

Culdoscopy

Culdoscopy is a diagnostic procedure that permits inspection of the pelvic viscera. It is useful in the study of infertility, particularly when Stein–Leventhal ovaries are suspected and for the diagnosis of obscure pelvic pathology such as minimal endometriosis. It is used with difficulty, and some danger, in the patient with endometriosis that involves the cul-de-sac of Douglas, and has been largely superceded by laparoscopy.

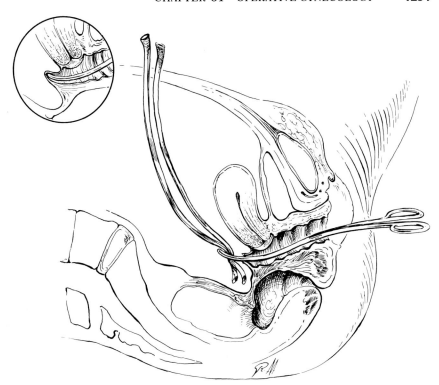

FIG. 61–19. Drainage of cul-de-sac through vagina during abdominal laparotomy. In inserting dressing forceps, assistant must be certain that tip of forceps does not accidentally enter urethra.

Basic Technique. 1) The knee–chest position is required. 2) Sedation is used, but not general anesthesia. 3) Outward traction is made on the cervix. 4) Local infiltration of the mucosa of the posterior fornix with an anesthetic is usually used. 5) A 5-mm incision is made through the vaginal mucosa over the ballooned-out area of the posterior fornix. 6) When it is certain that the lighting system of the culdoscope is properly functioning, the culdoscope with the obturator is placed against the mucosal incision and plunged boldly through the peritoneum. 7) When the obturator is removed, a gush of air can be heard to enter the instrument. 8) With the room completely dark, the culdoscope is introduced and the pelvic viscera visualized. 9) The patient is asked to exhale as forcefully as possible to force out intraperitoneal air when the instrument is removed; this will minimize shoulder pain when she sits up. 10) Manual pressure on the abdomen until the patient is placed prone aids in preventing reentry of air. 11) Suture of the incision in the vaginal mucosa is not necessary except to control bleeding.

Laparoscopy

Laparoscopy is a surgical diagnostic and operative endoscopic technique performed under anesthesia in the operating room under full aseptic conditions.

Diagnostic Laparoscopy. The gynecologic indications for diagnostic laparoscopy include all conditions in which visual examination of the pelvic organs might enable definitive diagnosis. Examples are ectopic pregnancy, infertility, or menstrual dysfunction due to adnexal disease, endometriosis, genital tuberculosis, pelvic inflammatory disease, and pelvic masses incidental to the first 3 months of pregnancy. In selected cases of ovarian cancer, laparoscopy has been used at the time of laparotomy to examine the inferior surface of the diaphragm for evidence of lymphatic involvement. The procedure is being used increasingly as a preliminary to the "second-look" operation in order to evaluate the efficacy of prior therapy; if residual tumor is found by laparoscopy, the second-look laparotomy is unnecessary, but if no tumor is found the full exploratory laparotomy is needed.

Its use is contraindicated in patients with generalized peritonitis or intestinal obstruction. It is also contraindicated in the presence of circulatory and respiratory deficiencies that would be aggravated by the Trendelenburg position and by pneumoperitoneum. Examples of such conditions are large diaphragmatic, abdominal, umbilical, or crural hernia; extensive intra-abdominal adhesions incidental to previous abdominal operations; certain infections; and, intra-abdominal malignancy.

Complications of the technique include hemorrhage

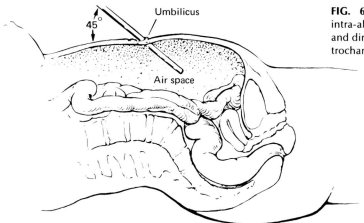

Umbilicus

45°

Air space

FIG. 61-20. Laparoscopy. Diagrammatic demonstration of intra-abdominal air space resulting from pneumoperitoneum and direction of thrust of trochar. Mentally visualized, thrust of trochar should be toward center of pelvic cavity.

from perforation of a blood vessel of the anterior abdominal wall or of the posterior iliac vessels owing to improper use or overpenetration of the gas needle or trochar, perforation of the intestine or bladder, gas embolism, subcutaneous emphysema, mediastinal emphysema, and accidental pneumothorax.

The required apparatus includes an appropriate laparoscope, a light source, a flexible glass fiber light guide, a carbon dioxide or nitrous oxide gas source, a uterine cannula and locking cervical vulsellum, a special automatic gas needle (Drapier or Verres), aspiration syringes, and a gas insufflation apparatus.

Basic Technique. 1) General anesthesia is induced (local anesthesia is used in selected cases). 2) The vagina and abdomen are prepared for surgery. 3) An intrauterine cannula is introduced and fixed with a vulsellum to the cervix. 4) A site is selected for puncture; the infraumbilical rim or the lateral border of the rectus is suitable if there is a midline scar. 5) A Verres or a Drapier needle is inserted beneath the skin for about 3 cm, then downward into the peritoneal cavity. 6) Aspiration is done with a 10-ml syringe and the aspirate is checked for fluid or malodorous gas. 7) About 10 ml air is injected; it should pass freely without pressure and produce no subcutaneous swelling. 8) Carbon dioxide (preferable) or nitrous oxide is insufflated at an initial rate of 0.5 liter/minute; the patient is observed for global distention of abdomen by tympanitic percussion and disappearance of liver dullness. 9) Speed of gas insufflation is increased to 1 liter/minute until firm abdominal distention is obtained, usually at 3 to 6 liters. 10) A 1-cm incision is made through the skin and subcutaneous fascia of the lower border of the umbilicus. 11) After ascertaining that there is no abdominal viscus beneath, the laparoscope trochar is introduced beneath the skin for about 3 cm, then at a downward angle of 45° toward the pelvic cavity (Fig. 61–20); both hands are used to prevent overinsertion

from sudden thrust when the trochar passes through the peritoneum, as indicated by a hollow sound. 12) The trochar is withdrawn, the laparoscope inserted, and the light source attached. 13) The pelvic viscera are inspected in semidarkness. 14) Tubal patency is tested by injection of 5 to 10 ml aqueous 2% methylene blue solution or indigo carmine through the uterine cannula. 15) Dilatation and curettage are done.

Operative Laparoscopy. For operative laparoscopy using electrocauterization it is essential that the patient be appropriately grounded and that instruments be of fiberglass nonconductive material. By means of special cutting, aspiration, and electrocoagulation equipment, a variety of intra-abdominal pelvic procedures can be performed: tubal cauterization for sterilization, ovarian biopsy and coagulation for control of bleeding, lysis of fine adhesions by coagulation or cutting, aspiration of benign ovarian cysts, and ventrosuspension of the uterus. The procedure can also be used to retrieve an intra-abdominal IUD.

Basic Technique. 1) Satisfactory diagnostic laparoscopic setup is achieved. 2) With the laparoscope light, an avascular area is demonstrated in the lower anterior abdominal wall. 3) A small skin incision is made and the operating trochar and cannula are introduced. 4) The operating trochar is removed and an appropriate operating instrument is introduced. 5) The operating instrument is guided to the operative site under direct vision (Fig. 61–20).

Electrocauterization of Fallopian Tubes for Sterilization. 1) The patient is checked for appropriate grounding and the instruments for proper function and nonsparking. 2) Coagulating grasping forceps are introduced and the fallopian tube is grasped at the point of narrow diameter about 3 cm lateral from the uterine cornu. 3) The fallopian tube is stretched

slightly upward to isolate it from the mesosalpinx. 4) The location of the intestine is checked to be certain it is well away from all instruments and from the fallopian tube coagulation site. 5) Cauterization current is induced and maintained until the tube site is blanched for a distance of about 3 cm. 6) A segment of the coagulated tube can be removed by drawing the tube against the serrated cutting edge of the forceps sleeve; however, experience has shown that this step is not required and may even be undesirable.

This technique for electrocauterization of the fallopian tube illustrates the fundamental principles required for other types of operative laparoscopy.

Improvements in instrumentation have been made recently. The development of an angulated laparoscope with a center channel for introduction of the operative instruments permits operative laparoscopy with a single abdominal puncture technique. Also under development and found to be practical are bipolar cautery instruments in which one electrode is placed in one arm of the grasping forceps and the opposite electrode in the other arm of the grasping forceps. With this instrument the ground plate can be eliminated, thereby preventing accidental burns and intra-abdominal sparking. When the current is applied, cauterization occurs only in the area within the grasp of the forceps. With the instrument insulated over all surfaces except the opposite sides of grasping prongs there is little danger of injuring adjacent viscera.

Repair of Inverted Uterus

Complete inversion of the uterus is rare, and surgery is required only if the fundus cannot be reinverted by nonsurgical manipulations performed under anesthesia. Inversion of the fundus is usually a complication of the puerperium, but occasionally a pedunculated submucous myoma may cause inversion of the nonpregnant uterus. Because the fundus is larger than the constricting ring of cervix, repositioning by manual pressure may be difficult or impossible.

The objective of all of these operations is to incise the cervix to release the constricting tension so that the fundus can be replaced in its normal position. The Kustner procedure is performed vaginally.

Application of Radium

The application of radium is employed in conjunction with external radiation as primary treatment for carcinoma of the cervix and occasionally as primary treatment for carcinoma of the corpus. The modalities and the techniques of application vary, not only with the sites treated but, because of variations in anatomy, with different patients. The rationale and technique of radiation therapy are discussed in Chapter 60.

After radium is applied, a gauze pack, which should

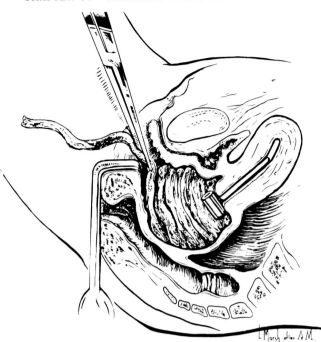

FIG. 61-21. Vaginal tamponade, used principally for control of cervical bleeding or for immobilizing intracavitary radium. If vaginal pack is to be used, it should be placed systematically and tightly and be very wet.

be sopping wet when it is inserted, is carefully and systematically placed in the vagina to immobilize the radium in the correct position and to move the adjacent structures to a safe distance from the radium sources. Figure 61–21 shows such a pack in place.

Vaginal Hysterectomy

Removal of the uterus by the vaginal approach gives superior results in certain specific situations: uterovaginal prolapse, carcinoma in situ, and extreme obesity. It is contraindicated when the diagnosis is obscure, when symptoms suggest involvement of other systems, when the uterus is excessively enlarged or excessively adherent, in the presence of large benign or malignant neoplastic ovarian cysts, and in the presence of other genital tract malignancy. In combination with anterior and posterior colporrhaphy and repair of relaxation of the vaginal vault, vaginal hysterectomy has as its objective definitive cure of symptoms and physical defects relating to attenuation of endopelvic supporting fascia. In carcinoma in situ a wide cuff of cervicovaginal mucous membrane can be more assuredly excised with vaginal hysterectomy than with abdominal hysterectomy, and there is probably less danger of injury to the bladder and ureters because the vaginal dissection is done under direct vision. Al-

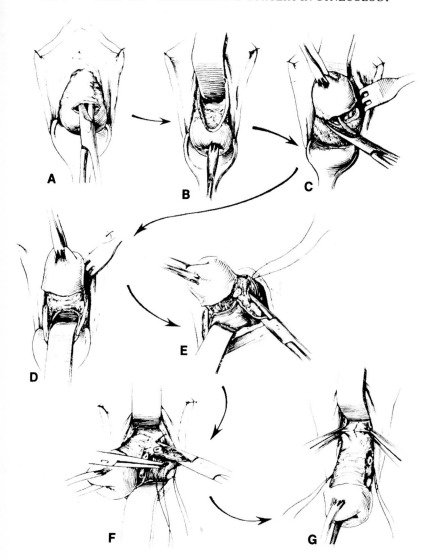

FIG. 61–22. Vaginal hysterectomy. *A.* Transverse incision above cervix through mucous membrane. *B.* Connective tissue between cervix and bladder (elevated by retractor). *C.* Continuation of transverse incision around cervix. *D.* Posterior cul-de-sac entered; Heaney retractor inserted. *E.* Left uterosacral ligament clamped, cut; suture placed. *F.* Left cardinal ligament with uterine artery clamped, cut; suture placed. *G.* Anterior vesical peritoneum grasped. *H.* Uterus delivered through posterior cul-de-sac. *I.* Left broad ligament clamped. *J.* Left broad ligament clamped, cut; suture placed. *K.* Uterus removed; broad ligament pedicles above; suture placed through left posterior vaginal mucosa, left uterosacral ligament, posterior peritoneum, right uterosacral ligament, and finally back through right posterior vaginal mucous membrane. *L.* Suture approximating broad ligaments and anterior vesical peritoneum. *M.* Suture approximating uterosacral ligaments and broad ligaments. *N.* Transverse closure of mucous membrane of vault of vagina. (Edwards EA: Vaginal hysterectomy, Chap IX–3. In Meigs JV, Sturgis (eds): Progress in Gynecology, Vol III. New York, Grune & Stratton, 1957)

(*Continued on next page*)

though the technique of vaginal hysterectomy is designed primarily to extirpate the uterus, the fallopian tubes and ovaries can usually be excised with little additional effort. Moderate increase in uterine size due to myomas of the uterus is not a deterrent to the technique because morcellation of the uterus can usually be easily accomplished. In extreme obesity, vaginal hysterectomy is the technique of choice because the danger of abdominal wound dehiscence is eliminated and postoperative morbidity is decreased. The steps in the technique are shown in Figure 61–22.

In vaginal hysterectomy performed for uterovaginal prolapse, little difficulty is encountered in mobilizing the uterus. However, in patients with normal support, uterine mobility is difficult until the uterosacral ligaments are detached in their entirety from the cervix. Numerous variations in technique are used to avoid the most common complication of the operation—sub-

sequent vaginal prolapse. High ligation of the uterosacral ligaments and their approximation in the midline provides the best focal point for attachment of the vaginal mucosa to prevent subsequent vault prolapse (Fig. 61–23). Subsequent stress urinary incontinence may occur from excessive elevation of the base of the bladder in patients who have undergone surgery because of uterovaginal prolapse. When myomas obstruct delivery of the uterus through the vagina, morcellation becomes necessary. This procedure is performed by cutting out wedge-shaped areas of the uterus beginning with the cervix and proceeding upward. If possible, the uterine vessels first should be cut and ligated. Excessive bleeding rarely occurs with myomectomy so long as the incisions angulate toward the midline. After the uterus is bisected, each broad ligament is clamped and ligated in the usual fashion.

Radical vaginal hysterectomy (Schauta's operation)

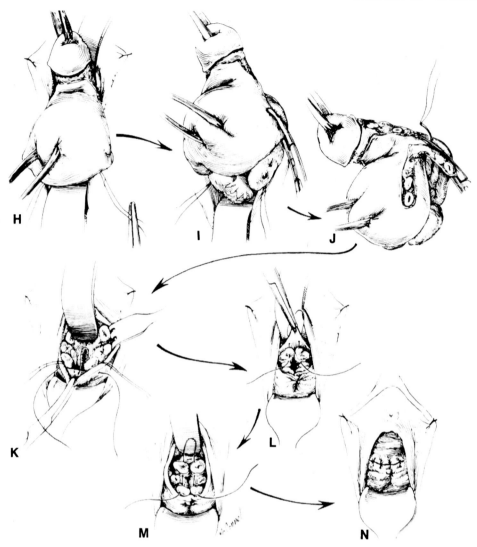

FIG. 61-22. (Continued)

is performed for carcinoma of the cervix. In this technique the bladder, ureters, and rectum are widely libberated, and the paracervical tissue is widely excised. The pelvic lymph nodes are not excised as part of the primary operation.

OPERATIONS BY THE ABDOMINAL ROUTE

Abdominal Incisions

Gynecologic abdominal operations are performed through vertical or transverse skin incisions (Fig. 61–24).

Vertical Incisions. These are generally slightly off-center or paramedian, extend from the umbilicus to slightly above the symphysis, and involve an area of the abdominal wall supplied by terminal arteries,

veins, and nerves (Fig. 61–25). All abdominal wall components are incised vertically, and the uncut rectus muscles are displaced laterally by retraction. No blood vessel of significant size is encountered. Only terminal branches of nerves are disturbed. Above the linea semilunaris, the posterior sheath of the rectus muscle is incised and below this level the transversalis fascia. When the vertical incision in the peritoneum is made, the bladder must be empty and care can be exercised to avoid incising the bladder.

Transverse Muscle-splitting Incision (Pfannenstiel). The skin is incised in the line of skin cleavage at the level of the transverse abdominal fold in the upper area of pubic hair (Fig. 61–26). The method has the advantage of leaving very little scar. At the level of the anterior sheath of the rectus muscle, the incision may be made either transverse (preferred) or vertical without

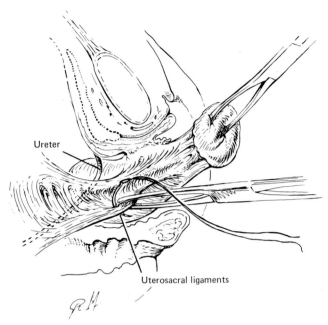

FIG. 61-23. High ligation of uterosacral ligaments to prevent recurrence of prolapse following vaginal hysterectomy. Under traction, uterosacral ligaments feel like cords, but appear as grooves. Techniques can be used only if location of ureters is accurately known. Ureter and upper level of uterosacral ligament run parallel and in close proximity.

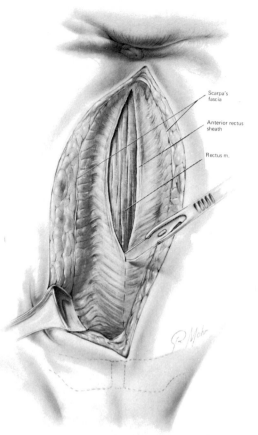

FIG. 61-25. Lower abdominal paramedian incision, made slightly off-center, extends from umbilicus to slightly above symphysis. Rectus muscle is retracted laterally. Few blood vessels and nerves are encountered in this area because incision is in area of embryonic body closure.

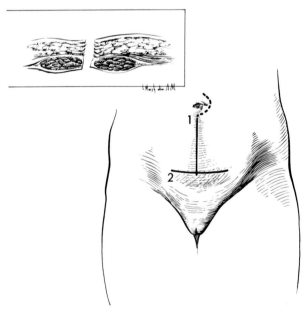

FIG. 61-24. Location of abdominal skin incisions. Incision *1* is vertical and slightly paramedian. *Inset* shows how abdomen can be entered without actually cutting muscle tissue. Incision *2* is transverse (Pfannenstiel's incision). Vertical incisions are used for all layers of abdominal wall except skin.

cutting the underlying rectus muscle. The upper and lower flaps of anterior rectus sheath are liberated above and below the incision, and dissection is carried through the peritoneum in the vertical direction. The method has the disadvantage of limiting exposure and should not be used for operations that require extensive intra-abdominal manipulation.

Transverse Muscle-cutting Incision (Cherney). The skin incision extends along a line between the anterior superior iliac spines (Fig. 61–27). The anterior fascia over the external oblique and rectus muscles is cut transversely. The external oblique muscle fibers are separated by blunt dissection in the direction of the fibers. The rectus muscles are cut transversely in the fibers of the pubic tendons. The pyramidalis muscles are cut from their midline attachments and displaced downward. The deep inferior epigastric vessels are cut between clamps and ligated with transfixion sutures.

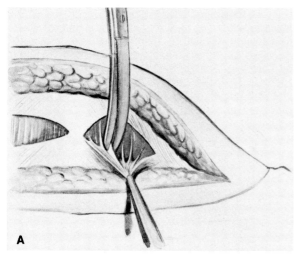

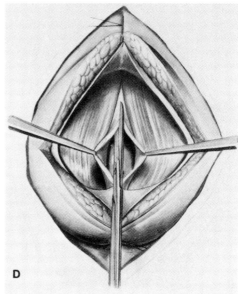

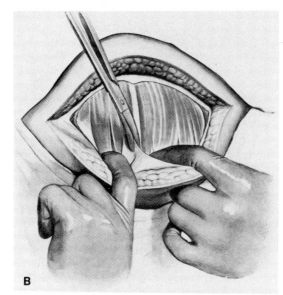

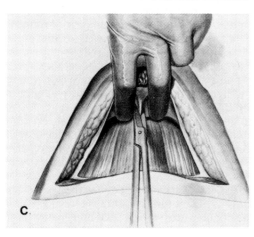

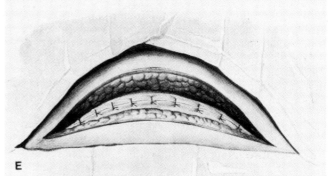

FIG. 61-26. Pfannenstiel's incision. *A.* Skin and subcutaneous fat have been incised by transverse semilunar incision superior to symphysis. Anterior rectus sheath has been opened transversely to right and left of linea alba. Rectus muscles are visible through openings. Right rectus is being freed from its loose attachment to anterior wall of sheath. *B.* Linea alba is placed on tension and incised with scissors in longitudinal direction parallel to skin surface. *C.* Preparation of caudal premuscular aponeurotic flap. *D.* Aponeurotic flaps may be sutured, as shown, or held away by retractors. Mesial edges of rectus muscles are separated and anterior parietal peritoneum incised. *E.* Closure. Peritoneum has been sutured. Rectus muscles are allowed to come together without suture. Fascia is closed with interrupted single or figure-of-eight chromic catgut sutures, usually 0 or 2-0. Subcutaneous fascia is closed with 3-0 plain catgut. Since major use of incision is cosmetic, skin is closed with subcuticular suture. (Peham HV, Amreich J: Operative Gynecology. Translated by LK Ferguson. Philadelphia, JB Lippincott, 1934)

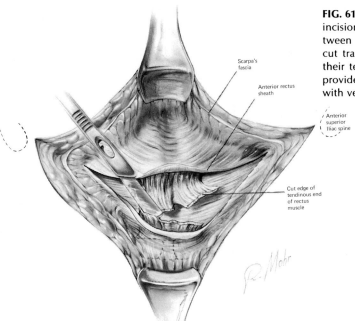

Scarpa's
fascia

Anterior rectus
sheath

Anterior
superior
Iliac spine

Cut edge of
tendinous end
of rectus
muscle

FIG. 61–27. Transverse muscle-cutting incision (Cherney). Skin incision follows along lines of skin cleavage and extends between anterior superior iliac spines. Anterior rectus sheath is cut transversely. Rectus muscles are cut transversely through their tendinous insertions into symphysis pubis. This incision provides excellent exposure of pelvis, and skin incision heals with very little scar.

The transversalis fascia and peritoneum are incised transversely. This method is used to advantage when the operative procedure involves extensive lateral dissection, as in radical hysterectomy or pelvic evisceration. It has the disadvantage of requiring the ligation of two major (but not vital) arteries and the cutting of two major muscles (rectus). It is a time-consuming procedure, and incidental blood loss is more than is encountered with incisions made near the midline. However, it heals well and causes little disability. The skin scar is minimal.

All incisions may be satisfactorily closed in layers with interrupted sutures of nonabsorbable plastic, silk, cotton, or metal wire. The time-honored opinion that absorbable suture must be used in gynecologic operations because of the danger of infection has been disproved. However, many surgeons prefer continuous or running absorbable suture for closure of abdominal incisions to save time.

Abdominal Hysterectomy

Abdominal hysterectomy is preferred over vaginal hysterectomy 1) when the diagnosis is questionable, 2) when abdominal exploration is needed, 3) when the uterus is excessively large, 4) when appendectomy or other bowel surgery is needed, 5) when there is a history of severe inflammatory peritonitis or extensive endometriosis, 6) in the presence of ascites, 7) in the presence of neoplastic ovarian cyst, and 8) during pregnancy.

Abdominal hysterectomy is indicated for myoma that has enlarged the uterus to the size of a 3-month pregnancy, when there is evidence of rapid growth, excessive bleeding, or pain. Other indications are carcinoma in situ of the cervix, carcinoma of the corpus, extensive adenomyosis and endometriosis, tuberculosis of the endometrium, carcinoma of the ovary, old salpingitis complicated by extensive hydrosalpinx, or pyosalpinx requiring the extirpation of the ovaries. Except in rare instances when, in the judgment of the operator, excision of the cervix would be dangerous, corpus and cervix should be removed. Supracervical hysterectomy is seldom performed.

Many individual variations in technique are employed in hysterectomy. Some gynecologic surgeons unite the round ligaments with the cut edge of the vaginal vault, while others allow the round ligaments to fall free. Some use nonabsorbable sutures while others use absorbable material. Which is used makes little difference as long as knots are secure.

The technique of abdominal hysterectomy used at the Henry Ford Hospital is shown in Figures 61–28 and 61–29.

The preliminary steps of supracervical (subtotal, supravaginal) hysterectomy differ little from those of complete hysterectomy. After the uterine arteries have been ligated, the anterior and posterior peritoneum is liberated slightly, and the cervix is amputated by means of a transverse wedge at the level of the cervical isthmus. The uterine stump is closed with interrupted absorbable sutures, and peritonealization is carried out as in total hysterectomy.

points usually prevents hemorrhage, and antibiotic therapy usually controls infection.

Myomectomy

In a woman in the early years of childbearing, myomectomy with preservation of the uterus is the treatment of choice. Myomectomy is particularly indicated if a previous pregnancy ended in premature delivery and if severe pain and rapid enlargement of the myoma were noted.

If possible, the uterine cavity should not be entered, but one should not be hesitant if this is needed. All palpable myomas should be excised, regardless of size.

Basic Technique. 1) A vertical incision is made through the serosa over the area of maximal distention by the myoma. 2) The incision is continued through the overlying myometrium until the capsule of the myoma has been entered. 3) The myoma is removed by blunt dissection. 4) The uterine defect is closed by interrupted sutures; care must be taken to control all active bleeding. 5) The serosa should not be excised until the cavity is closed; myometrial contraction occurs rather forcefully once the myoma is removed, and frequently little or no serosa need be excised. 6) The serosa is closed by an inverting continuous suture.

Pedunculated myomas are removed by means of elliptical incision around the base with closure as noted above. Myomectomy during pregnancy is best avoided unless symptoms are extreme because of the danger of hemorrhage and the possibility of inducing premature labor. If myomectomy becomes mandatory during pregnancy, the technique is unchanged, but extreme care must be taken to ensure complete hemostasis.

Excision of Uterine Septum (Strassmann Operation)

Infertility and frequent spontaneous abortion may be caused by a congenital intrauterine septum. Unification of the uterus by excision of the septum should be undertaken if complete evaluation has disclosed no other cause of infertility. Occasionally a septate uterus is associated with abnormal uterine bleeding and dysmenorrhea.

Initially, Strassmann recommended a transverse fundal incision for excision of the septum. Currently, most gynecologists use elliptical, wedge-shaped incisions directed anteroposteriorly.

Basic Technique. 1) The fundus is palpated manually to determine the size of the septum. 2) Beginning posteriorly in the midline below the lower limit of the septum, elliptical incisions are begun bilaterally and carried over the fundus to a similar midline point anteriorly, with excision of the septum in a wedge-shaped segment of uterus. 3) The defect is closed by a

first row of interrupted sutures of No. 0 absorbable material placed in the myometrium subendometrially. 4) A second row of interrupted sutures is passed through the myometrium. 5) A third serosal inverting layer of sutures is placed. 6) Prior to abdominal closure, the uterus is returned to the pelvis and the suture line draped with large bowel and omentum.

Should pregnancy occur, most gynecologists advise delivery by cesarean section, although often this is not necessary because the uterus is solidly healed. The major complication from the operation is intestinal obstruction from adherence of small bowel to the suture line.

Uterine Suspension

Indications for primary uterine suspension are extremely vague. Seldom done by the modern gynecologist, uterine suspension in former years was extensively performed; over 50 techniques have been described. The indications ran the gamut of subjective ailments of the female. Improved knowledge of menstrual physiology and the realization that in the vertical state of the biped the uterine fundus is a highly mobile organ that deftly responds to the forces of gravity have gradually changed concepts about symptoms that signify disease. In the quadruped, the uterine fundi (they are usually bicornuate) fall inferiorly because of gravity. In the erect human this inferior position becomes anterior or ventral. The ultimate position of the fundus, therefore, depends upon which side of the uterus, dorsal or ventral, is most affected by the force of gravity. An ill-advised uterine suspension in a patient with congenital retroversion causes the bladder to be displaced forward and favors the development of stress urinary incontinence. Acquired retrodisplacement may follow delivery and results from attenuation of the posterior cervical support. Defying gravity and sometimes causing retrodisplacement of the uterus are adhesions incidental to uterosacral endometriosis and pelvic inflammation. Experience has shown that symptoms are caused by the pelvic disease and not the retrodisplacement of the fundus.

Today uterine suspension is generally performed as a secondary procedure incidental to operation for endometriosis and pelvic adhesions in order to protect the fundus from being drawn toward the cul-de-sac by the contracting scar tissue in the uterosacral ligaments and posterior pelvis. It is improper to designate the intention of an operative procedure as restoring the uterus to a "normal anterior position," because a ventral tilt of the fundus is normal only in the quadruped. The Gilliam–Doléris and the Baldy–Webster techniques are most frequently employed.

Basic Technique, Gilliam–Doléris Procedure. 1) In performing the abdominal incision, the superficial fat and fascia over the anterior rectus sheath are cleared bila-

of cervix. Strong upward traction with first set of cornu clamps aids identification of uterosacral ligaments. Usually uterosacral ligaments can be cut free without ligation because there is seldom active bleeding. *E.* Before Kelly clamps are placed over cervical branches of uterine artery, pubocervical fascia is detached from anterior surface of cervix. This is facilitated by making upward and anterior traction with forefinger pressing from behind cervix. By means of scissors followed by blunt dissection with gauze-covered finger, broad attachment of pubocervical fascia is separated from anterior surface of cervix. *F.* After pubocervical fascia is separated from its cervical attachment and displaced downward, cervical branches of uterine vessels are clamped by placing blades of Kelly forceps inside cut edge of pubocervical fascia. Ureters and bladder lie on anterior surface of pubocervical fascia and are protected from injury by first detaching pubocervical fascia from cervix. *G.* Uterus is removed by cutting vaginal mucosa close to cervix; this may be done with scissors or scalpel. Usually bleeding is slight. Previous

application of clamps to vaginal mucosa is seldom necessary. Bleeding vessels are singly ligated. *H.* Cut ends of round ligament are approximated to lateral sides of vaginal cuff. This tends to compress lateral vascular pedicles and obliterate dead space, reducing chance of hematoma formation. It also gives some support to vaginal vault. *I.* Vagina is closed anteroposteriorly with running suture of No. 2-0 absorbable material. To prevent granulation tissue from forming in vaginal vault, cut edges of vagina are carefully approximated by placing sutures through paravaginal tissues rather than through vaginal mucosa. *J.* When vagina is closed, cut edge of pubocervical fascia is approximated to retrocervical tissue including cut ends of uterosacral ligaments. With these tissues united over vaginal cuff, hematoma formation is reduced by obliteration of dead space, and added support is provided for vaginal vault. *K.* Peritoneum is closed with running suture of No. 2-0 absorbable material. As peritoneum is closed, ligature stumps on fallopian tubes and ovarian ligaments are inverted.

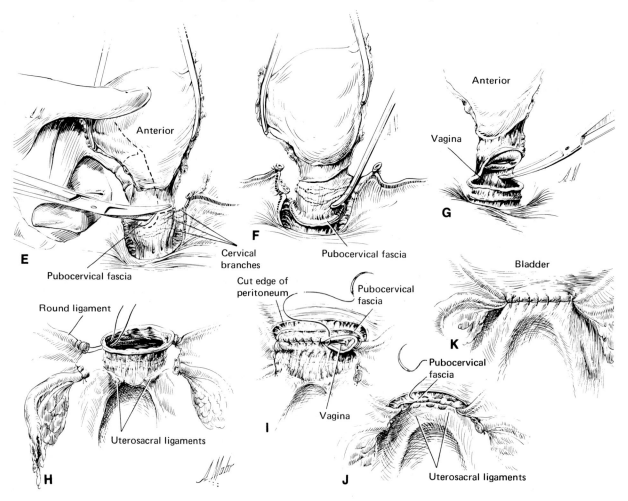

FIG. 61-29. Total abdominal hysterectomy. *A.* First clamps are placed upon cornu of uterus including round ligament, fallopian tube, and true ligament to ovary. To prevent bleeding from uterine artery, tip of Kelly forceps must be placed in avascular area of broad ligament. Upon reaching uterus, uterine artery turns upward between leaves of broad ligament to anastomose by inosculation with ovarian artery. If tip of Kelly forceps hugs uterus too closely, uterine artery will lie outside clamped area, where it may be cut accidentally. Utero-ovarian arterial anastomosis is indicated in drawing. *B.* Second set of clamps includes fallopian tube and true ligament of ovary. Tip of Kelly forceps extends to, but does not include, round ligament. If fallopian tube and ovary are to be removed, forceps are placed upon infundibulopelvic ligament lateral to ovary. Ureter is identified by snapping it between thumb and forefinger before placing for-

ceps on infundibulopelvic ligament. After tie has been placed around it, round ligament is cut and allowed to retract laterally; frequently, round ligament can be cut without ligating. *C.* Peritoneum is cut across just below level of internal os of uterus. Peritoneum can be separated easily from underlying tissue by opening and closing scissors in proper tissue plane. Posteriorly, peritoneum is cut with scissors to junction of uterosacral ligament. When traction is made upward with uterine cornu clamp, uterine vessels can be identified. Vessels are clamped just below level of internal os of uterus, and tip of forceps should extend directly to lateral side of cervix. Uterine vessels are cut between clamps and lower stump of vascular pedicle ligated with figure-of-eight suture of No. 0 absorbable material. *D.* After uterine vascular pedicles are clamped and tied on each side, uterosacral ligaments are dissected from posterior surface

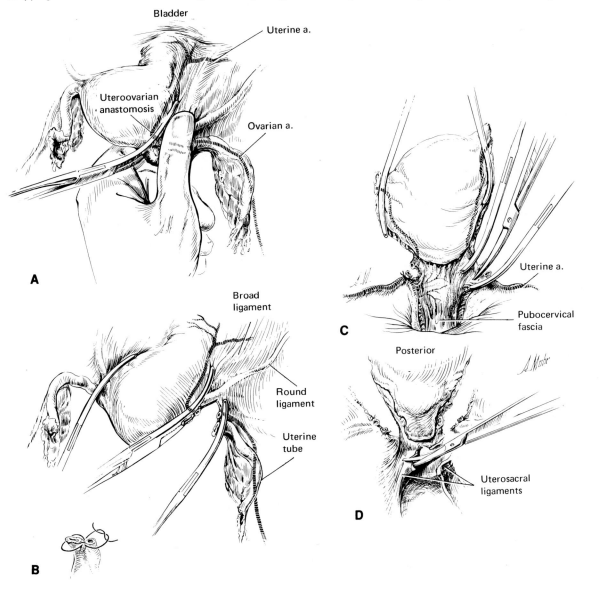

Radical Hysterectomy

Radical hysterectomy is employed for Stage I and early Stage II carcinoma of the cervix and for carcinoma of the corpus located at or near the internal cervical os. Some reserve its use for those patients with squamous cell cancer that incompletely responds to radiation therapy. Adenocarcinoma of the cervix frequently fails to respond to radiation; in dealing with this lesion, some gynecologists prefer primary radical surgery to radiation.

Radical hysterectomy (modified Wertheim operation), according to present day standards, implies the following: 1) excision of the internal, external, and common iliac lymph nodes; 2) excision of the obturator lymph nodes; 3) ligation of the ovarian vessels in the infundibulopelvic ligament; 4) ligation of the uterine arteries at the level of their branching from the anterior branch of internal iliac arteries; 5) excision en bloc of the parametrial and paracervical tissue containing the uterine veins; 6) division of the uterosacral ligaments at least 3 cm from the cervix; and 7) excision of the upper one-third of the vagina.

Basic Technique. 1) The procedure is suitable only for patients with Stage I or early Stage II cancer of the cervix, who are not obese, are in good general health and under 65 years of age, and who have not previously been subjected to total irradiation. 2) A lower paramedian incision is made with lateral paraumbilical extension or a transverse muscle-cutting abdominal incision of the Cherney type (Fig. 61–27). 3) The ovarian vessels are ligated well above the ovaries in the infundibulopelvic ligament after the ureter has been excluded. 4) The round ligament is ligated at least 3 cm from the uterus. 5) An incision is made in the peritoneum from the infundibulopelvic ligament ligature anteriorly to the vesicouterine reflection and posteriorly to the uterosacral ligament; care must be taken to exclude the ureter. 6) Dissection is continued to the common iliac artery. 7) An incision is made through the fibrous sheath of the common iliac artery and carried forward to the inguinal ligament. 8) In the plane of the arterial sheath, dissection is carried medially with removal of all lymph nodes. 9) The obturator fossa is dissected, with preservation of the obturator nerve. 10) The uterine artery is ligated where it branches from the internal iliac artery; frequently it comes off the internal iliac artery in common with the obliterated hypogastric artery; the latter forms the lateral umbilical ligament. 11) Medial dissection of the parametrial and paracervical tissue is carried out, with isolation of the ureter to its entrance into the bladder. 12) The paracervical tissue containing the uterine veins is ligated at the lateral pelvic wall; frequently the uterine veins divide to surround the ureter, while the uterine artery is always superior. 13) The bladder and

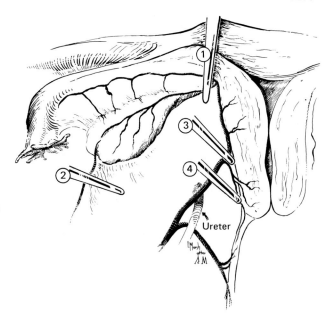

FIG. 61–28. Placement of clamps for abdominal hysterectomy. Clamp *1* interrupts utero-ovarian artery at uterine cornu. If fallopian tube and ovary are not to be removed, clamp *2* is not applied.

ureters are elevated from their attachments to the anterior cervix. 14) The uterosacral ligaments are ligated at least 3 cm from the cervix, and the peritoneum of the cul-de-sac of Douglas is excised. 15) Liberal dissection of the rectovaginal septum with posterior displacement of the rectum is carried out. 16) The bladder is elevated from the anterior vaginal wall for at least 5 cm. 17) The upper one-third of the vagina is excised as the final step in extirpation of the uterus, both fallopian tubes and ovaries, and the attached paracervical and parametrial tissue. 18) All bleeding points are ligated. 19) The vagina is not closed. 20) The pelvic floor is peritonealized by uniting the anterior and posterior peritoneal flaps after first placing retroperitoneally at least two soft rubber catheters (No. 21) with multiple holes cut in the distal one-third; these catheters are subsequently attached to suction pumps.

The major complications of radical hysterectomy are the formation of ureteral fistula and lymphocysts, pelvic infection, and hemorrhage. Most of these complications are preventable. Ureteral fistulas are infrequent if the ureters are not excessively separated from the peritoneum, if they are not handled roughly or placed over traction tapes, and if the small ureteral arteries above the level of the broad ligament are not severed. Mechanical suction has largely eliminated lymphocysts. Detailed technical attention to bleeding

(*Text continues on p. 1262.*)

terally for a distance of 4 cm from the midline on a line about 4 cm above the symphysis. 2) After the abdomen is opened by blunt dissection with the point of an artery forceps, tunnels are made about 4 cm above the symphysis and 4 cm from the midline bilaterally, through the anterior rectus sheath, rectus muscle, transversalis fascia, and peritoneum. 3) The midpoint of the round ligament is grasped with the forceps and drawn through the tunnel. 4) Each round ligament is swung toward the midline, where they are sutured to each other and to the anterior sheath of the rectus muscle.

Basic Technique, Baldy–Webster Procedure. 1) By blunt dissection an opening is made in the vessel-free area of the broad ligament just lateral to each side of the upper third of the uterus. 2) A clamp is passed from behind forward through the opening, and the midpoint of the round ligament is doubled through the opening to the posterior surface of the corpus where it is attached to the corpus with interrupted sutures of No. 2-0 absorbable material. 3) By means of fine absorbable sutures, the openings in the broad ligaments are closed anteriorly and posteriorly to prevent herniation of bowel.

The major complication of all intra-abdominal hysteropexy operations is intestinal obstruction. Care must be taken to close the openings of all tissue tunnels. Suture lines must be shielded as far as possible to prevent intestinal attachment by fibrinous adhesions. Uterine suspension by the Gilliam–Doléris operation usually withstands the pressure of pregnancy, but recurrence of retrodisplacement usually follows pregnancy when the suspension was performed by the Baldy–Webster technique.

OPERATIONS ON THE FALLOPIAN TUBES

ANATOMIC CONSIDERATIONS

The fallopian tube is considered to extend from the intrauterine stoma to the terminal fimbria and is divided into the interstitial portion (within the myometrium), the isthmus (the narrow segment adjacent to uterus), the ampulla (the widened portion lateral to isthmus), and the fimbriated extremity or infundibulum (ovarian end). It is made up of serous, muscular, and mucous membrane layers and extends from the uterus in the upper border of the broad ligament between folds of peritoneum. Except for the inferior surface, which faces between the layers of the broad ligament, and the interstitial portion, the fallopian tube is covered with peritoneum. This relation is important in tubal pregnancy because sometimes the tube ruptures into the broad ligament and may give rise to an extrauterine intraligamentous pregnancy. The mucous membrane is lined by columnar ciliated and nonci-

liated cells disposed over highly intricate rugae. Interrugal adhesions from salpingitis forming blind canals are supposed to be a major cause of tubal pregnancy.

OPERATIONS

Salpingectomy

Salpingectomy is performed for ruptured ectopic pregnancy, acute and chronic salpingitis, hydrosalpinx, hematosalpinx, and as an incidental procedure in combination with oophorectomy and hysterectomy. In the operation of salpingectomy the entire tube is removed. A cornual stump must not be left, for it invites nidation in this very hazardous area if subsequent pregnancy occurs.

Basic Technique. 1) The fallopian tube is elevated upward to stretch out the mesosalpinx. 2) Beginning at the fimbriated end, the mesosalpinx is clamped, cut, and ligated until it is liberated to the uterus. 3) By means of the sharp scalpel, the interstitial portion of the tube is removed by parallel incisions in the myometrium. 4) The myometrium is closed with interrupted sutures. 5) The uterine defect left by excision of the fallopian tube is peritonealized with a portion of the round ligament.

Frequently the fallopian tube and ovary are removed together. Some feel that ovarian function is disturbed by interference with blood supply when the fallopian tube alone is removed, giving rise to subsequent ovarian cystic enlargement; others believe that the ovary should not be removed unless it is diseased. This is a moot point. If it is deemed necessary to excise the ovary simultaneously, the technique must be modified to include ligation of the ovary vessels in the infundibulopelvic ligament above the ovary.

Segmental Resection and Reconstructive Operations

Infertility caused by mechanical obstruction of the oviduct may be relieved by salpingoplasty. If the obstruction is in the isthmic portion, excision of the area of obstruction and direct anastomosis may reestablish tubal patency. Microsurgical techniques have greatly improved the results of reconstructive operations and are still undergoing modifications that will increase the success of the procedures.

Sterilization operations on the fallopian tubes all have as their objective the permanent interruption of ovum transport. Although many techniques have been described, an occasional failure has been reported with each method. The operation may be performed upon different segments of the fallopian tube: interstitial (cornual resection), isthmic (Irving technique), ampullar (Madlener and Pomeroy techniques), fimbriated portion (Aldridge technique). The Pomeroy

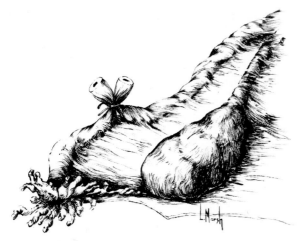

FIG. 61–30. Modified Pomeroy technique for sterilization.

technique is used most commonly. The Irving technique is said to be virtually 100% successful in producing permanent tubal occlusion.

Basic Technique, Modified Pomeroy. 1) The midportion of the tube is picked up with a medium clamp and elevated to form a sharp kink. 2) At a distance of about 2.5 cm from the kink, the ascending and descending portions of the tube are firmly crushed with heavy tissue forceps, such as Kocher clamp. 3) The crushed areas are ligated with a figure-of-eight suture of No. 1 absorbable material to intentionally produce local tissue reaction. 4) After the tube is tied, the loop portion of the tube is excised. 5) Some advise burying the Madlener loop and the Pomeroy tube ends beneath folds of peritoneum to reduce the chance for adhesion formation with intestinal loops. The Pomeroy technique (Fig. 61–30) is simple, effective, and widely used. The operation should be performed at the junction of the middle and outer thirds of the tube.

Basic Technique, Irving Procedure. 1) The tube is cut and the ends ligated about 3.5 cm from the uterine cornu. 2) A stab incision is made in the myometrium posterior to the cornu. 3) The uterine end of the tube is drawn into the myometrial defect and buried. 4) The opposite end is buried beneath the folds of the broad ligament.

Salpingorrhaphy

Salpingorrhaphy with preservation of the fallopian tube is occasionally possible in tubal pregnancy. If the tube has ruptured and bleeding can be well controlled, the remains of the ovular sac are removed from the tube and the defect closed with No. 4-0 absorbable sutures. If the tube is unruptured, an incision is made over the maximal bulge and the ovular sac extracted by finger pressure. Care must be taken to ligate bleeding points using very fine suture material. The procedure is especially indicated when only one tube remains. A number of successful pregnancies have been reported subsequent to salpingorrhaphy.

OPERATIONS ON THE OVARY

ANATOMIC CONSIDERATIONS

The ovary differentiates from an aggregation of undifferentiated cells on the anterior aspect of the genital ridge and descends into the pelvis attached to the müllerian ducts, which fuse to form the fallopian tubes, uterus, and upper vagina. The caudal end of the ovary remains attached to the uterine cornu by the true ligament of the ovary. The cephalic end of the ovary is loosely attached to the fold of peritoneum known as the infundibulopelvic ligament, which contains the ovarian arteries and veins that ascend to their point of origin near the level of the kidneys. The peritoneal folds of the infundibulopelvic and broad ligaments contain remnants of the wolffian system, which gives rise to paragenital cystic structures. The ovary gains its blood supply from secondary arteries arising from the main trunk of the shuntlike utero-ovarian artery, which inosculates near the uterine cornu. The ovary has no peritoneal covering: it is a true intraperitoneal organ.

OPERATIONS

Hemisection

Hemisection is performed for purposes of exploration and biopsy, if indicated, in patients with suspected ovarian disorders such as intersexuality, dermoid cysts, or polycystic disease (Stein–Leventhal syndrome). Physiologic function will not be disturbed providing the blood supply from the hilum is not compromised. Because the ovary has no peritoneal covering, it holds sutures poorly; special suturing is necessary to control bleeding.

Basic Technique. 1) The ovary is held between the index and middle fingers straddling the mesovarium. 2) With the sharp scalpel the ovary is bisected from the antemesovarium border to the hilum. 3) The cut surfaces are inspected and suspicious areas biopsied or excised. 4) The cut surfaces are reapproximated and bleeding controlled by deep through-and-through mattress sutures of No. 2-0 absorbable material tied firmly but not sufficiently hard as to incise the ovary. 5) A second row of finer sutures is used to approximate the cut edges.

Wedge Resection

Polycystic ovaries of the Stein–Leventhal type, associated with infertility, are treated by excision of a wedge of ovarian stroma. In this syndrome the tunica propria of the ovary is greatly thickened, and small follicular cysts can frequently be observed to line up against this membrane. Ovulation and pregnancy rather frequently follow wedge resection.

Basic Technique. 1) With the ovary grasped between the index and middle fingers, a wedge constituting about one-third of the ovary is excised with the sharp scalpel. 2) Because there is no peritoneum over the ovary, it holds sutures poorly, and to approximate the cut surfaces and arrest bleeding, deep suturing near the hilum is necessary. 3) A second row of sutures is used to close the cut edge. 4) Small ovarian retention cysts bulging through the surface should be punctured with a saber-pointed scalpel blade.

Management of Periovarian Pyogenic Infection

Pelvic suppurative inflammation extrinsically involving the ovary usually responds to antibiotics and drainage. Excision of the ovary in acute infections is not necessary unless irreparable damage has been sustained. In chronic infections associated with extensive adhesions, the ovary is subject to painful enlargement from the development of retention cysts, and extirpation of ovaries, fallopian tubes, and uterus is necessary to effect permanent cure.

Basic Principles. Operative steps cannot be outlined for procedures of this type, but awareness of certain principles may prevent accidental injury to the bowel or bladder. 1) Good anesthesia, good light, and adequate exposure are essential. 2) Adhesion planes should be carefully dissected with the sharp edge of a scalpel between lines of gentle traction until the uterine fundus is exposed. 3) The uterine cornu and the proximal portions of the broad ligament are exposed until clamps can be placed on the uterine cornu to include the utero-ovarian anastomosis. 4) Traction on the uterine cornu helps to define the location of supporting uterine attachments. 5) It is always necessary to be certain that adhesions have not drawn the bladder high over the anterior fundus. 6) Posteriorly, dissection must be kept close to the midline of the uterus until dissection has reached the lower level of the cervix. 7) Uterosacral ligaments are identified by upward traction on the uterine cornu. 8) Adherent adnexa are freed from the posterior surfaces of the broad ligament, and constant watch is kept for the ureter. 9) The ovary is freed from adhesions to peritoneum of the ovarian fossa. 10) Extirpation procedures should not be started until uterus and adnexa are fully identified and freely mobile. 11) In difficult dissections in which precise identification is necessary, the sharp scalpel is much safer than scissors. Before scissors can cut, they must pinch; the blades cut everything included in the pinch, and this may be the ureter. The sharp scalpel exposes as it cuts and pushes away rather than pinches.

Management of Ovarian Abscess

Intraovarian pyogenic infection presents as a pelvic mass of considerable size in association with signs and symptoms of acute pyogenic pelvic infection. Its major characteristic is failure to respond to adequate antibiotic therapy. The diagnosis is usually confused with pyosalpinx and cul-de-sac abscess.

Physical signs of infection limited to the pelvis, a confined pelvic mass of relatively stable size, increasing signs of systemic intoxication as indicated by temperature and pulse curves characteristic of sepsis and high leukocyte counts with more than 90% polymorphonuclear leukocytes, suggest a confined suppurative process likely to be ovarian abscess. Rapid recovery follows oophorectomy.

Basic Technique. 1) An adequate lower abdominal incision is made. 2) Fibrinous adhesions are separated by manual dissection, and the enlarged ovary is liberated. 3) Salpingo-oophorectomy is done. 4) The abdomen is closed without drainage.

Oophorectomy

A persistent pelvic tumor suspected of being ovarian in origin is an indication for abdominal surgery if it is larger than 4 cm in diameter, regardless of whether it produces symptoms. If ovaries can be palpated in the postmenopausal woman, they are presumed to be enlarged and should be removed. Unilateral oophorectomy, with or without salpingectomy, is indicated for benign cysts and solid neoplasms. All ovarian tumors and cysts should be opened in the operating room for gross inspection. With few exceptions, if malignancy is grossly present, the operation should be extended to bilateral salpingo-oophorectomy and complete hysterectomy, regardless of the patient's age. Suspicious malignant lesions should be subjected to immediate pathologic examination. A suspicion of ovarian malignancy is such a dangerous diagnosis that it allows no clinical or operative compromise. On the other hand, small (1 to 2 cm) physiologic or retention ovarian cysts require no operative treatment and, when discovered, should be left alone.

Ovarian cysts should be removed intact, employing a longitudinal incision that should be extended as needed. An ovarian cyst too massive to be delivered through a generous abdominal incision may require decompression, but care must be taken to prevent intraperitoneal spill of the cyst fluid. Once decom-

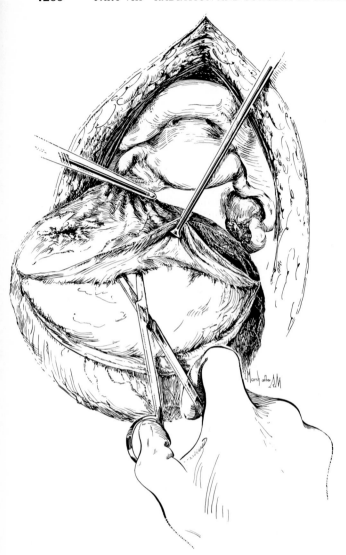

FIG. 61–31. Ovarian cystectomy.

pressed, a tense cyst is easily removed unless it has developed adhesions to surrounding structures. The cyst wall should not be handled with sharp instruments. Particular care must be used in handling ovarian cysts with twisted pedicles. It is best to deliver the cyst before the pedicle is untwisted, and a careful search should be made to locate the ureter. In twisting, the peritoneum over the ureter is sometimes taken up and involved in the twist. If the ureter is not in the pedicle, a clamp should be placed across the base of the twisted area before the cyst is untwisted; shock has been observed following absorption of material from an untwisted ovarian cyst. If the ureter is in the twisted pedicle, dissection should be carried above the involved

area and the ovarian veins ligated under direct vision.

Oophorectomy consists of the application of clamps across the mesovarium and ligation with figure-of-eight sutures of No. 0 absorbable material. The stump may be buried beneath the folds of peritoneum with a running suture. Occasionally salpingectomy must be done also.

Ovarian Cystectomy

This is performed for benign cysts, such as teratoma (dermoid cyst), which arise deep in the ovarian stroma. The operation is indicated if the patient is interested in future childbearing; it is a highly successful procedure not associated with complications, providing malignancy is ruled out (Fig. 61–31).

Basic Technique. 1) A shallow incision is made over the full diameter of the ovarian cyst into the overlying ovarian tissue. 2) In one area of the incision careful dissection with the sharp scalpel is continued until the wall of the cyst is identified. 3) Then, by opening and closing the blades of dissecting scissors, the cyst is easily separated from the wall of ovarian tissue. 4) The cyst is enucleated without encountering major blood vessels, except occasionally in the area of the hilum. 5) The cyst contents are examined immediately for areas suggestive of malignancy. 6) Closure of the cyst defect is accomplished by through-and-through mattress sutures of fine absorbable material.

Parovarian cysts arise from remnants of the wolffian system and may be intraligamentous or extraligamentous (hydatid of Morgagni), single or multiple, large or small. They are separate from the ovary. Usually they arise within the layers of the broad ligament and are important because they may greatly distort the position of the ureter. If they arise below the ureter, the ureter may be displaced to an extreme medial or a lateral position, where it may be cut or ligated because it is mistaken for a blood vessel.

Basic Technique. 1) The position of the ureter is determined. 2) The peritoneum is incised over the cyst, and the cyst is bluntly dissected from its bed. 3) Blood vessels are ligated separately; injury to the ovarian blood vessels should be avoided. 4) The peritoneum is repaired without kinking the ureter.

POSTOPERATIVE COMPLICATIONS

Postoperative complications include hemorrhage, shock, infection, thrombophlebitis and phlebothrombosis, pulmonary embolism, urinary retention, urinary infection, abdominal distention, intestinal obstruction, wound disruption, evisceration, fecal fistula and urinary fistula.

Hemorrhage

Hemorrhage may be arterial, venous, or capillary; delayed or immediate; confined or unconfined; obvious or occult; precipitous or gradual. The blood may be clotted or liquid.

Intraperitoneal bleeding is unconfined and usually occurs as immediate, precipitous, and occult hemorrhage. As a rule it is of arterial origin and, although initially clotted, the blood may become liquid and unclottable because of fibrinogen depletion. Generally, bleeding results from slipping of an insecure ligature and may occur incidental to either abdominal or vaginal hysterectomy. Usually intraperitoneal hemorrhage occurs within the first few hours of surgery, often before the patient has recovered from the effects of the anesthetic. Diagnosis, therefore, may be difficult because the early physical manifestations of hemorrhage may not be detectable. The predominant clinical picture is one of progressive shock that only temporarily responds to blood transfusions. The patient demonstrates skin pallor, lowered blood pressure, rapid pulse (usually above 120/minute) and, if sufficiently recovered from the general anesthetic, restlessness and air hunger. The most reliable signs are evidences of peripheral circulatory failure: very cold hands and feet and nondetectable or barely detectable peripheral pulses. Treatment is immediate circulatory support, as outlined in Chapter 38, followed as quickly as possible by transabdominal laparotomy and ligation of the bleeding vessel.

Retroperitoneal hemorrhage is confined by the peritoneum and usually manifests itself as an increasing pelvic mass. It may be arterial, venous, or capillary in origin, and initially the blood is generally clotted. Retroperitoneal hemorrhage is usually less precipitous and less severe than intraperitoneal hemorrhage because bleeding tends to be self-limited. It may go undetected until late in the postoperative period and then become manifest because of low-grade fever or spontaneous drainage of dark liquid blood. If detected immediately, the wound should be reopened and the bleeding point ligated. If detected late, evacuation of the hematoma, free drainage, and prevention of infection by administration of antibiotic usually suffice.

Wound hemorrhage is confined, usually self-limited, and of capillary, venous, or arterial origin. It manifests itself as localized pain, swelling, ecchymosis of the skin, and oozing between sutures. Immediate opening of the wound, ligation of bleeding points, and reclosure should be performed if the hemorrhage is detected early. Usually it is observed late, at which time drainage by opening the incision is sufficient treatment.

Cervical hemorrhage following cauterization, amputation, or biopsy may be profuse, recurrent, and even fatal. Usually it occurs several days after the procedure. Occasionally after treatment with cautery, suture, or packing it recurs with increased vigor. Finding a precise bleeding point may be impossible. If bleeding is severe and recurrent, the patient should be kept at complete bedrest until the hemorrhage is staunched by packing, cautery, or suture. The application of bovine-thrombin-soaked oxycellulose to the cervix may greatly aid local hemostasis. In recurrent hemorrhage, local necrotizing infection seems to play a causative role, and the concurrent administration of antibiotics in high doses is beneficial.

In all instances of hemorrhage, blood volume should be maintained by adequate transfusion of whole blood. A reliable sign of adequate therapy is the return of normal peripheral circulation, as indicated by warm hands and feet, pink skin, palpable pulses, and stabilization of vital signs.

Infection

The subjects of postoperative infections and antibacterial therapy are discussed in Chapter 13. Infections may be acute, delayed, local (wound, retroperitoneal spaces, abdominal cavity, urinary system), or systemic (septicemia). The bacterial organisms responsible may be pyogenic (exotoxic) or nonpyogenic (endotoxic), aerobic or anaerobic. Clinical manifestations may be primarily local (wound) or general.

Local infections, if superficial, are manifested by inflammation in the wound, *i.e.*, skin erythema and increased local heat, swelling, and pain. Deep infections in the retroperitoneal spaces or between the fascia layers of the abdominal wall initially may produce few local symptoms. Urinary tract infections are signaled by dysuria, hematuria, and flank tenderness to fist percussion. Systemic signs of local infection (fever, leukocytosis) are usually proportional to the severity of the infection.

Infections caused by exotoxic pyogens produced marked fever, leukocytosis with shift to the left, and signs of systemic reaction. Septicemia from endotoxic bacteria produces profound shock with slight pyrogenic response, although there is usually marked leukocytosis with shift to the left. Treatment of septic shock must be aggressive, as outlined in Chapter 38.

In the cellulitis phase, superficial infections should be treated initially by bedrest, the application of massive hot, wet compresses, and the systemic administration of antibiotics; later, abscesses should be drained as they appear. Deeper infections may not be detected until the swelling indicative of abscess formation becomes evident.

Signs of systemic infection call for the use of antibiotics in liberal dosage until the nature of the infection becomes apparent. Gynecologic infections are usually of mixed bacterial origin. If the true nature of the infection cannot be determined, antibiotic therapy

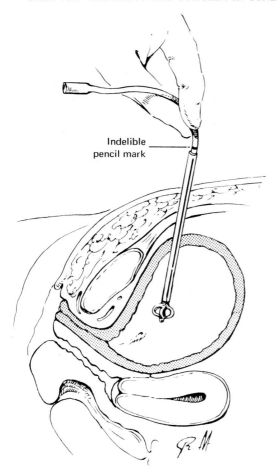

Indelible
pencil mark

FIG. 61–32. Suprapubic trochar cystostomy.

should be inclusive to combat both exotoxic and endotoxic organisms.

Urinary Infection and Retention

Bacteriuria following gynecologic operations may be symptomatic or occult, incidental or catheter-induced, and temporary or persistent. Bacteriuria may follow vaginal plastic operations. The use of an indwelling catheter should be avoided, but not at the expense of overdistention of the bladder. Failure to void following operations is directly related to neither the type nor the magnitude of the operation: pain from hemorrhoidectomy, repair of an enterocele, or perineotomy may be associated with recalcitrant urinary retention. Relaxation of the skeletal muscles of the pelvic floor is essential for voluntary voiding, and if this action is restricted because of pain, voluntary voiding will not occur.

The treatment of postoperative bacteriuria must include the elimination of urine retention. Constant

free-catheter drainage during the period of postoperative edema and pain is preferred over repeated, frequent catheterizations, particularly in the presence of bacteriuria. Sometimes the voiding process can be hastened by gentle dilatation of the urethra, sitz baths, and the administration of cortisone to reduce the postoperative inflammatory reaction. When the residual urine reaches 50 ml, routine catheterization should be stopped. Bacteriuria should be treated by administration of the appropriate antibiotic as determined by urine culture and antibiotic sensitivity tests.

Bladder Drainage by Transurethral Catheter. The indwelling transurethral balloon-tipped catheter has been the conventional technique for bladder drainage following gynecologic surgery. Many disadvantages are associated with its use: very high incidence of bacteriuria, pain, urethral trauma, a need for detailed nursing care and, following removal of the catheter, intermittent catheterization until voiding has become reestablished.

Bladder Drainage by Suprapubic Trochar Cystostomy. Bladder drainage by suprapubic trochar cystostomy (Fig. 61–32) circumvents many of the disadvantages of transurethral catheter drainage. It is associated with a reduced incidence of bacteriuria, minimal pain, no urethral trauma, minimal nursing care, and elimination of postoperative catheterization.

Basic Technique. 1) The lower abdomen is prepared for surgery. 2) A site is selected 3 cm above the symphysis in the midline; in the presence of a lower median incision, a site 1 cm lateral to the incision is selected. 3) The bladder is filled with 500 ml normal saline. 4) A spinal needle is directed toward the pelvis at an angle approximately 30° from the vertical until the bladder is entered and a free flow of fluid is obtained. 5) A Malecot catheter, No. 12 F, is threaded on a metal stylet. 6) The catheter is measured above the level of the winged tip against the length of the cannula and marked with sterile indelible pencil. 7) Following the same angulation as the spinal needle, a trochar and cannula are pushed through the abdominal wall into the bladder. 8) When a distinct give indicates bladder puncture, the operator should be prepared immediately to arrest further thrust of the trochar. 9) The trochar is removed from the cannula and the free flow of fluid is arrested with the finger; if a free flow of fluid is not obtained, the cannula is not in the bladder; the cannula should be removed and the status of the patient reappraised because either the bladder is empty or the trochar has been misdirected, overinserted, or underinserted. 10) If free flow of fluid is obtained, the stylet-armed Malecot catheter is inserted up to the indelible pencil mark and the metal stylet is removed. 11) After the metal stylet has been removed, the Mal-

FIG. 61–33. General types of catheters for suprapubic cystostomy. *Left to right:* standard rubber catheter; Foley; Malecot; curved tip. The Malecot and curved-tip catheters are most reliable.

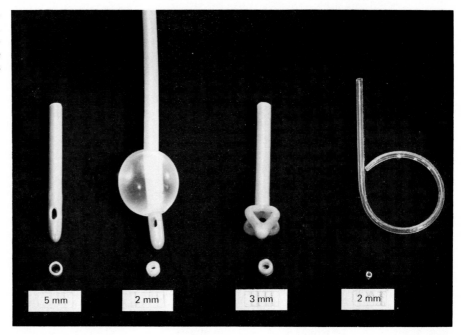

cecot catheter is cut off to permit removal of the cannula. 13) The catheter is tied in place with two skin sutures. 14) The catheter is connected to a closed drainage system that has small-caliber drainage tubing.

When the time comes to initiate voiding, the catheter can be disconnected from the closed drainage system and a clamp applied. The patient can be taught a do-it-yourself catheter management program, measuring voided and residual urine volumes. The catheter can be removed when satisfactory voiding has become reestablished.

Although the above technique pertains to trochar cystostomy, the principles described apply to the introduction of all types of suprapubic catheters. Since suprapubic trochar cystostomy was first introduced, several types of catheter kits have been made available (Fig. 61–33). It is important to emphasize the physical characteristics of the catheters which are most satisfactory for suprapubic catheter drainage. Once introduced into the bladder, the catheter tip should be sufficiently bulbous to prevent its entering the inner urethra and causing obstruction. For this reason, all straight catheters are unsatisfactory because the functional tip of the catheter tends to enter the inner urethra when the bladder is collapsed.

Thrombophlebitis and Phlebothrombosis

Intravenous thrombosis may be acute or chronic, superficial or deep, inflammatory (thrombophlebitis) or noninflammatory (phlebothrombosis), clinically apparent or nonapparent, embolic or nonembolic, septic or nonseptic, and idiopathic or secondary to surgical operation, parturition, direct trauma, blood stagnation, blood hypercoagulability, or a specific vein lesion (endothelial irritation, vein wall ectasia, intrinsic or extrinsic vascular occlusion).

In phlebothrombosis, pain is the leading symptom and may be direct or indirect. Swelling and discoloration are observed less consistently. Acute, superficial, inflammatory thrombophlebitis manifests itself directly as a tender, red, cordlike involvement of the vein. Deep involvement of the pelvic and leg veins usually begins insidiously. In the early noninflammatory (phlebothrombosis) stage, it is manifest indirectly as pain from movement of, or pressure on, structures contiguous to the involved veins, such as tensing the gastrocnemius muscle (Homan's sign) or squeezing the calf. Low-grade fever and disproportionate elevation of the pulse rate are common clinical signs.

Treatment should be directed toward four objectives: 1) relief of symptoms, 2) arrest of extension, 3) prevention of embolization, and 4) reabsorption of clots. The first stages of treatment should include total body immobilization with elevation of the affected extremity. Inflammatory symptoms are lessened by the application of massive hot, wet compresses and the use of a bed cradle to support the weight of the bedclothes. Fluid intake should be adequate, diet should be low in protein, constipation should be avoided. Heparin and coumarin may be used for anticoagulant therapy, pro-

viding appropriate blood coagulation tests are employed to guard against overdosage. Protamine sulfate as an antidote for excessive heparin administration, and vitamin K for coumarin excess, should be available. Ambulation should not be permitted until all signs and symptoms of thrombophlebitis are absent and the pulse and temperature have been normal for 24 hours.

Ligation of the vena cava above the bifurcation of the common iliac veins, combined with ligation of the ovarian veins, is indicated for pelvic and lower-extremity phlebothrombosis and thrombophlebitis in patients having nonfatal pulmonary emboli, particularly if recurrent. Massive pulmonary embolism, if not immediately fatal, sometimes may be treated successfully by pulmonary embolectomy.

Abdominal Distention

Postoperative abdominal distention may result from mechanical bowel obstruction, from adynamic ileus caused by overdistention of the stomach and intestines with swallowed air, from bacterial and chemical peritonitis, from ascites, or from spinal nerve involvement. Gastric and intestinal suction should be promptly instituted as initial treatment until diagnosis is accurately established. Air swallowing is best prevented and best treated by the institution of gastric suction, and the patient should be warned against constant belching and retching. The application of hot, wet stupes to the abdomen, intravenous administration of fluids, reduction of dietary intake, and gentle administration of enemas usually are effective in relieving simple abdominal distention from adynamic ileus. When mechanical intestinal obstruction and peritonitis are suspected, appropriate diagnostic studies must be performed. Ascites should be treated by paracentesis.

Wound Disruption and Evisceration

Abdominal wounds fail to heal because they are improperly closed; because they are unduly strained from postoperative distention, obesity, coughing, vomiting, belching, ascites, or hematoma formation; because they become infected; and occasionally because of an allergic reaction to the suture material or poor tissue healing incidental to general debility and emaciation. Most of the factors can be anticipated, and wound disruption can often be prevented by institution of gastric and intestinal intubation and constant suction.

If wound disruption is suggested by local pain, slight bulging of the wound, and drainage of serosanguinous fluid from the wound, skin sutures are best removed in the operating room with the patient under spinal anesthesia. If wound disruption is first detected when skin sutures are being removed with the patient in bed, the procedure should be stopped, and long, wide, abdomen-encircling strips of flamed adhesive should be firmly applied directly over the skin incision. Then the patient may be transferred to the operating room for secondary closure.

Precipitous wound disruption with eviseration of the intestine occasionally occurs without warning. If erect, the patient should be immediately placed flat in bed. The intestines should be replaced in as clean a manner as possible, and, with the wound edges firmly held together, flamed adhesive strips should be applied as noted above. With the wound well strapped, and if the patient's condition warrants, she may be transferred to the operating room for secondary wound closure. However, if the wound is firmly strapped together, time may be taken to institute appropriate treatment for shock, intestinal obstruction, hemorrhage, and infection. Surgery for secondary wound closure should be delayed until vital signs have stabilized and the patient's general condition has improved sufficiently to permit adequate anesthesia and the employment of operative techniques. There should be no attempt to close in layers; instead, through-and-through sutures of silver or steel wire or heavy nylon should be placed at intervals of about 2 cm and allowed to remain for 3 weeks. In the severely ill patient secondary wound repair may be postponed indefinitely; when the skin has healed and the patient's physical state permits, the wound may be repaired as a ventral hernia.

Fistula

Acute fecal and urinary fistulas appearing in the immediate postoperative period frequently heal spontaneously if diverting procedures are promptly employed. The introduction of a ureteral catheter to a level above a ureteral fistula usually leads to prompt healing. If a ureter is completely ligated, drainage of the renal pelvis by nephrostomy will usually preserve renal function until definitive operative measures to correct the ureteral obstruction can be undertaken later. For bladder fistula, the prompt installation of a retention catheter will favor spontaneous healing.

A fecal fistula is usually accompanied by extensive infection. The objectives of the diverting colostomy procedure should be to eliminate fecal bulk and fecal bacteria. These objectives are best served by an isolation loop colostomy rather than a simple loop colostomy over a glass rod. This permits complete isolation of feces and prevents continued bacterial contamination of the lower bowel segment. Experience has shown that local instillation of antibiotics into the distal stoma of the lower bowel segment aids in establishing bowel antisepsis; spontaneous healing of large fecal fistulas has been observed. A fistula involving the small intestine requires enterostomy performed above the level of the involved bowel segment.

REFERENCES AND RECOMMENDED READING

Ball TL: Gynecologic Surgery and Urology. St Louis, Mosby, 1959

Burch JC: Urethrovaginal fixation to Cooper's ligament for correction of stress incontinence, cystocoele, and prolapse. Am J Obstet Gynecol 81:281, 1961

Durfee RB: Anterior vaginal suspension operation: Report of 110 cases. Am J Obstet Gynecol 78:628, 1959

Gray LA: A Textbook of Gynecology. Springfield Ill, Charles C Thomas, 1960

Joel-Cohen S: Abdominal and Vaginal Hysterectomy, 2nd ed. Philadelphia, JB Lippincott, 1977

MacLeod D, Howkins J: Bonney's Gynaecological Surgery, 7th ed. New York, Harper & Row, 1964

Marshall VF, Marchetti AA, Krantz KE: Correction of stress incontinence by simple vesicourethral suspension. Surg Gynecol Obstet 88:509, 1949

Mattingly RF: Te Linde's Operative Gynecology, 5th ed. Philadelphia, JB Lippincott, 1977

McCall ML, Bolten KA: Martius' Gynecological Operations, Boston, Little Brown, 1954

Nichols DH, Randall CL: Vaginal Surgery. Baltimore, Williams & Wilkins, 1976

Ridley JH ed: Gynecologic Surgery: Errors, Safeguards, and Salvage. Baltimore, Williams & Wilkins, 1974

Rob C, Smith R (eds): Operative Surgery. In Roberts DWT (ed): Gynecology and Obstetrics, London, Butterworths, 1977

Steptoe PC: Laparoscopy in Gynecology. Baltimore, Williams & Wilkins, 1967

Tovell HMM, Dank LD (eds): Gynecologic Operations. Hagerstown, Harper & Row, 1978

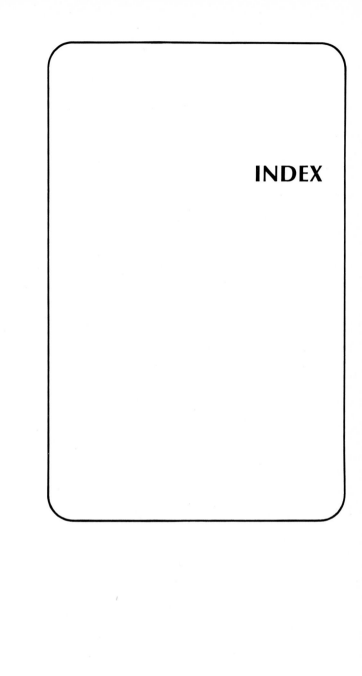

INDEX

Numbers in *italics* represent figures; numbers followed by a "t" represent tabular material.

in newborn, in ABO and Rh hemolytic disease, 438, 440
Biopsy
  breast, 1203–1204
  endometrial, abnormal bleeding
    and, 911
    for proof of ovulation, *938, 942*
    for tuberculosis, 989
    infertility and, 936, *937, 938*
  of cervix, 1247–1248, *1248*
    for cervical intraepithelial neopla-
      sia, 1058–1059
  of vulvar lesions, 1023–1024, 1027,
    1233, *1024, 1233*
  punch, for cervical cancer, 1059,
    1060
  technique of, 1233–1234, 1233
Biparietal diameter
  gestational age and, 806–807, *808,*
    807t
  in growth adjusted sonographic age,
    808
  multiple pregnancy and, 562
  See also Fetal head; Intrauterine
    growth retardation
Birth(s)
  future, 282, *284*
  illegitimate, 285, *285, 285t*
  live, definition of, 281
  registration of, 282
  time of, 652
Birth asphyxia, 839
  breathing and, 840
  in newborn vs. adult, 852
  moderate, 844–845, *845*
  prolonged, cardiac massage and,
    845
  respiratory responses with, 841,
    841
  severe, 845
  survival and brain damage after,
    851–853
Birth control. *See* Contraception
Birth defects. *See* Fetus and newborn,
    abnormalities of; Genitalia,
    ambiguous; Malformations
Birth injuries, 876–879, *877–880*
Birth rate, definition of, 282, *283*
Birth weight
  for classification of perinatal mor-
    bidity and mortality,
    283–284, 284t, 798, *853*
  gestational age and, 849, *850*
  maternal weight gain and, 537
  renal transplants and, 228, *228*
Birthing rooms, 642
Bladder. *See* Urinary bladder
Blastocyst, 93, 297, *298*
Bleeding
  anovulatory, in adolescence, 911
    in childbearing age, 911
  entrance to hospital for labor and,
    643
  in late pregnancy, 443
    differential diagnosis of, 453t
    other causes of, 454
  marginal sinus, 449, *449*
  nasal, in pregnancy, 489

postmenopausal, 178–179
  rectal, endometriosis and, 1009
  uterine, abnormal, 907–908
    endometrial disease with, 907,
      908t, 1009
    types of, 907
    dysfunctional, 908–910, *909, 910*
      at menopause, 1101, *1102*
      causes of, *909*
      endometrial cancer and, 1100
      follicular and luteal phase de-
        fects with, 908–910, *909, 912*
      management of, 911
    in puerperium, 661
    in renal disease, 226–227
    myoma and, 1087
    See also Menstruation
  vaginal, abortion and, 383, 385
    with abruptio placentae, 449–452
    with anovulation, 910, *910*
    with circumvallate placenta, 452
    with IUD use, 272–273
    with placenta previa, 443–449
    with rupture of uterus, 452–454
    with ruptured vasa previa, 454
Block
  caudal, 670, 672, *672*
  lumbar epidural, 672–673, *673*
  paracervical, 670, *671*
  pudendal, 670, *671*
  regional, contraindications to, 674
  spinal, 670
  subarachnoid, 670
Blocking antibody, abortion and, 225,
    392
Blond Heidler saw, for destructive op-
    erations, 785
Blood
  in amniotic fluid, 429
  in preeclampsia, 466–467
  in pregnancy, 331–333, 332t, 333t,
    482t
    disorders of, 537–541
  maternal-fetal exchange, 308–309
  menstrual, 169–170
  placental intervillous space, 307
Blood analysis
  fetal, labor and, 318
Blood cells, red. *See* Erythrocytes
Blood coagulation
  in abruptio placentae, 451
  mechanism of, 741, *742,* 741t
  missed abortion and, 389
  plasma transfusion and, 752
  pregnancy and, 487
  tests for, 467, 742–743
  with stored blood, 749
Blood composition
  contraceptives and, 205, 260
  fetal breathing movement and,
    831
  in hemostasis, 740–741
  in puerperium, 789
  menstrual, 169–170
  use and characteristics of, 747, 751,
    748, 751t
Blood count
  in prenatal care, 364

Blood flow
  through umbilical cord, 312–313
  uterine, in pregnancy, 330
Blood mole, 383
  tubal, 411, 417, *411*
Blood pressure
  in labor, 329
  in preeclampsia-eclampsia syn-
    drome, 459
  in pregnancy, 328–329, *328, 329,*
    330, 331, 329t, 365
Blood test
  for adrenal function, 145
  for septic abortion, 387, 387t
Blood transfusions, 747
  emergency, 750
  for septic shock, 757
  for sickle cell disease in pregnancy,
    538–539
  hazards of, 749–750, 752–754
  in septic abortion, 387
  in utero, for Rh hemolytic disease,
    430–432, 434–437
  indications for, 747
  massive, 749–750
  of erythrocytes, 747–749
  of noncellular plasma components,
    751–752, 751t
  of platelets, 750–751
  reactions to, 752–754
  to restore volume, 749
Blood vessels
  in colposcopy of cervical cancer,
    1067, 1070–1071, *1071*
  in pregnancy, 330–331, 487
  in umbilical cord, 312
Blood volume
  in preeclampsia-eclampsia, 466
  in pregnancy, 331
  in puerperium, 789
  replacement of, 749–751
Bloody show, 641, 643
Blundell, James, 9
Body temperature
  in newborn infant, 842
  birth asphyxia and, 839, *840*
Boeck's sarcoid, 547
Bone
  absorption of radiation by, 1220
  coxal, 46, 48, *47*
  of pelvic cavity, 46, 48, *47, 49*
Bone marrow, in refractory anemia of
    pregnancy, 485
Bone metastases, radionuclide imag-
    ing of, 1188
Bowel
  carcinoma of, in pregnancy, 515
  function of, in pregnancy, 370
  radiation tolerance of, 1222
Bowen's disease, of vulva, 1035, *1036*
Brachial plexus palsy, 878, *879*
Brachystasis, uterine, 578, 593, *578,*
    597
Bradycardia, fetal, with paracervical
    block, 670
Brain damage
  birth asphyxia and, 851–853